Nursing Adults
The Practice of Caring

Edited by

Chris Brooker
BSc MSc RGN SCM RNT
Author and Lecturer, Norfolk, UK

Maggie Nicol
BSc(Hons) MSc PGDipEd RGN
Senior Lecturer, Clinical Skills, City University,
St Bartholomew School of Nursing & Midwifery, London, UK

Foreword by
Dinah Gould
BSc MPhil PhD RGN RNT
Professor of Applied Health Science,
Department of Applied Biological Sciences,
City University, London, UK

Illustrations by
Graeme Chambers

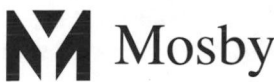 Mosby

EDINBURGH   LONDON   NEW YORK   OXFORD   PHILADELPHIA   ST LOUIS   SYDNEY   TORONTO 2003

MOSBY
An imprint of Elsevier Limited

First published 2003

ISBN 0 7234 3157 4

British Library Cataloguing in Publication Data
A catalogue record for this book is available from the British Library

Library of Congress Cataloging in Publication Data
A catalog record for this book is available from the Library of Congress

Notice
Medical knowledge is constantly changing. Standard safety precautions
must be followed, but as new research and clinical experience broaden our
knowledge, changes in treatment and drug therapy may become necessary
or appropriate. Readers are advised to check the most current product
information provided by the manufacturer of each drug to be administered
to verify the recommended dose, the method and duration of administration,
and contraindications. It is the responsibility of the practitioner, relying on
experience and knowledge of the patient, to determine dosages and the best
treatment for each individual patient. Neither the Publisher nor the editors
assume any liability for any injury and/or damage to persons or property
arising from this publication.

The Publisher

The
publisher's
policy is to use
**paper manufactured
from sustainable forests**

Printed in China

Nursing Adults

For Mosby:

Senior Commissioning Editor: Sarena Wolfaard
Project Development Manager: Mairi McCubbin
Project Manager: Derek Robertson
Designer: Judith Wright
Illustrations Manager: Bruce Hogarth
Page Layout: Kate Walshaw, Alan Palfreyman

Contents in brief

Contributors   *vii*

Foreword   *xi*

Preface   *xiii*

Acknowledgements   *xiii*

Getting the best from this book   *xiv*

Contents   *xvii*

Section 1 Nursing, quality and communication   *1*

1 Adult nursing: setting the scene   *3*

2 Quality management and standards of care   *23*

3 Communication in adult nursing   *39*

Section 2 Common nursing issues   *57*

4 Circadian rhythms and sleep patterns   *59*

5 Temperature regulation   *75*

6 Stress   *93*

7 Pain   *111*

8 Problems associated with fluid, electrolyte and acid–base balance   *133*

9 Shock, systemic inflammatory response and multiple organ dysfunction   *153*

10 Tissue viability: managing chronic wounds   *173*

11 Nutrition   *201*

12 Maintaining continence   *229*

13 Infection control   *253*

Section 3 Nursing patients with common disorders   *271*

14 Nursing patients with neurological problems   *273*

15 Nursing patients with problems of the eye and vision   *331*

16 Nursing patients with problems of the ear and hearing   *367*

17 Nursing patients with endocrine and metabolic disorders   *393*

18 Nursing patients with blood disorders   *445*

19 Nursing patients with cardiovascular disorders   *481*

20 Nursing patients with respiratory disorders   *533*

21 Nursing patients with nose and throat disorders   *565*

22 Nursing patients with gastrointestinal disorders   *591*

23 Nursing patients with hepatic, biliary and pancreatic disorders   *621*

24 Nursing patients with urinary disorders   *653*

25 Nursing patients with sexual health and reproductive problems   *705*

26 Nursing patients with breast disorders   *771*

27 Nursing patients with musculoskeletal disorders   *793*

28 Nursing patients with skin problems   *841*

Section 4 Specific areas of adult nursing   *877*

29 Perioperative nursing   *879*

30 Nursing patients in the accident and emergency department   *923*

31 Nursing critically ill patients   *947*

32 Nursing older adults   *967*

33 Nursing patients with cancer   *985*

34 Nursing patients who need palliative care   *1021*

35 Nursing patients with chronic (long-term) illness and disability   *1047*

Appendix: Normal values   *1067*

Glossary   *1069*

Index   *1079*

Contributors

Sheila Adam BNurs MSc RGN JBCNS100
Nurse Consultant, The Middlesex Hospital, London, UK
9 Shock, systemic inflammatory response and multiple organ dysfunction

Tanya Andrewes BSc(Hons) PGDip RGN
Senior Lecturer, Learning and Teaching,
Bournemouth University, Bournemouth, UK
33 Nursing patients with cancer

Helen Barlow MSc RGN ONCCert ENBA11, 237 998, 931
Implementation Lead, Nursing and Leadership Development,
Directorate of Health and Social Care North, Leeds, UK
26 Nursing patients with breast disorders

Ruhi Behi BSc(Hons) MSc CertMHS RGN RNT
Sub-Dean, Faculty of Health, University of Wales at Bangor,
Bangor, UK
2 Quality management and standards of care

Chris Brooker BSc MSc RGN SCM RNT
Author and Lecturer, Norfolk, UK
1 Adult nursing: setting the scene

Iain Bowie MA BA (Hons) RGN Dip N (Lond) Cert Ed RNT OND
Florence Nightingale School of Nursing and Midwifery,
King's College London, London, UK
14 Nursing patients with neurological problems

Linda Bywater BA(Hons) MSc RN
Cancer Directorate Manager, Radiotherapy Department,
Churchill Hospital, Oxford, UK
18 Nursing patients with blood disorders

Jacky Cotton MHS RM RGN
Head of Nursing: Gynaecology,
Birmingham Women's Hospital, Birmingham, UK
25 Nursing patients with sexual health and reproductive problems

Kate Davies MSc RGN
Lecturer in Pain Management, University of Wales,
Department of Anaesthetics, College of Medicine, Cardiff, UK
7 Pain

Sharon Edwards MSc DipN(Lond) PGCEA RGN
Senior Lecturer, Department of Nursing and Paramedic Science,
University of Hertfordshire, Hatfield Campus, Hertfordshire, UK
5 Temperature regulation

Glenda Esmond BSc(Hons) MSc PGCertEd DipN(Lond) RGN
Lecturer in Respiratory Nursing, City University,
St Bartholomew School of Nursing and Midwifery,
London, UK
20 Nursing patients with respiratory disorders

Lindsay Etherington BSc(Hons) RGN ENB199, 998 ATNC
Project Lead, Reforming Emergency Care, Chelsea and
Westminster Healthcare NHS Trust, London, UK
30 Nursing patients in the accident and emergency department

Hilary Fanning BSc(Hons) RGN
Senior Nurse, Renal Service, Department of Nephrology,
University Hospital Birmingham NHS Trust,
The Queen Elizabeth Hospital, Birmingham, UK
24 Nursing patients with urinary disorders

Madeleine Flanagan BSc(Hons) MA CertEd(HE) DPSN RGN
Principal Lecturer, Department of Post-Registration Nursing,
University of Hertfordshire, Hatfield, UK
10 Tissue viability: managing chronic wounds

Jacqui Fletcher BSc(Hons) PGCert RGN
Senior Lecturer, Tissue Viability,
Department of Post-Registration Nursing
University of Hertfordshire, Hatfield, UK
10 Tissue viability: managing chronic wounds

Peter Griffiths BA (Hons), PhD, RGN
Senior Lecturer, Primary and Intermediate Care Section,
Florence Nightingale School of Nursing and Midwifery,
King's College London, London, UK
35 Nursing patients with chronic (long-term) illness and disability

Hilary Harkin BSc(Hons) RGN
ENT Nurse Practitioner, Guy's and St Thomas' NHS Hospital
Trust, London, UK
16 Nursing patients with problems of the ear and hearing

Paul Hateley BSc MPH RGN RMN
Head of Nursing, Pathologies and Patient Services,
St Bartholomew's Hospital, London, UK
13 Infection control

David Howard MEd PhD Cert Ed DipN(Lond) RMN RGN
Health Lecturer, School of Nursing, University of Nottingham,
Lincoln, UK
6 Stress

Mark Jones MSc RN BSc(Hons) DipEd DipN
Programme Leader, Adult Nursing, Undergraduate Studies,
City University, St Bartholomew School of Nursing and
Midwifery, London, UK
25 Nursing patients with sexual health and reproductive problems

Kathy Martyn BSc BEd DipPNS SRN RNT
Senior Lecturer, INAM, Westlain House, Brighton, UK
11 Nutrition

Anthony McGrath BA MSc PGCE RMN RGN RNT
Senior Lecturer, Gastroenterology and Stoma Care Nursing,
City University, St Bartholomew School of Nursing and
Midwifery, London, UK
22 Nursing patients with gastrointestinal disorders

Shirley McKeon BSc DPSN
Lead Nurse, St John's Institute of Dermatology,
St Thomas Hospital, London, UK
28 Nursing patients with skin problems

Julienne Meyer BSc MSc PhD Cert Ed (FE) RN RNT
Professor of Nursing: Care for Older People, City University,
St Bartholomew School of Nursing and Midwifery,
London, UK
1 Adult nursing: setting the scene

David Morris MSc DipN(Lond) CertEd RGN RNT RCNT ENB176
Senior Lecturer, School of Health Care Practice,
Anglia Polytechnic University, Chelmsford, UK
29 Perioperative nursing

Maggie Nicol BSc(Hons) MSc PGDipEd RGN
Senior Lecturer, Clinical Skills, City University,
St Bartholomew School of Nursing and Midwifery,
London, UK
1 Adult nursing: setting the scene

Jill Peters BSc(Hons) DipNP RGN CMS ENB393 934 998 870 A33
Dermatology Nurse Practitioner, Dermatology Department,
Primary Care Trust, Ipswich Hospital, Suffolk, UK
28 Nursing patients with skin problems

Fiona Pringle RGN FETC
Clinical Nurse Manager, Oxford Fertility Unit, Level 4,
Women's Centre, Oxford Radcliffe NHS Trust, Headington,
Oxford, UK
28 Nursing patients with skin problems

Denise Quinton BA(Hons) DipN RGN ONCCert ENB998 931 285
Nurse Specialist, Peterborough District Hospital,
Peterborough, UK
34 Nursing patients who need palliative care

Elizabeth Rawlings RGN BSc(Hons)
Senior Nurse, Haematology, Oxford Radcliffe Hospitals NHS
Trust, Oxford, UK
18 Nursing patients with blood disorders

Mary Reet MSc DipN RGN RSCN CertEd
Formerly Health Lecturer, University of Nottingham,
Boston, UK
4 Circadian rhythms and sleep patterns

Jillian Riley BA(Hons) MSc RGN RM
Senior Lecturer, Cardio-Respiratory Nursing,
Thames Valley University, London, UK
19 Nursing patients with cardiovascular disorders

Mary Shaw BA MSc OND CertEd RGN RNT RCNT
Ophthalmic Nurse Practitioner, University of Manchester,
Royal Eye Hospital, Manchester, UK
15 Nursing patients with problems of the eye and vision

Mandy Sheppard DipPerformanceCoaching (Business) RN ENB100
Training and Development Consultant, Kent, UK
31 Nursing critically ill patients

Mike Smith MSc PGDipEd RGN
Coordinator, Postgraduate Diploma of Clinical Nursing
(Orthopaedic), Professional Development Unit,
Royal Perth Hospital, Perth, Western Australia, Australia
27 Nursing patients with musculoskeletal disorders

Martin Steggall BSc(Hons) MSc DipN RN
Lecturer in Applied Biological Science and Urology,
Honorary Urology Nurse Specialist (ED), City University,
St Bartholomew School of Nursing and Midwifery,
London, UK
25 Nursing patients with sexual health and reproductive problems

Sue Stringer BSc(Hons) RGN ENB998 ENB338 ENB931
Upper GI Nurse Specialist, Endoscopy Unit, King's Mill Centre,
Sutton-in-Ashfield, Nottinghamshire, UK
21 Nursing patients with nose and throat disorders

Philippa Sully MSc CertEd FPACert CCRelate RN RM RHV RNT
Senior Lecturer, Interprofessional Practice, Institute of Health
Sciences, City University, St Bartholomew School of Nursing
and Midwifery, London, UK
3 Communication in adult nursing

Ann Taylor BN MSc DipBN(Wales) RGN
Senior Lecturer in Pain Management, Department of
Anaesthetics and Intensive Care Medicine, College of Medicine,
University of Wales, Cardiff, UK
7 Pain

Francis Vaz BSc(Hons) FRCS
Specialist Registrar ENT South Thames, ENT Department,
Guy's and St Thomas' Hospitals NHS Trust, London, UK
16 Nursing patients with problems of the ear and hearing

Karrie Ward MSc DipN CertEd RGN RMN RNT
Senior Lecturer, School of Health Care Practice,
Anglia Polytechnic University, Chelmsford, UK
29 Perioperative nursing

Maggie Watkinson MSc DipHE CertEd(FE) RN
Diabetes Clinical Nurse Specialist, Diabetes Centre,
Duchess Building, Musgrove Park Hospital, Taunton, UK
17 Nursing patients with endocrine and metabolic disorders

Roger Watson BSc PhD RGN CBiol FIBiol ILTM FRSA
Professor of Nursing, School of Nursing, Social Work and
Applied Health Studies, University of Hull, Hull, UK
32 Nursing older adults

Jane Watts RGN
Dermatology Nurse Practitioner, Barking,
Havering and Redbridge Hospitals NHS Trust,
King George Hospital, Ilford, Essex, UK
28 Nursing patients with skin problems

Anne Waugh BSc(Hons) MSc CertEd SRN RNT ILTM
Senior Lecturer, School of Acute and Continuing Care Nursing,
Napier University, Edinburgh, UK
8 Problems associated with fluid, electrolyte and acid–base balance

Mandy Wells MSc DipN(Lond) RN RM PGCMS
Senior Nurse Specialist, St Pancras Hospital,
Continence and Stoma Services, London, UK
12 Maintaining continence

Liz Williamson BSc(Hons) RGN
Senior Nurse Manager, Surgery, City Hospital,
Nottingham, UK
23 Nursing patients with hepatic, biliary and pancreatic disorders

Amy Winsor RGN
Dermatology Nurse Practitioner,
University Hospital, Lewisham, London, UK
28 Nursing patients with skin problems

Sue Woodward MSc PGCEA RGN
Head of Specialist and Palliative Care, King's College London,
Florence Nightingale School of Nursing and Midwifery,
London, UK
14 Nursing patients with neurological problems

Foreword

The concept of clinical governance was introduced in the Department of Health White Paper 'The New NHS, Modern, Dependable' in 1997. It heralded a number of significant changes to the structure and working of the health service in the UK. Most significantly, however, it changed thinking about service delivery and means of improving patient/client care through the introduction of clinical governance. Five years later this concept has had a major impact on the nursing profession. The need to take the changes brought by clinical governance into consideration must be realised in programmes of nurse education if they are to be effective in preparing future practitioners.

Essentially clinical governance is a means of ensuring that all health professionals, including nurses, receive the appropriate education and training to equip them with the skills and competencies necessary to deliver the care needed by patients/clients. It ensures that the processes, which seek to improve quality of care, are in place throughout all organizations which provide health care and uses risk management to identify and prevent potential problems. Techniques such as clinical audit are employed to monitor and improve existing practice and to ensure that wherever possible practice is based on evidence.

Professional bodies such as the Royal College of Nursing quickly recognize the potential of clinical governance to improve the quality of patient/client care (RCN 1998). Like the Department of Health (1997), the RCN emphasises the need to ensure that care is:

- Patient-focused: all elements of clinical governance should seek to improve the service received by service-users and their families.
- Transferable: clinical governance should apply to all aspects of health care whether it is delivered in the acute sector or the community.
- Partnership: clinical governance requires multidisciplinary cooperation between all members of the health care team.
- User involvement: service users, their families and the involvement of the wider public are required for successful clinical governance.

Nurses, midwives and health visitors have welcomed clinical governance, reflecting their key position as the patient/client advocate and their unique role in promoting holistic care.

To meet the challenge of clinical governance, all nurses must:

- Ensure that wherever possible, care is based on sound evidence.
- Identify areas of patient/client care that could be improved and strive to develop strategies which can realise improvement.
- Evaluate the care they deliver.
- Disseminate examples of good practice through local, and where appropriate, national networks.

The publication of 'Nursing Adults: The Practice of Caring' edited by Chris Brooker and Maggie Nicol represents an important step into helping aspiring members of the nursing profession meet the challenges of clinical governance in improving the delivery of health care.

This book is intended primarily for pre-registration students, but it would provide a useful resource for any nurse who needs updating. It provides a comprehensive introduction to the care of adult patients/clients and their families in a format that is attractive, interactive and user friendly. The 35 chapters are sensibly arranged in 4 sections.

Chapters in Section 1 are concerned with nursing and quality issues, communication, and interpersonal skills. These issues, which are clearly essential to meet the clinical governance agenda, set the scene for the rest of the book. Section 2 presents important nursing issues; stress; pain control; shock; fluid balance and nutrition are all here. Section 3, the largest in the book, introduces the nursing care of people with common disorders using a broad systems approach. Each chapter has a firm nursing focus incorporating patient assessment, management, teaching and health promotion. This demonstrates the importance of the holistic approach to care and its place at the heart of modern health service delivery. Finally, Section 4 of the book deals with specific areas of adult nursing, including: preoperative care; management of patients in the accident and emergency setting; the critically ill; and cancer patients.

Each chapter adopts the same format. Concise aims and key words are followed by refreshingly clear text which has been generously augmented with diagrams, special interest boxes, a list of further reading kept to a sensible length, suggestions for student activities and useful summary. Relevant anatomy and physiology are included as appropriate throughout. The emphasis on evidence-based care and reflection in action are important and valuable features throughout every chapter in this book and will be warmly welcomed by student nurses and their tutors. The text is well-referenced with up-to-date sources.

Overall this book shows evidence of competent writing in an attractive style that effectively engages and informs the reader. Individual authors are clearly experts in their field and the editors have done a sterling job in drawing together material related to a wide range of topics concerned with care of the adult patient/client and crafting them into a chapter sequence that is logical, giving the book a uniquely nursing focus. Altogether this new book should be welcomed by nursing students, educationalists and those who commission education programmes as a step forward in promoting patient/client-focused, evidence-based care.

REFERENCES

Department of Health 1997. The New NHS: Modern, Dependable. Stationery Office, London

Royal College of Nursing 1998. Guidance for Nurses on Clinical Governance. RCN, London

Preface

When planning this book, we wanted to produce a textbook that includes the kind of information nurses need to be able to provide sensitive and knowledgeable care to adult patients and clients, and their families. Each chapter has been written by experts from clinical practice or education. Modern nursing is holistic in nature and based on the best available evidence. Nurses do not necessarily provide all the 'hands-on' care themselves (that is often done by health care assistants and other carers) and so they also need the knowledge and skills to be able to teach and supervise others. Therefore, nurses need a wide range of knowledge and skills and to be able to think critically and reflect on their experience in order to develop professionally and personally. This book provides the starting point for that professional journey.

The first section of the book sets the scene and explores two issues that are fundamental to all aspects of nursing practice: quality assurance, and communication and interpersonal skills. The second section addresses clinical issues that are pertinent to the care of many patients and clients, for example, sleep, nutrition and infection control. Section 3 is the largest section and deals with a wide range of conditions, such as respiratory and cardiovascular disorders, that you are likely to meet when caring for adult patients, and the final section covers specialist aspects of nursing such as perioperative nursing and caring for the critically ill.

The book includes a number of features designed to make it easy to use and help you get the most from it. Each chapter opens with a few words from a patient, a nurse or a carer that illustrate an important aspect of the chapter. Although these are not real quotes from real people, they are based on our extensive experience of caring for patients and their families and working with students and registered nurses, and as patients ourselves! We feel that starting each chapter in this way will emphasize the patient/client-centred approach of this book. A number of guidelines for specific nursing activities are also included. As with all aspects of nursing care, it is important that you gain experience under the supervision of a registered nurse until competent.

Each chapter also includes specialist boxes, illustrations, recommendations for further reading and websites. Because nursing and health care are constantly changing, website addresses are included to enable you to check the latest information. This is a textbook for enquiring nurses wishing to understand more and improve their practice. Whether you are a student, an experienced nurse or a nurse returning to practice after a break, this book is for you. We hope that you will find it interesting and informative.

Norfolk and London, 2003

Chris Brooker
Maggie Nicol

Acknowledgements

The editors would like to thank their families and colleagues for their support and understanding throughout this mammoth task and the contributors whose hard work made *Nursing Adults: the Practice of Caring* possible.

Thanks also to Peta Cunnane, Janet Mardle and Graham Nickson who offered help and ideas and to all those at Elsevier who were involved in the book. In particular, we would like to thank Jill Northcott (who started the whole thing!), Jackie Curthoys, Kirsty Guest, Mairi McCubbin, Inta Ozols and Sarena Wolfaard for their tremendous support and enthusiasm throughout the project.

Getting the best from this book

This book is designed so that you can dip in and out and is structured to enable you to find what you need quickly. It is designed to help you develop the knowledge and skills you need to care for your patients and clients more effectively, and to prepare for new placements and write assignments and essays.

STRUCTURE OF THE BOOK

The book comprises 35 chapters arranged in 4 sections, plus a glossary, table of normal values and an index.

SECTION 1 NURSING, QUALITY AND COMMUNICATION

The chapters in this section will help you to understand what adult nursing means and why high-quality care, effective communication and well-developed interpersonal skills are so central to nursing care.

SECTION 2 COMMON NURSING ISSUES

This section includes chapters addressing the sort of clinical problems that you will meet in almost all areas of nursing. These are issues such as ensuring adequate nutrition, relieving pain, preventing infection, promoting continence, and managing fever and hypothermia.

SECTION 3 NURSING PATIENTS WITH COMMON DISORDERS

The focus in this section is on specific conditions that you will meet as a nurse, both in and outside of hospital. For clarity of presentation and to reduce repetition the common disorders are grouped under functional systems (for example, blood disorders, cardiovascular disorders and respiratory disorders) rather than specific physical problems or symptoms such as breathlessness, which could be due to anaemia, heart failure or chronic obstructive pulmonary disease. However, each chapter focuses primarily on the important nursing matters such as assessment, management, patient teaching and health promotion.

SECTION 4 SPECIFIC AREAS OF ADULT NURSING

The fourth section focuses on the specialized areas of nursing such as perioperative nursing, caring for older adults, patients with cancer, caring for the critically ill and patients with long-term illness.

GLOSSARY

This includes definitions for all the key words plus other useful words and nursing terms.

NORMAL VALUES

The table of normal values includes the 'average' reference ranges, in adults, for blood, cerebrospinal fluid and urine.

CHAPTER LAYOUT

At the beginning of each chapter there is a list of outcomes that the chapter is designed to help you achieve, and a number of key words that highlight the focus of the chapter. These words are also defined in the glossary. Where appropriate, each chapter includes an overview of anatomy and physiology, medical tests and investigations and health promotion activities. In order to help you understand the various conditions and provide support and information for your patients and clients, the causes, prevalence, symptoms, and medical and surgical management are summarized. However, the prime focus of each chapter is the nursing assessment and management. Nursing management has a distinctive heading to emphasize its importance and allow for easy identification.

SPECIALIST BOXES

Each chapter has a number of special boxes that are designed to summarize key points, highlight important issues, guide your practice, or make you stop and think and reflect on your experience. Some of the boxes suggest activities such as reading a journal article, finding out about local practice or thinking about a patient you have nursed. As your experience broadens, you may wish to re-visit some of these activities and see whether your views/opinions have changed.

These boxes are:

 ### ETHICAL ISSUES BOXES

These boxes contain discussion and questions about ethical issues such as who should receive treatment or allocating scarce resources. Examples include: 'Pain management rationing', 'Dialysis provision', and 'Maintaining confidentiality'.

 ### EVIDENCE-BASED PRACTICE BOXES

Effective nursing care is based on sound evidence. These boxes explore some of the evidence available to nurses in practice, for example, 'Hip protectors as protection against hip fractures in older people', 'The importance of handwashing in the surgical environment'.

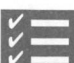 GUIDELINES FOR CARE PRIORITIES BOXES

These boxes provide a summary of best practice in a specific area and provide guidance for practitioners. The varied topics covered include 'Discharge criteria from recovery units following general anaesthetic', 'Physical examination and skin assessment', and 'Principles for safe blood transfusion'.

 HEALTH PROMOTION BOXES

Health promotion boxes illustrate the range of diverse activities directed towards promoting health and supporting patients who wish to change negative health behaviours, for example, stopping smoking. Other examples are 'Good practice in consent', 'Preparation for discharge', and 'Preventing burn injuries'.

 OLDER ADULT: NURSING PRIORITIES BOXES

Most adult patients in hospital and receiving nursing care in the community are classed as older adults. These boxes address the specific nursing needs of older people such as 'Dry skin', 'Breast cancer and older women', and 'Anaemia in older adults'.

REFLECTIVE PRACTICE BOXES

In order to develop as professionals and life-long learners, nurses need to be able to reflect on their experience. These boxes offer opportunities to reflect on a variety of situations in order to enhance your learning. In some of the boxes real patients have written about what happened to them and about the things that worried them. General examples of reflective practice boxes include: 'Sexuality and patients undergoing cytotoxic chemotherapy', 'Waiting for a diagnosis', and 'Performance ('league') tables'.

 SPECIAL ISSUES BOXES

These boxes highlight particularly important or less common aspects of the management of a particular condition or area of nursing. For example: 'Culture and the perioperative experience of patients', 'Bone marrow donation, and 'Proper positioning after a stroke'.

SUMMARY AND SELF-TEST

The summary of main points is designed to help you check your understanding of the major focus of the chapter, and the self-test is included to enable you to test your learning and identify areas in need of further reading or discussion.

 FURTHER READING

 USEFUL WEBSITES

 USEFUL ADDRESSES

REFERENCES

The areas above point you to specialist books and publications in the field to enable you to develop more specialist knowledge. All chapters are fully referenced and website addresses and other useful sources of information are also provided.

The clear and accessible information, illustrations, boxes and other features in *Nursing Adults: the Practice of Caring* will provide you with an excellent base for practice and for your professional development.

Contents

SECTION 1 NURSING, QUALITY AND COMMUNICATION   1

1 ADULT NURSING: SETTING THE SCENE   3

What is nursing?   4
The regulation of nursing   4
   Code of professional conduct   6
   Post-Registration Education and Practice (PREP)   6
Adult nursing   7
   Information-giving and informed consent   8
   Health and health promotion   9
     Sharing information   9
     Sharing skills   10
Nursing models   10
   The Activities of Living model   10
     Activities of living   10
     Influencing factors   11
Nursing process   11
   Assessment   11
     Nursing diagnosis   11
   Planning   12
     Goal-setting   12
     Integrated care pathways   12
   Implementation   12
     Primary nursing   12
     Team nursing   12
     Patient allocation   13
     Task allocation   13
   Evaluation   13
Evidence-based practice and research   13
   Types of knowledge   13
     Critical appraisal of evidence   13
   Guidelines for care   15
     Policies and protocols   15
Reflective practice   15
   Reflection – what is it?   15
     Using a model of reflection   16
     Writing a reflective journal (diary)   16
     Writing reflectively for assignments   16
Ethical issues   16
   The value of life   17
     Termination of pregnancy   17
     Euthanasia   18
   Goodness or rightness   18
   Justice or fairness   18

   Truth-telling or honesty   19
   Individual freedom   19

2 QUALITY MANAGEMENT AND STANDARDS OF CARE   23

Defining quality   24
Quality management in the health service   24
   Quality in the NHS   24
     Clinical governance   25
     NICE and CHI   25
   Evidence-based practice   26
   Quality in the private and voluntary sectors   27
   Quality and cost   27
   Benchmarking   27
   British Standards and The Patient's Charter   28
     British Standard (BS) 5750   28
     The Patient's Charter and the NHS guide   28
   Change management   29
Dimensions of quality in health care   29
   Use of models for quality in health care   29
     Maxwell's dimensions of quality   30
     Donabedian's structure–process–outcome model   30
   Standards and standard-setting   30
Making sense of quality interventions   32
   A hierarchical structure for quality interventions   32
     Quality control   32
     Quality assessment   32
     Quality improvement   32
     Quality assurance   32
     Quality management   32
     Total quality management   32
   Quality enhancement   32
     Quality circles   32
     Quality improvement teams   32
     Quality councils   33
Quality nursing care   33
   Evidence-based nursing   33
   Improving nursing standards   33
   Role of training and education   33
Monitoring, evaluating and auditing quality   34
   Monitoring and evaluating   34
   Audits   34

   Patient/carer feedback and satisfaction   35

3 COMMUNICATION IN ADULT NURSING   39

The nature of communication   40
   Verbal communication   40
   Non-verbal communication   40
   Paralinguistics   41
   Factors influencing communication   41
   Barriers to effective communication   41
Culture and communication   41
   Definition of culture   42
   Culture in nursing   42
The therapeutic relationship in nursing practice   43
   Nurses and power   43
   A model of helping   43
   The nurse–client relationship   44
     Self-awareness   44
     The helping relationship   45
Personality theories and communication   45
Communication and counselling skills   46
   Communication skills   46
   Counselling skills   46
   Counselling   47
   Boundaries   47
Communication and social contact   47
   Greeting skills   47
   Active listening skills   48
     Listening skills   48
   Questioning skills   48
     The value of questions   49
   Explanation skills   50
   Assertiveness skills   51
     Advocacy   51
     Contract-making skills   51
     Scripting skills   51
     Dealing with conflict   52
   Dealing with bad news   52
   Ending professional relationships   53
     Leave-taking   53
Communication in groups   53
   Group dynamics   53
   Roles in groups   54
   Teams   54
     Labelling

CONTENTS

SECTION 2
COMMON NURSING ISSUES 57

4 CIRCADIAN RHYTHMS AND SLEEP PATTERNS 59

Internal controls of sleep and rest **59**
The physiology of sleep 59
Stages of sleep 60
Neurochemical processes 60
Coma 61
Physical changes during sleep **61**
Body temperature 61
Cardiovascular system 61
Respiratory system 61
Renal system 62
Endocrine system 62
Purpose of sleep **62**
Sleep deprivation 62
The effect of shift work 63
Jet lag 63
Patients in hospital 63
Factors affecting normal sleep patterns **63**
Age 63
Culture 64
Individuality 64
Gender 64
Body mass 64
Genetics 64
Factors that interrupt sleep patterns **64**
External factors 64
Noise 64
Light 64
Internal factors 65
Pain 65
Diet 65
Drugs and alcohol 65
Exercise 65
Mental health 65
Disordered sleep patterns **65**
Insomnia 65
Nursing management of insomnia 65
Excess somnolence (narcolepsy) 66
Nightmares 66
Nursing management 66
Sleep terrors 67
Nursing management 67
Sleepwalking (somnambulance) 67
Nursing management 67
Sleep apnoea/hypopnoea syndrome 67
Medical management 67
Nursing management 67
Bruxism – grinding of teeth during sleep 67

Nursing interventions to promote sleep **67**
Assessment of sleep patterns and routines 68
Planning care 68
Helping patients to sleep 68
Evaluating the success of the planned care 68
Non-pharmacological means of promoting sleep 69
Darkness 69
Silence 69
Comfort 69
Physical activity 70
Food and drink 70
Temperature 70
Security 70
Daytime naps 70
Timing of regular medication 70
Complementary therapies 70
Pharmacological means of promoting sleep **70**
Analgesia 70
Hypnotics 70
Anxiolytics 71
Common disorders that affect sleep **71**
Breathing problems 71
Nursing management 71
Urinary system 72
Nursing management 72
Rhythmic pattern disorders 72
Seasonal affective disorder 72
Menstrual cycle 72

5 TEMPERATURE REGULATION 75

Physiology of temperature homeostasis **76**
Thermoregulation 76
Core and peripheral temperature 76
Heat regulation mechanisms 76
Heat transfer mechanisms 76
Heat loss mechanisms 77
Heat gain mechanisms 77
Factors affecting body temperature 77
Normal variations in body temperature 77
Abnormal variations in body temperature 77
Disorders of temperature regulation **78**
Pyrexia and hyperpyrexia 78
The stages and patterns of pyrexia 78
Beneficial and detrimental responses to pyrexia 79
Hyperthermia 79

Hypothermia 81
Accidental hypothermia 81
Therapeutic hypothermia 81
Frostbite 83
Nursing assessment of body temperature 83
Equipment 83
Glass mercury thermometers 83
Single-use chemical thermometers 83
Electronic thermometers 83
Tympanic membrane thermometers 83
Choosing the right thermometer 84
Taking the temperature 84
Time of day 84
Thermometer insertion time 84
Sites 85
Nursing management of raised body temperature 86
Management of pyrexia and hyperpyrexia 86
Management of hyperthermia, heat stroke and malignant hyperthermia 86
Cooling methods 86
Fluid management 87
Management of rigor 87
Nutritional needs during pyrexia and hyperthermia 87
Nursing management of hypothermia 87
Rewarming 88
Passive external rewarming 88
Active external rewarming 89
Active internal rewarming 89
Fluid replacement 89
Monitoring and observations 89
Observation of vital signs 89
Urine output 90
Blood glucose 90
Serum potassium 90
Acid–base balance 90
The electrocardiograph (ECG) 90
The consequences of hypothermia 90
Shivering 90
Rewarming shock 90
Impaired immunity 90
Acidosis 90
Nutritional needs 90
Pharmacokinetics 91
Nursing management of frostbite 91

6 STRESS 93

Concepts and models of stress **93**
A model of stress 94
Responses to stress **94**

Physiological responses 94
  The general adaptation syndrome 94
  The local adaptation syndrome 97
Psychological responses 97
  Mental defence mechanisms 97
Stressors **98**
Physiological stressors 98
Psychosocial stressors 98
Individual response to stress:
the stressful personality type 99
**Common stressors within
the health care system** **100**
Stress affecting patients 100
  Waiting for results 100
  Physical stress 100
Stress affecting health care
workers 100
  Burnout 101
  Post-traumatic stress disorder 102
Stress affecting carers 102
  Stress in patients' relatives 102
**Maladaption: stress-related
illness** **103**
The circulatory system 103
The immune system 103
Other vulnerable organs 103
  Gastrointestinal system 103
  Respiratory system 103
  Skin 103
  *Headache, backache and
  muscular aches* 103
  *Migraine and tension
  headaches* 104
  Substance misuse 104
Mental illness 104
  Anxiety 104
  Depression 104
Accidents or unsafe behaviour 104
  Nursing assessment 104
Measuring stress 104
  Physiological measures 104
  *Hospital anxiety and
  depression scale* 104
  Social readjustment rating scale 105
Self-reporting 105
**Reducing stress and
enhancing coping strategies** **105**
Pharmacological methods 105
  Anxiolytics 105
  Antidepressants 105
Complementary remedies 105
  Valerian 106
  *Hypericum perforatum
  (St John's wort)* 106
Non-pharmacological methods 106
  Diet 106
  Exercise 106
  Counselling 106
  Clinical supervision 106

  Time management 106
  Cognitive behavioural therapy 107
  Group therapies 107
  Relaxation methods 107
Reducing the stresses of nursing 107

7 PAIN **111**

Definitions of pain **111**
Types of pain **112**
Nociceptive pain 112
  Threshold and tolerance 112
Non-nociceptive pain 112
**The anatomy and physiology
of pain** **112**
The structures and
physiological processes
involved in pain perception 113
Stages of nociception 113
The placebo response 114
**Factors that affect pain
perception and management** **115**
Physiological factors 115
Psychosocial factors 115
Pharmacological factors 116
**The main adverse effects of
unrelieved pain** **116**
**Requirements for effective
acute pain management** **117**
Staff education 117
  *Lack of knowledge contributing
  to myths and misconceptions
  about pain and its management* 118
Patient information and
education 118
Acute pain assessment 119
A structured approach to pain
management and utilization
of resources 121
Use of an appropriate model
to direct care 121
Recommendations and
guidelines for practice 121
Managing acute pain **123**
Conventional analgesics 123
  Opioids 123
  Opioid antagonist (naloxone) 124
  NSAIDs and paracetamol 124
  Local anaesthetics 124
Conventional routes for the
administration of analgesia 125
  Oral administration 125
  Inhalation analgesia 125
  Transdermal administration 125
  Rectal administration 125
  Parenteral administration 125
  Patient-controlled analgesia 125
  *Epidural analgesia in acute
  pain management* 127

Non-pharmacological methods
of managing acute pain 127
Special considerations **128**
Acute pain management in
pre-existing substance misuse,
addiction or dependence 128
The patient with chronic
non-malignant pain 129

**8 PROBLEMS ASSOCIATED
WITH FLUID, ELECTROLYTE
AND ACID–BASE BALANCE** **133**

**Related anatomy and
physiology** **134**
Fluid compartments and
electrolyte concentrations 134
  Water distribution 134
  Electrolytes 134
Movement of water and
electrolytes 134
  Diffusion 134
  Osmosis 134
  Active transport 136
  Filtration 136
Formation of tissue fluid 136
  Oedema 137
Water and electrolyte balance 137
  Thirst 137
  *Hormonal control of fluid
  and electrolyte balance* 137
Disturbances of fluid balance 138
  Isotonic imbalances 138
  Osmolar imbalances 139
  Nursing assessment 139
Assessment of fluid and
electrolyte status 139
  The oral cavity 139
  Thirst 139
  Skin 139
  Oedema 139
  Sunken eyes 140
  *Confusion, lethargy and
  anxiety* 140
  Respiratory status 140
  Pulse 140
  Blood pressure 140
  Central venous pressure 140
  Jugular venous pressure 140
  Urinary output 140
  Bowel habit 140
Factors that predispose to
fluid and electrolyte imbalance 140
  *Drought or shortage of
  drinking water* 140
  Inability to respond to thirst 140
  Fasting 140
  Dysphagia 141
  Dyspnoea

CONTENTS

Alcohol 141
Reduced dexterity and mobility 141
Renal and cardiovascular disorders 141
Age 141
Fear of incontinence 141
Diuretic therapy 141
Terminal illness 142
Preventing dehydration 142
The relationship between thirst and dehydration 142
Oral rehydration solutions 142
Diagnostic tests and investigations 142
Blood tests: serum urea and electrolytes 142
Urine tests 142
24-hour urine collection 142
Urinalysis 142
Other investigations 143
Nursing management and interventions 143
Fluid balance charts 143
Fluid intake 143
Fluid output 143
24-hour fluid balance 143
Daily weight 144
Oedema 144
Helping patients with oral fluids 144
Types of oral fluids 144
Recommencing oral fluids after a period of fasting 144
Helping a patient to drink 144
Fluid restriction 145
Nasogastric tubes 145
Intravenous infusion 145
Maintaining safety and comfort during i.v. infusions 146
Complications of i.v. therapy 146
The role of the specialist i.v. nurse 147
Subcutaneous infusion 147
Rectal infusion 147
Common electrolyte disorders: management and nursing care 147
Hyponatraemia 147
Hypernatraemia 148
Hypokalaemia 148
Hyperkalaemia 148
Acid–base balance 148
pH regulation and buffers 149
The bicarbonate system 149
Assessment of acid–base status 149
Pulse oximetry 149
Arterial blood gases 149
Disorders of acid–base balance: causes and management 149
Metabolic acidosis 150
Metabolic alkalosis 150

Respiratory acidosis 150
Respiratory alkalosis 151
Mixed disorders 151

9 SHOCK, SYSTEMIC INFLAMMATORY RESPONSE AND MULTIPLE ORGAN DYSFUNCTION 153

Defining shock 153
Types of shock 154
Hypovolaemic shock 154
Cardiogenic shock 155
Distributive shock 155
Anaphylaxis 155
Septic shock 155
Obstructive shock 155
Spinal shock 155
Neurogenic shock 155
The stages of shock 155
Compensated shock 155
Progressive shock 155
Irreversible shock 155
Pathophysiological effects of shock 156
Cardiovascular system 156
Regulation of blood flow 156
Maintenance of blood pressure 156
Respiratory system 157
Hypoxia 157
Acidosis 157
Renal system 157
Decompensated shock 157
Cardiovascular system 157
Respiratory system 157
Renal system 157
Shock, the systemic inflammatory response and multiple organ dysfunction 157
Pathophysiology of SIRS 158
The inflammatory/immune response 158
Nursing assessment 159
Physical signs 160
Respiratory changes 160
Cardiovascular changes 160
Renal changes 160
Neurological changes 160
Monitored signs 160
Heart rate 160
Electrocardiograph (ECG) 160
Blood pressure 160
Temperature 160
Peripheral arterial oxygen saturation (pulse oximetry) 161
Central venous pressure (CVP) 161
Urine output 161
Arterial pressure monitoring and blood gases 161

Pulmonary artery catheters 162
Oesophageal Doppler 162
Blood lactate levels 162
Gastric tonometry 162
Nursing management of shock 162
Ensuring the patient has a patent airway 162
Supporting breathing 162
Determining circulatory status 162
Correcting hypoxaemia 163
Relieving anxiety and calming the patient 163
Ensuring adequate pain relief 163
Reducing body temperature 164
Supporting the patient's family 164
Correcting hypovolaemia 164
Choice of fluids for correcting hypovolaemia 164
Optimizing intravascular fluid volume 165
Correcting hypotension with drug infusions 166
Specific management for different types of shock 166
Management of hypovolaemic shock 166
Intravenous fluids 166
CVP measurement 166
Management of cardiogenic shock 166
Maintaining blood pressure 166
Intra-aortic balloon pump 167
Management of anaphylactic shock 167
Management of septic shock 167
Supporting haemodynamic status 167
Reducing oxygen demands 167
Managing hyperglycaemia 167
Treating and preventing infection 167
Multiple organ dysfunction 167
Manifestations 167
Renal failure 168
Acute respiratory distress syndrome (ARDS) 168
Disseminated intravascular coagulation 168
Gastrointestinal dysfunction 168
Cardiovascular dysfunction 168
Neurological dysfunction 168
Nursing and medical management 168
Metabolic support 168
Prevention of infection 169
Renal support 169
Nutrition and gastrointestinal support 169
Prevention of complications 169

10 TISSUE VIABILITY: MANAGING CHRONIC WOUNDS — 173

Anatomy and physiology of the skin — 173
Layers of the skin — 174
The epidermis — 174
The dermis — 174
The hypodermis — 175
Functions of the skin — 175
Protection — 175
Thermoregulation — 175
Sensation — 175
Metabolism — 175
Non-verbal communication — 175
The effects of ageing on the skin — 175
Principles of skin care — 176
Wound healing — 176
The physiology of wound healing — 177
The inflammatory stage — 177
The proliferative stage — 178
The maturation stage — 178
Factors influencing healing — 178
General health status and wound healing — 178
Lifestyle factors that may delay wound healing — 179
Principles of wound management — 180
Specific wound management objectives — 180
Wound assessment — 181
Wound measurement — 181
Wound cleansing — 181
Wound debridement — 181
Biosurgery — 182
Wound dressings — 182
The ideal dressing — 182
Dressing products — 182
Other dressing categories — 183
Selection of wound management products — 186
Professional factors influencing selection of dressing products — 186
Pressure ulcers — 187
Epidemiology and aetiology — 187
Pressure — 187
Shear — 188
Friction — 188
Risk assessment — 188
Pressure ulcer risk assessment tools — 188
Preventing pressure damage — 189
Positioning — 189
Classification of pressure damage — 190

Pressure ulcer prevention equipment — 191
Pressure-reducing equipment — 191
Pressure-relieving equipment — 192
Selection of equipment — 192
Practical issues — 192
Specialist additional features — 193
Prevention and management of leg ulcers — 193
Epidemiology and aetiology — 193
Patient assessment — 193
Venous leg ulcers — 194
Arterial leg ulcers — 194
Vascular assessment — 195
Principles of venous leg ulcer management — 196
Compression bandaging — 196
Compression hosiery — 197
Principles of arterial leg ulcer management — 197
Management of patients with ulcers of mixed aetiology — 198
Use of leg ulcer management protocols — 198

11 NUTRITION — 201

What is nutrition? — 202
Nutrients in food — 202
The nurse's role in health promotion — 202
Macronutrients — 203
Energy and energy balance — 203
Proteins — 203
Fats — 204
Saturated and unsaturated fats — 204
Lipid transportation — 204
Carbohydrate — 205
Monosaccharides — 205
Starch and non-starch polysaccharides — 205
Micronutrients — 205
Vitamins — 205
Vitamin A — 205
Vitamin D — 207
Vitamin E — 208
Vitamin K — 208
Vitamin B_1 (thiamin) — 208
Vitamin B_2 (riboflavin) — 208
Niacin — 208
Vitamin B_6 — 209
Vitamin B_{12} (cobalamins) and folic acid (folates) — 209
Biotin — 209
Pantothenic acid — 209
Vitamin C (ascorbic acid) — 209
Minerals — 209
Calcium — 209
Iron (Fe) — 210

Sodium, potassium and chloride (Na, K, Cl) — 210
Phosphorus (P) — 210
Zinc (Zn) — 210
Selenium (Se) — 210
Iodine (I) — 210
Magnesium (Mg) — 210
Copper (Cu) — 210
Chromium (Cr) — 211
Other minerals — 211
Nursing assessment and nutritional screening — 211
Psychological areas of nutrition and the nursing assessment — 211
Food preferences — 211
Sensory aspects of eating — 211
Sociological and cultural influences and the nursing assessment — 212
Sociological issues — 212
Physiological areas and the nursing assessment — 212
Alterations in food intake — 214
Altered gastrointestinal function — 214
Alterations in nutrient metabolism — 214
Assessing nutritional status — 214
Physical assessment — 214
Dietary history — 214
Anthropometric methods — 214
Body mass index — 214
Skinfold thickness — 214
Mid-arm muscle circumference — 214
Biochemical indicators — 214
Creatinine height index — 215
Twenty-four-hour nitrogen balance — 215
Serum proteins — 215
Nutritional screening tools — 215
Groups with specific nutritional needs — 216
Individuals with coronary heart disease — 216
The obese individual — 216
Helping with weight loss – the nurses' role — 217
Older adults — 217
Physiological changes — 217
Social changes — 217
Women of child-bearing age and vegetarians/vegans — 217
Patients with sepsis, trauma and cancer – the hypermetabolic patient — 217
Nutrition and wound healing — 218
Food allergy and intolerance — 219
Specific food intolerances

Nursing interventions 219
Food choice 219
In hospital 219
In the community 219
Environment 219
Eating 221
Staffing 221
Food fortification 221
Nutritional support **222**
Nutritional supplements
and sip feeding 222
Modifying textures 222
Sip feeding 222
Enteral feeding 222
Routes for enteral nutrition 222
Enteral feed regimens 223
Giving an enteral feed 224
*Complications of enteral
nutrition* 224
Parenteral nutrition 224
Managing parenteral nutrition 225
*Complications of parenteral
nutrition* 225
Drug–nutrient interactions **225**

**12 MAINTAINING
CONTINENCE** **229**
*Definition of urinary
incontinence* 229
**Anatomy and physiology
of the lower urinary tract** **229**
The bladder 230
Urethra 230
Pelvic floor 230
The levator ani 231
**Neurological control of the
lower urinary tract and
pelvic floor** **231**
The micturition cycle 231
Urinary incontinence **231**
The impact of urinary
incontinence 232
Continence care in hospital 232
Continence care at home 233
Causes of urinary incontinence 233
*Immobility/chronic
degenerative disease* 233
Congestive heart failure 233
Diabetes 234
Concurrent medication 234
Impaired cognition 234
Smoking 234
Environmental barriers 234
Faecal impaction 234
Obesity 234
Neurological disease/injury 234
Parity (number of children) 234
Oestrogen depletion 234

Urinary tract infection 234
Assessment of urinary
incontinence 234
Types of urinary incontinence 235
*Overactive bladder (also known
as detrusor instability and
urge incontinence)* 235
Stress incontinence 235
Mixed incontinence 235
Overflow incontinence 235
Voiding inefficiency 235
Nocturia and nocturnal enuresis 236
Investigations **236**
Urinalysis 237
Physical examination 237
Post-void residual volume 237
Frequency-volume chart 237
Urodynamic investigations 237
**Treatment of urinary
incontinence** **237**
Stress incontinence: pelvic
floor education 237
Assessment of the pelvic floor 238
Pelvic floor exercises 238
Vaginal cones 239
Biofeedback 240
Electrical stimulation 240
Voiding inefficiency 240
Overactive bladder 240
Caffeine and fluid manipulation 240
Bladder retraining 241
Pelvic floor exercises 241
Electrical stimulation 241
Acupuncture 242
Pharmacological treatment of
incontinence 242
Antimuscarinic drugs 242
Desmopressin 242
Oestrogen 242
Control of defecation **242**
Faecal incontinence 243
Causes 243
Assessment 243
Management 245
*Nursing management of
urinary and faecal incontinence* 246
Advice and education 247
Continence products 247
Incontinence pads 247
Continence appliances 248

13 INFECTION CONTROL **253**

Microbiology **254**
Methods of growing organisms 254
Identifying the organism 254
Antimicrobial resistance 254
Types of organism 254
Bacteria 254

Viruses 254
Classification of microorganisms 254
Resistance to antibiotics 255
*Methicillin-resistant
Staphylococcus aureus (MRSA)* 255
*Vancomycin-resistant
enterococcus (VRE)* 255
Clostridium difficile 255
*Mycobacterium tuberculosis
(MDRTB)* 255
Gram-negative organisms 255
Gram-positive organisms 255
Causes of infection **256**
Reservoir of infection 256
Mode of transmission 256
Host response 256
*Subclinical infection and
colonization* 256
Sepsis 257
Contamination 257
Pathogens 257
Endogenous infection 257
Exogenous infection 257
Hospital-acquired (nosocomial)
infection 257
Cross-infection 257
Principles of infection control **257**
**The role of the Infection
Control Nurse** **258**
Managing outbreaks of infection 258
Surveillance of infection 258
Outbreak recognition 259
Outbreak control 259
The role of the laboratory 259
Outbreak control measures 259
Prevention of infection **260**
Universal infection control
precautions 260
Handwashing 260
Handwashing technique 261
Social handwashing 262
Surgical hand disinfection 262
Hand towels 262
Alcohol hand rub 263
Protective clothing 263
Gowns 263
Gloves 263
Aprons 263
Masks 263
Eye protection 264
Prevention of cross-infection **264**
Isolation of patients 264
Source isolation 264
Protective isolation 265
Isolation facilities 265
Infectious disease units 265
Single room isolation 265
*Managing infectious patients
on open wards* 266

Categories of isolation nursing 266
Management of clinical waste and linen **266**
Linen disposal 266
Disposal of waste 266
Immunosuppressed patients **267**
Blood-borne infections **267**
Occupational transmission 267
Control measures for the prevention of infection by blood-borne viruses 268
Vaccination and immunization 268
Management of exposure to blood or body fluids 268

SECTION 3 NURSING PATIENTS WITH COMMON DISORDERS **271**

14 NURSING PATIENTS WITH NEUROLOGICAL PROBLEMS **273**

Anatomy and physiology – an overview **274**
The nerve impulse 275
Synapses 275
Central nervous system 276
Spinal cord 276
Brain 276
Blood–brain barrier 277
Blood supply to the brain 277
Cerebrospinal fluid and the meninges 277
Peripheral nervous system 279
Neurological nursing assessment **279**
Altered consciousness 280
Glasgow Coma Scale 280
Pupil response 283
Abnormal findings and what they may indicate 283
Limb movement 284
Changes in other observations 284
Blood pressure 284
Pulse rate 284
Temperature 284
Respiratory rate 284
Cognition and confusion 285
Cognitive problems and causes 285
Assessing cognitive function 285
Assessment of physical function – swallowing 286
General diagnostic tests and medical investigations **287**
Physical examination 287
Imaging 287
X-rays 287
Magnetic resonance imaging 287

Positron emission tomography 287
Ultrasound 288
Electroencephalography 288
Electromyography 288
Lumbar puncture 288
Biopsy 288
Blood tests 288
General disease prevention and health education **288**
Neurological impairment – general considerations **289**
Ethical and legal considerations 289
Nursing management of the unconscious patient 290
Common disorders affecting the nervous system **291**
Cerebrovascular disorders **291**
Stroke 291
Epidemiology and aetiology 291
Clinical presentation 292
Medical/surgical management 292
Nursing management 292
Subarachnoid haemorrhage 296
Pathophysiology 296
Epidemiology and aetiology 296
Clinical presentation 296
Specific investigations 296
Medical/surgical management 296
Nursing management 296
Trauma **297**
Brain injury (head injury) 297
Aetiology and epidemiology 297
Pathophysiology 297
Clinical presentation 298
Raised intracranial pressure 298
Pathophysiology 298
Clinical presentation 299
Specific investigations 300
Medical/surgical management 300
Nursing management 300
Cranial nerve disorders **303**
Bell's palsy 303
Clinical presentation 303
Management 303
Trigeminal neuralgia 304
Management 304
Demyelinating (inflammatory) disorders **304**
Multiple sclerosis 304
Epidemiology and aetiology 304
Pathophysiology 304
Clinical presentation 304
Specific investigations 304
Medical management 305
Nursing management 306
Tumours – benign and malignant **308**
Epidemiology and aetiology 308
Meningiomas 308

Glioma 308
Pathophysiology 308
Clinical presentation 308
Specific investigations 309
Medical/surgical management 309
Nursing management 309
Infections of the nervous system **310**
Meningitis – an overview 311
Bacterial meningitis 311
Aetiology and pathology – acute meningitis 311
Clinical presentation 311
Specific investigations 311
Medical management 311
Nursing management 311
Herpes zoster 312
Clinical presentation 312
Medical management 312
Nursing management 312
Creutzfeldt–Jakob disease 313
Aetiology, epidemiology and pathology 313
Clinical presentation 313
Nursing management 313
Seizures and epilepsy **313**
Epilepsy 313
Aetiology 313
Clinical presentation 315
Specific investigations 315
Medical management 315
Nursing management 315
Headache **316**
Types of headache 316
Nursing management 316
Nutritional and metabolic causes of neurological disorders **318**
Wernicke's encephalopathy 318
Pathophysiology and clinical presentation 318
Management 318
Wilson's disease 318
Pathophysiology and clinical presentation 318
Management 318
Degenerative disorders **318**
Parkinson's disease 318
Epidemiology and aetiology 319
Pathophysiology 319
Clinical presentation 319
Medical/surgical management 319
Nursing management 321
Alzheimer's disease 322
Nursing management 322
Motor neuron disease 323
Nursing management 323
Spinal cord disorders **323**
Spinal cord compression 324

CONTENTS

Spinal tumours 324
Nursing management:
spinal surgery 324
Spinal trauma 324
Aetiology 324
Clinical presentation 324
Management of the spinal
injury patient 324
Nursing management 324
Peripheral nerve disorders **326**
Polyneuropathy 327
Guillain–Barré syndrome 327
Epidemiology and aetiology 327
Pathophysiology 327
Clinical presentation 327
Specific investigations 327
Medical management 328
Nursing management 328

15 NURSING PATIENTS WITH PROBLEMS OF THE EYE AND VISION 331

Anatomy and physiology –
an overview **332**
Eyeball 332
Layers of the eyeball 332
Structures and cavities inside
the eye 333
Refraction, accommodation
and focusing 334
Refractive errors 335
Retinal physiology and the
visual pathway 335
Light and dark adaptation 336
Accessory structures 336
Eyelids, lashes and eyebrows 336
Lacrimal system 336
Conjunctiva 336
Extraocular (extrinsic) muscles 336
Nursing assessment of
ophthalmic patients **336**
Past medical history and
general health 336
History of present complaint 337
Examination of the eye 337
General diagnostic tests and
medical investigations **338**
Ophthalmoscopy 338
Slit lamp examination 339
Testing visual acuity 339
Colour vision testing 340
Gonioscopy 340
Visual field testing 340
Keratometry 340
Biometry 340
Focimetry 340
Goldmann applanation
tonometry 340

Corneal topography 340
Fluorescein angiography 340
Orthoptic examination 341
General disease prevention
and health education **341**
Visual impairment **341**
Registration as blind or
partially sighted 342
Nursing management: patients
with visual impairment 342
Nursing management:
ophthalmic medications 344
Painless visual impairment **348**
Cataract 348
Aetiology and epidemiology 348
Clinical presentation 348
Surgical management 349
Nursing management 349
Diabetic retinopathy 352
Aetiology 352
Specific investigations and
screening 352
Pathophysiology and
management 352
Nursing management 352
Age-related macular
degeneration 353
Pathophysiology, presentation
and management 353
Nursing management 353
Retinal detachment 354
Clinical presentation 354
Medical/surgical management 354
Nursing management 354
Primary open-angle glaucoma 355
Aetiology and epidemiology 355
Clinical presentation 355
Specific investigations 355
Medical/surgical management 355
Nursing management 356
Painful ocular conditions and
trauma **357**
Primary closed-angle glaucoma 357
Aetiology 357
Clinical presentation 357
Medical management 357
Nursing management 357
Enucleation 358
Nursing management 358
Corneal disorders –
an overview **359**
Corneal ulcers 359
Aetiology 359
Specific investigations 359
Medical management 359
Nursing management 359
Corneal damage due to
foreign body 359
Nursing management 360

Corneal abrasions 360
Chemical injury 360
Management 361
Conjunctival conditions **361**
Conjunctivitis 361
Clinical presentation 361
Management 361
Conditions of the uveal tract **362**
Uveitis 362
Aetiology 362
Clinical presentation 362
Management 362
Conditions affecting the
eyelids **362**
Blepharitis 362
Clinical presentation 362
Nursing management 363
Chalazion 363
Sty or external hordeolum 363
Ptosis 363
Dry eyes 363
Clinical presentation 364
Age-related disorders 364
Entropion 364
Ectropion 364

16 NURSING PATIENTS WITH PROBLEMS OF THE EAR AND HEARING 367

Overview: anatomy and
physiology of the ear **368**
Anatomy of the ear 368
External ear 368
Middle ear 368
Inner ear 369
Physiology of hearing 370
Nursing assessment 370
History-taking 370
Examination of the ear 371
Otoscopy – looking for
abnormalities 371
General otological
diagnostic tests and
medical investigations **372**
Calorics 372
Imaging 373
Electrocochleography 373
Hearing assessment and tests 373
Tuning fork tests 373
Audiometry 373
Tympanometry 373
Brain stem evoked responses 373
Nursing care of patients
undergoing hearing
investigations 373
General disease prevention
and health education **374**
Preventing noise damage 374

Hearing impairment 374
  Communicating with people
    with hearing problems 375
  Hearing aids 375
  Excess ear wax 376
    Pathophysiology 376
    Clinical presentation 376
    Specific investigations 376
    Medical/surgical management 376
    Nursing management 376
  Presbycusis 377
    Pathophysiology 377
    Clinical presentation 379
    Specific investigations 379
    Medical/surgical management 379
    Nursing management 379
  Otosclerosis 379
    Pathophysiology 379
    Clinical presentation 379
    Specific investigations 379
    Medical/surgical management 380
    Nursing management 380
  Noise-induced hearing loss 380
    Aetiology and epidemiology 380
    Pathophysiology 380
    Clinical presentation 380
    Specific investigations 380
    Medical/surgical management 380
    Nursing management 380
Trauma and foreign bodies 380
  Haematoma of the pinna 380
    Aetiology 380
    Pathophysiology 380
    Clinical presentation 380
    Medical/surgical management 380
    Nursing management 381
  Traumatic perforations of the
    tympanic membrane 381
    Aetiology 381
    Pathophysiology 381
    Clinical presentation 381
    Specific investigations 381
    Medical/surgical management 381
    Nursing management 381
  Foreign bodies in the ear 381
    Clinical presentation 381
    Medical/surgical management 381
    Nursing management 382
**Infections and inflammatory
conditions of the ear** 382
  Perichondritis 382
    Aetiology 382
    *Pathophysiology and clinical
    presentation* 382
    Medical/surgical management 382
    Nursing management 382
  Otitis externa 382
    Aetiology 382
    Pathophysiology 382

    Clinical presentation 382
    Specific investigations 383
    Medical/surgical management 383
    Nursing management 383
  Acute suppurative otitis media 383
    Aetiology 383
    Pathophysiology 383
    Clinical presentation 383
    Specific investigations 383
    Medical/surgical management 383
    Nursing management 384
  Chronic suppurative otitis media 384
    Tubotympanic 384
    Atticoantral 384
  Complications of suppurative
  otitis media 385
    Intracranial complications 385
    Temporal bone involvement 385
    Middle ear involvement 385
    *Nursing management of the
    patient undergoing ear surgery* 385
  Pre- and postoperative care 385
  Discharge advice for the patient 386
Disorders of balance 386
  Ménière's disease 386
    Aetiology 386
    Pathophysiology 386
    Clinical presentation 387
    Specific investigations 387
    Medical/surgical management 387
  Benign paroxysmal positional
  vertigo 387
    Aetiology and pathophysiology 387
    Clinical presentation 387
    Specific investigations 387
    Medical/surgical management 387
  Acute labyrinthitis 387
    Clinical presentation 387
    Medical/surgical management 387
    *Nursing management of patients
    with disorders of balance* 387
Tinnitus 388
    Aetiology 388
    Pathophysiology 388
    Clinical presentation 388
    Specific investigations 388
    Medical management 388
    Nursing management 388
Tumours 389
  Benign tumours of the
    external and middle ear 389
  Malignant tumours of the
    external and middle ear 389
    Clinical presentation 389
    Medical/surgical management 389
    Nursing management 389
  Tumours of the inner ear 389
    Acoustic neuroma 389
    Nursing care 389

**17 NURSING PATIENTS
WITH ENDOCRINE AND
METABOLIC DISORDERS** 393

**Anatomy and physiology –
an overview** 394
  Hormones 396
  Hypothalamus 396
  Pituitary gland 396
    *Anterior lobe
    (adenohypophysis)* 396
    *Posterior lobe
    (neurohypophysis)* 397
  Thyroid gland 397
    Thyroid hormones 398
  Parathyroid glands 399
    Parathyroid hormone 399
  Adrenal glands 399
    Adrenal cortex 399
    Adrenal medulla 399
    *Stress responses and the
    adrenal glands* 400
  The pancreas 400
    *Pancreatic hormones and
    glucose homeostasis* 400
Nursing assessment 401
**Diagnostic tests and medical
investigation – general** 401
  Diagnosis of diabetes mellitus 402
**General disease prevention
and health education** 403
**Disorders of the endocrine
pancreas** 403
  Type 1 diabetes 403
    Aetiology and epidemiology 403
    Pathophysiology 404
    Clinical presentation 404
    Specific investigations 404
    Medical management 404
    Nursing management 404
  Type 2 diabetes mellitus 415
    Aetiology and epidemiology 415
    Pathophysiology 416
    Clinical presentation 416
    Specific investigations 416
    Medical management 417
    Nursing management 418
**Acute complications of
diabetes** 421
  Hypoglycaemia 421
    Aetiology and epidemiology 421
    Pathophysiology 421
    Clinical presentation 421
    Specific investigations 421
    Medical management 422
    Nursing management 422
  Diabetic ketoacidosis 422
    Aetiology and epidemiology 422
    Pathophysiology 423

CONTENTS

Clinical presentation 423
Specific investigations 423
Medical management 423
Nursing management 424
Long-term diabetes complications 424
Aetiology and epidemiology 424
Pathophysiology 425
Clinical presentation 425
Specific investigations 426
Medical management 426
Nursing management 427

Disorders affecting the pituitary gland **428**
Pituitary tumours 428
Acromegaly and gigantism 428
Aetiology and epidemiology 428
Pathophysiology and clinical presentation 429
Specific investigations 429
Medical/surgical management 429
Nursing management 429
Prolactinomas 430
Aetiology and epidemiology 430
Pathophysiology and clinical presentation 430
Specific investigations 430
Medical/surgical management 430
Nursing management 430
Anterior pituitary hyposecretion 430
Aetiology and epidemiology 430
Pathophysiology and clinical presentation 430
Specific investigations 430
Medical and surgical management 431
Nursing management 431
Diabetes insipidus 431
Aetiology and epidemiology 431
Pathophysiology and clinical presentation 431
Specific investigations 431
Medical management 431
Nursing management 431

Disorders affecting the thyroid gland **431**
Graves' disease 432
Aetiology and epidemiology 432
Pathophysiology and clinical presentation 432
Special investigations 432
Medical and surgical management 432
Nursing management 433
Thyroiditis 434
Aetiology and epidemiology 434
Pathophysiology and clinical presentation 434
Special investigations 434

Nursing and medical management 434
Toxic multinodular goitre and toxic single adenoma 434
Aetiology and epidemiology 434
Pathophysiology and clinical presentation 434
Special investigations 434
Medical/surgical management 434
Nursing management 434
Hypothyroidism 435
Aetiology and epidemiology 435
Pathophysiology and clinical presentation 435
Special investigations 435
Nursing and medical management 435
Simple goitre 435
Thyroid cancer 435
Aetiology and epidemiology 435
Pathophysiology and clinical presentation 436
Specific investigations 436
Medical/surgical management 436
Nursing management 436

Disorders affecting the parathyroid glands **436**
Hypoparathyroidism 436
Aetiology and epidemiology 436
Clinical presentation 436
Specific investigations 437
Medical management 437
Nursing management 437
Hyperparathyroidism 437
Aetiology and epidemiology 437
Clinical presentation 437
Specific investigations 437
Medical and surgical management 437
Nursing management 437

Disorders affecting the adrenal glands **437**
Adrenal cortex insufficiency 437
Aetiology and epidemiology 437
Clinical presentation 438
Specific investigations 438
Medical management 438
Nursing management 438
Adrenal cortex hypersecretion – Cushing's syndrome 438
Aetiology and epidemiology 438
Pathophysiology and clinical presentation 438
Specific investigations 439
Medical and surgical management 439
Nursing management 439
Primary aldosteronism 440
Aetiology and epidemiology 440

Pathophysiology and clinical presentation 440
Specific investigations 440
Medical and surgical management 440
Nursing management 440
Phaeochromocytoma 440
Aetiology and epidemiology 440
Pathophysiology and clinical presentation 440
Specific investigations 441
Medical/surgical management 441
Nursing management 441
Adrenal sexual disorders: congenital adrenal hyperplasia 441
Aetiology and epidemiology 441
Pathophysiology and clinical presentation 441
Specific investigations 441
Medical/surgical management 441
Nursing management 441

18 NURSING PATIENTS WITH BLOOD DISORDERS **445**

Overview: anatomy and physiology **445**
Plasma 446
Blood cells 446
Red cells 446
White cells 446
Platelets 446
Blood groups 446
ABO system 446
Rhesus system 447
Haemopoiesis 447
Haemostasis 448
General nursing assessment **449**
Anxiety 449
Fatigue 449
Skin and mucosa 449
Appetite 449
Pain 450
Diagnostic tests **450**
Blood tests 450
Full blood count 450
Blood film 450
Erythrocyte sedimentation rate 450
Coagulation screen 450
Coombs' test or direct antiglobulin test 450
Bone marrow sampling 450
Blood donation and transfusion **451**
Blood donation 451
Types of blood product transfusion 451
Packed red cells 451
Platelets 451

Granulocytes	451
Fresh frozen plasma	452
Albumin	452
Factor VIII and factor IX	452
Cryoprecipitate	452
Apheresis	452
Blood transfusion	452
Pre-transfusion compatibility	
testing	452
Safe administration of blood	452
Complications of transfusion	452
Blood incompatibility	453
Circulatory overload	454
Febrile reactions	454
Allergic reactions	454
Acute bacterial reactions	454
Delayed complications of	
transfusion	454
Alternatives to blood	
transfusion	454

Disease prevention and
health education — 455

General health education	455
Diet	455
Smoking	456
Activity and exercise	456
Further information	456
Educating other professionals	456

Red cell disorders — 456

Anaemia – general points	456
Aetiology	456
General investigations	456
Clinical presentation	456
Haemorrhagic anaemia	457
Aetiology	457
Clinical presentation	457
Medical/surgical management	457
Nursing management	457
Iron deficiency anaemia	457
Aetiology	457
Special investigations	458
Clinical presentation	458
Medical management	458
Nursing management	458
Megaloblastic anaemias –	
general	458
Pathophysiology and aetiology	458
Megaloblastic anaemia due	
to vitamin B_{12} deficiency and	
pernicious anaemia	458
Aetiology and pathophysiology	458
Clinical presentation	459
Nursing management	459
Megaloblastic anaemia due	
to folic acid deficiency	459
Aetiology	459
Clinical presentation	459
Medical management	459
Anaemia of chronic disease	459

Polycythaemia	459
Clinical presentation	460
Medical management	460
Haemolytic anaemias – general	460
Pathophysiology	460
Clinical presentation	460
Autoimmune haemolytic	
anaemia	460
Aetiology	460
Medical/surgical management	460

Haemoglobinopathies — 460

Thalassaemia	461
Aetiology and pathophysiology	461
Clinical presentation	461
Medical/surgical management	461
Nursing management	461
Sickle cell disease	461
Aetiology and pathophysiology	461
Clinical presentation	462
Medical/surgical management	462
Nursing management	463

Disorders of the bone marrow — 463

Aplastic anaemia	463
Aetiology and pathophysiology	463
Special investigations and	
clinical presentation	463
Medical management	463
Nursing management	464
Myelodysplasia	464
Aetiology and pathophysiology	464
Medical management	464
Nursing management	464
Myeloma	464
Aetiology and pathophysiology	464
Clinical presentation	464
Medical management	464
Nursing care	465

White cell disorders — 465

Neutropenia	465
Aetiology	465
Medical management	465
Nursing management	465
Minimizing infection risk	466
Observing for signs of infection	466
Management of infection	466
Patient education and support	466
Acute leukaemia	466
Acute myeloid leukaemia	467
Acute lymphoblastic leukaemia	467
Nursing management:	
acute leukaemia	467
Chronic leukaemia	468
Chronic myeloid leukaemia	468
Chronic lymphocytic leukaemia	468
Nursing management:	
chronic leukaemia	469

The lymphomas — 469

Aetiology and pathophysiology	469
Clinical presentation	469

Special investigations	469
Hodgkin's lymphoma	469
Non-Hodgkin's lymphoma	470
Burkitt's lymphoma	470
Relapsed lymphoma	470

Nursing and medical
management of malignant
blood disorders — 470

Cytotoxic chemotherapy	470
Long-term central venous	
catheters	470
Administration of cytotoxic	
drugs	471
Side-effects of cytotoxic drugs	471
Haemopoietic stem cell	
transplantation (HSCT)	474
Graft-versus-host disease	475
Non-myeloablative stem	
cell transplants	475
Monoclonal antibodies	475
Nursing care	475

Disorders of haemostasis — 476

Thrombocytopenia	476
Aetiology	476
Clinical presentation	476
Medical management	476
Nursing care	476
Disseminated intravascular	
coagulation	477
Aetiology	477
Medical management	477
Nursing management	477
Haemophilia	477
Pathophysiology and clinical	
presentation	477
Multiprofessional management	477
Treatment	478
Nursing care	478

19 NURSING PATIENTS
WITH CARDIOVASCULAR
DISORDERS — 481

Anatomy and physiology:
an overview — 481

The heart	482
The heart wall	482
The heart chambers and valves	483
Coronary circulation	483
The electrical conduction	
system	483
The cardiac cycle	484
The vascular system	485
The arteries	485
The veins	485
Blood pressure	485

Nursing assessment — 486

Nursing history	486
Physical assessment	486

CONTENTS

Skin 486
Arterial pulses 486
Chest pain 487
Blood pressure 488
Central venous pressure 488
Pulmonary artery pressures 488
**General diagnostic tests and
medical investigations** **488**
The electrocardiogram 488
The 12-lead ECG 490
Bedside monitoring 490
Holter monitoring 490
Exercise test treadmill 490
Echocardiogram 490
Magnetic resonance scanning
(MRI) 491
Chest X-ray 491
Blood tests 491
Cardiac enzymes 491
Full blood count and erythrocyte
sedimentation rate 491
Coagulation studies 492
Blood lipid profile 492
Coronary angiography 492
Electrophysiology studies (EPS) 492
**General disease prevention
and health education** **493**
Hypercholesterolaemia 493
Drug therapy 494
Hypertension 494
Smoking 494
Lifestyle changes and exercise 495
**Cardiopulmonary arrest and
resuscitation** **495**
Aetiology 495
Pathophysiology and clinical
presentation 495
Nursing management 495
Assessment and resuscitation
of the airway and breathing 495
Steps in resuscitation 496
Assessment and resuscitation
of the circulation 496
Cardiopulmonary
resuscitation 496
Cardiovascular disorders **497**
**Disorders of the electrical
conduction system – atrial
arrhythmias** **497**
Sinus bradycardia 497
Aetiology 497
Clinical presentation 497
Medical management 497
Nursing management 497
Sinus tachycardia 499
Clinical presentation 499
Medical management 499
Atrial fibrillation 499
Pathophysiology 499

Clinical presentation 499
Medical management 499
Nursing management 499
Atrial flutter 500
Aetiology 500
Clinical presentation and
medical management 500
Nursing management 500
Premature atrial contraction,
atrial extrasystoles or atrial
ectopic beats 500
Clinical presentation 500
Medical management 500
Nursing management 500
Paroxysmal atrial tachycardia 500
Clinical presentation 501
Medical management 501
Nursing management 501
Supraventricular tachycardia
or narrow complex tachycardia 501
Aetiology and clinical
presentation 501
Medical management 501
Nursing management 501
**Disorders of the electrical
conduction system:
ventricular arrhythmias** **501**
Premature ventricular
contraction, ventricular
extrasystoles or ventricular
ectopic beats 501
Aetiology and
pathophysiology 501
Clinical presentation 502
Medical management 502
Nursing management 502
Ventricular tachycardia 502
Pathophysiology 502
Clinical presentation 502
Medical management 502
Nursing management 502
Ventricular fibrillation 502
Pathophysiology 502
Nursing management 502
Coronary heart disease **503**
Aetiology and epidemiology 503
Pathophysiology 503
Angina pectoris 503
Clinical presentation 503
Specific investigations 504
Medical and surgical
management 504
Nursing management 504
Unstable angina 505
Pathophysiology 505
Clinical presentation 505
Specific investigations 505
Medical management 505
Nursing management 506

Myocardial infarction 506
Epidemiology 506
Pathophysiology 506
Clinical presentation 506
Specific investigations 507
Medical management –
immediate care 507
Nursing management 507
Heart failure **510**
Cardiogenic shock 510
Aetiology 510
Clinical presentation 510
Medical management 510
Nursing management 510
Chronic heart failure 510
Aetiology 510
Pathophysiology 510
Clinical presentation 511
Specific investigations 511
Medical/surgical management 511
Nursing management 512
Valvular heart disease **514**
Acute rheumatic fever 514
Aetiology and epidemiology 514
Pathophysiology 514
Clinical presentation 514
Specific investigations 514
Medical management 514
Nursing management 514
Valvular heart disease 515
Nursing management 515
Infective endocarditis **516**
Aetiology and epidemiology 516
Pathophysiology 516
Clinical presentation 516
Specific investigations 517
Medical management 517
Nursing management 517
Disorders of the myocardium **518**
Myocarditis 518
Aetiology 518
Pathophysiology 518
Clinical presentation 518
Specific investigations 518
Medical management 518
Nursing management 518
Cardiomyopathy 518
Nursing management 518
Heart transplantation 518
Nursing management 519
Left ventricular assist devices 519
Nursing management 520
Disorders of the pericardium **520**
Pericarditis 520
Aetiology 520
Pathophysiology 520
Clinical presentation 520
Specific investigations 520
Medical management 520

Nursing management 520
Cardiac tamponade 521
  Aetiology 521
  Pathophysiology 521
  Clinical presentation 521
  Specific investigations 521
  Medical management 521
  Nursing management 521

Disorders of the vascular system **521**
Hypertension 521
  Aetiology 521
  Clinical presentation 521
  Medical management 521
  Nursing management 522
Aortic aneurysm and dissection 522
  Aetiology 522
  Clinical presentation 522
  Specific investigations 522
  Medical management 522
  Nursing management 523
Peripheral arterial disease 523
  Aetiology 523
  Pathophysiology 523
  Specific investigations 523
  Clinical presentation 523
  Medical and surgical management 523
  Nursing management 524
Raynaud's phenomenon and disease 524
  Clinical presentation 524
  Medical management 524
  Nursing management 525
Varicose veins 525
  Aetiology 525
  Pathophysiology 525
  Clinical presentation 525
  Medical management 525
  Nursing management 525
Deep vein thrombosis 525
  Aetiology 525
  Specific investigations 525
  Clinical presentation 526
  Medical management 526
  Nursing management 526
Pulmonary embolus 526
Thrombophlebitis 527
  Aetiology 527
  Clinical presentation 527
  Nursing management 527
Chronic venous insufficiency 527
  Aetiology 527
  Pathophysiology 527
  Clinical presentation 527
  Nursing management 528
Congenital heart disease **528**
  Nursing management 528

20 NURSING PATIENTS WITH RESPIRATORY DISORDERS **533**

Anatomy and physiology – an overview **533**
Control of breathing 534
  Respiratory centre 534
  Pulmonary stretch receptors 534
  Chemoreceptors 534
Gas transport 534
  Oxygen transport 535
  Carbon dioxide transport 535
  Ventilation and perfusion 535
Acid–base balance 535
Causes and predisposing factors of respiratory disease **535**
Smoking 535
  Smoking cessation 536
  Nicotine 536
  Nicotine replacement therapy 536
  Bupropion (Zyban) 536
  Behavioural change 536
Genetics 537
Microorganisms 537
Poverty 537
Allergens and trigger factors 538
Nursing assessment of respiratory status **538**
Physiological assessment 538
  Respiratory rate, rhythm and depth 538
  Chest movement 538
  Oxygen levels 539
Mental state 539
Causative factors 539
Symptoms 539
Impact on activities of daily living 539
Psychosocial factors 540
Respiratory investigations **540**
Respiratory function tests 540
  Peak expiratory flow rate 540
  FEV_1 and FVC 540
  Reversibility testing 541
Nursing role in respiratory function tests **541**
Pulse oximetry 541
Chest X-ray 541
Sputum 541
  Observation of sputum 541
Bronchoscopy 542
Common respiratory disorders **542**
Asthma 542
  Epidemiology 542
  Pathophysiology 542
  Treatment options for asthma 542
Acute severe asthma 543

  Nursing management: asthma 544
Chronic obstructive pulmonary disease 545
  Epidemiology 545
  Pathophysiology 545
  Treatment options for COPD 546
  Management of an acute respiratory exacerbation of COPD 548
Lung cancer 549
  Epidemiology 549
  Pathophysiology 549
  Clinical presentation 549
  Nursing management 550
Cystic fibrosis 550
  Epidemiology 550
  Pathophysiology 550
  Treatment 550
  Acute respiratory exacerbations of CF 551
  Nursing management 551
  End-stage management 552
  Gene therapy 552
Bronchiectasis 552
  Epidemiology 552
  Pathophysiology 552
  Treatment 552
Respiratory tract infections **552**
Pneumonia 553
  Epidemiology 553
  Pathophysiology 553
  Specific investigations 553
  Treatment 553
  Prevention of pneumonia 553
  Nursing management 553
Tuberculosis 555
  Epidemiology 555
  Pathophysiology 555
  Clinical presentation 555
  Specific investigations 555
  Treatment of pulmonary tuberculosis 555
  Role of the nurse in prevention and treatment of tuberculosis 556
Interstitial lung diseases 556
Respiratory failure 557
  Treatment 557
  Nursing management: patients receiving oxygen therapy 558
Pneumothorax 560
  Signs and symptoms 560
  Treatment 560
  Nursing management: underwater-seal drains 561
Pleural effusion 561
Haemoptysis 561
Aspergillus and allergic bronchopulmonary aspergillosis 562

21 NURSING PATIENTS WITH NOSE AND THROAT DISORDERS 565

Overview of anatomy and physiology 566
- The nose 566
- The paranasal sinuses 566
- The pharynx 566
- The larynx 567
- The trachea 567

Nursing assessment 568
- Nursing history 568
  - Patients presenting with nasal signs and symptoms 568
  - Patients presenting with signs and symptoms affecting the throat 568

General diagnostic tests and medical investigations 568
- Examination of the nose 568
  - The external nose 568
  - The internal nose 568
- Examination of the throat 569
  - Palpation of the neck 569
  - Internal examination 569
- General investigations 569
  - Blood tests 569
  - Radiology and scanning 569
- Specific investigation of nasal function and pathology 569
  - Rhinomanometry 569
  - Immunological investigations 569
  - Microbiological investigations 569
  - Investigation of olfaction 570
  - Investigation of mucociliary clearance 570
- Specific investigation of the throat 570
  - Swallowing analysis 570
  - Voice analysis 570

General disease prevention and health education 570
- Aetiology, prevention and early detection of nose and throat cancer 570
- Nose and throat disorders – general consideration 570

Infection and inflammation of the nose and sinuses 570
- Rhinitis 570
  - Aetiology and pathophysiology 570
  - Clinical presentation 570
  - Specific investigations 571
  - Medical/surgical management 571
  - Nursing management 571
- Sinusitis 573
  - Aetiology 573
  - Pathophysiology 573
  - Clinical presentation 573
  - Specific investigations 573
  - Medical/surgical management 573
  - Nursing management 574

Epistaxis and septal deviation 574
- Epistaxis 574
  - Aetiology and pathophysiology 575
  - Clinical presentation 575
  - Specific investigations 575
  - Medical/surgical management 575
  - Nursing management 576
- Deviated nasal septum 577
  - Aetiology 577
  - Pathophysiology 577
  - Clinical presentation 577
  - Specific investigations 577
  - Medical/surgical management 577
  - Nursing management 577

Nasal injuries 579
- Nasal fractures 579
  - Aetiology 579
  - Clinical presentation 579
  - Specific investigation 579
  - Medical/surgical management 579
  - Nursing management 579
- Septal haematoma 579
  - Aetiology and pathophysiology 579
  - Clinical presentation 579
  - Specific investigations 579
  - Medical/surgical management 579
  - Nursing management 579
- Septal perforation 579
  - Aetiology and pathophysiology 579
  - Clinical presentation 580
  - Specific investigations 580
  - Medical/surgical management 580
  - Nursing management 580

Nasal obstruction 580
- Nasal polyps 580
  - Aetiology 580
  - Clinical presentation 580
  - Specific investigations 580
  - Medical/surgical management 580
  - Nursing management 580
- Nasal foreign bodies 580
  - Clinical presentation 580
  - Medical/surgical management 580
  - Nursing management 580

Infections and inflammation of the throat 581
- Tonsillitis 581
  - Aetiology and pathophysiology 581
  - Clinical presentation 581
  - Medical/surgical management 581
  - Nursing management 581
- Peritonsillar abscess 582
  - Aetiology and pathophysiology 582
  - Clinical presentation 582
  - Medical/surgical management 582

- Nursing management 582
- Deep neck abscesses 582
  - Aetiology and pathophysiology 582
  - Clinical presentation 582
  - Specific investigations 582
  - Medical/surgical management 582
  - Nursing management 582
- Ludwig's angina 582
  - Aetiology and pathophysiology 583
  - Clinical presentation 583
  - Specific investigations 583
  - Medical/surgical management 583
  - Nursing management 583
- Pharyngitis 583
- Laryngitis 583
  - Aetiology and pathophysiology 583
  - Clinical presentation 583
  - Specific investigations 583
  - Medical/surgical management 583
  - Nursing management following direct laryngoscopy 583

Laryngeal obstruction 583
- Aetiology and pathophysiology 583
- Clinical presentation 583
- Specific investigations 584
- Medical/surgical management 584
- Nursing management 584
- Tracheostomy 584
  - Tracheostomy tubes 584
  - Nursing management 584

Vocal cord problems 585
- Paralysis 585
  - Aetiology and pathophysiology 585
  - Clinical presentation 585
  - Specific investigations 585
  - Medical/surgical management 585
  - Nursing management 585

Tumours of the nose and throat 587
- Sinuses 587
  - Aetiology and pathophysiology 587
  - Clinical presentation 587
  - Specific investigations 587
  - Medical/surgical management 587
  - Nursing management 587
- The external nose 587
- Benign laryngeal tumours 587
- Malignant laryngeal tumours 587
  - Aetiology, epidemiology and pathophysiology 587
  - Clinical presentation 587
  - Specific investigations 587
  - Medical/surgical management 587
  - Nursing management 587

22 NURSING PATIENTS WITH GASTROINTESTINAL DISORDERS — 591

Overview of the gastrointestinal tract — 591
Lining of the GI tract — 591
Adventitia — 592
Muscularis — 592
Submucosa — 592
Mucosa — 592
The mouth — 592
The tongue — 593
Oesophagus — 593
Stomach — 593
Functions of the stomach — 593
Gastric emptying — 593
Portal circulation — 594
Vomiting — 594
The small intestine — 594
Functions of the small intestine — 595
The pancreas — 595
The liver and gallbladder — 595
Large intestine — 595
Caecum — 595
Ascending colon — 595
Transverse colon — 596
Descending colon — 596
Sigmoid colon — 596
Rectum — 596
Anal canal — 596

Nursing assessment — 596
Assessment interview — 596
Nursing history — 596
Oral assessment — 597
Clinical presentation — 597
Abdominal pain — 597
Anorexia and weight loss — 597
Nausea and vomiting — 597
Flatulence — 597
Hiccups — 597
Abnormal stools — 598
Tenesmus — 598
Melaena — 598
Haematemesis — 598
Rectal bleeding — 598
Abdominal distension — 598
Jaundice — 598
Abdominal examination — 598

General diagnostic tests and medical investigations — 598
Gastric acid studies — 598
Urea breath test — 598
Endoscopy — 599
Biopsy — 599
Radiography — 599
Imaging techniques — 599
Plain X-rays — 599
Radioisotope studies — 599

Barium studies — 599
Blood tests — 600
Iron and folate levels — 600
Haemoglobin — 600
Erythrocyte sedimentation rate (ESR) — 600
Liver function tests — 600
Faecal occult blood (FOB) — 600

General disease prevention and health education — 600
Disorders of the gastrointestinal tract — 600
Disorders affecting the mouth — 600
Carcinoma of the mouth — 600
Stomatitis — 600
Xerostomia — 600
White patches in the mouth — 601
Oral candidiasis — 601
Ulceration — 601
Gingivitis — 601
Disorders of the tongue — 601
Vincent's angina — 602
Nursing management — 602
Disorders affecting the oesophagus — 602
Oesophageal diverticulum — 602
Hiatus hernia — 602
Achalasia — 602
Diffuse oesophageal spasm — 602
Oesophageal rings and webs — 603
Foreign bodies in the oesophagus — 603

Emergency situations – the acute abdomen — 603
Acute peritonitis — 603
Intestinal obstruction — 604
Intestinal ischaemia — 604
Nursing management — 604

Disorders of the upper GI tract — 604
Haemorrhage — 604
Oesophageal varices — 604
Medical/surgical management — 604
Oesophagitis — 604
Infective oesophagitis — 604
Medical/surgical management — 605
Corrosive oesophagitis — 605
Medical/surgical management — 605
Reflux oesophagitis — 605
Medical/surgical management — 605
Gastritis — 605
Pathophysiology — 605
Clinical presentation — 605
Medical/surgical management — 605
Carcinoma of the upper GI tract — 605
Carcinoma of the oesophagus — 605
Carcinoma of the stomach — 606
Medical/surgical management — 606

Nursing management: patients undergoing gastric surgery — 606
Peptic ulceration — 606
Specific investigations — 606
Medical/surgical management — 606
Pyloric stenosis — 607
Specific investigations — 607
Medical and surgical treatment — 607
Mallory–Weiss syndrome — 607
Nursing management: patients with acute GI haemorrhage — 607

Disorders of the lower GI tract — 607
Appendicitis — 607
Clinical presentation — 608
Medical/surgical management — 608
Nursing management — 608
Peritonitis — 608
Irritable bowel syndrome — 608
Investigations and management — 608
Constipation — 609
Diet and fluid intake — 609
Bowel habits — 609
Immobility and exercise — 609
Socioeconomic factors — 609
Medication — 609
Nursing management — 610

Bowel disorders including tumours and diverticular disease — 610
Hernia — 610
Hiatus hernia — 610
Inguinal hernia — 610
Incisional hernia — 610
Umbilical hernia — 610
Diverticular disease — 610
Clinical presentation — 611
Medical/surgical management — 611
Familial polyposis — 611
Colorectal cancer — 611
Aetiology — 611
Clinical presentation — 611
Investigations and management — 611
Bowel preparation — 611
Surgical management — 612
Nursing management — 612
Discharge preparation — 613
Inflammatory bowel disease — 613
Ulcerative colitis — 613
Crohn's disease — 613
Aetiology — 613
Clinical presentation — 614
Specific investigations — 614
Medical/surgical management — 614
Nursing management — 615
Pseudomembranous colitis — 616
Anorectal disorders — 616
Pruritus ani — 616
Medical/surgical management — 617

Anal fissure 617
  Medical/surgical management 617
Haemorrhoids 617
Anal fistulae 617
  Medical/surgical management 617
Pilonidal sinus 617
  Medical/surgical management 617
Perianal abscess 617
  Medical/surgical management 617
Rectal prolapse 617
  Medical/surgical management 617
Skin tags 617
Anal cancer 617
  Medical/surgical management 617

23 NURSING PATIENTS WITH HEPATIC, BILIARY AND PANCREATIC DISORDERS 621

Anatomy and physiology of the liver 622
Functions of the liver 622
  Bile production 622
  Metabolic functions 622
  Storage of energy 623
  Synthesis of blood components 623
  Destruction of erythrocytes 623
  Detoxification 623
  Heat production 623
The biliary system 623
  Bile concentration and storage 623
The pancreas 623
Nursing assessment 623
Patient history 623
  Nutrition 624
  Elimination pattern 624
  Pain or discomfort 624
  Personal and social history 624
  Culture and ethnicity 624
  Activity and lifestyle 624
  Occupational and environmental history 624
  Past medical history and illnesses 624
Physical examination 624
  General appearance 624
  Vital signs 624
  Height and weight 624
  Skin 625
  Physical signs of disease of the liver, gallbladder or pancreas 625
Diagnostic tests and medical investigations 625
Laboratory tests 625
  Blood tests 625
  Urine tests 626
  Tests on faeces 626
Endoscopic investigations 626

  Endoscopic retrograde cholangiopancreatography 626
Radiological investigations 626
  Plain and contrast X-rays 626
  Scintigraphy (nuclear imaging) 626
  Cholecystogram 626
  Computed tomography 626
Ultrasonography 626
Magnetic resonance imaging 626
Percutaneous biopsy 626
Disease prevention and health education 626
Nutrition 627
Environment 627
Lifestyle 627
  Smoking 627
  Alcohol 627
  Sexual practices 627
  Drug users 627
Clinical characteristics 627
  Jaundice 628
  Pruritus 629
Disorders affecting the liver 630
Hepatitis 630
Viral hepatitis 630
  Pathophysiology 631
  Clinical presentation 631
  Investigations and diagnostic procedures 631
  Medical management 631
  Nursing management 632
Alcohol-induced hepatitis 633
Drug-induced hepatitis 633
Toxic hepatitis 633
Cirrhosis 633
  Aetiology and epidemiology 633
  Pathophysiology 634
  Clinical presentation 634
  Investigations 634
  Medical management 634
  Nursing management 634
Liver failure and hepatic coma 636
  Aetiology and epidemiology 636
  Pathophysiology 636
  Clinical features 636
  Medical and surgical management 637
  Nursing management: liver failure 637
Liver tumours 637
  Aetiology and epidemiology 637
  Pathophysiology 637
  Clinical presentation 637
  Investigations 637
  Medical and surgical management 637
  Nursing management 637
Liver trauma 638

Diseases affecting the biliary system 638
Cholelithiasis 638
  Aetiology and epidemiology 638
  Pathophysiology 638
  Clinical presentation 639
  Investigations 639
  Medical and surgical management 639
  Nursing management 639
Acute cholecystitis 640
  Aetiology and epidemiology 640
  Pathophysiology 640
  Clinical presentation 640
  Investigations 640
  Medical and surgical management 640
  Nursing management 641
Chronic cholecystitis 641
  Clinical presentation 641
  Management 641
Acalculous cholecystitis 641
Choledocholithiasis and cholangitis 641
  Aetiology and epidemiology 641
  Clinical presentation 642
  Investigations 642
  Medical and surgical management 642
  Nursing management: bile duct stones 642
Tumours of the biliary tract and gallbladder 643
Disorders affecting the pancreas 643
Acute pancreatitis 643
  Aetiology and epidemiology 643
  Pathophysiology 643
  Clinical presentation 644
  Investigations 644
  Medical and surgical management 645
  Nursing management 645
Chronic pancreatitis 646
  Aetiology and epidemiology 646
  Pathophysiology 646
  Clinical presentation 646
  Investigations 646
  Medical and surgical management 646
  Nursing management 647
Tumours of the pancreas 647
  Aetiology and epidemiology 647
  Pathophysiology 647
  Clinical presentation 647
  Investigations 647
  Medical and surgical management 648
  Nursing management 648

Tumours of the islets cells **649**
Gastrinoma 649
Insulinomas 649

24 NURSING PATIENTS WITH URINARY DISORDERS 653

Anatomy and physiology – an overview **654**
Development and maturation of the kidneys and urinary tract 654
Kidneys – macroscopic structure 655
Blood supply to the kidneys 656
Nerve supply to the kidneys 656
The nephron and basic renal function 656
Glomerulus and glomerular capsule: glomerular filtration barrier 656
Juxtaglomerular apparatus 658
PCT 658
Loop of Henle 658
DCT and collecting duct 658
Summary: fluid and solute homeostasis 660
Renal contribution to acid–base balance 660
Renal contribution to calcium and phosphate homeostasis 661
The lower urinary tract 661
Ureters 661
Bladder 661
Urethra 661
Micturition 662
Prostate 662

Nursing assessment – urinary system function **662**
Assessment of fluid and electrolyte balance 663
Fluid balance charts 663
Daily weight 663
Skin turgor and mucous membranes 663
Arterial blood pressure 663
Skin temperature 663
Central venous pressure 663
Assessment of urine – urinalysis 663
Specific gravity 664
Blood 664
Glucose 664
Protein 664
pH 665
Ketones 665
Leucocytes and nitrites 665

General diagnostic tests and medical investigations **665**
Physical examination 665
Ultrasonography 665
Renal ultrasound 665

Bladder ultrasound 666
Angiography 666
Renal angiography 666
Computed tomography 666
Magnetic resonance angiography 666
Radionuclide scanning 667
Urography (pyelography) 667
Intravenous urography (IVU) 667
Retrograde urography (pyelography) 667
Antegrade urography (pyelography) 667
Cystography 667
Renal biopsy 667
Medical care 668
Nursing management 668
Cystoscopy 668
Urodynamic studies 669
Blood tests 669
Haematological tests 669
Biochemical tests 670
Urine tests 671

General disease prevention and health education **671**

Urinary system disorders **672**
Urinary tract infections: cystitis and pyelonephritis 672
Aetiology and pathophysiology 672
Clinical presentation 672
Investigations 672
Medical management: cystitis and pyelonephritis 673
Nursing management: cystitis and pyelonephritis 673
Reflux nephropathy (chronic pyelonephritis) 673
Infection associated with indwelling urinary catheters 674
Renal abscess 674
Cortical abscess 674
Corticomedullary abscess 674
Renal tuberculosis 674
Clinical presentation 674
Investigations 675
Medical management 675
Nursing management 675
Nephrolithiasis 676
Aetiology and pathophysiology 676
Clinical presentation 676
Specific investigations 676
Medical/surgical management 676
Nursing management: patients with a nephrostomy tube 676
Renal trauma 677
Malignant tumours of the kidney 677
Pathophysiology 677
Clinical presentation 677

Investigations 677
Medical/surgical management 677
Nursing management: the patient undergoing nephrectomy 677
Urothelial (transitional cell) tumours 678
Aetiology 679
Clinical presentation 679
Investigations 679
Medical/surgical management 679
Nursing management 679
Diabetic nephropathy 682
Epidemiology 682
Aetiology, pathophysiology and clinical presentation 682
Nursing and medical management 682
Glomerulonephritis 683
Pathophysiology 683
Clinical presentation 683
Investigations 683
Medical management 683
Nursing management 683
Nephrotic syndrome 684
Medical management 684
Nursing management 684
Tubulointerstitial disease – interstitial nephritis 684
Medical management 684
Polycystic kidney disease 684
Pathophysiology 685
Investigations 685
Clinical presentation 685
Medical management 685

Renal failure **685**
Acute renal failure 685
Aetiology 685
Pathophysiology 685
Investigations and medical assessment 686
Clinical presentation – course of ARF 686
Medical management 686
Nursing management 686
Chronic renal failure 686
Aetiology 687
Clinical effects of declining renal function 687
Renal replacement therapies 689
Haemodialysis 690
Peritoneal dialysis 691
Haemofiltration and haemodialysis in ARF 693
Renal transplantation 694
Nursing management 695

Disorders of the prostate gland **696**
Benign enlargement of the prostate 696

Aetiology and pathophysiology 696
  Clinical presentation 696
  Investigations 697
  Medical/surgical management 697
  Nursing management: TURP 697
Prostate cancer 699
  Aetiology 699
  Clinical presentation 699
  Investigations 699
  Medical/surgical management 700
  Nursing management: radical
  prostatectomy 701

25 NURSING PATIENTS WITH SEXUAL HEALTH AND REPRODUCTIVE PROBLEMS 705

Women's health **706**
Anatomy and physiology of the female reproductive system – an overview **706**
  Ovaries 706
    Female sex hormones 707
    Ovarian cycle and oogenesis 707
  Uterine/fallopian tubes 708
  Uterus 708
    Menstrual (uterine) cycle 710
  Vagina 711
  Vulva 711
Nursing assessment **711**
  Physical assessment 712
  Social assessment 712
  Psychological assessment 712
General diagnostic tests and medical investigations **712**
  Gynaecological examination 713
    Bimanual vaginal examination 713
    Speculum examination of
    the vagina and cervix 713
  Imaging techniques 713
    Ultrasonography 713
    X-rays 714
    CT/MRI 714
  Microbiology 714
    High vaginal swabs 714
  Cytology – cervical smear 714
  Colposcopy 714
  Laparoscopy 715
  Blood tests 715
General disease prevention and health education **715**
Common diseases/disorders affecting the female reproductive system **716**
Menstrual disorders **716**
    Aetiology, pathophysiology
    and clinical presentation 716
    Specific investigations 716
    Medical/surgical management 716

  Nursing management –
  an overview 719
Benign tumours of the female reproductive structures **719**
    Aetiology and pathophysiology 719
    Clinical presentation 719
    Specific investigations 719
    Medical/surgical management 719
    Nursing management 719
Malignant tumours of the female reproductive structures **720**
  Vulval cancer 720
    Aetiology and epidemiology 720
    Pathophysiology 720
    Specific investigations and
    clinical presentation 720
    Medical/surgical management 720
    Nursing management 720
  Cervical cancer 721
    Epidemiology 721
    Aetiology 721
    Pathophysiology 721
    Clinical presentation 721
    Specific investigations 721
    Medical/surgical management 721
    Nursing management 721
  Endometrial cancer 722
    Aetiology and epidemiology 722
    Pathophysiology 722
    Clinical presentation 722
    Specific investigations 722
    Medical/surgical management 722
    Nursing management 722
  Ovarian cancer 722
    Aetiology and epidemiology 722
    Pathophysiology 722
    Clinical presentation 723
    Specific investigations 723
    Medical/surgical management 723
    Nursing management 723
Uterine displacement and prolapse **724**
    Aetiology 724
    Clinical presentation 724
    Specific investigations 724
    Medical/surgical management 724
    Nursing management 725
Problems of early pregnancy **725**
  Spontaneous miscarriage 725
  Threatened miscarriage 725
    Aetiology and epidemiology 726
    Clinical presentation 726
    Specific investigations 726
    Medical/surgical management 726
    Nursing management 726
  Inevitable miscarriage 726
    Clinical presentation 726
    Management 726

Complete miscarriage 726
    Clinical presentation 726
    Medical/surgical management 726
  Incomplete miscarriage 727
    Clinical presentation 727
    Specific investigations 727
    Medical/surgical management 727
    Nursing management 727
  Blighted ovum 727
  Missed miscarriage 728
    Clinical presentation 728
    Medical/surgical management 728
    Nursing management 728
  Recurrent miscarriage 728
  Hydatidiform mole 729
    Aetiology and epidemiology 729
    Clinical presentation and
    investigations 729
    Medical/surgical management 729
    Nursing management 729
  Ectopic pregnancy 729
    Aetiology and epidemiology 729
    Pathophysiology 729
    Clinical presentation 730
    Specific investigations 730
    Medical/surgical management 730
    Nursing management 730
  Termination of pregnancy 730
    Medical/surgical management 731
    Late TOPs 731
    Nursing management 731
Infections of the female reproductive tract **732**
  Vaginitis 732
  Cervicitis and endometritis 732
  Salpingitis and pelvic
  inflammatory disease 732
  Toxic shock syndrome 733
    Nursing management:
    genital infections in women 733
Other gynaecological conditions **733**
  Endometriosis 733
    Aetiology and epidemiology 733
    Pathophysiology 734
    Clinical presentation 734
    Specific investigations 734
    Medical/surgical management 734
    Nursing management 734
  Polycystic ovary syndrome 734
    Aetiology and epidemiology 734
    Pathophysiology and clinical
    presentation 734
    Specific investigations 735
    Medical/surgical management 735
    Nursing management 735
Problems associated with the climacteric and postmenopausal problems **735**

Physiological events 735
Clinical presentation 735
Specific investigations 735
Medical management 735
Nursing management 736
Nursing management of patients undergoing gynaecological surgery 736
Preoperative assessment 736
Physical assessment 736
Psychological assessment 737
Social assessment 737
Spiritual assessment 737
Preoperative care 737
Postoperative care 738
Postoperative discharge advice 739
Postoperative complications 739
Men's health 741
Anatomy and physiology of the male reproductive tract – an overview 741
Testes 741
Testicular hormone production 742
Accessory glands and duct system 742
Penis 743
Physiology of penile erection 744
Nursing assessment 744
Physical assessment 744
Psychological assessment 744
Social assessment 744
General diagnostic tests and medical investigations 744
Disease prevention and health promotion 744
Testicular problems 745
Testicular cancer 745
Epidemiology and aetiology 745
Pathophysiology 746
Clinical presentation 747
Specific investigations 747
Medical/surgical management 747
Nursing management 747
Undescended testes 750
Torsion 750
Nursing management 750
Trauma 750
Varicocele 750
Hydrocele 750
Infection and inflammation 750
Epididymitis 750
Medical management 750
Orchitis 750
Prostatitis 750
Penile problems 751
Penile cancer 751
Epidemiology and aetiology 751
Pathophysiology 751
Investigations 751

Medical/surgical management 751
Nursing management 751
Phimosis and paraphimosis 752
Medical/surgical management 752
Problems with sexual function 752
Erectile dysfunction 752
Aetiology 752
Erectile dysfunction as communication 753
Nursing assessment 753
Medical/surgical management 754
Nursing management 756
Rapid ejaculation 756
Management 756
Sexual and reproductive issues and disorders affecting women and men 757
Sexual health issues 757
Contraception 757
Types of contraception 757
Nursing management 758
Infertility 758
Aetiology and epidemiology 758
Specific investigations 758
Medical/surgical management 759
Nursing management 759
Sexually transmitted infections 761
Genital warts 761
Clinical presentation 761
Management 762
Candidiasis (vaginal thrush) 762
Clinical presentation 762
Management 762
Trichomoniasis 762
Clinical presentation 762
Management 763
Chlamydia 763
Clinical presentation 763
Management 763
Genital herpes 763
Clinical presentation 763
Management 763
Gonorrhoea 763
Clinical presentation 763
Management 764
Syphilis 764
Clinical presentation 764
Management 764
Human immunodeficiency virus 764
Clinical presentation 765
Management 765

26 BREAST DISORDERS 771

Overview of anatomy and physiology 771
The normal breast 771
Nursing assessment 772

Physical assessment 772
Social assessment 772
Psychological assessment and coping skills 772
Role of the breast care nurse 773
Diagnostic tests and investigations 774
History 774
Clinical examination 774
Fine-needle aspirate 774
Imaging – mammography and ultrasound 774
Triple assessment 775
Other tests 775
Core biopsy 775
Open biopsy 775
One-stop clinics 775
General disease prevention and health education 775
Breast screening programme in the UK 775
Screening uptake 776
Benefits of breast screening 776
Breast awareness 776
High-risk patients – genetic issues in breast cancer 776
Common diseases/disorders affecting the breast 778
Breast pain 778
Aetiology, epidemiology and clinical presentation 778
Medical/surgical management 778
Nursing management 778
Infection 779
Aetiology, epidemiology and clinical presentation 779
Specific investigations 779
Medical/surgical management 779
Nursing management 779
Congenital breast disorders and variations in normal breast development 779
Aetiology and epidemiology 779
Specific investigations 779
Medical/surgical management 779
Nursing management 780
Benign tumours 780
Aetiology, epidemiology and clinical presentation 780
Specific investigations 780
Medical/surgical management 780
Nursing management 780
Nipple disorders 780
Aetiology, epidemiology and clinical presentation 780
Specific investigations 781
Medical/surgical management 781
Nursing management 781
Malignant tumours 781

CONTENTS

Aetiology and epidemiology	*781*
Pathophysiology	*782*
Clinical presentation	*782*
Specific investigations	*782*
Medical/surgical management	*782*
Nursing management	*784*

Metastatic spread and other problems — **785**
- Recurrent breast cancer — 785
- Lymphoedema — 785
  - *Pathophysiology* — *786*
  - *Clinical presentation* — *786*
  - *Medical/surgical management* — *786*
  - *Nursing management* — *786*
- Fungating lesions — 787
  - *Pathophysiology* — *787*
  - *Clinical presentation* — *787*
  - *Medical/surgical management* — *787*
  - *Nursing management* — *787*

Breast reconstruction — **788**
- Types of breast reconstruction — 788
  - *Flap reconstruction* — *788*
  - *TRAM flap* — *788*
  - *Implant surgery* — *789*
- Breast augmentation and reduction — 790
  - *Medical/surgical management* — *790*
  - *Potential problems and complications* — *790*
  - *Nursing management* — *790*

27 NURSING PATIENTS WITH MUSCULOSKELETAL DISORDERS — 793

Anatomy and physiology of the musculoskeletal system – an overview — **793**
- The skeleton — 793
  - Bone — 794
- Joints — 794
- Skeletal muscles — 795

Musculoskeletal conditions, mobility and nursing assessment — **796**
- The origins of musculoskeletal conditions — 796

General diagnostic tests and medical investigation — **797**
- Physical examination — 797
- X-ray — 797
- Computed tomography (CT scan) — 797
- Magnetic resonance imaging (MRI) — 797
- Ultrasound — 797
- Blood tests — 797
- Electromyography — 798
- Surgical diagnostic techniques — 798

General disease prevention and health education — **799**
General nursing considerations – patients with musculoskeletal disorders — **799**
- Nursing patients in traction — 799
- Nursing patients in a cast — 800
  - *General principles of care* — *800*
- Nursing patients fitted with orthotic devices — 801
- Nursing patients with a prosthesis — 802
- Bandaging and strapping — 802
  - *Stump bandaging* — *802*
- Use of mobility aids — 802
  - *Crutches* — *802*
  - *Wheelchairs* — *804*
- Care of patients with an external fixator — 804

Common diseases/disorders affecting the musculoskeletal system — **805**
Inflammatory disorders — **805**
- Bursitis — 805
  - *Pathophysiology and aetiology* — *805*
  - *Clinical presentation* — *805*
  - *Medical/surgical management* — *805*
  - *Nursing management* — *805*
- Tenosynovitis — 805
  - *Nursing management* — *805*
- Rheumatoid arthritis — 805
  - *Pathophysiology and aetiology* — *805*
  - *Clinical presentation* — *806*
  - *Specific investigations* — *806*
  - *Medical/surgical management* — *806*
  - *Nursing management* — *806*
- Ankylosing spondylitis — 807
  - *Clinical presentation* — *807*
  - *Medical management* — *807*
  - *Nursing management* — *807*

Metabolic disorders — **807**
- Gout — 807
  - *Pathophysiology and aetiology* — *807*
  - *Clinical presentation* — *808*
  - *Specific investigations* — *808*
  - *Medical management* — *808*
  - *Nursing management* — *808*

Muscle disorders — **808**
- Myopathies — 808
  - *Pathophysiology and aetiology – an overview* — *808*
  - *General clinical presentation – an overview* — *810*
  - *Specific investigations* — *810*
  - *Medical/surgical management – an overview* — *811*
  - *Nursing management of inheritable myopathies* — *811*
- Myasthenia gravis — 811

Joint disorders — **812**
- Septic arthritis — 812
  - *Pathophysiology* — *812*
  - *Clinical presentation* — *812*
  - *Specific investigations* — *812*
  - *Medical management* — *812*
  - *Nursing management* — *812*
- Osteoarthritis — 812
  - *Pathophysiology and aetiology* — *812*
  - *Clinical presentation* — *812*
  - *Medical/surgical management* — *812*
  - *Nursing management of the patient with OA* — *812*
- Hallux valgus — 813
  - *Pathophysiology, aetiology and management* — *813*
  - *Nursing management* — *814*

Entrapment neuropathy — **814**
- Carpal tunnel syndrome — 814
  - *Pathophysiology and aetiology* — *814*
  - *Clinical presentation* — *814*
  - *Medical management* — *814*
  - *Nursing management* — *814*

Back pain and problems — **814**
- Musculoskeletal back pain — 814
- Intervertebral disc degeneration and herniation — 814
- Spinal stenosis — 814
- Other causes of back pain and problems — 815
  - *Rheumatoid arthritis* — *815*
  - *Primary tumours* — *815*
  - *Infection* — *815*
  - *Osteoporosis* — *815*
  - *Disorders elsewhere in the body that may be mistaken for musculoskeletal syndromes* — *815*
- The patient with back pain — 815
  - *Specific investigations – back pain and problems* — *815*
  - *Management* — *815*
  - *Physiotherapy and occupational therapy* — *816*
  - *Surgical intervention* — *816*
  - *Nursing management* — *816*

Connective tissue disorders — **817**
- Systemic lupus erythematosus — 817
  - *Pathophysiology and epidemiology* — *817*
  - *Clinical presentation* — *817*
  - *Specific investigations* — *817*
  - *Medical management* — *817*
  - *Nursing management* — *818*

Bone disorders and infection — **818**
- Paget's disease (osteitis deformans) — 818
  - *Pathophysiology* — *818*
  - *Clinical presentation* — *818*
  - *Specific investigations* — *818*

Medical/surgical management 818
Nursing management 818
Osteogenesis imperfecta 818
Pathophysiology and aetiology 818
Clinical presentation 818
Specific investigations 819
Management (team approach) 819
Osteomalacia 819
Pathophysiology and aetiology 819
Medical management 819
Nursing management 819
Osteoporosis 819
Pathophysiology and aetiology 819
Medical/surgical management 819
Nursing management 819
Osteomyelitis 820
Pathophysiology and aetiology 820
Clinical presentation 820
Specific investigations 820
Medical/surgical management 820
Nursing management 820
Bone tumours **820**
Investigations 820
Benign tumours 821
Medical/surgical management 821
Nursing management 821
Malignant bone tumours 821
Types, pathophysiology and
management 821
Nursing management 821
Trauma – an overview **821**
Sports injuries **822**
Sprains and strains 822
Sprains 822
Strains 822
Medical/surgical management
of sprains and strains 823
Injuries to joints 823
Regional sports injuries –
upper limb 823
Rotator cuff tendinitis
and tears 823
Shoulder dislocation 824
Frozen shoulder
(adhesive capsulitis) 824
Fractured clavicle 824
Proximal humerus fracture 825
Epicondylitis 825
Acromioclavicular (shoulder)
separation 825
Biceps tendon tear 825
Fractures of the distal radius
and/or ulna 826
Regional sports injuries –
lower limb 826
Hip flexor injury
(iliopsoas injury) 826
Hamstring strain 826
Knee injuries – an overview 826

Problems affecting the
Achilles tendon – an overview 827
Ankle sprain 828
Ankle fracture 828
Nursing management of
the sports injury 828
Fractures **828**
Classification 828
Clinical presentation 829
Fracture healing 829
Complications of fractures 829
Overview of the management
of fractures 830
Indications for surgical
management of fractures 830
Fractures of the lower limb 830
Intracapsular fractures of
the femoral neck 830
Intertrochanteric fractures
of the femur 831
Nursing/surgical management
– hip fractures 831
Femoral shaft fractures 831
Supracondylar fractures of
the femur 831
Distal femoral fractures 831
Tibial plateau fractures 832
Fractures of the patella 832
Fractures of the tibia and fibula 832
Fractures of the ankle 833
Nursing management –
lower limb fractures 833
Upper limb injuries –
fractures and dislocations 833
Fractures of the clavicle 834
Shoulder dislocation 834
Fractures of the proximal
humerus 834
Fractures of the shaft of
the humerus 834
Supracondylar fractures
of the humerus 834
Fractures of the head of radius 834
Fractures of the olecranon
process of the ulna 835
Fractures of the shaft of
radius and ulna 835
Single forearm bone fractures 835
Injuries to the carpus and
metacarpus 835
Nursing management –
upper limb injuries requiring
surgical intervention 836

**28 NURSING PATIENTS
WITH SKIN PROBLEMS** **841**

**Anatomy and physiology –
an overview** **841**

Epidermis 842
Epidermal renewal and
keratinization 842
Normal pigmentation 842
Protective role of the skin 842
Skin appendages 843
Pilosebaceous unit 843
Sweat glands 843
Nails 843
Nursing assessment **843**
Collecting information 844
The physical examination 844
Distribution and configuration
of skin lesions 845
Changes in skin colour and
pigmentation 846
Documentation 846
**General diagnostic tests and
medical investigations** **846**
Microbiological investigations 846
Bacteriological investigations 846
Virology tests 846
Mycology 847
Wood's light examination 848
Ovasites and parasites
Sellotape test 848
Skin biopsy 848
Patch testing 848
Blood tests 848
**General disease prevention
and health education** **848**
Maintaining healthy skin 849
Inflammatory skin disorders **849**
Atopic eczema 849
Aetiology and epidemiology 849
Pathophysiology and clinical
presentation 849
Medical management 850
Nursing management 850
Stasis (gravitational or
varicose) eczema 851
Epidemiology and aetiology 851
Pathophysiology and clinical
presentation 851
Medical management 851
Nursing management 851
Contact dermatitis 851
Clinical presentation and
specific investigations 851
Medical management 851
Nursing management 851
Acne 851
Clinical presentation 851
Medical treatment 852
Nursing management 852
Rosacea 852
Medical management 852
Nursing management 853
Lichen planus 853

Clinical presentation	853
Nursing management	853
Pruritus	853
Aetiology	853
Pathophysiology and clinical presentation	853
Nursing and medical management	853
Urticaria	854
Aetiology	854
Medical management	854
Nursing management	854
Seborrhoeic dermatitis	854
Aetiology and epidemiology	854
Clinical presentation	854
Nursing and medical management	854

Infections and infestations of the skin — **854**

Bacterial skin infection	854
Medical management	855
Nursing management	855
Viral skin infections	855
Aetiology and clinical presentation	855
Nursing and medical management	855
Fungal infections	855
Dermatophytosis (tinea)	856
Nursing management	856
Superficial Candida infections (candidosis, candidiasis)	858
Pityriasis versicolor – Malassezia yeast infection	858
Nursing and medical management	859

Infestations — **859**

Scabies	859
Aetiology and pathophysiology	859
Clinical presentation	859
Medical management	860
Nursing management	860
Pediculosis	860
Head lice	860
Nursing management	860
Body and pubic lice	860

Benign skin changes — **861**

Cysts	861
Pathophysiology	861
Nursing and medical management	861
Keloids	861
Medical/surgical management	861
Nursing management	861

Disorders of keratin synthesis — **861**

Psoriasis	861
Aetiology	861
Pathophysiology	861
Clinical presentation	861

Medical management	862
Nursing management	862

Disorders of pigmentation — **862**

Albinism	862
Medical management	862
Nursing management	862
Vitiligo	863
Epidemiology and aetiology	863
Clinical presentation	863
Medical management	863
Nursing management	863
Chloasma	863
Freckles and lentigines	863
Nursing management	863

Vascular disorders — **864**

Haemangiomas	864
Telangiectasia (cherry angiomas)	864

Blistering skin disorders — **864**

Infective blistering disorders	864
Bullous impetigo	864
Bullous cellulitis	864
Eczema herpeticum	864
Nursing management: infective blistering disorders	865
Autoimmune blistering disorders	865
Bullous pemphigoid	865
Pemphigus	865
Nursing management: autoimmune blistering disorders	865
Dermatitis herpetiformis	866
Clinical presentation	866
Medical management	866
Nursing management	866
Epidermolysis bullosa	866
Nursing management	866
Stevens–Johnson syndrome and toxic epidermal necrolysis	866
Pathophysiology	866
Nursing and medical management	866

Skin tumours — **867**

Benign tumours – seborrhoeic keratoses	867
Clinical presentation	867
Nursing and surgical management	867
Malignant tumours – skin cancers	868
Basal cell carcinoma	868
Pathophysiology and clinical presentation	868
Surgical management	868
Squamous cell carcinoma	868
Clinical presentation	868
Medical/surgical management	868
Nursing management: non-melanoma skin cancers	868

Malignant melanoma	868
Pathophysiology	868
Clinical presentation	868
Medical/surgical management	869
Nursing management	869
Kaposi's sarcoma	869
Nursing and medical management	869

Abnormal hair growth — **869**

Alopecia	869
Medical management	869
Nursing management	869
Hirsutism	869
Nursing management	870
Hypertrichosis	870
Nursing management	870

Nail and nail fold problems — **870**

Paronychia	870
Nursing management	870

Skin reactions with systemic disorders — **870**

Xanthomas	870
Drug eruptions	870

Burn injuries — **871**

Types of burns	871
First aid	871
Assessment of burns	871
Depth	871
Body surface area	872
Initial management	872
Nursing and medical management	872
Surgical management	873
Body image	873

**SECTION 4
SPECIFIC AREAS OF
ADULT NURSING** — **877**

29 PERIOPERATIVE NURSING — **879**

The context and classification of surgery — **880**

Day surgery	880
Issues likely to influence suitability and acceptance for day surgery	882
Pre-admission assessment and admission	882
Postoperative pain management in day care	884
Criteria for discharge	885

General preoperative care — **885**

Preoperative assessment	885
Establishing fitness for surgery and anaesthesia	885

Assessing the potential for and preventing postoperative complications 887
   Infection and skin preparation 887
   Malnutrition and nutritional assessment 888
   Deep vein thrombosis 888
   Chest infection 889
Psychological preparation for surgery 889
   Physiological effects of stress and anxiety on surgical patients 890
   Nursing management: stress and anxiety 890
Consent 891
   Age and factors reducing potential for informed consent 892
Preoperative safety measures 892
   Fasting prior to surgery 892
   Bowel preparation 894
   Immediate preoperative measures 894
   Premedication 894
Patient transfer, safety and identification issues 895
   Identification 895
Intraoperative care **895**
Anaesthesia 896
   Local anaesthesia 896
   Regional anaesthesia 896
   Nursing management: following spinal and epidural anaesthetic 897
   General anaesthesia 898
Patient movement and issues of immobility 900
   Patient positioning 901
Dignity 902
Pressure ulcer prevention 902
Intraoperative prevention of deep vein thrombosis 902
Hypothermia 902
   Nursing management 903
Procedural safety issues 903
   Accounting for swabs, needles and instruments 904
   Haemostasis 904
Preventing infection in the operating theatre 905
   Skin preparation 905
   Handwashing and surgical scrub 905
   Surgical gloves 905
   Surgical clothing 905
   Surgical environment 906
   Sterile instruments 906
Sutures 906
Posoperative care **907**
Immediate postoperative care – recovery unit 907

Airway and breathing assessment 908
Temperature and shivering 908
Circulatory assessment 909
Assessing consciousness 909
Discharge from recovery unit 909
Managing postoperative pain 910
   Patient-controlled analgesia (PCA) 910
   Management of postoperative nausea and vomiting 911
Paralytic ileus – nasogastric intubation 911
Fluid balance maintenance and monitoring 912
   Intravenous infusions 912
Post-surgical nutrition and fasting 913
Postoperative renal/urinary issues 913
Constipation 913
Postoperative deep vein thrombosis 914
Postoperative chest infection 914
Wound management 914
   Wound assessment 915
   Wound dressings 915
   Wound drainage 915
   Wound drains 915
   Nursing management: wound drains 917
   Wound infection 917
   Wound dehiscence 918
   Nursing management: wound dehiscence 918
Mobility and ambulation 919
Discharge planning 919

30 NURSING PATIENTS IN THE ACCIDENT AND EMERGENCY DEPARTMENT **923**

The role of the A&E department **924**
Who uses A&E? 924
Prehospital care 924
Caring in the A&E department 925
The process of nursing in A&E **925**
Nursing assessment in A&E **925**
Triage 925
   Triage standards 926
   The skills of patient assessment 926
Health promotion and the prevention of accidents **927**
Accidents 928
Protecting children 928
Managing the A&E department **928**
Directing the traffic 928
Directing the team 928

Matching the person with the job 928
Sharing the skills 928
The role of the emergency nurse practitioner in A&E **929**
Resuscitation in the A&E department **929**
The environment 929
The team 930
Health and safety 930
The patient 930
   Witnessed resuscitation 931
Caring for the patient with major trauma **931**
Nursing roles within trauma management 932
Assessment and management 932
   The primary survey 932
   The secondary survey 933
   The definitive care phase 933
Caring for the patient with minor trauma **934**
Assessing minor trauma 934
   Acute wound management 934
   Discharging the patient with minor trauma 935
Social issues in the A&E department **936**
Alcohol-related attendance 936
Drug dependence 937
Victims of violence 937
   Domestic violence 937
   Rape and sexual assault 937
The homeless person 938
Dealing with challenging behaviour **938**
Handling aggression 938
Mental health problems in A&E **938**
Causes of disturbed behaviour 939
   Schizophrenia 940
   Depressive illness 940
   Acute anxiety state 940
Recognizing the patient with an acute mental health problem 940
   Deliberate self-harm 940
   Caring for the acutely disturbed patient 940
Sudden death in A&E **941**
The role of the nurse in caring for the bereaved 941
   Viewing of the deceased by relatives 941
   Contacting absent relatives 941
   Respecting religious and cultural values 941
   Liaising with the coroner 941
   Ensuring accurate documentation 942
   Ensuring follow-up and support 942

Caring for the carers 942
Major disasters **942**
The role of the hospital and
A&E department 942
*Communication and the
multidisciplinary team* 942
Support and debrief 942

31 CRITICALLY ILL PATIENTS 947

Development of critical care **947**
**Classification of critically ill
patients** **948**
Categories of organ
monitoring and support 949
Critical care outreach teams 949
Early warning systems 950
**Nursing management of the
critically ill patient** **951**
Communication 951
The multidisciplinary team 951
Nurses 951
Surgeons 951
Anaesthetists 951
Physicians 952
Physiotherapists 952
Speech therapists 952
Dieticians 952
Radiographers 952
*Microbiologists, pathologists
and haematologists* 952
Technicians 952
Decision-making and
informed consent 952
Personal care 952
Eye care 952
Oral hygiene 952
Effects of immobility 953
Nutrition 953
**The effects of the
environment on the patient** **954**
Physiological overview **954**
Respiratory system 954
Cardiovascular system 955
Cardiac output 955
Blood pressure 955
Monitoring and assessment **956**
Principles of monitoring and
assessment 956
Patient history 957
Sensory observations 957
Touch 957
Respiratory monitoring and
assessment 957
*Respiratory rate, pattern
and depth* 957
Tidal volume 957
Breath sounds 958

Pulse oximetry 958
Arterial blood gas analysis 958
Cardiovascular monitoring
and assessment 958
Blood pressure 959
*Nursing management: the
patient with an arterial line* 959
**Key clinical scenarios in
critical illness** **960**
Mechanical ventilation 960
*Indications for intubation
and mechanical ventilation* 961
*Principles of mechanical
ventilation* 961
Non-invasive ventilation 961
Nursing management 961
Inotrope therapy 962
Indications for inotrope therapy 963
Nursing management 963
Renal replacement therapy 963
*Indications for renal
replacement therapy* 963
Nursing management 963

32 NURSING OLDER ADULTS 967

Ageing **967**
The purpose of ageing 968
Heterogeneity of ageing 968
The ageing experience **968**
Images of ageing 968
Ageism 970
Consequences of ageing 970
Inequality and ageing 971
Families and older people 971
**Social, psychological and
biological aspects of ageing** **971**
Psychosocial theories of ageing 972
*Disengagement, activity and
continuity theories* 972
Erikson's theory of life span 972
Intelligence and personality 972
Memory 972
Dementia 973
Depression in old age 974
Biological theories of ageing 974
Hereditary theories 974
Physiological theories 974
Cellular theories 974
Physiological changes with
ageing 975
Ageing of organs 975
Frailty 975
*Immobility, instability,
incontinence and mental
impairment* 975
Implications of biological
ageing for individuals and
carers 976

The ageing skin 976
Medicines and the older adult 976
Pharmacokinetics 976
Compliance with drug regimens 976
Health and health promotion **977**
Falls 978
Sexual health 978
Nutrition and health 978
*Nursing management of
older adults* 979
Long-term care 979
*Institutionalization,
autonomy and paternalism* 979
Nutrition in long-term care 979
The oldest old 980
Caring for the carers **980**
Abuse 981
**Bereavement and dying in
old age** **981**
Spiritual aspects of old age **981**

33 NURSING PATIENTS WITH CANCER 985

Aetiology **986**
What is cancer and how does
it occur? 986
*Differences between normal
and cancer cells* 987
Carcinogenesis 988
Stages in tumour development 988
Natural history of cancer **988**
Modes of spread and
pathophysiological effects 989
**Factors that predispose to
cancer** **989**
Stress, emotion and cancer 989
Carcinogens 989
Tobacco 990
Diet 990
*Body weight, body mass
index and physical activity* 990
Alcohol 990
Occupational exposure 990
Pollution 990
Radiation 990
Drugs 991
Infection 991
Host characteristics and cancer 991
Age 991
Gender 991
Ethnicity and race 991
Preventing cancer **991**
Promoting healthy behaviour 991
Identifying warning signs 992
**Types and classification of
new growths** **992**
Benign and malignant tumours 992
Haematological malignancy 993

Acute leukaemia 993
Chronic leukaemia 993
Solid tumours 993
Lung cancer (Ch. 20) 994
Breast cancer (Ch. 26) 994
Cancer of the cervix (Ch. 25) 994
Colorectal cancer (Ch. 22) 994
Testicular cancer (Ch. 25) 994
Prostate cancer (Ch. 24) 994
Bladder cancer (Ch. 24) 994
Epidemiology **995**
Common cancers 995
Incidence and survival 995
Screening and early detection **996**
Principles of screening for cancer 997
Genetic screening 998
Screening for specific cancers 998
Lung cancer 998
Breast cancer 998
Cancer of the cervix 999
Colorectal cancer 1000
Testicular cancer 1000
Prostate cancer 1000
Bladder cancer 1001
Diagnostic procedures **1001**
Diagnostic tests 1001
Aspiration cytology 1001
Lymph node biopsy 1001
Breast biopsy 1001
Skin biopsy 1001
Endoscopy 1001
Bone marrow aspiration and biopsy 1002
Lumbar puncture 1002
Liver biopsy 1002
Imaging 1002
Isotope scanning 1002
Laparoscopy 1002
Grading 1002
Staging 1003
Treatment modalities for cancer **1004**
Surgery 1004
Principles of surgical treatment 1004
Radiotherapy 1005
Pathophysiology 1005
Treatment modalities 1005
Side-effects 1005
Safety issues 1005
Chemotherapy 1006
Pathophysiology 1006
Treatment schedules 1007
Side-effects 1007
Safety issues 1008
Immunotherapy/biological response modifier therapy 1008

Principles of BRM treatment 1008
Side-effects 1009
Emotional responses to a diagnosis of cancer **1009**
Nursing management and interventions **1011**
Communication 1011
Identifying patients' needs (Ch. 3) 1011
Addressing spiritual needs 1011
Patient teaching 1012
Preparing patient information materials 1012
Dealing with the side-effects of treatment and disease 1012
Nausea and vomiting 1012
Fatigue 1013
Diarrhoea 1013
Pancytopenia (Chs 13 and 18) 1013
Lymphoedema 1014
Oncological emergencies 1014
Septic shock (Ch. 9) 1014
Spinal cord compression 1014
Dealing with changes in body image 1015
Promoting adaptive responses 1015
Psychosexual issues 1016
Rehabilitation and survival 1016
Supporting family and friends 1016
Management of cancer pain **1016**
Pharmacological strategies 1017
Non-pharmacological strategies 1017
Specialist cancer nurse roles **1017**
Ethical dilemmas in cancer nursing **1017**
Ethical principles 1017
Cancer patients and research 1018

34 NURSING PATIENTS WHO NEED PALLIATIVE CARE **1021**

Concepts of palliative care **1021**
Historical background 1021
The development of palliative care in the 20th century 1021
The care team 1022
Settings for palliative care **1022**
Hospices 1022
Hospitals 1023
Day centres 1023
Home care 1024
General practitioners 1024
District nurses 1025
Macmillan nurses 1025
Marie Curie organization 1025
Occupational therapists 1025
Social workers 1025

Family 1025
Emotional responses to terminal illness **1025**
Stages of the emotional response 1025
Emotional support for all those involved **1026**
Supporting the family 1026
Needs of relatives 1026
Supporting health care professionals 1027
Ethical issues in palliative care **1027**
Advance directives 1027
Terminal dehydration and rehydration 1028
Nutritional support 1028
Euthanasia 1028
Nursing assessment **1028**
Areas for assessment 1028
Breathing 1028
Oral assessment 1029
Eating and drinking 1029
Skin condition and hygiene needs 1029
Elimination 1029
Mobility, activity and leisure 1029
Pain 1029
Sleep 1030
Understanding of illness and self-image 1031
Communication, mood and behaviour 1031
Assessing family needs – social and financial 1031
Assessing spiritual needs 1031
Nursing management and interventions **1031**
Symptom control 1031
Principles of symptom control 1032
Pain 1032
Types of cancer pain 1032
Management of pain 1032
Parenteral drug administration 1034
Mouth problems 1035
Coated tongue 1035
Dryness 1035
Stomatitis 1035
Oral pain 1035
Taste disturbances 1035
Halitosis 1035
Nausea and vomiting 1035
Physiology of nausea and vomiting 1035
Causes of nausea and vomiting 1036
Non-pharmacological interventions 1036

Pharmacological
interventions   *1036*
Cachexia and anorexia   1037
Management   *1037*
Constipation   1038
Causes   *1038*
Management   *1038*
Intestinal obstruction   1038
Management   *1038*
Breathing problems   1038
Cough   *1038*
Hiccups   *1038*
Dyspnoea   *1038*
Fungating wounds   1039
Management   *1039*
Psychological problems   1039
Agitation   *1039*
Anxiety   *1039*
Confusion   *1039*
Depression   *1039*
Emergencies in palliative care   1040
Fractures   *1040*
Haemorrhage   *1040*
Hypercalcaemia   *1040*
Superior vena cava
obstruction   *1040*
Spinal cord compression   *1040*
Seizures   *1040*
Role of specialist palliative
care nurses   **1040**
Referrals   1041
Reasons for referrals   *1041*
Care around the time
of death   **1041**
Nursing management   1041
Environment   *1041*
Skin care and hygiene   *1041*
Coping with restlessness   *1042*
Noisy respiration   *1042*
Medication   *1042*
Spiritual, religious and
cultural needs   1042
After death   1042
The official aspects of death   **1042**
Registering a death   1043

Reporting a death to the
coroner   1043
Funeral directors   1043
Organ donation   1043
Follow-up support and
counselling   **1043**
Grief and bereavement   1043
Abnormal grief   *1044*
Presentation of
unresolved grief   *1044*
Help during bereavement   1044
Bereavement counselling   *1044*
Support organizations   *1044*

35 NURSING PATIENTS WITH
CHRONIC (LONG-TERM)
ILLNESS AND DISABILITY   **1047**

What is illness, sickness and
disability?   **1048**
Definitions of chronic illness   1048
Definition of disability and
handicap   1048
Prevalence and impact of
chronic illness and disability   **1049**
Common causes of disability   1049
The impact of chronic illness   1049
Multiple pathology   1050
Common features of chronic
illness   1050
Prevention and rehabilitation
in chronic illness and disability   1051
Developmental, psychological,
social and cultural factors
in disability and chronic
illness   **1051**
Types of stigma   1052
Physical deformity   *1052*
Self-inflicted conditions   *1052*
Prejudice   *1052*
Responses to stigma   1052
Disregard   *1052*
Resistance   *1053*
Isolation   *1053*
Secondary gains   *1053*

Passing   *1053*
Covering   *1053*
Cultural variations   1053
Coming to terms with
chronic illness   1053
Stages of adaptation   *1054*
Psychological, social
and cultural factors   *1054*
Developmental factors   1054
Adolescence   *1054*
Young and middle-aged adults   *1054*
Older adults   *1055*
Health policy   **1056**
Care settings for those with
chronic illness and disability   **1056**
Hospital wards   1056
Rehabilitation settings and
intermediate care   1057
Community nursing and
practice nursing   1057
New nursing roles in
chronic disease management   1058
Long-term care   1058
Assessment of chronic illness
and disability and its impact
on the individual and family   **1058**
Models of nursing   1058
Assessment of impairment   1059
Secondary prevention   1059
Functional assessment   1059
Barthel index   *1059*
Ten-item abbreviated
mental test   *1060*
Assessment of coping and
well-being   1060
Nursing priorities for older
adults: assessment of social
and role functions   **1060**
Nursing care for those with
chronic illness and disability   **1060**
The care team   1061
Psychological support –
facilitating adaptation   1062
Promoting physical activity   1063
Sexual dysfunction   1063

SECTION 1

Nursing, quality and communication

Contents

1 Adult nursing: setting the scene   3

2 Quality management and standards of care   23

3 Communication in adult nursing   39

1 Adult nursing: setting the scene

Maggie Nicol, Chris Brooker, Julienne Meyer

> 'What is nursing? I thought that was obvious – it's about looking after ill people.
> But nursing is much more than that; it's about preventing people becoming ill as well.
> And it's not just about being kind to people – you need to know an awful lot to be able
> to care intelligently.'
>
> (Student nurse)

THIS CHAPTER WILL HELP YOU

- Understand what is meant by adult nursing
- Discuss definitions of health and health promotion, and their relevance to adult nursing
- Explore the role of the nurse in identifying and meeting the needs of adult patients and clients
- Identify the stages of the nursing process and the purpose of nursing models
- Understand the role of research and evidence-based practice in adult nursing
- Explore what is meant by reflective practice and its role in professional development as a nurse
- Explore ethical principles and ethical decision-making and their relevance to everyday nursing practice.

KEYWORDS

Adult nursing	Holistic care
Evidence-based practice	Nursing & Midwifery Council
Ethics	Nursing models
Health	Nursing process
Health promotion	Reflection

INTRODUCTION

The purpose of this chapter is to examine what is meant by adult nursing and to introduce some of the concepts and issues that are fundamental to the nursing care of adults.

In the UK all nurses must register with the Nursing & Midwifery Council in order to practise. There are currently four separate programmes or 'branches' of nurse education, designed to prepare nurses to care for different client groups: adults, children, those with mental health problems and those with learning disabilities. Adult nursing involves caring for those over the age of 18 years, although some teenagers are nursed on adult wards, if this is felt to be more appropriate to their individual needs. Each 'branch' has a separate programme of preparation leading to registration on different parts of the Nursing & Midwifery Council (NMC) register, although all four branches share a common foundation programme for the first year. The branch structure is currently under review and may be broadened to include specialist branches for the care of older adults and community nursing.

As with all forms of nursing, the nature of adult nursing is hard to define as it is constantly altering in response to the changing needs of society. Nowadays, due to the ageing population, most adult patients are over the age of 65 years. Thus care for older adults is a vital aspect of adult nursing. Older people often have more than one thing wrong with them and require complex care. The adult nurse needs to be able to identify their individual needs and plan and coordinate complex packages of care that involve a wide range of health and social care professionals, across a variety of different settings (e.g. hospital and community).

There are other changes in society that impact on adult nursing. *The NHS Plan* (Department of Health 2000a) is the government's framework to modernize and reform the NHS, and break down the traditional barriers between the professions. Care will be centred on the needs of patients and clients rather than on the needs of the system and this has called for new skills and roles in nursing. For instance, changes in the number of hours that junior doctors work have led to nurses expanding their role to undertake a wider range of tasks that were previously only performed by doctors. These include the right to make and receive referrals, admit and discharge patients, order investigations and diagnostic tests, run clinics and prescribe medication (Department of Health 2000a). In order to take on these new roles, work that was once the traditional role of nurses (e.g. personal care) is now sometimes delegated to non-registered carers (e.g. health care assistants, HCAs) or student nurses. This, together with the fact that chronically ill patients now live longer and need to have more responsibility for managing their own care, means that adult nurses now need to act as coordinators of care, taking on greater education roles to support and enable others to provide care. This may be patients themselves, their unpaid carers (relatives, neighbours and friends), volunteers, HCAs, student nurses and other health professionals.

Adult nursing is concerned with those who are healthy as well as those who are sick. Promoting good health and preventing ill health are important aspects of nursing and require nurses to be able to see patients as individuals and care for them in a holistic manner. Holism requires nurses to be attentive not only to the physical aspects of care, but also to the social, spiritual, mental, emotional and societal aspects. To do this, nurses use nursing models to help them identify their patients' individual needs and problems. In order to plan, deliver and evaluate care systematically, they use a shared system, such as the nursing process or integrated care pathways. In planning care, adult nurses need to draw on research findings to inform how best to provide effective care (evidence-based practice), and where evidence does not exist (or does not suit the specific needs of the individual patient), they need to draw on past experience of what works best.

Adult nursing, like all forms of nursing, throws up many exciting challenges. There are not always easy answers and nurses sometimes have to make hard decisions, in collaboration with the rest of the multidisciplinary team. To do this, they need to have a sound understanding of ethical principles to inform their decision-making. Patients should always be at the centre of this decision-making and adult nurses need to ensure that patients not only understand the nature of their illness, but are also concordant with (i.e. able to make informed choices that concord with their wishes) the care being proposed. These issues are explored in this chapter and throughout the book.

WHAT IS NURSING?

Adult nursing, like other types of nursing, has proved difficult to define. *The Chambers Dictionary* (1998) describes a nurse as 'a person who has care of the sick, feeble or injured, esp. one who is trained for the purpose', and nursing as 'the profession or practice of caring for the sick, feeble or injured'. Such definitions might go some way towards describing nursing, but they do not really reflect the diversity of roles within the different specialties and the role of nurses who work in schools and colleges and those whose primary role is health promotion. Neither do they provide any insight into what nurses actually do. Another problem is that caring for the 'sick, feeble or injured' is not exclusively the role of registered nurses. Non-registered

1.1 What nursing means

This chapter is all about nursing and the key concepts and core issues. Think back to when you first started nursing.

● What was your idea of what nursing was all about? Has that changed?
● What qualities do you think a nurse should have?
● If you were a patient, how would you like the nurse to behave?
● Imagine you are receiving nursing care at home. Would you expect the nurse to act any differently?

nurses such as HCAs, unpaid carers (e.g. family or friends), parents and volunteers do this every day of the week. Furthermore, many patients care for themselves.

A widely cited definition of nursing is that by Virginia Henderson, an American nurse theorist who in 1966 defined nursing in terms of the role of the nurse:

> The unique role of the nurse is to assist the individual, sick or well, in the performance of those activities contributing to health and its recovery (or to a peaceful death) that he would otherwise perform unaided if he had the necessary strength, will or knowledge. And to do this in such a way as to help him gain independence as rapidly as possible.

Although this definition has gained acceptance by many nurses because they can see how the definition 'fits' their role, it does not really explain what nurses actually *do*. It explains *how* they should do it, i.e. 'in such a way as to help him gain independence as rapidly as possible', but it does not define what nurses actually do apart from assist the patient. Perhaps it is impossible to be more explicit; nursing is a complex and dynamic activity (see Reflective Practice box 1.1).

Advances in medicine and changes in the way in which health care is delivered mean that whilst caring remains central to the role, nurses must also be multiskilled and adaptable, with highly developed technical and communication and interpersonal skills to enable them to support vulnerable people and their families at a critical time in their lives. Nurses need the skills to provide education and enhance coping strategies etc. to enable individuals to take charge of and improve their health and thus prevent them becoming patients (health promotion). They also need the skills to provide training to enable those with chronic conditions (e.g. diabetes or asthma) to manage their own lives and live independently. Nurses also need the skills and confidence to enable them to speak up or act on behalf of patients if necessary, and to communicate effectively with other members of the multidisciplinary health care team.

THE REGULATION OF NURSING

In the UK, entry to the professional register is restricted to those who have completed a programme of education (usually 3 years) and achievement of specific outcomes and competencies laid down by the Nursing & Midwifery Council (NMC, see below). There are two sets of outcomes: one for the first year foundation programme and another for the 2-year branch programmes. They are grouped into four 'domains' and are the same for all branches of nursing. Box 1.1 provides an outline of the outcomes and competencies (UKCC 2001). All programmes of nurse education have to demonstrate how they will enable students to achieve these competencies (see Box 1.1).

Box 1.1 Requirements for pre-registration nursing programmes (adapted from UKCC 2001)

Professional/ethical practice

Outcomes to be achieved for entry to the branch programme
- Discuss in an informed manner, the implications of professional regulation for nursing practice
- Demonstrate an awareness of the UKCC *Code of Professional Conduct*
- Demonstrate an awareness of and apply ethical principles to nursing practice
- Demonstrate an awareness of legislation relevant to nursing practice
- Demonstrate the importance of promoting equity in patient and client care by contributing to nursing care in a fair and anti-discriminatory way

Competencies for entry to the register
- Manage oneself, one's practice and that of others, in accordance with the UKCC *Code of Professional Conduct*, recognizing one's own abilities and limitations
- Practise in accordance with an ethical and legal framework that ensures the primacy of patient/client interest and well-being and respects confidentiality
- Practise in a fair and anti-discriminatory way, acknowledging the difference in beliefs and cultural practices of individuals or groups

Care delivery

Outcomes to be achieved for entry to the branch programme
- Discuss methods of, barriers to and boundaries of effective communication and interpersonal relationships
- Demonstrate sensitivity in interaction with and provision of information to patients and clients
- Contribute to enhancing the health and social well-being of patients/clients by understanding how, under the supervision of a registered practitioner, to:
  — contribute to assessment of health needs
  — identify opportunities for health promotion
  — identify networks of health and social care services
- Contribute to the development and documentation of nursing assessments by participating in comprehensive and systematic nursing assessment of the physical, psychological, social and spiritual needs of patients/clients
- Contribute to the planning of nursing care, involving patients/clients and where possible their carers, demonstrating an understanding of helping patients/clients to make informed decisions
- Contribute to the implementation of a programme of nursing care, designed and supervised by registered practitioners
- Demonstrate evidence of a developing knowledge base that underpins safe nursing practice

- Demonstrate a range of essential nursing skills to meet individuals' needs, which include:
  — maintaining dignity, privacy and confidentiality
  — effective observational and communication skills, including listening
  — safety and health, including moving and handling
  — essential first aid and emergency procedures
  — administration of medicines
  — emotional, physical and personal care
- Contribute to the evaluation of the appropriateness of nursing care delivered
- Recognize situations in which agreed plans of nursing care no longer appear appropriate and refer these to an appropriate accountable practitioner

Competencies for entry to the register
- Engage in, develop and disengage from therapeutic relationships through the use of appropriate communication and interpersonal skills
- Create and utilize opportunities to promote the health and well-being of patients, clients and groups
- Undertake and document a comprehensive, systematic and accurate nursing assessment of the physical, psychological, social and spiritual needs of patients, clients and communities
- Formulate and document a plan of nursing care, where possible in partnership with patients, clients, their carers and family and friends, within a framework of informed consent
- Based on best available evidence, apply knowledge and an appropriate repertoire of skills indicative of safe nursing practice
- Provide a rationale for the nursing care delivered that takes account of social, cultural, spiritual, legal, political and economic influences
- Evaluate and document the outcomes of nursing and other interventions
- Demonstrate sound clinical judgement across a range of differing professional and care delivery contexts

Care management

Outcomes to be achieved for entry to the branch programme
- Contribute to the identification of actual and potential risks to patients/clients and their carers, to self and others
- Participate in measures to promote and ensure health and safety
- Demonstrate an understanding of the role of others by participating in interprofessional working practice
- Demonstrate literacy, numeracy and computer skills needed to record, enter, store, retrieve and organize data essential for care delivery *(continued)*

Box 1.1 (continued)

Competencies for entry to the register
- Contribute to public protection by creating and maintaining a safe environment of care through the use of quality assurance and risk management strategies
- Demonstrate knowledge of effective interprofessional working practices that respect and utilize the contributions of members of the health and social care team
- Delegate duties to others, as appropriate, ensuring they are supervised and monitored
- Demonstrate key skills:
  - Literacy: interpret and present information in comprehensible manner
  - Numeracy: accurately interpreting numerical data and their significance for safe delivery of care
  - Information technology and management: interpret and utilize data and technology, taking account of legal, ethical and safety considerations, in the delivery and enhancement of care

- Problem-solving: demonstrate sound clinical decision-making which can be justified even when made on the basis of limited information

Personal/professional development
Outcomes to be achieved for entry to the branch programme
- Demonstrate responsibility for one's own learning through the development of a portfolio of practice and recognize when further learning may be required
- Acknowledge the importance of seeking supervision to develop safe nursing practice

Competencies for entry to the register
- Demonstrate a commitment to the need for continuing professional development and personal supervision activities in order to enhance knowledge, skills, values and attitudes needed for safe and effective nursing practice
- Enhance the professional development and safe practice of others through peer support, leadership, supervision and teaching

The nursing and midwifery professions are regulated by the NMC, whose role is to maintain a register of practitioners (currently around 640 000 entries), to set standards for nursing and midwifery practice and to safeguard the public. Part of that role includes hearing cases of alleged professional misconduct and, if found guilty, cautioning, imposing conditions or removing the practitioner from the professional register to prevent him or her practising. In this way the NMC monitors and regulates the profession to ensure that high standards of professional practice are maintained. Nurses are required to re-register every 3 years. Until April 2002, the UKCC maintained the professional register, but this is now undertaken by the NMC along with the work previously undertaken by four national boards (one for each country in the UK). Box 1.2 summarizes the central aims of the NMC.

Student nurses are not accountable to the NMC, because they are not yet registered practitioners. However, they will come into close contact with patients and clients. The NMC/UKCC provides guidance for students in clinical placements in the leaflet *Guidance on Clinical Experience for Students* (UKCC 1998). This

is available from the NMC, in university libraries and on the internet at www.nmc-uk.org. The guidance addresses issues of accepting responsibility, confidentiality, identifying yourself and respecting patient and client wishes. As the NMC/UKCC guidance makes clear, patients do have a right to refuse to allow student nurses (and medical students) to care for them. This is rare but their rights must be respected if they do so. The NMC stresses that at all times the rights of patients and clients supersede a student's rights to knowledge and experience (see Guidelines for Care Priorities box 1.1).

CODE OF PROFESSIONAL CONDUCT

As professionals, nurses, midwives and health visitors are governed by a code of conduct. The NMC published a new *Code of Professional Conduct* in 2002; an overview is provided in Box 1.3. The code acts as a guide for nurses. It is not law, but is a framework for behaviour and a statement about how the profession considers its members should behave (Rumbold 1999). Registered nurses are accountable to the NMC, which means that they can be called to account for their behaviour and judged against that expected in the *Code of Professional Conduct*. Nurses found guilty of misconduct may have their names removed from the register, thus preventing them from practising as a registered nurse.

Box 1.2 Central aims of the Nursing & Midwifery Council (NMC 2002)

- To treat the health and welfare of patients as paramount
- To collaborate with and consult key stakeholders
- To be open and proactive in accounting to the public and the professions for its work
- To deal effectively with individuals who pose unacceptable risks to patients
- To set and monitor standards of professional training, performance and conduct
- To link registration with evidence of continuing professional development

POST-REGISTRATION EDUCATION AND PRACTICE (PREP)

Nurses, like other professionals, have a professional duty to keep up to date with new knowledge and practices through continuing professional development (CPD). Good nurses have always done this and clause 6 of the *Code of Professional Conduct* requires nurses to maintain their professional knowledge and skills. However, in order to strengthen this requirement and be able to monitor compliance, the UKCC introduced

GUIDELINES FOR CARE PRIORITIES

1.1 NMC/UKCC guidance on clinical experience for students

The NMC/UKCC guidance on clinical experience for students is summarized here. The full text is available from libraries and the NMC website (www.nmc-uk.org).

At all times you should work only within your level of understanding and competence and always under the direct supervision of a registered nurse, midwife or health visitor. The principles underpinning this guidance reflect the standards that will be expected when you become a registered practitioner.

Accountability

As pre-registration students, you are never professionally accountable in the way that you will be after registration. So far as the UKCC is concerned, it is the registered practitioners with whom you are working who are professionally accountable for the consequences of your actions and omissions. This does not mean that you can never be called to account by your university or by the law.

The wishes of patients and clients

Respect the wishes of patients and clients at all times. They have a right to refuse to allow you to care for them and you should make it clear that you are a student right at the outset. You should leave if they ask you to do so. Their rights as patients or clients supersede at all times your right to knowledge.

Identifying yourself

Introduce yourself at all times and make it clear that you are a pre-registration student.

Accepting appropriate responsibility

Do not participate in any procedure for which you have not been fully prepared or during which you are not adequately supervised.

Patient and client confidentiality

Patients and clients have a right to confidentiality. If you wish to refer to real-life situations in a written assignment, do not provide any information that could identify a particular patient or client. Any written entry you make in the patient's records must be countersigned by a registered practitioner.

Handling complaints

Be aware of local procedures for dealing with complaints. If patients or clients indicate to you that they are unhappy with the treatment that they are receiving, report the matter immediately to your supervisor.

Box 1.3 The *Code of Professional Conduct* (NMC 2002)

Each of the clauses listed here is accompanied by subclauses that explain the purpose of the code and expand on what they mean. The full document is available from the NMC, in libraries and on the NMC website (www.nmc-uk.org).

The *Code of Professional Conduct* states that registered nurses and midwives are personally accountable for their practice and in caring for their patients and clients must:

- Respect the patient as an individual
- Obtain consent before you give any treatment or care
- Protect confidential information
- Cooperate with others in the team
- Maintain your professional knowledge and competence
- Be trustworthy.

---

post-registration education and practice (PREP), which means that in order to re-register every 3 years, nurses are required to maintain a portfolio of professional experience and to demonstrate a minimum of 5 days' (30 hours) updating activity. This does not have to be a course or study days – spending time in the library, a ward teaching session or a visit to another hospital are all valid examples of CPD. PREP also requires that a reflective account of the learning activity, which identifies the learning achieved and its relevance to practice, is kept in a professional portfolio and can be produced, if requested, at re-registration. The NMC checks a random sample every year.

Professional self-regulation is one of the cornerstones of clinical governance and so it is important that the NMC is able to demonstrate ways in which it is ensuring minimum levels of safe practice. PREP will ensure that all nurses not only update their practice but also reflect on that updating to identify their learning and future learning needs.

ADULT NURSING

As discussed earlier, adult nursing concerns the care of people from 16–18 years of age onwards, although some adolescents may be nursed in an adult ward if this is felt to be more appropriate. However, it should be noted that most adults who are nursed are over the age of 65 years. The National Beds Inquiry (Department of Health 2000b) found that two-thirds of all hospital beds are occupied by patients over 65 years. Adult nursing takes place in many settings (e.g. the person's home, other community settings such as nursing homes, community hospitals, rough sleepers' hostels, prisons, the workplace, and hospitals) both in the NHS and in the private sector.

Adulthood means reaching a stage in the life cycle: the person is first a child, then a youth or adolescent and then an adult. There is no one single age that defines an adult as the age-related restrictions associated with activities such as voting, getting married, buying alcohol or cigarettes vary between 16 and 18 years of age. However, one of the key concepts of being an adult is responsibility, i.e. not being childish and being responsible for oneself, one's deeds and development (Rogers 1996). For some, as they get older, their cognitive ability declines and they are less able to be responsible for themselves. However, it should not be assumed that this is the case for many older people. The vast majority are well able to make their own decisions and are living full and independent lives. Unfortunately, we are living in an ageist society, which seems to value youth above the wisdom of old age, and this sometimes affects the way in which care is delivered. It is a well-known fact that standards of care for older people are sometimes poor and that there is inequality in the way in which services are provided (SNMAC 2001). The Department of Health is trying to address this, through the National Service Framework for Older People, which is the first ever strategy to ensure fair, high-quality, integrated health and social care services for older people (Department of Health 2001). Nurses need to be aware of their own attitudes towards all age groups and ensure that they see their patients or clients as individuals and not as stereotypes. The poem in Older Adults: Nursing Priorities box 1.1 was found in the bedside locker of an older woman after she had died. It sadly demonstrates how the nurses who had cared for her had stereotyped her.

We are living in an ageing society. Since the early 1930s the number of people aged over 65 has doubled and today a fifth of the population is over 60. Between 1995 and 2025 the number of people over the age of 80 is set to increase by almost a half, and the number of people over 90 will double (Department of Health 2001). Adult nurses need to be sensitive to the special needs of older people, who can have complex pathologies that impact on their social situation. However, we need to guard against being paternalistic and promote older people's independence and individuality. This means that, like other adults, they should be treated as autonomous (self-governing) individuals who have the right to make decisions about their own health. In order to do this, all patients/clients require knowledge and information to enable them to make informed decisions.

INFORMATION-GIVING AND INFORMED CONSENT

An important part of the nurse's role is to ensure that patients understand what is happening, or going to happen, to them, for legal as well as ethical reasons. Informed consent means that patients/clients have received sufficient information to enable them to make a decision about a proposed treatment or investigation. Rumbold (1999) differentiates between *informed* and *educated* consent, the latter meaning that not only has the information been received, but it has been given in such a way that the patient can understand and make a reasoned decision. Once patients have made a decision based on accurate and relevant information, nurses must support them in that decision, even if it goes against their advice. The role of the nurse is to make sure that patients understand the issues involved and the benefits and potential disadvantages of any proposed treatment. If patients are mentally competent and choose not to act on that advice (e.g. they refuse to have an operation or a treatment that is risky but potentially life-saving), it is important that the health care team respect that decision and do not try to persuade

 OLDER ADULTS: NURSING PRIORITIES

1.1 Crabbit old woman (by Anon.)

What do you see nurses, what do you see?
Are you thinking when you look at me –
A crabbit old woman, not very wise,
Uncertain of habit with faraway eyes,
Who dribbles her food and makes no reply,
When you say in a loud voice, 'I do wish you'd try.'
I'll tell you who I am, as I sit here so still,
As I rise to your bidding, as I eat at your will.
I'm a child of ten, with a father and mother,
Brothers and sisters who love one another.
A bride soon at twenty my heart gives a leap.
Remembering the vows that I promised to keep.
At twenty-five now I have young of my own,
Who need me to build a secure happy home.
At fifty, once more babies play round my knee,
Again we know children, my loved one and me.
Dark days are upon me, my husband is dead,
I look to the future, I shudder with dread.
My young are all busy rearing young of their own,
And I think of the years and the love that I've known.
I'm an old woman now and nature is cruel,
'Tis her jest to make old age look like a fool.
The body it crumbles, grace and vigour depart,
There is now a stone where I once had a heart.
But inside this old carcase a younger girl still dwells,
And now and again my battered heart swells.
I remember the joys, I remember the pain,
And I'm loving the living all over again.
And I think of the years all too few – gone too fast,
And accept the stark fact that nothing will last.
So open your eyes, nurses, open and see,
Not a crabbit old woman; look close – and see me.

patients to agree with their views. Nurses do sometimes have to advocate on behalf of patients who are unable to do so for themselves, but providing information and giving time to explain and answer questions help to empower patients to act as their own advocates.

Informing patients to ensure understanding regarding the investigations and procedures that they are undergoing is also important. It is usually a doctor's responsibility to obtain patient consent prior to an invasive investigation or operation, although increasingly nurses and other health professionals are undertaking diagnostic procedures such as endoscopy, in which case it is their responsibility to obtain consent. Because nurses provide a 24-hour service, 7 days a week, they are in an excellent position to ensure that patients understand what they have been told. Patients may not want to 'bother' the doctor with questions and often feel much more comfortable asking the nurse to explain.

The nursing assessment should always include asking patients about their understanding of their condition or treatment. The nurse can clarify misconceptions and explain the terms used. For example, women undergoing hysterectomy may not understand that the uterus is another name for the womb, nor what the terms malignant and benign mean. The language we use is very important. Like any profession, nursing and medicine use a lot of jargon and we have to be careful to use ordinary language when explaining things to patients. If there are language difficulties (e.g. English is not the first language), we need to use interpreters and make sure that key literature is produced in the languages that are common in the local area. Some patients will require large-print literature or an audio version. Nurses can be imaginative in the way they provide information and answer questions, e.g. using web-based information, e-mail and telephone helplines.

HEALTH AND HEALTH PROMOTION

Nurses spend a lot of time caring for people who are ill, but an equally important, though often less visible, part of their role is health promotion. Health is notoriously difficult to define. The subjective feelings about health mean that definitions may be very different between individuals and will vary from place to place and time to time and between cultures. Health is sometimes defined negatively as merely the absence of disease, injury or disability, but in 1948 the World Health Organization (WHO) defined health more positively as 'a state of complete mental, physical and social well being and not merely the absences of disease or infirmity'. The development of holistic thinking has broadened definitions of health beyond the individual to include societal dimensions such as environmental and economic influences. Any holistic definition of health needs to include an individual's social, spiritual, mental and emotional reserves in addition to physical capacity. Nurses may work mainly with individuals but they also have a role and a responsibility to ensure that the society in which we live also promotes health, e.g. by lobbying for better services.

The importance of health promotion in nursing is recognized (Delaney 1994) and many authors and the regulatory and advisory bodies for nursing emphasize that nurses should be at the forefront of health promotion initiatives (NHS Executive 1998, Norton 1998, Whitehead 2000). There are many definitions of health promotion; however, the definition used by the *Ottawa Charter* (WHO 1986), which describes health promotion as '... the process of enabling people to increase control over, and to improve, their health' seems well suited to what nurses do.

The *Ottawa Charter* highlighted the following activities as important for health promotion:

- building healthy public policy
- creating supportive environments
- strengthening community action
- developing personal skills for health, including information and coping strategies
- reorientating health services away from treatment to prevention and improving access to health services.

Health promotion is an inclusive term used to describe measures that aim to improve the health of individuals, communities or populations. It includes many approaches, including:

- education and information to enable people to make informed decisions about their lifestyle

 HEALTH PROMOTION

1.1 Promoting health

The chapter makes the point that nurses are in an ideal position to promote health and every nursing interaction presents an opportunity for teaching. Imagine that you are a patient in hospital and enjoy smoking cigarettes. The nurses are concerned that this is affecting your health.

- How do you think the nurse should approach you about this issue?
- What might help you to consider stopping smoking?
- What support would you need to help you stop smoking?

- personal counselling to support and help people change their lifestyle or health behaviours
- legislative and fiscal measures, e.g. seatbelt legislation, tax on tobacco, free eye tests, social security benefits
- enabling communities to become involved in decisions that affect them and their health, e.g. through community profiling, needs assessment and community development (Brooker 2002).

Nurses are in an ideal position to promote health through advocacy, mediation and enablement. Every nursing interaction presents an opportunity for teaching (see Health Promotion box 1.1). For example, patients recovering from a heart attack are likely to be interested in reviewing their diet to reduce the risk of another heart attack or they may wish to give up smoking. Nurses are clearly well placed to be involved in the first two approaches (education and information, and counselling and support) and these are discussed below.

However, nurses should also be involved in local and national government to promote the other two approaches (legislative and fiscal measures and enabling communities to influence decisions that affect their health). Nurses are increasingly being invited to join government 'think tanks' as well as non-governmental organizations (NGOs) but they should not wait to be invited; they should be lobbying to be included. Nurses have a lot to offer and the skills to communicate this to others. What is needed is the confidence to take on this role and the improved academic preparation of nurses is now helping them to develop the confidence they need to speak on behalf of others. Health promotion on an individual basis mostly involves sharing information and skills, and supporting patients to adapt to changes in lifestyle as a result of their condition.

Sharing information

The aim of health education is to help individuals to make and maintain healthy actions and provide them with the knowledge and skills to exercise choice. It may include a wide range of activities at different levels. For example, it may involve advice on how to follow a treatment regimen (e.g. a special diet or exercise programme) following discharge from hospital. Nurses should be mindful that people's health behaviour may be a response to, and maintained by, their particular circumstances and the environment in which they live; for example, alcohol misuse may be a way of tolerating homelessness. Understanding individuals' health beliefs and perceptions about their own susceptibility and the seriousness of their disease is an important task of health education. The nurse's role is not to persuade patients and clients to comply but to support them in deciding what is right for them (concordance).

Nurses are in an excellent position to be involved in information-giving (e.g. what makes a healthy diet) and skills teaching (e.g. teaching patients or their carers how to administer an injection or change a dressing). In order to do this, they need highly developed communication skills to enable them to explain things clearly and concisely. However, it is important that nurses recognize that their role is to support patients to make lifestyle changes that they wish to make. Simply giving information about risks is not enough. Telling a patient that eating too much fat will increase the risk of another heart attack is unlikely to be effective unless the nurse also explores existing negative health behaviours or means by which the patient might introduce positive lifestyle changes. The nurse's role is to provide information, when appropriate, in a language and format that patients can understand, which enables them to make a choice, and then to support them in their decision, even if it is not the one the nurse would recommend or make personally.

Sharing skills

Nurses also have an important role in helping patients, carers and unpaid carers (e.g. families) to develop the skills they need to be able to manage their condition independently. These skills may include the use of equipment, which can range from something as simple as a peak flow meter used in the management of asthma to measure breathing effectiveness, to highly complicated dialysis equipment for those with kidney failure. Alternatively, it may involve techniques such as blood glucose monitoring or urine testing to enable them to manage their diabetes, or changing a stoma bag on a colostomy.

In addition to helping patients and clients and their families and carers develop the skills they need for independent living, nurses must also use these skills to teach HCAs and student nurses in order to help the next generation develop the knowledge and skills that they need. This is emphasized in clause 6.4 of the *Code of Professional Conduct*, which states that nurses '... have a duty to facilitate students of nursing and midwifery and others to develop their competence' (NMC 2002). Thus teaching skills are an important part of the repertoire of any nurse.

NURSING MODELS

A nursing model is based on nursing theory and provides an abstract representation of what nursing is or should be. Together with the nursing process (see p. 11), nursing models guide nurses as they assess, plan, implement and evaluate care (Aggleton & Chalmers 2000). The purpose of nursing models is to guide nursing practice, generate new ideas and distinguish the focus of nursing from other professions (Chinn & Kramer 1995). There are a large number of different models and theories (George 2001 lists 21) and discussion of each is clearly beyond the scope of this book. Authors such as Pearson et al (1996) and Aggleton & Chalmers (2000) offer a good starting point to find out more about models, whilst Fawcett (1995) and George (2001) offer a more advanced discussion.

There is one model that is widely used by adult nurses in the UK: the 'Activities of Living' model, first formulated in 1980 (Roper et al 1996). A brief overview of this model will serve to illustrate the function of nursing models. The model has been simplified here and we recommend that you consult Roper et al (1996) in order to gain a full understanding.

THE ACTIVITIES OF LIVING MODEL

The Activities of Living model (Roper et al 1996) is the only model to have been developed in the UK, although it is based on the work in the 1960s of the American nursing theorist Virginia Henderson. It uses more straightforward language than some of the models, making it more easily understood, and this may explain its popularity with nurses in the UK. It is based on the belief that the person is an individual engaged in certain 'activities of living' (ALs) that enable them to live and grow (see Box 1.4). Individuals' ability to be independent in these activities may be affected by illness or disease but also by their position on the life span from conception to death. For example, newborn babies are dependent on others for most of the ALs and will gradually become independent in these activities as they mature and develop. Illness, an accident or pregnancy may mean that someone who was previously independent in all ALs may now become dependent in some and require the assistance of others. Equally, as we become older, we may become increasingly dependent on others for certain activities (e.g. mobilizing and eliminating) while remaining completely independent in others, such as breathing and communicating. According to this model, the aim of nursing is to assist patients as necessary in order to restore independence and meet the goals planned in partnership with them. Nursing interventions will also be needed to implement the medical care plan (e.g. administering medications and other treatments) and health promotion activities to enable patients to prevent or avoid ill health.

Activities of living

The nursing beliefs are based on Henderson's definition of nursing (see p. 4), and the 12 ALs (Box 1.4) have been developed from the 14 activities of daily living originally identified by Henderson (1966). Breathing must be considered to be of prime

Box 1.4 The 12 Activities of Living (Roper et al 1996)

- Breathing
- Maintaining a safe environment
- Communicating
- Eating and drinking
- Eliminating
- Personal cleansing and dressing
- Controlling body temperature
- Working and playing
- Mobilizing
- Sleeping
- Expressing sexuality
- Dying

importance because it is essential for all other activities (Roper et al 1996), but the other ALs are not in any fixed order of priority. Nurses should vary the order according to the needs and priorities of their patients. The model provides a framework or 'aide-mémoire' for holistic assessment and nurses work in partnership with patients (or family members/significant others in the case of patients who are unable to participate) to assess their level of independence and any needs or problems in relation to each of the activities.

Influencing factors

The model identifies five factors that influence each activity:

- physical
- psychological
- sociocultural
- environmental
- politico-economic.

The influencing factors are crucial to the assessment process so that nurses do not simply focus on the physical needs of patients but consider all the other factors as well. For example, take the activity 'eating and drinking'; eating meets a physical need for food, but psychological aspects such as the appearance of the food and the amount presented are also important. There are also psychological conditions such as anorexia nervosa and bulimia that will obviously affect this activity of living. Eating and drinking is also a social activity and so people who are recently bereaved may fail to eat because their partner is no longer there to be cooked for, or alternatively to cook for them. Cultural, religious and ethical issues may influence the type of food eaten or the way in which it is prepared (e.g. kosher diet, halal meat, vegetarian diet, etc.). Environmental and politico-economic factors also need to be considered, e.g. if explaining about healthy eating to a low-income family living in bed-and-breakfast accommodation or an older person who is unable to leave the house to go shopping.

NURSING PROCESS

In order to ensure that patients receive appropriate and timely care, irrespective of who is providing that care, it is necessary to have a care plan that is available to all involved, including the patients themselves. To organize patient care in a systematic way, nurses use a problem-solving approach called the nursing process. This has four stages:

- assessment
- planning
- implementation
- evaluation.

Some nurses use a five-stage process that includes 'nursing diagnosis' between assessment and planning (Christendon & Kenny 1995). The nursing process is cyclical in nature (see Fig. 1.1), which means that evaluation will lead to reassessment and the process starting again if the problem is not resolved. Evaluation is an important stage that enables nurses to determine whether the plan was appropriate and whether the care that was implemented has been effective.

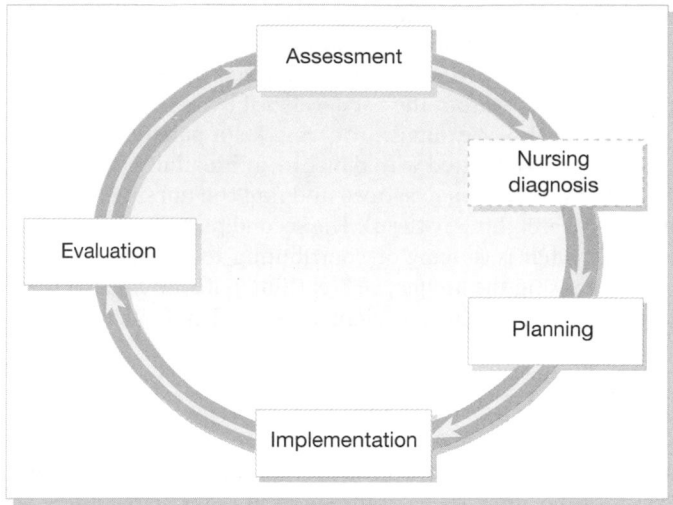

Figure 1.1 The nursing process.

ASSESSMENT

Assessment is the first stage and is crucial to the whole nursing process. This involves collection of data from a variety of sources – patient history, visual observations, touch, listening, etc. – and is structured according to the nursing model being used. For example, if the Activities of Living model is used (Roper et al 1996), it will involve assessing the patient's usual routines and level of dependence in the 12 ALs. This enables the nurse to plan care that is appropriate to the individual patient. It must be individualized to respond to that patient's needs, not the needs of that 'type' of patient or condition. Although there will clearly be similarities in the way that different people respond to the same disease, condition or situation, there will also be fundamental differences. The challenge of nursing is to make every patient feel like an individual. In order to do this, nurses must discover their patients' problems and personal preferences and consider their physical, psychological and social needs. An effective assessment enables the nurse to plan care that is appropriate and sensitive to individual needs and preferences.

Nursing assessment is a highly skilled activity that requires professional knowledge and a range of highly developed communication and interpersonal skills. It is the responsibility of registered nurses and should not be delegated to unsupervised student nurses and HCAs. A full assessment may not be possible immediately after admission if a patient's condition is unstable, but it should be completed as soon as possible. In order to improve the assessment of older adults, the 'single assessment process' is being introduced. This is designed to ensure that the scale and depth of assessment are appropriate, that health and social care agencies do not duplicate each other's assessments, and that professionals contribute to assessments in the most effective way (Department of Health 2002).

Nursing diagnosis

A nursing diagnosis is a clinical judgement about individual responses to actual or potential health problems and provides the basis for selection of appropriate nursing interventions. The North American Nursing Diagnosis Association (NANDA 2001) has developed nursing diagnoses in the USA. After thorough assessment of the patient or client, including information from physical examination and diagnostic tests, the nurse selects a nursing diagnosis from the list developed by NANDA (Ackley & Ladwig 1999). For example, if caring for a patient with acute asthma who is admitted with difficulty in breathing (dyspnoea), the nurse will look up dyspnoea and find the nursing diagnosis 'ineffective breathing pattern'. The second part of the diagnosis concerns what is causing or contributing to the diagnosis (i.e. what is causing the ineffective breathing pattern) and the third part describes the signs and symptoms, or 'defining characteristics' as NANDA call them.

The NANDA nursing diagnoses have not been widely adopted in the UK. However, increasingly nurses include 'nursing diagnosis' or 'nursing opinion' as part of the nursing process. This is because although the medical diagnosis is clearly important, there may be other issues that require nurse-initiated interventions. Nursing diagnoses explain the effect of the medical diagnosis, e.g. the medical diagnosis may be chest infection, while the nursing diagnosis will be 'ineffective breathing pattern'. Each of the NANDA diagnoses is accompanied by a list of recommended nursing interventions. Having established the nursing diagnosis, the nurse then selects appropriate nursing interventions in order to plan care.

PLANNING

Planning means identifying problems or needs, setting goals and planning the care that is necessary to meet those goals. Planning also involves prioritizing the care according to individual patient needs and setting goals and may include the use of an integrated care pathway.

Goal-setting

Goals should be SMART, i.e.:

- Specific – which means that they must state clearly what is to be achieved. For example, instead of stating 'encourage fluids', a SMART goal would say: 'For [patient's name] to drink 1.5 litres of fluid by 20.00 hours'
- Measurable – the goal must be quantifiable in some way and if it concerns something that is not measurable, e.g. anxiety, it should focus on how the patient expresses it. For example, the goal might say: '[Patient's name] will state that she knows what to expect and feels less anxious before the premedication is administered'
- Achievable and Realistic – it must be something that can be achieved by the patient. For example, if a woman suffers from chronic pain, it would be unrealistic to expect her to be pain-free at all times. An achievable and realistic goal would be for the patient to state that her pain is at an acceptable level 30 minutes after the administration of analgesics.
- Time-orientated – there must be an indication of when the goal should be achieved so that it is possible to evaluate whether this has happened.

Integrated care pathways

Integrated care pathways outline the expected pathway of care for any patient with a particular condition. Clearly not all patients will follow the expected pathway, as it is based on what is likely to happen for most people. However, it allows individual patient care to be compared with what can be reasonably expected and, where there is variance, for adjustments to be made. This means that problems are easily detected and dealt with quickly. An integrated care pathway makes it clear what the plan of care for a particular condition is expected to be. This enables the multidisciplinary team to work more closely together, with clear guidance on what to do in respect of each other's roles and responsibilities. It also ensures that best evidence-based practice is followed. The use of care pathways do not prevent clinicians implementing their own treatments, but it does require them to document the rationale for any deviation from the pathway (Benton 1999).

IMPLEMENTATION

This stage involves implementing the plan of care by providing appropriate evidence-based nursing interventions in order to meet the goals. Adult nursing in the hospital setting is usually organized in one of three ways: primary nursing, patient allocation or team nursing. A fourth system called task allocation, which involves nurses being allocated to various tasks and doing these for all patients that require them (e.g. observations or dressings), is no longer recommended.

Primary nursing

Primary nursing is a method of organizing nursing care so that a named nurse (the primary nurse) is responsible for the care of individual patients. Nurses are categorized as either primary nurses or associate nurses. The primary nurse provides the overall direction of nursing care, and when not available, care is provided by an associate nurse who follows the care plan developed by the primary nurse. Primary nurses are responsible for their patients and because the number of patients is small, a good relationship and real knowledge and understanding of individual patients can develop. Primary nursing is based on the key requirements for quality nursing care (Ersser & Tutton 1991):

- comprehensiveness of care
- accountability for care
- continuity
- coordination of care.

It requires a relatively large number of experienced nurses to act as primary nurses and so has been difficult to implement in areas with a high turnover of registered nurses.

Nurses caring for adults in the community use a similar system. Each nurse has a caseload of patients and a small team of nurses and care assistants to help deliver the care. The community nurse is responsible for assessing each patient's nursing and personal care needs. The nursing staff will provide nursing care such as changing dressings, bandaging leg ulcers or administering insulin to patients unable to do this themselves. In the main, care assistants provide personal care such as assistance with bathing and dressing.

Team nursing

Team nursing is a system in which the nursing staff is divided into a number of teams (usually two or three) who are then responsible for the care of a designated group of patients. Each team has an experienced nurse as leader, who is responsible for overseeing the care of the patients allocated to that team throughout their stay. Team leaders are also responsible for supervising the nurses and HCAs in the team and for planning professional development and performance review for the members of the team. Team nursing has some of the features of primary nursing, but the responsibility for the group of patients is shared within the team rather than falling to one primary nurse. This makes issues of responsibility for aspects of care and accountability less clear.

Patient allocation

Patient allocation involves the allocation of a group of patients to one or more nurses. Individual nurses are accountable for the care they provide, but the nurse in charge maintains overall control (Ersser & Tutton 1991). This system is similar to team nursing in that patients are cared for by a smaller number of nurses. However, unlike team nursing, the allocation of patients is usually only for the duration of a shift or a short period of time.

Task allocation

Task allocation is a system in which nursing care is broken down into smaller tasks. Each nurse is given responsibility for a task or group of tasks (e.g. observations or dressings) that are appropriate to that nurse's level of ability. The responsibility for planning care rests with the nurse in charge and the patient receives care from a variety of nurses, each providing a particular aspect. This means that patient care becomes fragmented, which is why this system is no longer recommended. However, it is an efficient means of organizing care, because it is planned by experienced nurses and then delivered by staff according to their level of experience and competence.

EVALUATION

The evaluation stage is when the nurse reviews the care plan to see whether the goals have been met or are on the way to being met, and whether the care that was planned was appropriate and effective. This may be every hour for acute problems such as bleeding or pain; every shift for others such as bowel activity; every day or week for goals such as weight gain or reduction; and every month for long-term goals such as rehabilitation. Evaluation is a crucial stage in the nursing process; without it there is no evidence that the planned care has been implemented or whether it has been effective. If the problem has not been resolved, reassessment is necessary to determine why. It may be that the initial assessment was incorrect or the care that was planned was not effective, or it may be that the goal was unrealistic. It may also be that the patient's condition has changed and what was appropriate is no longer so. For example, in a patient who suffers a mild stroke with only mild weakness in one leg, the goal of returning to full mobility would be realistic. If that patient then suffers another stroke, which leaves him or her with a dense weakness on one side, reassessment will be required.

Nursing interventions need to be evidence-based, i.e. based on the best available evidence as to their effectiveness. Nurses need to be reflective and analytical in their approach to make sure that their care is up to date and not simply the way it has always been done. Evaluation enables nurses to reflect on their care and seek out evidence to support their practices.

EVIDENCE-BASED PRACTICE AND RESEARCH

The term evidence-based practice describes the use of interventions that are based on systematic analysis of the research and other information regarding the effectiveness (including cost-effectiveness) of the intervention (Brooker 2002). The NMC's *Code of Professional Conduct* requires every nurse and midwife to 'protect and support the health of individual patients and clients' (NMC 2002, clause 1.2). In order to be able to do this, nurses need to know that their practice is based on sound knowledge and evidence. This is one of the key principles of the government's plans for quality assurance in the NHS, 'clinical governance' (NHS Executive 1999). Evidence includes scientific research findings, but there are many other forms of knowledge and evidence that can be used to develop good practice.

TYPES OF KNOWLEDGE

Research leads to the development of empirical knowledge and is important in the development of an evidence base for nursing. However, other forms of knowledge are also important, such as learning from experience (Eraut 1994). It is important to pass on such knowledge to colleagues, and students should be encouraged to question experienced nurses so that the knowledge is shared (Joyce 2000). When considering the types of evidence that are relevant to nursing decisions, Le May (1999) suggests the following:

- Theoretical knowledge – knowledge that is generated through logical thought
- Empirical knowledge – knowledge generated through research
- Practical knowledge – knowledge that emerges from the practice of nursing; it may be generated by research or logical thought
- Experiential knowledge – knowledge that is accumulated through our everyday experiences
- Interpersonal knowledge – knowledge that is gained through interacting with people (patients, clients, peers, carers and other professionals)
- Rituals – the traditions of practice may provide a safe level of care but often the effectiveness goes unquestioned and unevaluated. As discussed above, it is important not to simply do it the way it has always been done, unless there is good evidence to support that approach
- Intuitive knowledge – knowledge that we 'just knew' that seems to appear without logical thought.

Guidelines, policies and protocols incorporate a number of types of knowledge and evidence and these are discussed later.

Critical appraisal of evidence

Not all nurses will be actively engaged in research, but they will need to read research in order to keep up to date and answer

- To establish scientifically defensible reasons for nursing activities
- To provide nurses with an increased repertoire of scientifically defensible nursing intervention options
- To find ways of increasing the cost-effectiveness of nursing actions
- To provide a basis for standard-setting and quality assurance
- To provide evidence of weaknesses and strengths in nursing
- To provide evidence in support of demands for resources in nursing
- To give the term evidence-based practice scientific credence
- To satisfy the academic curiosity of thinking nurses
- To facilitate interdisciplinary collaboration in nursing and nursing research
- To earn and defend a professional status for nursing

Box 1.6 Sources of evidence for nursing practice

- *Evidence-based Nursing* – now also available online (ebn.bmjjournals.com/)
- *Evidence-based Medicine* – published by the BMJ
- The Cochrane Library (www.cochrane.co.uk) which includes:
  — the Cochrane database of systematic reviews (CDSR) – reviews of controlled trials and a meta-analysis of those studies that meet their strict inclusion criteria (that this is regarded as the highest level of evidence)
  — database of abstract reviews of effectiveness (DARE) which is a database of research reviews of the effectiveness of health care interventions
  — the Cochrane controlled trials register (CCTR) which is a bibliography of controlled trials
- NHS Centre for Reviews and Dissemination (York) – www1.york.ac.uk/inst/crd
- The Scottish Intercollegiate Guidelines Network (SIGN) – www.sign.ac.uk

specific clinical questions or in connection with a course of study or project. Nurses need to be able to evaluate evidence about the effectiveness of interventions. Box 1.5 summarizes the main purposes of research identified by Hockey (2000). Critical appraisal means being able to weigh up the evidence and make a judgement. Critical appraisal is not about criticizing; it involves assessing the quality of a piece of research and considering its usefulness and effectiveness in the nurse's area of practice (McCaughan 1999). Not all knowledge is valid; some may have dubious sources and be nothing more than ideas with little evidence base (Joyce 2000). The best evidence is that which has been synthesized from several sources of data, confirming the same findings. Clinical guidance issued nationally by the National Institute for Clinical Excellence (NICE, see p. 15) is based on the best available evidence. In order to be able to appraise research critically, nurses need an understanding of the purposes of research (see Box 1.5) and the methods used. A brief overview is presented below.

When reading research studies, it is important to consider whether the population under investigation was similar to the patients in your area of practice. The findings for a different population may be very different. For example, the Norton Score, a pressure ulcer risk assessment tool (Norton et al 1972), was developed for use with older adults and is not reliable if used in the assessment of younger patients. The environment in which the study took place is also important. The findings from research conducted in a nursing home cannot be assumed to be applicable to patients in an intensive care unit and vice versa.

All research studies have weak areas or limitations and a robust study will highlight these. Critical appraisal involves deciding whether the limitations are serious enough to affect the reliability of the findings (Crombie 1996). Nurses do not have to do everything themselves. There are now several sources of evidence that have already been critically appraised and put together in a 'user-friendly' form to help the busy professional (see Box 1.6). There are many and varied sources of evidence available to nurses, they just need to look. As Chambers (1998) so elegantly put it, the greatest obstacle to discovering the truth is being convinced that you already know it.

Research methods

In order to appraise research findings critically, it is necessary to know a little about the different research methods, to be able to decide whether the method used was appropriate to the topic being studied. Because nursing is both an art and a science, Docherty (2001) argues that it does not lend itself to any one particular process of enquiry. There are two major approaches to research, quantitative methods and qualitative methods, although in practice many studies include both approaches. Porter & Carter (2000) define them as follows:

- Quantitative research is a formal, objective, systematic process for obtaining quantifiable information about the world, presented in numerical form and analysed through the use of statistics. It is used to describe and test relationships and to examine cause-and-effect relationships. Quantitative research methods include randomized controlled trials (RCTs), experimental studies, questionnaire surveys and meta-analysis (e.g. Cochrane reviews).

- Qualitative research uses human speech or writing as data, rather than numbers. More generally, qualitative research is an umbrella term for those strategies that seek to explain human behaviour in terms of the reasons people have for behaving in the way they do. Qualitative research seeks to uncover the understanding and motives that lead to certain actions. Qualitative research methods include participant and non-participant observation, in-depth interviews, oral histories, case studies, focus groups, document research and conversational analysis.

Detailed discussion of each of the various research methods is beyond the scope of this book and the reader is advised to consult research textbooks such as Cormack (2000), Parahoo (1997) and Bowling (1997). Most research is published and change depends on practitioners reading about the findings and adjusting their practice accordingly. However, there is one type of research, action research (Meyer 2000), that focuses on involving practitioners in changing their practice and monitoring the process and outcomes of changes. Practice development through action research is becoming increasingly popular in health care settings (Hart & Bond 1995).

GUIDELINES FOR CARE

National guidelines provide a 'state of the science' of a particular disease or treatment and provide a concrete example of how clinically effective and patient-focused care can be delivered (Benton 1999). However, guidelines must be adapted to reflect local circumstances and should not simply be followed blindly. Nurses must think critically about their practice and use theory to inform rather than replace clinical judgement (Flanagan 2000). The range of professional guidelines available to assist nurses in their practice is increasing steadily, especially in response to clinical governance initiatives and the drive towards evidence-based care. Clinical guidance and protocols for many clinical topics are now regularly available from NICE, which was set up as a special health authority in 1999 to generate and distribute guidance based on the best available evidence.

Each chapter in this book includes guidelines that are relevant to that area of practice. There are also a number of professional guidelines that are designed to guide nurses rather than nursing. These range from codes of conduct and other professional requirements from the NMC (see p. 7), to policies and protocols that are developed by individual health care trusts.

Policies and protocols

The use of national guidelines and protocols is increasing as nurses seek to base their care on sound evidence. The Cochrane Library (see p. 14) offers systematic reviews of a range of topics with the aim of providing practitioners with a sound evidence base for their practice. Government organizations such as NICE produce clear guidance for clinicians about which treatments work best for which patients. In addition, the government sets national standards through national service frameworks, which detail how services can best be organized to cater for particular patient groups (e.g. cardiac patients and older adults), and indicate the standards that services have to meet. These standards are monitored by the Commission for Health Improvement (CHI), which is a national framework for assessing performance, and an annual national survey of NHS patient and user experience (Department of Health 1998).

Policies and protocols are important because they make a statement about the way in which the employer expects a particular activity to be performed. For example, there will be a policy for dealing with patients' property and a policy for handling complaints. There will also be policies for clinical activities such as moving and handling, infection control and intravenous therapy, which detail how these activities should be performed, who should perform them, etc. Failure to follow the employer's

policy may mean that the employer refuses to accept responsibility for the nurse's actions in the event of a complaint. This responsibility that an employer bears for the faults of their employees is called vicarious liability. However, the employer is only liable if the employee is within the 'course of employment', i.e. working in the way expected or authorized by the employer (Dimond 1995). Policies and protocols authorize employees to work in certain ways and thus it is important that nurses are familiar with these in their area of practice.

REFLECTIVE PRACTICE

Reflective practice is the key to professional development as a nurse. Nursing is a practice-based profession, which means that clinical practice is the central focus. Students of nursing cannot learn from books alone, but must be provided with opportunities to learn from clinical experience. Working in clinical placements provides an excellent opportunity to learn how to care for patients and clients, but in order to make the most of it, nurses need to be able to reflect on their experience in a structured way. Reflection helps them to determine what they did well, what they could do differently and what knowledge they require to be able to deal with such situations in the future. Reflective practice boxes are included throughout the book to encourage readers to reflect on and learn from their own experiences.

REFLECTION – WHAT IS IT?

'Reflection is an important human activity in which people re-capture their experience, mull it over and evaluate it. It is working with experience that is important in learning' (Boud et al 1985, p. 19). Reflection needs to take place at a conscious level in order to allow us to make decisions about our learning. It is only by consciously considering our thoughts and ideas that we are able to evaluate them and make choices about what we should do next (Boud et al 1985). In nursing, students spend 50% of their time in practice placements. Just being there in the practice setting is useful and enables students to gain experience and learn how to do things by observing others, but reflection involves examining that experience in order to learn more from it.

'Reflection in the context of learning is the generic term for those intellectual and affective activities in which individuals engage to explore their experiences in order to lead to new understandings and appreciations' (Boud et al 1985, p. 19). Reflection on all learning experiences (e.g. lectures and seminars, etc.) is a good idea but it is most powerful in helping students gain maximum benefit from their clinical placements. Despite their supernumerary status, nursing students are expected to, and indeed should, get involved in providing care for patients and helping to 'get the work done'. It is in this way that they learn the art and science of nursing, by observing and learning from expert nurses and under their supervision, developing their own skills. Reflection helps you to look back at your experience and determine what you have learnt, what knowledge you were applying and what you do not understand. This helps you to identify learning needs to enable you to perform better in the future.

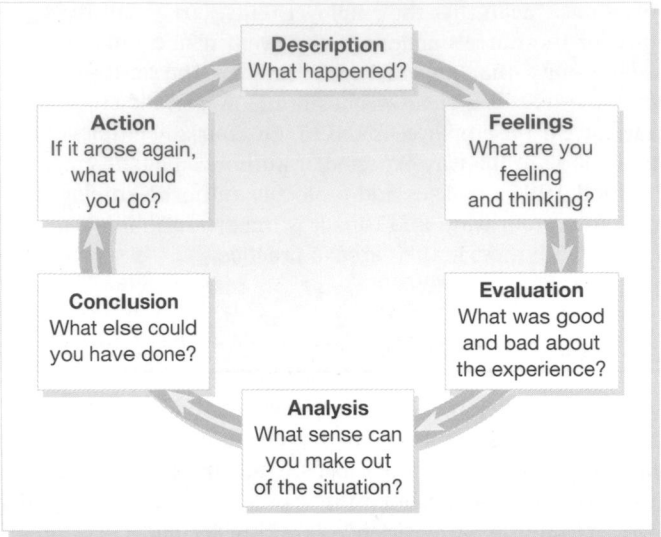

Figure 1.2   Gibbs' (1988) model of reflection.

Using a model of reflection

Using a framework for reflection can help nurses examine what happened and how they felt about it, and help them to think through what they might do differently if a similar situation were to arise again. It will also help to identify what knowledge they need to learn to be able to deal with such situations. There are several models or frameworks for reflection available, e.g. Boud et al (1985), Johns (1996) and Gibbs (1988; see Fig. 1.2). It is important to choose a model that is easy to use and get into the habit of regularly reflecting on experience. This will enable any negative emotions to be dealt with in a more positive and objective way, and enable the nurse to learn from the experience. It is a good idea to reflect on positive experiences as well as negative ones, as they are equally good sources of learning. Thinking beyond surface thoughts can be very fruitful and uncover a lot of learning that would otherwise remain hidden. Nurses can reflect alone or with others and are likely to need some help to get started. Clinical mentors are ideally placed to help, and so are lecturers who visit the clinical areas or facilitate reflection sessions in the university.

Writing a reflective journal (diary)

Writing a reflective journal can seem like a bit of a chore but it can really help nurses to learn from experience. Also, looking back over the journal can help them to see just how much they have learnt over time. It is important not to be too hard on yourself when reflecting, but to focus on what happened and why, in order to learn from the experience and be able to deal with similar situations in the future. Box 1.7 is an example of how a student nurse reflected on an incident in which a patient had a fall in the lavatory. Read that now and try to think of other options that the student could have considered. Note that the names have been changed to maintain confidentiality. As discussed below, it is vital to ensure that no patient or client could be identified from the entries in your journal or from essays and assignments.

It is only by reflecting on a situation that you are truly able to learn from it in a positive way and use the experience to develop your professional knowledge and skill. When writing

down such an incident in your reflective journal, work through what happened and try to think about what you have learnt from a particular experience. That way you are not just having the experience, you are also learning from it. That is the key to development as a professional.

Writing reflectively for assignments

Many assignments in both pre-registration and post-registration courses require you to reflect on clinical experience because, as discussed above, it is such an important part of learning from everyday practice. When writing reflectively, a model of reflection is a good idea because it will provide structure for your essay. It is important to use the literature to support your discussion and have a good academic style, but reflective essays are usually written in the first person ('I felt ...' or 'I did ...') instead of the third person ('the author felt ...'), which is more common for academic work. This is because reflection is a very personal activity and if it were written in the third person it would lose some of its richness (Webb 1983).

Written reflection such as that shown in Box 1.7 forms the basis of your essay but you need to expand it and use the literature to support it. For example, when referring to staff or patients, you would say that the names have been changed to preserve confidentiality. This could be followed by the reference 'NMC 2002' to indicate that the *Code of Professional Conduct* requires nurses to protect patient confidentiality. Likewise, when writing about the things that you could have done or would do differently another time, you could use the literature on the complications of immobility as evidence to support your discussion about the need for patients to be mobile. You might be able to find something about the type and ideal position of grab rails in lavatories to enable patients to be more independent. When discussing whether one should stay with the patient while she used the lavatory, you could refer to the literature on the need for dignity and privacy.

Reflection and reflective writing are important for all nurses because lifelong learning is not just about fulfilling PREP requirements and the competency required by the *Code of Professional Conduct*; there is also an ethical dimension. It is unethical to provide care that is neither reflective (i.e. has benefited from previous experience and formal learning opportunities) nor evidence-based.

ETHICAL ISSUES

Most nurses have to deal with ethical or moral issues on a daily basis. Sometimes these are very difficult issues (e.g. choosing the right time to tell someone that he or she is dying), but often they are much less dramatic and less obviously ethical in nature, e.g. how to prioritize care when busy. Nurses are required to provide equal and non-judgemental care for all patients, regardless of their own values and beliefs. This is stressed by the NMC/UKCC in the branch competencies, which require nurses to 'practise in accordance with an ethical and legal framework that ensures the primacy of patient and client interest and well-being and respects confidentiality' (see Box 1.1).

It is important that nurses are aware of their own values and beliefs (self-awareness) so that they can be alert to the possibility

Box 1.7 Reflective journal entry

I had a horrible day today. Everything was going fine until I took Mrs George* to the lavatory. She was fine so I left her and went to help Mrs Patel* wash her back and her feet. She can't reach those and loves it when I do it for her. I went back to help Mrs George walk back from the lavatory and found her on the floor! She said she slipped when she was trying to pull up her underwear. I panicked. I didn't know what to do so I just ran and got Anne*, my mentor. I was really scared. I thought Mrs George would be injured and it would all be my fault because I left her too long. I felt awful and just wanted to go home and never come back! I wanted to leave nursing – it was too difficult!

Anne was brilliant. She was so calm. She checked that Mrs George had not hurt herself by asking her if she could move her arms and legs and whether it hurt anywhere. Mrs George said she was fine; she just slipped and sort of slid down the wall. She just couldn't get herself up again. Anne then told her how to get up by getting onto her hands and knees and then holding onto the toilet to stand up. It really worked, just like we had been taught in school! There wasn't much room in there but she managed and then Anne asked me to get a wheelchair to take Mrs George back to bed because she was obviously a bit shaken.

The amazing thing was – no one blamed me! Mrs George said she should have waited for me to come back like I'd told her, and Anne said I did the right thing by coming to get her straight away. She was brilliant. I felt like crying it was such a relief! Anne said I should write about it in my journal and tomorrow we are going to discuss what I could do if something like that happened again. I have been thinking about that – what I could do differently.

If I didn't take Mrs George to the lavatory (give her a commode instead) she wouldn't fall, but it's good for her to walk and nicer to use the lavatory because there's more privacy. If I stayed in the lavatory with her, that wouldn't be very nice for her, having me watching, feeling like she's got to hurry. Maybe if I stand just outside so that she has privacy but I'm there as soon as she's finished and needs help. She was only struggling by herself because I wasn't there. It must be pretty horrible just sitting there, waiting for someone to appear, especially if you don't know if they have forgotten. I might ask Anne about grab rails in the lavatory. There is one on one side but not the other. She might have been OK if there were two; maybe one of those bars that come down from the wall, like they have in disabled lavatories.

This has made me realize that I need to try and not leave patients waiting in the bath or the lavatory. It's hard because obviously I've got others to look after. But thinking about it, Mrs Patel was in bed and not in any hurry so I could have left her a few more minutes. Maybe just straightened Mrs George's bed and then gone straight back, sorted her out and then helped Mrs Patel. I didn't really think about it before, I just thought: 'They'll have to wait, I'm busy.' But that's not really fair; also if they try and help themselves to save bothering you, they can end up in trouble and so can you! I need to look at my notes again about getting someone up off the floor. It was really effective. I'd still need someone to check that they were OK but next time I don't think I'd panic.

(*Names changed to preserve confidentiality.)

---

of unconscious actions on their part that may discriminate against a patient whose beliefs and/or lifestyle do not concur with their own, e.g. leaving a young intravenous drug user until last because 'he brought this on himself'. Nurses will also be involved in caring for patients undergoing treatments that they may consider morally wrong, e.g. termination of pregnancy. Nurses need to understand the ethical and professional issues involved to enable them to provide equally high-quality care. Nurses also need to understand issues such as patients' rights in order to act as advocates (i.e. on behalf of) for their patients if necessary.

In order to act in a moral and ethical way, it is necessary to do the 'right' thing. However, beliefs about what is right will vary between individuals and between different cultures. What we consider to be right or wrong is based on our beliefs and moral codes, often grounded in religious or spiritual beliefs. Thiroux (1980) established a set of principles that are designed to guide us. They are not a rigid set of rules and will not provide the answers to difficult situations, but they may help to guide thinking towards achieving a consensus and should be considered when deciding on action (Tschudin 1991). These principles are as follows:

- the value of life
- goodness or rightness
- justice or fairness
- truth-telling or honesty
- individual freedom.

THE VALUE OF LIFE

According to these principles, humans should revere life and accept death. That does not mean life at any cost, nor does it mean that we should ignore the quality of life. It means that we should neither kill nor preserve life without the person's consent unless there is a very strong justification (Tschudin 1991). This principle is relevant when nurses consider issues such as termination of pregnancy and euthanasia. Both could be considered wrong without 'a very strong justification'; however, as discussed below, neither issue is as clear as this would suggest.

Termination of pregnancy

When exploring the issue of termination, one has to consider the rights of the unborn child and the mother. The issue revolves around whether it is acceptable to sacrifice one life (the fetus) in order to preserve the life or health of the other (the mother). If it is deemed acceptable, does this just refer to physical health or does it also include mental health? As you can see, the principle of valuing life appears straightforward until we begin to apply it in different circumstances. In the UK, termination of pregnancy is permitted for a variety of reasons, including mental distress of the mother (Ch. 25). In some countries, termination of pregnancy is used as a method of birth control and is available on demand. Nurses will have their own views as to whether this is 'right', but as nurses we have a duty to care for our patients and clients even if their beliefs and moral codes are different from our own. Nurses are not obliged to assist in operations and treatments to terminate a pregnancy, but they are required to care for the patient before and afterwards in the way that they would care for all other patients. Clause 2.5 of the *Code of Professional Conduct* (NMC 2002) states that as a nurse you must 'report to a relevant person or authority, at the earliest possible time, any conscientious objection that may be relevant to your professional practice. You must continue to provide care to the best of your ability until alternative arrangements are implemented' (see Ethical Issues box 1.1).

Euthanasia

The term euthanasia is derived from the Greek and means a gentle and easy death, but it has come to mean the painless killing of a person to end his or her suffering, a so-called mercy killing (Rumbold 1999). It is illegal in the UK. Doctors and nurses have clear responsibilities to try to preserve life, but should this be done with no regard to the quality of that life? Nurses will be faced with some of these issues and that is why ethics is such an important part of the nursing curriculum. There are usually no 'right' answers. What is important is that the values and beliefs of the patient and the family are respected. Nurses will care for people who have made their wishes clear in an advance directive ('living will'). This is a written declaration made by mentally competent individuals describing their wishes with regard to life-prolonging medical interventions if they are incapacitated by an irreversible disease or are terminally ill, which prevents them making their wishes known to health professionals at the time. An advance directive is legally binding if it is in the form of an advance refusal and the maker is competent at the time.

GOODNESS OR RIGHTNESS

This principle requires that we:

- promote goodness over badness
- cause no harm or badness
- prevent badness or harm.

When doing good is not possible, we should at least try to do no harm (Tschudin 1991). This is implicit in the principles of beneficence and non-maleficence, which means that we have a duty not to harm patients or clients (Rumbold 1999). This is emphasized in clause 1.4 of the *Code of Professional Conduct* (NMC 2002), which states that nurses 'have a duty of care to your patients and clients, who are entitled to receive safe and competent care'. However, deciding what is best for patients and clients is not always as easy as it sounds.

When patients are conscious and able to understand, we can ask them what their wishes are. But even this is not as straightforward as it seems. Patients' decision-making will be heavily influenced by the information that they receive, and providing information to enable patients to make informed choices is an important part of the nurse's role (see p. 8). However, the information provided may be slanted towards what the doctors and nurses consider to be best for patients, and they may not even be aware of this. Nurses and other health care professionals must strive to ensure that information is provided in an unbiased way. As discussed earlier, the nurse's role is not to persuade patients and clients but to support them in deciding what is right for them. Paternalism can leave patients feeling patronized and prevented from making informed decisions about their care. As Rumbold (1999) points out, the duty of beneficence must be tempered by respect for autonomy.

JUSTICE OR FAIRNESS

Being good requires us to be just and fair. That sounds simple enough, but it becomes more difficult when there is not enough

---

 ETHICAL ISSUES

1.1 Caring for patients undergoing termination of pregnancy

Jo is a student nurse on placement in operating theatres. Jo's cultural and religious beliefs mean that she believes terminating a pregnancy to be wrong. While working in theatres, there will be women undergoing termination of pregnancy.

- What should Jo do?
- When working on the ward, can Jo refuse to care for patients undergoing termination of pregnancy?

As discussed above, nurses who have a conscientious objection to termination of pregnancy are not obliged to assist in treatments and operations to terminate a pregnancy, but they must care for patients before and afterwards in the way that they would care for all other patients.

Think of an aspect of care that you might not agree with. How would you ensure that that you 'practise in a fair and anti-discriminatory way, acknowledging the difference in beliefs and cultural practices of individuals or groups' (UKCC 2001)?

Reference
UKCC. Requirements for pre-registration nursing programmes – competencies for entry to the register. Online. Available: www.nmc-uk.org. 2001.

'goodness' to go around, e.g. when there are more patients than treatments available. The distribution of resources and availability of treatments for all patients remain controversial issues within the health service. For example, is it fair that one patient receives a treatment costing thousands of pounds while others have to wait for much cheaper treatments? Citing the work of Seedhouse (1988), Rumbold (1999) argues that justice must be considered on three levels:

- to each according to his rights
- to each according to what he deserves
- to each according to need.

The third level is probably the most pertinent to the work of nurses and other health care workers. Each patient is treated according to his or her need. This does not mean caring for every patient in the same way – far from it. It means treating people as individuals, finding out what their needs are and planning care to meet those needs. Justice and fairness mean treating all patients equally, i.e. with equal respect and courtesy and care that is appropriate to their needs. As Tschudin (1991) points out, the only entirely fair way to allocate resources would be to hold a lottery and draw names from a hat. That way everyone would be treated the same and have an equal chance of being chosen. However, that would not be just, because one person's need may be much greater than another's.

TRUTH-TELLING OR HONESTY

Truth-telling is necessary for a trusting relationship, but in any caring relationship it is natural to want to prevent unnecessary anxiety and distress. As discussed above, doctors and nurses may sometimes be tempted to omit detailed information about the risks involved in an operation or treatment 'so as not to worry the patient'. However, although this may appear to be in the best interests of patients, i.e. protecting them from additional anxiety, if they are not in possession of all the facts, they will be unable to make truly informed decisions about their care.

Equally, patients who are not told that they have a terminal condition will not be in a position to make decisions about what they wish to do with the time they have left. Patients' families are also faced with the problem of wanting to protect their loved ones from harm by withholding information. Giving sensitive information clearly needs to be carefully negotiated, but it is important to remember that patients always have the right to know.

The evidence that is available suggests that patients do indeed want to know and one study (Kerrigan et al 1993) showed that having side-effects explained prior to an operation did not increase the level of anxiety (see Evidence-based Practice box 1.1). In fact, providing information prior to stressful procedures has been shown to improve recovery.

When nurses are faced with difficult questions such as 'I'm not going to die am I?', telling the truth can be difficult. It is clearly not acceptable to give false reassurance if the patient is in fact likely to die. On the other hand, simply to answer truthfully is likely to cause additional distress. One way to deal with such a situation is to deflect the question with a response such as 'You are clearly anxious' and give the patient time to expand on his or her concerns. If patients really want to know whether they are dying, they will ask again and you will gain their trust if you sensitively tell the truth (if you are in a position to do so) or offer to get a more senior nurse to talk to them.

INDIVIDUAL FREEDOM

This means the freedom to choose to live in the way that we choose and according to our own moral beliefs. This means that we have the freedom to choose to kill or steal – it is our moral judgement that leads us to choose (or not) a more worthwhile path. As Tschudin (1991) puts it, nurses are paid to care, but they can also care in a way that shows that they want to care. Ethics is part of every nurse's practice: no-one can withdraw from moral and ethical decision-making and so an understanding of ethical principles is important for every nurse (Rumbold 1999).

 EVIDENCE-BASED PRACTICE

1.1 Who's afraid of informed consent?

It is sometimes argued that patients undergoing treatments and operations should not be given all the facts 'so as not to worry them unnecessarily'. However, Kerrigan et al (1993) found that providing patients with detailed information prior to surgery did not increase their anxiety. In a study, 96 men undergoing elective repair of inguinal hernia under general anaesthesia were asked to complete an anxiety scale and then randomly assigned to two groups. Both groups were provided with written information about the operation and left to read it for an hour; one group was given detailed information about possible complications of the surgery; and the other group simple information, the kind that was usually provided by house officers when obtaining consent. Both groups then completed the anxiety scale again.

The results showed that there was no change in anxiety among the group that had received the detailed information, whereas those who received the superficial information were significantly less anxious afterwards. The authors concluded that a detailed account of what might go wrong did not increase patient anxiety and enables patients to make a fully informed choice before they consent to surgery. It could be argued that superficial information prohibits informed consent if it serves to reduce anxiety by understating the risks involved.

Reference
Kerrigan D, Thevasagayam R, Woods T et al. Who's afraid of informed consent. Br Med J 1993; 306: 298–300.

SUMMARY: MAIN POINTS

- Nursing adults requires a holistic approach that takes account of physical, psychological, emotional, social and spiritual aspects.

- The Nursing & Midwifery Council's Code of Professional Conduct informs the profession of the standard of professional conduct required and informs the public and others of the standard that they may expect.

- The nursing process is a problem-solving approach that ensures that care is planned and its effectiveness is evaluated in a systematic way.

- Nursing models are used in conjunction with the nursing process to guide practice, generate new ideas and distinguish nursing from other professions.

- All nurses are likely to care for older adults and some will choose to specialize in the field of medicine and rehabilitation of older adults.

- Health promotion enables people to increase control over and improve their health. Nurses should be at the forefront of health promotion initiatives.

- Evidence-based practice is grounded in research and other information regarding the effectiveness. There are many sources of evidence available to nurses.

- Reflection is central to professional development as a nurse. It involves re-capturing an experience, mulling it over and evaluating it in order to learn from that experience.

- Ethics and moral decision-making are part of every nurse's practice and so an understanding of ethical principles is important for every nurse.

 FURTHER READING

Mulhall A, Le May A (eds). Nursing research: dissemination and implementation. Edinburgh: Churchill Livingstone; 1999.

Naidoo J, Wills J. Health promotion. Foundations for practice, 2nd edn. London: Baillière Tindall; 2000.

NHS Executive. Achieving effective practice: a clinical effectiveness and research information pack for nurses, midwives and health visitors. London: Department of Health; 1998.

 USEFUL WEBSITES

www.nice.org.uk – National Institute for Clinical Excellence (NICE)

nmc-uk.org – Nursing and Midwifery Council (NMC)

REFERENCES

Ackley B, Ladwig G. Nursing diagnosis handbook: a guide to planning care, 4th edn. St Louis: Mosby; 1999.

Aggleton P, Chalmers H. Nursing models and nursing practice, 2nd edn. Basingstoke: Macmillan; 2000.

Benton D. Clinical effectiveness. In: Hamer S, Collison G, eds. Achieving evidence-based practice: a handbook for practitioners. Edinburgh: Baillière Tindall; 1999.

Boud D, Keogh R, Walker D. Reflection: turning experience into learning. London: Kogan Page; 1985.

Bowling A. Research methods in health. Buckingham: Open University Press; 1997.

Brooker C (ed). Churchill Livingstone's dictionary of nursing, 18th edn. Edinburgh: Churchill Livingstone; 2002.

Chambers R. Clinical effectiveness made easy: first thoughts on clinical governance. Oxford: Radcliffe; 1998.

Chinn PL, Kramer MK. Theory and nursing: a systematic approach, 4th edn. St Louis: Mosby; 1995.

Christendon P, Kenny J. Nursing process: application of conceptual models, 4th edn. St Louis: Mosby; 1995.

Cormack D (ed). The research process in nursing, 4th edn. Oxford: Blackwell Science; 2000.

Crombie I. The pocket guide to critical reviews. London: The BMJ Publishing Group; 1996.

Delaney FG. Nursing and health promotion: conceptual concerns. J Adv Nurs 1994; 20(5): 828–835.

Department of Health. A first class service: quality in the new NHS. London: Department of Health; 1998.

Department of Health. The NHS plan: a plan for investment, a plan for reform. London: Department of Health; 2000a.

Department of Health. Shaping the future NHS: long term planning for hospitals and related services. Consultation document on the findings of The National Beds Inquiry – supporting analysis. London: Department of Health; 2000b.

Department of Health. National service framework for older people. London: Department of Health; 2001.

Department of Health. Single assessment process. Health services circular/local authority circular (HSC 2002/001; LAC (2002)1). London: Department of Health; 2002.

Dimond B. Legal aspects of nursing, 2nd edn. London: Prentice Hall; 1995.

Docherty B. An evidence base for nursing practice. Prof Nurse 2001; 16: 1355–1358.

Eraut M. Developing professional knowledge and competence. London: Falmer; 1994.

Ersser S, Tutton E. Primary nursing in perspective. London: Scutari; 1991.

Fawcett J. Analysis and evaluation of conceptual models of nursing. Philadelphia: FA Davies; 1995.

Flanagan M. The responsibility is yours. J Wound Care 2000; 9(8): 357.

George J. Nursing theories: the base for professional practice, 5th edn. Upper Saddle River, NJ: Prentice Hall; 2001.

Gibbs G. Learning by doing: a guide to teaching and learning methods. Oxford: Further Education Unit, Oxford Brookes University; 1988.

Hart E, Bond M. Action research for health and social care. Buckingham: Open University Press; 1995.

Henderson V. The nature of nursing: a definition and its implications for practice, research and education. New York: Macmillan; 1966.

Hockey L. The nature and purpose of research. In: Cormack D, ed. The research process in nursing, 4th edn. Oxford: Blackwell Science; 2000.

Johns C. Using a reflective model of nursing and guided reflection. Nurs Stand 1996; 11(2): 34–38.

Joyce L. Translating knowledge into good practice. Prof Nurse 2000; 16: 960–963.

Kerrigan D, Thevasagayam R, Woods T et al. Who's afraid of informed consent. Br Med J 1993; 306: 298–300.

Le May A. Knowledge for dissemination and implementation. In: Mulhall A, Le May A, eds. Nursing research: dissemination and implementation. Edinburgh: Churchill Livingstone; 1999.

McCaughan D. Developing critical appraisal skills. Prof Nurse 1999; 14: 843–847.

Meyer J. Using qualitative methods in health-related action research. Br Med J 2000; 320: 178–181.

NANDA. Nursing diagnosis: definitions and classification 2001–2002. Philadelphia: NANDA; 2001.

NHS Executive. Consultation on a strategy for nursing, midwifery and health visiting. London: Department of Health; 1998.

NHS Executive. Clinical governance: quality in the new NHS. London: Department of Health; 1999.

Norton L. Health promotion and health education: what role should the nurse adopt in practice. J Adv Nurs 1998; 28(6): 1269–1275.

Norton D, McLaren R, Exton-Smith A. An investigation of geriatric nursing problems in hospital. Edinburgh: Churchill Livingstone; 1972.

Nursing & Midwifery Council (NMC). The code of professional conduct. London: NMC; 2002.

Parahoo K. Nursing research: principles, process and issues. Basingstoke: Macmillan; 1997.

Pearson A, Vaughan B, Fitzgerald M. Nursing models for practice, 2nd edn. Oxford: Butterworth Heinemann; 1996.

Porter S, Carter D. Common terms and concepts in research. In: Cormack D, ed. The research process in nursing, 4th edn. Oxford: Blackwell Science; 2000.

Rogers A. Teaching adults, 2nd edn. Buckingham: Open University Press; 1996.

Roper N, Logan W, Tierney A. The elements of nursing, 4th edn. Edinburgh: Churchill Livingstone; 1996.

Rumbold G. Ethics in nursing practice, 3rd edn. Edinburgh: Baillière Tindall; 1999.

SNMAC. Caring for older people: a nursing priority. Integrating knowledge, practice and values. Report of the Nursing and Midwifery Advisory Committee. London: Department of Health; 2001.

The Chambers Dictionary. Edinburgh: Chambers Harrap Publishers; 1998.

Thiroux JP. Ethics, theory and practice, 2nd edn. Encino, CA: Glencoe Publishing; 1980.

Tschudin V. Ethics in nursing, 2nd edn. London: Butterworth; 1991.

United Kingdom Central Council. Guidance on clinical experience for students. Online. Available: www.nmc-uk.org 1998.

United Kingdom Central Council. Requirements for pre-registration nursing programmes. London: UKCC; 2001. (Online. Available: www.nmc-uk.org)

Webb C. The use of the first person in academic writing: objectivity, language and gate keeping. J Adv Nurs 1983; 17: 747–752.

Whitehead D. What is the role of health promotion in nursing? Prof Nurs 2000; 15(4): 257–259.

World Health Organization (WHO). Ottawa Charter for Health Promotion. Geneva: WHO; 1986. (Online. Available: www.who.int/hpr/archive/docs/ottawa.html.)

2 Quality management and standards of care

Ruhi Behi

'It was good to see that complaints actually do get dealt with and not just put in the bin. When I was in hospital last time, I complained that the hot drinks came too early in the evening. And now they've got a new system and I can help myself to a drink anytime I like.'

(Patient)

THIS CHAPTER WILL HELP YOU

- Describe the common features in various definitions of quality and their implications for nursing

- Explain how clinical governance can ensure quality care

- Understand the relationship between quality services and spending on resources and how nurses can contribute to efficiency

- Appraise the contribution benchmarking makes to improving nursing care

- Discuss the usefulness of the charters and British Standard BS 5750 to quality nursing care

- Understand how to manage change

- Describe common models (e.g. Maxwell's and Donabedian's) and appraise their usefulness in standard-setting

- Discuss the quality assurance spiral and the role of standard-setting within it

- Explain how quality enhancement can be achieved

- Discuss how evidence-based nursing contributes to quality nursing care

- Explain monitoring, evaluating and auditing of quality

- Understand the role of empowerment and education in ensuring quality.

KEYWORDS

Access	Outcome
Audit	Process
Benchmarking	Quality
Clinical governance	Quality assurance
Effectiveness	Quality enhancement
Efficiency	Standard
Equity	Structure
Evidence-based nursing	

INTRODUCTION

A basic understanding of the quality of nursing and standards of care issues is applicable to all areas of practice. What you learn here should be linked and applied to the other chapters. The emphasis is on nursing in the UK. The organizations mentioned and the examples used are also specific to the UK. However, the principles discussed and the procedures and systems described are applicable to quality health care in most countries of the world.

Nurses are central to the physical, psychological, social, emotional and spiritual care received by patients and clients in the National Health Service (NHS) and in the independent health care sector. More importantly, nurses are crucial in ensuring quality care and quality services to patients. We are required as professional nurses to give evidence-based nursing that contributes to high standards of care. Anything less is unacceptable and unprofessional. On reading the *Code of Professional Conduct* (NMC 2002) and various other guidelines for professional practice produced by the Nursing and Midwifery Council, one has no doubt regarding the expectation that nurses must ensure quality. A major thrust of all recent UK government initiatives in improving the NHS has been the achievement of high-quality care and outcomes for patients. These initiatives have been collectively termed 'clinical effectiveness' in recent years, but of late the term 'clinical governance' has been adopted.

In the UK the NHS Executive described clinical effectiveness as 'the extent to which specific clinical interventions when deployed in the field for a particular patient or population do what they are intended to do, i.e. maintain and improve health and secure the greatest possible health gain for the available resources' (Department of Health 1996).

The UK Department of Health (DoH 1998) has very clearly shown the importance it ascribes to quality by stating that: 'High quality care should be a right for every patient in the NHS. The Government wants a NHS that is both modern and dependable. Such a NHS should guarantee fair access and high quality to patients wherever they live.'

The consumers of health and nursing care, namely patients and clients, and their families, carers and significant others, just like consumers of any other service or product, expect the best that resources, technology and professional skills can reasonably be expected to provide. Nursing care can no longer be acceptable where it is based on tradition, trial and error, and individual preferences. Muddling along trying to do our best without proven validated evidence to support our care activities, actions and interventions is unacceptable. Unless research-based evidence is used to inform, guide and improve nursing care, practice will be very variable, which at best will be ineffective, and at worst harmful. Research, and the evidence it produces, needs to be of high quality. However, not all aspects of nursing practice have been researched, or investigated in a way that produces evidence that is reliable and credible. Practice cannot be influenced and changed on the basis of poor-quality research.

This chapter will, with a broad-brush approach, provide you an understanding of quality, standard-setting, quality assurance, measurement and monitoring. You will also find out about the means by which quality can be improved and enhanced. Specific initiatives in the NHS to guarantee the continuing importance of quality and its achievement, such as clinical governance, the National Institute for Clinical Excellence (NICE) and the Commission for Health Improvement (CHI), are described and discussed.

Quality cannot just happen, it has to be managed, and so there is a consideration of Total Quality Management (TQM), including a discussion of how change management can help the process. Evidence-based practice is explained. The chapter also includes a discussion of patient involvement, patient feedback (satisfaction and complaints), audits, and training and education, as contributory factors in the dynamic processes and systems needed to achieve quality enhancement. Readers practising outside the UK should, where appropriate, refer to local documents, systems and organizations, in order to make the principles discussed more relevant and useful.

DEFINING QUALITY

Quality is a term with many definitions; there are general definitions, health care definitions and definitions specific to nursing. A generally agreed definition, therefore, does not exist. However, many of these definitions share several common features and elements. Koch (1992) believes that it is pointless to try to define quality, because individuals, with their personal attitudes, values and beliefs, will influence and construct their own idea of what it is, and additionally believes that it is socially influenced and constructed. For example, a manager may prefer a definition that emphasizes cost-effectiveness and efficiency, whilst a nurse is more likely to prefer one that focuses on high standards of patient outcomes and effectiveness. Therefore, it is more important that nurses understand and appreciate the common features that will enable them to work in a way that assures quality care for patients.

Quality has the following common features:

- Quality is not an absolute concept, it is relative, being influenced by personal, political and social values.
- Quality is the responsibility of all health care professionals and their managers.
- Quality is perceived differently by professionals and by service users and customers.
- Quality is meeting service users' requirements.
- Quality is more likely to be achieved when professionals receive appropriate education and training.
- Quality requires striving for excellence in what we do.
- Quality is achieved when agreed standards of care are met.
- Quality is a process by which attempts are made to achieve excellence or agreed standards.
- Quality is dependent upon material, financial and human resources (called structures) to support the process.
- Quality is dependent upon research evidence to guide practice.
- Quality is ultimately about effective and efficient patient outcomes.

QUALITY MANAGEMENT IN THE HEALTH SERVICE

This section briefly describes the development of quality initiatives in the NHS and independent sector. Recent important developments and issues such as clinical governance, NICE, quality and cost, benchmarking, charter documents, and British Standards are discussed.

QUALITY IN THE NHS

Several authors, e.g. Sale (1996), have pointed out that Florence Nightingale, by systematically collecting data and information on patients and the care they received, was in effect one of the first to study quality. Of course, one could argue that at that time she was an exception, rather than the rule. It is also interesting that many of the quality initiatives that have been launched have often been as a result of media publicity following the exposure of errors in treatment and care, or of continuing poor-quality care in a given area of nursing or medical practice, e.g. stricter and more closely monitored guidelines for cervical smears (see Ch. 25) following extensively publicized errors that caused great concern and harm to large numbers of women. Patients and clients, as taxpayers and consumers of the NHS, have often been the catalysts for, and instigators of, changes to the standards being achieved in the health service.

Important and extensive efforts have regularly been applied in the health service from the 1960s to the present day, all of which were based on the need to improve effectiveness (achieving the right outcomes for patients) and efficiency (cost-effectiveness) of the service. For example, in the 1960s, Robb (1967) and Cohens (1964) questioned the quality of care given in the health service. There was a lack of clearly stated criteria and standards for quality. This meant that there was a general lack of methods, systems and processes for measuring whether quality was being achieved or not.

The NHS saw further developments in the 1970s and 1980s that highlighted and kept the quality issue in the spotlight. For example, the Royal College of Nursing (RCN) was in the fore-front with its work on standard-setting in nursing care. *Towards Standards* (RCN 1981) was one of the reports produced by a working group set up by the RCN to consider standards of care. An important element in this report was the unambiguous expectation that individual nurses are accountable for their own individual actions. Good-quality (and poor-quality) care is that individual nurse's responsibility. The report also recommended that the nursing process could be effectively used as a model on which standards of care could be based.

The early 1980s saw the introduction of general management and its implied ideology, principles and practices applied to the NHS. This had a knock-on effect on nursing and nursing practice. This was seen to be the way to overcome the continuing lack of monitoring and evaluation of NHS performance in relation to quality and standards and to achieve value for money (VFM). This was also a period when the internal market was introduced into the NHS with greater emphasis on competition between NHS providers of services. The intention was to purchase and commission services from providers who gave the best VFM, i.e. the highest possible quality of provision for the least cost (see 'Quality and cost', p. 27).

Frequent changes became the norm in the NHS. These were usually rationalized (although often there were political motivations for them) on the basis that they were needed to further ensure quality and VFM. Of course, when these two latter reasons were truly the case, then the changes were to be encouraged, welcomed and implemented (see 'Change management', p. 29). The 1990s brought more substantial changes in the UK NHS, and it is some of the most recent of these that have undoubtedly taken the issues of quality and evidence-based practice even further, by introducing the concept of clinical governance (DoH 1998, 1999).

Clinical governance

Clinical governance is a system by which goals for quality health care and treatments are going to be set, delivered and monitored. Where quality falls short of the expected or agreed standards, then clinical governance holds certain individuals to be ultimately responsible and answerable for it in any individual NHS Trust and provider of services. Chief executives of NHS Trusts are legally responsible for clinical quality. Such a clear indication and expectation of legal responsibility has never before been the case. There is no doubt that the introduction of such responsibility will sharpen the chief executives' focus on quality assurance and, through them, that of all staff employed in the NHS.

'Clinical governance is a key part of a concerted ten year programme of work throughout the NHS to improve the quality of patient care' (DoH 1999). Clinical governance applies to all UK NHS Health Authorities, NHS Trusts, Primary Care Trusts (England), Local Health Groups (Wales) and Local Health Care Co-operatives (Scotland). DoH (1999) identifies the following expectations for the implementation of clinical governance:

NHS organizations, and individuals working within them, need to monitor and improve quality in a number of ways. They must have:

- Clear lines of responsibility and accountability for the overall quality of clinical care;
- A comprehensive programme of quality improvement activities;
- Clear policies aimed at managing risk; and
- Procedures for all professional groups to identify and remedy poor performance.

It is useful to conceptualize clinical governance as an umbrella term to cover some new requirements in the way the NHS is expected to achieve high standards, such as the chief executive being legally responsible, but it also covers many of the existing principles and processes of quality improvement, which are also discussed in this chapter. For example, Scally & Donaldson (1998) suggest that existing methods of improvement, such as utilizing research findings in practice, education and training for health care professionals, measuring performance against standards, and dealing with and learning from complaints by patients, are brought together by clinical governance. Nurses are familiar with many such existing elements that have become part of clinical governance, such as dealing with and managing poor performance, risk management, clinical supervision, good management and leadership skills, reflective practice and clinical audit (see p. 34).

One of the new requirements is that NHS service providers must appoint a senior clinical professional such as a nurse or doctor to have responsibility for all the quality issues. To ensure quality care, clinical governance requires standard-setting and monitoring systems by NHS Trusts at a local level. At the national level, similar functions are the responsibility of NICE and CHI.

NICE and CHI

Recent initiatives concerning clinical governance resulted in the establishment of the NICE and the CHI. Since service providers are expected to meet acceptable levels of quality, the government has indicated that there must be national standards. One of the common complaints and unacceptable aspects of the NHS is the variability in level, type and quality of care and treatment offered to patients, such variability being a function of where patients live. This is unacceptable and is the reason why national standards are needed. NICE was set up to develop such standards.

NICE is a part of the UK NHS. It provides the NHS with 'authoritative, robust and reliable guidance on current best practice'. Its important activity is to give guidance on the clinical management of specific conditions and on pharmaceuticals, medical devices, diagnostic techniques and procedures.

To know whether these national standards and frameworks are being implemented, the CHI has the authority to review clinical governance arrangements across the NHS by undertaking audits. Such audits are on a rolling programme, so every individual NHS Trust can expect a visit from the CHI after a certain number of years. However, an annual clinical governance report has to be submitted by each health care organization. The Department of Health uses these annual reports to publish performance tables for health authorities and NHS Trusts. Patients can then compare the standards being achieved by the different health care providers, although it is important that the tables comprise only one of many sources used to make such comparisons.

Professional regulation is a complementary mechanism to clinical governance in maintaining high standards. Those professionals who fall short of the standards or who are guilty of misconduct, e.g. those who abuse patients, are reported to professional regulatory bodies. Severe sanctions can be imposed, including removal from the professional register. Employers can also discipline, suspend or dismiss individual employees who regularly and repeatedly have low standards.

The success of clinical governance undoubtedly rests with NHS staff, especially health care professionals and managers. Smith (1998) argues that 'a radical change is needed in the behaviour of clinicians and managers if clinical governance is going to work'. She also suggests shared governance as a means of achieving the change needed for clinical governance. Brooks et al (1998, p. 56) explain that 'shared governance is a system of network that attempts to move away from the traditional hierarchical style of nurse/midwifery management. It aims to increase the formal participation of nurses in the decision-making process, and to give them higher levels of professional autonomy.' The survey by Brooks et al (1998) found that staff believed that quality of care, improved communication and increased involvement in decision-making were associated with shared-governance.

EVIDENCE-BASED PRACTICE

There are several definitions of the term evidence-based practice but they are not that dissimilar in their implied meaning, which we will consider later. Basically, evidence-based actions are those that are backed by the findings of scientific research. It is, in reality, not that novel an idea. One can argue that nursing in the past was evidence-based, in that it was based on rationality and research evidence. However, often the nursing profession (like the medical) was guilty of giving care that was ineffective, wasteful of resources and of poor (and possibly dangerous) quality. This was because it was based on tradition and ritual (e.g. observations every 4 hours whether needed or not) and trial and error (e.g. trying untested and unproven products for pressure ulcer treatment in an unscientific way). Evidence-based practice aims to prevent such ineffectual, possibly harmful, and often expensive practice (Lockett 1997).

The essence of evidence-based practice is that professional practice should be based on validated (systematically reviewed and critically appraised) research findings. Of course, this is not possible in situations where a certain aspect or type of practice has not yet been sufficiently investigated scientifically.

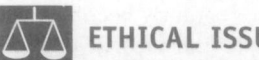 **ETHICAL ISSUES**

2.1 Lack of research findings

Ethical principles applicable to nursing care include the following: doing good for patients (beneficence); not causing harm to patients (non-maleficence); fairness for all (justice); the awareness that professionals don't always know what is best for patients (non-paternalism); the right of the patient to health and health care (human rights); and freedom on the part of the patient to choose to receive or refuse care (autonomy).

Student activities
Use any relevant ethical principles described above to write down supportive ethical reasons to give or withhold a particular complementary therapy, such as aromatherapy. You will need, at the same time, to take into account the existence or lack of relevant evidence to support the complementary therapy of your choice.

Consequently there can be a lack of findings to apply in practice (see Ethical Issues box 2.1). This decision about whether there is validated evidence can be made after a systematic, critical appraisal of the published literature in a given area of practice. There are several centres that make such systematically reviewed evidence easily available, especially on the internet and on CD-ROM, such as the Cochrane Library of Systematic Reviews. The most useful sources for objective unbiased evidence, particularly on the internet, are those that are independent of other bodies, e.g. not funded by companies that supply products or drugs to the health service.

Systematic appraisal of the literature by individual professionals has been made easier by the almost instantaneous availability of all the relevant references through the advances in information technology. The use of computers, electronic sources, CD- and DVD-ROMs and online databases of the literature, the internet and worldwide search facilities have increased access to all the literature on a given subject. Remember, though, that even the best of databases, such as CINAHL and MEDLINE, can miss potentially useful and important references. The excuse of non-availability or non-accessibility of the evidence is no longer acceptable for poor-quality care. Ignorance has never been, and is even less likely to be now, an excuse for unacceptable standards of care. Of course, the information overload resulting from the extensive availability provided by these various sources means that we have to become very discerning and selective in choosing the information we use. Even expert users can find it difficult to sort out the worthwhile research from the rubbish.

Clinical effectiveness is another term that is sometimes used synonymously with evidence-based practice, and sometimes is seen as the outcome of evidence-based practice. It refers to achieving effective outcomes for patients, i.e. doing more good than harm. Of course, it also means giving quality treatment and care.

QUALITY IN THE PRIVATE AND VOLUNTARY SECTORS

The statutory and other regulations that apply to the private and voluntary health care sectors are different from those that apply to the NHS. This does not mean that care given in these sectors is allowed to be of poor quality. Where it does fall below acceptable levels, there are regulations that allow a regulatory body to deal with it, e.g. through the recommendations made by inspectors of care homes, which can include removing registration from the establishment. There has been much dissatisfaction about the effectiveness of regulations in ensuring quality, particularly as they often involve vulnerable groups such as older adults. Statutory regulations relating to these sectors must be regularly reviewed so that they may be updated as necessary to ensure quality care for their customers. The UK government has recently introduced several initiatives, the Care Standards Act (2000), the National Care Standards Commission (NCSC) and the Social Care Institute for Excellence. One could argue that the same principle of clinical governance should be applied to these sectors, especially the need to have a clear indication of the individual(s) who are responsible and accountable in the organization.

The Care Standards Act (2000) replaces the Registered Homes Act 1984 and establishes the NCSC, an independent regulatory body (DoH 2001). The NCSC will use national minimum standards (published by the DoH) as the basis for the registration of care homes.

Quality has to be very high on the agenda of private sector health care providers because, as private businesses, they cannot afford to lose customers due to poor standards of care. As Nazarko (1997, p. 75) points out: "The [nursing] home's reputation will suffer if the care it offers is considered inadequate. In a competitive market this may lead to a reduction of referrals and a corresponding fall in occupancy, and the home could cease to be economically viable. This will threaten the jobs of all members of staff." It makes very good business sense to ensure quality provision. Otherwise, the customers will purchase their services elsewhere. The voluntary sector, which is dependent upon charity and goodwill, can suffer in similar ways if the quality of its work is unacceptable to the people it serves and the people who support it.

QUALITY AND COST

There is a close relationship between quality and cost. It would be wrong to assume, however, that this always means higher costs for higher standards of care. The relationship is more complicated and exercises the minds of many health economists. This subject does not fall within the remit of this chapter and some brief discussions on it can be found in Ellis & Whittington (1993) and Joss & Kogan (1995). It is useful, though, to consider some of the basic cost issues related to ensuring quality care. The first obvious cost implication is in establishing the systems, processes and structures needed for quality assurance. These take up much staff time (both managerial and clinical) and resources. There is, therefore, an initial high cost, following which there are costs associated with maintaining the whole system, including regular monitoring, evaluation and audit (see p. 34). It is important, however, to consider such costs in relation to the savings to the organization that undoubtedly follow from a quality service provision – less compensation, for example, because of less litigation. Fewer complaints consequent to quality care provision mean that the costs in dealing with them are lower. Additionally, there will be increased patient satisfaction and an increase in staff satisfaction and morale, which can create cost savings through lower sickness and absenteeism rates, and there will be lower recruitment, induction and training costs due to better staff retention.

There are often increased costs when quality provision is dependent upon new and better treatments, new drugs and equipment, specialist staff and their education, and new developments in general. The availability of such new and improved services, however, is dependent upon whether or not the health service can afford them. It is possible to show improved services without necessarily incurring extra costs. Different service providers sometimes spend different amounts of money on similar levels of standards of care and treatment. Some Trusts are more efficient than others.

Efficiency can simply be defined as doing things in such a way that money and resources are not wasted (Maxwell 1984) and maximum benefit is gained from minimum effort. Therefore, one can try to increase standards and the quality of services by becoming less wasteful of time (e.g. not carrying out unnecessary tests or observations on patients) and resources (e.g. drug wastage due to expiring use-by dates as a result of poor stock rotation). When quality is increased by such cost-efficiency measures, then VFM is achieved. Mason (1994, p. 174) supports the need for efficiency by arguing that 'because the cost of implementing the standards is vital in an era of limited resources and funding, you need to identify the combination of interventions and observations within each procedure and unit of care that requires the fewest resources and shortest time to implement yet results in the same positive outcomes for patients'.

BENCHMARKING

Most organizations determine internally what levels of quality and standards to aim for. However, sometimes these levels may be determined using an inappropriate yardstick for guidance and comparison. Benchmarking is the system of comparing an organization's standards against those of an external, but similar, organization which is chosen especially for excellence in quality. The aim of benchmarking is to strive towards achieving improvements continuously. Lam (1994, p. 48) points out another important distinguishing feature of benchmarking, which is that, it 'involves comparisons between practices that have actually been achieved; practices are not held up against an idealized model, which is often the case with many other initiatives that go under the "quality" banner'.

Benchmarking in the NHS is mainly a development of the 1990s. It is seen as another tool in the armoury against poor-quality practice and will help NHS organizations to learn from each other and contribute to VFM initiatives. Benchmarking depends on measurement and audit, and contributes to the cycle of quality improvements in the NHS.

Camp (1989), whose work is extensively and regularly referred to by other authors (e.g. Lam 1994, Williams 1998), suggests several steps in the process of benchmarking:

- The planning phases include identifying what is to be benchmarked and the organization for comparison, and collecting the data for comparison using an agreed method of data collection.
- In the analysis phase, the gap (if one exists) is determined and standards for the future agreed.
- The next phase of integration attempts to gain acceptance through good communication and establishes goals that can be achieved.
- Action is the next phase, with action plans, specific actions taken and monitored and, if necessary, amendments made to the benchmarks.
- The final phase, called maturity, is reached when the organization achieves the position of leadership (i.e. is used as a yardstick for benchmarking by other similar organizations) and full integration of practices.

BRITISH STANDARDS AND *THE PATIENT'S CHARTER*

Standards relating to quality systems within organizations and charters that relate to the rights of individuals are means by which quality can be assured for customers and consumers and, in the case of nursing, for patients and clients.

British Standard (BS) 5750

The British Standards Institution (BSI), an independent non-profit-making body, facilitates the writing of British Standards for effective quality systems in manufacturing and service industries such as health care. There are different sets of standards which are given specific numbers; BS 5750 (discussed below) is one that is very relevant to health care services. The institution is the body that inspects an organization's quality systems to determine whether they meet the agreed set of criteria before deciding to grant the BS5750 kitemark to that organization. There is an equivalent international standard accredited by the International Organization for Standardization (ISO 9000).

Some definitions of quality expect excellence, but excellence is often impossible to achieve because of reasons that are difficult to overcome, e.g. high costs and lack of resources. Instead, it has been suggested that an alternative approach is to take the customer's or service user's viewpoint, which, according to Jackson & Ashton (1993, p. 12) is 'another view of quality' that 'avoids the trap of an unattainable excellence and focuses on the needs of a group on which any business entirely depends – the customer'. British Standard 5750 takes this view as the basis of what it is supposed to be doing, i.e. meeting the customer's requirements. In the health services, it is about ensuring that the services we offer and the standards we achieve are 'fit for purpose', i.e. related to patients' needs and outcomes. BS 5750 is not concerned with specific products or services, but it is applicable to a 'quality system' that is formal and documented (Jackson & Ashton 1993).

When, for example, an NHS Trust, applies for and gains BS 5750 from the BSI, it means that the Trust has in place the processes and procedures, which can be changed as necessary, to assure quality. The assumption, therefore, is that the Trust will also have standards that meet patients' expectations and can deal with difficulties as they arise. Jackson & Ashton (1993,

p. 23) explain when a quality system is judged to be effective: 'An effective system, therefore, is not just a set of rules for quality production. It is recognized that problems will occur, but the system tries to ensure that they do not keep reoccurring. This is done by procedures for problem identification (e.g. auditing), investigation (e.g. corrective action), and long-term rectification (e.g. controlled procedural change).'

Many NHS Trusts have opted for BS 5750, but it is not sufficient in itself for total quality management (Joss & Kogan 1995). Joss & Kogan also express reservations about the usefulness of BS 5750 for NHS Trusts when it is employed as a stand-alone means of achieving quality, suggesting (p. 111) that 'it can become little more than a mechanistic document-driven system implemented for marketing purposes'.

The Patient's Charter and the NHS guide

In 1991, the UK government introduced *The Patient's Charter* (DoH 1991) to monitor the achievement by NHS Trusts of certain key, mostly time-related, standards involving patients. Patients had recognized rights and expectations: rights referred to standards that should always be available to patients; and expectations referred to those standards that NHS providers try to achieve, which may not always be available to patients.

The standards within the charter were monitored closely and continuously, e.g. waiting times for patients. Unfortunately, these standards were mainly quantitative and appropriate to acute services. They did not measure the qualitative aspects of those numerically measured standards. For example, whether patients have to wait for 15 minutes or half an hour before being seen by a nurse may be less important than how they are dealt with and their experience during that waiting period. Patients may be happier to tolerate a longer period of 'better quality waiting time' than to be seen in a shorter time but where the waiting experience is one of uncertainty and distress. Some of *The Patient's Charter* standards relevant to the community were introduced in 1995 (DoH 1995). These were only quantitative measures, such as home visits by a community nurse being carried out within 4 hours for urgent cases and within 2 days for non-urgent cases. Some separate qualitative standards were mentioned, such as respecting patients' religious and cultural beliefs, dignity and privacy.

One could argue that the most useful aspect of such a charter and its ongoing development is that it lays down in easily understood terms what patients can expect from the services. Users of health care provision also become aware of their rights, which empowers them. Health service providers could take this initiative and increase its contribution to quality provision by developing their own detailed charters, especially if they included qualitative measures as well.

Publication of the levels of achievement of the target standards by all NHS Trusts was supposed to give patients comparative data by which to judge the quality of services available to them – a 'league' table of good and bad quality Trusts. However, the system of publishing the easily quantifiable and measurable, i.e. numerical, data sometimes led to false conclusions about how well a Trust was doing. This is because it lacked the other important ingredient – qualitative data – and therefore did not reflect the total experience of patients (see Reflective Practice box 2.1).

REFLECTIVE PRACTICE

2.1 Performance ('league') tables

Performance tables are produced by the Department of Health that detail how well each health authority and NHS Trust performs using several criteria, e.g. emergency readmission to hospital within 28 days of discharge and time spent waiting in accident and emergency (A&E) for emergency admission.

Student activities
- These tables are popularly referred to as 'league' tables. Reflect on the consequences of viewing the data in this way.
- In terms of achieving high-quality care, what are the advantages and disadvantages of publishing these data?
- Reflect on whether the tables increase consumer choice and empowerment.
- Reflect on whether the data are equally accessible to all consumers.

Further reading
NHS Executive. Quality and performance in the NHS Performance indicators. London: HMSO; 2000 (Online. Available: www.doh.gov.uk/nhsperformanceindicators).

SPECIAL ISSUES

2.1 Activities for the successful change implementation (Plant 1987)
- Helping individuals or groups face up to change, understand and accept it, because of its value
- Communicating extensively with all concerned, upwards and downwards in hierarchical structures, explaining roles and responsibilities of staff
- Gaining energetic commitment to change, especially by showing that it was crucial to the success of the service, and important to staff
- Involvement of staff from all relevant groups as early as possible
- Turning perception of threat into opportunities, encouraging staff to be innovative and creative
- Avoiding over-organizing and too much control; flexibility helps.

What *The Patient's Charter* did do, though, was to increase consumer pressure on the health service to ensure quality.

In 2001, the UK government introduced the publication *Your Guide to the NHS*. This document replaces *The Patient's Charter* and aims to inform members of the public about what they can expect from the NHS. Areas covered include patients' rights and responsibilities, the standards and service that can be expected, accessing advice and treatment, and the procedures for voicing concerns or complaining when things go wrong.

CHANGE MANAGEMENT

The dynamic, cyclic nature of quality assurance and quality initiatives means that there is an inevitable and continuous string of changes that need to be implemented. Developments like the introduction of quality systems, charters and standards need to be implemented in a planned and systematic way, using the principles of good change management. Otherwise, real change will not occur, time and resources will be wasted, and quality will not be improved. A brief explanation of these principles is given below. It is important to note that this short section can only consider the subject in a very limited way and that there are many different models of change management, details of which can be found in a number of books and journal articles (see 'Further Reading'). For example, there are the top-down and bottom-up approaches to change management, the change through confrontation model, and the classic three-phase (unfreezing, moving and refreezing) model (Lewin 1958). Moreover, as Dunning (1998) points out: 'the literature

on management of change in the NHS is diverse, with no agreed practice model'.

Close (1997) brings many of these principles of change management together, specifically relating to ways in which 'to achieve successful implementation of a quality strategy'. Resistance from those staff who are likely to be affected by change is a common reaction because of the perceived threat and fears concerning their workload, working relationships and future job security. Therefore, it is important that managers reduce resistance by involving people, giving information, making support available and reducing uncertainty and anxieties. Key people in the organization, such as managers of resources, opinion leaders (those who can influence others to change) and those with appropriate knowledge and expertise, should be identified and used to support the change (Close 1997).

Plant (1987) suggests six activities for successful change implementation (see Special Issues box 2.1).

DIMENSIONS OF QUALITY IN HEALTH CARE

Quality in health care and its audit (analysis of the quality of care) can be managed in many ways. One method can be unsystematic, disorganized and reactive, while another can be systematic, organized, planned and proactive. Of course, it is the latter that should be used in health care.

USE OF MODELS FOR QUALITY IN HEALTH CARE

Models for quality or approaches to quality in health care are useful in understanding many of the issues underpinning quality. However, it is important to realize that models are only means of understanding quality issues, not ends in themselves. They are also useful frameworks for standard-setting and audit (see pp. 30, 34). Two common approaches are considered.

EVIDENCE-BASED PRACTICE

2.1 Maxwell's dimensions of quality

These dimensions group together the important issues by which quality of service provision can be planned and audited:

- *Access.* This dimension is about accessibility to services for patients, and can relate to waiting times, where the services are available, and the actual buildings that patients have to use.
- *Equity.* Patients should have services available to them irrespective of their social, cultural or racial background. A patient's need for health care should be the paramount determinant of the appropriate provision.
- *Relevance to need.* The health care needs of the whole community should be met. There should be no shortfalls in provision of services to meet the needs of the community being served by the relevant NHS services.
- *Social acceptability.* Services need to be in tune with social, cultural and religious values in order to be generally acceptable to the community. Care and treatments must meet the expectations of patients.

- *Efficiency.* The discussion about cost relates to this dimension. Services need to be cost-effective, i.e. delivered at as high a quality as possible within the resources available.
- *Effectiveness.* Health care provision should result in beneficial patient outcomes. Effectiveness is also about health care benefits for the population that is being served. Inappropriate and harmful treatments and care are seen as ineffective.

Joss & Kogan (1995, p. 31), in a brief review of the literature related to Maxwell's dimensions, draw the conclusion that 'these dimensions have been helpful in taking stock of services at the macro level, but they have proved less helpful in defining the more pragmatic aspects at operational levels'. These dimensions are not very useful when trying to define standards for individuals receiving individual care and treatment.

The problem can be overcome by using the Donabedian (1966) model, which has been used extensively by nurses to set and monitor standards.

Maxwell's dimensions of quality

Maxwell (1984) suggested a model in which quality is seen to have six dimensions (see Evidence-based Practice box 2.1):

- access
- equity
- relevance to need
- social acceptability
- efficiency
- effectiveness.

Donabedian's structure–process–outcome model

The Donabedian (1966) model can be easily used to set standards in relation to both the nursing care of individuals and the organization itself. The model uses three specific sets of criteria for quality and standards:

- *Structure* – the answer to the question 'What do we need to have to be able to achieve quality?' identifies the structures. For example, we need staff with appropriate skills and qualifications and in sufficient numbers to reach certain care standards. Other structures involve the equipment, drugs, buildings and so on that are needed for specific standards to be met. The structure relates to the environment, the resources and the documentation guiding staff that are needed for the delivery of care.
- *Process* – the answer to the question 'What do we need to do to achieve quality?' identifies the process aspects. For example, how we provide care and services is a process issue; nursing practices and procedures, monitoring and evaluation are also examples.
- *Outcome* – the answer to the question 'What do we need to achieve?' identifies the outcomes. For example, the result

of a nursing procedure carried out on a patient is an outcome. It is generally assumed to be a consequence of the structures and processes working together to deliver health care.

STANDARDS AND STANDARD-SETTING

Mason (1994, p. 1) describes a standard as a 'valid definition of the quality of health care. To guarantee quality, every standard must be valid – that is, health care administered according to a standard will result in positive outcome(s) for patients. A standard is not valid unless it is precise; that is, all staff implementing and evaluating care understand the meaning of the standard.' To be precise, a standard must be a level of performance that is agreed in advance and it should be measurable, because otherwise quality is too all-encompassing a term and is not directly quantifiable. Standards have to be achievable and realistic in relation to the available resources. When a standard is not directly measurable, it needs to be divided into parts that are measurable. Such measurable components are called 'criteria' and they give us the actual measurements that make it possible to determine whether or not the standard has been achieved. Box 2.1 gives an example of a standard using the structure–process–outcome approach.

Standard-setting is crucial to, and precedes, auditing of practice by professionals. However, standard-setting alone is not sufficient to achieving, maintaining and enhancing quality. TQM (managing quality with a continuing drive for improvements by involving all departments and staff at all levels in an organization), for example, is recommended by many experts in this field as the best overall way forward (e.g. Joss & Kogan 1995). Their comments are especially true when quality issues across the whole organization are being considered rather

Box 2.1 Example of a standard using Donabedian's model

Standard: Patients admitted with fractures will have their pain under control within half an hour of admission to hospital.

Structure

- Medical and nursing staff know the policies for administration of analgesia for fractures
- Assessment procedures are known and relevant paperwork is available
- Frequently used analgesic drugs for fractures are stocked for quick availability

Process

- The responsible doctor will assess and initiate treatment within the specified time
- The nurse or doctor will administer the analgesic
- Medical and nursing staff monitor pain and effectiveness of analgesia

Outcome

- Patient's pain is under control within half an hour

---

than focused specialized areas of nursing which have been well served by standard-setting programmes such as the RCN's Dynamic Standard Setting System (DySSSy) since the mid-1980s (RCN 1990).

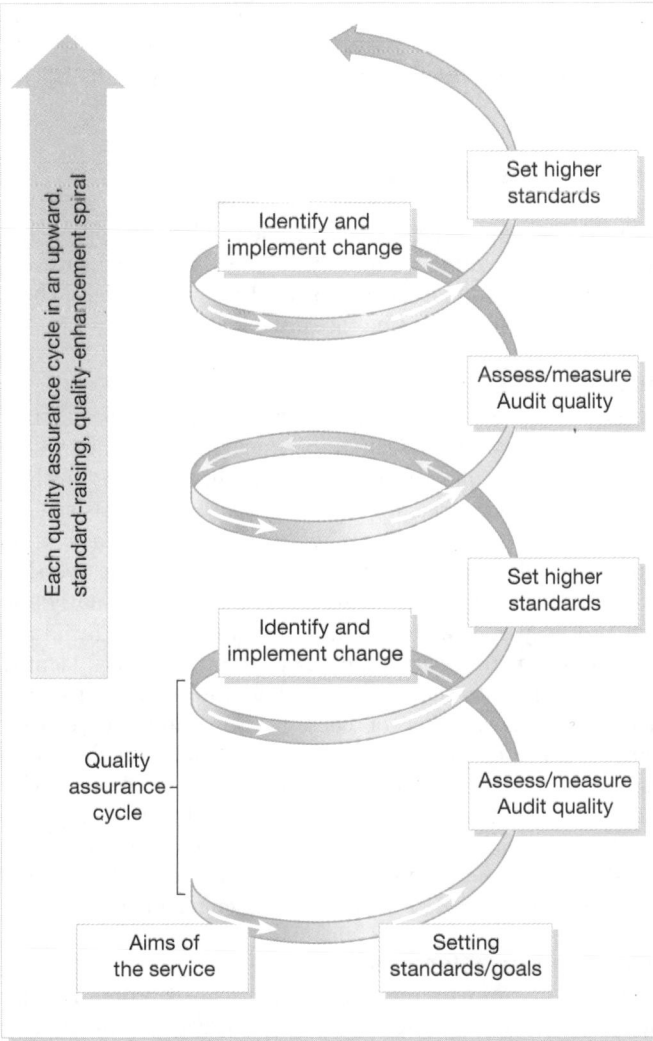

Figure 2.1 Quality enhancement. Spiralling quality assurance cycles for quality enhancement.

In the DySSSy one can see the strong influence of the Donabedian model and the quality assurance cycle. The cyclic process consists of identifying goals and values for the service, followed by standard-setting, auditing and measuring care given, which in turn indicates actions to be taken, acting on these and feeding this back into the system by changing standards accordingly (see Fig. 2.1). The system is designed so that nurses are in control of standard-setting and quality assurance. It encourages team-working and a bottom-up approach to standard-setting (staff at the grass roots level, rather than middle and senior managers, taking the lead), which is a positive mechanism (involvement by all stakeholders) for managing change. In a review of the DySSSy, Morrell et al (1997, p. 29) concluded that, to strengthen the system further, there was a need for some changes, for example, 'a continuous focus on ways to achieve true multiprofessional collaboration and involvement of patients in clinical audit'.

Whatever the model used, standard-setting should agree standards for nursing that are achievable by nurses, acceptable to all stakeholders, affordable by the NHS generally, and the health care provider specifically. It should also be relevant to the needs of patients, understandable by all concerned, and measurable for monitoring, evaluating and audit purposes (see Reflective Practice box 2.2).

R|Я REFLECTIVE PRACTICE

2.2 Using standards

Identify one area of care that has a standard in your clinical placement or setting.

Student activities

- Reflect on how this can be achieved in practice.
- Identify, through reflective analysis, the important criteria by which the standard can be measured.
- Give special consideration to the differences in what may be acceptable to people of different ages or from different ethnic, cultural and religious groups.
- List the criteria that can be used to audit whether this standard is being achieved.

MAKING SENSE OF QUALITY INTERVENTIONS

Writers and gurus on the subject of quality use so many different ideas and terms that, to a novice, it can be very confusing and unhelpful. Terms such as quality control, quality assessment, quality assurance, quality management, TQM, quality circles, quality councils and quality enhancement are some of the more commonly used ones and the sections below explain the basics of these by considering them as two groups of related concepts. The first group considers a hierarchical structure to understand terms to do with quality interventions, and the second group considers terms referring to methods for quality enhancement.

A HIERARCHICAL STRUCTURE FOR QUALITY INTERVENTIONS

The first group uses a hierarchical structure for different levels of management effort and interventions related to quality which also have different aims.

Quality control

Quality control 'is essentially the activities and techniques employed to achieve and maintain the quality of a product, process, or service' (Oakland 1993, p. 15). In the health service, therefore, it is about being able to have the mechanisms by which control of the service at the agreed standards is maintained. Quality control occurs at the level of service delivery to individual patients, e.g. when a patient is actually receiving care such as wound care or drug administration.

Quality assessment

At a different level, quality assessment aims to assess the degree of quality existing in an organization. Usually this type of assessment is carried out so that management can make decisions about what actions are needed, as part of a general quality management strategy to identify areas for quality improvement within a quality assurance system.

Quality improvement

Quality improvement is a term whose meaning is clearly self-evident, and is the next level in the hierarchy of efforts by all concerned. This can involve managers and practitioners. Improvements made by nurses can have effects on others. For example, changing the times of drug administration may affect the quality of another service, such as the meals service, because the time that patients eat at can be determined by their drug regimen.

Quality assurance

Quality assurance is further up the hierarchy of management interventions. It is generally seen to be a planned, dynamic and cyclic system that is able to ensure that problems can be identified through monitoring and measurement and that options for solutions can be considered so that the best one is chosen to be acted upon, thereby assuring quality. Measurement is against the agreed standards, so that corrective actions can be taken where they are not met. It could be argued that it is even better if

we consider quality assurance as a spiral, rather than a cycle – one that seeks to spiral upwards towards increasingly better standards for patients and clients (see Fig. 2.1). Quality assurance is one of many important systems and actions that are part of good quality management, which is the next and broader range of efforts by managers.

Quality management

Quality management includes planning and managing, acting upon and implementing, and regularly evaluating and reviewing quality issues and initiatives. It has to do with managers always keeping quality issues at the forefront of their considerations and decisions, and ensuring resources are used to optimize quality outcomes.

Total quality management

Total quality management, the highest level in this hierarchical approach, applies to all levels of an organization and to all staff within it, e.g. all those who work for an NHS Trust. It also includes external organizations that deal with the Trust, e.g. companies that supply equipment and drugs, or other service providers such as the ambulance service. It is an all-encompassing, all-embracing approach. Every part of an organization affects and is affected by all the other parts. The aim of TQM is to make each part of an organization become effective in playing its role in ensuring quality.

QUALITY ENHANCEMENT

The second group of terms mainly relates to helpful approaches for staff to use to enhance quality. In effect, this means raising standards of care and treatment by health care providers. Three of the more common methods are discussed below.

Quality circles

The idea of quality circles is Japanese in origin and is a system to help small groups of staff to be involved in enhancing the quality of the specific service or product that they are involved in. In the health service, a quality circle usually consists of six to eight members of staff, e.g. ward nurses. Having a small and manageable group is important. The group membership should be voluntary and the group should meet regularly and frequently, say once a fortnight. A recognized leader facilitates the group, e.g. the ward sister. The group members identify problems related to the quality of their care and service, and then undertake analysis of each problem and the relevant issues, looking for solution options. The quality circle is also responsible for choosing what option to act on, implementing it and monitoring its success. Additional benefits accruing from quality circles include better change management, greater team cohesion, improved relationships between staff and a general increase in the awareness of, and time given to, quality issues.

Quality improvement teams

A quality improvement team (QIT) consists of a group that has the necessary appropriate experience and expertise, including knowledge, to work on a specific project or to solve a particular problem. The group is established by management and should include individuals who have various functions; it is often multidisciplinary. Often the team is brought together to analyse and solve a problem identified by a quality council (see below). For example, in the health service, a small quality team could be formed to include knowledgeable and skilled nurses, doctors and other appropriate health care professionals (e.g. a radiographer), and managers to identify ways in which outpatient waiting times can be reduced. Once the options for action and change have been identified, the team is no longer needed, because it usually isn't the team's responsibility to implement the change. A different problem at some other time would require a different mix of staff and expertise.

Quality councils

Total quality management requires a substantial amount of time and commitment from senior members of an organization. The establishment of a quality council is one way of dealing with the continuous issues of quality. The chief executive should chair it, and it should include top management. The objectives of such an important council are to agree and take forward TQM strategy; agree, monitor and amend implementation plans for quality; and give projects to QITs and review their progress. The council needs to meet regularly and frequently to do its job, e.g. monthly. It should keep the quality strategy under constant review and monitor the progress of quality implementation and improvement.

QUALITY NURSING CARE

Earlier sections have discussed quality in a general sense, with some examples and applications to the health service. The transferable ideas and principles for achieving high quality should be applied to the practice of nursing. In this section some more specific issues crucial to achieving quality nursing care are discussed. Evidence-based nursing is a profession-specific example of evidence-based practice. This requirement by the health service and its relationship to quality are explained.

EVIDENCE-BASED NURSING

Evidence-based nursing is an essential factor, together with evidence-based medicine, in ensuring quality nursing care, quality medical treatments and quality health care. It is also a major contributor to clinical governance. Reading the RCN's brief guide to clinical effectiveness (RCN 1996), it becomes obvious that quality nursing care for patients is not possible if the relevant and appropriate evidence to guide practice is not used or is not available. The RCN guide states that (p. 3): 'clinical effectiveness is about doing the right thing in the right way for the right patient at the right time'. To know what is right, one has to find the supportive evidence mainly from the research literature.

RCN (1996) also includes useful guidance on the sorts of questions a nurse needs to ask to start becoming clinically effective and evidence-based, e.g.:

- What evidence is being used?
- How can one involve patients in making decisions about their care?

- How does a nurse update knowledge and skills?
- How does one plan and implement change in practice?
- Nurses must also consider how the care given is evaluated and monitored.

To be evidence-based in their nursing practice, nurses should know how to use that evidence to set higher standards and achieve better quality care, i.e. how to improve standards.

IMPROVING NURSING STANDARDS

Nursing care is such a major part of most patients' experience that improving nursing standards of care can make a substantial difference to patient satisfaction levels. The role of nurses in improving standards should be clearly understood, encouraged and expected as part of their accountability, in terms of both uniprofessional and multiprofessional standards. Nurses must learn the models, systems and processes (such as those described above) to help them develop and improve standards and contribute to quality enhancement. In essence, every concept discussed so far has to do with improving standards.

How models and systems can be helpful is seen in the example of the use of the DySSSy and its review by Morrell et al (1997). They showed that the standards developed by the use of this model 'resulted in continuous improvement; and could solve local problems' (p. 31). Some believed it was a good system for improving standards because it was designed by nurses for nurses; and there were those who believed the system was useful because it encouraged the development of multiprofessional standards. Most importantly, Morrell et al also found that (p. 32): 'the development of clinical practice was described as the overriding benefit of involvement with the system. Evidence from successive audits showed progress in clinical care in many areas.'

ROLE OF TRAINING AND EDUCATION

It would be difficult to imagine how improving standards and quality, with all that entails, could realistically and effectively be achieved unless nurses were given continuing education and training in relevant topics. Glen (1998, p. 95) argued that improvement in practice also depends on the nurses' emotional and motivational tendencies, and that 'in essence, professional development implies personal development'. The development of appropriate personal qualities in nurses is essential to providing quality nursing care. Scally & Donaldson (1998) believe that 'development of staff will make a major contribution' to clinical governance. The UKCC and the National Boards, which were replaced by the Nursing and Midwifery Council (NMC), played an important part in ensuring that professional development takes place, e.g. through the requirement for proof of regular updating by nurses before re-registration every 3 years. The NMC establishes the standards for professional development at different levels, e.g. for specialist level practice and advanced level practice, or for preceptorship of newly qualified staff.

The NMC, as the statutory regulatory body for nursing, midwifery and health visiting, is responsible for professional self-regulation, and so is every individual nurse. Professional self-regulation requires registered practitioners to monitor themselves. Self-regulation is guided and supported by three principles (UKCC 1999):

- promoting good practice
- preventing poor practice
- intervening in unacceptable practice.

Joss & Kogan (1995) suggest that resources should be made available for effective education and training, on which TQM is dependent. They also differentiate between education and training as follows (p. 83): 'education is used to emphasize the attitudinal and cultural changes required, while training usually refers to providing specific tools and techniques'. Knowledgeable and skilled practitioners with the right attitude are needed, and training and education together can develop such practitioners. The failure of programmes for quality has often been due to a lack of resources invested in education and training (Joss & Kogan 1995).

Empowering staff is very important and is crucial in the internal chain of staff that is essential to TQM. Motivation and remotivation of staff are achieved through empowerment (Joss & Kogan 1995). For example, helping a less experienced nurse take responsibility for, and succeed in dealing with, a difficult aspect of care will increase that nurse's motivation to deal with difficult situations in the future. Empowerment is about giving staff the knowledge, skills and attitudes through education and training to be able to take on their professional responsibilities. Having educated and trained nurses, empowerment can be facilitated by allowing and trusting them to do what is right to achieve quality. Shared governance also empowers because it involves all nurses in a less hierarchical system, and empowers them to use their professional autonomy and accountability when giving care. The achievement of self-confidence, self-reward and self-satisfaction from successfully giving quality care will maintain motivation and achieve continuing self-empowerment.

MONITORING, EVALUATING AND AUDITING QUALITY

Quality assurance requires that agreed standards are monitored on a frequent and regular basis to give staff regular feedback about the quality of care being achieved, so that corrective actions can be taken as and when necessary. Audit and evaluation are needed at specific regular, but not very frequent intervals, e.g. annually, and provide a measure and value of what has been achieved over the period of time the audit or evaluation covers, e.g. the previous year.

MONITORING AND EVALUATING

Any quality management system such as TQM needs to be monitored. This implies having mechanisms and measures that make possible continuous checking of the system. Monitoring is usually an ongoing check to see whether systems are functioning as they should. Of course, monitoring of quality and standards of nursing care are needed so that problems are immediately identified and rectified. This is a very effective way of ensuring continuous ongoing quality.

Evaluation, as the term implies, is to assess and determine the value of something. For example, monitoring might ensure that the agreed standards are being met as time passes, but one could at a specific time evaluate whether a quality management system or some specific nursing care is of value or not. The nursing process requires evaluation of the care given to any individual patient to determine whether that care has been effective.

Unfortunately, in the literature on quality, the terms monitoring, evaluating and auditing are often used interchangeably to mean measuring and collecting data to enable decisions to be made about whether quality and standards have been achieved.

AUDITS

Kogan & Redfern (1995, p. 1) assert that the definition of audit, like many of the other terms in this chapter, 'has acquired different meanings. It has been defined in the specific sense as assessing or measuring quality of care. It is often used, though, more broadly as measuring quality and changing practice when improvement to care or treatment is required.' Therefore, the specific restricted meaning is that an audit measures and assesses the standards of care and reports on this to the relevant body, often an external one, e.g. the commissioning Primary Care Trust. The second and broader sense in which it is used is similar to what is expected in the quality assurance cycle or quality enhancement spiral (see Fig. 2.1). Audit is conceptualized as the whole process of quality assurance, and not just the measurement and assessment of standards achieved or not achieved. This second definition is more widely used, especially internally in organizations, and is one that ensures that quality measures are achieving what they are intended to achieve.

The NHS has many different types and levels of audit, e.g. there is medical audit and nursing audit. Many patient outcomes are dependent on several different professionals, and in this context clinical audit is used, which is usually multidisciplinary (though sometimes it is used synonymously with medical audit). Other types of audit are support services audit, management audit and even a complete organizational audit. The Health Quality Service (previously known as King's Fund Organizational Audit) is a voluntary accreditation system used by UK health organizations and has encouraged many quality improvement initiatives within the whole organization. In addition, because of the need for joint working between health and social services, and for them to collaborate for the benefit of patients and clients, joint health and social services audits are essential.

Nursing audit, according to Malby (1995, p. 12), 'differs from medical audit in one important aspect – it is used as a managerial function to evaluate the cost-effectiveness of nursing, as well as for the professional development of practice and education'.

Measurement is central to monitoring, evaluating and auditing. This is done either by organizations developing specific measurement scales and tools for their own needs or by using off-the-shelf quality measurement tools, or both. The important consideration for any measurement audit tool is that it should be reliable (i.e. accurate and consistent) and valid (i.e. it actually measures quality and achievement of standards). Off-the-shelf packages for nursing audit include QUALPACS (Wandelt & Ager

R|Я REFLECTIVE PRACTICE

2.3 Audit tools

Identify one audit tool that has been used in an area of practice that you have worked in, e.g. the Health Quality Service (previously known as King's Fund Organisational Audit), an educational audit or a patient satisfaction audit.

Student activities

- Find out what aspects of care provision, educational activities or patient satisfaction were being audited.
- For the audit you have chosen, list the criteria used to measure the achievement of quality care provision, effective educational provision or levels of patient satisfaction.
- Did the audit include both qualitative and quantitative criteria and measures?
- Identify why both qualitative and quantitative measures are necessary.
- If in your area no audit is used (or as an additional reflective practice activity), consider the various aspects of care in that area and identify one aspect that should be audited. Identify the criteria you would use to audit that aspect of practice.

⚖ ETHICAL ISSUES

2.2 When consumers and professionals disagree

Patients and their families often have great faith in certain treatments or drugs, especially if they believe a treatment has benefited them or someone they know in the past. The professional may well know that treatment to be ineffective, potentially dangerous and not justified, but the patient may still demand it, e.g. wanting antibiotics for the common cold. This can create conflicts and dilemmas.

Student activities

- Discuss which ethical principles (see Ethical Issues box 2.1) would support the patient's demand to receive the treatment.
- Discuss which ethical principles would support the professional's attempts to convince the patient that the treatment should not be given.

1974), the Phaneuf Nursing Audit (Phaneuf 1976) and Monitor (Goldstone et al 1983) (see Reflective Practice box 2.3). These nursing tools mainly audit a list of nursing care activities (e.g. giving hands-on care such as wound care) and related structure and process items (e.g. availability of skilled nurses and record-keeping). Not many patient outcomes are included in these tools. Patient outcomes, both quantitative and qualitative, should be audited in order that a more complete picture of the quality and effectiveness of nursing care can be seen.

Patient/carer feedback and satisfaction

The active involvement of patients and carers in evaluation of the health services is essential in ensuring that their needs are met and their rights guaranteed, and that they are satisfied with the standard of care they have received. Patients and carers as individuals or groups (e.g. the Patients Association, Carers UK) should be involved at all stages of quality assurance and quality enhancement, from agreeing standards of quality care and treatment to auditing. Feedback from patients and carers and patient/carer satisfaction questionnaires are commonly used to measure quality of care for audit purposes. The common and appropriate aspects that can be surveyed involve the quality of care they have received, activities of daily living issues, facilities and resources made available to them, whether their rights and need for privacy, confidentiality and dignity were met, effectiveness of communication with and interpersonal skills of nurses and other health care professionals, and other similar aspects. However, these types of survey should be planned carefully because of the potential unreliability of responses from patients who may be unwilling to give honest negative views because they may be afraid of staff reaction. They may feel that their care may suffer, or that they may be

considered awkward and difficult patients. It is best to ask for their opinions after their episode of treatment and care is over, e.g. following discharge from hospital or from a community nurse's caseload.

The usefulness of such feedback for auditing and improving services and care has led to an increase in the use of other means of gaining feedback. For example, patients' forums, pressure groups, citizens' panels and focus groups are regularly used to identify and highlight important issues to patients and carers, and often also to identify solutions and ways of improving services.

Joss & Kogan (1995) found that TQM helped the most in making patients' views on quality count. They state (p. 73) that 'there had been a significant shift from professional and technical definitions of quality towards "customer-oriented" views of quality'. This sort of shift is to be commended and encouraged. Empowering patients will enable them to have greater and more effective involvement in their care, leading to a higher quality of care (see Ethical Issues box 2.2). This is in line with TQM's customer-driven philosophy.

CONCLUSION: ACHIEVING STANDARDS

Clinical governance and evidence-based practice are now central to ensuring cost-effective quality care. Quality management in the UK NHS is dependent on using the principles and practices highlighted in this chapter, within the framework of clinical governance and evidence-based practice. Failure to do so is unacceptable, wasteful of resources, unprofessional and unethical.

This chapter, along with the vast amount of information available in the literature on quality, aims to help you achieve the highest possible standards of care, with which all stakeholders will be satisfied, i.e. patients and their unpaid carers (family and friends), health care professionals, providers and commissioners of care, and tax-payers. The other chapters in this book provide you with the evidence for good quality nursing practice for patients with specific disorders.

SUMMARY: MAIN POINTS

- Common features emerging from the many definitions of quality are helpful to nurses implementing quality care.

- Clinical governance can ensure quality care for patients and clients and NICE and CHI contribute to this effort. There is an important relationship between quality services and spending on resources and how nurses can contribute to efficiency.

- Benchmarking is an activity that contributes to improving nursing care.

- The NHS guide and BS 5750 can prove useful to quality nursing care if genuinely implemented.

- Managing change effectively is a necessary skill in quality management.

- Maxwell's dimensions of quality and Donabedian's structure–process–outcome model are two common examples of standard-setting frameworks. Standard-setting has a crucial function in the quality assurance spiral.

- There are many methods by which quality enhancement can be achieved, e.g. quality circles and quality improvement teams.

- Evidence-based nursing contributes to quality nursing care.

- Monitoring, evaluating and auditing of quality are also crucial to quality enhancement.

- Empowerment and education of staff and patients creates a culture in which achieving quality is facilitated.

SELF-TEST: CRITICAL THINKING ACTIVITIES

1 Choose one aspect of nursing care in your area of practice that you believe could be improved. Plan how you can achieve your aim using one of the quality enhancement approaches, e.g. a quality circle.

2 Find out from your place of work the policies, systems, structures and procedures that are in place to achieve clinical governance. Review these to draw your own conclusions about whether they are effective in doing so. Can you identify anything else that should be done?

 FURTHER READING

Clark JE, Copcutt L (eds). Management for nurses and health care professionals. New York: Churchill Livingstone; 1997.

Cooke H. The role of the patient in standard setting and audit. Br J Nurs 1994; 3(22): 1182–1188.

Dale BG (ed). Managing quality, 2nd edn. New York: Prentice Hall; 1994.

Harvey G. Relating quality assessment and audit to the research process in nursing. Nurs Res 1996; 3(3): 35–46.

Hogston R. Quality nursing care: a qualitative inquiry. J Adv Nurs 1995; 21: 116–124.

Irwin P, Fordham J. Evaluating the quality of care. Edinburgh: Churchill Livingstone; 1995.

Oakland JS. Total quality management: the route to improving performance, 2nd edn. Oxford: Butterworth Heinemann; 1993.

Morton-Cooper A, Bamford M (eds). Excellence in health care management. Oxford: Blackwell; 1997.

Mulhall A. Changing practice: the theory. NT monograph no 2. London: Emap Healthcare; 1999.

Parsley K, Corrigan P. Quality improvement in nursing and healthcare: a practical approach. London: Chapman and Hall; 1994.

Sale D. Quality assurance for nurses and other members of the health care team, 2nd edn. Basingstoke: Macmillan; 1996.

Swage T. Clinical governance in healthcare practice. Oxford: Butterworth-Heinemann; 2000.

Zwanenberg TV, Harrison J (eds). Clinical governance in primary care. Abingdon: Radcliffe Medical; 2000.

 USEFUL WEBSITES

www.rcn.org.uk – for many useful links.

www.york.ac.uk/inst/crd – NHS Centre for Reviews and Dissemination.

www.bsi-global.com – British Standards Institution.

www.cochrane.co.uk – The Cochrane Library.

www.hfht.org/chiq – Centre for Health Information Quality.

www.man.ac.uk/rcn – RCN Research and Development Coordinating Centre).

www.nmap.ac.uk – internet resources in nursing, midwifery and the allied health professions.

www.nice.org.uk – National Institute for Clinical Excellence.

www.chi.nhs.uk – Commission for Health Improvement.

www.nmc-uk.org – Nursing and Midwifery Council.

www.nelh.nhs.uk – for a vast range of information and links.

REFERENCES

Brooks F, Martin M, Pugh J. Shared governance as a way to involve staff in decision-making. Nurs Times 1998; 94(46): 56–57.

Close A. Quality management in health care and health care education. In Morton-Cooper A, Bamford M, eds. Excellence in health care management. Oxford: Blackwell; 1997, 75–112.

Camp RC. Benchmarking: the search for industry best practices that lead to superior performance. White Plains, NY: Quality Research; 1989.

Cohens G. What's wrong with hospitals? Harmondsworth: Penguin; 1964.

Department of Health. The patient's charter. London: HMSO; 1991.

Department of Health. The patient's charter. London: HMSO; 1995.

Department of Health (NHS Executive). Promoting clinical effectiveness – a framework for action in and through NHS. London: HMSO; 1996.

Department of Health. A first class service: quality in the new NHS. London: HMSO; 1998.

Department of Health. Clinical governance: quality in the new NHS. London: HMSO; 1999.

Department of Health, National Care Standards Commission (NCSC). Care homes for older people. 2001. Online. Available: www.doh.gov.uk/ncsc/carehomes.htm March 2001.

Donabedian A. Evaluating the quality of medical care. Millbank Fund Quarterly 1966; 44(2): 166–206.

Dunning M. Securing change: lessons from the PACE programme. Nurs Times 1998; 94(34): 51–52.

Ellis R, Whittington D. Quality assurance in health care: a handbook. London: Edward Arnold; 1993.

Glen S. The key to quality nursing care: towards a model of personal and professional development. Nurs Ethics 1998; 5(2): 95–102.

Goldstone LA, Ball JA, Collier MM. Monitor: an index of nursing care for acute medical and surgical wards. Newcastle-upon-Tyne: Newcastle upon Tyne Polytechnic; 1983.

Jackson P, Ashton D. Implementing quality through BS5750 (ISO 9000). London: Kogan Page; 1993.

Joss R, Kogan M. Advancing quality: total quality management in the National Health Service. Buckingham: Open University Press; 1995.

Koch T. A review of nursing quality assurance. J Adv Nurs 1992; 17: 785–794.

Kogan M, Redfern S. Making use of clinical audit: a guide to practice in the health professions. Buckingham: Open University Press; 1995.

Lam E. Benchmarking best practice. Nurs Times 1994; 90(46): 48–51.

Lewin K. Group decision and social change. In: Maccoby E, ed. Readings in social psychology. New York: Holt Rinehart and Wilson; 1958.

Lockett T. Evidence-based and cost-effective medicine. Oxford: Radcliffe Medical Press; 1997.

Malby R (ed). Clinical audit for nurses and therapists. London: Scutari Press; 1995.

Mason EJ. How to write meaningful standards of care, 3rd edn. Albany: Delmar; 1994.

Maxwell R. Quality assessment in health. Br Med J 1984; 288: 1470–1472

Morrell C, Harvey G, Kitson A. Practitioner based quality improvement: a review of the Royal College of Nursing's dynamic standard setting system. Qual Health Care 1997; 6(1): 29–34.

Nazarko L. A few home truths. Nurs Times 1997; 93(39): 74–76.

Nursing and Midwifery Council. Code of Professional Conduct. London: NMC; 2002

Oakland JS. Total quality management: the route to improving performance, 2nd edn. Oxford: Butterworth Heinemann; 1993.

Phaneuf M. The nursing audit. New York: Appleton-Century Crofts; 1976.

Plant R. Managing change and making it stick. London: Fontana; 1987.

Robb B. Sans everything: a case to answer. London: Nelson; 1967.

Royal College of Nursing. Towards standards. Report of a working party. London: RCN; 1981.

Royal College of Nursing. Quality patient care: the Dynamic Standard Setting System. Harrow: Scutari; 1990.

Royal College of Nursing. Clinical effectiveness: a Royal College of Nursing guide. London: RCN; 1996.

Sale D. Quality assurance: for nurses and other members of the health care team, 2nd edn. Basingstoke: Macmillan; 1996.

Scally G, Donaldson I. Clinical governance and the drive for quality improvement in the NHS in England. Br Med J 1998; 317: 61–65.

Smith S. Model behaviour. Nurs Manage 1998; 5(6): 19–24.

United Kingdom Central Council for Nursing, Midwifery and Health Visiting. Professional self-regulation and clinical governance. London: UKCC; 1999.

Wandelt M, Ager J. Quality patient care scale. New York: Appleton-Century Crofts; 1974.

Williams M. Benchmarking: simply the best. Br J Theatre Nurs 1998; 8(2): 19–24

3

Communication in adult nursing

Philippa Sully

'I knew my operation was pretty serious but I had no idea what to expect. So I was really scared. I was too scared to ask the doctor in case she thought I was stupid because I couldn't remember what they told me in the clinic. The nurse was really good, she listened to what I was worried about, explained everything and even came back when my daughter was there to see if she had any questions!'

(Patient)

THIS CHAPTER WILL HELP YOU

- Describe the elements of communication

- Discuss the importance of communication in professional nursing practice and the barriers to effective communication

- Examine the nature of therapeutic relationships

- Explore the effect that culture has on verbal and non-verbal communication

- Explain the differences between communication skills, counselling skills and counselling

- Explore the nature and value of professional boundaries and make simple working contracts

- Discuss the importance of active listening skills

- Explore the skills of dealing with bad news

- Relate the theory of communication within groups to your experiences of groups in professional practice

- Reflect upon your ability to apply the skills of effective communication to adult nursing practice.

KEYWORDS

Active listening	**Power in nursing**
Assertiveness	**Reflective practice**
Counselling	**Self-awareness**
Culture	**Teams**
Groups	**Therapeutic relationships**
Non-verbal communication	
Paralinguistics	**Verbal communication**

INTRODUCTION

The development of effective working relationships underpins all aspects of nursing practice. Whether we are exploring the best way to arrange shift cover or discussing with patients and their families the most appropriate community care, how we communicate depends on our professional relationships with all those involved.

Making, maintaining and ending professional relationships require a number of verbal and non-verbal skills. Those that form the foundations for effective communication and counselling skills are addressed in this chapter. The elements of communication – the sender, receiver and the message – and how these influence our relationships in professional practice will be explored. The reader is referred to the list in 'Further reading' for more information on specialist or advanced skills.

Skilled practitioners will continue to develop their communication skills throughout their careers, applying them flexibly and creatively. Self-awareness and reflection are integral to this process. Therefore the principle that underpins all aspects of the chapter is as follows: the way we communicate depends on the nature of the relationships we intend to make.

THE NATURE OF COMMUNICATION

We communicate much of who we are and our intentions when we approach situations without ever having to say anything. Our capacity as nurses to consciously observe people's demeanour is an essential skill. Alongside this skill of observation, we need to be aware of our own manner, as those around us can readily perceive this whether they are conscious of doing so or not. The process of communication can be described as a cycle comprising the following (Macmillan 1996) (see Fig. 3.1):

■ *History* – what both the sender and recipient bring to the encounter, consciously and unconsciously. This includes personal history, society's history and the individual's own history in society.
■ *Intention* – what the sender intends to communicate and what the recipient expects from the encounter. This, too, is both conscious and unconscious.
■ *Interaction* – how the sender gives the message and how the recipient perceives it. This includes the words chosen, the tone used and the body language. Unconscious intentions influence these choices and perceptions.
■ *Consequences* – these are a result of the interventions made and what impact they have on the participants. Senders may not be aware of the consequences they hoped to invoke. Likewise, recipients might respond to the message in ways of which they are unaware.

This model works well for verbal and non-verbal as well as conscious and unconscious processes of communication. We can observe much from other people's body language as well as the tone of voice. Likewise, we give away much about ourselves without necessarily intending to do so, i.e. unconsciously. We do this by our posture and the words we choose, e.g. by using words like 'tell' and 'demand' instead of 'ask'.

VERBAL COMMUNICATION

This can be defined as the language – written and spoken – which we use to convey information to others. The way in which we use language varies according to the situations we are in and with whom we are communicating. Sign language used by deaf people is verbal communication. As with any language, it has its own vernacular, social conventions and dialect.

The way we talk or write to people who are intimates in our personal lives is different from the way in which we communicate in a professional or formal relationship. In nursing practice we need to weigh our words – written or spoken – to ensure that they convey the meaning we intend (the 'intention' of the cycle).

When people are anxious or distressed, it is more likely that they will hear our message within a frame that is intimately personal and not necessarily from the perspective from which we intend. As nurses we need to choose carefully the language we use, in order to demonstrate some understanding of how the world may seem to the frightened, angry patient or the person in pain. This is where non-verbal communication – or body language – becomes so important.

NON-VERBAL COMMUNICATION

Non-verbal cues express our emotions, sense of occasion, status and sense of who we are and of whom we are relating to. How close (proximal) are we to those with whom we are making a relationship? Do they seem comfortable near us or do they move away? Each of us has a sense of the space around us. The parameters of this are arguably culturally determined, particularly in relation to gender, age and social status. The space around us has been described as (Grasha 1995):

■ *Intimate* – from bodily contact up to 18 inches. We allow only those most intimate to us this close, unless there are exceptional circumstances, such as when we have a professional relationship that crosses this space, as between nurse and patient
■ *Personal* – ranges from 18 inches to 4 feet. This is evident in small groups, such as at parties
■ *Social* – ranges from 4 to 12 feet and is evident in formal situations, such as interviews
■ *Public* – the area beyond 12 feet, such as giving a lecture or watching a sporting event.

Should others around us behave inappropriately within these parameters, our verbal and non-verbal responses will be very evident, although they vary between individuals. For example, if people enter our intimate space uninvited, we back away from them.

The importance of non-verbal cues is very clear in our use of idiom and metaphor. Phrases such as someone's handshake 'was like a wet fish' and 'we jumped for joy' convey sensual as well as linguistic messages. We can feel the handshake and visualize the joy.

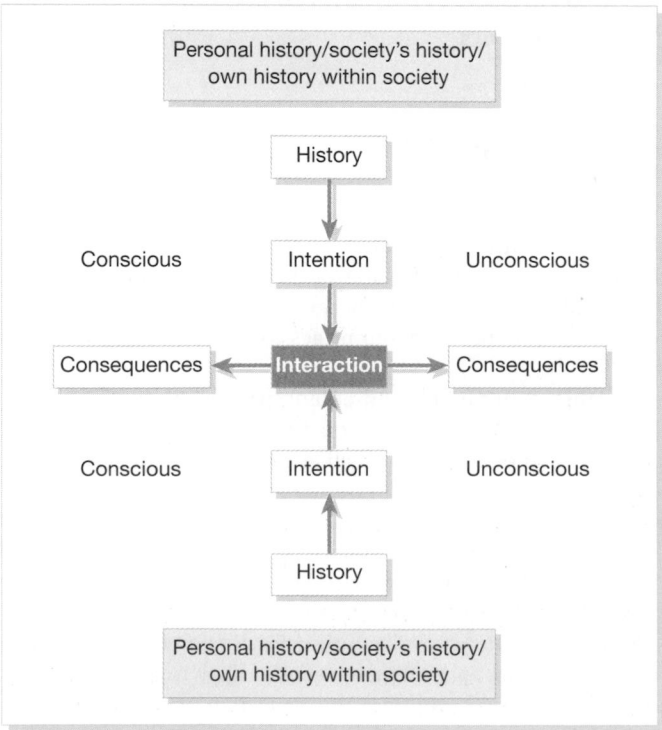

Figure 3.1 Macmillan model of communication. (Reproduced with kind permission from Macmillan 1996.)

How we look at each other, our gestures, facial expressions and frequency of eye contact express much more than words. How we present ourselves, e.g. our posture, dress, the way we move, whether we smile or shake hands on greeting, gives clues to others about who we are and how we might be feeling. The ways in which these cues are interpreted depends on a number of factors. They also vary in place, time and situation. For example, in some cultures it is rude to look your superior in the eye, while in others it is rude not to make eye contact with the person talking to you, regardless of status.

Nurses' uniforms are an integral part of the nursing profession's culture. This non-verbal cue gives a very clear identification of who we are and where we are in the hierarchy of the profession. It is also a mark of our status in wider society.

PARALINGUISTICS

Paralinguistics, the tone and pitch of our voice and the emphasis we put on words or phrases, also convey meanings. The variety of accents and regional phrases also adds richness and colour to our heritage of language, whatever languages we speak. However, this can be confusing to those who are not familiar with them. How paralinguistics are used and interpreted can also be influenced by other factors, as discussed below. Conscious and unconscious communication and shared and different psychological defences can be manifest in our paralinguistics as well as our verbal and non-verbal cues.

FACTORS INFLUENCING COMMUNICATION

From the discussion above, it is clear that the messages we give and receive are influenced by a number of factors. Whaley & Wong (1991) identify these as:

- perceptions – how we view others' appearance, behaviour or status. For example, we might automatically think all consultants are men
- values – e.g. whether we think nurses on duty should chew gum
- development – e.g. an older person is at a different developmental stage than a teenager and life experiences will influence how they communicate
- personal space – the distance between the nurse and the patient. Close proximity can feel comforting or threatening
- emotions – our feelings at the time of the interaction
- sociocultural background – e.g. our personal upbringing will influence how we introduce ourselves
- knowledge – our understanding of the issue we are dealing with
- roles and relationships – e.g. if we are talking to a colleague we are likely to use different language from that used when talking to partners or children
- environment – where the interaction takes place will affect how we conduct ourselves and how we communicate our message. Noise and lack of privacy can make it difficult to hear and understand what someone is telling us.

Whenever we meet people, whether for the first time or whether they are old acquaintances, these factors will influence our communication and thus the nature of the relationship we make. In nursing practice, when we meet clients or colleagues, the impression or the verbal message we intend to give will influence our intervention, how it is received and the consequences. Therefore, it is important to give some thought to how, when, where and with whom we are communicating and what relationship we intend to make with them.

BARRIERS TO EFFECTIVE COMMUNICATION

These can be divided into three different sources which overlap and are closely linked to the factors that influence communication:

- those originating from within ourselves, e.g. our age, race, social class, gender, feelings, culture, any disabilities, physical state or experiences of similar encounters
- those originating from within others, e.g. how other people perceive us, their ages, races, genders, cultures, any disability such as hearing loss, expectations of us and the situation
- those originating in the environment, e.g. the situation in which the encounter is taking place, extraneous noise, temperature, whether it is private or public space and whose space it is.

If we are aware of our inner and outer worlds, we are more able to avoid or minimize barriers to our making effective professional (and personal) relationships. Nursing takes place in a multitude of environments, including the street. How all those involved in the processes of care experience it will depend on how they feel in the environment in which care is being delivered or discussed.

Nelson-Jones (1990) highlights the importance of being accepting of others in order to communicate and thus deliver care or work effectively with them as colleagues. He identifies the barriers to an accepting attitude as:

- strong feelings
- trigger words and phrases
- unfinished business
- anxiety-evoking topics
- prejudice
- anxiety-evoking people
- anxiety-evoking situations
- bringing the past into the present (also known as *transference*)
- information different from your own self-picture
- physical barriers.

The barriers to effective communication are closely linked with the factors that may lead us to be rigid and unaccepting of others. These also apply to other people's attitudes towards us.

CULTURE AND COMMUNICATION

Conscious and unconscious processes are integral to the ways in which we communicate (see Fig. 3.1). As members of different social and professional groups, we learn both conscious and unconscious ways of communicating, as these are inherent in our group cultures.

SPECIAL ISSUES

3.1 Self-awareness

Think about your cultural background.

- Considering your language use, dress and tone of voice, how were you encouraged to relate to:

  — the religious leader(s) in your local community, e.g. the priest, mullah and/or rabbi
  — the person who delivers your post
  — your neighbours
  — your teacher in primary school
  — your school friends
  — your work colleagues?

- What differences did you notice in the ways in which you behaved towards these members of your community?
- What might be the reasons for this?
- What themes do you notice in your answers?

DEFINITION OF CULTURE

Culture has been defined as (Helman 1990, p. 2):

> A set of guidelines (both explicit and implicit) which individuals inherit as a member of a particular society and which tells them how to view the world, how to experience it emotionally and how to behave in it in relation to other people, to supernatural gods and to the natural environment. It provides them with a way of transmitting these guidelines to the next generation by use of symbols, language, art and ritual.

(See Special Issues box 3.1.)

CULTURE IN NURSING

It is evident, from the definition of culture given above, that culture influences all aspects of human life – everything from religious beliefs to the colours we favour and the manner in which we greet each other. The purpose of this section is to explore the significance of culture in professional nursing practice. To consider culture from a broader perspective, you might find it helpful to examine specialist psychology and sociology texts (e.g. Billington et al 1991, Hayes 1994).

The culture of the profession in the West is influenced by nursing's origins in military service and Christian religious orders. It is arguable that the significance of uniform and hierarchy, which are integral to nursing culture, has its origins there. Likewise, when we are dealing with life-changing circumstances as part of our everyday practice, it is important that we know where we stand – as is evident from our uniform and place in the hierarchy – and to whom we can turn for guidance. It is important, too, for our clients and patients to be able to identify us, e.g. when we visit them at home. Thus our professional culture informs us implicitly or explicitly about how we should behave as nurses; it also influences how we are received by others, i.e. the professional relationships we make.

As culture influences all aspects of our lives, it therefore influences our unconscious perceptions of others. We may choose a metaphor to describe something and yet be totally unaware that it is offensive to the listener who is from a different culture.

Likewise, culture and how we use different words for the same thing, such as euphemisms, e.g. 'spend a penny' (to pass urine) or 'passed on' (meaning someone has died), can lead to confusion and misunderstanding (see the section on 'Explanation skills').

The use of jargon or technical terms is a way of making our status and profession known. Nurses may discuss a client's treatment by saying, 'Jason Cooper has been admitted for 24-hours obs'. If Mr Cooper overhears this, he might well be concerned about what 'obs' are. Jargon and technical terms are also tools for keeping our distance and excluding others. Patients often ask nurses to explain their diagnosis and treatment. If we use technical terms to cover our discomfort at having to talk about sensitive issues, such as the effect surgery might have on someone's sexual relationship, patients and relatives may feel they are being kept at a distance and unable to ask us to describe exactly what we mean.

Uniform is an integral part of nursing culture and acts as a boundary and a barrier. As a boundary, its formality can be helpful to clients and nurses; it can set the scene where a client might feel embarrassed or vulnerable when receiving care that feels intrusive. As a barrier, it can set us at an unreachable distance, so that people in distress 'don't want to bother the Sister who has so many responsibilities'.

One of the great benefits of nursing in the UK is the opportunity to meet many people from a variety of racial, cultural and religious backgrounds. At the heart of our professional culture is the belief that all people are equally precious and entitled to the best care we can offer, regardless of their circumstances. It is important, therefore, that we address the significance of culture in its broadest sense in nursing practice. In order to respect culture, we need to celebrate differences between people (see Reflective Practice box 3.1 and Special Issues box 3.2).

R|Я REFLECTIVE PRACTICE

3.1 Caring for people from different cultures

Reflect on your experiences of working with clients, patients and colleagues who have different cultures from your own, and address the following questions.

List the different cultures you have come across in practice:

- How were these cultural differences manifested?
- Why is it important for us as practitioners to be aware of cultural differences among those with whom we work?
- How did you think, feel and act when you were required to enter into a professional relationship with clients, patients and/or colleagues where you were aware of cultural differences?

SPECIAL ISSUES

3.2 Helping people feel special

Joseph Myandu is a new patient on your ward. He is an African aged 45 and has come in for emergency surgery. You are asked to admit him. You are aware that he is far away from his home and family. He comes to the hospital unaccompanied.

Consider the following:

- How do you greet him?
- What can you do to help him feel at ease?
- How do envisage your professional relationship developing?
- What reasons can you give for your choice of interventions?
- What consequences do you hope to achieve by the language and non-verbal cues you choose?

THE THERAPEUTIC RELATIONSHIP IN NURSING PRACTICE

When we look at the realities of nursing practice, we might sometimes feel that we are being asked to be all things to all people. Clearly, however much we want to help people, whatever their circumstances, we can't take on everything that comes our way. Indeed, it would be inappropriate to think that we could. Moreover, to do so is often not in the best interests of those who are requesting it. This section will examine how best we can fulfil our professional responsibilities without being overwhelmed by the demands life places on those for whom we care professionally, and thus the demands that nursing places on us.

The care we give patients and clients depends on the type of professional relationships we make with them. These relationships are founded on the ways in which we communicate with those in our care and those with whom we share the duty of care, such as members of the multidisciplinary health care team. Our capacity to use language and non-verbal cues influences positively or negatively the development of these relationships, which form the essential foundations for our professional practice.

NURSES AND POWER

In your reflective exercise on culture (Reflective Practice box 3.1), when you considered your relationships with members of your community, you may have identified social differences in power. Nursing puts us in a very privileged and powerful position. Much of what we do or say, because of our role, crosses normal social constraints. This makes us very powerful. How we exert that power depends on our commitment to ethical practice in general, and to the nature of any given working relationship in particular.

Box 3.1 lists the different types of power identified by Grasha (1995). Nurses may have all six types of power. Awareness of this will help practitioners think carefully about the purpose of their working relationships, what their intentions are when they communicate with others, and in what context.

Box 3.1 Sources of social power and influence (adapted from Grasha 1995; see also Raven 1992)

- *Expert power.* This is based on personal knowledge and expertise that others do not have to the same degree, e.g. expert skills in health care and nursing practice
- *Information power.* This is based on having information needed to be able to develop logical and/or persuasive arguments on why certain actions should be taken, e.g. nurses hold privileged information about those in their care and can also withhold information if they choose
- *Referrant power.* This is based on the ability to support and nurture others and the degree to which the person appeals to others. This is fostered by the values represented by the person and his/her role, e.g. compassion and nurture are integral to nursing practice – consequently, patients can feel very grateful and thus beholden to those who have cared for them
- *Legitimate power.* This is derived from the formal position one holds within the group, e.g. nurses' social standing gives them specific privileges and power
- *Reward power.* This is based on the ability to dispense rewards, e.g. money, positive feedback – nurses can give or withhold positive feedback to patients or disallow shifts a colleague may have requested
- *Coercive power.* This is based on the ability to impose sanctions on others, e.g. qualified nurses can refuse to pass a student nurse, or patients can be moved to a different part of the ward if the nurses find their behaviour 'difficult'

The English language has many phrases or metaphors that deride older people, e.g. calling someone 'a sour old maid' or 'dirty old man'. Older adults are often infantilized by terms of purported endearment, e.g. calling people old enough to be our grandparents names like 'sweetie' or 'darling' or using their first names without their consent. By being overfamiliar we diminish the older person's status in relation to us. In Western societies, the esteem in which older adults are held (their value) is reflected in the fact that they are not viewed as wise or as people who have enriched society (see Older Adults: Nursing Priorities box 3.1).

A MODEL OF HELPING

The purpose of any helping interview is to enable clients or patients to have a greater awareness of their difficulties and thus help themselves. A number of writers, e.g. Culley (1991) and Egan (1998), have described the helping process as occurring over three stages. The first stage is where clients explore the situation as it is with their helper; the second stage is where the helper explores how clients would prefer their circumstances to be, and what is hindering their capacity to change these circumstances; and the third stage is where clients are helped to find ways to move on and achieve their desired outcomes (Egan 1998).

Throughout any interview with patients or clients, it is important to be aware of their physical state and the situation they are in. It is important not to expect very sick or breathless

OLDER ADULTS: NURSING PRIORITIES

3.1 Power and nursing attitudes to the elderly

Mr Michael Urquart is 78. He was involved in a road traffic accident and is in your orthopaedic ward. At report one morning, you hear a colleague describe him as 'the little old chap in the side bay'. You know he is almost 6 feet tall and that, up until his accident, he was organizing the fixtures and keeping the books of the bowls team at the local sports club. When you go in to greet him, you notice he has a towel tucked around his neck, his unfinished breakfast is pushed away from him and his personal pyjamas are in his locker. He is wearing a theatre gown but he is not scheduled for any investigations. He seems subdued and is not his usual optimistic self.

- What does your colleague's language tell you of her ideas about older people?
- How much control over his environment and situation does Mr Urquart have? Consider the non-verbal cues described.
- How do you perceive power to have been used in the nurse–patient relationship?
- What would you do to demonstrate respect for Mr Urquart and to help him have more control over his care?

patients to give lengthy explanations. Rather, choose a carefully worded, closed question, or one which is open but very specifically focused.

THE NURSE–CLIENT RELATIONSHIP

Without a sense of who we are, in relation to those to whom we offer nursing care, and what we might represent for them, we are at risk of behaving inappropriately. If we say or do something inappropriate, we may influence our working, or therapeutic, relationship by causing a withdrawal of collaboration or trust, or at worst causing deep offence (see Reflective Practice box 3.2).

REFLECTIVE PRACTICE

3.2 What sort of nurse do I want to be?

This exercise can be revisited throughout your career, so it is worth recording it in your reflective journal. Write down your answers to the following question: what sort of nurse do I want to be? Think about this in the context of three themes: attitudes, knowledge and skills.

When you have finished, you may find you have learned something new about yourself or, alternatively, clarified what you were aware of but had never put into words. Whatever the situation, this exercise is about your awareness of who you are and what attributes you would like to develop and bring to nursing practice.

	Known to self	Not known to self
Known to others	**Open area** (our 'public self': the person we and others see)	**Blind area** (our 'blind self': aspects of ourselves others can see but we cannot)
Not known to others	**Hidden area** (our 'private self': aspects of ourselves we are aware of but choose not to disclose to others)	**Unknown area** ('unconcious self': unknown to others and to ourselves)

Figure 3.2 The Johari window. (Adapted from Luft 1969.)

Self-awareness

To every reflective process we bring the 'self, critical thought and action' (Benner 2000). So, starting with who we are is a sound place from which to consider what we bring to our professional relationships and how we communicate within them. Awareness of who we are and what attributes we have enables us to use effectively our lived experience and our talents in our development as professional practitioners. Who we are is where we start from in our professional relationships and practice. How we see ourselves and how others see us are described by the Johari window (Luft 1969) (see Fig. 3.2).

The more we learn new skills, listen to feedback and notice how others respond to what we offer in our relationships – both professional and personal – the more we are able to use our knowledge, skills and attitudes appropriately. We can therefore choose to use our 'private' self in public and reduce the likelihood of our 'blind' and 'unconscious' selves negatively influencing our development as nurses.

Revisit your answers to the exercise in Reflective Practice box 3.2 and see whereabouts in the Johari window you would put your responses. For example, you might not have realized that you wanted to be an assertive as well as a caring nurse. In this situation, part of your unknown self, i.e. 'unconscious' in your communication with yourself, became 'conscious' and available for you to use in your dealings with others.

The more we know about ourselves and who we are, the more we are able to use our talents in the pursuits that matter to us, i.e. in our lifelong development as nurses. Wright (1992) describes self-awareness as having three aspects:

- self-concept – which develops as a consequence of our processing of other people's responses to us and our view of ourselves and our life experiences
- values and beliefs – these are learned and they influence all we do; culture has a strong influence on our values and beliefs and can lead to stereotyping and prejudice
- life-given experiences – how these influence us at any time, and how we deal/have dealt with difficulties and problems, affect how we respond to others; therefore it is important for us to recognize issues which are significant to us

How those in our care perceive us depends on the histories they bring to the relationship. This is likely to be influenced by the factors which are listed above but also by their personal cultural expectations of nurses, their unique experiences of being dependent, cared for or not when they are vulnerable, and the responses they expect from those around them when they are distressed. Often we are unaware of the expectations we have of others, i.e. these are unconscious, so our patients and clients might not realize that their behaviour seems inappropriate to us within the nurse–client relationship. A recurrent example of this is patients alluding to nurses being sexy or sexually available.

The helping relationship

The essential conditions of helping relationships are defined by Rogers (1957) as empathy or accurate empathic understanding, acceptance or unconditional positive regard, and openness and genuineness. Without these conditions being present, he argues, those in our care cannot be helped to deal with their distress. They are defined as follows:

- empathy or accurate empathic understanding – the demonstration of understanding of other people's thoughts, feelings and experiences from their point of view. This is achieved by being genuine and respectful and through the appropriate use of active listening skills
- acceptance or unconditional positive regard – an attitude that other people are valuable because they are human. It is demonstrated by the use of active listening skills and is essential in any therapeutic relationship
- openness and genuineness – being with other people as you are, without playing a role or adopting a stance that is alien to you.

It is by demonstrating these core conditions that we offer support to others, allowing them their experiences without the imposition of our perspective. The nurse–client relationship is a professionally intimate one. In order to be effective, it needs to reflect the above factors as well as trust, caring or love, hope, autonomy and mutuality (Sundeen et al 1998). In order to build these relationships, we need to consider the communication skills we use and what effect they will have. We need to explore how we can use communication skills –verbal, non-verbal and paralinguistic – to develop the relationships we intend to make.

PERSONALITY THEORIES AND COMMUNICATION

As we explore the nature of communication within our professional relationships, it will become evident that how we regard people and the way we learn to make, maintain and end relationships of all sorts depend on the values and beliefs we hold about human beings, the ways in which we develop and learn to relate to one another.

There are three main theoretical frameworks in the psychology of the nature of personality: conflict, fulfilment and consistency theories. They offer explanations about how we develop, behave socially, the nature of our inner lives and what motivates us to behave as we do (Maddi 1989). Each school of thought is underpinned by different value systems; for example, Freudian

theory is sometimes described as regarding human beings as 'sad, bad and mad'. All these models identify the importance of motivation and how we respond to situations in the light of previous experience and current demands. Clear sets of values therefore underpin these theories of who we are and why we behave the way we do.

Values are also inherent in our motivation to become nurses, as well as part of the culture we enter into when we join the profession. The fact that these values might differ from those of the people we care for, or work alongside, can be a cause of communication difficulties. In order to deal with the stress this causes, as well as the stress of situations that put us in touch with the immediacy of life, human distress and death, we use psychic defences which are unconscious. These are particularly important when others in our care are relying on us to help them cope with the situation.

Sigmund Freud identified unconscious defences such as denial, projection and rationalization as means of dealing with the anxiety that arises out of the conflicts that exist between our instincts and the demands of society. These defences can be observed in our own and others' behaviour and can also be shared by groups of people, e.g. professions (Obholzer & Roberts 1994). As nurses, it is important that we are aware of our own means of defending ourselves from the conflicts precipitated by the demands of our work, as well as being able to recognize in our patients and colleagues when their (or our) defences might be influencing our capacity to communicate effectively with them. An example of a defence against the anxiety of not being able to relieve patients' distress is when we do things like fill shelves instead of comforting a distressed patient, or when we say that we 'don't have time' to sit with patients. We always make time to deal with major care priorities but we cannot relieve every discomfort (see Reflective Practice box 3.3).

The responses in the exercise in Reflective Practice box 3.3 all demonstrate the following:

- a set of values
- some ideas of what motivates people
- some ideas of the influences of culture, society and loving/supportive relationships.

If you argued that you don't make assumptions because everyone is different, that too is an assumption, based on the value that everyone is unique and therefore it is best not to categorize them. All these responses also imply where we as nurses

R|Я REFLECTIVE PRACTICE

3.3 Values and assumptions

The importance of being self-aware is discussed in the text. The essential ingredient we bring to all nursing relationships is ourselves. In order to clarify some of your values about people, it is worth considering the following question: what assumptions do you make about people's ability to solve their own problems?

Write down your answers. You may then like to discuss the exercise with your supervisor or a friend.

R|Я   REFLECTIVE PRACTICE

3.4 Personality and self-awareness

Look at your responses to the exercise on values and assumptions (Reflective Practice box 3.3). What consistent themes run through your ideas of what sort of nurse you want to be and the ideas you have of people's self-efficacy as identified here? How do they relate to the different personality theories?

You might find that you have thoughts and values that match all of them or you may believe that essentially people develop and are motivated by one school of thought, e.g. human beings are motivated to reach their full potential and circumstances in living might intervene to inhibit this life force – in which case you would hold the values of the humanistic psychologists. There are no right or wrong answers, only views or perspectives.

Now return to the Johari window (Fig. 3.2). Look at each of the four aspects of yourself – your open, hidden, blind and unknown areas. Have any of these areas opened wider? You might have learned something new about yourself, making an aspect of your blind and/or unknown areas open like a window. An example might be that, until you did this exercise, you had not realized you held a particular view of humanity. Now that you are aware of this, your unknown self may have diminished a bit and your view of your hidden self may be clearer, sharper, or indeed your concept of yourself may have been reassuringly reconfirmed.

might be in relation to those in our care because of the expertise we have (Reflective Practice box 3.4). These values and beliefs will influence how we use language, how we perceive people's responses to us and how we work with them. The rest of this chapter will address the skills we need to communicate effectively and how these are determined by the nature of the relationships we intend to make such as with colleagues, clients and other carers.

COMMUNICATION AND COUNSELLING SKILLS

The relationships between communication skills, counselling skills and counselling are well illustrated in Figure 3.3. The hierarchy also illustrates the direct link between training, increased self-awareness for client and practitioner and the purpose of these skills. Clients and patients can also be helped to become more self-aware, and thus make more informed choices, when nurses use counselling skills appropriately.

COMMUNICATION SKILLS

The purpose of communication skills is to make social contact. They are fundamental to all professional practice. How we use them will depend on the relationships we intend to make with others and what we want to convey to them.

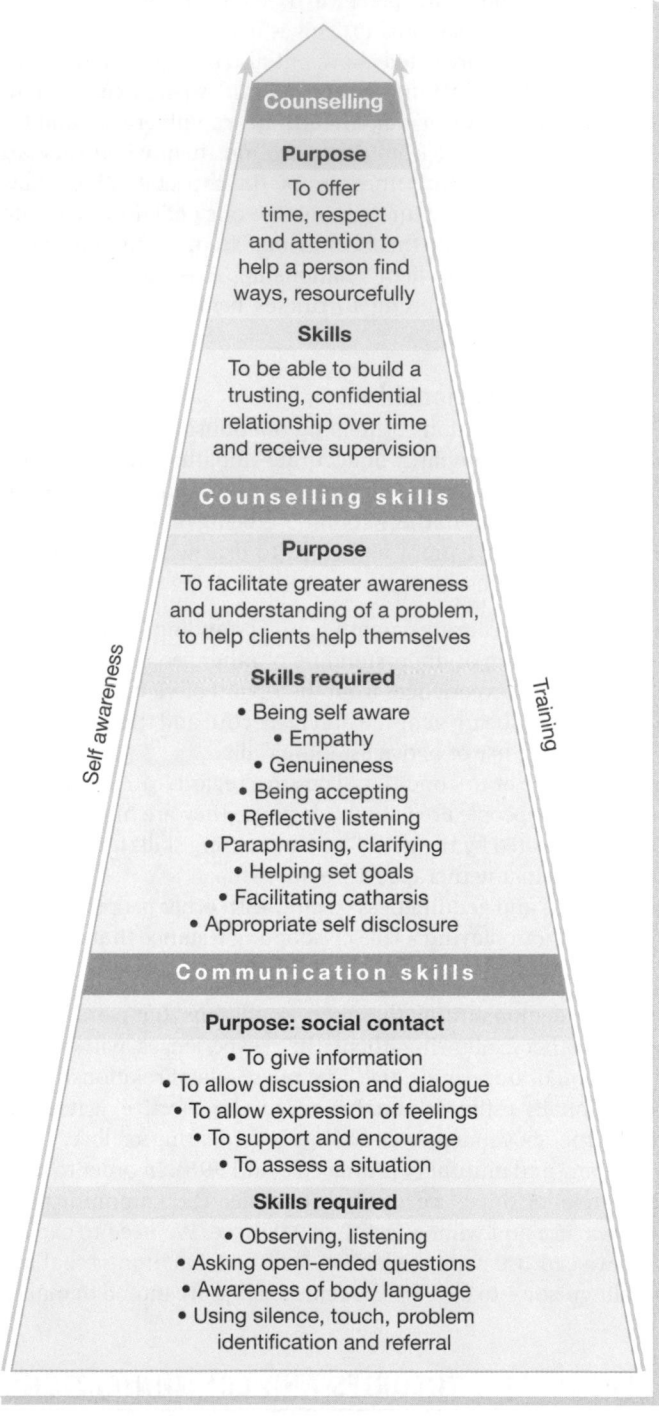

Figure 3.3 Communication skills, counselling skills and counselling. (Adapted from Clark & Jesson 1991.)

COUNSELLING SKILLS

Practitioners in a variety of disciplines or situations use counselling skills. They are used to enable clients to have a greater awareness of their strengths and difficulties and so be able help themselves. Nurses often use counselling skills in their practice but this does not make them counsellors.

COUNSELLING

Egan (2002, p. 43) describes as 'collaborative' the process of the helping (or counselling – writer's parenthesis) relationship. Its purpose is to enable clients, by means of this exclusive relationship, to grow and achieve outcomes they choose for themselves. Nurses who are counsellors are most likely to have had extra training, obtaining a recognized counselling qualification; they usually receive regular supervision for their case work and often agree to abide by a code of ethics for counsellors, such as that published by the British Association for Counselling and Psychotherapy.

If we consider the issues that influence how we are perceived and how we perceive ourselves in relation to others, it is possible for us to use communication and counselling skills to enable those with whom we work to collaborate with us, and ideally to trust us. We will also be able to set limits, or boundaries, on what we are able and willing to do, in order to fulfil our responsibilities as professional practitioners.

BOUNDARIES

Boundaries not only set limits on behaviour, but also contain behaviour, just as a jar holds honey and prevents it from spilling and being spoiled or wasted. Similarly, professional boundaries enable us to focus on the primary tasks of nursing practice and prevent other influences from distracting us from our roles and responsibilities.

Boundaries enable clients and patients to know what they can expect from nurses and others who care for them. They are a means of ensuring professionals practise ethically, within the law and within their own specialist areas. In this way, nurses can take on or refuse duties and can clarify their roles in relation to other practitioners as well as their clients, in order to ensure safe practice. Because boundaries define the extent and limits of professional practice, nurses need to be sure of their own individual skills and limits, what they can deal with themselves and what needs to be referred to others.

In professional practice, boundaries are manifest explicitly as well as implicitly. An explicit boundary is uniform: it makes clear the status of the nurse both within the ward and in wider society. An implicit boundary is one which practitioners in a team adhere to but which they have probably never discussed. An example is the practice of never using doctors' first names in front of patients, although nurses' first names are used. This implies that there is a different status for doctors and nurses and there are limits to the informality in all these professional relationships (see Guidelines box 3.1).

Uniform and hierarchy also provide boundaries, in the way they identify who people are in relation to each other. However, these are also examples of implicit boundaries because they are not necessarily negotiated and the rules of how the relationships are conducted are not always clear or consistent.

In order to use professional boundaries effectively, so they are helpful and containing, we need to be aware of them, their value and be able to communicate them clearly to others. When people have a clear idea of what to expect from each other, they are in a better position to choose for themselves, discuss options and, if necessary, negotiate to get their needs met. Patients who are

GUIDELINES FOR CARE PRIORITIES

3.1 Professional boundaries

- Self-awareness – of feelings, actions, thoughts and limitations to our own role and abilities
- The ability to negotiate explicit working contracts which include the limits to the relationship, e.g. confidentiality, personal responsibility, time and possibly place of work
- Assertive language skills, e.g. making 'I' statements
- Setting and keeping to time limits, e.g. stating the time and duration of a home visit and keeping to this arrangement
- Observation of process skills, e.g. stating what you observe is happening or has happened in a given situation
- Active listening and immediacy skills (addressing the here and now)
- Empathy, as opposed to identification, with other people and their situation. This means being alongside someone in distress but not allowing your own intense feelings, evoked by the situation, to confuse your thoughts and actions
- Problem-solving and decision-making skills
- Effective use of professional supervision in which constructive feedback and support can be sought and given
- Skills in leaving the issue behind, e.g. choosing to do so, changing clothes, leaving the place where the issues are dealt with, changing activities then or later.

very frightened and unsure of who is going to care for them will be reassured to be told who the allocated nurses are and what their responsibilities will be. This can be seen as an informal contract, which helps patients' anxieties to be contained, as they have specific points of reference, such as an individual practitioner or relevant information (verbal or written), to which they may turn. Guidelines box 3.1 lists some of the skills we need to do this.

This list is not meant to be comprehensive but focuses on the skills more specifically related to this aspect of helping relationships. In order to use these skills effectively, they are best demonstrated within relationships where the practitioners are respectful and accepting, warm and genuine, both to those with whom they work and to themselves.

COMMUNICATION AND SOCIAL CONTACT

The skills we use to make social contact are those of greeting and leave-taking, questioning, explaining, assertiveness, active listening, reporting and referring. Our non-verbal messages of gesture, facial expression, proximity, touch and self-presentation can all be used to enhance our verbal skills.

GREETING SKILLS

When we initiate therapeutic relationships, there is a series of processes we need to go through to do this effectively (Nelson-Jones 1982). These may be summarized as follows:

- introductions – 'meeting, greeting, seating'
- presenting concerns – enabling patients to tell us what concerns them, such as worries about investigations that may identify that they have cancer
- reconnaissance – exploring the issue(s) in a wider context and clarifying details or issues
- contracting
- summarizing and agreeing goals
- agreeing a contract of working
- termination – clarifying practical details and parting, e.g. at the end of a shift or when the patient leaves the clinic.

ACTIVE LISTENING SKILLS

The acquisition, application and evaluation of information is essential to nursing practice. In order to acquire information from other people or situations we need a range of skills.

Listening skills

When we consider the value of the information we receive, we perceive it through our own processes, i.e. where we are in the situation. It is therefore important that we start from ourselves. On listening to and questioning ourselves, we gain clues that raise our awareness to what might be going on in any given situation. We can also learn more about our own responses and the responses of others to us. Here it might be helpful to refer to the Johari window (Fig. 3.2) to review how self-awareness can be described and developed. We also question ourselves when we read and review written information such as research or nursing reports. The most commonly used active listening skills are described below.

Paraphrasing

This means repeating concisely in your own words what you have understood. Paraphrasing is often used to demonstrate empathy, to encourage the other person to explore certain issues and to clarify understanding – both one's own and the other person's. Consider, for example, the following exchange:

Client: 'When I came to outpatients I didn't expect to see the consultant, so when I was taken to her room I knew something was wrong. I knew something terrible had happened and I was right. She told me I had cancer.'

Nurse: 'As you weren't expecting to see the consultant, when you were taken to see her you knew something was terribly wrong and she told you then you had cancer.'

Reflecting

This means acting as a mirror for other people by restating their phrases or describing their non-verbal cues. The purpose is to enable the person to feel heard and encouraged to continue to talk, but it can also be a way of offering a different perspective. As such, it can be intrusive and needs to be used with caution. Consider the following:

Client: 'I am hurt by what my girlfriend said.'

Nurse: (gently and encouragingly) 'You're feeling hurt by what she said.'

Clarifying

This is the skilful use of paraphrasing, preferably without questions or with open-focused ones, in order to enable other people to have a clearer idea of what their issue or difficulty is. Consider the following:

Client: 'I am angry about what happened, because if I'd been told Janice was already in the ward I wouldn't have wasted all that time hanging about in accident and emergency. I could have gone straight up to her.'

Nurse: 'You're angry because you wasted time waiting in the wrong place when you could have been with Janice.'

Client: 'You see, don't you? If someone had told me, I wouldn't have felt so helpless and out of it, you know. I could have been supporting her.'

Nurse: 'If you'd been with her, you would have felt you were able to be there for her and not so helpless.'

Client: 'Yes, I felt so helpless you see, and there she was ... it was awful.' (*weeps*)

Nurse: 'You felt helpless and it was awful for you.'

Client: (*nods*) 'Yes, that's it really, it was awful for me, too, and I felt so helpless.'

Summarizing

Summarizing is drawing together the salient points of an interview into a short statement. Some uses are to enable reflection during a difficult interaction, to demonstrate empathy and to wind up an interview before leave-taking, e.g.:

Nurse: 'Not being able to be with Janice in the ward, supporting her when you could have been, has emphasized how helpless and awful you feel about her illness.'

Silence

The effective use of silence demonstrates respect by 'being with' other people, e.g. when they have just been given bad news. It also allows room for the expression of feelings and for reflection.

Self-disclosure

This is an effective use of offering one's own perspective on another person's situation, with the aim of demonstrating sincerity and empathy, or raising the person's awareness to another viewpoint. However, inappropriate use of this skill can feel intrusive and, indeed, can move the focus away from the client to the helper.

Self-awareness

Being aware of our thoughts, feelings and behaviour, such as tone of voice, during an interview can inform us about other levels of communication which may be going on and which are not necessarily verbal (see section on 'Self-awareness', p. 44).

QUESTIONING SKILLS

Skilful questioning enables the other person to feel valued and to disclose relevant information. Questions can be used to challenge a particular viewpoint and also to move an interview on. Nurses have a social standing which enables them to ask potentially intimate and intrusive questions. Therefore it is important that we look at how and why we use questions. The effective use of questions is a powerful communication skill. Practitioners might find them useful when they:

- need more specific information
- hope to encourage others to contribute to or participate in the situation
- want to demonstrate respect for others' opinions
- want to demonstrate empathy
- are assessing the extent of a client's or colleague's knowledge
- hope to direct attention to particular feelings or behaviour
- need to clarify the understanding they or others have
- want to test the accuracy of their perceptions.

The above examples (Lewars M 2000, personal communication) show that asking the right question at the right time can be very powerful, with significant consequences for some or all of the people involved in the transaction. Questioning skills are essential to the active listening process (see Reflective Practice box 3.5). There are a number of different types of questions.

Closed questions

These are valuable where there is only a very specific answer, such as 'yes' or 'it's 6 o'clock'. They are also useful if the patient is very breathless or weak, as closed questions only require short answers. However, they can be experienced as controlling by recipients, as only limited answers are required and they are not given the opportunity to discuss their experiences, e.g. during history-taking.

Open questions

These are useful for exploring issues and seeking a wider picture. There are no specific answers, e.g. 'How do you feel about the results of your tests?'.

Open focused questions

These are useful if you wish to focus on particular experiences or feelings, e.g. 'What were your reasons for choosing to make that decision?'.

 REFLECTIVE PRACTICE

3.5 Questioning skills

Think of a recent situation when you wanted information from someone.

- Who was the person?
- What was your relationship with the person?
- How did you go about acquiring the information?
- What communication skills did you use?

Think about the verbal and non-verbal skills you used, such as the choice of language and whether or not you made an appointment to see the person. How successful were you in learning what you wanted to know? Identify what helped and hindered the transaction, e.g. time, place, who, how, what you wanted to know and the overall context of the situation.

Multiple questions

The following is an example of multiple questioning: 'What was your reason for postponing your visit to Mrs Grainger? When will you be going to see her and have you considered other priorities for her care?' These questions give recipients so many options for a reply that they might become confused or indeed choose not to answer any of them. Multiple questions enable people to avoid answering specifically. This can be to the detriment of third parties such as patients or their relatives.

Disguised advice

An example of disguised advice is as follows: 'Have you considered eating more fruit and vegetables?'. Questions like these imply the course of action the questioner thinks should be followed but may be regarded as somewhat manipulative, because the intention is to give advice without saying so explicitly.

Leading questions

A leading question is one which may lead a recipient towards the answer the questioner wants to hear, such as: 'You're feeling relieved about the postponement of your treatment, aren't you Mr Blackman?'. Such questions may be regarded by recipients as an attempt to control them, i.e. to make them say 'the right thing'.

Rhetorical questions

These do not require a response in the sense of an answer and are often asked when people are in acute distress. e.g. 'Why did it have to happen to my child?'. The caring response here would be words recognizing the parent's distress rather than a philosophical discussion.

The value of questions

Questions can therefore help people to:

- focus on important experiences
- examine issues they had avoided
- clarify feelings and opinions
- identify areas where more information is needed
- feel valued because their opinions have been sought.

However, questions can also be very intrusive and threatening if they are used inappropriately. The 'tick the box' approach to taking nursing histories, i.e. by the use of closed questions, means that patients and clients are not given the opportunity to express in detail their experiences. Consequently they might feel controlled and powerless to state their needs.

How we ask questions can be linked to how we feel about the issues involved. The question 'Why did you do that?' could result in the recipient feeling criticized and defensive. Your reason for wording the question that way might have stemmed from a belief that what the other person had done was wrong. The use of the word 'why' therefore needs to be approached with caution (Stein-Parbury 1993). It may be better to phrase the question differently, e.g. 'What made you feel you should stop taking your tablets?'.

Active listening skills have a variety of functions. When we seek to acquire information, enable others to explore their experiences or wish to demonstrate we value their views, if we link the skills we use to information we have or to the preceding conversation, we keep them relevant, purposeful and focused. The effective use of active listening skills is essential if we want to demonstrate the core conditions of empathy, respect, warmth and genuineness. Inappropriate questioning can feel threatening or intrusive to the recipient, and overuse of paraphrasing, reflecting and jargon encouragers, such as 'I hear you', can appear condescending and insincere.

It is therefore important to prepare before we begin the interview, by considering who it is with, its purpose and what we intend to do once it is complete. If we think about what we need to know before or during the interview, what we intend to do with the information once we've received it and the purpose of the skills we use, we are more likely to engage the other person and develop a respectful partnership in the interaction. This approach is integral to developing any effective professional relationship. Thus the way in which we use active listening skills, for what purpose and in what context are integral to the relationship we have, or intend to have, with the person we are addressing.

Having completed this section, you might now find it helpful to return to Reflective Practice box 3.5 and review how you might alter your approach to obtaining information, e.g. by altering the wording of questions, asking them in a different context or relating them to different aspects of the situation (see also Ethical Issues box 3.1).

EXPLANATION SKILLS

The skills of careful explanation are needed for much of what we do in nursing practice and care management. Explanation enables us to clarify our thinking, helps others to understand the reasons for our decisions and is essential to the teaching of others. Patients and clients might need information about issues such as their diagnosis, treatment or discharge planning. Students and colleagues might need help to understand a new technique or policy. The effective use of questions is an important part of skilled explanation (see Health Promotion box 3.1).

In order to explain something effectively, it is important to prepare before you begin by:

- identifying any equipment that might be needed
- ensuring you are thoroughly versed in what it is you intend to explain
- choosing, whenever possible, when and where you will give the explanation
- reflecting on the type of relationship you have with the person – are you having to account for your actions to the primary care manager, or is this an explanation of a patient's discharge plan for her and her husband?
- deciding on the essential information and how it is interrelated
- clarifying a starting point with the other person – find out what he or she already knows
- providing a context for the explanation which the other person can understand
- talking logically through the information, from the agreed starting point to the end

 ETHICAL ISSUES

3.1 Dealing with interruptions

This is the first time you have worked with an interpreter for deaf people. Joan Randall is 25 and has been deaf from birth. She has been admitted to your ward for surgery. You are the student nurse assigned to her care and are taking a nursing history with the interpreter, Susan Georgiou. Susan is well known on the ward, having worked there for the last 3 years.

You draw the curtains and arrange the seating round Joan's bed (there is no private interview room on the ward), so Joan can see you and Susan without obstruction. After 5 minutes, the charge nurse comes behind the screens to say hello to Susan, interrupting the interview. A few minutes later, when you are mid-sentence, the staff nurse and the health care support worker come by and talk to Susan. She looks most discomfited and tries politely to keep only to a smile as a greeting.

- What are your views on this scenario?
- What is the focus of nursing in this situation?
- What messages might the staff be giving Joan?
- How does power in relationships influence this situation?
- What are the ethical issues here?
- How do they inform your choices in the way you would intervene?

 HEALTH PROMOTION

3.1 Avoiding hypoglycaemia

Mr Catchpole is an older man on Rachel Oliver's ward. He calls her over and says: 'Nurse, I don't understand what the doctor meant when she said I'm hypoglycaemic. She talked about sugar and said I was to eat half an hour after my insulin, because there was not enough sugar in my blood after the injection, but she said I wasn't to eat sweets instead of bread. When I asked her why, she said because sweets weren't the right sort of sugar. I just don't understand about sweets not being the right kind of sugar.'

It is clear that Mr Catchpole doesn't fully understand the nature of diabetes and its management. Write out an explanation for him of his illness and treatment, with particular focus on the importance of carbohydrate and blood sugar levels. What questions might you ask before and during your explanation?

- checking understanding regularly by asking the other person to paraphrase what has been understood and by using open focused questions
- reframing the information when the person doesn't understand, using age-, culture- and situation-appropriate metaphors. A suitable metaphor might be that sweets and bread are both forms of fuel for the body but, in the same

way that wood and coal burn differently in a fire, sweets and bread burn differently in the body. Use adjectives and descriptions that the other person can relate to (see the section on 'Culture and communication', p. 41).

At the end of the explanation, ask the other person to repeat what they have understood. Give them written information to support your explanation, e.g. on how to take their medication, an appointment card confirming the date of the next appointment, who it is with, its venue and if necessary a map. In the case of accounting to your manager for your practice you might need to support this with your case records.

ASSERTIVENESS SKILLS

Assertiveness means being able to state confidently our needs, views and arguments while respecting the others involved. This means we need to avoid being subservient, aggressive or apologetic. Nelson-Jones (1996) defines non-assertive, aggressive and assertive behaviour as follows:

Non-assertive behaviour is passive, compliant, submissive and inhibited. The individual doesn't like what is happening but colludes in allowing it to continue. For example, you may feel resentful because your clinical mentor is seldom able to work with you, but you don't raise this with your mentor or the nurse-in-charge. Instead you put up with the situation and struggle on.

Aggressive behaviour is self-enhancing at the expense of another person. It is unfriendly, quarrelsome and unnecessarily hostile. For example, consider a patient's relative who is angry because she has waited with her husband in the outpatient department for over an hour. She goes to the reception desk, leans forward over the counter and says loudly: 'This is outrageous. We have waited an hour and no-one has had the courtesy to tell us what is going on. Are you always so incompetent? I expect my husband to be seen at once!'

Assertive behaviour reflects confidence and respect for both yourself and others. It entails responding flexibly and appropriately strongly to different situations. For example, consider a colleague who starts talking to you about a client while you are standing in the bus queue. You may regard this as inappropriate because she is breaking confidentiality by discussing the client in public. You refuse to engage in conversation by saying in a courteous but firm tone: 'I know you have had a demanding day, but I do not think it is appropriate to discuss this here. If you like, we can talk about this in the office tomorrow morning.'

Advocacy

Advocacy is defined by Kohnke (1982) as 'the implementation of the role of informing the client and supporting the client's decision'. The ability to be assertive is particularly important when we are acting as advocate for those in our care and looking after their interests. Often people are too ill or disorientated to be able to think on their feet. One of the greatest privileges and responsibilities nurses have is to stand between the system and those for whom they provide professional care. This is perhaps what Benner (2000) describes as the 'being there' responsibility of the nurse (see Reflective Practice box 3.6).

R|R REFLECTIVE PRACTICE

3.6 Advocacy

Consider the following situation in which a woman is losing a pregnancy. The doctor asks her if he may examine her in front of three medical students. You are aware, from what she has told you, that she is feeling an awful sense of loss. She has told you that she has found the whole process of having to describe what has happened to her extremely embarrassing and she is very shy because the doctor is a man. It seems to you that this distress will only be exacerbated by a teaching session around her bed while she is bleeding and being examined vaginally.

You stand up for your patient's interests, i.e. you behave as her advocate, and state your view about what is in the best interests of your patient. You might say something like: 'I am not happy that three medical students should observe this examination. Jasmine has said she is finding this whole experience extremely distressing. I have noticed that she has cried a lot. As her doctor, I am sure you understand that the intimacy of this examination is very stressful. I know it is important for students to learn but I don't think it is in her best interests that anyone other than you are involved in this examination. She is desperately sad that she is losing her baby. Together we can help her by ensuring her privacy.'

The communication skills you have used here are those of assertiveness, as follows:

- making 'I' statements
- owning your opinions
- stating the situation as you see it
- using concise sentences and avoiding theorizing
- seeking collaboration with the doctor, which can help to avoid aggressive responses to challenge
- empathizing with the doctor's position.

Contract-making skills

Contracts in helping relationships are 'specific agreement(s)' between you and your clients and patients. They provide a focus and guidelines for the care you give and how you give it. Rather than patients having things 'done to them', contracts 'invite their cooperation', enabling them to share responsibility with you for their care (Culley 1991).

When we greet patients and clients for the first time, we usually do so in order to clarify our role in relation to them, i.e. who we are, how they like to be addressed, what their main concerns are at the time and what we have to offer. They may be in emotional or physical pain, may need information or may simply need help to walk to the bathroom. If we are scheduled to work with them that shift/session, it is important that we clarify through contracting how we will go about this. The skills of scripting can help when we make contracts with our patients and clients.

Scripting skills

Before addressing a potentially difficult situation, it is good practice to structure and rehearse what you intend to say, especially when you are endeavouring to address the needs of people who are vulnerable and less able to help themselves because of their situation, e.g. when breaking bad news. The skill of scripting outlines well the Macmillan model of communication (see Fig. 3.1). The language you use and how you approach the situation, as in Reflective Practice box 3.6 when you were standing between Jasmine and 'the system', will depend very much on the type of relationship you have or intend to make with the doctor as well as with the patient. Lindenfield (1989) describes this under four headings:

- Explanation:
  — explain the situation as you see it
  — be objective
  — keep to the point
  — be brief
  — don't theorize
- Feelings:
  — acknowledge your own
  — empathize with the other person
- Needs:
  — say what you want
  — be selective
  — offer a compromise if appropriate
- Consequences:
  — outline the positive results if they comply with your wishes
  — note the negative consequences if they don't comply.

Dealing with conflict

It is best to try to anticipate situations that are likely to give rise to conflict and prevent them through discussion with the others involved. How you go about this depends on the type of relationship you have or hope to have with the others involved and the power differentials, if any, within the relationship. For example, should you need to renegotiate your working arrangements with your manager, she or he may well hold all the types of power described earlier. Consequently, you might feel at a disadvantage when considering your position.

Negotiating skills

Scripting can be very useful when we need to confront a situation where there is conflict but, before we put our case using a script, it is worth considering the skills of negotiation. Negotiation is a search for a meeting of minds between two parties, each of whom would like this meeting to take place in a different location (Moore et al 1974). According to Honey (1988), the skills of negotiation are:

- focusing on interests not positions
- exploring proposals rather than counter-proposing
- attacking the problem not the person
- sticking to the facts rather than exaggerating
- disagreeing constructively
- being open about thoughts and feelings
- asking questions
- summarizing.

Should conflict arise, it is worth trying to learn from it through reflection and discussion with others.

DEALING WITH BAD NEWS

How would we define bad news? What is it we are apprehensive about when we work with people who are about to be, or have already been, given bad news? What is bad news to one person may be a relief to another. It is therefore very important that we don't assume that the patient or client is going to react in a particular way. Examples of bad news are as follows:

- being told there is no bed for you when you are due for surgery
- learning that the clinical nurse specialist in whom you have so much confidence is leaving
- hearing that your partner's treatment has to be delayed because of their physical state
- learning that you have an untreatable condition or that a loved one has died.

This fourth example of bad news is perhaps the one that most of us fear having to give, because it may be the one we most fear receiving. The reality is that it is usually doctors rather than nurses who give this sort of information to patients and their relatives, although nurses usually accompany the doctor in order to be there with the distressed person. When people receive bad news that is life-changing, they are likely to begin the process of mourning. For a detailed discussion of mourning and how to help, see Worden (1991).

Possible reactions to hearing bad news include stunned silence, anger, disbelief, acute distress, guilt or blaming (Fallowfield & Lipkin 1995) (see also Evidence-based Practice box 3.1). It will be an advantage to both the nurse and the person who has received bad news if they already have an established working relationship. This familiarity can provide reassurance and comfort. In these situations people try to elicit meaning from what they have learned. As nurses we can help by:

- making time to be with the distressed person in a private and quiet environment
- allowing the person to express his or her feelings, however intense, and avoiding false reassurance and soothing platitudes such as 'Don't worry, you'll be fine'
- allowing other loved ones to be with the distressed person if this is what is wanted
- recognizing the difference between the rhetorical 'why' and 'how' questions and those requiring answers, i.e. give information when it is asked for
- being aware of our own feelings throughout the interview, so that we can avoid imposing our own perspectives and allow the other person to experience the situation in an individual way
- ensuring that the person has access to follow-up care – if necessary, making the appointments, giving contact numbers and writing down the crucial information for the person to take away
- ensuring, wherever possible, that the person is not leaving the hospital or surgery alone, or, if this is unavoidable, trying to arrange for someone to be with the person at home
- taking time, after the interview is over, to acknowledge our own feelings, and to reflect and put our experiences of the situation into context.

EVIDENCE-BASED PRACTICE

3.1 The effect of bad news on our ability to remember

Remembering and forgetting are active processes. When people are frightened or shocked by news, they might not hear it clearly, not take in what they are told or forget a significant amount of what is said to them. Motivated forgetting is a well-documented response to painful or traumatic experiences. The factors that influence adults' capacity to learn are the environment, who is informing us and how, how we are ourselves, and the relevance of the information to our life situations. It is therefore important to help people manage their situations by ensuring that:

- the environment is psychologically safe and private
- wherever possible, clients or patients already know and have a positive relationship with the professional giving the news, because emotions influence our capacity to learn and to remember
- the information is straightforward so as not to overwhelm clients
- the news is related to what clients already know about their situation/illness
- written information, such as contact numbers, treatment details and follow-up appointments, is given to clients so they can refer to it later.

- Set the parameters of our working relationships at the start, e.g. when we greet patients and their loved ones for the first time, we may say: 'I'll be working with you for the shift today but then I will be on study leave for the rest of the week'
- Make time for the ending
- Be sensitive and polite – avoid implying rejection
- Use clear language in which the closure is self-evident; avoid phrases like 'see you later' when you are unlikely to see the person again
- Take care not to encourage inappropriate dependence. If appropriate, allow patients to keep in touch with the unit or surgery by letter or telephone (this might be necessary for clarifying continuing treatment or support, e.g. if they are terminally ill). Never give private telephone numbers or addresses
- Recognize when, how and why you should refer patients and clients elsewhere; clarify this with them
- End the relationship with the client's family and friends appropriately as well
- Acknowledge the importance of the relationship by valuing expressed feelings and owning your own, e.g. 'I feel very lucky to have worked with you, Mr Abrahams'
- Allow the opportunity for the others involved to offer you feedback on their experiences of their care
- Say good-bye; be culturally sensitive in how you do this, e.g. by shaking hands or bowing
- If practicable, see the people out by opening your office door for them or escorting them to the ward or surgery door.

ENDING PROFESSIONAL RELATIONSHIPS

Ending our professional relationships is an easily neglected skill. Many of the people with whom we work will not be seen again. Some may have been an integral part of our working lives over many months. They might be professional colleagues, patients or carers. Endings often bring sadness and a sense of loss, as well as new hope and/or relief – the latter in cases where we haven't got on well with other people or where we are pleased that they are able to move on to better things. Endings offer the opportunity to reflect on what has been gained from the relationship, but they can also remind us of other relationships that we have lost. The future can be considered as well as paradoxical feelings evoked by the ending. It is natural for patients to feel pleased when the services of a health care team are no longer required, but there may also be a sense of sadness at saying goodbye to those who have made a difference to one's life.

Endings can also precipitate separation anxiety in ourselves and in those whom we have cared for. It is important, therefore, that wherever possible nurses negotiate when the ending will happen. It is necessary to assess the needs of everyone involved and to plan ahead, whilst also recognizing the loss of the relationship. It is important to acknowledge the loss of the support that was offered to clients and to discuss how they feel about this.

Leave-taking

In order to be skilful at this, we need to:

COMMUNICATION IN GROUPS

We are all members of groups, although their significance in our lives may vary. For instance, patients' groups may take on a particular significance for people who are ill and far away from their families, who cannot therefore provide support on a regular basis. How groups develop and the ways in which we behave within them also vary according to the nature of the group and its purpose. Some groups are transient (e.g. people in a bus queue), while others (e.g. a family group) are more permanent.

The way that we communicate with each other in groups and teams depends on how we see ourselves in relation to others within that group and how they perceive us. It is crucial that we have a clear idea of the purpose of our professional task. If we acknowledge the roles of other members, the defences, values and power within the team, we are better able to make and maintain creative and task-focused working relationships.

Working in groups and teams is an integral part of professional practice. Conscious and unconscious processes are inherent in all group functioning. If teams are not able to focus on the tasks they have been established to perform, some group processes can develop which are unhelpful or indeed destructive (see Health Promotion box 3.2).

GROUP DYNAMICS

Each time we attend a new practice placement, we influence the group of people we will be working with. These are open groups

HEALTH PROMOTION

3.2 Safety in the home

As part of your experience in your community placement, you and another student are invited to teach a local women's group of different cultures about safety in the home. They meet weekly at a local community centre.

- What issues would you need to consider?
- How would you address the variety of cultural needs represented in the group?
- What type of relationship would you intend to make with each other and with the group?
- How would this differ from working with a group of your course peers?
- How would you engage the group's attention?

Student activity

Write short teaching notes for the session, bearing in mind what you know about effective explanation. Identify what teaching aids you might use in the session.

---

because the membership changes as people join and leave. This movement of people leads to a readjustment of roles and relationships within the group. Such readjustment of behaviour, i.e. the development of small groups, is described by Tuckman (1965) as follows:

- *Forming* – the group depends heavily on the leader to give guidance. This is evident in the manner in which students new to a course rely on the course director, often for information that they could readily find for themselves, and indeed, in other circumstances, they would do so
- *Storming* – here group members jostle for positions and roles. Sometimes the group leader is the focus of group conflict
- *Norming* – group relationships and behaviour are more stable, and spoken and unspoken rules are adhered to
- *Performing* – here the group focuses on the task it has been convened to do, e.g. to develop a new nursing protocol or to reflect on clinical practice
- *Adjourning* (Alladin 1988) – here the group members begin to disengage and there may be feelings of sadness, loss and anger alongside the excitement at moving on.

People tend to develop particular roles within groups. This will depend on the nature and purpose of the group and the personalities of the members. Someone might be the supporter in one group but the questioner in another. Roles are also interchangeable, with individuals taking on different roles that require different communication and observation skills and characteristics.

ROLES IN GROUPS

People's roles in groups can be divided into (Kindred & Kindred 1998):

- *Task roles* (those who enable the group to complete their task):
  - the proposer, e.g. someone who makes suggestions about how to go about a task
  - the information-seeker, e.g. the person who asks the critical question when the group cannot resolve a problem
  - the information-giver, e.g. the person who feeds back new research findings
  - the summarizer/ builder, e.g. someone who describes and links succinctly the work achieved at the end of a meeting
- *Maintenance roles* (those who 'look after people' so the group is able to function effectively):
  - the encourager, e.g. someone who makes an opportunity in the discussion for a timid person to contribute
  - the gatekeeper, e.g. the person who stops the discussion from wandering off course
  - the harmonizer, e.g. someone who pours oil over troubled waters when there is heated dissent in the group
  - the process observer, e.g. the person who describes the group's behaviour, in order to help members think about what they are doing or not doing.

Throughout our nursing careers, we will be members of different groups – our course peer group, the primary health care team, the specialist practice group, the multidisciplinary team, the management and community groups. If we understand the behaviour of groups, it enables us to function more effectively within them.

TEAMS

Reid & Hammersly (2000) define a team as a group of people who:

- work together regularly towards agreed common goals
- while in the team, regard their team identity as a main feature of their workplace identity
- have largely open communication among themselves
- are in the team because of their individual characteristics, although some teams are formed out of whoever is available
- usually adopt a variety of different roles within the team.

According to Roberts (1994), in order to be an effective team member, we need to:

- be clear about the task we have to do
- be able to mobilize sufficient resources, internal and external, to achieve the task
- have some understanding of how our task relates to both the task of the system in which we work and the task of the institution as a whole.

Labelling

If people become labelled as being of a particular type or as having a particular function in a group, it can lead to the restriction of their functioning, their acting out of their label, role-stereotyping and at worst scapegoating. Culture also affects the labelling process in groups, e.g. in the use of metaphors in the description of others. The label 'fussy old woman', for example, illustrates how in Western society older adulthood and women are devalued.

Labelling affects the ways in which we respond to individuals and how they respond to us, as exemplified by the maxim 'give a dog a bad name and hang him', which reflects how, once labelled, whatever a person does may never be regarded as acceptable. How we label patients, e.g. describing them as 'good' or 'difficult', can also be self-fulfilling, so that they behave in the ways we expect them to. Nurses need to be aware that groups, e.g. the ward team and indeed society, can directly influence how others see themselves and therefore the way they behave. For a detailed discussion of this phenomenon, see Obholzer & Roberts (1994) and Baron & Byrne (2000).

CONCLUSION

Nursing is an intimate, human and highly skilled service that is based on the establishment, maintenance and ending of a complex array of working relationships that are underpinned by conscious and unconscious processes, values and power. Sound therapeutic relationships are based on the core conditions of empathy, respect, openness and genuineness. In order to provide the best possible nursing care it is important to bear in mind who we are, the purpose of nursing, and the types of relationship that we intend to have.

SUMMARY: MAIN POINTS

■ Communication involves verbal, non-verbal, paralinguistic, conscious and unconscious communication and is fundamental to and affects all aspects of human relationships.

■ The core conditions of effective therapeutic relationships are warmth, empathy, respect and genuineness.

■ The recognition of diverse cultures within different professional disciplines as well as in society generally allows us to celebrate difference and learn from each other as well as those in our care.

■ Being able to communicate assertively is an essential nursing skill.

■ The differences between communication skills, counselling skills and counselling are evident in the

nature of the professional relationships in which these skills are used. Many nurses will use counselling skills but not all will have the training and skills to provide counselling.

■ The development, maintenance and ending of professional relationships depends on the application of active listening skills, assertiveness skills, explanation and negotiation skills.

■ Self-awareness and personal reflection are fundamental to continuing our development as professional practitioners, and effective communication skills are integral to this process.

■ Nurses have the power to influence people's lives significantly. How we use that power is based on our values and our intentions as practitioners.

SELF-TEST: CRITICAL THINKING ACTIVITIES

1 The core conditions of all therapeutic relationships are discussed in this chapter. What do you understand them to be?

2 Describe a situation from practice when a practitioner demonstrated these skills particularly well.
— What verbal and non-verbal skills were used?
— How did the patient, client or colleague respond?

3 Professional relationships of all sorts have spoken and unspoken parameters or boundaries. Consider a situation from practice where professional boundaries had been crossed.
— How did it become evident that they had been crossed?
— What did you and/or your colleagues do to deal with the situation?
— What communication skills were used effectively?
— What was the outcome for the professional relationships involved?

4 Making contracts is a significant part of nursing practice. Think of a situation involving a patient, colleague or relative where you think things might have been less stressful if a clear contract of working had been negotiated.
— What do you think made the situation difficult?
— How would the skills you have learned from this chapter have helped?
— What would you have done differently?

5 Diversity in language, culture and lifestyle is one of the riches of society in the UK.
— How have you benefited from nursing people from a variety of backgrounds?
— What changes would you make in your personal Johari window (see Fig. 3.2) to describe your learning?
— How has this influenced the way in which you communicate with people from backgrounds that differ from your own?

FURTHER READING

Baron RA, Byrne D. Social psychology, 9th edn. Boston: Allyn and Bacon; 2000.

Belbin RM. Management teams. London: Heinemann; 1981.

Billington R, Strawbridge S, Greensides L, Fitzsimmons A. Culture and Society. London: Macmillan; 1991.

Bion WR. Experiences in groups and other papers. London: Tavistock; 1961.

Douglas T. Survival in groups: the basics of group membership. Buckingham: Open University Press; 1995.

Douglas T. Scapegoats transferring blame. London: Routledge; 1995.

Faulkner A. When the news is bad. A guide for health professionals. Sheffield: Stanley Thomas; 1997.

Hayes N. Foundations of psychology: an introductory text. Walton-on-Thames: Nelson; 1994.

Lo B. Caring for patients with life-threatening or terminal illness. In: Lipkin M Jr et al, eds. The medical interview, clinical care, education and research. New York: Springer; 1995, ch. 25.

Maddi SR. Personality theories: a comparative analysis, 5th edn. Pacific Grove: Brooks/Cole; 1989.

Macmillan. Professional relationships. London: Macmillan; 1996.

Nelson-Jones R. Relating skills. New York: Cassell; 1996.

Palmer S, McMahon G. Handbook of counselling, 2nd edn. London: Routledge; 1997.

Zimbardo P, McDermott M, Jansz J, Metaal N. Psychology: a European text. London: HarperCollins; 1995.

REFERENCES

Alladin W. Cognitive-behavioural group therapy. In: Aveline M, Dryden W, eds. Group therapy in Britain. Milton Keynes: Open University Press; 1988, ch. 6.

Baron RA, Byrne D. Social psychology, 9th edn. Boston: Allyn and Bacon; 2000.

Benner P. From novice to expert: excellence and power in clinical nursing practice. Commemorative Edition. Menlo Park: Addison Wesley; 1984.

Clark JM, Jesson A. Progression into counselling. Nurs Times 1991; 87(9): 41–43.

Culley S. Integrative counselling skills in action. London: Sage; 1991.

Egan G. The skilled helper. A systematic approach to effective helping, 6th edn. Pacific Grove: Brooks/Cole; 1998.

Egan G. The skilled helper, 7th edn. Belmont, CA: Brooks/Cole; 2002.

Fallowfield LJ, Lipkin M. Delivering sad or bad news. In: Lipkin M, Putman SM, Lazare A, eds. The medical interview, clinical care, education and research. New York: Springer; 1995, ch. 26.

Grasha A. Practical applications of psychology, 4th edn. New York: HarperCollins; 1995.

Helman C. Culture, health and illness. London: Wright; 1990.

Honey P. Improve your people skills. Wimbledon: Institute of Personnel Management; 1988.

Kindred M, Kindred M. Once upon a group. Dover: Smallwood; 1998.

Kohnke MF. Advocacy: risk and reality. St Louis: Mosby; 1982.

Lindenfeld G. Super confidence. London: Thorsons; 1989.

Luft J. On human interaction. Palo Alto, CA: National Press; 1969.

Macmillan. Professional relationships: influences on health care. London: Macmillan; 1996.

Maddi SR. Personality theories: a comparative analysis. Pacific Grove: Brooks/Cole; 1989.

Moore S and the editors of Time-Life Multi-media in consultation with Dr Chester L Karrass. Negotiating successfully. USA: Time-Life Films Inc; 1974.

Nelson-Jones R. The theory and practice of counselling psychology. London: Cassell; 1982.

Nelson-Jones R. Human relationship skills, 2nd edn. London: Cassell; 1990.

Nelson-Jones R. Relating skills. London: Cassell; 1996.

Obholzer A, Roberts VZ. The unconscious at work. London: Routledge; 1994.

Raven BH. A power/interaction model of interpersonal influence: French and Raven thirty years later. J Social Behaviour Personality 1992; 7: 217–244.

Reid M, Hammersley R. Communicating successfully in groups. London: Routledge; 2000.

Roberts VZ. The organization of work: contributions from open systems theory. In: Obholzer A, Roberts VZ, eds. The unconscious at work. London: Routledge; 1994, ch. 3.

Rogers C. The necessary and sufficient conditions of therapeutic personality change. J Consult Psychol 1957; 21: 95–103.

Stein-Parbury J. Patient and person: developing interpersonal skills in nursing. London: Churchill Livingstone; 1993.

Sundeen SJ, Stuart GW, Rankin EAD, Cohen SA. Nurse-client interaction: implementing the nursing process. St Louis: Mosby; 1998.

Tuckman BW. Developmental sequence in small groups. Psychol Bull 1965; 63: 384–399.

Whaley LF, Wong DL. Nursing care of infants and young children. St Louis: Mosby; 1991.

Worden JW. Grief counselling and grief therapy, 2nd edn. London: Tavistock; 1991.

Wright B. Skills for caring: communication skills. Edinburgh: Churchill Livingstone; 1992, ch. 2.

SECTION 2

Common nursing issues

Contents

4 Circadian rhythms and sleep patterns   59

5 Temperature regulation   75

6 Stress   93

7 Pain   111

8 Problems associated with fluid, electrolyte and acid–base balance   133

9 Shock, systemic inflammatory response and multiple organ dysfunction   153

10 Tissue viability: managing chronic wounds   173

11 Nutrition   201

12 Maintaining continence   229

13 Infection control   253

4 Circadian rhythms and sleep patterns

Mary Reet

> 'I never sleep very well away from home so I was tired all the time as well as feeling lousy from the pain and sickness. Those periods after lunch when the ward was quiet and there were no visitors was an absolute life-saver.'
>
> (Patient)

THIS CHAPTER WILL HELP YOU

- Identify the normal physiology of sleep
- Describe circadian rhythms and their physiological effect
- Critically discuss the impact of shift working on circadian rhythms
- Explain the factors which may affect sleep and describe their effects
- Describe how sleep should be assessed and managed by nurses
- Identify and describe disorders of sleep and identify nursing strategies to manage these disorders
- Assess a patient's normal sleep pattern and plan the care to reflect individual needs
- Identify a range of pharmacological and non-pharmacological interventions to promote sleep
- Identify where sleep may be altered by disease processes and plan care to minimize the disturbance.

KEYWORDS

Circadian rhythm	Shift work
Diurnal variation	Sleep
Electroencephalogram (EEG)	Sleep hygiene
Electromyogram (EMG)	Sleep inversion
Electro-oculogram (EOG)	Sleep latency
Internal desynchronization	Somnambulance
Jet lag	Ultradian rhythm

INTRODUCTION

This chapter focuses on the mechanisms that control the body in terms of waking and sleeping. The role of circadian and ultradian rhythms is examined as well as their impact on bodily functions. The importance of sleep and rest for the promotion of healing and reduction of stress is also discussed. This is applied to the care of adults in a range of situations in order to promote understanding of its importance in the delivery of nursing care.

INTERNAL CONTROLS OF SLEEP AND REST

Sleep has been a source of interest to scientists for many years, but it is only within the last 100 years that understanding of the control mechanisms of sleep has been advanced. This has been made possible by advances in monitoring techniques. Development of the electroencephalogram (EEG), which monitors electrical brain activity via a series of electrodes placed on the scalp, has enabled scientists to study this activity during sleep and wakefulness. The electro-oculogram (EOG), which records electrical activity in the eye muscles, the electromyogram (EMG), which records electrical activity in the skeletal muscles, and techniques for the measurement of blood chemicals have further advanced our understanding. These experiments have been conducted in sleep laboratories where healthy volunteers are monitored and hypotheses tested. This has enabled scientists to identify and treat certain sleep problems. The monitoring of sleep using EEG, EOG and EMG is known as polysomnography.

THE PHYSIOLOGY OF SLEEP

Sleep is a recurrent, natural condition in which consciousness is temporarily lost and bodily functions partially suspended. It is reversible, either by a natural return of consciousness or by external stimulation, e.g. by an alarm clock. The maintenance of the sleep–wake cycle is thought to be controlled by the reticular activating system (RAS) of the brain, which consists of fibres projecting from the reticular formation through the thalamus to the cerebral cortex (Tortora & Grabowski 2000).

Two mechanisms, circadian and ultradian rhythms, and neuro-chemical processes control sleep and wakefulness (Cooper 1994a). The circadian rhythm is the body's ability to operate an approximate 24-hour cycle in terms of wakefulness and sleep. In experiments that have removed the time-setters, such as clocks, radios, newspapers, live television and daylight or dark, subjects still followed a sleep–wake pattern that on average was found to equate to 25 hours (Folkard 1991). Thus where there are no external controls of time, the individual body clock naturally settled to a circadian rhythm of around 25 hours. However, within these experiments there was a wide range of individual rhythms. The ultradian rhythm describes a subdivision of time within the circadian rhythm. Ultradian rhythms control the ability to fall asleep or resist sleep at certain times during the day. These rhythms last for about 90 minutes on average and explain the times in the day when sleep is more likely and those where alertness is foremost.

STAGES OF SLEEP

Sleep consists of five main stages, four of non-REM (rapid eye movement) sleep and one of REM sleep. Movement between these stages is indicated by specific changes on an EEG. The five stages are as follows:

- *Stage 1*. The subject becomes drowsy and begins to fall asleep. Breathing slows and becomes regular. The EEG shows alpha waves that are associated with the waking state.
- *Stage 2*. The subject is now asleep, although sleeping lightly. An unusual sound will disturb and arouse the subject quite easily. Breathing is regular and slow. The EEG shows the appearance of slow waves called K-complexes and bursts of rapid waves known as sleep spindles (Borbély 1987). Stage 2 comprises 45–55% of total sleep time in young adults (see Fig. 4.1, which gives the proportion of each stage of sleep; note that stage 1 isn't included as sleep is not fully established during this stage; Cooper 1994a).
- *Stage 3*. This is the beginning of slow wave sleep, which comprises 3–8% of total sleep. The subject is more deeply asleep and more difficult to arouse. The EEG shows slow waves that become larger, known as delta waves (Borbély 1987).
- *Stage 4*. This is the stage of deepest sleep during which the subject is most difficult to arouse. The EEG shows an increased number of delta waves. Sleepwalking and enuresis (bedwetting) occur during this stage of sleep, which comprises 10–15% of the total.
- *REM sleep*. This stage is characterized by rapid eye movement, which can be picked up by an EOG. The subject sleeps more lightly, with a change in the EEG to waves more associated with wakefulness. This is the stage of sleep where dreaming is thought to occur. In many people this stage is characterized by sleep paralysis, where they are unable to move. REM sleep comprises 20–25% of total sleep time.

Subjects move in and out of these various stages throughout the night (assuming sleep takes place at night; if not, this happens during the period of sleep) depending on how long they have been asleep, and the pattern of movement forms a visible ultradian rhythm (see Fig. 4.2). Sleep begins with stage 1 and,

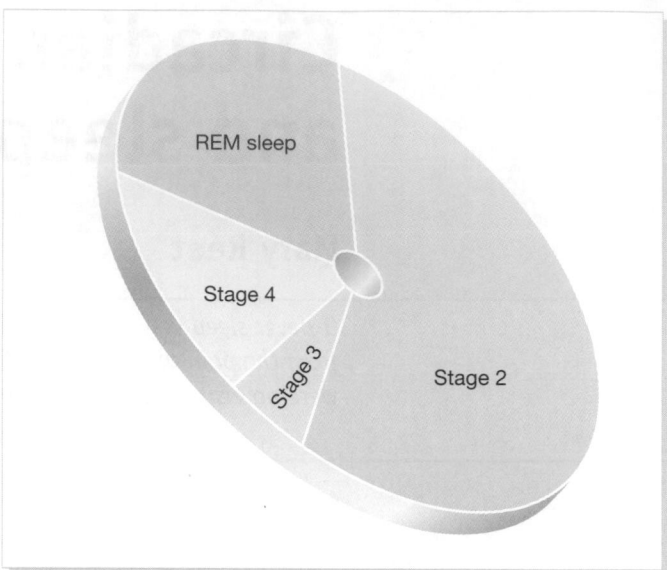

Figure 4.1 Proportion of each stage of sleep.

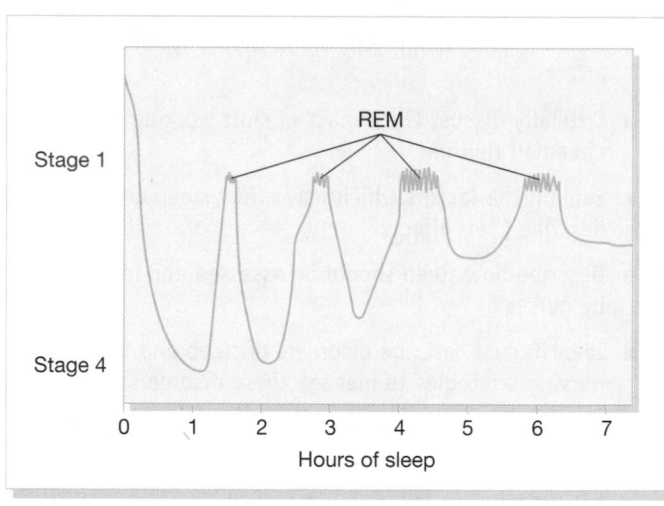

Figure 4.2 Sleep pattern in young adults. (Based on Reet 1998.)

once established, progresses through stages 2, 3 and 4; there is then a sudden shift to stage 2 followed by a period of REM sleep, a process which usually takes about 90–100 minutes. The pattern then repeats, but as the night progresses, less time is spent in stages 3 and 4 and more time is spent in REM sleep. Therefore the early part of the night is more important for sleep stages 3 and 4 and the latter part of the night is more important for REM sleep.

Patients who are unable to sleep or who can only doze for short periods may not be getting the amount of sleep they require for health or healing. This is explained more fully later on in the chapter.

NEUROCHEMICAL PROCESSES

The neurochemical processes in the brain which control the sleep–wake cycle are not very well understood due to the difficulty of measuring and analysing them. There are several neurotransmitters currently being investigated and many display a circadian-like cycle, although their connection with sleep and wakefulness is not fully understood. Zoltoski & Gillin (1994) identified the following:

- serotonin (5-hydroxytryptamine) – thought to have a role in the initiation and maintenance of sleep
- noradrenaline – has a relationship to REM sleep
- dopamine – increased during the wakeful state and is thought to be active in the waking state
- acetylcholine – thought to have a role in the generation of REM sleep
- adenosine – has a sedative effect that enhances deep sleep and REM sleep
- histamine – thought to have a role in the alert state
- gamma-aminobutyric acid (GABA) – thought to aid vigilance in the waking state
- melatonin – a major hormone released by the pineal gland which is increased in darkness and is thus associated with sleep latency
- interleukin-1 (IL-1) – it is thought that sleep and the immune system are interrelated.

One part of the controlling 'body clock' is thought be located in the area of the brain known as the suprachiasmatic nucleus, which is close to the hypothalamus just above the optic nerve (Zoltoski & Gillin 1994). This is strongly influenced by light and dark on the retina, and this influence provides the basis for the understanding and treatment of jet lag and the effect of shift work. The suprachiasmatic nucleus establishes patterns of sleep and is influenced by the release of melatonin from the pineal gland. During sleep the plasma levels of melatonin rise 10-fold and decrease again before waking (Tortora & Grabowski 2000). Melatonin is thought to increase sleep quality and in experiments with older adults it appeared to have some benefits in terms of quality if not quantity of sleep (Haimov et al 1994, Garfinkel et al 1995). However, Middleton et al (1996) suggested that the indiscriminate use of melatonin, e.g. as a treatment for jet lag, may have deleterious long-term effects on sleeping patterns despite offering initial help.

The activation of the RAS results in arousal. This can be activated by sensory stimuli such as bright light, an alarm clock, touch pressure on the skin, sudden limb movements or pain. Stimulation of the RAS leads to stimulation of the cerebral cortex, arousal occurs and consciousness is established. Interestingly, little stimulus is received by the RAS from the olfactory system (the sense of smell) and strong odours do not awaken sleepers. This is why house fires during the night often prove fatal, because people succumb to smoke inhalation and die without knowing there is a fire; hence the need for smoke detectors that emit a loud noise or, for the hearing-impaired, a bright flashing light.

Coma

Coma is a different phenomenon from sleep. Although some evidence of sleep-like states may be observed in the EEG in some types of coma, the arousal threshold is absent or markedly reduced. The extent to which this happens will be dependent on the point along the spectrum of unconsciousness at which the patient is situated (Cooper 1994b). The persistent vegetative state is a condition of altered consciousness where patients are unaware of and unresponsive to their inner needs and external environment (Cooper 1994b), despite sometimes appearing awake with open eyes. Although alternating patterns of apparent sleep occur in these patients, the normal sleep structure is disrupted.

PHYSICAL CHANGES DURING SLEEP

A number of physical changes occur during sleep. These are described below.

Body temperature

There are two rhythms that affect body temperature: the cyclical pattern of activity and sleep, and an endogenous rhythm that causes a fall in body temperature of up to 1°C during the night, with the lowest point between 4.00 and 6.00am. The two rhythms are normally in phase but if the sleep cycle is inverted (i.e. sleeping in the day and working at night) the two tend to cancel each other out (Kronauer 1994). Thermoregulation is thought to remain intact during NREM sleep but is inhibited or impaired during REM sleep.

Cardiovascular system

Systemic blood pressure and heart rate are lower during sleep. Thus, nurses undertaking observations should remember that changes observed during sleep may not be an indication of clinical change. Nurses should also remember that measuring blood pressure during sleep can cause sleep arousal and may affect the values recorded (Davies et al 1994). It has been shown that abnormal electrical activity peaks at around 4.00am in patients suffering from coronary heart disease (Centre for Sleep Research 1999).

Respiratory system

During NREM sleep there is a reduction in tidal volume rather than rate. During REM sleep there is variability in ventilation, often causing an increase in rate and tidal volume (Douglas 1994a). Breathing can be rapid and shallow during REM sleep and the relative hypoxaemia (low oxygen level in the blood) and hypercapnia (increased level of carbon dioxide in the blood) can seriously affect those who are compromised in these areas when awake. Most normal subjects maintain their oxygen saturation at more than 90% during sleep. In people with asthma, morning peak flow rate measurements typically demonstrate a dip. Sleep is also responsible for the depression of the cough response to inhaled irritants and suppresses the spontaneous cough (Douglas 1994a).

The reasons for the decrease in breathing during sleep include:

- decreased basal metabolic rate
- increased airflow resistance due to hypotonia of the upper airway muscles
- changes in thoracic contribution to ventilation and decreased ventilation drive during sleep, particularly during REM sleep

(see Reflective Practice box 4.1).

4.1 The effect of breathing difficulties on sleep

Think of a patient you have nursed with a breathing disorder.

- How did his/her medical condition affect the ability to rest and sleep?
- How did you help the patient to be comfortable and to sleep?
- What other strategies could you have used to aid the patient's sleep? Are there any strategies that might prove harmful in patients with breathing disorders?

Renal system

The volume of urine and plasma concentrations of potassium and sodium are at their lowest between 4.00 and 8.00am (Cooper 1994a). Plasma renin and aldosterone levels both peak between 8.00am and 12.00pm, declining slowly thereafter and reaching their lowest levels between 8.00pm and 4.00am. During sleep, therefore, there is a concentration of urine in order to maintain homeostasis (due to not taking fluids). This is reversed in the morning when drinking is resumed.

Endocrine system

Catecholamines – adrenaline (epinephrine) and noradrenaline (norepinephrine) – fall during sleep (Yamasaki et al 1998). Cortisol levels are clearly demonstrated to have a circadian rhythm, being at their peak in the early hours of the morning just prior to wakening and at their lowest in the early hours of sleep (Lutchmansingh et al 1994). The pituitary hormone with the most recognized link to a circadian rhythm and sleep is the growth hormone. The peak of secretion occurs in the early hours of the night and is in closest correlation to slow wave sleep. The relationship between sleep and growth hormone remains when sleep is inverted, and during sleep deprivation growth hormone is not secreted (Lutchmansingh et al 1994). Growth hormone is important to adults for tissue repair and reproduction. Although the adult is no longer growing, cellular growth by mitosis is continuous and the hormone promotes healing in cells damaged by trauma or disease.

Lutchmansingh et al (1994) report few links between thyroid hormone and sleep stages, although thyroid-stimulating hormone (TSH) does demonstrate a circadian rhythm, with the highest plasma concentration during the late evening hours prior to sleep onset, and has an ultradian rhythm of about 3 hours. When sleep is inverted (i.e. sleeping during the day and awake at night), TSH continues to rise with prolonged wakefulness and sleep inhibits the release of TSH. Slight rises in TSH are correlated with sleep stages 3 and 4.

PURPOSE OF SLEEP

Many theories about the purpose of sleep have been proposed as more and more research has been carried out. It is believed that during NREM sleep, due to a raised output of growth hormone particularly during stages 3 and 4, the body is repairing itself.

The importance of growth hormone to the maintenance and repair of body tissues adds weight to the theory. This emphasizes the importance of the promotion of sleep and rest as part of therapeutic management.

REM sleep is thought to be important for the health of the brain. An increased blood flow to the brain during sleep suggests that these tissues receive more nutrition and that there is an increased removal of waste products during sleep, thus improving brain function. Much of dreaming is thought to occur during REM sleep, which contributes to the notion that this sleep stage is important for the brain tissues. Dreaming is thought to help the brain deal with problems faced by the individual during waking hours (Griffin 1997) and is probably where the advice to 'sleep on a problem, as it will appear better in the morning' originates. People with anxiety or depression may show improvement with improved sleep patterns.

SLEEP DEPRIVATION

Some of our knowledge about sleep comes from the examination of the effects of sleep deprivation on subjects willing to undergo a period of enforced wakefulness. After 72 hours, subjects report hallucinations, have poor coordination, become overly suspicious (paranoid) and do and say strange things. Subjects also experience the overwhelming desire to sleep and would fall asleep if undisturbed, even if walking down a street (Oswald & Adam 1983)! It is now known that people who have been deprived of sleep for some time may indulge in 'microsleeps', periods of sleep which last a few seconds, as a way of staying alert (Horne 1988). This, of course, could be dangerous if the person is driving or in control of moving machinery, or indeed is a nurse in charge of patient care!

Hodgson (1991), in her review of the literature on sleep deprivation, found that the physiological changes reported included a fall in body temperature and poor thermoregulation, slight changes in cardiorespiratory function, slight hormonal changes (thought to relate to stress – see Ch. 6), changes in control of eye movements and, for some people, an increase in epileptic-like EEG activity. However, overwhelming tiredness was the most significant finding. The psychological effects included increased aggressiveness, irritability and increasingly antisocial behaviour. Tests that required speed and/or prolonged concentration were more poorly performed by sleep-deprived subjects.

The longest recorded sleep deprivation study involved a 17-year-old student called Randy Gardener who in January 1964 went 264 hours without sleep as part of a science fair (Horne 1988). Initially he was supervised by friends but after 150 hours he was supervised by a doctor from a sleep laboratory. At the end of the period of deprivation he slept for 14.75 hours and woke up feeling well and only a little sleepy. During the study he did not appear to experience any serious physiological problems. Although he experienced some psychological effects, these were quickly resolved after he had slept. Interestingly, he only replaced about 24% of the sleep he'd missed and this was mostly made up of stage 4 and REM sleep.

In other examples of long periods of sleep deprivation, the subjects have not been so fortunate. A radio DJ in New York attempted to prove that sleep was not necessary by going without it and continuing to perform his normal radio broadcasts. He developed severe psychological disturbances and eventually experienced severe paranoia (Bangura 1998). Recent cases of deaths caused by drivers who fall asleep at the wheel after a period of sleep deprivation have highlighted the dangers to self and others of operating machinery in this state.

The effect of shift work

Internal desynchronization is a phenomenon whereby 'some of the body's biological rhythms are out of phase with others so that their sensitively attuned rhythmical system becomes disordered' (Borbély 1987, p. 184). This can happen during shift work when working hours change and the sleep–wake cycle has to change suddenly, but hormones and metabolic rhythms take longer to adjust. Thus the person is sleeping yet the body's hormone secretions are at levels that would be normal for someone who was awake. Compared to the sleeping norm, therefore, the temperature is elevated, there is a higher level of adrenaline (epinephrine) in the blood, and kidney function is increased, thus causing disturbance due to the need to void urine; the secretion of melatonin is decreased (Borbély 1987). Problems associated with shift work, however, are not just related to desynchronization but also to the social effect of working 'unsocial hours'.

An awareness of the effects of sleep deprivation should prompt nurses to consider their own health in relation to shift work and how they maintain their requirement for sleep, as a failure to get enough sleep can have a seriously deleterious effect on the health of patients in their care (Bangura 1998). Sleep-deprived nurses may become less efficient, especially with cognitive tasks such as drug calculations or manipulative skills such as preparing and administering intravenous drugs. Nurses may also become irritable, which may affect their relationships with patients, relatives, colleagues and members of the multidisciplinary team (see Evidence-based Practice box 4.1). In recent years there has been a move away from the long rosters of night duty towards shorter internal rotations, as these have been shown to have a less negative effect on individuals through reduced effects of sleep inversion (Brugne 1994).

Jet lag

Jet lag is another example of the body being affected by desynchronization. It can take up to 2 weeks for the effects of jet lag to be overcome and resynchronized by the body when major time zones have been crossed. Travelling from west to east is particularly difficult (Borbély 1987). The timing of maintenance medication during travelling needs to properly considered and managed, particularly for patients with diabetes or asthma, whose medication must reflect their own needs rather than sticking to a strict timetable.

Patients in hospital

In the hospital setting, desynchronization can occur as a result of illness or altered routines. Where patients are treated uniformly, there is an accompanying tendency for poor quality of sleep to be reported (Webster & Thompson 1986). This may be more pronounced in areas of critical care (see Ch. 31) where noise levels are difficult to minimize. A study performed under laboratory conditions demonstrated poor sleep quality in people subjected to noise levels equivalent to those of a critical care unit at night (Topf et al 1996). The nurse's role in relation to the minimization of noise at night is discussed later in the chapter.

FACTORS AFFECTING NORMAL SLEEP PATTERNS

Several factors are known to affect sleep patterns: age, culture, individuality, gender, body mass, genetics and physical activity.

Age

It is well known that the need for sleep changes with age (Table 4.1). A young adult may require as much as 8–10 hours per night, whereas an older adult may only need 5–6 hours. Other changes to the pattern occur, such as young adults only sleeping during the night, while elderly adults often nap during the day as well as sleeping at night. Increased awakenings are another way in which sleep patterns change as we age. Empson (1989) suggests that this is due to lengthening of the circadian

 EVIDENCE-BASED PRACTICE

4.1 Effect of night duty on nurses

A survey by Humm (2000) found that a third of nurses working night shifts believed they were a potential danger to patients. Many respondents, particularly those in acute areas, felt that they had less support from senior staff and doctors when on night duty, which increased their feelings of responsibility and made working more stressful. Many also complained of minimal staffing levels and feelings of isolation.

In the survey, in which 279 nurses responded, 68% reported having experienced some ill effects when working night shifts. Chronic fatigue was the most commonly reported effect. Other effects included periods of depression, mood swings, inability to concentrate, irritability, gastrointestinal problems (constipation, indigestion, appetite disturbance and

abdominal pain), fluid retention, skin problems, headaches and increased predisposition to minor infections. However, while large numbers reported some ill effects, almost a third of respondents did not report any, while 18% indicated a preference for night duty.

Citing research into shift-work patterns by Knauth (1997), Humm (2000) recommends short spans of night duty and, if rotating between days and nights, a night shift should be followed by at least 2 days off. There should be a minimum of 11 hours' rest between shifts.

References

Humm C. A hard day's night. Nurs Times 2000; 96(20): 28–31.
Knauth P. Changing schedules: shift work. Chronobiol Int 1997; 14(2): 159–171.

Table 4.1 How patterns of sleep alter with age

	Age		
	3 years	**25 years**	**75 years**
Amount of sleep in 24 h	13 hours	8 hours	5 hours
Pattern of sleep	Night sleep and daytime naps	Night sleep only	Night sleep and daytime naps

rhythms of temperature and other physiological variations. In the older female, the onset of the menopause may be accompanied by night sweats, which can disturb sleep.

Culture

The sleep patterns we adopt are culturally influenced. For example, in the countries around the Mediterranean and in Central and South America there is a period of daytime napping known as a 'siesta'. The Chinese also have a custom of napping after lunch, which is understood as a right and is provided for by employers (Borbély 1987). The 24-hour availability of services has had an effect on the cultural sleep patterns adopted in many countries, and electricity has meant that sleep is not so greatly influenced by day/night light patterns. Most of us now choose a pattern of sleep that suits our individual lifestyles, but whether this will have an effect on health is not yet known.

Individuality

The requirement for sleep varies enormously between individuals and it is impossible to generalize about an appropriate amount of sleep. It is also inappropriate to generalize about the way in which individuals sleep, e.g. some may prefer to sleep in a chair or even on the floor.

Gender

The literature indicates that there is little difference between the sexes in relation to sleep patterns, apart from perceptions of sleep quality and complaints about sleep. It appears that women have a tendency to complain more about their sleep, although men tend to have more episodes of sleep disturbance (Oswald & Adam 1983).

Body mass

Oswald & Adam (1983) found that people with greater body mass sleep better than those with less, spend more time in REM sleep and have longer ultradian rhythms. They also found that weight loss can be associated with an accompanying loss of sleep, e.g. in those who have anorexia nervosa (see Ch. 11).

Genetics

It is thought that genetic factors can influence the length of sleep and the subjective judgement about the quality of sleep (Borbély 1987). Individual circadian rhythms can be considered responsible for the two main personality types, although these are on a continuum and are not as polarized as they might appear (Borbély 1987). 'Morning types' are those who are alert and bright in the morning; they often do their best work in the

morning and by early evening become tired and less efficient. 'Evening types', on the other hand, are those who find rising in the morning a chore and do not begin to function at their best until the afternoon. Many perform at their best in the early evening and will often work late into the evening and settle late.

FACTORS THAT INTERRUPT SLEEP PATTERNS

There are a variety of external and internal factors that can interrupt an individual's sleep pattern.

EXTERNAL FACTORS

Noise

Noise is a factor that has been identified in several studies investigating the sleep environment in hospital (Closs 1988, Southwell & Wistow 1995). On busy wards it can be difficult to keep the night hours peaceful and quiet, although nurses can help in the following ways:

- wearing quiet shoes that do not squeak or click
- ensuring that trolleys are regularly serviced so that trolley noises are reduced to a minimum
- using separate admissions areas – some hospitals have tried to address the issue of noise caused by admissions at night by using separate admissions wards, to which patients are admitted overnight and then transferred to the appropriate area in the morning
- using flashing lights instead of a bell to indicate a ringing telephone
- reducing unnecessary chatter in patient areas – this is an important and easy way to reduce noise
- using single rooms and four-bedded bays – this helps to create a quieter, more homely atmosphere, although many patients will not be used to sharing a room with other sleepers at all. Conversely, patients who are used to sleeping with their partners may have difficulty adjusting to sleeping alone.

Light

The nurse's need for light, however dim, to enable observation during the night may create difficulty for patients who require absolute darkness to sleep. Southwell & Wistow (1995) found that lights were often dimmed for the minimum amount of time and little allowance was made for the increased need for sleep and rest in those who are ill. The need for sleep has to be balanced against the need for observation and, where possible, flexibility should be encouraged, perhaps by letting patients fall asleep in darkness and putting the night light on after they are asleep.

Hill (1989) suggested that we should allow critically ill patients more normal patterns of sleep and avoid continuous disturbance throughout the night wherever possible. Topf et al (1996) provide evidence of the effect of noise in a coronary care unit and the long-term effect on patients' sleep. The reduction of noise in these units and the promotion of diurnal variations in light and movement can benefit patients in respect of their sleep (see Chs 19 and 31).

INTERNAL FACTORS

There are several physical problems that can affect sleep patterns, including dyspnoea (pain and discomfort with breathing), which also increases anxiety about sleeping and may require unusual sleep positions; restless legs (disturbance in sensation, often felt in the legs); raised intracranial pressure; hormonal disorders (or natural changes, e.g. during pregnancy or the menopause); and nocturia (having to wake up to empty the bladder in the night), which may be due to excess alcohol, hormonal changes or prostate disease. Other causes are discussed below.

Pain

Pain is an important cause of difficulty in sleeping. The pain may be the result of patients having to adopt an unusual position due to their medical condition. Such discomfort as a cause of sleep disturbance was highlighted by Southwell & Wistow (1995). Nurses should promote comfort when settling a patient to aid rest and sleep. This is an essential skill for all nurses working with patients of all ages and with all conditions. It may involve settling a patient in a chair rather than in bed, or providing extra pillows for support and comfort. The use of soft sheets ('cuddlies') may also improve comfort. Some patients may want to try using their own pillowcases. Following the patient's individual pre-sleep routine (e.g. warm bath, milky drink or 'nightcap') may assist, particularly if it is possible to adopt the patient's preferred sleep position when settling. Frequent movement of patients who are unable to move themselves should not be forgotten as a benefit to sleep; it is not just important for skin integrity.

Diet

Food can have an impact on sleep, sometimes exacerbating pre-existing problems with sleep. Indigestion (e.g. following a heavy meal or during pregnancy) or hunger may prevent or disturb sleep. Eating a large meal creates a desire to sleep, which is thought to be a result of the effects of the metabolic enzymes. An easily digestible bedtime snack promotes better, more restful sleep (Oswald & Adams 1983).

Drugs and alcohol

The use of certain drugs which act as stimulants will cause problems with sleep patterns. Nicotine, for example, is a stimulant, increasing depth of breathing, raising blood pressure and increasing the output of adrenaline (epinephrine). Caffeine is also known to be a potent stimulant (Oswald & Adam 1983). Alcohol in small amounts can aid sleep, but large amounts may have the opposite effect and cause nocturia.

Exercise

It is known that physical exercise can help to promote sleep when taken in moderation and not directly before settling. Strenuous exercise immediately before settling causes the body to take longer to relax from the stimulation.

Mental health

Mental health problems such as anxiety or depression can have a deleterious effect on sleep. In adult nursing, one of the most important of these to consider is anxiety (see Chs 3 and 6). Patients with an uncertain diagnosis or facing investigations or surgery can be most at risk, although no one is immune (Southwell & Wistow 1995). Patients may also feel insecure; most people are used to locking their front door and preventing other people having free access to them while they are sleeping. The change in circumstances can heighten anxiety and increase difficulties. They may also feel insecure about the other sleepers sharing their room, who may be noisy or confused.

Depression can have a serious effect on sleep patterns and cause additional distress for the sufferer. Patients are often unable to fall asleep (toss and turn, unable to settle) or wake frequently throughout the night. Even if they do manage to sleep, they often wake up feeling that they have not slept.

DISORDERED SLEEP PATTERNS

The variation seen within normal sleep patterns is very great, as discussed above. However, some people's sleep patterns are disordered and they require intervention to assist in the establishment of a more acceptable pattern.

INSOMNIA

Insomnia is a symptom or group of symptoms that constitutes a sleep problem rather than a disorder in itself. It can take different forms. It can affect sleep latency (the ability to fall asleep) or it can consist of frequent night awakenings or early awakening with difficulty falling asleep again (Bearpark 1994). Insomnia may be temporary, lasting a few nights, or long-term, lasting months or even years. In treating insomnia, the cause has to be established as this is an important part of choosing the right treatment. For example, some people may have difficulty sleeping because their minds are turning over the events of the day just finished or worrying about the day to come. This anxiety causes a higher physiological arousal, which reduces sleep latency. Another common cause of insomnia is jet lag, referred to earlier in the chapter. Figure 4.3 illustrates some of the many and varied causes of insomnia.

Once the cause of the insomnia is established, treatment should involve suggesting patterns to avoid the problem. Medication may be used to establish a sleep pattern in the first instance. This is discussed later.

▶ Nursing management of insomnia

In hospital patients may be unable to sleep because of anxiety about their condition, impending investigations or treatment, worries about their family and home, pain and discomfort, lack of exercise or the strange environment in which they find themselves. As the nurse caring for these patients, it is important to identify the cause of the insomnia in order to effect appropriate management. It is not appropriate to routinely issue all patients with night sedation as a solution to their insomnia problems, as this may result in dependency (Halfens et al 1994). It is better to discuss any sources of anxiety and to try to ameliorate these, as this may enable patients to settle naturally. The nurse may be able to promote sleep using non-pharmacological means,

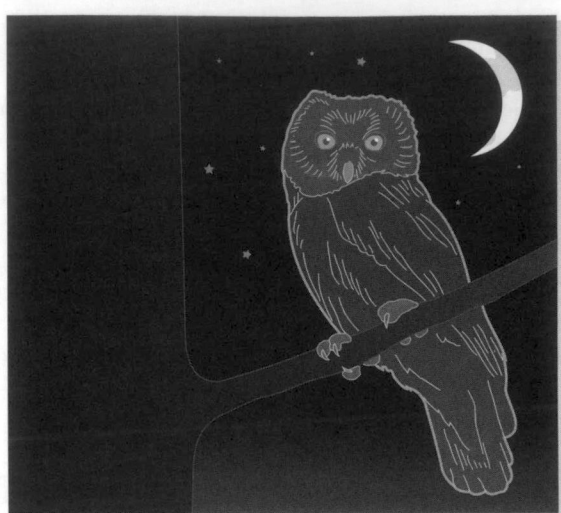

- Pain/discomfort
- Anxiety/fear
- Depression
- Bereavement
- Change in routine
- Too much/too little exercise
- Gender
- Genetics
- Excitement
- Light
- Noise
- Unfamiliar environment
- Too hot/too cold
- Hunger or over-eating
- Stimulants, e.g. caffeine, alcohol, nicotine
- Full bladder

Figure 4.3   Possible reasons for insomnia.

as discussed later in the chapter. As Ashton (1994) stresses, chronic insomnia is usually secondary to other conditions and treatment of the primary cause plus attention to sleep hygiene measures is important (see Health Promotion box 4.1).

EXCESS SOMNOLENCE (NARCOLEPSY)

Narcolepsy is a condition in which sufferers slip into REM sleep in an instant at any point during the day. There is a variety of symptoms, including sleep paralysis (the sufferer is alert but unable to move any muscles), hallucinations (seeing things that are not physically present) and insomnia. The condition can be severely debilitating and can result in sufferers having frequent accidents as well as losing their job. Some medications, which involve stimulants for daytime use, are in the process of being developed but are only 70% effective (Cooper 1994b). As narcolepsy is a lifelong condition, it is felt that the use of night

HEALTH PROMOTION

4.1 Managing insomnia

Borbély (1987) suggests the following to promote sleep:

- Avoid naps.
- Establish a regular bedtime.
- Reserve the evening hours for leisure activities and relaxation.
- Avoid caffeine, alcohol and nicotine in the hours before sleep.
- Create favourable conditions for sleep.
- If unable to sleep, get up and do something relaxing rather than lying in bed worrying about being unable to sleep.

Childs-Clark (1990) looked at the stimulus control technique using the following 'rules':

- Go to bed only when tired.
- If not asleep within 10–15 minutes, get up again and retire again when sleepy.
- Do not read, listen to the radio, watch television, eat, drink or smoke in bed.
- Get up at the same time each morning.
- No daytime catnapping.

The results of this study were encouraging as the sleep quality was increased with very little nursing support and without the use of sleep medication.

sedation should be kept to a minimum because of possible long-term effects of these drugs on the liver and renal system. Good sleep hygiene (measures to enhance sleep management) is crucial for these patients.

NIGHTMARES

Nightmares occur predominately during REM sleep. These are dreams that evoke a powerful emotional arousal that will often awaken the individual (Schatzman & Fenwick 1994). It has been suggested that the type of food eaten the previous evening may contribute to nightmares, but Griffin (1997) believes that they are more likely the result of events occurring in the evening or traumatic events in life. Repeated nightmares about the same subject may cause the individual to be frightened of going to sleep (Griffin 1997). This may be a symptom of post-traumatic stress (see Ch. 6).

▶ Nursing management

For most people, nightmares are unusual but can be rationalized and dealt with by the individual. As a nurse it may be necessary simply to provide some reassurance, reminding patients where they are and telling them that they are safe, as they may be disorientated when they wake up. Sometimes a cup of tea or a short chat helps to calm their fears and an increase in the amount of light may help.

SLEEP TERRORS

Sleep terrors are a phenomenon that commonly occurs in stage 4 sleep. Individuals wake up screaming and clearly terrified but are unable to vocalize the source of the fear. They may have some recollection but it is usually very brief and quickly forgotten. However, the arousal is sudden and causes the body to respond physiologically as in a fight-or-flight response, with an elevated heart and respiratory rate and the strong feeling of fear (this also occurs in nightmares).

▶ Nursing management

When caring for a person suffering night terror, it is important to remain calm and reassuring with a quiet, steady voice. It is best to be careful about the use of touch, because, if the person is not fully aroused, you may be mistaken as the protagonist of the piece and the person may become aggressive. It is best to be sure that the person is alert and knows who you are prior to touching or comforting.

SLEEPWALKING (SOMNAMBULANCE)

Sleepwalking occurs during stage 4 sleep and mostly affects children. Adults can also be affected, particularly as a result of anxiety or stress, and may resume sleepwalking as they once did as a child (this can be a symptom of regression). It is a myth that people who are sleepwalking never harm themselves. The main focus of management is to prevent injury whilst they are walking. Some sleepwalkers will perform quite complicated tasks whilst sleepwalking. One sleepwalker was known to walk to the fridge, pour a glass of orange juice and drink it before going back to bed. He remained completely unaware of the event.

▶ Nursing management

There are many myths about the right thing to do with sleepwalkers and whether or not to waken them. There is a limited amount of research into sleepwalking, mostly looking into the use of sleepwalking as a defence for crimes committed whilst asleep (Thomas 1997, Guilleminault et al 1998, Schenck & Mahowald 1998). It is best to simply watch sleepwalkers to ensure their safety (and that of others) and perhaps guide them gently back to bed, rather than trying to wake them up. It should be remembered that, as this happens in stage 4 sleep, sufferers will be difficult to wake. Attempting to do so could frighten them and cause a degree of shock. It is important for nurses on night duty to be aware of the potential for sleepwalking so that such behaviour does not surprise them.

SLEEP APNOEA/HYPOPNOEA SYNDROME

Sleep apnoea is a condition whereby a person stops breathing (apnoea) several times during sleep, due to occlusion of the upper airway. Hypopnoea is where there is a severe reduction in air flow without apnoea, due to the critical narrowing of the airway which restricts air flow. If the upper airway narrows subcritically, i.e. without causing hypopnoea or apnoea, turbulent flow occurs and the vibrating sound of snoring is produced

(Douglas 1994c). Airway patency relies on the upper airway opening muscles. During sleep, a loss of muscle tone is experienced and thus the upper airway is prone to narrowing. Normal breathing is restored following a brief arousal, as a result of negative intrapleural pressure, caused by the airway obstruction or partial obstruction. Patients are often unaware of awakening, although can be detected by EEG. Contributing factors to the condition are small mandibles, which rely on soft tissue functioning to maintain airways, and obesity, where fat deposits in the upper airway cause additional lack of muscle tone. Patients often complain about poor sleep and feeling tired all the time. This is due to the loss of sleep during the brief arousals throughout the night. Their partners may report very loud snoring and disturbances to their own sleep as a result.

Medical management

Treatment of sleep apnoea involves the promotion of weight loss, avoidance of alcohol in the evening and avoidance of sedatives. If severe, continuous positive airway pressure (CPAP) may be considered. This is where the patient receives a continuous gentle flow of air into the upper airway through a mask, which creates a positive pressure and maintains a patent airway. Some patients find this unacceptable due to the pressure of the mask or the noise of the machine, but in many patients it is very successful (Douglas 1994c). Upper airway surgery may be performed, involving resection of the uvula and soft palate, but it has been argued (Douglas 1994c) that this is less successful and may result in the patient being unable to use CPAP afterwards as an alternative.

▶ Nursing management

The management of uncomplicated snoring involves the promotion of weight loss in patients who are overweight, which may prevent more advanced problems of sleep apnoea. The avoidance of alcohol in the evening should be encouraged as this can add to the loss of muscle tone. If the sleep apnoea is posture-related, there are various techniques to prevent patients sleeping on their back. These range from sewing a golf ball into the back of pyjamas to prevent sleepers rolling onto their back, to propping them on their side by the use of a pillow wedge. If patients are having difficulties in hospital, it may be because sleeping on their side is not possible due to their medical condition; minimizing disturbance to other patients, e.g. by using a side ward for the snoring patient, may be the best option.

BRUXISM – GRINDING OF TEETH DURING SLEEP

This disorder is more common in children. In adulthood, some forms of drug treatment, stress or the persistence of a childhood habit can stimulate bruxism. No treatment is required, although dentists may suggest the use of a tooth guard if the patient's teeth are being worn away.

NURSING INTERVENTIONS TO PROMOTE SLEEP

There are a number of interventions that nurses can use to promote sleep (see Reflective Practice box 4.2). There is a growing

REFLECTIVE PRACTICE

4.2 Insomnia in hospital patients

Think of a preoperative patient you have nursed or someone awaiting investigations or results who had difficulty sleeping.

- What steps did you take to assist the patient to sleep?
- Were these effective in assisting the patient?
- Thinking back, could you have anticipated and/or prevented this patient's insomnia?

use of sleep clinics run by practice nurses or health visitors as a way of helping people with sleep problems (Childs-Clarke 1990). The following sections offer some suggestions for helping patients who are having difficulty sleeping.

ASSESSMENT OF SLEEP PATTERNS AND ROUTINES

It is important that patients are properly assessed and information gathered about their usual bedtime rituals or expectations about sleep (see Box 4.1). This information must reflect the patients' culture and social circumstances, as it should be an individualized assessment reflecting their beliefs and expectations. If the assessment is incomplete or inadequate, it is likely to be difficult to plan care that reflects individual needs and preferences. Partners or carers may be able to provide extra information, e.g. if a patient has had a cerebrovascular accident (see Ch. 14) and is unable to communicate (see Ch. 3).

PLANNING CARE

In the care plan (which should be negotiated with the patient) there should be an emphasis on maintaining the usual bedtime rituals. Patients should be encouraged to say what they want to happen to them in hospital. As far as possible, they should retain control over their own routine. Older patients may want to 'fit in' with the ward routine and not 'make a fuss' because the nurses are busy. They may be adopting the 'patient role' as a result of their previous experiences of hospital stays, particularly if they have not been in hospital since the 1960s or 1970s when much of the care was routinized and patients were

---

Box 4.1 Factors to consider in the assessment of sleep routine (Hodgson 1991)

- Age
- Normal pattern of sleep during health
- Current pattern of sleep
- Emotional status
- Day- and night-time symptoms
- Sleeping environment
- Sleep-related rituals
- Occurrence of dreams or nightmares
- Current medication
- Waking time behaviour

---

expected to follow the ward pattern. They may regard the accompanying lack of sleep as an expected by-product of the hospital stay – clearly an undesirable option for most people who are ill. At times it will not be possible to follow the patients' normal routine and the change should be discussed with those patients who can contribute to the formation of an alternative plan. If patients are unable to contribute initially (due to their condition) then this should be done as soon as their condition permits.

HELPING PATIENTS TO SLEEP

This involves being aware of and knowledgeable about the environment in which nurses work and patients try to sleep. It requires nurses to look critically at the care they give to patients and to make sure they are not acting without consideration of the patients' need for sleep and rest. For example, the ritual of waking all patients at 6.00am for routine observations or administration of medicines that could be scheduled for a more appropriate time should no longer occur.

EVALUATING THE SUCCESS OF THE PLANNED CARE

It is important that we respect patients' own reports of the quality of their sleep as part of our evaluation. It is a subjective matter and nurses cannot judge the quality of someone else's sleep. Hence, patient reports form an essential part of the evaluation process. Nurses may well report that patients appeared to be asleep all night, but some of these patients will report that they 'haven't slept a wink'. Other patients may avoid telling nurses they are not sleeping because the nurses are 'so busy' and they do not want to bother them.

As part of this process there should be a re-evaluation of the planned care and subsequent adjustment made to promote a better night's sleep. This process should be under continual review whilst patients are dependent on nursing care. Remember that this plan does not just relate to patients in hospital but can also relate to patients being cared for in their own homes who are receiving support from nurses working in the community.

 GUIDELINES FOR CARE PRIORITIES

4.1 Promoting sleep

In promoting sleep, nurses should:

- take a full assessment of normal routine
- plan care that enables individuals to maintain as much of their normal routine as possible
- ensure that the environment is conducive to sleep as far as is possible for each patient and that pain is well controlled
- ensure that sleep and rest are evaluated in light of the patient's report as well as nursing observation
- think of alternatives to promote sleep rather than using medications routinely
- foster an atmosphere in which patients can report problems they are having with sleep

NON-PHARMACOLOGICAL MEANS OF PROMOTING SLEEP

Nurses have considerable influence on the use of medication as a means of assisting sleep in the hospital setting, but there are numerous ways in which sleep can be promoted before resorting to the use of medicines (see Fig. 4.4; see also Evidence-based Practice box 4.2). Some of the alternatives to medication are discussed below.

Darkness

Darkness is a prerequisite for many people to fall asleep. It is not always possible to achieve in the hospital or nursing home setting, but reducing the quantity of light to a minimum will help in most cases; curtains for additional shade are also useful. Some patients find eyeshades helpful.

Silence

Silence, or at least very low noise levels, is also desirable. Thinking of ways in which to decrease the night-time noise levels in an institution is an important role of the nurse, particularly as it is often the nurses who are guilty of making the most noise! Some of the ways in which this might be achieved are discussed above.

Comfort

Relaxation and a comfortable position are important for settling, especially where beds and bedding are unfamiliar. If patients are

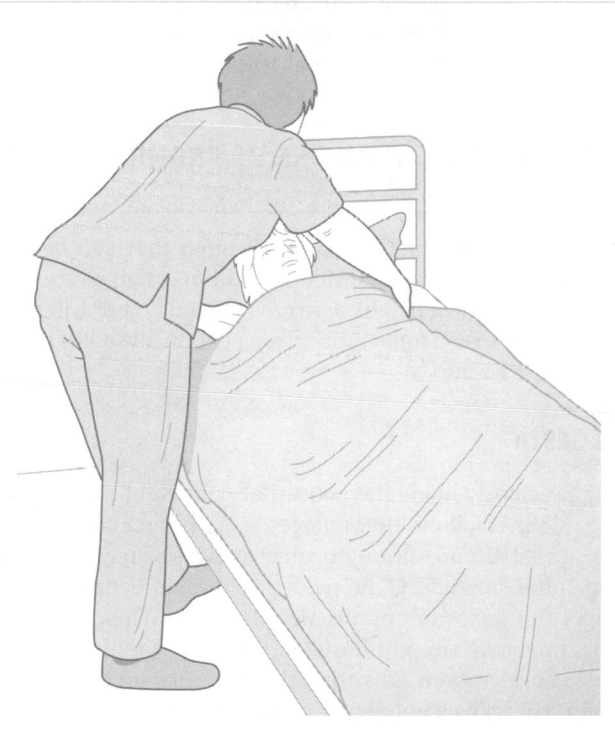

- Darkness
- Silence/reduced noise
- Relaxation
- Comfort/positioning
- Physical activity promoting tiredness
- Food/drink at bedtime
- Fresh air
- Security
- Familiarity
- Reading
- Day time activities
- Timing of medications, e.g. analgesia, diuretics
- Complimentary therapy, e.g. massage, aromatherapy

Figure 4.4 Non-pharmacological methods of promoting sleep.

 EVIDENCE-BASED PRACTICE

4.2 Use of sleep medication

A study by Halfens et al (1994) looked at the use of sleep medication in Dutch hospitals and its effect on patients' habits on leaving hospital. They found that patients who had used sleep medication for at least 5 days in hospital continued to use the medication at home, whereas those who had not had sleep medication in hospital did not use medication at home. As all participants in the study had not had any sleep medication prior to hospital admission, this highlights a worrying trend and calls into question the routine use of sleep medication before trying alternative non-pharmacological ways to assist sleep.

A further study undertaken by Duxbury (1994) examined the style of ward management and concluded that, where patients were cared for by team nursing, up to three times as much night sedation was administered than in those ward areas managed by primary nursing. The philosophy of care seemed to be an important aspect of care. The primary nursing team demonstrated more autonomy and used sleep medication as one of a range of methods for promoting sleep rather than as a first resort. It appeared that nurses working within the primary nursing system of care provided care for patients that was patient-centred and encouraged by individual responsibility for care.

Student activities
- Why do you think that primary nursing was shown to reduce the need for night sedation?
- When on practice, look at the systems of care in place and evaluate for yourself the extent to which they are patient-centred, and in particular consider how this affects care related to sleep and rest.

References
Duxbury J. An investigation into primary nursing and its effect upon the nursing attitudes about administration of p.r.n. night sedation. J Adv Nurs 1994; 19(5): 923–931.
Halfens R, Cox K, Kupper-Van Merwijk A. Effect of the use of sleep medication in Dutch hospitals on the use of sleep medication at home. J Adv Nurs 1994; 19(1): 66–70.

having difficulty, the use of their own bedding, particularly pillows and pillowcases, may prove helpful; this should be considered especially for those patients who are likely to be admitted for a long period. Positioning is important and with totally dependent patients the ability to position them appropriately is an essential skill for nurses to learn. Timing analgesia so that it is taken just before retiring will also aid sleep.

Physical activity

Feeling tired is an important component of going to sleep and patients in an institutional setting, especially if they are used to being very active, may find that they do not get tired enough to sleep. Nurses may help patients by suggesting activity according to their mobility and medical condition. If a patient has limited mobility, then remembering to assist that person with mobilization would be one method of aiding exercise.

Food and drink

The consumption of food and drink can be an important part of the bedtime ritual. A snack or nourishing drink such as hot malted milk prior to bed may enable some patients to sleep more soundly. This can be difficult to provide in hospitals, as many wards do not have access to catering facilities in the late evening. However, if there are drinks machines, most will have the facility to produce hot chocolate. As discussed earlier, avoiding large meals that may cause indigestion will also aid sleep.

Temperature

A warm environment will encourage sleep in some patients, while others like fresh air. Managing the temperature to suit everyone sharing a room is not an easy task. The use of warm clothing and the provision of extra blankets are ways of getting around the problem. Warm baths in the evening may also promote sleepiness and lead to a better night's sleep for some patients. There will be times, however, when a patient's area is too hot, in which case cooling measures such as a fan will be required.

Security

Feeling secure will help those patients who are nervous and anxious. The walk round by night staff in order to meet patients before they settle can promote this feeling of security, as the patients then know who is responsible for their care overnight. Familiar surroundings can also help and therefore family photographs or other personal effects from home should be encouraged as appropriate. This is particularly important in older adults in nursing homes, as it is most common for disorientation to occur during the night. Reading will help some to settle and a supply of reading material should be kept handy for those who haven't brought any into hospital with them.

Daytime naps

A good night's sleep can also be promoted by encouraging patients to avoid daytime naps. This may involve the provision of some kind of entertainment during the day to prevent boredom. This strategy of stimulation during the daytime in order to promote a better sleep pattern is increasingly being used in nursing and residential homes and a wide range of daytime activities is often available (Horne 1991).

Timing of regular medication

The administration of medication is an important consideration in the daytime routine. For example, it is more appropriate to give diuretic drugs in the morning so that the effects will have worn off prior to the patient settling (Horne 1991). On the other hand, drugs with drowsiness as a side-effect (e.g. certain types of analgesia, antidepressants) are best administered in the evening so that patients can sleep off the effect and be alert the following day. This will not only promote sleep but also reduce the likelihood of daytime naps.

Complementary therapies

There are a number of complementary therapies that can aid sleep. Mantle (1996) offers a useful summary of these, including massage and aromatherapy, hypnosis, acupressure and acupuncture. Several studies have investigated the use of complementary therapies in sleep and rest management in hospital (e.g. Cannard 1995, Dunn et al 1995, Ersser et al 1999).

PHARMACOLOGICAL MEANS OF PROMOTING SLEEP

There are a number of types of medication that can be used to promote sleep and rest. Although it is important to consider non-pharmacological means, for some patients there will be no alternative but to use some form of medication, even if it is only a temporary measure.

ANALGESIA

Having previously made the point that pain can be an impediment to sleep, it follows that analgesia can be an effective medication to aid sleep. Although some analgesia may also have a sleep-enhancing effect, the reduction of pain is undoubtedly an important factor in improvement in sleep. When caring for patients unable to sleep in hospital, analgesia should be one of the first considerations. Ensuring that patients are comfortable and pain-free is an essential part of the nurse's role.

HYPNOTICS

Hypnotic drugs act on the nervous system to promote sleep. These include nitrazepam, temazepam, chloral hydrate and clomethiazole. Benzodiazepines are the most commonly prescribed hypnotics, e.g. nitrazepam, temazepam and loprazolam. They induce sleep by depressing the reticular formation, which is responsible for alertness. Benzodiazepines also reduce nocturnal disturbances, thus increasing total sleep time (Ashton 1994). They tend to increase stage 2 sleep whilst stages 3 and 4 and REM sleep are reduced.

One of the difficulties with sleep medication is that, if given late at night, the patient will remain sleepy in the morning hours. It is not possible, therefore, to 'wait and see' and only administer the medication if the patient is unable to sleep. Rebound insomnia can occur following withdrawal from such medication, particularly if taken in large doses or for long periods and patients will often experience vivid dreams and nightmares when these drugs are stopped. Ashton (1994) found

OLDER ADULTS: NURSING PRIORITIES

4.1 Sleep and the older adult

Morgan (1987) suggested that the changes in the sleep patterns of older adults may be due to a number of factors:

- changes in bladder function
- disordered breathing – sleep apnoea, snoring
- increased limb movements
- pain and discomfort
- depression
- dementia – where sleep becomes short, shallow and desynchronized
- bereavement
- living alone – lack of security, reassurance and comfort
- financial hardship – leading to inadequate diet and cold
- noise due to institutionalization – auditory awakening thresholds decrease with age.

Kearnes (1989) found that an established bedtime routine, prevention of anxiety and the promotion of relaxation were key considerations for the promotion of sleep. Warner (1997), in a small study of residents in a nursing home, found that on the whole their bedtime rituals were respected, although a few residents reported having adopted new rituals since coming to the home. The study found that sleep quality was improved without the use of sleep medication. In older adults who experience a reduction in sleep quality, anything that nurses and carers can do to promote sleep is going to be of benefit. This means looking for ways to avoid the use of hypnotics which can have many side-effects in this age group.

References

Kearnes S. Insomnia in the elderly. Nurs Times 1989; 85(47): 32–33.
Morgan K. Sleepless and unsettled. Nurs Times 1987; 92(23): 46–47.
Warner J. Bedtime rituals of nursing home residents: a study.
  Nurs Stand 1997; 11(20): 34–38.

ETHICAL ISSUES

4.1 Should I wake patients for their night sedation?

You are on night duty. At 10.00pm, while you are administering the medicines, a patient collapses and requires your assistance. When you resume the medicine round at 10.45pm, many of the patients at the other end of the ward have fallen asleep. Some of them are prescribed essential medications as well as night sedation if required, while others normally only have night sedation.

What should you do? Should you wake the patients for their medication? What if you decide not to wake the patients and they wake up at midnight saying they are unable to sleep?

ANXIOLYTICS

These are tranquillizers and are usually administered throughout the day to reduce anxiety and promote relaxation (Burton 1992). They include beta blockers which reduce the physical effects of the anxiety, e.g. atenolol, oxprenolol and propanolol. Some of the hypnotics have an anxiolytic effect as well, which can prove useful (e.g. benzodiazepines such as diazepam and lorazepam).

COMMON DISORDERS THAT AFFECT SLEEP

Many disorders suffered by adults are likely to disturb their sleep. A few are discussed here in detail, but it should be stressed that sleep and rest are an important part of nursing assessment for all patients.

BREATHING PROBLEMS

Remembering the effect of sleep mechanisms on breathing described early on in this chapter, it is clear that getting to sleep and staying asleep can be a problem for those with disorders of the respiratory system, especially asthma, chronic obstructive airways limitation and heart failure. Many asthmatics suffer problems with the onset of sleep, with nocturnal wheezing or coughing (Douglas 1994b).

▶ Nursing management

Patients who have compromised airway or lung function prior to sleep are likely to have more difficulties during sleep. Position is important for efficient airway maintenance. Oxygen therapy may be instigated and it is important to remember that the oxygen should be humidified and warmed if possible to promote an ambient environment for sleep. Cold oxygen can trigger an allergic reaction in people with asthma and many will experience exacerbations of their asthma in cold weather. Many will need to sleep in an upright position, often wearing an oxygen mask or nasal cannulae, which can prove uncomfortable.

that when patients stopped taking benzodiazepines they experienced more slow wave and REM sleep and the symptoms of withdrawal sometimes lasted several weeks. Benzodiazepines are metabolized by the liver, which becomes less efficient in the older adult and in those with liver disease (see Ch. 23). Thus care must be taken when prescribing for these patients (see Older Adults: Nursing Priorities box 4.1; Ashton 1994).

Hypnotics can also cause a 'hangover effect' and impair performance the following day, which is most marked in the older adult. It can cause drowsiness, poor coordination, ataxia leading to falls and fractures, poor memory and mental confusion (see Ethical Issues box 4.1). Benzodiazepines can also create dependence when used over a long period and primary care practitioners are working to reduce such long-term use of these drugs.

Barbiturates are similar to benzodiazepines in their action, but are no longer widely used because of their toxicity (particularly their depressing effect on the respiratory centre in the brain), increased drug interactions and the susceptibility of users to dependence and abuse (Ashton 1994).

Patients of all ages are at an increased risk of developing skin integrity problems in the sacral area, buttocks or heels from prolonged sitting. Care must be taken to promote skin integrity, otherwise the patients will be disadvantaged if they develop a sore which inhibits their ability to choose the optimum position for their breathing. There are a number of devices that will help the patient in this area (see Ch. 10).

Patients with breathing difficulties may be afraid to go to sleep, in case they do not wake up. The apprehension is often worse at night without the daily hustle and bustle to distract them. Nurses must remember that such fears are real to patients and should not be dismissed, and patients should be reassured as much as possible, but always truthfully. A light may enhance their feelings of security and they may be comforted by the knowledge that the nurse will be returning to check on their condition frequently during the night.

URINARY SYSTEM

Disorders of the urinary system may disturb sleep, particularly if nocturia is one of the features of the condition. Older people usually find that their bladder requires to be emptied more frequently anyway. This is especially true for older men with prostate disease.

▶ Nursing management

Nursing management focuses on making special provision for the patient with urinary problems. For those who are confined to bed, this will mean changing their bottle frequently during the night, and for those who are ambulant, this will mean locating their bed near a toilet, so that the amount of time out of bed is limited. The need to respond quickly to a patient's request for assistance is paramount at night, as such patients may not be able to hold on for very long before voiding. Encouraging patients not to drink fluids late in the evening may reduce their need to pass urine during the night, but it is important in this case that their daytime fluid intake is adequate to prevent dehydration.

RHYTHMIC PATTERN DISORDERS

Two rhythmic pattern disorders known to affect sleep are seasonal affective disorder (SAD), which affects a number of people particularly in the northern hemisphere, and the menstrual cycle.

Seasonal affective disorder

This is a type of depression that is pronounced during the winter months when the daylight hours are shorter. It is thought to be a result of the overproduction of melatonin (Zoltoski & Gillin 1994) and there is evidence to suggest that melatonin is secreted in a seasonal pattern throughout the year (Wehr 1991) as well as in a circadian rhythm. The sufferer, who feels tired and depressed during the winter months, improves with the coming of spring (Kronauer 1994). The therapy of choice for this disorder is exposure to an artificial source of bright light that mimics sunlight. This has been found to bring relief to many sufferers without the need to resort to medication. For people with jet lag,

exposure to several hours of bright light to inhibit the production of melatonin has been shown to speed recovery (Tortora & Grabowski 2000).

Menstrual cycle

The hormones that control the menstrual cycle have been shown to undergo diurnal variation in their levels, although the reasons for this have not been fully explained (see Ch. 25).

Changes in the menstrual cycle can disturb sleep, and women experiencing the onset of menopause may find that their sleep patterns are altered, e.g. they may find themselves waking frequently during the night. This can occur with or without night sweats.

CONCLUSION

The importance to patients of sleep and rest, whether in the hospital environment, in their own home or within a care environment such as a nursing home, is self-evident. The role of nurses in promoting sleep for people in their care is clearly an important one and should not be diminished in any way. Nurses should take every opportunity to ensure that their patients are assisted to the best possible night's sleep, whilst at the same time respecting their individuality and cultural preferences.

SUMMARY: MAIN POINTS

- Sleep is a natural phenomenon, which every person requires whether well or ill.

- The main control mechanism is thought to be in the reticular activating system.

- Circadian rhythms dictate the daily routine of sleep and activity.

- Culture is an important aspect of sleep habit and should be considered for all individuals.

- Nurses can assist patients to improve their sleep in hospital, at home or in other care settings.

- Assessment is the key to nursing management of sleep in any setting and should incorporate patients' subjective report of the quality of their sleep.

- Sleep deprivation is associated with difficulties in concentration, ability to perform complex tasks and ability to remain alert.

- Nurses may suffer sleep deprivation as a result of working in shifts and need to ensure that their own needs for sleep and rest are met.

- Biological rhythms have an effect on temperature, blood pressure, pulse and respiration rates, as there are normal diurnal variations.

- Many disease processes disturb sleep or make it more difficult and nurses need to recognize this and instigate measures to improve sleep where possible.

SELF-TEST: CRITICAL THINKING ACTIVITIES

1 Consider a patient whom you have recently admitted:
— How did you assess the need for sleep and plan the care to promote sleep?
— Do you think your plan was successful? What made it a success? What could have improved it?
— Who was the true evaluator of success? Were that person's views sought?

2 An older adult is going to be moving into a nursing home. With particular regard for sleep and rest, state the important issues to be considered to ensure a smooth transition and the least disturbance. If you were working in the nursing home, how would you plan to meet the needs of this client?

3 One of the patients in a four-bedded bay begins to snore in the night and disturbs the other patients in the bay.
— How should the night nurse manage this situation?
— What might the long-term strategy to help the snoring patient involve?

4 One of the nurses you are working with boasts of working extra shifts for an agency to earn money to pay off debts. She reveals that she has worked eight nights in a row and has worked some day shifts as well and had not had a day off in 3 weeks.
— What would be your main concerns, and why?
— Imagine you are the ward manager and come to hear about this. How do you think this situation should be managed?

 ## FURTHER READING

Borbély A (Schneider D, trans). Secrets of sleep. Harlow: Longman; 1987 *offers a scientific explanation about sleep in an easy-to-digest format. There is discussion about the methods used to investigate sleep and some consideration about how sleep problems are diagnosed and treated.*

Cooper R (ed). Sleep. London: Chapman and Hall; 1994 – *aimed at medical staff; however, it offers a technical insight into the present understanding of sleep research for those who want a more detailed and technical explanation.*

Hodgson LA. Why do we need sleep? Relating theory to nursing practice. J Adv Nurs 1991; 16; 1503–1510 – *a discussion about sleep relating the theory to practice in a clear way.*

McMahon R (ed). Nursing at night: a professional approach. Harrow: Scutari Press; 1992 – *this edited book offers the reader insight into professional issues about night nursing. It discusses the promotion of sleep as well as quality and management issues.*

Webster RA. Sleep in hospital. J Adv Nurs 1986; 11: 447–457 – *offers a review of the literature and is a useful insight into sleep in hospital.*

 ## USEFUL WEBSITES

www.lut.ac.uk/departments/hu/groups/sleep – the sleep website of the university of Loughborough which provides information on research presently being undertaken by Professor J. Horne and his team.

www.unisa.edu.au/sleep – website for the Centre for Sleep Research in South Australia which gives some useful information and research updates.

www.sleepnet.com/index.shtml – this website offers links to other sites, which provide evidence of sleep research. It is user-friendly and regularly updated. There are reviews of many sites available worldwide.

REFERENCES

Ashton H. The effects of drugs on sleep. In: Cooper R, ed. Sleep. London: Chapman and Hall Medical; 1994: 175–211.

Bangura K. Dying for a snooze. Nursing Times 1998; 94(21): 29–30.

Bearpark HM. Insomnia: causes, effects and treatment. In: Cooper R, ed. Sleep. London: Chapman and Hall Medical; 1994: 587–613.

Borbély A (Schneider D, trans). Secrets of sleep. Harlow: Longman Scientific and Technical; 1987.

Brugne JF. Effects of night work on circadian rhythms and sleep. Prof Nurse 1994; 10(1): 25–28.

Burton E. Something to help you sleep? Nurs Times 1992; 88(35): 52–53.

Cannard G. On the scent of a good night's sleep. Nurs Stand 1995; 9(34): 21.

Centre for Sleep Research. Biological rhythms and body clocks. Shiftwork Executive Summary. Online. Available: www.unisa.edu.au/sleep/course_us/us_bio/ us_bio_course.html; 1999.

Childs-Clarke A. Stimulus control technique for sleep onset insomnia. Nurs Times 1990; 86(35): 52–53.

Close SJ. A nursing study of sleep on surgical wards. Report prepared for the Scottish Home and Health Department. Edinburgh: Nursing Research Unit, Department of Nursing Studies; 1988.

Cooper R. Normal sleep. In: Cooper R, ed. Sleep. London: Chapman and Hall Medical; 1994a: 3–46.

Cooper R. Neurology and sleep disorders. In: Cooper R, ed. Sleep. London: Chapman and Hall Medical; 1994b: 412–466.

Davies RJO, Jenkins NE, Stradling JR. Effect of measuring ambulatory blood pressure on sleep and on blood pressure during sleep. Br Med J 1994; 308: 820–823.

Douglas NJ. Breathing during sleep in normal subjects. In: Cooper R, ed. Sleep. London: Chapman and Hall Medical; 1994a: 76–95.

Douglas NJ. Breathing during sleep in patients with lung disease. In: Cooper R, ed. Sleep. London: Chapman and Hall Medical; 1994b: 301–325.

Douglas NJ. The sleep apnoea/hypopnoea syndrome. In Cooper R, ed. Sleep. London: Chapman and Hall Medical; 1994c: 272–292.

Dunn C, Sleep J, Collett D. Sensing an improvement: an experimental study to evaluate the use of aromatherapy, massage and periods of rest in an intensive care unit. J Adv Nurs 1995; 21: 34–40.

Empson J. Sleep and dreaming. London: Faber and Faber; 1989.

Ersser S, Taylor H, Wiles A et al. Measuring the sleep patterns of older people. Nurs Times 1999; 95(1): 46–49.

Folkard S. Circadian rhythms and hours of work. In: Warr P, ed. Psychology of work, 3rd edn. Harmondsworth: Penguin Books; 1991: 30–52.

Garfinkel D, Laudon M, Nof D et al. Improvements in sleep quality in elderly people by controlled release melatonin. The Lancet 1995; 346: 541–544.

Griffin J. The origin of dreams. Hailsham: The Therapist Ltd; 1997.

Guilleminault C, Leger D, Philip P et al. Nocturnal wandering and violence: review of a sleep clinic population. J Forensic Sci 1998: 43(1): 158–163.

Haimov I, Laudon M, Zisapel N et al. Sleep disorders and melatonin rhythms in elderly people. Br Med J 1994; 309: 67.

Halfens R, Cox K, Kupper-Van Merwijk A. Effect of the use of sleep medication in Dutch hospitals on the use of sleep medication at home. J Adv Nurs 1994; 19(1): 66–70.

Hill J. A good night's sleep. Senior Nurse 1989; 9(5): 17–19.

Hodgson LA. Why do we need sleep? Relating theory to nursing practice. J Adv Nurs 1991; 16: 1503–1510.

Horne JA. Why we sleep: the function of sleep in human and other mammals. Oxford: Oxford University Press; 1988.

Horne LA. No more wakeful nights: helping elderly people sleep properly. Prof Nurse 1991; 6: 383–385.

Kronauer RE. Circadian rhythms. In: Cooper R, ed. Sleep. London: Chapman and Hall Medical; 1994: 96–134.

Lutchmansingh P, Poland RE. Sleep neuroendocrinology. In: Cooper R, ed. Sleep. London: Chapman and Hall Medical; 1994: 375–411.

Mantle F. Sleepless and unsettled. Nurs Times 1996; 92(23): 46–47.

Middleton BA, Stone BM, Arendt J. Melatonin and fragmented sleep patterns. The Lancet 1996; 348(9026): 551–552.

Oswald I, Adam K. Get a better night's sleep. London: Martin Dunitz; 1983.

Reet M. In: Mallik M, Hall C, Howard D, eds. Nursing knowledge and practice: a decision-making approach. London: Baillière Tindall; 1998.

Schatzman M, Fenwick P. Dreams and dreaming. In: Cooper R, ed. Sleep. London: Chapman and Hall Medical; 1994: 212–242.

Schenck CH, Mahowald MW. An analysis of a recent criminal trial involving sexual misconduct with a child, alcohol abuse and a successful sleepwalking defence: arguments supporting two proposed new forensic categories. Med Sci Law 1998; 38(2): 147–152.

Southwell MT, Wistow G. Sleep in hospital: are patients' needs being met? J Adv Nurs 1995; 21(6): 1101–1109.

Thomas TN. Sleepwalking disorder and mens rea: a review and case report. J Forensic Sci 1997; 42(1): 17–24.

Topf M, Bookman M, Arand D. Effects of critical care unit noise on the subjective quality of sleep. J Adv Nurs 1996; 24(3): 545–551.

Tortora GJ, Grabowski SR. Principles of anatomy and physiology, 9th edn. New York: John Wiley; 2000.

Warner J. Bedtime rituals of nursing home residents: a study. Nurs Stand 1997; 11(20) 34–38.

Webster RA, Thompson DR. Sleep in hospital. J Adv Nurs 1986; 11: 447–457.

Wehr TA. The durations of human melatonin secretion and sleep respond to changes in daytime length (photoperiod). J Clin Endicrinol Metab 1991; 73(6): 1276–1280.

Yamasaki F, Schwartz JE, Gerber LM et al. Impact of shift work and race/ethnicity on the diurnal rhythm of blood pressure and catecholamines. Hypertension 1998; 32(3): 417–423.

Zoltoski RK, Gillin JC. The neurochemistry of sleep. In: Cooper R, ed. Sleep. London: Chapman and Hall Medical; 1994: 135–174.

5 Temperature regulation

Sharon Edwards

'I know my temperature was up because I was burning hot. I felt terrible. The nurses gave me some tablets to bring down my temperature, but the best bit was the refreshing wash and clean sheets that they gave me.'

(Patient)

THIS CHAPTER WILL HELP YOU

- Understand the physiological principles of thermoregulation
- Identify the factors affecting temperature
- Understand the types of abnormal temperature and their aetiologies
- Critically discuss the factors involved in temperature measurement and assessment
- Determine the appropriate evidence-based nursing intervention(s) for patients with abnormal temperature.

KEYWORDS

Afebrile	Hyperthermia
Core temperature	Hypothermia
Febrile	Peripheral temperature
Hyperpyrexia	Pyrexia

INTRODUCTION

A change in body temperature is a common occurrence in patients both in the community and in hospital. Such a change may alert nurses to the presence of infection, thermoregulatory dysfunction, deterioration in a patient's condition or hypothermia, and therefore its detection is vitally important in order that early therapeutic intervention may be instigated. Accurate monitoring of temperature is also important, as both abnormally high and abnormally low values can have deleterious effects on the body.

This chapter provides a review of the physiology of temperature homeostasis and thermoregulation. It explores issues around normal body temperature and the factors that affect it. Clinical data in relation to patients at risk from abnormal temperatures are discussed with special reference to older adults and those with specific illnesses. The main disorders of temperature regulation are pyrexia, hyperpyrexia, hyperthermia, hypothermia and frostbite. The difference between hyperpyrexia and hyperthermia and the aetiology of each are discussed, as well as the physiological benefits and detrimental responses to pyrexia. Hypothermia is also explored, and the different types, definitions and physiological processes involved, including frostbite, are outlined.

Assessment of a patient's body temperature is necessary to determine the specific nursing interventions required. Taking a patient's temperature, the sites and instruments used in current practice and the reliability of these instruments are discussed. Temperature regulation and management are complex issues and require an understanding of the physiological processes and the specific nursing practices involved. This chapter emphasizes the importance of nursing care in relation to patients suffering from a high temperature or hypothermia, and the knowledge and skills that are necessary for safe practice. It stresses the contribution nurses make in caring for patients with temperature abnormalities and the complexity and skill required in an area which is sometimes dismissed as 'basic' nursing care.

PHYSIOLOGY OF TEMPERATURE HOMEOSTASIS

The maintenance of body temperature within the normal range is necessary for life. The temperature is controlled by the hypothalamus, which maintains temperature homeostasis. This includes the ability to increase heat production and to conserve heat or increase heat loss, thus ensuring that body temperature remains between 35.5 and 37.5°C, a process known as thermoregulation.

THERMOREGULATION

This homeostatic process, whereby the body temperature is kept within acceptable limits regardless of the environmental conditions, is governed by anatomical and physiological mechanisms within the body. The temperature is regulated almost entirely by nervous feedback control mechanisms, and almost all of them operate through a temperature-regulating centre located in the hypothalamus. These feedback mechanisms consist of three parts:

■ a receptor – a sensor that is sensitive to particular changes in body or environmental temperature. These are found in the skin, spinal cord, abdomen and other internal structures of the body that transmit signals to the hypothalamus
■ a control or integration centre (the hypothalamus) – this receives and processes the information supplied by the receptor
■ an effector – a cell or organ that responds to the commands of the control centre and whose activities serve to reduce or increase body temperature.

To maintain set point temperature, receptors are continually sending information about environmental and body temperature to the hypothalamus (control centre). In extreme heat or cold, when the body temperature may be higher or lower than set point temperature, the hypothalamus maintains the desired level by interpreting the information received and passing regulatory commands to the effector cell, which then activates either heat loss or heat conservation mechanisms to adjust the body temperature so that it matches the set point temperature.

CORE AND PERIPHERAL TEMPERATURE

The temperature of the body is not the same all over: the skin and peripheries are normally several degrees cooler than the core (organs, blood and deeper tissues) (Fig. 5.1). The temperature of the skin will vary according to the temperature of the environment and thus if the air temperature is high, the peripheral temperature will also rise and may be almost equal to that of the core. This has an effect on heat transfer mechanisms, which is described below. The ability of the blood vessels near the surface of the skin to constrict or dilate is important to thermoregulation and monitoring the difference between peripheral and core temperature is indicated in the management of some patients. This difference may also be used to give an indication of the effectiveness of warming procedures in cases of hypothermia.

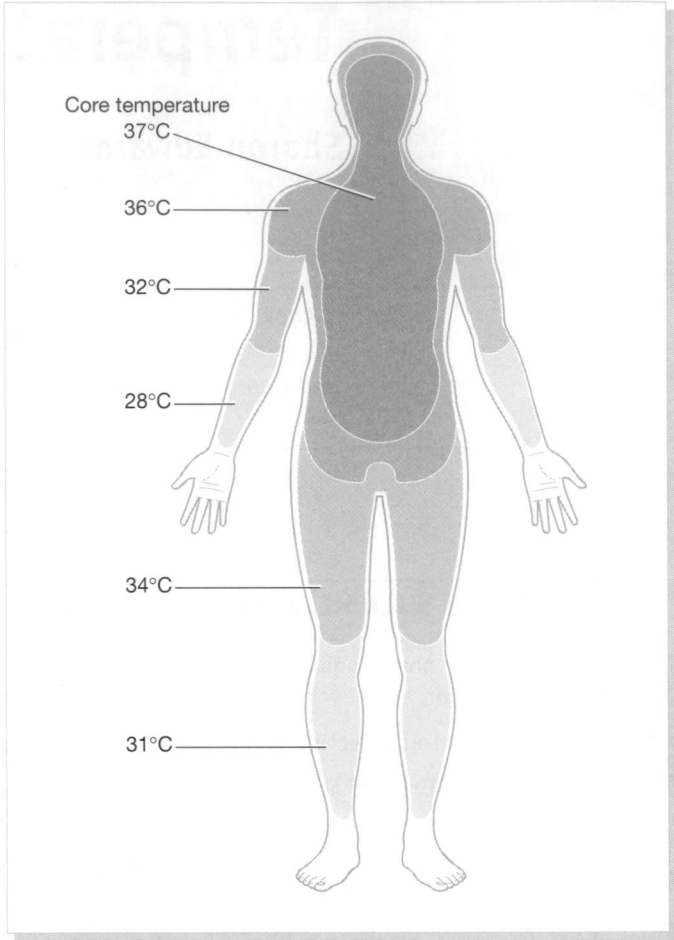

Figure 5.1 Body temperature at different sites.

HEAT REGULATION MECHANISMS

The body is continuously producing heat as a by-product of metabolism and this heat must be lost to the environment at the same rate as it is produced if body temperature is to remain constant. When environmental conditions are either too warm or too cold, the body must control the gains or losses to maintain homeostasis. This is achieved through heat transfer, heat loss and heat gain mechanisms.

Heat transfer mechanisms

Heat transfer mechanisms serve to maintain a balance between heat production and heat loss. There are four processes involved: radiation, conduction, convection and evaporation.

Radiation

Loss of heat by radiation comprises energy loss in the form of infra-red heat rays. This is heat lost from the body to any surroundings that are cooler than the body itself. This loss increases as the temperature of the surroundings decreases. Over half the heat that is lost is as a result of radiation. The exact amount varies with body temperature and skin temperature. Little heat will be lost through radiation if the air temperature is equal to, or higher than, skin temperature.

Conduction

The direct transfer of energy through physical contact, e.g. sitting on a cold chair, is referred to as conduction heat loss. Although heat loss through direct contact is not a very effective mechanism, loss of heat by conduction to air does represent a sizeable proportion of the heat lost under normal conditions.

Convection

Convection is heat transfer through a fluid (liquid or gas) via the movement of molecules from cool regions to warmer regions of lower density. Thus warm air (or liquid) next to the body is cooled as it is replaced by cooler air further away. This cooler air is then warmed by heat from the body (assuming, of course, the air temperature is lower than the skin temperature) and again replaced by cooler air, i.e. a convection current is set up. In warming the cooler air, the body itself loses heat and therefore cools. Fan therapy works by increasing heat loss through convection because the warmed air is being replaced more rapidly by cool air. Conversely, the use of a space blanket creates a layer of warm air around the body, thus reducing heat loss.

Evaporation

When water evaporates, it changes from a liquid to a vapour causing heat to be lost. Water evaporates from the skin and lungs at a rate of about 600 mL/day. This is termed insensible loss and at rest accounts for roughly one-fifth of the body's heat loss. The sweat glands responsible for perspiration have a tremendous scope of activity, ranging from virtual inactivity to secretory rates of 2–4 L/hour. When the body becomes overheated, large quantities of sweat are secreted onto the surface of the skin by the sweat glands to provide rapid evaporative cooling of the body. Heat loss through evaporation becomes increasingly important when the ambient temperature is the same as the skin temperature, because little or no heat is lost through radiation, conduction or convection.

Heat loss mechanisms

When temperatures rise above the set point, e.g. when information coming in via the sensory nerves informs the hypothalamus that the environment is too warm, the hypothalamus reduces the stimulation to the sympathetic nervous system in an attempt to increase heat loss. The thermostatic area of the hypothalamus increases the rate of heat loss from the body in the following ways:

- sweat glands are stimulated to increase their secretory output, perspiration flows across the body surface and evaporation heat loss accelerates
- depth and rate of respiration are increased, causing increased heat loss through evaporation from the lungs
- peripheral vasodilatation takes place, causing warm blood to flow closer to the surface of the body, greatly increasing loss of heat from the skin through radiation and convection
- heat production activities are decreased, e.g. a decrease in muscle tone.

Heat gain mechanisms

When the core temperature falls below the normal range, special mechanisms are set in motion to conserve the heat already in the body and to generate heat production to maintain core temperature.

Heat conservation mechanisms

Heat is conserved in the following ways:

- peripheral vasoconstriction decreases blood flow to the dermis of the skin, thus reducing heat loss through radiation, convection and conduction, and the skin cools
- hairs on the body stand on end (piloerection), trapping air next to the skin so that the transfer of heat via radiation is reduced
- sweating ceases, thus reducing heat loss through evaporation
- through voluntary behavioural measures, such as wearing warm clothing.

Heat generation mechanisms

There are three heat generation mechanisms:

- shivering – the stimulation of shivering increases the tone of the skeletal muscles throughout the body, causing muscle shaking, and body heat production during severe shivering can rise as high as four to five times normal
- chemical heat production (thermogenesis) – this results from the release by the sympathetic nervous system of adrenaline (epinephrine) and, to a lesser extent, noradrenaline (norepinephrine), which cause an increase in cellular metabolism (thermogenesis); the effects are immediate
- hormonal heat production – the hormone thyroxine increases the rate of cellular metabolism throughout the body, but unlike thermogenesis, this does not occur immediately.

There are occasions, when changes in temperature occur, when the homeostatic mechanisms described above are unable to generate enough heat or cause enough heat to be lost to maintain normal temperature, as a result of which the body temperature either increases (pyrexia, hyperpyrexia or hyperthermia) or decreases (hypothermia). These conditions may require hospital treatment and can be fatal.

FACTORS AFFECTING BODY TEMPERATURE

Normal variations in body temperature

Body temperature usually varies slightly according to the time of the day, influenced by circadian rhythms (Enright & Hill 1989). The diurnal variation is generally between 0.2 and 0.3°C. For example, temperature normally drops during sleep and peaks in the late afternoon between 5.00 and 7.00pm (Fig. 5.2). The process of digesting food produces heat and so causes a rise in core temperature. Hormones also influence the body temperature; during the ovulation phase of the menstrual cycle, for example, the metabolic rate increases, which causes the body temperature to rise. Exercise, emotional stress, pain, malaise, fatigue and headache also affect normal body temperature (Cunha et al 1984).

Abnormal variations in body temperature

Abnormal variations in body temperature arise as a result of the following:

Severe cold (hypothermia)

See page 81.

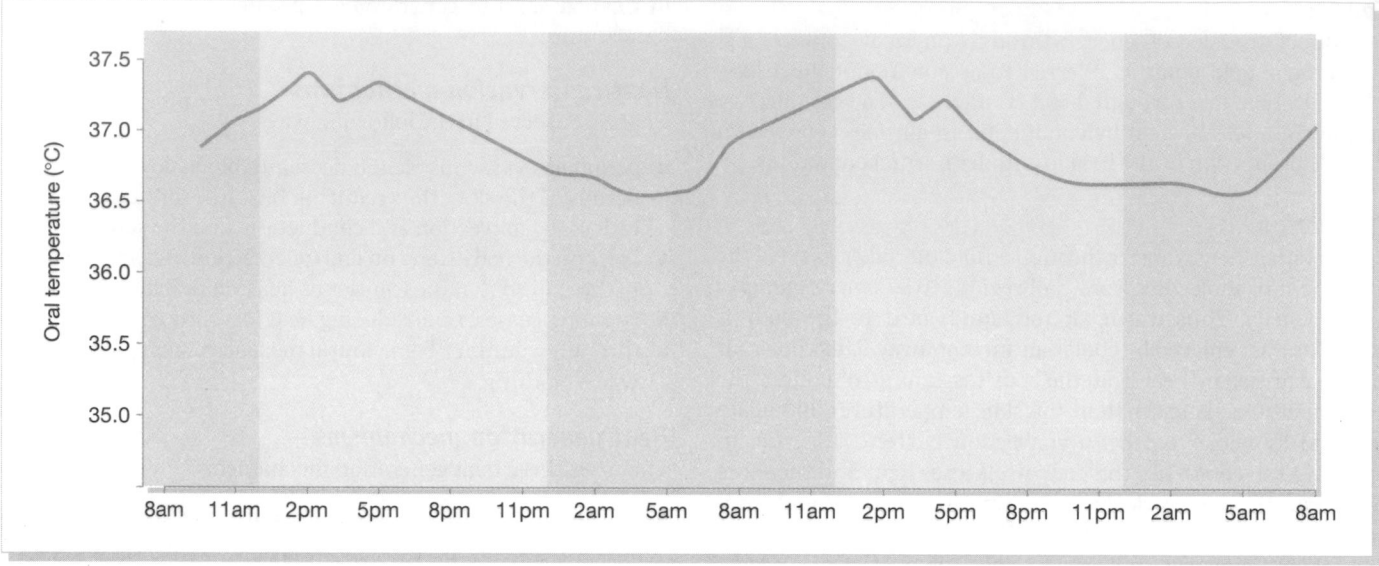

Figure 5.2 Changes in body temperature due to circadian rhythms.

Overheating (hyperthermia)

See page 79.

Clinical conditions

Infection This is the most common cause of pyrexia (see detailed discussion below).

Restricted circulation Conditions in which circulation is restricted, e.g. heart failure, where the heart's ability to pump blood around the body is impaired, are often associated with fever. A restricted circulation causes a reduction in the supply of nutrients to body tissues, circulatory stasis and pulmonary congestion, all of which increase circulatory congestion and vasoconstriction. Because the blood vessels are vasoconstricted, one of the body's heat loss mechanisms, that of vasodilatation, is not available to help with the reduction of body temperature.

Impaired sweat gland activity Conditions that impair sweat gland activity, such as drug reactions and some skin conditions, can result in pyrexia.

Hypothalamic injury Damage to the hypothalamus in the brain causes overheating of the body, which overwhelms heat loss mechanisms (Holtzclaw 1993). This is observed in situations in which the set point temperature of the hypothalamus is altered (e.g. neoplasms, surgery and conditions affecting the central nervous system) or where the body is unable to lose heat through normal means. These conditions are critical and may develop quickly because there is a malfunction of the temperature thermoregulating mechanism (Walton 1994).

DISORDERS OF TEMPERATURE REGULATION

There are four disorders of temperature regulation:

- pyrexia and hyperpyrexia
- hyperthermia
- hypothermia
- frostbite.

PYREXIA AND HYPERPYREXIA

Pyrexia (body temperature between 37.6 and 40°C) and hyperpyrexia (temperature > 40°C) are conditions in which the thermoregulatory mechanisms are intact but the body temperature is high. Infection is the most common cause of pyrexia but there other causes as well (Cunha et al 1984). A number of drugs have been associated with pyrexia, e.g. diuretics, anti-seizure therapy, analgesics, antiarrhythmics and antibiotics (Rang et al 1995). Other causes of pyrexia include neoplasm, surgery, acute myocardial infarctions, heart failure, haemolysis (seen in reactions to blood transfusions) and hyperthyroidism (Krickler & Dodge 1987).

The stages and patterns of pyrexia

There are four stages associated with pyrexia:

- The *chill stage* is the cold stage when the hypothalamic thermostat is reset to a higher level – the patient feels chilly, has goosebumps, is cool to touch and pale.
- The *plateau* is the hot stage when the body temperature has been raised to a level equal to the hypothalamic set point – the patient feels hot, warm to touch, is flushed, and has raised heart and respiratory rates.
- The *difervescence stage* is that stage when the temperature returns to normal, heat is dissipated through the heat loss mechanisms, the skin remains warm to touch and flushed, and eventually there is a drop in body temperature to a normal level.
- The *crisis stage* occurs if the temperature fails to respond to treatment, the microorganism responsible is unable to be eradicated and thermoregulation mechanisms can no longer control heat loss; death may ensue.

These stages account for the discomfort experienced by patients with high temperatures. They also explain why a patient with a high temperature may initially feel cold and want to wrap up rather than be uncovered.

Table 5.1 The patterns of a high temperature

Type	Clinical features	Causes
Intermittent – the temperature will return to normal at least once during a 24-hour period	Shaking chills (rigor) Exhaustion	Potent pyrogens Antigenic drugs Blood transfusions Pneumococcal pneumonia
Remittent – temperature pattern rises and falls throughout the day, but is less drastic than intermittent and does not return to normal	Feeling hot, sweating	Endocarditis Viral pulmonary infections Influenza Tuberculosis Pneumococcal pneumonia
Recurrent – the temperature remains high for a few days then returns to normal before the next episode (a normal temperature may be observed for weeks or even months)	Feeling hot, with periods of normality	Hodgkin's disease Malaria Parasitic infections
Sustained – the temperature remains consistently high and lasts for more than 24 hours	Temperature readings do not vary any more than 1–2°C throughout the day Hot and sweating	Central nervous system disorders Pneumococcal pneumonia Scarlet fever

In addition to the stages of pyrexia, different patterns, which exhibit recognizable changes in temperature over time, have been identified (Cunha et al 1984, Bruce & Grove 1992) (see Table 5.1). These patterns are influenced by circadian rhythms (Enright & Hill 1989) and thus vary according to the time of day, which may influence decisions regarding when to monitor body temperature (discussed later on in the chapter).

There is a lack of consensus in the literature regarding the importance of the patterns of pyrexia. Research undertaken in the late 1970s and early 1980s suggested that they were not significant (Cunha et al 1984); however, Bruce & Grove (1992) disagreed, arguing that they may be helpful in determining the cause of pyrexia, the severity of the underlying problem and the efficacy of treatment. It is becoming evident, though, that a variety of patterns may occur in one condition and hence their significance in the management of pyrexia remains uncertain.

Beneficial and detrimental responses to pyrexia

Pyrexia can be beneficial and is an important host defence mechanism. A body temperature of 40.9°C will kill some *Pneumococcus* and *Gonococcus* organisms. The high temperature causes a reduction in serum levels of iron, zinc and copper, which inhibits the replication of certain microorganisms (Cuhna 1985). Pyrexia as a result of viral infection increases interferon production by the infected cells, which then enters non-infected cells to inhibit infiltration by the invading virus. The activity of phagocytes and leucocytes is increased at temperatures between 38°C and 40°C, thus improving the infection-fighting ability of the immune system (Bruce & Grove 1992). Furthermore, high temperatures cause the breakdown of lysosomes (involved in the intracellular digestive system, which allows cells to digest and remove unwanted substances such as bacteria) in infected cells, thereby destroying cells and preventing them from initiating viral replication.

However, pyrexia can also be detrimental to the patient, whose basal metabolic rate will be increased, eventually leading to exhaustion. As a result, the glycogen stores in the liver become reduced and lead to nitrogen wastage (as protein is used for energy) and, if prolonged, may result in debility, impaired healing and delirium. If patients have compromised cardiopulmonary function, the effects of increased metabolic, heart and respiratory rates can be quite dangerous. These effects can lead to an increase in carbon dioxide production and oxygen consumption (Enright & Hill 1989).

Dehydration may result from fluid loss during sweating and from the lungs due to increased respiratory rate, leading to hypovolaemia and electrolyte imbalance (Bruce & Grove 1992), which can be life-threatening. In addition, the patient will feel uncomfortably hot and sweaty, with a loss of appetite, weakness and malaise, apathy and confusion (Bruce & Grove 1992). Special Issues box 5.1 summarizes the beneficial and detrimental effects of pyrexia. The question as to whether the pyrexia should be treated to make the patient feel better or left to run its course remains open to discussion.

HYPERTHERMIA

Hyperthermia is defined as an increase in body temperature, with increased cellular metabolism, oxygen consumption and carbon dioxide production, but where the body fails to activate compensatory cooling mechanisms (Morgan 1990). This condition is caused by problems of the central nervous system and does not respond to antipyretic therapy.

Hyperthermia causes cerebral metabolism to increase and the brain has great difficulty keeping up with the increase in carbon dioxide production. Cerebral vasodilatation occurs which may increase intracranial pressure and is thus dangerous in neurologically compromised patients. A temperature between 41°C and 43°C produces nerve damage, coagulation, convulsions and death. Unless effective cooling measures are initiated, irreversible brain damage and death will occur (Holtzclaw 1993).

SPECIAL ISSUES

5.1 Risks and benefits of pyrexia

Risks of pyrexia

- Increased basal metabolic rate, which will eventually cause exhaustion
- Glycogen stores in the liver become reduced and lead to nitrogen wastage (as protein is used for energy)
- Debility, impaired healing and delirium
- In patients with compromised cardiopulmonary function, the effects of increased metabolic, heart and respiratory rates can be quite dangerous
- An increase in carbon dioxide production and oxygen consumption
- Dehydration from fluid loss during sweating and from the lungs due to increased respiratory rate
- Hypovolaemia and electrolyte imbalance
- Temperature changes affect the slope of the oxygen–haemoglobin saturation curve
- Patient feels hot and sweaty, with a loss of appetite, weakness and malaise, apathy and confusion and is uncomfortable

Benefits of pyrexia

- An important host defence mechanism
- A body temperature of 40.9°C will kill some *Pneumococcus* and *Gonococcus* organisms
- There is a reduction in serum levels of iron, zinc and copper which inhibits the replication of some microorganisms
- Pyrexia as a result of a viral infection increases interferon production
- Activity of phagocytes and leucocytes are increased at temperatures of 38–40°C
- Hyperpyrexia will break down lysosomes in infected cells

Nursing assessment and actions

The patient's temperature should always be treated with an antipyretic if:

- there is an underlying problem such as liver failure, heart disease, respiratory failure or anaemia
- the patient is dehydrated or malnourished
- it is causing the patient discomfort
- it arises following surgery
- there is an open wound, e.g. varicose ulcer, trauma, broken limb

Hyperthermia also presents in five other conditions: heat cramps, heat exhaustion, heat stroke, malignant hyperthermia and neuroleptic malignant syndrome (NMS) (see Table 5.2). Heat cramps and exhaustion, even though they can be severe, do not generally warrant admission to hospital and those at risk can be taught ways to avoid it (see Health Promotion box 5.1). However, heat stroke, malignant hyperthermia and NMS must be recognized quickly, as, untreated, they may be fatal.

Table 5.2 The conditions that present with a hyperthermia

Condition	Clinical features	Causes
Heat cramps	Sweating Sodium loss when an individual has consumed large quantities of water but not taken any salt replacement	Strenuous physical exercise in high temperatures
Heat exhaustion	Profound vasodilatation Profuse sweating Decrease in blood volume Dehydration Hypotension	Malfunction of the thermoregulatory system
Heat stroke	Skin becomes hot and dry Sweat glands are inactive Body temperature climbs to 41–45°C Destruction of brain, liver, skeletal muscle and kidney cells	The thermoregulatory system ceases to function Excessive heat storage
Malignant hyperthermia	High temperature above 40°C Temperature does not respond to anti-pyretic drugs	Inherited muscular disorder Administration of drugs (anaesthetics, neuromuscular blocking agents, diuretics, analgesics, antibiotics)
Neuroleptic malignant syndrome	High temperature above 40°C Muscular rigidity Akinesia Impaired consciousness	Rare Psychotropic drugs used to treat psychosis (phenothiazines, butyrophenones)

HEALTH PROMOTION

5.1 Avoiding heat cramps

Advice for preventing heat cramps in people exercising in hot environments include:

- importance of drinking fluids
- taking salt – this will prevent the loss of water into the cells or by micturition; the presence of salt in the extracellular fluid will draw more water into the extracellular space to maintain adequate circulation
- showering after exercise – this will cool the individual down allowing heat to be lost through heat exchange mechanisms and thereby reducing the risk of heat exhaustion

Student activities

A friend (who is not a nurse) returns from the gym complaining that she developed cramp when running on the treadmill. How would you explain the physiology of heat cramps and how to avoid them?

HYPOTHERMIA

Hypothermia is defined as a core temperature of less than 35°C and affects virtually all metabolic processes in the body (Fritsch 1995). Degrees of hypothermia are classified as follows:

- mild (body temperature, 32–35°C)
- moderate (28–31.9°C).
- severe (20–27.9°C)
- profound (< 20°C).

In acute hypothermia, peripheral vasoconstriction shunts blood away from the cooler skin to the core in an effort to decrease heat loss. This peripheral vasoconstriction leads to peripheral tissue ischaemia, which causes the hypothalamus to stimulate shivering in an effort to increase heat production. Severe shivering occurs at core temperatures below 35°C and will continue until the core temperature rises or drops further to 30–32°C. At 34°C, thinking becomes sluggish and coordination is impaired.

At 31°C the individual becomes lethargic, heart and respiratory rates decline, cardiac output is diminished, and there is confusion, hyperactivity and exaggerated tendon reflexes (Holtzclaw 1993). Cerebral blood flow is decreased. Metabolic rate declines, further decreasing core temperature. This has an effect on drug metabolism as the drug half-life is increased (Fritsch 1995). Sinus node depression occurs with slowing of conduction through the atrioventricular node, and premature ventricular contractions (ectopics) are common. There is also an increased risk of atrial fibrillation and other dysrhythmias.

In severe hypothermia, pulse and respirations may be un-detectable and the blood coagulates more easily. Dehydration is common after a lengthy exposure to the cold (Danzl & Pozos 1994). Loss of consciousness and the absence of neurological reflexes follow. As the temperature falls below 20°C, hypothermic patients become unable to regulate their body heat and the thermoregulatory mechanisms fail (Holtzclaw 1993). Ice crystals form on the inside of cells, causing them to rupture and die.

Attention must be paid to the degree and time period of exposure of the patient (Fritsch 1995). Thus, the length of time hypothermia has taken to occur is significant in that it can influence outcomes. After 12 hours there will be significant fluid loss from the blood, due to shifts of fluid from extracellular to other fluid spaces and from cold-induced diuresis (Danzl & Pozos 1994). In addition, there is a marked increase in mortality. It is also significant when rewarming patients as the time span of hypothermia will determine the best method of achieving this (see Guidelines for Care Priorities box 5.2, p. 88).

Accidental hypothermia

Accidental hypothermia is defined as a core body temperature below 35°C that results from sudden immersion in cold water or prolonged exposure to cold environments. Environmental causes are common in older adults, the very young, those who have suffered trauma, homeless people, overdose patients and drug and alcohol misuse which diminishes the conscious perception of cold, and those with mental health problems. It may occur in accidents involving immersion in cold water or near drowning.

Older adults This group is particularly at risk of accidental hypothermia, as they have poor responses to extremes of environmental temperature as a result of slowed blood circulation, structural and functional changes in the skin, and overall decrease in heat-producing activities (Moddeman 1991). They also have a decreased shivering response (delayed onset and decreased effectiveness), slowed metabolic rate, decreased vaso-constrictor response, diminished or absent sweating and a decreased perception of heat and cold. If they also have psychological problems (e.g. a recent bereavement and/or loneliness), a sedentary lifestyle, low income, poor nutritional intake and a reduced ability to care for themselves, the risks are further increased.

Therapeutic hypothermia

The term therapeutic hypothermia generally refers to a deliberately induced state of hypothermia which is used to slow a patient's metabolism and thus preserve ischaemic tissue during some types of major surgery, thereby preserving function (Heidenreich et al 1992). However, hypothermia that occurs inadvertently during surgery is also termed therapeutic hypothermia because it presents during a therapeutic procedure. Both types of hypothermia can sometimes extend into the post-operative period. Therapeutic hypothermia is therefore classified into the following three categories:

- induced hypothermia
- inadvertent, intraoperative or unintentional hypothermia
- post-anaesthesia or postoperative hypothermia.

Induced hypothermia

Induced hypothermia is the intentional lowering of a patient's body temperature. It is generally used in neurosurgery and to treat hyperthermia, and during cardiac surgery to decrease metabolic rate and tissue oxygen demands, protect the brain, decrease the risk of ischaemic tissue damage to the heart and thereby protect other vital organs from hypoxia (Dennison 1995).

Inadvertent hypothermia

Major surgery often induces significant hypothermia (termed inadvertent hypothermia) because of the exposure of body cavities to the relatively cool operating room environment. In addition, procedures often involve irrigation of body cavities with room temperature solutions, infusion of room temperature intravenous solutions, inhalation of unwarmed anaesthetic agents, and the use of drugs that impair thermoregulatory mechanisms (Rich 1983, Blackburn 1994). Older adults are at a greater risk than other patients of suffering from this type of hypothermia (Moddeman 1991).

Dennison (1995) found that hypothermia occurs in 77% of patients undergoing surgery and develops within the first hour because anaesthetized surgical patients do not adapt quickly enough to cool intraoperative environments. In addition, patients are often transported along cold draughty corridors before being exposed to operating theatres that have an ambient temperature of between 18 and 21°C (Dennison 1995). Skin preparation may include the use of volatile fluids, or fluids that must be allowed to dry on the skin, which leads to an increase in heat loss by evaporation (Marta 1985). Medications such as muscle relaxants, narcotics, and inhaled anaesthetics also contribute to decreasing body temperature as they affect the temperature regulation mechanisms and prevent body movement (Marta 1985). The ability of patients to produce heat is blocked and they become dependent on the temperature of the environment. Once surgery begins, the use of intravenous solutions and blood at temperatures below that of the patient's body can compound the problem.

Effective means of preventing inadvertent hypothermia have been sought (Blackburn 1994, Tudor 1994a) (see Guidelines box 5.1). Table 5.3 shows a scoring checklist devised by Tudor (1994b) as an assessment tool to help nurses identify those patients at risk. A score of six or more indicates the use of heat-retaining devices, e.g. blankets, towels and hats, while a score of 10 or more indicates the use of heat-generating devices, e.g. blood warmers, humidifiers and warming blankets.

Post-anaesthesia hypothermia

Clinicians have also recognized hypothermia in the post-anaesthesia phase of the surgical procedure (Stevens 1993). Post-anaesthesia hypothermia may be an extension of the

 GUIDELINES FOR CARE PRIORITIES

5.1 Preventing hypothermia during a surgical procedure

- Apply warm blankets as soon as the patient arrives in the operating room
- Limit the amount of skin surface exposed when positioning the patient and when preparing the skin
- Minimize the time between completion of the skin preparation and application of sterile drapes
- Maintain the integrity of dry sterile drapes around the operative site to provide insulation, prevent heat loss and maintain asepsis
- Cover the patient with a warm blanket as soon as the sterile drapes are removed
- Warmed intravenous and irrigation fluids can help maintain temperature

- Warming and humidification of inspired gases are helpful in reducing the heat loss through evaporation
- Warming gel pad keeps the bed cushioned at a comfortable temperature of 39–41°C
- Keep theatre temperature at above 24°C
- Use warmed convection systems that force warm air through a plastic disposable blanket lying directly on the patient
- A warm blanket transfers heat through conduction to the patient's outer surface
- Radiant heat lamps are an effective surface skin warmer
- Cover exposed areas, e.g. head and legs, with thermal draping systems or warmed blankets
- Relay the patient's temperature to post-anaesthesia care unit for determination of appropriate treatment methods

Table 5.3 Score checklist for patients at risk from inadvertent hypothermia (Tudor 1994b)

Factor	Score 1 if	Score 2 if	Score
The patient is:	70–80 years old	Over 80 years old	
The patient is:	Thin	Very thin	
The operation is:	Intermediate	Major	
The operation site is:	Extra-abdominal/thoracic	Intra-abdominal	
Blood loss may be:	300–500 ml	Above 500 ml	
Surgery may last:	1.5–2 h	Over 2 h	
Cold fluids will be:	Infused or irrigated	Infused and irrigated	
The room temperature will be:	Between 21 and 24°C	Below 21°C	
The anaesthetic will be:	A regional block	A spinal or general anaesthetic	
Total score			

A score of six or more indicates the use of heat-retaining devices, e.g. blankets, towels and hats.
A score of 10 or more indicates the use of heat-generating devices, e.g. blood warmers, humidifiers and warming blankets.

induced hypothermia used for a particular surgical procedure or of hypothermia that occurred inadvertently during a surgical procedure. Post-anaesthesia hypothermia is of clinical concern, particularly for older patients in whom cardiac function and temperature regulation are less efficient (Holtzclaw 1990). Problems occur with monitoring blood pressure, assessing respiratory rate and auscultating cardiac sounds in patients who are hypothermic immediately after surgery.

Fat is an insulator, and as body weight increases, temperature loss during surgery is minimized (Dennison 1995). A person with a large amount of adipose tissue is well insulated because fat acts as a thermal buffer against heat loss. Thus, it is thin, older adults in particular who are at high risk of developing post-anaesthesia hypothermia, especially as they may also have poor circulation and be taking antihypertensive medication (Holtzclaw 1990).

FROSTBITE

Frostbite is a localized cold injury to the surface of the body rather than to its core (as in hypothermia). It results from exposure to sub-freezing temperatures and causes temporary or permanent tissue damage (Strohecker & Parulski 1997). When exposed to extreme cold, the body tries to protect vital internal organs by reducing the blood flow to the periphery, thus preventing cooling of the blood. Because of the lack of warm blood supply, skin tissue freezes and dies. Frostbite occurs in tissues that reach and maintain temperatures of −6°C (21°F), including the epidermis, dermis, subcutaneous tissue, muscle and bone, as well as nerves, lymph tissue and blood vessels (Sullivan 1993).

The body parts at greatest risk from localized cold damage are the fingers, toes, hands, feet and face, especially the nose, ears and cheeks (Jackson 1995). The people most at risk are those wearing clothing that is wet, poorly insulated and constricts movement, who postpone the search for shelter and warmth. Fatigue and dehydration also increase risk. Conditions such as diabetes mellitus (see Ch. 17), blood vessel disease such as Raynaud's disease (see Ch. 19), peripheral neuropathy (see Ch. 14) and traumatic injury also increase the risk. Drugs can affect circulation and thus alter the body's normal response to cold. Alcohol produces a sense of warmth because it dilates the capillaries. However, excessive alcohol impairs judgement as well as the body's ability to generate heat through shivering and can therefore contribute to the risk of frostbite.

▶ Nursing assessment of body temperature

Assessment of temperature is necessary to identify abnormalities in temperature regulation, to ensure the correct treatment is promptly instigated.

EQUIPMENT

There are four types of thermometer in common use, which are described below.

Glass mercury thermometers

Glass mercury thermometers are cheap but require disinfection after use and may take longer to use (minimum of 2 minutes orally, 3 minutes axilla). There is a risk of cross-infection but disposable covers are available to minimize this, and they may break, exposing people to small amounts of mercury vapour. Glass thermometers are unsuitable for oral temperature recording in patients who have seizures, as well as those who are unconscious or confused as they may bite on the thermometer causing it to break in their mouth.

Single-use chemical thermometers

These thermometers have small temperature-sensitive dots that change colour with increasing temperature (see Fig. 5.3). The thermometer is left in place for 1 minute for oral recordings and 3 minutes for axilla and is ready to read seconds after removal. It will record temperatures between 35.5 and 40.5°C. The use of this type of disposable chemical thermometer is increasing and they are particularly suitable for people with badly fitting dentures or sore mouths. Single-use thermometers require no cleaning, thus reducing the risk of cross-infection.

Electronic thermometers

Electronic thermometers use an electronic probe to measure oral and axilla temperatures, providing a reading in digital format. The disposable cover over the probe is changed between patients. A signal indicates when the maximum temperature has been reached, to prevent premature removal of the thermometer. These thermometers are accurate and easy to use, but they are more expensive than glass or single-use thermometers.

Tympanic membrane thermometers

Tympanic membrane thermometers use infra-red reflectance thermometry that detects heat radiated as infra-red energy from the tympanic membrane of the ear, which correlates well with

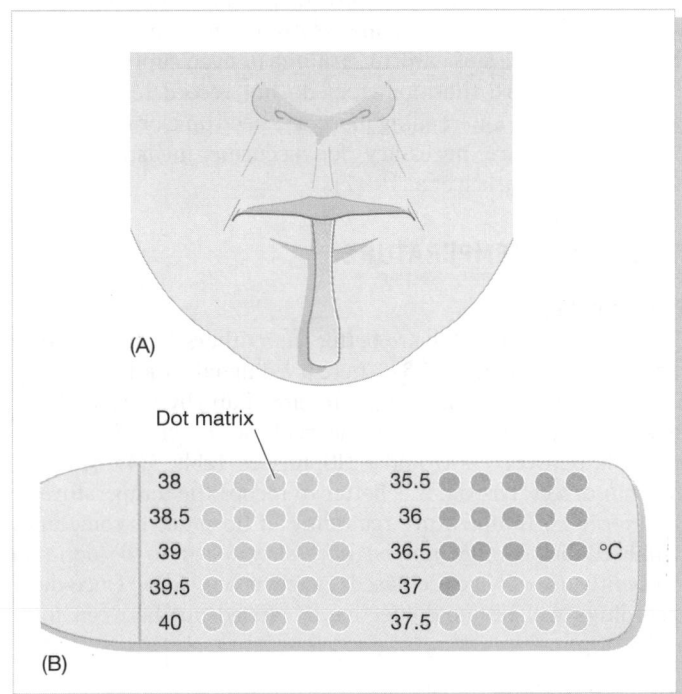

Figure 5.3 (A) Single-use thermometer. (B) Recording oral temperature with a single-use thermometer.

pulmonary artery temperature. The probe is inserted into the ear so that is close to, but not touching, the tympanic membrane and a digital recording is obtained in a matter of seconds. Otitis media or the presence of cerumen (wax) or hair in the ear canal may influence recordings. If the patient has been lying on one ear, causing more heat to be retained, this may also influence the recording. Tympanic membrane thermometry can be undertaken quickly, with little inconvenience and no discomfort to the patient.

CHOOSING THE RIGHT THERMOMETER

There is a continuing debate as to which type of thermometer is the most appropriate for ward or community use. In a study of 1246 readings over 12 months in seven clinical areas, Takacs & Valenti (1982) found that although the electronic type takes less time to use, nurses often went about other tasks rather than wait for the thermometer to register. They suggested this was because nurses are used to waiting for up to 3 minutes for an accurate temperature with a glass thermometer and so often use that time to do something else. A study by Pugh-Davies et al (1986) showed that great variations exist between glass mercury thermometers and electronic thermometer readings. In addition, when glass thermometers are broken, mercury spills out, releasing a toxic vapour which may be inhaled or absorbed through the skin and can remain in the environment for months. Despite this, glass thermometers are still used, but this is likely to change as a recent European Directive banning the use of mercury is implemented.

In terms of patient comfort, the single-use chemical thermometer is the preferred choice. Some patients find it uncomfortable to have an oral temperature taken using a glass thermometer or electronic thermometer, and they can be unsafe for patients who are restless, disorientated or shivering. While tympanic membrane probes are relatively safe and comfortable, there is a slight risk of eardrum trauma or even rupture.

Many standard thermometers do not record temperatures below 35°C, and low-reading mercury, electronic or light-reflect thermometers are necessary for accurate measurement of hypothermia (Haskell et al 1997).

TAKING THE TEMPERATURE

Time of day

Certain times of the day are better than others for temperature recording (Holtzclaw 1993). There is a diurnal variation in body temperature in humans, owing to circadian rhythms, and it is most likely to be elevated at the peak of the circadian cycle, which is between 5.00 and 8.00pm (see Table 5.4). Thus, in order to detect pyrexia, it is better to record the temperature in the evenings. Temperature recording in hospitals is sometimes ritualized but it may not be necessary for it to be done so frequently (see Evidence-based Practice box 5.1). Once-daily recordings will be most effective if carried out between 5.00 and 8.00pm.

Thermometer insertion time

Table 5.5 shows the recommended insertion times for each type of thermometer and site of reading. There is a lack of consensus

Table 5.4 Temperature changes during the day

Time of day	Changes in temperature
At night	Body temperature falls between 1 and 2°C and so a pyrexia may not be detected
Early evening: 5.00–8.00pm	During this period, the body temperature peaks, and as such it is the best time to take a patient's temperature
Afternoon/ during the day	Patient temperatures are often lower during this period, and so it is not the best time to observe a pyrexia

 EVIDENCE-BASED PRACTICE

5.1 Ritual temperature-taking: frequency and time of day

The frequency of temperature recording in the clinical area is generally 4-hourly following admission, which continues until the patient goes home or until the temperature has been normal for a period of time and a senior member of staff reduces the frequency to twice or once a day. The 4-hourly temperature is usually recorded at 6.00am, 10.00am, 2.00pm, 6.00pm and 10.00pm; the twice-daily temperature at 6.00am and 6.00pm; and the once-a-day temperature may be at any time.

Angerami (1980) studied temperature recordings over a period of 15 hours on a total of 255 adult patients in a range of hospital wards. The results indicated that the time at which pyrexia, if present, is most likely to register is between 6.00 and 8.00pm. Therefore, the accuracy of a temperature is dependent on the time of day, and the majority of the time the patient's temperature may not be at its peak and the reading is therefore not a true record of the temperature.

Reference
Angerami E. Epidemiological study of body temperature in patients in a teaching hospital. Int J Nurs Stud 1980; 17(2): 91–99.

Table 5.5 Recommended insertion time according to thermometer and site of reading

Site	Mercury	Single-use	Electronic	Infra-red
Oral	3 min	1 min	1 min timed signal	NR
Rectal	NR	3 min	NR	NR
Axilla	4 min	3 min	1 min timed signal	NR
Eardrum	NR	NR	NR	1 s timed signal

NR, not recommended.

in the literature, particularly in relation to the insertion times for mercury thermometers. Nichols & Kucha (1972) suggested that the average time required for an accurate temperature in 90% of patients is 8 minutes for men and 9 minutes for women at room temperatures of 18–24°C. However, in a more recent study, Pugh-Davies et al (1986) found that there was no clinical advantage in leaving it longer than 3 minutes.

Sites

The pulmonary artery temperature is the most accurate measure of core body temperature. However, this form of temperature measurement is extremely invasive and only available in critical care settings (see Chs 29 and 31). Temperature sites in close proximity to the brain (e.g. tympanic membrane, mouth) best reflect the thermal environment of the brain. This is particularly relevant to the oral temperature, as it is in close proximity to the sublingual artery, which is in direct contact with the brain and hypothalamus. None of the sites discussed is ideal in every respect, and the notion that one site is a more accurate reflection of core temperature than another is erroneous. The type of information required and the patient's safety, comfort and convenience will influence the choice of site.

Normal body temperature varies between 35 and 37.5°C, and also varies from site to site. The difference between core temperature and oral and ear temperatures is about 0.5°C. The temperature in the axilla is approximately 1°C below core temperature. Thus, if the core temperature is 37°C, the temperature in the mouth and ear would be 36.5°C, and that in the axilla 36°C. The temperature should not be recorded immediately after bathing or physical exercise because it will be raised in response to heat production.

Oral

The mouth is the most common and most accessible site for temperature recording. The oral temperature will be affected by factors such as recently taken hot or cold drinks. Similarly, smoking involves the inhalation of heat, which increases the temperature in the mouth and upper respiratory tract, and lingers after the cigarette is finished.

Erickson (1980) examined 50 patients with pyrexia and 50 with normal temperatures in order to determine the most appropriate placement of the thermometer. The findings indicate that, for the greatest accuracy, the bulb of the thermometer should be placed under the tongue to the right or left of the frenulum. This is close to the sublingual artery and so will reflect the temperature of the blood.

Axilla

The axilla is a convenient site and is comfortable for the patient. However, it is used less commonly than the mouth because it is thought to be a less accurate reflection of core body temperature. Recordings can be inaccurate in thin patients, because of poor contact between the thermometer and the skin in the axilla, and in obese people, because the presence of adipose tissue prevents close contact with the blood supply. However, it is a valuable site if the thermometer is used correctly (Heidenreich et al 1992). The temperature in the axilla is generally 0.5°C below oral temperature and so if this site is used, it should be noted on the chart.

Rectal

While some authors have suggested that core temperature is most accurately reflected in the rectum (Fisher & Raper 1987), heat being produced there from the waste substances of metabolism, others have argued that rectal temperatures are affected by heat generated by faecal bacteria and consequently might be inaccurate (Fulbrook 1993). This lack of agreement on the value of rectal temperature, in conjunction with the fact that taking the temperature there can be uncomfortable and embarrassing for the patient as well as possibly causing rectal trauma (Holtzclaw 1993), means that in the UK, this site is usually used only for patients who are acutely ill or unconscious. A small probe, which is designed to remain in place continuously, provides a constant recording. Care must be taken to ensure that the patient is not lying on the probe or cable, as this will cause pressure sores.

Tympanic membrane

This site has a number of advantages. It is close to the hypothalamus and so gives an accurate reflection of core temperature. It provides a rapid recording and is convenient and comfortable for the patient. The probe should not touch the tympanic membrane and so the risk of trauma is small, but as discussed earlier, the presence of ear wax or hairs and the position of the patient may affect the accuracy. Care when positioning the thermometer probe is also important. It should fit snugly in the ear canal to prevent air affecting the reading (Jevon & Jevon 2000) (see Fig. 5.4).

Peripheral temperature

When a patient's circulation is impaired, changes occur in the peripheral blood flow to the extremities. This is reflected in the peripheral skin temperature (normally several degrees lower than the core temperature), which provides a good indication of the presence and severity of a circulatory defect. The toe temperature provides a valuable, inexpensive and non-invasive way of monitoring tissue perfusion and is a useful guide to

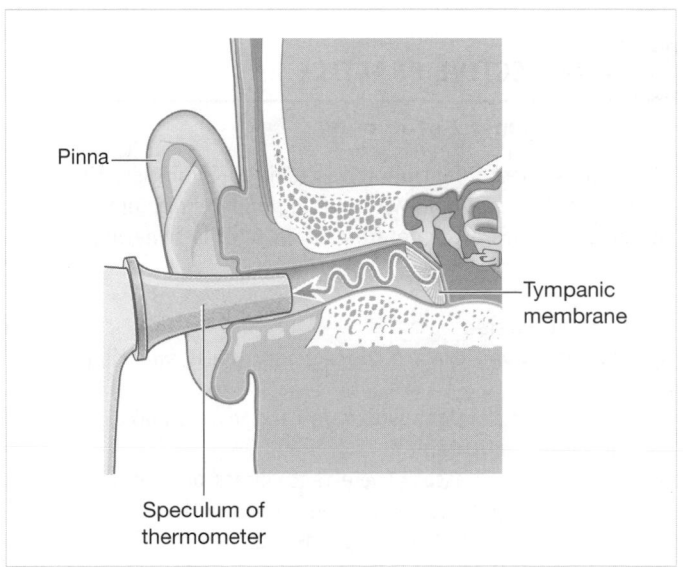

Figure 5.4 Using a tympanic thermometer.

determining the severity of shock. During hypovolaemic shock, circulation to the major organs and central temperature need to be maintained (see Ch. 9).

Nurses are responsible for assessing and intervening in states in which the body temperature is affected, and therefore effective monitoring is vital. Managing temperature is important for patient comfort, as patients with pyrexia are likely to feel hot and exhausted. Frequent washes with a cool face cloth will greatly improve the feeling of comfort, as will a change of linen, providing fresh, cool sheets. A pyrexic patient will be sweating and may become dehydrated and so, if the condition allows, frequent drinks should be offered; if patients are unable to take oral fluids, frequent mouthwashes should be given or they should be encouraged to suck on ice chips.

MANAGEMENT OF PYREXIA AND HYPERPYREXIA

As discussed earlier, some researchers suggest that instead of routinely treating a high temperature, it should be allowed to run its natural course. Cuhna et al (1984) advise against treating pyrexia unless there are cardiopulmonary complications, the temperature exceeds 41°C or the patient is extremely uncomfortable, in which case antipyretic treatment is recommended (Cunha 1985) (see Reflective Practice box 5.1). Whilst recognizing that a high temperature is uncomfortable for the patient, these researchers hold that a compelling reason not to lower the temperature is that it will deprive the patient of an important host defence mechanism. They even suggest that bringing temperatures down has more to do with reducing the apprehension of medical personnel than with helping the patient.

A traditional means of managing an abnormally high temperature is with cooling methods such as tepid sponging or fanning. However, these methods have been criticized by some researchers (e.g. Bruce & Grove 1992) who argue that ultimately they are of no use, as they stimulate a compensatory

response by the hypothalamus which provokes heat-generating activities such as shivering. Such heat-generating activities may well compromise unstable patients by depleting their metabolic reserve and can create a new temperature spike that is as high as, or even higher than, the original one, a response that will further compromise the patient. Krikler & Dodge (1987) also advise against the use of fanning or tepid sponging, arguing that they make the patient feel weak, especially during the early stages when the temperature is still rising.

This view is not supported by Fisher & Raper (1987), who suggest that physical methods of cooling (e.g. tepid sponging) are useful as they improve patient comfort. Howie (1989) advises that cooling methods should be used before the onset of the temperature spike (38.5°C) so that the benefits will not be lost.

Such opposing views can be confusing and it becomes difficult to decide what is in the patient's best interest. On the one hand, a high temperature is a normal body response and so should not be treated, while on the other hand, this natural response can be physiologically and psychologically detrimental; yet management by cooling and tepid sponging may serve to increase the temperature further, causing the patient discomfort and possible harm. On balance, the strategy suggested by Bruce & Grove (1992) is recommended: that the best way to treat a high temperature is to use antipyretics such as aspirin or paracetamol, which prevent the hypothalamus from synthesizing prostaglandin E and thus inhibit the set point of temperature from rising further.

MANAGEMENT OF HYPERTHERMIA, HEAT STROKE AND MALIGNANT HYPERTHERMIA

Cooling methods

Artificial cooling methods are valuable in hyperthermia, heat stroke and malignant hyperthermia because the body fails to activate compensatory cooling methods. Moreover, these conditions generally do not respond well to antipyretic therapy (Morgan 1990). Aggressive cooling should be commenced early, as temperatures of above 41°C cause cell, tissue and eventually organ damage (Bruce & Grove 1992).

Cooling techniques commonly used include packs of iced water, cold water, water with 70% isopropyl alcohol with paracetamol administered orally, cooling mattresses, fanning, immersion in cold water and tepid water sponging. Dyer & Bagnall (1970) evaluated the application of cold or iced water and found that they lowered the local and systemic temperatures rapidly. In addition, temperatures continued to drop 35–50 minutes after the cold application was removed. Although iced water and alcohol in water solutions reduced the temperature more rapidly than tepid water, the latter afforded significantly better comfort for the patient.

Kielblock (1986) investigated the use of a combination of cold packs to the neck, groin and axillae, immersion in cold water, cooling mattresses and fanning, which cools the patient through increased heat loss by convection and radiation. This study found that the combination of cold packs and fanning produced the best cooling rates. However, Hickey (1986) found that cooling mattresses and blankets reduced the temperature in the shortest amount of time.

R|Я REFLECTIVE PRACTICE

5.1 Management of pyrexia

Mary has a chest infection and is taking antibiotics. She is being cared for at home with nursing and general practitioner support. She has a temperature of 38.6°C, is sweating and feels hot.

Student activities
- How would you explain to Mary why she is sweating and feeling hot?
- What nursing actions would you suggest to make Mary feel more comfortable?
- How would you assess the effectiveness of your actions?
- Think about a person you have nursed with a chest infection – what other problems did they have?
- Why do you think these problems occurred?

Immersion in cold water causes shivering which generates heat and thus increases the temperature. It is associated with convulsions, is uncomfortable for the patient and reduces hyperthermia too quickly, and so is generally not recommended.

When evaluating cooling methods, issues of cost, resources available, nursing time and comfort to the patient all have to be taken into consideration (Morgan 1990). The cooling blanket is the cheapest in relation to nursing time. However, cooling blankets are expensive to buy or rent and can cause shivering, which is an adverse effect of any method of cooling but more so with this one. Cooling blankets are also uncomfortable and so are generally used on comatose patients. Tepid sponging is cheap (although it does require nursing time) and comfortable for the patient, and is the best cooling method for hyperthermia, heat stroke and malignant hyperthermia.

In malignant hyperthermia the above methods of cooling may be beneficial, but the addition of dantrolene sodium will give a more marked improvement (Donnelly 1994). In heat stroke, cooling methods are the intervention of choice because heat production in the body is higher than heat loss, creating an increase in temperature which is overwhelming the regulatory system. Neuroleptic malignant syndrome (NMS) is a life-threatening condition that requires cooling methods and may also require additional resuscitative measures.

Fluid management

Intravenous fluid therapy with colloid and crystalloid fluids (see Chs 8 and 9) is necessary to maintain haemodynamic stability. Circulating volume has to be increased to compensate for the vasodilatation caused by high temperatures and for the fluid lost during sweating and from the lungs due to the increased respiratory effort to maintain oxygen transport. Colloid solutions bring about this improvement in circulating volume and also tissue perfusion. However, during a high temperature, dehydration and/or endothelial damage may occur, causing sodium to leak into the surrounding cells, carrying with it extracellular water. Therefore, crystalloid solutions containing sodium are required to restore extracellular fluid volume. A failure to do this will increase the risk of mortality and morbidity. Blood transfusion may be necessary to maintain clotting factors and haemoglobin levels and to prevent haemodilution.

MANAGEMENT OF RIGOR

A rigor occurs when the hypothalamic set point temperature has risen in response to a microorganism and the body is attempting to achieve that temperature by generating heat through excessive shivering. In this instance, it is best to apply extra clothing and allow the body temperature to rise.

NUTRITIONAL NEEDS DURING PYREXIA AND HYPERTHERMIA

The normal daily energy expenditure in adults is generally 1700–2500 kcal (30–35 kcal/kg; see Ch. 11). An increased basal metabolic rate results in an increased demand for energy, which, if not available, will result in weight loss (see Evidence-based Practice box 5.2).

 EVIDENCE-BASED PRACTICE

5.2 Nutritional needs of a person with pyrexia

Until recently it was assumed that patients suffering from pyrexia in hospital or at home increased their basal metabolic rate (BMR). An increased BMR increases heart rate, liver function, blood pressure and skeletal muscle tone and results in a greater demand for energy, which, if not available, will cause weight loss. If there is higher energy expenditure, a higher carbohydrate and fat intake will be necessary.

However, Elia (1995) has shown that the energy requirement of disease is overestimated. The recommendation that more energy should be provided to take into account the effects of pyrexia and other illnesses is now suggested to be inappropriate. The energy requirement of patients with pyrexia is similar to or less than that of healthy subjects. This is because patients who have had pyrexia or other illness for some time may have a reduced BMR, due to not eating a sufficient amount of calories (a normal body response to protect diminishing energy stores). If given a normal or higher calorie intake, they may be at serious risk of developing some of the problems identified with an increased carbohydrate and lipid diet. An excess carbohydrate intake can cause hepatic steatosis and abnormal liver function, and can lead to excess carbon dioxide production, which can precipitate respiratory failure. An excess of lipids may cause deposits in the lung and impair diffusion of gases, and produce infusional hyperlipidaemia (Elia 1995). Hypocaloric feeding reduces the risk of liver and lung complications and metabolic instability and their consequences. An increase in calorie intake should take place in the recovery phase, when the patient is no longer at risk.

Reference
Elia M. Changing concepts of nutrient requirements in disease: implications for artificial nutritional support. Lancet 1995; 345: 1279–1284.

► **Nursing management of hypothermia**

Accidental hypothermia is more likely to occur in the community than in hospital. It will, however, require a stay in hospital. Advanced age is a known risk factor. Older patients often experience more severe temperature drops and rewarming difficulties due to limited cardiac reserve, reduced cardiac output, a diminished muscle mass, lower basal metabolic rate and impaired sweating ability. All contribute to alterations in heat generation, conservation and dissipation (Moddeman 1991). An ageing autonomic nervous system often results in a decreased shivering response, low resting peripheral flow, reduced vasomotor tone and decreased peripheral vascular reactivity to cold. In addition, many older patients take daily doses of antihypertensive medications, which have a vasodilating effect that can increase the loss of body heat (Dennison 1995).

Hypothermia in older adults is usually preventable (see Older Adults: Nursing Priorities box 5.1). Nurses in the community

5.1 Risk factors for accidental hypothermia and early recognition in the community

Age-related changes
Many older adults lose the ability to regulate temperature and to feel the cold and so may fail to recognize when to put on warm clothing. They may also get wet due to incontinence or be exposed to the cold if they fall and are unable to get up unaided.

Assessment of factors
- A cold flat or house
- Insufficient income to pay for heating
- No insulation in the house or flat to hold in the heat
- Nutritional status – body mass index, dietary intake, biochemical investigations
- Recent illness or bereavement
- Looking very thin, pale and lethargic
- Physical ability to cook own meals at home

Nursing action
- Discuss the availability of help with paying the bills and assist in the completion of forms to claim available benefits
- Refer to a social worker
- Recommend installation of additional heating if necessary
- Check that there is warm clothing available
- Discuss meals on wheels if the person's diet inadequate, or home help to assist with shopping
- The person may require to move to a more appropriate dwelling
- Contact any family members who may be able to help
- Recommend installation of any aids that might help with cooking and/or bending down to light or switch on the fire
- Recommend moving the bed downstairs to a warm room

can aid prevention by, for example, giving advice on obtaining financial assistance with heating bills, involving a social worker, and discussing meals on wheels or cooking aids.

REWARMING

Restoring the hypothermic patient to normothermia is vital to prevent the complications associated with hypothermia, which can be fatal (Stevens 1993). However, raising body temperature to normal can double a patient's oxygen consumption, and prompt and effective assessment and evaluation of the patient's physiological response to being cold enables the nurse to individualize treatment. The instigation of appropriate rewarming techniques is a critical intervention to minimize hypothermic shivering, which increases metabolic rate, oxygen consumption and myocardial workload (Murakami 1995).

The process of rewarming should proceed no faster than 1–2°C per hour (Murakami 1995). If a patient is rewarmed too rapidly, oxygen consumption, myocardial demand and vasodilatation increase faster than the heart's ability to compensate and death can result. Taking account of the patient's core temperature and the duration of the hypothermia, rewarming should be started with intravenous fluid administration, monitoring of blood results and the electrocardiograph (ECG). Urine output should be measured and any drugs administered with caution as the half-life of many drugs is greatly extended. There are three methods of rewarming a hypothermic patient: passive external, active external and active internal rewarming (see Guidelines for Care Priorities box 5.2).

Passive external rewarming
This method involves warming patients using normal metabolic heat production while insulating with blankets to prevent further heat loss to the environment. Patients may be covered with

GUIDELINES FOR CARE PRIORITIES

5.2 Principles of rewarming following hypothermia
- Remove all wet clothing
- Gently dry the patient
- Insulate with blankets
- Place in a warm room
- Use convective warming therapy if available
- Give a hot bath if condition allows
- If ventilated, administer warmed gases to the respiratory tract
- Administer warmed intravenous fluids

Nursing actions
- Fluid balance chart and close observation of fluid intake
- Avoid vigorous movement to prevent cardiac arrest
- Measure vital signs, e.g. central venous pressure, blood pressure, heart rate, temperature, urine output and peripheral temperature
- The rewarming process should proceed no faster than 1–2°C/hour
- All actions are designed to reduce the time the patient's core temperature is below 32.2°C

a space blanket and placed in a warm room. Space blankets are made of reflective material and trap warm air around the body, preventing heat loss by radiation, but not that lost by conduction or convection. Space blankets may cause sparks and so care must be taken if oxygen is used. Considerable heat is lost from the head and the back and so these should be insulated as well.

Passive external rewarming is recommended for both mild (32–35°C) and moderate (28–31.9°C) hypothermia with an onset of less than 12 hours. Passive rewarming treatment will be sufficient for an unconscious hypothermic patient suffering from deep hypothermia and may have limited value in profound hypothermia (< 20°C) (Danzl & Pozos 1994, Larach 1995).

Close observation of patient temperature is necessary to ensure that nursing interventions are effective. This should be at least half-hourly in the first instance, then every 1–2 hours until the temperature is above 35°C. Other vital signs such as blood pressure, heart rate and respiration, cautious use of intravenous fluids and avoidance of vigorous movement to prevent cardiac arrest are essential. Movement contributes to heat loss through convection and may reduce temperature further if not closely monitored. If the patient's temperature fails to rise, active external rewarming should be commenced.

Active external rewarming

This type of rewarming is achieved by using hot baths, hot air blowers or radiant heat. This method can also be used as an adjunct to active internal rewarming. One of the most effective methods of active external rewarming is convective warming therapy (Fritsch 1995), in which warm air is blown directly onto the patient's skin through a disposable blanket.

This method should be used when the hypothermia has occurred slowly, i.e. over a period longer than 12 hours, and is mild or moderate in nature. It is not recommended for use alone in the treatment of severe hypothermia (Fritsch 1995). The patient's vital signs and peripheral temperature must be closely monitored, as rewarming shock may occur in the severely hypothermic patient if the peripheries are warmed before the core (Larach 1995). Peripheral rewarming promotes vasodilatation, causing cold blood to be returned to the heart, which may cause myocardial (heart muscle) depression. To minimize this effect, it is recommended that only warming of the trunk is undertaken (Fritsch 1995). If the patient has a persistently low blood pressure or if the core temperature continues to fall, active internal rewarming should be started.

Active internal rewarming

In active internal rewarming, warming is achieved by using invasive procedures such as:

- warm fluid for gastric and peritoneal lavage
- mediastinal and pleural irrigation
- continuous arteriovenous or venovenous rewarming
- cardiopulmonary bypass.

These techniques are highly invasive and are only indicated in extreme cases. The use of warmed gases to the respiratory tract via an endotracheal tube if the patient is ventilated, and warmed intravenous fluids via a blood warmer are the easiest methods (Fritsch 1995). If warmed oxygen is used, it should be humidified as well. The aim is to reduce the risk of cardiac arrest, by reducing the time that the patient's core temperature is below 32.2°C.

All three methods of rewarming allow the deep tissues of the body to be warmed safely, as they allow the lungs and heart to be rewarmed first. The advantage of active internal rewarming is that it avoids the peripheral vasodilatation associated with

surface rewarming, and allows correction of any fluid deficits (see Ch. 8). A disadvantage is that after-drop may be observed after internal active rewarming is discontinued – a decrease in temperature of as much as 2°C may occur as blood circulates to the peripheries, cools and then returns to the core (Fritsch 1995). Thus, when active internal rewarming methods are discontinued, passive and active external rewarming are necessary to prevent such an after-drop. Active internal rewarming is most effective when the hypothermia has developed in less than 12 hours, and is moderate or severe in nature (see Reflective Practice box 5.2).

FLUID REPLACEMENT

During hypothermia, there is peripheral vasoconstriction in order to maintain body temperature by preventing heat loss from skin. The circulating volume in the body does not change but the changes in the peripheral blood supply cause a decrease in oxygen consumption, heart rate and an increase in blood pressure. However, when the patient is warming, vasodilatation occurs and consideration needs to be given to support the circulation. There needs to be effective management of fluid replacement in response to peripheral vasodilatation, increasing temperature and corresponding heart rate, central venous pressure, and blood pressure. This is maintained through the administration of warmed intravenous fluids containing sodium. Potassium and other electrolytes may be required as indicated by regular biochemical analysis (Fritsch 1995).

MONITORING AND OBSERVATIONS

Regular observations and blood tests are necessary to monitor the patient's condition, particularly blood glucose levels, potassium and arterial blood gases.

Observation of vital signs

Respiratory observation during hypothermia is vital in order to detect hypoxia leading to inadequate cerebral perfusion. There may be changes in a person's behaviour and/or level of consciousness. Very early signs of cerebral underperfusion include

5.2 Postoperative hypothermia

Jack has just had major surgery and has been on the operating table for over 6 hours. His postoperative observations showed an axilla temperature of 32.9°C, he feels cold to touch and is shivering.

Student activities
- Why do you think Jack has such a low temperature?
- What nursing actions are needed to reduce the shivering experienced by Jack?
- What might be the consequences for Jack if his shivering continues?

the inability to think abstractly or perform simple mental tasks, restlessness, apprehension, uncooperativeness and irritability. Short-term memory may also be impaired. There may be changes in blood pressure, pulse rate and the colour of mucous membranes. Oxygen saturation measurement using a probe on the patient's finger will indicate whether saturation is normal, i.e. between 98 and 100%. However, a patient may experience a significant drop in oxygen supply but with minimal effect on oxygen saturation and so careful observation is important.

Urine output

Hypothermia initiates a cold diuresis. Peripheral vasoconstriction shunts blood to the core, creating a relatively hypervolaemic state which suppresses antidiuretic hormone (ADH) secretion. As a result, urinary output is increased, leading to hypovolaemia. Renal function is dependent on adequate renal perfusion, determined by the blood pressure, cardiac output and vascular tone, and acute tubular necrosis and renal failure may result (Fritch 1995). If the hourly urine output falls below 0.5 mL/kg for more than 2 hours, this may indicate that cardiac output is low and the doctor needs to be informed. The urinary output should be at least 30 mL/hour. Patients may need to be catheterized to enable accurate measurement of urine output at hourly intervals.

Blood glucose

Blood glucose levels should be closely monitored. As body temperature decreases and shivering stops (at around 30°C), hyperglycaemia occurs, insulin secretion decreases and the cells become more resistant to insulin that is present (Fritsch 1995). Hyperglycaemia may be resistant to treatment, until the patient's core temperature is above 30°C, as below this temperature, glucose and insulin utilization is minimal; if insulin is administered, rebound hypoglycaemia may occur during rewarming and so this is generally avoided in the hypothermic patient (Danzl & Pozos 1987). However, if hypoglycaemia occurs during rewarming, it should be corrected.

Serum potassium

Frequent estimations of serum potassium should be made, as alterations in potassium levels may occur as temperature decreases. Alterations in the sodium–potassium pump within body cells may result in an increased potassium level outside the cell (extracellular) during hypothermia. During rewarming, the sodium–potassium pump returns to normal and the potassium moves back inside the cell (intracellular) and hypokalaemia may follow (Fritsch 1995). If the patient's cardiac signs are being monitored, changes to the T wave are an early warning sign of hypokalaemia.

Acid–base balance

Arterial blood gas analysis is necessary because, as temperatures fall, acid–base changes occur (see Ch. 8). Hyperventilation occurs during early hypothermia causing respiratory alkalosis. As the temperature decreases, respiratory failure leads to a progressive respiratory and metabolic acidosis (Holtzclaw 1993). However, measurement of arterial blood gases is invasive and requires puncturing an artery or obtaining a specimen from an arterial line.

The electrocardiograph (ECG)

The ECG should be monitored, as a slow heart rate and unusual QRS and T complexes are common in hypothermia. In addition, the incidence of cardiac arrest increases with decreasing temperature and active internal rewarming is indicated; continuous basic life support may be necessary. Ventricular and atrial fibrillation, asystole and electromechanical dissociation have all been reported as cardiac arrest rhythms due to hypothermia (Berry & Hash 1996). Defibrillation may not be successful at lower body temperatures but should still be attempted (Resuscitation Council 1998).

THE CONSEQUENCES OF HYPOTHERMIA

There are a number of consequences of hypothermia which need to be considered in the management of patients.

Shivering

In acute hypothermia, peripheral vasoconstriction shunts blood away from the skin to the core in an effort to decrease heat loss. This peripheral vasoconstriction produces peripheral tissue ischaemia. When this occurs, the hypothalamus stimulates shivering in an effort to increase heat production. It may also occur during rewarming. Body movement increases, the muscles become tense and energy is used to produce heat. Shivering causes a raised metabolic rate, leading to increased oxygen consumption (400–500%) and increased carbon dioxide production and myocardial work. It increases blood viscosity and there is a risk of disseminated intravascular coagulation (DIC). It is important that nurses monitor and control shivering to avert the increased metabolic demand and the discomfort this creates.

Rewarming shock

Shock may occur if peripheral warming occurs before central warming and cold acidic blood is returned to the heart causing myocardial depression. It may also occur during rewarming if the patient's circulating volume is inadequate. Vigilant temperature and haemodynamic monitoring is imperative to avoid this.

Impaired immunity

Hypothermia may cause impaired immunity. Vasoconstriction and the consequent decrease in oxygen supply to the tissues reduce the body's ability to kill microorganisms; wound healing may also be affected. Leucocytosis is also impaired on the first postoperative day in hypothermic patients.

Acidosis

Acids from the waste products of metabolism accumulate in the stagnant blood in the periphery and then return to the heart during rewarming (Stevens 1993). These acids cause a fall in blood pH as a result of the sudden increase in lactic acid concentration, caused by a reduction in oxygen and resulting in a metabolic acidosis. Systemic acidosis depresses the activity of all vital organs, especially the cardiovascular system.

Nutritional needs

Postoperative patients who suffer from some form of hypothermia do not advance to solid food intake as quickly as do normothermic patients and this may delay healing and lengthen the stay in hospital. Collagen formation is reduced due to a reduction in nutrients and poor wound healing ensues. In addition, loss of nitrogen and protein increases the patient's risk of wound infection and prolonged recovery (McNeil 1998).

Pharmacokinetics

Temperatures of 30°C have effects on the half-life of drugs (Danzl & Pozos 1994). In hypothermic patients there is increased protein binding of administered drugs, with the result that their effects are often diminished. However, as the core temperature rises, the drugs are released from the protein binding, which may lead to toxicity during rewarming (Fritsch 1995). Most authors suggest that the use of all drugs should be restricted and carefully monitored during the rewarming process (Danzl & Pozos 1994, Fritsch 1995).

▶ Nursing management of frostbite

The severity of frostbite is often difficult to determine (Sullivan 1993). Superficial damage affecting the skin and subcutaneous tissues only is often very painful. With appropriate treatment most cases of mild frostbite will make a full recovery, although the healing process may take 6–12 months. If there is no pain or sensation, this means that deeper damage has occurred. Grave injuries will have developed necrosis and look black. In severe cases, amputation of the affected part is often required.

The most severe tissue damage comes with rewarming of the tissues (Strohecker & Parulski 1997). Reperfused capillaries, with their damaged endothelium, leak fluid and protein, leading to oedema. Blisters form, and prostaglandins and thromboxanes in the blister fluid cause platelet aggregation. This cuts off the blood supply to the affected area, resulting in death of the tissue. Therefore, it is imperative that rapid thawing and rewarming are instigated quickly. This is now the acceptable practice (Strohecker & Parulski 1997).

Thawing is achieved by immersing the affected parts in warm water, but immersion is contraindicated if the core temperature is less than 32°C (Day 1998). The affected part is immersed in a temperature-controlled (37.7–41.1°C) whirlpool bath (Strohecker & Parulski 1997). The skin is very vulnerable to damage and so must be dried very carefully. Warm intravenous fluids may be prescribed together with analgesics, including narcotics, to relieve severe pain.

Following thawing, the viability of the affected area should be determined by radioactive scan of blood flow. This also provides a baseline against which to compare future healing (Sullivan 1993). Nursing observations of frostbite damage should include frequent monitoring of the circulation to the affected tissues, sensation, numbness, tingling, pain, pressure, presence or absence of pulses, colour, discoloration, texture, patterns and shape of tissues. A well-balanced diet and good fluid intake are encouraged to aid healing and improve circulation to the extremities. Extremities are elevated to reduce oedema, or kept in a neutral position if there are concerns about arterial blood flow. If the affected limb, toe or finger can be moved and the swelling is not causing too much pain, movement should be encouraged to aid circulation.

SUMMARY: MAIN POINTS

- A change in body temperature is a common phenomenon and may alert the nurse to the presence of infection, thermoregulatory dysfunction or hypothermia.
- Administration of aspirin or paracetamol is the best way to treat pyrexia.
- Prevention of hypothermia during and after surgery is particularly important in older adults who are at greater risk than other patients.
- There is a variety of types of electronic and single-use thermometers available. Mercury thermometers are being phased out because of the risk of exposure to mercury vapour if the thermometer breaks.
- Daily temperature recordings are best measured between 5.00 and 8.00pm to detect pyrexia.
- The difference between core body temperature and oral or ear (tympanic membrane) temperature is about 0.5°C, and temperature in the axilla is 1°C below core temperature.
- Cooling methods such as tepid sponging provide patient comfort but need to be used with care to ensure they do not cause vasoconstriction and thus a rise in temperature.
- Hypothermia requires careful rewarming, which should proceed no faster than 1–2°C/hour.

SELF-TEST: CRITICAL THINKING ACTIVITIES

1 Imagine you are on placement in the community with the district nurse and go to visit an elderly woman who has regular leg ulcer dressings. It is bitterly cold. There is no response when you ring the doorbell and a neighbour who has a key lets you in. You find the woman sitting in a chair in front of an unlit fire wearing her nightdress and dressing gown. She is confused and does not know where she is, but is able to cooperate with you. What is the likely cause of her confusion and what is the district nurse likely to do and why?

2 Think of all the times you have measured patients' temperatures. What types of thermometer have you used? Which was easiest to use and which did the patients like best. Why did those patients need to have their temperatures recorded? Were they recorded at the most effective times of day?

3 What methods have you seen used to warm or cool patients? Thinking of the ways that heat is lost or preserved (e.g. radiation), identify how those methods of warming or cooling work.

FURTHER READING

Guyton AC. Body temperature, temperature regulation, and fever. In: Guyton AC, ed. Textbook of medical physiology, 9th edn. Philadelphia: WB Saunders; 1996.

Hickey JV. The clinical practice of neurological and neurosurgical nursing, 2nd edn. London: JB Lippincott; 1986.

Hinchliff S, Montague S, eds. Physiology for nursing practice, 2nd edn. London: Baillière Tindall; 1998.

McCance KL, Huether SE. Pathophysiology: the biologic basis for disease in adults and children, 2nd edn. St Louis: Mosby; 1998.

Marieb EN. Human anatomy and physiology, 4th edn. Redwood City, CA: Benjamin/Cummings Publishing; 1998.

REFERENCES

Angerami E. Epidemiological study of body temperature in patients in a teaching hospital. Int J Nurs Stud 1980; 17(2): 91–99.

Berry RG, Hash VW. Hypothermia: risk factors and electrocardiographic confirmation. Consultant 1996; 36(11): 2428–2432.

Blackburn E. Prevention of hypothermia during anaesthesia. Br J Theatre Nurs 1994; 4(8): 9–14.

Bruce J, Grove S. Fever: pathology and treatment. Crit Care Nurse 1992; 12(1): 40–49.

Cunha B. Significance of fever in the compromised host. Nurs Clin North Am 1985; 20: 163–168.

Cunha B, Digamon-Beltran M, Gobbo P. Implications of fever in the critical care setting. Heart Lung 1984; 13: 460–465.

Danzl DF, Pozos DS. Multicenter hypothermia study. Ann Emerg Med 1987; 16: 1042–1055.

Danzl DF, Pozos DS. Accidental hypothermia. New Engl J Med 1994; 331(26): 1756–1760.

Day MW. Action stat. frostbite. Nursing 1998; 28(1): 33.

Dennison D. Thermal regulation of patients during the perioperative period. AORN J 1995; 61(5): 827–832.

Donnelly AJ. Malignant hyperthermia: epidemiology, pathophysiology, treatment. AORN J 1994; 59(2): 393, 395, 398–405.

Dyer E, Bagnall HK. Local tissue and general temperature changes in dogs produced by temperature applications. Nurs Res 1970; 19(1): 37–40.

Edwards SL. High temperature. Prof Nurse 1998; 13(8): 523–526.

Edwards SL. Hypothermia. Prof Nurse 1999; 14(4): 253–258.

Edwards SL. Measuring temperature. Prof Nurse Study Suppl 1997; 13(2): S5–S7.

Enright T, Hill M. Treatment of fever. Focus Crit Care 1989; 16: 96–102.

Erickson R. Oral temperature differences in relation to thermometer and technique. Nurs Res 1980; 29(3): 157–164.

Fisher M, Raper R. Fever in the intensive care unit. Br J Hosp Med 1987; 38(2): 109–111.

Fritsch DE. Hypothermia in the trauma patient. AACN Clin Iss 1995; 6(2): 196–211.

Fulbrook P. Core temperature measurement in adults: a literature review. J Adv Nurs 1993; 18(9): 1451–1460.

Haskell RM, Boruta B, Rotondo MF et al. Hypothermia. Advanced practice in acute critical care. Clin Iss 1997; 8(3): 368–382.

Heidenreich T, Giuffre M, Doorley J. Temperature and temperature measurement after induced hypothermia. Nurs Res 1992; 419(5): 296–300.

Holtzclaw BJ. Temperature problems in the postoperative period. Crit Care Nurs Clin North Am 1990; 2: 589–597.

Holtzclaw BJ. Monitoring body temperature. Clin Iss Adv Pract Acute Crit Care 1993; 4(1): 44–55.

Howie J. How and when should I respond to post operative fever? Am J Nurs 1989; 95(3): 52.

Jackson L. Emergency! Quick response to hypothermia and frostbite. Am J Nurs 1995; 95(3): 52.

Jevon P, Jevon M. Using a tympanic thermometer. Nurs Times 2001; 97(9): 43–44.

Kielblock AJ, Van Rensburg JP, Franz RM. Body cooling as a method for reducing hyperthermia. S African Med J 1986; 69: 378–380.

Krickler JA, Dodge GH. What to do about temperatures. Nurs Stand 1987; 14(25): 37–38.

Larach MG. Accidental hypothermia. Lancet 1995; 345: 493–498.

McNeil BA. Addressing the problems of inadvertent hypothermia in surgical patients: part 1: addressing this issues. Br J Theatre Nurs 1998; 8(4): 8–14.

Marta MR. Intraoperative hypothermia: a review of measures to protect patients. AORN J 1985; 42(2): 240–242.

Moddeman G. The elderly surgical patient – a risk of hypothermia. Am Op Room Nurs J 1991; 53(5): 1270–1272.

Morgan SA. Comparison of three methods of managing fever in the neurologic patient. J Neurosci Nurs 1990; 22(1): 19–24.

Murakami WM. External re-warming and age in mildly hypothermic patients after cardiac surgery. Heart Lung 1995; 24(5): 347–358.

Nichols GA, Kucha DH. Oral measurements. Am J Nurs 1972; 72(6): 1091–1092.

Pugh-Davies S, Kassab J, Thrush A, Smith PA. A comparison of mercury and digital clinical thermometers. J Adv Nurs 1986; 11(5): 535–543.

Rang D, Dale M, Ritter J. Pharmacology, 3rd edn. Edinburgh: Churchill Livingstone; 1995.

Resuscitation Council. 1997 resuscitation guidelines for use in the United Kingdom. London: Resuscitation Council; 1997.

Rich J. Hypothermia in surgical patients. Br J Nurs 1983; 1(11): 539–435.

Stevens T. Managing postoperative hypothermia, re-warming and its complications. Crit Care Nurs Quart 1993; 16(1): 60–77.

Strohecker B, Parulski CJ. Frostbite injuries of the hand. Plastic Surg Nurs 1997; 17(4): 212–216.

Sullivan SA. How severe is this frostbite? Am J Nurs 1993; 93(2): 59–64.

Takacs KM, Valenti WM. Temperature measurement in a clinical setting. Nurs Res 1982; 31(6): 368–370.

Tudor M. Scaling the patient's temperature – part 1. Br J Theatre Nurs 1994a; 3(11): 20–23.

Tudor M. Scaling the patient's temperature – part 2. Br J Theatre Nurs 1994b; 3(12): 14–15.

Walton J. Nurse-aid management of hyperthermia. Br J Nurs 1994; 3(5): 239–242.

6 Stress

David Howard

'It wasn't a bit like me – I can always cope. I'm the one that everyone else relies on. But when they changed the theatre list for the 4th time, I just burst into tears! Charge nurse was brilliant, he sent me for a cup of coffee and then in the afternoon we talked through what happened and how to manage the stress that things like this cause.'

(Registered nurse)

THIS CHAPTER WILL HELP YOU

- Understand the different concepts and models of stress
- Explain the physiological and psychological responses to stress
- Identify physiological, psychological and social stressors
- Describe how individuals react to stress and ways in which this can be measured
- Discuss how stress affects patients, health care workers and carers
- Identify the nature of stresses in your own life
- Understand the relationship between stress and related illnesses
- Describe appropriate methods of measuring stress within the nursing assessment
- Identify optimal methods for individuals to reduce the amount of stress they experience
- Assist individuals to enhance their coping strategies.

KEYWORDS

Assessment of stress	Stress
Burnout	Stressors
Distress	Stress-related illness
Eustress	Stress management
Post-traumatic stress	

INTRODUCTION

Although used as an everyday term for feeling pressured, stress, as defined and used clinically, refers to a condition that has profound effects on an individual's physical and psychological well-being. It is therefore important for nurses to understand the processes associated with these effects as it will help them to manage the stresses that occur in their own lives, and also enable them to help patients recognize how stress can contribute to their illnesses. Later on in this chapter, the causes and effects of stress in the individual are explored. Methods of assessing stress during the nursing assessment are compared and a description of stress management techniques is given. Owing to the ambiguity of the use of the term stress in the vernacular, however, it is appropriate to begin by defining precisely what is meant by it. Consequently, this chapter opens by exploring fundamental concepts that underpin all definitions of stress, from which a composite model of stress for use within this chapter will emerge.

CONCEPTS AND MODELS OF STRESS

Selye (1984) argues that stress is the response of an organism to any demand made upon it. It is generally associated with negative effects on health, but a certain amount of stress is necessary for survival, a concept first introduced by Hebb in 1954 (reproduced in Hebb 1971) in the arousal curve (Fig. 6.1). Thus, contrary to the popular conception of stress as a negative phenomenon, the arousal curve demonstrates that as the level of stress increases there is a corresponding increase in the individual's performance. For example, people engaging in sporting contests often 'psyche' themselves up immediately before competing to maximize their potential. What Hebb discovered, though, was that performance only improves up to a certain level of stimulus. Beyond this point, performance begins to deteriorate and, if the stress continues to increase, individuals experience adverse health effects. Consequently, people living

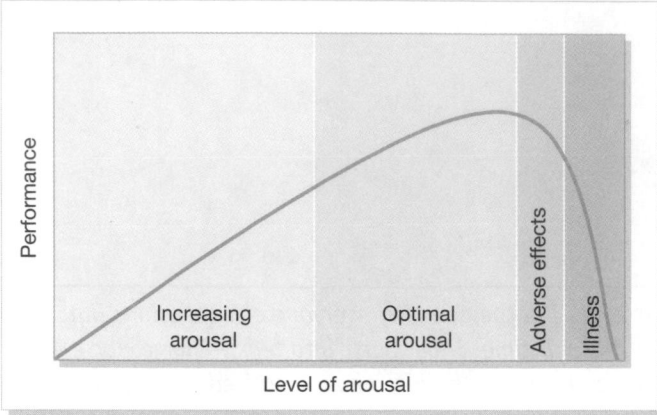

Figure 6.1 The arousal curve (Hebb 1971; note that Hebb's original article was published in 1954).

excessively stressful lives are likely to experience stress-related illnesses (Cooper et al 1996).

The ability of accumulated stressors in people's lives to bring about illness in this way is sometimes referred to as the engineering model of stress. This is because of the simple mechanistic assumption that stress increases in a linear fashion until breaking point is reached, in the same way that engineers test models (Cox 1978). This view was challenged by Sutherland & Cooper (1990), who found that people in monotonous, tedious jobs experienced similar stress-related diseases as those with highly pressured jobs traditionally associated with stress. They concluded that understimulation is just as damaging as overstimulation and represented this as the inverted U hypothesis (Fig. 6.2), which illustrates that stress does not follow a simple linear pathway. Consequently, there must be other aspects of stress contributing to the effect it has on individuals.

Both Hebb (1971) and Sutherland & Cooper (1990) consider stress from a negative viewpoint. This is not always the case (see Reflective Practice box 6.1); for example, many people expose themselves to stressful activities for pleasure, such as going on a rollercoaster, and feel good about doing so. Therefore, the single term stress, implying only negative aspects, is inadequate. This issue was developed by Selye (1984) who identified both positive and negative types of stress. He defined positive stress as eustress, which is associated with excitement and euphoria, and

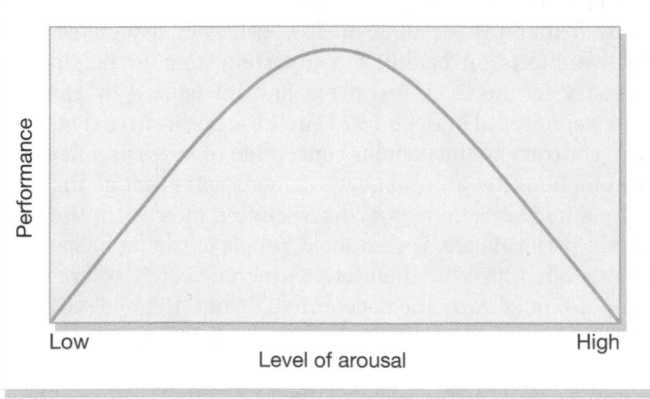

Figure 6.2 The inverted U hypothesis (Sutherland & Cooper 1990).

contrasted it with negative stress, i.e. distress. He found that similar physiological changes occur on exposure to both types of stress; however, the long-term effects of distress are far more damaging than those of eustress.

The experiences of eustress and distress are elaborated by Brown (1986) who notes that the severity of the effects of stress can be correlated with the level of control individuals feel they have over the object of stress (stressor). Where individuals feel they have little control over stressors, they experience damaging results. Conversely, where individuals retain control, negative outcomes are less intense. Contemporary research supports Brown, associating distress attributed to external locus of control with poor self-esteem and a suppressed immune response (Brosschot et al 1998, Pruessner et al 1999) and to burnout (Janssen et al 1999).

A MODEL OF STRESS

By integrating these theories concerning the nature of stress, it is possible to construct a composite model which will be used for the remainder of this chapter. Individuals require a certain amount of arousal to perform optimally. This occurs in response to stressors, which remain, to a great extent, within the individual's control and results in eustress stimulation. Therefore, in eustress stimulation, individuals feel positive and ultimately exhilarated. Although this is partly due to endorphins (chemicals that promote feelings of well-being) and improved self-esteem, it is mainly due to retaining control of the stressor. If stressors become too great, they extend beyond the individual's immediate control and eustress is rapidly replaced by distress. Thus the damaging effects of stress occur when there is little control of stressors.

RESPONSES TO STRESS

Models of stress examine the physical, psychological and social changes that occur in response to stressors. Understanding how stress affects individuals and the implications for nursing practice requires that these processes are understood.

PHYSIOLOGICAL RESPONSES

The General Adaptation Syndrome

The physiological responses to stress were described by Selye (1984) in the General Adaptation Syndrome (GAS), which is illustrated in Figure 6.3. On exposure to the stressor, the limbic system (the part of the brain surrounding the brain stem that is responsible for the emotional aspects of behaviour needed for survival) is stimulated. In turn, the limbic system stimulates the hypothalamus which causes the autonomic nervous system (ANS) to initiate the immediate physiological responses: the alarm and resistance reactions.

Alarm reaction

The immediate physiological response to stress is the alarm reaction, activated by the ANS. Its function is to prepare the body for defensive action to counter the stressor. Before an impending stressful event (for example think of how you feel prior to an examination or visiting the dentist), a paradoxical fear may be generated which causes substantial activation of

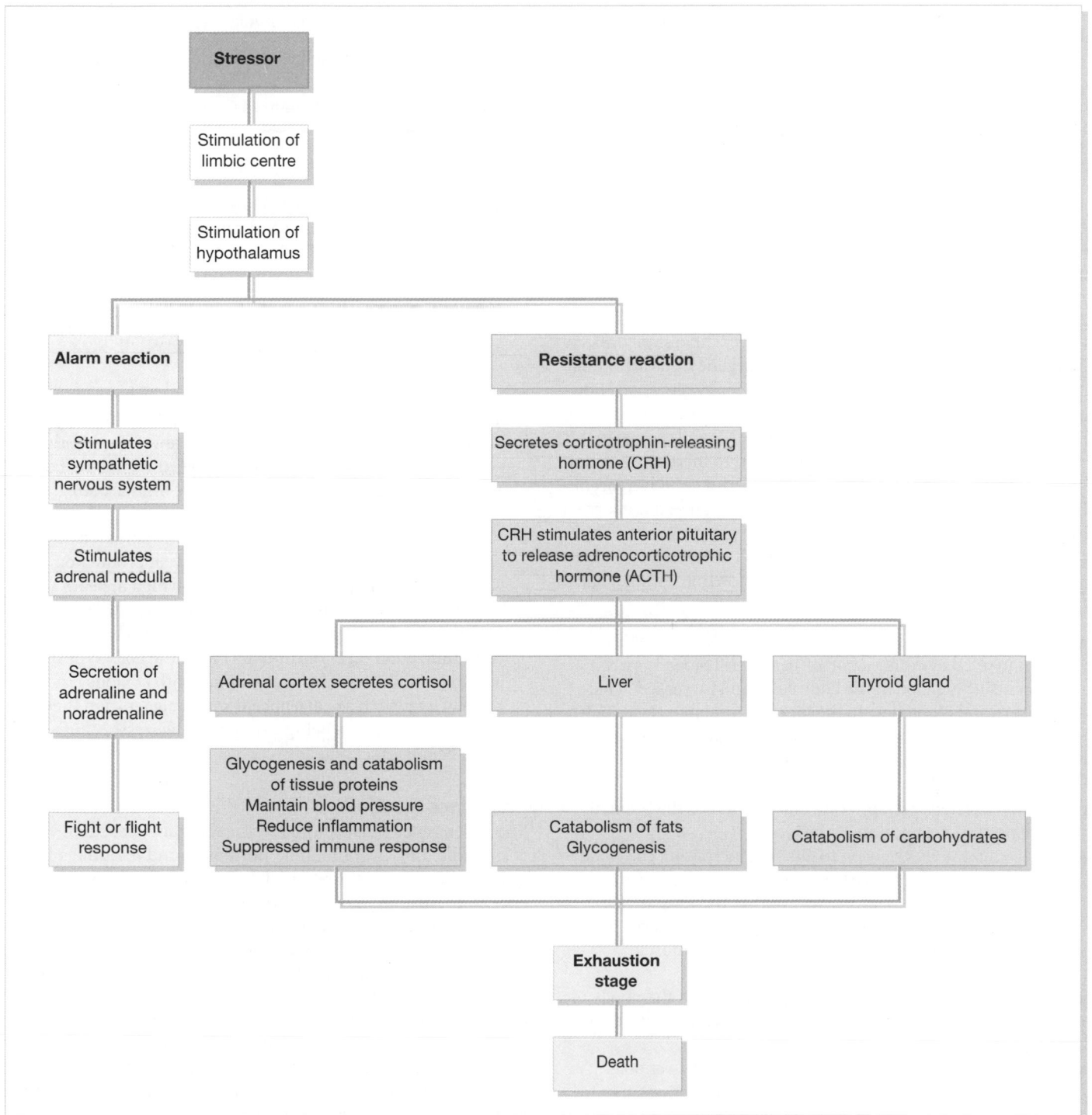

Figure 6.3 The general adaptation syndrome. (Adapted from Selye 1984.)

Table 6.1 Physiological changes associated with the fight/flight response

System	Effect
Circulatory system	Increased heart rate and force of contraction Increased blood pressure Peripheral vasoconstriction
Respiratory system	Increase in respiration rate Dilation of bronchi
Liver	Increased conversion of glycogen to glucose
Eyes	Pupil dilation
Digestive system	All secretions within the digestive tract diminished or stopped Decreased peristaltic activity
Skeletal muscles	Increased tension
Skin	Sweat gland activation Erection of body hair by pilomotor contraction

R|Я REFLECTIVE PRACTICE

6.2 Baseline observations on admission

Immediately on admission most patients have baseline observations of temperature, pulse, respiration and blood pressure recorded.

Student activities
Reflect on the advantages and disadvantages of this procedure (refer to the General Adaptation Syndrome).

- How accurate are baseline observations taken on admission?
- How might the disadvantages be addressed?

the parasympathetic division of the ANS. This mainly affects elimination and individuals experience urgency and frequency of urination and defecation. In an emergency situation, however, the fight-or-flight response is invoked. This occurs through the dominant sympathetic division of the ANS and to sustain this response the adrenal medulla is stimulated to increase secretion of the catecholamines adrenaline (epinephrine) and noradrenaline (norepinephrine). The fight-or-flight response, summarized in Table 6.1, prepares the body for intense physical action either to fight against or to escape from the object of stress.

The alarm response has the following physiological characteristics:

- Heart contractions increase in rate and volume. This is accompanied by constriction of peripheral blood vessels, concentrating blood in the body core, and increased blood pressure and blood flow to the large skeletal muscles which will be used either in fighting or running away. This has significant implications for nursing practice (see Reflective Practice box 6.2).
- An increase in respiration rate and dilation of the bronchi increase the oxygenation of the blood.
- The liver converts glycogen to glucose, increasing the blood glucose level, and adipose tissue converts triglycerides (triacylglycerols) into fatty acids. Within the muscle cells, glucose and fatty acids are oxidized to produce energy in the form of adenosine triphosphate (ATP) for muscle contraction.
- To enable the person to identify danger quickly, the pupils dilate, which allows more light into the eyes and results in better vision.
- In paradoxical fear, where danger is expected, to enable rapid reaction the body loses as much weight as possible. Excess fluid is removed by producing more urine, resulting in the frequent desire to urinate. Further fluid and gut content are removed by increasing peristalsis which often

results in diarrhoea. A full stomach also entails extra weight; thus vomiting may occur and a feeling of a lump in the throat and a dry mouth dissuade the individual from eating, so preventing the accumulation of body weight. The flight-or-fight response, however, is an emergency and all non-essential gastrointestinal activity ceases, resulting in suspension of peristalsis and inhibition of all gastrointestinal secretions.

- Skeletal muscle tone increases, preparing the body for immediate physical action. Skeletal muscles work in antagonistic pairs, i.e. flexors and extensors. When both muscles contract, the joint will not move until one relaxes. This, however, provides a faster response than if both muscles were relaxed.
- Vast amounts of heat are generated by the increased muscle activity. Therefore, the body increases sweat production to begin cooling. Piloerection also occurs, which appears contradictory as it is usually used to conserve heat (Ch. 5). In this instance, though, it is a form of non-verbal communication (Ch. 3). Humans have little body hair so it is not really observable, but animals with copious amounts of body hair, such as cats, appear much bigger than they actually are, the idea being to make the aggressor think twice before attacking.

Resistance reaction

The alarm reaction is followed by the resistance reaction, which is stimulated by hypothalamic hormones and continues for as long as the stressor threatens. The resistance reaction provides energy to sustain the stress response and protects the body by compensating for any damage occurring during the alarm reaction. Corticotrophin-releasing hormone (CRH) stimulates the anterior pituitary gland to secrete adrenocorticotrophic hormone (ACTH) which causes the adrenal cortex to increase cortisol secretion. This glucocorticoid has several functions. It increases glycogenesis and catabolism of body proteins to provide glucose. This maintains the high blood glucose level, providing energy to sustain skeletal muscle demands. Cortisol also suppresses the inflammation response to enable the body to continue action if it is damaged. It delays the formation of connective tissue and consequently delays wound healing (Ch. 10);

this is significant for postoperative patients who are anxious, e.g. those with an uncertain prognosis (Ch. 29). These are issues that nurses ought to assess so that they may provide support to minimize patients' distress and promote recovery.

Finally, cortisol enhances peripheral vasoconstriction to maintain blood pressure. This is augmented by increased secretion of aldosterone (mineralocorticoid), which, by stimulating the renal tubules to increase sodium reuptake, leads to water retention. Consequently, if the body were damaged, these actions would partially compensate for severe blood loss (Ch. 9).

Exhaustion

The final reaction to stress, according to Selye (1984), is the exhaustion stage. This occurs following prolonged excessive distress and, if continued, will lead to illness and eventually death. Thus, repeated instigation of the GAS, as occurs in stressful environments from which there is no escape, will have negative health consequences.

The Local Adaptation Syndrome

Although the GAS releases corticoids which reduce inflammation, Selye (1984) noticed that when tissue was subject to direct injury, inflammation occurred locally. This is the Local Adaptation Syndrome (LAS) and its function is to protect damaged tissue. Selye found a symbiotic relationship between the LAS and the GAS, in which the LAS defends the body against localized damaging stressors, such as an infection or wound site, while the GAS protects the body from overreaction.

PSYCHOLOGICAL RESPONSES

Psychological responses to stress vary according to the level of threat from the stressor. The model of stress outlined above suggests a pathway from eustress to distress. Eustress stimulation is accompanied by feelings of well-being and increased alertness, a confident posture and positive outlook (Hebb 1971, Selye 1984, Sutherland & Cooper 1990). As eustress becomes distress, however, the feelings of well-being are replaced by those of losing control and being overwhelmed. Individuals become restless, demanding and sometimes aggressive. Indeed, within stressful departments such as accident and emergency (A&E, Ch. 30), patients or relatives may act out their distress by behaving aggressively. Consequently, defusing aggression focuses on addressing those factors contributing towards the distress being experienced.

Continued exposure to distress makes individuals unable to concentrate and problem-solving becomes impossible. Consequently, their ability to function decreases (Brown 1986) and they drift undirected between tasks. Interpersonal relationships deteriorate, further worsening their difficulties and individuals become locked into a stress cycle.

Mental defence mechanisms

Some individuals adopt mental defence mechanisms to cope with psychological distress. These mechanisms were initially identified by Freud (1936), who found that individuals used them to defend the self against conflict, and this early work has since been developed by many other researchers (see Box 6.1).

Box 6.1 Mental defence mechanisms

- *Denial* – if the reality is too unpleasant, individuals may deny that it really exists
- *Displacement* – anger is redirected towards another object when it is impossible to address the actual cause of stress
- *Intellectualization* – using intellectual powers of thinking, analysis and reasoning to detach oneself from emotional issues
- *Projection* – individuals blame someone else for how they are feeling
- *Rationalization* – finding an acceptable explanation for an act that is unacceptable
- *Reaction formation* – individuals conceal what they really feel by thinking and acting in the opposite way
- *Regression* – engaging in behaviours from an earlier, more secure life stage
- *Repression* – painful thoughts are forced into the unconscious; they may, however, resurface in dreams
- *Sublimation* – redirecting the energy from unacceptable sexual or aggressive drives into another socially acceptable activity

---

In the short term, the use of mental defence mechanisms is a healthy response as they help individuals to survive the immediate period following exposure to distress. Mental defence mechanisms do not alter the cause of distress, however, but simply create an illusion. Consequently, they involve a degree of self-deception and the individual remains vulnerable to the stressor. Prolonged use of mental defence mechanisms is therefore unhealthy (see Ethical Issues box 6.1).

 ETHICAL ISSUES

6.1 Maud and George

Maud is 78 years of age and has widespread metastases following a primary carcinoma of the left breast, which was removed 3 years ago. She is extremely ill, requiring in-patient care, and is likely to die within a matter of weeks. Her husband George, aged 80 years, is very frail himself. He refuses to accept his wife's prognosis and is pressurizing staff to discharge Maud home.

Student activities

- Which mental defence mechanism is George using?
- What are the consequences of confronting George?
- What are the consequences of colluding with him?
- What ethical issues are involved with either confronting or colluding with George?

See Chapters 3 and 34 for more information.

STRESSORS

A stressor is any stimulus that invokes the stress response and it follows that stressors encompass both physiological and psychosocial phenomena.

PHYSIOLOGICAL STRESSORS

The GAS prepares the body to defend itself against stressors and to compensate for any injuries. Thus, physiological stressors such as extreme temperature, hunger or, more acutely, blood loss or pain will invoke the stress response and are of particular concern when caring for patients. There are less obvious environmental factors, however, that affect both nurses and patients, particularly in the hospital environment. Stressors such as chemicals, solvents, poor lighting, poor heating, inadequate ventilation and excessive noise all contribute to the stress experienced in this setting (Levi & Lunde-Jensen 1996), and patients in critical care units have been known to experience extreme psychological distress due to the surrounding life-supporting technology and persistent lighting (see Ch. 31). It is difficult to isolate these factors from psychological influences; for example, if someone experiences pain, it is impossible to detach the physiological factors from the psychological ramifications that accompany it (see Ch. 7).

PSYCHOSOCIAL STRESSORS

The origin of the fight-or-flight reaction is to protect the individual from danger. Although physiological stressors may invoke the stress response, in this context it is a reactive strategy and would not ensure an individual's survival for long. On the other hand, where the fight-or-flight reaction originates in response to psychosocial stressors, this is usually a proactive strategy to protect the individual. Potential dangers are appraised before they occur and retaliatory or evasive action taken. Consequently, many stressors are psychosocial in origin and arise in response to a potential threat.

What individuals perceive as a threat forms a major part of research into psychological stress. Early research focused on quantifying psychological stressors, such as the seminal research of Holmes & Rahe (1967) who developed the social readjustment rating scale. By studying the relationship of life events to the amount of stress experienced by individuals, they were able to rate them according to severity, resulting in an inventory of life events (Table 6.2). Using this inventory enables an individual's level of stress to be assessed by indicating which events occurred during the previous year. The scores for the events are then summated to produce an index of stress. In their research Holmes & Rahe found that individuals who returned scores >300 were likely to develop a stress-related illness. In everyday use, however, higher scores indicate elevated stress and provide a focus to explore ways for reducing that stress.

A common observation is that following exposure to the same additional stressor, some people appear to cope whilst others are unable to do so. By combining the Hebb (1971) model of arousal and the social readjustment rating scale (Holmes & Rahe 1967) it is possible to explain why this happens. Holmes

Table 6.2 Social readjustment rating scale (Holmes and Rahe 1967)		
Rank	Life event	Rating
1	Death of spouse	100
2	Divorce	73
3	Marital separation	65
4	Jail term	65
5	Death of close family member	63
6	Personal injury or illness	53
7	Marriage	50
8	Loss of job	47
9	Marital reconciliation	45
10	Retirement	45
11	Change in health of family member	44
12	Pregnancy	40
13	Sex difficulties	39
14	Gain of new family member	39
15	Business readjustment	39
16	Change in financial state	38
17	Death of close friend	37
18	Change to different line of work	36
19	Change in number of arguments with spouse	35
20	Mortgage over $10,000	31
21	Foreclosure of mortgage or loan	30
22	Change in responsibilities at work	29
23	Son or daughter leaving home	29
24	Trouble with in-laws	29
25	Outstanding personal achievement	28
26	Wife begins or stops work	26
27	Begin or end school	26
28	Change in living conditions	25
29	Revision of personal habits	24
30	Trouble with boss	23
31	Change in work hours or conditions	20
32	Change in residence	20
33	Change in school	20
34	Change in recreation	19
35	Change in church activities	19
36	Change in social activities	18
37	Mortgage or loan of less than $10,000	17
38	Change in sleeping habits	16
39	Change in the number of family get togethers	15
40	Change in eating habits	15
41	Holiday	13
42	Christmas	12
43	Minor violations of the law	11

& Rahe argue that the effects of stress are cumulative. Therefore, according to Hebb (1971), should one individual experience many stressful life events over 1 year and another experience comparatively few, exposure to the same stressor could push the first individual into overload while the second individual would have sufficient coping reserve (Fig. 6.1). Consequently, the second individual would appear to cope with the stressor while the first would not.

Although the social readjustment rating scale was developed over 30 years ago, it remains a reliable instrument and enjoys extensive contemporary use (Hobson et al 1998). There are,

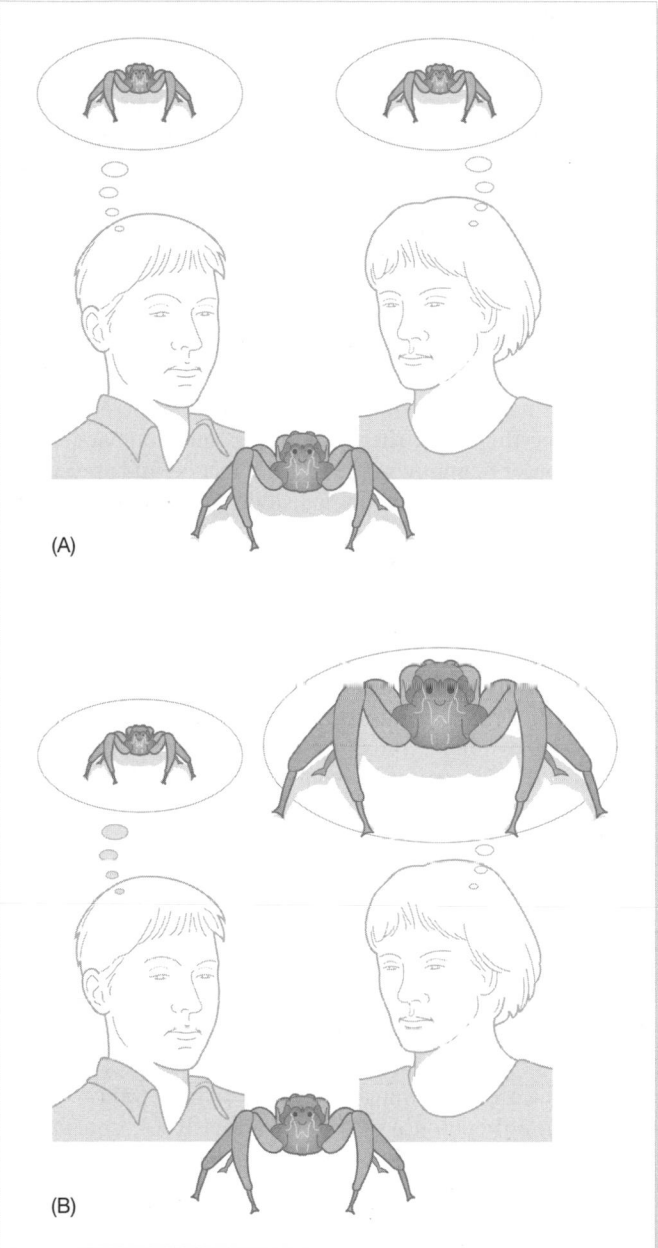

Figure 6.4 (A) Viewing the stressor identically. (B) How the subjects each perceive the threat.

OLDER ADULTS: NURSING PRIORITIES

6.1 Social and cultural norms and the stress response in older people

Think about how gender and cultural factors might affect the amount of distress experienced by older people in the following situations:

- receiving a blood transfusion
- being admitted to a mixed gender ward
- selling their house and moving into a nursing home.

Reflect on the distress you have observed in older patients or clients during your clinical placements. What measures could you have taken to reduce their distress?

is interpreted identically by both subjects 1 and 2. Cox (1978) argues that this is too simplistic and that to gain a true understanding of the nature of stress, the stressor must be appraised in the context of the perceived threat it poses to the individual. Consider Figure 6.4(B) in which subjects 1 and 2 are exposed to the same stressor as before but, because of the meaning subject 2 attaches to the spider in this particular context, the perceived threat is greater for subject 2 than for subject 1.

Thus, while the social readjustment rating scale is useful in providing an overview of stressors the individual has experienced, it is only by assessing the meaning of the stressor to the individual that it becomes possible to understand the severity of the stress response. This is particularly significant in the context of social and cultural norms (see Older Adults box 6.1).

INDIVIDUAL RESPONSE TO STRESS: THE STRESSFUL PERSONALITY TYPE

In their research into the relationship between coronary heart disease and stress, Freidman & Rosenman (1974) classified individuals into two groups according to personality characteristics. The first group, those with a type A personality, are typified by extreme competitiveness and inability to place stress in perspective. They are unable to delegate and find it difficult to refuse additional work. Consequently, they have insufficient time to complete tasks and, instead of problem-solving and prioritizing, they juggle them, switching in an undirected manner from one task to another without completing any. Type A individuals often appear aggressive, reacting to minor irritations with temper tantrums.

The second personality type, type B, is the antithesis of type A. Individuals with type B characteristics remain totally relaxed and almost unconcerned when confronted by stressors. Types A and B are, in reality, two extreme points on the same scale. Most people exhibit traits from both personality types and are situated on a point along this scale somewhere between the two extremes. But there does seem to be some correlation between health and personality type; for example, Friedman & Rosenman found that people who were less susceptible to heart disease had a greater number of type B characteristics than type A, observations shared by Levi & Lunde-Jensen (1996) (see Health Promotion box 6.1).

however, two major limitations of the scale. First, it only addresses long-term stressors, failing to take into account short-term stressors such as being late for work. Such stressors, or 'hassles', invoke a severe stress response but only for a short period (Lazarus et al 1985); being out of the individual's control, however, they invoke distress and ultimately result in similar damaging effects as those resulting from long-term distress.

The second shortcoming of the scale is highlighted by Cox (1978) who argues that it is difficult to generalize people's unique experiences of stress. Holmes & Rahe (1967) assume that the object of stress is external to the individual and causes more or less the same amount of stress for everyone. This is the engineering model of stress (Cox 1978) and it is demonstrated in Figure 6.4(A) in which the stressor, in this case a spider,

HEALTH PROMOTION

6.1 Leigh

Leigh, aged 45, attends a well man's clinic. He is found to be overweight and hypertensive with a blood pressure of 195/110 mmHg. He works long hours as an accounts manager in a local building firm. On being questioned about his lifestyle, he states that he has little time for exercise or to eat properly, particularly since his wife left him 3 years ago. During the day he takes snacks at work and his main meal is in the evening, usually a takeaway on his way home from work. He smokes 30 cigarettes a day to help with the stress of work, and drinks approximately 70 units of alcohol each week. He appears restless, stating that the time he is spending at the clinic answering questions could be better spent finishing his work, as nobody else in the office can be trusted to do it properly. He's concerned that, yet again, it will be 7.30pm before he finishes work.

Student activities

- What are the likely consequences for Leigh if he continues this lifestyle?
- What advice could the nurse give to Leigh to encourage him to adopt a healthier lifestyle?
- Leigh possesses many characteristics of a type A personality. Consider ways in which your suggestions may be made acceptable to him.

COMMON STRESSORS WITHIN THE HEALTH CARE SYSTEM

STRESS AFFECTING PATIENTS

Being ill makes physiological and psychological demands on patients and generates stress. Even if the prognosis is good, being ill removes a patient's internal locus of control and may result in adverse psychological reactions. These may manifest physically through the action of the GAS or as psychological distress, which is most likely to result in a change in behaviour. Two common stressors that trigger these responses in patients are considered below.

Waiting for results

Waiting for results is a particularly distressing time for patients. The insecurity of the situation inhibits positive thought, and this is often exacerbated by denial on the part of the patient, particularly if the tests are to confirm a potentially life-threatening disease. The uncertainty moves the stressor out of the control of patients and they become distressed which, by invoking the fight-or-flight response, may also cause aggression. At this time, nurses should acknowledge the patient's distress and offer crisis interventions that address the immediate symptoms. It is only when the test results are known that the stressor can be isolated and positive steps taken to secure control in the long term.

Physical stress

Many patients will suffer physical damage as a result of their illness or damage due to medical or surgical intervention. Moreover, falling ill is a major life event with psychological and social implications (Holmes & Rahe 1967) that cause psychological distress and thus augment the severity of the stress response. These are prolonged stressors and patients are likely to have progressed through the alarm stage to the longer-term resistance stage, which seeks to sustain the body and minimize further injury through the secretion of cortisol (Fig. 6.3). Unfortunately, cortisol also suppresses the construction of connective tissue and the immune system. In patients recovering from surgery, this is particularly significant as it delays wound healing and makes them more susceptible to postoperative infections. During this stage, therefore, nurses must be particularly vigilant in order to minimize the risk of infection and prevent the occurrence of postoperative complications (see Chs 13 and 29).

STRESS AFFECTING HEALTH CARE WORKERS

Many investigations into the effects of stress have focused specifically on health care workers. Perhaps the most consistent stressors found to affect this group are those highlighted by Dewe (1987), identified in interviews with nurses who reported experiencing psychological distress as a result of being overwhelmed with work pressures, role conflict, lack of support and working with seriously ill or dying patients (see Evidence-based Practice box 6.1).

 EVIDENCE-BASED PRACTICE

6.1 Stressors affecting nurses

Harris (1989) developed the Nurse Stress Index from interviews with charge nurses and ward sisters (ward managers). Although use of the instrument is widespread, its focus is mainly on clinical and managerial issues, which limits its usefulness in those working in other grades, such as student nurses. Rhead (1995) investigated the experiences of student nurses and identified coursework, practice placements and confrontation with mortality as particularly distressing. Howard (1999), in addition, identified financial difficulties, time management and relationship problems as significant causes of distress. It is difficult to generalize all experiences of stress in clinical areas to all grades of health care staff. However, certain core issues – mortality, work load and role conflict – are consistently cited.

References
Harris PE. The nurse stress index. Work Stress 1989; 3(4): 335–346.
Howard DJ. Psychological, social and emotional changes experienced by student nurses undertaking the Project 2000 system of training. PhD thesis. Nottingham: Nottingham Trent University; 1999.
Rhead MM. Stress among student nurses: is it practical or academic? J Clin Nurs 1995; 4(6): 369–376.

Burnout

The causes of work-related stress vary according to the grade of a person's job, but all health care workers spend intense, prolonged, stressful periods working with ill people. This has been found to be a powerful stressor in the caring professions, and as a result workers in this area are highly susceptible to developing burnout (Maslach 1982), particularly when the distress is prolonged, continuous and outside the individual's locus of control (Janssen et al 1999). According to Maslach (1982) there are three main symptoms of burnout:

- emotional exhaustion – the individual feels emotionally drained and unable to give more
- depersonalization – the individual becomes isolated and hardened towards others
- decreased sense of personal accomplishment – the individual is unable to deal with problems positively and may trivialize any achievements.

Similar symptoms are reported by Welch et al (1982), who placed them into the following categories: physical, intellectual, emotional, social and spiritual (Box 6.2). Unlike Maslach, who defines burnout as a single pathology, Welch et al identified two types: short-term and long-term. Short-term burnout is a temporary condition in which individuals experience primarily physical effects and generally feel run-down. It is quickly reversed by either a break from work, such as a holiday, or a change in the work environment, such as a new project. In contrast, long-term burnout comprises the profound psychological and social changes identified in Box 6.2. Individuals become emotionally blunted, their cognitive ability decreases, they find it difficult to mix with others and consequently become isolated. Thus, although burnout arises from work-related issues, the ramifications filter through to individuals' personal lives. Relationships with their family and others deteriorate and this, in turn, worsens the situation. In contrast to short-term burnout, the effects of long-term burnout are devastating and the recovery is long and difficult.

Box 6.2 Symptoms of burnout

Physical
Lack of energy and persistent feeling of fatigue, which often leads to a lack of exercise and poor nutrition

Intellectual
Loss of problem-solving and cognitive abilities
Lack of creativity and interest in hobbies

Emotional
Feelings of helplessness and depression
Over-investment in work to the exclusion of other interests

Social
Inability to share problems with others; withdrawal from others
May act aggressively towards those whom they feel threatened by

Spiritual
Individuals feel unfulfilled, cheated, resentful and cynical

Causes of burnout in health care workers

Burnout occurs in response to continued distress. High workload, time pressure, pressure from patients, insecure career path, resource cuts, poor communication, constant change and poor management are the most significant factors in its development in health care workers. Commonly, those who are affected feel that it results from a weakness in their own character and suffer poor self-esteem (Burnard 1991, Janssen 1999). It should be remembered, however, that burnout occurs as a result of factors outside the individual's control; 'No one burns out except in a climate that encourages burnout' (Welch et al 1982, p. 9).

To help individuals experiencing distress, many employers make counselling services available. The uptake of this type of service is likely to be small, however, and will only really be used by those who are desperate (Maslach 1982, Welch et al 1982). Indeed, to utilize these services requires a degree of assertiveness. As individuals suffering adversely from occupational stress are also likely to have low self-esteem, they are unlikely to avail themselves of this support (Janssen et al 1999). Moreover, although counselling interventions are effective for those who do use the service (Cooper et al 1996), by definition the intervention comes after the event. To deal with burnout effectively, it is the causes that require to be minimized. One recent proactive development to address work-related stress in nursing has been the introduction of clinical supervision (see Evidence-based Practice box 6.2).

Many employers ignore workplace stress and argue that individuals are responsible for managing their own stress. This is called victim blaming and it is common in insecure, competitive work environments where there is minimal support; the employer's financial gains are therefore maximized at the expense of the quality of the employees' lives. Maslach (1982) reported that some employers deliberately introduce competitiveness into the workplace to achieve this. For example following the recession of the early 1980s, many European organizations underwent mergers and restructuring, which introduced job insecurity and often increased workloads, consequently increasing the distress of many employees (Cooper et al 1996).

One of the reasons that stressful workplaces are allowed to evolve is that stress and stress-induced conditions are not

 EVIDENCE-BASED PRACTICE

6.2 Clinical supervision and the management of work-related stress

For health care workers, clinical supervision has a valuable role in the management of work-related stress. It has been shown to develop self-confidence and to help individuals take control of their situations (White et al 1998).

Student activities
- Find out how clinical supervision is implemented in your area of work.
- Do the staff receiving clinical supervision in your area agree with White et al's findings?
- How could clinical supervision be improved?

classified as industrial diseases. Traditionally, industrial injuries have warranted compensation only when the employer's negligence has resulted in physical injury to an employee. Earnshaw & Cooper (1994) noted that where injuries are not directly measurable, such as repetitive strain injury, the success of employees in seeking redress from employers is limited. Therefore, those individuals unable to work through stress-induced illness, even though their employer may have invoked it, find it difficult to obtain compensation. Recently, however, the way in which stress-induced disease is viewed by the legal establishment has altered and, increasingly, claims against employers have succeeded in securing compensation for this type of disease (Earnshaw & Cooper 1994). Should this trend continue, the costs to employers and their insurers of continuing to ignore employee stress in the workplace are potentially enormous.

Post-traumatic stress disorder

Post-traumatic stress disorder (PTSD) is a condition that occurs within 6 months of exposure to a triggering event and is defined as (WHO 1992, p. 147): 'a delayed and/or protracted response to a stressful event or situation (either short or long lasting) of an exceptionally threatening or catastrophic nature, which is likely to cause pervasive distress in almost anyone'. The trigger is therefore any major psychological event outside the range of usual day-to-day experience, e.g.:

- natural disasters – earthquakes, floods, hurricanes
- man-made disasters – major car/air/maritime accidents, industrial accidents
- intentional man-made disasters – witnessing violent death, victim of rape/torture/assault, prolonged combat.

Extreme experiences can occur within many areas of health care, such as in A&E, thus making staff working in these departments particularly vulnerable. PTSD has five major features:

- Flashbacks – individuals relive the experience during nightmares. Additionally, when awake, they may experience a type of *déjà-vu* and feel that the situation is about to recur
- Emotional numbing – individuals repress the distressing experience and the feelings they associate with it. This leads to emotional blunting and detachment from others
- Hypervigilance – individuals are very restless, as if on a constant lookout for danger. They also have an enhanced startle reaction, reacting in an exaggerated way to unexpected events
- Avoidance – individuals avoid anything reminiscent of the triggering event
- Confusion, anxiety and depression – individuals become confused, anxious or depressed and suicidal attempts may occur. Additionally, many individuals blame themselves for the incident and the resultant guilt augments their symptoms.

There are also a number of associated symptoms that can occur with PTSD, including insomnia, headaches, peptic ulcers and circulatory problems. Furthermore, to compensate, individuals may misuse alcohol or other drugs (both prescribed tranquillizers and illegal substances), which may lead to dependence.

The most effective treatment for PTSD is early counselling (Sims & Owens 1993). This focuses on patients' unique problems, enabling them to make some sense out of their experience, adopt a problem-solving strategy and move through the initial period of crisis. This should be supplemented by debriefing exercises following traumatic incidents, clinical supervision and peer support.

STRESS AFFECTING CARERS

Many patients are now cared for within the community, a consequence of changes to UK health care policy that has deliberately involved greater use of informal carers. Although the goal of community-based care was set during the 1950s, this rapidly accelerated in the 1980s following the redefinition of community care in the *Growing Older* report (DHSS 1981), which stated that 'care in the community must increasingly mean care by the community'.

The focus of government policy has been to replace formal care with informal (non-paid) care, and the role of the statutory services has changed so that they have become facilitators rather than providers of care. The Griffiths report on community care (DHSS 1988) advocated that more care be delivered in the community, making greater use of voluntary, not-for-profit and commercial sectors instead of statutory services, proposals which were subsequently embraced in the NHS & Community Care Act (DoH 1990).

Stress in patients' relatives

Many carers are immediate family members and the stress they experience as a result of the patient's illness may manifest as guilt at not being able to cope or anger that the patient is ill at all; this is part of the grieving process (see Ch. 34). In cases where patients formerly cared for at home are admitted to a nursing home or hospital, the guilt felt by some former carers leads them to avoid visiting the patient. This may appear callous and uncaring, but can be the result of denial or a flight response provoked by the stress of the situation.

Similarly, the fight-or-flight response can explain why other relatives may be aggressive. This aggression is often directed at the nurse: relatives are acrimonious and constantly find fault with the care given. This may, in turn, result in the relative being labelled as troublesome and being treated with hostility by other staff. In the community this may lead to shorter or less frequent visits by nursing staff. This reaction may be understandable, but nevertheless it will exacerbate the situation. This emphasizes the importance of understanding stress mechanisms so as to be able to recognize the distress experienced by relatives and to implement actions to ameliorate their concerns.

Following the UK general election in 1997, two documents were published in which the reliance on carers was recognized. The discussion document *Partnership in Action* (DoH 1998) looked to improve collaborative care, and within it health authorities were expected to consult local interested parties via health improvement programmes. This was reinforced in *Caring about Carers* (DoH 1999a), which identifies specific measures intended to assist carers. What both papers fail to address, however, is whether informal carers actually want to, or are able to, adopt the caring role, because where the care demands exceed their capacity to care, they will experience profound psychological distress. With increased involvement of informal carers in providing care for patients, it is imperative to recognize the pressures and to identify the signs of excessive distress. This is particularly important in the community, where the nurse provides support for both patients and their carers.

MALADAPTION: STRESS-RELATED ILLNESS

The GAS is invoked whenever individuals perceive themselves to be in danger. (A similar response is invoked each time a stressful event occurs, e.g. a job interview or admission to hospital.) It prepares the body for intense physical action to either escape or fight the stressor. Two physiological systems in particular are extremely susceptible to the destructive effects of prolonged stress however: the circulatory and immune systems.

THE CIRCULATORY SYSTEM

The fight-or-flight response causes the heart rate to increase and peripheral vasoconstriction. In the long term the heart and arteries are damaged as they attempt to compensate. Thus, circulatory conditions such as hypertension and coronary heart disease are frequently associated with periods of psychological distress and these conditions are often referred to as stress-related illnesses (Friedman & Rosenman 1974, Totman 1990, Cooper et al 1996). Indeed, Levi & Lunde-Jensen (1996) carried out a study on 1600 Swedish workers which reinforces this association. The study looked at two groups. In the first group, members of which had stressful employment over which they had little control, 20% developed circulatory disorders, whereas members of the second group, who had employment with minimal stress over which they enjoyed a high degree of control, none developed circulatory disease. Thus, it can be seen that the physiological consequences of long-term distress may ultimately be life-threatening.

THE IMMUNE SYSTEM

In the resistance reaction of the GAS, inflammation is suppressed to enable the body to continue action if it is damaged (Fig. 6.3). An undesirable effect of this, however, is suppression of the immune system, which in turn leaves an individual more susceptible to disease. This was confirmed by Brosschot et al (1998) who found that when individuals were exposed to stressors they were unable to control, they became immunosuppressed. Similarly, Pruessner et al (1999) reported that individuals placed in situations in which they experienced high distress and low self-esteem had higher serum cortisol than would be expected, which in turn would suppress their immune systems.

Individuals suffering prolonged distress in the medium term become more susceptible to minor infections such as colds. You may have noticed this phenomenon in yourself. Often when you are stressed, or due for a holiday, you pick up minor infections more easily and probably find it takes longer than usual to recover. Many managers use this phenomenon as an indicator of a stressful workplace (Levi & Lunde-Jensen 1996). In the long term, however, suppression of the immune system can enable malignancies to develop (Totman 1990, Cooper et al 1996), reinforcing the seriousness of long-term exposure to stress.

OTHER VULNERABLE ORGANS

Due to the integral relationship between psychological, social and physiological systems, any organ may be adversely affected as a result of continued exposure to psychological distress. Although the circulatory and immune systems are particularly affected, some illnesses affecting other systems are also seen as stress-related (WHO 1992).

Gastrointestinal system

Peptic ulcers These occur in people with a genetic predisposition towards hypersecretion of gastric hydrochloric acid. Under prolonged distress this manifests as peptic ulceration. Typically, people who develop these ulcers are hardworking and have often been promoted to senior positions within their profession.

Ulcerative colitis This is another stress-related disease and people prone to developing it often have underlying obsessive personalities. They become anxious when not in total control of situations and have difficulties in forming relationships. Although they crave support from others, they fear the loss of control associated with rejection so they do not become involved with other people. Similarly, when they become angry, they internalize the anger so as to remain in control. Consequently, ulcerative colitis is often exacerbated by stressful events in patients' lives (Neese 1994).

Irritable bowel syndrome This may affect people who are tense and anxious. They are often conscientious individuals who worry excessively, e.g. about money or their health.

Respiratory system

Many people who suffer from asthma find their symptoms are worse during periods of psychological stress. When patients suffer an attack, addressing their fears and providing reassurance helps to reduce the severity and forms an integral part of nursing care (Ch. 20).

Skin

The skin is influenced by a wide variety of emotions. In the fight-or-flight response, sweating occurs, goose bumps appear and individuals become pale as their peripheral capillaries constrict; likewise, when people become embarrassed, they blush. These are all transient responses, but persistent skin conditions can arise in response to stress. Although eczema and psoriasis are conditions that occur in response to an irritant (Ch. 28), they are often exacerbated during periods of psychological distress.

Headache, backache and muscular aches

The tension of antagonistic muscles causes muscles and joints to ache. Most people experience these symptoms following long periods of acute distress, such as at the end of a stressful day. Similarly, relaxation is associated with a reduction in muscle tone, which can occur quite rapidly. Imagine, for example, that you are waiting for examination results to arrive by letter and the letter finally arrives; think of how the tension in your body mounts just prior to opening it and how it will melt away when you discover that you have passed. Thus tense muscles are associated with psychological distress and relaxed muscles with tranquillity, which is why massage and progressive muscle relaxation therapy are used as part of stress management programmes (discussed on pp. 108 and 107).

Migraine and tension headaches

People with obsessive, competitive personalities are more prone to migraine and tension headaches, which affect around 20% of the population (Neese 1994). Migraine disturbances are frequently unilateral or temporal and may occur after certain foods are eaten (Ch. 14), but stress is highly influential in the history of attacks. Significant reciprocal relationships between psychological stress and the onset of both migraine and tension headache symptoms have consistently been reported (Spierings et al 1996, Holm et al 1997). Furthermore, Reid & McGrath (1996) found that migraine symptoms abate following psychological intervention, confirming the significance of psychological stress in the aetiology.

Substance misuse

People experiencing stress sometimes turn to alcohol, nicotine and, in a minority, various illegal substances to relieve their symptoms. Although these substances are likely to provide short-term relief, the underlying causes of the stress are not being addressed. Continued misuse of the substance may then progress to addiction, and as tolerance develops, increasing amounts are required to achieve the same effect, which can lead to deterioration of health.

MENTAL ILLNESS

Although the onset of many mental illnesses can be traced back to an increase in stressful life events, the most common mental disorders that arise from psychological distress are anxiety and depression.

Anxiety

Anxiety is the emotional response to distress. It is normal to feel anxious when exposed to stressors, but what differentiates clinical anxiety from everyday anxiety is that the emotional response associated with the former is inappropriate to the threat posed by the stressor and continues after the threat is removed (Sims & Owens 1993). Clinical anxiety that occurs when there is no apparent danger is called generalized anxiety and the individual complains of feeling anxious all of the time.

Panic attacks are related to anxiety. These are periods of intense fear, which often occur despite no obvious cause. During a panic attack, the somatic symptoms of the fight-or-flight response are exaggerated, in particular increased heart and respiration rates. The individual experiences palpitations, arrhythmias (such as occasional ectopic beats, Ch. 19), hyperventilation and dizziness. Sufferers often think they are having a heart attack and are about to die, which serves to reinforce the panic.

Depression

The low self-esteem of individuals undergoing prolonged psychological distress is associated with negative thinking, which can lead to clinical depression. Although many will be helped by support from mental health services, for some the depression may not resolve and they may become so desperate that they attempt suicide. Brenner (1983) demonstrated a relationship between suicide and unemployment, reflecting the complex interaction between life events, psychological distress and mental illness. One group of particular concern are young males, in whom suicide is the second most common cause of death (DoH 1999b); this group has been targeted for specific health promotion intervention.

ACCIDENTS OR UNSAFE BEHAVIOUR

Increasing levels of arousal make it difficult for individuals to concentrate and this in turn leads to an increase in accidents (Cooper et al 1996). Roseman & Booker (1995) examined nurses' errors in administering medication and found the most significant factor to be increased workload. In an attempt to meet tight deadlines, individuals sometimes ignore safe working practices, thus exposing themselves, and others, to risk. This is in line with Hebb's (1971) assertion that individuals are unable to process excessive arousal, instead losing concentration and thereby making mistakes.

▶ Nursing assessment

MEASURING STRESS

While psychological stress is an issue frequently addressed by mental health nurses, the ramifications vis-à-vis a patient's physical health and recovery, seen in the GAS, emphasize the importance of incorporating these issues into patients' nursing care plans in all branches of nursing. By understanding how individuals respond to stress, it becomes possible to utilize this knowledge as a basis of assessment. Although individuals respond to stress in their own unique way according to age, culture, gender and past experience, some responses are universal and measuring these allows an assessment of stress to be incorporated within the care plan.

Physiological measures

The relationship between psychological stress and physiological disturbance makes it possible to assess stress levels using physiological measurements. For example, one effect of stress is increased perspiration; this leads to greater electrical conductivity of the skin surface, which can be measured using a galvanometer. Heart rate and blood pressure are also indicators, as these become elevated in a person under stress. The disadvantage of all physiological measures, however, is that, in the absence of qualitative data, the meaning of the stressor to the individual is impossible to determine. For example, Selye (1984) found that the immediate physiological effects of eustress and distress were identical; hence similar physiological recordings would be obtained for both positive and negative stressors.

Hospital anxiety and depression scale

The hospital anxiety and depression scale (Zigmond & Snaith 1983) is widely used to identify anxiety and depression. It is a self-administered questionnaire and consists of 14 questions assessed on a Likert-style agree/disagree scale. Seven questions measure traits of anxiety, e.g. 'Worrying thoughts go through my mind', and seven traits of depression, e.g. 'I have lost interest in my appearance'. A maximum score of 21 is attainable for each scale, with a score greater than eight indicating a pathological state. Although patients must have sufficient insight into their problems to complete this instrument, its strength lies in the fact that it helps to differentiate between anxiety and depression as the predominant problem. When used within the nursing assessment, this enables the nurse to optimize subsequent interventions.

Social readjustment rating scale

As described earlier, the social readjustment rating scale (Holmes & Rahe 1967; see Table 6.2) lists a fixed number of life events and assumes that these invoke similar stress responses in everyone. Its main use is to gain insight into major life events contributing to a patient's background level of stress and it is possible to use this instrument within a nursing assessment providing the scores are removed on the patient's copy (so their responses are not influenced). As it only lists a limited number of events, it is inappropriate to use this instrument alone, as it may not record all the salient factors that invoke stress. Furthermore, because the stressors are ascribed a generalized score, the instrument assumes an engineering model of stress (discussed on p. 98), consequently failing to measure the severity of the stress as it is experienced by the patient. If this instrument is used, it must therefore be supplemented in two ways: with additional information about how patients interpret the threat posed by the stressors; and with the identification of any stressors not listed.

SELF-REPORTING

All of the preceding instruments attempt to generalize the individual experience of stress. However, because patients' experience of stress is based on their unique interpretation of threat, using these instruments alone is not generally considered an accurate mode of assessment. Stress is a psychological construct, and because only the individual experiencing it knows its true meaning, using a rigid model of assessment becomes difficult. A self-reporting method may prove more effective.

Dewe (1989) argued that to gain insight into the phenomenon of stress from an individual's perspective, instruments should measure the nature, frequency and intensity of the experience. This was addressed by research into the stresses experienced by student nurses during the Project 2000 course (Howard 1999). Students were asked to record how stressed they felt on a 10-point scale and to list the main reasons why they felt that way in a diary. This was repeated weekly for a period of 1 year during which time patterns of stress became apparent, identifying particularly stressful periods of the Project 2000 course. When these data were supplemented by the diary entries, it became evident that the major causes of distress on the Project 2000 course were assessments, lack of time, financial problems, inappropriate theory and a deterioration of interpersonal relationships.

The universal measures identified earlier have a place in the assessment of stress, but it is self-reporting that provides insight into patients' experiences. Both methods should therefore be part of the nursing assessment, in order to determine the degree of distress experienced and also to discover what the stress means to the patient. This allows effective care planning that addresses the individualistic concerns of each patient.

REDUCING STRESS AND ENHANCING COPING STRATEGIES

In this chapter, ways of reducing stress have been divided into two major categories: pharmacological and non-pharmacological. Although it is usual to utilize non-pharmacological methods to arrive at a permanent resolution of stress-related problems, it is likely that in a crisis many patients will take medication.

PHARMACOLOGICAL METHODS

The routine use of drugs as part of stress management is not advocated, but in severe instances where pathologies develop, the use of medication is helpful. Two categories of drugs are commonly prescribed: anxiolytics such as diazepam or lorazepam and antidepressants such as amitriptyline or fluoxetine.

Anxiolytics

These drugs provide immediate relief from the unpleasant feelings associated with stress. This is a very short-term solution, although in periods of crisis they may be prescribed for a brief period to reduce the anxiety level and facilitate the return of problem-solving thinking. Counselling may be used to aid this process, because if the underlying problems responsible for the anxiety are not addressed, the unpleasant feelings will return when the drug is discontinued. The danger is that as the underlying problems remain unresolved, the individual will continue to take the drug to avoid the symptoms of stress. This quickly becomes a self-perpetuating cycle and may ultimately lead to dependence.

Antidepressants

These drugs are sometimes prescribed when individuals experience prolonged periods of distress. Some antidepressants also have a sedative effect and in the very short term this helps to reduce the level of discomfort experienced by the patient. When individuals experience prolonged periods of distress, however, they also experience low self-esteem. The main reason antidepressants are prescribed is to help improve this feeling of low self-esteem, enabling patients to think more positively and thus empowering them to address the cause of their problems.

COMPLEMENTARY REMEDIES

Increasing use is being made of non-prescribed preparations, particularly herbal remedies, which are claimed to possess similar properties to traditional prescribed medication. Generally, herbal preparations have been the subject of little empirical research and their exact mode of action remains unknown. Furthermore, the quality of herbal preparations is variable as the active ingredients are often mixed with other preparations, making it difficult to draw conclusions about the benefits or side-effects (Linde 1996, Wong 1998). In particular, the safety of these preparations in pregnancy and during lactation is not established and therefore pregnant women and breast-feeding mothers should not take them, nor should they be taken around the time of conception. Despite these cautions, however, herbal remedies remain popular. The two most frequently used in the management of stress are valerian and hypericum.

Valerian

Valerian is used as an anxiolytic. While it is reported to possess sedative properties, valerian may also interact with other medication, particularly other sedatives, including alcohol. When taking this preparation, therefore, it is prudent to observe similar precautions as are observed with other sedative medications, such as caution when driving, avoiding alcohol, and interaction with other medication.

Hypericum perforatum (St John's wort)

Hypericum has a long history of use as an antidepressant and it is the most investigated of the herbal remedies (Wong 1998). Linde (1996) notes that it is widely prescribed in Germany for the treatment of anxiety and depression. Within the UK, its use is mainly by self-medication. It is thought to work in a similar way to selective serotonin reuptake inhibitors (SSRIs) such as fluoxetine, and studies comparing hypericum to both placebo and antidepressant medication have reported its success in treating mild depression (Linde 1996). Within stress management, the rationale for its use is therefore similar to conventional antidepressants. Generally, hypericum has fewer side-effects than conventional antidepressants, but skin sensitivity to the sun, gastrointestinal disturbance, dry mouth, restlessness and sedation have all been reported (Wong 1998).

NON-PHARMACOLOGICAL METHODS

While pharmacological methods are useful in a crisis, they only react to a situation that has already got out of control. In contrast, non-pharmacological stress management methods both assist in managing a crisis and encourage adoption of a healthier lifestyle. As a result, these methods may also help to prevent future problems.

Diet

Stress may lead to changes in eating habits. Some individuals regress to a more secure developmental stage and consume a greater amount of comfort foods with a high sugar and fat content, while others drastically reduce the amount they eat or eat inappropriately (e.g. binge eating). Some individuals crave the sedative properties of alcohol and increase their consumption. Indeed, alcohol may even replace a balanced diet, resulting in a depletion of essential nutrients. During the resistance stage of the GAS, the body retains sodium by excreting high levels of potassium. Left unchecked, this can lead to exhaustion and illness (Ch. 8). Although this is an extreme example, because of the disturbances in nutritional intake and the adoption of unhealthy eating habits, a well-balanced diet (Ch. 11) is central to all stress management programmes (see Special Issues box 6.1).

Exercise

Exercise is often advocated as a part of stress management. Engaging in sport has a distracting quality, as the person's attention is focused on the activity and not on the worrying recurrent thoughts that sustain the underlying stress. It also increases physical fitness, particularly of the cardiopulmonary system, which counteracts some of the damaging effects of the GAS syndrome. Playing sport also provides a safe, socially acceptable

 SPECIAL ISSUES

6.1 Diet and stress management

Cooper et al (1996) suggest that employers should assist in the management of stress by providing healthy canteen menus. Referring to the guidelines for healthy eating in Chapter 11 (p. 202), look at the staff menu in your local canteen and see if it is possible to adhere to these guidelines. Do the same for the patients' meal choices.

outlet for the aggressive drives that manifest as part of the fight-or-flight response. Using sport as a method of stress management requires caution, however, as the individuals most susceptible to the negative effects of stress are those with the highly competitive type A personality (Friedman & Rosenman 1974). They may set themselves ever-increasing goals that they will be unable to achieve, failure to do so contributing to rather than alleviating the stress. To counter this effect, some contemporary authors advocate taking part in non-competitive sports, but then, a convincing argument can be made that all sport is competitive. What is important, therefore, is that individuals diminish the competitive element of the sport and play for enjoyment rather than achievement.

Counselling

When used as part of stress management, counselling aims to enable individuals to gain control of stressful situations by developing problem-solving strategies for coping with the distress invoked by the stressor. There are times when this may seem idealistic. For example, a patient admitted following a myocardial infarction will probably be distressed about the condition and the prognosis. It is impossible to generalize, but it is likely that this person will use mental defence mechanisms to cope, particularly denial. In a case like this, counselling would focus on helping the person accept the situation and any limitations that arise out of it. From this base the patient would be encouraged to build his or her life positively, using a problem-solving approach, and to take control of events where possible to minimize distress.

Clinical supervision

For practitioners, clinical supervision provides a method to discuss with a supervisor events that occur during clinical practice, to explore feelings towards these events and to learn from the experience. These sessions take place on a one-to-one or a group basis. The supervisor is usually an experienced professional who helps supervisees reflect on issues that occur in practice and consider alternative perspectives, thus also helping them to develop their knowledge, confidence and self-esteem. While this enables practitioners to improve their practice, by maximizing their feeling of control over the stressors they encounter, it also acts as a stress management tool (White et al 1998).

Time management

When under stress, individuals often find that they have little time for anything other than work and work-related issues.

Their ability to organize is usually curtailed as they attempt to sustain an ever-increasing workload in an ever-decreasing amount of time, a situation often compounded by working unsocial hours or shifts. The finite amount of time means that tasks have to be prioritized, which may leave little time for family and social commitments. Life loses structure and the stressed person becomes overwhelmed.

It is essential that individuals under stress continue to maintain social contact with friends and family, in order to retain a proper perspective on the new stressors in their lives. Effective time management is therefore a fundamental part of stress management. By rigorously allocating time to each and every commitment, it is possible to take control over stressors and decide what will and will not be achieved.

Cognitive behavioural therapy

Cognitive therapy aims to put a stop to negative, destructive thoughts and replace them with positive, constructive ones. It was originally used in the treatment of depression, but like those who are depressed, individuals who feel overwhelmed through excessive stress also experience feelings of low self-esteem and have negative thought processes. Cognitive therapy can be successful with such individuals and therefore has a part to play in the management of stress (Sims & Owens 1993).

Group therapies

There are many kinds of group therapy that may be utilized in a stress management programme. Local community mental health teams frequently facilitate these and they commonly include:

- *Anxiety management groups* that use education, social skills and self-help techniques – the aim of these groups is to provide individuals with an understanding of the nature of stress and anxiety and to help them learn more effective coping skills
- *Social skills groups* which help individuals to deal with low self-esteem and possible isolation, by regaining their ability to interact socially – these groups are also useful for people with type A personality traits (Friedman & Rosenman 1974), who are often impatient and aggressive, as they can be helped to develop more appropriate interpersonal skills; this can also lead to an improvement in their physical health (see Evidence-based Practice box 6.3)
- *Self-help groups* attended by people with similar problems – these groups meet under the supervision of a trained facilitator, the intention being for members to offer each other support and learn alternative ways of coping with problems. Self-help groups are not confined to patients and are frequently run for carers by service providers or agencies such as Age Concern (http://www.ageconcern.org.uk)
- *Assertiveness groups* – these can help individuals in whom low self-esteem is accompanied by poor assertiveness skills, traits that can lead, for example, to people agreeing to take on additional work they know they can't handle. Assertiveness skills enable individuals like this to take more control of their lives, which allows better management of commitments and consequently of stress. Assertiveness

EVIDENCE-BASED PRACTICE

6.3 Benefits of adopting a more relaxed approach to life

Both Friedman & Rosenman (1974) and Levi & Lunde-Jensen (1996) found a relationship between stressful personality types and coronary heart disease. Friedman & Rosenman used a behaviour modification programme to enable these individuals to adopt a more relaxed approach to life. This intervention reduced the probability of recurrence of their heart problems.

Student activities
- What physiological changes associated with stressful personality types are implicated in an increased risk of heart disease?
- How do you think behaviour modification programmes might reduce the probability of a recurrence of heart problems?

groups can also be helpful for people with type A personalities, teaching them less aggressive and more assertive modes of interaction. However, the presence of dominant type A individuals in groups containing people with low self-esteem should be carefully considered, as their behaviour could become extremely destructive to the group process.

Relaxation methods

Relaxation techniques are used in the control of the symptoms of stress. Although this is a reactive measure, these techniques are sometimes used to prevent a stressful period in an individual's life from developing into a crisis.

Meditation

Individuals adopt a relaxed, balanced posture so that no muscular correction is needed to maintain position. Breathing is controlled to slow deep breaths, a counter to the increased shallow respirations common in the stress response. They try to empty their minds of all thoughts or alternatively focus on a single object, such as a lighted candle. In effect, this stops the recurrent worrying thoughts that often occupy people under stress and helps to promote a sense of calm. Once in a relaxed state, individuals may then be better able to apply problem-solving strategies to deal with their stressors; if the anxiety returns, the techniques of meditation can once again be applied to control these feelings.

Progressive muscle relaxation

Any prolonged increase in muscle tone, such as that associated with the fight-or-flight response, leads to tension, perpetuating the feeling of stress. In progressive muscle relaxation, individuals are asked to contract and then relax one muscle group at a time, to compare the difference and to remember the feeling of relaxation. This usually takes place with the person lying in a quiet room, with relaxing music playing in the background.

Each major muscle group is addressed in turn, leading to an overall reduction in muscle tone. Relaxed muscles are incompatible with feelings of tension and progressive muscle relaxation thereby results in the individual feeling relaxed. The initial relaxation sessions are usually led by a trained therapist. This is necessary because some patients may react to the feelings of relaxation with panic as they feel a loss of control, while others may require additional instruction. Relaxation requires practice and patients are often given a tape to use at home. Eventually, most patients become proficient; however, while the therapy can provide relief from the physical symptoms of stress, it does not address the causes. Therefore, it is usually used as a supplement to other interventions that focus on managing stressors.

Massage

This is an alternative method of muscle relaxation, this time combined with touch. Touch is a form of non-verbal communication and suggests that the person performing the massage cares about the person receiving it (see Ch. 3). Massage may be enhanced by the use of aromatherapy oils. Olfactory receptors are excited by these oils and in turn stimulate the limbic centre to produce endorphins which promote a sense of well-being. The effect of massage is often to relax individuals sufficiently to enable them to discuss anxieties; from this foundation, problem-solving strategies may be developed.

Biofeedback

This is a behavioural technique that uses operant conditioning, a method of unconscious learning, to teach the patient how to manage the stress symptoms. There are several variations to this method, all of which utilize the physiological symptoms of the fight-or-flight response. At its simplest, patients are told to monitor their heart rate or concentrate on their breathing. Using methods of stress management similar to those used in meditation, individuals are asked to try to reduce their pulse or respiration rate. As these fall, so does the level of stress.

A more technical variation uses a galvanometer to measure the electrical conductivity of the skin. As part of the fight-or-flight response, the rate of perspiration increases in proportion to the level of stress. This increases the electrical conductivity of the skin (i.e. reduced resistance), which is measured by the galvanometer and represented audibly through a loudspeaker tone. A high tone indicates low resistance and vice versa. Again, using methods of stress management similar to those used in meditation, the individual attempts to reduce the pitch of the galvanometer and maintain it at the low level. The feedback thus provided helps the user learn to relax.

REDUCING THE STRESSES OF NURSING

The methods of stress assessment and management discussed in this section do not apply solely to patients. Nursing is an extremely stressful occupation. In a climate of financial restrictions, conflicting demands on time and pressure from patients, often combined with career uncertainty, many nurses suffer extreme, prolonged, psychological distress. In such a climate, nurses are highly susceptible to developing burnout, with its consequent negative effects on both their work and home lives.

It is important, therefore, that nurses monitor their individual levels of stress, and that of their colleagues, and use the strategies identified within this chapter proactively to prevent a stress crisis from occurring.

SUMMARY: MAIN POINTS

- Stress is the response of the body to physical, psychological and social stressors.

- Depending on the locus of control, the stressors and the level of threat, stress can have positive or negative consequences.

- The body responds to stressors physically, through the general adaptation syndrome (GAS) and via various psychological mechanisms.

- The significance of stressors depends on the individual's interpretation of threat and the number of concurrent stressors. The precise nature of the response is unique.

- Continued exposure to excessive stress can precipitate illness and delay healing.

- Even if patients' problems are mainly physical, the amount of distress experienced significantly affects recovery.

- Caring (professional and unpaid) is physically and psychologically demanding. Therefore, the amount of stress carers experience requires monitoring by the nurse and appropriate support strategies implemented to minimize adverse consequences for both carers and patients.

- There are several ways of recording stress that can be incorporated into a nursing assessment; however, an understanding of the nature of the stressor from the individual's perspective is essential.

- The overall purpose of stress management is to empower the individual to gain control over stressors and minimize the distress they invoke.

SELF-TEST: CRITICAL THINKING ACTIVITIES

Reflect on your life at work and at home:

1 Overall, how stressed do you feel?

2 What are the stressors and do they invoke eustress or distress?

3 What coping mechanisms do you use?

4 What support facilities are available to you?

5 Could you reduce the amount of distress in your life? How?

6 How can this knowledge enhance your professional role?

FURTHER READING

Muir J. Stress in the community: teaching relaxation. Nurs Stand 1997; 11(51): 36–38.

O'Brien S. Staff wellness program promotes quality care. Am J Nurs 1998; 98(6): 16B–16D

Payne RA. Relaxation techniques: a practical handbook for the health care professional. Edinburgh: Churchill Livingstone; 1995.

White E, Butterworth T, Bishop V, Carson J, Jeacock J, Clements A. Clinical supervision: insider reports of a private world. J Adv Nurs 1998; 28(1): 185–192.

Wilkinson G. Coping with stress. London: BMA; 1997.

REFERENCES

Brenner MH. Mortality and economic instability: detailed analysis for Britain and comparative analysis for selected countries. Int J Health Service 1983; 13: 563–620.

Brosschot JF, Godaert GLR, Benschop RJ, Olff M, Ballieux RE, Heijnen CJ. Experimental stress and immunological reactivity: a closer look at perceived uncontrollability. Psychosom Med 1998; 60(3): 359–361.

Brown R. Social psychology, 2nd edn. New York: Free Press; 1986.

Burnard P. Coping with stress in the health professions. London: Chapman & Hall; 1991.

Cooper CL, Liukkonen P, Cartwright S. Stress prevention in the workplace: assessing costs and benefits to organisations. Loughlinstown: European Foundation for the Improvement of Living and Working Conditions; 1996.

Cox T. Stress. London: Macmillan; 1978.

Department of Health. National Health Service and Community Care Act. London: HMSO; 1990.

Department of Health. Partnership in action: new opportunities for joint working between health and social services. London: HMSO; 1998.

Department of Health. Caring about carers: a national strategy for carers. London: HMSO; 1999a.

Department of Health. Saving lives: our healthier nation. London: HMSO; 1999b.

Department of Health and Social Security (DHSS). Growing older. London: HMSO; 1981.

Department of Health and Social Security (DHSS). Community care: agenda for action (Griffiths report). London: HMSO; 1988.

Dewe PJ. Identifying the causes of nurses' stress: a survey of New Zealand Nurses. Work & Stress 1987; 1(1): 15–24.

Dewe PJ. Stressor frequency, tension, tiredness and coping: some measurement issues and a comparison across nursing groups. J Adv Nurs 1989; 14: 308–320.

Earnshaw J, Cooper CL. Employee stress litigation: the UK experience. Work and Stress 1994; 8(4): 287–295.

Freud A. The ego and the mechanisms of defence. London: Chatto & Windus; 1936.

Friedman M, Rosenman RH. Type A behaviour and your heart. New York: Knopf; 1974.

Hebb DO. Drives and the conceptual nervous system. In: Bindra D, Stewart J, eds. Motivation, 2nd edn. Harmondsworth: Penguin; 1971 (note that Hebb's original article was published in 1954).

Hobson CJ, Kamen J, Szostek J et al. Stressful life events: a revision and update of the social readjustment rating scale. Int J Stress Man 1998; 5(1): 1–23.

Holm JE, Lokken C, Myers TC. Migraine and stress: a daily examination of temporal relationships in women migraineurs. Headache 1997; 37(9): 553–558.

Holmes TH, Rahe RH. The social readjustment rating scale. J Psychosom Res 1967; II: 213–218.

Howard DJ. Psychological, social and emotional changes experienced by students undertaking the project 2000 system of training. PhD thesis. Nottingham: Nottingham Trent University Library; 1999.

Janssen PPM, Schaufeli WB, Houkes I. Work-related and individual determinants of the three burnout dimensions. Work Stress 1999; 13(1): 74–86.

Lazarus RS, Delongis A, Folkman S, Gruen R. Stress and adaptational outcomes: the problem of confounded measures. Am Psychol 1985; 40: 770–779.

Levi L, Lunde-Jensen P. A model for assessing the costs of stressors at national level: socio-economic costs of work stress in two EU member states. Dublin: European Foundation for the Improvement of Living and Working Conditions; 1996.

Linde KM. St John's wort for depression – an overview and meta-analysis of randomised clinical trials. Br Med J 1996; 313(7052): 253–258.

Maslach C. Burnout: the cost of caring. Englewood Cliffs, NJ: Prentice-Hall; 1982.

Neese JB. The hospitalised person. In: Varcarolis EM, ed. Foundations of psychiatric mental health nursing, 2nd edn. Philadelphia: WB Saunders; 1994: 747–778.

Pruessner JC, Hellhammer DH, Kirschbaum C. Low self-esteem, induced failure and the adrenocortical stress response. Personal Indiv Diff 1999; 27(3): 477–489.

Reid GJ, McGrath PJ. Psychological treatments for migraine. Biomed Pharmacother 1996; 59(2): 58–63.

Roseman C, Booker R. Workload and environmental factors in hospital medication. Nurs Res 1995; 44(4): 226–230.

Selye H. The stress of life. New York: McGraw-Hill; 1984.

Sims A, Owens D. Psychiatry, 6th edn. London: Baillière Tindall; 1993.

Speirings EL, Sorbi M, Hainowitz TR, Tellegen B. Changes in daily mood and sleep in the 2 days before a migraine headache. Clin J Pain 1996; 12(1): 38–42.

Sutherland VJ, Cooper CL. Understanding stress. A psychological perspective for health professionals. London: Chapman Hall; 1990.

Totman R. Mind, stress and health. London: Souvenir Press; 1990.

Welch ID, Medeiros DC, Tate GA. Beyond burnout: how to enjoy your job again when you've just about had enough. Englewood Cliffs, NJ: Prentice-Hall; 1982.

White E, Butterworth T, Bishop V et al. Clinical supervision: insider reports of a private world. J Adv Nurs 1998; 28(1): 185–192.

Wong AHC. Herbal remedies in psychiatric practice. Arch Gen Psychiatry 1998; 55(11): 1033–1044.

World Health Organization. The ICD-10 classification of mental and behavioural disorders. Geneva: WHO; 1992.

Zigmond AS, Snaith RP. The hospital anxiety and depression scale. Acta Psych Scand 1983; 67(6): 361–370.

7 Pain

Kate Davies, Ann Taylor

'I thought the pain would be a lot worse. Having the button that you press when it starts to hurt was great, and I was able to walk round the ward the next day – which really surprised my visitors!'

(Patient)

THIS CHAPTER WILL HELP YOU

- Define types of pain
- Understand the basic physiological principles thought to be responsible for the perception of pain
- Identify factors responsible for inadequate pain management
- Provide information about the causes and effects of pain
- Demonstrate how pain can be accurately assessed/measured and safely managed from a biopsychosocial perspective
- Reflect on the value of evidence-based nursing in pain management
- Plan individualized strategies using the requirements for effective pain management and consider the relevant ethical issues.

KEYWORDS

Acute pain	Pain
Analgesia	Pain assessment
Biopsychosocial	Pain threshold
Chronic pain	Pain tolerance
Neuropathic pain	Somatic pain
Nociception	Visceral pain

INTRODUCTION

Pain is associated with many conditions. Some are addressed here, but it is impossible to cover all the conditions that may cause pain. Opportunities to extend your understanding of pain management are offered in the texts listed in 'Further reading'. As you read other chapters, consider how pain affects individuals with specific conditions and think about how holistic management could improve care and reduce the impact of pain on individuals and families.

Pain is multidimensional. It is an experience of the whole person with a variety of factors influencing its perception and severity. If we only address the physical aspects of pain, we may be denying psychological involvement, leading to inaccurate identification of the cause and hence inappropriate pain management.

Effective management of all aspects of pain requires the skills and knowledge of many disciplines. As nurses have frequent and regular contact with patients in pain, they are well placed to act as their advocate. This chapter addresses the role of nurses in pain management and the areas in which their particular expertise can benefit patients in pain.

Unrelieved pain can have detrimental physical, psychological, emotional, spiritual and social consequences, and it is therefore essential that all available interventions are implemented to prevent adverse suffering of this kind.

This chapter concentrates on acute pain, with chronic pain mentioned briefly as a special consideration. The rationale for this approach is that trying to cover both will do neither justice. However, it is important to understand the similarities and differences between acute (nociceptive) and chronic non-malignant (neuropathic) pain.

DEFINITIONS OF PAIN

The International Association for the study of pain (IASP) defines pain as 'an unpleasant sensory and emotional experience associated with actual or potential tissue damage, or described in terms of such damage' (Merskey & Bogduk 1994).

Although rather complex, it highlights that pain always has a subjective component with a physiological sensation and an emotional reaction. McCaffery (1968) proposed a definition that reminds nurses of the subjectivity of pain: 'pain is what the patient says it is and exists when he says it does'. However, its simplicity belies the complexities of pain perception and assumes that everybody can verbalize their pain (Ch. 3).

TYPES OF PAIN

Pain may be either nociceptive (acute) or non-nociceptive (chronic non-malignant); however, this only describes its physical nature. It is important to remember that pain affects individuals in many ways and the emotional and spiritual aspects of pain must be considered. Although spiritual pain is not a recognized 'type' as defined by the IASP (Merskey & Bogduk 1994), it must be considered. Spiritual pain can incorporate religion, but it can equally include philosophical and cultural ideas of belief and meaning of life (Elsdon 1995).

NOCICEPTIVE PAIN

Nociceptive pain is the 'normal' reaction to a painful stimulus transmitted through intact neural pathways. It is the process that transmits pain from the injury to the brain and is normally referred to as acute pain. Acute pain usually ceases once the injury has healed or the disease has been treated. It often responds to treatment with analgesics and management of the cause (Duarte 1997).

Nociceptive pain can be subdivided into somatic and visceral pain. Somatic pain is experienced in superficial structures, muscle and fascia and is usually described as dull or achy, well localized and consonant with the underlying lesions, e.g. metastatic bone pain (Ch. 34) and postoperative pain (Ch. 29). Visceral pain arises in hollow organs and is usually poorly localized, deep, squeezing and cramp-like. Examples include intestinal obstruction (Ch. 22) and myocardial infarction (Ch. 19). It is frequently associated with autonomic sensations, e.g. nausea, and often has referral sites. A bizarre property of visceral pain is that it is perceived to be in sites distant from the injury, e.g. cardiac pain is referred to the arm or jaw. The explanation for this lies in the embryonic development of the central nervous system (CNS) and various tissues. For instance, diaphragmatic pain can be felt at the shoulder tip and one explanation is that both structures originate in the same area of the embryo. As the diaphragm descends it carries its original nerve supply with it. Since pain impulses from both areas enter the spinal cord at the same level, the brain is 'fooled' into believing that the pain originates at the shoulder tip (Melzack & Wall 1988).

Threshold and tolerance

Nociceptive pain has a threshold defined as an intensity of stimulation below which it is not perceived. The pain perception threshold is relatively constant and not, as is commonly thought, something that varies widely between individuals and races. However, the maximum amount of pain an individual will stand is the pain tolerance threshold (Melzack & Wall 1965). This may vary both between and within individuals at different times and will be influenced by cultural, emotional and psychological factors.

NON-NOCICEPTIVE PAIN

Non-nociceptive pain is subdivided into neuropathic and psychogenic pain (Duarte 1997). Neuropathic pain (chronic pain, non-malignant and benign pain) is the pain of neural injury or irritation. It persists long after the precipitating event and may be due to abnormal pain transmission (Duarte 1997). The most common descriptors are burning or stabbing pains. Non-painful stimuli may be perceived as painful (allodynia), e.g. light touch. Spasms of electrical sensations may also be experienced. Neuropathic pain serves no useful biological purpose. In some cases, psychological factors are significant in its perception. An example of neuropathic pain is phantom pain where, after amputation, there exists some physical 'memory' of the sensations or pain that existed in the amputated part (Portenoy 1997). Another example is post-herpetic neuralgia which is prolonged pain after herpes zoster (shingles); the viral infection leads to chronic changes in the affected nerves which then fail to transmit normal pain impulses or nociception. Note, however, that not all patients with shingles will develop post-herpetic neuralgia.

Psychogenic pain is presumed to exist when no nociceptive or neuropathic mechanisms are identified and there are sufficient psychological symptoms to meet the criteria for such pain (Duarte 1997). As pain has a large subjective component, psychogenic pain is very difficult to diagnose and should be evaluated by psychiatrists or psychologists. Examples of psychological symptoms that meet the criteria are depression, somatoform disorders (emotional distress and conflict are converted into physical complaints) and hysterical personality.

Classifying pain from a pathophysiological perspective (nociceptive and non-nociceptive) provides information about possible origins of the pain and can direct health care professionals towards appropriate pain management interventions.

THE ANATOMY AND PHYSIOLOGY OF PAIN

The link between pain and injury seems so obvious that it is widely believed that pain results from physical damage and that pain intensity relates to injury severity. Sometimes, the relationship between pain and injury does equate, but not always. The 'gate control theory' postulated by Melzack & Wall (1965) provided a biopsychosocial rationale for pain perception. It allows for a diverse range of factors to influence pain experience and enables holistic pain management. Prior to 1965, pain was considered to be a hard-wired system similar to an electrical circuit. By the 1950s, through Beecher's (1959) work, it was becoming apparent that pain was not just a physical sensation and that there were higher centre controls (brain) modulating pain – controls that are affected by psychosocial factors. Therefore, consideration of both the physical and psychosocial aspects of pain is required for effective pain management.

Various anatomical structures are involved in generating, propagating and integrating pain impulses: sensory receptors, nerve fibres, spinal cord and brain. In addition there are numerous locally produced chemicals that influence pain perception.

THE STRUCTURES AND PHYSIOLOGICAL PROCESSES INVOLVED IN PAIN PERCEPTION

Receptors are modified nerve endings that convert the stimulus into electrical potentials which are propagated along the nerve fibres. Injury to tissue normally results in inflammation, and strong noxious stimuli cause local tissue damage and the release of local chemicals, such as histamine, bradykinin, prostaglandins and 5-hydroxytryptamine (5-HT). The chemicals activate receptors and initiate reactions that are ultimately perceived as pain (see below).

Several types of nerve fibres function in pain transmission: $A\beta$, $A\delta$ and C fibres. The $A\delta$ fibres conduct rapidly and appear to give rise to distinct, sharp, well defined and localized pain; they conduct initial pain impulses. Thin unmyelinated C fibres conduct slowly and appear to give rise to diffuse, dull, aching and unpleasant pain that continues after the initial sensation. Activation of $A\beta$ fibres reduces painful stimuli; these fibres can be activated through rubbing of the painful area, massage, acupuncture and transcutaneous electrical nerve stimulation (TENS).

In the spinal cord, the nerve fibres of the dorsal columns (tracts) carry sensations from the periphery to the brain. The modifying mechanism in the spinal cord is called gate control (Melzack & Wall 1965). The mechanism may completely inhibit the upward transmission of pain impulses or, alternatively, may amplify it to make the pain more severe. Tiredness, anxiety and depression will all amplify the pain.

Nociception is transmitted towards the brain in various ascending tracts. Some tracts carry precise information about localization of painful stimuli and others carry information about pain position and quality. All nociceptive ascending transmission can be modified by descending control from the brain. Modification occurs mainly at spinal cord and brain stem levels and most pain impulses never reach conscious level. Modification involves the activation of inhibitory pathways and the release of inhibitory chemical transmitters; for example, when you pick up a very hot dish, but one that is very expensive, the ability to hold onto it until you can put it down safely without breaking it is due to such modification.

Each spinal cord mechanism has its own chemical transmitters and research effort has concentrated on developing drugs to mimic the inhibitory effects. Many substances have been isolated, including substance P, somatostatin and cholecystokinin.

The spinal cord passes into the skull to become the brain stem, which is responsible for processing and integrating pain sensations. The brain summates the sensory inputs and compares them to previous experiences to provide a basis for the rational behaviour of the individual (mostly related to survival and avoiding damage). Parts of the brain exchange information between various parts of the body and formulate coordinated responses. Other parts convey information about the precise location and nature of noxious stimuli and influence the discriminative and motivational aspects of pain.

There is also considerable evidence to suggest that a neural system exists at brain stem level which, when activated, results in a reduction in perceived pain (Melzack & Wall 1999). Specifically, endogenous opioid neurotransmitters capable of reducing pain perception are released from brain tissue, e.g. endorphins, enkephalins and dynorphins.

STAGES OF NOCICEPTION

Nociception refers to the electrochemical events occurring between the site of tissue damage/activation and pain perception. There are four stages to the nociceptive process:

- Transduction – noxious stimuli registering at receptors are translated into electrical activity in sensory nerves
- Transmission – impulses are propagated through the sensory nervous system (nerve fibres → ascending tracts of spinal cord → brain)
- Modulation – transmissions are modified by neural influences (pain gate) and chemical inhibitors
- Perception – transduction, transmission and modulation are developed into the subjective sensory and emotional pain experience.

A key component of the four stages is the physiological 'gating' mechanism as described in Melzack & Wall's (1965) gate control theory. The amount of stimulation passing through the 'gate' that may result in pain is dependent on the response intensity in the conducting fibres and on descending influences from the brain which may reduce pain. The gate is thought to be situated in the dorsal horn of the spinal cord. When the amount of information passing through the gate reaches a certain level, it activates the neural areas responsible for pain experience and response. Pain perception can be modified by reducing or increasing the stimulation, i.e. 'closing' or 'opening' the gate, through ascending and descending neural mechanisms (Box 7.1).

Further work has been undertaken since the 1960s and three important aspects have been postulated (Melzack & Wall 1999) which will influence patient care:

Central sensitization Excitation of pain pathways can lead to a type of 'wind up' phenomenon. In association with nerve injury, changes can occur in the neural mechanisms that lead to heightened excitation and the perception of pain long after the initial injury has ceased to be a causative factor. This explains why pain can continue long after the acute damage/activation and become chronic.

Naturally occurring opiates Endogenous opioid peptides produced naturally within the body can modify pain transmission rather than altering pain perception or tolerance and inhibit prostaglandin synthesis (inflammatory pain mediator) during an inflammatory response.

The 'inflammatory soup' Substances such as substance P, prostaglandins and leukotrienes are released during stimulation of nociceptive fibres involved in the transmission stage (i.e. C fibres) and from local tissue. These substances activate the release of more substances and together they form the 'inflammatory soup'. Both local inflammation and C-fibre activation and sensitization occur, heightening the pain experience. Many drugs used for acute pain, e.g. the non-steroidal anti-inflammatory group of drugs, inhibit the formation of the inflammatory soup, thus reducing pain potential.

In summary, it can be seen that the anatomy and physiology of pain perception can be altered at each of the four stages mentioned (Box 7.1). Using a combination of therapeutic approaches aimed at all four levels will result in better management of a patient's pain. When combining approaches, drugs and therapies

---

Box 7.1 Perception and modification of pain

Transduction

During transduction, pain can be modified by:

- Non-steroidal anti-inflammatory drugs (NSAIDs) – these reduce synthesis of prostaglandins and leukotrienes
- Local anaesthetics – used to infiltrate wound edges which blocks nociceptor transduction

Transmission

During transmission, pain can be modified at peripheral or central levels by:

- Local pressure
- Cryotherapy
- Local anaesthetics
  — regional blocks
  — epidural and spinal
- Heat
- Neurolytic agents (phenol sympathetic blocks)

Conditions such as diabetes, multiple sclerosis, spina bifida and injury can also modify the transmission of pain

Modulation

During modulation, pain can be modified by:

- Acupuncture – this probably stimulates branches of Aδ afferents which synapse onto the inhibitory interneuron and have a positive effect on it

- Transcutaneous electrical nerve stimulation (TENS) – this causes stimulation of Aβ fibres, increasing activity in the interneuron which closes the pain gate
- Opioids – these mimic the action of enkephalin at the pain gate
- Antidepressants – these increase the levels of serotonin and enhance activity in interneurons
- NSAIDs – these probably affect modulation in the spinal cord and brain

Perception

During perception, pain can be modified by:

- Psychoactive drugs – e.g. opioids, tricyclics, benzodiazepines
- Cognitive techniques
- Relaxation
- Hypnotherapy

The quality and intensity of pain can also be modified at this level by:

- The individual's previous experiences of pain
- Anxiety
- Social and cultural background
- The individual's personality
- The circumstances in which the pain occurs

---

can work together (synergy) to maximize pain relief, reduce the amount of each individual drug and reduce the side-effects. It is important to have a basic understanding of pain physiology when nursing patients holistically.

THE PLACEBO RESPONSE

By now it will be apparent that pain is not a simple mechanism akin to switching on a light. It is a complex process in which pain perception modification depends on several factors. One such factor is the placebo response, which may have a major effect on pain perception. The power of suggestion in relation to pain has been clearly demonstrated by studies involving placebo control (Melzack & Wall 1988). Giving a placebo (non-analgesic substance in this case) in place of morphine or other strong analgesic drugs can relieve severe pain, such as postoperative pain. The placebo response can range from 0 to 100%, but 35% is a commonly quoted figure (Beecher 1959). This is a strikingly high percentage because morphine, even in large doses, relieves severe pain in only 75% of patients (Melzack & Wall 1988).

The placebo response phenomenon is the reason why rigorous analgesic studies incorporate the double blind method (neither researchers nor subjects know whether the active drug or placebo has been given). Patients responding to a placebo are termed 'placebo responders'. This does not mean, however, that such patients do not have pain; it is not a test for psychogenic pain or malingering. Prescribing a placebo with strong analgesics may improve pain management, but unfortunately this can be misused. Staff may label placebo responders negatively

and active analgesics may be withheld. For this reason, although the practice may be useful, it is not advocated. However, when nursing patients in pain, it is important to utilize the placebo response. For instance, be positive about analgesics but make sure you assess the patient regularly to check that the drugs are effective (see Reflective Practice box 7.1).

R|R REFLECTIVE PRACTICE

7.1 Myfanwy

Myfanwy has been diagnosed with cancer and has undergone a radical hysterectomy. Identify the main physiological and psychosocial processes that contribute to her perception of pain.

Student activities

- List the treatment strategies that could be used to modify the experience of pain.
- Identify where in the physiological process these strategies modify pain, e.g. transmission, transduction, modulation, perception.
- Think about specific nursing actions that could modify the perception of pain and identify their mode of action.

After completing these activities, reflect on how a basic knowledge of pain physiology can inform nursing practice and improve pain management.

FACTORS THAT AFFECT PAIN PERCEPTION AND MANAGEMENT

It can be seen from the chapter so far, that pain is a multidimensional phenomenon that cannot be explained solely from a physiological perspective. Psychosocial factors must be considered if the total pain experience is to be understood.

PHYSIOLOGICAL FACTORS

The degree of acute postoperative pain experienced by individuals varies enormously. The duration of severe postoperative pain is generally short and analgesia requirements usually reduce significantly within 48–60 hours after surgery. Some patients, however, have prolonged pain and they should be investigated for problems, e.g. infection (Chs 13 and 29). Where no abnormality is detected, the patient's report of pain should be believed and appropriate interventions utilized. The operation site has been implicated as a factor that may determine the severity of acute pain. Thoracic and abdominal incisions are considered to be the most painful, particularly when the serous membrane has been breached. The rationale behind this is that patients need to cough and breathe deeply, which affects the abdominal muscles. However, it is dangerous to assume that major surgery equates with severe pain and minor surgery with mild pain. This belief has caused problems in day surgery where minor surgery

has produced severe pain in some patients who either suffer at home or require admission to hospital. Whilst the type of surgery and site provide a guide for pain management strategies, it is only through individual patient assessment that effective pain management is achieved.

PSYCHOSOCIAL FACTORS

Psychological factors account for some of the differences between people's perception of pain. Previous pain experiences, anxiety, depression, ethnicity and culture all interact and influence pain. Staff attitudes in their interaction with patients can also affect the pain that these patients suffer. There are a great many psychosocial factors that influence pain perception and only a few are mentioned here:

- *Age.* The effect of age on the pain experience is not easily identified and studies undertaken to date have been inconclusive. Overall, there seems to be good evidence that age has an important effect only on optimal analgesic dosing. However, the differing behaviour of staff towards individuals of different ages may affect the anxiety and stress they feel and can heighten their pain. For example, some health care professionals assume that pain is part of the ageing process and do little to alleviate pain in older adults (see Older Adults box 7.1; see also Ch. 32). Such ageist attitudes will only provide barriers to good pain management (Corran & Melita 1998).

 OLDER ADULTS: NURSING PRIORITIES

7.1 Pain management

- Findings from surveys, clinical and experimental studies demonstrate the high prevalence of persistent and chronic pain during the later years of life (McCaffery & Beebe 1994, Melzack & Wall 1999)
- Older adults do not feel less pain than younger individuals
- Pain should not be dismissed as just a consequence of ageing and reports of pain must be investigated
- There has been a lack of attention to research and management of pain in the older adult
- Older adults in hospital environments will behave in the way they think you want them to; if you treat them like children they will act like children.

Assessment in the older adult
In addition to the assessment criteria covered in the chapter, assessment in the older adult should include:

- A description of the individual's normal daily activities (to establish normal functional capacity) and any consequent difficulties in performing the activities of daily living (ADL)
- Physical or mental impairments
- Any recent changes in the patient's life that could heighten anxiety and/or spiritual dimensions of pain
- Chronic painful condition
- Current drug therapy.

Nursing management
This should include:

- Caring for pain and functional disability together where possible
- Finding out whether older adults want family and/or friends involved in their care where possible
- Psychological therapies, especially patient-led or encouraged biographies (discussion of previous positive life events), as these can be powerful distractors
- The use of appropriate interventions – the more sophisticated techniques such as patient-controlled analgesia (PCA) should not be precluded by age alone.

Administration of analgesics
- Administer small doses regularly
- Use a preventative approach – treat when reported pain is mild
- Titrate to effect by slowly and carefully increasing the dose
- If preparing the patient for discharge home and analgesics are still required, schedule administration around significant times of the day to increase compliance
- NSAIDs are contraindicated in the frail older population because the side-effects are more prominent in this group
- Monitor carefully for common side-effects in this age group, e.g. constipation, and use preventative strategies
- Confusion and anxiety could be the result of unrelieved pain rather than the common misunderstanding that they are analgesic side-effects – careful assessment is therefore required.

■ *Gender.* The evidence regarding the role of gender in the perception of pain is conflicting. Glynn et al (1976) found that pain scores amongst chronic pain patients were higher for females than males, whilst Khun et al (1990) found no such difference amongst postoperative patients. Nayman (1979) found that males experience less pain. However, staff gender, the individual's culture and the expectation of what male and female responses should be may all affect pain perception. As with investigations into other factors involved in pain perception, gender differences are mainly supported by dated research.

■ *Culture.* While some patients do have different pain expressions related to their culture, others exhibit less distinctive behaviours because cultures have merged as international travel has grown. Zborowski (1952) found that 'old' Americans (early immigrants) had an accepting, matter-of-fact attitude towards pain and consequently a muted pain expression, whereas Jewish and Italian immigrants tended to be vociferous in their complaints and openly seek support and sympathy. However, this research is dated and cultural determinants may have changed significantly.

Figure 7.1 illustrates the main psychosocial factors involving both patient's and nurse's experience of the patient's pain. Readers requiring more information are directed to the 'Further reading' list.

PHARMACOLOGICAL FACTORS

Pharmacological factors include the way in which drugs act on individuals and the way in which they are excreted. Differences in these are responsible for the wide variations between patients in the efficacy of pain interventions. For instance, older adults are more sensitive to the side-effects of opioids and the dose to relieve pain can be reduced. Reductions in muscle bulk and fat stores in these patients mean that drug concentrations are raised after a standard dose, and the analgesic properties and side-effects are prolonged (see Older Adults box 7.1).

THE MAIN ADVERSE EFFECTS OF UNRELIEVED PAIN

Despite increases in the knowledge and availability of sophisticated techniques and drugs with which to manage pain, an alarming number of patients suffer from unrelieved pain. Two audits of postoperative pain found incidences of moderate or severe acute pain of 87% (n = 2755) (Bruster et al 1994) and 76% (n = 1076) (Harmer & Davies 1998). Unrelieved pain increases a patient's susceptibility to develop detrimental physical, psychological, spiritual and social effects.

Absolute evidence proving that unrelieved pain results in specific adverse events is not available – no ethical committee would approve a study which allowed patients to have unrelieved pain.

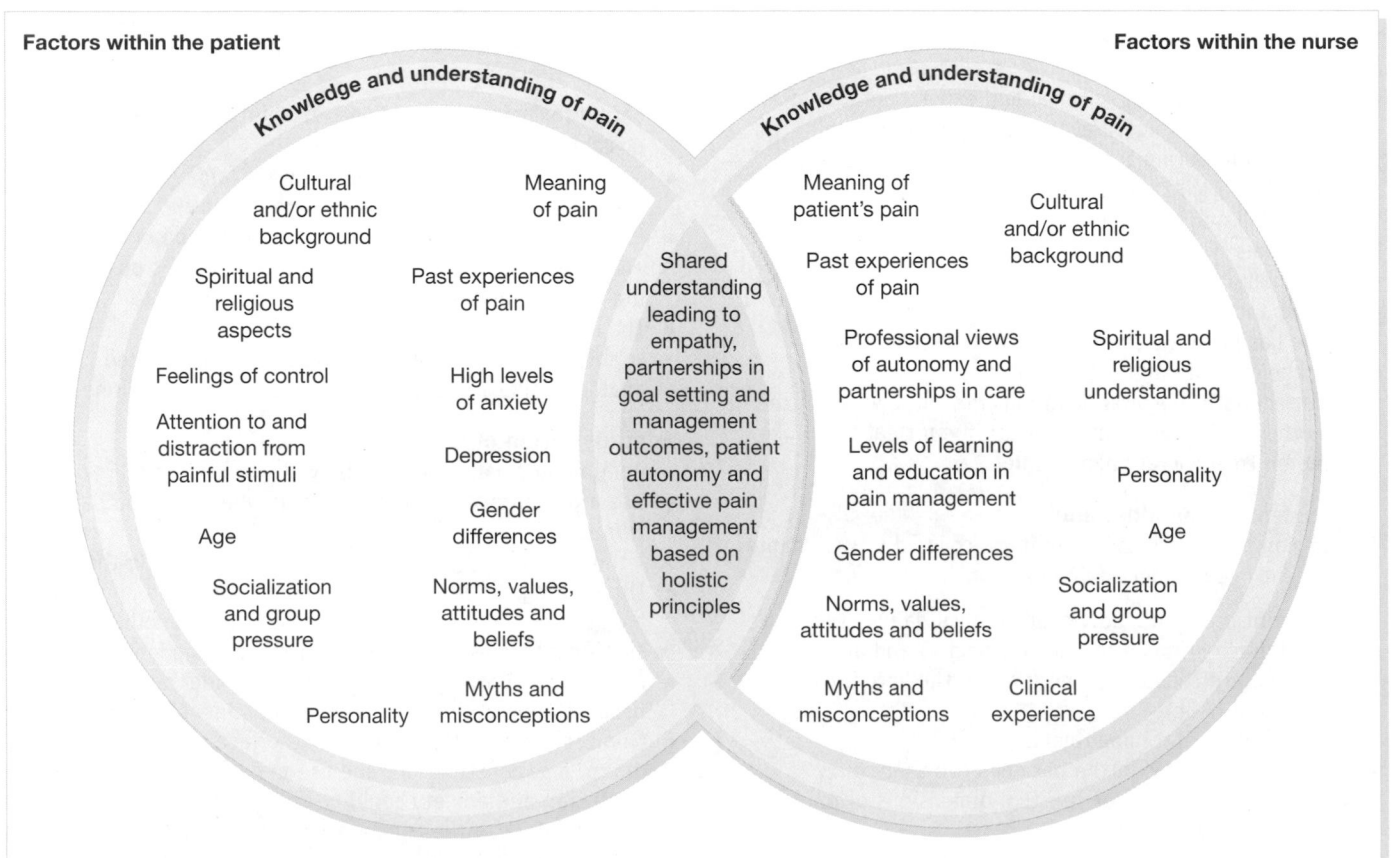

Figure 7.1 Psychosocial factors involved in pain perception and management.

However, the consensus of opinion regarding acute postoperative pain is that good management, which enables mobility, deep breathing, coughing and early return of gut motility, reduces the risk of adverse physiological events such as deep vein thrombosis and pulmonary atelectasis (Ch. 29). Other effects, such as hypertension and tachycardia, can hasten myocardial infarction and ischaemia in susceptible patients (Ch. 19).

Preventing these complications avoids prolonged hospital stays, which has cost implications for the NHS. There is also some evidence that improved acute pain management reduces the risk of patients developing chronic pain (Notcutt 1997), which has implications for both patients and the health services.

The main adverse events of unrelieved acute pain are outlined in Box 7.2, but in addition to these, it is important to be aware of other consequences. Pain and its management are used as quality indicators and those commissioning care are increasingly requesting specific services and standards of care. This could have a profound effect on providers of care if their standards are not sufficient to meet the requirements of purchasers, who may take their business elsewhere.

There are additional financial considerations for health care providers who do not treat serious pain appropriately. In the United States, a health care provider was held liable for failure to treat serious pain in terminal illness appropriately and the family were awarded substantial damages (*Estate of H. James vs. Hillhaven Corp.* 1991). Although this case involved terminal illness, there are implications for health care staff and managers responsible for postoperative care.

The provision of good pain management strategies is therefore important not just for humanitarian reasons, but also because of the biopsychosocial and financial consequences of poor pain management for patients, families and health services.

Box 7.2 Effects of unrelieved pain [Adapted from The Royal College of Surgeons of England and the College of Anaesthetists (1990) and Wilson & Smith (1993)]

Respiratory effects
- Reduced vital capacity and inhibition of cough – leading to retention of secretions and chest infections
- Hypoxia
- Respiratory failure

Cardiovascular effects
- Tachycardia and hypertension which may lead to myocardial ischaemia and infarction, particularly in susceptible patients
- Increased circulatory catecholamines

Gastrointestinal effects
- Decreased bowel motility leading to constipation, nausea and vomiting and prolonged need for intravenous fluids
- Nausea caused by inappropriate analgesia which may lead to dehydration and restricted dietary intake

Neuroendocrine response
- Metabolic and endocrine changes increase secretion of catecholamines and catabolic hormones, which in turn increase metabolism and oxygen consumption, and promote sodium and water retention. These changes are not caused exclusively by pain, but unrelieved pain may increase the extent of the changes

Effects of reduced mobility
- Deep vein thrombosis
- Reduced musculoskeletal function
- Pressure ulcers

Psychological effects
- Fear and anxiety
- Helplessness
- Depression
- Fatigue

Social effects
- Isolation and withdrawal from family/friends
- Inability to function within the family unit
- Inability to maintain normal roles within society

REQUIREMENTS FOR EFFECTIVE ACUTE PAIN MANAGEMENT

There are a number of barriers that prevent pain from being effectively managed. If we, as health care professionals, are to manage pain effectively, we need to address and overcome these barriers. The primary barriers to the effective management of pain are summarized below:

- gaps in health care staff's knowledge/education and inaccurate perceptions leading to misconceptions regarding pain and its management
- inadequate education/information for patients and relatives contributing to misconceptions regarding pain and its management
- poor assessment of pain
- lack of a structured formal approach to the management of pain and limited resources (staff, equipment, etc.)
- use of the biomedical model of care rather than a biopsychosocial one.

STAFF EDUCATION

The knowledge, expertise and experience of health care professionals influence the quality of pain management (Acute Pain Management Guideline Panel 1992). To minimize the incidence and severity of acute pain, staff are required to possess the appropriate knowledge and to apply this in practice. Knowledge is also required if staff are to educate patients about the benefits of good pain relief and the methods used to achieve it.

Research-based evidence identifying educational and training needs in acute pain management in the UK is limited. The low priority that has been given to pain management and inadequate staff education are perhaps the primary reasons for this lack of evidence. In 1990, a report from the Royal College of Surgeons & College of Anaesthetists stated that formal education in pain management for nursing and medical staff is often deficient and frequently fails to prepare staff adequately to assist patients with postoperative pain.

Since this report, interest in managing postoperative pain has grown. There are now pain management courses available and specialist acute pain teams can be found in many hospitals in the UK (Windsor et al 1996). There is also an abundance of published literature addressing the difficulties of pain management and offering possible solutions. Inadequate care can no longer be blamed on lack of information or knowledge, but rather on the fact that this knowledge is not reflected in practice.

Lack of knowledge contributing to myths and misconceptions about pain and its management

A lack of knowledge is not the only factor that limits appropriate pain management. Inaccurate perceptions of pain and its management are also implicated. Fears of addiction and of unwanted drug effects, such as respiratory depression, act as powerful deterrents to appropriate provision of certain analgesics. This has led to patients receiving minimal doses of analgesia at maximum time intervals, resulting in ineffective pain relief (Closs et al 1993) (see Reflective Practice box 7.2).

These misconceptions, together with inadequate knowledge, have influenced attitudes to pain and its management. Pain is considered by many staff to be a normal occurrence after surgery. It is accepted that complete relief from pain is not necessarily achievable or desirable in the initial postoperative period – low pain intensity prevents over-exertion. However, pain that is severe, prolonged or which limits activity can be detrimental (see p. 112).

Improving acute pain management requires that educational programmes identify and address knowledge deficits. Staff need to attain and maintain up-to-date knowledge about pain. They

REFLECTIVE PRACTICE

7.2 Pain management: myths and misconceptions

Zahid complains of severe abdominal pain, which is possibly due to appendicitis but this has not yet been diagnosed. He appears to be comfortable when watching the ward television and frequently leaves the ward for a cigarette. As a result, his complaints of pain are not believed. Zahid is, in fact, so worried about the prospect of surgery and the meaning of his pain that he is desperately trying to take his mind off the pain and the situation by diverting his attention elsewhere.

Student activities

There are many myths and misconceptions associated with pain and its management (see McCaffery & Beebe 1994, pp. 13–26, 75–80).

- Why do you think these myths and misconceptions have continued to influence practice despite the lack of evidence to support them?
- Do you think these myths and misconceptions affect nursing practice? If yes, to what extent.
- How can these myths and misconceptions be corrected? Think about strategies you can use to prevent the perpetuation of these myths and misconceptions.

also require information and practical experience relating to the current methods for preventing and managing pain. Outdated attitudes must be challenged and staff should be made aware of realistic treatment goals. The adverse effects of poor pain management, as well as the benefits of good pain management, should be reinforced in order that staff may achieve appropriate and acceptable pain relief for patients. Knowledge should be applied to practice according to the needs of individual patients and the skills of the practitioner.

In summary, health care staff should have information about:

- causes of pain and the main factors influencing pain
- effects of unrelieved pain
- appropriate methods of assessing pain
- pharmacological interventions according to individual needs
- potential complications of pain relieving methods and monitoring, preventing and treating them
- appropriate non-pharmacological interventions.

PATIENT INFORMATION AND EDUCATION

Many patients who experience acute pain because of trauma or surgery (in-patient or day case) will require hospital admission. Patients have little knowledge of what is expected of them and what they should expect and also limited awareness of the environment. Under these circumstances, hospitalization can cause anxiety. Hayward (1994) describes surgical patients who not only face the social and environmental pressures of admission, but also the direct physical threat of surgery. Radcliffe (1993) suggests that when patients are facing surgery, the fear of potential death, disfigurement and unsatisfactory outcomes often increases anxiety levels.

Increased preoperative anxiety can lead to greater postoperative pain, partly because anxiety may lower the patient's pain threshold, but also because anxiety induces prolonged muscle spasm at the pain location and at trigger points, as well as vasoconstriction, ischaemia and the release of pain-producing substances (Keefe & Gil 1986).

Providing information in the preoperative period has been implicated in anxiety reduction and hence pain reduction (Hayward 1975, Kanto et al 1990, Wong 1990). The level and amount of information provided must be appropriate to individuals and should enable patients to prepare adequately for postoperative recovery.

Patients require the following types of information:

- procedural information about the surgical procedure
- descriptions of equipment that may be in situ postoperatively
- the methods used to assess and treat pain and their potential side-effects
- the limitations of normal activities that may occur and the anticipated recovery programme
- sensory information about possible sensations and feelings, including pain.

It is important to discuss what sensations may occur, so that patients have a realistic expectation of pain, but it is essential to advise patients about what levels of pain are acceptable and what levels are not. This should enable patients to request analgesia or assistance in accordance with their individual needs.

Patients should also be advised as to the importance of deep breathing, coughing and mobilizing and given some instruction (Ch. 29).

Although the provision of procedural and sensory information is important, there is a risk that this information will increase anxiety by reinforcing the expectation of pain and discomfort. If information is to be beneficial, it must be accompanied by education to give patients the skills to cope with pain and to give them a sense of control. Teaching relaxation or distraction strategies has been shown to decrease postoperative pain scores (Janssen & Arntz 1996), as patients develop individual coping strategies.

In summary, patients require appropriate preoperative information and education to assist in developing active cognitive and behavioural strategies that help them to cope with and manage postoperative pain. It is important that nurses use their expertise to assist patients to become knowledgeable about pain and its management. Informed and educated patients are given some control over health outcomes, which enables them to participate actively in their care.

ACUTE PAIN ASSESSMENT

If a patient is in pain, or has the potential to experience pain, an accurate assessment of the pain must be made. As accountable practitioners, nurses would not care for patients with diabetes without regularly assessing their blood glucose level, yet assessment of patients in pain is often inadequate. Pain, unlike blood glucose, has no way of being measured accurately. In addition, pain is influenced by many factors and can be further modified by the individual's ability to perceive and tolerate it. We therefore need to acknowledge and use the most reliable and accurate method of assessment: patients' self-report of pain. The person in pain can describe pain quality, locality, intensity and the things that make it better or worse. No instrument could give such accurate data.

Melzack & Katz (1994) proposed that the main aims of pain assessment are to:

- determine pain intensity, quality and duration
- aid diagnosis
- determine the most appropriate therapy
- evaluate the relative effectiveness of different therapies
- monitor standards of clinical practice.

Pain assessment is also valuable because it provides patients with the means to verbalize their pain and takes account of their personal experience. If pain relief is provided following an assessment showing an unacceptable level of pain, patients will realize that staff believe their description, which will increase their confidence and feelings of security.

Pain assessment is often confused with pain measurement – most tools available for postoperative use simply measure intensity. They do not assess the total pain experience and are more accurately described as measurement tools. Any tool has to be reliable, valid, easy to use, and appropriate to the patient's developmental status (Acute Pain Management Guideline Panel 1992) (see Evidence-based Practice box 7.1).

A variety of tools have been developed, including the visual analogue scale (VAS – usually a 10 cm line with the words

EVIDENCE-BASED PRACTICE

7.1 Validity and reliability of pain assessment/measurement tools

Definitions
- *Validity* – the extent to which measurements reflect the true situation
- *Reliability or reproducibility* – the extent to which the same results would have been obtained if a different observer had taken the measurements at a different time

Desired characteristics of a pain assessment/measurement tool
- Valid
- Reliable
- Easy to use
- Subjective
- Able to rank highest and lowest pain scores
- Individualized
- Multidimensional
- Appropriate for the patient's developmental, physical, emotional and cognitive status
- Guidelines for suggested intervention are included

Student activities
A description of a variety of pain assessment/measurement tools can be found in Thomas (1997, pp. 70–92). This chapter provides some detail of the strength of evidence supporting the use of these tools in practice. Critically examine the literature to evaluate whether the assessment tools commonly used in practice are valid and reliable and whether they fulfil the desired characteristics listed above. This will help you in appraising your current practice and in planning for future developments.

Reference
Thomas VN. Pain, its nature and management. London: Baillière Tindall; 1997.

'no pain at all' at one end and 'worst pain possible' at the other; patients mark the position that best represents their current pain), the numeric rating scale (NRS), the verbal rating scale (VRS) and various questionnaires, e.g. the McGill Pain Questionnaire. One of the most commonly used tools in the postoperative period is the categorical verbal rating scale. Although this tool does not assess pain quality, Gould et al (1992) found it to be simple to use and effective in assessing postoperative pain. However, to make it easier to record the outcome, they combined it with a numerical rating scale and attributed a number to each verbal rating, e.g. none = 0, mild = 1, moderate = 2, severe = 3. This pain measurement tool has been incorporated into an observation chart to make the process of recording vital signs including pain assessment easier (Fig. 7.2). Pain should be assessed on movement rather than at rest. It is relatively easy to obtain low pain scores at rest and the aim of pain management is to enable patients to mobilize appropriately, breathe deeply and cough.

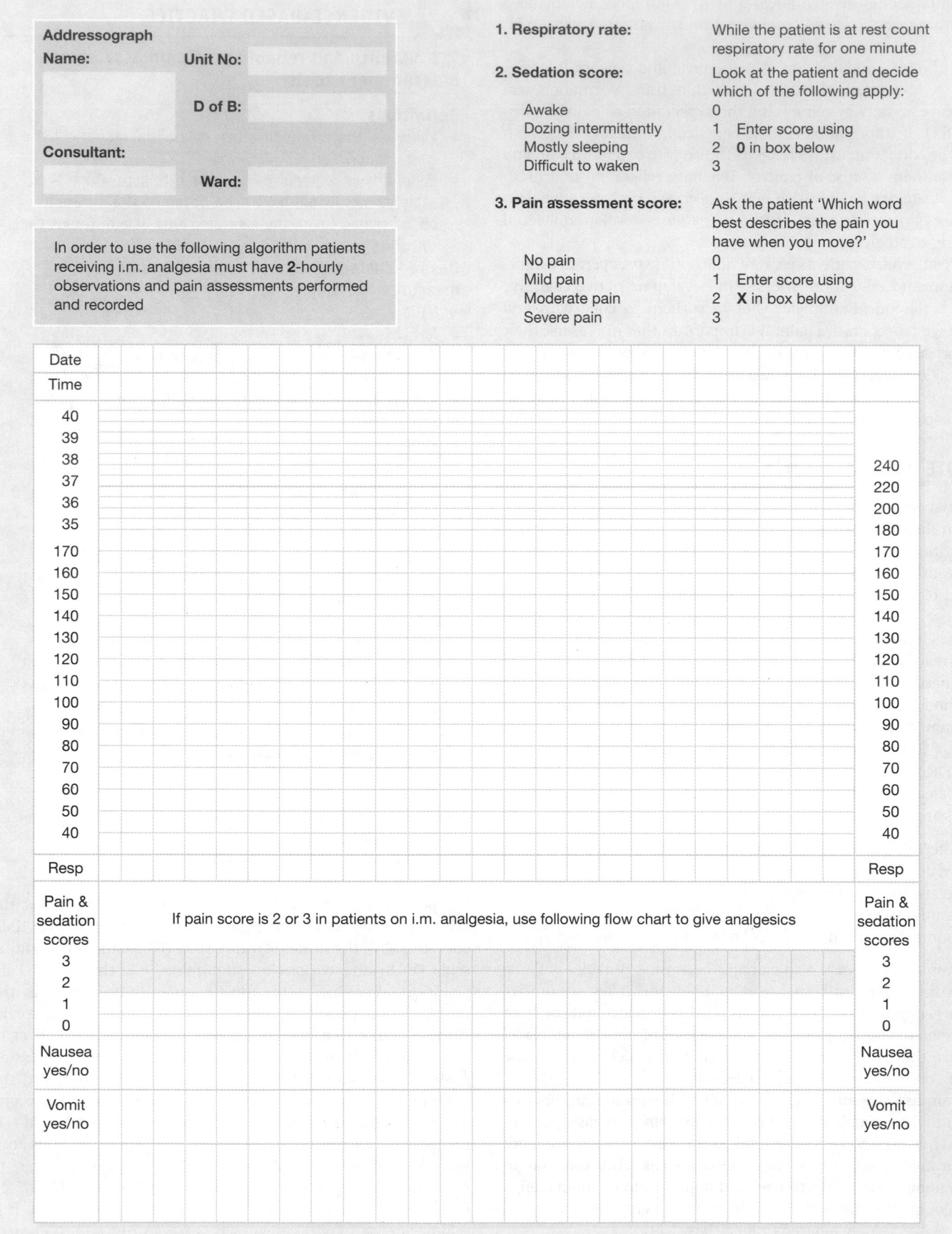

Figure 7.2   Postoperative pain assessment and observation chart incorporating the categorical verbal rating scale.

The advantages of the categorical verbal rating scale are as follows:

- it is simple, quick and easy to use
- it is accepted as a standard research tool (Max & Laska 1991)
- it can be easily incorporated into postoperative observation charts
- there is good correlation with other scales, e.g. VAS (Max & Laska 1991)
- it is reliable and consistent (Jenson et al 1986).

Disadvantages include the following:

- it assumes pain is unidimensional (Melzack & Katz 1994)
- it forces decisions into categories (Max & Laska 1991)
- it is less sensitive to small changes than the VAS (Breivik et al 1994).

The most reliable indicator of pain presence and severity is the patient's description. However, there are some patients who cannot describe their own pain, e.g.:

- infants or adults with poorly developed language skills
- patients with mental health problems or neurological disorders
- critically ill patients.

Under these circumstances, behavioural signs (e.g. crying) and physiological signs such as tachycardia can be used as indicators of pain. However, these signs are not accurate (e.g. the physiological signs may have causes other than pain) and provide no detailed information, but in the absence of self-reporting they may assist in detecting pain.

Although pain measurement is a valuable tool in the management of postoperative pain, it is only effective if prompt action is taken when unacceptable pain is identified. To assist practitioners, guidelines need to be developed that suggest appropriate action corresponding to the patient's individual report of pain. Assessments should be performed frequently whilst the patient is in pain – the frequency will depend on the patient's condition, self-report of pain and response to treatment. Continuous monitoring and recording of pain levels provide evidence of treatment efficacy, as well as evidence that pain control may need adjustment. They also ensure that patient safety is monitored during and after administration of analgesia.

A STRUCTURED APPROACH TO PAIN MANAGEMENT AND UTILIZATION OF RESOURCES

An unstructured approach to pain management can lead to inequalities in education and care. This can result in the use of a vast range of techniques, drugs and equipment, and lead to confusion and errors. The establishment of a multidisciplinary acute pain team assists in:

- formalizing staff and patient education
- organizing and monitoring acute pain management
- safely introducing new techniques and maximizing the potential of existing ones
- standardizing pain assessment
- formulating and introducing practice guidelines
- auditing service efficacy (Ch. 2).

Acute pain services have been established in many of the hospitals in the UK. These services have been shown to improve the quality of care and reduce the incidence of unrelieved pain and associated suffering (Wheatley et al 1991, Gould et al 1992). To be effective, a pain service must have sufficient resources (staff, equipment) to meet the needs of the patient group and there must be some responsibility for addressing problems out of hours – usually the on-call anaesthetist.

Where no pain team exists, experienced clinicians should initiate regular assessment of postoperative pain and sedation combined with specific guidelines and protocols for junior doctors to prescribe simple analgesics correctly. These changes have been shown to help patients with postoperative pain (Gould et al 1992).

USE OF AN APPROPRIATE MODEL TO DIRECT CARE

The biomedical model assumes a cause-and-effect relationship between stimulus and pain intensity. This model attributes pain to either psychological or organic causes. It is unidimensional and fails to see the total pain experience or take into account the many factors influencing pain. In essence, it is problem-centred rather than person-centred.

The biopsychosocial model reflects many of the components of the gate control theory and enables nurses to use a holistic approach to gain insight into the acute pain experience. It also allows socioeconomic influences to be considered. This information enables the provision of appropriate care based on individual needs and should help to improve outcomes for postoperative patients.

RECOMMENDATIONS AND GUIDELINES FOR PRACTICE

Decisions about care should be based on valid, reliable evidence that supports the selection of a specific intervention over an alternative. Without the use of evidence-based medicine to guide clinical decisions, there is a potential for immense variation in care. Guidelines for practice can be utilized to ensure that standards of pain management are attained and maintained (Table 7.1, Guidelines for Care Priorities box 7.1). Guidelines should be flexible enough to allow variation in response to individual needs, but rigid enough to maintain quality. These guidelines must be based on reliable evidence and need to be realistic and achievable.

Battista & Hodge (1993) have suggested that the main goals of practice guidelines should be:

- to assess and assure quality of care by:
  — assisting clinical decision-making by patients/ practitioners through reducing uncertainty
  — educating the public, practitioners and managers
- to guide resource allocation
- to reduce the risk of negligent care and ensuing liability.

The efficacy of practice guidelines should be continuously monitored and, if necessary, adapted in line with current evidence-based information. This can be aided by:

- critically reviewing rigorous studies, systematic reviews and meta-analyses (e.g. Cochrane Collaboration) and reflecting the results in practice in line with clinical governance initiatives

Table 7.1 Nursing standard for acute pain management

Topic: Individualized patient care
Sub-topic: Acute pain management
Care group: Surgical patients and patients with acute pain

Standard statement: Each patient will achieve an acceptable level of comfort with minimal complications and side-effects associated with pain and its management

Structure criteria	Process criteria	Outcome criteria
• Staff education re. pain management and pain-relieving methods (e.g. care of patients receiving i.m., PCA and epidural analgesia, advice re. positioning and supporting wound, etc.) • Research literature • Patients' individualized assessment forms and care plans • Patient information sheets • Pain assessment and observation charts • An algorithm which provides guidelines for the safe administration of postoperative analgesia • Appropriate prescribed analgesia • Acute pain service • Equipment to administer analgesia (e.g. pumps, PCA machines)	**Preoperative action** • Staff are educated with regard to: —different methods of pain relief —the importance of ongoing assessment • The nurse explains and discusses with the patient postoperative pain management, and briefly explains the different methods of pain management that the patient may receive • Potential side-effects are discussed (if appropriate) and methods of overcoming them are explained • The nurse ensures that the patient (and carers, if appropriate) understands what has been said and has been given the opportunity to ask questions **Postoperative action** • Observations of vital signs continue at a minimum frequency of 2-hourly while the patient is still requiring opioid analgesia • The nurse liaises with the patient and completes the pain assessment charts with routine postoperative observations initially (half-hourly and hourly), then 2-hourly until the patient is no longer experiencing pain after surgery • Guidelines for analgesic administration are used correctly to ensure that postoperative analgesia is administered safely • Appropriate analgesia is given as prescribed • The acute pain service visits each patient with epidural analgesia and all patients who have commenced PCA within the last 24 hours • The acute pain service is contacted if advice or information is required	• Staff are knowledgeable about pain-relieving methods and how to detect and prevent possible complications • The patient is knowledgeable about pain management and achieves a relative state of comfort that is acceptable to him or her • The patient's movement is not restricted by pain • The patient is free from or has minimal complications associated with the treatment of pain • Any side-effects are effectively managed

GUIDELINES FOR CARE PRIORITIES

7.1 Pain management standards: main points

Table 7.1 presents an example of a nursing standard for acute pain management. When formulating standards, guidelines and/or protocols for pain management, the main points to consider are that it is:

- valid
- reliable
- clinically applicable
- clinically flexible
- clearly worded
- reflecting multidisciplinary practice
- reviewed or audited on a regular basis
- well documented
- based on the best knowledge available.

Further reading

Audit Commission. Anaesthesia under examination: a study of the efficiency and effectiveness of anaesthesia and pain relief services. Abington: Audit Commission Publications; 1997.

Duff LA, Kitson AL, Seers K et al. Clinical guidelines: an introduction to their development and implementation. J Adv Nurs 1996; 23: 887–895.

Dukes J. Patient protocols: a review for those who commission, design and use them. Oxford: Oxford Health Care Management Institute; 1993.

Fennessey G. Guidelines and protocols. Pract Nurs 1998; 9: 14–16.

Royal College of Nursing. Protocols and nursing: guidance for good practice. London: RCN Issues in Nursing Series; 1993: 21.

The Royal College of Surgeons of England and the College of Anaesthetists. Commission on the provision of surgical services. Report of the Working Party on Pain After Surgery. London: HMSO; 1990.

- keeping up to date with reports published by the National Institute of Clinical Effectiveness (NICE), which aims to ensure that practice is informed by the best evidence possible
- requesting guidelines and information from centres of excellence in acute pain management.

MANAGING ACUTE PAIN

This section describes the delivery methods and analgesics commonly used to manage acute pain. Readers should consult a pharmacology book or national formulary for further information about conventional approaches to pain management and drugs.

It is important that nurses understand the properties and side-effects of the analgesics they are administering and impart appropriate aspects of this knowledge to patients. This assists patients in making informed decisions about their care, increases compliance and ensures that patients are active in reporting inadequate analgesia or side-effects.

CONVENTIONAL ANALGESICS

Opioids

Opioid analgesics interact with various opioid receptors to produce analgesia at the spinal and supraspinal (brain) levels. They can be classed as pure agonists, mixed agonists/antagonists and partial agonists depending on how they act on receptors. It is important not to administer an agonist, partial agonist and full antagonist simultaneously, as this may increase the pain and side-effects and can cause withdrawal in long-term opioid users. Opioid analgesics mimic the actions of naturally occurring endogenous opioid peptides and attach to the same receptor sites. Opioids such as morphine attach to μ-receptors and consequently cause side-effects (see below).

Morphine

Morphine (an agonist) is the standard opioid analgesic and remains the most popular opioid at present. It is the 'gold standard' analgesic and will be described here in some detail. Most other agonist opioids have similar effects to morphine and it is only the differences that will be acknowledged when the other opioids are discussed. Morphine is effective for nociceptive pain due to tissue damage, but neuropathic pain may not respond. An important aspect of morphine analgesia is mood elevation, which often reduces fear or anxiety about pain (Ch. 34). At high doses, morphine can produce muscular rigidity and convulsions.

After intramuscular (i.m.) or subcutaneous (s.c.) administration, peak plasma levels are attained within 30–45 minutes. After this, there is a decline in analgesia that reinforces the need for regular assessment – the effects of morphine usually cease within 3 hours, but this is variable (Macintyre & Ready 1996). Therefore, morphine 4- to 6-hourly p.r.n., for instance, will not provide effective pain management. For effective use, the prescription needs to be flexible enough to allow patients to receive morphine regularly after expressing moderate to severe pain on movement (see Fig. 7.3, p. 126).

The side-effects of morphine include:

- sedation
- nausea and vomiting
- respiratory depression
- bradycardia
- postural hypotension
- euphoria
- constipation
- pruritus
- urinary retention.

Nausea and vomiting are by far the most troublesome side-effects experienced with all opioids including morphine (see Special Issues box 7.1). There is little point in withholding an opioid because it causes nausea and vomiting, as severe pain has the same effect. Prolonged severe pain and opioids can also cause sedation, respiratory problems, hypotension, etc. Therefore, as with nausea and vomiting, just stopping the analgesia in the presence of side-effects will make little difference. Alternative

 SPECIAL ISSUES

7.1 Postoperative nausea and vomiting

Nurses usually see postoperative nausea and vomiting (PONV) as 'just a passing thing'. It is usually self-limiting, never life-threatening in itself, can be exacerbated by anxiety and, being subjective, is very difficult to assess. It hampers the management of acute pain quite severely at times and therefore it is an important aspect to consider in the management strategy (Chs 8 and 29)

Causes of PONV
Pain, dehydration, starvation, anaesthetic and analgesic drugs, gastric irritants, type and duration of surgery, anxiety, failure to starve preoperatively, and inappropriate or no use of preventative strategies

Other factors which influence PONV
Age, gender, weight (obesity), phase of menstrual cycle, history of motion sickness or previous PONV and movement

Impact on the patient
Dehydration, electrolyte imbalance, damage to operation site, depression and interference with oral therapy

Prevention and management
- Frequent assessment of nausea and evaluation of interventions
- Establish the causes (if possible)
- Administer appropriate anti-emetics
- Consider altering analgesic regimen
- Consider adding opioid-sparing analgesics
- Correct dehydration
- Provide regular mouth care
- Assist in providing anxiety and stress-reducing strategies
- Monitor oral intake and ensure palatable diet when able to eat and drink

opioids, the inclusion of opioid-sparing drugs, e.g. non-steroidal anti-inflammatory drugs (NSAIDs), and preventative strategies need to be considered. All opioid prescriptions must be accompanied by an effective anti-emetic. If, despite good hydration, regular anti-emetics and adequate pain control, the patient still has nausea and vomiting, the medical staff should be encouraged to change to an alternative opioid, e.g. pethidine.

The incidence of respiratory depression with opioids tends to be exaggerated. With good assessment procedures, for instance when the i.m. algorithm is used, the incidence of respiratory depression is very small and early detection of increased sedation alerts the nurse. A protocol and/or guidelines should be in place that supports the staff in managing acute pain. All opioid prescriptions should be accompanied by one for naloxone (reverses opioid effects on μ-receptors) and a suitably qualified and skilled nurse should be prepared to give the first dose if the respiratory rate is < 9/min and the patient is mostly sleeping or difficult to wake. Patients receiving regular opioid analgesia in acute settings must have an intravenous (i.v.) cannula in situ for the administration of naloxone if required. Most opioid side-effects are self-limiting – the longer the patient receives opioids, the fewer the side-effects experienced. However, constipation and a dry mouth are lasting problems and need nursing and medical management.

Diamorphine

Diamorphine may cause more euphoria than morphine and less nausea. It is more soluble than morphine and can be injected in smaller volumes, which is an advantage in cachectic patients (Ch. 34) and for subcutaneous administration.

Pethidine

Pethidine is an effective analgesic but some of its clinical effects differ from morphine. It is shorter acting and has local anaesthetic properties. Hypotension and tachycardia may occur. This is especially important for postoperative patients who may already have hypotension and tachycardia due to hypovolaemia and/or infection. The active metabolite may accumulate and increases the risk of convulsions. Oral pethidine is extensively metabolized in the liver. This reduces drug availability and therefore should not be used for severe pain.

Fentanyl

Fentanyl is much more potent than morphine and acts rapidly. It can be stored in the body and subsequently be released, causing secondary peaks in plasma levels with the potential for respiratory depression. As much smaller doses are needed, side-effects such as constipation may be lessened.

The high lipid solubility of fentanyl has encouraged the development of transdermal patches. However, transdermal fentanyl is not licensed for acute pain management and only chronic patients who have had opioids for a prolonged period should receive it.

Codeine and dihydrocodeine

Codeine is less effective than morphine and is used for mild to moderate pain (Ch. 34). Despite the fact that it is a weaker drug, it still retains the same side-effects as morphine and these need to be assessed, prevented or managed.

Dextropropoxyphene

Dextropropoxyphene is a mild analgesic and is normally combined with paracetamol for mild to moderate pain. It is widely used postoperatively when parenteral opioids are no longer needed.

Tramadol

Tramadol is a useful analgesic with minimal sedation and misuse potential. It is weaker than morphine and is useful for mild to moderate pain.

Opioid antagonist (naloxone)

Naloxone is a competitive antagonist to the analgesics described above. A single dose can reverse opioid-induced respiratory depression, but a repeat dose or infusion may be needed, as most opioids have longer elimination half-lives than naloxone (opioid effects take longer to wear off than the naloxone).

NSAIDs and paracetamol

Non-specific anti-inflammatories have anti-inflammatory, analgesic and antipyretic properties. Commonly used NSAIDs include ketorolac and diclofenac. Most are given orally or rectally, although some can be given by injection. They are not suitable for sole use after major surgery. However, they are very suitable for use with opioids as both NSAIDs and paracetamol are opioid-sparing. Nurses administering NSAIDs should be aware of their disadvantages and contraindications, e.g. with aspirin-sensitive asthma. Other side-effects include interference with platelet function, renal impairment and peptic ulceration. Side-effects are most common in older patients. Paracetamol can be used where NSAIDs are contraindicated. Although paracetamol is a mild analgesic, it is useful in combination with opioids.

Local anaesthetics

Local anaesthetic agents can be administered by bolus injection or infusion to block sensory pathways and are increasingly used to manage postoperative pain. Regional anaesthesia can be very effective in peripheral nociception. The correct regional block can provide good-quality analgesia perioperatively, but few local anaesthetic agents last long enough to extend the block postoperatively and catheters inserted into the nerve plexus/large nerves may be needed to enable infusions or 'top-up' doses.

Local anaesthetics can also be given epidurally and intrathecally. To obtain epidural analgesia or anaesthesia, drugs are administered into the epidural space. An epidural catheter allows for repeated doses or drug infusion. Drugs administered into the cerebrospinal fluid (CSF) and used for intrathecal analgesia are more commonly given as single doses through a spinal needle at the time of spinal anaesthesia. Drug doses required for intrathecal analgesia are much smaller than for epidural analgesia because of direct contact with the CSF.

Adverse effects from local anaesthetics can be caused by excessive doses, abnormal reactions to normal doses, or toxicity or vital centre depression after inadvertent injection into the bloodstream or CSF. The anaesthetist should always secure i.v. access before a block is performed in case of complications. Resuscitation equipment and drugs should be immediately available. The CNS is particularly sensitive to the effects of local anaesthetics. Early signs of toxicity are shivering, confusion, and twitching and tremors followed by generalized seizures. Nursing assessments should include observation for these signs. Eventually, with large doses, generalized CNS depression ensues, with cessation of seizures, respiratory arrest and hypoxia. Treatment comprises anticonvulsants and oxygenation, with endotracheal intubation and respiratory support if necessary.

The cardiovascular system is more resistant to local anaesthetics, but vasodilatation leading to hypotension, myocardial depression and arrhythmias can occur which lead to cardiac arrest and circulatory collapse (Ch. 19).

CONVENTIONAL ROUTES FOR THE ADMINISTRATION OF ANALGESIA

Opioids tend to be the mainstay of acute pain management where the goal is maximal pain relief with minimal or no analgesia side-effects. Opioids can be supplemented with nursing interventions, e.g. relaxation, information and drugs (NSAIDs), and local anaesthetic techniques. Preoperative patients should be prepared for surgery and pain management. Preoperative analgesia may be used. However, postoperative pain relief should commence in the recovery room and will usually be i.v. bolus doses of opioids titrated until patients are comfortable. Where qualified and skilled nurses provide this service, protocols and/or guidelines should exist and the i.v. analgesia is usually given through an i.v. cannula. It is important that a patient's pain is controlled before leaving the recovery unit especially if commencing patient-controlled analgesia (PCA). A therapeutic plasma level of an opioid must be established because only small increments are delivered via PCA, which are insufficient to manage severe pain without previous titration.

Oral administration

Oral administration is the most convenient and economical route. However, it is not useful until patients are taking oral fluids. Often this is after several days of parenteral opioid administration. It is difficult to predict who will require parenteral opioids. However, patients who have major abdominal surgery, for instance, may be unable to eat or drink for several days or may require strong opioids for adequate pain relief.

Inhalation analgesia

Fifty per cent nitrous oxide in oxygen (Entonox) has been used in midwifery and by paramedics for many years. It can be effectively used in ward areas for the management of procedural pain, e.g. drain removal. Entonox is quick to administer, is patient-controlled and side-effects wear off within seconds of ceasing inhalation. Other gas mixtures (isoflurane) are being manufactured for managing procedural pain.

Transdermal administration

Transdermal administration of drugs provides sustained levels of analgesia. The incidence of side-effects is low because small concentrations of drugs are used and this contributes to high patient compliance. Research has largely been in the area of palliative care because transdermal preparations are not suitable for patients who have not received long-term regular opioid

analgesia (Ch. 34). There is no short-term control with fentanyl, which is the current analgesic used transdermally. However, study sites are researching PCA iontophoretic preparations for transdermal administration.

Rectal administration

Absorption of drugs from this route can be unpredictable. Some drugs can irritate the rectal mucosa and patients may be unhappy with this route for cultural reasons. However, it is useful for some NSAIDs and for administering paracetamol in patients who are not drinking or who have severe nausea and vomiting. Informed consent should always be obtained before administration.

Parenteral administration

Parenteral administration may be required to ensure absorption of the active drug and may be the only suitable route, especially when patients are not drinking. Absorption after i.m. injection is usually more rapid and predictable than after oral administration.

If opioids are administered as required via the i.m. route to treat pain, they are often underprescribed and/or under-utilized. It becomes difficult to achieve effective analgesia and avoid side-effects. Gould et al (1992) provide one of the best examples of a strategy which combines a simple pain assessment to direct analgesia administration with an algorithm. This allows nurses to administer up to hourly analgesia depending on the patient's pain and vital signs (Fig. 7.3).

Observations are performed 2-hourly unless the patient is unstable (Fig. 7.2). A high pain score enters the patient into the algorithm, which then involves a checklist of sedation level, pulse rate and blood pressure, and a duration >1 hour since the last injection allows further opioid administration. In practice, most patients have analgesia administered 2-hourly, but flexibility exists to increase frequency if pain persists. Close monitoring when administering opioids ensures patient safety. This technique takes i.m. analgesia to its current limit; the control of analgesia is transferred safely to nurses but it is time-consuming. It is useful in intermediate levels of surgery or where PCA or epidural regimens are unavailable or inappropriate. Repeated injections can be avoided by using i.m. cannulae inserted into large muscles. Pethidine cannot be used through a cannula as it is an irritant and drug uptake is affected.

The algorithm can be used for s.c. administration, but drugs that cannot be given regularly through an i.m. cannula cannot be given subcutaneously. Subcutaneous injections may be less painful.

The desired plasma concentration of drugs can be achieved more rapidly and precisely by i.v. administration. Intravenous bolus provides the most rapid onset and shortest duration of analgesic action. Continuous opioid i.v. infusion can be used postoperatively, but dosage needs careful control and the patient must be well monitored to avoid excessive sedation and respiratory depression. This technique is advisable only in a critical care environment (Ch. 31).

Patient-controlled analgesia

Patient-controlled analgesia (PCA) allows patients to self-administer analgesic drugs to achieve analgesia. PCA is

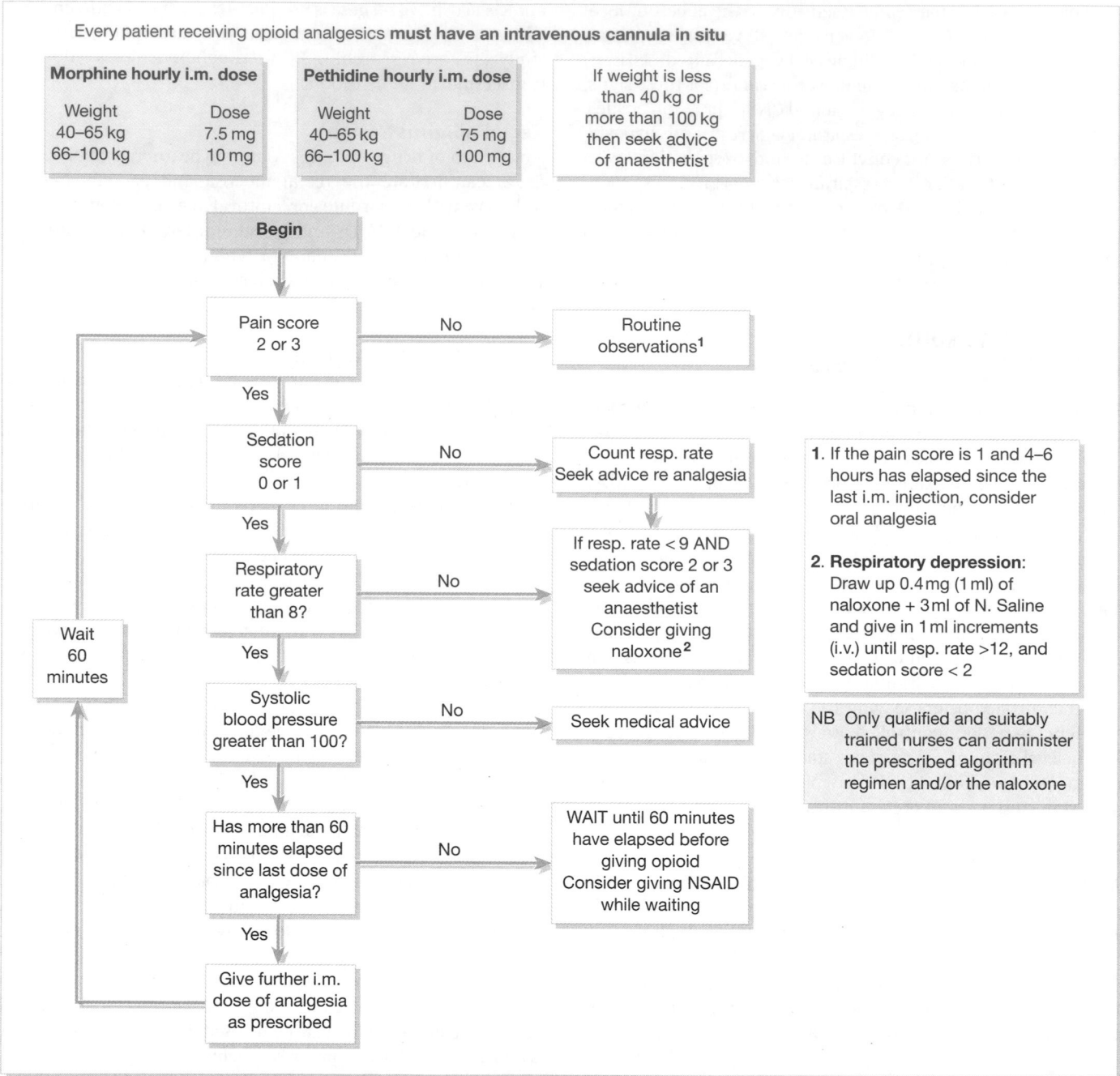

Figure 7.3 Algorithm presenting guidelines for postoperative analgesia in adults.

particularly indicated following operations where there is a likelihood of parenteral opioid analgesia being required for 24 hours or more. PCA is not a panacea for all pain, but used to full potential it is extremely beneficial. Preoperative information on effective use is important, as is patient selection. Patients should be able to understand the idea of self-administration of pain relief and be capable of pressing the button for drug delivery. Clinically, it appears that the best that can be achieved safely is no pain or mild pain, both at rest, and mild to moderate pain on movement. Where pain intensity exceeds this, the nurse ascertains that the device is being used properly. If it is, the analgesia needs to be reviewed carefully.

PCA is most commonly used for i.v. demand dosing, although it can also accommodate s.c., inhalation and epidural administration (Macintyre & Ready 1996). With i.v. PCA a background constant-rate infusion can supplement patient demands. PCA comprises loading doses, bolus dose, lockout interval and sometimes a background infusion. PCA can only be used optimally with regular, expert nurse and medical supervision. Patients should be continually reassessed to ensure that they understand the system and are using it properly and that adequate pain relief on movement is obtained with tolerable and well managed side-effects. Side-effects or problems may be related to the drug, the device or operator error. Mechanical or operator problems include:

- *Siphoning* – when the contents of the syringe empty into the patient via the giving set. Using an anti-siphon valve can prevent this (Fung 1998). One-way valves also need to be inserted in i.v. giving sets to prevent the opioid travelling up the maintenance fluid side of the giving set (Fung 1998). This can result in a bolus dose being given when the infusion rate is increased. Static electricity and mobile telephone use reprogramming the system have also been reported as producing a non-fatal overdose (Fung 1998).
- *Misprogramming* (Macintyre & Ready 1996) is a particular problem that can only be prevented by scrupulous protocols and programming checks by two nurses or doctors.
- *Poor patient understanding* of PCA can be rectified by thorough assessment of their ability to receive PCA and by education and patient information sheets (Fung 1998). Problems can occur with other people pressing the button – only the patient presses the button. Patients do not use PCA properly for several reasons, including poor retention of information on how to use it, as well as fear of using it and fear of addiction; re-education and reassurance must be offered by the nurse.

Epidural analgesia in acute pain management

Patients receiving epidural analgesia should only be nursed in ward areas when the nurses have appropriate education and can give knowledge-based care. If an epidural infusion is working well, a patient following major surgery can be pain-free at rest and on movement, or have only minimal discomfort. This speeds recovery because complications such as chest infections and deep vein thrombosis are much less likely where patients are able to cough and move.

Local anaesthetics and opioids are used either alone or, more frequently, in combination. Total spinal anaesthesia caused by excessively high spread of local anaesthetic in the intrathecal space upwards towards the brain may occur following a dural puncture, the inadvertent introduction of an epidural dose of local anaesthetic into the intrathecal space. Signs of a total spinal include apnoea, hypotension, loss of consciousness and convulsions. Excessive motor blockade causes muscle weakness and immobility, which is contrary to what is usually desirable postoperatively. While adverse events are uncommon, patients need careful monitoring.

Epidural morphine may produce unpredictable late respiratory depression because of slow absorption. This is more likely in older patients or if there has been concomitant opioid use by different routes. Morphine complications, even at reduced doses for epidural analgesia, include the side-effects seen with administration via other routes, but the incidence may be lower. Diamorphine acts quickly with a similar duration of action to morphine. The use of pethidine has never been particularly popular, perhaps because its duration of action is short. Fentanyl is absorbed rapidly from the epidural space and CSF. Therefore, it does not remain in the intrathecal space for long and quickly enters the systemic circulation. It is unlikely to travel upwards to the brain so the side-effects are fewer.

Both local anaesthetics and opioids individually cause their own characteristic side-effects. The two drugs act differently and combination of both drugs should lead to synergism of effect, reduced doses and fewer side-effects.

Continuous and patient-controlled epidural administration (PCEA) seems to provide far superior analgesia in selected patients when compared with other routes (Ellis et al 1990). PCEA provides an exciting development in epidural analgesia but there is inadequate evidence to suggest how best to use the technique.

NON-PHARMACOLOGICAL METHODS OF MANAGING ACUTE PAIN

Non-pharmacological interventions can be an asset to motivated nurses and patients keen to use these approaches. Some complementary therapies are commonly being used for chronic pain within the NHS, e.g. acupuncture, but not for acute pain. The 'Further reading' section provides texts for you to consult and the Evidence-based Practice box 7.2 allows you to explore this issue.

 EVIDENCE-BASED PRACTICE

7.2 Complementary therapies in pain management

In 1993, the National Association of Health Authorities and Trusts (NAHAT) published a report of a survey undertaken on the use of complementary therapies within the NHS (Cameron-Blackie 1993). Over 50% of the respondents (who included DHAs, FHSAs and GP fundholders) considered that some complementary therapies should be available on the NHS. Those who did not were influenced by:

- lack of proven effectiveness
- lack of proven cost-effectiveness
- resource constraints and priorities
- fears about uncontrolled demands on NHS resources
- lack of demand from the public or from GPs.

In evaluating the evidence to prove effectiveness, the studies to date have been difficult to generalize from because of the nature of the methodologies chosen. However, it is difficult to undertake double blind studies on acupuncture, chiropractic, aromatherapy, etc., as a sham comparison is not possible. Therefore, the strength of evidence provided is not great (Ernst & White 1998). However, individual patients must be having some benefit, as in 1996, the *British Medical Journal* quoted from a survey by the Research Council for Complementary Medicine that 1 in 10 people in Britain consults a practitioner of complementary medicine each year. Therefore, there seems to be a patient-driven initiative for these therapies. It is important for the nursing profession to be aware of any practical, legal and professional implications of facilitating complementary therapies within the NHS.

References
Cameron-Blackie G. Complementary medicine in the NHS. Birmingham: National Association of Health Authorities and Trusts; 1993.
Ernst E, White AR. Acupuncture for back pain: a meta-analysis of randomised controlled trials. Arch Intern Med 1998; 158: 2235–2241.
British Medical Journal. News item. Br Med J 1996; 313: 131–133.

Patient comfort is very important for good pain management. Time should be taken to position the patient to maintain comfort and support. Analgesia may be needed before movement and positioning. Cold packs may reduce joint swelling and pain, and advice should be sought from either the acute pain team or the physiotherapist. Patients may want to use supportive measures, e.g. magnets or relaxation tapes. Advice should be sought from senior nurses and/or the acute pain team regarding safety issues.

Information-giving, simple relaxation, imagery and bio-feedback (Ch. 6) may help patients understand their pain and allow them to be active in assessment and management (Carter 1998). These interventions aim to change perceptions of pain, alter pain behaviour and provide patients with a greater sense of control. Cognitive behavioural approaches (changing behaviour) in the acute setting are intended to supplement, not replace, conventional approaches.

There are both strengths and limitations to using simple cognitive behavioural techniques, e.g. information-giving, distraction and simple relaxation (McCaffery & Beebe 1994). Strengths include:

- increase in pain tolerance
- increase in self-control and confidence
- decrease in pain intensity, anxiety and muscle tension
- improved sleep and rest
- strengthening of the nurse/patient relationship
- increase in the effectiveness of other pain interventions.

Limitations include the following:

- patients may misinterpret and perceive that nurses think their pain is 'psychological'
- the techniques may increase pain awareness
- others may doubt the pain is 'real' because it responds to simple interventions
- they may confirm disbelief in patients' reports of pain because of response to simple interventions
- they may be substituted for conventional methods
- once the pain is severe, relaxation is unlikely to work
- patients may need time to develop their chosen technique (and there is limited time in acute settings).

Nurses need to assess a patient's suitability for simple relaxation and distraction techniques. These interventions are appropriate for patients who:

- find such interventions appealing
- express anxiety or fear
- may benefit from avoiding or reducing drug therapy.

Giving patients information about what to expect is an intervention to reduce anxiety and pain (see pp. 115 and 116).

Psychological coping skills should be assessed by asking how patients cope in stressful situations. Nurses should be able to provide practical suggestions for managing pain, e.g. relaxation or distraction, and teach patients how to use them preoperatively (see Health Promotion box 7.1).

Relaxation is the most widely evaluated cognitive behavioural approach to postoperative pain management (Acute Pain Management Guideline Panel 1992). However, individual studies on relaxation have all shown some improvement in

 HEALTH PROMOTION

7.1 Teaching relaxation

You will need to undertake this with patients a few times in order for them to memorize the following steps:

- Touch your thumb to your index finger. As you do, go back in time to a period when you felt secure and content. Take deep breaths in through your nose and out through your mouth and think about how it felt.
- Touch your thumb to your middle finger. As you do so, go back to a time when you felt at peace. Close your eyes and remember how that made you feel.
- Touch your thumb to your ring finger. As you do so, go back to a time when you felt relaxed, when your whole body felt heavy, warm and at ease. Take time to tense and relax each part of your body starting with your feet and ending with your face.
- Touch your thumb to your little finger. As you do so, go back to the most beautiful place you have ever been and dwell there for a while; carry on deep breathing with your eyes closed.

The five-finger exercise takes less than 5 minutes and can help patients to relax and distract their thoughts from the source of pain.

acute pain, but study quality means that findings should be viewed cautiously. Hence, while relaxation should be used, it should be carefully evaluated and not used as the main measure for management in acute settings (Seers & Carrol 1998). Relaxation and imagery techniques need not be complex to be effective. Strategies for use with acute pain need to be quick and easily remembered to be useful. However, periodic reinforcement through encouragement, coaching and family support is advisable. Audio-taped and written information can be provided locally or the patient/relatives can buy relaxation tapes.

Music can be used informally and effectively for relaxation but headphones are required to avoid disturbing other patients.

Humour has been reported to be useful for pain relief. Laughter may release endorphins and has been described as internal jogging, promoting hope and optimism (Stevensen 1995). However, humour must be appropriate and patient-led.

Other cognitive behavioural strategies, such as hypnosis and biofeedback, require expert professional involvement.

SPECIAL CONSIDERATIONS

ACUTE PAIN MANAGEMENT IN PRE-EXISTING SUBSTANCE MISUSE, ADDICTION OR DEPENDENCE

Substance misuse or addiction is the compulsive use of a drug, alcohol and/or tobacco resulting in physical, psychological or social harm and where the user continues to use the substance despite the harm. Pseudo-addiction refers to people who received inadequate pain relief, which results in drug-seeking behaviour to avoid pain. Unfortunately, these patients are often labelled incorrectly as addicts. Dependence refers to the situation where sudden discontinuation or antagonist administration produces a withdrawal syndrome. This differs from tolerance, which refers to decreased effects of a drug despite stable or increasing doses.

A person with tobacco dependence may require nicotine replacement postoperatively to prevent agitation and patients who misuse alcohol may require clomethiazole. Requirement for these interventions should be assessed by a doctor and contraindications evaluated prior to drug administration.

The majority of concerns relate to drug misuse. Addiction to analgesic drugs, e.g. opioids, is rare in previously opioid-naive patients, but fears of addiction continue to influence the provision of adequate analgesia. Patients who misuse drugs suffer even more, as a misconception exists that they are already receiving analgesic drugs and providing drugs postoperatively is often restricted. These patients need appropriate analgesia for pain and their report of pain should be believed (see Ethical Issues box 7.1).

Addiction to opioids should be distinguished from tolerance, dependence and pseudo-addiction as this affects pain management.

To establish the required dose of postoperative analgesia it is important to know what opioids (type and quantity) are used by the patient. However, this may be difficult as doses of non-prescription opioids may not be calculable. Caring for a drug addicted person is challenging, but it is important to be aware that everyone has the same right to pain control. Addiction rehabilitation can be offered, but may not be realistic. The major concerns should be treating pain and preventing withdrawal symptoms.

Readers requiring more information are directed to the recommendations produced by The US Department of Health and Human Services (Acute Pain Management Guideline Panel 1992).

 ## ETHICAL ISSUES

7.1 Pain relief and substance misuse

John is 32 years old and is a substance misuser. He is admitted to your ward following surgery. He has severe pain on movement, has not passed urine, has moderate nausea, is tachycardic and hypotensive and complains of being exhausted and anxious. He was given 7.5 mg of morphine 3 hours ago. Despite his physical signs and complaints of pain, the health care staff are reluctant to provide additional analgesia. After reading the special consideration section on substance misuse, what are your views on this scenario?

Student activities
Find out if your local health care trust has any policies or guidelines to inform practice. You may also want to contact other health care trusts and consult the literature for further information. Consider the ethical dilemmas involved here and think about how you would prevent this situation from occurring again.

THE PATIENT WITH CHRONIC NON-MALIGNANT PAIN

Chronic non-malignant pain covers a large heterogeneous group of painful conditions which includes back and neck pain, post-incisional pain, atypical face pain, central pain and phantom limb pain. Highlighting two of these may provide some indication as to why chronic non-malignant pain is so difficult to manage. Central pain, for instance, can follow any injury to the CNS and in approximately 90% of cases is the result of a stroke. The patient may experience superficial or deep pain that is usually constant but is sometimes intermittent (Hamilton 1998). Pain may increase with movement, cold, warmth, emotion and other factors. Complete pain relief is seldom attainable (Hamilton 1998).

Phantom limb pain is also difficult to manage once it is established. The pain is variously described as cramping, pressing, crushing or burning in the absent limb. However, phantom pain is not just associated with a limb; it may also occur after mastectomy or bowel surgery.

Such a multiplicity of conditions require an equally wide range of management approaches and hence it is impossible to do justice here to this subgroup of painful conditions. Pain management interventions include:

- conventional analgesics
- adjuvant analgesics – anticonvulsants (e.g. carbamazepine), antidepressants (e.g. amitriptyline) and systemic local anaesthetics (e.g. mexilitine)
- regional and central blocks
- cognitive behavioural management
- drug delivery via a permanent intraspinal catheter
- spinal cord stimulation via electrodes or a catheter with electrodes placed alongside the spinal cord; these are stimulated by a device that may be patient-controlled
- surface and deep brain stimulation where electrodes are stimulated by subcutaneously implanted pulse generators
- ablation techniques of the spinal cord where selected tracts are destroyed either temporarily or permanently
- physical therapies, e.g. exercise, TENS
- complementary therapies, e.g. acupuncture.

Unfortunately, in many cases, the reasons for the pain will have long ceased to be the cause. Many chronic non-malignant pain syndromes do not have an identifiable cause and patients may exhibit pain behaviours. These, coupled with pain complexity, lead to patients being labelled as malingerers, attention-seekers or mentally ill by uninformed health care professionals. Further research on the gate theory has provided some relatively sound explanations for chronic non-malignant pain development (Melzack & Wall 1999). However, why some patients develop chronic non-malignant pain and others do not is not readily explained.

Chronic non-malignant pain destroys the lives of many sufferers – it affects work, hobbies, sexual and social relationships, sleep and the person's role within society and the family. With continual pain and loss of control, patients can become depressed, isolated and helpless. Therefore assessment and evaluation must incorporate all activities of daily living. A realistic goal may not

ETHICAL ISSUES

7.2 Pain management rationing

Evidence suggests that a multidisciplinary pain management programme helps patients with intractable chronic pain. Such a programme offers multidisciplinary and interdisciplinary evaluation and treatment. The cohesive team approach is directed towards understanding and managing pain and suffering. The philosophy behind such an approach is rehabilitation and it involves physiotherapy, psychology, occupational therapy, medical and nursing support. These programmes can be in-patient or outpatient led. However, they are costly to run. The initial cost prevents many NHS Trusts from establishing them, but these costs can be offset by considering how much is involved in managing patients with chronic pain within the health care system. The cost is not just financial; there are emotional, physical and social costs to the individual, his or her family and society.

What are your views on the provision of in-patient or outpatient chronic pain management programmes?

Student activities
Find out about the provision of such services from centres of excellence around the UK. Waddell (1998) has discussed the implications to the individual, to the NHS and to society in his book and it is worth consulting this when formulating your views.

Reference
Waddell G. The back pain revolution. Edinburgh: Churchill Livingstone; 1998.

---

be pain reduction which could prove difficult, but instead may be increasing function so that patients are better able to undertake the activities of daily living (see Ethical Issues box 7.2).

The major contributions that nurses can make in the case of patients with chronic non-malignant pain are:

- listening to their concerns
- liaising with a multidisciplinary, multiprofessional team to provide holistic care
- always believing the patient.

As this section is extremely limited, some texts on chronic non-malignant pain are recommended in the 'Further reading' section.

SUMMARY: MAIN POINTS

- Pain is multidimensional and influenced by many factors.
- Management strategies need to reflect this and use a range of strategies which are appropriate to individuals.
- Effective acute pain management is achievable for the majority of patients if current knowledge is reflected in practice and available resources meet patient needs.
- All health care professionals contribute to the care of patients in pain. A multiprofessional collaboration ensures effective management of acute pain

---

SELF-TEST: CRITICAL THINKING EXERCISES

1 Identify a patient who has had moderate to severe pain. Examine the nursing and medical documentation. Where appropriate, talk to the patient about his or her experiences.

2 Does the patient's pain management reflect the practices advocated in this chapter?

3 Which components of care are managed well? Justify with evidence from the chapter and any additional reading.

4 Which components of care could be improved?

5 Propose interventions and changes in nursing practice to address any required improvements identified.

 FURTHER READING

Aronoff GM. Evaluation and treatment of chronic pain, 3rd edn. Baltimore: Williams & Wilkins; 1999.

Ashburn MA, Rice LJ. The management of pain. New York: Churchill Livingstone; 1998.

Carter B. Perspectives on pain: mapping the territory. London: Arnold; 1998.

Dimond B. The legal aspects of complementary therapy practice, a guide for health professionals. Edinburgh: Churchill Livingstone; 1998.

Ferrell BR, Ferrell BA. Pain in the elderly. Seattle: International Association for the Study of Pain Press; 1996.

Fordham M, Dunn V. Alongside the person in pain: holistic care and nursing practice. London: Baillière Tindall; 1994.

Harrison J, Burnard P. Spirituality and nursing practice. Aldershot: Avebury; 1993.

Main C, Spanswick C. Pain management. An interdisciplinary approach. Edinburgh: Churchill Livingstone; 2000

McQuay H, Moore A. An evidence-based resource for pain relief. Oxford: Oxford Medical Publications; 1998.

Melzack R, Wall P. The textbook of pain. Edinburgh: Churchill Livingstone; 1999.

Stein JM. Phantom limb pain. In: Warfield CA, ed. Manual of pain management. Philadelphia: JB Lippincott; 1991.

REFERENCES

Acute Pain Management Guideline Panel. Acute pain management: operative or medical procedures and trauma. Clinical practice guideline. AHCPR Pub. No. 92-0032. Rockville, MD: US Department of Health and Human Services; 1992.

Battista RN, Hodge MJ. Clinical practice guidelines: between science and art. Can Med Assoc J 1993; 148: 385.

Beecher HK. Measurement of subjective responses. New York: Oxford University Press; 1959.

Breivik EK, Bjornsson GA, Skolund LA. Comparison of 4 different pain scales in acute post-operative pain after wisdom teeth surgery. Proceedings of the 18th Annual Meeting of the Scandinavian Association for the Study of Pain, 1994.

Bruster S, Jarman B, Bosanquet N et al. National survey of hospital patients. Br Med J 1994; 309: 1542–1546.

Carter B (ed). Perspectives on pain: mapping the territory. London: Arnold; 1998: 186–194.

Closs SJ, Fairtlough HL, Tierney AJ et al. Pain in elderly orthopaedic patients. J Clin Nurs 1993; 2: 41–45.

Corran TM, Melita B. Pain in later life. In: Carter B, ed. Perspectives on pain: mapping the territory. London: Arnold; 1998.

Duarte RA. Classification of pain. In: Kanner R, ed. Pain management secrets. Philadelphia: Hanley & Belfus; 1997.

Ellis DJ, Millar WL, Reisner LS. A randomised double blind comparison of epidural versus IV fentanyl infusion for analgesia after caesarean section. Anesthesiology 1990; 72: 981–986.

Elsdon R. Spiritual pain in dying people: the nurses' role. Prof Nurse 1995; 10: 641–643.

Fung DL. Postoperative pain. In: Gershwin ME, Hamilton ME, eds. The pain management handbook. New Jersey: Humana Press; 1998.

Glynn CJ, Lloyd JW, Folkland S. The diurnal variation in the perception of pain. Proc Royal Soc Med 1976; 69: 369

Gould TH, Crosby DL, Harmer M et al. Policy for controlling pain after surgery: effect of sequential changes in management. Br Med J 1992; 305: 517–522.

Hamilton ME. Pain by etiology. In: Gershwin ME, Hamilton ME, eds. The pain management handbook. New Jersey: Humana Press; 1998.

Harmer M, Davies KA. The effect of education assessment and a standardised prescription on postoperative pain management. The value of clinical audit in the establishment of acute pain services. Anaesthesia 1998; 53: 424–430.

Hayward J. Information: a prescription against pain. London: RCN; 1975.

Hayward J, Boore JRP. Research classics: information – a prescription against pain. Prescription for recovery. London: Scutari Press; 1994.

Janssen SA, Arntz A. Anxiety and pain: attentional and endorphinergic influences. Pain 1996; 3031: 145–150.

Jenson MP, Karoly P, Braver S. The measurement of clinical pain intensity: a comparison of six methods. Pain 1986; 27: 117–126.

Kanto J, Laine M, Vuoriasslo A et al. Preoperative preparation. Nurs Times 1990; 86(20): 39–41.

Keefe FJ, Gil KM. Behavioural concepts in the analysis of chronic pain syndromes. J Consult Clin Psychol 1986; 54: 776–783.

Khun S, Cooke K, Collins M et al. Perceptions of pain relief after surgery. Br Med J 1990; 300: 1687–1690.

Macintyre PE, Ready LB. Acute pain management, a practical guide. London: WB Saunders; 1996.

Max M, Laska E. Single dose analgesic comparisons. In: Max M, Portenoy L, Laska E, eds. Advances in pain research and therapy. New York: Raven Press; 1991: 55–95.

McCaffery M. Nursing practice theories related to cognition, bodily pain and man-environment interactions. California: University of California at Los Angeles; 1968.

McCaffery M, Beebe A. Pain, clinical manual for nursing practice. London: Mosby; 1994.

Melzack R, Katz J. Measurement in persons in pain. In: Wall P, Melzack R, eds. Textbook of pain, 3rd edn. Edinburgh: Churchill Livingstone; 1994: ch. 18.

Melzack R, Wall PD. Pain mechanisms: a new theory. Science 1965; 150: 971–979.

Melzack R, Wall PD. The challenge of pain, 2nd edn. London: Penguin Books; 1988.

Melzack R, Wall P. The textbook of pain, 4th edn. Edinburgh: Churchill Livingstone; 1999.

Merskey N, Bogduk N (eds). Classification of chronic pain. Task Force on taxonomy, 2nd edn. Seattle: IASP Press; 1994.

Nayman J. Measurement and control of postoperative pain. Ann Roy Coll Surg 1979; 61: 419–426.

Notcutt WG. What makes acute pain chronic? Curr Anaesth Crit Care 1997; 8: 55–61

Portenoy RK. Neuropathic pain. In: Kanner R, ed. Pain management secrets. Philadelphia: Hanley and Belfus; 1997: 122–144.

Radcliffe S. Preoperative information: the role of the ward nurse. Br J Nurs 1993; 2(6): 305–309.

Royal College of Surgeons of England and the College of Anaesthetists. Commission on the Provision of Surgical Services. Report of the Working Party on Pain After Surgery. London: RCS/COA; 1990.

Seers K, Carroll D. Relaxation techniques for acute pain management: a systematic review. J Adv Nurs 1998; 27: 466–475.

Stevensen C. Non-pharmacological aspects of acute pain management. Comp Ther Nurs Midwif 1995; 1: 77–84.

Wheatley RG, Madej TH, Jackson JB et al. The first year's experience of an acute pain service. Br J Anaesth 1991; 67: 353–359.

Wilson IG, Smith G. The management of acute pain. Hospital Update 1993; 4: 214–222.

Windsor AM, Glynn CJ, Mason DG. National provision of acute pain services. Anaesthesia 1996; 51: 228–231.

Wong CA. Preoperative patient preparation. J Post-anaesth Nurs 1990; 5(3): 149–156.

Zborowski M. Cultural components in responses to pain. J Soc Iss 1952; 8: 16–30.

8 Problems associated with fluid, electrolyte and acid–base balance

Anne Waugh

'The district nurse said I need to drink something every hour so the catheter tube doesn't block but I got fed up with cold drinks. Then she suggested that I ask my neighbour to make me a flask of tea when she pops in every morning. That's worked really well – it keeps hot until at least mid-afternoon.'

(Patient)

THIS CHAPTER WILL HELP YOU

- Explain the relevance of extracellular fluid (ECF), intracellular fluid (ICF) and electrolytes in relation to the nursing management of patients

- Describe the four mechanisms of impaired tissue fluid formation that predispose to development of oedema

- Distinguish between isotonic and osmolar disorders of fluid balance

- Identify clients at risk from fluid and electrolyte imbalance

- Describe the assessment of a patient with actual or potential disorders of fluid and electrolyte balance

- Explain the investigations used to identify disorders of fluid, electrolyte and acid–base balance

- Discuss the nursing care required for actual and potential problems related to fluid overload and dehydration

- Outline the role of the specialist i.v. nurse

- Describe the principles of subcutaneous fluid administration

- Outline how hydrogen ions are produced and excreted from the body and identify acid–base disorders using arterial blood gas results.

KEYWORDS

Acidosis	Hypodermoclysis
Alkalosis	Ion
Buffer	Insensible loss
Colloid	Oedema
Crystalloid	Osmosis
Diffusion	Skin turgor
Electrolyte	Urinalysis

INTRODUCTION

Human beings are dependent on a supply of clean drinking water for their survival – without this, dehydration will occur within a day or two in temperate climates and more quickly in hotter climates. The ability to drink is closely associated with eating, and together these activities serve an important social function. Our culture largely determines when, what and with whom we eat and drink, and wide variations occur (see Ch. 11). During childhood, independence in managing one's dietary intake is established, although electrolyte and acid–base balance are not usually considered when choosing food and fluids. In health these balances may be upset; for example, in hot weather or when exercising, fluid and electrolyte imbalance or acid–base disorders may occur. This chapter examines how these balances are maintained or restored and explores the related nursing implications. It is important to remember that because problems with fluid, electrolyte and acid–base balance are interrelated, they often occur in combination.

RELATED ANATOMY AND PHYSIOLOGY

In this section, an overview of relevant physiology is provided although this is not intended to replace your relevant textbook on the subject. A simple introduction can be found in Waugh & Grant (2000) and a more detailed discussion in Tortora & Grabowski (2000).

FLUID COMPARTMENTS AND ELECTROLYTE CONCENTRATIONS

The amount of water and electrolytes within the body compartments is controlled so that conditions that will allow normal body function are maintained. In this section we will explore how this occurs.

Water distribution

Water makes up about 60% of human body weight in the average man, accounting for some 40 litres in a 70 kg male adult. Fat (adipose tissue) contains little water and therefore the proportion of body water is lower in obesity and also in females, who have a higher proportion of body fat than males. This is found mainly in the breasts and around the hips. The proportion of body water decreases with age. Age and gender differences in the proportions of body water are shown in Figure 8.1. Body water is found in two compartments: the intracellular fluid (ICF) accounts for two-thirds of the total body water and the extracellular fluid (ECF) the remaining one-third. ICF consists of the watery cytosol within all body cells. ECF includes the plasma in the circulatory system and fluid in the spaces between tissue cells known as tissue or interstitial fluid. Figure 8.2 shows the water distribution within the two compartments. Homeostasis of many factors, including water and electrolytes in the fluid compartments, is essential for life and health.

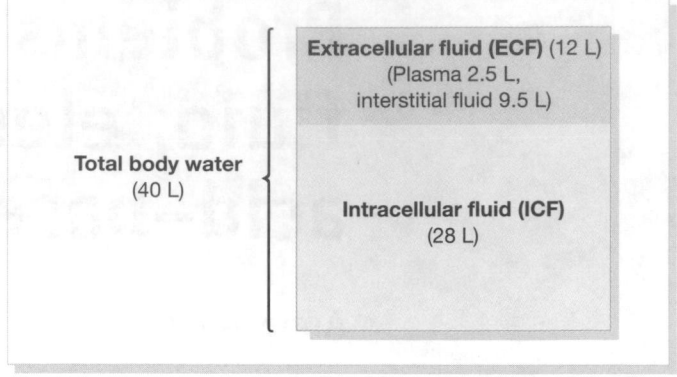

Figure 8.2 Distribution of body fluid in a 70 kg adult male.

Electrolytes

The term 'electrolyte' describes a compound that dissociates into charged particles, called ions, in solution. Ions carry an electrical charge: cations are positively charged and anions negatively charged. For example, sodium chloride (table salt) is described in chemical notation as NaCl, but when in solution it dissolves, forming an equal number of Na^+ ions and Cl^- ions. The main electrolytes are sodium, potassium, calcium, magnesium, chloride, bicarbonate and phosphate. While water can move freely between the fluid compartments, electrolytes cannot. Sodium is found mainly within the ECF while potassium is nearly all in the ICF. Electrolytes constitute the major solutes in body fluids and contribute to their osmotic pressure. They are essential for transmission of nerve impulses and many metabolic activities in the body. The normal serum levels of the common electrolytes, their function and the effects of abnormal levels of these electrolytes are summarised in Table 8.1.

MOVEMENT OF WATER AND ELECTROLYTES

Water and other small molecular substances can normally pass freely across the membranes that surround body cells and separate them from capillary membranes. A number of processes are involved: diffusion, osmosis, active transport and filtration.

Diffusion

This takes place when a difference in concentration of substances, known as a concentration gradient, exists. Gases and solutes move from an area of high concentration to one of low concentration until the concentration is the same and equilibrium is reached. No chemical energy is required and therefore transport is described as passive. Diffusion also occurs across a semi-permeable membrane, such as the plasma membrane, and some solutes can also cross it. Water can move freely while large molecules such as proteins are too large to cross membranes.

Osmosis

This is the movement of water across a semi-permeable membrane down its concentration gradient from an area of high water concentration to one of low water concentration. It occurs when equilibrium cannot be achieved by the movement of solute molecules (e.g. salt or sugar) across the semi-permeable

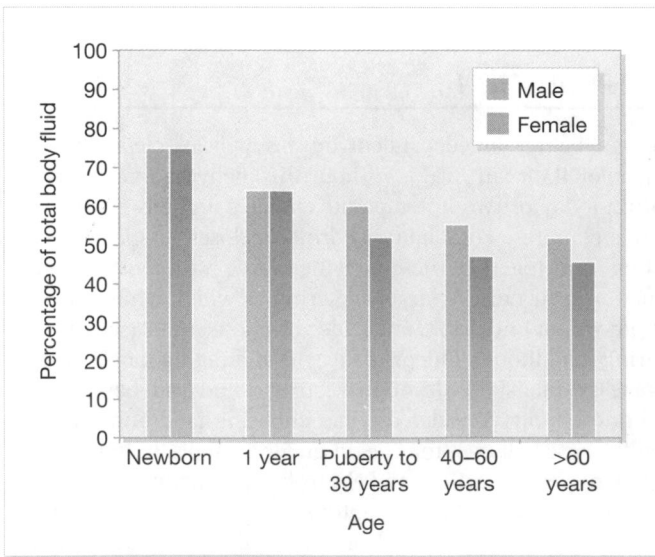

Figure 8.1 Percentage of total body fluid in relation to age and gender (based on Metheny 1996).

Table 8.1 Common electrolytes and disorders of electrolyte imbalance

Electrolyte	Disorder	Causes	Signs and symptoms
Sodium (Na$^+$), normal range 135–143 mmol/L • Most abundant cation in ECF • Provides plasma with up to half its osmotic pressure • Required for action potentials in neurons and muscle • Levels regulated by the hormones aldosterone, antidiuretic hormone and atrial natriuretic peptide • Exchanged for K$^+$ ions when Na$^+$ crosses cell membrane • Average dietary intake usually exceeds daily requirements • Kidney can conserve sodium if necessary • Sweating increases loss of sodium	Hyponatraemia (low serum sodium)	Diuretic therapy, profuse sweating, diarrhoea, hypovolaemia, cardiac failure, acute renal failure (diuretic phase), hyperglycaemia (osmotic diuresis)	Muscle weakness, abdominal cramps, headache, dizziness, tachycardia and hypotension, altered mental state
	Hypernatraemia (high serum sodium)	Excessive water loss without sodium, diabetes insipidus, water deprivation, sodium gain	Profound thirst, fatigue, lethargy, irritability, hypertension, weight gain, altered mental state
Potassium (K$^+$), normal range 3.3–4.7 mmol/L • Most abundant cation in ICF; 98% intracellular (Forrest et al 1995) so serum levels do not accurately reflect total in body • Plays key role in resting membrane potential, repolarization of neurons and muscle cells, and maintains ICF volume • Exchanged for Na$^+$ ions when K$^+$ crosses cell membrane • Levels regulated by the hormone aldosterone • K$^+$ lost mainly in urine and small amount in faeces and sweat • Kidneys cannot conserve K$^+$ in the same way as they conserve Na$^+$	Hypokalaemia (low serum potassium)	Excessive diuresis due to, e.g., diuretic drugs, acute phase of acute renal failure, uncontrolled diabetes mellitus, prolonged vomiting or diarrhoea, laxative abuse, alkalosis	Confusion, fatigue, malaise, muscle cramps and weakness to paralysis, nausea and vomiting, ECG abnormalities, cardiac arrest
	Hyperkalaemia (high serum potassium)	Excessive K$^+$ supplements, acidosis (H$^+$ cross from ICF to ECF), reduced urinary output, e.g. renal failure, hypercatabolic states (widespread release of K$^+$ from cells to ECF)	Anxiety, confusion, muscle weakness and abdominal cramp, diarrhoea, paraesthesia, bradycardia, ECG abnormalities, cardiac arrest
Calcium (Ca^{2+}), normal range 2.1–2.6 mmol/L • Most abundant mineral in the body. Majority is combined with phosphate as salts • In its ionized form (Ca^{2+}) it is mainly extracellular • Ca^{2+} is essential for blood clotting, release of neurotransmitters, excitability of nerves and muscles • Levels controlled by parathyroid hormone and calcitonin	Hypocalcaemia (low serum calcium)	Hypoparathyroidism, burns, metabolic and respiratory alkalosis, diarrhoea, diuretics	Lethargy, muscle tremors and cramps, paraesthesia of fingers, tetany
	Hypercalcaemia (high serum calcium)	Hyperparathyroidism, renal disease, malignancy, Paget's disease, alkalosis, immobility	Fatigue, lethargy, muscle weakness, anorexia, nausea, vomiting, polyuria, paraesthesia, depression
Magnesium (Mg^{2+}), normal range 0.75–1.0 mmol/L • Half of body magnesium found in bone matrix as magnesium salts • Remainder is ionized (Mg^{2+}) and found mainly in ICF • Magnesium is a co-factor required for enzyme action and sodium–potassium pump	Hypomagnesaemia (low serum magnesium)	Severe malnutrition, malabsorption, diarrhoea, alcohol excess, diuretic therapy, renal disease, pancreatitis	Muscle weakness and tremors, irritability, tetany, confusion, anorexia, nausea, vomiting, paraesthesia
	Hypermagnesaemia (high serum magnesium)	Rare – renal failure, Addison's disease, high intake of magnesium-containing antacids, acidosis	Hypotension, muscle weakness, nausea, vomiting, confusion, convulsions *(continued)*

Table 8.1 *(continued)*

Electrolyte	Disorder	Causes	Signs and symptoms
Chloride (Cl⁻), normal range 97–106 mmol/L • Most common extracellular anion (Cl⁻) • Crosses cell membrane freely in exchange for bicarbonate	Hypochloraemia (low serum chloride)	Excessive diarrhoea and vomiting	Muscle spasms, metabolic alkalosis, decreased respiratory rate
	Hyperchloraemia (high serum chloride)	Renal failure, dehydration, hypoaldosteronism	Vomiting, metabolic acidosis
Phosphate, normal range 0.8–1.4 mmol/L • Found as a salt in bones and teeth and in nucleic acids and adenosine triphosphate (ATP) • Small proportion ionized, mainly as HPO_4^{2-} • Principally found in the ICF • Levels controlled by parathyroid hormone and calcitonin • Ionic forms of phosphate ($H_2PO_4^-$ and HPO_4^{2-}) have a role in phosphate buffer system	Hypophosphataemia (low phosphate)	Hyperparathyroidism, metabolic and respiratory alkalosis	Muscle pain and weakness, lethargy, confusion, fits, coma
	Hyperphosphataemia (high phosphate)	Chronic renal failure, massive cell necrosis, e.g. crush injury, malignancy	Anorexia, nausea, vomiting, muscle weakness, tetany, tachycardia
Bicarbonate (HCO_3^-), normal range 22–28 mmol/L • Second most common extracellular cation (HCO_3^-) • Essential for homeostasis of blood pH through bicarbonate buffer system • Levels regulated by kidneys in response to pH of blood	Acidosis (abnormally high level of hydrogen ions – see p. 150)		
	Alkalosis (abnormally low level of hydrogen ions – see p. 150)		

membrane. The pressure needed to oppose this movement of water across membranes is called osmotic pressure and is related to the size of the concentration gradient. The concentration of osmotically active particles in a litre of fluid is known as the osmolality of the solution.

Osmosis continues until equilibrium is reached and the water concentrations on each side of the semi-permeable membrane are the same. The solutions are then said to be isotonic. In the body, isotonic means having the same osmolality as plasma. Solutions with a higher concentration of solutes than plasma are hypertonic and those with solute concentrations less than plasma are hypotonic. This is an important consideration in intravenous (i.v.) fluid replacement (see p. 145).

Active transport

This is transport of substances against their concentration gradient and is described as active because chemical energy in the form of adenosine triphosphate (ATP) is needed to drive the process. The sodium–potassium pump is an active transport mechanism and is present in cell membranes to maintain homeostasis of sodium and potassium. As sodium is mainly extracellular and potassium intracellular, there is a tendency for sodium ions to diffuse inwards and potassium ions outwards along their concentration gradients. Homeostasis is maintained as excess sodium is driven out of the cell in exchange for potassium by the sodium–potassium pump.

Filtration

This mechanism is also important in the movement of fluids in the body but it relies on pressure differences rather than concentration differences as described above. When a pressure gradient exists, the higher (hydrostatic) pressure causes water and other small molecules to be pushed through membrane pores to an area of lower pressure. This process is important in the formation of tissue fluid and in filtration of blood by nephrons in the kidney (see Ch. 24).

FORMATION OF TISSUE FLUID

Hydrostatic pressure is the pressure a liquid exerts against the walls of its container. In capillaries, this is the pressure blood exerts against the walls. Capillary walls are only one cell thick and there is movement of water and dissolved solutes across the walls that is determined by the balance between the hydrostatic and osmotic pressures. The effect of hydrostatic pressure is movement of water and dissolved solutes out of the capillary, while the effect of osmotic pressure is movement of water into the capillary.

As blood enters the arterial side of a capillary bed, the hydrostatic pressure is about 35 mmHg; it then drops to about 15 mmHg at the venous side (see Fig. 8.3). Plasma proteins (albumin and globulin) are too large to leave through the walls of normal capillaries and contribute to plasma osmotic pressure.

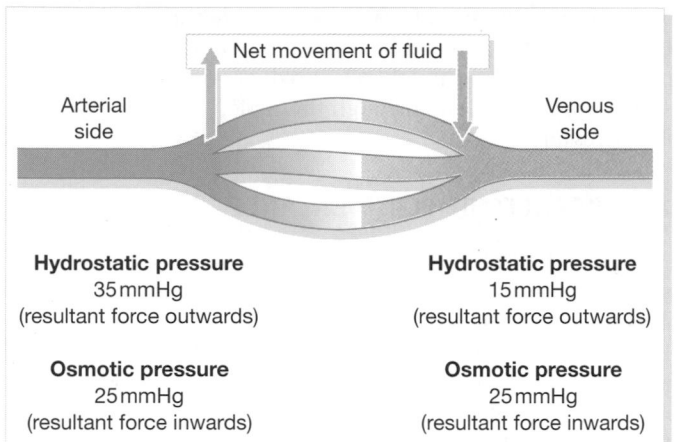

Figure 8.3 Formation of tissue fluid in capillary bed.

The osmotic pressure of plasma remains constant around 25 mmHg. This means that hydrostatic pressure exceeds osmotic pressure on the arterial side of the capillary bed and there is net movement of fluid and dissolved substances, including nutrients, from the capillaries into the tissue fluid. Within the tissue fluid, substances move by diffusion along their concentration gradients. On the venous side of the capillary bed, the osmotic pressure exceeds the hydrostatic pressure and there is net movement of fluid and dissolved substances, including waste products, from the tissues into the capillaries.

Oedema

Oedema is the retention of excess interstitial fluid due to disruption of the normal process of tissue fluid formation. It is usually most apparent in dependent areas (e.g. ankles) and is caused by a number of mechanisms, as described below.

Increased venous hydrostatic pressure

Congestion of the venous system increases venous hydrostatic pressure. On the venous side of capillary beds this means that the difference between outward hydrostatic pressure and inward osmotic pressure is reduced and therefore less fluid returns to the circulation. Excess fluid accumulates in the tissues. This is common in fluid volume excess (see below), cardiac failure (see Ch. 19) and renal disorders (see Ch. 24).

Decreased plasma osmotic pressure

The osmotic pressure of the plasma is decreased when there is depletion of plasma proteins. This means that more fluid remains in the tissues because the inward flow of fluid at the venous side of the capillary beds is reduced. Situations in which the osmotic pressure of the blood is reduced include glomerulonephritis (see Ch. 24), nephrotic syndrome (see Ch. 24), liver failure (see Ch. 23) and protein-energy malnutrition (see Ch. 11).

Impaired lymphatic drainage

Normally, less fluid returns to the venous side of a capillary bed than leaves at the arterial side, and the remainder returns to the circulation through the lymphatic system. When lymphatic drainage is impaired at any point between the peripheral tissues and the circulation, oedema develops. This may be due to blockage of lymph nodes by disease, e.g. malignancy (see Ch. 33), chronic inflammation or following surgical removal of lymph nodes, e.g. radical mastectomy (see Ch. 26).

Increased capillary permeability

The chemical mediators of inflammation act locally, increasing capillary permeability. Plasma proteins are then able to escape from the circulation and enter the tissues in the affected area, raising the tissue osmotic pressure. This draws fluid into the area causing localized swelling, characteristic of inflammatory conditions.

WATER AND ELECTROLYTE BALANCE

This is regulated mainly by the kidneys and is under hormonal control. In health this is carried out independently with fluid coming not only from what we drink but also from food when it is broken down and (a smaller volume) from chemical reactions that occur in the body (metabolic water). Electrolytes are ingested in the fluids we drink and food we eat. Fluid and electrolytes are lost from the body in urine and faeces and through insensible perspiration and sweat. Water is also lost from the lungs during respiration. Average daily volumes are shown in Table 8.2.

Thirst

The sensation of thirst is an important mechanism in the regulation of fluid intake. It is a natural response to fluid depletion and normally causes people to increase their fluid intake, thereby maintaining or restoring homeostasis. Rising osmolality of the blood accompanies water depletion and stimulates sensory receptors, called osmoreceptors, in the hypothalamus, giving rise to the feeling of thirst. Thirst is accompanied by decreased secretion of saliva and dryness of the oral mucosa. When reduced blood volume or hypotension activates the renin–angiotensin mechanism, there is conservation of fluid by the kidneys. When unable to respond to thirst, people are at risk of fluid depletion; susceptible groups include young children, unconscious patients and the elderly, especially if they are confused (see Older Adults: Nursing Priorities box 8.1).

Hormonal control of fluid and electrolyte balance

Hormones play a vital role in homeostasis of fluid and electrolyte balance through their effects on the kidneys. The kidneys filter 180 litres of blood daily. They reabsorb nearly all the filtrate, with the remainder (~1.5 L) being excreted as urine.

Table 8.2 Daily water balance			
Input (mL)		**Output (mL)**	
Oral fluid	1700	Lungs	500
Breakdown of food	1000	Skin	900
Metabolic water	300	Faeces	100
		Urine	1500
Total	3000	Total	3000

OLDER ADULTS: NURSING PRIORITIES

8.1 Dehydration in older adults

Watson (1996, p. 26) states that 'dehydration is a serious but eminently preventable condition' in institutions and urges that provision of an adequate fluid intake be made a care priority.

Student activities

- Reflect on the times of day when drinks are routinely offered to patients or clients in your clinical area.
- Assess how many of your clients achieve the recommended daily fluid intake of 1.5–2 L.
- Identify changes in practice that would enable all your clients to achieve the necessary daily fluid intake.

Aldosterone

This hormone is a mineralocorticoid secreted by the adrenal cortex and is the principal hormone involved in the regulation of sodium and water balance. It causes the renal tubules to excrete potassium and to reabsorb sodium with concurrent reabsorption of water. Low renal blood flow is caused by decreased blood volume or low serum sodium levels and both stimulate the kidneys to secrete the hormone renin. This converts angiotensinogen, a plasma protein, to angiotensin I. Angiotensin-converting enzyme (ACE) then converts angiotensin I to angiotensin II, which stimulates the secretion of aldosterone. In turn, this increases reabsorption of sodium and water by the renal tubules, reversing the original imbalance, and suppresses secretion of aldosterone and renin through a negative feedback mechanism. Angiotensin 2 causes potent vasoconstriction that also increases blood pressure. ACE inhibitors are a group of drugs that inhibit the effects of ACE and are widely used in the treatment of hypertension (Ch. 19).

The adrenal cortex secretes other steroid hormones that are structurally similar to aldosterone but they have only limited mineralocorticoid action (Ch. 17). In conditions where there is excessive secretion of cortisol or when high doses of hydrocortisone or prednisolone are administered, their effects can be widespread and include fluid retention by mimicking the effects of mineralocorticoids.

Antidiuretic hormone (ADH)

This hormone is secreted by the posterior pituitary gland in response to raised serum osmolality. ADH acts on the distal tubules and collecting ducts of nephrons, increasing the reabsorption of water and decreasing urine output. Therefore, in response to increased serum sodium or dehydration, more water is reabsorbed and less urine is produced, lowering the serum osmolality towards the normal range again. Once the serum osmolality is normal, a negative feedback mechanism causes ADH secretion to cease.

Atrial natriuretic peptide (ANP)

This hormone is secreted by the atria of the heart in response to their distension. ANP acts on the kidneys, increasing renal excretion of sodium and water. Atrial distension is associated with increased venous return. Secretion of ANP decreases the intravascular volume and therefore reduces venous return. ANP is also a vasodilator and through this action decreases systemic blood pressure.

DISTURBANCES OF FLUID BALANCE

These may be isotonic or osmolar. Isotonic imbalances occur when water and electrolyte levels are increased or decreased in proportion to their levels in the ECF. In osmolar imbalances there is loss or gain of water only affecting the concentration of electrolytes, mainly sodium, and therefore the serum osmolality. The principal differences are shown in Figure 8.4. Although described separately, the disorders below often occur in combination.

Isotonic imbalances

Fluid volume deficit

In this condition there is loss of electrolytes and water in proportion to their levels in the ECF and therefore serum levels remain normal (Fig. 8.4A[ii]). This should not be confused with dehydration, which correctly describes an osmolar imbalance (see below). It is usually the result of loss of fluid from the gastrointestinal tract from vomiting, diarrhoea, fistulae or nasogastric or other drainage tubes. Other causes are polyuria, fever, sweating and third space events (Metheny 1996).

Third space events occur when fluid is effectively lost from the circulation (ECF) due to a pathological condition. Susceptible patients include those with major trauma, burns or surgery, intestinal obstruction, sepsis and pancreatitis. The effective fluid loss can amount to several litres and may accumulate in the pleural, peritoneal or pericardial cavities. Its movement there is largely due to increased capillary permeability. Although still present in the body, this fluid is unable to contribute to ECF or plasma volume. As fluid is lost to the 'third space' from the circulation, the patient shows signs of fluid volume deficit, including tachycardia and hypotension, falling central venous pressure (CVP), oliguria and loss of skin and tongue turgor (Ch. 9). The physiological response to these events is conservation of sodium and water by the kidneys. If the condition continues untreated, acute renal failure will follow.

Careful monitoring and observation are required so that when the 'lost' fluid does return to the circulation, early signs of fluid overload are detected. These include increased urine

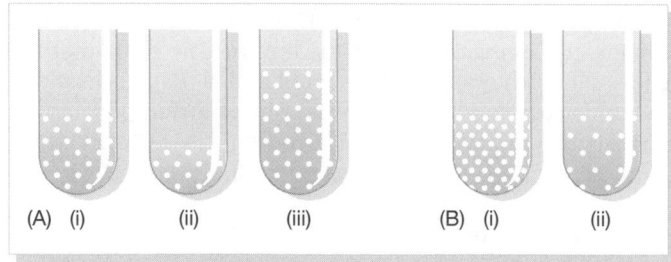

(A) (i) (ii) (iii) (B) (i) (ii)

Figure 8.4 Water imbalance. (A) Isotonic imbalance: (i) normal; (ii) fluid volume deficit; (iii) fluid volume excess. (B) Osmolar imbalance: (i) hypernatraemic; (ii) hyponatraemic.

output, raised systolic blood pressure, distended neck veins and dyspnoea if pulmonary oedema occurs. When there is return of fluid to the circulation, corrective measures must be instituted.

Signs of fluid volume deficit are as follows:

- mild (< 2 L) – thirst, concentrated urine
- moderate (2–3 L) – dizziness, weakness, oliguria (< 400 mL urine/day), postural hypotension
- severe (> 3 L) – confusion, hypotension, tachycardia, reduced skin turgor, poor peripheral circulation and cold extremities.

Fluid volume excess

This condition arises when there is retention of electrolytes and water in proportion to the levels in the ECF (Fig. 8.4A[iii]). It is usually the result of sodium retention that is accompanied by retention of water. Fluid moves into the interstitial spaces and accumulation leads to oedema (see above). Causes include congestive cardiac failure, renal failure, cirrhosis of the liver, excessive corticosteroid levels and over-transfusion with i.v. fluids containing sodium.

Osmolar imbalances

Hyperosmolar imbalance

Dehydration, or water depletion, is one form of this condition and occurs when there is water loss without significant loss of electrolytes (Fig. 8.4B[i]). There is an increase in the serum sodium level and osmolality. This results in movement of fluid out of cells and into the circulation to maintain blood volume. As the cells become dehydrated, their function is impaired. The kidneys respond by secreting less urine in an attempt to conserve body fluid. Thirst is the natural response to fluid depletion and occurs as the osmolality of the blood increases. This abnormality may occur with a nearly normal ECF volume or may be accompanied by a fluid volume deficit or excess.

Signs of hyperosmolar imbalance include a dry and furred tongue, loss of skin turgor, sunken eyes and often lethargy. The urine is dark in colour, of high specific gravity and volumes are small. When untreated, dehydration progresses and the blood volume and blood pressure decrease until the kidneys are no longer able to secrete waste products. Renal failure and death may follow.

Hypo-osmolar imbalance

This is also known as water excess and it effectively dilutes the ECF (Fig. 8.4B[ii]). Movement of fluid is from the ECF into the ICF. It is caused by excessive water intake – 'water intoxication', a severe mental health problem also called psychogenic polydipsia – or abnormally high levels of ADH (see SIADH and diabetes insipidus, Ch. 17).

NURSING ASSESSMENT

Monitoring for actual and potential nursing problems associated with fluid and electrolyte balance requires an understanding of the physiology of the mechanisms that normally maintain homeostasis. This enables the nurse to anticipate situations where problems are likely to arise in patients, especially those with disordered states.

ASSESSMENT OF FLUID AND ELECTROLYTE STATUS

This requires review of the patient's history together with nursing observations. During the assessment interview, a history of the patient's normal eating and drinking patterns is sought together with any recent changes in habits. This includes approximate daily volumes and preferred types of drinks. Understanding the history enables anticipation of potential nursing problems in addition to the detection of actual nursing problems. The following should be assessed.

The oral cavity

The oral cavity and the structures within it are normally moist and shiny. Assessment of the oral cavity in terms of general health is discussed in Chapter 22. When mouth breathing or unhumidified oxygen therapy causes dryness, the areas inside the cheeks where the gums meet the tongue usually remain moist. Dryness in these areas is a sign of dehydration or other problems. Some drugs, e.g. atropine and scopolamine, anticholinergic agents sometimes used as preoperative premedication, have side-effects that include dryness of the mouth.

Pain or oral discomfort when drinking suppresses a person's wish to take fluids. This may be due to ulceration of the tongue, which may be caused by the sharp edge of a broken tooth or trauma due to ill-fitting dentures. Toothache is another potential problem. Dental caries causes a dull toothache, while a throbbing toothache may arise from a dental abscess which is exacerbated resulting in an acute stabbing pain when the exposed nerve is stimulated by hot or cold fluids. Oral candidiasis (Ch. 22) may cause pain that also reduces oral intake.

Thirst

The sensation of thirst is an important indicator of fluid depletion (see above). This often exists in people with increased fluid losses due to pyrexia, diarrhoea, vomiting and hyperglycaemia and also in those with swallowing problems.

Skin

When pinched up, the skin of a healthy person returns immediately to its normal position when released, due to the recoil of elastic tissue. This is referred to as turgor. When turgor is reduced, the skin remains elevated for some seconds after release, e.g. when a patient has fluid volume deficit. The skin is more susceptible to development of pressure sores when turgor is reduced and careful assessment of the pressure ulcer risk using a rating scale is required (Ch. 10). Turgor is reduced in elderly people, as there is less elastic tissue present. It may be difficult to assess turgor in patients who have recently lost weight because the skin can be loose.

Oedema

As discussed earlier, this is present when there is retention of excess interstitial fluid and is especially apparent in dependent areas. The feet and ankles commonly swell when sitting and the sacrum may also be affected if the patient is in bed. After lying flat overnight, the eyes may be puffy due to periorbital oedema. When the oedematous tissue remains indented after firm digital pressure is applied, it is referred to as 'pitting oedema'.

Affected areas require special vigilance and care to avoid the development of pressure ulcers (Ch. 10) as the swollen tissue is easily traumatized. The swelling can also damage adjacent tissues. In severe cases of oedema, fluid may also collect in the pleural cavity, causing a pleural effusion, or in the abdominal cavity causing ascites. Oedema is often improved by careful positioning and the use of gravity to assist drainage of excess tissue fluid. Daily weight may be carried out to evaluate fluid loss following treatment. Acute pulmonary oedema is a medical emergency (see Ch. 20).

Sunken eyes

These are a sign of moderate or severe fluid volume deficit and occur as a result of loss of interstitial fluid around the orbit.

Confusion, lethargy and anxiety

These non-specific symptoms often accompany fluid loss and acid–base disorders. In elderly people, the presence of confusion is an indicator that all is not well and more detailed inquiry is required to identify the underlying cause. Without thorough assessment, this may be missed and the use of sedatives considered, especially if the patient is noisy and disturbing others. Sedatives should only be used after a diagnosis has been made and then care taken to prevent over-sedation.

Respiratory status

Respiratory rate, depth and effort are assessed and recorded, providing baseline information. Abnormalities or trends may indicate an underlying disorder of fluid, electrolyte or acid–base balance. Fluid volume excess and cardiac failure may lead to pulmonary oedema. This is the result of fluid movement from the capillaries to the interstitial fluid in the lungs and causes cyanosis, dyspnoea and expectoration of white or clear frothy sputum (Ch. 20).

Pulse

Tachycardia is usually the first sign of decreased intravascular volume but this is not always present in older adults.

Blood pressure

When the blood pressure is recorded with the patient lying down and then when standing up, a sustained decrease when standing is known as postural hypotension. This often accompanies fluid volume deficit. In more severe cases, hypotension occurs even when lying flat due to reduced blood volume. Rising blood pressure may be indicative of fluid overload.

Central venous pressure

This is measurement of the pressure in the right atrium and is an indicator of blood volume, cardiac contractility and vasomotor tone (Ch. 9). CVP measurements are interpreted together with pulse, blood pressure, respiratory rate, fluid intake and urine output. A trend in any or all of these values is often of significance. Low CVP occurs when blood volume is decreased, venous return is reduced and there is vasodilatation. Raised CVP occurs when there is increased blood volume, increased venous return and vasoconstriction. Intravenous fluid administration is often titrated against CVP measurements. In critically ill patients, when evaluation of more accurate data is required, a pulmonary artery catheter is used (Chs 9 and 31).

Jugular venous pressure

The jugular veins in the neck provide an indicator of CVP as the blood volume determines the level of filling and distension of these veins. Assessment of jugular venous pressure (JVP) is explained in Kumar & Clark (1998) and Metheny (1996).

Urinary output

The volume and colour of urine can provide important clues about abnormalities and more information is gained by urinalysis (see below). The ability of the kidneys to concentrate urine in the elderly is reduced and therefore more fluid is required to excrete waste products in this age group.

Bowel habit

Normally around 100 mL of water is lost daily in the faeces depending on the consistency.

Constipation

Recent development or worsening of constipation may be an indicator of fluid volume deficit or dehydration. This may cause patients to take laxatives, but when used in excess they are also a cause of electrolyte imbalance. Elderly people are prone to using laxatives rather than dietary modification to treat constipation.

Diarrhoea

Normal water loss from faeces is greatly increased during episodes of severe diarrhoea or paralytic ileus, leading to fluid depletion and electrolyte and acid–base imbalance.

FACTORS THAT PREDISPOSE TO FLUID AND ELECTROLYTE IMBALANCE

Patients with increased losses due to pyrexia, diarrhoea, vomiting, hyperglycaemia and burns are at risk of dehydration or fluid volume deficit, as are those with inadequate intake who may be debilitated or unable to respond to thirst. In other conditions, fluid and electrolyte restriction may be required to restore homeostasis. This section considers factors and situations that may disrupt fluid and electrolyte balance.

Drought or shortage of drinking water

In developed countries running water is taken for granted, but in many developing countries a long daily journey is required to get drinking water. In areas without an adequate supply of fresh water, diseases such as dysentery and cholera are a common cause of fluid depletion.

Inability to respond to thirst

This may occur in people suffering from depression, nausea or fatigue and in those who are fasting or debilitated. Clients with learning disabilities and the elderly infirm often fall into this category, too, as they may be unable to get themselves drinks independently.

Fasting

This is important in some religions, e.g. for Muslims during the month of Ramadan, although there are other situations where fasting is also practised (Jogee & Lal 1999). Fasting may result in fluid volume deficit, especially in susceptible groups, including

EVIDENCE-BASED PRACTICE

8.1 Fasting times

Seminal research by Hamilton-Smith (1972) and a more recent study by Hung (1992) concluded that excessive preoperative fasting was widespread. Anaesthetists and nurses both recognized dehydration as the most likely complication of prolonged fasting (Hung 1992) and hypovolaemia is a major cause of perioperative death. Appropriate fasting times are 6–8 hours for food and 2–4 hours for clear fluids (Jester & Williams 1999) although there is no evidence to support widespread change in this practice over the past 30 years.

Student activities
- Identify how long patients in your clinical area are fasted for preoperatively or prior to investigations.
- Discuss the practice in your clinical area in relation to the findings above.

References
Hamilton Smith SH. Nil by mouth? London: RCN; 1972.
Hung P. Pre-operative fasting. Nurs Times 1992; 88(48): 57–60.
Jester R, Williams S. Pre-operative fasting: putting research into practice. Nurs Stand 1999; 13(39): 33–35.

the elderly. Many medical investigations and procedures require fasting beforehand, but to prevent fluid depletion this period should not be longer than necessary (see Evidence-based Practice box 8.1).

Dysphagia
Dysphagia (difficulty in swallowing) is a common consequence of cerebrovascular accident (CVA or stroke) and in such cases food and oral fluid are withheld until a speech therapist has carried out a swallowing assessment (Ch. 11). This will prevent choking or inhalation (aspiration) of fluid into the lungs resulting in aspiration pneumonia (Ch. 20). Dysphagia may be due to the position a patient has to adopt, e.g. it is difficult to swallow when lying down. When dysphagia is present, the patient is at risk of dehydration and fluid volume deficit.

Dyspnoea
Dyspnoea (breathlessness) is associated with many conditions and poses potential problems with fluid balance in two ways:

- Increased insensible fluid loss occurs during mouth-breathing.
- The effort of breathing is so great that there is little reserve for drinking, and fluid intake may be neglected.

Alcohol
There are wide variations in the use of alcohol. It is forbidden by some religions, e.g. Islam, and forms part of the rites of others, e.g. Christian communion (Jogee & Lal 1999). Its use forms an intrinsic part of celebrations and social activities in many cultures worldwide. Alcohol has a diuretic effect and excessive use causes cirrhosis of the liver (Ch. 23) (see Reflective Practice box 8.1).

8.1 Drinking alcohol in hot weather

After a long walk with friends on a summer's day, it is suggested that you retire to the pub on the way home.

Student activities
Consider how alcohol affects hydration and suggest the best types of drink to consume.

Reduced dexterity and mobility
Lack of manual dexterity required for preparing drinks and inability to carry them due to reduced mobility predispose to low fluid intake and are common problems for the elderly at home. Safety is an important issue especially when considering hot drinks. In rheumatoid arthritis, for example (Ch. 27), the hands may be deformed making it difficult to hold drinking vessels.

Renal and cardiovascular disorders
People with renal and cardiovascular disorders may require their fluid intake to be restricted, in order to avoid fluid overload. Sodium and potassium intake may also need to be restricted (see Chs 19 and 24).

Age
Older adults are susceptible to dehydration as their body water is lower than that of younger age groups (see Fig. 8.1). Watson (1996) identifies further causes, citing reduced concentrating ability of the kidneys and decreased perception of thirst, although there is no evidence to suggest that this age group require a lower daily fluid intake than others. Older adults are also more prone to the effects of other factors within this section. Dehydration is a common reason for hospital admissions in older people (Bennett 2000). The effects of dehydration in the elderly include urinary tract infection, confusion and drowsiness, renal failure, collapse and death (see Older Adults: Nursing Priorities box 8.1).

Fear of incontinence
This may lead people to restrict their fluid intake in order to reduce the need to visit the toilet or avoid the embarrassment of asking for a bed pan in hospital. Bladder control is often reduced in the elderly and may be lost when other predisposing factors are present, e.g. urinary tract infection, diabetes mellitus and the use of diuretic or sedative drugs (Coni & Webster 1998). The ability to perceive a full bladder declines as part of the ageing process and is often accompanied by increasing urgency of micturition (Redfern 1998).

Diuretic therapy
Diuretic drugs are those that increase the production of urine by the kidney. When prescribed once daily they are normally given in the morning so that diuresis occurs during the day. The resulting increase in the number of trips to the toilet may cause some older people to omit them when going on outings, in order to spare them inconvenience or embarrassment. Omission may

ETHICAL ISSUES

8.1 Intravenous hydration in the terminally ill patient

Bennett (2000) reviews the advantages and disadvantages of dehydration and concludes that:

- dehydration is a situation that should normally be prevented or reversed
- in terminal illness, however, dehydration may have beneficial effects. In the last days of life, withholding artificial hydration may reduce pain and other unpleasant symptoms.

Gray (1999) provides an interesting reflective account of the care given to a patient that she nursed and questions her assumptions regarding the traditional practice of administering fluids to terminally ill patients. Reading this article may help you consider this issue in a new light.

Student activities
In the light of the findings above, discuss practice that you have seen in your placements.

References
Bennett J. Dehydration: hazards and benefits. Geriatr Nurs 2000 21(2): 84–87.
Gray R. Palliative care. To hydrate or not to hydrate. Nurs Times 1999; 95(23): 36–37.

exacerbate the underlying problem and even result in admission to hospital. Many diuretics, particularly thiazides and loop diuretics such as furosemide (frusemide) and bumetanide, cause electrolyte imbalance, especially potassium depletion, and are therefore prescribed with potassium supplements.

Terminal illness
In the absence of i.v. therapy in terminal illness, dehydration occurs, which may in fact have a beneficial effect (see Ethical Issues box 8.1).

PREVENTING DEHYDRATION

The relationship between thirst and dehydration
Dehydration may already be present when thirst becomes apparent, especially in the heat or during exercise. This predisposes to heat exhaustion and heat stroke (Ch. 5). During exercise, muscular activity generates heat and the body compensates by sweating to prevent overheating. To prevent dehydration, it is therefore recommended that about 500 mL of fluid is taken in the hour or two before exercise and every 20 minutes during exercise. In recreational exercise lasting up to an hour, water is suitable for this purpose.

Athletes usually avoid alcohol, tea, coffee and cola because their diuretic effect increases dehydration. In more strenuous activity carried out over a longer period, fluid intake and the type of fluid require more consideration. Sports drinks containing a weak carbohydrate solution, usually less than 5% glucose, are often used.

Oral rehydration solutions
Commercially prepared sachets can be readily bought from chemists and are useful for managing diarrhoea, especially in cases of 'travellers' tummy' on holiday. When these are not available, it can be made by taking 1 litre of clean water and dissolving in it 8 teaspoons of sugar and half a teaspoon of salt. Ideally, half a teaspoon of baking soda (sodium bicarbonate) and one-third of a teaspoon of potassium chloride (e.g. Lo Salt) should also be included in the solution.

DIAGNOSTIC TESTS AND INVESTIGATIONS

BLOOD TESTS: SERUM UREA AND ELECTROLYTES
Normal electrolyte levels are shown in Table 8.1. Urea is the end-product of protein catabolism and has a normal range of 3.5–6.6 mmol/L. Levels are influenced by dietary intake and the volume of urine produced. Raised levels may be due to a high-protein diet, renal failure or the presence of a catabolic state such as trauma, major burns or septicaemia. Abnormally low levels arise when dietary protein intake is low, e.g. in anorexia and malnutrition (Ch. 11), and in liver failure (Ch. 23). The causes and effects of abnormal electrolyte levels are explained below.

URINE TESTS

24-hour urine collection
The bladder is emptied at the beginning of this investigation and the urine passed is discarded. All urine passed in the next 24 hours is saved. At the end of the 24 hours, the bladder is emptied again and this specimen is saved to complete the collection.

This investigation is used to calculate glomerular filtration rate (Ch. 24) by measuring creatinine levels over the 24-hour collection period. Metabolites of hormones can also be measured to assess endocrine function (Ch. 17).

Urinalysis
A fresh specimen of urine is tested using reagent strips. Specific gravity and pH are measured along with protein, glucose, ketones, blood and bilirubin. A brief overview is presented here. Wells (1997) discusses the implications of abnormal findings in more detail.

Proteinuria, the presence of protein in the urine, is an abnormal finding that is usually caused by a urinary tract infection or renal disorder (Ch. 24).

Haematuria is the presence of blood in the urine, another abnormal constituent. This may be visible to the naked eye (frank haematuria) or 'microscopic' when it is only found on testing. A smoky appearance may be indicative of haematuria. The cause is bleeding in the urinary tract usually due to the presence of infection, stones (calculi) or trauma (Ch. 24). Female patients between puberty and the menopause should be

EVIDENCE-BASED PRACTICE

8.2 Evaluating results of investigations

Using the information in this chapter, relate actual and potential nursing problems to suspected abnormalities of the following types of investigations:

- blood tests
- urinalysis
- arterial blood gases.

Explain to patients the nursing implications of results of their investigations.

asked if they are menstruating as this may cause a false positive for blood.

Glycosuria, the presence of sugar in the urine, is an abnormality indicative of diabetes mellitus (Ch. 17).

Ketones are a product of fat metabolism and ketonuria is found in starvation and uncontrolled diabetes mellitus (Ch. 17).

Urinary pH is usually around 6 with a normal range of 4.5–8. This is affected not only by the amount of hydrogen ions being excreted but also by the numbers of bicarbonate ions excreted when there is compensation for acid–base imbalances.

Specific gravity is a measure of urine concentration. Distilled water has a specific gravity (SG) of 1.000 and urine has a normal range of 1.003–1.035. This can be interpreted with urine volumes to determine the likely cause of reduced urine output. When the specific gravity and urine volumes are both reduced, this suggests impairment of renal function. A low urine output together with increased specific gravity suggests fluid deficit, as do small volumes of dark urine.

OTHER INVESTIGATIONS

These include pulse oximetry and arterial blood gas analysis. These are discussed later and also in Chapters 9 and 31 (see also Evidence-based Practice box 8.2).

▶ **Nursing management and interventions**

Maintaining fluid balance means the patient will have sufficient blood pressure and blood volume to supply body organs with oxygen and nutrients and to remove waste products. This is especially important for the vital organs, the brain, heart and kidneys, and interruption of their blood supply will result in rapid damage.

FLUID BALANCE CHARTS

A fluid balance chart is used when there is an actual or potential problem in maintaining fluid balance. This provides a record of all fluid intake and output for a 24-hour period (normal values are shown in Table 8.2). It is of diagnostic significance and maintaining accuracy is an important nursing responsibility. A sign above the patient's bed may be used as an aide memoire for members of the care team, the patient and their relatives.

Fluid intake

Fluid intake includes fluid from all sources, including drinks, nasogastric tube, infusions and medicines. The total daily intake is agreed with the medical staff and the nursing care plan is designed to meet requirements and the frequency of drinks calculated. The terms 'push fluids' and 'encourage fluids' are unhelpful as they are imprecise. Patients are taught about their involvement in maintaining the chart, which they may either do themselves or with the support of the nursing team. When appropriate, patients are given a list indicating the volumes to be recorded for cups of tea, glasses of juice, bowls of soup and milk added to cereals and puddings.

Fluid output

Fluids lost include urine, vomit, gastric aspirate, losses from wounds or drainage tubes and from diarrhoea if this is profuse. Accurate estimation also requires inclusion of an estimate of insensible and sensible losses. Patients need to know about arrangements for measuring urine. It is crucial that urine left for nurses to measure is clearly labelled with the patient's name.

Insensible loss

Insensible losses include losses due to perspiration, which evaporates from the body surface, amounting to around 600 mL daily, and losses due to water vapour in expired air. Such losses increase when un-humidified oxygen therapy is administered (see Ch. 20) and during hyperventilation.

Sensible loss

This is related to sweating which the individual is aware of, e.g. during exercise and high environmental temperatures. Such losses can be considerable, amounting to 1 L/h, but act as an important cooling mechanism (Ch. 5). Pyrexia increases water loss by approximately 200 mL/day for each 1°C rise in temperature above normal (Forrest et al 1995). Although sweat is hypotonic, it contains significant amounts of sodium (20–70 mmol/L) and potassium (10 mmol/L).

Accurate measurement of losses

When measuring small volumes of fluid, an appropriate container is used to ensure accuracy, e.g. wound exudates. A urimeter enables hourly urine measurements in catheterized patients who are at risk of oliguria (low urine output). Vomit and losses from diarrhoea should be measured whenever possible, and occurrence of the event recorded on the fluid balance chart when measurement is not possible. Weighing of wet and soiled incontinence pads provides a good estimate of losses when they cannot be measured directly. Each gram of additional weight is equal to 1 mL of fluid (see Reflective Practice box 8.2).

24-hour fluid balance

This is calculated at the same time each day and is the difference between the total intake and output. It may be negative or positive. Negative balance arises when more fluid has been lost than taken in, and is the aim when there is fluid overload. Positive balance means that more fluid has been taken in than lost and is the aim when managing dehydration and fluid volume deficit. A record of daily balances is also kept to enable assessment of trends or changes in fluid status from day to day and over several days.

R|Я REFLECTIVE PRACTICE

8.2 Fluid balance charting in practice

'There are innumerable possibilities for error in the measurement and recording of fluid gains and losses, however some errors occur much more frequently than others' (Metheny 1996, p. 31).

Student activities
- Think of situations in which it may be difficult to assess a patient's fluid losses accurately and how these might be overcome.
- Reflect on the accuracy of charting fluid intake and output in your practice area and how this might be improved.

Reference
Metheny NM (ed). Fluid and electrolyte balance, 3rd edn. Philadelphia: Lippincott; 1996.

 HEALTH PROMOTION

8.1 Reducing ankle oedema

Nursing advice would include:

- Mobilizing or exercising the ankles and feet when possible, which uses the skeletal muscle 'pump' in the legs to promote venous return
- Elevating the feet when sitting to promote drainage of excess fluid by gravity
- Using support stockings, which also promotes venous return
- Avoiding socks and other hosiery with tight bands which will impair venous return below the band
- Wearing flat, fairly tight-fitting shoes rather than sandals with straps, as excess fluid will collect around the straps.

Student activities
Consider how you would explain to a patient what oedema is and ways to minimize ankle oedema.

DAILY WEIGHT

Measurement of daily weight often provides a more accurate estimation of fluid balance over a period of days because fluid balance charts may not be accurate. In the absence of a cause of rapid tissue loss, changes in body weight reflect body water changes rather than changes in body mass. The following principles are used:

- Use the same weighing scales.
- Measure at the same time each day after emptying the bladder and before breakfast.
- Ensure the patient is dressed in the same or similar clothing.

OEDEMA

The aim of care is to facilitate drainage of excess fluid and, if appropriate, elevation of the affected area(s) will often help. Use of a pressure area assessment tool will determine the care required to maintain skin integrity (see Ch. 10). The patient may feel self-conscious or embarrassed about areas affected by oedema. Swollen ankles and legs become uncomfortable due to the tightness caused by the stretched skin. When ankle oedema is a long-term problem, patients can be educated about actions that will reduce swelling and promote comfort (see Health Promotion box 8.1).

HELPING PATIENTS WITH ORAL FLUIDS

The oral route is used for fluid replacement whenever possible as it is non-invasive and free of the discomforts and complications of enteral and i.v. routes. This is not possible when there is vomiting, paralytic ileus, obstruction of the alimentary tract or dysphagia (Ch. 22) or when the swallowing reflex is in doubt.

Types of oral fluids

The volume and types of oral fluids offered require consideration. In cancer patients and others with increased calorific requirements, high-calorie drinks may be provided with advice from a dietician. Some of these also contain other nutrients and vitamins. Milk is encouraged when a patient is at risk of osteoporosis (Ch. 27). Thickened fluids are sometimes used for clients with dysphagia. In electrolyte disorders, fluids with substantial electrolyte content may be encouraged or restricted. Stock cubes and Bovril are high in sodium while fruit juice is rich in potassium. Iggulden (1999) provides other examples.

Recommencing oral fluids after a period of fasting

Following surgery or after a period of fasting, a patient starts on small, prescribed hourly drinks of 15 mL of water, which are gradually increased as peristalsis is re-established (Ch. 22). When the patient can manage over 90 mL hourly, other fluids may be introduced and a normal fluid intake pattern restored. A light, easily digestible diet follows shortly afterwards.

Helping a patient to drink

The aim is to provide individualized nursing care that meets the nursing goals. Safety is a prime consideration for patients being prepared for discharge and those living at home in the community. Home assessment is undertaken by the occupational therapist and includes the ability to boil a kettle and to make tea or coffee independently. Where appropriate, aids can be provided to assist in undertaking these activities safely. These include beakers, modified drinking cups and straws, especially the flexible type.

From early childhood, independence in drinking is taken for granted and therefore nursing patients experiencing decreasing independence requires tact and empathy. When help is required, the nurse should sit level with the patient and have any aids, e.g. a straw, at hand. The patient should sit upright whenever possible to facilitate swallowing. Drinks should be within the patient's reach and fluids are usually most acceptable when they are what the patient likes. Cold drinks should be served cold, or iced, and hot ones hot! Hochreiter (1999) includes other practical tips to enable people to achieve their planned fluid intake (see also Health Promotion box 8.2).

HEALTH PROMOTION

8.2 Helping patients to achieve planned daily fluid intake

The nurse plays a key role in managing patients' fluid intake.

Student activities

- Devise a plan with a client to provide a fluid intake of 1.5–2 L/day.
- Prepare a poster or patient leaflet that could be used at home or in hospital to help patients record their daily fluid intake. It should show a variety of containers, e.g. a cup, mug and various glasses.
- Devise a plan with a client to provide an acceptable intake when fluids are restricted to 500 mL in 24 hours.

Fluid restriction

If the patient's fluid intake has to be restricted, the volume of fluid prescribed is discussed with the patient and compared with the usual intake pattern and preferred times of drinks. A plan showing when fluids will be offered is drawn up, with fluids spaced over the 24-hour period. This should include the patient's preferred types of fluid and, when taken, the volume is recorded on the fluid balance chart. Many patients enjoy crushed ice or ice cubes to suck, to keep their mouth moist while minimizing the fluid ingested.

NASOGASTRIC TUBES

A nasogastric tube is passed via the nose and oesophagus into the stomach to aspirate gastric contents or for fluid replacement and/or enteral feeding (Ch. 22) when a patient is unable to take food orally. The principles of care are explained in Mallett & Dougherty (2000) and Nicol et al (2000).

INTRAVENOUS INFUSION

An intravenous infusion is used to administer sterile fluid into the circulation when the enteral route is not appropriate, e.g. pre- and postoperatively and following major trauma. The fluid may be infused for several reasons:

- to maintain fluid and electrolyte balance
- to restore fluid and electrolyte balance
- for nutritional purposes, when it is referred to as parenteral nutrition (see Ch. 11)
- for administration of drugs.

In this section, replacement of fluid and electrolytes will be considered. Fluids infused are described as either crystalloid or colloid. Colloid solutions contain solute particles that remain in the bloodstream, as they are too large to cross capillary membranes. They include blood and blood products – plasma, plasma expanders and platelets (see Chs 9 and 18). Crystalloids are clear fluids that readily cross cell membranes and pass between the circulation and the tissue fluid. They are used to manage fluid and electrolyte balance (see Table 8.3).

Table 8.3 Intravenous fluids – crystalloids		
Solution	Content	Comments
5% dextrose	Water, glucose 50 mg/mL	Isotonic solution used to replace water deficit – enters ICF. Glucose is metabolized, providing 170 cal/L, effectively leaving only infused water in the cells Over-transfusion causes over-hydration and hyponatraemia Never mix with blood as haemolysis will occur Contraindicated in hyperglycaemia More concentrated solutions (10 and 20%) are used to treat hypoglycaemia (Ch. 17) and in parenteral nutrition (Ch. 11)
0.9% saline (normal saline)	Water, sodium 150 mmol/L, chloride 150 mmol/L	Isotonic solution used to correct sodium depletion and all expands ECF, not only the intravascular volume – does not enter ICF Sodium content predisposes to fluid retention and circulatory overload Hypertonic solutions (1.8 and 3%) are used to treat hyponatraemia
4% dextrose 0.18% saline	Water, glucose 40 mg/L, sodium 30 mmol/L, chloride 30 mmol/L	An isotonic solution that enters ICF and ECF used in combined sodium and water depletion Less widely used but has the advantages of both fluids above
Hartmann's solution (Ringer's lactate)	Water, sodium 131 mmol/L, potassium 5 mmol/L, chloride 111 mmol/L, calcium 2 mmol/L, lactate 29 mmol/L	Isotonic solution containing near physiological electrolyte concentrations used to correct electrolyte imbalance and mild metabolic acidosis Lactate is metabolized to bicarbonate in the liver and excess causes mild alkalosis. Contraindicated in liver disease
Sodium bicarbonate 1.26%	Water, sodium 150 mmol/L, bicarbonate 150 mmol/L	Isotonic solution used to correct acidosis
Sodium bicarbonate 8.4%	Water, sodium 1000 mmol/L, bicarbonate 1000 mmol/L	Hypertonic solution used to correct severe metabolic acidosis during cardiac arrest

The tonicity of i.v. fluids is important as it affects their destination within the fluid compartments. Isotonic fluids, e.g. normal saline, have the same concentration of solutes as plasma. They maintain ECF volume and prevent movement of water from the ECF to the ICF. Hypotonic solutions, e.g. 5% dextrose, have a lower osmolality than plasma and infusion results in movement of water into the body cells (ICF). In contrast, hypertonic solutions have a greater concentration of solutes than plasma and infusion causes movement of water from the body cells (ICF) to the ECF.

Normal daily requirements of fluids and electrolytes are met by providing 1 litre of 0.9% saline and 2 litres of 5% dextrose plus 60 mmol potassium chloride. More is required to compensate for losses due to pyrexia, diarrhoea and intestinal obstruction.

Maintaining safety and comfort during i.v. infusions

A cannula is inserted into a peripheral vein, usually in the forearm or dorsum of the hand, and secured in place according to local policy. The fluid container is connected to an administration set and connected to the cannula. The system must be patent and kept closed to avoid introducing contaminants. Aseptic technique and universal precautions are required when the system is open. Intravenous fluids should be changed every 24 hours using aseptic technique. The giving set is changed every 72 hours for i.v. fluids and every 24 hours for parenteral nutrition (Scales 1997). The site is checked regularly for signs of complications (see below). Intravenous fluids and any additives must be prescribed and volumes recorded on the fluid balance chart.

Accurate calculation and control of the flow rate are the nurse's responsibility. Flow rate is checked at least hourly. The formula for calculating the flow rate for i.v. infusions in drops per minute (drops/min) is as follows:

$$\text{Flow rate (drops/min)} = [\text{volume of fluid to be infused (mL)}/\text{infusion time (min)}] \times \text{drop factor}$$

The drop factor is:

- *For standard giving sets* – 20 drops/mL for crystalloids and 15 drops/mL for colloids
- *For microdrop giving sets (burettes)* – 60 drops/mL.

Common causes of obstruction or inadequate flow rate are as follows:

- the height of the infusion container is too low and the infusion stand needs to be raised
- kinking of the giving set tubing
- position of the cannula in the vein – altering the position of the hand or forearm may improve the flow.

Infusion control devices (pumps) are used to regulate the flow rate for accuracy when small volumes are prescribed or drugs are added and when there is danger of rapid over-infusion. Audible alarms indicate when the infusion is complete or if the flow is impeded. The nurse is responsible for using this equipment safely and requires training for each type of pump used in the clinical setting to ensure familiarity with correct use.

Complications of i.v. therapy

These can be minor or major with serious consequences. Complications increase the length of admission and therefore the nursing care and hospital resources required to manage the patient. The effects of complications are local or systemic and are examined in detail by Dougherty & Lamb (1999). A brief overview is presented here.

Local complications

- *Infection* is caused by contamination of any part of the system.
- *Infiltration* of the tissues occurs when fluid infuses into the tissues instead of the circulation, causing swelling around the cannula site. The site may also appear pale and can be painful. The infusion may stop but this does not always happen.
- *Extravasation* occurs when irritant solutions enter the tissues. They can cause severe damage including tissue necrosis. Such substances may be hypertonic, e.g. 8.4% sodium bicarbonate, or contain vasoconstricting drugs, e.g. dopamine (Ch. 31), and are normally given through a central line to minimize this potential problem.
- *Phlebitis*, which is inflammation of the inner layer of the vein (see Special Issues box 8.1).

 SPECIAL ISSUES

8.1 Minimizing phlebitis associated with intravenous infusions

Phlebitis is inflammation of the inner layer of the vein. Its cause may be:

- mechanical – caused by the cannula in the vein
- chemical – caused by the substances infused
- bacterial – caused by local infection.

Signs
- Inflammation often with pain and redness at the site
- Redness may track from the cannula along the course of the affected vein towards the heart
- In thrombophlebitis there is also an intravascular blood clot usually associated with a palpable cord.

Causes
- Cannula is too large to be appropriate and/or not in a suitable vein and/or inserted using poor technique
- Cannula moving within the vein
- Infusion of irritant solutions (e.g. hypertonic, acid, alkaline, containing drugs)
- Contamination of the system.

Prevention or early detection
- Secure cannula firmly in place to avoid movement in the vein
- Infuse irritant solutions slowly. Dilute irritant solutions whenever possible
- Inspect the site frequently for signs of inflammation
- Remove cannula if phlebitis is present and re-site if necessary
- Maintain aseptic technique to minimize the risk of contaminating the system.

Student activities
Prepare a tutorial outlining the nursing measures taken to prevent and manage phlebitis.

Systemic complications

- *Circulatory overload* occurs when fluid, especially normal saline, is infused too quickly, increasing the blood volume and venous pressure. This may result in cardiac failure and acute pulmonary oedema. Infusion control devices are therefore used in susceptible patients. Regular checks of the flow rate are made to detect this potential problem which often happens when the cannula is 'positional', i.e. when the position of the arm affects the flow rate.
- *Fluid volume deficit* due to overly slow infusion of fluid.
- *Septicaemia* occurs when pathogenic bacteria are spread from a local infection and invade the bloodstream. This is especially dangerous when large numbers of virulent bacteria are present in a host with compromised immunity (Ch. 13).
- *Pulmonary embolism* is a rare but life-threatening complication that arises when a dislodged blood clot travels in the venous circulation to the right atrium, through the right ventricle and then lodges, blocking a pulmonary artery. Occurrence is minimized by using a filter to administer blood or particulate solutions and using only gentle pressure to flush a cannula if resistance is encountered.
- *Air embolism* is another rare and potentially life-threatening complication. It arises when an air bubble travels through the venous system as above and, when it reaches the right ventricle, interferes with its pumping activity. This is most likely to happen during insertion of a central line.
- *Allergic reactions and speed shock* are rarely associated with infusion of crystalloid fluid but may occur during intravenous drug administration or blood transfusion (Dougherty & Lamb 1999).

The role of the specialist i.v. nurse

Nurses working either alone or as part of a team may provide a specialist intravenous service. In both cases, training in relevant skills, including i.v. cannulation and other techniques, is undertaken before these skills are used. Willis (1999) advocates the development of national minimum standards of care and training to enable transfer of these skills between NHS Trusts. The role of these nurses is varied and may include administration of parenteral nutrition, cytotoxic therapy and venepuncture in both hospital and community settings (Dougherty 1996). They use standardized procedures, which have several advantages including a reduction in side-effects and increased cost-effectiveness. Patients and other nurses value the support and service these specialists provide.

SUBCUTANEOUS INFUSION

Subcutaneous fluid administration is also called hypodermoclysis. It is used in palliative care and in the care of older adults for one of the following reasons:

- to maintain hydration when adequate oral intake is not possible
- to correct mild dehydration in patients who are able to take some oral fluids.

A suitable site is selected and discussed with the patient, taking into account mobility, comfort, skin condition and ease of access. Suitable sites include the anterior chest wall and the scapular area, but several others may also be used. The infusion is given via a butterfly needle inserted into the subcutaneous tissues and secured in place with a semi-permeable occlusive dressing for easy inspection. The site should be changed every 24 hours. Intravenous administration sets and isotonic i.v. fluids are used. It should be noted that fluids are only licensed for i.v. use and therefore formulation of a local policy for safe practice is advised. Rates of infusion are up to 125 mL/h or 2 litres in 24 hours through one site and occasionally more than one site is used. Absorption of the fluid into the circulation takes about an hour. The flow rate may be set or the fluid infused by gravity alone. Infusion by gravity reduces the risk of local oedema formation (Noble-Adams 1995). Hyaluronidase may be used to prime the butterfly needle, as it increases the subcutaneous absorption rate.

Side-effects are fairly uncommon but include local oedema and occasionally local infection, bruising and pain (Gluck 1982). Infection rates are lower than those with i.v. infusion and phlebitis does not occur. As with i.v. infusions, fluid overload is a potential problem if infusion is too rapid.

The advantages of this route are well recognized in North America and New Zealand and it is increasingly being used in the UK. Advantages include suitability for use in a variety of settings including the patient's home. The route is cost-effective, as nurses set up and manage the infusions, thereby saving doctors' time. Subsequent care takes less nursing time than an i.v. infusion. It is also convenient for patients. Fluid can be administered overnight, allowing the patient to be independent and mobile during the day or, for patients who are restless at night, it can be given during the day.

RECTAL INFUSION

This is also called proctoclysis. A nasogastric catheter is inserted about 40 cm into the rectum to administer fluids. Bruera et al (1998), in a study of terminally ill cancer patients, reported that this technique was safe, inexpensive and maintained hydration effectively.

COMMON ELECTROLYTE DISORDERS: MANAGEMENT AND NURSING CARE

Normal serum electrolyte ranges and the causes and manifestations of electrolyte disorders are summarized in Table 8.4. Management of the most common conditions is explained below and for others the reader is referred to Metheny (1996) or Mirpuri & Patel (1998).

Hyponatraemia

Vital signs are recorded, a fluid balance chart is maintained and sodium replacement started orally whenever possible. In more severe cases, parenteral replacement with sodium chloride (0.9%) or hypertonic saline (1.8 or 3%) is sometimes used. Diuretic therapy should be reviewed, as this may be not only a contributing factor but also part of the treatment. Fluid restriction may also be required. Serum and urine sodium and osmolality are measured daily and further treatment prescribed according to the results.

Table 8.4 Acid–base disorders: changes in blood gas values (from Haslett et al 1999)

Disorder	[H⁺]	Paco₂	HCO₃⁻
Metabolic acidosis			
Acute	Raised	Normal	Lower than normal
Compensated (by increased ventilation)	Slightly raised or normal	Lower than normal	Lower than normal
Metabolic alkalosis			
Acute	Lower than normal	Normal	Raised
Compensated (by reduced ventilation)	Slightly reduced or normal	Raised	Raised
Respiratory acidosis			
Acute	Raised	Raised	Normal
Compensated (by renal retention of CO₂)	Slightly reduced or normal	Raised	Raised
Respiratory alkalosis			
Acute	Lower than normal	Lower than normal	Normal
Compensated (by ↑ renal excretion)	Slightly reduced or normal	Lower than normal	Lower than normal

Hypernatraemia

Vital signs are recorded, a fluid balance chart is maintained and daily weight measured. When there is excess water loss, this is replaced orally or intravenously using 5% dextrose. When there is excess sodium, the cause is identified and treated. Serum and urine sodium and osmolality are measured daily and further treatment is determined by the results. Neurological assessment is undertaken to detect early signs of cerebral oedema caused by too rapid a shift of fluid from the ECF to the ICF.

Hypokalaemia

In mild cases, oral replacement is used together with increased dietary intake of fruit, fruit juice, chocolate, coffee, milk and animal protein. Patient education also includes advice about the correct use of laxatives and diuretics if these are a potential cause. In patients receiving digoxin, the pulse is monitored and, if below 60 beats/min, the drug is withheld and the doctor informed. Bradycardia is a sign of digoxin toxicity and this is potentiated by hypokalaemia. In more severe cases, cardiac monitoring is carried out and potassium replacement given intravenously (see Guidelines for Care Priorities box 8.1).

Hyperkalaemia

This condition can cause bradycardia and cardiac arrest. In moderate cases, potassium-containing foods are restricted (see above) and an exchange resin, e.g. calcium resonium, is given either orally or rectally. In more severe cases, cardiac monitoring is implemented and fast-acting treatments are given intravenously to lower serum levels. These include:

- calcium gluconate – this diminishes the effect of hyperkalaemia on the myocardium for 30–60 min
- sodium bicarbonate – this is used in metabolic alkalosis and causes short-term movement of potassium into the cells
- dextrose and insulin – insulin promotes the uptake of potassium by tissue cells.

Hyperkalaemia is effectively treated by haemodialysis, haemofiltration and peritoneal dialysis (see Ch. 24) but these techniques require specialist facilities which are not always available where and when they are required.

 GUIDELINES FOR CARE PRIORITIES

8.1 Intravenous potassium supplements – safe practice

The aim is to prevent rapid administration of a concentrated solution containing potassium, as it will cause cardiac arrest.

Main points

- Use commercially prepared solutions when possible.
- Ampoules of potassium are always diluted and the solution mixed thoroughly before use.
- Potassium is an irritant solution that causes pain at the insertion site and concentrations should not exceed 60 mmol/L via a peripheral line.
- Infusion rate should not exceed 10–20 mmol/h.
- In order to prevent hyperkalaemia, potassium supplements should be given with caution to patients with low urine output (oliguria).
- Potassium ampoules should be kept separate from others (e.g. sodium chloride) to prevent accidental use.
- Slowing pulse, return of muscle tone and bowel sounds accompany increasing potassium levels.

If a more rapid infusion is required:

- A flow control device must be used.
- Continuous cardiac monitoring is required and the ECG should be observed for signs of hyperkalaemia.
- Regular serum potassium measurements are made to evaluate treatment.

ACID–BALANCE BALANCE

An acid is a substance that can donate hydrogen ions (H⁺). A base, or alkali, is a substance that can accept hydrogen ions. The acidity of a solution is measured using the pH scale which ranges from 1 (strongly acidic) to 14 (strongly alkaline) with a midpoint of 7, which is neutral. The pH scale is logarithmic, meaning that a change of one on the scale represents a 10-fold change in the concentration of H^+. For example, a solution of pH 7 has 10 times more H^+ than a solution of pH 8. This is important when considering the pH of blood, as the concentration of H^+ must remain within a narrow range (pH 7.35–7.45) for homeostasis to be maintained.

A strong acid readily dissociates into its constituent ions, e.g. hydrochloric acid:

HCl (hydrochloric acid) → H^+ (hydrogen ion) + Cl^- (chloride ion)

A strong alkali does the same, e.g. sodium hydroxide forms sodium and hydroxyl ions:

NaOH (sodium hydroxide) → Na^+ (sodium ion) + OH^- (hydroxyl ion)

Alkalis accept hydrogen ions. Salts are formed when an acid and an alkali combine:

HCl (hydrochloric acid) + NaOH (sodium hydroxide) → NaCl (a salt) + H_2O (water)

Weaker acids and bases dissociate less readily into their constituent ions.

In health, the pH of the ECF is in the range of 7.35–7.45. Outwith this range, physiological dysfunction rapidly occurs. On a daily basis the amount of H^+ excreted by respiration and in the urine must balance H^+ taken in the diet and produced by metabolic processes:

H^+ intake in food + H^+ generated by metabolism – H^+ excreted in urine + H^+ lost from lungs as CO_2

Effective mechanisms are therefore necessary to prevent accumulation of hydrogen ions and maintain homeostasis. The most important are:

- Buffer systems – these quickly bind H^+ keeping the pH up but do not remove excess H^+ from the body
- Excretion of CO_2 by the lungs – when the rate and depth of breathing are increased, the lungs excrete more CO_2, raising an acid pH in 1–3 minutes, removing excess H^+. Raised arterial Pa_{CO_2} is a potent stimulus for increasing the rate and depth of breathing. Excretion of CO_2 takes place through the series of reactions below:

H^+ + HCO_3^- (bicarbonate ion) → H_2CO_3 (carbonic acid) → H_2O (water) + CO_2 (carbon dioxide excreted by the lungs)

- Renal excretion of hydrogen ions – carbonic acid (H_2CO_3) is secreted by the renal tubules and dissociates into H^+ and HCO_3^-. The HCO_3^- is reabsorbed for recycling and the H^+ is excreted in the urine:

H_2CO_3 (carbonic acid) → H^+ (hydrogen ion, excreted by kidneys) + HCO_3^-

This mechanism removes excess H^+ over many hours and also explains why urine usually has a slightly acidic pH.

pH REGULATION AND BUFFERS

A buffer is a substance which can accept H^+ from an acid solution and donate H^+ to an alkaline solution. It can therefore minimize changes in pH by compensating for either a shortage or excess of H^+. The main buffering systems are the bicarbonate system, the phosphate system and plasma proteins, including haemoglobin. The bicarbonate system is the major system and is outlined below. The other systems operate in a similar way and the reader is advised to consult a physiology text for detailed explanation.

The bicarbonate system

This system is based on the bicarbonate ion, which can act as a weak base, and carbonic acid, which can act as a weak acid. Bicarbonate ions are present in both ICF and ECF. When there is an excess of H^+ (an acid environment), bicarbonate ions act as a weak base and remove the H^+:

H^+ + HCO_3^- (bicarbonate ion, weak base) → H_2CO_3 (carbonic acid) → H_2O (water) + CO_2 (carbon dioxide)

In the lungs, carbonic acid dissociates into carbon dioxide and water and the CO_2 is exhaled. When there is a shortage of H^+ (an alkaline environment), carbonic acid acts as a weak acid and donates its H^+, thereby lowering the pH:

H_2CO_3 (carbonic acid, weak acid) → H^+ + HCO_3^-

ASSESSMENT OF ACID–BASE STATUS

Acid–base balance is assessed using arterial blood gas (ABG) analysis. The variables measured are pH, HCO_3^-, Pa_{O_2}, Pa_{CO_2} and oxygen saturation. Pa_{O_2} (normal range 10.0–13.3 kPa) indicates oxygenation levels of the blood and Pa_{CO_2} (normal range 4.6–6.0 kPa) reflects the effectiveness of ventilation. Hypoxaemia is present when the Pa_{O_2} is lower than normal. The normal pH of arterial blood is 7.4 (range 7.35–7.45) and, if outside these limits, disruption of homeostasis occurs. Enzyme action is particularly susceptible to changes in pH. When evaluation of ABGs has been carried out, a pulse oximeter may be used for continuous monitoring of oxygen saturation levels.

Pulse oximetry

This is a non-invasive procedure that enables continuous transcutaneous measurement of oxygen saturation levels of haemoglobin (S_pO_2). This is the percentage of haemoglobin saturated with oxygen. The value reflects arterial Pa_{O_2} and is used to evaluate respiratory status, O_2 therapy and other interventions, e.g. tracheal suction, exercise or physiotherapy. For most patients the normal range is 95–98%. A sudden decrease or downward trend requires evaluation together with the vital signs and the patient's general condition. Using this equipment reduces the need for repeated ABG analysis (see Ch. 9). Jevon & Ewens (2000a,b) explain the nursing care required.

Arterial blood gases

If the patient is in a high-dependency or intensive care unit, there may be an arterial line in situ that can be used for this purpose (see Ch. 9), otherwise intermittent arterial puncture is required.

DISORDERS OF ACID–BASE BALANCE: CAUSES AND MANAGEMENT

Acid–base disorders are described as either respiratory or metabolic according to their cause. Acidosis (acidaemia) is present

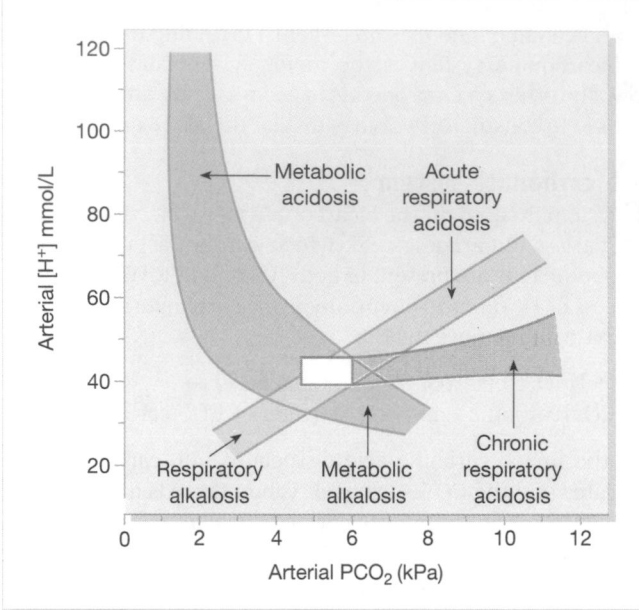

Figure 8.5 The Flenley acid–base nomogram. The white box shows the approximate limit of arterial pH and P_{CO_2} in normal individuals. (Based on Kumar & Clark 1998.)

when arterial blood pH is less than 7.35 and alkalosis (alkalaemia) when the arterial blood pH exceeds 7.45. When they occur, homeostatic mechanisms attempt to restore normal blood pH. This is either through alterations in the amount of CO_2 excreted by the lungs (which is rapid) or changes in the levels of bicarbonate (normal range 22–26 mmol/L) secreted by the kidney tubules (which is slow to take effect). The Flenley acid–base nomogram (see Fig. 8.5) can be used to identify which acid–base disorder is present when arterial H^+ concentration and P_{aCO_2} are known. Table 8.4 summarizes the changes in ABG values that occur in the acid–base disorders explained below.

Metabolic acidosis

This condition arises when there is an increased hydrogen ion concentration (low pH) and low serum bicarbonate. It develops following increased production of hydrogen ions or loss of bicarbonate. Compensation takes place in the lungs and hyperventilation lowers P_{aCO_2} and raises the hydrogen ion concentration. Bicarbonate levels remain reduced. It is potentiated by renal failure.

Signs and symptoms

Deep rapid respirations are characteristic of this condition. There may also be nausea and vomiting, headache, confusion and drowsiness. When the H^+ concentration exceeds 70 nmol/L, myocardial function is impaired and arrhythmias can occur, which may be life-threatening, e.g. ventricular fibrillation (Ch. 19). This is accompanied by drowsiness and confusion. The underlying cause is identified and treated.

Causes

These include:

- Failure to excrete H^+ at a normal rate as a result of acute or chronic renal failure (Ch. 24)

- Excessive loss of bicarbonate – this may occur in acute renal failure and during diuretic therapy when carbonic anhydrase inhibitors are used, e.g. acetazolamide. It can also accompany diarrhoea and losses from gastrointestinal fistulae (Ch. 22)
- Lactic acidosis – this arises when anaerobic metabolism occurs in cells because they have insufficient O_2 for aerobic metabolism. This results in the production of lactic acid, which causes a marked reduction in pH. It is common in patients with poor tissue perfusion, e.g. in severe shock (Ch. 9), in cardiac or respiratory conditions and major sepsis. This condition also occurs in diabetic ketoacidosis (Ch. 17). A less severe form is also the cause of muscle cramps in athletes.

Metabolic alkalosis

In this condition the hydrogen ion concentration is low and the bicarbonate level is raised. Compensation is by hypoventilation and conservation of carbon dioxide occurs, increasing P_{aCO_2} and raising the hydrogen ion concentration. The bicarbonate level remains raised. It is often accompanied by hypokalaemia as the kidneys conserve hydrogen ions by exchanging them for potassium. Signs and symptoms are not apparent.

Causes

This is commonly caused by excessive loss of hydrogen ions from the gastrointestinal tract through vomiting, gastric aspiration or gastrointestinal obstruction and is accompanied by ECF depletion. Others causes include diuretic therapy inducing potassium depletion, e.g. furosemide (frusemide), thiazides; excessive mineralocorticoid production, e.g. hyperaldosteronism and Cushing's syndrome (see Ch. 17); and ingestion of large amounts of bicarbonate-containing antacids.

Treatment

This is aimed at reversing the underlying disorder, including surgery for gastrointestinal causes. ECF depletion is corrected by i.v. infusion of normal saline with potassium supplements.

Respiratory acidosis

This condition may be acute or chronic. In acute respiratory acidosis, the P_{aCO_2} and hydrogen ion concentration are raised initially while bicarbonate remains normal. The lungs fail to excrete the CO_2 that is being produced and its accumulation in the plasma results in rising hydrogen ion concentrations. The acute form is especially dangerous and bicarbonate remains in the normal range until renal compensation slowly takes effect. In chronic respiratory acidosis, renal retention of bicarbonate compensates for chronically increased P_{aCO_2} and the cause is usually chronic obstructive airways disease (Ch. 20).

Signs and symptoms

In the acute condition, increases in pulse, respiratory rate and blood pressure occur.

Causes

Hypoventilation is the underlying cause and may be brought about by acute conditions that depress the respiratory centre, including over-sedation with opiate drugs or severe impairment of gaseous exchange in the lungs, e.g. acute pulmonary oedema, pneumothorax, severe pneumonia (Ch. 20) and cardiac arrest

(Ch. 19). The chronic, or compensated, form of respiratory acidosis often accompanies chronic lung disease.

Treatment

The aim is to increase ventilation by alleviating the underlying cause, including reversal of opiate-induced cases by the intravenous administration of an opiate antagonist. Mechanical ventilation may be required (Ch. 31). In chronic conditions, treatment of exacerbating conditions such as bronchospasm or pneumonia is indicated.

Respiratory alkalosis

In this condition, hyperventilation results in increased loss of CO_2 accompanied by a reduction in hydrogen ion concentration. Bicarbonate levels remain normal until renal compensation occurs. At this point, bicarbonate levels are reduced and the hydrogen ion concentration returns to normal.

Signs and symptoms

In episodes of anxiety, palpitations, sweating, dry mouth, nausea and vomiting and visual disturbances may occur accompanied by dizziness and inability to concentrate. In severe cases, the patient may faint; hyperventilation then stops and breathing returns to normal.

Causes

The most common cause is anxiety or panic attacks. Other causes include septicaemia, severe pyrexia, pneumonia, pulmonary emboli and excessive mechanical ventilation.

Treatment

When caused by a panic attack, the patient is asked to breathe slowly into a closed system, e.g. into a paper bag, as rebreathing air high in CO_2 increases the arterial blood level.

Mixed disorders

In mixed disorders, there is a combination of the above events, which usually occurs in seriously ill patients. For example, following cardiac arrest (Ch. 19) there is mixed respiratory and metabolic acidosis, hypoxaemia causes lactic acidosis with a decrease in bicarbonate, and respiratory arrest results in retention of CO_2.

SUMMARY: MAIN POINTS

- Homeostasis of water, electrolytes and acid–base balance is essential for health.

- Fluid and electrolyte imbalance is associated with deficiency caused by reduced intake and/or increased excretion, or excess caused by increased intake and/or decreased excretion.

- Disturbances of fluid balance may be isotonic or osmolar, or both.

- Abnormalities of serum sodium are accompanied by changes in water volume and its distribution within the body.

- Serum potassium deficiency or excess causes life-threatening arrhythmias.

- Accumulation of tissue fluid causes oedema.

- Administration of appropriate intravenous fluids will maintain or re-establish the composition of the ECF and ICF, enabling normal cellular function.

SELF-TEST: CRITICAL THINKING ACTIVITIES

1 Most patients have their urine tested at some point. What would the presence of each of the following indicate: protein, glucose, ketones, blood and bilirubin?

2 Weighing patients is often the responsibility of junior nurses or care assistants. How would you explain to a junior nurse the reasons for weighing patients and how to do this to ensure accuracy?

3 Explain what is meant by diuretic therapy and what advice you might give a patient who is taking diuretics every day.

4 When caring for patients receiving i.v. therapy, what are the common complications that can occur?

 FURTHER READING

Ahern-Gould K, Stark J. Quick resource for electrolyte imbalance. Crit Care Nurs Clin North Am 1998; 10(4): 477–490.

Brown MK, Worobec F. Hypodermoclysis: another way to replace fluids. Nursing 2000; 30(5): 58–59.

De Ridder D, Gastmans C. Dehydration among terminally ill patients: an integrated and practical approach for caregivers. Nurs Ethics 1996; 3: 305–316.

Eccles R. Electrolytes, body fluids and acid base balance. London: Edward Arnold; 1993.

Edwards S. Regulation of water, sodium and potassium: implications for practice. Nurs Stand 2001; 15(22): 36–42.

Fox ET. IV hydration in the terminally ill: ritual or therapy. Br J Nurs 1996; 5(1): 41–45.

Jamieson EM, McCall JM, Blythe R, Whyte LA. Clinical nursing practices, 3rd edn. New York: Churchill Livingstone; 1997.

McVicar A, Clancy J. Principles of intravenous fluid replacement. Prof Nurse 1997; 12 (suppl 8): S6–9.

Malone N. Hydration in the terminally ill patient. Nurs Stand 1994; 8(43): 29–32.

Mansfield S, Monaghan Hall J. Subcutaneous administration and site maintenance. Nurs Stand 1998; 13(12): 56–62.

Sims J. Making sense of tonicity and intravenous therapy. Nurs Times 1996; 92(14): 42–43.

REFERENCES

Bennett J. Dehydration: hazards and benefits. Geriatr Nurs 2000; 21(2): 84–87.

Bruera E, Pruvost M, Schoeller T, Montejo G, Watanabe S. Proctoclysis for hydration of terminally ill cancer patients. J Pain Symptom Manage 1998; 15(4): 216–219.

Coni N, Webster S. Lecture notes on geriatrics, 5th edn. Oxford: Blackwell Science; 1998.

Dougherty L. The benefits of an IV team in hospital practice. Prof Nurse 1996; 11: 761–763.

Dougherty L, Lamb J (eds). Intravenous therapy in practice. Edinburgh: Churchill Livingstone; 1999.

Forrest APM, Carter DC, Macleod IB. Principles and practice of surgery, 3rd edn. Edinburgh: Churchill Livingstone; 1995.

Gluck S. Hypodermoclysis revisited. J Am Med Assoc 1982; 248(11): 1310–1311.

Haslett C, Chivers ER, Hunter JAA, Boon NA. Davidson's principles and practice of medicine, 18th edn. Edinburgh: Churchill Livingstone; 1999.

Hochreiter J. How do you ensure your clients drink the amount of fluid calculated by the dietician? J Gerontol Nurs 1999; 25(5): 46–48.

Iggulden H. Dehydration and electrolyte disturbance. Elderly Care 1999; 11(3): 17–22.

Jevon P, Ewens B. Pulse oximetry – 1. Nurs Times 2000a; 96(26): 43–44.

Jevon P, Ewens B. Pulse oximetry – 2. Nurs Times 2000b; 96(27): 43–44.

Jogee M, Lal L. Religions and cultures, 5th edn. Edinburgh: Edinburgh and Lothian Racial Equality Council; 1999.

Kumar P, Clark M. Clinical medicine, 4th edn. Edinburgh: WB Saunders; 1998.

Mallett J, Dougherty L (eds). The Royal Marsden manual of clinical nursing procedures, 5th edn. Oxford: Blackwell Science; 2000.

Metheny NM (ed). Fluid and electrolyte balance, 3rd edn. Philadelphia: Lippincott; 1996.

Mirpuri N, Patel P. Mosby's crash course: renal and urinary systems. London: Mosby; 1998.

Nicol M, Bavin C, Bedford-Turner S, Cronin P, Rawlings-Anderson K. Essential nursing skills. Edinburgh: Mosby; 2000.

Noble-Adams R. Dehydration: subcutaneous fluid administration. Br J Nurs 1995; 4(9): 488–494.

Redfern S. Nursing elderly people, 3rd edn. Edinburgh: Churchill Livingstone; 1998.

Scales K. Practical and professional aspects of IV therapy. Prof Nurse 1997; 12 (suppl 8): S3–5.

Tortora GJ, Grabowski SR. Principles of anatomy and physiology, 9th edn. New York: John Wiley; 2000.

Watson R. Thirst and dehydration in elderly people. Nursing Older People 1996; 8(3): 23–26.

Waugh A, Grant A. Ross and Wilson's anatomy and physiology in health and illness, 9th edn. Edinburgh: Churchill Livingstone; 2000.

Wells M. Urinalysis. Prof Nurse 1997; 13 (suppl 2): S11–13.

Willis J. IV therapy: an expanding role with implications for education. Nurs Times 1999; 85(25): 48–49.

9 Shock, systemic inflammatory response and multiple organ dysfunction

Sheila Adam

'I was doing the post-op observations and realised that something was not right; her skin was cool and sweaty and her pulse had gone up again. When I looked under the bedclothes I nearly died – the dressing and the bed were soaked with blood! She had to go back to theatre in the end. Thank goodness I decided to do her obs a bit early.'

(Student nurse)

THIS CHAPTER WILL HELP YOU

- Understand the term 'shock' and explain the physical manifestations of shock in patients

- Recognize shock in a patient you are caring for and respond appropriately

- Understand the patient experience during a period of shock and multisystem failure and identify their needs for comfort and support

- Describe the potential triggers of inflammatory response and multiple organ dysfunction

- Outline the principles and priorities of management of shock and multiple organ dysfunction

- Understand the consequences of shock and outline the process of systemic inflammatory response syndrome and multiple organ dysfunction syndrome

- Describe nursing interventions to promote patient comfort and prevent complications from shock.

KEYWORDS

Aerobic metabolism	Hypoxaemia
Anaerobic metabolism	Hypoxia
Anaphylactic shock	Ischaemia
Cardiogenic shock	Multiple organ dysfunction and failure
Hypovolaemia	Perfusion
Hypovolaemic shock	Shock

INTRODUCTION

Nurses have a key function in preventing, recognizing and initiating early management of shock. They are responsible for observing, monitoring and assessing their patients in order to recognize the changes associated with early shock, allowing prompt, potentially life-saving intervention. If shock is recognized and treated adequately, it is possible to prevent deterioration into multiple organ dysfunction. Recent research (McQuilland et al 1998, McGloin et al 1999) suggests that the quality of care on the ward and the timing of interventions can influence the patient's ability to survive a period of critical illness. It may also modify the patient's requirement for intensive care. Lundberg et al (1998) have shown that the mortality of patients who develop septic shock on the ward is 70%, compared with 39% for those who develop it in intensive care, despite the fact that patients on the ward are generally younger and less seriously ill.

Nurses are in a key position to detect and respond to early indications of deterioration in ward patients. They are also vital in intervening to improve patient comfort and the ability to respond to their illness, as well as in acting to prevent further complications. Nurses can also help patients and their family cope with the frightening and unexpected nature of a life-threatening situation by demonstrating a calm, competent and alert approach (Burfitt et al 1993) as well as ensuring that both patient and family are informed, comforted and reassured (Molter 1979, Leske 1991) (see Reflective Practice box 9.1).

DEFINING SHOCK

The physiological definition of shock is 'acute circulatory failure with inadequate or inappropriately distributed tissue perfusion resulting in generalized cellular hypoxia' (Hinds & Watson 1999). An increased understanding of cellular mechanisms has modified the original concept of shock, from purely a product of

153

9.1 Providing support

Think about how you would respond if a close friend were suddenly to become critically ill.

- What sort of support would you want from nursing and other staff?
- How would you expect them to respond to you?
- If you were required to support others, what would you see as potential obstacles to your being able to do so?

low blood flow to one of dysfunction affecting the ability of the cell to acquire adequate oxygen for its metabolic requirements. In order to fully understand what is happening in shock, it is useful to review the body's requirement for oxygen and the consequences of the oxygen supply to the cell being interrupted (see Ch. 20).

If delivery of oxygen to the cells of the body is interrupted, anaerobic rather than aerobic metabolism will take place. Anaerobic metabolism produces only two adenosine triphosphate (ATP) energy bonds, compared with aerobic metabolism which produces 38 ATP bonds. If the amount of energy produced is insufficient for the energy needs of the cells or anaerobic metabolism continues for a long period, the cells will die (see Fig. 9.1). If the cause of shock is not corrected, vital organ function will be impaired and multiple organ dysfunction syndrome will occur. Ultimately, if shock remains uncorrected the patient will die.

TYPES OF SHOCK

There are a number of causes of shock, but the final effect is always to reduce the ability of the cells to adequately acquire or possibly utilize oxygen.

HYPOVOLAEMIC SHOCK

Hypovolaemic shock is caused by loss of circulating blood volume. The loss can be either external, as in haemorrhage or burns, or internal, as in plasma loss through altered permeability of the blood vessels or leakage into body cavities such as the peritoneum (see Box 9.1).

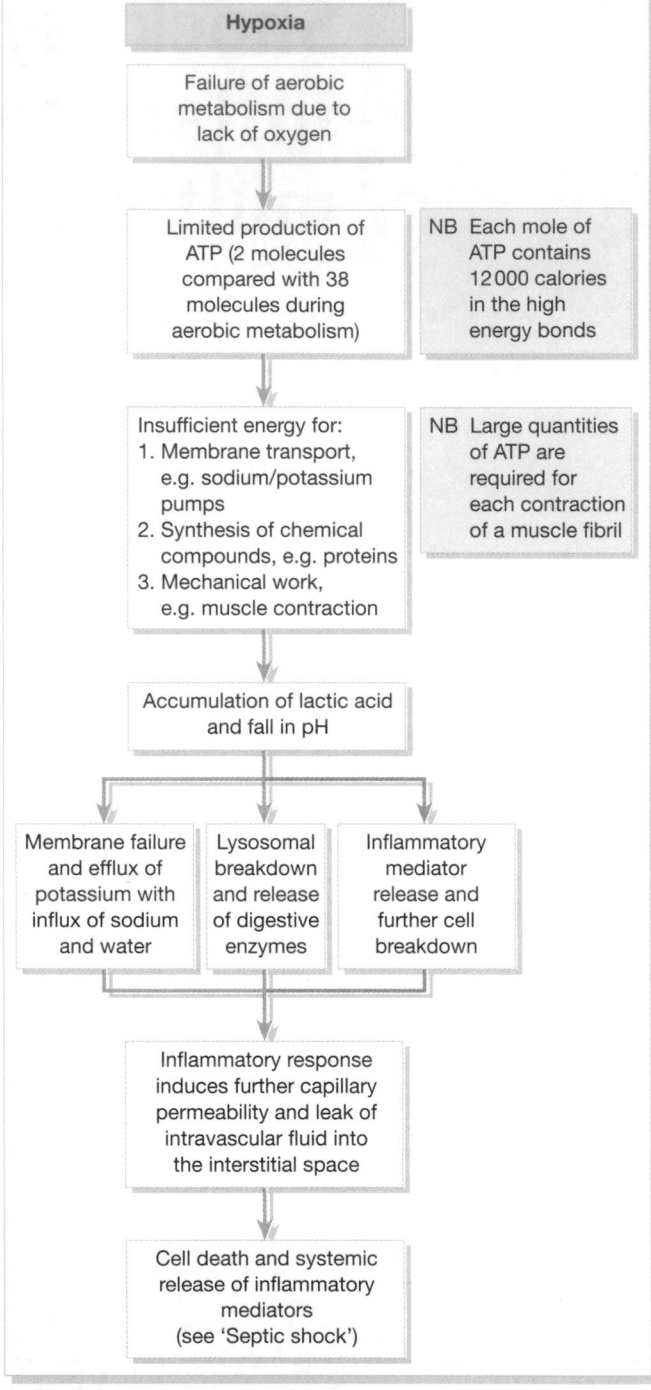

Figure 9.1 Effects of hypoxia on the cell.

Box 9.1 Causes of loss of circulating blood volume

External fluid loss
- Bleeding from trauma/wounds
- Vomiting/diarrhoea
- Burns
- Diabetes insipidus (inadequate secretion of antidiuretic hormone from the posterior pituitary gland – see Ch. 17)

Internal fluid loss
- Haemothorax – a collection of blood in the pleural space
- Retroperitoneal bleeding – bleeding into the space behind the peritoneum lining the back of the abdominal cavity
- Paralytic ileus/intestinal obstruction (see Ch. 22)
- Gross ascites – free fluid in the abdomen leaked as a result of high portal vein pressures in the liver from cardiac failure or hepatic obstruction

CARDIOGENIC SHOCK

Cardiogenic shock is caused by failure of the heart to pump an adequate volume of blood through the circulation. The failing pump produces a low cardiac output and this will induce the peripheral vasoconstriction associated with baroreceptor and renin–angiotensin–aldosterone responses (see p. 156 and Ch. 24). The vasoconstrictive response increases resistance to blood flow and increases the ventricular workload, thus adding to the cardiac failure. A degenerative spiral then ensues unless intervention occurs.

Causes of cardiogenic shock include acute myocardial infarction, valvular incompetence or stenosis, arrhythmias and intracardiac shunts (ventricular/atrial septal defects that allow blood to pass directly through the heart without entering the pulmonary circulation) as well as cardiomyopathies or myocarditis (see Ch. 19). Acute cardiogenic shock is associated with a mortality rate of between 70 and 80% (Col et al 1994).

DISTRIBUTIVE SHOCK

Distributive shock is caused by abnormalities of peripheral circulation, i.e. inappropriate vasodilatation of the capillary beds, thereby increasing the capacity of the system. This results in effective hypovolaemia because the volume of blood is distributed through a greatly increased systemic volume, resulting in inadequate venous return (Hinds & Watson 1999). Causes of distributive shock are anaphylaxis and sepsis.

Anaphylaxis

Anaphylaxis is derived from the Greek and means 'against protection'. It is a normal inflammatory response designed to render foreign substances inactive and to amplify the response to recruit other immunoresponsive cells. It involves a highly complex mechanism which, in true anaphylaxis, requires involvement of IgE immunoglobulin (Henderson 1998). This response becomes life-threatening when it is grossly exaggerated and produces generalized inflammatory responses. The principal effect producing the shocked state is the action of inflammatory mediators (substances released as part of the immune/inflammatory response), particularly histamine, on the vascular endothelium (the lining of the blood vessels). This causes greatly increased capillary permeability with immediate loss of intravascular fluid into the interstitial space.

Septic shock

Septic shock manifests as hypotension (systolic blood pressure < 90 mmHg or reduced by more than 40 mmHg from baseline without other cause), which is associated with infection and is unresponsive to fluid resuscitation. There are also indications of organ hypoperfusion such as oliguria (low urine output, < 0.5 mL/kg per hour) and altered mental state (Task Force of the American College of Critical Care Medicine 1999). The cause of the hypotension is vasodilatation of peripheral blood vessels, which is induced by the systemic inflammatory response to the infection and, in the later phase, to extravascular fluid losses due to alterations in capillary permeability. The term toxic shock has been used to apply to septic shock associated with the organism *Staphylococcus aureus* and was originally identified as a syndrome associated with tampon use during menstruation.

OBSTRUCTIVE SHOCK

Obstructive shock is caused by a central mechanical impediment (such as an embolus) to the flow of blood around the circulation. It causes increased resistance to blood flow and thus increased cardiac workload and produces a similar picture of hypotension although central venous pressure will be increased. Causes of obstructive shock include pulmonary embolus and cardiac tamponade (see Ch. 19).

SPINAL SHOCK

Spinal shock applies to all phenomena surrounding physiological or anatomical transection of the spinal cord that results in temporary loss or depression of spinal reflex activity below the level of the lesion (Atkinson & Atkinson 1996). This produces loss of peripheral sympathetic tone (the neural signals maintaining the level of constriction of the capillaries – see p. 156), diminished venous return and venous pooling with varying degrees of involvement in other circulatory venous reservoirs (such as the gastrointestinal blood vessels) depending on the level of the spinal injury. Reflexes will return in time, but those deriving directly from the area of injury may not.

NEUROGENIC SHOCK

Neurogenic shock is caused by sudden cessation of sympathetic impulses from the central nervous system to the peripheral vascular system. The result is similar to spinal shock as there is loss of sympathetic tone and diminished venous return due to venous pooling of blood. However, this is usually short-lived. This is occasionally seen with epidural analgesia where block of the pain receptors also causes block of the sympathetic impulses (Anderson 1999).

THE STAGES OF SHOCK

Compensated shock

Compensated shock is seen when the body's normal physiological responses are able to cope with the reduction in circulating blood volume, usually until about 750 mL or 15% of total blood volume has been lost. Providing further loss of volume does not occur, the compensatory mechanisms described below will cope until the circulating blood volume is restored.

Progressive shock

Further sustained loss of circulating blood volume will result in damage to vital organs and their ability to compensate for or recover from the effects of poor perfusion and ischaemia begins to fail. This damage to vital organs and the consequent multiple organ dysfunction then becomes self-perpetuating even if the initial cause of shock is corrected. The patient will require prolonged organ support and intensive care (see Ch. 31) in order to survive.

Irreversible shock

When damage sustained by vital organs is so severe and comprehensive that no support or treatment will induce recovery, a descending spiral of abnormal physiology and cell death will occur. The patient will die in spite of all therapeutic intervention.

PATHOPHYSIOLOGICAL EFFECTS OF SHOCK

Shock will primarily affect the cardiovascular, respiratory and renal systems but will have secondary effects on many others. It is these responses that provide the compensatory mechanisms in compensated shock.

CARDIOVASCULAR SYSTEM

The initial phase common to all types of shock is the reduction in circulating blood volume for whatever reason. This will result in alterations in the flow of blood to the tissues but may not initially result in a decreased blood pressure. This is because the body has a number of compensatory mechanisms which will maintain blood pressure at first. The initial cardiovascular response to a low circulating blood volume will be to attempt to maintain pressure at the expense of blood flow to less vital tissues such as the skin and the gastrointestinal tract. Thus the patient appears pale, with cold peripheries (limbs) which may also appear mottled.

Regulation of blood flow

The main regulators of blood flow to the different tissues are the arterioles and their smooth muscle walls respond to two regulatory stimuli.

Autoregulation

This is a response to the local requirements of tissues when oxygen or nutrient supply falls below need or exceeds demand. Matching of blood flow to tissue requirements is stimulated by oxygen need (except in the brain and the kidney). Thus blood flow increases to tissues with increased oxygen uptake, e.g. the muscles during exercise.

Autonomic signals

The sympathetic nerves supply a stream of signals to the arterioles, veins and arteries moderating the state of vasoconstriction. In the hypovolaemic state, these signals will increase, thus increasing the level of vasoconstriction and overriding the autoregulation associated with oxygen lack.

Maintenance of blood pressure

There are three normal regulatory mechanisms, as described below.

Neural control of contractility and vasoconstriction and the baroreceptor feedback mechanism

Central neural control of blood pressure occurs from the vasomotor centre (VMC) in the brain stem. This is regulated mainly via the sympathetic nervous system. Increased signals cause vasoconstriction of the arterioles, increased heart rate and increased contractility of the heart. Decreased signals cause vasodilatation and decreased heart rate and contractility.

Receptors sensitive to the degree of stretch (baroreceptors) are located in the vessel wall of the aortic arch and carotid sinus. They send signals which inhibit the sympathetic outflow of the

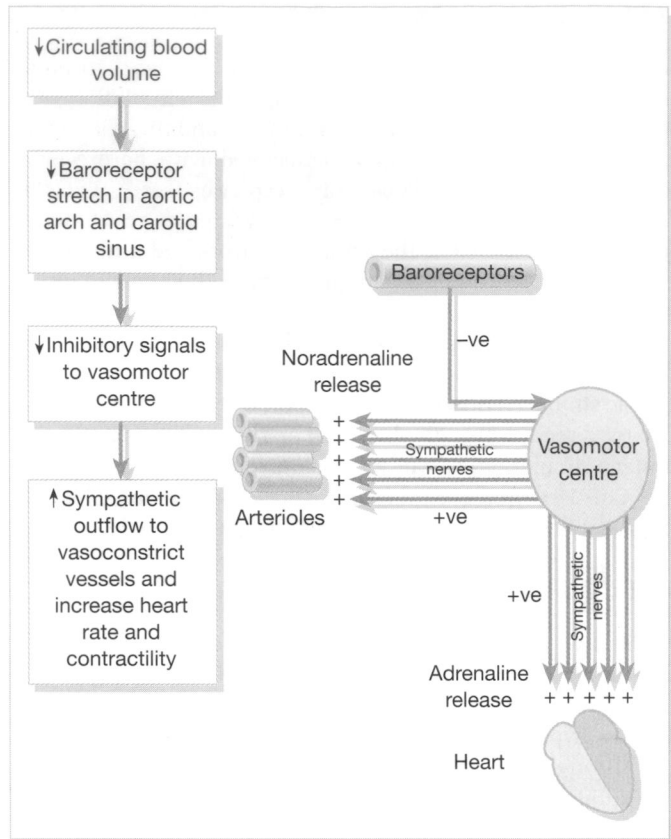

Figure 9.2 Normal physiological response to decreased circulating blood volume.

VMC. When blood pressure falls, the degree of stretch on the wall is reduced and the receptors decrease their inhibitory signals to the VMC. This results in increased sympathetic effect, i.e. vasoconstriction, increased heart rate and contractility.

Increased sympathetic stimulation induces adrenaline (epinephrine) and noradrenaline (norepinephrine) release from the adrenal medulla. Adrenaline will directly affect myocardial rate and contractility, resulting in increased cardiac output. Noradrenaline will induce vasoconstriction (see Fig. 9.2).

Capillary fluid shift

This mechanism for maintaining circulating blood volume depends on the changes in hydrostatic pressure associated with the systemic blood pressure in the capillaries. If systemic blood pressure falls, capillary hydrostatic pressure will also fall, resulting in a decreased pressure counteracting the pressure exerted by plasma proteins (oncotic pressure) which retains fluid in the capillaries (see Ch. 8). This will result in a net fluid attraction across the capillary wall by osmosis from the interstitial space into the capillaries. The interstitial space will therefore become relatively fluid-depleted.

Renal excretory and hormonal mechanisms

The renin–angiotensin–aldosterone (RAA) system will also respond to falls in blood pressure which reduce renal perfusion (see Ch. 24). Angiotensin II (a hormone produced by this system) is a potent vasoconstrictor which increases blood pressure. It stimulates the adrenal cortex to secrete aldosterone, which acts on the distal tubules and collecting ducts of the kidney to increase reabsorption of sodium and water. This will increase retention of fluid and result in a decreased urine output. The posterior pituitary gland will also release antidiuretic hormone, which stimulates an increase in renal water reabsorption as well. Adrenaline (epinephrine) will stimulate the anterior pituitary gland to release adrenocorticotrophic hormone (ACTH) which will act on the adrenal cortex to release glucocorticoids (hydrocortisone) and mineralocorticoids, stimulating further release of aldosterone.

RESPIRATORY SYSTEM

The respiratory physiological response will occur at two levels, with a tissue hypoxia response at capillary level and a more generalized response to hypoxaemia (low blood oxygen) causing an increase in respiratory rate and depth, tachycardia and peripheral cyanosis.

Hypoxia

Hypoxia is a lack of oxygen for energy production for cellular work. Low levels of circulating blood volume will produce a hypoxic state in many tissues and the normal response to tissue hypoxia is to increase blood flow to these areas. However, in shock this may be insufficient to overcome the intense vasoconstriction in the peripheral and gastrointestinal (splanchnic) circulation, which is a response to hypovolaemia (see above) and hypoxia will continue.

The low circulating blood volume will also affect blood flow to the lungs directly, resulting in an imbalance between ventilation and perfusion in the alveoli known as ventilation/perfusion (V/Q) mismatch (see Ch. 20). Gas exchange will be decreased and blood oxygen levels will reduce. Low blood oxygen levels will stimulate the chemoreceptors in the carotid arteries and aortic arch to increase ventilatory effort. Low blood pressure will also stimulate an increased ventilatory rate via the same baroreceptors that trigger an increased heart rate, contractility and vasoconstriction. Patients will therefore increase their rate and depth of breathing (hyperventilation) and may appear distressed and short of breath.

Acidosis

Lack of oxygen will cause anaerobic metabolism to occur in the cells and this will result in a build-up of lactic acid which cannot be broken down unless there is aerobic metabolism (see Ch. 8). The increase in lactic acid means an increase in hydrogen ions in the body and thus a metabolic acidosis will occur. Initial compensation for this will be by increased rate and depth of breathing to reduce carbon dioxide levels (see Ch. 20) and increasing bicarbonate availability to neutralize the hydrogen ions. Renal mechanisms of acid–base balance will compensate in the longer term as long as renal function is still adequate (see Ch. 24).

RENAL SYSTEM

Production of urine by the kidneys depends on a relatively high renal capillary perfusion pressure to support glomerular filtration. Renal autoregulation will maintain capillary perfusion pressure if the mean arterial pressure (MAP) drops below 80 mmHg. When the MAP falls below 80 mmHg, the renal blood flow starts to decrease, but dilatation of the efferent arterioles will ensure that this does not affect perfusion pressure. If perfusion pressure continues to fall, the renin–angiotensin–aldosterone (RAA) mechanism is activated (see above) and post-glomerular vasoconstriction occurs.

The decrease in renal perfusion and glomerular filtration will increase reabsorption of sodium and water by the proximal tubules, allowing circulating blood volume to increase. Urine output will therefore decrease to a minimum and the patient will become oliguric (urine output < 0.5 mL/kg per hour).

DECOMPENSATED SHOCK

If shock has remained undetected, or inadequately managed then decompensation will rapidly occur. This is often the point when patients will be referred to intensive care.

Cardiovascular system

If the compensatory mechanisms fail to correct the low blood pressure and/or hypoperfusion then a degenerating spiral will occur. The switch to anaerobic metabolism in poorly perfused tissues will lead to a build-up of lactic acid, energy production will be insufficient for normal cell processes (maintenance of sodium pump, cell membrane function, etc.) and the cells will die, releasing lysosomal enzymes which will damage surrounding tissues.

Respiratory system

The hypoxia associated with poor perfusion will induce increased respiration and the patient will appear breathless and tachypnoeic. Cyanosis will increase and may be compounded by pulmonary oedema from increased capillary permeability. Fluid accumulates in the interstitium, and neutrophils adhere to the capillary endothelium resulting in poor perfusion and gas exchange (shunt). Alterations in conscious level will also affect the ability of patients to protect their airway, which may increase the respiratory difficulties. If high-flow, high-concentration oxygen therapy is insufficient, the patient will rapidly require intubation and ventilation (see Ch. 31).

Renal system

The continuation of poor renal perfusion means that the tubular cells themselves will become starved of oxygen. Tubular cells are very vulnerable to ischaemia and hypoxia as they have very little oxygen reserve. They will therefore quickly become damaged or die, leading to acute renal failure as a result of acute tubular necrosis. Unless the circulating blood volume is increased and renal perfusion improved, irreversible damage will result and the acute renal failure will not resolve.

SHOCK, THE SYSTEMIC INFLAMMATORY RESPONSE AND MULTIPLE ORGAN DYSFUNCTION

A systemic inflammatory response syndrome (SIRS) is invoked by a number of triggers (see Box 9.2), but the common feature of underlying pathophysiology is decreased organ perfusion. The

Box 9.2 Triggers of the systemic inflammatory response syndrome (SIRS)

- Trauma
- Pancreatitis
- Major burns
- Major surgical procedures
- Infection
- Haemorrhage/major blood transfusion
- Ischaemic tissue
- Periods of inadequate tissue perfusion

Box 9.3 Defining criteria for systemic inflammatory response syndrome and septic shock

Systemic inflammatory response syndrome (SIRS) is manifested by two or more of the following conditions:

- Temperature > 38°C
- Heart rate > 90 beats/min
- Respiratory rate > 20 breaths/min or hyperventilation with a Pa_{CO_2} < 4.3 kPa (32 mmHg)
- White blood cells > 12×10^9/L or < 4×10^9/L or 10% immature neutrophils

Definition of septic shock (American College of Chest Physicians/Society of Critical Care Medicine 1992)

Sepsis-induced hypotension (systolic BP < 90 mmHg or reduced by > 40 mmHg from baseline without other cause) which is unresponsive to fluid resuscitation with manifestations of hypoperfusion such as oliguria, altered mental state, etc.

term SIRS has replaced non-specific and somewhat misleading older terms such as sepsis and septicaemia. The terms sepsis and septic shock now refer exclusively to an infective cause of SIRS. SIRS is defined by a collection of physiological criteria (see Box 9.3) which are broad in order to cover the range of the syndrome but which require considerable further assessment and monitoring of the patient in order to confirm any diagnosis.

When SIRS is triggered, any organ may be affected by the generalized inflammatory response, even those not directly involved in the trigger.

PATHOPHYSIOLOGY OF SIRS

The triggers associated with SIRS initiate a common pathway of response, i.e. the inflammatory/immune response, resulting in the release of inflammatory mediators.

The inflammatory/immune response

This is a series of complex, interactive pathways which would normally be subject to extensive inhibitory regulators. These inhibitory systems may fail once generalized activation has occurred (see Fig. 9.3). This can follow a period of hypoperfusion or shock. Initial immune responses designed to protect the body trigger plasma enzyme cascades such as complement, coagulation and kallikrein/kinin. These cascades produce proteins which induce further inflammatory responses, activate phagocytic cells, prepare foreign particles (antigens or organisms) for binding to phagocytic cells and cause rupture of some target cell membranes.

Cellular responses from macrophages, neutrophils and lymphocytes as well as mast cells, platelets and vascular endothelium

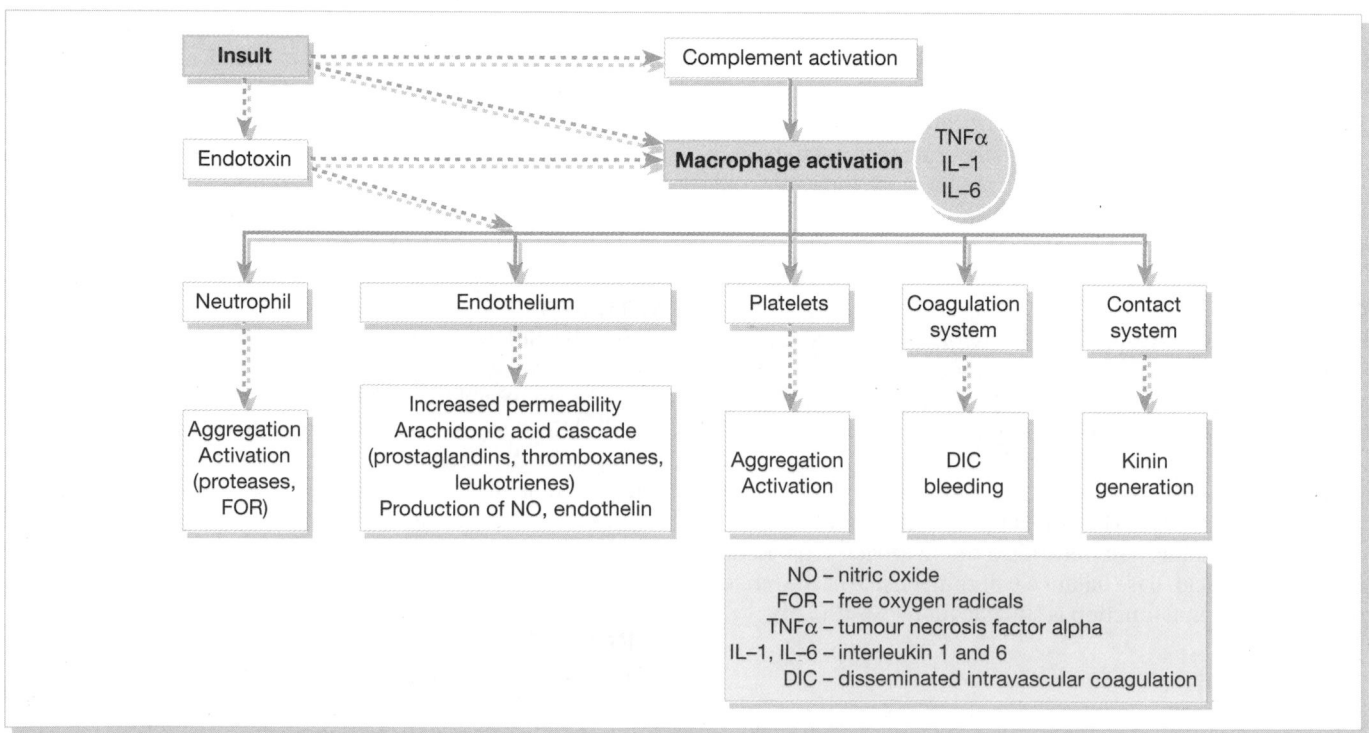

Figure 9.3 The inflammatory response. (Reproduced from Adam & Osborne 1997, *Critical Care Nursing: the Science and Practice* by permission of Oxford University Press.)

all act to increase the inflammatory response by releasing inflammatory mediators. These highly reactive molecules have a profound effect on the body, the vascular endothelium and the cells of the tissues themselves. Three major pathological changes occur as a result, as described below.

Maldistribution of circulating blood volume

The inflammatory mediators induce capillary permeability and vasodilatation causing movement of intravascular fluid into the interstitial space. White cell clumping and platelet aggregation cause obstruction of the vascular flow and normal peripheral vascular autoregulation of flow is disrupted. This results in shunting of blood around the damaged tissues and further hypoxia.

Imbalance of supply and demand

Available oxygen supply does not always seem to be utilized by the tissues and this is thought to be due to one of the following:

- mitochondrial dysfunction
- impaired oxygen diffusion
- maldistribution of circulating blood volume.

Catabolic alterations in metabolism

Inflammatory mediators have a profound effect on the metabolic response, inducing hypermetabolism (greatly increased metabolic rate), catabolism (breakdown of protein and fat stores), hyperglycaemia and gluconeogenesis (production of glucose from non-carbohydrate sources by the liver), alterations in zinc and trace element mobilization from the tissues. It is assumed that most of these alterations are to support tissue repair, immune cell proliferation and the immune response. The effect is one of accelerated malnutrition (see Ch. 11).

▶ **Nursing assessment**

One of the most important features of the nursing role in caring for patients at risk of shock is the ability to recognize indicators of the shocked state as early as possible (see Table 9.1). Early intervention can be vital in limiting the effects of shock and reducing the likelihood of organ dysfunction. Therefore the nurse should be able to recognize the early symptoms and ensure that medical staff are informed. Instigating appropriate supportive measures such as oxygen therapy as early as possible is also vital.

Table 9.1 Patients at risk of shock/systemic inflammatory response syndrome

Types of shock	Types of patient problem	See also Chapter
Hypovolaemic shock	Trauma victims	30
	History of gastrointestinal bleeding, e.g. oesophageal varices, gastric/duodenal ulcers	22
	Patients post-major surgery	29
	Burns victims	28
	Postpartum patients	
	Prolonged uncontrolled diarrhoea & vomiting	
Cardiogenic shock	Recent myocardial infarction	19
	Dilated cardiomyopathy	19
	Cardiac failure	19
	Arrhythmias	19
Distributive shock, septic shock	Immunosuppressed patients, e.g. receiving cytotoxic therapy, post-organ transplant	
	Pancreatitis	23
	Major overwhelming infection	13
	Presence of invasive vascular cannulae, particularly central venous cannulae	
Anaphylactic shock	Patients undergoing radiological investigation requiring contrast medium	
	Patients with known allergies, e.g. plaster, antibiotics	
	Patients receiving intravenous drugs for the first or second time	
Obstructive shock	Patients following cardiac surgery or thoracic trauma who may develop:	
	pericardial tamponade (accumulation of blood or fluid in the pericardial sac compressing the myocardium and restricting the ability of the heart to pump)	19
	Patients who develop pulmonary embolus	20
	Patients who have severe pulmonary hypertension	20
	Patients with constrictive pericarditis	19
Neurogenic shock and spinal shock	Patients with neurological disorders likely to affect sympathetic outflow from the vasomotor centre such as trauma to the brain stem, or spinal anaesthesia progressing up the spinal cord to the brain stem	14
	Patients following spinal cord trauma	

When assessing your patient, bear in mind that fit young patients may compensate for decreased circulating volume with little appearance of tachycardia, low blood pressure or oliguria until severely compromised.

PHYSICAL SIGNS

The patient in shock will exhibit the following clinical signs:

- the skin appears pallid or grey, there may be peripheral pallor or cyanosis (blue or mottled fingertips and toes)
- mucous membranes (in the mouth) will appear dusky or purple
- the patient's peripheries will feel cold and the level of peripheral shutdown can be monitored by feeling for the point where warmth returns in the legs or arms – this is due to vasoconstriction of blood vessels in the skin and peripheral circulation associated with angiotensin II and adrenaline (epinephrine) release
- the patient may be sweating and anxious or distressed – this is due to the increased levels of sympathetic stimulation and high amounts of circulating adrenaline (epinephrine).

Respiratory changes

The patient may be tachypnoeic, dyspnoeic or using accessory muscles in order to increase the vital capacity of each breath, and hyperventilating to reduce the levels of carbon dioxide (see Ch. 8). Accessory muscles of respiration include the shoulder and neck muscles in inspiration and the abdominal muscles to force expiration, and the patient will appear stiff at the neck with the shoulders moving up and down with each breath. The abdomen will move in and up with expiration. Respiration will appear laboured with nostrils flaring on inspiration. This is due to the hypoxic response and the need to try and compensate for the metabolic acidosis associated with poor tissue perfusion and anaerobic metabolism.

Cardiovascular changes

Heart rate will rise and blood pressure may fall, although initially it can be maintained by the compensatory responses described earlier. This is due to the need to maintain cardiac output in the presence of either a reduction in circulating blood volume (e.g. hypovolaemia) or an increased requirement for circulating blood volume (e.g. septic shock). In decompensated shock, the patient will be hypotensive and tachycardic. Confounding factors should be taken into consideration, such as the effects of beta-blockers (heart rate will remain slow) and anaemia, where there may be insufficient haemoglobin to produce the required 5 g of reduced haemoglobin needed to exhibit a blue tinge to the blood.

Renal changes

The patient may complain of thirst initially due to the loss of circulating blood. Urine output will decrease to less than 0.5 mL/kg per hour in a catheterized patient or less than 500 mL in 24 hours in an uncatheterized patient. This is due to the decrease in renal perfusion as a result of hypovolaemia.

9.2 Caring for patients in shock

Review your recent practice caring for patients at risk of shock. Could you identify those at risk, and which observations did you monitor for signs of shock?

Neurological changes

Decreased cerebral perfusion may result in confusion, loss of reasoning, agitation, inability to carry out routine tasks and irritability, and in extremis the patient will be unresponsive.

MONITORED SIGNS

Some of these techniques will only be available in specialist units with higher staff:patient ratios and monitoring facilities (see Reflective Practice box 9.2).

Heart rate

The pulse rate will be > 100 beats/min or will have increased by at least 40 beats/min. The radial pulse may feel weak and ectopic beats or irregular rhythms may be felt. Ectopic or premature beats are triggered by an area in the heart other than the normal pacemakers and occur before the next normal heartbeat would be expected. Patients complain that their heart has 'thumped' or 'skipped', which they may find distressing (see Ch. 19).

Electrocardiograph (ECG)

The patient will have a tachycardia (heart rate >100 beats/min) and there may be evidence of myocardial strain such as raised ST segments and frequent ventricular ectopic beats (see Ch. 19). In some patients, arrhythmias such as atrial fibrillation or supraventricular tachycardia may occur. These must be treated urgently, particularly if they are affecting the patient's blood pressure, and medical staff should be informed immediately.

Blood pressure

The blood pressure may initially remain within normal limits, but it should be monitored frequently if there are other signs of shock. Once compensatory mechanisms are overcome the blood pressure will fall. Non-invasive blood pressure measurement is less accurate in hypotensive patients and oscillometry (automated cuff pressure measurement) may be unable to detect low blood pressure.

Normal blood pressure measurement may only allow detection of the systolic pressure in hypotensive patients as the diastolic sound is inaudible. Ideally, direct pressure measurement via an indwelling arterial cannula is the method of choice for monitoring blood pressure in shocked patients. However, the potential risks of exsanguination from accidental disconnection or removal mean that the technique is only appropriate in specialist units with a higher ratio of staff to patients and monitoring facilities.

Temperature

Peripheral temperature, as a sign of peripheral perfusion, should be assessed and the gradient between that and the core temperature (tympanic membrane, oral, nasopharyngeal, rectal or axilla) can be monitored to indicate peripheral perfusion. However, this can be affected by other factors (such as ambient temperature) and cannot always be relied upon. If the patient is suffering from septic shock, the peripheries may feel warm due to the vasodilatation invoked by the inflammatory response (see above).

Peripheral arterial oxygen saturation (pulse oximetry)

Pulse oximetry monitors the oxygen saturation of the arterial blood. It measures the variations in light absorption across the vascular bed, associated with arterial pulsation. It can provide immediate detection of hypoxaemia. If the patient has poor peripheral perfusion, the pulse oximeter may be unable to detect the changes in light absorption and the low perfusion alarm will sound. Finger and toe probes can be problematic in the restless patient and the use of a central site for monitoring, such as the bridge of the nose, may be helpful in the shocked patient (Adam & Osborne 1997).

Normal levels of arterial oxygen saturation are 95–100%. If saturations are less than 92% when the patient is breathing air and less than 95% when the patient is breathing an oxygen mixture, medical staff should be informed.

Central venous pressure (CVP)

The patient in shock will have a decreased circulating blood volume and this can be monitored through a central venous catheter with the tip placed in the superior or inferior vena cava or the right atrium. The pressure in these central venous vessels will reflect the volume of circulating blood providing that:

- right ventricular function is normal
- the tricuspid (right atrioventricular) valve between the atrium and the ventricle is not leaking or stenosed
- pulmonary outflow from the right ventricle is unobstructed
- there is no external pressure on the heart as in pericardial tamponade (Adam & Osborne 1997).

The normal insertion points for CVP monitoring are the internal jugular vein or the subclavian vein (Anderson 1999). Normal CVP measurements are between 3 and 10 mmHg if the pressure is measured via an electronic transducer, or 2 and 7 cmH$_2$O if measured by a water manometer. A decreased circulating blood volume can result in a negative CVP reading.

The pressure must be measured at the same level as the right atrium of the heart. Thus, a device such as a spirit level or laser pointer is necessary to level the monitor to the correct point (see Fig. 9.4). The landmark used for this is the fourth intercostal space in the mid-axilla with the patient lying supine or at an angle of up to 30° from the horizontal (Potger & Elliott 1994). The CVP can be used to monitor the response to the infusion of fluid to ensure that the patient receives the optimum amount. For a more detailed explanation of CVP monitoring, see Edwards (2000).

Urine output

One of the most sensitive indicators of poor perfusion is the urine output. If the patient has a urinary catheter in place then output should be measured hourly. Normal output will be > 0.5 mL/kg per hour, which is 30–35 mL/h in a 60–70 kg

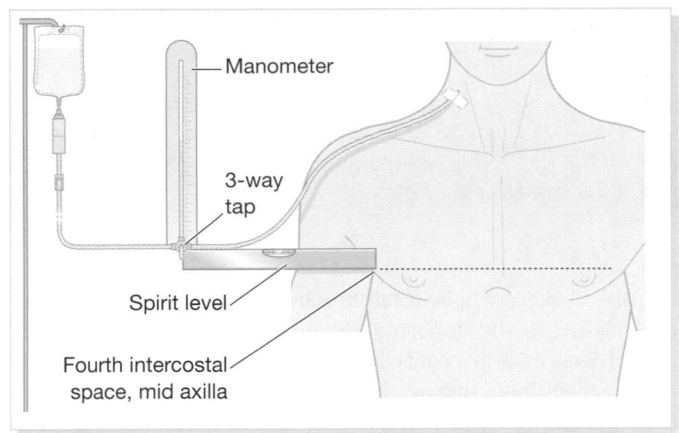

Figure 9.4 Central venous pressure measurement using a water manometer.

person. If there is no urinary catheter, accurate recording of urine output can still be very useful in assessing the patient's fluid status. In this case, the 60–70 kg patient should produce more than 240–280 mL of urine over a period of 8 hours.

If hypovolaemia is suspected but there are no clear physiological signs, urinary electrolytes can be measured. Providing renal function is not yet affected, the kidney will retain sodium in order to retain fluid (see Ch. 24) and therefore urinary sodium can give an indication of the hydration of the patient. Normal values of urinary sodium are 30–50 mmol/L, but if this falls below 20 mmol/L then the kidney is retaining water. Care must be taken that the patient has not received loop diuretics (e.g. furosemide [frusemide]) in the previous 24 hours as this will affect the ability of the kidney to conserve sodium and give a misleading result.

Arterial pressure monitoring and blood gases

Samples of arterial blood can be taken either by direct arterial puncture or from an indwelling arterial cannula. The indwelling cannula is attached to a high-pressure (300 mmHg) system allowing a continuous flush of heparinized saline through the cannula at 3 mL/h to prevent clotting. The high-pressure system includes a transducer (which converts pressure changes to an electrical trace on a monitor) allowing continuous monitoring of arterial pressure. These should only be used in specialist units such as high dependency, intensive care and coronary care units, as there are risks of exsanguination (severe blood loss) if there is undetected disconnection. Arterial lines should always be attached to a transducer and monitor with appropriate alarm settings to ensure that staff are alerted to any possible disconnection.

Arterial blood can be analysed to measure the partial pressure of oxygen (Pao_2), carbon dioxide ($Paco_2$), blood pH, and bicarbonate (HCO_3) and base excess (see Box 9.4), which reflect the buffering action of bicarbonate in the blood on hydrogen ions. Any increase in acidosis (e.g. the lactic acid produced in poor tissue perfusion during shock) will cause a reduction in available bicarbonate as it will be bound into buffering the extra hydrogen ions (see Ch. 8). In the early stages of compensated shock, the arterial blood gases may show little change other than a slight reduction in $Paco_2$ and bicarbonate/base excess. As the shock

---

Box 9.4 Normal values of arterial blood gases

- pH   7.35–7.45
- Pco_2 4.6–6.0 kPa
- Po_2 10.0–13.3 kPa
- HCO_3^- 22–26 mmol/L
- Base excess   –2 to +2

---

progresses, there will be a fall in Pao_2 and the pH will decrease towards 7.0 as the buffering responses to the increased levels of hydrogen ions are overwhelmed. The patient may continue to hyperventilate, thus reducing $Paco_2$ further, in an effort to compensate for the increasing metabolic acidosis. As decompensation sets in, acidosis will increase and the pH will decrease to < 7.2, the Pao_2 will drop further and the $Paco_2$ will rise, as the patient is no longer able to maintain compensatory hyperventilation.

Pulmonary artery catheters

In order to determine the cause of shock, it is sometimes necessary to insert a monitoring catheter into the pulmonary artery. The catheter (once known as a Swan–Ganz catheter) has a small balloon near the tip which, when inflated, allows measurement of the pressure in the pulmonary artery. This is known as the pulmonary artery occlusion or wedge pressure (PAOP/PAWP) and reflects the pressures on the left side of the heart, in particular the left ventricular pressure at the end of diastole. High pressures will indicate left ventricular failure and the shock is likely to be due to cardiac causes. If the pressure in the pulmonary artery is normal or low then the cause of shock is due to sepsis, hypovolaemia, etc. (see Table 9.2). Pulmonary artery catheters can also measure the cardiac output (the volume of blood expelled by the ventricles over 1 minute) which provides a useful measure of intravascular fluid status as well as myocardial function.

The pulmonary artery catheter also allows the measurement of cardiac output and the calculation of stroke volume, cardiac index, systemic vascular resistance and pulmonary vascular resistance. More detailed information is available in Adam & Osborne (1997).

Oesophageal Doppler

Doppler ultrasound can be used to measure cardiac output by monitoring blood flow through the aorta by placing the probe in the oesophagus. The oesophageal Doppler is used to monitor trends such as patient responses to fluid challenges and alterations in therapy.

Blood lactate levels

Lactate is produced during anaerobic metabolism and measurements of blood lactate levels can be used as an indicator of ischaemia (see Chs 8, 17 and 20). Lactate levels > 2 mmol/L reflect increased lactate production which is often associated with tissue hypoxia. However, there are other recognized causes of raised lactate levels, such as altered lactate metabolism, and these measurements should always be taken in clinical context.

Gastric tonometry

This is a method of monitoring regional (gastric) tissue perfusion. As gastrointestinal (splanchnic) blood flow is one of the earliest venous reservoirs to vasoconstrict in response to hypovolaemia, any change in gastric tissue perfusion should be reflected early in incipient shock (Sato et al 1998). A thin semipermeable silicone balloon on a fine-bore nasogastric tube is placed in the patient's stomach and filled with air. Carbon dioxide from the gastric mucosal cells equilibrates with the air inside the balloon and is monitored. Changes in these levels will reflect initial decreased perfusion and the patient's ensuing response to fluid volume resuscitation.

▶ Nursing management of shock

The principal aim of nursing (and medical) management is to restore oxygen delivery to the tissues and correct the underlying problem/cause of the shock (see Guidelines box 9.1). As with any other patient emergency, the order of priority will be airway, breathing and circulation. Immediate responses are determined by a swift assessment of the patient, ensuring a patent airway, supporting breathing and determining the circulatory status. If the patient has problems with any of these, an immediate call for assistance is essential.

ENSURING THE PATIENT HAS A PATENT AIRWAY

The patient's ability to breathe should be assessed by observing chest movement and listening for sounds of obstruction (gurgling, whistling and noisy inhalation and exhalation). In complete obstruction of the airway, there will be no sounds, no chest movement will be visible and the patient will quickly become cyanosed and unresponsive. Any mechanical obstruction must be cleared away either by suction – if it is sputum, vomit or fluids – or by a finger sweep if it is solid. If the obstruction is caused by the base of the tongue falling back to occlude the pharynx, the airway can be maintained by the jaw thrust or chin lift manoeuvre (see Ch. 19).

SUPPORTING BREATHING

If the airway is patent but breathing is compromised, the patient should be resuscitated with a manual inflation bag (Ambubag), with reservoir supplying 100% oxygen, and mask (see Ch. 19).

DETERMINING CIRCULATORY STATUS

If the patient has a pulse (palpated at the carotid or femoral artery), the heart rate and blood pressure should be checked

Table 9.2 Causes of shock and associated haemodynamic parameters

Cause	Cardiac output	Pulmonary artery wedge pressure
Hypovolaemia	Decreased	Decreased
Cardiogenic	Decreased	Increased or unchanged
Inflammatory	Increased	Decreased
Obstructive	Decreased	Increased or unchanged
Anaphylactic	Increased	Decreased

GUIDELINES

9.1 The patient in shock

- Oxygen therapy and airway management – to maintain circulating levels of oxygen in the blood at the level required by the patient
- Ensuring the appropriate type of oxygen mask is correctly placed with the right percentage of oxygen and correct gas flow (see Ch. 20)
- Positioning of patient to improve respiratory function – semi-recumbent for optimal matching of ventilation/perfusion (Field 2000)
- Reassurance of the patient to reduce anxiety – providing comfort, remaining with the patient where possible, providing sensory and procedural information (Suls & Wan 1989)
- Close/accurate monitoring of respiratory rate and oxygen saturation as well as other indicators of poor organ perfusion (conscious level, urine output, heart rate and blood pressure) should be maintained
- Alerting other staff – this is not a situation which can be managed by the nurse alone. The medical team should be informed as soon as there are indicators of shock – both compensated and decompensated
- Circulatory support – fluid therapy – to correct hypovolaemia and maintain cardiac output
- Ensuring the correct amount of intravenous fluid is delivered as fast as possible to the patient. Assess the response to each fluid 'challenge' using pulse rate and blood pressure as well as CVP where available
- Position the patient to aid venous return and assist cerebral perfusion (legs at the same level as the body; if hypotensive, lay the patient flat, or semi-recumbent if this is not tolerated)
- Circulatory support – vasoactive drugs, e.g. adrenaline (epinephrine), dobutamine – to maintain blood pressure. These may be required but are generally used in specialist units with continuous arterial pressure monitoring

and abnormalities (heart rate > 130 or < 55 beats/min, systolic BP < 90 mmHg) reported at once to either a senior colleague or to medical staff. If there is no pulse, a cardiac arrest call should be made and cardiopulmonary resuscitation commenced (see Ch. 19).

CORRECTING HYPOXAEMIA

If shock is present but the patient is maintaining airway and respiratory status, only oxygen therapy will be required. If there are problems maintaining the airway or respiratory function then intubation and mechanical ventilation may be necessary (see Ch. 20). Oxygen therapy should be administered via a high-flow air entrainment (Venturi effect) system so that accuracy of the oxygen percentage delivered is ensured. If the patient requires more than 60% oxygen, a reservoir bag will be necessary. Where possible, the oxygen should be humidified to counteract the drying effects of the gas on the respiratory mucosa.

Ideally, the response to oxygen therapy should be monitored using pulse oximetry or arterial blood gas analysis and patient requirements adjusted accordingly. In conjunction with increasing the oxygen supply, reduction in the tissue demand should also be supported. There are many nursing interventions that can assist with this goal and these are described in the following section.

Relieving anxiety and calming the patient

There is a clear physiological pathway between perception of an event as threatening or stressing and physical responses. Anxiety has been shown to activate the hypothalamic–pituitary–adrenal (HPA) axis resulting in the production of adrenaline (epinephrine) and noradrenaline (norepinephrine) as well as cortisol (Hibbert 2000) (see Ch. 6). This affects the cardiovascular, gastrointestinal and metabolic functions of the body, resulting in increased heart rate, increased blood pressure, increased oxygen consumption and other metabolic alterations such as increased blood glucose levels. This can also affect the patient's respiratory rate and distress associated with breathing (De Vito 1990).

It is therefore particularly important that patients with shock are not further compromised by the physical manifestations of acute anxiety. A calm environment and the presence of a nurse who appears competent have been shown to be important to patients (Burfitt et al 1993) and it is likely that this will reduce the levels of anxiety. From a meta-analysis of the effects of information on coping with stressful medical procedures and pain, Suls & Wan (1989) suggest that combined sensory (what the patient will feel) and procedural (what will happen to the patient) information is most useful. For example, the nurse should explain about the feel of the oxygen mask and the dryness of the gas flow as well as why it is needed, before placing it on the patient.

Ensuring adequate pain relief

Pain (like anxiety) is thought to stimulate the HPA axis, resulting in increased cortisol, adrenaline (epinephrine) and noradrenaline (norepinephrine) production. It is also likely to have an amplifying effect on the patient's anxiety and stress (Puntillo 1994). Therefore, assessment and intervention to alleviate the patient's pain are vital. In the past, nursing assessment of the level of pain experienced by patients has been inadequate (Seers 1987, Tittle & McMillan 1994); to deal with a patient's pain properly requires assessment, intervention and reassessment to ensure that the intervention has been adequate (see Ch. 7 for details of assessment tools). Opiate analgesia may be contraindicated if patients are hypovolaemic and/or hypotensive, as it is likely to decrease blood pressure due to its vasodilatory effects.

The mode of delivery of analgesia in the shocked patient may also need review as the decreased perfusion to the peripheries makes the absorption of intramuscular injections highly variable. Similarly, oral analgesia may not be well absorbed when gastrointestinal perfusion is decreased by the hypovolaemic response. The intravenous route is probably most effective, although great care will be required in monitoring blood pressure following administration. Alternative methods of managing pain should also be considered, such as 50% nitrous oxide (Entonox) inhalation (see Ch. 7 for further information).

EVIDENCE-BASED PRACTICE

9.1 The most effective method of treating fever in the critically ill

Studies have compared antipyretics with physical cooling and compared different types of physical cooling. Although sample sizes are very small, two studies in critically ill adults showed improved cooling in patients treated with both antipyretics (paracetamol) and physical cooling (cooling blankets, tepid sponging, ice packs) (Henker et al 1997, Poblete et al 1997). Care must be taken not to promote shivering, as oxygen consumption will be further increased rather than decreased (Manthous et al 1995). A study comparing temperature settings of cooling blankets in 89 patients found that cooling blanket temperatures of 18–29°C are just as effective as lower settings of 7–13°C in reducing body temperature and are more comfortable for patients (Caruso et al 1992). Innovative approaches such as wrapping extremities to warm peripheral skin sensors have shown a decrease in shivering time when reducing fever in oncology patients (Holtzclaw 1990).

Although limited evidence is available to support the use of physical cooling methods to reduce fever in combination with paracetamol, further large-scale clinical studies are required.

References
Caruso CC, Hadley BJ, Shukla R et al. Cooling effects and comfort of four cooling blanket temperatures in humans with fever. Nurs Res 1992; 41: 68–72.
Henker R. Evidence-based practice: fever-related interventions. Am J Crit Care 1999; 8: 481–487.
Holtzclaw BJ. Control of febrile shivering during amphotericin B therapy. Oncol Nurs Forum 1990; 17: 521–524.
Manthous CA, Hall JB, Olson D et al. Effect of cooling on oxygen consumption in febrile critically ill patients. Am J Resp Crit Care Med 1995; 151: 10–14.
Poblete B, Romand JA, Pichard C et al. Metabolic effects of iv propacetamol, metamizol or external cooling in critically ill febrile sedated patients. Br J Anaesth 1997; 78: 123–127.

Reducing body temperature

Pyrexia increases a patient's metabolic rate by 13% for each 1°C rise (Holtzclaw 1992). It will therefore increase the requirements for oxygen to fuel the metabolic processes and increase the level of tissue hypoxia. Vigorous shivering can increase a patient's energy expenditure (and therefore need for oxygen) by up to 400% (Holtzclaw 1992). If body temperature can be reduced without shivering, this may be beneficial for the patient who is shocked. The most effective method is a combination of antipyretic medication, e.g. paracetamol (acetaminophen) and cooling blankets (see Evidence-based Practice box 9.1).

Supporting the patient's family

The patient's family members will be experiencing feelings of severe anxiety, fear and distress. They will need support, comfort, information and explanation (Leske 1991) and, where possible,

 EVIDENCE-BASED PRACTICE

9.2 Family needs in the critical care environment

There is a moderate body of evidence identifying the needs of families with a critically ill relative. Most of the research highlights the importance of communication and permission to be present at the patient's bedside. However, there are still places where visiting times are restricted and families are discouraged from attending.

A meta-analysis of 32 papers using the Molter family needs inventory was carried out by Leske (1991). It identified five common factors:

- the need for support
- the need for comfort
- the need for information about the patient
- the need for proximity to the patient
- the need for assurance.

Reference
Leske J. Internal psychometric properties of the critical care family needs inventory. Heart & Lung 1991; 20: 236–244.

should be allowed access to the patient and repeated information regarding progress, interventions and plans (see Evidence-based Practice box 9.2). This is time-consuming and may be best given by other members of the nursing team to allow the nurse at the bedside to concentrate on the patient. Support workers such as counsellors, chaplains and voluntary workers trained to work with relatives can be invaluable in meeting some of these needs.

CORRECTING HYPOVOLAEMIA

Optimization of the intravascular fluid volume is vital in patients with reduced perfusion, but care must be taken with those in cardiac failure or cardiogenic shock. Intravascular fluid volume must be restored to the level appropriate for optimal cardiac function and oxygen delivery. Ideally, this should be monitored by oesophageal Doppler or pulmonary artery catheter, but at the very least CVP measurement should be used to monitor the patient's response.

Choice of fluids for correcting hypovolaemia

The type of fluid used to correct hypovolaemia is usually an artificial plasma substitute or human albumin solution (known collectively as colloids). Blood may be used depending on the cause of the hypovolaemia and the haemoglobin level (Dreger 1998). Bleeding, whether internal or external, will result in a fall in haemoglobin levels which must be corrected by transfusion.

Current recommendations suggest using blood to maintain a haemoglobin level of 8–10 g/dL in the critically ill unless there are cardiovascular limitations (Hebert et al 1999). Crystalloid fluids (Ringer's lactate, 0.9% saline, 5% dextrose, etc.) can be used, but due to their almost immediate distribution to the interstitial space, the volume required is two to four times that of colloid solutions and there may be considerable tissue and

Table 9.3 Distribution of colloid and crystalloid solutions

Type of fluid	Volume given	Intravascular	Interstitial	Intracellular
Colloid	1000 ml	1000 ml (approx.)	0 ml	0 ml
Saline	1000 ml	330 ml	670 ml	0 ml
5% glucose	1000 ml	125 ml	440 ml (approx.)	440 ml (approx.)

pulmonary oedema as a result. In order to increase circulating blood volume, colloid fluids which are retained in the intravascular compartment are preferable (see Table 9.3). This will depend on molecular size, ability to cross the capillary membrane and fluid composition.

Colloids

Gelatin solutions are considered appropriate for first-line fluid resuscitation. Where there is the likelihood of increased capillary permeability, e.g. in patients with acute respiratory distress syndrome or septic shock, hydroxyethyl starch (see below) is considered a more suitable alternative due to its larger average molecule size.

Gelatin solutions

Two solutions made from gelatin bases are currently available: Gelofusine and Haemaccel. The risk of contamination by bovine spongiform encephalitis (BSE) is very small due to stringent requirements by the European Medicine Evaluation Agency (Baron 2000). Their molecular weight is 30 000 Da and the solutions remain in plasma for 4–6 hours although this is considerably shortened by increased capillary permeability such as that occurring in SIRS (Weinbren & Soni 1997).

Hydroxyethyl starch (Hetastarch)

This is a modified starch compound in a 6% solution with physiological saline. It is composed of a range of molecule sizes with an average molecular weight of 450 000 Da. The larger molecules remain in the intravascular compartment and may exert an effect for up to 36 hours following administration. It is therefore extremely useful in situations such as SIRS where there is an increased capillary permeability (see p. 157) (Weinbren & Soni 1997).

Albumin

Human albumin solution (HAS) is an aqueous solution of either 4.5% or 20–25% proteins from either pooled plasma or normal human placentas. It is sterilized by filtration and heating at 60°C for 4 hours in order to prevent any risk of disease transmission. The ability to remain in the intravascular fluid compartment varies greatly and is greatly reduced where there is increased capillary permeability. Albumin 20–25% reportedly increases plasma volume by four to five times the volume of albumin infused. This is due to the greatly increased colloid oncotic pressure exerted by the plasma proteins in the intravascular space which draws fluid from the interstitial space (see Ch. 8 for further detail).

Dextran

Dextran is a solution of glucose polymers that is not routinely used as a colloid any longer because it affects clotting and interferes with cross-matching of blood. There are also reported incidents of mild to severe allergic reactions (Baron 2000).

Optimizing intravascular fluid volume

Optimizing intravascular fluid volume will correct preload and this is the most essential and commonly the most appropriate intervention in shock. The volume of blood ejected at each ventricular contraction (i.e. stroke volume) will depend on three factors: preload, afterload and contractility.

Preload

Preload refers to the degree of stretch of the myocardial fibres at the end of diastole and is directly related to the volume of blood filling the ventricle. Starling's law of the heart states that the force of myocardial contraction is determined by the length of muscle cell fibres. Larger volumes of blood will stretch the muscle cell fibres more, producing an increase in the force of contraction. This can be likened to stretching elastic; the more the elastic is stretched, the stronger the recoil when it is released. However, there is an optimal range of stretch, beyond which further increases in volume will reduce the force of contraction (see Fig. 9.5). The aim of fluid optimization is to reach the peak of contractility without overstepping the optimal range of stretch.

Afterload

Afterload is the resistance to outflow of blood that must be overcome by the ventricle during systole and is primarily related to vascular resistance. The more constricted the peripheral circulation, the higher is the resistance to outflow. Thus a patient who is in cardiac failure and who has greatly increased vasoconstriction of the peripheries will have a greatly increased afterload. If a vasodilator such as glyceryl trinitrate is given, the afterload (resistance to blood flow) will be reduced.

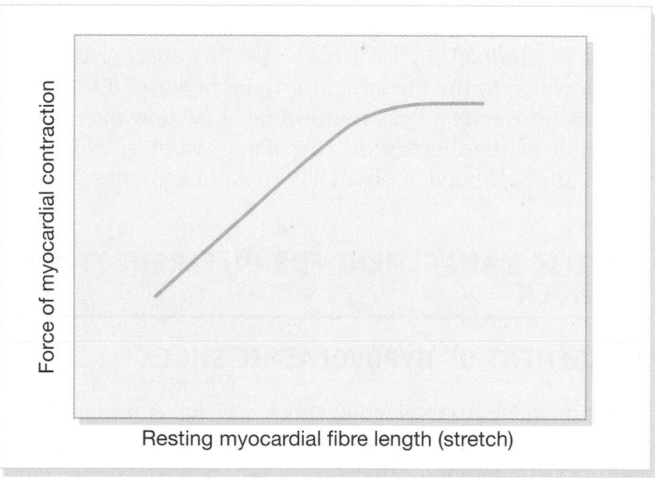

Figure 9.5 Graph to illustrate Starling's law of the heart.

Contractility

Contractility refers to the ability to shorten the myocardial muscle fibres without actually altering their length. This is controlled by neural stimuli and levels of circulating catecholamines (adrenaline [epinephrine] and noradrenaline [norepinephrine]) which alter the force of contraction. Preload and contractility will also be affected by the volume of blood returning to the heart (venous return).

Correcting hypotension with drug infusions

Optimization of the patient's intravascular fluid volume will frequently be sufficient to correct hypotension; however, if the cause is myocardial failure or a degree of intracellular acidosis then drugs which stimulate myocardial contractility (positive inotropes) may be required. If the hypotension is due to profound vasodilatation of the peripheral blood vessels, vasoconstrictive drugs may be required.

Positive inotropes

The most commonly used inotropes are dobutamine, adrenaline (epinephrine), dopexamine and dopamine. These drugs stimulate receptors located in the vascular smooth muscle, sinoatrial node, myocardium, and arterioles of heart, liver and skeletal muscle as well as the smooth muscle of the bronchioles.

There are two types of receptors: alpha and beta. Stimulation of alpha receptors primarily produces vasoconstriction of the vascular smooth muscle. Stimulation of beta receptors primarily produces vasodilatation and an increased heart rate and contractility. These drugs are given as infusions and (with the exception of dobutamine) require central venous access due to their profound vasoconstrictive effect in the peripheral blood vessels. The patient also requires continuous arterial blood pressure monitoring during the infusion of inotropes, in order to ensure responses to their effects are closely monitored.

Vasoconstrictive drugs

If the cause of hypotension is due to profound peripheral vasodilatation, as in septic shock, then vasoconstrictive agents may be required to maintain the peripheral vascular tone. The most commonly used drug in this situation is noradrenaline (norepinephrine) which has a predominant effect on alpha receptors in the peripheral blood vessels. This causes intense vasoconstriction and increases peripheral resistance, thus increasing blood pressure. The effect may decrease cardiac output due to the increase in afterload but it will have a positive effect on coronary blood flow due to the increase in arterial pressure during diastole. Hepatic, renal and gastrointestinal blood flow may also fall as a result of the increase in vascular resistance, which may increase the likelihood of organ failure in these organs.

SPECIFIC MANAGEMENT FOR DIFFERENT TYPES OF SHOCK

MANAGEMENT OF HYPOVOLAEMIC SHOCK

Management of hypovolaemic shock will focus principally on replacement of fluid volume and identification and management of the underlying cause. Oxygen therapy and optimization of cardiac function as well as prevention of complications (e.g.

arrhythmias) are also important. A central venous catheter should be inserted as soon as possible, to allow monitoring of the patient's response to the fluid delivered.

Intravenous fluids

Nurses are responsible for the delivery, monitoring and documentation of prescribed intravenous fluids. This is particularly vital in this situation, as the patient is highly dependent on accurate, immediate delivery of intravenous fluids, and assessment of response in order that the effects of hypovolaemia can be reversed. Fluid should be delivered as a series of aliquots (usually between 100 and 200 mL per aliquot) known as 'fluid challenges'. The patient's response to each aliquot should be monitored (see below). However, in extreme hypovolaemia it may be necessary simply to deliver a large volume of fluid without stopping to assess patient response. In this case, a pressure infusor bag will be needed to deliver fluid at very high flow rates.

CVP measurement

Monitoring of intravascular fluid volume should be carried out either by CVP measurement or by the use of oesophageal Doppler or pulmonary artery monitoring. If CVP measurements are used, the CVP should be measured after each aliquot of fluid. If a rise of greater than 2.5 cmH$_2$O (3 mmHg) occurs, no further fluid should be given and the CVP should be reassessed after 10 minutes. If the rise is sustained, the medical staff should be informed as further fluid may not be necessary. If the CVP has fallen again after 10 minutes then further fluid should be given. In hypovolaemia due to haemorrhage, large volumes of blood will be needed. Extra care should be taken with all the precautionary transfusion checks (see Ch. 18) as the need for speed of delivery can increase the likelihood of mistakes.

MANAGEMENT OF CARDIOGENIC SHOCK

Care must be taken with the optimization of fluid volume in patients with cardiogenic shock. The volume of fluid delivered with each 'fluid challenge' should be less than 100 mL and the patient's intravascular fluid status must be monitored with either an oesophageal Doppler or a pulmonary artery catheter. CVP measurements are not reliable as they may be falsely high if the patient has right-sided heart failure or pulmonary hypertension.

Maintaining blood pressure

Support of the blood pressure to maintain organ perfusion is essential but the patient may already have extreme vasoconstriction (greatly increased afterload) due to the compensatory response and it may be difficult to increase the pumping ability of the heart if the resistance to flow remains high. In the first instance, if the patient is hypotensive and vasoconstricted, inotropes with associated dilator activity (e.g. dobutamine, dopexamine, milrinone, enoximone) are appropriate, although some centres advocate the use of a peripheral vasodilator infusion such as glyceryl trinitrate (GTN) with adrenaline (epinephrine) to provide a combination of peripheral dilation and increased myocardial contractility. If the blood pressure is adequate and the fluid status has been optimized, afterload reduction (vasodilatation) may improve cardiac output using infusions such as GTN or in some cases diuretics such as furosemide (frusemide) which initially vasodilate and then increase diuresis.

Intra-aortic balloon pump

In circumstances where the above measures are ineffective, mechanical support of the heart may be necessary. The intra-aortic balloon pump (IABP) has been used to support patients with cardiogenic shock since 1967. It consists of a central catheter with a 25–40 mL polyurethane balloon (about 25 cm in length) which is inserted into the femoral artery and positioned in the descending aorta. The catheter is attached to a pump which inflates and deflates the balloon in response to ventricular contraction. The pump is triggered by the patient's ECG and inflation occurs during diastole.

The two main effects of the IABP are:

- reduction of ventricular workload by deflation of the balloon immediately prior to systole, which reduces resistance to blood flow
- increased coronary artery perfusion by inflation of the balloon, which increases pressure during diastole when coronary artery flow occurs.

Use of the IABP is a temporary measure until either cardiac surgery or myocardial recovery takes place.

MANAGEMENT OF ANAPHYLACTIC SHOCK

There may be physical signs associated with the cause of the anaphylactic response, e.g. an urticarial rash associated with contact with the cause, or angio-oedema (facial swelling) associated with ingestion of the allergen. The principal feature of management of anaphylaxis is the administration of adrenaline (epinephrine) which is effective for bronchospasm, angio-oedema and hypotension. It will induce bronchodilation, reduce the swelling associated with angio-oedema (facial swelling) and laryngeal obstruction, and vasoconstrict the peripheral blood vessels, restoring blood pressure (Henderson 1998). Patients may alert the nurse to their incipient anaphylaxis when they experience feelings of 'impending doom'. They can also exhibit profound distress associated with the onset of anaphylaxis, which requires comfort and support as well as management of the emergency.

Any drugs which have been administered immediately prior to the anaphylactic response should be suspected as the cause of the anaphylaxis and discontinued. Adrenaline (epinephrine) can be administered intramuscularly or subcutaneously, or, where the patient is in extremis, intravenously. Due to the powerful nature of the immediate response to intravenous adrenaline, this should be given with extreme caution by appropriately trained staff.

Colloid should be given as the fluid of choice for fluid resuscitation. The greatly increased capillary permeability (see p. 156) means that many more litres of crystalloid may be required to produce an adequate response. Antihistamines (e.g. chlorphenamine [chlorpheniramine]) are not always useful in anaphylactic shock, although some patients have responded to their use when other treatments have failed. They are principally of use as a preventative measure or in the early stages of an anaphylactic response. Corticosteroids (e.g. hydrocortisone) have not been shown to be of therapeutic benefit in anaphylactic shock. However, where bronchospasm continues, they may be useful.

MANAGEMENT OF SEPTIC SHOCK

Once again, nursing and medical interventions focus on maintaining oxygenation and circulation.

Supporting haemodynamic status

The cardiovascular effects of sepsis are vasodilatation, a relatively high cardiac output and a low blood pressure. These are managed by the correction of hypovolaemia and vasoconstriction using noradrenaline (norepinephrine) in order to maintain blood pressure. There may be some myocardial depression from the circulating inflammatory mediators and care must be taken not to over-constrict the peripheral circulation and increase the cardiac workload by increasing resistance to flow.

Reducing oxygen demands

Reduction of the demand for oxygen may also be accomplished by supporting the patient on mechanical ventilation (see Ch. 31). This will reduce the work associated with breathing (tachypnoeic patients use a lot of energy and oxygen) and help to improve the level of oxygen in the blood. Sedation and other methods of relieving anxiety will also reduce oxygen demand, but care is necessary as they may also reduce blood pressure.

Managing hyperglycaemia

Hyperglycaemia (high blood sugar), which occurs as a response to high circulating adrenaline (epinephrine) levels and a resistance to normal levels of insulin, may need treatment with insulin.

Treating and preventing infection

It is important to find and treat the source of infection so that the trigger for sepsis is removed. This is achieved through microbiological screening (sending samples for culture and antibiotic sensitivity), diagnostic testing such as echocardiography to look for endocarditis, and physical examination for foci such as abscesses. Prevention of secondary infection is vital and patients must be protected from cross-infection. Intravenous cannulae sites must be regularly inspected and changed where there are signs of infection such as reddening, oedema and pain (Elliott et al 1994).

MULTIPLE ORGAN DYSFUNCTION

MANIFESTATIONS

Multiple organ dysfunction is a process of progressive physiological failure of several interdependent organ systems (Smith & Bihari 1997). This develops either as a result of a systemic inflammatory response or following a direct episode of tissue injury (such as ischaemia) affecting a number of different organ systems simultaneously. Some organs, such as the kidneys, are more vulnerable to injury than others. The underlying physiology is decreased organ perfusion and will occur after an episode of shock if perfusion is not restored in time to prevent damage.

Treatment depends on identification and correction of the cause accompanied by support of the failing organs. Initially, following haemodynamic stabilization, any injuries are actively treated, which includes removal of necrotic tissue, debriding burn eschar (see Ch. 28) and stabilizing fractures (see Ch. 27). If this is not done, these injuries will remain a focus of the inflammatory response. Blood, urine, sputum and other cultures appropriate to the patient's condition should be taken to attempt identification of any infective source. Drainage of any infective focus such as an abscess should be carried out and antibiotics should be prescribed, either as a broad spectrum cover appropriate to the patient's condition or according to culture sensitivities.

Renal failure

Renal failure may occur at the time of poor tissue perfusion, as a result of direct damage, or at a later stage following the release of inflammatory mediators and toxins (see p. 157). Oliguria, rising creatinine and urea levels, as well as failure to control plasma potassium and blood pH, are all indicators of renal failure. Initial management will concentrate on restoring renal perfusion, but if this is too late then renal support with haemofiltration and haemodiafiltration may be necessary.

Haemofiltration is a continuous form of renal dialysis through a double-lumen venous cannula. Blood is pumped from the patient at a rate of 100–200 mL/min through a semi-permeable membrane (filter) which removes fluid and solutes, e.g. urea, potassium and creatinine. A physiologically compatible replacement fluid is then added to the blood before it is returned to the patient. For further information, see Chapter 24.

Acute respiratory distress syndrome (ARDS)

This is the term for the respiratory system involvement in multiple organ dysfunction syndrome. The patient usually shows evidence of respiratory failure (dyspnoea, tachypnoea, tachycardia and agitation) and arterial blood gases reveal a low Pao_2 (< 8.0 kPa) when the patient is breathing air (Brandstetter et al 1997). There may also be a high $Paco_2$ (> 6.5 kPa) and a pH of less than 7.25 in the absence of primary metabolic acidosis, such as diabetic ketoacidosis (see Ch. 17).

The chest X-ray will show diffuse fluffy white shadowing and gas exchange will be poor. On auscultation, the lungs will sound clear or there may be fine crackles or wheezes associated with alveolar fluid. The patient will require increasing inspired oxygen and then either continuous positive airway pressure support (CPAP), non-invasive positive pressure ventilation (NIPPV) or pressure-controlled mechanical ventilation (PCMV) (see Ch. 31).

Disseminated intravascular coagulation

Disseminated intravascular coagulation (DIC) is a pathological over-stimulation of normal coagulation occurring as a result of platelet activation and inflammatory mediator, e.g. tumour necrosis factor (TNF), production. It causes microvascular thrombi and bleeding. The bleeding occurs because the intravascular thrombi deplete normal stores of clotting factors and activate the fibrinolytic system, thus interfering with normal clotting mechanisms (see Ch. 18).

The patient will develop petechiae (small haemorrhagic spots under the skin or mucous membrane), purpura (extravasation of blood from the capillaries into the skin or mucous membranes), bruising or haematomas and there may be bleeding from the gums and mucous membranes. There may also be oozing from cannulae or wound sites. The diagnosis is made from measurement of fibrin degradation products and D-dimer

(one fraction of the disrupted fibrin) levels. There is no treatment other than supportive measures, including blood and clotting factor transfusion and early resolution of the cause.

Gastrointestinal dysfunction

Effects on gastrointestinal organs are frequently more prolonged due to the hypoperfusion associated with early compensatory vasoconstriction of the gastrointestinal blood supply. The integrity of the gut mucosa may be affected, allowing translocation of organisms from the gut to the blood (Adam 1994, Lipman 1995). The liver and pancreas may develop dysfunction resulting in deranged carbohydrate, protein and lipid metabolism as well as dysfunctional immune response, protein synthesis and impairment of detoxification processes in the liver. Patients may develop stress ulceration, pancreatitis, and symptoms of liver failure such as coagulopathy, encephalopathy and raised bilirubin levels (Marshall 1996).

Cardiovascular dysfunction

The heart may be directly affected by circulating inflammatory mediators and this may reduce the ability to respond to increased demands (Ognibene et al 1988). There is a decrease in the ventricular ejection accompanied by ventricular dilatation and response to a fluid challenge may show increased ventricular wall resistance, resulting in a rise in pressures but little improvement in function.

Neurological dysfunction

Decreased levels of consciousness ranging from confusion to coma are seen and may continue even after the patient is stabilized and in the recovery phase. There may be septic encephalopathy (altered conscious level with abnormal EEG changes), critical illness neuropathy (profound weakness and muscle wasting) and neuroendocrine failure (hypoadrenal response, disturbances in blood glucose, low triiodothyronine, etc.) (Sprung et al 1990).

▶ Nursing and medical management

Multiple organ failure has a profound effect on the patient with a very poor outcome. Mortality rates increase with the number of organs affected and the duration of organ failure (Smith & Bihari 1997). A recent review of outcome shows that hospital mortality rates for failure of three or more organs have improved to 84% in the USA (Zimmerman et al 1996), although hospital mortality for two or more organ failures has altered only slightly at 62.5% (see Ethical Issues box 9.1). As a result, the importance of prevention cannot be over-emphasized and should remain the main aim of caring for patients at risk of developing shock and consequent multiple organ failure.

Further interventions are designed to support the failing organs and prevent further dysfunction.

Metabolic support

Abnormal levels of pH, electrolytes, blood glucose, body temperature, etc. should be corrected as quickly as possible. Where these are as a result of renal failure, renal replacement therapy (haemofiltration or haemodialysis) may be necessary to achieve this (see Ch. 24).

 **ETHICAL ISSUES**

9.1 Mortality rates in patients with multiple organ failure

Patients with failure of three or more organs have an 84% mortality rate, yet their care consumes a significant proportion of resources particularly in intensive care. During winter in the UK, available intensive care beds become a scarce resource.

- Should these patients continue to be treated once three or more organs fail, knowing that they may be preventing others from receiving treatment as well as consuming large proportions of already limited budgets?
- What are the reasons for your decision?

Prevention of infection

Prevention of secondary infection is essential as these patients are highly vulnerable due to compromised immune response, invasive cannulae/catheters and wounds. The highest standard of infection control should be maintained.

Renal support

Optimization of intravascular fluid volumes and maintenance of renal perfusion pressures by maintaining mean arterial blood pressures above 60–70 mmHg should prevent further deterioration. If renal failure is evident from either metabolic acidosis, high levels of urea and creatinine and/or high potassium levels then renal support in the form of haemofiltration, diafiltration or dialysis will be needed.

Nutrition and gastrointestinal support

Enteral nutrition may have a role in protecting the gastric mucosa and, providing adequate perfusion has been restored, it is an essential part of protective management (see Ch. 11). Provision of appropriate amounts of carbohydrate, protein and fat as well as an adequate supply of electrolytes, vitamins and trace elements will ensure the nutrients needed for immune response and maintenance of gastrointestinal mucosal integrity are available, thereby preventing further infection. (Scott et al 1998).

Prevention of complications

The integrity of the patient's skin and mucous membranes rapidly become compromised in this situation. Great care must be taken to prevent the complications of immobility such as pressure sores or limb contractures (see Ch. 10). Oral hygiene, eye care and urinary catheter care are all vital in preventing secondary infection and painful sores and ulceration.

Oral hygiene

Hypovolaemia will decrease the volume of saliva produced, and intolerance or inability to take oral fluids will compound the damage to the oral mucosa. Currently, the use of soft toothbrushes to remove plaque and bacteria, accompanied by soft foam sticks to rehydrate the mouth and remove old saliva or debris, is considered appropriate (Somerville 1999). Oral care must be carried out regularly in order to be effective.

Eye care

Patients who are critically ill lose a number of the normal protective mechanisms and become vulnerable to eye damage and infection (Farrell & Wray 1993). The relatively dry flow of gas from around the oxygen mask may also dry the corneas. There may be decreased tear production as well as decreased resistance to infection. Eyes should be assessed regularly for signs of inflammation or drying of the cornea. Artificial tears such as hypromellose drops can be instilled and any discharge cleaned away with sterile water and gauze (Adam & Osborne 1997).

Urinary catheter care

If the patient has a urinary catheter in situ, there is an increased risk of urinary tract infection (Mulhall et al 1988). The patient with multiple organ failure will be vulnerable to infection and urinary catheter care is important in preventing this (see Ch. 24).

SUMMARY: MAIN POINTS

- Shock is a feature of a number of different pathophysiological states. It relates to inadequate or disordered tissue perfusion associated with abnormal cellular metabolism. Usually cardiac output and oxygen delivery do not meet tissue oxygen demand and anaerobic metabolism occurs.

- Nurses have a significant role in identifying and alerting medical staff to the early stages of shock and in providing immediate supportive care.

- Progression of shock moves from compensated via progressive to irreversible shock. Interventions to restore tissue perfusion and oxygen delivery are vital to prevent degeneration from one stage to the next.

- The systemic inflammatory response syndrome (SIRS) can be triggered by a number of factors, but most commonly it is due to the release of inflammatory mediators.

- Assessment of the patient's respiratory, cardiovascular, renal and neurological status is vital to ensure early detection of deterioration.

- The principal aims of nursing (and medical) management are to restore oxygen delivery to the tissues and correct the underlying problem or cause of the shock.

- The priorities of care are airway management and oxygen therapy, circulatory support and close/accurate monitoring of the patient.

- Reducing anxiety, relieving pain, decreasing pyrexia and supporting the patient and family are significant nursing interventions in this context.

- Multiple organ failure following a period of poor perfusion (shock) can affect the lungs, kidneys, brain, heart, liver, gastrointestinal tract and clotting system.

- The secondary aims of nursing (and medical) management are to prevent complications, such as those arising from infection, and immobility.

SELF-TEST: CRITICAL THINKING EXERCISES

1 Review the process of aerobic metabolism:
   — What does hypovolaemia mean and why does it affect the ability of the heart to deliver oxygen to the tissues?
   — How can nurses intervene to help patients reduce the amount of oxygen they are consuming?
   — How can a patient be in shock but maintain a normal blood pressure?

2 Review the physiological responses to a reduction in circulating blood volume:
   — Why would the administration of fluid assist in reducing tachycardia and increasing low blood pressure in a shocked patient?
   — What types of fluid loss are associated with the shocked state?

3 There are many nursing interventions which can assist the patient to cope with shock. What can nurses do to:
   — enhance the patient's ability to improve oxygenation
   — reduce the patient's requirement for oxygen
   — prevent complications associated with shock such as infection?

 ## FURTHER READING

Adam SK, Osborne S. Critical care nursing: the science and practice. Oxford: Oxford University Press; 1997: 398–421.

Huddleston VA. Multisystem organ failure: pathophysiology and clinical implications. St Louis: Mosby Year Book; 1992.

Manley K, Bellman L (eds). Surgical nursing: advancing practice. London: Churchill Livingstone; 2000.

Scott A, Skerratt S, Adam SK. Nutrition in the critically ill. London: Edward Arnold; 1998.

REFERENCES

Adam S. Aspects of current research in enteral nutrition in the critically ill. Care Crit Ill 1994; 10: 246–251.

Adam SK, Osborne S. Critical care nursing: the science and practice. Oxford: Oxford University Press; 1997: 398–421.

American College of Chest Physicians/Society of Critical Care Medicine. Consensus conference: definitions for sepsis and organ failure and guidelines for the use of innovative therapies in sepsis. Crit Care Med 1992; 20: 864–874.

Anderson I. Care of the critically ill surgical patient. London: Arnold; 1999: 57.

Atkinson P, Atkinson J. Spinal shock. Mayo Clin Proc 1996; 71: 384–389.

Baron JF. Crystalloids versus colloids in the treatment of hypovolemic shock. In: Vincent JL, ed. Yearbook of intensive care and emergency medicine. Berlin: Springer-Verlag; 2000: 443–466.

Brandstetter R, Sharma K, Dellabadia M et al. Adult respiratory distress syndrome: a disorder in need of improved outcome. Heart Lung 1997; 26: 3–14.

Burfitt S, Greiner D, Miers L et al. Professional nurse caring as perceived by critically ill patients: a phenomenologic study. Am J Crit Care 1993; 2: 489–499.

Col J, Hochman J, Lejemtel T. Cardiogenic shock: how should we revascularize? In: Vincent JL, ed. Yearbook of intensive care and emergency medicine. Berlin: Springer-Verlag; 1994: 304–309.

De Vito A. Dyspnea during hospitalizations for acute phase of illness as recalled by patients with chronic obstructive pulmonary disease. Heart Lung 1990; 19: 186–191.

Dreger V. Blood and blood product use in perioperative patient care. AORN J 1998; 67: 154–190.

Edwards S. Maintaining an adequate circulation. In: Manley K, Bellman L, eds. Surgical nursing. London: Churchill Livingstone; 2000: 507–537

Elliott TSJ, Faroqui MH, Armstrong R et al. Guidelines for good practice in central venous catheterization. J Hosp Infect 1994; 28: 163–176.

Farrell M, Wray F. Eye care for ventilated patients. Intens Crit Care Nurs 1993; 9: 137–141.

Field D. Maintaining effective breathing. In: Manley K, Bellman L, eds. Surgical nursing: advancing practice. London: Churchill Livingstone; 2000: 446–465.

Hebert PC, Wells G, Blajchman MA et al. A multicenter, randomised, controlled clinical trial of transfusion requirements in critical care. N Engl J Med 1999; 340: 409–417.

Henderson N. Anaphylaxis. Nurs Stand 1998; 12: 49–55.

Henker R. Evidence-based practice: fever-related interventions. Am J Crit Care 1999; 8: 481–487.

Hibbert A. Stress in surgical patients: a physiological perspective. In: Manley K, Bellman L, eds. Surgical nursing: advancing practice. London: Churchill Livingstone; 2000: 152–167.

Hinds CJ, Watson D. ABC of intensive care: circulatory support. Br Med J 1999; 318: 1749–1752.

Holtzclaw BJ. The febrile response in critical care: state of the science. Heart Lung 1992; 21: 482–501.

Leske J. Internal psychometric properties of the critical care family needs inventory. Heart Lung 1991; 20: 236–244.

Lipman TO. Bacterial translocation and enteral nutrition in humans: an outsider looks in. J Parent Ent Nutr 1995; 19, 156–165.

Lundberg JS, Perl T, Wiblin T et al. Septic shock: an analysis of outcomes for patients with onset on hospital wards versus intensive care units. Crit Care Med 1998; 26: 1020–1024.

Marshall J. Gut dysfunction in critical illness: definition and prevalence. In: Rombeau JL, Takala J, eds. Gut dysfunction in critical illness. Update in intensive care and emergency medicine, no. 26. Berlin: Springer-Verlag; 1996.

McGloin H, Adam S, Singer M. Unexpected deaths and referrals to intensive care of patients on general wards. Are some cases potentially avoidable? J Roy Coll Phys 1999; 33: 255–259.

McQuillan P, Pilkington S, Allan A et al. Confidential inquiry into quality of care before admission to intensive care. Br Med J 1998; 316: 1853–1858.

Molter NC. Needs of relatives of critically ill patients: a descriptive study. Heart Lung 1979; 8: 332–339.

Mulhall A, Chapman R, Crow R. The acquisition of bacteriuria and meatal cleansing. Nurs Times 1988; 84: 66–69.

Ognibene F, Parker M, Natanson C et al. Depressed left ventricular performance: response to volume infusion in patients with sepsis and septic shock. Chest 1988; 93: 903–911.

Puntillo KA. Dimensions of procedural pain and its analgesic management in critically ill surgical patients. Am J Crit Care 1994; 3: 116–122.

Sato Y, Weil M, Tang W. Tissue hypercarbic acidosis as a marker of acute circulatory failure (shock). Chest 1998; 114: 263–274.

Scott A, Skerratt S, Adam SK. Nutrition in the critically ill. London: Edward Arnold; 1998: 13–36.

Seers K. Perceptions of pain. Nurs Times 1987; 83: 37–38.

Smith SM, Bihari DJ. Multiple-organ failure. In: Goldhill D, Withington S, eds. Textbook of intensive care. London: Chapman & Hall; 1997: 171 177.

Somerville R. Oral care in the intensive care setting: a care study. Nurs Crit Care 1999; 4: 7–12.

Sprung CL, Peduzzi PN, Shatney CH et al. Impact of encephalopathy on mortality in the sepsis syndrome. Crit Care Med 1990; 18: 801–806.

Suls J, Wan CK. Effects of sensory and procedural information on coping with stressful medical procedures and pain: a meta-analysis. J Consult Clin Psychol 1989; 57: 372–379.

Task Force of the American College of Critical Care Medicine, Society of Critical Care Medicine. Practice parameters for hemodynamic support of sepsis in adult patients in sepsis. Crit Care Med 1999; 27: 639–660.

Tittle M, McMillan SC. Pain and pain-related side effects in ICU and on a surgical unit: nurses' management. Am J Crit Care Nurs 1994; 3: 25–30.

Weinbren J, Soni N. Crystalloids and colloids. In: Goldhill D, Withington S, eds. Textbook of intensive care. London: Chapman & Hall; 1997: 119–124.

Zimmerman JE, Knaus WA, Wagner DP et al. A comparison of risks and outcomes for patients with organ system failure: 1982–1990. Crit Care Med 1996; 24: 1633–1641.

10 Tissue viability: managing chronic wounds

Madeleine Flanagan, Jacqui Fletcher

'After my accident I was in a wheelchair for quite a while and my bottom began to get sore. The district nurse gave me a special cushion that looked very odd but did the trick. She also showed me how to lift my bottom off the chair and rock from side to side every now and then to relieve the pressure.'

(Patient)

THIS CHAPTER WILL HELP YOU

- Understand the normal physiological process of wound healing
- Understand the intrinsic and extrinsic factors that may delay wound healing
- Identify the optimal conditions required to promote wound healing
- Explore the performance characteristics of a range of wound management products
- Identify a range of factors which may increase the risk of pressure ulcer development
- Suggest criteria which may be used to select pressure ulcer prevention equipment
- Differentiate between the clinical signs and symptoms of venous and arterial leg ulcers
- Discuss the role of compression bandaging in the management of venous leg ulcers.

KEYWORDS

Arterial leg ulcers	Necrosis
Blanching erythema	Pressure-reducing equipment
Chronic wounds	
Compression therapy	Pressure-relieving equipment
Connective tissue	Pressure ulcers
Debridement	Primary intention
Eschar	Secondary intention
Exudate	Slough
Granulation tissue	Venous leg ulcers

INTRODUCTION

The assessment of wounds has always been the responsibility of nurses, who are the only members of the multidisciplinary team who regularly dress wounds and assess the condition of patients' skin. Nurses have a fundamental role in the prevention and management of an individual's tissue viability and need to base wound management on informed and rational decisions. In order to monitor the rate of wound healing and the effectiveness of prescribed care, a holistic and objective approach to the management of wounds is required. Accurate wound assessment is dependent on an understanding of the physiology of healing, the factors that delay this process and the optimal conditions required at the wound surface to maximize healing.

The term 'tissue viability' refers literally to the preservation of healthy tissues. It is a phrase that was first defined in the early 1990s to refer to the prevention and management of patients with skin damage, including those who have acute and chronic wounds. Tissue viability services have developed over the last 20 years as a result of technological advances in wound management. These services tend to concentrate on the management of patients with chronic, non-healing wounds such as pressure sores and leg ulcers. Specialist wound care units have emerged in the UK offering patients a comprehensive range of support services and the combined expertise of a wide range of health professionals. This chapter will focus on the management of chronic wounds; information related to the management of surgical wounds and aseptic technique can be found in Chapter 29.

ANATOMY AND PHYSIOLOGY OF THE SKIN

The skin is the largest organ of the body, accounting for approximately 15% of body weight and receiving a third of the circulating blood volume. Protection is one of the major homeostatic functions of the skin as it is constantly exposed to the traumas of its external environment. Therefore preservation or restoration of intact skin is of great importance. There are three main layers of the skin: the epidermis, the dermis and the subcutis (see Fig. 10.1).

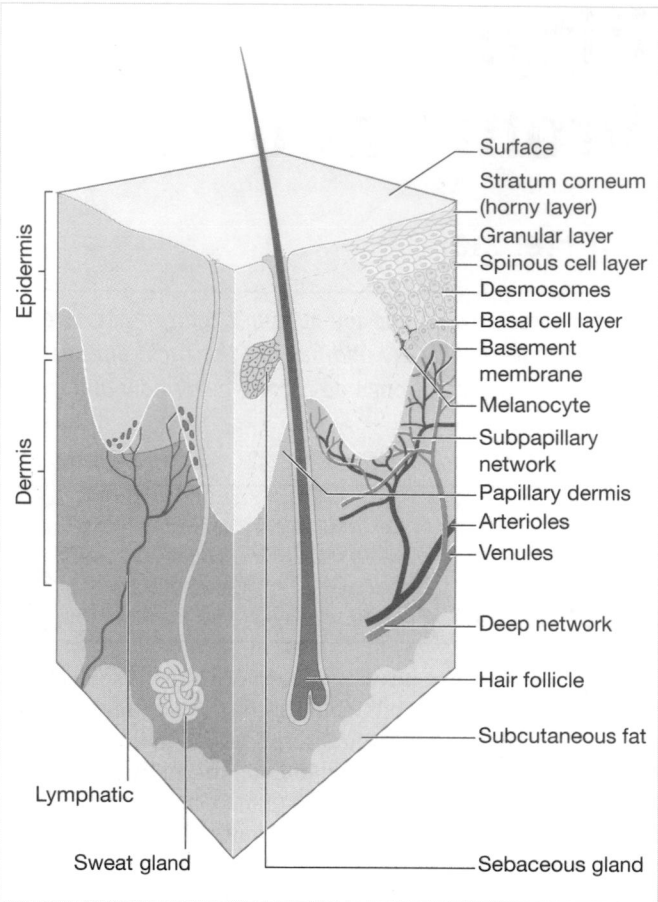

Figure 10.1 The skin. (Reproduced from Powell J. Physiology of the Skin. *SURGERY* 1999; 17: 3: v, by kind permission of The Medicine Publishing Company.)

The skin is transected by hair follicles and sebaceous glands which, despite being present as deeply as the hypodermis, are lined by epidermal cells. For this reason new islands of epithelial cells will be generated from the centre of a wound if the area initially contained hairs. The sebaceous glands secrete sebum which is responsible for maintaining the softness and pliability of the skin and hairs. Sebum also provides a degree of water-proofing and has some bactericidal activity.

LAYERS OF THE SKIN

The epidermis
The outermost layer of the skin, the epidermis, is cellular, avascular (without a blood supply) and varies in thickness. The epidermis is thicker in areas which are subject to greater levels of stress and require more protection, e.g. the palms of the hands and soles of the feet. A layer of epidermal cells lines the hair follicles, and sweat and sebaceous glands. In a healthy young adult, the epidermis is replaced approximately every 3 weeks. Within the epidermis there are five differentiated layers, as described below.

Stratum corneum
This is the outermost layer and is composed of dead keratinocytes, which are thin, flattened cells filled with keratin, a fibrous protein

which is insoluble and resistant to enzymatic digestion and changes in pH and temperature. Keratin is capable of absorbing large amounts of water and it is this capacity to absorb fluid which may lead to skin maceration and eventual breakdown with continuous exposure to moisture, e.g. in incontinent patients.

Stratum lucidum
The stratum lucidum is the second layer of the epidermis and it is not always present. In areas where the epidermal covering is very thin, e.g. the eyelids, it is usually absent. This layer is transparent and made up of dead cells with no visible nuclei. It serves a mainly protective function – hence its presence on areas such as the soles of the feet.

Stratum granulosum
The middle layer of the epidermis, the stratum granulosum is between one and three cells thick. It contains flattened cells which have all the organelles necessary for active metabolic functioning. The thickness of this layer is proportional and varies according to the thickness of the stratum corneum.

Stratum spinosum
The stratum spinosum contains living cells. They have spiny processes called desmosomes along their edges which form the area of contact between cells and are important in maintaining epidermal integrity. Their contact with other cells is what prevents the cells from being torn apart when subjected to normal stresses and strains.

Stratum basale
The innermost layer of the epidermis is the stratum basale. This layer is sometimes grouped with the stratum spinosum and called the stratum germinativum (or germinative layer) as together they are responsible for producing new cells by constant mitotic activity. The stratum basale is only one cell thick and as the epidermis is avascular receives its supply of oxygen and nutrients via the dermal blood supply.

The basement membrane zone
In between the epidermis and the dermis is an acellular layer referred to as the basement membrane zone or dermoepidermal junction. It has two layers, the lamina lucida and the lamina densa (these names simply refer to their visibility under an electron microscope). The basement membrane is a semi-permeable membrane with two main functions: it regulates the transfer of materials, particularly proteins, between the dermis and the epidermis and also acts as a mechanical supporting layer for the epidermis with anchoring fibrils which extend in to the dermis.

The dermis
The dermis is sparsely populated by cells and is between 2 and 5 mm thick. It is the dermis that gives the skin bulk. It has a good blood supply and is divided into two main layers, the papillary layer and the reticular layer. Some of the cells within the dermis, e.g. fibroblasts (which are responsible for the production of new connective tissue) and macrophages (which have a variety of roles including the production of a range of growth factors), are able to move around within the confines of a gelatinous fluid matrix. Use of dressing products that maintain a moist wound environment facilitate this process.

The papillary dermis is the uppermost layer. Being directly beneath the basement membrane, it forms finger-like structures known as dermal papillae, which maintain a close contact with the basement membrane. It is these dermal papillae that contain the capillary loops that provide the blood supply to the epidermis via the semi-permeable basement membrane. Small collagen and elastin fibres are present in this layer but are held within a less organized meshwork of ground substance. There is no clear division between the reticular layer and the papillary layer. The area becomes more densely packed with collagen and elastin fibres, which are laid down in an organized meshwork in a parallel plane to the surface of the skin. It is this meshwork that gives the skin its elasticity and strength.

Collagen is a major structural protein and accounts for approximately 30% of the volume of the dermis. It is an extremely tough biological material and is formed from the fibroblasts. Elastin is a fibre-forming protein secreted by the fibroblasts. It is this that provides the skin with elastic recoil which allows it to retain its shape.

The hypodermis

The final layer of the skin is the hypodermis. It is the thickest layer and provides the main support for the skin. It is made up largely from adipose tissue, connective tissue and blood vessels. The adipose layer forms a protective layer for underlying organs and also anchors the dermis to underlying structures.

FUNCTIONS OF THE SKIN

The skin has five main functions:

- protection
- thermoregulation
- sensation
- metabolism
- communication.

Protection

The skin is the first defence against invading microorganisms, chemical substances, dehydration, mechanical damage and radiation. This protection is provided by the stratum corneum, secretions from the sebaceous glands and the skin's immune system. In addition, the regular shedding of the surface layers prevents colonies of microorganisms becoming established. The majority of skin microorganisms, such as *Staphylococcus epidermidis*, are found in the superficial layers of the epidermis and upper regions of hair follicles and sweat glands, and even a superficial break in the skin may result in these bacteria penetrating the wound and initiating an infection (see Ch. 13).

Thermoregulation

The skin plays a major role in temperature control. This occurs via three main mechanisms:

- secretion and evaporation of sweat which cools the skin surface
- vasodilatation and vasoconstriction of the blood vessels within the skin, which releases or conserves heat
- insulator mechanisms such as the erectile function of hair which traps currents of warm air close to the skin.

Although there are other means of controlling temperature, approximately 97% of heat loss from the body occurs via the skin (see Ch. 5).

Sensation

The skin contains many sensory organs that are widely distributed throughout the dermis and allow it to respond to pain, temperature, touch, pressure and vibration. There are no nerve endings in the epidermis and, if removed, e.g. by friction on the skin, the area is extremely painful as the nerve endings in the dermis are left exposed. Messages from the nerve endings are transmitted to the sensory area of the cerebrum where the sensations of pain, touch and temperature are perceived.

Metabolism

The skin is responsible for synthesis of vitamin D in the presence of ultraviolet light from the sun. Excess vitamin D is stored in the liver.

Non-verbal communication

The skin expresses a great deal about an individual. It communicates emotions by changing colour, e.g. blushing, and also by the secretion of pheromones, chemical scents which are recognized subconsciously by others. Conscious communication also occurs through the use of facial expressions or touch. The condition of the skin may also be a visual communication of underlying health status; for example, dry inelastic skin may be seen in individuals who are dehydrated.

THE EFFECTS OF AGEING ON THE SKIN

Ageing results in changes to the skin structure and its ability to maintain its normal functions. These changes are progressive but are more noticeable from the age of 65. There is a reduction in the barrier function of the stratum corneum which results in an increased susceptibility to infection and increased risk of skin irritation. In addition, reduction in the numbers of sensory receptors, thinning of the epidermis and changes in the basement membrane make the skin more susceptible to trauma. Within the basement membrane there is a flattening of the structure and consequent reduction in the surface area in contact with the dermis. This means that there is an increased likelihood of the epidermis being sheared off the dermis by either trauma or friction such as vigorous rubbing. The reduction in contact between these two layers also means a reduced blood supply to the epidermis which slows down the rate of cell division and replacement, thereby increasing the healing time of wounds in the older adult (Desai 1997).

Changes also occur within the dermis, most noticeably to the dermal proteins, collagen and elastin. The fibre bundles become more compact as there is a loss of ground substance, the bundles of collagen may lose their structure and the elastin loses its elasticity. This means that the skin has less resistance to stretching and is more likely to tear. The amount of collagen produced decreases by 1% per year after the age of 20, becomes less soluble, has less ability to swell and is therefore more susceptible to exposure to moisture such as that from incontinence (Leaper & Harding 1998). There is also an increase in the time necessary to produce collagen molecules, increasing the time necessary for repair.

There is a reduction in the amount and density of hypodermis. This, together with a decrease in the number of sweat glands, reduced vascularity and a reduction in subcutaneous fat, results in a reduction in the protective and thermoregulatory function of the skin (Bryant 1992).

PRINCIPLES OF SKIN CARE

The aim of skin care is to retain the functions of the skin. To do this, the skin needs to remain intact and well hydrated. A simple skin care regimen, which keeps the skin clean without excessive use of chemicals (including soap), followed by the application of a simple moisturizing agent is sufficient to maintain good quality of skin. Mechanical damage from over-enthusiastic rubbing should be avoided as this may lead to a loss of skin integrity (see Special Issues box 10.1).

WOUND HEALING

Wound assessment must be underpinned by a thorough understanding of the physiology of the skin as well as the delicate process of tissue repair. Wound healing comprises a complex series of events that are interlinked and dependent on one another and can be defined as the physiological processes by which the body replaces and restores function to damaged tissues (Tortora & Grabowski 1996).

Primary intention is the term used to describe healing when the two edges of a wound are held together by sutures, staples or other methods of skin closure; these wounds are characterized by minimal tissue loss such as surgical incisions or lacerations. Wounds that have significant tissue loss, such as burns or pressure sores, cannot have their wound edges brought together; the term given to describe this type of healing is secondary intention.

Healing by secondary intention is usually a slower process, as healing occurs from the wound base with the growth of new capillaries and connective tissue. All tissues in the human body are capable of healing by one of two mechanisms: regeneration and repair. The process of regeneration is the more limited one and describes the replacement of damaged tissues by identical cells. In humans, complete regeneration is only possible to replace a limited number of cells, e.g. epithelial, liver and nerve cells. The main mechanism by which healing occurs is by tissue repair during which damaged tissue is replaced by connective tissue which then forms a scar.

In clinical practice, wounds are often classified as either acute or chronic. The characteristics of these types of wounds are described in Table 10.1.

Chronic wounds have a tendency to produce large amounts of wound fluid (exudate) containing inflammatory mediators that cause additional tissue damage at the wound margin such as skin sensitivities leading to excoriation and excessive dermal thickening (Fig. 10.2). The management of this type of exudate presents a challenge to health professionals as it prolongs the healing process and leakage and odour are often unpleasant for the patient.

 SPECIAL ISSUES

10.1 Skin assessment

Skin assessment should involve all areas of the body. It must be remembered that some people will feel very vulnerable during this examination, which must be performed with privacy and dignity. Assessment of the skin can reveal the following:

- excessive dryness, scaling and fissuring
- dermatological conditions such as eczema and psoriasis (see Ch. 28)
- allergic reactions, sensitivities, rashes and dermatitis (see Ch. 28)
- local infection – cellulitis, lymphangitis, phlebitis
- skin trauma caused by pressure, friction, shear, puncture, bruising
- dependent oedema.

Nursing assessment should involve the following senses:

- Touch – local temperature rises indicate inflammation and/or pressure damage
- Smell – abnormal odours may indicate infection or inability to maintain hygiene
- Sight – appearance can suggest dehydration, inflammation, excoriation, hyperpigmentation
- Hearing – surgical emphysema.

Accurate documentation of these findings is required to identify the extent, severity and possible causes of skin problems. It is often easier to describe skin condition by identifying the location of any lesions on an assessment chart that includes a diagram of the front and back of the body.

Table 10.1 Characteristics of acute and chronic wounds		
	Acute wounds	**Chronic wounds**
Examples	Surgical wounds, lacerations, burns	Leg ulcers, pressure ulcers, malignant wounds
Cause	Trauma (no underlying aetiology)	Various aetiologies, i.e. venous hypertension
Duration	Short (uneventful healing)	Prolonged (delayed healing)
Exudate secretion	Low (output associated with trauma)	Copious
Local inflammatory response	Normal	Hyperactive
Recurrence rates	Low (recurrence only if additional trauma)	Frequent and cyclical

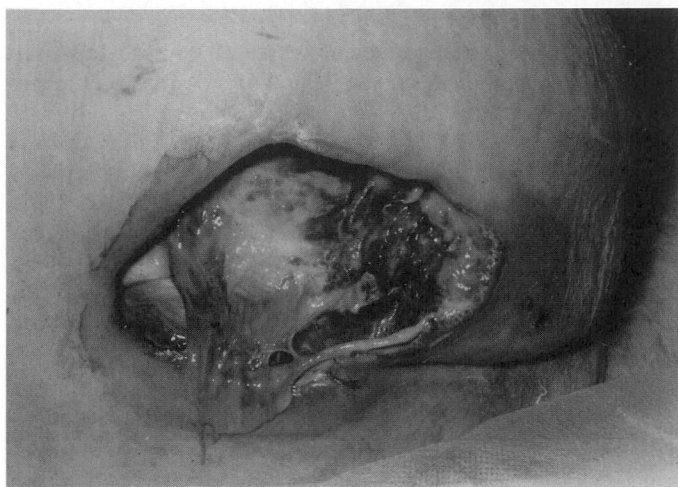

Figure 10.2 A pressure ulcer showing signs of damage to the surrounding skin.

THE PHYSIOLOGY OF WOUND HEALING

The process of wound healing can be divided into three stages: inflammatory, proliferation and maturation. These do not occur in isolation; there is considerable overlap between them and the time required by an individual to progress to the next phase of healing is dependent on a variety of factors (see Fig. 10.3).

The inflammatory stage

In acute wounds, the inflammatory stage lasts approximately 3–5 days, but in chronic wounds this process is prolonged. Injury to the dermis causes bleeding. The damaged blood vessels constrict, to minimize blood flow and initiate the clotting process, which is accelerated due to platelet aggregation and the release of growth factors required for tissue repair. The activation of clotting factors stimulates the release of inflammatory mediators such as histamine, which cause local blood vessels to become more permeable and dilated. This inflammatory response is normal and is necessary to initiate the rest of the healing process, and although the clinical signs are similar, they should not be confused with infection. The inflammatory response can be observed around an injured area by the presence locally of:

- oedema (swelling)
- erythema (redness)
- heat
- discomfort
- functional disturbance (loss of movement).

These signs are due to increased blood flow and accumulation of fluid in the soft tissues. The combination of discomfort and swelling usually restricts the movement of the injured part.

Neutrophils are the first type of white blood cell to be attracted into the wound, usually arriving within a few hours of injury, followed by macrophages. The activity of neutrophils essentially cleanses the wound bed of bacteria and cellular debris. The macrophages are active during all stages of wound healing as they produce a variety of cytokines (chemical messengers) that regulate tissue repair, e.g. platelet-derived growth factor (PDGF) and fibroblast growth factor (FGF) (Leaper & Harding 1998).

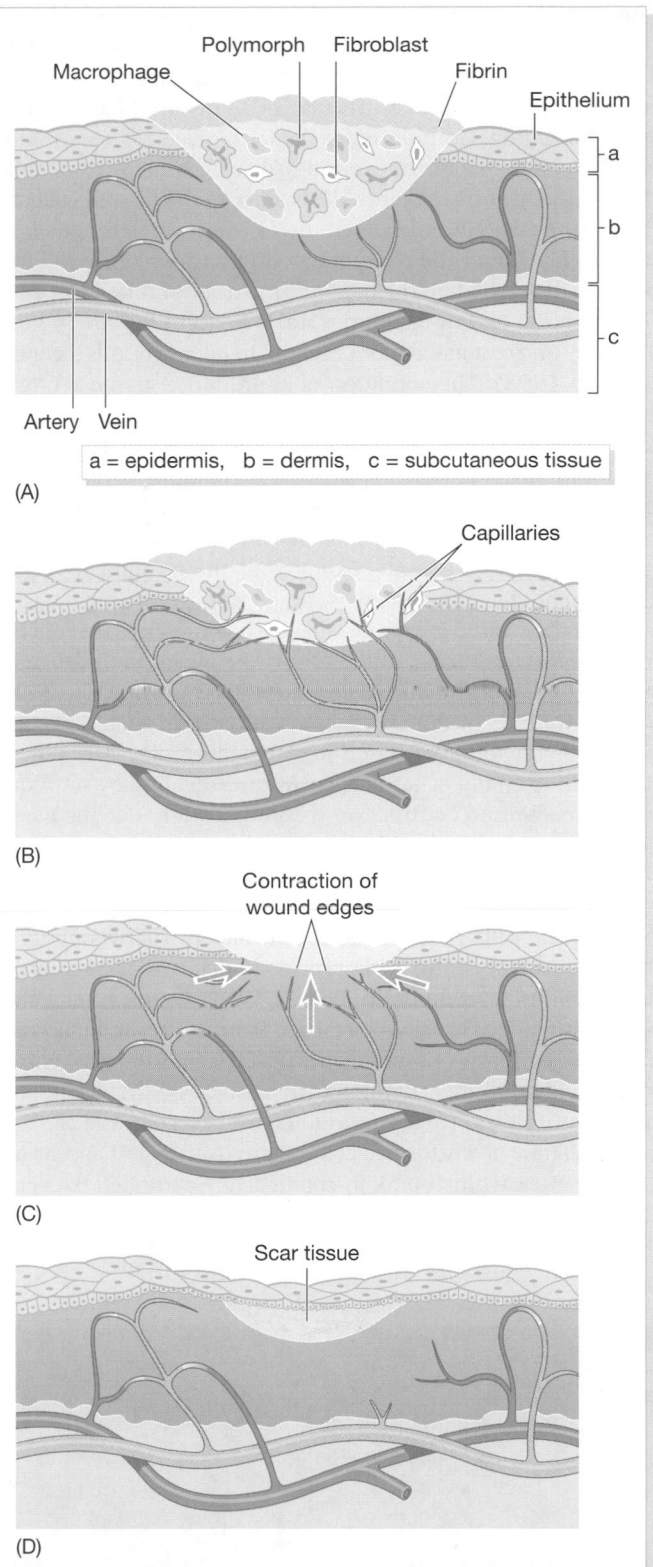

(A) a = epidermis, b = dermis, c = subcutaneous tissue

Figure 10.3 The stages of wound healing. (A) Inflammatory stage. (B) Proliferative stage – note the epithelial growth at the wound margins and extension of capillaries into the wound bed. (C) Maturation stage. (D) Mature stage (early) – note the complete re-epithelialization of the wound surface.

The proliferative stage

During this phase the wound is filled with new connective tissue. The main processes involved are the formation of new blood vessels (angiogenesis), contraction of the wound edges and re-epithelialization. Granulation is the term given to the formation of new capillaries in the wound bed, which helps to establish new connective tissue. Fibroblasts start to divide and collect at the wound edges in order to produce collagen to strengthen the wound. The larger the wound, the longer this process will take. It is also dependent on the patient's nutritional state.

Formation of new capillaries starts to occur within 36 hours of injury and can usually be observed in open wounds (Leaper & Harding 1998). The condition of granulation tissue is often a good indicator as to how the wound is healing. Healthy granulation tissue is bright red and moist and does not bleed easily. Granulation tissue that appears dark in colour is often a sign that a wound has a poor blood supply; if granulation tissue bleeds very easily this may indicate that the wound is infected. It is during this stage of healing that the amount of wound exudate should start to decrease and become more manageable.

Once the wound is loosely filled with connective tissue, fibroblasts begin to contract, pulling the edges of the wound together so that the size of the wound area is reduced. Contraction is minimal in wounds healing by primary intention, such as sutured wounds with minimal tissue loss, but does play a significant part in the healing of large open wounds healing by secondary intention. Wound contraction will only begin after the wound bed has filled with healthy granulation tissue. At this point the processes of wound contraction and re-epithelialization combine to reduce the overall size of the wound.

Epithelial cells grow across the surface of the wound in the final stages of healing. This process is delicate and requires a moist wound environment (Winter 1962, Dyson et al 1988). New epithelial cells originate either from the wound margin or from the remnants of hair follicles or sebaceous or sweat glands. They divide and migrate along the surface of the granulation tissue until they form a continuous layer of cells and close the wound. These newly formed cells have a translucent appearance and are often whitish-pink in colour. They can often be seen at the edges of open, clean wounds and as small islands on the wound surface originating from hair follicles (see Fig. 10.4).

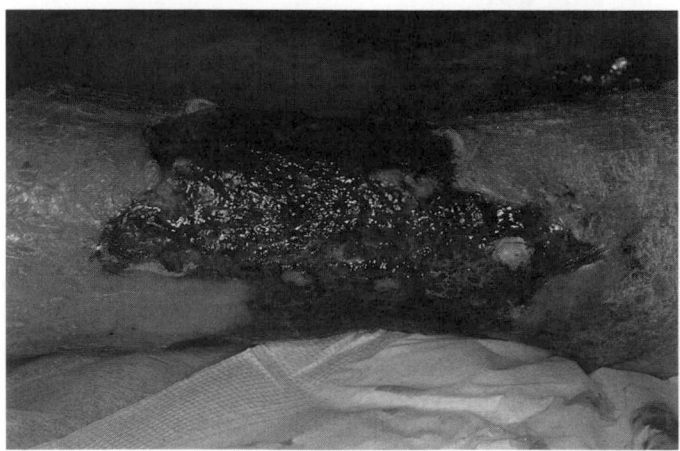

Figure 10.4 A leg ulcer showing islands of re-epithelialization.

The maturation stage

The end stage of healing begins when the wound has been closed by the combined processes of contraction and epithelialization, and continues in some instances for up to a year or longer. In Caucasian skin, scar tissue is initially raised and red in colour, and as it matures, the local blood supply decreases and the scar becomes flatter, paler and smoother. In darkly pigmented skin, however, the scar tissue usually has a lighter appearance than the surrounding skin (Eisenbeiss et al 1998). Mature scar tissue is avascular and contains no hairs or sebaceous or sweat glands (Tortora & Grabowski 1996).

The normal process of wound healing ensures that the majority of wounds heal quickly and without complication. However, nursing skills are often challenged by those patients with chronic wounds, such as leg ulcers and pressure sores, which can have a profound effect on the quality of life of an individual.

FACTORS INFLUENCING HEALING

Tissue repair is a complex physiological process that is easily disrupted even in healthy individuals. The process of normal wound healing depends on a healthy immune system, a balanced diet, sufficient sleep and a positive attitude. Wound healing may be impaired as a result of a combination of local and systemic factors (see Box 10.1). Even a healthy adult with a traumatic wound may experience delayed healing, due to the combined effects of a large irregular shaped wound, anxiety, loss of appetite and lack of sleep.

General health status and wound healing

In addition to the factors previously discussed, there is also a variety of general factors that can have a detrimental effect on the rates of healing (Box 10.1).

The general health of an individual has a direct influence on the person's ability to heal normally. Chronic diseases, e.g. diabetes mellitus and renal failure, affect the delicate process of wound healing by disrupting tissue perfusion and causing metabolic disturbances. Musculoskeletal diseases, such as rheumatoid arthritis and osteoarthritis, cause deformities which increase pressure on soft tissues and increase the risk of skin breakdown. Illness may also reduce an individual's appetite, increase anxiety and reduce mobility, all of which combine to prolong wound healing. Many chronic diseases disrupt normal healing. Some common ones are listed below:

- respiratory disorders, e.g. chronic obstructive airway disease, bronchitis, pneumonia, anaemia, as they all reduce oxygen saturation in the blood (see Chs 18 and 20)
- circulatory disorders, e.g. peripheral vascular disease, as the diminished blood supply causes reduced perfusion of the local tissues (see Ch. 19)
- metabolic disorders, e.g. diabetes mellitus, which affect the macro- and microcirculation. These vascular changes make the diabetic more susceptible to gangrene and formation of arterial leg ulcers (see Ch. 17)
- immune deficiency disorders, e.g. AIDS and conditions where the number and function of neutrophils and monocytes is depleted, will lead to prolonged wound

Box 10.1 Factors prolonging healing

Local factors

- *Impaired blood supply*
  — Disturbances to peripheral blood supply reduce tissue perfusion and limit the local supply of oxygen and nutrients required for repair
  — Reduced oxygen levels impair collagen synthesis and epithelial growth and lower tissue resistance to infection
- *Temperature fluctuations*
  — Mitotic activity of cells occurs most rapidly at body temperature. Extremes of temperature prolong tissue repair
- *Dehydration of wound bed*
  — Formation of granulation tissue and re-epithelialization occur at a faster rate in a moist than in a dry environment
- *Presence of necrotic tissue and foreign bodies*
  — Necrotic tissue impedes epithelial migration and impairs flow of nutrients to the wound bed
  — Foreign bodies such as fragments of dressing materials may cause tissue irritation which can prolong the inflammatory response and delay healing
- *Size of wound*
  — Large, irregular-shaped wounds with extensive tissue loss heal slowly as they require more tissue regeneration to fill the defect
- *Wound location*
  — Position of a wound affects its vascularity and will also determine the mobility of the wound site
  — Wounds on or close to joints are usually slower to heal
- *Duration of wound*
  — Chronic wounds are slow to heal as the inflammatory response is prolonged
- *Mechanical stress*
  — Mechanical stress delays healing by prolonging the inflammatory response
  — Unrelieved mechanical stress may cause localized necrosis due to ischaemia, resulting in rapid deterioration of the wound
- *Local infection*
  — Wound infection prolongs the inflammatory stage of healing and delays collagen synthesis and re-epithelialization
- *Skin maceration*
  — Wounds producing copious exudate are associated with damage to the surrounding skin. This can cause skin sensitivities and excoriation
- *Surgical technique*
  — Excessive handling of tissues during surgery, tight skin closure materials and inadequate wound drainage can all delay wound healing

General factors

- *Ageing*
  — Increasing age reduces the inflammatory response, the proliferative phase and the production of collagen as the immune system becomes less efficient
  — The process of repair starts later, is slower and there is a reduced resistance to infection
- *Dehydration and electrolyte imbalance*
  — Dehydration and electrolyte imbalance impair cellular function and may be markedly increased if wound drainage is significant, i.e. burns, fistulae
- *Nutritional state*
  — Proteins, fats, carbohydrates, vitamins and minerals all play a fundamental role in the process of wound repair and are required to produce collagen and connective tissue
- *General health status*
  — Many systemic diseases, such as diabetes, will prolong wound healing as they make additional demands on the immune system
  — Other diseases, such as anaemia and bronchitis, prolong healing by reducing local tissue perfusion
- *Body mass index*
  — Extremes of body build can influence healing rates. Cachexia and anorexia are indicative of poor nutritional status
  — Obesity can exert considerable tension on a wound, increasing the likelihood of dehiscence
- *Immunosuppression*
  — Consequences of radiotherapy and chemotherapy include inhibition of cellular division and suppression of cell growth
  — Irradiated skin is prone to loss of vascularity, ulceration and atrophy
- *Drug therapy*
  — Non-steroidal anti-inflammatory drugs (NSAIDs), corticosteroids, cytotoxic agents and anticoagulants all reduce healing rates by interrupting either cellular division or the clotting process
- *Stress*
  — Anxiety releases glucocorticoids, which have anti-inflammatory effects and inhibit fibroblasts, collagen synthesis and formation of granulation tissue
- *Lack of sleep/rest*
  — Tissue repair and rate of cellular division are enhanced by sleep
  — Healing of wounds, particularly near joints, will benefit from the reduction in tension and physical stress that occurs when resting

healing. People infected with HIV are prone to opportunist infections, which are often manifested in the skin, such as seborrhoeic dermatitis, herpes zoster and Kaposi's sarcoma (see Ch. 28).

Lifestyle factors that may delay wound healing

Wounds affect a person's lifestyle in many ways, ranging from minor inconvenience to severe disruption of daily activities of living. The environment in which the patient lives can also affect

10.1 Factors affecting wound healing

Mike is 48 and has recently lost his job. He smokes 20 cigarettes a day and enjoys a few pints of beer in the local pub most nights. He struggles to keep his weight under control, which he has found more difficult since losing his job. Ten days ago he was admitted to hospital with a ruptured appendix, which was surgically removed. His wound is now red, inflamed, painful and producing moderate amounts of serous fluid. Following suture removal the wound gaped open, revealing a cavity 2.5 cm deep.

Student activities
- Identify those factors you think contributed to Mike's wound breakdown.
- How would you manage Mike's wound?
- What other postoperative complications could Mike be at risk of developing (see Ch. 29)?

healing and is an important factor to consider when caring for patients in their own homes (see Reflective Practice box 10.1). The following factors can be particularly important when caring for patients with chronic non-healing wounds:

- Compliance is affected by many factors, including the length of time the wound has been present, success of previous treatments, the patient's health beliefs and confidence in professional carers. Non-compliance, such as interfering with planned treatment, e.g. removal of either dressings and/or bandages, can prolong wound healing.
- Cultural/religious beliefs may have a direct influence on diet, fasting, hygiene practices and uptake of medical intervention and technologies.
- Major life stressors such as bereavement and unemployment may have a cumulative negative effect due to anxiety, depression, lack of sleep and loss of appetite. Psychological stress has been shown to reduce healing rates by depressing the immune system.
- Activity levels and working patterns can influence care and the frequency of dressing changes. Sport and exercise make specific demands on types of dressings and bandages.
- Knowledge and understanding of both health professionals and patients directly influence the acceptance of the wound and its subsequent treatment. Failure to implement research-based practice may also be due to lack of awareness among health professionals.

PRINCIPLES OF WOUND MANAGEMENT

The principles of caring for acute and chronic wounds are similar and should be based on objective wound assessment. Wound assessment facilitates identification of specific management objectives and is an activity reliant upon complex decision-making skills and practical experience. Accurate wound assessment is dependent on an understanding of the physiology of

healing and those factors that delay this process as well as the optimal conditions required at the wound surface to maximize healing. Inappropriate wound management may occur if practitioners fail to differentiate between healthy and abnormal characteristics of healing. Wound assessment should always involve the multidisciplinary team and is not the sole remit of nurses, as the assessment process provides a baseline from which to plan appropriate wound management and to evaluate the effectiveness of treatment.

General wound management principles include:

- identification of the cause of the wound – is the wound caused by trauma or a chronic disease process?
- identification of factors responsible for delaying healing – is the individual well nourished? What is their general health status?
- provision of an optimum environment to maximize healing potential – has the wound a good blood supply? Is the wound bed moist?
- identification of realistic treatment objectives that promote quality of life – has the patient been involved in planning their care?
- prevention of any further wound deterioration or complications – is the wound being frequently evaluated using a relevant wound assessment tool?
- evaluation of the effectiveness of wound management interventions – are wound treatments being frequently evaluated using a relevant wound assessment tool?
- provision of psychological support to promote self-esteem and compliance – is the patient satisfied with the care given? Have they been given the opportunity to discuss any anxieties or concerns?

SPECIFIC WOUND MANAGEMENT OBJECTIVES

Once the general principles of wound management have been considered by the multidisciplinary team, attention can be focused on specific wound management treatment objectives. Members of the multidisciplinary wound management team include tissue viability nurse specialists, vascular surgeons, dermatologists, chiropodists, dieticians and physiotherapists. Wound management treatment objectives will vary depending on a multitude of factors, including the wound type, location and size as well as the patient's psychological response to the wound. Examples of specific treatment objectives for acute and chronic wounds are described below. However, in practice, many of these objectives are relevant to the care and management of both types of wounds.

Acute wounds
- Prevention and control of haemorrhage (see Ch. 29)
- Establishing the size and extent of tissue damage by cleaning the wound thoroughly and measuring it
- Removal of foreign bodies from the wound
- Prevention and control of wound infection.

Chronic wounds
- Management of wound exudate
- Removal of necrotic tissue from the wound bed (debridement)

- Promoting growth of granulation tissue from wound bed
- Controlling wound odour
- Protection of the surrounding skin.

WOUND ASSESSMENT

One of the purposes of wound assessment is to determine the aetiology of the wound, as this helps to determine the appropriateness of various treatment options. Factors identified as likely to prolong healing should become management priorities and improved if possible. If this principle is overlooked, the result may be a non-healing wound despite appropriate management.

An important objective of wound assessment is to provide the optimum environment that supports the process of tissue repair as this is known to be of utmost importance when trying to maximize the healing potential of a wound (Winter 1962). It has been widely acknowledged that control of the optimal local conditions in the wound can significantly reduce the time that it takes to heal. The work of Winter in 1962 demonstrated for the first time that moist wounds healed more rapidly than those exposed to the air or covered with traditional dry dressings. The progress of epithelial migration is significantly slowed in the presence of either necrotic or desiccated tissue, as epithelial cells are forced to burrow underneath the eschar (dehydrated exudate, fibrinogen and cellular debris) which forms a mechanical obstruction in the wound bed. Cellular activity within wounds is sensitive to fluctuations in temperature and is significantly slowed at extremes of temperature. It is therefore important that wound care practices do not disrupt the delicate physiological process of wound healing. All of the following are known to lower the temperature of the wound and allow it to dry out and therefore should be avoided:

- cleaning the wound with cold cleansing solutions
- exposing the wound for longer than necessary when applying a new dressing
- changing the dressing more frequently than necessary
- leaving the wound exposed and without the protection of a dressing.

Wound cleansing and dressing techniques should promote an optimal environment in order to maximize the wound's healing potential. However, the selection of appropriate wound dressings alone cannot compensate for unresolved systemic or local conditions known to impair rates of healing.

WOUND MEASUREMENT

There is a variety of methods available for measuring wounds, ranging from simple measurement of surface area to the use of sophisticated computer tools. Simple measurements of surface area are only relevant for superficial, shallow wounds and can be crudely calculated by measuring the widest and longest parts of the wound with a ruler. Although imprecise, especially for irregular shaped wounds or cavities, such measurements do at least provide a baseline for objective evaluation of healing. The circumference of the wound can be measured by tracing the wound margin on to a transparent material using a fibre-tipped pen. This can then be transferred onto a wound assessment chart and recorded with the date and wound details. Tracings made in this way do not consider the three-dimensional aspect of the wound bed, nor do they provide information relating to wound depth and volume but it is important to establish the relative change in wound size. Weekly tracings of wound circumference are usually sufficient, as measurements taken more frequently tend not to reflect changes in wound size.

WOUND CLEANSING

Both acute and chronic wounds may require cleansing for a variety of reasons:

- to remove debris from the surface of the wound including devitalized tissue, pus, excess exudate, foreign bodies and dressing residue
- to rehydrate the surface of a wound in order to provide a moist environment
- to keep the skin surrounding the wound clean and free from excessive moisture
- to facilitate wound assessment so that the size and extent of the wound can be visualized
- to minimize wound trauma when removing adherent dressing material
- to promote patient comfort and psychological well-being.

It is important to achieve the correct balance between the beneficial effects of wound cleansing as indicated above and the potentially harmful effects of unnecessarily disturbing the delicate conditions that naturally exist at the wound surface. The ultimate aim of wound cleansing is to remove both organic and inorganic debris whilst maintaining the optimum local environment to facilitate wound healing.

The decision to cleanse a wound should be based upon the following:

- the size, shape and location of the wound
- the condition of the wound bed and stage of healing
- the availability and effectiveness of different methods of cleansing
- the availability and effectiveness of different cleansing agents
- the patient's perceptions and needs.

WOUND DEBRIDEMENT

The objective of wound debridement is to remove slough and necrotic tissue from the wound bed. This allows the full extent of the wound to be visualized and facilitates the healing process. Wound debridement may be achieved in a variety of ways, the most efficient of which is surgical debridement, usually performed under anaesthetic. This has obvious cost implications and the associated risk of the patient undergoing a general anaesthetic. However, this method of debridement is much faster and may therefore reduce costs in the long term and reduce the risk to patients in other ways, e.g. reducing the risk of infection.

Some specialist nurses receive additional training to enable them to undertake sharp debridement, i.e. removal of adherent slough and necrotic tissue using a scalpel or scissors (Hampton

1997). However, the three most common forms of debridement used in clinical practice are:

- enzymatic – the use of dressing products containing proteolytic enzymes (streptokinase and streptodornase) which break down the structural proteins within the wound
- autolytic – debridement by the normal healing process which is facilitated by provision of a moist wound environment using dressings such as hydrogels or hydrocolloids
- biosurgery.

Biosurgery

The use of larval (maggot) therapy is again becoming popular. Larvae are used for their ability to debride even very dehydrated wounds quickly and efficiently. They are particularly useful in ischaemic wounds where a poor or diminished blood supply may reduce the potential for autolysis. Sterile blowfly larvae (*Lucilia serricata*) are used as they specifically feed on dead tissues. These larvae are specially bred in sterile conditions, currently in only two centres in the UK. The skin surrounding the wound should be covered with a hydrocolloid to protect it from the secretions of the larvae and to prevent the patient feeling their movement if they accidentally make their way onto healthy tissue. The larvae are held in situ with a fine mesh, which prevents them from leaving the wound area and which is changed after a maximum of 3 days. Larvae are not suitable for use in wounds where there is a high level of exudate as they will drown. They should be removed from the wound bed by irrigation and in some instances a repeat application is required. Patients may require additional psychological support during the period of application. Where there is accidental inoculation with larvae (i.e. the patient's wound is infested), it is safer to remove the larvae as they are of unknown origin and species.

SUMMARY

This section has highlighted some of the complex issues related to wound management and has emphasized the need to identify specific treatment objectives when planning care. Thorough wound assessment is required in order to maximize the wound healing potential of both acute and chronic wounds. Nurses need to relate their knowledge of the physiology of wound healing to everyday clinical practice and are in a unique position within the multidisciplinary team to assess patients' wounds. Health professionals caring for patients with wounds should take into account the delicate balance between the physical and psychosocial influences that can affect healing.

WOUND DRESSINGS

Prior to the work of Winter (1962) it was generally believed that, in order to promote healing, wounds should be exposed to the air and allowed to dry. However, following Winter's work on superficial wounds, which demonstrated an increased migration of epithelial cells in a moist environment, the concept of moist wound healing became slowly accepted (see Evidence-based

 EVIDENCE-BASED PRACTICE

10.1 Moist wound healing

A paper by Winter (1962) presents the first research into the use of occlusive dressings and is the basis on which most of the modern wound dressings have been developed. It was originally published in the *Nature* in 1962 and the original is now difficult to obtain. However, in 1995 it was reproduced in the *Journal of Wound Care*, accompanied by a critique by three experts.

In the study, small, superficial, acute wounds were created on the backs of young domestic pigs. The wounds were either left exposed to the air or covered with a polythene film and examined at regular intervals. In the wounds that had been covered with polythene, the epidermal cells were seen to migrate more quickly than those exposed to air. The author proposes that this is because the epidermal cells in the exposed wounds have to burrow beneath the dry scab that forms on the surface of the wound. In the wounds covered by polythene, formation of a scab is prevented and the rate of re-epithelialization is markedly increased.

Reference

Winter GD. Formation of the scab and the rate of epithelialisation of superficial wounds in the skin of the young domestic pig. Nature 1962; 193: 293–294 (reproduced in Journal of Wound Care 1995; 4(8): 366–367).

Practice box 10.1). Over the last 30 years there has been an explosion in the number and types of dressings available, often with little difference between competing brands of products. It can be difficult, therefore, to select the most appropriate dressing.

THE IDEAL DRESSING

The requirements of an ideal dressing identified by Scales (1956), prior to the adoption of the principles of moist wound healing by Winter (1962), were refined by Turner (1985) who defined what is now widely accepted as the minimum criteria for the optimum dressing products:

- maintain a high humidity at the wound/dressing interface
- remove excess exudate and toxic components
- allow gaseous exchange
- provide thermal insulation
- be impermeable to bacteria
- be free from particulate and toxic contaminants
- allow removal without causing additional trauma.

DRESSING PRODUCTS

There are currently over 300 dressing products available. However, they can be broadly broken down into two main categories, passive wound dressings and interactive wound dressings.

Passive dressings

Passive dressings, as the name suggests, are usually simple products that have no direct effect on the wound. They have a simple protective function and protect the wound by covering it. Gauze is an example of a passive dressing. This type of product has many disadvantages and does not generally meet the criteria of an ideal dressing.

These dressings have very little absorbency and will become rapidly saturated. Once this happens, leakage will occur and the dressing may fall off. In wounds that produce only a small amount of exudate, this will soak into the dressing and then dry out, resulting in adhesion of the dressing and a painful and traumatic dressing change. However, these passive products are suitable for use where there is minimal or no drainage (e.g. closed surgical wounds) or as secondary products to provide padding and protection.

Interactive dressings

Most modern dressing products are classed as interactive dressings as they interact with the wound in some way, providing an optimum environment at the wound/dressing interface. Many interactive dressings are also occlusive, i.e. they do not allow passage of fluid or gases, but not all. Some interactive dressings are not occlusive or even semi-occlusive.

Other dressing categories

In addition to being passive or interactive, dressing products are classified into broadly similar generic groups. Table 10.2 compares the characteristics and clinical indications of wound dressings. Most dressings will fit into a discrete generic group but increasingly manufacturers are developing dressings that combine two separate products, giving the benefits of both categories.

Table 10.2 Characteristics of wound dressings

Generic name	Properties	Clinical indications	Practice guidelines
Alginates	High absorbency Haemostatic Atraumatic removal	Moderate to heavily exuding wounds May be used on infected wounds Debridement in wet wounds	Only use on wet wounds If the dressing is adhered to the wound, irrigate with saline When dressing cavities, loosely fill; do not tightly pack as this impedes free drainage of exudate
Deodorizing products	Little absorbency Contain deodorizing agents capable of controlling/reducing offensive odours	Used for exuding malodorous wounds Can be used on infected wounds	Can be used in conjunction with other dressings Dressing changes should be frequent Some products should not be cut as the fibres leak into the wound
Foams	Varying absorbency between brands and presentations Available as flat sheets, extra absorbents, low absorbents, shaped products for tracheostomy and drain sites, pre-formed shapes for heels and sacrum, with or without adhesion As cavity dressings pre-formed or in a presentation which is made by the practitioner and sets to fit the shape of the wound Permeable to water vapour – prevent the wound from drying out	Low to heavily exudating wounds	Can be used on a wide range of wounds Retain absorbency even under compression bandaging Self-adhesive foams are waterproof, which allows bathing and showering Generally very acceptable to patients
Hydrocolloids	Varying levels of absorbency depending on presentation Available in flat sheets, shaped products for heels and sacral area, thin products and extra adhesive products On contact with exudate, form a soft viscous gel Facilitate autolytic debridement of slough and necrotic tissue Rehydrate dry wounds Promote pain relief by keeping nerve endings moist	Suitable for low to moderately exuding wounds Useful for debriding dry or moist devitalized tissue Can be used at all stages of healing	Produce a characteristic odour at dressing change Self-adhesive and waterproof Thinner versions are semi-transparent, allowing wound progress to be observed without dressing removal Some products change colour to indicate progress of gel formation

(continued)

Table 10.2 *(continued)*

Generic name	Properties	Clinical indications	Practice guidelines
Hydrogels	Donate fluid to the wound which rehydrates dry necrotic tissues and liquefies slough Varying levels of fluid absorbency between brands Promote pain relief by keeping nerve endings moist Available as sheet presentations and, more commonly, amorphous gels Sheet gels are easier to handle and some have an adhesive backing	Sheet gels; dehydrated to moderately exuding flat wounds Amorphous gels; any dehydrated to moderately exuding wounds useful for narrow cavities or sinuses Can be used at all stages of the healing	Amorphous gels are removed by irrigation Sheet gels may occasionally become dehydrated; they can be rehydrated by irrigation or soaking Rapid debridement may initially make the wound appear larger Amorphous gels tend to dissipate under pressure Sheet gels allow visualization of the wound through the dressing Use of hydrogels is sometimes associated with maceration of the wound margins
Semi-permeable films	No absorbency Exhibit varying degrees of water vapour permeability Impermeable to water and microorganisms Trap exudate at the wound surface, providing a moist environment	Wounds with a low level of exudate Prophylaxis to reduce friction damage Often used as a secondary dressing, e.g. to hold a hydrogel in place	Only use on lightly exuding wounds Use with care on fragile or blistered skin Not designed to be removed on a daily basis, the acrylic adhesive becomes less adherent over time Stretch and pull to remove, do not peel off Transparent, so allowing visualization of the wound Not recommended for clinically infected wounds
Silicone sheets (gels)	Chemically inert Soften and flatten scar tissue although the precise mode of action is unknown Non-adherent	Use on recently healed wounds for best effect, although may be used several years after healing Used to minimize scar formation and contractures	Comfortable and simple for the patient to self-manage Can be worn beneath pressure garments Wear time is gradually built up to allow the skin to acclimatize to the product Suitable for reuse for the same patient; wash between use in mild soap and water Contraindicated in known silicone allergy and on open wounds
Silicone sheets (wound contact layers)	Chemically inert Porous Non-adherent	Fragile or painful wounds Wounds with high levels of exudate	May be left in situ for 7–10 days Do not adhere to the wound bed A secondary product may be used to absorb exudate Contraindicated in known silicone allergy
Low adherent primary contact dressings (medicated)	Have low absorbency Contain 10% povidone-iodine Base is polyethylene glycol which is water-soluble	Prophylaxis and treatment of a wide range of microorganisms including bacterial and fungal infections	Change dressing when orange/brown colour changes to white Some sensitivity to the iodine has been reported Require removal with caution; may adhere to some wounds Require a secondary dressing Contraindicated in pregnant and lactating women owing to the possible side-effect of elevated serum iodine levels
Polysaccharide bead dressings (medicated)	Absorbent dressing: on contact with exudate, a moist gel is formed Available as a powder, paste or flat sheet Iodine is not released until moistened by exudate Reduce bacterial count by antimicrobial effect of the iodine and also by the process of capillary action as the beads swell	Low to heavily exuding sloughy wounds Can be used on infected wounds	Dressings change colour from orange/brown to white as the iodine is utilized Maximum weekly dosages are stipulated; these vary with the differing presentations Require the use of a secondary dressing

Alginate dressings

Alginate dressings are derived from seaweed. They form a moist gel in the presence of wound exudate. They are available in a variety of presentations, including flat sheets, ribbon or rope dressings for use in cavity wounds. There are also combination products mixed or layered, e.g. with carbon dressings. There are different types of alginate and these are classified by the amount of mannuronic or guluronic acid present in the product. These acids affect the type of gel formed by the dressing. Alginates rich in guluronic acid gel more slowly and form a firmer gel, while alginates with high amounts of mannuronic acid gel quickly and form a much softer, more fluid gel which may appear to have completely dissolved leaving a thicker viscous liquid. Alginates also have a haemostatic capacity which is initiated when calcium ions within the product exchange with sodium ions in the wound, activating the clotting process and stimulating platelets and clotting factors VII, IX and X (Sussman 1996) (see also Ch. 18). However, few alginate dressings carry a product licence for use as a haemostat because they may dry out and become very difficult to remove in the absence of moisture to form a gel.

Deodorizing dressings

There is a range of deodorizing dressings available which usually contain activated charcoal or activated carbon to adsorb odour. These dressings are often used in combination with other products. They are used on malodorous wounds such as fungating tumours or infected surgical wounds.

Foam dressings

These are polyurethane foam dressings which have a hydrophilic action, i.e. they absorb and retain fluid. These dressings have a contact layer of low adherence and some have a film backing which prevents strike-through of exudate. Fluid is absorbed into the dressing and either spreads throughout it or, in simpler foam dressings, travels directly to the outside. Foam dressings are soft and conformable and were initially designed as non-adhesive products for use on friable skin, although newer versions may now have adhesive borders. There are differing levels of absorbency, with some brands of foam being extra-absorbent versions. They may be used as a secondary or protective dressing in areas subject to repetitive trauma, such as the heels or over a pretibial laceration. Non-adhesive versions can easily be cut and moulded to fit even very awkward areas.

Hydrocolloid dressings

Hydrocolloids have three main parts: the base, an adhesive matrix (which holds the product in shape) and a backing or outer layer. The base consists of sodium carboxymethylcellulose (CMC) in most products, but gelatin and pectin are used in some brands which may not be acceptable to vegans. These base products are held together in a flat sheet presentation by an adhesive polymer matrix. Different brands have a variety of backings: all are waterproof, some are polyurethane films and others are polyurethane foams. All prevent strike-through of exudate on to the outer surface of the dressing and transmission of bacteria into and out of the wound. A dressing 1.5–2 cm larger than the size of the wound should be used. This will improve wear time and allow for the gelling action of the product.

Hydrogel dressings

These products all have a significant water content but other components of the product (CMC, agar, glycerol and pectin) may vary and will affect the absorbency properties. Their main use is debridement. Hydrogels are available in two presentations:

- amorphous gels, packaged in tubes or similar dispensers, which are squeezed into or onto the wound, taking the shape of the wound and making them particularly suitable for cavity wounds
- sheet gels, which are held together by a matrix, making them easier to handle and making them stay in place, even on areas such as heels where pressure from walking would squeeze an amorphous gel away from the wound area.

Semi-permeable film dressings

A semi-permeable film dressing is a transparent polyurethane film coated with an acrylic adhesive. Initially designed and still used to produce a sterile field through which to make surgical incisions, some more sophisticated films are now manufactured with differing moisture/vapour handling rates. Film dressings with higher moisture/vapour permeability (the ability to allow fluid to escape) are now available for venous access sites. These products differ from wound management dressings and are generally much more expensive. Semi-permeable films are most commonly used as secondary dressings to hold other products in situ, and a non-sterile version, designed to hold other dressings in place, is now available on a roll.

Silicone dressings

These are soft conformable products in two presentations: silicone gels and silicone wound contact layers. Silicone gel products are transparent, usually 3–4 mm thick, and are used for scar reduction and softening. These products are reusable for the same patient but are not suitable for use on open wounds. Silicone gel dressings require the patient to build up a level of tolerance to them otherwise minor irritation may occur. For this reason, the patient may initially require support from health care professionals when using the product, after which this is usually a self-administered product.

Silicone wound contact layers are silicone-coated, porous, non-adherent dressings. They are used as a contact layer directly on the wound and may be left in place for 7–10 days. Other dressing products are then used on top. This allows free drainage of any exudate from the wound through the contact layer into the secondary dressing, but does not require frequent change of the dressing that is in direct contact with the wound. Silicone contact layers are used mainly on wounds that are very painful or producing very large quantities of exudate.

Low adherent medicated primary contact layers

These are knitted viscose products impregnated with polyethylene glycol, which contains 10% povidone-iodine (equivalent to 1% available iodine). Although the use of topical antimicrobial agents is controversial (Gilchrist 1997), iodine has one of the broadest spectrums of activity and a low sensitivity rate. Use of topical antimicrobials should be carefully controlled until more information is available. Where wounds are clinically infected, a topical antimicrobial may be used as an adjunct to systemic therapy.

Polysaccharide bead dressings (medicated)

These products contain hydrophilic beads of cadexomer impregnated with 0.9% iodine. They are available as flat sheet products with a paste sandwiched between carrier sheets or as an amorphous paste delivered from a tube. As with the medicated contact layers, the use of topical antimicrobials should be carefully controlled and observed until more information about the mode of action is known. Current opinion suggests that in addition to the antimicrobial effect of iodine there may be an as yet undetermined effect on the inflammatory response (Gilchrist 1997). These products may initially feel greasy but newer presentations are easier to handle.

Combination dressing products

There are an increasing number of combination dressings being manufactured. These seek to provide the benefits of two combined generic groups and are often developed as a response to clinicians regularly combining products in clinical practice but with less than satisfactory results. By producing a prepared product, there is often a reduction in bulkiness and additional advantages such as ease of application and reduced costs.

Biotechnology

There is growing interest in the field of biotechnology, especially in the use of cultured skin replacements and growth factors. These products are in the early stages of development and are not yet widely used. They are generally expensive and are mainly used in specialist centres but it is likely that there will be an increasing amount of information generated about these products over the next decade.

SELECTION OF WOUND MANAGEMENT PRODUCTS

A greater understanding of the physiology of wound healing and tissue repair in the last 20 years has resulted in the development of various innovative treatment approaches. The clinical efficacy of modern wound dressings has yet to be empirically demonstrated, although improvements in patient comfort and acceptability have been seen. In clinical practice, the selection of wound dressing products is influenced by a wide range of factors. The significance of these factors needs to be recognized if the most appropriate dressing materials are to be selected to manage wounds. Inappropriate selection of wound dressings may be uncomfortable for the patient, at best; at worst it may prolong wound healing.

A study carried out by Flanagan (1992) found that the following factors influenced the selection of dressings by hospital nurses:

- clinical factors – wound characteristics, cost-effectiveness of dressings, patient needs
- educational factors – knowledge base, clinical experience, research-based practice
- personal factors – confidence, negotiation skills, assertiveness, conflicting opinions
- team dynamics – pressure to conform with established practices, objective decision-making, willingness to consult others.

Similar factors have been found to influence the decision-making processes of community nurses. Lucker et al (1998) reported that factors relating to patient compliance and acceptability, i.e. comfort and absorbency, are of primary importance to both district and practice nurses when choosing dressing products.

Professional factors influencing selection of dressing products

In some clinical settings, the selection of dressing products causes conflict between colleagues and different professional groups. Current philosophies of wound management reflect a major shift from the use of antiseptics to the promotion of an environment conducive to healing, using interactive dressings. This corresponds with the development of tissue viability services in the UK led by nurse specialists and the launch of nurse prescribing.

Some health professionals experience difficulties when trying to make wound management decisions using research-based practice, as decisions relating to the type of dressing may be linked to issues relating to power, status and leadership (Flanagan 1992, Lucker et al 1998). The influence of medical staff on the selection of wound dressing and bandages is variable and tends to be more prescriptive within the acute hospital setting. Issues of power and control also relate to the professional relationships that nurses have with each other. At some time in their career, most nurses will have experienced disappointment when colleagues have changed a patient's dressing regimen without prior consultation and often without supportive rationale.

In recent years, cost-effectiveness of wound management has assumed greater importance. In most clinical settings, dressing use is determined by local guidelines formulated by a multidisciplinary wound care team and reviewed regularly in the light of new developments. Selection of appropriate wound dressings depends on a combination of skills such as clinical decision-making and the application of theory to practice. Selection of a wound dressing needs to be made on an individual basis as no two patients' wounds are the same. The choice of dressing product to cover a laceration on a 17-year-old's shin is likely to be different from that required to manage the same type of wound on an elderly person's leg (see Older Adults: Nursing Priorities box 10.1).

The Medicinal Products Prescription by Nurses, Midwives and Health Visitors Act (Department of Health 1992) had significant implications for the improvement of tissue viability services in the UK. From April 1999, this Act allowed specific categories of community nurses to prescribe wound dressings and certain medicines from a limited list of products. This extension of nurses' prescribing rights and the adoption of a nationally accepted system through which community nurses can provide a limited range of dressing products, via protocols agreed with medical practitioners, will particularly benefit older adults and those suffering from chronic disabilities. Early indications are that nurse prescribing saves time, reduces costs and enhances the continuity of care.

Nurses have been instrumental in affecting changes in wound management practices over the years and in many cases are fostering the development of multidisciplinary wound management groups. These collaborative professional groups have spent an increasing amount of time and effort developing clinical practice guidelines for acute and chronic wound management,

OLDER ADULTS: NURSING PRIORITIES

10.1 Dressing selection and older adults

Age-related skin changes, such as the loss of elasticity and dehydration, make the skin of older adults more susceptible to skin damage. The selection of dressing products for older adults therefore requires careful consideration if trauma is to be minimized.

The following factors need to be considered:

- Is an adhesive dressing product necessary? Many adhesives are very effective but may tear delicate skin when removed. Remember, manufacturers provide useful application and removal tips to minimize skin trauma.
- Could an alternative method of securing the dressing be used, e.g. bandaging?
- Is the dressing too bulky? Thick dressings on the sacrum and/or heels can cause additional skin trauma due to the effects of shearing.
- The use of dressings with a high water content on highly exudating wounds can cause skin irritation due to the effects of maceration. Selection of a more absorbent dressing should minimize these effects.
- Will the dressing cause skin sensitivities? A range of products may cause skin irritation, including the adhesive components of dressings, tapes, skin creams, moisturizers and washing detergents.

OLDER ADULTS: NURSING PRIORITIES

10.2 Pressure ulcer risk status in older patients

Specific nursing actions required:

- *Skin assessment.* Age-related changes affect the resilience of the skin and therefore full skin assessment should include colour and texture of skin – look for areas of discoloration, dryness, rough texture, reduced elasticity, small breaks, evidence of maceration, excoriation or dehydration, thinning/paper-like skin. Skin conditions such as eczema should also be noted.
- *Assessment of risk status.* Most risk assessment tools will include the following factors:
  - level of mobility
  - condition of the skin
  - nutritional status
  - level of continence
  - medication which may affect skin condition.
- *Plan of prevention.* Develop and implement a plan of prevention which addresses all the factors (intrinsic and extrinsic) that combine to make the patient 'at risk'.

and the impact of such documents on the quality of care has been significant (RCN 1998).

PRESSURE ULCERS

Pressure ulcers (also known as pressure sores, bed sores, decubitus ulcers) affect all age groups and are costly in financial terms, use of resources and more importantly human suffering. A pressure ulcer is an area of localized damage to the skin and underlying tissue caused by pressure, shear or friction, or a combination of these (European Pressure Ulcer Advisory Panel [EPUAP] 1999a). Pressure ulcers are a largely preventable problem, and a thorough ongoing assessment and implementation of a holistic plan of prevention can reduce their frequency and the distress they cause to patients.

EPIDEMIOLOGY AND AETIOLOGY

Pressure ulcers remain common, the frequency of occurrence varying considerably between different patient groups and differing care settings. Estimates of the frequency vary between 2.7 and 66% and their true costs are not known, but estimates range from £60 million to £200 million per year (Department of Health 1993). The costs to the patient may include pain and suffering, embarrassment caused by odour or exudate leakage, loss of function within the family, an increased loss of income, if employed, a potential job loss due to an extended period of hospitalization and in some situations death. Costs to the health

care provider fall into two main categories: financial costs associated with the provision of dressing materials, specialist equipment, treatment for complications such as antibiotics or surgery; and lost opportunity costs associated with the potential use of the bed, nursing time and other resources (Department of Health 1993). It is likely that with an ageing population and increasing survival rates for even major disease processes, the number of patients at risk and those who develop pressure ulceration will continue to rise (EPUAP 1999b) (see Older Adults: Nursing Priorities box 10.2).

Many clinical areas attempt to measure their incidence of pressure ulcers but there is little consistency in the type and accuracy of data collected, making meaningful comparison of the numbers difficult (Fletcher 1997). It is, however, suggested that the incidence is higher in those who are elderly, immobile or have a range of concurrent disease processes.

Pressure ulcers are caused by three external forces: pressure, friction and shear. These external forces lead to occlusion of the blood supply to the skin, which in turn leads to hypoxia, ischaemia and eventually tissue death. In reality, pressure, friction and shear rarely occur in isolation and components of all three are involved in the development of most pressure ulcers (see Fig. 10.5).

Pressure

Application of pressure alone does not cause damage. The amount of pressure applied to the skin has to be sufficient to cause occlusion of the underlying blood vessels and has to be applied for enough time for damage to occur. Thus, there is a relationship between the amount of pressure and the time during which it is applied before tissue damage is irreversible. This varies between individuals and depends upon many intrinsic factors which allow the body to resist the effects of pressure.

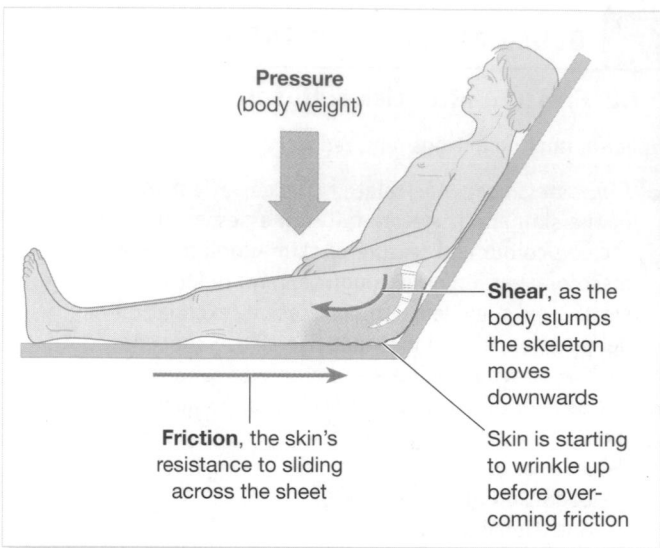

Figure 10.5 The relationship between pressure, shear and friction. The shaded area around the patient's buttocks is the area of highest risk – combined forces of pressure, shear and friction compress and stretch the tissue between the bone and surface.

Shear

Shear is an internal force caused when adjacent surfaces slide across each other, which results in twisting and tearing of the underlying blood vessels and leads to tissue ischaemia and localized tissue death. Shear commonly occurs when patients are semi-recumbent in bed. The body begins to slide and, before the frictional force of the skin on the bedclothes is overcome, the internal parts of the body, such as the skeleton, move down the bed, but as the skin does not move there is a stretching or tearing of the blood vessels.

Friction

Friction is the force caused when two touching surfaces move in opposite directions and may result in superficial scuffing or abrasion of the skin. This force is sufficient to tear the epidermis from its anchoring to the dermis and, if sufficient force is applied, may tear the dermis from the basement membrane, overcoming the anchoring forces of the desmosomes. This commonly occurs when patients are not moved appropriately or when they are not adequately supported and slide down the bed. Friction may also be generated by brisk rubbing of the skin, a practice which was previously felt to be beneficial because it stimulated blood supply, but which is now known to cause both friction and shearing forces, thereby causing tissue damage.

RISK ASSESSMENT

Although the true causes of tissue damage are pressure, shear and friction, there are other factors, known as intrinsic risk factors, which determine an individual's susceptibility to these external forces. Factors which increase an individual's risk include any concurrent disease process which affects either the blood supply, e.g. peripheral vascular disease and cardiac failure (see Ch. 19), or the quality of the circulating blood and therefore

its ability to provide adequate oxygen and nutrition to the tissues, e.g. any lung disease (see Ch. 20) and malabsorption syndromes (see Chs 11 and 22). A variety of intrinsic factors are thought to predispose to pressure ulcer development and those more frequently described include general medical condition, skin condition, immobility, nutritional status and incontinence (EPUAP 1999b).

To prevent the development of pressure ulcers, it is therefore important to identify those who are at increased risk of tissue damage. The most common way of doing this is to use a pressure ulcer risk assessment tool.

Pressure ulcer risk assessment tools

There is a range of risk assessment tools available to help identify individuals at risk of developing pressure ulcers. The first of these tools, the Norton Score (Norton et al 1962), was designed for use with the older adult and comprises five categories – physical condition, mental condition, activity, mobility and level of continence – each with a range of scores. Each broad category scores a maximum of four, indicating no risk, and a minimum of one, indicating a high risk. The scores from each category are totalled and a threshold score is described, beyond which the patient is deemed to be 'at risk' of pressure ulcer development.

Newer risk assessment tools further subdivide the total to denote differing levels of risk, e.g. the Waterlow Score (Waterlow 1985) suggests risk bands of 'at risk', 'high risk' and 'very high risk'. The terms used vary between the tools, with other systems suggesting 'low', 'medium' and 'high' risk levels. A more important difference between the systems is the direction of the numerical indicators. Norton (Norton et al 1962) and Braden (Bergastrom et al 1987) suggest that the lower the score, the greater the risk, whilst others, e.g. Waterlow (Waterlow 1985), suggest that the higher the score the higher the risk. This is obviously related to the way individual risk factors are weighted within the individual tools, but highlights that a number alone does not signify anything unless the tools from which the number was derived is known.

Different risk assessment tools include (and exclude) a host of risk factors (Table 10.3), with the majority concentrating purely on the intrinsic factors. There is little research evidence to support these decisions; however, the factors included would generally be supported by clinicians. Many new tools were developed because clinicians felt that existing tools did not address the needs of their particular patient group and therefore some were developed for use in very specific areas: for example, Walsall (Milward et al 1993) was designed for use in the community. Use outside of the area for which they were designed will affect the accuracy of the tools and lead to a tendency to under- or over-predict the level of risk.

Many clinical areas now routinely use these tools to assist in the decision-making process, particularly for the allocation of specialist equipment but also for the planning of general care. Many criticisms have been levelled at the tools but it must be remembered that they are used to support and not replace the clinical decision-making process. The accuracy of the tools may be improved by ensuring that they are appropriate to the patient group and that all those using the tools receive adequate educational preparation and support.

Table 10.3 A summary of risk factors included in different pressure ulcer risk assessment tools

	Norton (Norton et al 1962)	Braden (Bergastrom et al 1987)	PSPS (Lowthian 1987)	Waterlow (Waterlow 1985)	Gosnell (Gosnell 1973)	Medley (Williams 1992)	Walsall (Milward et al 1993)	Anderson (Hinton 1992)
Physical condition	✓		✓			✓	✓	
Medical condition	✓				✓			
Activity	✓	✓			✓	✓		
Mobility	✓	✓		✓	✓	✓	✓	✓
Continence	✓		✓	✓	✓	✓	✓	✓
Nutrition		✓		✓	✓	✓	✓	✓
Build/weight for height				✓				
Skin condition				✓		✓	✓	✓
Age				✓				✓
Sex				✓				
Sensory perception		✓		✓				
Moisture		✓						
Friction and shear		✓						
Sitting up			✓					
Conscious level				✓		✓	✓	✓
Tissue malnutrition				✓				
Major surgery				✓				✓
Medication				✓				
Carer involvement							✓	
Dehydration								✓
Pain						✓	✓	

As the patient's condition may change, regular reassessments are necessary. There is no defined time interval but recent guidance from the European Pressure Ulcer Advisory Panel suggests that assessment should be ongoing, with the frequency of reassessment being dependent upon changes in the patient's overall condition (EPUAP 1999b). This ensures that if the patient's level of risk increases, adequate preventative action is taken, and also, if their level of risk reduces, that the preventative strategies are altered accordingly. This ensures that resources are utilized effectively with the associated benefits for both patients and funding.

PREVENTING PRESSURE DAMAGE

Once a patient has been assessed as being 'at risk' of pressure damage, an appropriate plan of prevention must be initiated. This must address, where possible, all the factors (both extrinsic and intrinsic) that contribute to the level of risk (see Guidelines for Care Priorities box 10.1).

Positioning

Pressure ulcers more commonly occur over large bones or bony prominences where the blood vessels are compressed between a hard external surface (the bed or chair) and a hard internal force (the bone), which leads to occlusion of the underlying blood vessels. To reduce this risk, it is important to position the patient correctly. Patients should not be routinely placed directly on their sides or flat on their back, as these are high-risk areas. Use of positioning techniques such as the 30° tilt (Preston 1991), which uses pillows to support the patient, will redistribute the

GUIDELINES FOR CARE PRIORITIES

10.1 Pressure ulcer prevention

Main points
- Identify 'at risk' individuals needing prevention and the specific factors placing them at risk
- Maintain and improve tissue tolerance to pressure in order to prevent injury
- Protect against the adverse effects of external mechanical forces: pressure, friction and shear
- Improve the outcome for patients at risk of pressure damage through educational programmes.

Reference
European Pressure Ulcer Advisory Panel. Pressure ulcer prevention guidelines. Oxford: European Pressure Ulcer Advisory Panel; 1999.

weight over the large muscle masses and spread the pressure over a large surface area. This reduces the amount of pressure at any individual point on the body. Simply supporting the patient adequately whilst in the bed or chair, to evenly distribute the pressure, can significantly reduce the risk of pressure ulceration. Patients at high risk of pressure damage should not be allowed to sit out of bed for long periods (no more than 2 hours at any one time) as this concentrates the whole body weight on a small supporting area (EPUAP 1999b). Frequency of repositioning should be determined by assessing the individual's tolerance to

HEALTH PROMOTION

10.1 Avoiding pressure damage

Vikram is 19 years old and is paraplegic. It is a year since his injury (a diving accident) and he has asked what he can do to prevent his skin breaking down as he sits in his wheelchair for long periods. Advice should include the following:

- The importance of correct seat height and depth – the seat height should allow for the feet to be placed securely on the floor (or foot rests) with the knees and hips at right angles. This ensures pressure is distributed along the buttocks, backs of legs and the feet. The seat should be wide enough to be comfortable and not cause pressure on the hips, but not so wide as to allow the patient to lean sideways causing uneven distribution of pressure on to one side.
- The importance of the correct cushion – the cushion must provide an appropriate level of pressure reduction for the patient's needs and fit the chair securely. The effect of the dimensions of the cushion should be included in the overall assessment of the seat height and depth.
- The importance of regular checking and maintenance of the cushion – cushions should be checked for integrity of the cover, correct level of inflation (where appropriate), integrity of foam, etc.

- The role of position changes to relieve pressure – pressure relief when seated is achieved by lifting the buttocks clear of the seat for short periods on a regular basis. If there is not enough arm strength to achieve this, leaning forward for a short period may reduce the pressure on the sacrum. The plan of position changes may also include set periods in bed and must be negotiated individually with the patient.
- The importance of wearing the correct clothing – clothing must be comfortable and well-fitting, as tight clothing or prominent seams may cause additional pressure, as may excessively loose clothing. Natural fibres reduce sweating.
- The importance of regular skin checks – where possible, patients should be taught to inspect their own skin, using a mirror if necessary. Where this is not possible, a carer should be involved. Both parties should be taught to check the skin for changes in colour, texture and heat. Information should be given on who to contact and how to contact them. Pain, discomfort, discoloration and breaks in the skin should be brought to the attention of the appropriate health professional immediately.

---

pressure, which is simply done by visual inspection of the skin for signs of initial pressure damage (see Health Promotion box 10.1).

CLASSIFICATION OF PRESSURE DAMAGE

Should pressure damage occur, it is important to be able to quantify the extent of the damage, both to ensure adequate and accurate record-keeping and to improve communication between all the health care professionals involved in the patient's care. As with the risk assessment tools, there is a variety of classification or grading tools which may be used to describe the degree of tissue damage. There is little agreement between these tools, e.g. whether to include or exclude transient reddening of the skin as pressure damage, or how to classify a necrotic wound where the full extent of tissue damage may not be visible. Grades described range from 0 to 5 with some tools, and from 1 to 4 with others. This can lead to confusion in clinical practice with different practitioners using different tools (see Evidence-based Practice box 10.2).

During assessment, the skin is observed for signs of tissue hypoxia, which is usually characterized by erythema (redness). This redness is a normal physiological response and can be seen, for example, when healthy individuals have been sitting with their legs crossed. This initial redness, known as blanching erythema, is a result of a temporary occlusion of the blood supply and does not persist for any length of time. A simple way to test the extent of damage is to press the reddened area. In normal skin the redness will pale to white (blanch) under the finger pressure, as the underlying blood vessels are fully occluded, and when the finger is removed the blood supply will return to the area, giving an increased density of colour. The first stages of

EVIDENCE-BASED PRACTICE

10.2 Validity and reliability of pressure ulcer classification systems

A paper by Healey (1995) summarizes a research study that evaluated the reliability and utility in clinical use of three pressure ulcer classification systems: the Sterling, Torrance and Surrey classification systems. In the study, 109 qualified nurses were asked to use the scales to grade 10 photographs of pressure ulcers of varying severity. Ease of use of the scales was also discussed.

The study found that the Surrey classification system was the simplest and easiest to use and also the most reliable. Most agreement between users was found when rating the more severe sores, but the limitations of using photographs as opposed to grading real sores on patients is acknowledged. The Stirling classification system was found to be the least reliable.

Reference
Healey F. The reliability and utility of pressure sore grading scales. Journal of Tissue Viability 1995; 5(4): 111–114.

---

damage may be said to have occurred when the redness does not resolve even when the pressure is relieved for some time. This redness, when pressed with the finger, will not blanch and is known as non-blanching erythema. This condition is also characterized by a slight warmth and a hardening or induration of

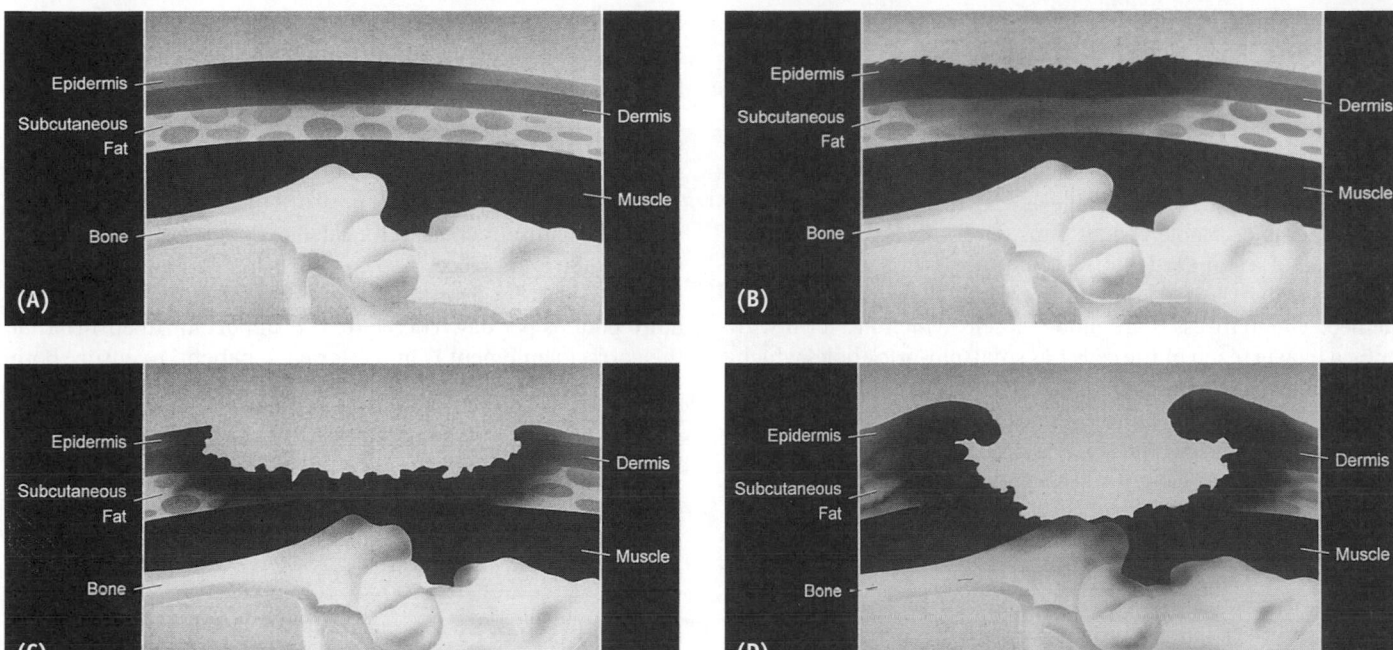

Figure 10.6 The European Pressure Ulcer Advisory Panel (EPUAP) four-grade classification tool. (A) Grade 1: non-blanchable erythema of intact skin. Discoloration of the skin, warmth, oedema, induration or hardness may also be used as indicators, particularly in individuals with darker skin. (B) Grade 2: partial-thickness skin loss involving the epidermis or dermis, or both. The ulcer is superficial and presents clinically as an abrasion or blister. (C) Grade 3: full-thickness skin loss involving damage to, or necrosis of, subcutaneous tissue that may extend down to, but not through, underlying fascia. (D) Grade 4: extensive destruction, tissue necrosis or damage to muscle, bone or supporting structures with or without full-thickness skin loss. (Reproduced with permission of Huntleigh Healthcare.)

the local area. In darker skin tones, it may not be possible to see the redness, with only differences in skin tone being visible, and in this instance palpation of the area for warmth and induration may provide evidence of tissue damage.

There are at least 14 classification tools in use (Reid & Morison 1994) and they describe tissue damage in a variety of ways. The grade of damage described usually refers to the layers of skin involved and relies upon the assessors to have an appreciation of the relevant anatomical structures. The EPUAP suggest the use of a four-grade classification tool (EPUAP 1999a) (see Fig. 10.6). As with the risk assessment tools, it is important to ensure that the individual using the tool has a good understanding of the terminology used.

PRESSURE ULCER PREVENTION EQUIPMENT

Part of any preventative plan of care should be the provision of equipment to reduce the risk of pressure ulcer development. There is a broad range of equipment available to prevent and assist in the treatment of pressure damage. Equipment to be considered usually includes a specialist mattress or bed and a cushion or chair. Other simpler pieces of equipment that should also be considered include the overhead trapezium (monkey pole), which allows patients to lift themselves and relieve pressure, and electronic bed frames and bedside rails, which may also help patients to reposition themselves. Equipment is described in a variety of ways but for simplicity will be categorized according to the definitions of pressure-relieving and pressure-reducing (Kenney & Rithalia 1999).

Pressure-reducing equipment

Pressure-reducing equipment works by increasing the amount of the body in contact with the support surface so that each point on the body supports less weight and is subjected to less pressure. Pressure reduction can be achieved in a variety of ways and this type of equipment varies from simple to extremely sophisticated.

Foam mattresses

The simplest pressure-reducing equipment is a good quality foam mattress or cushion with a stretch cover, which allows the foam to contour to the shape of the patient and increase the contact area. The stretch cover follows the shape of the foam, is usually made of a breathable fabric which reduces the likelihood of sweating and is waterproof, thus protecting the foam from contamination by fluids. These are suitable for patients at low risk of pressure damage.

Static overlays

Static overlays are designed for use on top of a standard mattress or cushion. They are made from a variety of materials including hollow core fibres, foam, gel and air. They provide an extra cushioning layer and are generally soft, which allows them to conform more closely to the body shape. As they are used in addition to the standard mattress/cushion, they increase the height of the bed or chair. This needs to be taken into consideration, as it may affect patients' ability to mobilize independently or their safety; for example, raising the height of the seat in relation to the arm rests may increase the risk of patients falling out of the chair. The additional height may also have implications for staff safety when moving and handling patients. Some of the air-filled overlays require setting for the individual patient's weight to obtain the maximum pressure reduction.

Low air loss systems

Low air loss systems are available as mattress overlays, mattress replacements or whole bed systems. Overlays are designed for use on top of a standard mattress; mattresses are placed directly on the standard bed frame and the whole bed system replaces the bed. The mattresses are made of cells which are filled with air by a blower; each of the cells has small pin-prick holes which, when subjected to the patient's body weight, allow the air to escape. The air is constantly replaced by the blower and the holes are so small that the surface simply becomes much softer and conforms very closely to the patient's body shape. In the more sophisticated whole bed systems, it is possible to set different zones of the bed, e.g. torso, head or heels, to different pressures to ensure comfort for the patient and also to achieve maximum pressure reduction for different patient weights. If there is an interruption in the power supply, these systems will deflate very quickly. This is an important feature when caring for critically ill patients who might suffer a cardiac arrest.

Air-fluidized systems

These systems are only available as whole bed systems. They are large 'bath-like' beds which are filled with micro-hemispheres of silicone through which warm air is constantly blown. This results in a constantly shifting surface which continually moves the pressure, ensuring that no area of the body is subjected to pressure for longer than a minute or so. This type of bed is suitable for patients at very high risk of pressure ulcers and also is the only system on which it is not necessary to turn the patient. This means it is also suitable for patients for whom movement is painful, e.g. patients with severe rheumatoid disease, carcinoma with bone metastases, etc. In an emergency (e.g. cardiac arrest) the power is disconnected and the surface becomes solid.

Pressure-relieving equipment

Pressure-relieving equipment alternately applies and then removes pressure to areas of the body. This type of equipment requires an electrical power supply or battery but will remain inflated for several hours should there be a loss of power. There is a mechanism for immediate deflation in the event of an emergency. This type of equipment is more commonly known as an alternating system. Such systems are available as overlays, mattress replacements and more recently as a whole bed system supplied with an electronic bed frame.

The systems are made up of a series of cells or cushions, which are filled with air and alternately inflate and deflate in a fixed cycle, so if one cell is fully inflated the next cell is fully deflated. It should be possible to slide a hand beneath the patient where the cell is deflated to check that that area is not subjected to any pressure. Different manufacturers produce systems with a different number of cells in the cycle, e.g. one cell deflated or two cells deflated, and with different cell cycle times. The time for a whole cycle, i.e. complete inflation, complete deflation and back to inflation, varies between 7.5 and 10 minutes. This cycle time is meant to mimic the frequency with which a healthy adult would change position during sleep. Alternating systems are suitable for patients with a medium to high risk of developing pressure ulcers.

SELECTION OF EQUIPMENT

There are currently over 200 pressure ulcer prevention devices available, with little research evidence to support the selection of any individual piece. The cost of using this equipment can vary considerably, from a few pounds a week to a hundred or more pounds per day. Therefore, it is important to ensure that the correct equipment is in use for each patient, to ensure both adequate prevention and best use of limited resources. The first criterion to consider is the patient's level of risk. Most manufacturers recommend a level of risk for which their equipment should be used and this is a useful start point. However, many different pieces of equipment are suitable for the same level of risk and therefore different criteria need to be considered during the selection (see Ethical Issues box 10.1).

Practical issues

Practical issues may limit the choice considerably. Most equipment has recommended maximum and minimum weight limits: for the majority of foam mattresses this will be between 38 and 114 kg, but for the more sophisticated equipment it may rise to 222 kg. Weight limits for cushions vary considerably dependent upon the type of material from which they are made. If patients are lighter than the minimum weight, the pressure exerted may be too high and would cause discomfort and potential tissue damage. If patients are heavier than the maximum weight, they would 'bottom out' the mattress, i.e. they would flatten the mattress to such an extent that they would be resting on the bed frame. Some companies now produce a bariatric (designed for obese patients) range of products for patients over 225 kg. This includes reinforced bed frames, as the weight limit for the majority of bed frames is 178 kg.

Some patients may initially dislike the movement of alternating systems but after a short time they become accustomed to it. Equally, a small number of patients may notice the movement of the air-fluidized systems.

 ETHICAL ISSUES

10.1 Pressure ulcers: health care rationing

Once a patient is assessed as being 'at risk' of developing pressure ulcers, preventative action should be taken. This usually involves the provision of specialist mattresses and/or cushions. Provision of this often costly equipment varies considerably between different hospitals, in the community and in the nursing home sector. In some care settings, provision of equipment is extremely limited.

- What are your views about how freely this equipment should be available?
- How would you prepare a case to justify the cost of a special bed for a patient you had identified as being at very high risk of developing a pressure ulcer?

Particular consideration should be given to the actual dimensions of the equipment. Cushion sizes vary considerably and different cushions will be needed for hospital chairs, chairs in the home setting and wheelchairs. A problem in the community setting is often the size of mattresses, especially when they need to be used on a double bed. Most equipment is considerably more than half the size of a bed, thereby leaving very little room for the partner to sleep. Some pieces of equipment, such as air-fluidized beds, are themselves very heavy and may weigh up to three-quarters of a ton. This places considerable limitations on where they may be used. It is unlikely, for example, that they would be used in a patient's home, and even in hospitals it is often not possible to transport them to anywhere other than the ground floor without the use of a special lift.

Specialist additional features

Many of the sophisticated systems also offer a range of other features. With some low air loss systems, it is possible to weigh the patient and rotate the patient to reduce the risk of chest infections. Some air-fluidized systems include the management of fluid (such as wound exudate or incontinence). The silicone hemispheres (beads) in the bed are very dry and any fluid that passes through the sheet is instantly absorbed and forms a clump of beads which then drops into a filter pan in the base of the bed and can be removed. The pH of the beads is such that they are actively bactericidal, so there is little risk of infection. The warm air also dries the sheet so that the patient's skin is not left wet. This can be useful when managing patients with large, heavily exuding pressure ulcers or large wet burns. It is also possible to control the temperature of the air-fluidized beds and they may be used to slowly warm a patient who is hypothermic (see Ch. 5). However, because the air around patients cared for on air-fluidized beds is continuously warm and dry, they have an increased requirement for fluids of approximately an extra 1–1.5 litres/day (see Ch. 8).

As there is a wide range of equipment available, it should be possible to select the most appropriate, taking care to assess the objectives of each patient's care while being aware of how equipment works and the benefits it can offer. Equipment should be a 24-hour provision and any patient who requires a mattress but spends time sitting in a chair should also be supplied with an appropriate level of seating.

The need for specialized equipment should be regularly reassessed and the appropriate equipment utilized as the patient's needs change. It should be stressed that use of equipment does not replace nursing care and patients will still require turning, although frequency may be reduced. The frequency of turning will be determined by checking the individual patient's tolerance to pressure as previously described.

PREVENTION AND MANAGEMENT OF LEG ULCERS

Ulceration of the lower leg is a common chronic condition that frequently recurs and causes a great deal of discomfort. All leg ulcers are caused by an insufficiency of the blood supply to the lower limb. The majority occur due to poor venous return, which causes oedema and eventual skin breakdown (venous ulcers). The remainder (arterial ulcers) result from an inadequate arterial blood supply to the foot, which causes ischaemia and a breakdown of the soft tissues. Leg ulcers have been defined as 'a loss of skin below the knee on the leg or foot that takes more than six weeks to heal' (Dale et al 1983). This definition takes no account of other common causes of non-healing wounds, such as pressure ulcers and pre-tibial lacerations, and may account for an over-estimation of the size of the problem.

EPIDEMIOLOGY AND AETIOLOGY

Leg ulcers are common. Prevalence is reported to be between 0.15 and 1%, particularly in older adults (Callum et al 1985), although this varies according to the population studied and methodology used. A wide range of leg ulcer healing rates are documented, ranging from 45 to 81% at 24 weeks for all ulcer types (Moffatt et al 1992). Direct comparison of leg ulcer healing rates is problematic as population sampling, methodologies and treatment protocols vary. A systematic review commissioned by the Department of Health suggests that there is no single treatment that is more effective than others and concludes that after-care should be a priority combined with optimum use of resources (NHS Centre for Reviews & Dissemination 1997).

Leg ulceration is characterized by alternating phases of ulceration, healing and recurrence. It is estimated that approximately 25% of all patients with leg ulcers will have open ulcers at any time (Moffatt et al 1992). Although good healing rates for leg ulcers can be achieved, recurrence is common and recurrence rates ranging from 22 to 69% at 12–18 months post-healing have been reported. A randomized trial (Moffatt & Dorman 1995) recruited 188 people with recently healed venous ulcers and demonstrated a 28% recurrence rate in those who complied with treatment consisting of compression hosiery and skin care, compared with 57% for those who were unable to tolerate stockings.

PATIENT ASSESSMENT

Assessment is the key to effective management of leg ulcers. Since the mid-1980s, studies have demonstrated that significant improvements in healing rates can occur when leg ulcer services are rationalized and grounded in research-based protocols (NHS Centre for Reviews & Dissemination 1997). However, some patients with leg ulcers have never been referred for specialist opinion, despite suffering from ulceration for many years, and subsequently may not have had the aetiology of their ulcer confirmed. Dedicated leg ulcer services consistently demonstrate that after-care is an important factor in the prevention of recurrence. The importance of leg ulcer after-care is recognized in some areas with the provision of healed ulcer clinics where recurrence at 6 months follow-up is reported to be low. Currently this type of service is only available in limited locations due to finite resources.

All leg ulcers have an underlying aetiology that determines which management strategy should be implemented. The first stage is a detailed holistic assessment that includes a comprehensive history, examination of the limbs, Doppler ultrasound assessment and other relevant investigations. A Doppler assessment is a non-invasive technique using a hand-held ultrasound probe which determines the volume of blood flow reaching the lower limbs. Accurate patient assessment is required when a patient presents for the first time with a leg ulcer, in order to determine:

- the underlying aetiology of the ulcer
- any associated factors that may prolong healing
- previous treatments which have been used
- the patient's social environment and support network.

It is also important to identify when the ulcer first occurred and whether the patient has a previous history of leg ulceration. If there is a history, the site of previous ulcers should be noted, together with the number of previous episodes of ulceration and the time the ulcers took to heal. All of this information should be carefully documented on an assessment form designed specifically to record relevant details of leg ulceration. Regular reassessment is important in order that the management plan can be modified according to the patient's response to treatment. In the UK this type of assessment usually takes place in the community and would normally be undertaken by a community nurse.

Effective treatment of leg ulcer patients depends upon accurate diagnosis and differentiation between venous insufficiency and arterial disease. Venous and arterial leg ulcers have different characteristics that can be identified by careful observation. However, caution is required when assessing patients with leg ulcers of mixed aetiology, i.e. ulcers caused by a combination of venous insufficiency and arterial impairment, as these ulcers often exhibit mixed characteristics.

Venous leg ulcers

Approximately 70% of leg ulcers are caused by chronic venous hypertension and are secondary to long-established disease of the deep veins in the lower limb (Cullum & Roe 1995). Damage to valves in the perforating veins linking the deep and superficial veins of the lower leg results in venous hypertension which causes the superficial veins to dilate. The resulting back-flow of blood and increased hydrostatic pressure is eventually transmitted to the capillaries in the skin around the ankle. The capillaries become stretched, which increases their permeability and causes abnormal leakage of fluid into the subcutaneous tissues. Oedema quickly forms and characteristic dark brown staining of the skin occurs as red blood cells leak through damaged

capillary membranes and release haemoglobin as they disintegrate. These changes frequently cause a variety of skin problems, including eczema, hypersensitivities and excessive dryness (see Fig. 10.7).

Venous ulcers are generally large and shallow and are located between the ankle and the calf. They produce copious amounts of exudate which may cause surrounding skin damage and sensitivities. Skin changes characteristic of venous hypertension are often associated with venous ulcers and include dark brown pigmentation and a hardening of the subcutaneous tissues around the ulcerated area (lipodermatosclerosis); sometimes white mottling of the skin occurs (atrophe blanche). Venous leg ulcers are associated with ankle oedema and aching legs.

Arterial leg ulcers

Arterial or ischaemic leg ulcers are caused by an inadequate arterial blood supply. Arterial insufficiency is often caused by peripheral vascular disease where the deposition of fatty plaques (atheroma) on the inside of arterial walls causes narrowing and eventually a blockage. The tissues of the lower leg and foot gradually become underperfused with oxygenated blood, resulting in ischaemia, necrosis and ulcer breakdown (Cullum & Roe 1995). These wounds are often very painful and restrict patient mobility. Arterial leg ulcers are often small but relatively deep and are most commonly found on the feet or toes (see Fig. 10.8). Where appropriate, vascular surgery may help to heal the ulcer by restoring the local blood supply, but there are no controlled studies to support the effectiveness of this approach.

Arterial ulcers are typically small, but deep, and are found on the foot or toes. They are often dry and covered with a scab or produce minimal to moderate amounts of exudate. The skin changes associated with this type of ulcer occur due to ischaemia of the limb. In the early stages, the limb will be pale and cool; as the ischaemia worsens, the affected leg will become reddish and mottled; eventually it takes on a purplish/blue appearance before finally becoming black and necrotic. One of the most reliable indicators of arterial ulceration is intense pain associated with the ulcer. This pain is worse on walking and is typically worse at night. Patients will often resort to sleeping in a chair at night so that they can maximize arterial blood flow to their feet which reduces the pain. A comparison of the clinical signs and symptoms associated with leg ulcers is summarized in

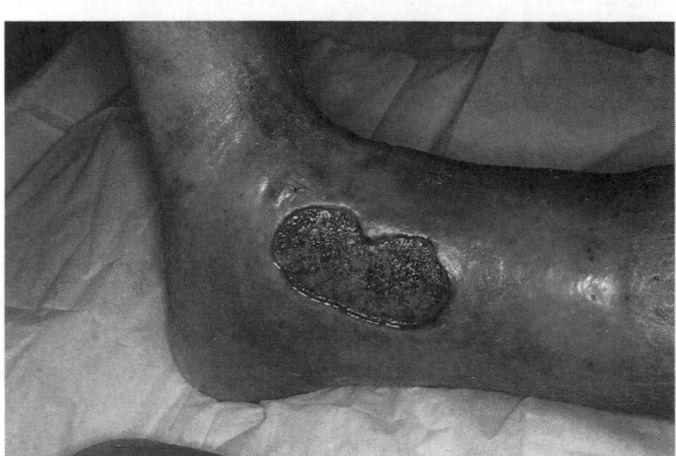

Figure 10.7 A venous leg ulcer.

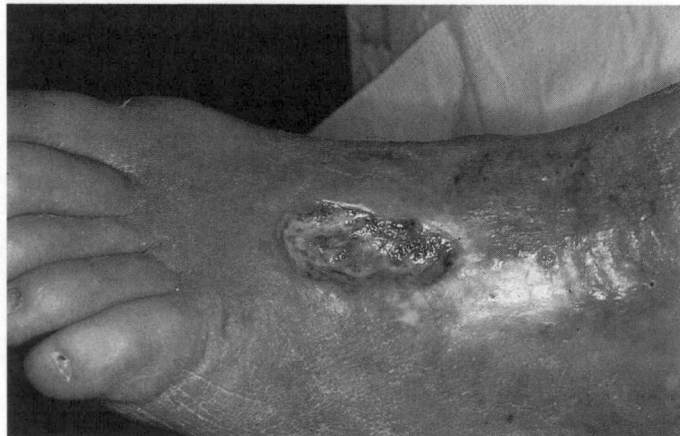

Figure 10.8 An arterial leg ulcer.

Table 10.4 Comparison of clinical signs and symptoms of venous and arterial leg ulceration

	Venous ulceration (Fig. 10.7)	Arterial ulceration (Fig. 10.8)
Previous medical history	Deep vein thrombosis (DVT), varicose veins or family history of leg ulcers	Cerebrovascular accident (CVA), angina, peripheral vascular disease, hypertension, diabetes
Site/position	Often near the ankle or between the ankle and knee	Usually on the foot and between the toes, or close to the ankle
Appearance	Typically large, shallow wounds producing copious exudate	Often smaller, deep wounds producing less exudate
Surrounding skin condition	Characteristic pigmentation – lipo-dermatosclerosis (brown staining), atrophe blanche (white patches) Contact dermatitis and eczema are common	Hairless, shiny skin Skin colour ranges from white to dusky pink and purple Dusky pink feet turn pale when raised above the heart In darker-skinned individuals, ischaemic skin ranges from a paler colour to a dark mottled appearance Thickening of nail beds is sometimes seen
Pain/discomfort	Aching or heaviness in legs often related to localized oedema Localized pain, tenderness of ulcer	Intermittent claudication (pain on exertion) Rest pain, severe, constant pain, often worse at night

Table 10.4 and is intended as a framework to help identify the significance of the symptoms of vascular disease.

Vascular assessment

The use of a vascular assessment method such as the Doppler ultrasound can increase the accuracy of patient assessment. The Doppler test produces a reading which is the index of the brachial systolic blood pressure divided by the ankle-systolic blood pressure. This reading is called the ankle brachial pressure index (ABPI). An ABPI reading of 1.0 is normal and indicates that 100% of blood flow is reaching the extremities, whereas a value of 0.8 indicates reduced peripheral tissue perfusion as only approximately 80% of blood flow is reaching the affected foot. Although approximately 70% of leg ulcers are of venous origin, it is recognized that many of these patients, especially older adults, will have coexisting arterial disease and an ABPI reading of below 0.9. Some ulcers have a combined aetiology resulting from venous insufficiency and arterial impairment and have the combined features of both types of ulcer (see Reflective Practice box 10.2).

R|Я REFLECTIVE PRACTICE

10.2 Which type of ulcer?

Mr Ballard has a small, dry ulcer near his toes. Despite its size, the ulcer is extremely painful and has recently been keeping him awake at night. On initial nursing assessment you note that his leg is pale and cool and you find it difficult to palpate a foot pulse. He has some mild oedema in his foot which make his slippers pinch across the toes.

- Which type of leg ulcer do you suspect Mr Ballard has?
- Explain the rationale for your decision.
- What further actions should be taken to confirm your provisional assessment?

If Doppler ultrasound techniques are not available, nurses have to rely on the palpation of pedal pulses in the feet to determine the vascularity of the lower limb. This is a crude and unreliable method of assessment which can result in inappropriate care (Moffatt & O'Hare 1995). The use of a Doppler assessment in isolation is of no value. The aetiology of the ulcer should be established on the basis of the patient history and physical assessment. Doppler assessment aids the management of venous ulcers by indicating whether or not standard compression therapy can be applied. Ulcers that appear to be venous in origin may be associated with some degree of arterial impairment. It is therefore important to determine the status of the arterial circulation of the limb prior to application of compression bandages. The force applied by compression bandages on people with ischaemic legs may cause additional skin damage, as the arterial vessels become occluded. For patients with arterial ulcers, the Doppler reading provides an indication of the severity of the arterial disease. It is currently best practice that patients with Doppler readings of 0.8 and below do not have compression bandaging applied (RCN 1998).

Experienced nurses may perform Doppler assessment provided they are competent in this procedure. All patients with leg ulcers should have their ABPI calculated prior to commencement of treatment. As arterial impairment can occur over time it is important to reassess this every 3 months (Vowden et al 1996). In addition, the following tests should be routinely performed on initial assessment of patients presenting with ulceration of the lower leg:

- patch testing to determine the presence of skin sensitivities or allergies (see Ch. 28)
- urine test to exclude undiagnosed diabetes (see Ch. 17)
- full blood count – haemoglobin levels may be low and are relatively easily corrected, depending on the cause. A raised erythrocyte sedimentation rate (ESR) may indicate infection.

Whatever the cause of the ulcer appears to be, it is important to exclude the less common causes of ulceration such as malignancy, especially if the ulcer has been slow to heal or has an atypical appearance. Patients should always be referred to medical staff for more detailed assessment if any of the following conditions apply:

- The patient is a younger and more mobile person who may benefit from vein surgery.
- Ulcers have not responded to treatment within 3 months or have failed to heal within a year.
- The patient is an individual with severe ischaemic disease (ABPI below 0.6).
- There is contact dermatitis suggested by a reaction to dressings, creams or bandages.
- The aetiology of ulceration is uncertain.

Specialist advice is important for those patients with arterial disease, including those with diabetes mellitus and rheumatoid arthritis, as a more comprehensive vascular assessment is required to determine the extent of vascular disease and appropriate management.

PRINCIPLES OF VENOUS LEG ULCER MANAGEMENT

The primary aim of venous leg ulcer management should focus on the reversal of venous and capillary hypertension. General management principles for patients with venous leg ulcers include:

- accurate assessment of the underlying ulcer aetiology
- reduction of the high pressure exerted on the superficial venous system
- improving venous return to the heart
- maintenance of patient compliance with treatment
- prevention of complications associated with ulcer pathology.

Compression bandaging

It is widely accepted that sustained graduated compression from the toes to the knee is the treatment of choice for uncomplicated venous leg ulcers (ABPI must be ≥ 0.8) (Vowden et al 1996) (see Evidence-based Practice box 10.3). Compression therapy can be provided using a variety of different methods but needs to be sustained for at least a week. Choice of method will depend upon:

- resources available, including availability of equipment and training
- locally determined treatment protocols/clinical practice guidelines
- patient mobility
- the size and shape of the patient's leg
- patient preference.

Compression is usually applied using bandages or hosiery and has been shown to improve venous ulcer healing rates compared with treatment without compression. However, there is little reliable evidence demonstrating the clinical efficacy of one method of compression over another (RCN 1998). There is a variety of compression bandages available, such as long stretch, short stretch and multilayer bandaging techniques. Whichever system of compression is used, it is important that it is correctly applied.

 EVIDENCE-BASED PRACTICE

10.3 Compression therapy for venous leg ulcers

NHS (1997), a systematic review, summarizes the results of research on:

- the methods of diagnosing venous ulceration
- the effectiveness and cost-effectiveness of different forms of compression therapy for the treatment of venous ulceration
- interventions to prevent recurrence
- organization of care.

The main findings of this systematic review revealed that provision of care for people with leg ulcers is costly, fails to utilize research findings and is largely ineffective. The following recommendations were made:

- Assessment of arterial status by qualified nurses to determine suitability of compression therapy is more accurate when using Doppler ultrasound than it is using palpation of foot pulses.
- Routine application of compression therapy using multilayer, short-stretch bandages or compression stockings is the most effective treatment for venous leg ulcers.
- The application of all compression therapy systems requires training, supervised practice and regular updates. This is a qualified nurse's responsibility.
- Compression stockings should be worn once the ulcer is healed in order to minimize the risk of recurrence. Health promotion plays a fundamental role in preventing further ulcer breakdown.

Reference

NHS Centre for Reviews and Dissemination, Compression Therapy for Venous Leg Ulcers. Effective Health Care Bull 1997; 3(4): 1–12.

Factors affecting the efficacy of compression bandaging

If the ulcer is of venous origin with a Doppler reading of greater than 0.8, standard compression should be applied that exerts a sub-bandage pressure of 30–40 mmHg at the ankle. Three factors affect the amount of pressure exerted onto a limb by a compression bandage: number of layers, limb radius and bandage tension (NHS Centre for Reviews & Dissemination 1997).

Number of layers

Bandage tension depends on the amount of extension or stretch used by the person applying the bandage to the patient's limb. Two layers of bandage exert twice the amount of pressure on the limb than a single layer. Therefore a consistent number of bandage layers must be applied to the leg to maintain uniform pressure. Most compression bandage application techniques use two layers, as each turn of the bandage usually overlaps the previous turn by 50%. Many compression bandaging systems utilize a layer of padding between the skin and the bandage in order to redistribute the pressure and protect the skin from local pressure points.

Limb radius

This is an important variable affecting the magnitude of pressure exerted upon a limb. As long as bandage tension and the number of layers applied to the limb remain constant, a compression bandage will exert a higher pressure on the diameter of a smaller limb than on a larger one. This ensures, in a typically shaped leg, that at constant tension a compression bandage is capable of producing a higher pressure at the ankle than at the calf. As the diameter of the calf increases, the pressure exerted by the compression bandage decreases. This allows the natural shape of the lower limb to facilitate the application of graduated compression, which reduces venous hypertension and helps to control oedema. Prior to application of any compression bandage, it is therefore important to measure the ankle circumference, as the size of the patient's ankle will influence the level of compression exerted by the bandage.

Bandage tension

Another variable affecting the amount of tension applied by a compression bandage relates to the amount of elastomeric fibres within the bandage. The force generated by these fibres when the bandage is applied to the leg causes pressure to be exerted on the limb. This pressure squeezes the veins underneath the skin and pushes the stagnant peripheral blood flow towards the heart, thus improving venous return. It is important to read the bandage manufacturer's instructions, as indications are provided as to how much pressure on average can be exerted by a particular bandage when applied at a given tension.

Compression hosiery

Once a venous ulcer is healed, it is important that the patient should wear a below-knee support stocking to prevent ulcer recurrence. Compression hosiery maintains a compression force of 30–40 mmHg at the ankle and therefore continues to maintain venous return. However, some patients find high-compression stockings uncomfortable and prefer to wear stockings that provide lower levels of support. Hosiery must be fitted correctly and patients need to be accurately measured before being supplied. All stocking manufacturers provide instructions and sizing charts to aid measurement.

Hosiery should be applied with care to prevent skin damage and trauma. The ability of patients to apply and remove their stockings should be assessed. Those who are unable to apply stockings will require assistance from relatives, friends or other carers, who will need training to apply the hosiery correctly. All patients will require follow-up assessments for a minimum of 1 year after the ulcer has healed, to minimize the risk of recurrence (Moffatt & Dorman 1995) (see Health Promotion box 10.2). During this time, they will need to have their Doppler readings reassessed to ensure that their arterial blood supply has not deteriorated.

PRINCIPLES OF ARTERIAL LEG ULCER MANAGEMENT

Management of these patients is usually conservative and is concerned with relief of symptoms. If arterial insufficiency is due to local arterial occlusion, surgical intervention may be appropriate. Arterial ulcers are common in patients with diabetes due to a combination of peripheral vascular disease and diabetic neuropathy. It must be remembered that Doppler ABPI

 HEALTH PROMOTION

10.2 Minimizing the recurrence of venous leg ulcers

Hosiery
- Wear compression hosiery during the day
- Apply and remove hosiery carefully to avoid skin damage/irritation
- Renew compression hosiery every 6 months.

Exercise
- Walk as much as possible
- Avoid prolonged standing
- Move toes and ankles several times an hour even when resting
- Avoid sitting with legs crossed.

Skin care
- Wash legs in warm water
- Use emollient creams in the water and apply to skin after washing
- Take special care of feet and toenails. Podiatry (chiropody) referral may be necessary.

Elevation
Position ankles higher than the buttocks by:

- resting on a bed with feet on a pillow
- sitting on the sofa with feet resting on one of the arms
- using a stool and pillows.

readings are difficult to interpret in this group of patients as falsely high readings may occur due to calcified arteries which make it difficult to obtain accurate blood pressure readings (Vowden et al 1996).

Treatment objectives for patients with arterial ulcers focus on symptom relief, local wound management, patient education and psychological support. The management principles of caring for patients with arterial ulcers are:

- daily examination of the legs and feet, looking for any skin breaks or signs of ischaemia
- regular foot and nail assessment by a podiatrist
- maximization of arterial blood flow to the feet by avoiding constrictive clothing or shoes and resting the legs in a dependent position
- avoidance of mechanical trauma and prevention of any further deterioration in the condition of the limb
- effective pain control
- maintenance of skin hygiene and rehydration of dry skin.

These patients require adequate pain relief. Analgesia needs to be regularly evaluated to monitor its effectiveness. Patients with severe arterial impairment will adopt a position that minimizes their pain, which often means that they prefer to sleep in a chair with their legs hanging down. Patients who can be encouraged to stop or reduce smoking usually benefit by experiencing some degree of pain relief. A period of rest each day should be encouraged in the early stages of disease, although gentle exercise, limited by patient tolerance, is a good idea in order to encourage the development of a collateral circulation.

Skin hygiene and protection of vulnerable areas are of utmost importance to prevent further deterioration of the limb. Feet should be kept clean and dry and moisturizing creams used to prevent excessive scaliness. It is important to ensure that footwear fits correctly. If this is too tight, local pressure is likely to cause further ulcers, and if it is too loose, friction can cause blisters that result in tissue breakdown.

Under no circumstances should any type of compression therapy be applied to a limb with an ankle pressure index of 0.8 or below without medical supervision as worsening of ischaemia can occur.

MANAGEMENT OF PATIENTS WITH ULCERS OF MIXED AETIOLOGY

Patients with ulcers of mixed aetiology exhibit characteristics of both arterial and venous ulcers which can make assessment and treatment problematic. The use of Doppler ultrasound is important to determine the ratio of venous to arterial involvement. The Doppler ABPI will usually be between 0.8 and 0.6. It must be remembered that the vascular status of a limb is dynamic and can change quickly, and therefore regular reassessment is recommended (Vowden et al 1996).

Treatment objectives will depend on whether venous or arterial disease is predominant. The primary aim of management of this type of ulcer is to:

- determine the vascular status of the limb
- manage the limb in accordance with the predominant aetiology
- regularly reassess the vascular status of the limb.

In this group of patients, treatment is usually directed at the venous component of the ulcer and some form of reduced compression may be used without impairing the already compromised arterial circulation. This requires the specialist knowledge of a leg ulcer specialist nurse as close monitoring of the patient is required. Once the ulcer is healed, some form of reduced compression needs to be maintained in the form of low-grade compression stockings or modified compression bandaging.

Use of leg ulcer management protocols

Since the mid-1980s, numerous studies concerned with the organization of leg ulcer services have concluded that the most effective treatment outcomes result from a coordinated approach. This has led to the development of leg ulcer protocols based upon published evidence at both local and national levels (RCN 1998) in an attempt to standardize 'best practice' in both acute and community settings. A systematic review of leg ulcer research (NHS Centre for Reviews & Dissemination 1997) has formed the basis for many of the recommendations made in such guidelines, which emphasize the need for comprehensive patient assessment, a coordinated multidisciplinary approach and the use of graduated high-compression therapy for uncomplicated venous ulcers. Figure 10.9 summarizes the principles of chronic leg ulcer assessment, management and follow-up.

Leg ulcer management protocols aim to rationalize treatment regimens in order to improve healing rates and minimize recurrence and to disseminate evidence-based practice to a wide multidisciplinary audience. Many areas are currently maximizing the

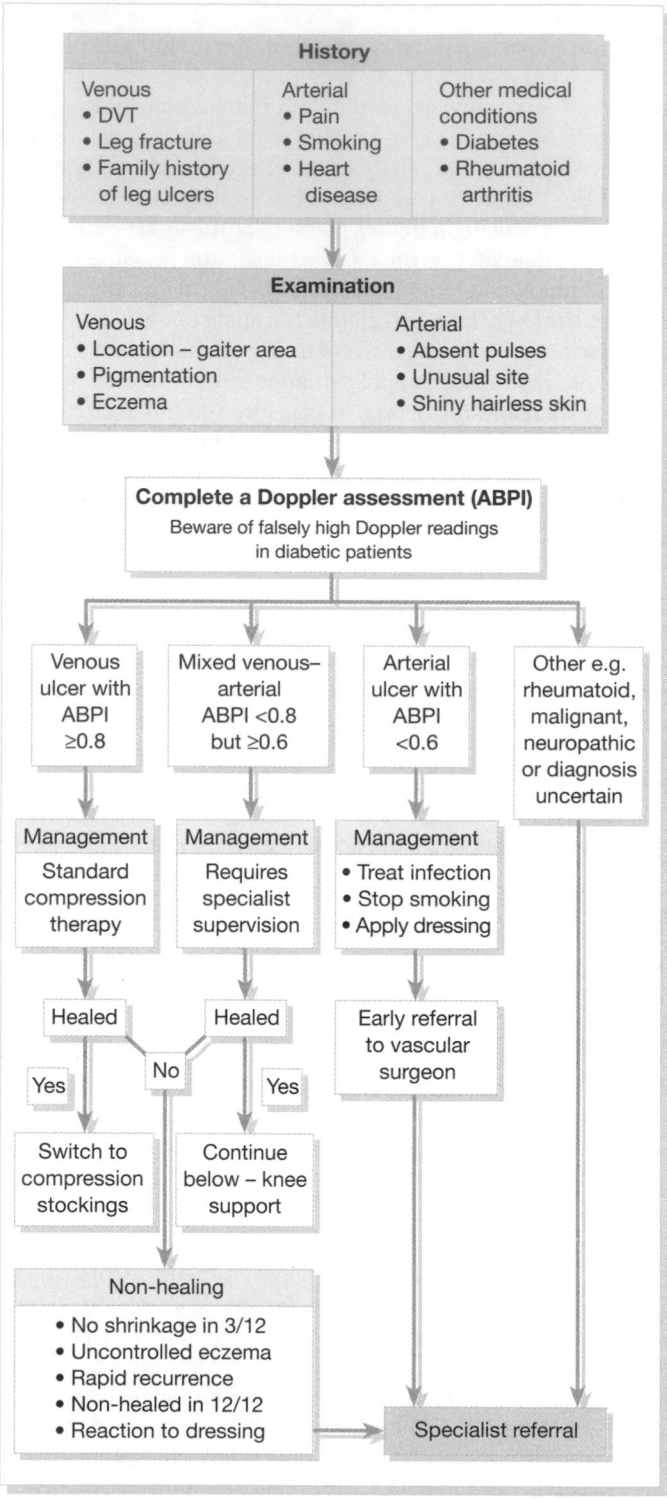

Figure 10.9 Chronic leg ulcer assessment and management.

use of local resources by providing care within the framework of leg ulcer protocols which encourage evidence-based decision-making and continuity of care. Management protocols of this type are supported by the implementation of educational programmes for practitioners and the value of this approach is usually evaluated by local clinical audit (see Guidelines for Care Priorities box 10.2).

GUIDELINES FOR CARE PRIORITIES

10.2 The management of venous leg ulcers

The RCN (1998) clinical practice guidelines for the management of venous leg ulcers may be summarized as follows:

Patient assessment
- Clinical history and observations
- Clinical investigations
- Doppler assessment
- Referral criteria

Management principles
- Pain assessment and relief
- Compression therapy
- Prevention of recurrence

Wound management
- Cleansing
- Debridement
- Dressings
- Contact sensitivity

Education and training issues
- Reducing variations in practice
- Impact of different training programmes

Quality assurance issues
- Meaningful performance indicators
- Reliable outcome measures

Reference

Royal College of Nursing Clinical Practice Guidelines: The Management of Patients With Venous Leg Ulcers. London, RCN.

SUMMARY: MAIN POINTS

- Wound management is a rapidly expanding and dynamic specialty. Rapid advances in the management of wounds have led to the recognition that tissue viability is a specialty within its own right.

- Wound assessment is a complex activity which requires an understanding of the physiological processes involved in tissue repair and a thorough understanding of the physiology of the skin.

- Nurses are well placed to identify the intrinsic and extrinsic factors that can prolong wound healing rates but the management of wounds should reflect a multidisciplinary perspective.

- The application of the principles of wound management facilitates clinical decision-making and the choice of treatment interventions such as wound debridement, and the selection of pressure-relieving equipment.

- Newer wound dressings are technologically advanced and are designed to promote the principle of moist

wound healing and provide the optimal local environment for healing.

- An important correlation exists between wound healing and psychological needs, although the exact relationship between the two is not fully understood.

- Health promotion is important in promoting compliance for patients with compromised tissue viability, e.g. those at risk of pressure ulcers.

- Pressure ulcers are costly to the individual and the health care system. They are largely preventable if risk assessment is carried out and appropriate preventative strategies initiated.

- Leg ulcers cause immobility, social isolation and low self-esteem. Good healing rates for leg ulcers can be achieved if the accurate aetiology of the ulcer can be determined. Application of compression therapy is proven to improve healing rates of venous leg ulcers.

SELF-TEST: CRITICAL THINKING ACTIVITIES

1 Wound assessment forms the basis of wound management but is a complex activity that requires the documentation of a wide range of patient-related information. If you were designing a wound assessment chart, what type of information would it include?

2 What are the three intrinsic causes of pressure ulcers and how might these risk factors be minimized.

3 What are the key differences between venous and arterial ulcers?

 FURTHER READING

Boulton A, Connor H, Cavanagh PR. The foot in diabetes. Chichester: Wiley; 1994.

Fletcher J. Pressure sore grading. J Wound Care 1997; Resource File.

Miller M, Glover D (eds). Wound management. London: NT Books; 1999.

Moffatt C, Harper P. Leg ulcers: access to clinical education series. Edinburgh: Churchill Livingstone; 1997.

USEFUL WEBSITES

cebm.jr2.ox.ac.uk – Centre for Evidence Based Medicine, Oxford
nice.org.uk – National Institute for Clinical Excellence
www.smtl.co.uk – Surgical Materials Testing Laboratory
This address is a universal resource locator which enables you to address the following groups: World Wide Wounds (Electronic Journal of Wound Management Practices); European Pressure Ulcer Advisory Panel; European Tissue Repair Society; European Wound Management Association.

www.woundcaresociety.org – The Wound Care Society
This address is a universal resource locator, which enables you to address the following groups: Medical Device Agency; The Wound Care Institute; Trauma on Line.
woundsresearch.com – WOUNDS: a compendium for clinical research and practice

REFERENCES

Bergastrom N, Braden B, Laguzza A, Holman V. The Braden scale for predicting pressure sore risk. Nurs Res 1987; 36(4): 205–210.

Bryant RA. Acute and chronic wounds: nursing management. St Louis: Mosby; 1992.

Callum M, Ruckley V, Harper D, Dale J. Chronic ulceration of the leg: extent of the problem and provision of care. Br Med J 1985; 290: 1855–1857.

Cullum N, Roe B. Leg ulcers and nursing management: a research-based guide. London: Scutari Press; 1995.

Dale J, Callum M, Ruckley C. Chronic ulcers of the leg: a study of prevalence in a Scottish community. Health Bull (Edinburgh) 1983; 41: 310–314.

Department of Health. Pressure sores: a key quality indicator. London: Department of Health; 1993.

Department of Health. The Medicinal Products Prescription by Nurses, Health Visitors and Health Visitors Act. London: Department of Health; 1992.

Desai H. Ageing and wounds. Part 2: healing in old age. J Wound Care 1997; 6(5): 237–239.

Dyson M, Young S, Pendle CL. Comparison of the effects of moist and dry conditions on dermal repair. J Invest Dermatol 1988; 91: 435–439.

Eisenbeiss W, Peter FW, Bakhtiari C. Hypertrophic scars and keloids. J Wound Care 1998; 7: 255–257.

European Pressure Ulcer Advisory Panel (EPUAP). Pressure ulcer treatment guidelines. Oxford: European Pressure Ulcer Advisory Panel; 1999a.

European Pressure Ulcer Advisory Panel (EPUAP). Pressure ulcer prevention guidelines. Oxford: European Pressure Ulcer Advisory Panel; 1999b.

Flanagan M. Wound management. Edinburgh: Churchill Livingstone; 1997.

Flanagan M. Variables influencing nurses' selection of wound dressings. J Wound Care 1992; 1(1): 33–43.

Fletcher J. Accurate data collection. J Wound Care 1997; 6(8): 388–400.

Gilchrist B. Should iodine be reconsidered in wound management? J Wound Care 1997; 6(3): 148–150.

Gosnell D. An assessment tool to identify pressure sores. Nurs Clin North Am 1987; 22(2): 399–416.

Hampton S. Sharp debridement. J Wound Care 1997; 6(3): 151.

Hinton C. Pressure sore responsibilities of an ambulance service. Second European conference on Advances in Wound Management. London: Macmillan Magazines; 1992.

Kenney L, Rithalia S. Technical aspects of support surfaces. J Wound Care 1999; Sept: 1–8.

Leaper DJ, Harding KG. Wounds biology and management. Oxford: Oxford Medical Publications; 1998.

Lowthian P. The practical assessment of pressure sore risk. Care: Sci Pract 1987; 5(4): 3–7.

Lucker K, Hogg C, Austin L, Ferguson B, Smith K. Decision-making: the context of nurse prescribing. J Adv Nurs 1998; 27: 657–665.

Milward P, Poole M, Skitt T. Tissue viability. Pressure sore prevention: scoring pressure sore risk in the community. Nurs Stand 1993; 7: 50–55.

Moffatt C, Dorman M. Recurrence of leg ulcers within a community ulcer service. J Wound Care 1995; 4(2): 56–62.

Moffat CJ, O'Hare L. Ankle pulses are not sufficient to detect impaired arterial circulation in patients with leg ulcers. J Wound Care 1995; 4(3): 134–137.

NHS Centre For Reviews & Dissemination. Compression therapy for venous leg ulcers. Effect Health Care Bull 1997; 3(4): 1–12.

Norton D, McLaren R, Exton-Smith AN. An investigation of geriatric nursing problems in hospital. Edinburgh: Churchill Livingstone; 1962.

Preston K. Positioning for comfort and pressure relief: the 30 degree alternative. Care: Sci Pract 1991; 7(4): 116–118.

Reid J, Morison M. Towards a consensus: classification of pressure sores. J Wound Care 1994; 3(3): 157–160.

Royal College of Nursing (RCN). Clinical practice guidelines. The management of patients with venous leg ulcers. London: RCN; 1998.

Scales JT. Development and evaluation of a porous surgical dressing. Br Med J 1956; 2: 962–981.

Sussman G. Alginates: a review. Primary Intention 1996; Feb: 33–37.

Tortora GJ, Grabowski SR. Principles of anatomy and physiology, 8th edn. New York: Harper Collins College Publications; 1996.

Turner TD. Which dressing and why? In: Westerby S, ed. Wound care. London: Heinemann Medical Books; 1985.

Vowden K, Goulding V, Vowden P. Hand held Doppler assessment for peripheral arterial disease. J Wound Care 1996; 5(3): 125–128.

Waterlow JA. A risk assessment card. Nurs Times 1985; 81(48): 49–55.

Williams CA. Comparative study of pressure-sore prevention scores. J Tissue Viability 1992; 2: 64–66.

Winter G. Formulation of the scab and the rate of epithelialisation in the skin of the domestic pig. Nature 1962; 193: 293–294.

11 Nutrition

Kathy Martyn

'I thought the domestic staff did the meals so nurses didn't need to worry but Sister told me how important it is to make sure your patients can eat. And feed them if they can't do it themselves. Now I always check my patients at mealtimes to make sure they are able to reach their food and open everything and then see what food they've eaten. Some eat lots more if you help them a little bit.'

(Student nurse)

THIS CHAPTER WILL HELP YOU

- Understand the complexity of human nutrition
- Describe the role of the nurse in ensuring that dietary needs are met
- Describe a healthy diet and recognize how it may change during illness
- Describe the food groups: macronutrients and micronutrients
- Outline metabolic changes occurring during stress and trauma
- Outline the importance of nutritional screening and the use of nursing assessment and nutritional screening tools
- Recognize the impact of age and physical, social and psychological factors on nutritional status
- Provide nutritional support
- Recognize the role of dieticians and the multidisciplinary team in providing nutrition to patients/clients.

KEYWORDS

Anabolic	Mineral
Catabolic	Nutrition
Carbohydrate	Protein
Fat	Vitamin
Lipid	

INTRODUCTION

Nutrition is important at all stages of life. Eating food is essential not only as a source of nutrients but also because of complex social and psychological interactions. This is evident in health, yet during illness the importance of diet may be secondary to other activities and medical interventions. Nurses are in an ideal position to ensure that the nutritional needs of individuals are met, both in the community and in hospital, through:

- assessing nutritional status
- giving dietary advice and health education
- monitoring effects of specific diets
- feeding patients/clients
- overseeing food provision and delivery
- referral to members of the multidisciplinary team.

In the community, recognizing the long-term impact of diet on health may reduce the incidence of health problems in later life, whilst in hospital, addressing nutritional needs can both promote recovery and reduce the incidence of complications, such as pressure ulcers and poor wound healing (Ch. 10).

Early writings by authors such as Florence Nightingale make reference to diet and its importance in patient recovery. However, in recent years, the drive towards professionalism, expansion of the nursing role and the increased use of technology has seen a decline in the importance of nutrition. Lennard-Jones (1992) described patients as being 'hungry in hospital', citing a failure to recognize patient needs and to plan appropriate interventions as contributing factors. This study identified factors that had been recognized 20 years before in the USA when there was a call for nutrition to form part of the therapy regimen.

Other studies have measured the level of under-nutrition of patients in hospital and in the community setting in the UK. McWhirter & Pennington (1994) found that 27% of hospitalized patients were malnourished and that many left hospital more malnourished than on admission. Edington et al (1997, 1996) identified that 11% of surgical patients were malnourished 6 weeks after surgery, 10% of cancer patients and 8% of patients

11.1 Meeting nutritional needs in hospital

The main causes of an inadequate diet for patients in hospital have been identified by Lennard-Jones (1992) as:

- prolonged periods of fasting
- inability to access food
- inability to eat due to poor position, poor dentures, reduced dexterity and confusional states
- inappropriate food
- failure to recognize nutrition as part of the therapy of the patient.

Student activities

Reflect on your clinical area:

- In the past week, have any patients had inadequate food intake?
- What were the causes?
- What actions by the nurse could prevent this happening in the future?
- Which members of the multidisciplinary team should be involved?

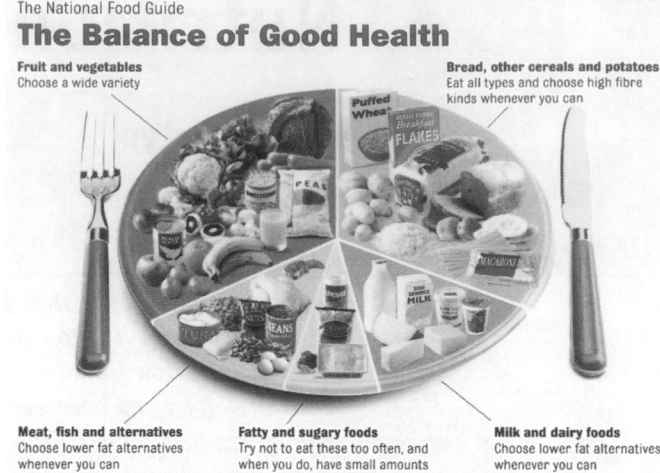

Figure 11.1 The balance of good health. (Reproduced with kind permission from the Health Education Authority 1994.)

with chronic diseases. In 1993, the Royal College of Nursing and the United Kingdom Central Council clearly identified the nursing role in meeting patients' nutritional needs. Fulfilling this role and being part of the multidisciplinary team require that nurses have a sound knowledge base. Recently, standards for meeting nutritional needs have been set for hospitalized patients (Sizer 1996) and it has been suggested that nutrition should be a quality standard by which NHS Trusts are measured (Ch. 2) (see Reflective Practice box 11.1).

WHAT IS NUTRITION?

Nutrition is the composition of food and the relationship between diet and health. In understanding nutritional needs, it is necessary to explore the physiological effects of nutrients and the sociological and psychological impact of eating.

NUTRIENTS IN FOOD

The nutrients in food are divided into macronutrients (fats, carbohydrates and protein) and micronutrients (vitamins and minerals). Water is required in addition to these nutrients. Health is maintained when the relative amounts of each of the nutrients meet individual requirements. Ill health may influence both nutrient requirements and the ability to utilize nutrients.

A typical diet consists of differing amounts of macro- and micronutrients from a variety of sources. Concerns over the health of the population have led to the publication of guidance as to what constitutes a healthy diet and to the formulation of dietary reference values (DRVs) for the UK (Department of Health 1991). These recommendations are based on the study of populations and observing the effects of nutrient deficiency or excess.

DRVs include the reference nutritional intake (RNI) and the lower reference nutrient intake (LRNI) for specific nutrients. These figures are based on population studies and assume that individuals within the population will be normally distributed. The RNI is the amount of a nutrient required by 97.5% of the population to maintain health. The LRNI is the lowest amount of a nutrient that is required to ensure that only 2.5% of the population will show signs of deficiency. These specific amounts are used in food processing and for measuring an individual's nutritional status, but are of little use in guiding food choices, most foods being composites of more than one nutrient in differing amounts. In 1994 the Health Education Authority (HEA) developed the 'Balance of Good Health' which represented the nutritional requirements in the form of a plate (Fig. 11.1). This has also been supported by health education programmes aimed at specific populations, including the campaign to increase the consumption of fruit and vegetables (National Heart Forum 1997).

Dietary recommendations are not unique to the UK and are produced under the guidance of the World Health Organization (WHO), which is concerned with nutrition at a global level.

The healthy diet aims to increase the intake of fruit and vegetables, starch and carbohydrate, whilst reducing the intake of processed foods, meat and dairy products (Fig. 11.1). This should reduce the intake of saturated fats as a proportion of the total energy intake and increase fibre intake. By reducing processed foods, it is hoped to reduce the intake of salt and sugar, which are often 'hidden' or added during preparation.

THE NURSE'S ROLE IN HEALTH PROMOTION

Nurses have an important role in promoting a healthy diet in a variety of health care settings and in the community. Targets have been identified for reducing the incidence of coronary heart disease (CHD), stroke and cancer (DoH 1999). Dietary changes will play a crucial role in meeting these targets. Nurses will need to understand dietary recommendations and work with individuals, families or groups to encourage fundamental

⚖ ETHICAL ISSUES

11.1 Healthy eating advice

Consider the ethical implications of giving 'healthy eating' advice to individuals or groups where there is very little opportunity for them to follow the advice. For example:

- Maria, aged 19 years, is unemployed and lives alone on a housing estate with few food shops. She has no car and is some miles from the nearest supermarket.
- Anwar lives with his son and daughter-in-law. He is 85 years old and has very poor vision. All his meals are prepared by his daughter-in-law who decides what the family will eat.

Apart from one-to-one advice and counselling, how might health professionals help individuals and groups to improve their access to 'healthy eating' choices?

changes in lifestyle and diet. Advice can be complicated by the media, who promote 'cure all' diets which may conflict with the information conveyed by nurses.

Successful health advice is advice that is appropriate to individuals (see Ethical Issues box 11.1). The timing of such advice is critical, e.g. acutely ill patients may not be receptive to information, whilst patients with chronic disorders may feel unable to change or be disillusioned by the advice. Conversely, healthy individuals may not see the benefits of making changes to their diet. Factors that need to be considered include:

- complete assessment of the individual
- using appropriate language in small practical amounts
- planning achievable and realistic changes with the person
- where possible, giving advice that applies to the whole family or social group
- involving all members of the multidisciplinary team.

MACRONUTRIENTS

Macronutrients include proteins, fats and carbohydrates. Each has an important role and the relative amounts of each consumed will influence the quality of the diet. Macronutrients comprise carbon, oxygen and hydrogen in different proportions. In addition, proteins contain nitrogen and some also contain sulphur and phosphorus.

ENERGY AND ENERGY BALANCE

The macronutrients are potential energy sources. Energy is measured in joules (J) or kilojoules (kJ). Previously, energy was measured in calories or kilocalories (kcal) (or large Calorie). The term calorie is still used in nutrition and can be seen on food packaging. The conversion between kilocalories and kilojoules is as follows:

1 kcal = 4.186 kJ
1 kJ = 0.239 kcal

The most important body energy source is carbohydrate, 1 g of which produces 16 kJ (3.75 kcal). Fat is more energy-dense, producing 37 kJ/g (9 kcal/g), and it is important that sufficient fat is consumed to meet cellular requirements and provide adequate stores of fuel. However, in the typical diet, the proportion of fat eaten is too great and excess energy intake causes obesity (see p. 216). Protein produces 17 kJ/g (4 kcal/g), but protein is not normally used for energy in health (see below). Alcohol contains large amounts of carbohydrate and yields 29 kJ/g (7 kcal/g). However, alcohol is not a nutrient and consumption should be in moderation (Ch. 23).

Energy requirement depends on age, size, health and activity level. It is calculated from the basal metabolic rate (BMR) and physical activity levels (PAL), as follows:

Energy demand = energy expenditure = BMR × PAL

The BMR is the amount of energy required for biosynthesis, active transport and mechanical work whilst the body is at rest. Prediction equations allow the calculation of BMR for males and females of different ages (MAFF 1995). BMR is influenced by body mass, gender and age. Over-nutrition causes an increase in metabolically active tissue, increasing BMR, and in under-nutrition there is a loss of metabolically active tissue and a decrease in BMR.

The PAL is the energy required for all other work. It takes into account dietary-induced thermogenesis and physical activity. The former is the energy required for digestion, absorption and transport of nutrients, and accounts for about 10% of food energy ingested. By multiplying the BMR by a figure derived for activity, the total energy requirement of an individual can be calculated. In the UK, the average PAL is 1.4, representing very little physical activity at work or during leisure time. Values for moderate activity are 1.6 for women and 1.7 for men, whilst for high levels of activity the figures are 1.8 for women and 1.9 for men (MAFF 1995).

PROTEINS

Proteins supply amino acids for tissue synthesis by anabolic reactions (building up where simple substances are used to make complex molecules). Proteins are therefore essential for cellular function, growth and repair. They can be used as an energy source during catabolic states where complex molecules such as protein are broken down for energy (see p. 217).

We obtain amino acids from proteins either by eating plants or by eating animals (and their products) which have consumed plants. In the Western diet, the main sources of protein are considered to be meat, fish, eggs and dairy produce. However, cereal products such as bread or pasta, whilst having lower protein content, contribute a significant proportion of the protein in the diet because of the large volumes consumed. Fish accounts for only a relatively small proportion of protein in the diet.

Each protein is composed of different amino acids arranged in different sequences, which determine the properties of the protein. Changing the sequence or a single amino acid will change its properties. The amino acid content will determine the quality or biological value of the protein as a component of the diet. Twenty amino acids are important in the diet and, of these, nine are essential (indispensable) in the diet because they cannot be synthesized in the body. The essential amino acids are histidine, isoleucine, leucine, lysine, methionine, phenylalanine, threonine, tryptophan and valine. In infancy, a 10th amino acid, arginine, is also considered to be essential because it is only synthesized in small amounts. The remaining amino acids – alanine, asparagine, aspartate, cysteine, glutamate, glutamine, glycine, proline, serine and tyrosine – are required by the body but are not essential (dispensable) in the diet because they are synthesized by the liver.

Protein containing all the essential amino acids, in the required amounts, will be completely usable for tissue protein synthesis. In reality, proteins do not contain all the essential amino acids in sufficient quantities and the value of protein is limited by the essential amino acid that is present in the lowest amount relative to requirements. In cereals, the limiting amino acid is lysine, and in animal proteins and most other vegetable proteins it is the sum of methionine and cysteine (synthesized from methionine). The total value of protein in the food is increased by combining proteins from different sources, such as bread and cheese, and rice pudding (rice and milk).

FATS

The main dietary fat is triacylglycerol (also known as tri-glycerides). Other fats such as phospholipids and cholesterol are important but can be synthesized in the body. Phospholipids are important in the structure and function of cell membranes. Cholesterol is a component of cell membranes and is essential in steroid production. Synthesis of cholesterol in the body is influenced by dietary fat intake. All these fats, as well as others, belong to a large group of molecules called lipids.

Saturated and unsaturated fats

Animal fats are generally sources of saturated fats, whilst oily fish and vegetables are sources of unsaturated fats. The building blocks of triacylglycerols are: a glycerol backbone and three fatty acids (Fig. 11.2). The fatty acids are normally different, thus creating a wide diversity of triacylglycerols. It is these fatty acids that are saturated or unsaturated. In a saturated fatty acid, the carbon atoms are attached to as many hydrogen atoms as possible, whereas in unsaturated fatty acids, there are one or

more double bonds between carbon atoms, which cannot attach to hydrogen; those with one double bond are monounsaturated and those with two or more double bonds are polyunsaturated.

Heating or hydrogenating unsaturated fatty acid changes the structure. It can become the *trans* form in which the fatty acid molecules pack tightly together to form a solid fat. *Trans* fatty acids are present in some fat spreads which would normally be oils at room temperature and in processed foods such as biscuits. In the body, *trans* fatty acids are metabolized in the same way as saturated fats and are linked to ill health (Troisi et al 1992).

The dietary sources of fat are diverse, each fat containing differing amounts of fatty acids (Fig. 11.3). Triacylglycerols are a source of the essential fatty acids and of the fat-soluble vitamins A, D, E and K (see pp. 205–208). The essential fatty acids are n-6 polyunsaturated fatty acid (PUFA) (linoleic acid) and n-3 PUFA (alpha linolenic acid). The main sources of n-6 PUFA are vegetables, cereal products, fat spreads and meat and meat products, and the main sources of n-3 PUFA are vegetables and vegetable oils, fish oils, fat spreads, meat and meat products. Arachidonic acid is synthesized in the body from linoleic acid. Monounsaturated fatty acids (n-9 oleic acid) are found in olive oil, which is a common ingredient in the Mediterranean diet.

Although more energy-dense than carbohydrate, fats are not generally used as an immediate energy source. Triacylglycerols provide a major reserve of metabolic fuel stored in fat cells (adipocytes). Current dietary advice is to reduce the total fat in the diet from 40 to 30%. The fat intake should also be a mixture of polyunsaturated and monounsaturated fats, with saturated fats forming only 15% of the total intake. It is important that there is a mixture of the polyunsaturated fats in the diet: n-3 polyunsaturates are beneficial in CHD (see Ch. 19), n-6 poly-unsaturates are important for immune function, and both are important for neurological development (see Ch. 14).

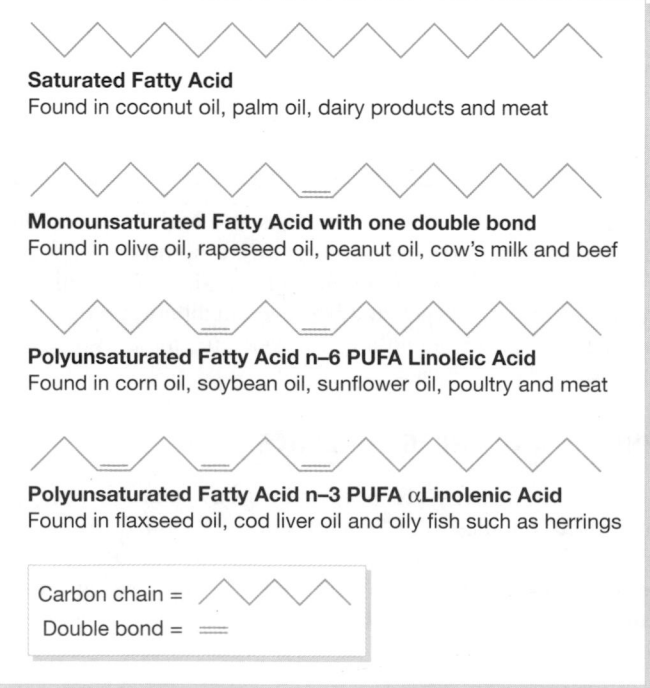

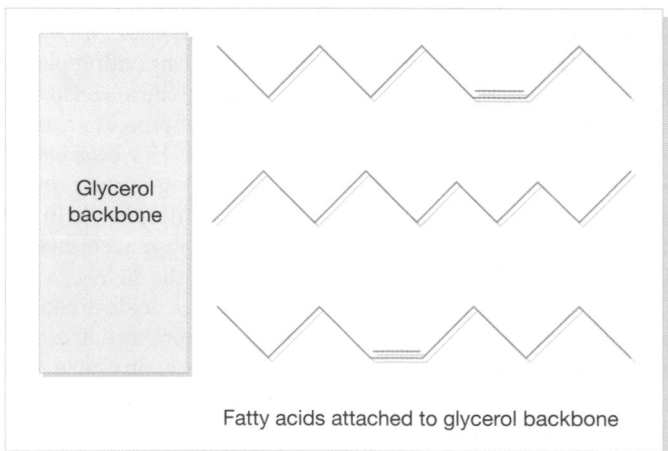

Fatty acids attached to glycerol backbone

Figure 11.2 Basic structure of a triacylglycerol (triglyceride).

Figure 11.3 Fatty acids – basic structure and source.

Lipid transportation

After absorption, triacylglycerols are reassembled and transported in the blood as lipoproteins (lipid joined to a protein). The protein component enables the molecule to be recognized by cell receptors and cleared from the blood. Most cholesterol in the blood is carried by low-density lipoproteins (LDLs). High circulating levels of LDLs have been linked to CHD (Ch. 19). Other molecules, called high-density lipoproteins (HDLs), also carry cholesterol, retrieving it from places where it has accumulated, for disposal by the liver (see p. 216).

CARBOHYDRATE

Carbohydrates are used as an energy source. They are the cheapest source of energy worldwide. The simplest carbohydrates are sugars, which are present as single units (monosaccharides), double units (disaccharides) or chains of between three and 10 units (oligosaccharides). Simple sugars are found in fruit, jam, honey, sugar and milk, and are added to many processed foods, e.g. baked beans. Complex carbohydrates are called polysaccharides and are found in cereals and flour-based foods, e.g. chapatis, and pulses and potatoes.

Monosaccharides

Monosaccharides (glucose, galactose and fructose) and disaccharides (maltose, lactose and sucrose) are divided in two groups: intrinsic sugars found within the plant cell wall, and extrinsic sugars found in solution within foods. Extrinsic sugars in the diet are considered more harmful as they provide a source of sugar for bacterial fermentation and have been linked to dental caries.

Glucose is the essential source of energy in the body. Nervous tissue and red blood cells rely on a blood concentration of between 3.5 and 6 mmol/L to meet their energy requirements. Other cells can, in the presence of insulin, utilize glucose at other concentrations (Ch. 17). Galactose and fructose are converted to glucose in the liver for cellular use.

Starch and non-starch polysaccharides

Polysaccharides contain many monosaccharide units arranged in straight, branched or coiled chains. Based on structure, they are divided into starches and non-starch polysaccharides (NSP). Starch is composed of linked glucose units arranged either in straight (amylose) or branched (amylopectin) chains. Most starchy foods, such as potatoes, cereals and pulses, contain 75% amylopectin and 25% amylose. Amylose is more resistant to digestion and forms an important part of starch that passes into the colon undigested, where it becomes available for bacterial fermentation. Some amylopectin enclosed within the plant wall also resists digestion and passes into the colon. Processing starchy foods disrupts the starch granules or the cell wall and increases their digestibility. Starches that are not broken down completely by enzymes in the small intestine are called resistant starches.

NSPs are divided into cellulose and non-cellulose polysaccharides. Cellulose is insoluble and is the main component of the plant cell wall resistant to digestion. This increases the faecal mass in the colon. Non-cellulose polysaccharides, including fruit pectins, glucans in cereals and gums in food additives, are soluble.

Both resistant starch and NSPs become available for fermentation in the colon by commensal bacteria there. During fermentation, short-chain fatty acids (SCFAs) are produced, which reduces colonic pH and provides an additional energy substrate that is absorbed and utilized by the body. NSPs are considered beneficial to health, through the speeding up of faecal transit time and production of energy. The decreased transit time means that faecal toxins spend less time in contact with colonic cells. The production of SCFAs provides an energy source for colonic cells and helps to maintain their health. Resistant starch also provides a source of slow-release glucose, which is beneficial to people with diabetes because it helps to maintain blood glucose levels without sudden swings (Ch. 17).

MICRONUTRIENTS

Vitamins and minerals (including trace elements) are important micronutrients and daily amounts are required for cellular function and health (see Tables 11.1 and 11.2). The amount required of each varies from micrograms to grams and reflects the activity of the substance, its toxicity and evidence of disease caused by deficiency. Recommended daily amounts of vitamins and minerals have been calculated and take into account age and bioavailability (MAFF 1995). Vitamins and trace elements are usually only required in minute quantities.

VITAMINS

Vitamins are organic compounds mainly consumed as part of the daily diet. However, vitamin K is made by commensal bacteria in the intestine and vitamin D is also synthesized in the body and is more like a hormone in its mode of action. Vitamins are found in both plant and animal foods and are named alphabetically and by their structure. Gaps in the alphabetic nomenclature occur either because the substance was originally given another name or because different substances have similar structure and function, e.g. the B group of vitamins. Vitamins may be described as fat-soluble (A, D, E and K) or water-soluble (B group of vitamins and C). It should be noted that severe toxicity can occur when some vitamins are taken in excess.

Vitamin A

Many substances have vitamin A activity, including retinol, retinaldehyde and retinoic acid. These are only found in animal foods, particularly in liver, which is a store of vitamin A in animals. The body also converts provitamin carotenoid pigments (mainly beta-carotene) into vitamin A. Carotenes are found in yellow, red and green vegetables as well as meat and dairy sources. Many of the carotenes are metabolized in the intestinal mucosa, producing retinol.

Vitamin A is best known for its function in vision (it forms part of rhodopsin found in the rod cells of the retina). Vitamin A deficiency is a major problem worldwide and is the most preventable cause of blindness in developing countries. The main action of vitamin A, however, is the control of cell differentiation and turnover through the regulation of transcription genes. The carotenes also have an important role as antioxidant nutrients because they prevent oxidative damage to cells, which is linked to the development of heart disease and cancer (see Chs 19 and 33).

Table 11.1 Some important vitamins

Vitamin	Function	Sources	Deficiency
Vitamin A	Visual pigments in retina Cell growth and replication Antioxidant	Liver, meat and meat products Milk and milk products Vegetables especially carrots, red and orange fruits Margarine	Night blindness Skin disorders
Vitamin D	Calcium homeostasis	Fatty fish (herring, sardines) Margarine and low-fat spreads Eggs, evaporated milk Breakfast cereals Action of sunlight on skin	Rickets (children) Osteomalacia (adults)
Vitamin E	Lipid-soluble antioxidant Prevents cell membrane damage	Vegetable oils and margarine Wholegrain cereals, eggs, dark green vegetables, nuts	Rare, neurological dysfunction Deficiency may occur in malabsorption or poor utilization
Vitamin K	Synthesis of procoagulant factors	Green leafy vegetables, dairy produce, vegetable oils, cereals and meat	Impaired clotting
Vitamin B_1 (thiamin)	Coenzyme for carbohydrate metabolism Nerve impulse conduction	All cereals, especially bread and breakfast cereals Potatoes, vegetables and meat Yeast extract	Peripheral nerve damage or CNS alterations Wernicke–Korsakoff syndrome Beri-beri
Vitamin B_2 (riboflavin)	Coenzyme for the metabolism of fuel molecules	Milk and milk products, eggs Fortified breakfast cereals Yeast extract	Lesions at the corner of the mouth, lips and tongue Corneal vascularization
Niacin	Energy metabolism	Meat and meat products Bread and fortified breakfast cereals Yeast extract	Pellagra Depressive psychosis
Vitamin B_6	Amino acid metabolism	Many foods; meat, fish, eggs, nuts, vegetables, potatoes and breakfast cereals	Convulsions Disorders of amino acid metabolism
Vitamin B_{12} (cobalamins)	Folic acid utilization Red blood cell production Nerve myelination	Meat and liver products Eggs and milk products Yeast extract	Pernicious anaemia Spinal cord degeneration
Folic acid	DNA synthesis Red blood cell production	Green leafy vegetables Milk and milk products Fortified breakfast cereals Yeast extract	Megaloblastic anaemia
Vitamin C	Collagen synthesis Antioxidant Iron absorption	Citrus fruit and juices Green vegetables and fruit Potatoes	Scurvy Delay in wound healing

In the UK, vitamin A deficiency is rare but it can occur with protein energy malnutrition (PEM). People with PEM may be unable to synthesize plasma retinol binding proteins which normally transport vitamin A from reserves in the liver to its site of action. This deficiency can impair immune function which requires rapid cell differentiation and turnover. The immune response may also be reduced due to the under-nutrition. Early recognition by nurses of under-nutrition is important, especially in older adults whose recovery can be slower due to the ageing process.

Vitamin A requirements are based on the amount needed to maintain a liver concentration of 20 µg retinol/g. This will maintain adequate plasma levels. Signs of deficiency may not be evident for some time because liver reserves maintain adequate plasma levels even when the diet contains no vitamin A for many months. Lack of vitamin A leads to night blindness and skin problems.

Dietary intakes in excess of that required to maintain the liver reserve will not increase the total reserve but will be metabolized and excreted from the body. Vitamin A toxicity occurs once the intake is increased to a level at which the ability to metabolize and excrete the metabolites is exhausted. Excessively high concentrations of free unbound vitamin A accumulate in the liver and other tissues. This can lead to liver and bone damage, hair

Table 11.2 Some important minerals and trace elements

Mineral[a]	Function	Sources	Deficiency
Calcium	Strengthening bones and teeth Neuromuscular function Intracellular function Blood coagulation	Milk and milk products Bread, soya beans, lentils, sesame seeds Sardines Hard water	Reduced peak bone mass Osteoporosis
Magnesium	Skeletal development Neuromuscular function Cofactor for many enzymes	Cereals and cereal products Potatoes, green vegetables Nuts and seeds	Neurological problems Cardiac arrhythmias
Sodium and chloride	Maintains extracellular fluid compartment Neuromuscular function Acid–base regulation	Common salt Cereal products Meat products, canned vegetables, sauces, pickles Prepared meals and snack foods	Cramp (usually with water depletion)
Potassium	Major intracellular mineral Neuromuscular function Acid–base regulation	Vegetables, potatoes, bananas Meat and milk products	Muscle weakness Reduced peristalsis Cardiac arrhythmias Confusion and apathy
Iron	Constituent of haemoglobin and myoglobin Required for many enzymes	Meat and meat products Cereal products, pulses, vegetables, dried fruit and potatoes Eggs	Iron deficiency anaemia
Zinc	Cofactor required for many enzymes Needed for insulin storage	Meat and meat products Milk, eggs Cereals, bread, pulses, nuts	Delayed puberty Wound healing delayed
Phosphorus (phosphates)	Present in bone and teeth Needed for many enzymes Present in all cells in organic biomolecules, such as proteins	Many animal and vegetable protein foods, e.g. meat, milk and nuts	Deficiency extremely rare
Iodine	Required for thyroid hormones	Seafood, milk and dairy products Eggs and meat	Goitre Hypothyroidism
Selenium	Enzyme pathways Antioxidant	Meat and fish Cereal and cereal products	Deficiency uncommon
Copper	Enzyme pathways Catecholamine synthesis Antioxidant	Cereals and bread Vegetables Meat	Anaemia Fragile bones and non-elastic elastin
Chromium	Required for insulin function and lipid metabolism	Widespread in foods such as meat, cereals, beans and nuts	Poor glucose tolerance Possible link with CHD

[a] Plus cobalt, fluoride, manganese and molybdenum

loss, vomiting and headaches. Vitamin A is teratogenic (harmful to the fetus) and pregnant women should be advised to limit their intake by avoiding foods rich in it, such as liver and liver products. High levels of carotene are not known to have toxic effects other than yellow discoloration of the skin.

Vitamin D

Vitamin D is not strictly a vitamin. Its action is similar to that of hormones and it is mainly obtained by synthesis in the body. The action of ultraviolet light upon the provitamin 7-dehydrocholesterol (a sterol), present in the dermis, forms pre-vitamin D. This is converted to cholecalciferol and is absorbed into the bloodstream. Both synthesized and dietary cholecalciferol are then hydroxylated by the liver to form 25-hydroxycholecalciferol before being converted in the kidney to active calcitriol (1,25-hydroxycholecalciferol) or inactive 24-hydroxycalcidiol.

Dietary sources of vitamin D are few, only fish, eggs, butter and margarine having significant amounts. In temperate zones, where there is little winter sunshine, the main source is dietary. Vitamin D is often added to other foods such as margarine as a method of supplementation. Nursing assessments should recognize those factors that lead to reduced exposure to sunlight and a deficiency in vitamin D, such as old age, living in nursing/residential homes, immobility and cultural objections to exposing the limbs and body. Dietary preferences or low-fat diets and kidney disease can also lead to deficiency.

Vitamin D is important in maintaining calcium homeostasis. When serum calcium levels fall, parathyroid hormone is released which stimulates the kidney to produce active calcitriol. The calcitriol causes more calcium to be absorbed from the bowel.

Vitamin D deficiency occurs in two forms: rickets in children and osteomalacia in adults. In rickets, the bones become weakened due to poor calcium absorption and bowed as body weight increases. It also occurs in adolescents, who are already marginally deficient in vitamin D, as the demand for calcium increases during growth spurts. Osteomalacia in adults occurs due to demineralization. Women whose exposure to sunlight is limited or who have had multiple pregnancies are at increased risk of osteomalacia. It is more common in older adults, as activity decreases with more time indoors and the production of 7-dehydrocholesterol in the dermis may reduce with age. Nurses need to be aware that older adults have an increased reliance on dietary sources of vitamin D.

There are no DRVs for vitamin D for children over 4 years or adults under 65 years as skin synthesis is the major source, but at-risk groups may need a dietary source. However, during pregnancy, lactation and for those aged over 65 years, the RNI is 10 μg/day. Fortifications of food or supplements are important for older adults, as they are increasingly reliant on dietary sources.

Toxicity is rare, but high levels of vitamin D intake may lead to hypercalcaemia (Chs 8 and 17) with calcium deposition in the kidney and other organs. Infants are most at risk and toxicity has been observed with fortified infant foods.

Vitamin E

Vitamin E activity is shown by two groups of molecules. The most important are the tocopherols, especially alpha-tocopherol. Vitamin E is an important antioxidant that limits the oxidative free radical damage to PUFAs within cell membranes.

Dietary requirements are unknown as deficiency is rare. Requirements depend on PUFA intake, and foods high in PUFAs are also rich sources of vitamin E. However, in cases of severe fat malabsorption, cystic fibrosis and some chronic liver diseases, deficiencies may occur. This is due to failure either to absorb the vitamin or to transport it around the body. In such cases, free radical damage to nerve and muscle membranes can occur.

There is some evidence to suggest that a high intake of vitamin E can protect against the development of ischaemic heart disease (Stephens et al 1996). This is thought to be due to the inhibition of the oxidation of PUFAs in the plasma lipoproteins. This oxidation process initiates the development of atherosclerosis. The amount required for this effect can only be achieved by supplementation. Few toxic effects have been observed from consuming large amounts of vitamin E.

Vitamin K

Several compounds have vitamin K activity. The important dietary source is phylloquinone, which is found in green leafy vegetables. Vitamin K is required for the proper formation of various protein coagulation factors, e.g. prothrombin. Lack of vitamin K or the presence of an antagonist, such as warfarin, means that an abnormal precursor to prothrombin is formed

and blood coagulation is not initiated. Another protein, osteocalcin, is also dependent on vitamin K. This protein is essential for normal bone formation. Pregnant women treated with warfarin are at high risk of having infants with severe bone disorders. For this reason, if deep vein thrombosis occurs during pregnancy, an alternative to warfarin is used.

Requirements for dietary vitamin K are hard to establish, as the menaquinones, synthesized by intestinal bacteria, have a similar mode of action. The absorption of vitamin K depends upon the presence of bile in the intestine. People with biliary obstruction may require parenteral supplements (Ch. 23).

Vitamin B$_1$ (thiamin)

Thiamin is an important coenzyme in the metabolism of carbohydrate. It is also important in the conduction of nerve impulses, by activation of chloride ion channels in the nerve membrane (Ch. 14). The main sources of thiamin are cereals, vegetables and meat (especially pork). Requirements for thiamin depend on the proportion of the energy derived from carbohydrate. Thus, requirements may increase in diets that are low in fats or which are predominantly carbohydrate.

There are two known disease states associated with deficiency: beri-beri and Wernicke–Korsakoff syndrome. Beri-beri is associated with long-term dietary deficiency and is a major problem in South-east Asia. It is characterized by heart failure and ascending neuritis. In Western countries, Wernicke–Korsakoff syndrome may result from chronic alcohol misuse leading to deficient intake and reduced absorption and metabolism of thiamin. There is often damage to the central nervous system and Korsakoff's psychosis with poor recent memory and confabulation (making up stories). Thiamin deficiency can occur quickly following binge drinking with little food intake. Alcohol is a source of carbohydrate and in these situations pyruvate and lactate accumulate in the blood to cause life-threatening acidosis (Ch. 8).

It is important that nurses recognize the impact of alcohol on thiamin intake and utilization. Once damage to the nervous system has occurred, supplementation with thiamin is of little use.

Vitamin B$_2$ (riboflavin)

Riboflavin is an important coenzyme involved in the metabolism of fuel molecules: carbohydrates, fatty acids and amino acids. It is found in milk and milk products, meat and eggs. Riboflavin deficiency is common, but does not usually cause serious conditions because most diets contain enough riboflavin to maintain metabolic processes. Signs of deficiency include angular stomatitis, cheilosis, seborrhoeic skin lesions and corneal vascularization.

Niacin

Niacin, whilst considered a vitamin, can be synthesized from the essential amino acid tryptophan (see p. 209). Deficiency results from a lack of tryptophan. Its main biological role is the metabolism of fuel molecules, but it also activates DNA repair mechanisms and is concerned with intracellular calcium concentrations.

Niacin deficiency leads to pellagra, which is characterized by a sunburn-like rash on exposed areas, diarrhoea and depressive psychosis. Untreated pellagra is fatal because energy-yielding metabolism is disrupted. Depressive psychosis occurs because tryptophan is required for the formation of serotonin 5-hydroxy-tryptamine (a neurotransmitter). This is not usually a problem in a mixed Western diet, which contains adequate tryptophan to meet requirements. Determining niacin requirements is difficult as the diet can contain both pre-formed niacin and the essential amino acid tryptophan.

Niacin toxicity can occur following prolonged intakes of >500 mg/day. Toxic effects may include vasodilatation, skin irritation and liver damage. For this reason, there is strict control over tryptophan supplementation.

Vitamin B$_6$

Vitamin B$_6$ is a group of compounds that are converted to pyridoxal phosphate in the body. The main function is as a cofactor for enzymes involved in a variety of amino acid reactions including transamination. It is also a cofactor of glycogen phosphorylase in muscle and liver, and helps to regulate the action of steroid hormones. Vitamin B$_6$ is found in meat, wholegrain cereals, vegetables and nuts, and deficiency is extremely rare. When it occurs, there is an increased sensitivity of target tissues to the action of low concentrations of steroid hormones, such as the oestrogens, androgens, cortisol and vitamin D. It can also lead to convulsions and altered tryptophan and methionine metabolism.

Controversy exists over the relationship between oral contraceptives and vitamin B$_6$ deficiency. There is, however, no research to support the use of vitamin B$_6$ to counteract the side-effects of oral contraceptives.

Vitamin B$_6$ toxicity can occur with large intakes of several hundred milligrams per day and the effects include peripheral nerve damage and partial paralysis that is only partially reversed by reduced intake. At lower doses (50–100 mg/day) the effects are less serious, e.g. tingling sensations, and they cease on reduction of intake. This has led to stricter regulation of the sales of vitamin B$_6$.

Vitamin B$_{12}$ (cobalamins) and folic acid (folates)

The metabolic functions of vitamin B$_{12}$ and folic acid are linked, and it is important to consider them together. Vitamin B$_{12}$ is essential for rapidly dividing red blood cells (erythrocytes) and myelination of nervous tissue. It is only present in food of animal origin. Absorption in the terminal ileum is dependent on the presence of intrinsic factor (produced by the stomach). Intrinsic factor can decrease with age and vitamin B$_{12}$ deficiency is associated with old age (see p. 217 and Ch. 32). Deficiency is also associated with a failure to produce intrinsic factor which causes pernicious anaemia (Ch. 18).

Folic acid is found in a variety of foods, including green leafy vegetables, pulses, yeast extract, fortified cereals and fruit. Folic acid is required for the synthesis of DNA and deficiency affects rapidly dividing cells such as erythrocytes and hair. Only about half the folic acid ingested is absorbed and folic acid deficiency is common. It can occur through insufficient dietary intake or secondary to vitamin B$_{12}$ deficiency. Vitamin B$_{12}$ plays an important role in folic acid metabolism. Folic acid is converted to an intermediary and cannot be reconverted to folic acid without vitamin B$_{12}$ and functional deficiency can occur. Folic acid deficiency can also lead to an increase in homocysteine, which is linked to an increased risk of cardiovascular disease (Ueland & Refsum 1991).

A deficiency of vitamin B$_{12}$ or folic acid will lead to megaloblastic anaemia (Ch. 18). In addition, vitamin B$_{12}$ deficiency leads to irreversible degeneration of the spinal cord in around a third of patients even where there are no signs of anaemia.

Folic acid supplementation at doses of 400 µg/day, to prevent neural tube defects, is important for woman prior to conception and during the first 28 days of pregnancy. Supplementation after this time will have no effect, as the neural tube has already formed. In many countries, flour is fortified with folic acid.

Biotin

Biotin is widely distributed in foods such as offal, egg yolk, milk and milk products. As such, deficiency is virtually unknown, only occurring after major intestinal resection (Ch. 22) and during parenteral nutrition (see p. 224). It acts as a cofactor in fatty acid synthesis and gluconeogenesis (production of glucose from non-carbohydrate sources, e.g. lactate).

Pantothenic acid

Also widely distributed in animal products, legumes and cereals and deficiency is rare. Pantothenic acid is important for energy release from carbohydrate and fat.

Vitamin C (ascorbic acid)

Vitamin C is needed for collagen synthesis and for maintaining connective tissue. This makes it essential in the prevention of scurvy and wound healing (Ch. 10). It has an important anti-oxidant role in trapping extracellular free radicals and enhancing vitamin E activity. Vitamin C is found in fresh raw fruits and vegetables, but is destroyed by oxidation and sunlight. The RNI is 40 mg/day for adults. Higher intakes have been linked to protection against cancer and treatment of influenza, but the research is limited. A high intake of vitamin C will increase absorption of non-haem iron (see p. 210).

MINERALS

Inorganic mineral elements that have a function within the body must be present in the diet. The minerals in food often represent the environmental conditions and mineral content of the soil. The more varied the diet from differing regions, the less likely there is to be mineral deficiency (see Table 11.2, p. 207). Readers should also refer to Chapter 8 where electrolyte imbalances are discussed in more detail.

Calcium (Ca)

Calcium is an important mineral in bone and teeth. An adult can have 1.2 kg of calcium, of which 99% will be in bone. During pregnancy, infancy, adolescence and lactation, calcium requirements increase to support the rapid growth. Calcium also has an important role in muscle contractility, cell structure, cellular responses to neurotransmitters and hormones, and blood coagulation. It is found in milk and cheese, bread, sardines and hard water and absorption from the diet is dependent on calcitriol (active vitamin D).

Calcium deficiency in childhood leads to a reduced rate of bone growth and loss of mineral and organic structure. Peak bone mass (PBM), occurring at around 30 years of age, is dependent upon earlier calcium intake. Calcium deficiency in adulthood leads to osteoporosis. This occurs earlier in women due to the reduction in bone mass that follows the loss of oestrogen hormones at the menopause; however, older men also develop osteoporosis due to reduced levels of androgens.

Iron (Fe)

Iron is required for the formation of oxygen-carrying haem in haemoglobin and for many enzymes. The most prevalent condition associated with iron deficiency is anaemia, because of the reduced synthesis of haem (Ch. 18). In the UK, dietary sources of iron, both non-haem (inorganic salts in vegetables) and haem forms (in meat), are plentiful. Despite this, there is evidence of deficiency in pre-school children (Gregory et al 1995), adolescents (MAFF 1994), and in inner city and Asian communities.

Deficiency occurs mainly due to insufficient absorption. Only about 10% of dietary iron is absorbed, haem iron being better absorbed than non-haem iron, which is affected by physiological and dietary factors. Inorganic iron salts are only absorbed in their reduced ferrous (Fe^{2+}) state and the presence of reducing agents, such as gastric acid and vitamin C, improves absorption. Iron absorption is reduced by phytates found in wholegrain cereals, some types of dietary fibre, tannic acid (found in tea) and calcium.

Absorbed iron accumulates in intestinal mucosal cells, binding to the protein ferritin. Once all the ferritin is bound with iron, no more can be absorbed from the intestines.

Nursing assessments need to recognize those individuals most at risk of developing iron deficiency anaemia. These include individuals who make sudden changes in dietary intake, such as deciding not to eat meat products, those with diets high in wholegrain products, and cases where blood loss is high (10–15% of women have a menstrual loss of iron greater than can be met from normal dietary intake; Bender 1999). Nurses should encourage vegetarians and those taking iron supplementation to drink orange juice or other products high in vitamin C to maximize iron absorption. Optimum iron absorption is achieved with an intake of 25–50 mg of vitamin C with each meal.

Sodium, potassium and chloride (Na, K, Cl)

Sodium, potassium and chloride are essential in maintaining the composition of intracellular and extracellular fluids. The gradient (maintained by active pumps) of sodium and potassium across cell membranes is essential for cell function, especially for nerve and muscle activity.

Sodium (as common salt) is consumed in excess from a variety of sources. Sodium is often a 'hidden' component of processed foods, the natural content of most foods being relatively low. It is estimated that in the UK we consume 2.5 times the required amount.

Excess sodium intakes have been associated with hypertension, but there is considerable debate about its physiological impact. The controversy surrounds whether reducing salt intake alters the blood pressure of normotensive individuals. In older, hypertensive individuals, salt reduction has been shown to reduce blood pressure. In general, the Department of Health (DoH 1991) recommends a gradual reduction in salt intake.

Potassium is found in many foods, especially fruit (bananas, dried fruit) and potatoes.

Phosphorus (P)

Most phosphorus (as phosphates) is present within bones, where it contributes (with calcium) to bone rigidity. It is a constituent of the organic biomolecules, such as proteins and adenosine triphosphate (ATP), and is involved in many enzyme reactions. Phosphorus is present in most foods of both animal and vegetable origin.

Zinc (Zn)

Zinc has a wide range of biological functions and is a cofactor for several enzymes. Although it is present in many foods, meat, milk and milk products are a good source because the availability of zinc is reduced when bound to the phytic acid (as phytates) in cereals.

Zinc deficiency is commonly associated with developing countries where it can delay puberty. In the UK, mild to moderate zinc deficiency has been linked to reduced wound healing (Ch. 10). A number of clinical situations can also lead to zinc deficiency, including liver disease, malignancy, diabetes, burns and trauma. In burns, the deficiency is associated with loss of body proteins (Ch. 28). King (1996) found that a minority of young people may have zinc intakes less than the LRNI, influencing bone mineralization and a failure to reach PBM.

Selenium (Se)

Selenium is a component of several enzyme pathways. It has an important role in the antioxidant defence system and in the formation of the active thyroid hormone T_3. Selenium deficiency is linked to the development of cardiomyopathy (Ch. 19), altered lipid and glucose metabolism and impaired leucocyte function.

Selenium is present in a variety of foods, but the amounts reflect the selenium content of the soil. Since 1978, it has been noted that in the UK the selenium level in cereals has decreased, amounts in meat have increased and amounts in dairy products have remained constant (Butcher et al 1995). It is possible that individuals on low incomes or eating a vegetarian diet will suffer from selenium deficiency. It is, however, toxic at doses above 450 µg/day.

Iodine (I)

Iodine is required for the synthesis of the thyroid hormones. Deficiency of iodine will lead to a goitre and reduced metabolic rates. In the UK, iodine is widely available in the diet, with milk and dairy produce being major sources. The average daily intake is in excess of the RNI for adults of 140 µg.

Magnesium (Mg)

Magnesium is a cofactor for some enzymes and in DNA replication and transcription. It is required for skeletal development and for the proper function of nerve and muscle membranes. Nutritional deficiency is rare, but hypomagnesaemia occurs with diarrhoea and vomiting. Magnesium salts given intravenously are beneficial immediately following a myocardial infarction (Bender 1999).

Copper (Cu)

Copper plays an important role in the synthesis of catecholamines and in protection against oxygen radical damage. In copper deficiency, the bones are more fragile and elastin is less elastic. This can lead to fractures or ruptures of major arteries such as the aorta. Anaemia may be a feature of copper deficiency.

Chromium (Cr)

Chromium is involved in the interaction between insulin and cell surface insulin receptors. Chromium deficiency is associated with impaired glucose tolerance, similar to that seen in diabetes mellitus. It also plays a role in lipid metabolism, which may be significant as a risk factor for coronary heart disease.

Other minerals

Several other minerals – cobalt (Co), fluoride (F), molybdenum (Mo) and manganese (Mn) – have a function in the body. Still others, such as silicon, vanadium, nickel, tin and lithium, have been shown to have an effect on the body but their function or essentiality has yet to be demonstrated. However, such detailed information is beyond the scope of this chapter and readers are directed to DoH (1991).

NURSING ASSESSMENT AND NUTRITIONAL SCREENING

Assessment is essential in identifying problems or needs and in planning appropriate interventions. It is the role of the dietician to complete nutritional assessments, whilst nurses complete a nursing assessment and nutritional screening. The nursing role includes:

- recognition of malnourished patients (see Evidence-based Practice box 11.1)

 EVIDENCE-BASED PRACTICE

11.1 Malnutrition in hospital

The consequences of malnutrition have been demonstrated in controlled clinical studies and include:

- delayed wound healing
- increased risk of pressure ulcers
- loss of muscle strength
- increased incidence of postoperative complications
- impaired immune responses
- increased risk of death.

Despite this, the incidence of malnutrition in hospital remains high and nutrition is still neglected as part of treatment. It is hoped that the introduction of nutritional screening tools will reverse this situation.

Further reading

Edington J, Kon P, Martyn C. Prevalence of malnutrition in patients in general practice. Clin Nutr 1996; 15: 60–63.

Ward, J, Close J, Little J et al. Development of a screening tool for assessing risk of undernutrition in patients in the community. J Hum Nutr Diet 1998; 11; 323–330.

Lennard-Jones J (ed). Positive approach to nutrition as treatment: report of a working party. London: Kings Fund; 1992.

- identification of patients at risk of malnutrition
- making appropriate referrals to the dietician
- ensuring that dietary intake is sufficient to meet nutritional needs.

The use of nursing frameworks or models provides the focus for assessing individuals holistically and determining nursing interventions (Ch. 1). Assessment can explore nutrition in the context of three broad areas: psychological, sociological and physiological. The importance of each and the order in which they are addressed will reflect the nature of the illness, the health care environment and the framework chosen. Understanding the relationship between the different factors that influence an individual and nutrition is important and each aspect is considered separately.

PSYCHOLOGICAL AREAS OF NUTRITION AND THE NURSING ASSESSMENT

Eating is an essential human activity that reflects lifestyle, feelings and understanding of food and society. Over the years, different theories have been proposed to explain eating behaviour, fuelled by increasing concerns about diet and disease, such as obesity, heart disease and cancer, and various food 'scares', e.g. bovine spongiform encephalopathy (BSE). Understanding why we eat and why we make particular food choices is important for implementing effective strategies to improve the nation's diet.

Food preferences

Food preferences arise from a combination of innate and learned behaviours, starting in infancy and continuing through to adulthood. Learning and experience, coupled with peer, socio-cultural and adult pressures, modify a person's eating patterns. In adulthood, illnesses such as cardiovascular disease are associated with a lifetime of poor dietary intake. Recognizing the powerful influence on eating behaviours of parents and peer groups, and the strength of the resistance to change is important in planning interventions to improve dietary intake and health.

Association of food with unpleasant situations or symptoms will influence learned preferences, such as associating a particular food with the nausea of pregnancy. These aversions may persist long after the event. Patients with cancer (Chs 33, 34) may also develop food aversions, as the taste of food can be associated with 'tumour-induced malaise' or taste disturbance. Negative views of school or hospital meals may reflect the individual's experience; low expectations of food quality, e.g. in hospital, may weaken the appetite even before the meals are presented.

Sensory aspects of eating

The integration of sensory information, sight, smell, sound, taste, texture and temperature is important and allows us to construct images of familiar food. This has an important physiological as well as psychological component and is referred to as the cephalic phase of eating (Ch. 22). During periods of ill health this sensory information is diminished and responses to food or appetite are affected. Alternatively, the diet may be modified, either in texture or in taste, leading to dissonance between the food expected and what is received. Encouraging people to eat in these circumstances is difficult. Nurses need to take responsibility for ensuring that dietary needs are met. This may involve food presentation, including portion size, or suggestions for alternatives to replace unpalatable foods.

In assessing individuals, the nurse could consider the following:

■ What foods do they like?
■ Will they eat unfamiliar foods?
■ What foods did they like when they were in hospital?

SOCIOLOGICAL AND CULTURAL INFLUENCES AND THE NURSING ASSESSMENT

Eating is a social activity. Beliefs and attitudes about food will vary between cultures. Food often symbolizes hospitality, wealth, status, or religious beliefs. Society has strong beliefs about which foods are desirable and which are offensive. For many, food acceptability and eating behaviour are associated with religious beliefs. The moral links to food are more overt in groups who have retained strong, universal religious beliefs, such as Hindus and Muslims. This may extend from the food itself to those who prepare it and the time at which it is eaten, e.g. Muslims fast between sunrise and sunset during Ramadan.

In the UK, our multi-faith society can make giving nutritional advice complex. Often foods considered acceptable for one cultural group are unacceptable to another. Recognizing this diversity and seeking advice from other professionals are important if the nurse is to be effective in improving dietary intake.

Sociological issues

Social disadvantage has been linked to increased levels of ill health (Townsend et al 1988). The number of individuals living in poverty (income < 40% of average income) in the UK is estimated at 8 million (Howarth et al 1999). Poverty can influence nutritional status in several different ways:

■ it restricts access to shops, limits income available for food purchase and limits food choices
■ it limits access to cooking facilities leading to further restriction of choice
■ it limits access to education and advice on healthy eating.

Furthermore, poverty is associated with increased ill health, which may alter nutritional requirements. Nurses must ensure that dietary advice is practicable (see Reflective Practice box 11.2). Having an awareness of the resources available within the local community is important. These may include social services, religious organizations, meal clubs, day centres, charities and self-help groups.

In assessing sociological issues and nutrition, the following questions may be valuable:

■ What food do you normally buy?
■ Do you like cooking?
■ What food do you prepare for yourself?
■ What food can you store at home?
■ Where do you shop?
■ What benefits do you receive?
■ Do you live alone?
■ What cooking facilities do you have?

R|Я REFLECTIVE PRACTICE

11.2 Helping a patient in the community to improve nutritional status

John is a 28-year-old lone parent caring for two children of pre-school age. He lives in a small, damp flat with only one electric ring to cook on. He is very thin, pale and tired looking. Both children are pale with runny noses.

John has recently attended the GP surgery and has been diagnosed as having bronchitis and iron deficiency anaemia. The health visitor is also concerned about the development of the children.

Student activities

● What practical advice can you offer John to improve his and his children's nutritional status?
● How could the effectiveness of the advice be assessed?
● What factors may prevent John from making changes to his diet?
● What other members of the multidisciplinary team could be involved?

PHYSIOLOGICAL AREAS AND THE NURSING ASSESSMENT

Disease states will influence nutritional status either directly (see below) or indirectly by altering the patient's ability to ingest and utilize nutrients. Many signs and symptoms common to a variety of conditions can indicate a change in nutritional status before advanced under-nutrition is evident. Assessment should explore the following areas:

■ alterations in food intake
■ altered gastrointestinal function
■ alterations in nutrient metabolism.

Alterations in food intake

Food intake is dependent on both liking food and being able to eat. Factors that can influence food intake include the following.

Altered taste

Cancer and liver disease can lead to alterations in taste, and certain drugs, including chemotherapy and antidepressants, can cause a metallic taste. Dehydration and oral infections, such as candidiasis (Ch. 22), both reduce taste sensations.

Nausea and vomiting

Underlying physiological conditions, such as intestinal obstruction, cancer and infection, can lead to nausea and vomiting. Anaesthesia and drugs such as the narcotic analgesics, chemotherapy and antibiotics can cause nausea and vomiting. Pain, anxiety, odours and taste can also cause nausea.

Chewing and swallowing

Common reasons for people not eating are ill-fitting dentures and poor dental care. Speech problems can indicate difficulty with chewing or swallowing, as many of the same muscles are used. Coughing or choking can indicate dysphagia (swallowing difficulty). In this case, a swallowing assessment by a speech and language therapist (SLT) or appropriately trained nurse will be required. Using a flow chart (Fig. 11.4) will ensure that dietary needs are recognized with the minimum of delay.

Mobility

Certain conditions, such as rheumatoid arthritis, stroke or fractures, can reduce mobility and manual dexterity and make the handling of cutlery and cups more difficult. In the community this can cause problems with shopping. Changes in coordination and balance, e.g. following a stroke, may result in reduced food intake as both the preparation and eating of food become more difficult. Kyphosis or osteoporosis can cause problems with lifting the head, which in turn makes eating and swallowing hard.

Altered consciousness and mental state

Changes in the level of consciousness can reduce nutritional intake, as awareness and independence are altered. Confusion and disorientation may make sitting and eating more difficult.

Excess intake

Excess dietary intake of the macronutrients is an increasing problem in the developed world leading to obesity (see p. 216). This can also occur as a result of medications such as prednisolone which increase the appetite.

Insufficient intake

Rapid weight loss due to either eating disorders (of concern in young adults) or loss of appetite (anorexia) may result from physical disease, treatment, anxiety, depression, pain or drug therapy (see below).

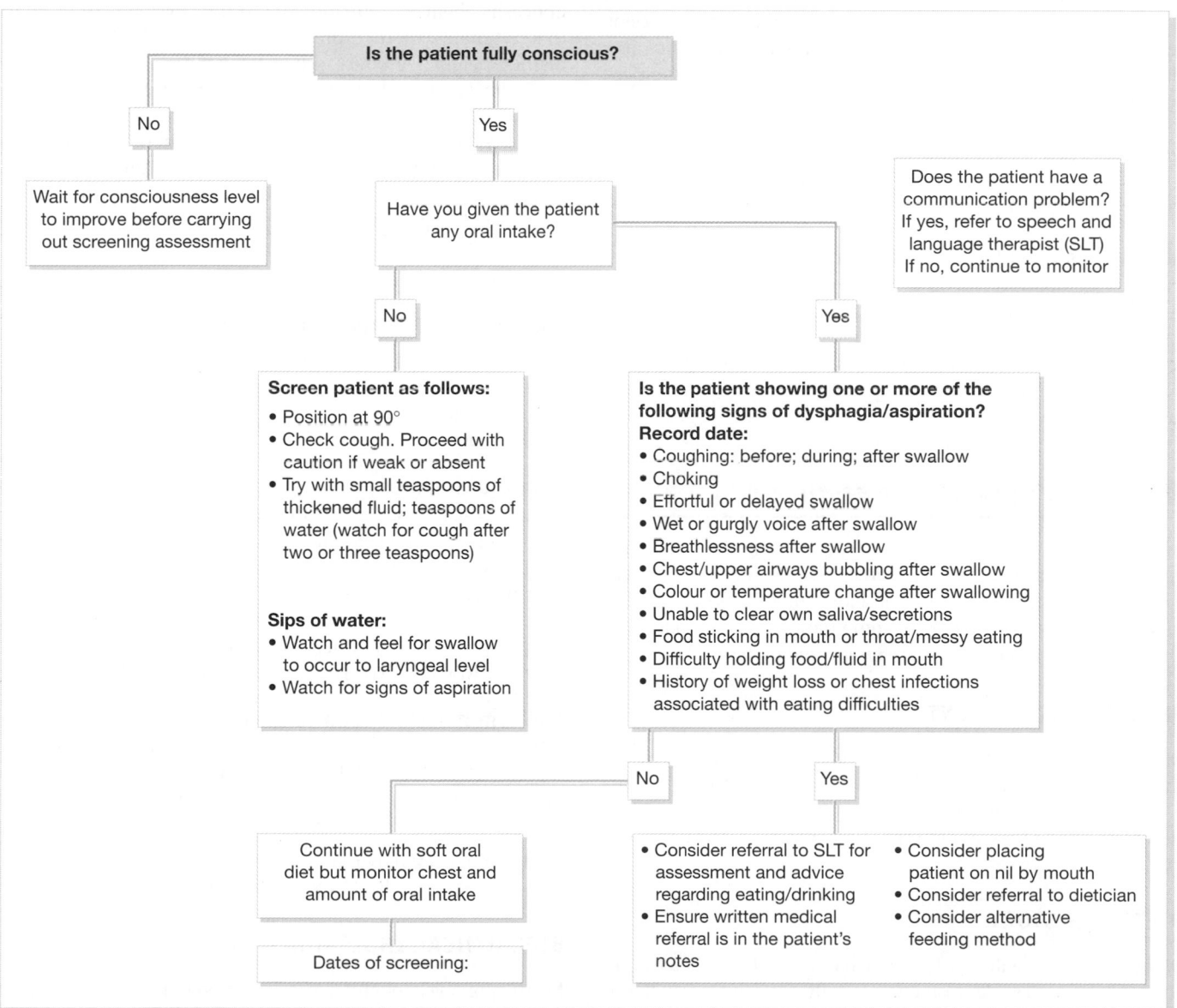

Figure 11.4 Screening assessment for dysphagic patients. (Reprinted with permission from Portsmouth Healthcare NHS Trust Speech and Language Therapy Department. The dysphagia flow charts were designed by speech and language therapists in Portsmouth Healthcare NHS Trust [Ruth Sullivan, Lynn Dangerfield]. They are designed for use by nurses trained by SLTs using a structured training package.)

Altered gastrointestinal function

The ability to absorb and utilize nutrients may be impaired by factors such as age and disease.

Poor nutrient absorption

Nutrient absorption is essential to maintain nutrition. Any condition that alters gastrointestinal (GI) function can influence nutrient absorption. For example, patients with inflammatory bowel disease, cystic fibrosis or following surgical resection of the GI tract may have poor nutrient absorption. Older adults may have altered GI function, such as reduced intrinsic factor, which is essential for vitamin B_{12} absorption. Many drugs interfere with nutrient absorption, such as laxatives which may prevent the absorption of fat-soluble vitamins. The interaction between drugs and food is covered later in the chapter.

Increased nutrient loss

Patients with diarrhoea are at increased risk of micronutrient deficiency, particularly of sodium and potassium. They are also at risk of dehydration (Ch. 8). Where diarrhoea is due to infection, patients may have the additional problems of needing more nutrients because they are hypermetabolic and do not feel like eating, as well as having nutrient loss.

Patients with gallbladder disease may become deficient in fat-soluble vitamins due to biliary obstruction (Ch. 23).

Alterations in nutrient metabolism

Nutrient metabolism can be affected by specific diseases such as diabetes mellitus, liver disease and pancreatic disorders. Acute illness and chronic immune conditions can also alter nutrient requirement and metabolism. Many drugs compete with nutrients in metabolic pathways, e.g. methotrexate which antagonizes folic acid.

ASSESSING NUTRITIONAL STATUS

Assessment of nutritional status requires a multidisciplinary approach, which includes subjective assessment (e.g. physical appearance), anthropometric and biochemical methods. Accuracy is increased by using a combination of methods, and changes in nutritional status are monitored with serial testing.

PHYSICAL ASSESSMENT

Observation of the skin, hair, nails and oral mucosa can provide subjective information about nutritional status. Obvious thinness, pallor and weakness should be noted. Micronutrient deficiency states can present with specific symptoms (see Tables 11.1 and 11.2).

DIETARY HISTORY

Dietary histories will provide information on food choices and eating behaviours. Assessment of daily food intake will not give a true representation of food intake that varies from day to day, whilst long-term dietary records may not be sustained over time. A dietary history can provide an overview of dietary intake, which helps in encouraging dietary changes. The value of dietary histories is limited by their reliance on patient/client compliance and recall and interpretation of food consumed. In care settings, keeping an accurate record of dietary intake is essential to monitor nutritional status and ensure that intake is sufficient to meet nutrient need.

ANTHROPOMETRIC METHODS

Weighing patients on admission to hospital, at discharge and in the community provides an accurate record of changes. A loss of 10% or more in less than 3 months, for those who are not on a weight-reducing diet, is associated with an increased risk of illness. Anthropometry allows the estimation of body fat. Three methods are used: height-for-weight ratio or body mass index (BMI), skinfold thickness and mid-upper arm circumference.

Body mass index

Concerns about malnutrition led to the development of charts that estimate whether an individual's weight is correct for his/her height. A chart produced by the Health Education Authority (1994) takes into account frame size and produces an optimal range of weight to height. The BMI is calculated using the same data and is used to estimate the amount of fat tissue. It is widely employed to encourage the attainment of optimal body weight. The BMI is calculated as the weight (in kg) divided by the height squared (m²), e.g. a woman weighing 65 kg who is 1.78 m tall will have a BMI of:

$$65/(1.78^2) = 20.5$$

The BMI value is interpreted as follows (MAFF 1995):

< 20 = underweight
$20-24$ = desirable
$25-30$ = overweight
> 30 = obese.

Skinfold thickness

Skinfold thickness, first identified in the 1960s, is still used to assess body composition. The accuracy is questionable as the original data did not consider age changes and assumed that subcutaneous fat stores are representative of total body fat. Triceps skinfold (TSF) measurements are taken at the midpoint of the upper arm using a set of skinfold calipers. The normal range for women is 10–16.5 mm and for men is 7.5–12.5 mm.

Mid-arm muscle circumference

Estimation of skeletal muscle mass is done using the mid-arm muscle circumference (MAMC). A tape measure is used to determine the upper arm circumference at the same point used for the TSF. MAMC is calculated using the following equation:

$$\text{MAMC (cm)} = \text{upper arm circumference (cm)} - [0.314 \times \text{TSF (mm)}]$$

BIOCHEMICAL INDICATORS

Measuring levels of nutrients in the body tissues can indicate nutritional status. The accuracy and reliability of measurements reflect the dynamic nature of the individual, body stores, metabolism and excretion. Serial measurements over a specified period of time are recommended to increase reliability.

Creatinine height index

Creatinine, produced during muscle protein turnover, is excreted by the kidneys in urine. Urinary excretion rate is proportional to the individual's muscle mass. A 24-hour urine collection allows the daily excretion of creatinine to be measured and compared with standard tables. This provides an estimate of skeletal muscle loss; 60–80% of the standard suggests moderate malnutrition and less than 60% severe malnutrition.

Twenty-four-hour nitrogen balance

There is a constant turnover of protein in the body which can increase during times of ill health such as infection, trauma and surgery (see p. 217). Where protein intake matches protein demand, the individual is said to be in nitrogen balance. Nitrogen is measured as the amino acids that make up proteins are broken down. If amino acid breakdown is greater than dietary intake then the patient is in a catabolic state (breaking down complex molecules).

Serum proteins

Individual plasma proteins can provide an estimation of nutritional status by measuring protein stores. The most commonly used is albumin which is synthesized by the liver and there is a large body reserve. Serum albumin can be influenced by administration of blood products, altered liver mass, changes in extracellular volume and catabolism associated with trauma. Its reliability as a predictor of nutritional status can be questioned. Hypoalbuminaemia (low serum albumin) is associated with sepsis, trauma and long standing PEM. Other proteins can be measured including transferrin and prealbumin.

NUTRITIONAL SCREENING TOOLS

Nutritional screening tools have been devised to provide specific information related to nutritional status (McLaren & Green 1998). Their simplicity ensures that they can be used by all members of the health care team, but they should not replace a nursing assessment. Screening tools are often devised for specific clinical areas. In general they consider factors that include diet, weight, appetite, swallowing and social factors (Fig. 11.5). They often include a scoring system with a series of actions dependent on the score.

Using screening tools as part of managed nutritional care can ensure that those patients who are undernourished are

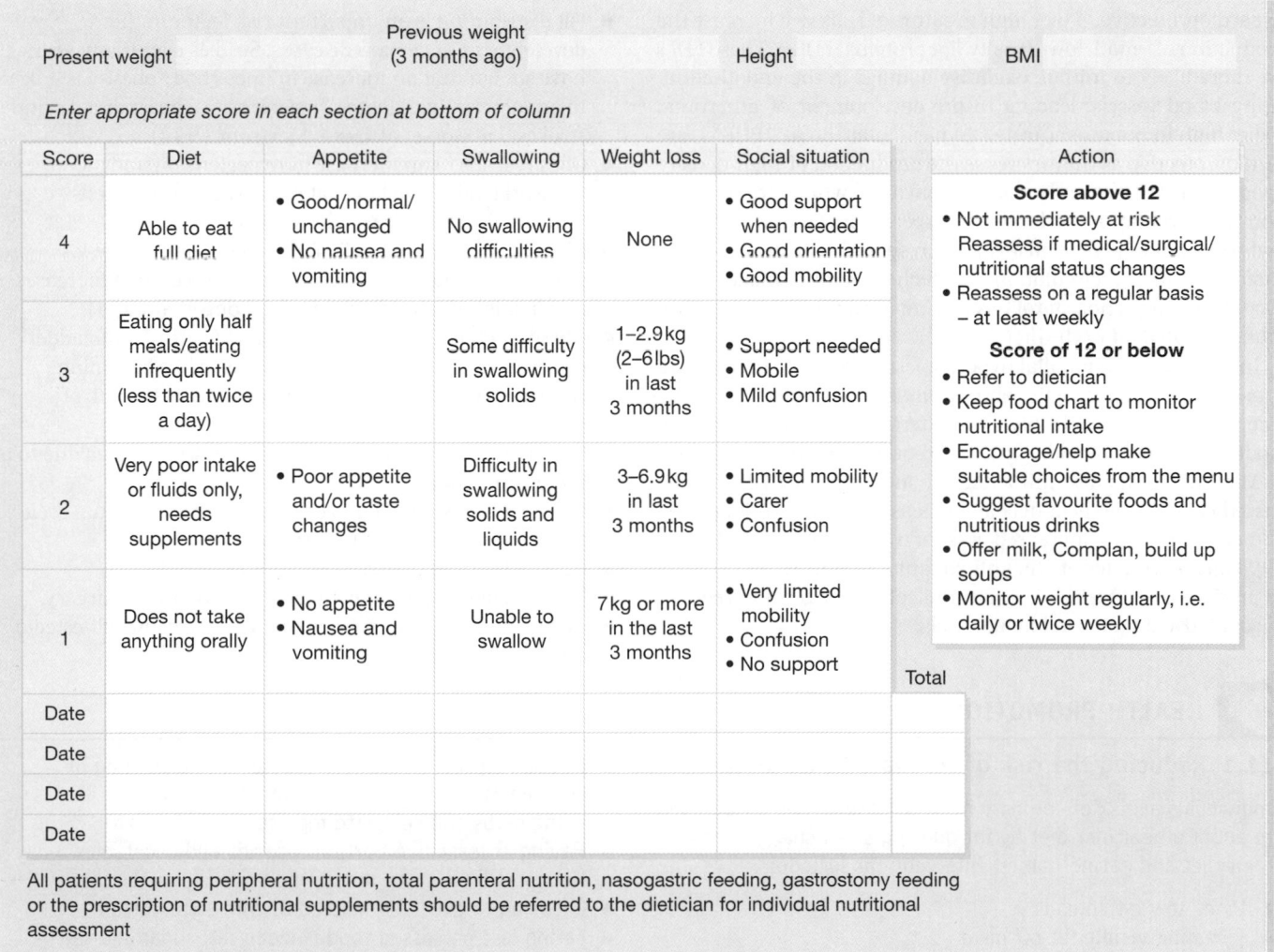

Present weight		Previous weight (3 months ago)			Height		BMI

Enter appropriate score in each section at bottom of column

Score	Diet	Appetite	Swallowing	Weight loss	Social situation	Action
4	Able to eat full diet	• Good/normal/ unchanged • No nausea and vomiting	No swallowing difficulties	None	• Good support when needed • Good orientation • Good mobility	**Score above 12** • Not immediately at risk Reassess if medical/surgical/ nutritional status changes • Reassess on a regular basis – at least weekly
3	Eating only half meals/eating infrequently (less than twice a day)		Some difficulty in swallowing solids	1–2.9 kg (2–6 lbs) in last 3 months	• Support needed • Mobile • Mild confusion	**Score of 12 or below** • Refer to dietician • Keep food chart to monitor nutritional intake • Encourage/help make suitable choices from the menu
2	Very poor intake or fluids only, needs supplements	• Poor appetite and/or taste changes	Difficulty in swallowing solids and liquids	3–6.9 kg in last 3 months	• Limited mobility • Carer • Confusion	• Suggest favourite foods and nutritious drinks • Offer milk, Complan, build up soups
1	Does not take anything orally	• No appetite • Nausea and vomiting	Unable to swallow	7 kg or more in the last 3 months	• Very limited mobility • Confusion • No support	• Monitor weight regularly, i.e. daily or twice weekly
Date						Total
Date						
Date						
Date						

All patients requiring peripheral nutrition, total parenteral nutrition, nasogastric feeding, gastrostomy feeding or the prescription of nutritional supplements should be referred to the dietician for individual nutritional assessment

Figure 11.5 Nutrition assessment chart (reprinted with kind permission from Brighton Health Care NHS Trust).

referred to the dieticians. They can aid communication between all members of the multidisciplinary team, which is essential to ensure that nutritional care is coordinated and effective.

Lennard-Jones (1992) recommended the development of nutritional teams that include dieticians, nurses, catering managers, pharmacists and doctors. The development of nutritional teams will facilitate the development of a protocol to be followed after assessment and enable nutritional standards to be set and audited.

GROUPS WITH SPECIFIC NUTRITIONAL NEEDS

INDIVIDUALS WITH CORONARY HEART DISEASE

The incidence of coronary heart disease (CHD) is influenced by dietary intake (Ch. 19). Obesity and a high-fat diet increase the risk of CHD, whilst a diet high in polyunsaturated fats, vitamin E and other antioxidants may be cardioprotective. Intervention and population studies have also demonstrated that dietary modification may influence the mortality and morbidity associated with CHD (Stephens et al 1996).

Dietary fats have long been associated with CHD, some fats predisposing to the development of atheroma whilst others may be cardioprotective. A diet high in saturated fats will increase the production of small, low-density lipoproteins (LDLs). These LDLs are more likely to initiate oxidative damage in the endothelium lining blood vessels, leading to the development of atheroma. A diet high in polyunsaturates, in particular the n-3 PUFAs, are cardioprotective as they increase the production of high-density lipoproteins (HDLs) and large LDL particles which are removed from the circulation by binding to specific receptors. The LDLs and HDLs (more beneficial form) are responsible for transporting cholesterol in the circulation. Most cholesterol is made in the liver and dietary cholesterol has less impact on serum cholesterol than saturated fat in the diet.

Individuals with familial hypercholesterolaemias (high serum cholesterol) have genetic abnormalities that affect the LDL receptors. These types of high cholesterol are resistant to dietary modification and the individual will require lipid-lowering drugs.

Micronutrients also influence the incidence of CHD. As discussed earlier, folic acid deficiency is associated with increased homocysteine and increased risk of CHD (Ueland & Refsum 1991). High intakes of the antioxidant vitamins (E and C) may be protective. Vitamin E is a free radical scavenger and reduces the oxidative damage in blood vessels.

All patients with a history of CHD or with CHD in their family should be encouraged to eat a healthy diet (see Health Promotion box 11.1), increasing their consumption of fruit, vegetables and starch and decreasing their total fat intake. The total fat should have a greater percentage of polyunsaturated and monounsaturated fats than of saturated fats. Overweight individuals should be encouraged to reduce their total energy consumption, which when coupled with exercise leads to weight reduction. Decreasing total salt intake will also benefit those with hypertension by helping to reduce blood pressure.

THE OBESE INDIVIDUAL

It is estimated that in the last decade the number of obese adults has doubled and that childhood obesity is increasing. Obesity results from many factors and as such is difficult to control. The basic mechanism of obesity is an imbalance between energy intake and energy expenditure, resulting in a positive energy balance. Excess energy is converted to fat and stored in adipose tissue as an available energy source for later. The number of adipose cells increases in those individuals whose weight is $\geq 75\%$ above the desirable weight. People with more modest obesity are more likely to have an increase in fat cell size (Bray 1996).

Obesity is associated with an increased incidence of illness:

- Fat distribution is an important risk factor in the development of certain diseases. Studies over many years have shown that an increase in upper body obesity is linked to an increase in diabetes, hypertension, heart attacks and strokes (Larsson et al 1984, Sjostram 1992).
- Obesity leads to an increase in hypertension and increases the workload of the heart at rest, even in normotensive individuals (Drenick & Fisler 1992).
- Obesity increases the risk of diabetes. With weight loss, glucose tolerance can improve, insulin secretion increases and insulin resistance is reduced (Long et al 1994).
- Obese women have an increased incidence of gallbladder disease. Cholesterol production leads to bile becoming saturated with cholesterol which increases the risk of gallstones (Bray 1996).
- Obesity has been linked to obstructive sleep apnoea due to an increase in pharyngeal fat (Ch. 4).
- Obesity has been linked to changes in the menstrual cycle and a reduction in free testosterone.
- Obesity is linked to increased joint wear.
- There is an increase in complications following surgery.
- The obese individual may be isolated, have low self-esteem and be stigmatized by society.

 HEALTH PROMOTION

11.1 Reducing the risk of coronary heart disease

Individuals at risk of coronary heart disease can be encouraged to adopt a healthier diet by introducing small changes into their diet and eating habits. Interventions include:

- Using low fat spreads
- Trimming visible fat off meat
- Grilling food instead of frying

- Not adding salt to cooked foods or in the cooking of vegetables
- Using herbs and spices to replace salt
- Having at least five portions of fruit and vegetables a day
- Not spreading fat on bread when making sandwiches
- Choosing thick-sliced instead of thin-sliced bread
- Eating less processed food (hidden fat, sugar and salt)
- Keeping alcohol intake within safe limits

Helping with weight loss – the nurses' role

Most overweight people will have tried many diets and it is important to identify the individual's knowledge of dieting and a healthy diet. The majority of people who are overweight are simply consuming more energy than is required. Encouraging a healthy diet, by increasing consumption of fruit, vegetables and starch whilst reducing intake of fat and processed foods, will reduce total calorie intake. It is important that the diet is balanced for all nutrients and advice from dieticians should be sought where appropriate. Measures that encourage and maintain weight loss include:

- ensuring that patients are informed and knowledgeable about all aspects, e.g. that initial weight loss is due to water loss rather than loss of fatty tissue
- gradually decreasing calorie intake whilst increasing activity
- setting achievable targets with the person – no more than 1.5 kg/week weight loss
- not encouraging crash diets, as successful weight loss requires changes in lifestyle to be maintained
- support groups and family support.

OLDER ADULTS

The older population is increasing in number. It has been estimated that by 2025 the older adults will account for 21.5% of the total population and that, of these, a third will be over the age of 80 years (Kinsella 1996). This demographic change will influence the health requirements of the population (Ch. 32). Old age is associated with specific physiological and social changes that can predispose to micro- or macronutrient imbalances. Although data about nutritional requirements for the very old is limited, it is known that nutrient requirements alter with age.

Physiological changes

As one ages, there is a reduction in lean body mass and activity which reduces energy demand. Obesity can occur in older adults if their intake of energy-dense foods (those containing sugar or fat) is high. In contrast, protein requirements can remain unchanged or increase, as utilization of dietary proteins is less efficient. Chronic wounds such as leg ulcers can further complicate the dietary requirements (Ch. 10).

Taste acuity diminishes with age, often limiting food choices and appetite. It can also lead to an increase in the intake of salt to compensate for the lack of taste. Poor dental care or ill-fitting dentures will affect food intake and may lead to nutrient deficiencies, e.g. it may be difficult to eat fresh fruit.

Reductions in GI motility and function are associated with changes in body composition. Coupled with a diet low in fruit, vegetables or fluid can cause constipation. This in turn can lead to an increase in the production of bacterial toxins in the bowel, which may contribute to confusion.

The secretion of gastric intrinsic factor reduces or even ceases. Insufficient absorption of vitamin B_{12} leads to anaemia and nerve damage. Where intrinsic factor is insufficient, it is necessary to administer vitamin B_{12} parenterally.

Ageing is associated with multiple pathology and older adults are often affected by stroke, heart disease, cancer, arthritis, osteoporosis and infections. These conditions may limit mobility, dexterity, access to food, nutrient intake and absorption. Multiple pathology often means multiple prescription medications and polypharmacy is a recognized risk factor for under-nutrition as drugs inhibit nutrient absorption or compete with nutrients for metabolic pathways (see p. 225).

Social changes

Older adults are at increased risk of living alone or being reliant on others for their care. Bereavement and isolation are factors that contribute to poor nutrition. Many older adults are reliant on state pensions and have a reduced income. This leads to reduced food choices and increases the risk of micronutrient deficiency, as the disposable income is used on food products with low nutritional value. The diet can become imbalanced with a greater ratio of energy content to nutrient content.

WOMEN OF CHILD-BEARING AGE AND VEGETARIANS/VEGANS

Iron deficiency anaemia is one of the most common nutrient deficiencies. It occurs primarily as a result of difficulties in absorbing iron. Although iron is found widely in the diet, only about 10% of ingested iron is absorbed. Individuals with regular blood loss, such as during menstruation, or restricted dietary intake are particularly vulnerable. This is due to both the loss being greater than amounts absorbed and the reduced bioavailability of iron in the diet. Vegetarians rely on the absorption of iron from non-haem sources and the bioavailability may be further reduced by the presence of phytates in the diet.

Pregnancy can increase the likelihood of anaemia by increasing iron requirements and the need for folic acid has already been discussed (see p. 209).

Vegetarians and vegans may be deficient in essential amino acids. This is likely to happen where individuals simply stop eating meat and fish and do not have another protein source. It is important that nurses provide information and encourage a diet that provides a wide variety of proteins, e.g. beans on toast, lentil curry and rice. The total biological value of the proteins is then enhanced.

PATIENTS WITH SEPSIS, TRAUMA AND CANCER – THE HYPERMETABOLIC PATIENT

Illness is associated with an increase in energy demand and it is important that energy requirements are met. During illness, appetite can be reduced and the body will mobilize stores of energy by glycogenolysis (breakdown or catabolism of stored liver glycogen) and later by lipolysis (breakdown of stored fat). The utilization of fat for energy is limited and catabolism of muscle protein will take place to provide amino acids for gluconeogenesis (production of glucose from non-carbohydrate sources). This ensures the constant supply of glucose for tissues such as the brain.

Ensuring adequate energy intake will conserve body proteins. Where this does not occur, PEM will become evident. Patients with acute (sepsis, trauma and burns) and chronic illnesses (cancer, AIDS, chronic lung disease and autoimmune disorders) can develop severe wasting, which contributes to mortality and morbidity. This extreme catabolism of tissue leads to a condition known as cachexia. Cachexia is characterized by anorexia, early satiety, weight loss, debility, anaemia and oedema. Development is thought to be due to a systemic inflammatory response with increased production of various inflammatory chemicals, e.g. acute-phase proteins (Ch. 9). These chemicals increase inflammation and modulate metabolic rate and energy demand, and increased secretion of catecholamines can lead to insulin resistance. Simple re-feeding does not reverse cachexia. Current views suggest that attenuation of cachexia is best achieved by modulating the inflammatory response and various supplements are being studied, such as n-3 PUFAs for patients with pancreatic cancer.

NUTRITION AND WOUND HEALING

Nutritional status has been shown to influence wound healing (Ch. 10). During hypermetabolic states, increased nutrient availability is essential to meet energy requirements and support immune function. Even in mild PEM there is evidence of organ protein depletion, suboptimal immune function and reduced wound healing. Problems with healing have been noted where there was brief preoperative illness or reduced nutrition in the immediate postoperative period. In elective surgery, nutritional assessment and planned care should be started at preoperative assessment to:

- increase the likelihood of achieving optimum nutritional status before surgery
- increase the understanding of nutritional needs resulting from surgery, including dietary changes and/or food restrictions.

The amount of time a patient is nil-by-mouth preoperatively can have a direct impact on nutritional and fluid status. Current recommendations suggest that patients should go no longer than 6 hours without solid food or 2 hours without water preoperatively (American Society of Anesthesiologists 1997). This varies between NHS Trusts, but it is clear that extended periods of time without food or drink are detrimental. Nurses

R|Я REFLECTIVE PRACTICE

11.3 Fasting for surgery

You are on a busy surgical ward. The theatre list is delayed due to the admission of three patients following a road traffic accident, each of whom requires emergency surgery. There are four patients awaiting surgery on your ward and each one has been fasted since 6.00am; it is now 6.00pm. Their operations have been cancelled until tomorrow morning. The last evening meal has been served in the hospital.

Student activities
- What should your actions be?
- Is there a protocol in your local NHS Trust on ensuring that meals are available?
- When would you fast these patients again?

have a responsibility to monitor the fluid and nutritional intake of patients during the perioperative period (Ch. 29). Clear protocols should be in place for those occasions when surgery is delayed or operations are suddenly cancelled. Liaison between wards, theatre, catering department and dieticians is important to ensure food availability during these times (see Reflective Practice box 11.3).

It is also essential that nutritional intake is monitored postoperatively. Standard intravenous (i.v.) fluids are not intended to meet nutritional requirements. The nutrient content of standard i.v. fluids is limited to glucose for energy. Early return to oral feeding helps to prevent perioperative malnutrition and increased mortality and morbidity in the following:

- older adults
- operation delays and prolonged fasting
- face, neck and gastric surgery
- prolonged nausea and vomiting
- pancreatic or bowel cancer
- fracture of the neck of femur.

Specific nutrients each play a role in the wound healing process (Table 11.3). Patients with chronic wounds, such as leg ulcers, may have other nutritional needs (Ch. 10). Obesity may increase the risk of leg ulcers and influences wound healing. Often obese individuals will be inactive and suffer from micronutrient deficiencies such as iron, zinc and vitamin C.

Infected wounds will also increase nutrient demand. This may be an increase in protein demand due to the loss of protein-rich exudate. Patients may also be pyrexial and hypermetabolic, further increasing energy demand whilst reducing nutrient intake.

Table 11.3 Specific nutrients and wound healing

Nutrient	Role and comments
n-6 linoleic PUFAs	Proinflammatory and as such are important in mediating the immune response
Exogenous amino acids, e.g. arginine, ornithine, glutamine and alpha-ketoglutarate	Improve nitrogen balance in trauma and sepsis. Arginine has also been demonstrated to have a pharmacological effect on promoting normal wound repair in humans
Vitamin A	Enhances the inflammatory response in wounds by increasing the influx of macrophages into the damaged area. Collagen synthesis by fibroblasts is also increased
Vitamin C	An important antioxidant scavenging free radicals produced by macrophage activity. It is also important in collagen synthesis. Vitamin C levels are rapidly depleted in trauma and sepsis
Zinc	Surgical trauma can decrease serum zinc concentrations. Zinc deficiency can reduce fibroblast proliferation and collagen synthesis. Overall wound strength is reduced and epithelialization is delayed

FOOD ALLERGY AND INTOLERANCE

Many foods contain substances that cause allergic reactions, including peanuts, strawberries and shellfish. An allergic reaction occurs immediately on contact with the food and is normally mediated by immunoglobulin (IgE). The cause is often easy to identify and once removed from the diet (or immediate environment) the allergic response will cease. In some instances, the reaction is severe and can lead to anaphylaxis.

In contrast, food intolerance or sensitivity is less easy to define. It is estimated that as many as 30% of individuals will have experienced intolerance to a food (Chandra 1997), but identifying the cause is difficult. Altering the diet and eliminating specific foods are the main tools for diagnosis. An elimination or exclusion diet may involve:

- exclusion of a single food or food constitute
- exclusion of a number of foods commonly associated with adverse reactions such as dairy produce
- having a very limited diet that contains a few selected foods with little or no ability to trigger a reaction, e.g. pears and rice
- withdrawal of all food and replacement with a formula or elemental diet.

An accurate diagnosis is made when symptoms and physical signs:

- improve when the food is excluded
- recur when the suspect food is added
- show sustained improvement when the suspect food is excluded long term.

Signs and symptoms associated with food intolerance can affect many different tissues and include skin irritation, dry itching eyes, abdominal pain and bloating, diarrhoea, insomnia, muscle aches, hypertension, fluid retention and palpitations.

Specific food intolerances

Lactose intolerance

Individuals who are lactose-intolerant lack the enzyme (lactase) to digest milk sugar (lactose). Undigested lactose will then pass into the colon where it can cause diarrhoea and cramping pain. Sufferers may be able to tolerate fermented milk products such as yoghurt and cheese.

Coeliac disease

Coeliac disease (gluten-sensitive enteropathy) is an unpleasant reaction to gluten (cereal protein) that may damage the intestinal villi. Symptoms may be mild or more severe with abdominal bloating and progressive weight loss. Management involves avoiding products containing gluten, which is found, for example, in wheat, rye and barley-based foods.

▶ Nursing interventions

Nurses must be actively involved in ensuring that the nutritional needs of patients are being met. Multidisciplinary nutritional teams in hospital (dieticians, nurses, doctors, pharmacists and catering managers) ensure that nutritional provision is coordinated. The development of similar community-based teams could influence nutritional provision across a wide spectrum of health care settings. Where teams are established, there is evidence that nutritional support, advice and provision are improved and coordinated as communication within and between professional groups is enhanced.

Recently there has also been a move towards clinical nurse specialists with a specific interest in nutrition. Their role is to provide advice for multidisciplinary team members and to liaise with dieticians to ensure specific regimens are met. It is important that nurses who develop a specialist role have sufficient education and training to ensure that nutritional advice is evidence-based and appropriate. In this way nutrition becomes part of the managed care for the patient (Fig. 11.6).

Nursing interventions begin at a very practical level. Many interventions are applicable to both the community and hospital settings.

FOOD CHOICE

The more varied the diet, the more likely it is that the recommendations for a balanced diet (HEA 1994) will be met. Nurses can assist individuals to choose appropriate food, whilst considering factors such as age and general health.

In hospital

Guidance and support in choosing from a menu may be needed. This should take into account dietary restrictions, evidence of deficiencies and personal preferences. Extra help may be needed to overcome communication problems and nurses must ensure that spectacles and functioning hearing aids are worn.

Ensuring that patients have sufficient calories to meet energy demand is important. Therefore, it may be better for patients to eat a less balanced diet, increasing energy content and decreasing the fruit and vegetable content, during an acute phase of their illness. Advice should be sought from the dietician if nurses are concerned.

In the community

In the community, advice is given on shopping, food storage and food preparation. The basic diet should reflect the advice given by the HEA (1994). Nurses can discuss with individuals the food purchased and how its nutritional value can be improved (see p. 221). Older adults or those who are housebound need to be advised about what foods can be stored for long periods, to be used when they are unable to shop. Nurses can advise older adults about ways to improve food intake (see Older Adults: Nursing Priorities box 11.1).

ENVIRONMENT

Nurses can ensure that mealtimes are pleasant. Simple activities that improve the environment and encourage eating include:

- removing commodes, bed pans, vomit bowels and sputum pots, etc.
- offering handwashing facilities
- ensuring that ward rounds, appointments or other interventions do not disrupt mealtimes; or if meals are missed that they are replaced

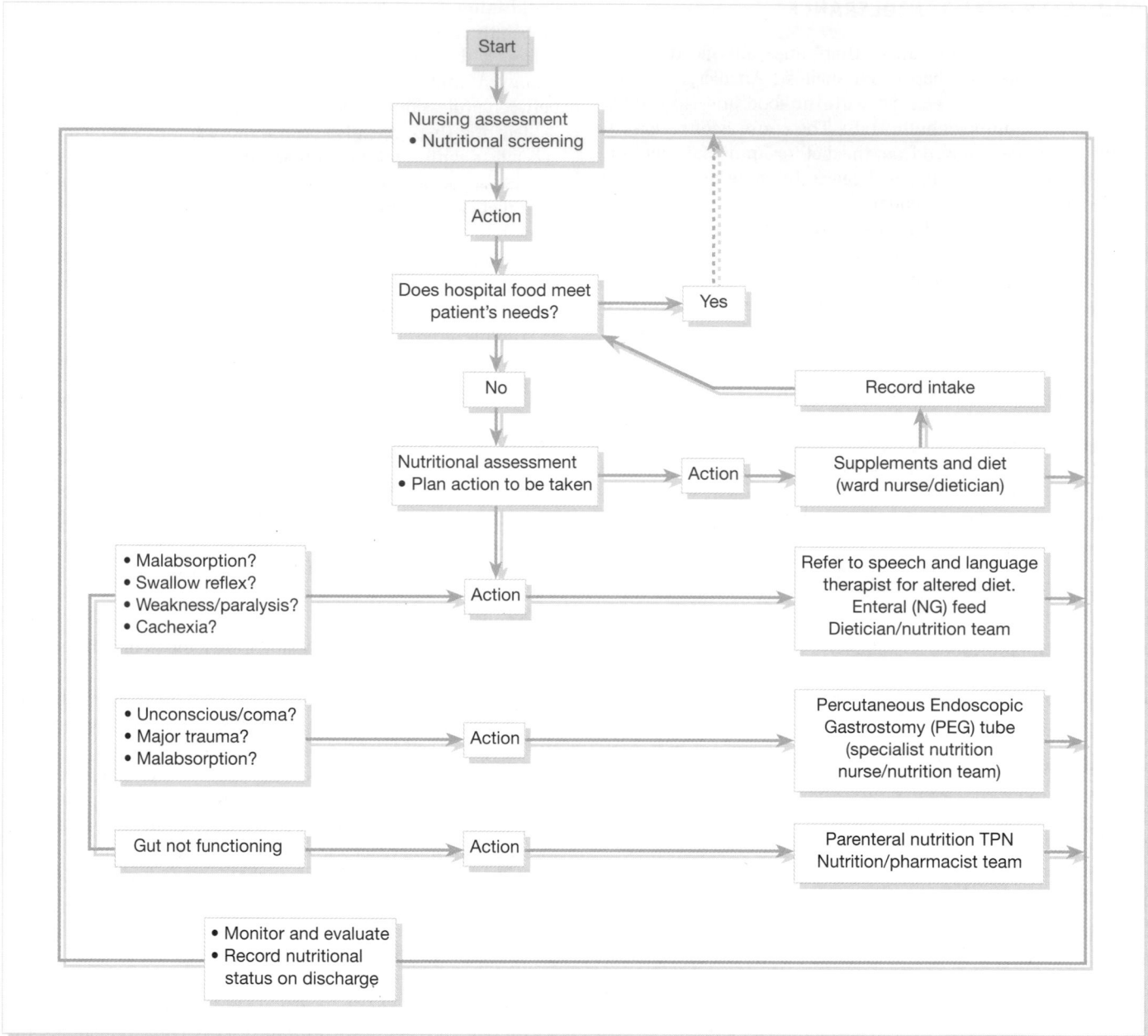

Figure 11.6   Managed nutrition flow chart.

65 83 / 50 71   OLDER ADULTS: NURSING PRIORITIES

11.1 Increasing food intake

- Identify what individuals normally eat and what they understand about what they should be eating
- Find out what they like to eat
- Identify what facilities they have for cooking/shopping/eating
- Identify any difficulties in eating, e.g. swallowing, dentures, posture, dexterity
- Encourage them to eat frequent meals or snacks between meals if appetite is small

- Encourage them to eat at least one hot meal a day
- Consider using full-fat and more energy-dense foods, but not refined food products
- Explore the possibility of eating out at day centres, church clubs, meal clubs, hotels or restaurants
- Discuss foods that could be stored for long periods for times when they cannot shop, e.g. packet soups, tinned fish, dried milk powder, pasta, frozen complete meals

- encouraging the use of a separate dining area, if available, to normalize mealtimes
- stressing the importance of having time to eat to patients at home
- using mealtimes to socialize by exploring the possibility of eating with friends, at day centres and meal clubs
- providing help during mealtimes.

EATING

As with your own meals, it is important to prepare for eating. Sitting upright to eat makes swallowing and using cutlery much easier. Nurses will need to devise individual adaptations where sitting upright is not an option, such as:

- using pillows to support the back and shoulders
- making sure both arms are free and that the hands can reach the mouth
- making sure that the table is the correct height
- ensuring that food can be reached and eaten without stretching.

Choosing the correct cutlery, plates and cups will also improve intake. If you are unsure then referral to the occupational therapist for assessment will help:

- Choose cutlery with thicker handles. Where special cutlery is unavailable, covering the handles with foam can help.
- Cups with two handles, plate guards, non-slip mats and beakers with straws can be useful, but care must be taken to maintain the person's dignity.
- Offering drinks at mealtimes can improve the intake of food and fluids.

Oral hygiene can also improve intake. It is important that teeth and dentures are cleaned regularly and are well maintained:

- Do not allow dentures to become dry and warped.
- Encourage the use of denture fixative.

- Refer to a dentist if you are concerned about the patient's mouth, teeth or dentures.

STAFFING

In care settings there must be sufficient staff available to support individuals at mealtimes; staffing levels may need to be reviewed or staff meal breaks reorganized. All staff who handle food must be aware of food hygiene regulations, and where food handling is part of daily nursing activities, a food handling certificate must be obtained. In the community, liaison with relatives, friends, social services and neighbours may enable someone to assist during mealtimes.

- Ensure food intake is monitored and recorded.
- Offer supplements to individuals who are not eating sufficient food (see section on nutritional supplements, p. 222)
- Assist with feeding where individuals are having difficulties with eating (see Guidelines for Care Priorities box 11.1)
- Ensure food is served at the correct temperature.

FOOD FORTIFICATION

Except in health promotion or specific disease states, nutritional advice may involve the fortification of food to modify its nutrient quality. General advice to individuals who are malnourished or those at risk of malnutrition should include:

- Eat small frequent meals.
- Have high energy protein snacks between meals, e.g. whole milk yoghurts, fortified cereals with whole milk, cheese and biscuits or toast and peanut butter.
- Use full-fat dairy products.
- Add milk powder to fortify ordinary milk, drinks, cereals and puddings.
- Add milk, cream, cheese or milk powder to bought soup.
- Add energy, e.g. sugar, honey, jam and dried fruit, to cereals and puddings.

 GUIDELINES FOR CARE PRIORITIES

11.1 Feeding patients

Feeding patients is a basic nursing intervention, but one that requires skill to do well. Prior to feeding a patient it is important that you are competent and that there is time set aside for the activity.

- Wash hands
- Ensure the food is what patients will like and that, where possible, they have been able to choose it
- Make sure the food is of the correct consistency and temperature
- Position patients so that the head, neck and trunk are supported in an upright position
- Make sure the teeth are clean and that dentures fit and are in place
- If the mouth is dry, offer sips of water prior to feeding

- Choose appropriate feeding utensils; be careful with forks as they can be uncomfortable
- Sit facing patients so that you can communicate with them
- If communication is difficult, establish a method by which patients can give you information such as 'that is enough' or 'a drink please'
- Describe the food prior to feeding
- Offer small amounts, allowing plenty of time for chewing and swallowing
- Offer drinks
- Allow time for feeding but do not offer food that has become cold and unpalatable
- Record all food and fluids consumed
- Evaluate and reassess whether nutritional intake can be maintained totally from feeding

NUTRITIONAL SUPPORT

NUTRITIONAL SUPPLEMENTS AND SIP FEEDING

The emphasis on improving nutritional status should always be on encouraging a normal diet. Nutritional supplements are used where food fortification or dietary modification has not improved intake sufficiently to meet nutritional needs. Nutritional products are numerous and many are available from chemists and supermarkets. They can, however, be expensive, and when recommending nutritional supplementation the cost must be considered.

A range of products are normally available in hospital and community via the dietetic service or pharmacy. Following assessment, supplements should be given in addition to food according to local protocols or regimens.

Modifying textures

Individuals with chewing problems or dysphagia may improve nutritional intake by changing the texture and consistency of food. Assessment of swallowing is done by a speech and language therapist (SLT). Where a SLT is unavailable, a specifically trained nurse can use a dysphagia flow chart (see Fig. 11.4, p. 213).

Changing the consistency of food alters the flavour and palatability. It is important to ensure that foods are well prepared and attractively presented. Where patients have dysphagia, the nurse should consider the following:

- Check oral condition, teeth and dentures.
- Offer drinks with meals.
- Ensure food is not too dry and crumbly.
- Mash, liquidize or purée food.
- Prepare each food separately to retain its colour.
- Thicken liquids.

Sip feeding

Sip feeding is a term used to describe nourishing drinks taken at regular intervals, instead of food, to meet nutritional needs. Dietetic assessment and advice are essential to ensure that an adequate diet is prescribed. Proprietary feeds are nutritionally complete and may have added vitamins and minerals. Many are formulated to take into account specific disease states such as renal failure.

Nursing interventions include the following:

- Monitor and record daily intake.
- Continue nutritional screening for evidence of change in condition, e.g. weight change, decreased lethargy.
- Store feeds safely according to manufacturers' guidelines and expiry dates.
- Provide psychological support to encourage maintenance of the dietary regimen.

ENTERAL FEEDING

Enteral feeding describes the feeding of an individual via a tube in the GI tract. Increasingly, enteral feeding is being used in situations where parenteral feeding previously would have been considered. The benefits of the enteral route include the following:

- It can be additional to oral intake, which maintains normality and is associated with fewer complications (Kudsk et al 1992).
- Mucosal integrity is maintained by encouraging normal gut function (Keithley & Eisenberg 1993). The incidence of bacterial translocation and sepsis is reduced (Raper & Maynard 1992).
- It is significantly safer and cheaper than parenteral nutrition.

The only absolute contraindication to enteral feeding is mechanical obstruction and the general criteria for enteral nutrition are that:

- the individual has some GI tract function
- the individual is able to take in sufficient nutrients by this route.

Before enteral feeding is commenced, a dietetic referral and nutritional assessment are essential. In emergencies, many care settings will have a protocol for an emergency feeding regimen that can be commenced in advance of an assessment being completed (see Special Issues box 11.1). The responsibility of the nurse is to ensure that referral and assessment are completed and a feed regimen prescribed. An additional requirement is that an adequate nutritional intake is maintained through administration of the prescribed feeding regimen. This is particularly important in situations where hypermetabolic states can occur.

Routes for enteral nutrition (Fig. 11.7)

The nasogastric route

This is readily accessible but is only suitable for short-term use. Complications such as local irritation, epistaxis and sinusitis make it unpopular with patients and reduces compliance. Feeding tubes generally of small bore should be used in preference to

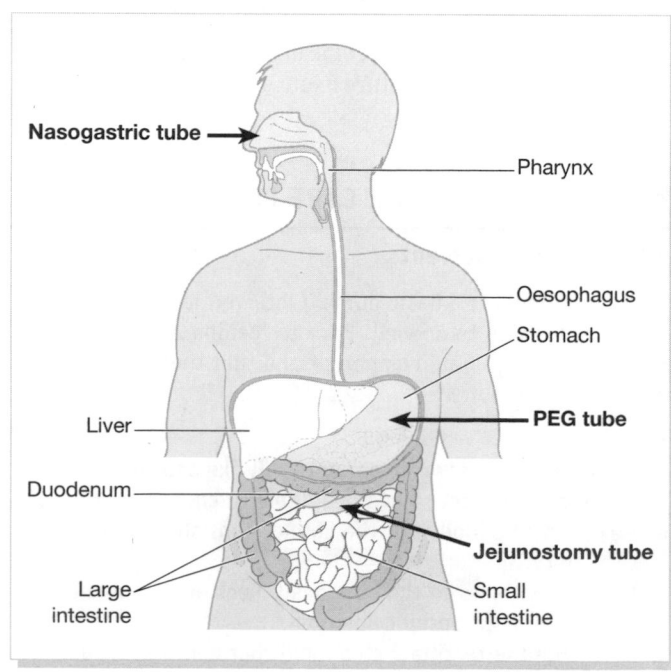

Figure 11.7 Routes for enteral feeding: nasogastric tube, PEG (percutaneous endoscopic gastrostomy) and jejunostomy tube.

SPECIAL ISSUES

11.1 Example of an emergency enteral feeding regimen for interim use when a dietician is unavailable

- This feeding regimen must be approved and clearly documented by medical staff before being commenced
- This feed may not be suitable, e.g. for liver or renal failure
- The feed is not nutritionally complete and should only be used for 1–2 days, until the patient is seen by a dietician for an individualized feeding regimen

- Phosphate and serum urea and electrolytes are checked so that the most appropriate feeding regimen can be advised
- The tube should be flushed with 25 mL water before and after feeding and any medication
- Additional fluid will be needed i.v. or in flushes to ensure adequate hydration
- Medication must be checked as some should not be given within 2 hours of feeding

Feeding regimen	Pump flow rate	Total feed	Nutritional value of regimen				
			Energy (kcal)	Protein (g)	CHO (g)	Sodium (mmol)	Potassium (mmol)
Osmolite	50 mL/hour	1000 mL over 20 hours, 4-hour rest period	1000	40	136	39.1	37.9

traditional nasogastric tubes used to aspirate gastric contents. Small diameter tubes are better tolerated than larger nasogastric tubes. Before insertion of a feeding tube, it is essential that a full explanation is given and informed consent obtained. The inserted tube will sit in the fundus of the stomach and the correct position is checked radiographically. Bedside checking of the position of the tube by testing for the gastric enzyme trypsin may be possible in the future (Colagiovanni 1999).

Nasoduodenal or nasojejunal tubes

These are inserted under endoscopic or fluoroscopic guidance. For their correct positioning, gastric motility may be required to help pass the tube into the small intestine. The preferred position of the tube is the third portion of the duodenum. Medication can assist in the positioning of smaller tubes beyond the pylorus by increasing peristalsis.

Percutaneous endoscopic gastrostomy (PEG)

This route is used for long-term feeding. The tube is inserted into the stomach through the abdominal wall. Less obvious than routes via the nasal passages, this is often the method of choice for home feeding. The tubes are inserted endoscopically and are held in place with a balloon or flange.

Jejunostomy

This is similar to a PEG but the tube is inserted into the jejunum. It can be used after major upper GI surgery where the stomach and duodenum have been removed or bypassed. Feeding via a jejunostomy can achieve a better nitrogen balance with nutrient absorption than parenteral nutrition. Jejunostomy feeding is contraindicated in Crohn's disease, malabsorption syndromes and radiation enteritis where nutrient absorption can be reduced.

Enteral feed regimens

Prior to commencement of enteral feeding the nurse needs to ensure clean procedures and that manufacturers' guidelines are followed. The feeds need to be stored correctly, used before their expiry date and administered at the correct temperature. Enteral feeding can be delivered by bolus, gravity or pump-controlled methods.

Bolus delivery

Bolus delivery via a syringe through the feeding tube can be a reliable delivery method if the prescribed volume of feed is given. A bolus feed of 200–400 mL may be needed at any one time to meet nutritional requirements. Inserting this volume of feed into the GI tract can cause discomfort. Large volumes are absorbed more slowly in the small intestine, increasing the likelihood of a high residual volume (feed remaining in the stomach at the commencement of the subsequent feed).

Gravity feeding

Gravity feeding is delivered by an intermittent or continuous drip method. In this system the route of delivery is not precise. Without careful monitoring of input, the amount delivered can be insufficient to meet needs. There may be serious complications, such as gastro-oesophageal reflux and aspiration of stomach contents into the lungs.

Closed enteral feeding systems

These systems allow the delivery of a specified amount via a giving set with a drip chamber. The method is similar to gravity feeding with the same complications.

Pump feeding

Pump feeding allows controlled feeding on either an intermittent or a continuous regimen. It is the preferred method of delivering enteral feeds, as it is easier to regulate the volume given. Most feeding regimens allow for continuous feeding for 20 hours with 4 hours' rest at night. This method is associated with fewer episodes of aspiration and diarrhoea than intermittent feeding. Continuous feeding is essential through a jejunostomy tube because bolus infusion into the jejunum can lead to abdominal distension, cramps, hyperperistalsis and diarrhoea.

Giving an enteral feed

1. Wash hands and prepare feed following the manufacturer's guidelines.
2. Check feeding tube position according to local protocols and that the patient is comfortable.
3. If a nasogastric tube is used, aspirate remnants of previous feed and record the residual volume.
4. Return aspirate to the stomach (not doing so reduces total feed volume and nutrient intake). Where residual volume is greater than 100 mL, the rate of the next feed should be slowed down. Do not stop the feed because of one high residual volume.
5. Clean tube by flushing with drinking water.
6. Commence feed according to regimen and method of delivery. Many care settings will have a 'starter regimen' which involves gradually increasing the strength of the feed to ensure it is tolerated.
7. At the end of the feed, flush the tube with clean water.
8. Flush tube before and after administration of medications.
9. Check that medications are suitable for tube administration and will not interact with the feed.
10. Record volume of feed given.

Complications of enteral nutrition

The complications associated with enteral feeding can be unpleasant for the patient. The nurse not only needs to be able to recognize their occurrence but also to act accordingly to ensure that nutritional status is not compromised by a delay in feeding. The most common complications are outlined in Table 11.4.

PARENTERAL NUTRITION

Parenteral nutrition is the administration of nutrients outside the GI tract and should only be used where the enteral route is unsuitable. Intravenous feeding can be supplemental nutrition or total parenteral nutrition (TPN). The most common route is centrally, through the subclavian vein into the superior vena cava. Alternatively, peripherally inserted central catheters (PICCs)

Table 11.4 Common complications of enteral feeding (Pennington 1991, Payne-James 1995)

Complication	Possible causes	Action
Diarrhoea	Rapid infusion rate Hyperosmolar feed	Slow infusion rate Slowly introduce feed Refer to dietician Increase fibre content of feed
	Formula bacterial contamination	Review hygiene standards at commencement of feed Change giving set every 24 hours Do not allow feed to hang for more than 12 hours Treat feed system as a closed system
Nausea and vomiting	Drug interactions Anxiety Large gastric residuals	Review prescription Give information and allow time for discussion Check gastric residuals every 4–6 hours Delay feed by 2 hours if residual is greater than 100 mL Use continuous rather than bolus feeding
	Patient position	Elevate the head of the bed 30–45° throughout the feeding period Before placing patient in recumbent position, stop feed and aspirate gastric residual
	Cold feeding	Ensure feed is at room temperature
Constipation	Dehydration Low residue formula	Ensure free fluids are given Maintain fluid input/output chart Refer to dietician
Dehydration	Fever or infection Inadequate fluid intake Excessive fluid loss	Increase fluid input Monitor intake and output Refer to physician
Tube obstruction	Tube kinked. Coagulation of formula, obstruction by medication, precipitation of incompatible drugs	Check positioning of tube. Flush feeding tube with water before and after giving medication or enteral feed. Flush tube after gastric residual has been aspirated as acid contents of stomach will cause the formula to coagulate. Use elixir forms of medication instead of crushing tablets
Nasal irritation	Improper taping of tube	Check tape, ensure that tube is not pressing against nasal passage Change tape as required Check nasal passage each day

are sited through the basilic vein (in the arm) to the superior vena cava via the right subclavian vein.

Intravenous catheters are inserted using aseptic procedures. PICC lines can be inserted by appropriately trained nurses. Central lines via the subclavian vein are normally inserted by a physician. The position of the catheter is confirmed radiographically.

Large veins are required for administrating feeds containing amino acids, glucose, fat emulsions, minerals and vitamins. Infusing concentrated solutions into smaller veins can lead to inflammation of the endothelial lining. Large veins ensure that feeds are rapidly transported and diluted by blood flow into the circulation. Parenteral nutrition is prescribed by a dietician to ensure dietary needs are met either by proprietary feeds or by those prepared in the pharmacy department.

Managing parenteral nutrition

The nurse's role in managing parenteral nutrition is to maintain the feed infusion and monitor for signs of complications. Monitoring consists of observing the i.v. site for inflammation (daily and before commencing a feed), blood pressure, fluid balance and serum urea, electrolytes and glucose. Other important aspects of care include:

- maintaining aseptic technique during i.v. site handling and feed preparation
- checking that feeds are in date and stored at correct temperature
- protecting infusion from sunlight to prevent vitamin degradation
- changing the administration set according to local protocols
- flushing the line before and after feeding according to local protocols
- care of the i.v. site dressings and keeping the site dry – see Nicol et al (2000) for a detailed description
- making sure that medication or other additives are not added to the feed. This reduces the risk of infection and incompatibility (see p. 226); separate i.v. lines should be used for their administration. Where a multi-port line is in use,

ensure that the feed has a dedicated route that is not used for drug administration or taking blood.

Complications of parenteral nutrition

Complications must be reported immediately to ensure that appropriate action is taken. The most common complications are outlined in Table 11.5.

DRUG–NUTRIENT INTERACTIONS

When food and drugs are mixed together they may interact to prevent the utilization of important nutrients or alter the action of some drugs (Table 11.6). People taking more than one type of medication (prescribed and over-the-counter), such as older adults, are at increased risk of drug–nutrient interactions.

- Some drugs will interfere with the uptake of nutrients, e.g. antacids containing magnesium and aluminium hydroxide may lower vitamin A. Mineral oil, sometimes used as a laxative, prevents the absorption of fat-soluble vitamins (A, D, E and K).
- Some foods may reduce drug absorption, such as dairy products and tetracycline.
- Some nutrients may increase drug absorption. Foods rich in vitamin C enhance the absorption of iron.
- Drugs can also decrease the appetite and intake by causing nausea, vomiting and alterations to taste.
- In contrast, other drugs increase the appetite. Insulin, corticosteroids and certain antihistamines can all improve appetite.
- Alcohol (although not strictly a nutrient) should be avoided when taking any type of medication. It increases drowsiness with antihistamines or sleeping pills. Alcohol may cause flushing, headaches, nausea, vomiting and chest pain in conjunction with oral hypoglycaemics and some antibiotics. Alcohol may dissolve the coating on time-release pills, causing sudden release and a potentially toxic dose.

Table 11.5 Complications of parenteral feeding		
Complication	Cause	Action
Infection at the intravenous site	Poor aseptic technique and management	Maintain aseptic technique at all times Ensure i.v. site is protected Observe daily for signs of infection (redness, swelling and pain) Document and report occurrence
Thrombophlebitis	Irritation by parenteral feed More common if peripheral veins are used, but can occur at central vein sites as well	Follow local protocol Report and document
Parenteral refeeding syndrome	Rapid uptake of potassium, magnesium and other electrolytes as energy source switches from endogenous lipids (stored body fat) to exogenous carbohydrate (from feed)	Daily monitoring of serum electrolytes and minerals Observe for signs of potassium depletion (apathy, muscle weakness) Report and document
Hyperglycaemia	Insulin resistance can occur due to the hypermetabolic state of the patient	Daily monitoring of serum glucose Report if glucose is >6 mmol/L (or according to local protocol) Give prescribed insulin
Psychological distress	Absence of normal eating behaviour	Give information and listen to the patient Support patient and relatives as appropriate

Table 11.6 Nutrient recommendations and patient teaching for some common drugs

Drug name	Vitamin and mineral recommendations	Patient-teaching points
Tetracycline	Riboflavin (B_2), vitamin C	Take on an empty stomach 1 hour before or 2–3 hours after meals Avoid milk or other dairy products and supplements within 1 hour before or within 2 hours after drug dose Avoid iron products and zinc Eat citrus fruits, baked potatoes, broccoli, and wholegrain breads and cereals
Warfarin	Consistent vitamin K intake Avoid excessive vitamin K intake	Eat consistent amounts of foods containing vitamin K, such as spinach, liver and cabbage Excess vitamin K may reduce anticoagulant effects
Hydralazine	Vitamin B_6	Avoid natural liquorice and monosodium glutamate (MSG) Take with food to increase bioavailability Eat wholegrain breads and cereals, leafy vegetables and meats
Aspirin	Vitamins B_{12} and C, folic acid, iron	Take with a large glass of water or milk Eat wholegrain breads and cereals, citrus fruits, baked potatoes, broccoli, organ meats and green leafy vegetables Drink juice
Cholestyramine, colestipol	Folic acid, vitamins A, D, K	Take with food or milk and a full glass of water Eat a high-fibre diet Eat green leafy and deep yellow vegetables, citrus fruits and broccoli Drink low-fat milk
Chlorpromazine, thioridazine and other phenothiazines	Riboflavin	Avoid alcohol and caffeine-containing foods and beverages, such as coffee, tea, soft drinks and chocolate Eat wholegrain breads and cereals, organ meats, leafy vegetables and citrus fruits Drink milk
Phenytoin	Folic acid, vitamins D, K	Take with food or milk Eat citrus fruits and broccoli Drink milk
Primidone	Vitamin K	Take on an empty stomach 1 hour before or 2–3 hours after meals Eat green leafy vegetables
Isoniazid	Vitamins B_6, D, niacin	Take with food if gastrointestinal irritation occurs Avoid fish, cheese, alcohol and chocolate Eat wholegrain breads and cereals, organ meats, leafy vegetables and citrus fruits Drink milk
Rifampicin	Vitamins B_6, D, niacin	Take on an empty stomach 1 hour before or 2–3 hours after meals Take with food if gastrointestinal irritation occurs Avoid alcohol Eat wholegrain breads and cereals, organ meats, leafy vegetables and citrus fruits Drink milk
Griseofulvin		Avoid vitamin A supplements Eat a variety of foods Take with food or milk
Isotretinoin		Take drug without regard to meals
Hydrochlorothiazide, furosemide	Folic acid, potassium, zinc, magnesium	Take with food or milk Eat bananas, nuts and baked potatoes Drink orange juice and milk
Antacids	Folic acid, thiamin (B_1), calcium, phosphate	Eat wholegrain breads and cereals, leafy vegetables, citrus fruits and dairy products Drink milk

(continued)

Table 11.6 *(continued)*

Drug name	Vitamin and mineral recommendations	Patient-teaching points
Cimetidine	Thiamin	Eat wholegrain breads and cereals, leafy vegetables, citrus fruits and dairy products Drink milk
Indomethacin	Iron, vitamin B$_{12}$	Take with food or milk Eat deep yellow vegetables and organ meats
Oestrogen and progesterone (oral contraceptive)	Folic acid, vitamin B$_6$	Eat wholegrain breads and cereals, organ meats, leafy vegetables and citrus fruits Drink milk Avoid high doses of vitamin C (1 g or more)
Prednisone	Folic acid, thiamin, vitamin D, calcium	Take with food or milk Eat a low-sodium diet Eat wholegrain breads and cereals, leafy vegetables, citrus fruits and dairy products Drink milk Potassium supplements may be prescribed
Mineral oil	Vitamins A, D, K	Take on an empty stomach 1 hour before or 2–3 hours after meals Eat green leafy and deep yellow vegetables and dairy products Drink milk

SUMMARY: MAIN POINTS

- Nutrition is one of the most important aspects of daily living.

- Poor nutritional care during illness by nurses and other health care professionals is of great concern. It is important that nurses redress the balance and consider the nutritional needs of individuals both in health and during illness.

- In the UK there are many people who suffer from nutrient deficiency and nutrient excess. The challenge for health promotion is to improve dietary intake in an increasingly diverse, multicultural and dynamic society.

- Poor nutrition causes disease and nutrients may function by modifying individual responses to disease.

- It may be that, as knowledge of individual nutrients increases, nutrition will become an integral part of therapeutic regimens.

SELF-TEST: CRITICAL THINKING ACTIVITIES

1 Complete a nursing assessment or nutritional screening of a patient/client, focusing on nutritional status and nutritional need.

2 Complete a plan of care to ensure that nutritional needs are met.

3 Critically evaluate your plan. Consider issues such as staffing levels, skill mix, organizational and resource constraints, and ethical and legal dilemmas.

 FURTHER READING

Barker H. Nutrition/dietetics for healthcare, 10th edn. Edinburgh: Churchill Livingstone; 2002

British Association for Parenteral and Enteral Nutrition. Organisation of nutritional support in hospitals. Silk, D (Chairman). Report of the BAPEN. London: BAPEN; 1994.

Dudek, SG. Nutrition handbook for nursing practice, 3rd edn. New York: Lippincott; 1997.

Edington, J. Problems of nutritional assessment in the community. Proc Nutr Soc 1999; 58(1): 47–51.

Fox BA, Cameron AG. Food science nutrition and health. London: Arnold; 1995.

Morgan SL, Weinsier RL. Fundamentals of clinical nutrition, 2nd edn. London: Mosby; 1998.

Nicol M, Bavin C, Bedford-Turner S, Cronin P, Rawlings-Anderson K. Essential nursing skills. London: Mosby; 2000.

USEFUL WEBSITES

www.nutrition.org.uk.
www.springnet.com.

www.bsg.org.uk/clinical/data/gans.htm.

REFERENCES

American Society of Anesthesiologists. Practice guidelines for preoperative fasting and the use of pharmacologic agents for prevention of pulmonary aspiration: application to healthy adults undergoing elective procedures. Park Ridge, IL: American Society of Anesthesiologists; 1997.

Bender D. Introduction to nutrition and metabolism, 2nd edn. London: Taylor and Francis; 1999.

Bray G. Obesity. In: Ziegler E, Filer L, eds. Present knowledge in nutrition, 7th edn. Cardiff: Cardiff Academic Press; 1996: 19–32.

Butcher M et al. Current selenium content of foods and an estimation of average intake in the United Kingdom. Proc Nutr Soc 1995; 54: 131A.

Chandra RK. Food hypersensitivity and allergic disease. A selective review. Am J Clin Med 1997; 66: 526–529S.

Colagiovanni L. Taking the tube. Nurs Times 1999; 95(21): 63–70.

Department of Health. Dietary reference values for food, energy and nutrients in the UK. Report of the panel on Dietary Reference values of the Committee on Medical Aspects of Food Policy. Report on Health and Social Subjects 41. London: HMSO; 1991.

Department of Health (DoH). Saving lives – our healthier nation. London: The Stationery Office; 1999.

Drenick E, Fisler J. Myocardial mass in morbid obese patients and changes with weight reduction. Obes Surg 1992; 2: 19–27.

Edington J, Kon P, Martyn C. Prevalence of malnutrition in patients in general practice. Clin Nutr 1996; 15: 60–63.

Edington J, Kon P, Martyn C. Prevalence of malnutrition after major surgery. J Hum Nutr Diet 1997; 10: 111–116.

Gregory JR, Collins DL, Davies PS et al. National diet and nutrition survey of children aged $1\frac{1}{2}$–$4\frac{1}{2}$ years. London: HMSO; 1995.

Health Education Authority. The balance of good health. London: HEA; 1994.

Howarth C, Kenway P, Palmer G. Monitoring poverty and social exclusion. York: Joseph Rowntree Foundation; 1999.

Keithley J, Eisenberg P. The significance of enteral nutrition in the intensive care unit patient. Crit Care Clin North Am 1993; 5: 23–29.

King JC. Does poor zinc nutrition retard skeletal growth and mineralization in adolescents? Am J Clin Nutr 1996; 64, 375–376.

Kinsella K. Demographic aspects in epidemiology in old age. In: Ebrahim S, Kanlache A, eds. Epidemiology in old age. BMJ in collaboration with WHO; 1996.

Kudsk KA, Croce MA, Fabian TC et al. Enteral versus parenteral feeding. Effects on septic morbidity after blunt and penetrating trauma. Ann Surg 1992; 215: 503–513.

Larsson B, Svardsudd K, Welin L et al. Abdominal adipose tissue distribution, obesity and risk of cardiovascular disaese and death: 13 year follow up of men born in 1913. Br Med J 1984; 288: 1401–1404.

Lennard-Jones J (ed). Positive approach to nutrition as treatment: a report of a working party. London: Kings Fund Centre; 1992.

Long S, O'Brien K, Macdonald K et al. Weight loss in severely obese subjects prevents the progression of impaired glucose tolerance to type II diabetes. Diabetes Care 1994; 17: 372–375.

MAFF. The dietary and nutritional survey of British adults – further analysis. London: HMSO; 1994.

MAFF. Manual of nutrition, 10th edn. London: The Stationery Office; 1995.

McClaren S, Green S. Nutritional screening and assessing. Nurs Stand 1998; 12(48): 26–29.

McWhirter J, Pennington CR. Incidence and recognition of malnutrition in hospital. Br Med J 1994; 308: 945–948.

National Heart Forum (Sharp I, ed). At least five a day – strategies to increase vegetables and fruit consumption. London: The Stationery Office; 1997.

Nicol M, Bavin C, Bedford-Turner S, Cronin P, Rawlings-Anderson S. Essential nursing skills. London: Mosby; 2000.

Payne-James J. Peripheral administration of total parenteral nutrition in artificial nutrition support. In: Payne-James J, Grimble G, Silk D (eds). Artificial nutrition support in clinical practice. London: Arnold; 1995.

Pennington CR. Parenteral nutrition: the management of complications. Clin Nutr 1991; 10: 133–137.

Raper S, Maynard N. Feeding the critically ill patient. Br J Nurs 1992; 1(6): 273–280.

Sizer T. Standards and guidelines for nutritional support of patients in hospitals. A report by a working party of the British association for parenteral and enteral nutrition. Maidenhead: BAPEN; 1996.

Sjostram LV. Morbidity of severely obese subjects. Am J Clin Nutr 1992; 55, 508–515S.

Stephens NG, Parsons A, Schofield PM et al. Randomised controlled trial of vitamin E in patients with coronary disease: Cambridge Heart Antioxidant Study (CHAOS). Lancet 1996; 347: 781–786.

Townsend P, Davidson P, Whitehead M. Inequalities in health: the Black report and the health divide. Harmondsworth: Penguin; 1988.

Troisi R, Willett WC, Weiss ST. Trans-fatty acid intake in relation to serum lipid concentrations in adult men. Am J Clin Nutr 1992; 56: 1019–1024.

Ueland P, Refsum H. Plasma homocysteine, a risk factor for vascular disease: plasma levels in health, disease and drug therapy. J Lab Clin Med 1991; 114(5): 475–501.

12 Maintaining continence

Mandy Wells

> 'I was always so particular about keeping clean – now every time I cough or laugh I leak a bit and I'm convinced that I smell. The Practice Nurse was good. She suggested panty liners because they don't show, and gave me some exercises to do to strengthen the muscles down there. I am seeing the specialist nurse next month but I think it's a bit better already.'
>
> (Patient)

THIS CHAPTER WILL HELP YOU

- Describe the prevalence of urinary incontinence and the impact this has on the individual

- Understand how the bladder and the bowel work to maintain continence

- Apply concepts of assessment to practice

- Identify the symptoms of the different types of incontinence

- Explain the treatment of incontinence symptoms

- Discuss the role of the nurse in continence care delivery

- Describe the range of products that can be used in the management of incontinence.

KEYWORDS

Detrusor muscle	Mixed incontinence
Catheterization	Urinary incontinence
Continence	Overactive bladder
Faecal incontinence	Stress incontinence
Intermittent catheterization	Pelvic floor
	Pelvic floor exercises
Micturition	

INTRODUCTION

Incontinence, both urinary and faecal, is a problem that affects all age groups. It is commonly under-reported by patients and goes unrecognized by nurses, especially those working in acute care settings. Continence problems also tend to be viewed negatively by the nursing professions and its care can be seen as a chore. However, both urinary and faecal incontinence can be treated successfully if the correct strategies are used. Since incontinence can have a major impact on patients' well-being, the role of the nurse in correctly assessing need and being proactive in developing strategies for care is becoming increasingly important. Maintaining continence is an area of care that has recently been highlighted by several Department of Health guidelines (Department of Health 2001). This chapter provides an overview of urinary and faecal incontinence issues and describes everyday treatment and management that will lead to improved outcomes for the patient.

Most nurses can provide the strategies outlined. However, the role of the nurse specialist is also paramount. Continence nurse specialists can provide advice and support to ward-based and community nurses. They can also provide training in all aspects of bladder and bowel care, to enhance the knowledge of general nurses in order to provide more effective care.

Definition of urinary incontinence

Urinary incontinence is defined by the International Continence Society as 'a condition where involuntary loss of urine is a social or hygienic problem and is objectively demonstrable'. Other definitions have been suggested which incorporate other aspects of the problem, such as time periods, e.g. 'any uncontrolled urine loss in the previous 12 months, without regard to severity' (Abrams et al 1988).

ANATOMY AND PHYSIOLOGY OF THE LOWER URINARY TRACT

The lower urinary tract consists of the ureters, the bladder, the urethra and the pelvic floor muscles (see Fig. 12.1). Urine enters

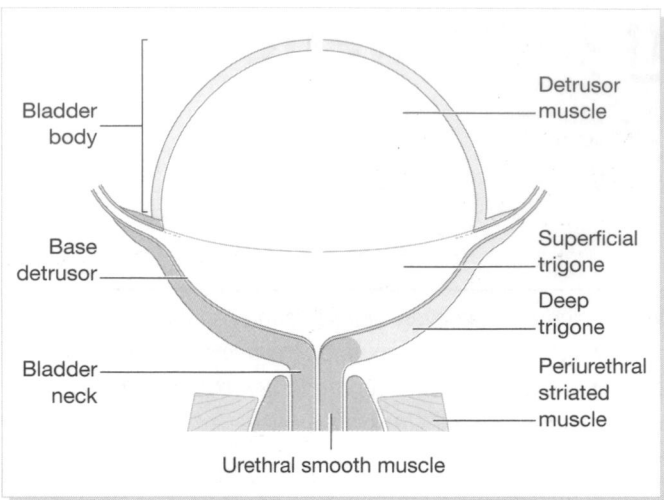

Figure 12.1 Lower urinary tract.

the bladder from the kidneys at a rate of 0.5 ml–5ml per minute (average 1 ml per minute), via the ureters, which are hollow muscular tubes approximately 25 cm long and 0.5 cm in diameter. The ureters enter the bladder near its base in a small triangular area known as the trigone. The oblique angle at which the ureters enter the bladder effectively acts as a valve, which prevents reflux of urine back to the kidneys.

THE BLADDER

The bladder is a hollow vessel that can be divided into two areas: the base, which includes the trigone and bladder neck; and the bladder body, or dome. The trigone is an area of specialized smooth muscle and is located in the bladder base and the vesical neck, extending into the urethra. The trigone undergoes little change in size; it is very sensitive to stretch, owing to the large number of sensory nerve endings it contains.

The bladder wall is made up of four layers:

- The innermost layer (mucosa) is extensively folded into rugae when it is not full and consists of mucus-secreting transitional cell epithelium, which aids stretching. These two features allow considerable distension to take place during filling.
- The second layer (submucosa) is formed of connective tissue, which links the mucosa to the third layer.
- The third layer is made up of muscle fibres that are collectively known as the detrusor muscle, which includes both longitudinal and circular fibres that form an interlacing meshwork. The outer layer of detrusor muscle is predominately longitudinal muscle fibres, which on the anterior surface continue past the bladder neck into the pubovesical muscles and into the tissues of the pelvic wall near the symphysis pubis. Contraction of the detrusor muscle causes the bladder to reduce in length and diameter so that it empties effectively.
- The fourth and outermost layer, the serosa, is composed of peritoneum and covers only the upper surface of the bladder.

The bladder has a dual function: for the majority of the time it acts as a highly compliant storage vessel for urine from the kidneys, but periodically the bladder acts as a contractile organ, expelling its contents via the urethra. The bladder is unique in that it is the only organ comprising smooth muscle that is under voluntary control. Effective emptying of the bladder requires the coordinated activity of the urethral sphincter and the detrusor muscle and relaxation of the urethral sphincter preceding detrusor contraction (see below). As the bladder reaches functional capacity, sensory impulses initiate the urge to void. This can be voluntarily suppressed so that bladder emptying can occur at a convenient time and place.

URETHRA

At the base of the bladder is the bladder neck, which leads into the urethra, and its function is to convey urine from the bladder to the external urethral meatus. It is approximately 3–5 cm long in women and 23 cm in men. The muscle structure of the urethra comprises an inner longitudinal smooth muscle layer and an outer circular striated muscle layer. This forms the external sphincter and is under voluntary control (Flynn 1999).

In females, the urethra lies embedded in the lower third of the anterior vaginal wall, and so the support of the lower third of the vagina and the urethra are identical. The bladder neck is supported by ligaments arising from the pelvic bone and fascia (Flynn 1999). Contraction of the levator ani, the deep muscle of the pelvic floor, supports the proximal urethra and pulls the bladder neck anteriorly, compressing it closed. Relaxation of the levator ani allows the bladder neck to descend and open during micturition.

PELVIC FLOOR

The pelvic floor is a complex structure that can be divided into three areas: the endopelvic fascia, the levator ani muscles and the superficial perineal muscles. The perineal membrane attaches the lateral walls of the vagina and the perineal body to the ischiopubic rami (Flynn 1999). The endopelvic fascia has an important role as it gives attachment to and also envelopes the pelvic floor muscles and the pelvic organs. The vagina and urethra pass through the fascia and pelvic floor musculature (see Fig. 12.2).

The fascia is composed of smooth muscle, elastin, collagen and blood vessels (Flynn 1999). The deep layers of muscle are known collectively as the levator ani and consist of three muscles: the puborectalis, pubococcygeus and iliococcygeus. The levator ani lie superior to the superficial muscles and are of great importance in the maintenance of continence. The pubococcygeus muscle arises anteriorly on either side of the symphysis pubis and passes posteriorly on either side of the urethra, vagina and anus and attaches to the coccyx. There are some loops of muscle fibres that pass posteriorly behind the urethra; some loop behind the vagina and some behind the anus, and their muscle fibres are called the pubovaginalis and the puborectalis. The iliococcygeus arises from the arcus tendineus and is suspended between the pubic bone and the ischial spine. These muscles form a type of hammock and it is through this that the urethra, vagina and anal canal pass; it is important for its supportive function.

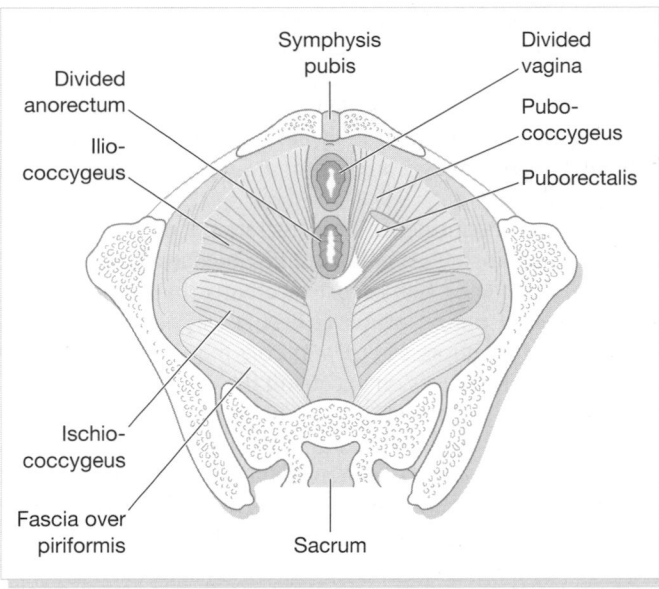

Figure 12.2 Pelvic floor muscles.

Urinary continence can be compromised if the bladder neck is not supported in its correct anatomical position. If weakness occurs in the surrounding supporting structures, allowing the bladder neck to descend when increased intra-abdominal pressures are exerted (e.g. coughing or sneezing), the bladder will empty because there is no corresponding pressure on the bladder neck to keep it closed.

The levator ani

This muscle provides contractile support and forms a sheet originating from the back of the body of the pubis, continuing around the lateral walls of the pelvis as far posteriorly as the ischial spines. Fibres from this muscle attach to the perineal body in males to form the levator prostatae, and in females the medial fibres attach to the lateral vaginal wall to form the pubovaginalis. This muscular sheet plays an important role in supporting the position of the pelvic organs, and contraction of the muscle compresses the urethra, assisting the urethral sphincter in maintaining continence during increases in abdominal pressure. The levator ani receives its nerve supply from sacral roots S2–4, with the majority of fibres originating from S3. These nerve fibres travel in the pudendal nerve, which carries both motor and sensory nerves from the sacral plexus.

NEUROLOGICAL CONTROL OF THE LOWER URINARY TRACT AND PELVIC FLOOR

The exact mechanism of continence remains unclear but it is known that complex neuromuscular coordination is required to regulate between urine storage and elimination. The autonomic nervous system (parasympathetic and sympathetic) is involved in the control of micturition (passing urine). The parasympathetic outflow arises from the spinal cord as the pelvic nerve between S2 and S4 and is known as the spinal micturition

centre. This area receives information of bladder activity from the sensory nerves and relays outgoing motor nerve impulses to the relevant areas. The spinal micturition centre also links via nerve fibres to the micturition centres in the pons and cerebral cortex of the brain, relaying information to higher centres and allowing voluntary inhibition of the micturition reflex.

The somatic nervous system is essential for the maintenance of continence. The pudendal nerve arises from S2–S4 and is the somatic nerve supply to the pelvic floor muscles. The pudendal nerve also joins the pelvic nerve to supply the external urethral sphincter (Flynn 1999). It is because the bladder is so closely linked to the brain and spinal cord that any neurological and spinal disease or injury can lead to bladder symptoms.

THE MICTURITION CYCLE

At birth, both the bladder and bowel are completely controlled by reflexes, some of which are learned to be controlled during 'potty training'. Reflexes play an important role in the normal control of the micturition cycle.

The normal micturition cycle includes a filling and storage phase and a contraction and emptying phase (Doherty 1997). During the filling and storage phase, the control is subconscious; tension receptors within the bladder wall transmit information via the afferent fibres to the spinal cord at the S2–S4 level. To maintain the compliance of the bladder, the rugae flatten and the bladder volume increases with very little change in the internal pressure. Efferent impulses are transmitted to the bladder, which make it relax, and impulses are also sent to the urethral sphincter and the pelvic floor muscles to increase tone (Getliffe & Dolman 1997, Flynn 1999). Total bladder capacity varies, but on average is between 400 and 600 mL, and as the bladder fills it first becomes spherical and then 'pear-shaped' as it rises up out of the pelvic cavity (Getliffe & Dolman 1997). The first sensation of the desire to void usually occurs at approximately 200–300 mL, or 50% of bladder capacity, and if bladder function is normal, an individual should be able to resist the desire to void until it is convenient to do so. This urge represents the micturition threshold (Doherty 1997).

URINARY INCONTINENCE

Urinary incontinence refers to the involuntary loss of urine. It is not uncommon in adults, particularly women, and the incidence increases with age (Milsom et al 2001, Stewart et al 2001). This does not mean that it is just a problem of old age; a study by Wolin (1969) found that, in a sample group of young nurses who had never had a baby, 51% reported involuntary loss of urine at sometime in their life.

Milsom et al (2001), using a definition of overactive bladder symptoms (frequency, urgency and nocturia, with or without urge incontinence), estimated the prevalence in the UK as being 5.15 million. Another study (Stewart et al 2001) estimated an overall prevalence of overactive bladder symptoms as being 16.9% in women and 16.0% in men, the incidence increasing with age. One study found a mean prevalence of 24.5% in elderly women and 55.7% in those in care settings (Thuroff et al 1998).

12.1 Nursing skills to reduce embarrassment

Imagine that you have urinary incontinence and have finally got up courage to go and see the practice nurse for advice.

- What can the nurse do to make you feel less embarrassed?
- What information would be helpful at this stage and what format is likely to be most effective (e.g. verbal, written leaflets, websites, etc.)?

There is also an increase in prevalence for people who have cancer, diabetes, congestive heart failure and neurological disorders, those who have had a stroke and men with an enlarged prostate. Not only is incontinence caused by other underlying conditions but it can be associated with considerable other problems. For instance, there is a significant increase in the risk of falling and fracturing limbs. Incontinence in the younger female population, associated with childbirth, has been well documented, showing that between 1 in 3 and 1 in 5 women report problems following childbirth. Bladder problems become more common as maternal age increases and there is also a significant increase in women following a forceps delivery compared with those having a normal delivery.

Many people only report their symptoms to a health professional when they find them particularly worrying or can no longer cope. This seems particularly true for the older age group. Norton et al (1988) found that the proportion of women aged 65 and over who delayed more than 5 years before discussing urinary problems with a health professional was twice that of women aged under 35 years. The reluctance to consult on these problems may stem from beliefs of inevitability and that nothing can be done, as well as the embarrassing nature of the problem. Elderly women in particular are thought to delay consulting professionals for fear of surgery. Many elderly people use multiple strategies to prevent the sight and smell of urine from being detected (see Reflective Practice box 12.1).

Coordinated, socially acceptable micturition is dependent upon many factors and is susceptible to damage or injury at many levels. Most commonly, neurological damage results in urinary incontinence due to an impaired ability to store urine. Impaired voiding can also result and, when this occurs with disrupted storage, bladder dysfunction can be particularly severe.

THE IMPACT OF URINARY INCONTINENCE

The impact of incontinence on the emotional, social, physical and economic well-being of individuals and their carers should not be underestimated. The experience of incontinence has a profound impact on an adult's psychological well-being. Control of bowels and bladder is fundamental to the developmental stage shift from infant to child. To lose control over the most intimate of bodily functions is humiliating and distressing at any age. Fear of this loss of control being witnessed by others leads people to curtail their social and public activities. People who are

incontinent describe a range of emotions, including increased levels of depression, irritability, anxiety and feelings of hopelessness. One study of women attending a specialist continence clinic found 25% to be as depressed, anxious and phobic as psychiatric patients (McCauley et al 1991). Increased levels of social isolation may compound the psychological impact (Grimby et al 1993).

People with incontinence tend to remain near home and often feel uncomfortable about travelling too far or using public transport. This factor has been exacerbated by the reduction in the number of public lavatories over recent decades. Lack of ease of access to lavatories in GP surgeries may be significant for some people in their decision to consult the GP.

Living with a person who is incontinent can be distressing and physically exhausting. Studies in the USA have shown that incontinence has not only been a significant factor in the decision by carers to place their demented relative in a nursing home, but also, as demonstrated in one (O'Donnell et al 1992), a predictor of institutionalization.

CONTINENCE CARE IN HOSPITAL

There is a lack of research-based evidence in the UK relating to the management of incontinence in hospital wards. Studies in the USA (Hancock et al 1996, Schultz et al 1997) have shown that ward-based nurses fail to recognize continence problems on assessment and suggest that this is because other clinical problems are perceived as more pressing. Also there is a general lack of knowledge concerning appropriate management and treatment measures than can be implemented. Nurses often resort to 'throwing a pad' at the problem or catheterizing the patient, often unnecessarily. In addition, treatment of the problem is often related to the knowledge and skills of the nurses on duty at the time of admission or the one who has overall responsibility for the duty of care.

Few patients are actually admitted to hospital for the treatment of urinary incontinence; it usually presents as an unrelated or secondary condition. Because of this, the nurse's energies are expended on nursing strategies directed towards the main presenting diagnosis. Factors such as shortened length of stay in hospital can interfere with the identification of continence problems. Consequently, continence issues tend to be sidelined.

In order to investigate the extent to which urinary incontinence was identified as a problem, and the nature of its assessment and management, Cheater (1993) carried out a retrospective survey of 229 nursing and medical records of patients identified as incontinent by nurses in 14 acute medical wards and 26 elderly care wards. The results showed that the recording of incontinence was inconsistent and that there was a paucity of information that might have contributed towards its assessment (see Evidence-based Practice box 12.1).

Incontinence is a symptom that can be extremely difficult to monitor and may go unrecognized, even in hospital. A number of factors within the context of the work environment, such as staff turnover or shift system, can obstruct effective communication and hence awareness of patient problems (Cheater 1993). In addition, it is not uncommon for nursing staff to consider that continence is mainly an issue of old age. Schultz et al

EVIDENCE-BASED PRACTICE

12.1 The assessment of urinary incontinence and its management in elderly hospitalized patients

A retrospective survey of 229 nursing and medical records of patients in acute medical wards and elderly care wards (Cheater 1993) revealed the following:

- Causes of incontinence were rarely recorded, and in approximately half the nursing and medical records examined there was a complete absence of any information related to a management plan. In addition, where recorded, interventions reflected predominantly palliative measures, such as routine toileting regimens and the use of continence aids.
- The patient's usual micturition habits were recorded in less than a quarter of the nursing records. Specific information concerning the duration, pattern, type and cause of the incontinence prior to admission was recorded in only 10 cases. Details concerning the patient's usual living circumstances prior to admission, e.g. the provision and location of toilet facilities within the home, availability of carers or the patient's customary method of coping with incontinence, were absent in all the nursing records examined.

- With respect to the management of incontinence, of the nursing records, 96 had at least one written entry relating to an aspect of this. The most frequent method prescribed in the nursing records related to some type of routine or fixed-interval toileting – e.g. '2-hourly toileting' (51%), 'frequent' or 'regular' toileting (47.9%). Other strategies related to the use of continence aids, such as pads and pants (42.7%), sheath drainage appliances (25%) and indwelling urethral catheters (4.2%). Strategies such as the use of bladder-training regimens, behavioural modification techniques or intermittent catheterization (all accepted as appropriate continence care treatments) were not mentioned in any of the records examined. The use of pelvic floor exercises, another proven and accepted treatment regimen, was documented in one medical record only.

Reference

Cheater F. Retrospective document survey: identification, assessment and management of urinary incontinence in medical and care of the elderly wards. J Adv Nurs 1993; 18: 1734–1746.

(1997) stress the fact that nurses should be identifying people across the whole age band who might experience incontinence. Ward-based nurses are in an exceptionally strong position to be able to identify symptoms when they carry out assessments on admission. If a patient's length of stay in hospital is short, ward-based nurses need to ensure that the person is directed towards appropriate specialist services. For patients who have a longer stay in hospital, management and treatment plans should be commenced and reinforced. These can then be continued in the community setting by a community nurse, the general practitioner or a specialist centre.

CONTINENCE CARE AT HOME

The Audit Commission (1999) carried out a national pilot audit to review district nursing services in England and Wales in relation to two conditions: leg ulcers and incontinence. These conditions were selected because of their prevalence, their prominence in district nurses' caseloads, their costs to the National Health Service and the existence of evidence-based clinical practice guidelines. In addition, comprehensive, accurate assessment is a major determinant of successful patient outcomes in both conditions.

This study found that district nurses often implemented a conservative care plan focused on managing the problem rather than treating the underlying cause. Assessment documentation was more complete than that for patients with leg ulcers, but often this was because the documentation was required as a prescription for pads; the assessment bore little relationship to the care actually provided (Audit Commission 1999). They concluded that if health care trusts were to contain expenditure on

continence products, assessments needed to be comprehensive and should lead to an appropriate evidence-based care plan.

CAUSES OF URINARY INCONTINENCE

The causes of urinary incontinence are complex, demonstrating the interplay between the following associated factors.

Immobility/chronic degenerative disease

Poor mobility due to such conditions as osteoarthritis can mean the difference between being continent and incontinent. Individuals with overactive bladder symptoms who are mobile are more likely to get to the toilet in time than those who are immobile. Consequently, those with immobility problems are more likely to be incontinent. Similarly, osteoarthritis can lead to dexterity problems and this can affect an individual's ability to undo clothing and zips quickly.

Congestive heart failure

Congestive heart failure in itself cannot cause urinary incontinence; however, aspects of the condition can lead to it. The most common problem tends to arise in individuals with swollen legs. When going to bed, the fluid in the legs goes back into the circulation and into the kidneys. This leads to nocturia (frequency of micturition at night), which in turn leads to lack of sleep and can be very distressing. In addition, diuretics are the common medication for congestive heart failure. Diuretics, especially when given in large doses, lead to an increased diuresis. Individuals may find it difficult to cope with the frequency and urgency that occurs as a result of diuretic medications and may be incontinent if they cannot get to the toilet in time.

Diabetes

Autonomic neuropathy, which is associated with diabetes, can lead to voiding inefficiency (see below). All individuals with diabetes who have symptoms of continence problems require an estimation to be made of residual urine measurements.

Concurrent medication

The effect of medication is discussed in more detail later in this chapter (see p. 236). It is important to review concurrent medication as numerous medicines have an effect on continence status.

Impaired cognition

Individuals who are confused or suffer from dementia have a high likelihood of developing continence problems because they are unable to interpret the sensation of needing to void. Impaired cognition can lead to inappropriate voiding and abnormal behaviours.

Smoking

Smoking does not actually cause incontinence; however, someone suffering from stress incontinence who has a smoker's cough is likely to have worse symptoms than someone who does not smoke.

Environmental barriers

Environmental barriers, e.g. when an individual has mobility problems and the only toilet is upstairs, can lead to urinary incontinence becoming a problem in a way that it might not if the toilet was downstairs. It is important that an occupational therapy referral is made if any environmental problems are identified, so that an appropriate package of care can be delivered.

Faecal impaction

Faecal impaction can cause urinary incontinence. If the impaction is high up, it can cause the bowel to press on the bladder, leading to overactivity. Faecal impaction lower down in the bowel can cause an obstruction and lead to voiding inefficiency.

Obesity

Although, like smoking, obesity cannot cause incontinence, it can worsen the symptoms and put additional strain on the pelvic floor. For those with stress incontinence, being overweight can worsen their symptoms.

Neurological disease/injury

Individuals who have neurological diseases, such as multiple sclerosis and Parkinson's disease, cerebrovascular accidents or a cerebral or spinal injury are more prone to incontinence because the bladder is controlled by the central and autonomic nervous systems. For individuals with multiple sclerosis, it can in fact be the presenting symptom and most people with the disease will have incontinence at some point during the course of the illness.

Parity (number of children)

Although the number of children a woman has is not important to the treatment of incontinence, it is relevant to the assessment of stress incontinence. It is generally recognized that incontinence can occur during pregnancy and following childbirth. Factors relevant to developing incontinence after childbirth are if the baby was large, if the labour was long, if the birth was traumatic and whether or not the woman had an assisted delivery using Ventouse extraction (suction) or forceps.

Oestrogen depletion

Oestrogen depletion occurs in women after the menopause and can lead to frequency and urgency of micturition as well as urinary tract infections. This is because lack of oestrogen can lead to atrophic changes, which results in rigid, inelastic and easily inflamed tissues. Because of this it is important to perform a vulval examination on all postmenopausal women.

Urinary tract infection

Overactive bladder symptoms are sometimes caused by the wall of the bladder becoming irritable as a result of a urinary tract infection. It is therefore important to perform urinalysis in individuals with frequency and urgency with or without urge incontinence.

ASSESSMENT OF URINARY INCONTINENCE

A complex interaction of factors contributes to the development of urinary incontinence, especially in the frail older person. Identification and management of problems such as an inability to undo clothing in time at the toilet need as much attention as the diagnosis of underlying pathology and point to the need for systematic assessment of all potential factors, preferably using a single assessment protocol based on evidence-based guidelines and customized to the particular area (see Older Adults: Nursing Priorities box 12.1).

A thorough assessment is crucial. This should preferably be multidisciplinary using a single evidence-based assessment protocol or care pathway (Baylis et al 2001). The following key aspects of assessment should be covered:

The presenting symptoms and history of incontinence. A detailed exploration of the symptoms is important, as is clarifying the most bothersome symptoms. This will help lead to a preliminary nursing diagnosis of what type of incontinence problems the patient might have.

Impact on the person's quality of life, e.g. reducing social contact outside the home, impact on sexuality, evidence of depression.

Past medical history, e.g. whether the onset was during or following childbirth and how many children the woman had, or whether it was following surgery such as a prostatectomy or hysterectomy. Other medical history is also relevant, such as congestive heart disease which requires treatment with diuretics and could lead to continence symptoms. If an individual has asthma and a related cough, this may worsen stress incontinence symptoms.

Associated disease, e.g. dementia, diabetes, neurological disease (multiple sclerosis, Parkinson's disease, cerebral vascular disease), can lead to incontinence symptoms. Spinal cord disease or injury can also be a predisposing factor. Arthritis can lead to mobility problems that may influence whether an individual can reach the toilet in time when the urge to void is felt.

Environmental factors, e.g. if the toilet is too low or too high. Furthermore, in individuals with mobility problems, toilets

OLDER ADULTS: NURSING PRIORITIES

12.1 Assessment of urinary incontinence in older adults

A 78-year-old woman is admitted to your ward with pneumonia. She rings the bell every half hour because she wants to pass urine but by the time you get to her she has already been incontinent. You are giving her incontinence pads to contain the situation until you assess it more fully.

In order to assess the cause of her frequency and incontinence, you will need to:

- Test her urine in case she has diabetes
- Test her urine for leucocytes, nitrites and blood and send a midstream specimen if the urine dipstick test is positive to any of these findings. If she has a urinary tract infection, discuss treatment with the medical staff
- Assess for constipation, which may occur if she is not drinking or eating well or if her mobility is poor. Discuss treatment of constipation with the rest of the nursing team and medical staff
- Perform an in/out catheterization or bladder scan to ensure she is emptying her bladder fully. If the residual is above 150 mL, she may have a voiding problem
- Keep frequency and fluid intake charts for 3 days, as small frequent volumes could mean that she has an overactive bladder. If she is passing small volumes of urine, liaise with your local continence or urology nurse specialists
- Note the medications she is taking. Many medications have side-effects that could cause frequency or urinary incontinence. Discuss this with the medical staff.

Catheterization should not be considered without further discussions with continence or urology nurse specialists.

located some distance from where they are sitting, or upstairs, can lead to them having difficulty reaching it on time and thus maintaining continence. Many people with continence symptoms find it difficult to leave the house due to the lack of public toilet facilities.

Current medications and drug use, e.g. diuretics, sedatives, antiparkinsonian drugs, alcohol consumption, and smoking. Table 12.1 illustrates the medications that can affect the individual with continence problems.

Dietary intake and fluids, e.g. how much and what type of fluids are drunk. Caffeine, alcohol, fizzy and diet drinks are known to aggravate continence symptoms. In addition, many people with continence symptoms tend to restrict their fluid intake, which can lead to urine becoming concentrated and cause bladder irritation. Conversely, if they drink large quantities of fluids this can also aggravate bladder symptoms.

TYPES OF URINARY INCONTINENCE

There are a number of different types of urinary incontinence as classified by the International Continence Society (Abrams et al 2002).

Overactive bladder (also known as detrusor instability and urge incontinence)

The overactive bladder is a symptomatic diagnosis that comprises the symptoms of frequency of micturition (more than eight times in a 24-hour period) and urgency with or without urge incontinence, occurring either singly or in combination. Patients with an overactive bladder may or may not have a neurological cause for their symptoms (Milsom et al 2001).

The overactive bladder is a chronic condition defined by urodynamic investigations as detrusor overactivity, and characterized by involuntary bladder contractions during the filling phase of the micturition cycle (Abrams et al 2002). Urge incontinence is the most common cause of urinary incontinence in the elderly (Malone-Lee 1994).

Stress incontinence

Stress incontinence is defined as urine loss coincident with an increase in intra-abdominal pressure, in the absence of a detrusor contraction or an overdistended bladder. Clinically it presents as the involuntary loss of urine on coughing, sneezing, laughing or performing physical activities. It occurs in about 85% of women presenting with incontinence (Cardozo 1991). It is usually associated with bladder outlet incompetence due to weakness of the supporting pelvic floor muscles and insufficiency of the urethral sphincter. In women this is usually, but not always, due to childbirth; in men it can occur following prostate surgery.

Mixed incontinence

It is not uncommon for people to complain of both urge and stress symptoms. This is termed mixed urinary incontinence. This is particularly common in postmenopausal women. The most important aspect of this type of incontinence is identifying which is the most 'bothersome' symptom that should then be targeted.

Overflow incontinence

This term is used to describe the involuntary loss of urine associated with overdistension of the bladder. It can be caused by a number of different conditions, including bladder outlet or urethral obstruction, which is most commonly seen in men with prostatic hyperplasia. This type of incontinence is less common in women but may occur as a complication following surgery to correct incontinence or because of severe pelvic organ prolapse.

An underactive or acontractile detrusor muscle can also lead to overdistension and overflow. The causes include neurological disorders such as strokes or multiple sclerosis, diabetes and medication side-effects. In some individuals it is idiopathic.

Voiding inefficiency

Voiding inefficiency means that the bladder fails to empty completely, leading to the involuntary loss of urine associated with overdistension. Voiding inefficiency is a common problem in individuals with neurological problems such as multiple sclerosis or Parkinson's disease or those who have had cerebrovascular accidents. Individuals who have diabetes can also have voiding inefficiency due to autonomic neuropathy (see Ch. 14). Benign prostatic hypertrophy in men (see Ch. 24) may lead to obstruction which can cause voiding inefficiency, and women may have an obstruction due to a pelvic organ prolapse.

Table 12.1 Drug therapy and urinary incontinence

Drug	Use	Effect
Antidepressants (e.g. amitriptyline, lofepramine, imipramine)	Depression	Voiding difficulties
Calcium channel blockers (e.g. nifedipine)	Angina, arrhythmia, hypertension	Nocturia Increased frequency
Cytotoxic drugs (e.g. cyclophosphamides, ifosfamide)	Malignancy	Haemorrhagic cystitis
Diuretics		
Loop diuretics (e.g. furosemide [frusemide], bumetanide, metolazone)	Management of pulmonary oedema, heart failure, oedema	Urinary urgency Urge incontinence
Thiazides (e.g. bendrofluazide, cyclopenthiazide, amiloride, tramterent, spironolactone)	Diabetes insipidus, oliguria due to renal failure, ascites, nephritic syndrome	Urinary urgency and frequency Urge incontinence
Hypnotics		
Barbiturates (e.g. amobarbital, phenobarbital) and chloral derivatives (e.g. chloral hydrate, chloral betaine)	Sedation	Decreased awareness, drowsiness and impaired mobility
Alcohol	Social – mood enhancing Alcohol abuse	Impairs mobility, reduces sensation, increases urinary frequency and urgency, induces diuresis
Anticholinesterase (e.g. neostigmine)	Myasthenia gravis, irritable bowel spasm, gut spasm	Bladder sphincter muscle relaxation causing involuntary micturition Contraction of smooth muscle, increased peristalsis
Antimuscarinic (anticholinergic) drugs (e.g. benzhexol, procyclidine, hyoscine, propantheline)	Parkinson's disease, drug-induced parkinsonism	
Drugs with antimuscarinic side-effects (e.g. antihistamines, pizotifen, promethazine)	Allergies, hay fever, rashes, migraine, travel sickness	Voiding difficulties Reduced awareness
Antipsychotics (e.g. chlorpromazine, thioridazine)	Schizophrenia and psychotic illness, nausea, vomiting, agitation	Voiding difficulties Reduced awareness
Xanthines (e.g. theophylline, caffeine)	Asthma, stimulant	Increased diuresis, aggravates detrusor instability causing urge incontinence
Sedatives		
Benzodiazepines (e.g. diazepam, lorazepam, nitrazepam, temazepam)	Sedation	Decreased awareness
Phenothiazines (e.g. chlorpromazine, thioridazine)	Anxiety	Drowsiness
Antipsychotics[a] (e.g. droperidol, haloperidol, pimozide)		Impaired mobility
Opiate analgesics (e.g. diamorphine, morphine)	Pain control, drug abuse	Bladder sphincter spasm causing difficulty in micturition and urge incontinence

[a] These are also above.

Nocturia and nocturnal enuresis

Nocturia is a complaint where individuals have to wake up one or more times at night to void. Nocturnal enuresis is when individuals wet the bed at night. Nocturia can be a normal phenomenon in the elderly due to the fact that they have small bladder capacities and a reduced excretion of antidiuretic hormone overnight. In addition, congestive cardiac failure can lead to an increased diuresis at night if they have oedematous legs, as the fluid in these extremities goes back into the circulation when they are elevated and this is voided overnight. Nocturnal enuresis occurs commonly in children; however, sometimes this continues into adulthood. In addition, those individuals who have overactive bladders can have nocturnal bedwetting if they sleep through the impulse to void.

INVESTIGATIONS

There are a number of baseline investigations that need to be carried out in order for an accurate picture to be obtained of a patient's symptoms. These include urinalysis, physical examination, post-void residual urine and frequency–volume chart.

Urinalysis

Urinalysis is performed to detect conditions that are associated with, or contribute to, urinary incontinence, such as haematuria (suggestive of infection, stone, renal disease or cancer) and glycosuria (glucose in the urine), which may cause polyuria (excretion of excessive amounts of urine) and contribute to symptoms. Dipstick methods are available to detect infection and the urine should be tested for leucocytes and nitrites as well as blood, as the presence of these is indicative of infection and antibiotic therapy may need to be considered. If blood is present and there is no infection, it is important to send a urine sample for cytology testing in case there is a malignancy.

Physical examination

Physical examination is imperative and will usually be carried out by a doctor or a specialist nurse. Vaginal examination is necessary to detect genital atrophy, pelvic organ prolapse and pelvic mass, and to assess paravaginal muscle tone. Rectal examination is required to rule out constipation or impaction and, in men with suspected outlet obstruction, to assess prostate size and consistency. A general examination for neurological abnormalities is also indicated.

Post-void residual volume

Measurement of post-void residual volume is an essential component of the assessment of urinary incontinence. This can be estimated using abdominal palpation and percussion, by urethral catheterization, or by using portable ultrasound equipment usually available from continence services or urology departments. In clinical practice, it is generally accepted that a residual volume below 100 mL in the younger adult and below 150 mL in the older adult is normal.

Frequency–volume chart

Detailed information about the pattern of frequency, volume of voiding and fluid intake is obtained through a 3-day frequency–volume chart. Charting will provide more objective information about the number of incontinent episodes, the frequency of micturition (diurnal and nocturnal) and functional bladder capacity. These types of chart can be used to inform treatment decisions as well as monitor progress.

This type of assessment lends itself to protocol development by professionals to ensure all aspects are covered. There are numerous locally developed assessment tools and it is best to find out the type that is being used locally and initiate any new assessment using this. Referral for more specialist evaluation, such as urodynamic investigations, may be necessary although this is not appropriate in every situation and may not be desired by the patient. It should be considered in the following circumstances:

- uncertain diagnosis
- difficulties in developing an appropriate treatment plan
- failure to respond to the treatment/management plan after an appropriate period
- the presence of other complicating morbidity.

Urodynamic investigations

Urodynamic investigation (cystometry) involves computerized studies that are undertaken in order to diagnose the exact cause of continence symptoms. It is an invasive procedure that involves the insertion of a catheter and a transducer line into the bladder through the urethra, and a rectal line into the rectum. The bladder is then filled with normal saline and any bladder symptoms that occur during the investigation are shown and analysed on the computer. Urodynamic studies used to be carried out on most patients who were referred to specialist units; however, they are now only performed following initial failed treatment or if the patient has unusually complex problems. This is because the investigation is uncomfortable, undignified and there is a high incidence of associated urinary tract infections.

TREATMENT OF URINARY INCONTINENCE

The primary aim of the treatment and support of incontinence is to reduce the impact of the symptoms and other factors that occur in relation to it, including depression and, especially in the elderly, the avoidance of social isolation (Fonda et al 1999). The evidence base for continence treatment and management is lacking in many aspects. A number of consensus guidelines have been produced (Button et al 1998) to assist clinicians in their decision-making when assessing and treating urinary incontinence. The treatment categories are:

- behavioural – e.g. bladder retraining, fluid manipulation, pelvic floor exercises, biofeedback, electrical stimulation
- pharmacological – e.g. antimuscarinic drugs, desmopressin, oestrogen
- surgical – e.g. colposuspension, tension-free vaginal tape, prostatectomy.

STRESS INCONTINENCE: PELVIC FLOOR EDUCATION

Stress incontinence is usually treated conservatively through teaching pelvic floor exercises as part of a programme of education. Unfortunately, like so much of continence management, there is a paucity of robust evidence concerning pelvic floor education. However, a large number of studies investigating the value of this technique have consistently found an improvement in the level of stress incontinence following a programme of pelvic floor education, both after childbirth and in later years. One randomized controlled trial conducted on older women found that they will accept and maintain a regimen of pelvic floor exercises and that beneficial effects are maintained for at least 6 months after completion of the initial intervention (Burns et al 1993).

The effect of pelvic floor exercises is known to be long term, with individuals maintaining improvement for at least 5–10 years following initial treatment. There is no consensus regarding the form that pelvic floor education should take, and many studies do not detail the exact form of any pelvic education used. The types of exercise regimens described include: 15 contractions twice a day; or five contractions performed 10 times a day. It used to be thought that the use of muscles other than those of the pelvic floor would render the pelvic floor exercises ineffectual. However, two studies (Laycock et al 2001, Sapsford et al 2001) have shown that it is normal to utilize abdominal muscles when undertaking pelvic floor re-education.

Assessment of the pelvic floor

Prior to prescribing a regimen of pelvic floor exercises, it is imperative that a specialist nurse, physiotherapist or doctor undertakes a detailed assessment of the pelvic floor. This includes assessing the strength of the pubococcygeal muscle and the condition of the local surrounding tissue, and identifying whether the patient has a cystocele, rectocele or vaginal vault prolapse. However, the most important element is the assessment of the individual's ability to identify and isolate the correct muscle group and perform effective contraction of the muscles. Despite this, the vast majority of people will not have access to a practitioner trained in pelvic floor assessment. It is therefore beneficial to instruct them verbally and advise them that if this does not work they should seek specialist help.

Pelvic floor exercises

For women

It is important to isolate the pelvic floor muscles to know which muscles to work. The Continence Foundation provides the following guidance for women in their fact sheet.

1. Sit comfortably with your knees slightly apart. Now imagine that you are trying to stop yourself passing wind from the bowel. To do this you must squeeze the muscle around the back passage. Try squeezing and lifting that muscle as if you really do have wind. You should be able to feel the muscle move. Your buttocks and legs should not move at all. You should be aware of the skin around the back passage tightening and being pulled up and away from your chair. Really try to feel this squeezing and lifting.

2. Now imagine that you are sitting on the toilet passing urine. Picture yourself trying to stop the stream of urine. Try doing it now while you are reading this. You should be using the same group of muscles that you used before, but don't be surprised if you find this harder. (Do not try to stop the stream when you are actually passing water as this may, if repeated, cause problems with proper emptying.)

3. Now try to tighten the muscles around your back passage, vagina and front passage and lift up inside as if trying to stop passing wind and urine at the same time. It is very easy to bring other, irrelevant, muscles into play, so try to isolate your pelvic floor as much as possible by not pulling in your tummy (though you may feel your lower tummy tensing), not squeezing your legs together, not tightening your buttocks and not holding your breath. In this way most of the effort should be coming from the pelvic floor.

It is important to assess a woman's lifestyle and motivation prior to prescribing a course of pelvic floor education. If her motivation is low, adherence to a complicated regimen is likely to be poor and a simple regimen is likely to be more effective. The Continence Foundation has developed a factsheet and a regimen of pelvic floor exercises that a woman can perform without requiring full assessment (see Health Promotion box 12.1).

For men

One of the main causes of stress incontinence in men is sphincter damage following transurethral resection of the prostate (TURP) or radical prostatectomy. Emberton et al (1996) found that one-third of men who were continent before surgery reported some incontinence post-surgery.

 HEALTH PROMOTION

12.1 Pelvic floor exercises for women (Source: The Continence Foundation – www.continence-foundation.org.uk)

Exercise 1: Your pelvic floor muscles need to have stamina. So: sit, stand or lie with your knees slightly apart. Slowly tighten and pull up the pelvic floor muscles as hard as you can. Try lifting and squeezing them as long as you can. Rest for 4 seconds and then repeat the contraction. Build up your strength until you can do 10 slow contractions at a time, holding them for 10 seconds each with rests of 4 seconds in between.

Exercise 2: Your pelvic floor muscles also need to react quickly to sudden stresses from coughing, laughing or exercise that put pressure on the bladder. So practise some quick contractions, drawing in the pelvic floor and holding it for just 1 second before relaxing. Try to achieve a strong muscle tightening with up to 10 quick contractions in succession.

Aim to do a set of slow exercises (exercise 1) followed by a set of quick contractions (exercise 2) six times each day. It takes time for exercise to make muscles stronger. You are unlikely to notice any improvement for several weeks – so stick at it! You will need to exercise regularly for several months before the muscles gain their full strength.

Tips to help

- Get into the habit of doing your exercise with things you do regularly – every time you turn on a tap if you are at home; every time you answer the phone if you are at the office ... whatever you do often.
- If you are unsure that you are exercising the right muscles, put your thumb or one or two fingers in the vagina and try the exercises, to check. You should feel a gentle squeeze as the pelvic floor contracts.
- Use the pelvic floor when you are afraid you might leak: pull up the muscles before you cough, laugh, sneeze or lift anything heavy. Your control will gradually improve.
- Drink normally – at least 6–8 cups every day, avoiding caffeine if you can. And don't get into the habit of going to the toilet 'just in case'. Go only when you feel that the bladder is full.
- Watch your weight – extra weight puts extra strain on your pelvic floor muscles.
- Once you have regained control of your bladder, don't forget your pelvic floor muscles. Continue to do your pelvic floor exercises a few times each day to ensure that the problem does not come back.

Digital rectal examination must be undertaken to assess strength of pelvic muscles prior to prescribing a regimen of pelvic floor exercises. Men can be encouraged to tighten and lift the pelvic floor muscles as if controlling flatus or preventing the flow of urine, and should practise in front of a mirror to observe a lift at the base of the penis and scrotal lift (Dorey 2000a).

Following assessment, men can also undertake the same sort of pelvic floor education as women in the amount of exercises they do, how often they contract and how long they hold for (Dorey 2000b). Men can also be taught 'the knack' of tightening the pelvic floor muscles prior to coughing, sneezing, rising from sitting, or lifting (see p. 241).

The Continence Foundation also has a fact sheet on pelvic floor exercises for men. The commonest cause of a weak pelvic floor in men is following a prostectomy operation. It is important to correctly identify the muscles that need to be exercised. To achieve this, the Continence Foundation recommends that men do the following:

1. Sit or lie comfortably with muscles of the thighs, buttocks and abdomen relaxed.
2. Tighten the ring of muscle around the back passage as if trying to control diarrhoea or wind. Relax it. Practise this movement several times until sure that the correct muscle is being exercised. Try not to squeeze the buttocks or tighten the thighs or tummy muscles.
3. Imagine passing urine, trying to stop the flow midstream, then restarting it. Only do this to learn which muscles are the correct ones to use and then no more than once a week to check progress, otherwise it may interfere with normal bladder emptying. If the technique is correct, each time the pelvic floor muscles are tightened, the base of the penis should move up slightly towards the abdomen.

If the pelvic floor exercises (see Health Promotion box 12.2) do not lead to an improvement in symptoms, a course of pelvic floor re-education by an expert practitioner is recommended.

Vaginal cones

The use of vaginal cones has been advocated as an adjunct to pelvic floor training for strengthening the pelvic floor muscles. The woman holds onto a cone in her vagina for increasing lengths of time, gradually improving pelvic floor strength.

The efficacy of vaginal cones is much debated and the research evidence on their effectiveness is limited. They may help to increase the strength of the muscle contraction and provide proprioceptive feedback, and are considered a low-risk therapy for stress incontinence (Agency for Health Care Policy and Research 1996) with some evidence of objective improvement in symptoms (Peattie et al 1988). However, Bo et al (1999) reported that many women found them difficult to use and that their use as an additional part of a treatment programme did not improve outcomes. Vaginal cones are advertised widely in

---

 HEALTH PROMOTION

12.2 Pelvic floor exercises for men (Source: The Continence Foundation – www.continence-foundation.org.uk)

1. Tighten and draw in strongly the muscles around the anus and the urethra all at once. Lift them up inside. Try and hold this contraction strongly as you count to five, then release slowly and relax for a few seconds. You should have a definite feeling of 'letting go'.
2. Repeat ('squeeze and lift') and relax. It is important to rest in between each contraction. If you find it easy to hold the contraction for a count of five, try to hold for longer – up to 10 seconds.
3. Repeat this as many times as you are able up to a maximum of 8–10 squeezes. Make each tightening a strong, slow and controlled contraction.
4. Now do 5–10 short, fast but strong contractions, pulling up and immediately letting go.

Do this whole exercise routine at least 4–5 times every day. You can do it in a variety of positions – lying, sitting, standing, walking.

While doing the exercises:

- DO NOT hold your breath
- DO NOT push down instead of squeezing and lifting up
- DO NOT tighten your tummy, buttocks or thighs.

Do your exercises well. The quality is important. Fewer good exercises will be more beneficial than many half-hearted ones.

Make the exercises a daily routine

Once you have learnt how to do these exercises, they should be done regularly, giving each set your full attention. It might be helpful to have at least five regular times during the day for doing the exercises – e.g. after going to the toilet, when having a drink, when lying in bed. You will wish to tighten your pelvic floor muscles also while you are getting up from a chair, coughing or lifting. Some men find that by tightening before they undertake such activities they assist themselves in regaining control.

Good results take time. In order to build up your pelvic floor muscles to their maximum strength you will need to work hard at these exercises. You will probably not notice an improvement for several weeks and you will not reach your maximum performance for a few months. When you have recovered control of your bladder, you should continue doing the exercises twice a day.

Other tips

- Share the lifting of heavy loads
- Avoid constipation and prevent any straining during a bowel movement
- Seek medical advice for hay fever, asthma and bronchitis to reduce sneezing and coughing
- Keep your weight within the right range for your height and age.

the press and women may purchase them unaware of the mixed outcomes of research into their efficacy. The use of cones in women who have overactive bladder symptoms has not been researched and they could well be ineffectual in these cases.

Biofeedback

Biofeedback is where information about what is normally an unconscious physiological process is shown to the patient and/or practitioner as a visual, auditory or tactile signal. Because many women, especially those with stress urinary incontinence, are not aware of the pelvic floor muscles and are unable to produce a voluntary contraction, biofeedback is a useful method of re-education.

The most common method of biofeedback involves the woman being attached to a computerized machine. The woman performs a specific exercise programme and a vaginal probe relays information on the function of the pelvic floor to the computer monitor, providing the woman with immediate feedback on how well her pelvic floor is exercising. A programme of several sessions of biofeedback is usually provided so that the woman can monitor her progress. This acts as reinforcement and acts as a motivational tool (Laycock 1994).

Electrical stimulation

Electrical stimulation as part of the treatment of stress urinary incontinence is well documented. Its mode of action is that it contracts the striated pelvic floor musculature, including the external urethral sphincter. Electrical stimulation can be given using either office-based computer systems or a home unit. A probe is inserted into the vagina and a small electrical current, similar to that provided by a transcutaneous electrical nerve stimulation (TENS) machine, causes the pelvic floor muscles to contract. Improvement of symptoms in 60–90% has been reported in individuals using electrical stimulation (Miller et al 1998).

One theory behind the success of electrical stimulation is that its use helps the patients to correctly identify how to contract the correct pelvic floor muscles and that it also 'kick-starts' them. It is a useful adjunct to a course of pelvic floor re-education if the patient finds it difficult to perform a voluntary contraction.

VOIDING INEFFICIENCY

When a patient presents with symptoms of voiding inefficiency, it is important to exclude faecal impaction and, in men, prostatic enlargement. Physical examination is important. Faecal impaction needs to be treated with oral medication, suppositories or an enema (see Ch. 22) and the patient then reassessed. If prostate enlargement is found, the patient should be referred to a urologist.

Voiding inefficiency due to detrusor failure with a post-micturition residual urine of over 150 mL responds well to a programme of clean intermittent catheterization. This is a procedure that has been found to be effective in managing voiding inefficiency problems for many years. It is usually carried out every 3–6 hours. In the elderly, however, as the fluid output tends to be lower, a less frequent regimen of twice-daily catheterization may prove adequate. It is performed using clean

(non-sterile) catheters by patients themselves or their carer. If the procedure is performed by the patient, gloves are not necessary, but if a health care professional is performing the task, gloves are necessary to prevent cross-infection. A catheter is inserted into the bladder through the urethra and the urine drained. The catheter is then immediately removed.

Patients need to be motivated and have good manual dexterity, and they need to be taught by a confident and experienced health care professional. For many older people, this procedure may have to be performed by community nursing staff. Some patients may have concurrent detrusor overactivity in conjunction with voiding inefficiency. It is important that a regimen of intermittent catheterization is commenced in addition to any other treatment.

OVERACTIVE BLADDER

A programme of non-pharmaceutical treatment is the first option to treat detrusor overactivity. Conservative measures such as caffeine restriction, fluid manipulation and bladder retraining are commonly advocated behavioural techniques in the management of patients with this condition. This is particularly true for older patients who are more likely to experience side-effects of a medication due to co-morbidity (the presence of multiple illnesses) and the interaction of drugs. Associated voiding inefficiency should be excluded through investigation of residual urine volumes.

Caffeine and fluid manipulation

People with urgency and urge incontinence tend to reduce their fluid intake in order to reduce the severity of their symptoms (Pearson & Kelber 1996). These patients need to be reminded of the importance of drinking approximately 1.5–2 litres of fluid a day. In addition, patients need to be made aware of the diuretic effect of constituents in everyday drinks such as caffeine and alcohol. James et al (1989) found that caffeine abstinence significantly helped to reduce the incidence of urinary incontinence among psychogeriatric patients.

Caffeine causes a mild diuresis by acting on the renal tubules. This may be the cause of increased urinary frequency. It is also possible that caffeine has a direct effect on the bladder muscle, increasing its activity (Arya et al 2000). A North American study (Gilbert 1984) identified that 60% of caffeine was consumed in coffee, 16% in soft drinks, and approximately 2% in chocolate. In the UK, a large amount of caffeine is likely to be consumed in tea.

Some studies have highlighted the effect of caffeine in relation to the amount and type of fluid taken. Creighton & Stanton (1990) found that during urodynamic investigation, patients who were administered caffeine had a significant increase in detrusor pressure on bladder filling compared with those who were not. Arya et al (2000) found that women who had a high caffeine intake had a significant association with detrusor instability symptoms compared with those with a minimal caffeine intake (see Health Promotion box 12.3).

Patients are often routinely advised to drink between 1.5 and 2 litres/day, but Abrams & Klevmar (1996) recommend that fluid intake should be linked to patients' weight – the less they weigh, the less they need to drink. For example, someone

HEALTH PROMOTION

12.3 Caffeine restriction

When restricting caffeine, patients can get withdrawal symptoms. Headache is the most common symptom, with fatigue, anxiety and irritability also occurring. These withdrawal symptoms usually occur 12–24 hours after the last intake of caffeine, peak at 20–48 hours, and take up to a week to resolve (McKimm & McKimm 1993). It is therefore important to ensure that the patient is motivated to give up caffeinated drinks. This can be particularly difficult with older people who often say they have 'the pot on the brew all day'.

Because of the length of time of withdrawal effects of caffeine, it is advisable to withdraw it slowly. One way to minimize side-effects and maintain motivation and adherence is to substitute one cup of decaffeinated fluid for one cup of caffeinated every 5–7 days depending on how the person feels. This is more likely to be effective than stopping drinking caffeinated fluids all at once. However, in an Australian study linking the effects of caffeine to frequency, urgency and urge incontinence (Bryant et al 2000), 28% of patients were lost to follow-up even though they were to reduce their caffeine intake slowly. Of those patients who completed the study, a significant improvement in the occasions of leakage of urine per day was shown.

References

McKimm EM, McKimm WA. Caffeine: how much is too much? Can Nurse 1993; 89(11): 19–22.

Bryant CM, Dowell CJ, Fairbrother G. A randomised trial of the effects of caffeine upon frequency, urgency and urge incontinence. J Neurol Urodyn 2000; 19(4): 501–502.

---

weighing 90 kg should drink 6 glasses/mugs of fluid per day (1200 mL), while someone weighing 140 kg would need to drink 10 (2000 mL).

Bladder retraining

Bladder retraining was first introduced in the 1960s (Jeffcoate & Francis 1966) and involves the patient learning to resist the desire to void, thus stretching the bladder and reducing its activity. A retraining programme gradually increases the time between voiding, aiming for periods of 3–4 hours (Button et al 1998). There are two main types of programmes taught, although there is no evidence of superiority of one over the other. The first encourages the person to resist the desire to void as long as they possibly can, with the aim of getting the frequency of voids down to six a day. The second has the same aim but instructs patients to gradually extend the length of time they wait before they pass urine once they have felt the urge. Bladder retraining is only carried out during waking hours.

Sampselle et al (1997) have described how individuals can readily understand the mechanism of bladder retraining when it is framed as a 'mind over bladder' situation. One useful tip for patients to assist them to 'hold on' is for them to sit down on a hard surface. They suggested that such techniques should be used in conjunction with deliberate relaxation, such as slow, deep breathing, to combat a stressful rush to the toilet when the first urge to empty the bladder is perceived. Patients may also find it useful to employ techniques such as doing a crossword or watching television to take their mind off the desire to void.

Both methods use a bladder chart or urinary diary. These provide a permanent record for baseline and subsequent evaluation of symptoms (Robinson et al 1996). They are useful to patients in that they provide a feedback of improvement in their frequency and in their incontinent episodes, aiding motivation. Bladder diaries should only be used for a short time, otherwise patients tend not to complete them accurately. A period of 3 days appears to be optimum. In addition, patients should measure how much they void, if possible. This will give them feedback as to whether they are able to hold on longer and pass larger amounts of urine as the programme progresses.

Pelvic floor exercises

Although generally equated with the treatment of urinary stress incontinence pelvic floor exercises (see p. 237) can also be a useful adjunct to bladder retraining and fluid manipulation in the management of overactive bladder symptoms (Elser et al 1999, Janssen et al 2001). By contracting the pelvic floor, the patient will be able to compress the urethra against the back of the pubic bone, delaying voiding and reducing the amount of leakage. This manoeuvre has become known as 'the knack' (Ashton-Miller & DeLancey 1996). It is also believed that contracting the pelvic floor initiates a feedback mechanism to the hypogastric nerves, which calm the bladder down if there is a bladder contraction.

Electrical stimulation

Electrical stimulation, already described for the treatment of urinary stress incontinence (see p. 240), is also used for overactive bladder symptoms although the precise mechanism of action remains unproven. Lindstrom et al (1983) have suggested that electrical stimulation improves urinary incontinence by inhibiting the parasympathetic excitatory neurons in the pelvic nerve and activating the sympathetic inhibitory neurons in the hypogastric nerve. This leads to an inhibition of detrusor muscle activity and an increase in urethral sphincter contractility.

Although the efficacy of electrical stimulation is debated because its mode of action in the treatment of overactive bladder is not fully understood, there is good evidence to indicate that it is effective, with an overall improvement/cure rate of 50% (Brubaker 2000). Clinicians tend to vary in the frequency of treatment and duration that they give. Stimulation is given using either office-based computer systems or home units. With home units patients are able to treat themselves, usually twice daily for 20 minutes each. Electrical stimulation should only be performed by practitioners who specialize in its use and are proficient in setting treatment parameters.

Although electrical stimulation is inappropriate for certain types of patients, specifically those women who have atrophic vaginitis, the side-effects are far fewer than those of drug treatment. The main side-effect is encountered when individuals turn up the intensity of the stimulation too far and too fast and experience pain on treatment.

Acupuncture

Acupuncture has been used with some success in people with overactive bladder symptoms. Three studies (Ping et al 1984, Chang 1988, Philp et al 1988) have demonstrated favourable outcomes but despite its early promise, acupuncture is not recognized as an alternative treatment modality. Its use needs to be investigated in greater depth. There may be benefits for those patients who prefer to use complementary therapy options to conventional medicine.

PHARMACOLOGICAL TREATMENT OF INCONTINENCE

There are several drugs in general use for the treatment of the overactive bladder. As more and more research is being undertaken, these will increase in number. It needs to be noted, however, that the use of these drugs in the elderly requires special consideration.

Antimuscarinic drugs

The side-effects of many antimuscarinic drugs (e.g. oxybutynin and tolterodine) include a dry mouth, constipation, reflux oesophagitis (the usual reason for withdrawal of the medication, see Ch. 22), dry skin, blurred vision, constipation, nausea, abdominal discomfort, facial flushing, some minor ankle swelling and difficulty with micturition (Wagg & Malone-Lee 1998). Contraindications include intestinal obstruction, severe ulcerative colitis, bladder outlet obstruction, glaucoma and myasthenia gravis. In older people, caution should be exercised in the presence of hepatic or renal impairment, severe cardiac disease and autonomic neuropathy. Special care should be taken with hiatus hernia, especially in the elderly if associated with reflux oesophagitis.

Desmopressin

Desmopressin (DDAVP) is a synthetic form of antidiuretic hormone (ADH) with no effect on blood pressure but a strong antidiuretic effect. It has been primarily used in the treatment of nocturia and nocturnal enuresis in children and adults. It is safe for long-term use, is effective and well tolerated, reducing the frequency of nocturnal voids and nocturnal diuresis. However, its use with the elderly has to be treated with caution due to the risk of hyponatraemia. If the patient continues to drink freely, this can cause dilution of the plasma and lead to headaches or even convulsions or coma. If prescribed DDAVP, older people need their urea and electrolyte levels checked 1 week after commencing treatment and regularly thereafter. If hyponatraemia does develop, the medication must be discontinued.

Oestrogen

The role of oestrogen replacement therapy in the treatment of urinary incontinence remains unclear with few controlled studies reported (Cardozo 1997). Data regarding the effect of the medication is incomplete despite widespread anecdotal evidence. It does, however, have an important physiological effect on the female lower urinary tract. It can improve frequency and urgency in postmenopausal women. Another instance where it might be considered useful is in the management of recurrent urinary tract infections (Stapleton & Stamm 1997) when it tends to reduce the incidence.

CONTROL OF DEFECATION

The lower bowel comprises the sigmoid colon, rectum and anal canal (see Ch. 22). The nerve supply to the internal sphincter is from the sympathetic part of the pelvic plexuses. The external sphincter is under voluntary control and is supplied by the inferior rectal nerve, a branch of the pudendal nerve.

When compared with the bowel's absorptive and digestive functions, relatively little is known about the processes that regulate bowel transit and defecation. The human colon is approximately 1.2–1.5 metres in length. Its most proximal aspect is joined to the small intestine at the ileocaecal valve. This valve permits gastrointestinal contents to move from the small to the large bowel, and prevents movement of bacteria-laden fluids backwards. After entering the large bowel, these contents move through the ascending colon and into the transverse colon, which is a major site for mixing colonic contents. At its termination, the transverse colon turns sharply into the descending colon where it terminates in the rectum. The descending and sigmoid colons are principally storage compartments for stool before evacuation.

The final segment of the gastrointestinal tract comprises the rectum and anal canal. The rectum, in turn, terminates in the anal canal. It maintains continence through the actions of the internal sphincter, consisting of circularly arranged smooth muscle, and the external sphincter, made up of circular and longitudinally orientated striated muscle.

The primary function of the colon is the absorption of water and electrolytes from the intestinal contents. It also plays a minor role in the absorption of nutrients, but the small bowel handles most of this task. Under normal circumstances, the colon absorbs 1–2 litres of water per day, but it is capable of absorbing up to 6 litres when faced with severe dehydration. Absorption of water and electrolytes relies on two factors: the ability of the gut lining cells to extract them from ingested materials within the gut, and the motility of the bowel wall.

Digestive contents move through the rectum via a process of peristalsis. When a bolus of digestive materials enters the normal colon, a period of 8–15 hours elapses before it enters the rectum as soft, formed stool. Constipation occurs when the transit time through the colon is increased, leading to excessive absorption of water and hardening of the stool. Normal ageing does not increase transit time, but many diseases are associated with dysmotility and an abnormal increase in transit time.

The process of defecation relies on the storage of sufficient stool within the sigmoid colon to cause rectal distension and to alert the person to the need to defecate. Sensory receptors in the proximal anal canal sense rectal distension and stool consistency (solid, liquid or gaseous). This distension causes a reflex relaxation of the internal sphincter and contraction of the external sphincter as well as adjacent pelvic floor musculature. If defecation is postponed, this desire is ultimately inhibited until further distension again leads to sensory awareness of the desire to evacuate the bowels. However, if the person elects to defecate, the internal and external sphincters are reflexively relaxed. This relaxation is mechanically enhanced when the individual assumes a squatting position that straightens and promotes movement of stool into the rectum. Stool evacuation is accomplished by increasing abdominal pressure and it may be complemented by peristalsis.

FAECAL INCONTINENCE

The impact of faecal incontinence mirrors and amplifies those described for urinary incontinence. Underestimates of prevalence are common because of reluctance to admit to this symptom. People tend to find it a distasteful topic to discuss; it is a taboo subject that is often hidden by patients.

Prevalence studies show faecal incontinence to be more common than health care professionals previously realized, especially in the female population, often the result of damage to the anal sphincters during childbirth (Kamm 1994). A UK study of 15 904 adults over the age of 40 by the Medical Research Council Incontinence Study Team (Perry et al 1998) found that 8% of those aged 65–84 and 16% of those aged over 85 reported faecal incontinence. Double incontinence (urinary and faecal) was also found to be common. The Royal College of Physicians (1995) defines faecal incontinence as the 'involuntary or inappropriate passing of liquid or solid stool'; however, there is a lack of consensus regarding the definition (Perry et al 1998). A consensus definition of faecal incontinence is needed to avoid inconsistencies in epidemiological studies and to aid treatment.

Causes

Faecal incontinence is more common in women than in men and more common in older adults. It is not, however, a normal part of ageing. Faecal incontinence can have several causes, as described below.

Damage to the anal sphincter muscles

Faecal incontinence is most often caused by injury to one or both anal internal and/or external sphincters that lie at the bottom of the anal canal. The sphincters keep stool inside. When damaged, muscle weakness leads to stool or gas leaking out. In women, this damage most often happens during childbirth. The risk of injury is greatest in instrumental delivery or if a midline episiotomy is performed. Surgery for haemorrhoids can also damage the sphincters.

Damage to the nerves of the anal sphincter muscles or the rectum

If the sensory nerves are damaged, there is no sense that stool is in the rectum and faecal leakage occurs. Nerve damage may be caused by childbirth, a long-term straining to pass stool, stroke and chronic conditions affecting the nerves, such as diabetes and multiple sclerosis.

Loss of storage capacity in the rectum

Rectal surgery, radiation treatment, and inflammatory bowel disease can cause scarring of the rectal walls, which makes them stiff, and less elastic. The ability of the rectum to hold stool is then compromised, and faecal incontinence may result.

Diarrhoea

Diarrhoea, or loose stool, is more difficult to control than solid stool that is formed. Even people who don't have faecal incontinence can be incontinent of faeces when they have diarrhoea.

Pelvic floor dysfunction

This includes decreased perception of rectal and anal sensation, rectal prolapse and generalized weakness of the pelvic floor. This may be more pronounced in later life. When the cause of pelvic floor dysfunction is childbirth, incontinence does not usually present until the fifth decade.

Constipation

The most common cause of faecal incontinence in older adults is believed to be constipation (Petticrew et al 1998). Recent studies of the prevalence of constipation in adults in the UK demonstrated that 20% of people over the age of 65 were affected (Petticrew et al 1998). The common definition of constipation is defecation less frequently than every third day (Wald 1994). However, there are people who believe daily defecation is normal and important for maintenance of health, and any other pattern for them represents constipation. Others believe they are constipated if they have to strain to defecate (Whitehead et al 1989). The actual diagnosis of constipation should be based on the diagnostic criteria devised by a working group on bowel disease, known as the 'Rome' criteria (Thompson et al 1992):

- straining at defecation for at least a quarter of the time
- lumpy and/or hard stools for at least a quarter of the time
- a sensation of incomplete evacuation for at least a quarter of the time
- two or fewer bowel movements per week.

Constipation interferes with daily living and impairs well-being (O'Keefe et al 1995). Approximately 6% of the frail, community-living elderly population have counted constipation as one of their top three health concerns (Wolfson et al 1993). In addition, constipation is known to affect 50% of pregnant woman and 37.9% of these still have the problem 8 weeks postpartum. Given these statistics, it is not surprising that in 1997 the cost to the NHS for the treatment of constipation was estimated to be £47 million (Petticrew et al 1998).

Assessment

The key elements of assessment reflect those of assessment of urinary continence (see p. 234). A detailed understanding of type of stool and frequency of problems is aided by pictorial stool charts such as the Bristol Stool Chart (see Fig. 12.3). Bowel habit diaries are also essential in the assessment of stool symptoms.

A stepwise progression in dealing with constipation is advocated by many commentators and supported in a systematic review of the effectiveness of laxatives in older adults (Petticrew et al 1998). There is little robust evidence on best prevention and management options and guidance tends to develop from expert consensus. Baylis et al (2001) have developed a specific care pathway package for the assessment and treatment of bowel problems (Figs 12.4 and 12.5).

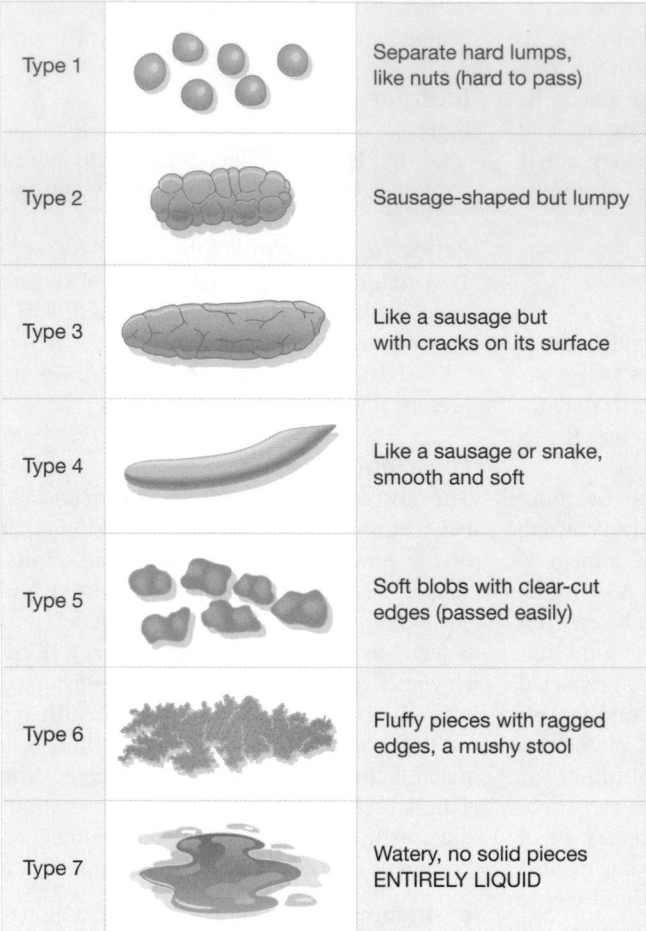

Type 1		Separate hard lumps, like nuts (hard to pass)
Type 2		Sausage-shaped but lumpy
Type 3		Like a sausage but with cracks on its surface
Type 4		Like a sausage or snake, smooth and soft
Type 5		Soft blobs with clear-cut edges (passed easily)
Type 6		Fluffy pieces with ragged edges, a mushy stool
Type 7		Watery, no solid pieces ENTIRELY LIQUID

Figure 12.3 The Norgine Bristol Stool Form Scale. (Reproduced by kind permission of Dr KW Heaton, Reader in Medicine at the University of Bristol. © 2000 Norgine Ltd.)

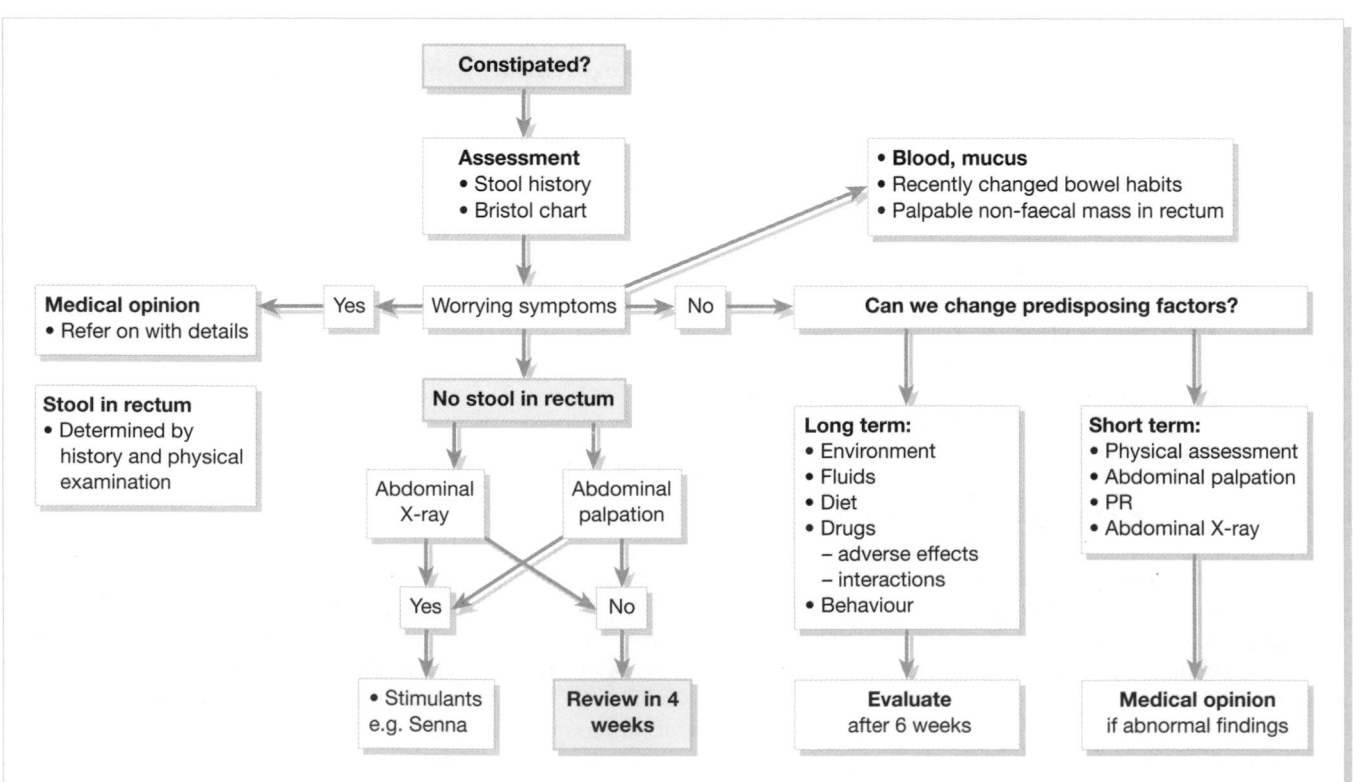

Figure 12.4 Assessment of constipation.

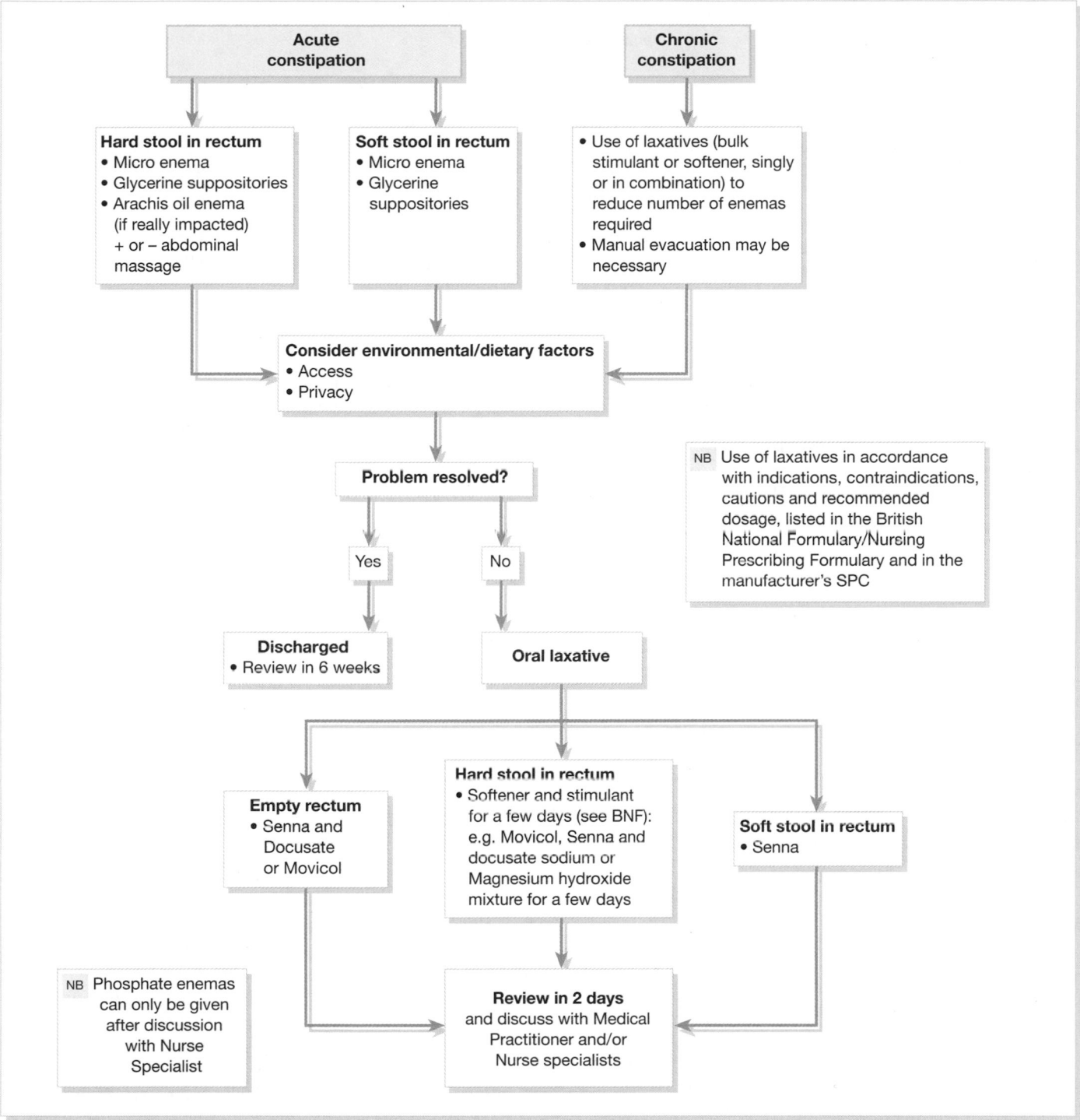

Figure 12.5 Management of constipation.

Management

The management of faecal incontinence will depend on the cause. If this is constipation, the initial aim is to empty the rectum and colon. This can be achieved by the use of oral aperients, rectal suppositories or, in some cases, an enema. Prevention and management of constipation then becomes the aim.

Faecal incontinence may also be due to faecal impaction, when a watery or mushy stool seeps around the obstructing faecal mass. In this instance, the initial aim of treatment is to empty the rectum and colon by a combination of enemas and aperients. Prevention and management of constipation then becomes the aim. Figure 12.6 provides an overview of the type of treatment programme that could be followed.

The treatment options for faecal incontinence remain fairly limited and under-researched but include bowel habit training and drug therapy for liquid stools once the cause has been established.

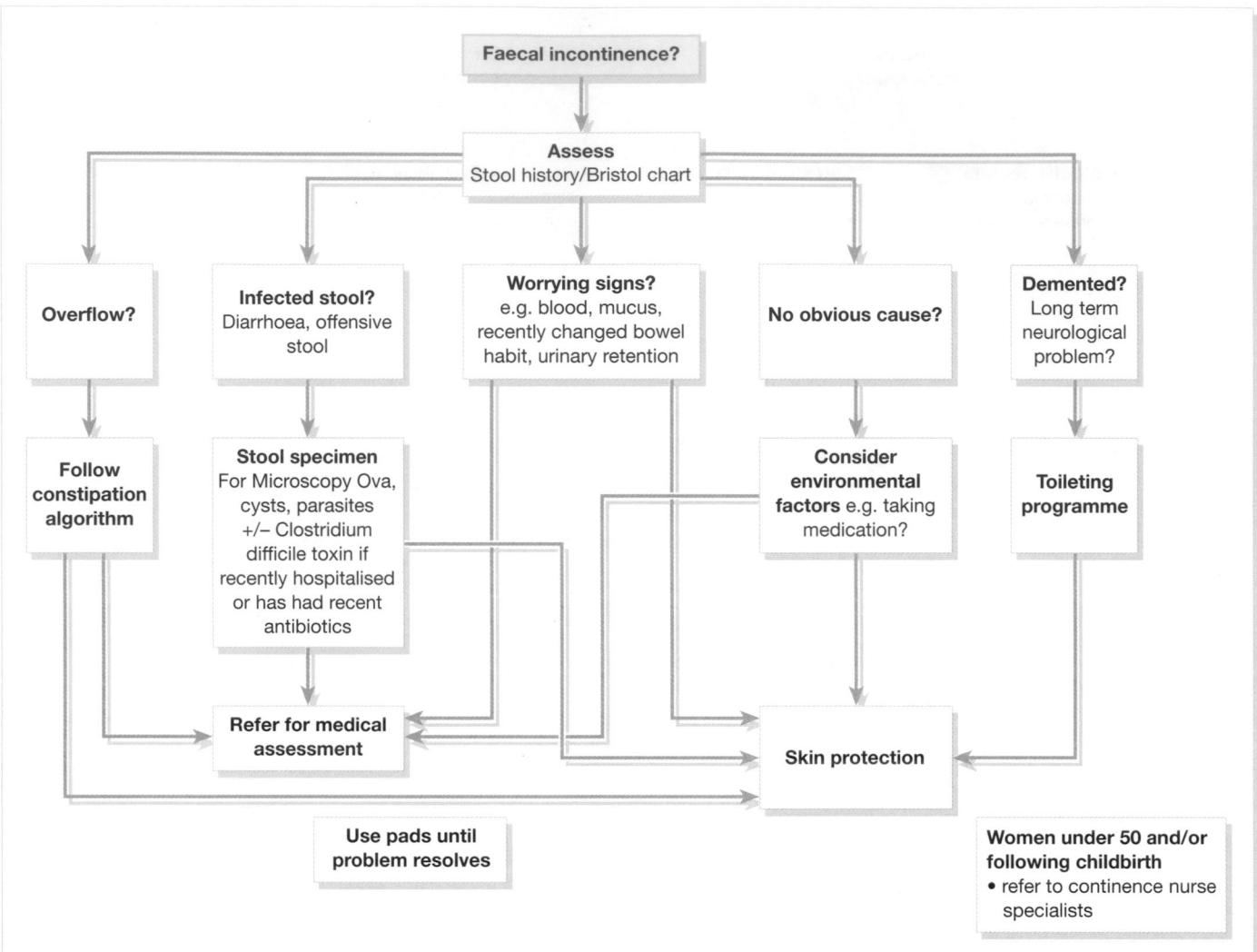

Figure 12.6 Management of faecal incontinence.

Bowel training

Bowel training is the first-line, non-invasive treatment of choice and includes:

- a regular schedule for sitting on the toilet, in line with the person's previous habits
- a fluid intake of at least eight cups/glasses of fluid a day to prevent constipation and ensure that the faeces remain soft and easy to pass
- a diet including a minimum of five portions of fruit and vegetables a day (in addition to potatoes) and adequate dietary fibre. Fibre adds bulk to the stool as well as stimulating gut motility
- as much exercise as possible within the constraints of the individual's ability, as this also stimulates gut motility.

Pharmacological treatment

Loperamide and codeine phosphate help to deal with incontinence by making the stool firmer. There is also some evidence that loperamide directly reduces the sensation of urgency and increases resting anal pressure (Goke et al 1992). Both drugs can be individually titrated to reach their maximum effect. For some patients in whom passive leakage is a major problem, they can stop spontaneous evacuation by using these drugs to constipate themselves. Artificial means such as suppositories or enemas can then be used to empty the bowel at a planned and convenient time (Glickman & Kamm 1996).

Bowel problem management has been detailed by the Continence Foundation (see Guidelines for Care Priorities box 12.1).

▶ Nursing management of urinary and faecal incontinence

Alongside, and in some instances instead of, the treatment options, patients and their carers need advice and help on the associated management of the problem. Most Trusts now employ a continence nurse specialist who can give advice and support to clinicians, patients and carers. It is a good idea to spend some time with them to find out about their role and about how to put patients and carers in contact with them.

GUIDELINES FOR CARE PRIORITIES

12.1 Management of bowel problems
(Adapted with kind permission from *A Brief Guide to Faecal Incontinence in Adults*, The Continence Foundation. www.continence-foundation.org.uk)

Anal sphincter weakness or damage
Causes
- Childbirth
- Anal surgery
- Direct trauma
- Rectal prolapse

Usual symptoms and treatment
- Urgency/urge incontinence (external anal sphincter) → sphincter exercises if weak
- Passive soiling (internal anal sphincter) → surgical repair if disrupted

Intestinal injury
Causes
- Infection
- Inflammatory bowel disease
- Irritable bowel syndrome
- Drug-induced

Usual symptoms and treatment
- Frequency, urgency, urge incontinence, loose stool → treat underlying cause; constipating agents

Impaction with overflow
Causes
- Immobility
- Physical or mental frailty
- Medication
- Dementia

Usual symptoms and treatment
- Passive loss of 'spurious diarrhoea' or of solid stool → disimpact then keep rectum empty

Neurological disease or damage
Causes
- Spinal injury
- Multiple sclerosis

Usual symptoms and treatment
- Reflex incontinence or impaction with overflow → regulate bowel habit; control evacuation with laxatives or evacuants

---

In line with benchmarking, a number of continence nurse specialists now have support and user groups. 'Incontact', the consumer charity for people with bladder and bowel problems, has a list of areas where there are such groups. These can be beneficial to both the patient and the carer to obtain advice, meet others and receive support (see p. 250).

ADVICE AND EDUCATION

Advice and education are important for the person with urinary and/or faecal incontinence and their family members and carers. The more cognitively or physically impaired the patient, the more carers and family members will need advice and support. This should include discussion of:

- appropriate fluid intake and diet – including fibre intake. This may need more detailed exploration to identify and eliminate foods (e.g. green vegetables, lentils and brown rice) which may cause excessive foul-smelling flatus
- continence aids – containment products and their use
- skin care, including frequent washing and the use of barrier creams – in order to prevent excoriation and, in less mobile people, pressure ulcers
- the correct disposal of clinical waste and the arrangements between the local authority and the health authority
- the importance of laundering soiled clothes in hot, soapy water to remove the residue and prevent offensive smells as well as criteria for access to local authority incontinence laundry services
- the use of plastic covers in beds and chairs to prevent spoiling these items and their becoming a source of offensive odour

- the use of disinfectant cleaning materials to clean urine and faeces from floors, walls and household items, in order to eliminate odour problems and minimize the risks of cross-infection. Fragrant sprays are also useful
- advice on handwashing and precautions for infection control for the individual and any other carers
- advice on odour management, particularly of faeces.

CONTINENCE PRODUCTS

Containment is one the most important issues to a person who has continence problems. Continence products include continence pads with pants and uro-sheaths. Continence products are funded through health authority budgets and usually provided by community health services. Urological products (catheters, drainage bags, sheaths) are prescription-only items and are included in the *Nurse Prescribers' Formulary*.

Incontinence pads

The total cost of National Health Service provision of absorbent incontinence products has been estimated at £69 million in England and £82.5 million in the UK as a whole (Continence Foundation 2000). McClish et al (1999) showed that in a group of 315 women with urinary incontinence, costs were greater for women with detrusor instability than in those with genuine stress incontinence. The increased cost was likely to be associated with greater use of special incontinence pads.

Incontinence pads are normally only provided after a member of the community nursing team has carried out a continence assessment. Occasionally products will be supplied within the in-patient setting; however, hospitals tend to keep a restricted

⚡ **SPECIAL ISSUES**

12.1 Provision of continence supplies

Product provision can be limited by local financial constraints, and anecdotal evidence suggests that rationing is widespread. The Department of Health Working Party for developing good practice in continence services (Department of Health 2000) was concerned about the gross difference in NHS Trust policies for the provision of continence supplies. This was also highlighted by Anthony (1998). In a survey of 173 NHS Trusts, he found that many were using arbitrary rules and policies to limit the supply of continence pads, rather than conducting individual assessments of need. The common pad allowance was five (47 Trusts) with one Trust only supplying a maximum of two pads in 24 hours. In addition, there were inflexible rules around the provision of either washable or disposable pads. The study concluded that many policies offered no more than the illusion of rationality and really served to provide a formal basis for the legitimization of controls over supply that owed more to the exigencies of local budgets than to patients' clinical needs (Anthony 1998).

As a result of these variations, the Department of Health (2000) issued the following guidance:

- Continence products should not be supplied before an initial continence assessment, which should be carried out without delay. Products may be needed temporarily by patients awaiting or undergoing treatment and by those whose incontinence has proved intractable to treatment. Incontinence pads have sometimes been perceived as a quick fix in the past, leading to misuse and overuse.
- Pads should be provided in quantities appropriate to the individual's continence needs. Arbitrary ceilings are inappropriate. Guidelines should be developed for the primary health care team to aid product choice, but these should not be seen as rules.

References

Anthony B. Provision of continence supplies by NHS Trusts. London: Middlesex University; 1998.

Department of Health. Good practice in continence services. London: Department of Health; 2000.

---

selection of pads and the majority discharge patients with only a few days' supply of pads. It is therefore important that a patient supplied with pads on discharge from hospital is reassessed by the community nursing team to prevent problems with supply. It can be extremely distressing for someone to run out of pads within a few days of arriving home.

In the UK, incontinence pads are provided free without prescription charges after assessment by nursing staff. The vast majority of budgets for incontinence pad provision are held by primary care trusts. The responsibility for budget control is usually delegated to the local continence nurse specialist or continence advisor (see Special Issues box 12.1).

It is not unusual for a general practitioner to refer a patient who complains of incontinence directly to community nursing services for pads. However, a drawback to free supply of pads might be that the use of pads is seen as a solution, enabling the patient to feel safe and reluctant to attempt a treatment programme. A culture can arise where the only solution is to provide a pad. The patient then comes to believe that a pad is the only answer.

Disposable body-worn pads

This is the most commonly used product for managing incontinence. Most pads have a non-woven cover stock and absorbent cellulose core. Considerable research and technology have gone into improving pad design by using different types of pulp, varying pulp distribution for maximum effect, channelling or compressing the pad to maximum absorbency and incorporating super-absorbent polymers. Likewise with the waterproof backing, which may be micro-embossed or covered with non-woven cover stock to minimize skin adherence (Evans & White 2000).

Continence appliances

Such appliances include uro-sheaths in men, catheters for intermittent catheterization and long-term catheters. The annual cost incurred in the provision of appliances in the UK has been estimated to be in the region of £59 million (The Continence Foundation 2000). The majority of these products are only available on prescription. Hospital nurses are able to order them from hospital supplies departments, but until recently, in the community, they had to be prescribed by a general practitioner. Doctors receive little, if any, education on product types and availability and have therefore been in a difficult position where prescribing is concerned. With the advent of nurse prescribing by community nurses, this situation is changing with nurses becoming more proactive in choosing products and prescribing for individual patients. Over the next few years, the categories of nurses who can prescribe them will expand to include hospital nurses.

The majority of individuals who use continence appliances do not have to pay prescription costs because they usually have illnesses or disabilities which exempt them, such as multiple sclerosis, diabetes or spinal injuries. Furthermore, the elderly are exempt from all prescription charges. However, a small section of the population will have to pay and affording this can be quite difficult for those on low incomes.

Catheters

The selection of urinary catheters tends to be based on expert opinion, although there are a few studies that measure encrustation and catheter blockage of the various types (Morris & Stickler 1999). There are several different materials used in the manufacture of urethral catheters and each is suitable in a different situation (Evans & White 2000):

- Latex – used for short-term catheterization (these and the 'siliconized' latex type are not suitable for patients with a suspected latex allergy)
- 'Siliconized' latex – where the silicone facilitates ease of insertion; used for short-term catheterization
- Plastic (PVC) – used when the urine contains a lot of debris, in particular postoperatively; for short-term use only
- Latex coated with an inert material such as Teflon or PTFE – used for short- to medium-term catheterization
- Silicone (silicone elastomer) coated or encapsulated catheters – used for long-term catheterization
- All silicone – used for long-term catheterization
- Hydrogel-coated or encapsulated catheters – used for long-term catheterization. Hydrogels (used to make soft contact lenses) facilitate insertion and have similar properties to all-silicone when in place.

For long-term catheterization, the catheter of choice is hydrogel-coated. As well as providing a smooth surface, minimizing trauma and urethral irritation, encrustation is also reduced. One hundred per cent silicone catheters should also be considered, especially if the patient may have a latex allergy. Cox et al (1998) and Morris & Stickler (1999) found that there is no significant difference between silicone or hydrogel catheters and their level of encrustation; both performed equally well.

A catheter valve can be used instead of a drainage bag. The patient simply opens the valve to drain out urine. It is very discreet and consequently liked by patients. However, their use is contraindicated in patients with an overactive bladder because a detrusor contraction can lead to bypassing. Research into their use is limited but it is believed that they can lessen catheter blockage because of the periodic 'flushing' effect of opening the valve to empty the bladder (Doherty 1999). Use of a valve rather than continuous drainage is also thought to reduce risk of trauma/erosion to the bladder wall because, as the bladder fills, the bladder wall moves further away from the catheter.

Uro-sheaths

A uro-sheath, also known as a penile sheath, condom urinal external catheter or incontinence sheath, is a soft rubber, latex or plastic sleeve, which fits over the penis like a condom and is then attached to a urine drainage bag. A uro-sheath is not suitable (Evans & White 2000) for:

- men with a very small retracted penis, as attachment is difficult and unreliable
- some very confused or demented men, who may pull the sheath off
- a few men with skin that is sensitive to the rubber in the sheath
- men with limited physical abilities who may not be able to manage putting on the sheath alone and can only use sheaths if a relative or other carer is willing to help.

It is important that the sheath is applied correctly to ensure that it stays in place. Prior to using the sheath, the penis should be measured using the guides provided by the manufacturer, otherwise it could be too tight or too big. Evans & White (2000) have produced guidelines for using a sheath (see Guidelines for Care Priorities box 12.2).

 GUIDELINES FOR CARE PRIORITIES

12.2 Application of a urinary sheath

- First wash and dry the genital area thoroughly. Long pubic hairs should be trimmed (there is no need to shave pubic hairs). Avoid using creams or powders on the penis, as these will prevent the sheath from sticking.
- If adhesive is used, apply this to the penis following manufacturer's instructions. Generally, adhesive strips should be placed about halfway along the penis and not overlapped unless made of elastic.
- Unroll the sheath over the penis. Make sure that the foreskin is not pulled back to expose the head of the penis. A gap of about 2.5 cm should be left between the tip of the penis and the outlet of the sheath to allow for sudden gushes of urine but prevent pressure on the penis itself. Too large a gap will risk the sheath becoming twisted. The sheath should be firmly held in position to allow the adhesive to work.

Leg drainage bags

Leg bags should be used for patients with uro-sheaths and catheters who are up and about. They come with male and female length tubing and different bag capacities ranging from 350 mL to 1.5 litres. They are easily hidden under clothing and can be attached to the leg either with straps or with special leg bag holders. There are also special leg bags for wheelchair users, which bend over the knee as the individual is in the sitting position.

Faecal collector

Faecal collection pouches look rather like a stoma bag and fit over the anus. They have been used successfully with acutely ill, terminally ill and bed-bound patients, where they can improve dignity and reduce the distress, pain and skin damage caused by frequent perineal cleansing.

SUMMARY: MAIN POINTS

- Bladder and bowel symptoms, including incontinence, occur frequently in the adult population.
- Bladder and bowel symptoms can lead to social isolation and depression, especially in the elderly.
- A full and appropriate assessment is necessary, not simply the use of pads and catheters.
- Behavioural programmes, including fluid manipulation, toileting programmes and pelvic floor exercises, can greatly improve an individual's continence status.
- There are a wide variety of products available to help manage incontinence symptoms. These need to be used appropriately.

SELF-TEST: CRITICAL THINKING ACTIVITIES

1 A patient on an older adult ward is complaining of frequency, urgency and some urge incontinence. What would you consider to be important components of any assessment you carry out and what questions would you ask?

2 Once you have assessed the patient, what treatment and management strategies might you use in order to improve

the symptoms? What barriers might you face, from either colleagues or the patient?

3 A patient is complaining of constipation – what lifestyle advice might you give?

 FURTHER READING

Doughty DB. Urinary and fecal incontinence, 2nd edn. St Louis: Mosby; 2000.

Getliffe K, Dolman M (eds). Promoting continence: a clinical and research resource. London: Baillière Tindall; 1997.

Laycock J, Haslam J (eds). Therapeutic management of incontinence and pelvic pain: pelvic organ disorders. London: Springer; 2002.

Roe B (ed). Clinical nursing practice: the promotion and management of continence. London: Prentice Hall; 1992.

Norton C (ed). Nursing for continence, 2nd edn. Beaconsfield: Beaconsfield Publishers; 1996.

Schussler B, Llaycock J, Norton P, Stanton S (eds). Pelvic floor re-education: principles and practice. London: Springer-Verlag; 1994.

 USEFUL ADDRESSES

Incontact
United House
North Road
London N7 9DP
Tel: 0870 770 3246
e-mail: info@incontact.org
www.incontact.org
A charity that provides information and support for people affected by bladder and bowel problems. They coordinate user support groups around the country

The Continence Foundation
307 Hatton Square
16 Baldwins Gardens
London EC1N 7RJ
Helpline: 020 7831 9831
www.continence-foundation.org.uk
A charity that produces a range of leaflets on various topics. They also run a national helpline staffed by nurses

PromoCon
Redbank House
St Chad's Street
Manchester M8 8QA
Tel: 0161 834 2001
A charity that offers advice and information on products that can help manage bladder and bowel problems

Radar
12 City Forum
250 City Road
London EC1V 8AF
Tel: 020 7250 3222
A charity that has information about keys for disabled toilet facilities, as well as information about holiday accommodation that caters for people with continence problems

REFERENCES

Abrams P, Klevmar B. Frequency volume charts – an indispensable part of lower urinary tract assessment. Scand J Urol Nephrol 1996; 179: 47–53.

Abrams P, Blaivas JG, Stanton et al. Standardisation of terminology of lower urinary tract function. Neurourol Urodyn 1988; 7: 403–407.

Abrams P, Cardozo L, Fall M et al. The standardisation of terminology of lower urinary tract function: report from the standardisation sub-committee of the International Continence Society. Neurol Urodyn 2002; 21: 167–178.

Agency for Health Care Policy and Research. Urinary incontinence in adults: acute and chronic management. Clinical practice guidelines, No. 2 1996 update. Washington: US Dept of Health and Human Services; 1996.

Arya LA, Myers DL, Jackson ND. Dietary caffeine intake and the risk for detrusor instability: a case-control study. Obs Gyn 2000; 96: 85–89.

Ashton-Miller JA, DeLancey JOL. The knack: use of precisely-timed pelvic muscle contraction can reduce leakage in stress urinary incontinence. Neurourol Urodyn 1996; 15: 392–330.

Audit Commission. First assessment: a review of district nursing services in England and Wales. London: The Audit Commission; 1999.

Baylis V, Davies L, Gunner C et al. North Hampshire bowel care pathway. London: GI Education, Norgine Ltd; 2001.

Bo K, Talseth T, Holme I. Single blind, randomised controlled trial of pelvic floor exercises, electrical stimulation, vaginal cones and no treatment in management of genuine stress incontinence in women. Br Med J 1999; 318(7182): 487–494.

Brubaker L. Electrical stimulation in overactive bladder. Urology 2000; 55: 17–23.

Burns PA, Pranikoff K, Nochajski TH et al. A comparison of effectiveness of biofeedback and pelvic muscle exercise treatment of stress incontinence in older community-dwelling women. J Gerontol 1993; 48: M167–174.

Button D, Roe B, Webb C et al. Consensus guidelines – continence promotion and management by the primary health care team. London: Whurr; 1998.

Cardozo L. Urinary incontinence in women: do we have anything new to offer? Br Med J 1991; 303(6815): 1453–1457.

Cardozo L. Discussion: the effect of estrogens. Urol. 1997; 50: 85.

Chang PL. Urodynamic studies in acupuncture for women with frequency, urgency and dysuria. J Urol 1988; 140: 563–566.

Cheater F. Retrospective document survey: identification, assessment and management of urinary incontinence in medical and care of the elderly wards. J Adv Nurs 1993; 18: 1734–1746.

Continence Foundation. Making the case for investment in an integrated continence service: a source book for continence services. London: Continence Foundation; 2000.

Cox AJ, Hukins DWL, Sutton TM. Comparison of in vitro encrustation on silicone and hydrogel-coated latex catheters. Int J Urol 1998; 61: 156–161.

Creighton S, Stanton S. Caffeine: does it affect your bladder? Br J Urol 1990; 66: 13–14.

Department of Health. Essence of care: patient-focused benchmarking for health care professionals. London: Department of Health; 2001.

Dorey G. Male patients with lower urinary tract symptoms 1: assessment. Br J Nurs 2000a; 9: 497–501.

Dorey G. Male patients with lower urinary tract symptoms 2: treatment. Br J Nurs 2000b; 9: 553–558.

Elser DM, Wyman JF, McClish DK, Robinson D, Fantl JA, Bump RC and the Continence Programme for Women Research Group. The effect of bladder training, pelvic floor muscle training, or combination training on urodynamic parameters in women with urinary incontinence. Neurourol Urodyn 1999; 18: 427–436.

Emberton M, Neal DE, Black N et al. The effect of prostatectomy on symptom severity and quality of life. Br J Urol 1996; 77: 233–247.

Evans D, White H. The continence products directory, 5th edn. London: Continence Foundation; 2000.

Flynn R. Structure and function in continence and incontinence. In: Luca M, Emery S, Beynon, eds. Incontinence. Oxford: Blackwell Science; 1999.

Fonda D, Benvenuti F, Castleden M et al. Management of incontinence in older people. In: Abrams P, Khoury S, Wein A, eds. Incontinence. First International Consultation on Incontinence. World Heath Organization and International Union Against Cancer. Plympton: Plymbridge Distribution; 1999, pp 731–733.

Getliffe K, Dolman M (eds). Promoting continence: a clinical and research resource. London: Baillière Tindall; 1997.

Gilbert RM. Caffeine consumption. In: Spiller GA, ed. The methylxanthine beverages and foods: chemistry, consumption and health effects. New York: Alan R. Liss; 1984, pp 185–214.

Glickman S, Kamm MA. Bowel dysfunction in spinal cord injury patients. Lancet 1996; 347: 1651–1653.

Godec C, Cass AS, Ayala GF. Electrical stimulation for incontinence: technique, selection and results. Urology 1976; 7(4): 388–397.

Goke M, Ewe K, Donner K et al. Influence of loperamide oxide on the anal sphincter: a manometric study. Dis Colon Rectum 1992; 35: 857–861.

Grimby A, Milsom I, Molander U et al. The influence of urinary incontinence on the quality of life of elderly women. Age Ageing 1993; 22: 82–89.

Hancock R, Bender P, Dayhoff N, Nyhuis A. Factors associated with nursing interventions to reduce incontinence in hospitalized older adults. Urol Nurs 1996; 16: 79–85.

James JE, Sawczuk D, Merrett S. The effect of chronic caffeine consumption on urinary incontinence in psychogeriatric inpatients. Psychol Health 1989; 3: 297–305.

Janssen CCC, Lagro-Janssen ALM, Felling AJA. The effects of physiotherapy for female urinary incontinence: individual compared with group treatment. BJU Int 2001; 87: 201–206.

Jeffcoate TNA, Francis WJA. Urgency incontinence in the female. Am J Obs Gyn 1996; 94: 604–618.

Kamm MA. Obstetric damage and faecal incontinence. Lancet 1994; 344: 730–733.

Laycock J. Biofeedback control. In: Schussler B, Laycock J, Norton P, Stanton S, eds. Pelvic floor re-education: principles and practice. London: Springer-Verlag; 1994.

Laycock J, Chiarelli P, Haslam J, Lavender R, Mann K, Naylor D. Pelvic floor exercises: are we teaching them correctly? Neurourol Urodyn 2001; 20: 427–428.

Lindstrom S, Fall M. The neurophysiological basis of bladder inhibition in response to intravaginal electrical stimulation. J Urol 1983; 1129: 381–389.

McClish DK, Wyman JF, Sales PG, Camp J, Earle B. Use and costs of incontinence pads in female study volunteers. Continence Program for Women Research Group. J Wound Ostomy Continence Nurs 1999; 4: 207–208, 210–213.

Malone-Lee J. Recent developments in urinary incontinence in later life. Physiotherapy 1994; 80: 133–134.

Miller K, Richardson DA, Sidgel SW, Karram MM, Blackwood NB, Sand PK. Pelvic floor electrical stimulation for genuine stress incontinence: who will benefit and when? Int Urogynaecol J 1998; 9: 265–270.

Milsom I, Abrams P, Cardozo L, Roberts RG, Thuroff J, Wein AJ. How widespread are the symptoms of an overactive bladder and how are they managed? A population-based prevalence study. Br J Urol Int 2001; 87: 760–766.

Morris NS, Stickler DJ. Encrustation of indwelling urethral catheters by *Proteus mirabilis* biofilms growing in human urine. J Hospital Infect 1999; 39: 227–234.

Norton PA, MacDonald LD, Sedgewick PM et al. Distress and delay associated with urinary incontinence, frequency and urgency in women. Br Med J 1998; 297: 1187–1189.

O'Keefe EA, Tally NJ, Zinsmeister AJ et al. Bowel disorders impair functional status and quality of life in the elderly: a population-based study. J Gerontol A Biol Sci Med Sci 1995; 50: 184–189.

COMMON NURSING ISSUES

12

Pearson BD, Kelber S. Urinary incontinence: treatments, interventions and outcomes. Clin Nurse Special 1996; 10: 177–182.

Peattie AB, Plevnik S, Stanton SL. Vaginal cones: a conservative method of treating genuine stress incontinence. Br J Obs Gyn 1988; 95: 1049–1053.

Pegne A, de Goursac F, Nyssen C, Barrat J. Acupuncture and the unstable bladder. London: Proceedings of the 14th Internal Continence Meeting; 176–177.

Perry SI, Shaw C, Mensah CW et al and the MRC Incontinence Study Team. The prevalence of faecal incontinence in a community-based population. Proceedings of the British Geriatrics Society Spring Meeting, Edinburgh; 1998.

Petticrew M, Watt I, Sheldon T. Systematic review of the effectiveness of laxatives in the elderly. Executive summary, Vol. 13. NHS Research and Development, Health Technology Assessment Programme. London: HMSO; 1998.

Philp T, Shah PRJ, Worth PHL. Acupuncture in the treatment of bladder instability. Br J Urol 1988; 61: 490–493.

Robinson D, McClish D, Wyman JF, Bump RC, Fanti JA. Comparison between urinary diaries completed with and without intensive patient instructions. Neurourol Urodyn 1996; 15: 143–148.

Royal College of Physicians. Incontinence – causes, management and provision of services. London: RCP; 1995.

Sampselle CM, Burns PA, Dougherty MC, Newman DK, Thomas KK, Wyman JF. Continence for women: evidence-based practice. J Obs Gyn Neonat Nurs 1997; 26: 375–385.

Sapsford RR, Hodges PW, Richardson CA, Cooper DH, Markwell SJ, Jull GA. Co-activation of the abdominal and pelvic floor muscles during voluntary exercises. Neurourol Urodyn 2001; 20: 31–42.

Schultz A, Dickey G, Skinner M. Self-support of incontinence in acute care. Urol Nurs 1997; 17: 23–28.

Stapleton A, Stamm WE. Prevention of urinary tract infection. Infect Dis Clin N Am 1997; 113: 719–733.

Stewart W, Herzog R, Wein A, Abrams P, Payne C, Corey R, Hunt T and the NOBLE Program Research Team. The prevalence and impact of overactive bladder in the US: results from the noble programme. Neurourol Urodyn 2001; 20: 406–408.

Thompson GW, Creed F, Drossman AJ et al. Functional bowel disease and functional abdominal pain. Gastroenterol Int 1992; 5: 75–91.

Thuroff JW, Chartier-Kastler E, Cocus J et al. Medical treatment and medical side effects in urinary incontinence in the elderly. W J Urol 1998; 16: S48–S61.

Wagg A, Malone-Lee J. The management of urinary incontinence in the elderly. Br J Urol 1998; 82: 11–17.

Wald A. Constipation and faecal incontinence in the elderly. Semin Gastrointest Dis 1994; 5: 179–188.

Wheeler JS, Peters MJ. Anatomy and physiology of voiding, Chapter 1. In: Doughty DB (ed) Urinary and fecal incontinence. Nurs Mgt 1991. St Louis: Mosby Yearbook.

Whitehead WE, Drinkwater D, Chesking LJ et al. Constipation in the elderly living at home. Definition, prevalence and relationship to lifestyle and health status. J Am Geriatr Soc 1989; 37: 423–429.

Wolfson CR, Barker JC, Mitteness LS. Constipation in the daily lives of frail elderly people. Archiv Family Med 1993; 2: 853–858.

Wolin LH. Stress incontinence in young healthy nulliparous female subjects. J Urol 1996; 101: 545–549.

13 Infection control

Paul Hateley

'I couldn't believe it – the timetable said hand washing! I thought I already knew how to do that but I now know that it's a bit different when you're a nurse. You have to wash your hands in a particular way to make sure you don't pass on infection or catch anything yourself. If only all the other skills were so easy to get right!'

(Student nurse)

THIS CHAPTER WILL HELP YOU

- Understand the principles of infection control in clinical practice

- Identify the pathogenic bacteria that cause hospital- and community-acquired infections

- Discuss the principles of infection control practice in managing outbreaks of infection

- Demonstrate safe and effective hand hygiene

- Discuss the issues relating to the prevention and control of methicillin-resistant *Staphylococcus aureus* (MRSA)

- Understand the principles of universal infection control precautions and source and protective isolation.

KEYWORDS

Antimicrobial	Inoculation injury
Bacteria	Isolation
Colonization	Microorganism
Contamination	Normal flora
Cross-infection	Nosocomial infection
Handwashing	Pathogenic
Hospital-acquired infection (HAI)	Sepsis
Infection	Universal precautions
	Virus

INTRODUCTION

Infection control in health care premises is both a legal and a moral obligation for all health care workers. Studies looking at rates of infection in hospital have shown that about 1 in 10 patients acquire an infection as a direct result of their hospitalization, with a similar number of infections acquired in the community and present upon admission to hospital (Meers et al 1981, Plowman et al 1999).

Although infections in hospital and in the community are common, they are largely preventable. Practising infection control safely will prevent the transmission of organisms between staff, from patients to staff, from staff to patients and from patient to patient. Routine infection control practices should be utilized in the care of all patients and they include key procedures that minimize the transmission of organisms, such as handwashing, protective clothing, the safe management of all body fluids and good hygiene and cleaning standards. Infection control nursing as a specialty is now over 40 years old, but the role of infection control teams is to provide expert advice; individual practitioners are responsible for the implementation of that advice to ensure their practice is safe. This is the key to ensuring a safe environment.

The most frequently seen infections in hospital are those of the urinary tract, surgical wounds, lower respiratory tract and skin. The frequency and severity vary according to many factors, including age, the surgical intervention, invasive procedures such as urinary catheters or intravenous cannulae, immuno-suppressive treatments and the patient's own ability to respond to exposure to pathogenic bacteria.

By the very nature of their work, health care professionals expose patients to microbiological risks. Just by entering a hospital, patients exchange their secure home environment, where most organisms are not disease-causing, for an environment which may not have the same standard of cleanliness and in which many organisms have developed a resistance to antibiotics. Sharing facilities, equipment and staff with other patients further compounds this risk.

MICROBIOLOGY

Microbiology is the study of living organisms, most of which are so small they cannot be seen with the naked eye, only under a microscope. Microbes live everywhere. They are able to survive almost every type of environment where many other plants and animals cannot. Some can withstand temperatures in excess of 95°; others live well below freezing point. Some require oxygen to survive (aerobic organisms), while others survive well without it (anaerobic organisms). Bacteria are identified through a system of classification. Various forms of classification have been in existence for almost 200 years.

Bacteria of a species can be further distinguished into different strains based on the identification of different characteristics. This subdivision often requires complex techniques undertaken within a laboratory, examining bacterial cells under a microscope, identifying important information in relation to the structure and shape of the organisms. The two main shapes are round, usually referred to as cocci, or oblong, which are bacilli or rods. Over 100 years ago, Christian Gram developed a method of staining cell walls with dyes which today is known as a Gram stain. It is a fairly straightforward practical procedure and classifies bacteria into Gram-positive and Gram-negative. The Gram-positive organisms absorb the dark blue dye and are identified as blue under a microscope. Gram-negatives do not absorb the dye but, when stained with a red dye, stain reddish-pink, thus differentiating between Gram-positive and Gram-negative bacteria. Microscopy (examining under a microscope) and Gram staining are two of the most frequently used methods for provisional identification.

METHODS OF GROWING ORGANISMS

Bacteria cannot reliably be identified under a microscope. Therefore they are grown (cultured) in special media and, depending on the type, a whole range of tests is used to identify each particular organism. The most frequently used media comprise a mixture of nutrients with blood agar containing horse blood. A change in the balance of chemicals within these media is utilized to reflect more closely the environment in which the pathogens would normally grow and facilitate the growth of pathogenic organisms over and above the normal flora, thus making them easier to identify. Organisms that usually live on or cause disease in humans grow best in a medium that would be similar to the secretions or tissues of that part of the human body. The agar is then incubated at body temperature for up to 40 hours to encourage the organisms to grow.

IDENTIFYING THE ORGANISM

Once the culture has taken place and the organism has grown (or cultured), further testing may then be undertaken to identify the exact species. There are many ways of doing this, but more recently there has been an increase in commercially prepared kits available on the market, which facilitate an accurate and quick identification. They are usually inoculated with a small amount of organism, incubated for between 12 and 24 hours, and then a colour change mapped against the control is used to identify the species.

ANTIMICROBIAL RESISTANCE

Once the organism has been identified, it is extremely important to establish whether or not it remains sensitive to the group of antimicrobial agents that are usually used to treat a systemic infection. Antibiotic sensitivity testing is undertaken by spreading the organism evenly over an agar plate. The organism is then exposed to small pieces of paper (discs) impregnated with antibiotic, and incubated for a further period, usually 18–24 hours. If the antibiotic is sensitive to the organism, it will eradicate organism growth around the disc. If it is resistant, a growth will occur up to and over the paper disc.

TYPES OF ORGANISM

Bacteria

Bacteria live in a variety of environments and require a variety of nutrients to survive. Whilst being fed by these nutrients, bacteria will continue to divide and replicate until the supply of nutrients is no longer available and then the cells may die off.

Fungi are essentially plants. They have eukaryotic cells but are lacking any type of the green pigment that other plants use for photosynthesis. Most fungi groups are filamentous and are often described as moulds. Others, however, may grow as ovid cysts and are referred to as yeasts. Many species of fungi can replicate either as a yeast or a mould, depending on the temperature and the supply of nutrients and oxygen available. The study of fungi is referred to as mycology.

Protozoa are relatively large organisms. They have a very tough outer cell membrane as opposed to a cell wall. Nutrients are obtained by ingesting solid food particles. The cells multiply by dividing in two. Many protozoa have life cycles, i.e. there are various stages of their development. They are motile in many of these stages and some are capable of forming dormant cyst-like formations which, when disturbed, are an important issue in their transmission.

Viruses

Viruses, unlike other organisms, are not cells. They are a piece of nucleic acid, either RNA or DNA, protected by an envelope of lipids. Viruses contain none of the structures necessary to synthesize the proteins encoded by their nucleic acid. Viruses are very small compared to other bacteria and can usually only be seen under an electron microscope, which uses a beam of electrons instead of light to create the visible image. Viruses can only multiply inside living cells.

CLASSIFICATION OF MICROORGANISMS

A process of identifying organisms and their relationship to each other has been developed. Organisms are placed into groups according to similar characteristics in their structure. This classification revolves around the genus and the species. The genus denotes the group (e.g. *Staphylococcus*) to which they belong and the species gives the organism a specific name within that group, e.g. *Staphylococcus epidermidis* or *Staphylococcus aureus*. Bacteria of a particular species can be further identified by using different strains.

RESISTANCE TO ANTIBIOTICS

The increase in microorganisms that are highly resistant to antibiotics is a major international problem. Many of these are associated with hospital-acquired infections, particularly when antimicrobial usage is high, resulting in frequent opportunities to spread between patients in the same areas. Antibiotic-resistant organisms commonly seen in the UK are methicillin-resistant *Staphylococcus aureus* (MRSA), vancomycin-resistant *enterococcus* (VRE), *Clostridium difficile* and multiple drug-resistant *Mycobacterium tuberculosis* (MDRTB).

Methicillin-resistant *Staphylococcus aureus* (MRSA)

The management and control of MRSA (see Special Issues box 13.1) is a typical example of an antibiotic-resistant microorganism. Work by the Combined Working Party of the British Society of Antimicrobial Therapy & Hospital Infection Society

 SPECIAL ISSUES

13.1 Management of methicillin-resistant *staphylococcus aureus*

Infections caused by *Staphylococcus* are an important cause of morbidity and mortality and are costly in terms of treatment and disruption due to outbreaks. Outbreaks are difficult to control and require strict adherence to local protocols. Precautionary measures must be instituted when the organism is first isolated or suspected. These measures can then be modified if the organism is found to be less aggressive (Horton & Parker 1997). Screening for MRSA usually includes taking swabs from the nose, perineum and throat plus any wounds or skin lesions. If patients are catheterized, a catheter specimen of urine should be obtained. If patients are expectorating sputum, a sputum specimen should be obtained.

- Educate patients and their visitors about the need for isolation/precautions
- Wear gloves and aprons for direct patient contact
- Wash and dry the hands thoroughly after every patient contact. Visitors do not need to wear protective clothing but must wash and dry their hands before they leave
- If a wound is infected with MRSA, keep it covered whenever possible, to prevent dissemination of MRSA into the environment
- Linen is infected. Use the appropriate used linen bag
- All waste must be discarded as clinical waste
- Administer the MRSA protocol as prescribed and administer antibiotics if prescribed
- Re-screen in accordance with local protocol
- Swabs for MRSA clearance must not be taken whilst the patient is on MRSA protocol

When in doubt, contact the infection control nurse.

Reference

Horton R, Parker L. Informed infection control practice. Edinburgh: Churchill Livingstone; 1997.

and Infection Control Nurses Association (MRSA Working Party Report 1998) has shown that MRSA is present in most hospitals in most countries, with new epidemic strains appearing in the UK in the early 1980s. Many epidemic strains are only sensitive to vancomycin or teicoplanin. In addition to hospital problems, the presence of MRSA in the community and the wider movement of patients and staff between both hospital and primary care facilities have further increased the difficulties in controlling it.

Vancomycin-resistant *enterococcus* (VRE)

The emergence of vancomycin-resistant *enterococcus* (VRE) has been causing much difficulty. New strains are increasingly being reported, and over the last decade VRE has caused devastation in the USA in relation to their infection control programmes, with some severe untreatable infections (Lucas et al 1998).

Clostridium difficile

Outbreaks of *Clostridium difficile*, also referred to as *C. diff.* or CDT, on hospital wards have also caused problems throughout the last two decades. This is associated with antimicrobial therapy use when the gut flora is destabilized, allowing an increase in *Clostridium difficile*, and therefore diarrhoea is an everyday occurrence to be dealt with by infection control teams (see Guidelines for Care Priorities box 13.1). Effective treatment of *Clostridium difficile* remains either oral metronidazole or oral vancomycin. However, despite both antibiotics remaining effective to *Clostridium difficile*, both have been found to cause *Clostridium difficile* diarrhoea in some patients, particularly when administered intravenously.

Mycobacterium tuberculosis (MDRTB)

In recent years, antibiotic-resistant strains of *Mycobacterium tuberculosis* (MDRTB) have been responsible for small outbreaks of hospital-acquired infection, most of which have been associated with immunocompromised patients, in particular those with HIV and AIDS. Prevention of spread to staff by the use of particulate filter respiratory masks has received much attention, especially in the USA. These masks filter microbes as small as 0.2 μm (microns), which includes all bacteria and most viruses.

Gram-negative organisms

Gram staining is a method of identification and classification of microorganisms; those that stain violet are referred to as 'Gram-positive' and those that stain pink are 'Gram-negative' (see p. 254). Gram-negative organisms caused major problems throughout the 1970s and 1980s and continue to do so today, particularly with the increase in invasive procedures. Outbreaks of infection are widely documented with Gram-negative organisms such as *Pseudomonas*, *Klebsiella*, *Enterobacter* and *Serratia marscessans*. Ventilated patients in intensive care units are particularly vulnerable to Gram-negative organisms, as well as those who have undergone major invasive surgery where devices such as drains, cannulae and catheters are used.

Gram-positive organisms

Gram-positive organisms also cause outbreaks of infection, the most frequent of which is MRSA. Other Gram-positive organisms such as group A *Streptococcus* also cause cross-infection, clusters and outbreaks.

GUIDELINES FOR CARE PRIORITIES

13.1 Managing *Clostridium difficile* diarrhoea

Educate patients and staff about the need for isolation and precautions. Ensure adequate fluid balance is maintained and, if possible, record the volume of diarrhoea being passed. Implement stool precautions as detailed below:

- Wash hands and dry thoroughly after contact with stool and/or before leaving room
- Wear gloves and aprons when in contact with stool. *Masks are not necessary*
- Bedpan washer – ensure it is heating to 80°C and holding for 1 minute
- Bedpan macerator lid must be kept closed for 1 minute after the cycle has finished to minimize aerosol dispersal
- Disposable crockery and cutlery are *not required*
- Change *all* bed linen daily – linen is infected; use red alginate bags
- Waste must be discarded into yellow bags
- Explain to patients the need for handwashing after using the toilet and before eating
- Visitors *do not need* protective clothing – but *must* wash and dry their hands thoroughly before leaving the patient area/room
- Stool specimens, if required for clearance, must not be obtained whilst still on treatment
- Stool precautions may be discontinued once the patient has had formed stools for 48 hours
- Decontaminate nursing/medical equipment as appropriate
- For disinfection of room after cleaning (*not* mattress or pillows), the infection control nurse will advise on the appropriate disinfectant
- Check terminal clean is satisfactory. When cleaned, the room/area can be used immediately.

CAUSES OF INFECTION

The occurrence and effects of exposure to potentially pathogenic bacteria and their ability to cause disease and infection depend upon four factors (Ayliffe et al 1992):

- the microorganism(s) – the organism and its ability to cause disease (pathogenicity)
- the host (patients and/or staff) and the response to exposure to pathogenic organisms
- the environment – this includes the microbial load and the ability for the organisms in the environment to cause disease in the host
- treatments – whether there are adequate agents available which continue to be effective against the organisms.

The source of infection in hospital is defined as a place where pathogenic microorganisms are growing or have grown and from which they are transmitted to patients, such as with wound infections.

RESERVOIR OF INFECTION

A reservoir is a place where pathogenic bacteria can survive or sometimes multiply outside the body and from which they can be transferred either directly, such as on unwashed hands, or indirectly through equipment or furniture which has not been thoroughly cleaned. For an organism to cause an infection, a variety of factors are required. Pathogenic organism must be present either on or in living tissue or in the environment or on inanimate objects. This becomes the reservoir. Patients carrying the organism may or may not be symptomatic and, if hospitalized and symptomatic, may be isolated. A portal of exit for the organism must be available, e.g. for infectious diarrhoeas it would be faeces and for a wound infection it would be the infected wound.

MODE OF TRANSMISSION

In order for cross-infection to occur, a means or mode of transmission and a portal of entry are required. In health care settings, the mode of transmission is often the hands of health care workers; the portal of entry will vary. For example, if organisms from infectious diarrhoea are on a health care worker's hands and those hands go around or inside the health care worker's mouth, the organisms could then be swallowed, ingested into the gut, and the health care worker become symptomatic within a period of hours. In the same way, a wound infection may be spread to another wound (portal of entry) on a health care worker's hands (mode of transmission).

Direct contact spread refers to the transfer of infection to a patient via direct contact with an infected person. Indirect contact refers to the acquisition of organisms, such as blood-borne pathogens, from needles and instruments, or microorganisms from bedding, dirt and dust or food and must also include the unwashed hands of hospital staff.

Regardless of the way in which organisms are spread, in order for pathogenic organisms to take hold and cause an infection, they require a susceptible host. This may be another patient, an informal carer or a health care worker.

HOST RESPONSE

The term 'infection' is used to describe the deposition and increase of bacteria and other organisms in tissues or on surfaces of the body which result in an associated tissue reaction (Ayliffe et al 1992).

Subclinical infection and colonization

If there is no tissue reaction in the host or it is subclinical (i.e. there are no overt symptoms of infection), it is termed 'colonization', meaning that the organism is carried but, as there is an absence of any host response, it may not be identified as being present. Colonization in a number of patients may indicate that an organism is spreading in a ward or unit, as seen in many outbreaks of MRSA. Colonized patients will spread the organism to both health care workers and other patients but this may go unnoticed unless somebody exposed to it becomes clinically infected.

Sepsis

Sepsis refers to the presence of inflammation, pus and other signs of infection. Infective illnesses are sometimes described using terms that refer to the site of infection, e.g. pneumonia for the lungs and tonsillitis for the tonsils, or, alternatively, as a specific disease, such as tuberculosis.

Contamination

Contamination refers to the presence of organisms on inanimate objects or living material that may have harmful infectious or unwanted matter.

PATHOGENS

Microorganisms capable of causing disease are called pathogens. Infection is the end result when pathogens have gained access to tissues and established themselves, increased in number and caused an adverse reaction in the host. Over the last century there have been major improvements in public health, sanitation and nutrition, and improvement in housing with fewer patients living with lower deprivation scores. This, coupled with extensive immunization programmes, has brought many infectious diseases, such as diphtheria and measles, under control. In addition, smallpox has been eradicated internationally, and tuberculosis is now fairly well controlled, particularly throughout western Europe.

There are two types of infection – endogenous and exogenous – as described below.

Endogenous infection

Endogenous infection (self-infection) is caused by microorganisms which originate from patients themselves. Some parts of the body such as the lower respiratory tract and the bladder, which are normally free from organisms, are particularly prone to exposure to organisms which may become pathogenic. Other areas, such as the gut, have a wide and varied natural flora (commensal) population of microbes. Normal flora are harmless in the area where they normally live, but migration may result in an infection elsewhere in the body, e.g. gut organisms are the commonest cause of urinary tract infections. The likelihood of a urinary tract infection due to gut flora increases dramatically if a urinary catheter is in situ because organisms can track along the catheter.

Exogenous infection

Exogenous infection is caused by the transfer of a microorganism to an individual. This will have originated either from another patient or health care worker or from the environment. Any hospitalized patient whose normal natural defences to infection are reduced (e.g. those with a surgical wound) will be particularly vulnerable to exogenous infections. This may be from a member of staff who is a *Staphylococcus* carrier, or who may have boils or septic lesions or, more commonly, have failed to wash his or her hands properly.

Pathogens can be subdivided into three types: conventional, conditional and opportunistic.

Conventional pathogens

Conventional 'pathogens' are capable of causing infection in somebody who has previously been healthy. These are organisms that do not form part of the normal flora. An example is β-haemolytic streptococci Lansfield group A (group A *Strep*), which can cause a range of diseases from a sore throat to endocarditis.

Conditional pathogens

Conditional pathogens are capable of causing infection but only under certain circumstances. They are part of the normal flora, but if disturbed from their normal site they can cause an immune response, resulting in infection elsewhere in the body. An example of this would be *Escherichia coli* (*E. coli*) causing a wound infection following bowel surgery.

Opportunistic pathogens

Opportunistic pathogens are pathogens that will only cause infection if the patient's immune defence system is impaired. An example commonly seen with patients who have HIV/AIDS is *Pneumocystis carinii* pneumonia.

HOSPITAL-ACQUIRED (NOSOCOMIAL) INFECTION

A hospital-acquired infection (HAI), also known as a nosocomial infection, is one that is acquired by patients during their hospitalization or by health care workers through their work in the hospital. It is not always possible to determine definitively whether an infection was indeed acquired by the patient in hospital or whether or not it was present prior to admission. The exception to this, of course, is infection of a surgical wound.

CROSS-INFECTION

Cross-infection is slightly different from hospital-acquired infection, and refers to infection acquired from other people, either patients or staff (exogenous), or from the patient's own organisms (endogenous). Endogenous infections are caused by organisms which are normally present, often as normal flora, but which have induced an immune response resulting in infection.

PRINCIPLES OF INFECTION CONTROL

Patients are afforded protection against infection in three principal ways:

- By applying the principles of asepsis to our practice and by high standards of hospital hygiene, the purpose of which is to remove the sources, or potential sources, of infection, i.e. to remove the disease-producing organisms; this includes the treatment of infected patients as well as the cleaning, disinfection and sterilization of equipment, contaminated materials and surfaces (Ayliffe et al 1992)
- By blocking the routes of transfer of bacteria from their potential sources and reservoirs to uninfected patients. Methods include isolation of infected or susceptible patients, applying the principles of asepsis (use of a non-touch technique and sterile gloves) and effective hand hygiene, and the use of protective clothing
- By enhancing the patient's resistance to infection, especially during surgical operations. This is achieved by careful handling of tissues and removal of slough (necrosed tissue)

and foreign bodies, and by enhancing the general defences with reinforcement of the immune system and, when indicated, prophylactic antimicrobial therapy, e.g. prior to bowel surgery. All of these factors, however, will be most widely influenced by the patient's overall physical health, including nutritional status and susceptibility to infection.

In 1968, the Medical Research Council proposed a way of categorizing methods used for the control of infection. Although originally proposed almost 40 years ago, these categories remain as relevant today as when first published. The categories are described by Bagshaw et al (1978) as follows:

- Established methods for which good evidence is available, e.g. handwashing
- Provisionally established methods for which there is some evidence, e.g. maintaining environmental standards
- Rational methods which are consistent with our knowledge of bacteria but which cannot be evaluated by experiments, e.g. maintaining air quality
- Rituals or methods that have been shown by experiment or observation to have no value or even to be harmful, e.g. the use of surgical gowns and overshoes for patients nursed in isolation.

There is a wealth of literature, science and research available on all aspects of infection control. We know that a significant number of infections can be prevented, reducing morbidity and mortality, by applying particular methods of infection control to our practice. The most simple is thorough washing and drying of the hands, yet health care workers consistently fail to do this. However, it should be pointed out that over the last two decades, surveys of infection rates in hospitals have consistently reported figures of around 10%. Given the increasing invasiveness of our interventions, this may in fact indicate a reduction in the overall rate, but there is clearly no room for complacency. There is a core group of patients in most hospitals who are highly susceptible to infection, e.g. those with severe immunosuppression, but in most cases cross-infection is the result of erratic and poor application of the principles of asepsis, coupled with poor standards of cleaning.

THE ROLE OF THE INFECTION CONTROL NURSE

The role of the infection control nurse (ICN) is to provide an advisory service on all aspects of the prevention and control of infection, utilizing methods that are evidence-based, practical and cost-effective. Audit, research and education are key aspects of this role. The ICN and team have a major role in managing outbreaks of infection.

MANAGING OUTBREAKS OF INFECTION

The Department of Health (1995) describes an outbreak of infection either as the occurrence of two or more related cases of the same infection or when the observed number of cases exceeds the number expected. Outbreaks frequently occur both in hospital and in community settings and most involve fairly small numbers. In most incidents or small outbreaks of infection within hospitals, it is the infection control doctor or infection control team who takes the lead in the investigation and implementation of effective control strategies. However, in a major outbreak, it may be more appropriate for the consultant in communicable disease control (CCDC) of the health authority to take the lead. This is particularly important when the outbreak may affect more than just hospital patients and staff, and where there are significant implications for the community, such as that involving a notifiable disease (see Box 13.1) or food poisoning.

Surveillance of infection

Effective surveillance involves the collection, collation, analysis and, most importantly, the dissemination of information. This is essential for the early identification of an increased incidence of alert organisms (organisms that are potentially pathogenic and are of concern to the infection control team), potential outbreaks and trends relating to the incidence of infectious diseases. In the USA, a study of the efficacy of nosocomial infection control (SENIC) conducted over a 6-year period in the late 1970s and early 1980s still provides some of the best evidence as to the value of an infection control team and the efficiency of surveillance of infections (Hayley et al 1995).

Box 13.1 Notifiable infectious diseases

The diseases notifiable in England and Wales are:

- Acute encephalitis
- Acute meningitis
- Acute poliomyelitis
- Anthrax
- Cholera
- Diphtheria
- Dysentery (amoebic and bacillary)
- Food poisoning (suspected or confirmed)
- Infective jaundice
- Lassa fever
- Leprosy
- Leptospirosis
- Malaria
- Marburg (Green monkey)
- Measles
- Meningococcal disease (septicaemia and/or meningitis)
- Mumps
- Ophthalmia neonatorum
- Paratyphoid
- Plague
- Rabies
- Relapsing fever
- Rubella
- Scarlet fever
- Smallpox
- Tetanus
- Tuberculosis
- Typhoid fever
- Typhus
- Viral haemorrhagic fever
- Whooping cough
- Yellow fever

Box 13.1 lists the notifiable infectious diseases in England and Wales. In Scotland the list is similar, but the laws and legislation vary slightly. The statutory notification system is the oldest established source of surveillance information. All formal notifications of food-borne alert organisms and respective diseases are sent to the local authority. Anonymized data are forwarded to the Central Public Health Laboratory and published in the Communicable Disease Report on a weekly basis to identify trends throughout England and Wales.

Outbreak recognition

A communicable disease or potential food-borne illness in the community or health service may come to the attention of many people. Part of an ongoing education campaign is to educate all staff members as to their role in reporting promptly all suspected clusters of cases so that the appropriate investigation and control measures may be implemented. If done in a timely, effective manner, this often prevents further spread. Experienced infection control practitioners will often have knowledge of the normal background level of infection in a particular ward or hospital and normal numbers of potential organisms. Therefore, they can ascertain whether this is an increased risk or whether it falls within normal limits. This factor, although crude, is often the first alert to a potential outbreak. Often an outbreak is not immediately apparent and the expertise of an infection control team is required to link together time, place and person.

Time

The incidence of cases that show symptoms within a short space of time may be the first indication of an outbreak. This may be two or three patients in a ward with diarrhoea and vomiting; two patients who are immunosuppressed and have symptoms of influenza; a sudden increase in the number of cases of diseases such as *Salmonella*; or postoperative wound infections occurring in a group of patients.

Place

Sometimes a cluster of cases occurs in which the same infection is linked by place. The classic example of this is a food-borne illness where a group of people who are all symptomatic have attended the same social event or eaten in the same restaurant.

Person

Often cases can be linked by personal characteristics, such as sex, age and race, particular membership of an organization, or common factors such as similar hobbies or recreational activities. An example of this was the AIDS epidemic, in which the first indication that there was a problem was when opportunistic infections and rare cancers, such as Kaposi's sarcoma, appeared in young homosexual men in California.

OUTBREAK CONTROL

As soon as there is suspicion that a major outbreak may be occurring, an outbreak control committee must be convened. This committee is responsible for deciding on the strategy of the group and the work plan. Any outbreak control committee will only be effective if clear guidelines and strategy are established, with each member of the committee having a specific role and being empowered to act within this capacity. Communication is a key issue when dealing with major outbreaks. Open and frank information must be delivered so that everybody identifies what is going on and believes the strategy is in place. If there is any misinformation or if any information is withheld, the infection control team may lose the trust and support of both staff and the public.

THE ROLE OF THE LABORATORY

Samples will be required for microbiological examination or virological examination to identify causative organisms. The role of the laboratory in early detection and identification is crucial. Advice relating to sampling as well as the expertise of a local infection control team can also be obtained from the Public Health Laboratory Service and their specialist reference laboratories.

The safe collection and handling of specimens is important (see Guidelines for Care Priorities box 13.2). All specimens should be collected immediately before the control measures are introduced. Nothing should be implemented that interferes with the investigation of the outbreak unless it is deemed essential for its control or for patient care. Close liaison with the laboratory at the outset is necessary to ensure that the laboratory staff make adequate arrangements to accommodate the increased workload and that their advice is sought in relation to appropriate specimens. For example, they may be able to confirm that a rectal swab will suffice if a stool specimen cannot be readily obtained. The identification and typing of isolates play a key role in determining whether or not a cluster of cases is in fact an outbreak. It may be that six cases of *Salmonella*, appearing to be a major outbreak, are in fact six different strains. This would indicate a cluster of *Salmonella* infections and not cross-infection.

OUTBREAK CONTROL MEASURES

The control measures necessary during an outbreak will vary according to the nature and source of the infection and its mode of spread and may include:

- systemic antimicrobial therapy or prophylactic therapy (treating a clinical infection or giving antimicrobial therapy to prevent a systemic infection)
- immunization/vaccination
- restriction of admissions into hospital or transfers to other wards to prevent 'seeding' of the outbreak, i.e. dissemination of pathogenic organisms to patients who move between wards and departments
- in some cases, treatment of water cooling towers or drinking water systems.

At the end of the outbreak, a report will be sent to the Communicable Disease Surveillance Centre. A final meeting of the group is then held to review the experiences, identify shortfalls and difficulties, revise the major outbreak policy and make recommendations regarding any improvements that are required to reduce the chance of recurrence of the outbreak. Wide dissemination of the information regarding the outbreak must be a priority. The more people that read it, the more lessons are learnt and the more likely it is that future outbreaks will be prevented.

13.2 Safe collection and handling of specimens

The decision to obtain a specimen for laboratory analysis is usually a medical one, but nurses are responsible for obtaining the specimen. The following points will ensure that good quality specimens arrive safely in the laboratory (Horton & Parker, 1997, p. 161):

- Use the correct container for the specimen. If unsure, check with the laboratory
- Label the container (not the lid) with the patient's details and date. If a series of specimens is required, number them sequentially
- Explain the procedure to the patient
- Wash your hands before and after obtaining a specimen
- If the specimen is to be obtained by needle or aspiration, clean the skin with an alcohol-impregnated swab or chlorhexidine or povidone-iodine in 70% alcohol
- Collect an adequate amount. The greater the quantity of material, the higher the chance of detecting the causative organism. Laboratory staff are more likely to incubate organisms from a sample of pus than from a wound swab
- Moisten a wound swab with sterile water or saline when taking swabs from dry wounds/body surfaces to ensure sufficient organisms are attached to the swab
- Close the container tightly so that it does not leak or become contaminated during transport to the laboratory
- Specimens should be taken before antibiotic therapy is started. If therapy is already in progress, specify the antibiotic(s) on the laboratory request form
- Complete the request form with the patient's details and the specimen site, the diagnosis, date, time and the test requested, e.g. culture and sensitivity
- Use a specimen bag that keeps the form separate from the specimen, preventing contamination
- Send specimens to the laboratory immediately to prevent overgrowth of non-pathogens and death of pathogens
- Refrigerate (at 4°C) specimens that cannot be transported immediately. The fridge should be for specimens only and should not contain food or medicine
- Blood cultures must be kept at body temperature and should be transported to the laboratory immediately and not refrigerated. An incubator should be available for 'out of hours' specimens.

Reference
Horton R, Parker L. Informed infection control practice. Edinburgh: Churchill Livingstone; 1997.

PREVENTION OF INFECTION

The prevention and control of infection are moral and legal obligations for all health care workers. Government initiatives and proposals for league tables of hospital-acquired infections within the NHS in England and Wales mean that the prevention of infection has never had a higher profile. There are a variety of methods that can be implemented to ensure safe and effective practice and reduce the risk of cross-infection to a minimum.

UNIVERSAL INFECTION CONTROL PRECAUTIONS

The risk of spread of hepatitis B, C and HIV viruses in hospitals, although a very low prevalence, has highlighted the importance of the safe handling of blood, bloodstained body fluids and needles and other sharp instruments. The Center for Disease Control (CDC) and the Hospital Infection Control Practices Advisory Committee (HICPAC) guidelines have combined to produce standard precautions, which are designed to reduce the spread from unrecognized sources. These guidelines have been adapted to form the universal infection control precautions (Wilson & Bredan 1990), which involve hand hygiene, the wearing of protective clothing such as gloves, as well as other precautions in handling blood and bloodstained body fluids from all patients (see Guidelines for Care Priorities box 13.3). Body substance isolation (preventing transmission through body fluids) extends to all secretions, not just blood and bloodstained body fluids.

HANDWASHING

Handwashing (also referred to as hand hygiene) is the single most important procedure related to infection control and yet we know it is still not carried out properly (Ayliffe et al 1992). Hateley & Jumaa (1999) conducted a study comparing the frequency and efficacy of handwashing after the use of a toilet in health care workers and the general public. The study found that although health care workers did wash their hands more frequently after using the toilet than the general public, there was not 100% compliance. The overall standard of hand hygiene was poor. Some health care workers will only wash their fingertips or one hand and even that did not involve thorough washing but merely running their fingertips or hand under a tap.

A key role of any infection control programme is effective handwashing and these strategies have been repeated widely by all infection control teams over many years. Hands are the most important vehicles of infection and this is emphasized in most published papers about infection but still requires constant reinforcement (see Evidence-based Practice box 13.1). Hands can become sore after repeated washing and this may account for some people being reluctant to wash their hands as often as they should. Careful drying and frequent use of a safely dispensed hand lotion (individual-use not multi-use pots) supplied in clinical areas should be encouraged. Hot air dryers are not recommended for clinical use (see p. 262).

GUIDELINES FOR CARE PRIORITIES

13.3 Universal infection control precautions

Taking universal precautions means the routine implementation of safe infection control practices based on assessment of the risks associated with the procedure about to be undertaken, not the patient's antibody status (Cockcroft & Elford 1994). The following guidelines are recommended by Horton & Parker (1997):

- Apply good hygiene practices with regular handwashing
- Cover any wounds or skin lesions with waterproof dressings
- Avoid invasive procedures if suffering from chronic skin lesions on the hands
- Protect the mucous membranes of the eyes, mouth and nose from splashes of blood and bloodstained fluids

- Avoid sharps usage wherever possible and institute safe procedures for the use and disposal of sharps when avoidance is not possible
- Institute approved measures for the sterilization and disinfection of instruments and equipment
- Clear up spillages of blood and other body fluids promptly and disinfect the surface
- Institute a safe procedure for the disposal of contaminated waste.

References

Cockcroft A, Elford J. Clinical practice and the perceived importance of identifying high risk patients. J Hosp Infect 1994; 28: 127–136.
Horton R, Parker L. Informed infection control practice. Edinburgh: Churchill Livingstone; 1997.

EVIDENCE-BASED PRACTICE

13.1 Nurses' handwashing practices

The hands of health care personnel are known to be the main means of transmission of microorganisms and effective hand decontamination is the most important means of prevention of infection. Handwashing or decontamination with alcohol hand rub is recommended after every patient contact, but it is recognized that this is impractical in most clinical areas. However, Gould et al (1996) regard it as mandatory in the following situations:

- Following contact with faeces, urine, vomit bowls, soiled bed linen, before and after urinary catheterization and when handling catheter bags
- After contact with blood or body fluids or items contaminated with them
- After extensive patient contact, e.g. bed bathing
- After handling equipment or objects likely to be heavily contaminated, e.g. waste bins, floor cleaning, etc.

- When moving from one patient to another
- After contact with own body secretions, e.g. after blowing one's nose
- After contact with any patient known to be infectious.

A study into nurses' hand decontamination practices (Gould et al 1996) involved 173 nurses in ITU, medical and surgical wards in two hospitals. Each was observed for a 2-hour period. The study found that the hands were washed after only 49.85% of activities that were likely to result in heavy contamination. Hand decontamination was often haphazard rather than being done at times when they were most likely to cause cross-infection. The study concluded that each nurse investigated had considerable potential to cause cross-infection.

Reference

Gould D, Wilson-Barnett J, Ream E. Nurses' infection-control practice: hand decontamination, the use of gloves and sharp instruments. Int J Nurs Studies 1996; 33(2): 143–160.

Handwashing technique

Research by Taylor (1978) showed that the areas most frequently missed during handwashing were between the fingers, the tips of the fingers and the thumbs. The procedure described by Ayliffe et al (1978) is recommended (see Fig. 13.1). Surgical hand disinfection should take 3 minutes and social (hygienic) hand disinfection 30–60 seconds. Thorough drying of the hands is important as moist environments encourage the growth of microorganisms.

For both hygienic hand disinfection and surgical hand disinfection, the same antiseptic soaps are used. The two most commonly used are chlorhexidine and iodine-based products. The difference is in the procedure and the length of time it takes (see p. 262). Alternatives to chlorhexidine and iodine-based products are hexachlorophane and triclosan. These are less frequently used but remain good alternatives if any member of staff shows

an allergic reaction to either chlorhexidine or iodine. Repeated use of antiseptic soaps reduces resident bacteria to low levels.

As previously discussed, hands are one of the main routes of spread of infection. Effective handwashing and disinfection therefore comprise probably the single most important infection control measure. Various studies over the last three decades have identified that health care workers do not wash their hands as often as they should (Ayliffe et al 1992). To improve compliance, it is essential that all products (liquid soap, antiseptic disinfectant, alcohol hand rubs or gels and hand towels) are acceptable to the users, otherwise they simply will not be used. Running water from elbow-operated mixer taps should be used so that the appropriate temperature can be maintained, and a hand towel that is soft and does not cause any trauma to the hands when drying them (see below).

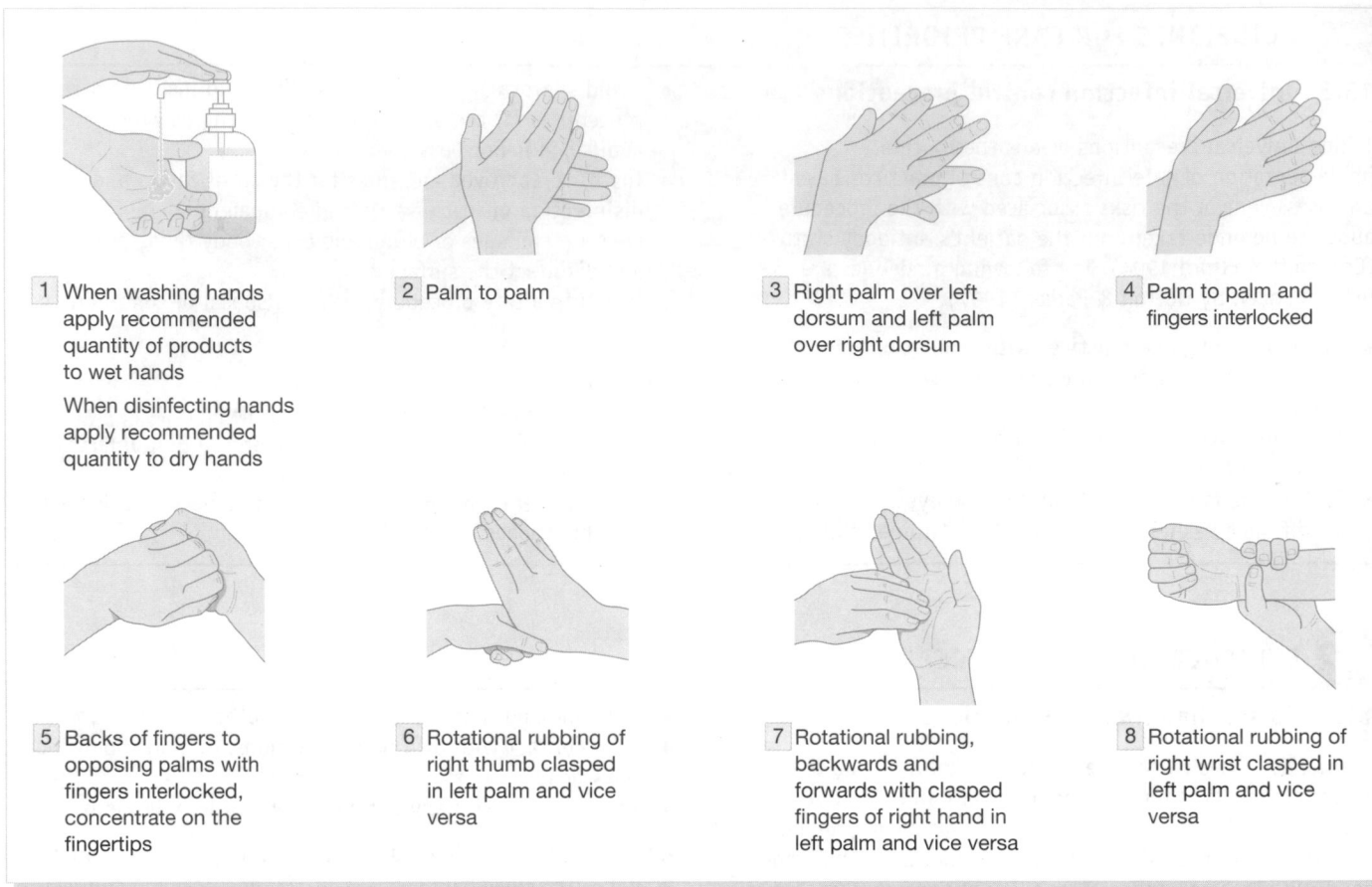

1. When washing hands apply recommended quantity of products to wet hands

   When disinfecting hands apply recommended quantity to dry hands

2. Palm to palm

3. Right palm over left dorsum and left palm over right dorsum

4. Palm to palm and fingers interlocked

5. Backs of fingers to opposing palms with fingers interlocked, concentrate on the fingertips

6. Rotational rubbing of right thumb clasped in left palm and vice versa

7. Rotational rubbing, backwards and forwards with clasped fingers of right hand in left palm and vice versa

8. Rotational rubbing of right wrist clasped in left palm and vice versa

Figure 13.1 Handwashing technique. This technique is based on the procedure described by Ayliffe et al (1978). Using this sequence every time you wash your hands ensures maximum effectiveness. (Reproduced from 'Handwashing technique', Shülke & Mayr UK Ltd, with permission.)

Social handwashing

Social (hygienic) hand disinfection involves washing the hands with a non-medicated soap or liquid soap and water. Hygienic hand disinfection results in the killing of transient organisms and their removal if an antiseptic detergent is used. Washing with soap or detergent and water removes dirt and dead skin cells and the bacteria that are present on them. Non-medicated liquid soap is usually adequate but if bar soap is used, it must be kept dry and not in a dish of fluid because it will quickly become colonized with Gram-negative organisms such as *Pseudomonas* and *Klebsiella*. Liquid soap and detergent are preferred but the dispensers must be regularly cleaned and maintained. Washing hands without a disinfectant is sufficient for most clinical procedures, as the microbial kill is high. However, an antiseptic detergent preparation is usually more effective in reducing transient microorganisms than washing with a non-medicated soap, although the differences are often minimal. Continued use of disinfectant liquid soaps often have an accumulative effect, particularly chlorhexidine (Ayliffe et al 1978). Social handwashing with a liquid soap complemented with an alcohol-based hand rub reduces the microbial load significantly.

Surgical hand disinfection

Surgical hand disinfection is carried out by surgeons and their assistants prior to operations and other invasive procedures.

This involves the killing of transient organisms and also a substantial microbial kill with the number of resident organisms. If an antiseptic detergent is used instead of liquid soap, it is associated with the removal of higher numbers of organisms (Newsome & Rowland 1988).

Hand towels

The type of hand towel is also important. Disposable hand towels must be used in health care facilities; reusable towels encourage bacterial growth as they remain moist and carry high levels of microorganisms from staff who do not wash their hands adequately and deposit organisms onto the towel when they dry them. Rough towels that make the hands sore are unlikely to be used properly. If the hands are not dried thoroughly, the moist environment may encourage colonization with Gram-negative bacteria (see p. 254). Hot air dryers are not recommended for use in clinical areas because they can disperse dirt and dust in the environment around large areas. If not maintained properly, they become dirty and dusty inside and blow organisms onto clean/disinfected hands. In clinical areas, clinical wash hand basins with soft paper towels must be readily available and alcohol-based hand rub is ideal for disinfecting hands where wash hand basins are not easily accessible or inconveniently placed. The infection control team should advise, in the form of a policy, when to wash or use hand rub to disinfect the hands.

Alcohol hand rub

Alcohol hand rubs contain 70% alcohol and emollients to counteract the drying action of the alcohol. They may also contain an antiseptic. Their use significantly reduces the microbial load of transient bacteria on the hands to much lower levels than ordinary handwashing (Pittet et al 2000). A small amount (3 mL) of solution is dispensed into cupped hands and rubbed all over the hands until dry, which takes approximately 30 seconds. As with handwashing, care is necessary to ensure that all areas of the hands receive adequate coverage of alcohol hand rub to ensure microbial kill. A recent study (Kramer et al 2002) found that alcohol-based gels were less effective than liquid hand rub and recommended that they should not be used.

For hands that are visibly soiled, washing with a liquid detergent soap and water is required before the application of any alcohol-based hand rub. The same technique is used for surgical scrub but the application must be extended to cover the forearms.

Alcohol-based solutions clearly have a place in hand hygiene but it must be noted that they have very little effect against some viruses, in particular entero-viruses, due to the minimal time of exposure of the agent to the hands. If contamination is likely with viruses then washing with soap and water prior to the use of an alcohol hand rub is advisable as the viral load is further reduced. However, one of the most common causes of viral diarrhoeal illness, particularly in children, is the rotavirus, against which 70% alcohol-based hand rub is extremely effective (Bellamy et al 1993).

PROTECTIVE CLOTHING

Gowns, gloves, aprons and facemasks have all been widely used to control infection and still have an important role to play although they are often over-used.

Gowns

Water-repellent gowns should be used for any procedures that are likely to cause significant contamination of skin or clothing with blood or bloodstained body fluids, such as in the operating theatre, in the accident and emergency department when dealing with a trauma case, or in the delivery suite. These will protect the skin from contamination and reduce the risk of infection to other patients from clothing.

Gloves

Gloves should be worn when in direct contact with blood or body fluids and for direct contact with non-intact skin or mucous membranes (Infection Control Nurses Association 1999) and the hands must be washed after removal of the gloves. It is important to do this because several studies have identified that, post-use, most surgical gloves have holes in them. Non-surgical gloves have a lower British Standard specification and therefore are likely to have more holes. In addition, the warm, moist environment that is created underneath the gloves encourages the growth of any microorganisms that are present on the hands. Thorough washing after removal will remove these. The choice of sterile or unsterile gloves will depend on assessment of the risks involved in the task being undertaken. The Infection Control Nurses Association (1999) makes the following recommendations:

Sterile gloves. These should be worn when there is a need to protect the patient from infection as well as the practitioner. This includes all aseptic procedures with potential exposure to blood or bloodstained body fluids, e.g. aseptic dressings, insertion of a central venous catheter or urinary catheter. Sterile gloves should also be used for sterile pharmaceutical preparations.

Unsterile gloves. These should be worn to protect the practitioner during:

- Non-aseptic procedures with potential exposure to blood or bloodstained body fluids, e.g. venepuncture.
- Procedures involving the use of 'sharps', e.g. injections, removal of sutures, etc.
- Handling of cytotoxic materials and disinfectants.

Aprons

The front of the body ('nipple to knee' area) is the area most frequently contaminated with body fluids and a disposable plastic apron usually affords adequate protection, e.g. when dealing with spillages and undertaking dressings. Plastic aprons should also be worn during all direct care procedures where contamination of staff clothing is likely, such as bed making and bathing patients. Care should be taken to avoid touching the hair or clothing when putting on and removing the apron, as this may result in contamination with high levels of microbes, which will then contaminate the hands the next time an apron is worn.

Masks

Masks should be worn when there is a risk of respiratory transmission of microorganisms such as tuberculosis. They should also be used when nursing patients with meningococcal meningitis for the first 48 hours following the commencement of antibiotics. This is because the causative organism, *Neisseria meningitidis*, is carried in the nasopharynx of the patient with the disease. Eradication is usually achieved within 48 hours of therapy commencement. A mask should also be worn where there is a danger of blood or bloodstained body fluids being sprayed or splashed into the mouth and nose, e.g. during surgical operations.

An ordinary surgical mask will substantially reduce any aerosol generated by a cough or a sneeze for a short period of time, although this period cannot be clearly defined as it depends on the volume of moisture generated by the wearer (Joint Tuberculosis Committee of the British Thoracic Society 1998). However, handling the masks and continuing to use them when wet from respirations increase the likelihood of contamination. When using a mask, it must be handled as little as possible, must fit snugly and be changed when wet. Once removed, it must never be re-used.

For resistant strains of tuberculosis, particulate filtration masks which will filter particles of 0.2 μm and provide greater than 95% filtration efficiency are recommended for multiple drug-resistant strains of tuberculosis (Belchin 1997). Patients with sensitive or resistant strains of tuberculosis are likely to require investigations and treatments that require them to visit other departments in the hospital. To reduce the risk of infection for those who are not immune to TB, these patients should wear surgical masks while outside their room.

Eye protection

Masks and eye protection should be worn during procedures in which blood, bloodstained body fluids or chemicals may be sprayed or splashed into the mouth or eyes. This includes patients involved in a surgical operation and those who are coughing or vomiting blood or bloodstained fluid. People who wear spectacles do not need to wear additional eye protection.

PREVENTION OF CROSS-INFECTION

There are a number of ways in which patients and staff can be protected from cross-infection, including:

- Universal infection control precautions – as discussed above, protective clothing such as gloves and aprons are used to reduce the risk of contact spread between patients and staff, as well as protecting the staff. The prevention of spread of gastrointestinal infections such as *Salmonella* depends primarily upon the implementation of effective universal infection control precautions
- Segregation or isolation in single rooms or cubicles – to reduce airborne spread to and from patients
- Cohort nursing – this may also be useful and involves putting a group of patients with the same infection together in a separate ward or section/bay of a ward. However, not all patients will become asymptomatic at the same time and there is a danger of re-infection of patients who become clear
- Negative pressure ventilation or ventilation that filters both incoming and outgoing air – this reduces the risk of airborne spread by removing the bacteria from the patient's room with negative pressure and also by the use of protective isolation facilities whereby air going into the room is filtered to protect patients from airborne bacteria outside. Cross-infection via the airborne route from respiratory infections, whether for source or protective isolation, is only really controlled when patients are confined to an isolation facility in a single room or an isolator. The term 'isolation' is usually used to define segregation of patients in a single room.

ISOLATION OF PATIENTS

It is important to minimize the risk of infection to other patients and staff. The spread of infection can easily be controlled by physical protection in terms of isolation, although the extent of this control varies through most hospitals (Garner 1996). However, it is not without problems. To nurse a patient in isolation safely, a risk assessment of the need for isolation must be undertaken. The decision as to the type of isolation should be tailored to the individual requirements of each patient and consider the following:

- the route of transmission of the organism
- the actual risk of spread to other patients and staff
- the severity of the infection and the availability of effective treatments
- the risk of sensory deprivation as a result of isolation
- best practice based on evidence in relation to the hospital policy.

13.1 The effects of isolation

Isolation in a separate room can be a frightening and anxious time for patients, their family members and visitors. Think back to a patient that you have nursed in isolation:

- How do you think your patient felt?
- What (if anything) did you do to minimize the psychological effects of isolation for your patient?

Gammon (1999) found that patients may feel confined, imprisoned and 'shut in' whilst in isolation, and may suffer from depression, disturbed sleep and even hallucinations. They may feel forgotten and worry that no one will respond when they need help. Because nurses need to put on aprons and gloves before entering the room, they are much less likely to 'pop in' to see that the patient is all right. Nurses need to recognize how the patient may be feeling and make a point of entering the room regularly and responding to the call bell quickly.

Reference
Gammon J. The psychological consequences of source isolation: a review of the literature. J Clin Nurs 1999; 8: 13–21.

The transfer from hospital to the community, particularly for patients colonized with MRSA, is often an answer to many of these problems (see Reflective Practice box 13.1).

One of the many problems associated with the isolation of patients is to ensure that members of staff are aware of the interventions necessary to nurse them safely. Isolation policies may encroach on issues such as confidentiality, because certain isolation information or precautions may suggest specific infections such as TB or HIV (see Ethical Issues box 13.1). Unnecessary precautions such as excessive use of disposable clothing or disinfectants add considerably to hospital costs.

There are two types of isolation: source isolation and protective isolation.

Source isolation

Source isolation, previously called barrier nursing, means removing the source of infection, i.e. the patient with the infection or infectious disease, to a single room either on a ward or in an isolation unit to prevent the patient acting as a source of cross-infection to health care workers and other patients. The emphasis on isolation in a single room has declined in recent years as a result of the introduction of universal infection control precautions, which aim to isolate body substances that are capable of carrying infective organisms and blood-borne pathogens. The Center for Disease Control (CDC) and the Hospital Infection Control Practices Advisory Committee (HICPAC) guidelines have combined these to produce standard precautions, which are designed to reduce the spread from unrecognized sources. These measures, which are discussed in detail on pages 261–264, involve wearing non-sterile gloves

ETHICAL ISSUES

13.1 Confidentiality and isolation

Isolation procedures are necessary to reduce the risk of infection to health care workers and other patients. However, by their very nature, they may indicate the type of infection. This can result in a breach of patient confidentiality.

- Who has the right to know why a patient is in isolation?
- Is the patient's right to confidentiality more important than the right of others to protect themselves?

The implementation of universal infection control precautions means that instead of relying on identifying those patients who present a risk to health care workers, the blood and body fluids of ALL patients is considered to be high risk. This means that the same precautions are used with all patients and so those known to be a high risk should not be treated any differently. This should help to preserve patient confidentiality in relation to blood-borne infections.

when handling blood and body fluid secretions, excretions and contaminated items such as dressings, followed by handwashing after removal of the gloves. Eye protection and plastic aprons are worn if splashing of blood or bloodstained body fluids is a possibility.

The HICPAC guidelines also include policies relating to airborne, droplet and contact isolation precautions. Many countries and NHS Trusts have adopted their own local policies based on the HICPAC guidelines. The most practical is the adaptation of these guidelines in the form of universal infection control precautions (Wilson & Bredan 1990).

Protective isolation

Protective isolation is often used for patients whose immune system has been suppressed with drugs such as cytotoxic therapy for the treatment of cancers and leukaemias. These patients have an increased susceptibility to infection due to their immunosuppression and therefore are in protective isolation to protect them from exposure to pathogens that may result in an infection. If exposed to infection, it may be far more severe and life-threatening in an immunosuppressed patient, but most clinical infections that immunosuppressed patients get, such as those who have had a bone marrow transplant, are usually from their own normal flora. Three main types of infection – bacterial, viral and fungal – may afford life-threatening risk to this group of patients. Precautions will have to be implemented to prevent the acquisition of exogenous organisms. Furthermore, not only is cross-infection clearly a big risk, but most patients who are immunosuppressed, particularly as a result of cytotoxic therapy, are also at a high risk of endogenous infections from their own flora. Prophylactic antimicrobial therapy is often prescribed to reduce the patient's own microbial load and therefore to reduce the risk.

A self-contained isolation facility with en suite shower/bath and toilet should be available with air changes ranging between eight and 10 per hour, particularly for patients with a low neutrophil count. High standards of handwashing and the use of protective clothing to prevent spread of infection are important.

Measures such as sterilization of linen, food and gut decontamination with prophylactic antimicrobial therapy are all questionable and are not supported by science. The evidence is conflicting and prophylactic antimicrobial therapy, with the exception of prophylactic cotrimoxazole in the prevention of *Pneumocystis* infection following bone marrow or liver transplant, is not routinely recommended. However, uncooked food such as salad and organically grown foods should be avoided by highly immunosuppressed patients.

ISOLATION FACILITIES

There are various types of isolation facilities and each affords a different degree of protection. They range from separate infectious disease isolation units to patients being nursed on an open ward with the implementation of precautions to prevent the spread of infection.

Infectious disease units

High-security infectious disease units with facilities for treating patients with highly communicable infections, such as the viral haemorrhagic fevers Lassa fever and Ebola fever, are very rare in the UK. Environmental control in such units is usually achieved with the use of negative pressure plastic isolators, located in regional isolation units.

Infectious disease units are now usually part of a ward or unit within a hospital, although historically many were in separate buildings. An isolation unit requires a separate ventilation system, and a team of health care practitioners who work only in that unit. Such units are usually available to treat all infections except the viral haemorrhagic fevers mentioned above. Many isolation units now have the provision of negative pressure facilities to enable them to treat sensitive and resistant strains of tuberculosis safely.

Throughout the UK, very few general hospitals have satisfactory isolation units. This is often because of the high cost of set-up and maintenance. Additionally the negative pressure or filtered air ventilation for patients, particularly for respiratory infections, is deemed to add a further cost of £30,000 per single room. However, this cost has to be weighed against that of an outbreak (Plowman et al 1999).

Single room isolation

Single room isolation on a general ward provides a much less secure isolation facility than the above methods because of the close proximity to other patients and the contact that both nursing and support staff will have with patients who are not infected. Single rooms have a valuable role to play in terms of isolation, but the overall standards afforded to the care delivered on that ward will really determine whether or not the infection is allowed to spread. Ideally, single rooms on general wards should have en suite facilities.

Managing infectious patients on open wards

Controlling infections on an open ward is probably one of the most difficult ways to deal with infection, but with the implementation of universal infection control precautions, it can be an extremely effective way of controlling those infections that are not spread by the air. A number of patients with infections caused by the same organism, e.g. MRSA, can safely be nursed with good standards of nursing care, implementation by all health care workers of universal infection control precautions and high standards of domestic services.

Ultra-clean wards are often deemed necessary for centres specializing in organ transplantation and the treatment of leukaemia, particularly bone marrow transplantation, and those other diseases associated with severe immunosuppression, making the patient extremely susceptible to infection. However, clear definitions of what is meant by an 'ultra-clean' ward are not available.

CATEGORIES OF ISOLATION NURSING

There are a variety of systems for categorizing patients into isolation. A widely used method is to subdivide them into categories according to the mode of spread in order to standardize the precautions required. The Center for Disease Control recommends that as few groupings as possible should be created, to reduce confusion amongst clinical and domestic staff. Commonly, the guidelines are categorized as follows:

- wound and skin precautions – for infections such as MRSA and wound infections caused by group A *Streptococcus*
- stool precautions – for all of the infectious diarrhoeas
- respiratory precautions – for colds and flu-like symptoms and tuberculosis
- blood precautions – for hepatitis B, C and HIV.

MANAGEMENT OF CLINICAL WASTE AND LINEN

The safe management of clinical waste and used linen is important in order to ensure a safe environment. The recommendations given are intended to protect the interests of patients, staff and the general public and revolve around emphasizing the need to:

- train and educate staff in safe practice
- safely segregate types of waste
- provide self-storage awaiting collection
- provide collection and transportation to the central disposal points.

LINEN DISPOSAL

Guidance for the safe handling and disposal of all used linen in contact with patients who have infections or infectious diseases must be compliant with the Health and Safety at Work Act 1974 and *Health Service Circular 95 (18): Hospital Laundry Arrangements for Used Infected Linen*. The principles of these recommendations are intended to protect the interests of patients, staff and used linen handlers. The emphasis is on training and education of staff in safe practice, segregation of different types of used linen, providing appropriate storage while awaiting collection and providing collection and transportation to a central disposal point. All staff have a responsibility to carry out safe practice.

Segregation using a colour coding system based on national recommendations is essential as it allows priority laundry to be immediately identified and processed. Infected linen should be placed in an alginate (soluble seam) bag and then into a red linen bag; soiled linen should be placed in a plastic bag and then into a brown linen bag; ordinary used linen is placed in a white/cream coloured linen bag or clear plastic bag. Priority is usually given to infected laundry, theatre laundry and staff clothing. Broad principles of safe practice include the following:

- Infected laundry must be sealed in a water-soluble (alginate) bag. This is placed directly into the washing machine and the bag or seam dissolves at high temperatures. Laundry workers never handle the infected laundry and so they are not at risk of infection.
- Bags must never be more than 75% full and must be securely tied.
- If any bag is leaking, it should be re-bagged in the appropriate colour-coded water-soluble bag.

For collection and transportation, all trolleys and carts used should be constructed so that all surfaces are smooth and impermeable. They should offer no harbourage to insects or rodents and must be easily cleaned and maintained on a regular basis. If laundry is transported over a public highway, between sites, or to and from a laundry room, dirty and clean laundry must never be transported together on the same vehicle.

DISPOSAL OF WASTE

Guidance for the safe handling and disposal of waste within health care premises must also be in accordance with the Health and Safety at Work Act 1974, the Environmental Protection Act 1990, and the Department of Health guidance on clinical waste. Different waste materials require different methods of disposal. It is essential that all staff are aware of the safe methods of waste disposal related to each category. It remains the responsibility of the individual manager to ensure that staff comply with the waste disposal legislation. Segregation must be by careful use of the correct colour-coded bags. All staff who may be required to move waste should comply with the following guidance.

- All bags must be securely sealed.
- Clinical waste bags have coded plastic closure tags that indicate the department or ward to allow tracing of the origin of the waste in the event of incorrect disposal.
- Bags should be handled by the neck only and it should be ensured that the bag is intact and the seal on the bag is unbroken prior to removing.
- Staff should know the procedure in case of spillages.

Types of waste include:

- *Domestic waste*, including glass, aerosols and batteries; this must be placed in black plastic bags

- *Clinical waste*, which is all non-domestic waste; this must be placed in yellow clinical waste bags and the source clearly identified. The bags must be closed with secure non-opening tags that identify the source of the waste
- *Used sharps* (needles and scalpel blades, etc.) – these must be placed in rigid plastic boxes conforming to British Standard. USED NEEDLES MUST NEVER BE RE-SHEATHED. To reduce the risk of needlestick injury, needles should not be removed from syringes prior to disposal. If this is necessary for some reason, the needle-removing device on the top of the sharps bin should be used for this purpose.

IMMUNOSUPPRESSED PATIENTS

Due to the very nature of the work undertaken in hospital, all patients admitted for treatment or investigations are in close contact with many staff and likely to undergo invasive procedures. This means that all patients are at risk of infection. However, this risk is dramatically increased when the immune system is not functioning normally because of the inability of the body to produce an immune response to fight off bacteria and viruses which may cause infection. Therefore, immuno suppressed patients are more vulnerable to hospital-acquired infection.

All interventions must be aimed at minimizing the risk of infection when a patient is neutropenic. The more severe infections, such as a Gram-negative bacteraemia, are more likely to occur when the neutrophils are very low. Wade & Schimpff (1989) identified that the level of neutropenia is a reliable indicator of the infection risk.

The need for protective isolation (see p. 265) in neutropenic patients is debatable and may even be detrimental to their overall well-being. Nauseef & Mackie (1981) undertook a study comparing two groups of neutropenic patients, in which one group received protective isolation and the other standardized hospital care. They found no difference in survival rates of the two groups, or in the acquisition of hospital-acquired infections. Good standards of handwashing, minimal use of invasive devices and the use of prophylactic antimicrobial therapy were found to be just as effective as protective isolation. Knowles (1993) identified some negative aspects of isolation in relation to sensory deprivation; however, Wilson (1995) argued that when a patient is isolated in a single room, this act alone reinforces to staff and visitors the importance of simple hygiene measures.

Communication is a key factor in the control of infection for immunosuppressed patients. It is most important that all staff, visitors and relatives are educated in the correct procedures. Visitors must be advised not to visit if they themselves have an infection as this may place the patient at great risk. Hands must be washed before entering and leaving the cubicle to prevent taking organisms in to the patient or bringing the patient's organisms out and subjecting others to the possibility of spread. There is little evidence to support the use of protective clothing; it is not beneficial and merely leads to unnecessary expense.

Many transplant units have HEPA filtered air which removes over 99% of particles of, or above, 0.3 μm in diameter (Ayliffe et al 1992). Air is forced through the room via the filters under a positive pressure. When filtration systems are in use, monitoring of the air quality is important. Infections acquired from air ventilation systems are not common amongst immunocompromised patients (Wilson 1995), although outbreaks of *Aspergillus* have been documented (Barnes & Rogers 1989). Mooney et al (1993) recommend regular air sampling to ensure adequate air quality for these vulnerable patients.

BLOOD-BORNE INFECTIONS

Blood-borne infections are defined as those where blood contains infectious agents or pathogens that can be transferred into the body of another person, giving rise to infection (Advisory Committee on Dangerous Pathogens 1995). Many factors are associated with the risk of transmission, including:

- the length of time that the infectious agent remains in the blood
- the volume or viral load that is actually present
- the virulence of the pathogen (its disease-causing ability)
- the susceptibility of the recipient.

Of particular concern are the blood-borne viral pathogens hepatitis B, hepatitis C and HIV, as there is a risk of occupational and patient exposure to all of these within health care settings.

OCCUPATIONAL TRANSMISSION

The risk of occupational transmission to health care workers occurs whenever there is exposure to blood or bloodstained body fluids. This is irrespective of the environment in which one works and does not just affect clinical practitioners, but support services and pathology workers as well. Therefore, an effective strategy to manage the exposure must be in place. This will include serum storage for testing at a later date, immunization if not already immunized against hepatitis B and, if exposure to HIV is deemed to be a risk, the commencement of oral antiretroviral therapy to prevent seroconversion. In a large percentage of those exposed to HIV, if antiretroviral therapy is taken within the first hour of exposure then seroconversion to HIV status is preventable.

Internationally, the incidence of occupationally acquired HIV is low, which reflects its low infectivity outside the main routes of transmission, which are unprotected sexual intercourse and intravenous drug users sharing used needles (Shanson 1999). Worldwide there are over 100 documented cases of seroconversion in health care workers infected with HIV through contact with patients. To date, few cases have occurred in the UK and inoculation injury (percutaneous or needlestick injury) was responsible for all of these. The risk of contracting hepatitis B following an inoculation injury is around 30%, whereas it is believed that the risk from HIV-infected blood is 0.36%. The risk from hepatitis C-infected blood is thought to be between 2 and 12% (Zuckerman 1995).

The risk of exposure to blood-borne pathogens during surgery is probably the most widely documented. This is illustrated in an outbreak of four cases of hepatitis B infection occurring amongst theatre and intensive care unit staff at a London teaching hospital. This followed emergency surgery on a road traffic accident victim who was hepatitis B-positive but who, at the time of admission, was asymptomatic (Shanson 1999).

The risk to patients is much lower than the risk to health care staff. However, patients can still be put at risk of exposure to contamination during invasive procedures if instruments and equipment have not been sterilized. Like hospital patients, they may also be at risk from infected health care workers during exposure-prone procedures (EPPs). These are procedures during which others can become exposed to a health care worker's blood and bloodstained body fluids. These interventions are mostly limited to staff working in the operating theatre or a labour ward during delivery. In 1998, the United Kingdom Expert Advisory Group on AIDS published a document entitled *Health Care Workers: Prevention of Exposure to Blood Borne Pathogens* (Department of Health 1998). This document sets out key recommendations on the management of infected health care workers. It highlights the need to protect patients whilst maintaining public confidence and safeguarding confidentiality for employees who carry blood-borne pathogens.

CONTROL MEASURES FOR THE PREVENTION OF INFECTION BY BLOOD-BORNE VIRUSES

It is not possible to identify all those who may be infected with a blood-borne virus and therefore guidance to protect health care workers against hepatitis viruses and HIV has been based on the concept of universal infection control precautions (Advisory Committee on Dangerous Pathogens 1995, Department of Health 1998). Historically, health care workers have relied on being able to identify high-risk patients. However, with the implementation of universal infection control precautions, all blood and bloodstained body fluids are now regarded as potentially infectious, and, based on the risk assessment, the appropriate interventions are made. These involve hand hygiene, the use of gloves, covering all non-intact skin with occlusive dressings, avoiding the use of sharp instruments whenever possible, and avoiding contamination with blood and bloodstained body fluids (see p. 261).

Invasive procedures are a necessary part of many health care interventions. Gloves are recommended for any invasive procedure that involves the use of needles, such as venepuncture, intravenous cannulation and intramuscular injection. Although gloves will not protect against a needlestick injury, Zuckerman (1995) argues that glove materials, irrespective of the type, will reduce the volume of blood inoculated in any needlestick injury by around 50%. However, this work does not specifically refer to hollow-bore inoculation injuries when the blood from inside the needle is injected into the recipient.

Intraoperative exposures have a higher risk of exposure to blood-borne pathogens and percutaneous inoculation injury rates depend greatly on the type of surgery being undertaken. Perforation rates for single gloves during surgical procedures range from 10% to over 50%, but when double gloving is undertaken, perforation of the inner glove is reported at around 2% (Jeffries 1995).

Commercially, the manufacturing world has risen to the challenge of making the working environment safer for health care workers. Many systems are being developed to reduce exposure risks, such as retractable needles and needle-free administration systems for intravenous therapy, although these have yet to be widely adopted throughout the UK.

Vaccination and immunization

There is currently no vaccine available to protect against hepatitis C or HIV, but hepatitis B is fully preventable. The need for immunization will be determined as part of a risk assessment based on the Control of Substances Hazardous to Health (COSHH) regulations from the Health and Safety Executive (1999). All health care staff potentially at risk of exposure to blood, tissues or other body fluid in the course of their work should be immunized against hepatitis B (Department of Health 1998). Those who have been vaccinated must have their antibody levels checked every 3–5 years and a booster must be given if required. However, up to 10% of people fail to develop adequate antibodies, even after four doses. They should be advised to have hepatitis B virus immunoglobulin if exposed to hepatitis B virus-positive blood.

Management of exposure to blood or body fluids

Immediate action following exposure should include:

- Wash off splashes on the skin with warm soapy water.
- If the skin has been punctured or broken, encourage bleeding by milking outwards whilst washing under warm running water (not by pressing or sucking the wound).
- Splashes into the eye (conjunctiva), nose or mouth should be washed out with large amounts of water – sterile water for the eye if available.
- The incident must be recorded and the source of contamination, i.e. name of the patient if known, type of fluid, the injury and how it occurred, should be recorded for legal reasons and reported in line with local policy.
- A risk assessment must be undertaken by either the occupational health department or a clinical virologist without delay in accordance with local Trust policy.

The risk assessment will determine whether exposure to a blood-borne pathogen has been likely, and if the source is known this makes it easier. The need for antiretroviral therapy will be based on the risk assessment and should be taken within 1 hour of the injury. Therefore speed is of the essence and expert advice should be sought without delay. Post-exposure prophylaxis should be considered whenever there has been exposure to material that is known or suspected to be infected with HIV. Local policies must be based on the Department of Health's comprehensive guidelines (Department of Health 1998) and risk assessment following an incident. Given the potentially serious health risks following exposure to blood-borne pathogens and the lack of vaccination programmes for both hepatitis C and HIV, the prevention of inoculation injuries is of great importance.

SUMMARY: MAIN POINTS

- Handwashing is the single most important factor in the prevention of cross-infection.

- Hospital-acquired infection (HAI) costs the NHS nearly £1 billion pounds each year in England alone (Plowman et al 1999).

- MRSA is present in most hospitals in the UK and throughout Europe. Strict adherence to MRSA protocols is vital to prevent outbreaks.

- Universal infection control precautions involve hand hygiene, protective clothing such as gloves, covering cuts and grazes with occlusive dressings and avoiding contamination with blood and bloodstained body fluids wherever possible.

- Blood-borne infections are those in which the blood contains infectious agents or pathogens that, if transferred into the body of another person, will give rise to infection.

- All health care workers that are at risk of exposure to blood, tissues or other body fluids should be immunized against hepatitis B.

- In the event of an inoculation injury (needlestick injury), the wound should be washed thoroughly under warm running water and encouraged to bleed by 'milking' outwards.

SELF-TEST: CRITICAL THINKING ACTIVITIES

1 Research has shown time and time again that nurses and other health care personnel do not wash their hands enough. What can be done to encourage them to wash their hands more frequently?

2 Most nurses and other health care workers are immunized against TB. How can you reduce the risk of infection if a patient with TB has to leave his room to visit other departments for tests and investigations?

3 The use of gloves is designed to protect the hands from contamination during invasive procedures:
   — Why do you need to wash your hands before and after wearing gloves?
   — In what situations do you need to wear sterile gloves?
   — When would you need to wear eye protection?

FURTHER READING

Ayliffe GAJ, Lowbury EJL, Geddes AM, Williams JD. Control of hospital infection: a practical handbook, 3rd edn. London: Chapman & Hall Medical; 1992.

Horton R, Parker L. Informed infection control practice. Edinburgh: Churchill Livingstone; 1997.

Infection Control Nurses Association London Regional Group. Information resources, 2nd edn. Hertfordshire: Decorum Printing Services; 1997.

Wilson J. Infection control in practice: the management of the infectious patient. London: Baillière Tindall; 1995.

USEFUL WEBSITES

www.icna.co.uk – Infection Control Nurses Association
www.his.org.uk – Hospital Infection Society
www.escmid.org/preview.html – European Society of Clinical Microbiology and Infectious Diseases

www.infectioncontroltoday.com – Infection Control Today
www.phls.co.uk/services/icu.htm – Public Health Laboratory Service (Infection Control Unit)

REFERENCES

Advisory Committee on Dangerous Pathogens (ACDP). Categorisation of biological agents according to hazard and categories of containment. London: HMSO; 1995.

Ayliffe GA, Babb JR, Quoraishi AH. A test for 'hygienic' hand disinfection. J Clin Pathol 1978; 31(10): 923–928.

Ayliffe GAJ, Lowbury EJL, Geddes AM, Williams JD. Control of hospital infection: a practical handbook, 3rd edn. London: Chapman & Hall Medical; 1992.

Bagshaw KD, Blowers R, Lidwell OM. Isolating patients in hospital to control infection. Br Med J 1978; ii: 609, 684, 744, 808, 879.

Barnes RA, Rogers TR. Control of an outbreak of nosocomial aspergillosis by lamina air flow isolation. J Hosp Infect 1989; 14(2): 89–94.

Belchin NL. The evolution of the surgical mask: filtering efficiency versus effectiveness. J Infect Control Hosp Epidemiol 1997; 18(1): 49–57.

Bellamy K, Alcock R, Babb JR, Davies JG, Ayliffe GA. A test for the assessment of 'hygienic' hand disinfection using rotavirus. J Hosp Infect 1993; 24(3): 201–210.

Department of Health. Hospital infection control – guidance on the control of infection in hospitals. Prepared by the DH/PHLS/ Hospital Infection working party. London: HMSO; 1995.

Department of Health. Guidance for clinical health care workers: protection against blood borne viruses. Recommendations of the expert advisory group on AIDS and the advisory group on hepatitis. London: HMSO; 1998.

Garner JS. Guideline for isolation precautions in hospitals. The Hospital Infection Control Practices Advisory Committee. Infect Control Hosp Epidemiol 1996; 17(1): 53–80.

Gould D, Wilson-Barnett J, Ream E. Nurses' infection-control practice: hand decontamination, the use of gloves and sharp instruments. Int J Nurs Studies 1996; 33(2): 143–160.

Hateley P, Jumaa PA. Handwashing is more common amongst healthcare workers than the public. Br Med J 1999; 7208: 519.

Hayley RW, Culver DH, White JW et al. The efficacy of infection surveillance and control programs in preventing nosocomial infections in US hospitals (SENIC study). Am J Epidemiol 1985; 121: 185–205.

Health and Safety Executive. Control of Substances Hazardous to Health Regulations (COSHH). London: HMSO; 1999.

Infection Control Nurses Association. Glove usage guidelines. ICNA: West Lothian; 1999

Jeffries DJ. Viral hazards to and from health care workers. J Hosp Infect 1995; 39(suppl 1): 40–55.

Joint Tuberculosis Committee of the British Thoracic Society. Chemotherapy and management of tuberculosis in the United Kingdom: recommendations. Thorax 1998; 53(7): 536–548.

Knowles HE. The experience of infectious patients in isolation. Nurs Times 1993; 89(30): 53–56.

Kramer A, Rudolph P, Kampf G, Pittet D. Limited efficacy of alcohol-based hand gels. Lancet 2002; 359: 1489–1490.

Lucas GM, Lechtzin N, Puryear DW et al. Vancomycin-resistant and vancomycin sensitive enterococcal bacteremia: comparison of clinical features and outcomes. Clin Infect Dis 1998; 26: 1127–1133.

Meers PD, Ayliffe GAJ, Emmerson A et al. Report on the national survey of infection in hospitals – 1980. J Hosp Infect 1981; 2(suppl): 1–53.

Mooney BR, Reeves SA and Larson E. Infection control and bone marrow transplantation. Am J Infect Control 1993; 21(3): 131–138.

MRSA Working Party Report. Revised guidelines for the control of methicillin-resistant Staphylococcus aureus infection in hospitals. J Hosp Infect 1998; 39(4): 335–338.

Nauseef WM, Maki DG. A study of the value of simple protective isolation in patients with granulocytopenia. N Engl J Med 1981; 304(8): 448–453.

Newsome SWB, Rowland C. Studies in perioperative skin flora. J Hosp Infect 1988; 11(suppl B): 21–26.

Pittet D, Hugonner S, Harbarth S et al. Effectiveness of a hospital wide programme to improve compliance with hand hygiene. Lancet 2000; 354: 1307–1312.

Plowman R, Graves N, Griffin M et al. The socio-economic burden of hospital acquired infection. London: Public Health Laboratory Service; 1999.

Shanson DC. Microbiology in clinical practice, 3rd edn. Oxford: Butterworth-Heinemann; 1999.

Taylor LJ. Evaluation of hand washing techniques, parts 1 and 2. Nurs Times 1978; 74: 54, 108.

Wade J, Schimpff BJ. Protective isolation: who needs it? J Hosp Infect 1989; 30(suppl): 218–222.

Wilson J. Infection control in practice: the management of the infectious patient. London: Baillière Tindall; 1995.

Wilson J, Breedon P. Universal precautions. Nurs Times 1990; 86(29): 67–70.

Zuckerman AJ. Occupational exposure to hepatitis and human deficiency viruses: a comparative risk analysis. Am J Infect Control 1995; 23(5): 286–289.

SECTION 3

Nursing patients with common disorders

Contents

14 Nursing patients with neurological problems 273

15 Nursing patients with problems of the eye and vision 331

16 Nursing patients with problems of the ear and hearing 367

17 Nursing patients with endocrine and metabolic disorders 393

18 Nursing patients with blood disorders 445

19 Nursing patients with cardiovascular disorders 481

20 Nursing patients with respiratory disorders 533

21 Nursing patients with nose and throat disorders 565

22 Nursing patients with gastrointestinal disorders 591

23 Nursing patients with hepatic, biliary and pancreatic disorders 621

24 Nursing patients with urinary disorders 653

25 Nursing patients with sexual health and reproductive problems 705

26 Nursing patients with breast disorders 771

27 Nursing patients with musculoskeletal disorders 793

28 Nursing patients with skin problems 841

14 Nursing patients with neurological problems

Iain Bowie, Sue Woodward

'I was unconscious for 3 days and when I woke up I couldn't move this side. I thought I'd never be able to walk again and if it wasn't for the nurses and the therapists I wouldn't – it was them that kept me going. Without them I couldn't have done it'

(Rehabilitation patient)

THIS CHAPTER WILL HELP YOU

- Describe the structure and function of the nervous system in simple terms
- Recognize the key points when planning care for neurological or neurosurgical patients
- List the main assessment strategies associated with neurological or neurosurgical patients
- Explain care to patients and carers
- Support patients and family members while preparing for discharge.

KEYWORDS

Amnesia	Hemiplegia
Ataxia	Intracranial pressure
Bradykinesia	Paraesthesia
Demyelination	Paraplegia
Diplopia	Phonophobia
Dysarthria	Photophobia
Dysphagia	Quadriplegia/tetraplegia
Dysphasia	Seizure
Flaccid	Spastic
Glasgow Coma Scale	Tremor
Hemiparesis	

INTRODUCTION

The care of patients with neurological disorders is a complex task involving many members of the multidisciplinary team. The nurse's role is increasingly more technical and demands skill and specialist knowledge. Many patients are nursed in specialist neurology or neurosurgery units, but many others are cared for in medical and surgical wards. This chapter explains some of the foundations for safe care. Many of the problems discussed have been dealt with quite generally, as specific care details will vary from place to place. In this chapter, you will find information on the structure and function of the nervous system, investigations commonly performed and also information about common disease processes that affect the nervous system. Readers needing information about less common conditions are directed to the suggestions for further reading (p. 329).

People with neurological disorders will present in many ways depending on the nature and location of the lesion. For this reason, not all neurological care appears in the first instance to be about the brain and spinal cord but is related to the functions that the nervous system supports. Some patients may have problems swallowing and have much in common with ENT patients. Others will have visual defects and may be referred to the ophthalmologists. Still others will have mobility problems affecting gait and may have a similar presentation to orthopaedic patients. Indeed, sometimes there are areas of overlap, as in the case of spinal injury, which is both orthopaedic and neurological. Of course, many other patients have behavioural problems because the nervous system determines behaviour. The neurological nurse should remember the following maxim: 'All behaviour is neurological unless proven otherwise'. Neurological disease is variable in its effect and nursing interventions may be minimal, or, as in the case of an unconscious patient, the patient may rely on the team for all aspects of care.

ANATOMY AND PHYSIOLOGY – AN OVERVIEW

The nervous system is really very simple. It does three things only (see Fig. 14.1):

- it gathers information
- it processes the incoming information
- it acts upon the information if necessary.

Only an overview of the nervous system, with an emphasis on the central nervous system (CNS), is provided here and readers needing more detailed information are advised to consult an anatomy and physiology book.

Information is gathered by sensory receptors monitoring the external and internal environments. Information about the internal environment includes temperature, blood pressure and blood chemistry. The external environment is detected in terms of heat or cold, wet or dry, hard or soft, light or dark, sweet or sour, quiet or noisy and so on. Action by the nervous system can also be described in terms of internal and external environments. The internal environment is modified by hormones, which are ultimately under neurological control, and by smooth and cardiac muscle. The external environment is moderated by the action of voluntary muscle.

The nervous system is classically described structurally as consisting of the CNS, comprising the brain and spinal cord, and the peripheral nervous system (PNS), which is formed by the cranial and spinal nerves throughout the body (see Fig. 14.2). Functionally it is described as consisting of the somatic nervous system, which is concerned with the external environment, and the autonomic nervous system (ANS), which is concerned with life support functions and homeostasis. The nervous system reacts to the information gathered and processed using the motor nerves. These are sometimes called efferent fibres because the nerve impulses leave the central nervous system. The sensory nerves are sometimes called afferent because they take information towards the central nervous system.

The nervous system consists of nerve cells or neurons (see Fig. 14.3) and glial cells. Neurons are excitable cells that react electrochemically to a stimulus and transmit a nerve impulse, i.e. they are said to show irritability. They are classified by their shape and function. The neurons vary in structure but all of them have a nucleated cell body and elongated processes (fibres) that are called either axons or dendrites depending on their shape and function. Some nerve fibres are covered with myelin (white fatty material) that insulates the nerve and allows faster transmission of the nerve impulse. The myelin sheath lies within the outer connective tissue covering the neurilemma.

Glial cells are not excitable cells; they do not show irritability. They support the neurons and act as intermediaries between the blood and neurons for the transport of oxygen, glucose, carbon dioxide and other waste. Glial cells actively divide within the nervous system, whereas neurons have very limited capability of cell division after the nervous system has matured. Glial cells may become malignant and most malignant primary

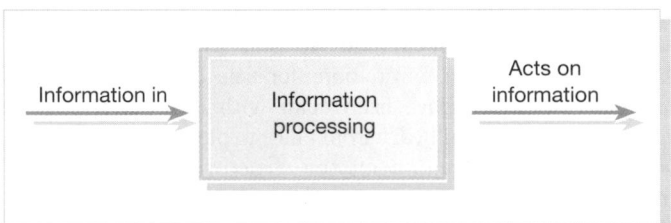

Figure 14.1 Functions of the nervous system.

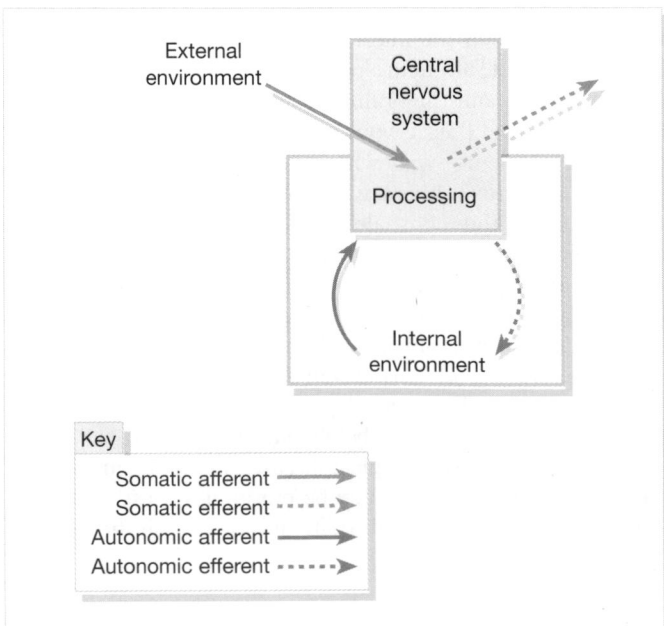

Figure 14.2 Conceptual diagram of the nervous system.

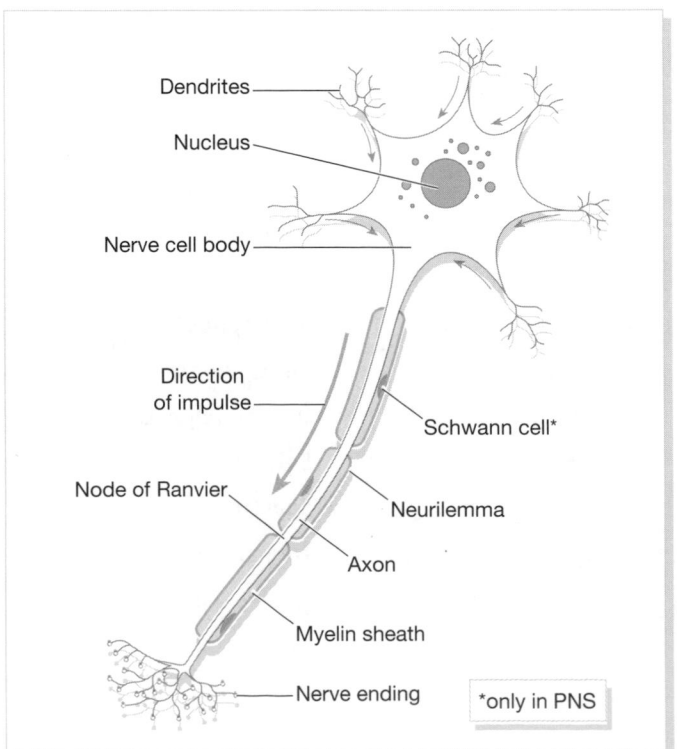

Figure 14.3 A neuron.

Table 14.1 Types of glial cells

Cell name	Basic shape	Function
Astrocytes ('star cell')	Cell bodies with numerous dendrite processes (like a star)	Form supporting framework for nerve cells Contribute to the blood–brain barrier. Act as 'filter' between blood vessels and neurons, facilitating the passage of oxygen, glucose, waste metabolites and other substances
Oligodendrocytes ('few dendrite cells')	Cell bodies with very few dendrites	Form the myelin sheath around myelinated fibres and facilitate the conduction of the nerve impulse
Microglia ('small glial cells')	Amoeboid cells	Scavenge cell debris and microorganisms
Ependymal cells	Endothelial cells	Production and absorption of cerebrospinal fluid

brain tumours in adults are gliomas (see p. 308). There are several different types of glial cell (see Table 14.1).

THE NERVE IMPULSE

The basic element of the nervous system is the action potential or nerve impulse (see Fig. 14.4). All cells have a protein-based cytoplasm that is electrically neutral within the cell. The protein molecules have an overall negative charge that is balanced by the intracellular positive ions (see Ch. 8). The extracellular fluid is also electrically neutral, but there is a difference between the intracellular charge and the extracellular charge. This occurs in all cells of the body. However, cells that display irritability make use of this potential difference in electrical charge between intracellular and extracellular fluids. These excitable or irritable cells are neurons and muscle cells.

During the action potential, extracellular cations (sodium) enter the cell through the membrane that is normally impervious to the passage of ions and so the intracellular charge rises.

The extracellular cations enter the cell because they are passing down a concentration gradient, i.e. from an area of high concentration outside the cell to an area of low concentration within the cell. When the intracellular concentration rises sufficiently, there is an electrical potential difference between adjacent areas of the intracellular contents and therefore a current is generated. This is known as depolarization.

After the peak in the action potential, the sodium ions are actively pumped out of the cell using energy and the potential difference is restored; this is called repolarization. The time taken for this process to occur prevents a second action potential being generated. This 'time out' is called the refractory period. Local anaesthetics work by preventing the cell membrane repolarizing so that they are unable to generate an action potential.

Limiting the areas where the passage of ions can take place increases the speed of the action potential. Some nerve cells have electrical insulation provided by myelin, which is produced by the oligodendrocytes in the CNS and Schwann cells in the PNS. Small gaps, called nodes of Ranvier in the peripheral nervous system, are left between the myelin insulation and this is where the exchange of ions takes place (see Fig. 14.3). A nerve fibre in the PNS looks a bit like a string of sausages with the Schwann cells as the sausages and the nodes of Ranvier as the links between them. As the gaps are separated from each other by a length of insulated nerve fibre, the message 'jumps' from node to node and thus speeds up the conduction as the exchange of ions does not have to take place along the entire length of the fibre. This 'jumping' is called saltatory conduction. Thus myelination facilitates faster conduction. In demyelinating diseases such as multiple sclerosis (see p. 304), the action potential cannot pass the nerve segment without myelin.

Synapses

When a nerve impulse reaches the end of a nerve, there is a small gap called the synaptic cleft. The action potential cannot pass across this cleft and so an alternative method of conduction is required. This is accomplished by the release of calcium ions and chemicals (neurotransmitters), which are released from one side and diffuse across the cleft. There are many different neurotransmitters, some of them occurring in minute quantities in very specific parts of the nervous system. The most common neurotransmitters are noradrenaline (norepinephrine) and acetylcholine. Others include gamma-aminobutyric acid (GABA), serotonin and glutamate.

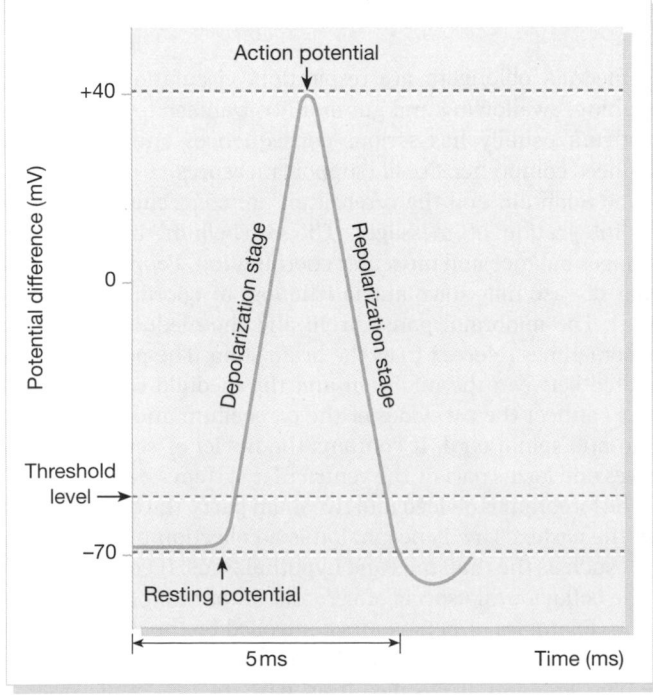

Figure 14.4 Action potential.

In addition to chemical synapses, there is a class of electro-synapses where small tubules connect one neuron to another. These allow the passage of the electrical potential difference to pass directly from cell to cell. They are found in smooth and cardiac muscle and in the CNS.

When an action potential reaches the terminal bulb at the end of the axon branch or dendrite, small vesicles containing the neurotransmitter move to the cell membrane adjacent to the synaptic cleft. The vesicles rupture on the surface and the neuro-transmitter diffuses across the cleft and 'locks' onto a specific receptor site on the membrane of the next neuron in the chain (or muscle cell). There are receptors for each type of neurotrans-mitter and sometimes there is more than one. For example, receptors for acetylcholine (cholinergic receptors) can be 'mus-carinic' or 'nicotinic'. Receptors for noradrenaline (adrenergic receptors) are classified by Greek letters, e.g. alpha (α) and beta (β). In fact the adrenergic receptors are subdivided and classified by number, thus α_1, α_2, β_1 and so on. The neurotransmitter sub-stance once locked onto the receptor site initiates the necessary change in the membrane to allow a new action potential to be initiated. Many drugs work by imitating or blocking the action of neurotransmitters. Beta-blockers are drugs that block the β-adrenergic receptors and therefore prevent the action of the sympathetic nerves that release noradrenaline (norepinephrine) at their synapses: as a consequence, the heart slows down (i.e. it is not speeded up!).

CENTRAL NERVOUS SYSTEM

Understanding the anatomical arrangement of the nervous system is also important in appreciating its functions and its relationships to the disordered function seen in neurological patients (see Fig. 14.5). The functional organization of the CNS (brain and spinal cord) reflects embryonic development. There are 'layers' of increasing complexity of neurological task, each one arranged above the preceding one in both an anatomical and functional order; in other words they form a hierarchy. The brain is contained within the skull in three cranial fossae – anterior, middle and posterior. The posterior fossa contains the cerebellum, pons varolii and medulla oblongata. The lowest part of the brain, the medulla oblongata, becomes the spinal cord as it leaves the cranial cavity through the foramen magnum (opening). The spinal cord is surrounded by the vertebral column.

Spinal cord

The most primitive organized part of the CNS is the spinal cord. In humans it is a relay tract taking messages from the brain to the peripheral nerves to the body, and information via sensory nerves from the body to the brain. However, it is capable of some filtering and 'decision' making in the form of reflex actions, e.g. muscle stretch reflexes and tendon reflexes as well as some primitive reflexes that are 'submerged' by later development and learned responses. Some of these primitive reflexes are released following neurological damage.

Brain (see Fig. 14.6)

In ascending order, the next part of the CNS is the medulla oblongata. This is an area of the brain that is responsible for the life support functions. Examples of functions controlled by

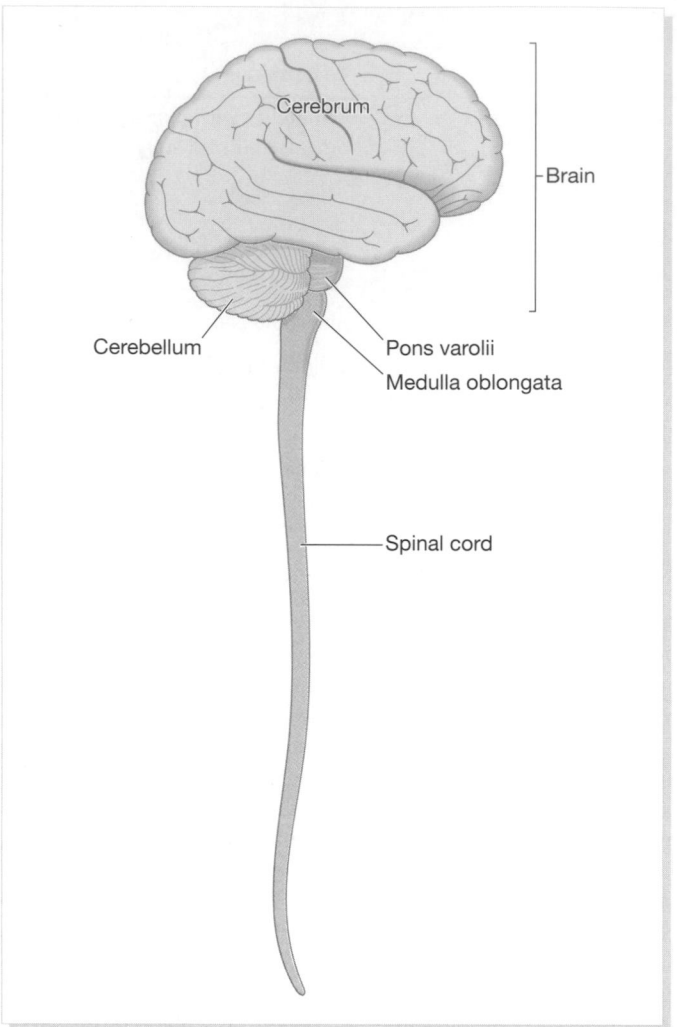

Figure 14.5 The central nervous system.

the medulla oblongata are respiration, circulation, vomiting, coughing, swallowing and gut motility. Damage to the medulla oblongata usually has serious consequences and the patient may need comprehensive life support measures.

The midbrain and the cerebellum are concerned with relay and integration of messages. The cerebellum, in particular, manages balance and muscular coordination. People with cere-bellar disease may have ataxia (the loss of coordinated move-ment). The midbrain, pons varolii and the medulla oblongata are sometimes referred to as the brain stem. The pons varolii is situated between the midbrain and the medulla oblongata; its fibres connect the two lodes of the cerebellum and connect the brain and spinal cord. It contains the nuclei of several cranial nerves and forms part of the ventricular system (see below).

The forebrain is divided into two main parts, the diencephalon and the cortex. The diencephalon is a collection of deep struc-tures such as the thalamus and hypothalamus. It controls many of the behavioural aspects of cerebral output and relaying sen-sation. Examples of behaviours controlled by the diencephalon are thirst, hunger and sexual behaviours. Some structures of the diencephalon are formed from parts of the limbic system, which is the part of the brain responsible for emotional behaviour

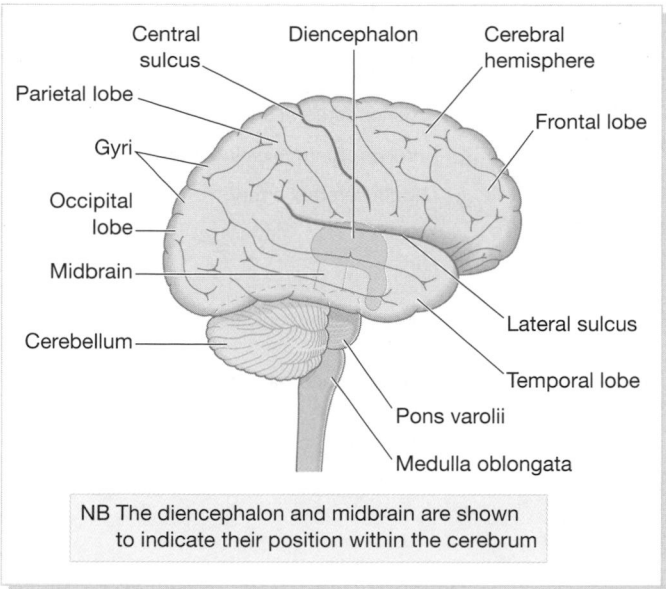

Central sulcus
Diencephalon
Cerebral hemisphere
Parietal lobe
Gyri
Frontal lobe
Occipital lobe
Midbrain
Lateral sulcus
Cerebellum
Temporal lobe
Pons varolii
Medulla oblongata

NB The diencephalon and midbrain are shown to indicate their position within the cerebrum

Figure 14.6 The brain.

such as anger, pleasure, fear, sexual behaviour and pain. The limbic system is placed by some authors in the limbic lobe, while others consider it to be formed from surrounding lobes of the cerebrum (see below). Regardless of whether the limbic system is a separate lobe or not anatomically, it is certainly a series of structures with discrete functions. People with damage to the diencephalon or limbic system may display extremes of emotion or behavioural disturbances.

The cortex is divided into lobes named after the bones of the skull that overlie each lobe – hence frontal, parietal, occipital and temporal lobes (see Fig. 14.6). The cortex is also divided into two hemispheres; motor control and sensory information cross over so that the left hemisphere controls the right-hand side of the body and vice versa. Simplifying the functions of the lobes greatly, the frontal lobe is concerned with personality and intellect as well as the conscious control of movement. The parietal lobe is mainly concerned with sensory data and the interpretation of sensation, i.e. perception. The occipital lobe receives its input from the eyes and then interprets the visual information. The temporal lobe receives its input from the ears and interprets acoustic information. This is an oversimplification and each lobe has many functions in addition to those listed above. The cortex has a convoluted surface that is formed of ridges, called gyri (singular gyrus), and clefts between them called sulci (singular sulcus). This arrangement increases the working surface area of the cortex.

The hierarchical arrangement of the nervous system generally involves inhibition downwards from the cerebral cortex, each 'layer' inhibiting the one below. For example, the sacral reflex that causes bladder emptying is inhibited from the cortex: this control over a reflex is learned during 'potty training'. Spasticity, an increase in muscle tone, occurs when inhibition of the spinal muscle-stretch reflexes is lost in some neurological conditions. The cortex also inhibits behaviours that are socially unacceptable, such as micturating inappropriately. Always remember the maxim: 'All behaviour is neurological unless proven otherwise'.

This maxim underlines the fact that people with brain damage who cannot control their behavioural responses (disinhibited) may display behaviour that is socially unacceptable.

Blood–brain barrier

The brain and spinal cord have a very sensitive chemical environment. These structures do not receive a direct blood supply but are separated from the general circulation by the special arrangement of astrocytes (glial cells) and the capillary endothelium. This arrangement forms the blood–brain barrier, which allows only certain substances into the nerve cells and normally maintains the sensitive environment. Not all drugs cross the blood–brain barrier, a point often noted in pharmacology reference texts. This inability to cross the blood–brain barrier may be significant in the treatment of neurological diseases. The choice of medication or the dose of some medication may need to be increased to ensure sufficient reaches the target cells.

Blood supply to the brain

The brain receives blood at a rate of 850 mL/min (around 20% of the cardiac output), which is disproportionate to its size. This volume of blood is needed to perfuse the brain with oxygen and glucose, without which it would not survive. Blood supply to the brain is mainly via the left and right internal carotid arteries and the vertebral arteries. These arteries unite inside the cranium at the base of the brain to form the circle of Willis (see Fig. 14.7). From the circle of Willis, the blood is distributed to the lobes of the cortex via the pair of anterior cerebral arteries, one to each lobe, which supply the frontal lobes and part of the parietal lobe. A pair of middle cerebral arteries supplies the sides of frontal lobes, temporal lobes and part of the parietal lobes. The posterior cerebral arteries supply the occipital lobe. The brain stem structures receive their supply from branches of the basilar artery, which is formed by the union of the vertebral arteries.

Venous blood leaves the brain in blood sinuses that return the blood to the internal jugular vein from where it enters the superior vena cava and so to the heart. The meninges have their own blood supply. It is often the meningeal blood vessels that rupture in head injuries.

Cerebrospinal fluid and the meninges

Cerebrospinal fluid (CSF) is formed by specialized capillaries (choroid plexuses) that line the brain ventricles; it enters the subarachnoid space and circulates around the brain and spinal cord (see Fig. 14.8). The purpose of CSF is to provide a shock-absorbing 'jacket' for the brain and spinal cord. Intracranial pressure (ICP) is maintained by the CSF. CSF is reabsorbed through arachnoid granulations that project into the venous sinuses. The skull is a closed box and the pressure within it is determined by the three components that fill the box, namely, the CSF, the blood in the intracranial vessels and the brain tissue itself. A change in any of these three components (e.g. swelling of the brain) will affect the ICP (see p. 298). There is physiological control over the production of CSF and the cerebral blood flow, but the volume of brain tissue cannot be altered.

The arrangement of membranes that cover the brain and spinal cord are called the meninges (singular meninx) (see Fig. 14.9). There are three meningeal layers; the first is the two-layer dura mater that forms a tough inner lining to the

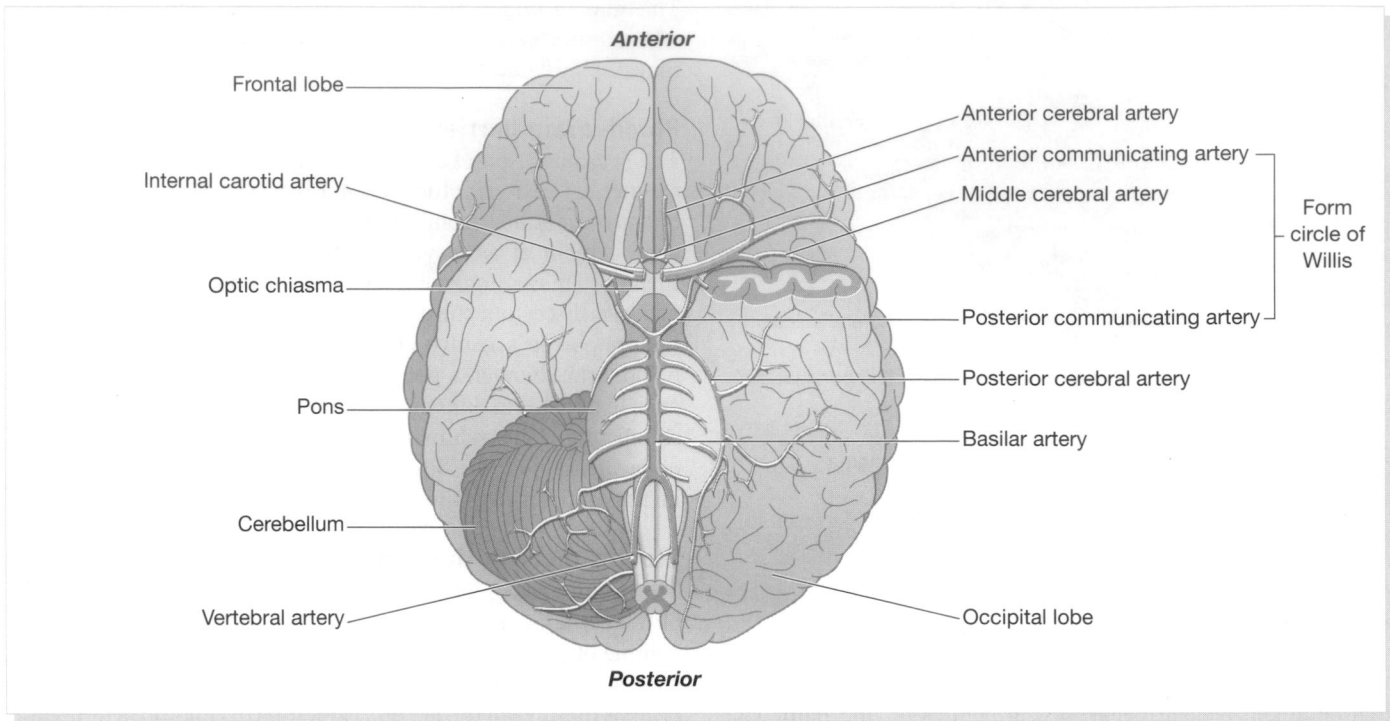

Figure 14.7 The circle of Willis.

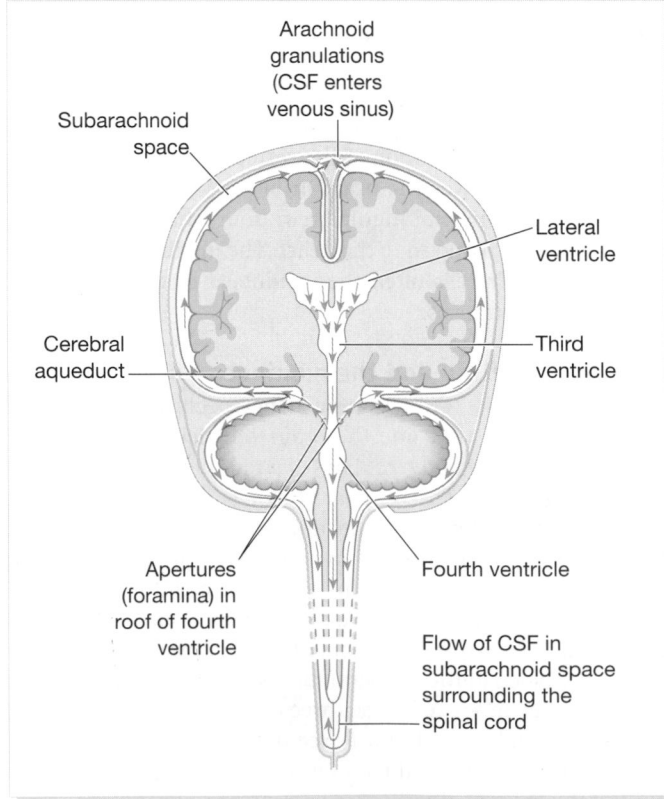

Figure 14.8 The ventricular system and the circulation of cerebrospinal fluid.

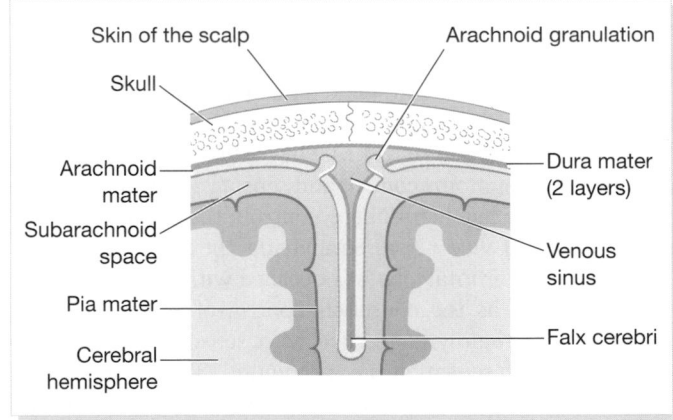

Figure 14.9 The meninges (simplified).

skull. The second is the arachnoid mater, which consists of fine filaments with numerous sensory nerve endings and a subarachnoid space filled with CSF. The arachnoid (named for its similarity to a spider's web) forms a connection between the dura and pia, the third meninx. The pia is a fine, diaphanous membrane that covers the surface of the cortex and dips down into the sulci. The meninges dip down into the longitudinal fissure between the two cerebral hemispheres to form the falx cerebri, a partition rather like those in a walnut. There is another of these meningeal partitions that runs in a horizontal plane and separates the cerebral cortex and diencephalon from the cerebellum and brain stem. This is the tentorium cerebelli and has important relevance in raised ICP as the supratentorial contents (i.e. those above the tentorium) may be pushed down and 'wedge' in the hole in the tentorium, compressing nerves, especially the third pair of cranial nerves (oculomotor) which normally constrict the pupil (see p. 283).

Blood vessels that supply the meninges may be damaged in accidents and bleeding may occur between the layers. Subdural haematoma refers to a collection of blood between the dura and arachnoid layer. Subarachnoid haemorrhage occurs when there is bleeding into the subarachnoid space. As this blood can flow around the space, subarachnoid haemorrhage tends to produce symptoms that are general, whereas subdural haematomas, because the pressure they cause is local, tend to have focal symptoms. Focal symptoms are ones that affect a specific area, e.g. paralysis of one arm or speech impairment. A large subdural haematoma may displace the brain enough to cause general symptoms and a rise in ICP. If the pressure is greater than arterial blood pressure, blood will not be able to enter the brain and it will become ischaemic.

PERIPHERAL NERVOUS SYSTEM

The PNS consists of the peripheral nerves, which are either cranial or spinal depending on whether they originate from the brain or spinal cord. The 12 pairs of cranial nerves originate from the brain and are identified by a Roman numeral and a name. They may be motor (five), sensory (three) or mixed (four) (see Table 14.2).

There are 31 pairs of mixed (motor and sensory) spinal nerves that arise from the spinal cord. They are named and classified by the level at which they exit the spinal cord. There are eight cervical (C1–C8), 12 thoracic (T1–T12), five lumbar (L1–L5), five sacral (S1–S5) and one coccygeal (see Fig. 14.10, see p. 280).

NEUROLOGICAL NURSING ASSESSMENT

A comprehensive and accurate nursing assessment is extremely important in the care of patients with neurological problems. It is vital that nurses are alert to the, sometimes subtle, changes in condition that may indicate a worsening of the patient's condition.

In addition to the assessment processes discussed below, nurses should always ascertain the presence of other signs and symptoms that may be indicative of a neurological problem. These are discussed at appropriate points in the chapter when particular conditions are covered and include:

- pain
- headache
- speech problems
- nausea and vomiting
- visual problems, e.g. double vision (diplopia)
- loss of balance, dizziness
- weakness and movement problems
- abnormal sensation, e.g. numbness
- sleep disturbance (see Ch. 4).

Table 14.2 The cranial nerves

Cranial nerve Name and number	Type	Functions
Olfactory (I)	Sensory	Smell (olfaction)
Optic (II)	Sensory	Vision
Oculomotor (III)	Motor	Controls four of the external muscles that move the eyeball, and the muscle that raises the upper eyelid Some fibres control the iris muscle that constricts the pupil, and the ciliary muscle, which changes lens shape
Trochlear (IV)	Motor	Controls the external muscle that moves the eyeball down and outwards
Trigeminal (V)	Mixed	Motor to the muscles of chewing (mastication) Sensory to the face, mouth, teeth and the nose
Abducens (VI)	Motor	Controls the external muscle that moves the eyeball outwards
Facial (VII)	Mixed	Controls the facial muscles. Autonomic fibres to the lacrimal (tear), nasal and some salivary glands. Taste. Supplies the stapedius muscle in the ear
Vestibulocochlear (VIII) (auditory or acoustic)	Sensory	Hearing (audition) and balance
Glossopharyngeal (IX)	Mixed	Controls the pharyngeal muscles involved in swallowing. Autonomic fibres to some salivary glands. Taste
Vagus (X)	Mixed	Autonomic fibres to heart, bronchi, lungs and gastrointestinal tract. Taste. Sensory nerves from the external ear, trachea, bronchi, lungs, heart, pharynx and gastrointestinal tract
Accessory (XI)	Motor	Controls muscles of the neck and shoulders (head movement and shoulder shrugging), and the pharynx and larynx
Hypoglossal (XII)	Motor	Controls the muscles of the tongue needed for tongue movement during speech and swallowing

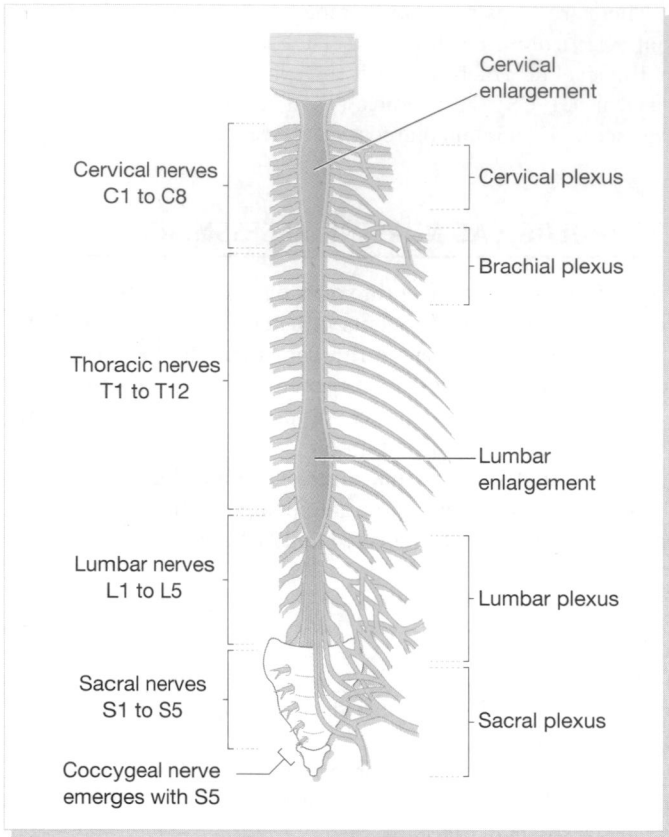

Figure 14.10 The spinal cord and spinal nerves.

ALTERED CONSCIOUSNESS

Consciousness is a state of wakefulness, alertness and aware-ness of self and the environment. It is generally considered as functioning of the cerebral cortex. Altered consciousness occurs due to abnormalities within the brain. Consciousness may deteriorate rapidly (e.g. due to a rapidly increasing extradural haematoma) or more insidiously (e.g. due to a more slowly expanding lesion such as a chronic subdural haematoma or brain tumour). As lesions within the brain expand, the ICP rises causing compression of the brain tissues and deterioration in the level of consciousness. If unrelieved, this will eventually lead to brain shifts, compression of the vital respiratory and cardiac centres within the brain stem, coning (see p. 299) and death. Deteriorating level of consciousness is the first sign of raised ICP.

Glasgow Coma Scale

The Glasgow Coma Scale (GCS) was first developed by Teasdale & Jennet (1974). It consists of a 14-point scale for assessing conscious level by evaluating three behavioural responses:

- eye opening (E)
- verbal response (V)
- motor response (M).

Each of these categories is assessed individually and the observed responses are recorded on a chart. Neurological assessment charts are familiar to almost every practising nurse, but only part of the chart constitutes the GCS (see Fig. 14.11). The rest of the chart is used to record other observations, such as respiration, which are useful in identifying the site of any neurological lesion and the cause of the neurological deteriora-tion. When documenting findings from the assessment on the chart, a series of joined-up dots should be used. This makes it easy to see any pattern developing and deterioration in level of consciousness.

Different levels of response in each of the above categories are afforded a numerical value, which may then be documented. On occasions these figures are summed and a 'coma score' is calcu-lated; however, it is better to document the score achieved from each of the subdivisions separately, e.g. E-4, V-5, M-5. The coma score is sometimes used to define specific levels of consciousness and a patient with a GCS of 8 or below and no eye opening may be defined as being in a coma.

The GCS has been extensively used and researched. Inter-rater reliability has been tested and it has proven to be a quick, accurate and simple tool for assessing consciousness (Teasdale et al 1978). It has also been adapted to a 15-point score with the addition of a further subdivision of abnormal flexion within the motor response category. This can cause confusion when patients are transferred between units where different forms of the scale are being used. The extra subdivision may be useful in clinical studies, but for routine care the 14-point score is sufficient (North & Reilly 1990). Most centres are still using the 14-point score and this is the one discussed here.

Assessing eye opening

Within this category, the subdivisions are eyes open sponta-neously, response to speech, to pain or no responses (see Table 14.3, see p. 282). When assessing consciousness it may be nec-essary to apply a painful stimulus to elicit a response. Painful stimuli should be applied with care and only after training, observation and supervised practice. Many methods used to apply pain will cause severe bruising.

When assessing level of consciousness, you are assessing CNS function and therefore a central painful stimulus should be used. This will also enable you to assess the response to pain if the patient has suffered a spinal injury (see p. 324), in which case a peripheral stimulus would have no effect, or to differenti-ate between localizing and flexion in terms of motor response. The methods used include supraorbital pressure and pressure at the jaw margin (Woodward 1997a) (see Guidelines for Care Priorities box 14.1, see p. 282).

Assessing verbal response

Within this category the subdivisions are orientated, confused, inappropriate words, incomprehensible words and none (see Table 14.4, see p. 282).

Assessing motor response

The subdivisions within this category on the 14-point scale are obeys commands, localizes to pain, flexion to pain and extension to pain (see Table 14.5, see p. 283).

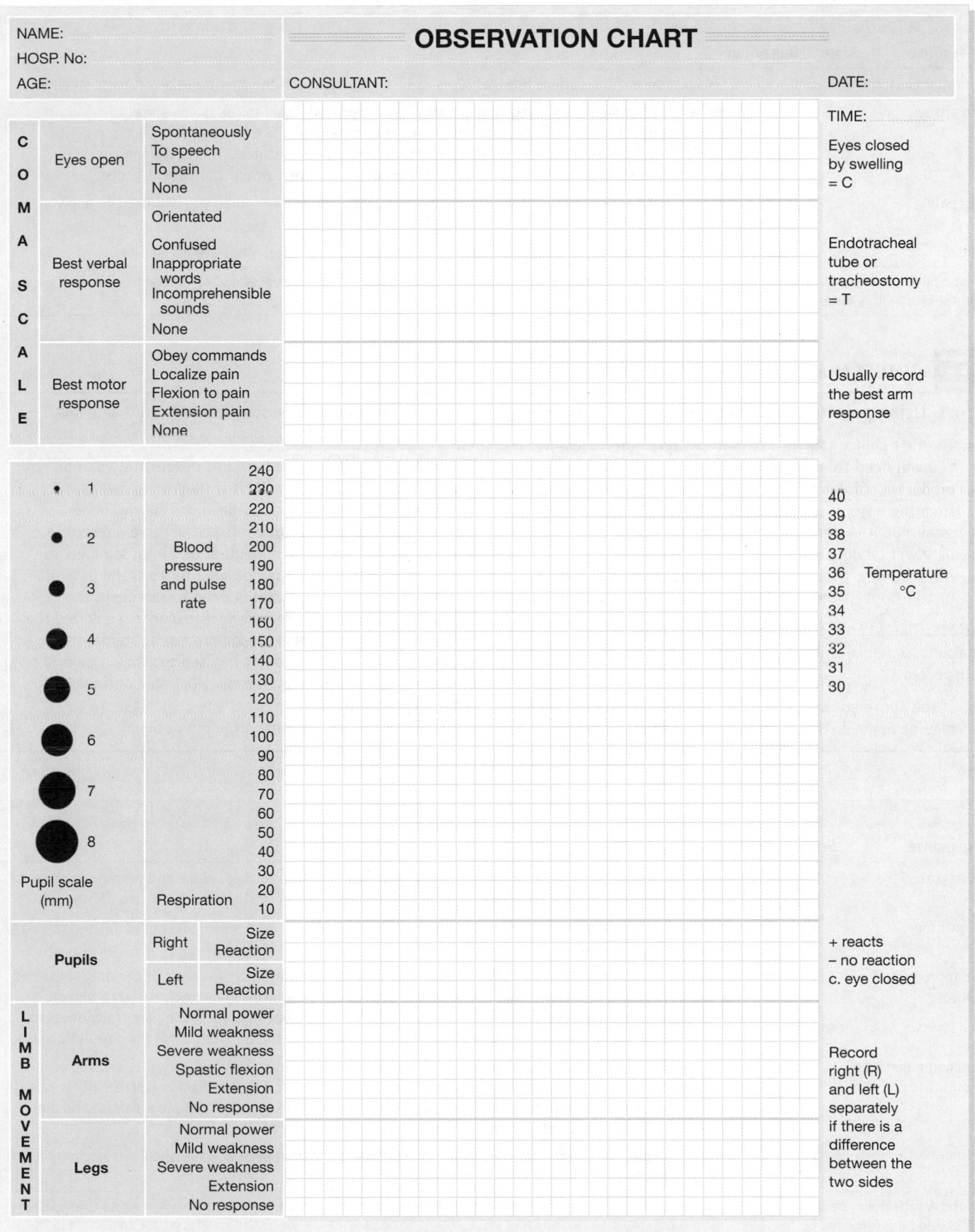

Figure 14.11   Neurological observation chart – Glasgow Coma Scale.

Table 14.3 Assessing eye opening

Response	Score	Behaviour
Spontaneously	4	Document this response if the patient has their eyes open as you approach them, without any further stimulation
To speech	3	This response will be recorded if the patient opens their eyes if you ask them to, or as you speak to them. Initially use your normal tone of voice, but do not be afraid to raise your voice and be persistent in order to elicit a response. It is also acceptable to gently shake the patient by the shoulder. This is the same level of neurological stimulation and overcomes a possible misinterpretation of response if the patient is deaf
To pain	2	If the patient has not opened their eyes when you touch or gently shake them, then you will need to apply a painful stimulus
None	1	Record this response if the patient does not open their eyes at all, even after you have applied pain

Note: Some patients will be unable to open their eyes due to periorbital swelling, rather than because of a reduced level of consciousness. This is recorded on the chart with a letter C.

 GUIDELINES FOR CARE PRIORITIES

14.1 Using painful stimuli to assess conscious level

- The first choice stimulus is that of supraorbital pressure. You will need to exert very little pressure in order to produce a painful stimulus. Feel along under the eyebrow from the nose, just under the orbital rim until you reach a small notch. A nerve runs through this notch and pressure here will produce pain.
- Alternatively, pressure can be applied at the jaw margin, just in front of the earlobe.

(**Note:** These two methods are contraindicated if the patient has facial injuries or if basal skull fractures are suspected.)

- If the above stimuli cannot be used then a trapezius pinch may be applied. This is done by taking approximately 5 cm of the trapezius muscle between the thumb and forefinger and twisting.

The first two sites described are both exquisitely painful and patients will respond to this if they are going to. Any stimulus should be applied once and for no longer than 30 seconds in order to elicit and observe a response. Many nurses do not apply enough of a painful stimulus to elicit a response, as they do not wish to harm the patient. In this instance, causing pain is done to safeguard the patient's well-being. If the incorrect response is elicited the patient's management may be compromised. Sternal rub causes bruising and should not be used to apply a painful stimulus in assessing consciousness. Debate continues regarding the suitability of other sites, such as nail bed pressure, for testing response to painful stimuli.

Table 14.4 Assessing verbal response

Response	Score	Behaviour
Orientated	5	In order to record that patients are orientated, they must be orientated to time, place and person. They must be able to tell you who they are, where they are and at the very least correctly identify the month and year
Confused	4	The person who is able to converse, but is unable to answer the above, even when questioned further will be recorded as confused
Inappropriate words	3	In this case, patients will answer using only one or a few words which make little sense. If the only response is swearing, then this is also considered inappropriate but needs to be taken in context. Patients who are woken repeatedly in the middle of the night may respond initially by swearing, but if they are really orientated then they will understand what you are doing and will usually respond appropriately once they are fully roused
Incomprehensible sounds	2	If you are unable to elicit any comprehensible words from a patient, but some vocalization is heard, i.e. moans/groans, then this will be the response recorded on the chart. You may elicit this response either when you speak to patients or, if their level of consciousness is slightly worse, when you apply a painful stimulus. Either way if any sounds are produced, this will be the response recorded
None	1	If no words or sounds are uttered from a patient in response to either speech or pain, then this response should be documented

Note: A patient may be unable to produce any verbal response due to the presence of a tracheostomy or endotracheal tube. If this is the case then a letter 'T' should be documented on the chart and no score should be calculated for this category. Some patients may be unable to respond due to damage to the areas of the cerebral cortex that control speech, causing dysphasia or aphasia. It is not acceptable, however, to record a letter 'A' or 'D' on the chart to denote this. Always score what you see, i.e. document the behaviour you actually observe in response to your stimulus.

Response	Score	Behaviour
Obeys commands	5	In order to assess whether patients are obeying commands, ask them to stick their tongue out. Always use a command that requires movement of muscle above the neck. It will be obvious to the observer if they have obeyed and it will enable you to assess patients who may have a spinal injury which prevents them from moving limbs. Be aware that asking patients to squeeze fingers to command may elicit a primitive grasp reflex from the touch of your fingers within the patients' palm, which may be confused with an appropriate response
Localizes to pain	4	If patients do not obey commands then you will need to apply a painful stimulus. If they are localizing to pain, they will purposefully move an arm in an attempt to remove the cause of the pain. If you have applied pain above the neck, this will be obvious. If other sites have been used, it will be more difficult to differentiate localizing from flexion. Patients may also be seen to be localizing in an attempt to remove uncomfortable nasogastric tubes, etc. If you have observed patients localizing to the painful stimulus when applied to assess eye opening, there is no need to inflict pain again to assess motor response
Flexion to pain	3	If patients do not localize, you may observe a purposeless general flexion of the arms in response to the painful stimulus. If this has not been observed, then increased pressure is required
Extension to pain	2	If patients have not flexed their elbow away from the painful stimulus, you may observe the arm being extended by straightening the elbow and sometimes internally rotating the shoulders and hands
None	1	If the arms do not move at all in response to speech or pain then this response is documented

Table 14.5 Assessing motor response

Note: Applying painful stimuli to the lower limbs may not be reliable in assessing consciousness. Any response elicited may be the result of a spinal reflex, rather than cortical function.
Abnormal flexion on the 15-point scale: describes a response in which patients will flex their elbows and wrists, while extending and internally rotating their legs.

PUPIL RESPONSE

There is usually space on a neurological observation chart to record pupillary responses. This is not part of the GCS and does not assess consciousness. It does, however, assist in identifying the location of an expanding mass lesion and is a later sign of increasing ICP, following deterioration in level of consciousness. When assessing pupil response the nurse should assess the size, shape and reaction to light of both pupils and record the findings on the chart (Woodward 1997b) (see Guidelines for Care Priorities box 14.2).

Abnormal findings and what they may indicate

A pupil that is becoming oval, enlarging or losing the ability to react to light may be an indication of rising ICP. This will often occur before a pupil becomes fixed and dilated (you may hear it said that the patient has 'blown' a pupil), although this process can be rapid and the intermediate stages can be missed.

The pupil response is controlled by two cranial nerves: optic (II) and oculomotor (III) (see Table 14.2). If there is an expanding lesion in the right cerebral hemisphere, which causes herniation of part of the temporal lobe through the tentorium,

 ## GUIDELINES FOR CARE PRIORITIES

14.2 Assessing pupil response

- Explain to the patient what you are going to do and why.
- Examine each eye separately, moving a bright pen-torch from the outer aspect of the eye towards the pupil and watch the pupil into which the light is being shone; then remove the light source. It should constrict briskly and then dilate to its usual size immediately on removal of the light source. This is known as the direct light response. Then repeat the above procedure, shining the light into the same eye as before. This time watch the reaction of the opposite (contralateral) pupil. It should respond in exactly the same way as the other pupil simultaneously. This is called the consensual light response. This procedure should then be repeated exactly, shining the light into the second pupil. The normal finding is that both pupils are equal in size and react briskly to light, both directly and consensually.

- The response from each is then documented separately. The size is measured in millimetres and the printed scale of pupil sizes on the chart is used to estimate the size of each pupil. Note the shape of each pupil (normally round).
- It may be necessary to darken the environment in which the observations are being performed in order for the nurse to be able to see a pupil constricting, especially if the patient has a darkly coloured iris or if the room is particularly brightly lit. It is easier to see if a larger pupil reacts or not.
- A brisk constriction to light is recorded with a plus (+) sign on the chart, while an unreactive pupil is documented with a minus (–) sign. Pupil size is recorded on the chart using the pupil scale (mm).
- Report any abnormal findings.

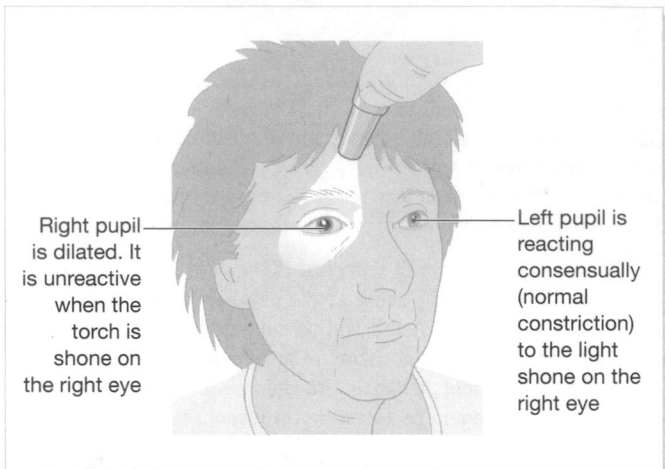

Right pupil is dilated. It is unreactive when the torch is shone on the right eye

Left pupil is reacting consensually (normal constriction) to the light shone on the right eye

Figure 14.12 Fixed and dilated pupil.

then the right oculomotor nerve will be compressed. This will result in loss of the ability to constrict the pupil in response to light and it will become fixed and dilated (see Fig. 14.12). If the pressure is unrelieved and continues to increase, the oculomotor nerve on the opposite side will also become compressed and the contralateral pupil to the side of the lesion will become fixed and dilated.

Pinpoint pupils may result from administration of narcotics, including codeine phosphate. Codeine is often used as an analgesic within neurosciences as it does not mask neurological signs; however, it does still have an effect on pupil constriction.

LIMB MOVEMENT

Limb movement is also documented on the neurological assessment/observation chart (Woodward 1997c). Whereas the GCS assesses the best arm response in order to assess consciousness, the limb movement section is used to assess the function of each limb individually, in order to localize any focal neurological limb deficits. A deficit (weakness or loss of limb movement) may be caused by either compression of the motor cortex within the brain or damage to the motor nerve pathways, often in the spine due to spinal lesions or injuries. Arms and legs are assessed separately. The subdivisions within the category assessing arm function are:

- normal power – this should be self-evident
- mild weakness – the patient can move the limb against gravity
- severe weakness – the patient is unable to move against gravity
- spastic flexion – the limb is flexed (e.g. bent at the elbow and the muscles are rigid)
- extension – the limb is straight
- no response.

Mild arm weakness may be difficult to identify in some cases. Where possible, ask patients to raise both arms above their heads and close their eyes. If they have normal power, their arms will stay still in space. If a mild weakness is present, then the affected arm will start to drift gently downwards.

The subdivisions within the category of assessing leg function are:

- normal power
- mild weakness
- severe weakness
- extension
- no response.

The power of patients' limbs can only be accurately assessed if they are able to initiate voluntary movement. The responses of flexion or extension or no response refer to the response to painful stimuli. Limb responses to pain may have been observed when assessing the GCS. It may not have been evident, however, possibly due to spinal injury. It is therefore useful to assess the response of each limb individually to pain in order to gain an indication of spinal cord function, to establish if patients have hemiplegia/paresis (paralysis or weakness on one side of the body) etc. This is done by applying pressure with a pen against the side of a finger or toe, adjacent to the nail bed. If patients are flexing to pain, they will bend their elbow and pull their hand away from the stimulus. Legs will not flex, but will extend in response to pain. This should be repeated on each limb, but remember that this may cause bruising, so the sites at which you apply the stimulus will need to be rotated, especially if these observations are being recorded frequently.

CHANGES IN OTHER OBSERVATIONS

Any change in the following observations will occur late in response to rising ICP.

Blood pressure
Unrelieved raised ICP causes brain hypoxia and compromises cerebral perfusion. The vasomotor centre (see Ch. 19) responds to this by attempting to increase cerebral blood flow by raising the mean arterial blood pressure. Serial blood pressure monitoring will show an upward trend in both diastolic and systolic blood pressures, and because the mean arterial blood pressure is rising there will be a widening gap between the diastolic and systolic pressures. It is more important to observe for this than for a global rise in blood pressure.

Pulse rate
At the same time, the pulse rate is usually observed to fall. Baroreceptors outside the skull detect what appears to be an abnormally rising blood pressure and attempt to reduce it by slowing the heart rate and therefore reducing cardiac output.

Temperature
The patient's temperature may increase in the end stages of unrelieved raised ICP. It is caused by loss of temperature control due to compression of the hypothalamus and is an ominous sign.

Respiratory rate
As the level of ICP rises, so does cerebral hypoxia and compression of the respiratory centre within the brain stem. The respiratory rate will begin to decrease, until in the end stages it will become shallow, slow and irregular.

COGNITION AND CONFUSION

Assessment of cerebral function not only encompasses assessment of consciousness, but also involves the measurement of a range of cognitive skills. Cognition refers to the psychological processes by which people become aware of objects of thought or perception, including all aspects of perceiving, thinking and remembering and the organization of the information. However, nurses do not often undertake formal cognitive assessments. Sometimes an informal assessment is made as indicated by a comment in the patient's notes, such as 'appears confused'. This indicates that the nurse has seen something suggesting that the patient is confused and behavioural indicators have been used to describe the patient's mental state, e.g. he or she is agitated.

Cognitive problems and causes

The word 'confused' has no clear definition and young people with cognitive deficits are taken more seriously than older people. Nevertheless, confusion is an altered state of consciousness. Cognitive functioning is complex and encompasses orientation, memory, attention, ability to evaluate, affect (mood), abstract reasoning and insight. When a patient appears confused the assessment performed should be able to identify if there is a neurological cause, or if it is due to something else. Too often behaviour is observed and hasty assumptions are made about the reason for that behaviour, without considering all the possibilities; for example, a female patient may be observed to be eating very little and the assumption may be that she is anorexic or apathetic. In reality, it may be that she is depressed, may have forgotten how to eat (as in the case of people with severe cognitive deficits) or may not be able to see all the food on the plate, as can be the case with those with visual field deficits. So when behaviour is observed, nurses need to consider if they are making the right assumption. We need to be able to differentiate between the three Ds – delirium, dementia (see also Ch. 32) and depression, which can often present in very similar ways.

Delirium is characterized by impaired consciousness and commonly accompanies physical illness. For example, delirium occurs in up to 15% of patients in general wards, and as many as 30% of patients in surgical intensive care units. Features of delirium include:

- reduced ability to maintain attention to external stimuli
- disorganized thinking – memory impairment, perceptual distortions and increased or decreased psychomotor activity
- possible paranoia
- possible hallucinations
- disturbed sleep–wake cycle – this is common, with patients often waking at night in a confused state
- disorientation in time and often in place
- mood changes are common.

Delirium may be caused by abnormalities within the brain (cerebral causes) or by factors outside the brain (extracerebral) affecting brain functioning (see Box 14.1).

Assessing cognitive function

There are many assessment tools available to assess cognitive function. Some are widely used, e.g. the Mini-Mental State

Box 14.1 Causes of delirium

Cerebral causes
- Post-epileptic states
- Trauma
- Transient ischaemic attacks
- Encephalitis
- Primary or secondary tumours
- Raised ICP

Extracerebral causes
- Drugs – all psychotropic drugs, antiparkinsonian drugs, anticonvulsants, analgesics
- Drug and alcohol withdrawal
- Metabolic causes – anorexia, hypoglycaemia, hypothyroidism, vitamin deficiencies (e.g. thiamine and B_{12}), hepatic failure, uraemia
- Infections – chest and urinary tract
- Constipation and urinary retention – may cause confusion especially in older people

Examination, which tests ability in ways that include counting backwards in 7s from 100, demonstrating orientation in time and place, identification of objects and writing a simple sentence (Folstein et al 1975). It is a simple tool and is easy and quick to use at the bedside. Other tools exist that can be more helpful in a critical care setting to assist in differentiating causes of confusion (Foreman 1984). It is also useful to involve the multidisciplinary team in assessing cognitive function, such as the occupational therapist (OT) who may perform more detailed assessments to identify specific deficits.

However, it may be necessary to perform a simple nursing assessment in cases where patients appear confused so that appropriate referrals can be made. This can easily be achieved without any specific assessment tools, by simply asking patients to read a newspaper and then discussing the headline story (having ascertained that they can read and can understand the language used). By doing this you can assess vision and motor ability as well as cognitive ability. Consider whether patients recognize the paper – can they hold it and read it; do they want to read it; can they remember what they have read; do they recognize faces; do they understand the story they have read; and can they discuss it with you and hold a conversation about the content including the implications of the events they have read about? Using this method, the main aspects of cognitive function have been assessed, i.e. attention, concentration, visual perception, initiation, memory, ability to evaluate, abstract reasoning and insight.

Having found that a patient may have a problem with cognitive function, the cause then needs to be identified and treated where possible, which will involve referral to other members of the multidisciplinary team. From a nursing viewpoint, some of the most important care relates to maintaining the safety of patients and those around them, while still respecting their dignity. If patients are conscious, then reorientation is also a priority.

ASSESSMENT OF PHYSICAL FUNCTION – SWALLOWING

A normal swallow is divided into three phases (sometimes described as four) and the nurse may observe problems associated with a particular phase:

- *Oral phase* – during which food is placed in the mouth and chewed and prepared for swallowing. This is a voluntary phase because you may decide to stop and spit out the food at any time during this phase. Poor lip closure may result in drooling. If the patient cannot control the tongue properly, there may be pocketing of food in the cheeks
- *Pharyngeal phase* – during which there are movements of the tongue and pharyngeal muscles. It is involuntary and cannot be stopped at will, although reflexes such as the cough reflex may 'reverse' the action. Food may become stuck in the pharynx which in turn may lead to aspiration and potential choking or pneumonia. In this case there will be excess mucus secreted, leading to a gurgly, wet voice. If the nose is not closed off during swallowing (by the soft palate), the nasal passages will remain open during speech and give a curious sound (hypernasal) to the voice as air is escaping down the nose. Food may lodge as a result in the nasal passages and block air passage, leading to loss of nasal resonance; this may be accompanied by nasal regurgitation of food or drink. The voice quality is usually called nasal by the public as it is similar in colds, but in reality it is hyponasal with loss of nasality. If the swallow happens before the respiratory tract has been closed off, the patient will cough and choke to clear the airway. This may also happen if there is a delayed or absent swallow as the respiratory tract opens 'too soon' before the food is clear
- *Oesophageal phase* – during which the food or fluid moves down the oesophagus to the stomach. Patients may complain of the sensation of a foreign body in the oesophagus. There may be regurgitation while lying down. Solid food is more difficult to swallow than fluids when a disorder of the oesophagus is present.

Problems with swallowing, such as dysphagia (difficulty in swallowing), are quite common in patients with neurological disease. It can accompany stroke, multiple sclerosis, Parkinson's disease and motor neuron disease, and sometimes follows head injury. Indeed, almost any neurological disease may have dysphagia as a sign. As swallowing is a sequence of events involving both voluntary and reflex activity, it is quite a complex event. Food, fluid and air for respiration share a common pathway in the pharynx. This means that poor swallowing may result in inhalation of food or fluid, which can lead to chronic or acute chest infection or even death by asphyxiation. For this reason the safety of the swallowing process is of crucial importance in all patients.

The muscles and nerves of swallowing are essentially the same as those used for speech. This means that patients with a language or speech problem such as dysphasia (disorder of language – expressive and/or understanding) or dysarthria (disorder of speech resulting from a problem in muscular control of speech mechanisms) are likely to have (but not necessarily) dysphagia as well. This means that the first clue that a patient may have dysphagia is a language or speech problem. Many hospitals and care homes have a swallowing assessment protocol (see Ch. 11) that leads the assessor through a series of questions and activities, including swallowing increasing amounts of clear water (which is less likely to cause problems if it is inhaled). If the patient fails the test, referral to a speech and language therapist (SLT) or other experienced professional for a full swallowing assessment is required before oral feeding is commenced.

There are, however, a number of indications and signs and symptoms that suggest the nurse should use caution before oral feeding is commenced. The most important ones are discussed below.

- It is important to obtain a history. Areas of relevance include the condition of the mouth, e.g. dryness, and disorders such as multiple sclerosis.
- The time taken to swallow should not be more than a couple of seconds and so if patients are having obvious difficulty and taking a longer time for each swallow, the SLT should be consulted. The swallowing assessment protocol should be followed soon after admission.
- Some reflexes protect the airway so it is vital to check for their presence. The cough reflex is most important as it clears debris from the larynx. Ask the patient to cough. The gag reflex is often thought to be important but it has been found that not all adults have a gag reflex (especially older adults) – swallowing can be safe in the absence of the gag reflex and unsafe in the presence of the gag reflex. Some so-called primitive reflexes (those found in infants but superseded by learned behaviour) may resurface in adults with profound neurological damage. Therefore, if the sucking, biting or rooting (the head turns, as if searching for a nipple, when the cheek is stroked) reflexes are found, it implies severe neurological damage, and extreme caution should be adopted with oral feeding.
- Needless to say, patients must be alert and responsive before a meal or drink is offered.
- Head, neck and trunk control are important if patients are to be able to control the movements that are necessary for eating and drinking. The ability to move the facial muscles is also necessary, so nurses should observe to see if patients can smile, frown and puff out the cheeks.
- Voice quality may be affected if patients cannot control the vocal organs. If there is constant irritation of the upper respiratory tract by food particles or fluids, then patients may have a wet and gurgly voice.
- Ask patients to swallow while you place a finger gently over the larynx (Adam's apple); it should bob up and down during the swallow.
- If any of the above signs are present, the SLT should be consulted.
- If patients already have problems, they may be pyrexial due to chest infection. Nurses should be alert to this and other signs of infection, such as increased respiration rate or cough (see Ch. 20).
- Some medications (e.g. sedatives) may affect swallowing and caution is needed when offering food or fluid.
- Some patients have none of the problems discussed above, but still require to be observed during their first meal. These patients have difficulty or pain with solids and fluids or the sensation of food being stuck. If there is nasal regurgitation, the meal should be stopped and the therapist informed.

GENERAL DIAGNOSTIC TESTS AND MEDICAL INVESTIGATIONS

PHYSICAL EXAMINATION

A full medical history and general physical examination will be undertaken. In addition, a specific neurological examination, which involves many different tests, is carried out during the examination of the neurological or neurosurgery patient. Many of these tests are functional tests. For example, reflexes are tested by seeing if they are present, absent, strong or weak. Tests of the reflexes demonstrate the conduction of peripheral sensory nerves, lower motor neuron and the integrity of the spinal cord or brain. Absent reflexes suggest lower motor neuron involvement. Exaggerated reflexes indicate upper motor neuron damage. Other functional tests involve sensations of touch, heat, taste and smell, which indicate the integrity of the nerve pathways for these functions. Sometimes cognitive tests of memory, intuition and orientation will demonstrate abnormal cerebral function. The scope of this text does not allow for a complete discussion of all these tests and readers requiring further information are advised to consult a neuroscience textbook (see 'Further reading', p. 329).

Another important test that is commonly used is ophthalmoscopy, because it allows the observer to visualize directly the blood vessels of the retina which are tributaries of the internal carotid arteries (see Ch. 15). Any vascular disease within the cranium is likely to be present in the retinal arteries as well. In some cases it is possible to see demyelination of nerve fibres in the retina and raised ICP when the optic nerve bulges forward into the cavity of the eye; this is called papilloedema.

IMAGING

X-rays

The brain is soft tissue and does not show up well on a plain X-ray but nevertheless this technique may be useful to detect skull fractures. There is a structure known as the pineal body which is found on the midline in the brain. It has calcium deposited in it and shows up as a small white mark in X-rays of adults. If there is a lesion, such as a tumour, pushing the brain to one side, the pineal body will also be displaced. Plain X-rays may also be used to show any defects of the spine and spinal cord.

- *Angiography* uses X-rays to visualize blood vessels following the injection of opaque contrast medium into an artery (arteriogram). It is used to show abnormal circulation or aneurysms (weaknesses/bulges in the artery wall).
- *Contrast medium* can also be introduced into the CSF but this has been largely superseded by the use of computed tomography (CT) or magnetic resonance imaging (MRI). The contrast medium may be injected into the brain ventricles (ventriculography), the CSF-containing cisterns at the base of the skull (cisternography), or the subarachnoid space of the spinal cord (myelography), depending on the area being investigated. Patients will usually require a rest following the procedure, as headache is common after procedures involving the injection of contrast medium into the CSF. Analgesia will usually be required and this must be prescribed – not all analgesics are suitable for people with neurological symptoms. Outpatients must be fully recovered before discharge home. Emergency contact information should be given to patients in case of prolonged or serious after-effects (e.g. increasing headache), together with after-care instructions and information about the next appointment.
- *Computed tomography* uses X-rays to produce images of tissues at different depths. A computer processes these 'slices' to produce a series of three-dimensional images. CT will show a certain amount of detail in soft tissue because the contrast between soft tissue and bone is shown. However, contrast medium may be injected intravenously during CT imaging to improve visualization of the structures and any disease processes.

The imaging techniques that involve the injection of contrast medium into the circulation or the CSF must be performed using aseptic conditions. The medical staff must ensure that patients are fully informed about the procedure and the potential risks, such as a stroke during angiography or adverse reactions to contrast medium. Written consent may be necessary. Many imaging departments have printed material, outlining the procedure, that the nurse can use to help patients understand what will happen and what to expect. There is a risk of adverse reactions to contrast medium and patients must be asked about any history of allergy or conditions such as asthma. The risk of adverse reactions and collapse during these invasive procedures means that resuscitation equipment should be readily at hand and the nurse should be aware of resuscitation policy and practice.

Magnetic resonance imaging

Magnetic resonance imaging (MRI) produces images of brain tissue and bone in great detail. The technique uses a strong magnetic field to cause hydrogen molecules to emit a radio signal that can then be detected and formed into an image. X-rays are not involved so radiological precautions are unnecessary. Sometimes marker substances are injected to identify specific areas, so patients will need to be prepared for an injection. The procedure can be frightening because the MRI scanner can be very claustrophobic. Panic buttons are given to patients and they can communicate via a speaker. The equipment is very noisy and patients should be warned of this. The magnetic field generated is very strong so metallic objects and items such as watches and credit cards, of both patients and staff members in attendance, need to be removed and stored securely. Any metallic prostheses and other metallic residues in the body will affect the scan and may prevent one being performed. The images produced are very clear and show anatomical and pathological detail. For instance, areas of demyelination in multiple sclerosis patients are evident.

Positron emission tomography

Positron emission tomography (PET) scanning is a technique used to identify areas of activity in the nervous system. The brain uses blood glucose, as it cannot store glucose like other tissues. Oxygen is also taken direct from the circulation. This arrangement can be used to provide an image of brain activity. If glucose with a radioactive marker molecule attached is administered to a patient, it will be metabolized by nervous tissue immediately. Therefore if the patient is asked to perform a verbal or mathematical task, active areas of the brain can be identified by the release of positrons (positively charged subatomic particles) from the marker as the glucose is metabolized in the brain. This can be used to locate lesions within the brain, such as brain tumours, that affect the metabolism of the surrounding tissues. Other markers such as ones that have a chemical affinity to dopamine (a neurotransmitter) can be used to identify dopamine concentrations within the brain: this is of use in Parkinson's disease (see p. 318). Some mental health conditions can show unusual PET scans. It is commonly used in research into brain function as well as disease processes. The scans produce 'slice' images that can give a three-dimensional picture. Colour is used to show intensity of activity (uptake and metabolism of the marker substance), with red showing most activity and blue showing the least. Radiological precautions will be used and patients will need preparation for an injection. Patients may be asked to avoid eating before the test to reduce the blood glucose level and ensure that the marked glucose is selected for uptake by the cells. The test may take up to an hour and the injection may be given up to an hour before the scan.

Ultrasound

Ultrasound employing echoes from high-frequency sound is non-invasive and can be used to demonstrate problems with the blood supply or flow and to determine risk of stroke when the carotid artery blood flow is affected.

ELECTROENCEPHALOGRAPHY

An electroencephalogram (EEG) is a recording of the electrical activity of the brain. This is especially useful in the diagnosis of epilepsy and sleep disorders, but other conditions such as tumours can also produce abnormal patterns. Patients have electrodes (up to 22) applied to specific locations on the scalp. The readings are taken and recorded onto folding paper, videotape or digitally. The reading is often done for about half an hour but sometimes a continuous record over a 24-hour period is needed. In this case, patients will have a portable transmitter attached and the information is gathered at a central point. This continuous technique is called EEG telemetry or just telemetry for short (but be aware that there are other meanings of the word telemetry). EEG requires patients to be relaxed during the recording, as tension in the scalp muscles can affect the recording. This is helped by patients having full information about the procedure (e.g. that it is not painful or invasive). They should have clean hair without any gels, spray or oil applied. Sometimes they will be asked to perform tasks, or lights will be shone into the eyes to observe the response of the brain.

ELECTROMYOGRAPHY

An electromyogram (EMG) records the electrical activity of a specific muscle or muscle group and the speed of nerve transmission and so can be used to investigate the action of peripheral nerves. There are two phases to an EMG. Electrodes are placed over the skin covering a muscle and an electrical stimulus is administered. This will enable the nerve conduction rate to be estimated.

In another part of the test, thin needle electrodes are placed into the muscle being studied and recordings are made of the electrical activity. EMG may be used in the diagnosis of disorders of peripheral nerves.

LUMBAR PUNCTURE

Lumbar puncture (LP) is performed to obtain a sample of CSF for chemical, cytological or bacteriological analysis. A spinal needle is introduced under local anaesthetic into the subarachnoid space between the third and fourth lumbar vertebrae and a sample of CSF withdrawn. A manometer can be applied to the spinal needle and the pressure of the CSF measured. Lumbar puncture is an invasive procedure that can be frightening. Patients will need to be prepared both physically and psychologically and be in a position to give informed consent. Usually patients will lie on their side with the knees drawn up and the neck flexed. This position opens up the spaces between the vertebrae and makes needle insertion easier. The skin is cleaned with a surgical skin preparation solution such as povidone-iodine and the procedure is carried out with aseptic precautions. Patients may be asked to straighten their legs and neck when the pressure is measured. Headache can occur after lumbar puncture and this is relieved by keeping patients lying down for 2 or more hours following the procedure. Analgesics can be administered if prescribed.

BIOPSY

The biopsy of peripheral nerves, muscle, meninges and even brain tissue may be undertaken to assist in diagnosis.

BLOOD TESTS

Patients with neurological problems will usually have blood tests that include full blood count and other routine haematological tests (see Ch. 18) and urea and electrolytes. Specific blood tests, such as vitamin B_{12}, copper level and antibodies, may be ordered in appropriate situations.

GENERAL DISEASE PREVENTION AND HEALTH EDUCATION

Many neurological problems have specific and preventable risk factors or determinants. Cerebrovascular disorders have well documented risk factors and the *National Service Framework for Older People* (Department of Health 2001) focuses on health promotion in the prevention of stroke. The risk factors that can be reduced include hypertension, smoking, high cholesterol levels and poor blood sugar control in diabetes.

Brain and spinal injuries are usually accident-related and many are preventable. Some legislation in the UK has reduced the risk of these injuries with the introduction of compulsory wearing of seat belts and crash helmets, although one cannot prevent individuals from choosing to ignore this and therefore increasing their risk. Alcohol is also implicated in many such injuries and the government has run many anti-drink driving campaigns in an attempt to reduce the incidence and severity of road traffic accidents.

Some nervous system infections are preventable through immunization programmes, e.g. poliomyelitis and some types of meningitis (see p. 311), and people should be encouraged to have themselves or their children vaccinated. Public awareness campaigns about the risks of bacterial meningitis and how to identify it have also appeared in the media.

Genetic counselling is also used with families who are known to have a hereditary neurological disorder, such as Huntington's disease (see 'Further reading', p. 329).

The difficulty for health promotion and disease prevention is that the cause of many neurological disorders is unknown (idiopathic). Much emphasis should therefore be placed on early detection of the disorders so that they can be treated early. This is important because many neurological problems are irreversible, but deterioration may be slowed or stopped if treated early, e.g. Wilson's disease (see p. 318).

NEUROLOGICAL IMPAIRMENT – GENERAL CONSIDERATIONS

Neurological impairment varies according to the function usually performed by the damaged part of the nervous system. Remember that the nervous system has three main functional divisions: sensory (input), central processing and motor (output). Therefore impairment will be in these main categories (see Box 14.2).

The management of these conditions will be discussed as they apply to the specific conditions outlined in the rest of the chapter.

ETHICAL AND LEGAL CONSIDERATIONS

There are many ethical and legal issues that may occur within a neurological setting, as patients are often not in a position to be able to make informed decisions for themselves. Nurses may be called upon to advocate for patients who are unconscious or cognitively impaired, particularly when issues of informed consent for procedures or discharge planning are being discussed.

There are also many issues relating to death and dying within the neurological setting. There has been much discussion in the media about people with advanced, progressive neurological disorders such as motor neuron disease who have gone to court to be allowed to undergo assisted suicide at a time of their choosing. This links into the debate about advance directives (see Ch. 34). There have also been landmark cases in this area, such as the one involving a young man in a permanent vegetative state whose relatives obtained a legal ruling allowing the medical team to stop feeding him enterally.

Other ethical and legal issues relate to the diagnosis of brain stem death and organ donation. These issues are usually resolved within an intensive care setting according to specific criteria for the diagnosis of brain stem death (see Ch. 31). However, many more opportunities exist for the procurement of cadaveric organs from patients who die as a result of neurological damage within a ward environment, so this should always be discussed sensitively with family members (see Ethical Issues box 14.1).

Box 14.2 Neurological impairment

Sensory impairments
- Visual field loss such as diplopia or hemianopia (loss of vision in the temporal or nasal half of the visual field of one or both eyes) in stroke
- Visual acuity loss occurs in optic neuritis (inflammation of the optic nerve)
- Hearing loss occurs with damage or tumours affecting the VIIIth cranial nerve
- Disturbance of balance associated with VIIIth cranial nerve damage
- Loss of sense of smell ( ) occurs in frontal lobe damage or disease
- Abnormal or impaired sense of taste (dysgeusia) can occur in some cerebral disorders
- Abnormal (e.g. paraesthesia, such as tingling) or loss of peripheral sensation (anaesthesia) associated with spinal disease or peripheral nerve damage
- Loss of proprioception (joint position sense)
- Neurogenic pain (see Ch. 7)

Processing impairments
- Changes in awareness, including level of consciousness
- Cognitive disturbance
- Memory loss (amnesia)
- Perceptual disturbances (agnosias)
- Hallucinations
- Seizures
- Dysphasia (aphasia) and language deficits
- Dyspraxia (the inability to initiate voluntary action)

Motor impairments
- Weakness (paresis) and paralysis (plegia) associated with either upper (spastic) or lower (flaccid) motor neuron lesions. This may affect one limb (monoparesis or monoplegia), one side of the body (hemiparesis or hemiplegia), the lower limbs (paraplegia) or all four limbs (quadriplegia or tetraplegia).
- Spasticity and clonus (a rhythmical jerking) associated with upper motor neuron lesions
- Ataxia (ill-timed and uncoordinated) movements associated with cerebellar disease
- Tremor, rigidity and bradykinesia (slowness of movement), associated with movement disorders, such as Parkinson's disease
- Dystonia, i.e. an abnormal posture produced by spasm of large trunk and limb muscles

ETHICAL ISSUES

14.1 Brain stem death

The definition of death in the past has presented few problems, but in the 20th century it became a more complex question. The reasons for this include the wider use of life-supporting treatments and equipment, the success of cardiopulmonary resuscitation and the question of organ removal for transplant. Where the confirmation of death is not clear-cut, the definition of brain stem death may be used. Brain stem death relates to the loss of functions supported by the brain stem, i.e. respiration, cranial nerve functions and heart rate. The definition of death as absence of heartbeat is inadequate because the heart may continue to beat for a period of days or even weeks after cessation of brain stem function if the patient is ventilated. This raises ethical and moral questions as many people feel that brain stem death is not really 'dead', as body functions continue if supported. A search of the internet will produce many websites arguing for the acceptance of brain stem death or for rejection of the notion. Guidelines have been produced by the Department of Health (1998) in conjunction with the Royal College of Physicians (London) that offer a code of practice and definition of death and brain stem death.

Readers may wish to consider this issue. Bear in mind how you would feel about accepting the diagnosis of brain stem death in a patient you have nursed and how you might feel if this were someone close to you personally. Is there a difference and, if so, what is the source of your uncertainty?

Further reading

Department of Health. A code of practice for the diagnosis of brain stem death including guidelines for the identification and management of potential organ and tissue donors. London: DoH; 1998. Online. Available: www.doh.gov.uk/pdfs/brainstemdeath.pdf.

▶ Nursing management of the unconscious patient

Patients may be unconscious for a variety of reasons and conditions, some of which are discussed in this chapter. There are general and essential aspects of care required by any unconscious patients. These are outlined here and discussed later in the chapter as relevant, but readers will also need to consult other chapters, e.g. Chapter 11 on nutrition.

Patients should always be positioned in such a way as to maintain their airway, preferably lying on their side to prevent the tongue from falling back and obstructing the airway. Sometimes insertion of a device may be required to ensure airway patency, such as a Guedel or nasal airway (see Ch. 29). Patients may require suctioning to clear oropharyngeal secretions, or humidified oxygen administration to maintain oxygen saturations.

Respiratory function, i.e. rate and depth, should always be assessed regularly. Chest auscultation should also be performed and oxygen saturation monitored using pulse oximetry, as patients are at risk of developing chest infections. Nurses should work in collaboration with the physiotherapist to prevent chest infections.

Serial neurological assessment and other vital signs (pulse and blood pressure) should be monitored frequently in order to detect changes that might indicate deterioration (see above). Changes in blood pressure, for example, may be due to deconditioning of the baroreceptors following prolonged bed rest or caused by raised ICP (see p. 280). Pulmonary emboli may also arise from deep vein thrombosis (DVT), which would result in cardiovascular and respiratory changes (see Chs 19 and 29). In some situations, anti-embolism stockings and subcutaneous heparin may be used in DVT prophylaxis.

Regular assessment of body temperature should be undertaken. Autoregulation of temperature may be affected, resulting in hyperthermia. Patients are also at risk of developing infections of the chest or urinary tract, which may present with pyrexia. For the care of a patient with alterations in body temperature, see Chapter 5.

Side rails (bed sides) may be used to prevent patients from falling off the bed; however, some NHS Trusts have strict policies governing the use of side rails, following incidents in which confused patients have fallen over the top. Even patients who are unconscious can still move limbs involuntarily.

Patients should be positioned carefully and in a neck-neutral position to minimize the risk of increasing the ICP. This is discussed in greater detail in the section on brain injury (p. 297). The limbs are positioned carefully, particularly so after a stroke (see p. 293). Patients should be repositioned on a regular basis to reduce the complications associated with bed rest, e.g. pressure ulcers, DVT and chest infection. The risk of pressure ulcer development should be ascertained using an appropriate tool and preventative measures commenced (see Ch. 10).

Unconscious patients will be unable to meet their hygiene needs and will need daily skin care and more frequent washes if they are pyrexial or cannot maintain continence. Mouth care and teeth cleaning, attention to hair and nails and eye care according to local protocols to prevent damage or drying will all be required (see Guidelines for Care Priorities box 14.3). Remember that family members may want to be involved in personal care.

Patients may need intravenous fluids in the short term and nurses should monitor the infusion and observe the cannula site for inflammation, etc. In the longer term, patients will have their nutritional and fluid needs met by enteral feeding (see Ch. 11). Nurses should keep meticulous records of fluid intake and output and observe the skin for signs of dehydration, e.g. loss of turgor (see Ch. 8).

A urinary catheter is usually required, e.g. for accurate measurements in critically ill patients or increased output when osmotic diuretics are given for raised ICP (see p. 301). The nurse should observe and measure the drainage, and follow local protocols regarding catheter care and maintenance of the closed drainage system. Unconscious patients must not be allowed to become constipated and nurses should monitor bowel action and, where necessary, give prescribed laxatives.

Communicating with unconscious patients and, of course, their family members is extremely important. Nurses must introduce themselves and explain nursing interventions in the

GUIDELINES FOR CARE PRIORITIES

14.3 Eye care for unconscious patients
(Supplied by Mary Shaw, see also Ch. 15)

Unconscious patients are at risk of drying of the eye or corneal damage (Mercieca et al 1999) leading to ulceration because the corneal (blink) reflex is absent, normal tear production is reduced and the eyes may not close completely. Nurses should assess the patient's eyes as soon as possible after admission and plan appropriate nursing interventions (Suresh et al 2000), including the following:

- Follow appropriate infection control protocols.
- Explain procedure to the patient in the normal way.
- Contact lenses, if worn, should be removed and stored safely.
- The eyelid itself is the best barrier to prevent corneal drying – the eyelids may be taped shut, usually with hypoallergenic tape placed horizontally. Padding should be avoided as the eyelids may not be completely closed beneath. The tape will usually be re-applied every 4 hours, after the pupil reaction has been assessed and the eyes examined. If the eye cannot be closed properly by this method, e.g. because of swelling, the ophthalmic surgeon may put a suture (Frost suture) in the upper lid to keep it closed. The suture is then taped to the cheek.
- 'Artificial tears', such as Lacri-lube, are applied, as prescribed, to prevent drying.
- Secretions and any other debris are cleaned from the eyelid margins with sterile swabs and sodium chloride 0.9% solution as often as required. Each swab is used once only and the eyelids cleaned from the inner to the outer aspect of the eye.
- Observe the eyes for signs of damage – redness, discharge, etc. (see Ch. 15).

References
Mercieca F, Suresh P, Morton A, Tullo A. Ocular surface damage in intensive care unit patients. Eye 1999; 13(part 2): 231–236.
Suresh P, Mercieca F, Morton A, Tullo A. Eye care for the critically ill. Intens Care Med 2000; 26(2): 162–166.

usual way. However, an important nursing role is getting the right balance between too much stimulation (overload) and too little (deprivation), by planning care that allows for periods of quiet and rest.

COMMON DISORDERS AFFECTING THE NERVOUS SYSTEM

CEREBROVASCULAR DISORDERS

These are neurological disorders characterized by some disruption to the blood supply to the brain (sometimes called cerebrovascular accident – CVA). They include various types of stroke and subarachnoid haemorrhage.

STROKE

The World Health Organization (1988) defines stroke as 'rapidly developing clinical signs of focal or global disturbance of cerebral function with symptoms lasting twenty-four hours or longer or leading to death with no apparent cause other than of vascular origin'. Although this is wordy, it does capture the essentials of stroke. 'Rapidly developing' distinguishes stroke from other conditions that usually have a slow onset. Head injury will have a rapid onset but it is ruled out of the definition by the phrase, 'with no apparent cause other than of vascular origin'. The diverse effects of cerebrovascular damage are captured in 'clinical signs of focal or global disturbance of cerebral function' and transient ischaemic attack (TIA) is ruled out by the phrase, 'symptoms lasting more than twenty-four hours ... or leading to death'. So a stroke is a disturbance of cerebral function that lasts longer than 24 hours and is of vascular origin.

Epidemiology and aetiology
Stroke accounts for 10–12% of all deaths in industrialized countries, and 88% of stroke deaths occur in those over 65 years of age (Bonita 1992). In a typical British health district of 250 000 people, 1500 have had a stroke and, of these, 730 will have significant problems such as paralysis or speech impairment, 400 will have a stroke within a year and 200 will die within the year. Stroke is a very costly condition and it accounts for 5% of the expenditure within each health district. It is the commonest cause of severe long-term physical disability and 50% of long-term nursing home residents have had a stroke.

Strokes are often described in terms of the damage done to the cerebral circulation, e.g.:

- Haemorrhagic (about 17%) when there is a bleed within the cranium. The haemorrhage can be into the substance of the brain (an intracerebral haemorrhage) or it can be into the subarachnoid space (subarachnoid haemorrhage). The latter are often dealt with as a separate diagnostic category.
- Ischaemic stroke (about 73%) either caused by a clot forming in a cerebral artery (cerebral thrombosis, thrombotic stroke) or a clot or other debris travelling from another part of the body, often the heart. This is called embolic stroke. Thrombotic stroke is more common than embolic stroke. Ischaemic strokes are sometimes divided into four main syndromes dependent on which cerebral blood vessels are affected.

Less common causes of stroke include cerebral venous sinus thrombosis (a clot within the venous drainage) which causes ischaemic damage and arterial venous malformation where a plexus of abnormal vessels fails to supply blood or ruptures, causing a haemorrhagic stroke.

Risk factors for stroke
- Hypertension (see Ch. 19)
- Current diagnosis of coronary heart disease (see Ch. 19)
- Congestive heart failure (see Ch. 19)
- Peripheral arterial disease (see Ch. 19)
- Diabetes mellitus (see Ch. 17)
- Other risk factors are associated with hypertension and vascular disease such as obesity and cigarette smoking

- Age – men have a higher rate of stroke in the younger age groups but women have a higher rate at the older end of the range
- Racial differences – e.g. there is a higher proportion of stroke in people of south Asian and African Caribbean origin.

Clinical presentation

The clinical presentation varies according to the type and severity of the stroke and the area of the brain affected (see Box 14.3).

Medical/surgical management

Sometimes surgery is used to improve cerebral circulation. Carotid endarterectomy is relatively common, where atheroma is removed from the artery wall to improve circulation. An arteriogram will be performed before this operation to establish the location and prognosis of surgery.

If the patient has had a thrombus, thrombolytic drugs can be administered in an attempt to reduce damage. Streptokinase and tissue plasminogen activator (tPa) are given as soon as possible but only when it is established that the stroke is not a haemorrhage, as thrombolytic drugs would extend the bleed and damage. A CT scan within 24 hours is recommended to identify the correct stroke type. This will usually differentiate between haemorrhagic and ischaemic stroke.

Not all the damage to brain tissue after stroke is due directly to ischaemia. Some is caused by the release of chemicals, such as glutamate from the ischaemic cells, that damage the non-ischaemic, healthy surrounding cells and these in turn release more chemicals and so extend the damage in a cascade effect. Some drugs, such as nimodipine (a calcium-channel blocker), are given as neural protectors because they prevent the chemical cascade and improve the outcome for the patient.

▶ Nursing management

The management of stroke patients is holistic and patient outcomes depend very much on the collaborative working of a multidisciplinary team of nurses, doctors, therapists (physical, OT and SLT), dieticians, and the patient, family and other carers.

Management of stroke patients can be difficult, because there is often a wide variety of symptoms and variation in severity among patients. Some may make full recoveries while others become dependent on care; still others may die within hours or days of the stroke. Patients come from diverse sociocultural backgrounds which present a challenge when care planning.

Care should aim to maintain the airway where consciousness is altered (see p. 290), maximize hydration, nutrition, communication, mobility and skin integrity (see Chs 3, 8, 10 and 11). Bowel and bladder function (see Ch. 12) need sensitive and careful intervention to promote continence, prevent complications and maintain dignity for patients. Sometimes a patient who cannot speak or move to the toilet and remove clothing will not be incontinent but will have difficulty with bowels and bladder. This is called functional incontinence.

Prevention of complications such as urinary tract infections, chest infections and constipation will involve maintaining hydration and improving movement and mobility.

The effects of hemianopia are usually permanent and patients have to learn how to overcome the deficit by turning the head or learning to scan the field of vision. Nurses should approach patients from the unaffected side. Another technique of use in hemianopia is learning to turn the dinner plate after each mouthful to ensure that the meal is completed. The visual deficit increases the potential for accidents and nurses must be mindful of environmental hazards.

Box 14.3 Clinical presentation of stroke (depends on type, severity and brain area affected)

- Alteration in consciousness (acute phase)
- Hemiplegia – the side will depend on which cerebral hemisphere is affected, as the left hemisphere controls the right side of the body and vice versa. As the two hemispheres are not identical in function, for instance language is most commonly situated in the left hemisphere, left hemiplegia and right hemiplegia are accompanied by different problems. Language problems (deficits) and dysphasia are associated with left hemisphere damage in most people and therefore dysphasia accompanies right hemiplegia
- Hemiparesis – rather than hemiplegia. The pattern of the weakness is the same distribution as the paralysis
- Dysphasia, or if there is complete loss of language (aphasia). This is different from dysarthria which is a problem associated with the production of speech, i.e. language is unimpaired and the person understands speech. In dysphasia, understanding and/or expression of speech can be affected; these are called receptive dysphasia and expressive dysphasia, respectively, and represent different areas of the brain supplied by the middle cerebral artery. Both types can occur together and this is called global dysphasia

- Loss of sensation as well as motor loss (paralysis). This may lead to poor coordination or even loss of the ability to move at all (without true loss of motor function), as the brain relies on sensory input to monitor the position of the body and its movements and without it movement is difficult or impossible
- Agnosias – various types of perceptual problem can occur in which patients have difficulty in recognizing or identifying objects, people or situations. These can be very disabling
- Hemianopia – various patterns of visual field loss depending on the part of the visual pathway affected. Hemianopia can be bitemporal with both temporal fields affected, binasal with both nasal fields affected, or homonymous, where one eye has lost the temporal field and the other eye has lost the nasal field
- Loss of the perceptual ability that underlies the sensation – patients are then said to have neglect or hemi-inattention. This is a troublesome symptom because patients may not even acknowledge the existence of a whole side of their body, world and universe
- Dysphagia – frequently accompanies stroke with dysphasia or posterior infarct
- Emotional lability

Neglect or hemi-inattention is very hard (if not impossible) for a person with normal perception to understand and it can be profoundly disabling. Intervention should aim to make patients aware of the neglected side by gradually spreading out from the midline, which is usually not affected. The patient's locker should be placed on the unaffected side.

Dysphagia needs to be carefully assessed by a qualified and experienced assessor, usually a SLT (see p. 286). Severe dysphagia may put patients at risk and they may require nasogastric or gastrostomy feeding. Oral feeding will often be of thickened puréed foods as these are generally easier to swallow. Positioning the patient's head and feeding in an upright position are the most common interventions to help with dysphagia.

Loss of sensation puts patients at increased risk of skin damage or burns. Pressure area assessment and care are vital, as is maintaining a safe environment, e.g. making sure that patients are positioned at a distance from radiators.

Spasticity is a common complication after the initial phases of stroke. This is an increase in muscle tone, where movement becomes difficult and the limbs become stiff. There are muscle stretch reflexes which, in unaffected people, are designed to regulate muscle activity in response to the task being performed. For example, more muscle power is needed to lift a heavy weight than a lighter one. In spasticity these reflexes are disconnected from cerebral control due to damage in the motor pathways and they overreact, causing the increase in tone. This can be serious because, if untreated, patients will not regain function and everyday tasks will be difficult or impossible. Spasticity can also be painful and, if an unusual posture is involved, the soft tissues such as muscles, ligaments and tendons may contract permanently, leading to contractures and deformity. Spasticity is controlled by physiotherapy, medication and careful positioning of the patient.

The goals of care are:

- protection from injury
- prevention of complications
- maximizing functional ability.

Recovery is a slow process and unpredictable. All activity should start with simple skills and progress. It is important to be methodical (DeLisa 1988) and there is said to be a progression in recovery of function:

- Reflex to voluntary control – the patient's reflexes will be present before functional voluntary movement is achieved. Some reflexes are unhelpful in patient care if they interfere with normal function, such as some neck reflexes that produce odd postures if the head is turned
- Gross to fine movement – large movements are possible before finer functional movement is achieved
- Proximal to distal – there is a tendency to recover control over the body near to the centre (proximal) before peripheral (distal) movement is regained. In other words, patients will regain the use of the shoulder and elbow before the wrist, hand and fingers, and likewise with the lower limbs.

Patients should be assessed for skills for daily living, such as meeting personal hygiene needs, that are intact and plans should be drawn up to develop those skills or compensatory strategies for those skills that are not intact and cannot be

regained. This will involve teaching patients and family members (see Health Promotion box 14.1, p. 294). Care must be planned with other members of the rehabilitation team. It is important that work done in the therapy departments is reinforced on the ward or in the patient's home to maintain progress. Patients also need general information about stroke; an example of a stroke education programme delivered in the rehabilitation setting is described by Barton et al (2002).

Positioning, movement and mobility

Positioning helps to prevent pressure ulcers, contractures and spasticity and allows passive movement. The positions recommended are aimed at reducing spasticity (see Fig. 14.13, p. 295). Although the evidence base for this is limited, experience of practitioners suggests that it is important. Nurses positioning patients must remember that proper positioning should be practised at all times to maintain optimal effect and reinforce therapy sessions (see Special Issues box 14.1, p. 294).

When patients are correctly positioned and spasticity is minimized, it will be possible for the multidisciplinary team to improve range of motion (ROM) for the joints. Patients will be able to build up the strength and endurance necessary to carry out daily activities. This should enable them to begin to regain trunk balance and head control necessary for ambulation.

To facilitate movement, ROM exercises need to be given to patients. In these exercises, each joint is supported both above and below and gently moved to the fullest range. This is called passive ROM exercise because the nurse or carer is performing the activity for the patient. Passive ROM should not be done when patients can move themselves, and it must never cause pain. Movement should be slow, careful and precise; each movement should be repeated five to 10 times and up to three times a day. Activities should always be coordinated with the therapy programme.

Strength and endurance can be developed and increased for patients. Nurses should plan rest and activity so that patients do not tire. The pulse rate may rise 20–50 beats/minute during activity, but should return to within 10 beats of the baseline rate within 2 minutes. If the pulse does not improve within 6 minutes, the activity should be stopped. Observe patients for signs of cardiovascular distress, such as breathlessness. If they have been lying down for a long period, the baroreceptors may not be sensitive to postural change and patients will be unable to maintain blood pressure (postural or orthostatic hypotension). The use of anti-embolism stockings can help if patients have orthostatic hypotension, as they prevent blood pooling in the dependent legs. Factors that can affect strength and endurance in patients are low oxygen saturation, nutritional deficiencies, anaemia, some medications and sleep disorders. Nurses should aim to increase sitting by 15 minutes a day and it should be done about two or three times a day. A daytime rest period of 60–90 minutes should be included. Remember to support the head and trunk during activities to prevent contractures, abnormal postures and spasticity.

ROM and strength and endurance will allow patients greater mobility in bed and improved sitting balance, which will allow for functional activity and social interaction. Transfers from bed to chair will improve. When nurses help patients with activity, it is important to prepare the area so that activity and movement

HEALTH PROMOTION

14.1 Dressing plan after a stroke

Dressing may be a problem for patients with a one-sided paralysis or weakness. The occupational therapist will work with patients and family members to enable maximum functional independence (Webster 2002). The following plan can be used as a general guide to dressing.

- Use clothing that is easy to use or modified if necessary, such as polo shirts that do not require doing up. Braces on trousers may be useful. Slip-on shoes are another example. Clothing should also be suitable for the patient so that it can be removed easily for toileting or perhaps frequent washing is necessary. Patients must be able to select their own clothing.
- Patients with unilateral neglect may find it easier if clothing is presented to them front down. It is usual to place shirts front upwards but this requires the patient to turn it over before putting it on. In neglect this ability may be lost and if clothing is presented front upwards they may end up dressed back to front. By placing the clothing front downwards it removes the 'rotate' operation. Clothing should be laid out in the order that it is put on, i.e. underwear first.
- Use assistive devices such as buttonhooks, zip pull rings, or sock applicators if necessary.
- Start the dressing in bed to maximize safety if balance is impaired.
- Upper limbs – use unaffected arm to pull the shirt sleeve up the weak arm above the elbow and then put unaffected arm into the other sleeve. Place the head through the neck opening and use the good arm to pull the back of the collar and the back of the shirt overhead. Readjust to remove wrinkles and folds.
- Lower limbs – when in a sitting position, use the unaffected arm to flex the affected knee. Pull pants or knickers over the foot and up to the ankles, pushing down the knee to straighten the leg. Place the unaffected foot into the other leg and pull the garment up as far as possible. When both legs are in the garment, pull it up with the good arm until it reaches the knees. Above the knees, the patient will need to roll from side to side to pull up the garment completely. Place the affected foot into sock or tights and pull up before placing the unaffected foot into sock or pulling tights right up. Trousers and skirts may be put on in the same way as underpants. If patients have standing balance, they can dress the lower limbs from a chair or a standing position. The affected leg can be crossed over the stronger leg for easier access. Close buttons, zips or Velcro before standing up where possible to prevent patients falling down. Button hooks and zip pull rings may be useful and clothing can be modified so that fastening is easier.
- Put shoes on using a shoe horn if necessary.

Teaching plans for patient dressing and undressing can be found in Alexander et al (1999).

References

Alexander TT, Hiduke RJ, Stevens KA. Rehabilitation nursing procedures manual, 2nd edn. New York: McGraw-Hill; 1999.

Webster J. Client-centred goal planning. Nurs Times 2002; 98(6): 36–37.

 SPECIAL ISSUES

14.1 Proper positioning after a stroke

- Neutral alignments should be selected, but the patient's comfort is important.
- Patients should be in a functional position, i.e. one that facilitates range of motion (ROM) exercises to maintain joint function and prevent contractures.
- The position should be changed frequently to ensure comfort and prevent pressure ulcer development. Position changes will need to be coordinated with the therapy programme – it is not helpful to position a patient lying down for rest just before a therapy session.
- Limbs that are weakened or paralysed should be supported with pillows or foam rolls to maintain the best position (see Fig. 14.13).
- Following a position change, always remember to check catheters, intravenous lines and monitoring wires.
- If splints or other orthotic devices are used, patients should be monitored for pressure and friction damage (see Ch. 27).
- The patient's head should be aligned to promote upright posture so that the patient looks straight ahead and the neck is aligned with the spine.
- Correct alignment might cause spasticity because, following stroke, some abnormal reflexes associated with head and neck movements govern abnormal limb postures. These are called the tonic neck reflexes. Legs should be placed to avoid contractures and abnormal postures that might limit normal standing and walking on recovery. The upper limbs should be supported to decrease contracture, increase functional use, strength and control as many normal daily activities, such as eating and washing, depend on the arms and hands.

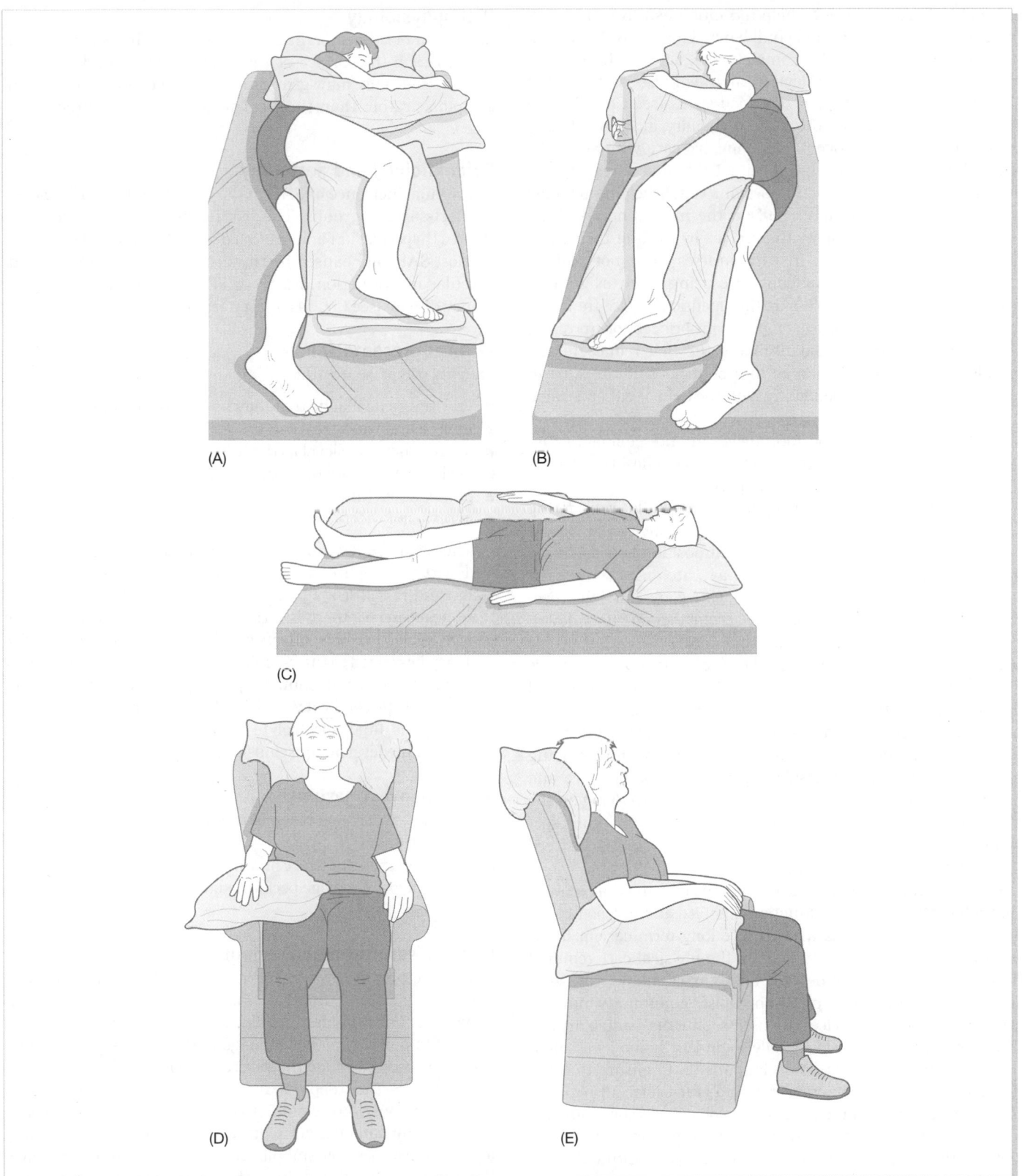

Figure 14.13 Limb positioning after a stroke (right-sided hemiplegia). (A) Side lying on the unaffected side. (B) Side lying on the affected side. (C) Lying supine. (D) Sitting in a chair (front view). (E) Sitting in a chair (side view).

are unrestricted. Try not to help too much as this can undermine a patient's practice and confidence. This involves allowing patients sufficient time to complete the activity. In may be necessary to use assistive devices such as hoists and mobility aids such as Zimmer frames or tripod sticks (see Ch. 27). The care plan is updated as the patient's ability increases. Safety issues in caring for stroke patients involve care with armrests, wheelchair footplates, bars and rails. Tubes and wires must be adjusted to prevent removal and pain. When helping patients to transfer, they must never pull on the nurse's neck – some patients may try to support themselves by putting their arms around the nurse's neck. In turn, nurses must not pull on stabilization devices that patients are using, such as Zimmer frames. Think of all transfers as therapeutic because they promote strength and balance, improve proprioception (position sense) and coordination and ultimately they will reduce nurses' workload. Patients will then be in a better position to start to be able to mobilize independently with the help of either a frame or a wheelchair.

Assessment for stroke positioning is a multidisciplinary activity and should involve all the team members. Residual deficits are varied, so a systematic holistic approach is needed.

Select the position for each patient carefully, considering staff available, equipment needed and the activity the patient is preparing to do. The semi-recumbent position is widely used for patients in bed for activities such as watching TV, receiving visitors, resting after activities, and during some nursing procedures, e.g. bed bathing and bladder care. The prone (face down) position is sometimes used to prevent contractures, but people with mobility problems may not be able to tolerate it and it is best used in the therapy department. Sitting in a chair is used during much of the day, while patients are out of bed and not in a therapy department. It is a position suitable for many functional activities such as eating, drinking, washing, reading and writing. Lying on the side is used to relieve pressure and as a resting position. There are differences between lying on the affected and unaffected sides for people with hemiplegia, especially for the paralysed shoulder which should be moved forward to prevent shoulder retraction.

With careful and planned care, patients may make a recovery that allows them the best functional ability and independence. There are many patients who require long-term care at home or in other community settings and the physical care required depends on their level of dependence. Nurses should work with the patient, family, OT, physiotherapist, community nursing service and social services to assess patients' suitability for discharge home. This will usually include a home assessment by a therapist and visits home by patients to ensure that the discharge is adequately supported and is feasible. All patients, families and carers will require psychological and social support following a stroke. Nurses can provide information about organizations that offer support and resources (see 'Useful websites', p. 329).

SUBARACHNOID HAEMORRHAGE

Subarachnoid haemorrhage (SAH) is a type of stroke but it is often dealt with separately because there are many differences from other types of stroke.

Pathophysiology

Subarachnoid haemorrhage occurs into the subarachnoid space, i.e. on the surface of the brain rather than deep in the brain tissue. This may give rise to more general neurological symptoms rather than the focal symptoms of an intracerebral bleed.

Epidemiology and aetiology

The annual incidence of SAH in the UK is about 15 in 100 000. It affects all age groups. The risk factors are similar to other strokes (hypertension and arterial disease (see pp. 291–292)).

Most SAHs are caused by rupture of an aneurysm or other vascular malformation. Rarely, it is associated with polycystic kidney disease (see Ch. 24) or even trauma.

Clinical presentation

Patients will present with:

- very severe headache that may have a sudden onset
- nausea and vomiting
- altered conscious level as the ICP increases
- neck stiffness (sometimes called nuchal rigidity or stiffness)
- photophobia (intolerance to light)
- pyrexia may occur.

There may be signs of nervous system damage such as localized paralysis. Ophthalmoscopy may show signs of haemorrhage and raised ICP. Up to 50% of patients will die, and for those who survive there is a risk of a second bleed. Vasospasm (spasm in blood vessels) affects nearly half of those who survive and may be related to the chemical changes that take place after bleeding has occurred. Some people will develop hydrocephalus, a dilation of the cerebral ventricles due to obstructed flow of the cerebrospinal fluid. Electrolyte imbalance can occur and this may affect the level of consciousness.

Specific investigations

- CT scan – will reveal blood in the subarachnoid space in most instances
- Lumbar puncture – the CSF will be bloodstained
- An angiogram may be performed to identify the vessel involved.

Medical/surgical management

Immediate care involves intravenous fluids to maintain normal blood pressure and thus ICP and to adjust any electrolyte imbalance. Calcium-channel blockers such as nimodipine may be used to prevent further damage and vasospasm. Analgesics should be prescribed for the severe headache, but not narcotic analgesics as they depress the nervous system further and changes in consciousness due to analgesia could mask deterioration. Many patients will require surgery to clip the bleeding artery. Sometimes coil embolization is performed; this involves the insertion of a coil into the blood vessel under X-ray visualization and control.

▶ Nursing management

Patients who have a subarachnoid haemorrhage will usually be transferred to a neurosurgical unit for management. Recovery rates vary with the extent and site of the bleed. Surgery is often carried out soon after diagnosis and initial stabilization and patients and family members will need careful explanation and support during this very distressing time.

Some people may make a full recovery while others will require rehabilitation and perhaps long-term care. The site of the bleed determines which functions are affected. Anterior cerebral artery bleeds may cause cognitive impairment whereas basilar artery bleeds may interfere with life support centres such as respiration and heart function. Patients will be nursed on bed rest and require very careful monitoring of neurological and general condition (see above). Many of the care problems for the longer-term care of patients with SAH are similar to stroke, e.g. such as management of swallowing, communication and mobility.

TRAUMA

BRAIN INJURY (HEAD INJURY)

Head injury refers to any injury to the scalp, skull or brain that is of sufficient magnitude to interfere with normal function and require hospital treatment. A more accurate term that describes such a major traumatic event is brain injury (Hickey 1997). Injuries are sometimes classified using the GCS as follows:

- mild brain injury – GCS 13–15
- moderate brain injury – GCS 9–12
- severe brain injury – GCS 3–8.

Brain injuries may also be classified according to location and type of injury under some systems. Acute brain injury can have a devastating impact, not only on the patient but also on family members. Brain injury can result in physical and cognitive problems for patients, as well as having an emotional, psychological and social impact on both patients and their family members, which can be immeasurable and devastating. It is not uncommon for brain-injured patients to have sustained other injuries such as chest injuries, cervical spine injuries, abdominal injuries, other fractures and lacerations.

Aetiology and epidemiology

In the UK, 1 person in 100 attends an accident and emergency department each year as a result of head injury and, of these, 300 per 100 000 are admitted to hospital and 9 out of every 100 000 patients affected will die from their injury, mostly within 24 hours (Lindsay et al 1997). Brain injury affects predominantly young men, the male:female ratio being 3:1, and over 50% of people sustaining an injury are under 20 years of age. It is the commonest cause of death in 15- to 24-year-olds. Around two-thirds of patients will survive severe brain injury, whereas 20 years ago only half survived. This improvement in survival has not been due to any advance in medical care or innovative technology, but rather to the legislation that made the wearing of seat belts and crash helmets compulsory. However, virtually all of these survivors have some degree of brain damage and the disability following a moderate injury is as bad as that following a severe injury. The charity Headway (www.headway.org.uk) estimates that the number of people with severe brain damage is in excess of 120 000 in the UK and that number is increasing by over 11 000 per annum.

The causes of brain injury in the UK include:

- road traffic accidents (most common) – occur most commonly in young men and alcohol is frequently involved; the injuries sustained are often more serious (Lindsay et al 1997)
- falls
- assaults
- sports and recreational injuries
- workplace injuries
- firearms or other blunt force.

Pathophysiology

The different types of injury that may be sustained include penetrating injury, crush injury, deceleration injury (the majority) and missile injuries. These can cause different categories of damage to the structures inside and outside the skull. This damage is categorized as either primary brain injury (i.e. occurring at the time of the impact) or secondary damage, which results from complications of the initial injury. Once a head injury has occurred, nothing can change the impact damage; therefore management is aimed at preventing and reducing the secondary sequelae.

Primary brain injuries
Cerebral contusions (coup and contre-coup)
These are in effect bruises on the brain. They are caused at the time of the injury as the brain tissue rocks backwards and forwards within the skull, hitting the surface of the brain against the inside of the skull. Coup and contre-coup injuries are sustained during deceleration when the brain has a forward momentum that will shake it backwards and forwards within the skull vault. Coup injuries are sustained across the frontal lobes of the brain as it hits the front of the skull due to forward momentum, then having hit the skull at the front the brain is bounced back and hits the back of the skull where contre-coup injuries are sustained across the occipital lobes. This kind of injury is often associated with cerebral oedema and raised ICP, which may result in brain herniation (see p. 299).

Haemorrhage
This also occurs at the time of the injury and bleeding can occur in several different layers within the brain and meninges, leading to clot formation (haematoma).

Extradural haemorrhage. This is the outermost haemorrhage and is often due to the rupture of the middle meningeal artery, lying between the skull and the dura mater. Often a result of arterial bleeding, they expand rapidly and cause pressure on the brain tissue underlying the haematoma. An extradural haemorrhage shows up on a CT scan as a bright white lesion near the surface of the brain, as fresh blood is denser than the surrounding brain tissue. The mortality rate for patients in deep coma is 20% (Trauma.org 2000).

Subdural haemorrhage. This may occur when the bleeding is due to rupture of the bridging veins between the cortex and the dura mater. As the bleeding is venous, the haematoma will often accumulate more slowly and the blood will spread out over the surface of the brain within the subdural space. Subdural haemorrhages are often associated with underlying contusions and the mortality rate may be as high as 60% (Trauma.org 2000). They may be detected in the acute phase when the patient presents with signs of raised ICP due to the contusions, or may not be identified until a few days/weeks after the initial injury, when the patient becomes increasingly confused, drowsy and may develop focal neurological deficits. These chronic subdural haematomas are not usually associated with contusions and will show up on CT scan as a darker area spreading out over the surface of the brain, as the blood clot dissolves and becomes less dense. They may be present and symptomatic for months.

Subarachnoid haemorrhage. This refers to bleeding into the subarachnoid space. It will show up with fresh blood (white on CT scan) within the ventricles, but is not usually life-threatening.

Intracerebral haemorrhage. This occurs within the substance of the brain tissue itself and may also bleed into the ventricular system.

Skull fractures

These may occur at any point from a blow to the skull. They may be associated with a wound overlying the fracture that increases the risk of infection. They may also become depressed if a fragment of bone is pushed downwards into the brain tissue underneath. Basal skull fractures are potentially very serious and patients are at increased risk of meningitis, as a route of entry for infection exists. The clinical signs associated with basal fractures are outlined in Box 14.4.

Shearing/diffuse axonal and white matter injury

This type of brain damage occurs as a result of mechanical forces causing shearing following deceleration. This results in disruption to and tearing of the axonal fibres. The brain stem may be affected and will often result in coma.

Concussion

This is a temporary disruption in cerebral function resulting from the injury. Consciousness may fluctuate and there may be other temporary loss in neurological function.

Box 14.4 Clinical signs – basal skull fracture

A basal skull fracture should be suspected if any of the following clinical signs are present:

- CSF rhinorrhoea (leak of CSF from the nose) – this can be differentiated from other nasal discharge as it tests positive for glucose
- Bilateral periorbital haematoma (bruising around the orbits)
- Subconjunctival haemorrhage (bleeding under the conjunctiva of the eye)
- CSF otorrhoea (a leak of CSF from the external auditory meatus) which may be associated with Battle's sign (bruising over the mastoid bone behind the ear, which may take up to 48 hours to develop)

Secondary brain injuries

Often nursing and medical management following brain injury are aimed at minimizing or preventing the secondary damage that can occur. Secondary sequelae include further bleeding, seizures, hydrocephalus, infection, hypoxia, infarction and cerebral oedema (swelling of the brain), many of which will result in raised ICP (see below). It is important to understand the mechanisms leading to cerebral oedema. Damage to any part of the body results in swelling and the brain is no exception. Normally the cerebral capillaries form a barrier between the brain tissue and the blood, the blood–brain barrier. When the brain is traumatized, the blood–brain barrier becomes disrupted, allowing water to move by osmosis into the brain tissue. This increase in fluid volume within the brain tissue results in swelling and increased ICP. It is considered to be proportional to the severity of the injury and reaches its maximal level within 72 hours. The raised ICP may lead to brain herniation syndromes, which are discussed later.

Clinical presentation

Patients with brain injury may present with a range of signs and symptoms that vary in severity, depending on the nature, mechanism and site of the injury. Signs and symptoms of concussion may include immediate unconsciousness, which is usually quite transient, headache, drowsiness, confusion, irritability, dizziness, gait disturbances and visual disturbances ('seeing stars') (Hickey 1997).

Patients with haematomas may lose consciousness at the time of the injury and then recover. However, if the haematoma is present and increasing in size then they will begin to show signs of raised ICP. Consciousness will deteriorate rapidly in the case of extradural haematoma, or more gradually in subdural haematoma. Hemiplegia or hemiparesis will become evident along with abnormal pupillary response (see p. 283) and possibly changes in vital signs.

Patients with late stage brain herniation may also vomit, often projectile vomiting, as the vomiting centre within the brain stem becomes compressed.

RAISED INTRACRANIAL PRESSURE

Apart from cerebral oedema following trauma and brain injury there are many other causes of raised ICP, including brain tumours, obstruction to the circulation of CSF, cerebral haemorrhage and abscess, and non-neurological causes such as liver failure.

Pathophysiology

The skull is a rigid box and the contents within it exert pressure. This is ICP, which is determined by the volumes of three components:

- brain tissue (70%)
- CSF (23–25%)
- blood volume (5–7%).

The average volume of these contents within the skull of an adult is between 1 and 1.6 litres. The intracranial contents are incompressible, but they are interchangeable. The cerebral blood volume is the most easily and rapidly altered. This becomes important if a patient develops an expanding mass lesion within the skull such as bleeding.

The intracranial contents provide resistance to the perfusion of the brain by compressing the intracranial arteries. Blood must therefore be perfused through the brain under pressure. This is known as the cerebral perfusion pressure (CPP). A minimum CPP of 60 mmHg is required for adequate perfusion of the brain. This can be calculated by the following equation: $CPP = MABP - ICP$ (where MABP is the mean arterial blood pressure). In effect, MABP needs to be sufficient to overcome the resistance caused by the ICP and still maintain cerebral perfusion.

Normally, ICP is approximately 10 mmHg, but this may be raised as high as 30 or 40 mmHg following trauma. You can then see that in order to overcome this increased resistance and maintain cerebral perfusion, the mean arterial blood pressure needs to increase. This is the natural mechanism the body uses to deal with raised ICP in the later stages in order to maintain cerebral perfusion.

Prior to this happening, the volume of the constituents within the skull alters. If the volume of brain tissue increases due to swelling, then the cerebral blood vessels will constrict in order to reduce the volume of blood within the skull and therefore reduce the ICP. This can only happen to a limited extent, otherwise the blood supply is so reduced that cerebral perfusion is compromised.

Furthermore, the volume of CSF within the skull can be reduced in an attempt to reduce the rising ICP by shunting CSF into the spinal subarachnoid space.

The mechanism of interchanging the volumes of the different components within the skull is called compensation, but it is limited and cannot continue indefinitely. When the point is reached where the volume occupied by the blood vessels and CSF within the skull can be reduced no further, the pressure within the skull starts to rise exponentially. This is known as decompensation and is very difficult to reverse once it begins.

Brain shifts (herniation syndromes) and 'coning'

As a lesion expands within the skull, the surrounding brain tissue becomes compressed. Pressure gradients are established and cause brain tissue to shift from an area of high pressure to one of low pressure. In other words, brain tissue will swell and be compressed against the point of least resistance (see Fig. 14.14).

An expanding lesion in the right cerebral hemisphere causes the brain to herniate under the falx cerebri (see p. 278). This is called subfalcine herniation. If the lesion expands further then the brain will also begin to herniate downwards. Firstly the medial part of the temporal lobe of the cerebrum (the uncus) will herniate through the gap in the centre of the tentorium cerebelli (see pp. 278–279) through which the nerve fibres from the cerebral cortex pass (tentorial hiatus). This is known as transtentorial herniation and will result in immediate compression of the midbrain and the third cranial nerve, resulting in loss of pupil constriction in response to light on the same side as the lesion.

Finally, if the pressure is unrelieved, the structures within the posterior fossa are compressed and begin to shift. The cerebellar tonsils (part of the cerebellum) will herniate downwards through the foramen magnum and compress the medulla

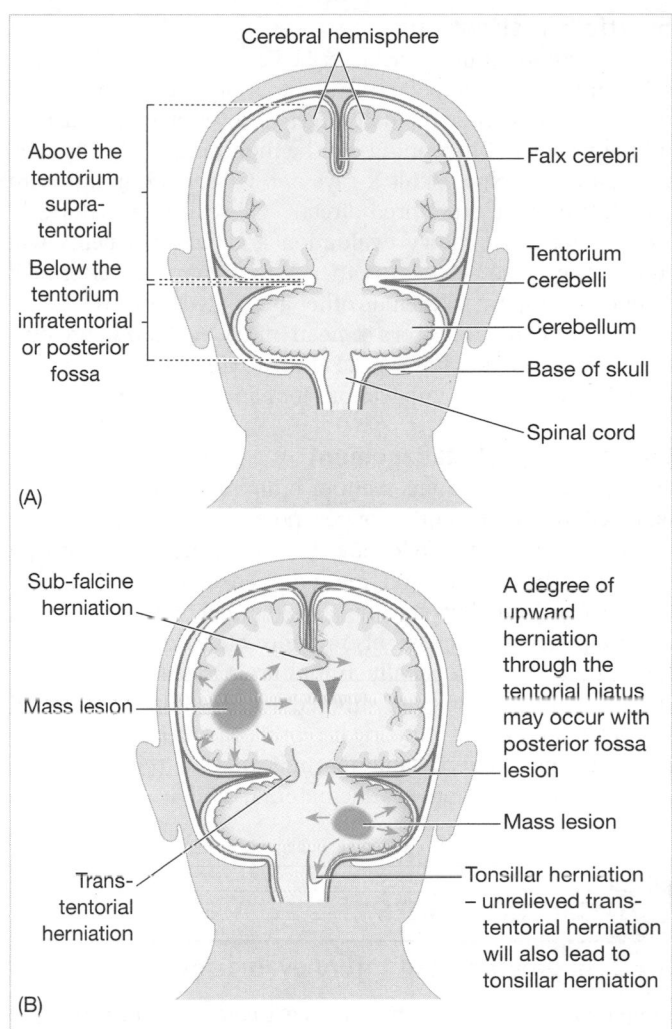

Figure 14.14 Normal structures, brain shifts. (A) Normal structures – note the gap between cerebral hemispheres and tentorium cerebelli, and between the base of the cerebellum and the floor of the skull. (B) Brain shifts.

oblongata. The blood supply to the medulla oblongata is interrupted and vital functions such as respiration will cease; the pupils will be fixed and dilated. This may occur as the final stage of a progressive cerebral lesion as described, or may occur alone due to an expanding lesion within the posterior fossa itself. The process described above is also known as coning.

Clinical presentation

- One of the earliest signs of raised ICP is deterioration in level of consciousness.
- Focal neurological deficits may also develop quite early on as specific areas of brain tissue become compressed, e.g. limb deficits.
- Later, changes in pupillary response to light will be evident and changes may be seen in systemic observations (see 'Neurological nursing assessment', p. 279). These, however, are late signs of raised ICP and indicate that brain herniation is occurring.

Specific investigations

Neurological assessment, as described earlier, is vital following brain injury. More importantly, it is serial assessment that is required so that trends and changes in level of consciousness and neurological functioning can be monitored. Other specific investigations include skull X-rays and CT scanning; in severe cases ICP may be monitored directly. CT scanning is the gold standard for head injury evaluation and many patients will require one at some point. Other X-rays may be performed, e.g. chest and spine, to exclude other associated injuries.

The most common errors in head injury evaluation are outlined in Special Issues box 14.2. Failure to undertake a complete evaluation clearly has implications for patient outcomes.

Medical/surgical management

The goals of acute management of brain injury are to focus on stabilization and prevention of secondary damage. In the early stages of resuscitation following the injury, the main aims are to protect the airway and maintain adequate oxygenation. Hypovolaemia and hypotension should be corrected (see Ch. 9). Any scalp lacerations may also require attention and wounds should be dressed aseptically. Initial brain resuscitation treatment for patients who have suffered a severe injury is directed at controlling ICP and reducing cerebral oedema and ischaemia. A neurosurgical referral may be indicated for removal of an expanding mass lesion or haematoma, and in severe cases

 SPECIAL ISSUES

14.2 Improving head injury evaluation

Trauma.org (2000) identifies the most common errors in head injury evaluation as a failure to:

- look beyond the obvious head injury
- assess baseline neurological status
- undertake careful repetitive observation
- identify other injuries that may produce shock
- consider other brain injury in patients with a history of trauma, but no focal signs
- maintain ICP adequately.

Student activities

Identify a patient admitted for observation following head injury, and thinking about the importance of 'assess baseline neurological status' and 'careful repetitive observation', look at the nursing observations and documentation.

- What observations were done on admission and how often were they repeated?
- Why do you think each observation was performed?
- What changes in the observations would you have reported to the registered nurse?
- Did you identify any areas for improvement?

Reference

Trauma.org. Traumatic brain injury. Online. Available: www.trauma.org/neuro/index.html. 2000.

patients may require ventilation in intensive care for a variety of reasons, not least of which is to manage raised ICP (see Ch. 31). The management of raised ICP is outlined in Box 14.5.

> ▶ **Nursing management**

Most of the following nursing care relates to patients who have suffered a moderate to severe injury that has impacted on conscious level and therefore the ability to carry out activities of living independently. Most patients who attend hospital after a head injury are able to be discharged home, with advice to contact A&E if they develop a worsening headache, nausea and vomiting or if they are noticed to become more drowsy or confused (see Health Promotion box 14.2).

Assessment

Holistic assessment is vital in the management of the acutely brain-injured adult. Patients can experience problems with any body system as a result of the injury, which may lead to complications that increase the risk of secondary brain damage.

Neurological assessment

Neurological assessment (including GCS) is the most important nursing assessment performed and must be documented accurately, with changes reported immediately. Clinical decisions are made on the strength of these nursing observations and patients can deteriorate rapidly and unpredictably. In the acute stages following injury, neurological observations should be performed at least half-hourly, but may then be reduced to hourly and even 2-hourly according to the patient's condition.

Patients who have suffered an apparently mild head injury can also deteriorate within the 24 hours following the injury and so may be admitted for observation. The above also applies. Patients may also experience headache, so pain assessment should be undertaken. Worsening headache, increasing drowsiness or vomiting should be reported immediately as this may indicate development or worsening of cerebral damage and haemorrhage.

Respiratory assessment

Respiratory assessment (see Ch. 20) is also important, as alterations in respiratory pattern can result in cerebral hypoxia. Respiratory rate and depth should be observed and pulse oximetry may be performed to monitor oxygen saturation. Patients are also at risk of aspiration, so should be positioned in such a way as to protect their airway. Patency of the airway should be assessed on a regular basis. Patients are also at risk of developing respiratory infections and pneumonia, as well as neurogenic pulmonary oedema. Respiratory auscultation should therefore be performed to assess air entry to all areas of the lungs. Suctioning may be required, but should be undertaken with caution as it can cause a rise in ICP.

Assessment of vital signs

Patients are at risk of cardiovascular problems following acute head injury. Cardiac arrhythmias and hypo/hypertension may develop for a variety of reasons. Assessment of vital signs is therefore important. Cardiovascular assessment is discussed in Chapter 19.

Box 14.5 Medical management of raised intracranial pressure

Osmotic diuretic therapy (e.g. mannitol)

- Raised ICP can be effectively managed in the short term by the use of intravenous mannitol given as a bolus dose
- It reduces ICP by establishing an osmotic gradient between the plasma and the brain tissue. It also reduces the blood viscosity and causes a reflex vasoconstriction and reduced ICP
- Mannitol can be used 6-hourly for up to 24 hours and 'buys time' for a patient who has brain herniation
- There is a reduced effect with repeated doses and a rebound rise in ICP when stopped

Ventilation

- Carbon dioxide (CO_2) dilates the cerebral blood vessels, increasing the volume of blood within them and therefore increasing ICP
- The cerebral vasculature is very sensitive to the level of CO_2 and a reduction in this causes hypocapnia and vasoconstriction. This will result in a reduction of the cerebral blood volume and therefore ICP
- ICP can fall within minutes of the onset of ventilation; however, if the level of CO_2 falls below normal limits then the cerebral vessels may constrict too much, reducing cerebral blood flow and therefore compromising cerebral perfusion, leading to ischaemia
- Previously hyperventilation was used routinely, but as there is a lack of evidence that this is beneficial, current practice is to ventilate to normocapnia (normal CO_2 level) (Trauma.org 2000)

Intravenous fluid therapy

- Patients with severe brain injury should be kept normovolaemic, as dehydration has little effect on cerebral oedema (Trauma.org 2000)
- Normal saline or Ringer's solution is usually used to hydrate brain-injured patients
- Dextrose/glucose solutions should be avoided as they can worsen cerebral oedema. The brain capillaries are very efficient at passing glucose into the brain tissue as this is essential to maintain cellular function. If extra dextrose is given intravenously, this moves into the brain tissue in a greater concentration than normal. This will increase the concentration gradient across the blood–brain barrier, which acts as a semi-permeable membrane, causing more water to follow by osmosis and therefore worsening cerebral oedema

Cerebrospinal fluid (CSF) removal

- Some patients develop hydrocephalus following brain injury. It may therefore be necessary to remove a volume of CSF to reduce the raised ICP that this causes
- This can be done by inserting a catheter into a ventricle and withdrawing a small amount of CSF. Although this will immediately reduce ICP, CSF is constantly being produced and so will soon return to previous levels. Continuous drainage via an external ventricular drain is usually preferred. The management of drainage devices is beyond the scope of this book and readers are advised to consult a specialist neuroscience book

 HEALTH PROMOTION

14.2 Discharge advice after mild head injury
(Adapted from Headway – The Brain Injury Association 2002)

Most patients who have mild head injuries are allowed home after assessment and treatment in the hospital A&E department. Nurses should ensure that patients will be discharged into the care of a responsible adult for the first 24 hours to monitor them. It is vital that nurses stress the importance of always seeking medical help if they are concerned in any way and to follow their instincts – especially where children are concerned.

The first 24 hours

Although unlikely, following discharge from hospital, it is possible that in the first 24 hours following the head injury, patients may have one of the following signs/symptoms indicating an unexpected complication. If this happens they should be taken back to hospital urgently for treatment.

- Drowsiness or loss of consciousness
- Sleep so deeply that they cannot be woken up
- Severe, continuous headache
- Repeated vomiting
- Irritability
- Altered behaviour
- Seizures.

Headache is common after head injury and patients may take paracetamol or similar medication but should not take anything containing aspirin. Patients with head injury who leave hospital in the evening should be woken up at least twice during the night to check that they are not developing complications.

After 24 hours

Complications can occur after 24 hours but they are much less likely. It is normal, depending on the severity of the injury, for patients not to feel well for up to 10 days or so. Headaches are not uncommon for the first 2 or 3 days and this may be worsened by physical activity. It might be difficult to concentrate for the first few days and people may be unable to work. People may find themselves becoming bad-tempered or irritable. Patients should not drive for the first 24 hours as reaction time is slowed and concentration affected.

If patients have not previously sought medical advice following a head injury – and one or more of the preceding symptoms occur – they should seek medical help urgently.

NB. Nurses should update their advice in line with clinical guidance to be published by NICE in 2003.

Nursing interventions to reduce raised ICP

A sudden transient rise on top of a sustained raised ICP can reduce cerebral perfusion. This can happen with some routine nursing activities. Common causes of raised ICP are coughing, suctioning and poor positioning of the patient. It has also been shown to rise when the patient is being discussed but is not included in the conversation, However, some studies have shown that there is no rise in ICP if patients are turned slowly and kept in a good position (Chudley 1994). A cumulative effect of activities has been noted, but it remains a controversial issue as to whether activities should be grouped together or spread out over time. One of the main problems is that most of the research studies have been fairly small-scale and it has not been possible to produce conclusive evidence as to which one practice should be based upon. However, professional consensus has been reached.

Positioning

Jugular venous pressure and ICP have been shown to rise when the head is turned through 90°, so patients should be positioned with the head and neck in neutral alignment with the body (see Evidence-based Practice box 14.1). This will also prevent the stimulation of tonic neck reflexes (abnormal reflexes that are released following brain injury and result in abnormal flexor and extensor posturing of the limbs). It is also recommended to position patients with the head elevated by 30°, i.e. on only one pillow. This is thought to assist venous and CSF drainage from the head and therefore to reduce ICP. Passive movements cause little rise in ICP, so it is safe to turn patients and is even advisable in order to reduce the risk of complications such as respiratory infection caused by fluid stasis within the lungs. Turning should always be carried out slowly, keeping the body in neutral alignment.

 EVIDENCE-BASED PRACTICE

14.1 Position for raised intracranial pressure

Most protocols for the care of patients with raised ICP advise that they should lie supine or on the side with the head raised to about 30°. The reasoning for this is that it allows sufficient drainage of venous blood. Venous blood drains passively from the cranium (i.e. it is not pumped) and gravity helps venous return. Of course gravity also impedes arterial blood flow if the head is raised and may reduce cerebral perfusion. For this reason the head tilt of 30° is selected as it maximizes venous return without greatly affecting arterial perfusion. The head must be in a neutral position, i.e. straight in relation to the neck and trunk, so that the veins of the neck are not bent or twisted and to provide optimal drainage (Walters 1998).

Reference

Walters FJM. Intracranial pressure and cerebral blood flow. Anaesthetic Updates 1998; 8: 4. Online. Available: www.nda.ox.ac.uk/wfsa/html/u08/u08_014.htm

Family contact

Presence of family members or touch has been shown to result in a fall in ICP (Chudley 1994). However, there has been no significant difference in effect shown between familiar and unfamiliar voices, such as the nurse, on ICP in comatose patients. This may be because a nurse caring for and communicating with the patient also becomes a familiar person. Touching the cheek of a comatose patient has been shown to be more effective than hand-holding. There is some evidence to support communicating with comatose patients, both verbally and through the use of touch. Family members and visitors should be encouraged to do the same.

Nutrition

Following a severe injury, the metabolic response is one of hypermetabolism, hypercatabolism and glucose intolerance. The increased metabolic rate results in increased energy needs and muscle mass protein is used to provide energy. Following a severe brain injury, the basal metabolic rate may be increased by up to 260%, similar to that following burns or major trauma. This hypermetabolic state may persist for up to a year post-injury and can result in malnutrition with sequelae of immunosuppression, delayed wound healing and loss of body mass. There is therefore a need to predict and meet the nutritional needs of patients, so nutritional assessment should be undertaken (see Ch. 11).

The aim of nutritional support is to provide sufficient calories and protein to maintain a positive nitrogen balance. Patients may be unable to take in sufficient nutrition orally, so enteral feeding, or rarely parenteral feeding, may be required. However, there may be poor tolerance of enteral feed due to ileus up to 2 weeks post-injury. The patient is therefore at increased risk of aspiration and gastric emptying should be checked if enteral feeds are administered. (See Chapter 11 for further information about the management of enteral and parenteral nutrition.)

Nurses are in a strong position to influence the nutritional support provided to patients following brain injury, by ensuring that attention is focused on nutrition early and not forgotten. Effects of malnutrition and complications of nutritional replacement therapies should also be monitored.

Hydration – fluid balance

Patients usually need to be hydrated intravenously, but not with dextrose/glucose solutions, as these may increase cerebral oedema. Dehydration should be prevented and normal fluid intake and output maintained. Patients may also develop problems with urinary continence due to loss of voluntary control over micturition. In order for an accurate fluid balance to be maintained, it may be necessary to catheterize the patient, but nurses should always consider alternatives to this (see Ch. 24). In critically ill patients, hourly urine measurements should be recorded.

Psychological care

Both patients and their families can become anxious and distressed following a brain injury and it can often be more devastating for family members. Brain injury can cause changes to a patient's personality and behaviour and it is often these psychological sequelae that are the most distressing, particularly for close family members. Patients are no longer the same as they were before the injury; some relatives have described it as if the patient had become suddenly old. Following a severe injury, many patients are not aware of these changes, but patients with a moderate injury do have insight and this in itself can lead to further loss of self-esteem.

Rehabilitation and long-term care

Of 100 000 patients in the UK who sustain a brain injury, 1000 will remain severely disabled and unable to work. Generally speaking, the older the patient, the worse the outcome. Access to services for head injury rehabilitation can be problematic and much of the responsibility for long-term care falls upon relatives (see Reflective Practice box 14.1). Some specialist units do exist, such as the brain injury rehabilitation unit at the Royal Hospital for Neurodisability in London. Specialist units provide services for patients requiring long-term ventilation or who remain in a permanent vegetative state. There are also some units that provide care for patients with neuropsychological problems following brain injury, but these are few and far between in the UK.

Voluntary organizations and self-help groups such as Headway can often be a useful source of support for brain-injured patients and their families.

R|Я REFLECTIVE PRACTICE

14.1 Long-term care for brain injury

Sometimes brain injury can be so severe that the patient requires 24-hour support and care. Long-term care provision in the UK is complex and varies in its provision between the constituent countries. Home care can be funded by social services and can include carers, services, structural changes to the home and equipment. Local authorities may also provide accommodation and care either in their own establishments or by funding places in private residential homes. The NHS also provides some long-term accommodation with nursing care or funds private placement. Usually patients will be expected to contribute to the care costs, which may involve releasing capital by selling property. Funding costs are also met by compensation awards by courts. Charities may help in funding placement or provision of equipment, carers or respite. The system is very complex. Further information is available from the Department of Health, The King's Fund and the voluntary sector (see 'Useful websites', p. 329).

Student activities
- What do you feel is the responsibility of central and local government, voluntary sector and the patient or family in provision of long-term care?
- Consider the responsibility of the family and carers in long-term care. Is it fair that family members may have to change their own lives to meet the patient's needs?
- Many head injuries occur in young adults. Does your view of long-term care differ for these patients from your views on provision of care for older people?

CRANIAL NERVE DISORDERS

Disorders of the cranial nerves associated with the eye (optic, oculomotor, trochlear and abducens nerves) are usually considered ophthalmological, and disorders of the vestibulocochlear (acoustic) nerve are considered the domain of the ear, nose and throat department. Two other conditions are fairly common and merit individual discussion: Bell's palsy and trigeminal neuralgia (pain in a nerve distribution). Neither of these two conditions is likely to require in-patient hospital treatment except when admitted for surgery. However, patients in any clinical or home care setting may have these conditions as well as another diagnosis.

BELL'S PALSY

Bell's palsy affects the facial (VII) cranial nerve, and usually only affects one side. It tends to affect older people more commonly and is uncommon in those under 60. Men and women are affected equally. There is some evidence that Bell's palsy may be caused by a reactivation of the herpes simplex virus in many cases. People with diabetes are more likely to be affected than those without.

Clinical presentation
The presentation includes:

- fairly abrupt onset with progressive paralysis of the facial muscles of one side of the face taking only a few hours or a couple of days
- drooping of the affected side of the face and inability to smile, pout or frown on that side
- pain — this may occur, especially in the bony prominence behind the external ear (the mastoid process) on the affected side
- excess tears
- some patients complain of painful sensitivity to sound
- altered sensation of taste
- the eye will not close completely during a blink or at night, which leads to drying of the eye surface
- increased production of saliva and incomplete closure of the lips, which may result in drooling.

Most (but not all) people recover well from Bell's palsy. There may be some residual problems such as facial weakness and excess tear production. Some patients may develop muscle contractures or unusual movements of the affected side of the face.

Management
Corticosteroids such as prednisolone are the usual treatment and recently aciclovir has been used with some good results, in line with the viral theory. Patients will need relief for the pain if present. Eye care is needed for people with poor eyelid closure. Artificial tears may be used during the day and ophthalmic lubricant ointment at night to prevent drying. Sometimes taping the lids shut, goggles or plastic eye shields can help to maintain humidity and prevent dehydration. The teaching of eye hygiene is important, as dabbing the eye with a used handkerchief or tissue may lead to infection. Drooling is embarrassing for patients and

they can be advised to keep their mouth clean and skin dry to prevent excoriation. Sometimes surgery is performed to decompress the facial nerve.

TRIGEMINAL NEURALGIA

Trigeminal neuralgia is a condition in which the patient has sudden, severe, spasmodic pain along the distribution of the trigeminal (V) nerve that is felt in the cheek and jaw. The pain is very acute, often passing off quickly, but can be repeated rapidly in succession. Touching or moving the face and mouth can trigger the pain, such as during eating and talking. Patients may become afraid of trigger activities and become withdrawn from social contact. Like Bell's palsy, it rarely affects people aged under 50 years, but the sex distribution is different: more women are affected than men. The condition is chronic and can last for years or it may resolve only to reappear years later. The condition is associated with pressure on the trigeminal nerve root at the base of the brain. This can be from blood vessels or tumours. For this reason patients should always be fully investigated. It needs to be stressed that the pain in trigeminal neuralgia can be very severe and debilitating, causing great distress to patients.

Management

Patients are encouraged to identify the trigger activities and take care when performing them. The condition responds to anti-epileptic drugs and carbamazepine is the drug of choice, but other drugs such as phenytoin or sodium valproate may be used in conjunction. Surgical treatments, such as decompression of the trigeminal nerve root or the partial severing of some of the pathways, may provide lasting and drug-free relief.

DEMYELINATING (INFLAMMATORY) DISORDERS

Demyelinating disorders are characterized by loss of the myelin covering the nerves in the CNS, and include multiple sclerosis.

MULTIPLE SCLEROSIS

Multiple sclerosis (MS) is a common demyelinating disease and is the commonest reason for chronic disability in young adults in the UK today.

Epidemiology and aetiology

Multiple sclerosis affects around 85 000 people in the UK. The peak age of onset is between 20 and 40 years and it affects more women than men (ratio 3:2). At the start, most individuals with MS follow a remitting relapsing course (MS Society 2001), with exacerbations followed by complete/partial recovery and periods of stability in between. Within 10 years, 50% of patients go on to develop secondary progressive MS, which is characterized by a gradual progression, while 15% follow this progressive course from the outset (primary progressive) (Goodkin 1998).

Prevalence of MS is high in the UK, Europe and North America, but low in Africa and Asia. It has been shown that people who move away from the UK before the age of 15 or 16 can reduce their risk, but immigrants who enter the UK from Asia or Africa before the age of 15 increase their risk to that of the indigenous population (Dean & Elian 1997).

The precise cause of MS is still unknown, but it is believed to be influenced by both environmental and genetic factors. The evidence from immigrant studies suggests an environmental factor is at work in some parts of the world, whereas twin studies have provided evidence for a genetic link. It has also been shown that there is a higher incidence where there are high standards of living, with women in social class 1 in the UK having the highest mortality from the disease (Dean & Elian 1997).

Viral and autoimmune factors are also thought to play a part. Abnormal antibodies and macrophages seem to recognize the body's own myelin as foreign and start to attack it, although the trigger for this process is not clear. The immune system is regulated, at least in part, by signalling molecules called cytokines, e.g. the interferons (alpha, beta and gamma). Gamma-interferon is thought to be instrumental in the damage processes in MS, but its effects are counteracted by beta-interferon. This is why so much research is currently directed towards the therapeutic use of beta-interferon and this is discussed in greater detail on page 305.

Pathophysiology

In MS, areas of myelin are attacked and become inflamed. The inflammation may destroy the myelin, leaving scar tissue or plaques; this process is called demyelination. The loss of myelin causes nerve conduction velocities to slow down, which can affect both the motor and sensory nerves, and symptoms vary considerably depending on which nerves are affected.

Plaques or areas of demyelination usually occur in the white matter around the ventricles within the brain, along the optic nerve, within the brain stem and spinal cord. Before a diagnosis of MS can be made, a patient must have symptoms due to plaques affecting multiple sites within the CNS and multiple attacks over time.

Clinical presentation

Presentation depends on the part of the nervous system affected. Visual disturbances are common and many people present initially with an episode of optic neuritis, characterized by diplopia. There may be unilateral visual failure and retrobulbar pain (at the back of the eye). Motor symptoms are common, with limb weakness and spasticity that often result in significantly reduced mobility and sometimes spastic paralysis. Sensory symptoms can also occur, with patients experiencing areas of numbness and paraesthesia, although these are often transient and worse after a hot bath. Urinary symptoms are common and patients may present with either urge incontinence or overflow incontinence and urinary retention (Woodward 1996) (see Ch. 12). Cranial nerve lesions occur that can affect swallowing and speech. Patients may be emotional, labile, extremely fatigued and become depressed.

Specific investigations

Diagnosis is made on the strength of the patient's history and clinical presentation, supported by various laboratory, radiological and neurophysiological findings. There is not a specific test to diagnose MS and findings can often only point to an inflammatory process affecting the CNS. To be given a diagnosis of MS, a

REFLECTIVE PRACTICE

14.2 Waiting for a diagnosis

After doing various tests the consultant said I would need an MRI scan. No-one said what they were looking for, or what might be wrong and I felt too scared to ask.

I had the awful MRI scan and went to see the consultant who said that I had a spinal lesion. When I asked what that meant and what would happen now, he calmly said: 'Oh you won't get any better.' Not surprisingly I was rather upset and asked what was wrong with me. I was shown the scan and the dark blur. This, he said, was the lesion, spinal damage. I asked what could be done. He was very unforthcoming and began to tell the nurse to arrange further tests. I was too confused to ask what all this meant; all I could think of was that I wouldn't get any better.

The tests all took place one day some months later; meanwhile my GP wouldn't commit himself to a diagnosis until they were completed. The lumbar puncture wasn't too painful, but I wasn't sure what was going on except I was told to stay flat on my back for 2 hours and left alone in a sort of storeroom attached to a ward. Eventually a nurse came

to say that I would soon be taken for the MRI. The day seemed to go on forever, all those tests, but never much explanation. Perhaps I should have asked more. Would I get worse? I still had no idea of what could be wrong.

Finally, another appointment with the consultant for the test results, but they weren't really explained and I felt that I wasn't being told everything. He went to great lengths to explain that I wouldn't be a candidate for beta-interferon, but nothing about a diagnosis. I came away confused – had I got MS or not?

By coincidence it was when MS and beta-interferon were much in the media. I clearly remember a TV documentary detailing the life story of an MS patient; I sat and cried about ending up disabled and totally dependent on others.

Student activities
Reflect on the experiences of this patient.

- Consider how explanations and information provision could have been improved during the time of uncertainty.
- How might the nurse have helped?

---

patient has to have had more that one episode affecting more than one part of the CNS (see Reflective Practice box 14.2).

Lumbar puncture is performed and the CSF examined for oligoclonal bands (antibodies present in the CSF that differ from those found in serum), but these will also be produced in the presence of CNS infections and are only indicative of inflammation. There may also be an elevated white cell count within the CSF.

Neurophysiological tests that may be performed include visual evoked potentials and auditory evoked potentials. These will display delayed conduction velocities along the axons in MS.

MRI is useful and will often show multiple lesions in the sites that are commonly affected.

Medical management

There is no curative treatment for MS and no surgical intervention is usually indicated. Treatment is directed by neurologists and takes a multidisciplinary approach (specialist nurses and therapists), aiming to reduce acute relapses and accelerate recovery, delay disability and control symptoms. Treatment may include:

- Corticosteroids, e.g. methylprednisolone
- Immunosuppression using azathioprine
- Intravenous immunoglobulin (i.v. Ig)
- Beta-interferon – there has been much controversy over the use of beta-interferon in recent years in the UK (see Evidence-based Practice box 14.2). Beta-interferon does not cure MS, but has been shown to reduce the frequency of exacerbations and slow the accumulation of the disability (Polman 1999). The debate has centred on the cost-effectiveness of the treatment, as the drug is extremely expensive and some argue that, although short-term quality of life gains are demonstrated, the cost of these is high (Parkin et al 2000)

 EVIDENCE-BASED PRACTICE

14.2 The use of beta-interferon – the story so far

In August 1999, the Department of Health asked the National Institute for Clinical Excellence (NICE) to appraise beta-interferon. A review of published evidence of clinical and cost-effectiveness was commissioned and the results of this were sent out for consultation in May 2000. The guidance issued in 2001 (and confirmed in 2002) was that on the grounds of clinical and cost-effectiveness beta-interferon was not recommended for the treatment of MS in England and Wales. However, several appeals were received against this appraisal and final guidance following the appeal process was issued. This was again sent out for consultation and the final decision regarding the use of beta-interferon has yet to be made, although there was no change in the overall recommendations from previously. NICE have been commissioned to produce full clinical guidance on the management of MS and this is due for publication in 2003.

References
National Institute for Clinical Excellence. Final appraisal determination – beta interferon and glatiramer for multiple sclerosis. Online. Available: www.nice.org.uk/Docref.asp?d=24036. 2001.

National Institute for Clinical Excellence. Beta interferon and glatiramer acetate for the treatment of multiple sclerosis. Technology Appraisal Guidance No. 32. Online. Available: www.nice.org.uk. 2002.

- Symptom control
  — spasticity is the most common symptom encountered by patients with MS. This can be painful and will limit mobility. Spasticity is often treated with oral medication in conjunction with physiotherapy. Drugs include baclofen, dantrolene sodium and tizanidine. In severe cases of spasticity that are resistant to oral preparations, intrathecal (in the meninges, usually the subarachnoid space) baclofen may be administered via a programmable pump into the lumbar region. By bypassing the blood–brain barrier in this way, much lower doses are used with the same efficacy but with fewer side-effects
  — fatigue is also a common and debilitating problem and amantadine (a dopaminergic drug) may be prescribed.
  — training, rehabilitation and devices (cooling vests and electromagnetic fields) have also been tried, as well as complementary therapies, including acupuncture and yoga (Branas et al 2000)
  — there is considerable interest in the use of cannabis for MS symptom control, and trials are ongoing
- Physiotherapy – the use of drugs is only one component of active management and there is a need to include rehabilitation strategies that improve quality of life. There is some evidence that specialist neurological physiotherapy helps to improve mobility, although there have only been a few scientific studies in this area (Freeman & Thompson 2001).

▶ Nursing management

Nursing management of MS is predominantly aimed at symptom control, preventing complications and providing information and support to patients and their families during the progression of symptoms. Community- and hospital-based nurses work closely with the multidisciplinary team to provide holistic care. Where they exist, specialist MS nurses are able to act as a valuable resource for patients and all those involved in their care (see Reflective Practice box 14.3).

Spasticity

Spasticity is one of the most debilitating symptoms experienced by people with MS. It results in reduced mobility, with the ensuing reduced functional ability and life satisfaction, pain and decreased sexual function, and can lead to contractures in the longer term, amongst other problems (Currie 2001). Nurses should assess the degree of spasticity and its impact on the patient. Treatment of spasticity requires a multidisciplinary

---

R|Я REFLECTIVE PRACTICE

14.3 The role of the specialist MS nurse in improving quality of life

Fortunately I had a visit from the hospital specialist MS nurse. Here at last was a down-to-earth person who explained the tests and what the results had meant. She reassured me that no two people's MS takes the same path and it was by no means a certainty that I would become completely helpless. She explained the unpredictability of MS and the difficulty in giving a diagnosis. We discussed ways in which I could help myself, particularly in planning rest times to minimize the inevitable fatigue. She explained that there were different types of MS and it could be some time before I had a complete diagnosis. I felt a lot brighter about my future, but still wanted a 'proper' diagnosis.

Following another episode, I contacted the nurse, who was very willing to come and see me. We discussed my loss of temperature perception and the need for a temperature-controlled shower to reduce the risk of scalding. Brain lesions have affected my memory and the nurse explained why and suggested that it would be a good idea to write things down and also to explain to friends that I might need reminders. Apart from a Filofax to note nearly everything down, a small electronic reminder is very useful. We also discussed the very odd phenomenon of 'word blindness' – I can read something and be convinced it says something completely different. I sing in a choir and it can be very interesting when I read and sing something that just isn't there.

It took four years and five different episodes before the consultant eventually said that I had primary progressive MS. Not finding him the easiest of people to talk to, I telephoned the nurse, as I was unsure of the difference between types of MS. She contacted the consultant, discussed the diagnosis and rang me back to explain. Finally, after so many years, I had an 'official label'. It was actually a relief to have a label, something I could research. I felt able to join the MS society now I was part of the club.

Life has changed in many ways and some for the better. I gave up going out to work as a full day left me tired and confused. I have been able to work on tasks at my own pace. If I had a bad day, I could have a day off. Of course, there are drawbacks – not knowing when, or if, I will have another episode and how I might be affected; the frustrations of having an episode when I'm particularly busy. I do have times when my walking or speech is affected, but explaining to people that I have MS means that now they know that I'm not drunk. Before I had a diagnosis it was hard to tell people what was wrong with me.

Being in contact with the MS nurse has proved invaluable. She is always at the end of a telephone to discuss symptoms and ways of coping, or just to listen to my concerns. She can reassure me as to whether I need to contact my doctor or whether what I'm describing is 'normal'. I am extremely grateful for her support.

Student activities
Reflect on the experiences of this patient.

- In what ways did the specialist MS nurse improve quality of life for this patient?
- Find out if a specialist MS nurse is available in your area and if so what services they provide?

approach and includes physiotherapy and drug therapy (see above). Patients need to be positioned in a way that breaks the pattern of spasticity, in a similar way to patients who develop spasticity following stroke. Sometimes splints are used to support a limb in a good position; however, care must be taken to ensure that they do not cause pressure ulcers. Pressure ulcers may develop due to the reduced mobility and nurses should assess the risk using a suitable risk score. Pressure areas should be assessed on a regular basis and appropriate preventative and/or treatment measures instituted (see Ch. 10).

Drug compliance

Nurses should educate patients/families about the need to take drugs on time, and where self-administration is not appropriate, the nurse should take responsibility for this. It is important to monitor the effectiveness of the skeletal muscle relaxants administered and for side-effects.

Comfort

Nurses should also work with physiotherapists and OT to promote comfort and functional stability.

Fatigue

As more effort is required to walk, patients become increasingly tired and fatigued. Sleep patterns can also be disturbed due to painful spasticity, which further exacerbates fatigue. The exact cause of fatigue is not known and it may be due to a problem with neurological transmission. Regardless of the cause, fatigue can have a significant effect on quality of life. The fatigue associated with MS has certain unique characteristics (see Special Issues box 14.3).

Cognitive impairment

At least 50% of patients with MS develop cognitive impairment that can significantly affect functional ability and quality of life. These problems can also have an effect on the patient's family. In-patient rehabilitation has been shown to be effective in restoration of some functions that can persist after discharge (Kraft 1999). Patients with cognitive deficits can present with difficulties with speed of information-processing, learning capacity and problem-solving behaviours. Patients should be assessed for cognitive impairment and, if this is suspected, they should be referred for further assessment and management as soon as possible to reduce the deleterious effects that can occur. OTs are particularly skilled in dealing with cognitive deficits.

Urinary problems

Patients often present with urinary problems, including urinary incontinence (see Ch. 12). This occurs mainly for one of two reasons. Some patients develop an unstable bladder with detrusor hyperreflexia, due to spasticity and unstable contractions of the bladder muscle. Patients will have frequency, urgency and urge incontinence, and treatment may be either behavioural or pharmacological. Bladder retraining may help, but patients are often treated with antimuscarinic drugs such as oxybutynin that block the unstable contractions of the detrusor.

Others may develop urinary retention due to detrusor/external sphincter dyssynergia. The bladder is unable to empty, as detrusor muscle contractions and relaxation of the external sphincter are uncoordinated. The main danger with this condition is that the pressure inside the bladder can increase as the detrusor muscle contracts, leading to back-pressure and reflux of urine up the ureters to the kidneys, which can cause kidney

---

 SPECIAL ISSUES

14.3 Fatigue and MS

The unique characteristics of fatigue in MS include the following (Hubsky & Sears 1992):

- It occurs more quickly than normal
- It is more severe and frequent than normal
- It is chronic
- It exacerbates other MS symptoms
- Its severity is not always related to neurological status or severity of other symptoms.

Fatigue occurs without warning and patients may have a sudden urge to sleep, which can obviously have a huge impact on self-care and everyday activities.

Rest periods interspersed with activity can help and should encompass both physical rest and psychological relaxation. A planned exercise programme may also be helpful and activities should be managed throughout the day; OTs can help with this planning.

Fatigue can prevent patients from going to work, but a change in working pattern can help. A workplace occupational health department or disablement resettlement office can often advise in this regard.

Fatigue also has psychological and cognitive effects. Patients may become anxious or depressed, forgetful and find concentrating difficult. Counselling may be helpful and further information about managing these symptoms can be obtained from the MS Society and other support networks, and patients and their families should be given information about these organizations.

Heat and humidity also exacerbate fatigue and other symptoms as heat will slow conduction velocities along already damaged neurons even further. It is important therefore that patients do not bathe in water that is too hot, avoid infections that could cause an increase in body temperature and reduce foreign travel to hot climates.

Student activities
- Access the MS Society website (www.mssociety.org.uk) and find out what information is available about fatigue.
- Think about ways you could use this information to plan and give care to patients with MS being cared for at home.

Reference
Hubsky EP, Sears JH. Fatigue in multiple sclerosis: guidelines for nursing care. Rehab Nurs 1992; 17(4); 176–180.

damage (see Ch. 24). It is vital therefore that the bladder is emptied, and self-catheterization is often the treatment of choice, always using a hydrophilic catheter to prevent urethral trauma and development of strictures in the longer term (see Chs 12 and 24).

Nutrition

Various diets have been tried to improve symptoms, such as diets high in polyunsaturated fatty acids or gluten-free diets. However, there is scant evidence to support their effectiveness in the management of MS. Many patients will supplement their diet with evening primrose oil, although there is no evidence to support this practice.

Nutritional management falls within the domain of nursing and nurses should take a lead in the assessment of nutritional status (see Ch. 11). Referral to a specialist nutrition nurse or dietician may be indicated if a nutritional assessment suggests that a patient is malnourished in any way. Patients should be encouraged to eat a healthy diet and reduce weight gain as this can exacerbate the problems of reduced mobility. A good fibre and fluid intake should be encouraged to reduce the incidence of constipation that accompanies reduced mobility. Patients may also experience feeding difficulties due to dysphagia. Swallowing should be assessed and patients referred to a SLT for advice (see p. 286).

TUMOURS – BENIGN AND MALIGNANT

Brain tumours may be benign or malignant, and may be primary (arising in the brain) or secondary (metastatic), spread from cancers elsewhere in the body (e.g. bronchus, gastrointestinal tract, kidney or breast). Primary tumours arise from structures that surround the neurons rather than the neurons themselves; these include gliomas (from glial cells), meningiomas (from the meninges), acoustic neuromas (cells around the vestibulocochlear VIII or acoustic nerve) (see Ch. 16) and the pituitary gland (see Ch. 17) or pineal gland. Gliomas are malignant whereas meningiomas, acoustic neuromas and pituitary tumours are benign. However, both benign and malignant intracranial tumours cause problems mainly due to compression and raised ICP.

This chapter concentrates on gliomas, including a discussion of the care needed following craniotomy (an operation to open the skull). The general principles will also be applicable to patients having craniotomy for other reasons.

Epidemiology and aetiology

Primary brain cancer is quite rare, but there are over 4300 new cases in the UK per annum (Cancer Research UK 2002). Brain tumours make up approximately 1.5% of all cancers in adults in England and Wales (Dinnes et al 2001). They commonly affect children and adults over 40 years of age, and are more common in men.

There are many factors known to cause brain cancer, including radiation, exposure to certain chemicals such as some pesticides, occasional hereditary influences, exposure to viruses and microwaves, plus the metastatic cancers that spread from elsewhere. In most cases no cause can be identified. Although

smoking has not been directly linked to the formation of a glioma, it can be indirectly causative, as it has been linked as a determinant of other primary tumours that spread to the brain.

MENINGIOMAS

Meningiomas account for 15% of intracranial tumours, are most common in adults and occur more frequently in females. They arise from the arachnoid mater, are slow-growing and benign. Meningiomas are easily identified from CT scan, as they always grow close to the inner surface of the skull and are almost always spherical in shape. Occasionally they may erode into the bone overlying the tumour. They are usually easily removed via a craniotomy and the prognosis is good. Sometimes patients will receive radiotherapy following surgery, especially after an incomplete excision or following a recurrence.

GLIOMA

Glioma is an umbrella term for a tumour arising from one of several types of glial tissue (see pp. 274–275).

Pathophysiology

Gliomas occur within the white matter of the brain tissue. They may be solid or cystic, often containing fluid. They may occur as a single solitary lesion or in multiple sites (secondary brain tumours are more likely to produce multiple deposits than primary brain tumours). Tumours are very vascular and are prone to haemorrhages. They also disrupt the blood–brain barrier, which results in cerebral oedema.

Gliomas are classified according to the glial cell of origin. Those that arise from astrocytes are called astrocytomas; from oligodendroglia are called oligodendrogliomas and so on. A glioblastoma multiforme is a poorly differentiated tumour (see Ch. 33), where the cell shape has changed so that the cell of origin cannot be identified. These are rapidly growing and highly malignant. The degree of malignancy and speed of growth are indicated by the grade of the tumour, from 1 (slow-growing) to 5 (fast-growing and highly malignant).

Prognosis depends on the type and site of the tumour. Less than 20% of patients with a glioblastoma survive longer than 1 year following diagnosis.

Clinical presentation

Gliomas manifest in one of three ways:

- With symptoms of raised ICP, i.e. headache (classically on waking in the morning, but resolves when the person gets up), vomiting, altered consciousness and visual disturbance
- With seizures – 30% of patients with a tumour in their cerebral hemispheres will present with seizures, so anyone presenting with seizure activity over the age of 30 should be investigated
- With focal neurological changes (e.g. hemiparesis, diplopia, poor memory) – these would obviously depend on the site of the tumour, and are usually progressive.

It is important to investigate the symptoms to determine the cause and identify if the patient does have a tumour or if the symptoms are being produced by another pathology such as a chronic subdural haematoma, cerebral abscess, encephalitis or venous thrombosis, all of which may have a similar presentation.

Specific investigations

The gold standard in identifying a space-occupying lesion (as brain tumours are often referred to) within the brain is a CT scan (with i.v. opaque contrast medium to enhance visualization of the tumour), although MRI is increasingly being used. Skull X-rays may also be taken to see if the tumour has infiltrated the bones of the skull, and scans and X-rays of other parts of the body may be performed if the tumour is suspected of being a secondary cancer in a patient with no history of a primary malignancy. It is important in these cases to identify the primary site, as this will also require treatment and may aid in both diagnosis and prediction of the likely outcome. Visual fields may also be charted as they can often be affected due to compression of the visual pathways from raised ICP.

Scanning will not identify the type of tumour, so to identify its nature more precisely, it will need to be biopsied and the cells looked at under the microscope by a pathologist. A biopsy is usually performed by a neurosurgeon, during which a small hole (burr hole) is drilled through the skull and a small amount of the tumour removed for closer inspection.

Medical/surgical management

Clinical guidelines have been produced for good practice in the management of adults with malignant cerebral gliomas (Davies & Hopkins 1997). These provide guidance for all health professionals from the time of investigation and diagnosis through to palliative care. Patients who have been diagnosed with a brain tumour are usually referred to a neurosurgeon for management. The neurosurgical consultant will often work closely with a neuro-oncologist in long-term management. Management strategies are summarized in Box 14.6.

Research is directed towards developing drugs that prevent cancer cells from growing, e.g. by reducing their ability to stimulate the growth of new blood vessels within the tumour that support its survival. Interferon-alpha, -beta and thalidomide have all been evaluated. Drugs that prevent cancer cells from invading the surrounding brain tissue are also being developed. The delivery of genes or gene products into cancer cells is also an area of interest and is likely to continue to receive much attention in the future (Levin 1999).

▶ Nursing management

It is difficult to be specific about the care of a patient who has been diagnosed with brain cancer, as so much of the care required will be dependent on the patient's specific neurological deficits in terms of physical needs. A sound and holistic nursing assessment of all activities of living is important before care can be planned (see Ch. 1). There are, however, some aspects of care that should be considered in more detail, irrespective of tumour location.

Pain management

Patients may experience headache either due to pressure from the tumour or following surgical removal via a craniotomy (see p. 310). The brain has no nociceptors (see Ch. 7) and does not feel pain, but there are pain-sensitive structures within the cranium, including the cerebral blood vessels and meninges. When these structures are stretched or compressed, as with raised ICP, or are cut during surgical intervention, they will cause the patient to feel pain.

Box 14.6 Management strategies – glioma

Drugs to reduce cerebral oedema and raised ICP
Dexamethasone (a powerful corticosteroid drug) and mannitol (see Box 14.5) are used to reduce cerebral oedema and raised ICP to improve level of consciousness and reduce focal neurological deficits. Dexamethasone reduces inflammation around the tumour and is also thought to have an effect on stabilizing the cell membranes within the blood–brain barrier. It is usually administered orally, but may also be given intravenously if the patient's conscious level dictates. Often a larger loading dose is administered and symptoms can improve within 24 hours

Anticonvulsant drugs
Used to reduce seizures in those patients who have presented with seizures. They may also be used prophylactically after craniotomy (opening into the skull)

Surgical interventions
The treatment of choice is excision of the glioma; however, this is not always possible as the tumour may be affecting vital centres within the brain, which would result in lasting damage and loss of function if it is removed. The brain does not regenerate, so tumours are often simply debulked, i.e. as much as possible is removed, to reduce the ICP. They will

therefore continue to grow following surgery. It is never possible to remove every single cancerous cell. If the glioma has caused obstructive hydrocephalus (literally 'water on the brain') a ventriculoperitoneal shunt can be inserted to drain CSF from the ventricles to the peritoneal cavity to relieve raised ICP

Radiotherapy
Also used to treat gliomas, although they are not very radio-sensitive. It is often used to destroy small numbers of cancer cells remaining behind following surgery, or for the palliative reduction of recurrent tumour. It is also known that over 20% of patients receiving radiotherapy will develop significant damage and neurocognitive deficits (Levin 1999). A specific type of therapy known as radiosurgery involves the delivery of a sphere of high-dose radiation, more localized than would be achieved with conventional radiotherapy, and is often described as a gamma knife

Chemotherapy
This may not be successful, as most cytotoxic drugs do not cross the blood–brain barrier. However, the drug temozolomide is available as a 'second-line' drug for certain patients with recurrent glioma

It is important that analgesia administered to treat the headache should not mask further neurological deterioration, so paracetamol, tramadol or codeine-based analgesia preparations are usually selected. These are usually extremely effective against headache and are widely used within neuroscience nursing practice. It is important to remember, however, that codeine-based drugs may cause constipation, which should be avoided at all costs. Patients will have additional factors that increase the risk of constipation, such as reduced mobility that accompanies the loss of neurological function. Constipation is to be avoided, as straining during defecation can increase ICP and cause neurological deterioration.

Psychosocial care

Patients may be affected by a number of psychosocial problems, such as time off work and financial difficulties, loss of a driving licence and personality changes. At the same time, they may be going through a process of bereavement and grieving at the permanent loss of function and changes in body image that occur. It has been reported that functional status is an indicator of quality of life and loss of function can be devastating (Hickey 1997). Patients may also be trying to come to terms with the diagnosis of a life-threatening illness, so psychological nursing care cannot be underestimated (see Chs 33 and 34). The responses of patients and their families are influenced by a number of factors, including details of the diagnosis (type, grade of tumour and presenting symptoms) and patient factors such as age, family dynamics and coping skills (of both the patient and family members) (Hickey 1997). Many of the needs of patients and family members relate to a lack of knowledge about their diagnosis and the prognosis for the future. The nurse can therefore provide accurate information in a way that the individuals involved will be able to understand and can also refer them to other sources of support in the community. Many agencies, such as BACUP, provide specific resources for patients with brain tumours and are available to support patients and families. Most of these organizations produce literature, have helplines, provide information and also have a web presence (see 'Useful websites').

Patients undergoing surgery need specific information and adequate preparation about what will happen, such as the need for head shaving in some cases, wound drains and pain relief postoperatively. Nurses should be able to reinforce information about the risks of surgery outlined by the surgeon.

Nurses may also find themselves in the role of patient advocate, especially if the tumour has affected the patient's cognitive abilities (see Ch. 3). It is often useful for a nurse to be present when patients and family members are given the bad news about their diagnosis, so that they can then continue to provide emotional and psychological support throughout the patient's illness. A range of psychological problems may be encountered, including fear, anxiety and fluctuations in mood, and nursing interventions need to be tailored towards each individual.

Referrals to other health professionals may be appropriate, such as a clinical psychologist, counsellor, clinical nurse specialist in neuro-oncology, or a palliative care nurse specialist (see Ch. 34).

Care of a patient following craniotomy

Many patients will undergo either a burr hole biopsy of their tumour or a craniotomy to debulk the lesion. This is an operative procedure that is not without risk. Following surgery, cerebral oedema can be worsened and bleeding may occur within the skull, leading to haematoma formation. These will both result in raised ICP and so neurological assessment including GCS is vital to detect this (see pp. 279–285). Any neurological deterioration or change in level of consciousness should be reported immediately.

Patients should be nursed in the same way as described for head-injured patients in terms of reducing the risk of raised ICP, i.e. positioned well in a neutral alignment, 30° head elevation and pain-free.

Patients will also have a scalp wound that should be dressed according to the surgeon's instructions. Asepsis should be maintained when changing dressings and removing clips from the wound. A wound drain attached to a suction device may have been inserted. This can usually be removed within 24–48 hours following surgery. Clips may remain in situ in a scalp wound following craniotomy for anything between 3 and 10 days, depending on the surgeon's preference. Burr holes are usually closed with a couple of sutures and these can usually be removed within a few days of surgery.

Some patients will have had an area of scalp shaved (depending on the surgeon's preference) and will need support as they adjust to the change in body image and advice regarding head covering or the use of a wig.

The general principles of care for patients undergoing surgery apply to those having a neurosurgical procedure (see Ch. 29). Readers needing more detail about neurosurgical nursing should consult the 'Further reading' section (p. 329).

Care of patients during radiotherapy

Patients undergoing radiotherapy to the head will become particularly fatigued and feel generally unwell. Nurses should plan care to reduce fatigue and encourage patients to have periods of rest. Patients may experience mucositis (sore mouth), which may lead to reduced appetite and intake, and malnutrition (see Ch. 33).

Patients usually experience hair loss as a result of radiotherapy and the skin of the scalp often becomes sore. It may therefore be more appropriate for soft head coverings to be worn in preference to a wig until this has settled down.

Patients will be required to have a clear plastic mask formed, which encloses and immobilizes their head so that treatment can be directed to the right location each time. This can be distressing for some patients and is something that they need to have explained to them.

INFECTIONS OF THE NERVOUS SYSTEM

Infections may affect the brain, spinal cord, nerves and meninges. They may be caused by bacteria, viruses, fungi, protozoa or, less commonly be due to helminths or prions (virus-like infectious agents consisting of protein but with no nucleic acids). These infections include meningitis, encephalitis (infection/inflammation of the brain), cerebral abscess, herpes zoster, rabies, tetanus, Creutzfeldt–Jakob disease (CJD) and poliomyelitis. Many of these conditions are uncommon and the intention is to discuss two that occur more commonly, namely meningitis and herpes zoster, and also CJD which, although rare, achieved a prominence due to the rise in the number of people affected in recent years.

MENINGITIS – AN OVERVIEW

Meningitis is inflammation of the meninges, and may be viral, bacterial or, more rarely, protozoal or fungal in origin. Viral meningitis is the most common type and is usually self-limiting and has no specific treatment. It occurs in both children and adults, causing severe headache, pyrexia and meningeal irritability (see below). Occasionally it is present with encephalitis when it is more serious, and will usually require treatment with an antiviral drug such as aciclovir or ganciclovir.

Infections by fungi and protozoa are rare, but immuno-compromised patients, such as those with HIV infection, may develop fungal meningitis caused by *Cryptococcus neoformans*.

BACTERIAL MENINGITIS

Bacterial meningitis may be caused by a number of micro-organisms, including *Neisseria meningitidis* (meningococcal), *Haemophilus influenzae*, *Escherichia coli*, *Streptococcus pneumoniae* (pneumococcal) and *Mycobacterium tuberculosis*, although the first two are less common now due to immunization in infancy. Meningitis is usually an acute disease, although *M. tuberculosis* meningitis tends to have a slower onset due to the slow growth of this microorganism.

Meningitis may lead to complications such as septicaemia, and long-term sequelae, including seizures or even death. For example, 95% of those with meningococcal meningitis will survive, whereas only 50% of patients who develop meningococcal septicaemia will survive (Meningitis Research Foundation 2002). It is therefore imperative that everyone is alert to the signs of infection and that early treatment is started.

Aetiology and pathology – acute meningitis

Acute meningitis sometimes follows septicaemia (an illness due to bacteria in the blood). It can, however, be caused by the direct spread of bacteria from infections of the sinus or the ear, or through a skull fracture.

The meninges are inflamed, pus forms and there may be cerebral oedema. Adhesions may form later and these can obstruct the circulation of CSF, leading to hydrocephalus.

Clinical presentation

The signs and symptoms vary according to which micro-organism is involved and the severity of infection. The onset may be very rapid, especially with meningococcal meningitis, where the person becomes desperately ill within a matter of hours. Typically, patients have headache, pyrexia and meningism. Meningism comprises meningeal irritation (demonstrated by a positive Kernig's and/or Brudzinski's sign) and neck stiffness. The two signs are demonstrated as positive when the hip is bent (flexed), when straightening (extending) the knee causes spasm in the hamstring muscles at the back of the thigh (Kernig's), and when neck flexion causes bilateral flexion of the hips and knees (Brudzinski's). Other presenting features may include:

- photophobia and phonophobia (intolerance of noise)
- alterations in conscious level, may be drowsy or unconscious
- nausea and vomiting
- a skin rash (dark red/purple) – petechial (small spots) or purpuric (larger spots) spots that do not blanch with pressure, disseminated intravascular coagulation (see Chs 9 and 18) and circulatory collapse are associated with meningococcal septicaemia
- seizures.

Specific investigations

- A lumbar puncture is performed in order to examine the CSF for changes including the presence of white blood cells, increased protein and reduced glucose. The CSF may look cloudy (turbid) if infection is present, and although microbiological tests (microscopy and culture) will be done to confirm the infective microorganism, treatment will be commenced without delay. As many of the microorganisms that cause meningitis are fragile outside the body, samples should be taken to the laboratory without delay.
- A CT scan may be performed to rule out other neurological infections.
- Blood culture is done if septicaemia is suspected.

Medical management

Treatment is with the appropriate antibiotics that cross the blood–brain barrier, e.g. cefotaxime and ceftriaxone. Increasingly, antibiotic resistance is a problem with some microorganisms. In the community, intramuscular penicillin is given to any suspected cases of meningitis. Management also involves supportive measures, which may include intravenous fluid replacement, reduction of cerebral oedema and respiratory support.

Family members and other contacts of meningococcal meningitis are offered prophylaxis with either oral rifampicin or ciprofloxacin.

▶ Nursing management

Patients with bacterial meningitis require skilled nursing, and they and their family need information and psychological support. The nursing management includes:

- liaison with the control of infection nurse regarding precautions to prevent spread to others. The risk to nursing and medical staff is minimal, and prophylaxis is generally not required
- observations – level of consciousness (GCS), temperature, pulse, respiration and blood pressure and the development of a rash or seizures, etc. All changes are immediately reported to the doctor and documented
- airway maintenance
- protection against injury if seizures occur such as falling out of bed
- administration of prescribed antibiotics and information for family members who are taking oral prophylaxis
- management of i.v. fluid administration including observations of the cannula site and accurate records of fluid intake and output. Oral fluids and diet are reintroduced gradually as the patient's condition improves

- administration of prescribed analgesia, antipyretic and antiemetic drugs and monitoring of effects
- measures to reduce pyrexia (see Ch. 5)
- providing a cool, quiet and reduced-light environment
- attention to hygiene needs, e.g. frequent cool washes and mouth care for patients who are hot, sweaty and vomiting
- general measures to reduce the risks of immobility, e.g. range of motion exercises as tolerated, pressure-relieving devices, etc.

Patients and family members should be made aware that full recovery may take some weeks or months, and that some patients will need rehabilitation if neurological deficits persist. In addition, nurses have an important role in providing information about the early recognition of the signs and symptoms of bacterial meningitis (see above) and about vaccination (see Health Promotion box 14.3).

HERPES ZOSTER

Herpes zoster (shingles) is caused by the reactivation of the varicella zoster virus (VZV) that has remained dormant in a nerve root ganglion since the person had varicella (chickenpox) during childhood. It usually affects middle-aged and older people and those who are immunocompromised, e.g. people with cancer or AIDS. The VZV can also affect the brain (encephalitis) or spinal cord (myelitis).

Clinical presentation

Shingles is characterized by continuous, severe pain along the distribution of the affected nerve. After a few days, vesicles and reddening are present. Commonly, the sensory nerves supplying the trunk are involved and there is pain and skin eruption on one side of the body. If the motor root is also involved, patients may have some muscle wasting. The trigeminal nerve ganglion may be affected and, if the ophthalmic branch is involved, the vesicles are present on the cornea and may lead to corneal ulceration (see Ch. 15).

Unfortunately some patients develop post-herpetic neuralgia after the initial pain and vesicles subside.

Medical management

Treatment is based on the early use of oral aciclovir. Immunocompromised patients may need i.v. aciclovir. Topical preparations of idoxuridine may be used on the vesicular skin rash or for corneal involvement; however, it is only effective if used at the start of the infection.

Post-herpetic neuralgia is difficult to treat and patients may need amitriptyline (tricyclic antidepressant) or referral to a specialist pain clinic.

▶ Nursing management

Nurses should be alert to the possibility that a client or patient in their care may have shingles, as early treatment is beneficial. This is likely to be in community settings and patients should be encouraged to seek medical advice. It is important to educate patients about the proper use of antiviral drugs. Patients with corneal involvement should be observed for corneal ulceration and specialist help sought as necessary (see Ch. 15). The nurse may offer advice regarding general skin care (e.g. avoiding factors that increase irritation) if patients are bothered by the vesicles.

 HEALTH PROMOTION

14.3 Protection against meningitis

Currently in the UK, immunization that protects against some types of meningitis is available during infancy, young adulthood and to individuals with a higher risk of infection.

Haemophilus influenzae type b (Hib)
Three doses starting at 2 months of age. Others who are at higher risk of infection, e.g. following splenectomy (removal of the spleen), are advised to have the vaccine. In addition, older children with sickle cell disease or cancer may be offered protection.

Meningococcal group C
This too is offered as three doses starting at 2 months of age. Young people (late teens/early 20s) are at risk and are currently offered the vaccine in a programme that aims to protect those groups who were not vaccinated as babies or children. Recently the UK government extended this to include those aged 20–25 years. People working in laboratories who have close contact with the microorganism may also be offered the vaccine.

Pneumococcal meningitis
There is no routine immunization programme, but individuals who are more susceptible to pneumococcal infection should be immunized, e.g.:

- after splenectomy and those with a poorly functioning spleen
- chronic kidney, lung, liver or heart disease
- diabetes
- coeliac disease
- sickle cell disease.

The current polysaccharide vaccine is not effective in young children, and a new vaccine that does work in this group is currently being introduced.

It is important for people to understand that the vaccines do not protect against all types of meningitis; for example, no vaccine against meningococcal group B is currently offered, and those travelling overseas still need protection against group A.

Nurses should ensure that people know the signs and symptoms of meningitis, and understand the importance of early recognition and obtaining urgent medical treatment when meningitis is suspected.

Patients who develop post-herpetic neuralgia may become depressed and will need psychological support, as well as help to understand the reasons for the pain (see Ch. 7). Some patients will derive relief from the use of transcutaneous nerve stimulation (TENS).

Nurses will also need to provide information about the link between shingles and chickenpox, i.e. that a patient with shingles can give someone else chickenpox, but that the reverse does not occur.

CREUTZFELDT–JAKOB DISEASE

Creutzfeldt–Jakob disease (CJD) is a rare but well-known condition, especially the new form variant CJD (vCJD). CJD is characterized by amyloid deposits in the brain, formation of microscopic holes (spongiform encephalopathy), loss of neurons and proliferation of astrocytes. A form of CJD called sporadic CJD has been recognized for many years. Variant CJD shares some clinical features but has different aetiological patterns.

Aetiology, epidemiology and pathology

Sporadic CJD is associated with older people and a rapid deterioration. It is found around the world and does not coexist in the same areas as endemic bovine spongiform encephalopathy (BSE) which is characteristic of vCJD.

Variant CJD is associated with younger onset and a slower deterioration, although there is an overlap of the two forms. There may be a connection between BSE and vCJD as the two conditions overlap in geographical area; both are caused by a similar prion and the histological pattern is similar. The incidence in Britain is low and the incidence of vCJD is falling. A prion protein causes CJD. Prion proteins have the same amino acid sequence as the normal form, but different 'folding' alters the molecular shape. They are abnormal and cannot be easily broken down by protease enzymes and are less soluble than normal protein. They can cause a chain reaction where other normal proteins take on the prion form.

Clinical presentation

Patients with CJD have a variety of symptoms and signs associated with the parts of the brain first affected. There may be psychiatric symptoms present. In the later stages, atrophy of the brain leads to dementia, sensory and motor failure and, ultimately, death.

▶ Nursing management

At present there is no cure for CJD and people affected will be totally dependent on others for their care. Nurses have an important role in providing support, information and education for families and other carers, and in working with other health and social care professionals to ensure that care provision continues to meet needs. Another important nursing function is that of providing unbiased information about CJD to the wider community who may have anxieties that originate from sensational media coverage of BSE, CJD and risk.

Key points in the care include:

- utilizing the skills of psychiatric nurses in the early stages
- providing total care in the later stages of disease

- palliative care during the final phase with symptom management (see Ch. 34)
- support for the family – especially in cases of vCJD, which has political and legal ramifications due to the supposed connection with BSE. The family and patient will need extensive help. Decisions regarding the end of life may have to be discussed, such as the decision to stop feeding or withdraw systematic support
- no special precautions are needed to care for patients with CJD; universal precautions regarding body fluids will suffice. However, as the prion is resistant to disinfection processes, certain products and instruments that come into contact with nervous or lymphoid tissue have restrictions. These include blood products, human growth hormone derived from donor pituitary material, donor corneas, etc. Some surgical instruments that come into contact with prion-infected tissue should be disposable.

SEIZURES AND EPILEPSY

A seizure occurs when cerebral neurons fire (i.e. generate impulses) abnormally. A seizure can be regarded as an electrical disturbance in the brain. The word 'fit' is not useful because seizures may not resemble the 'classic fit' of convulsions and loss of consciousness: seizure is a more suitable term. Seizures may or may not show clinical manifestations. Seizures may be caused by several triggers, e.g. hyperventilation, flickering light stimulation, sleep deprivation and migraine, as well as those causes occurring in people diagnosed with epilepsy (see p. 316).

EPILEPSY

Epilepsy is a condition characterized by recurrent seizures. The prevalence of epilepsy in the UK is about 600 people per 100 000. This makes epilepsy the second most common neurological condition after migraine (see below).

There are two main types of epilepsy (International League Against Epilepsy 1981):

- partial seizures
- primary generalized seizures.

Details of the different types of epilepsy are outlined in Table 14.6.

Aetiology

Epilepsy may be primary (idiopathic), when no cause is found, or secondary to conditions affecting the brain or other organs: the latter is more common.

There are many known causes of epilepsy, the most common being diseases of the nervous system, e.g. head injury, stroke, brain cancer, and infections such as meningitis. Other causes include:

- cerebral ischaemia and hypertensive encephalopathy (brain disease)
- neurological damage caused by injury or hypoxia around the time of birth
- hyperthermia
- hypoglycaemia (low blood sugar)

Table 14.6 Types of epilepsy and medication

Main type	Medication	Subgroup	Description
A. Partial seizures These occur when there is a specific point, a focus, on the surface of the brain. A common focus for partial seizures is the hippocampus, an area within the limbic system responsible for memory. Note that memory appears to be located in many sites within the nervous system and is not confined to the hippocampus	Partial seizures are treated with phenytoin, carbamazepine or primidone	*1. Simple partial seizures* In a simple partial seizure the electrical activity spreads across the surface but it does not affect consciousness	Patients may report an aura, a particular feeling that varies from person to person. An aura may be visual, auditory or even a taste or smell, as well as bodily sensations. The type of aura depends on the focus of the electrical activity. As this can be of use in diagnosis, a record should be made by asking the patient about the aura. As patients are conscious during an aura, and an aura may precede a more generalized seizure, the sensation can be used to warn them to lie down or summon help
		2. Complex partial seizure	In complex partial seizures, consciousness is affected. For example, someone may stop speaking, may smack the lips together, and may not respond to speech for up to several minutes. When the seizure has ended, the person will feel tired and have amnesia. Complex partial seizures commonly arise in the temporal lobe and were once called 'temporal lobe epilepsy'. Patients may report sensory, cognitive (such as memory, perception and thought) and affective (such as emotional) signs and symptoms
B. Primary generalized seizures These occur when there is bilateral, simultaneous electrical activity. Consciousness is usually lost. There are several patterns to primary generalized seizures	If the seizures are predominantly tonic-clonic then phenytoin or carbamazepine is usually prescribed. In absences, ethosuxamide is the preferred treatment. Myoclonic seizures are usually treated with sodium valproate or clonazepam	*1. Tonic-clonic*	In tonic-clonic seizures, patients have a general increase in muscle tone (in other words they become stiff) – tonic; and then have rhythmic limb jerking (contraction and relaxation of muscles) – clonic
		2. Tonic	Patients will stiffen as muscle tone increases but there is no clonic jerking of the limbs
		3. Clonic	There is jerking of the limbs
		4. Myoclonic	There is a sudden brief jerking of one or more limbs. This is often associated with degenerative neurological disorders Note that myoclonus may not be epileptic in origin and sometimes occurs as people are going to sleep. The sudden jerking will return them to wakefulness
		5. Atonic	Patients will be flaccid, i.e. they will have no muscle tone and be floppy
		6. Absence	Absence seizures occur when patients stop what they are doing and become unresponsive. They may remain standing or they may fall to the ground. Absences usually only last a few seconds although they may be repeated fairly quickly, sometimes hundreds or thousands of times a day

Status epilepticus describes a situation characterized by a continuous seizure or a series of repeated seizures. This condition can be life-threatening and patients should receive immediate care. They may not regain consciousness between the seizures. In status epilepticus, the most commonly used first-line drug is diazepam (often given rectally), although phenytoin and even the barbiturate drug phenobarbital may be used.

- hyponatraemia (low serum sodium)
- hypocalcaemia (low serum calcium)
- major organ failure – renal failure, liver failure, etc.
- certain drugs, and drug overdose and withdrawal
- eclampsia (during pregnancy).

Clinical presentation

The age at onset of epilepsy can be useful in the identification of causal factors. Idiopathic epilepsy is usually diagnosed in childhood or during the first decades of adulthood. Seizures associated with trauma are also more common in childhood and earlier adulthood because trauma tends to be associated with young people. Epilepsy caused by birth injury is usually diagnosed early in childhood and as children are more prone to infections than adults, post-infection epilepsy is usually diagnosed early in life. Epilepsy associated with stroke, metabolic disorders and tumours is diagnosed later in life because these illnesses are more common in older people.

The type of seizure described by onlookers and the presence of features such as an aura are also useful in diagnosis.

Specific investigations

An EEG is a very useful test as it can identify the site of the lesion and the nature of the seizure. Sometimes a video recording is taken simultaneously with the EEG which enables the outward signs of the seizure to be related to the EEG trace. The EEG can also be used to record evoked potentials following exposure to a stimulus. Patients are often exposed to a light or sound stimulus and the response of the brain can be seen as electrical activity. CT scan and MRI will identify lesions. Positron emission tomography may also be used because it shows the brain in action and can identify the focus of the seizures.

A full neurological examination that includes testing sensation, smell, etc. will also be useful.

Medical management

The treatment for epilepsy is usually in the form of anti-epileptic medication (see Table 14.6). Certain medications are more effective than others for different seizure types. Drugs (e.g. phenytoin, carbamazepine) with a narrow therapeutic range require that patients have regular blood tests to ensure that serum levels of the medication are sufficient to be effective without causing toxicity.

▶ Nursing management

Helping patients and their families to adjust to a diagnosis of epilepsy and all that entails is a key nursing role. Patients will need information about employment restrictions and the regulations regarding holding a driving licence after a seizure. Education of patients will also include advice about safe participation in certain sports and other leisure activities, such as only swimming in the presence of others who know that a seizure might occur. The need to consider safety at home should be discussed, e.g. safety guards around fires, only bathing when another person is in the house and not locking the bathroom door.

The nurse's role in administering medication is to ensure concordance and to be aware of dose irregularities and side-effects, e.g. gum hyperplasia (overgrowth) with phenytoin. It is important that nurses are familiar with the side-effects of anti-epileptic medication and readers are urged to consult a current national formulary or the manufacturer's literature. Nurses will also provide information for patients about the drugs and the need for blood level monitoring to ensure that self-medication is safe and effective.

Care during a seizure

The management of patients during a seizure is an important aspect of the care they receive. As patients with epilepsy may have very individual problems and seizure types, the management will need to be based on individual assessment of needs. However, some general points include:

- Stay calm, even though seizures can look very dramatic. Reassure onlookers.
- Do not put anything in the person's mouth as this may damage the patient's teeth (biting the tongue is an uncommon event).
- Protect patients from harm during the seizure. This may involve moving furniture, or moving them away from hazards or padding their head with a pillow during convulsions.
- After the convulsion is over place patients in the recovery position until they regain consciousness.
- If the seizure occurs in the community, do not call an ambulance immediately. Patients should be asked if they have had a fit before, and if it is a regular occurrence, they can usually return to everyday activities. If it is a first seizure, they convulse for more than 3–5 minutes or they do not regain consciousness within 10 minutes, an ambulance should be called. If they progress to status epilepticus, medical help is required.
- Patients should be observed carefully during the seizure. Noting the time of onset will help to identify whether the seizure is focal or generalized. Eye movements and pupil size can be used to monitor the location and progress of the seizure. Note if the limbs and trunk show tonic and clonic features. Sometimes speech may cease even if the seizure is of very short duration, although this is not always the case and patients may respond verbally during a seizure.
- Within health care settings, patients should have a care plan or protocol to follow in the event of a seizure. This may involve administering anti-epileptic drugs. However, during a seizure patients should not receive any medication by mouth, and in status epilepticus rectal diazepam is usually the drug of choice (see Guidelines for Care Priorities box 14.4). Intramuscular or intravenous drugs may also be used.
- After the seizure has ended, patients should be allowed to rest, as the experience can be exhausting.
- Stay with patients until they are fully recovered, because following a seizure patients may show unusual behaviour of which they are not aware. This is called automatism.
- It may be necessary to monitor consciousness and blood pressure, pulse and respiration after the seizure.
- Explain to the person who has had a seizure what has happened.

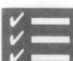

GUIDELINES FOR CARE PRIORITIES

14.4 Administration of rectal diazepam in status epilepticus

1. Explain proposed treatment to patient and family, so that they may give informed consent
2. Check the drug (preloaded in a tube) dose and prescription chart according to local protocols
3. Check the identity of the patient
4. Use standard infection control measures
5. Ensure privacy and maintain the patient's dignity
6. Position the patient on the left side
7. Lubricate the drug delivery tube prior to insertion into the rectum
8. Squeeze the tube to expel the contents into the rectum
9. Ensure that the patient is clean and dry
10. Dispose of drug tube and other equipment, and wash hands
11. Record the drug administration in the usual way.

HEADACHE

Headache may be defined as any ache or pain in the head that is caused by the stimulation of pain-sensitive structures in the cranium or the extracranial tissues in the head and neck. Headache is the commonest neurological symptom reported and is something that most people will experience. Headaches may be experienced as a one-off event or may be recurrent, acute or chronic.

Headaches can occur due to a number of different pathologies. They may be primary, e.g. tension headache or migraine, or secondary to a more serious underlying intracranial pathology such as bleeding or a tumour. Tension headaches are by far the most common, affecting up to 86% of women and 63% of men each year. For many people the occurrence of headaches decreases with age.

The exact mechanism of many headaches is unclear; however, there are a limited number of pain-sensitive structures in and around the head, and the brain tissue itself does not contain nociceptors (see Ch. 7). Intracranial pain-sensitive structures include the dura, venous sinuses and some other vessels.

Examples of extradural pain-sensitive structures include the scalp muscles, orbital contents, nasal mucosa, external and middle ear and the teeth and gums. Pain is predominantly conveyed by the Vth cranial nerve (trigeminal), but also by other cranial nerves and the upper three cervical nerve roots.

TYPES OF HEADACHE

Headaches may fall into one of the following categories, each having its own specific causes and mechanism of onset:

- tension headaches (most common)
- migraine
- cluster headaches
- temporal (giant cell) arteritis
- headache associated with raised intracranial pressure (see above)
- non-neurological headache (see specific chapters, such as Chs 15 and 16)

When assessing a patient's headaches, it is important to note the character, site and onset of the pain as well as the frequency, duration and timing. It should also be noted whether there are any accompanying symptoms such as vomiting, or precipitating factors that could aid in differentiating between the different types of headache.

Information about the aetiology, clinical presentation, mechanism, investigations and medical management of the main types of headache is provided in Table 14.7.

▶ Nursing management

Headaches can be an extremely distressing symptom. Patients experiencing cluster headaches will often describe wanting to hit their head against the wall and will not know what to do with themselves, the pain is so severe.

One of the main nursing interventions is assessment of the pain to assist in evaluation of the headache type and the effectiveness of treatment. It may be useful to assist the patient in keeping a headache diary, noting the time of onset, and any precipitating factors that may be associated with the onset. The nurse will also need to assess the pain itself, noting the quality, quantity and site. It may be useful to use a pain assessment tool to assist in this process (see Ch. 7).

Once a diagnosis has been made, the main nursing interventions include administration of prescribed medication and other

Table 14.7 Types of headaches

Type of headache	Aetiology and clinical presentation	Investigations and medical management
Tension headache	• Associated with tension, but no other physical symptoms • Affects four times as many women as men • Usually described as diffuse, dull, aching and band-like headaches • Often worse on touching the scalp • Aggravated by noise • Does not disturb sleep • May last for hours or even days and may be infrequent or occur daily (Lindsay et al 1997)	• Diagnosis usually based on the clinical presentation and history • Simple analgesia and reassurance that there is no serious underlying pathology • Often stress-related, and some patients benefit from stress management strategies (see Ch. 6). **NB.** Drug therapy (tranquillizers, etc.) is only used if other measures fail to bring relief

Table 14.7 *(continued)*

Type of headache	Aetiology and clinical presentation	Investigations and medical management
Migraine (two main forms: classical and common)	• Common familial disorder, affecting 5–10% of the population • Usually begins in childhood or early adulthood • The exact mechanism of migraine is unclear, but is associated with constriction of cerebral blood vessels during the aura phase, followed by vasodilatation and resultant stimulation of pain fibres leading to the headache • Approximately 20% of those affected report an association with certain foods, such as cheese, chocolate and citrus fruits • Migraine may also be exacerbated by taking the oral contraceptive pill (Williams 1999) • Classical migraine presents with an aura (flashing lights, fortification spectra, scintillating scotoma), vomiting and headache • Common migraine does not present with an aura; there may be vomiting and the headache is poorly differentiated • Migraine headache is usually unilateral, throbbing, paroxysmal, worsened by bright light and relieved by sleep. It is often associated with nausea and vomiting (Lindsay et al 1997)	• Usually diagnosed from the clinical presentation, especially if there is a family history of migraine and often travel sickness as a child. Patients may often be investigated with an EEG and CT scan as migraine may present similarly to other neurological conditions such as focal epilepsy, stroke and dilated cerebral aneurysm • There may be some improvement if suspect foods are avoided • Patients who have frequent, recurrent attacks are prescribed drug prophylaxis to prevent migraine. These include pizotifen and beta-blockers, such as atenolol. It is thought that these can be effective as the pathophysiological processes that lead up to a migraine can begin up to 48 hours before the onset of the pain (Williams 1999) • In an acute attack, patients may be treated with analgesics, and sumatriptan has been shown to be effective. These analgesics often need to be given parenterally as gastric emptying is delayed in migraine, leading to nausea and vomiting. This means that the drugs would not pass through into the intestinal tract and absorption is therefore delayed
Cluster headache	• Less frequent than migraine • Affects five times as many men as women • Age of onset in early middle age • The exact mechanism of cluster headaches is unclear although there is evidence of increased histamine release, with resultant vasodilatation • Many patients find that attacks are triggered by intake of alcohol • Headaches are characterized by distinct episodes of excruciating pain, usually around one eye. Accompanied by lacrimation, nasal stuffiness and drainage and can last from 10 minutes to 2 hours • They usually occur during the night, waking the patient up, and occur in clusters of attacks separated by weeks or even years (Williams 1999)	• History and clinical presentation are usually diagnostic, but sometimes a CT scan is performed, as some pituitary lesions (see Ch. 17) can present with similar symptoms • Antihistamines have been used prophylactically, but are often ineffective • Ergotamine may be used prophylactically • During an acute attack, the administration of 100% oxygen can help • Corticosteroids are also prescribed during bouts of attacks, with up to 40 mg prednisolone being administered daily for 7–10 days, reducing the dose over the second week to zero
Temporal (giant cell) arteritis	• Generally affects older people and may involve any extra- or intracranial vessel, although it usually occurs within the superficial temporal artery • It occurs as the artery walls thicken and become infiltrated by 'giant cells'. The arterial lumen narrows with resultant ischaemia and stimulation of the pain fibres • The headache, overlying the affected vessel, is severe and throbbing • The affected artery is not pulsating and will feel thickened and tender. The condition is intractable until treatment is commenced • May also be associated with double vision or blindness and systemic symptoms	• The erythrocyte sedimentation rate (ESR) is raised, as this is essentially an inflammatory condition • Temporal artery biopsy • Untreated, this condition can lead to blindness and brain stem stroke, so treatment is urgent • Treatment is usually with corticosteroids, e.g. prednisolone. Treatment may be required for life
Headaches due to raised intracranial pressure	• Caused by stretching and tension on the intracranial pain-sensitive structures • Headaches are usually generalized • Worse in the morning, on awakening and may disturb sleep • Aggravated by bending and coughing	See relevant sections covering raised intracranial pressure, tumours, subarachnoid haemorrhage, meningitis, etc.

therapies and patient education. This is aimed at preventing and minimizing the frequency of attacks, such as avoiding precipitating factors. However, during an attack, patients often appreciate a dark, quiet environment in which to rest until the analgesia begins to relieve the pain.

Tension headaches are stress-related, resulting in muscle tension around the temples and back of the neck, so psychological support is important. Patients often benefit from relaxation and stress management techniques. This type of headache can also be precipitated by poor posture, so advice about this aspect can be useful. Some patients find relief from gentle massage to the shoulders and neck, often given by a partner or family member.

Migraine sufferers have been found to have lower levels of magnesium, a mineral that is thought to help regulate swelling of the blood vessels in the head. As well as dietary advice about foods to avoid (having identified the precipitating factors by using the headache diary), nutritional advice about good sources of magnesium can also be given, e.g. green leafy vegetables, legumes, seafood, nuts, seeds and whole grains. Nurses can also advise patients to cut down on exposure to bright or fluorescent lighting and to adopt a regular routine. Patients who have a regular routine of going to bed, waking and eating have found that the frequency of their headaches reduces.

Some patients have also reported benefit from complementary therapies such as acupuncture and acupressure, which are thought to release endorphins, the body's natural painkillers.

NUTRITIONAL AND METABOLIC CAUSES OF NEUROLOGICAL DISORDERS

The nervous system does not store nutrients and is therefore completely dependent on the circulation for all its requirements. For instance, patients with diabetes are likely to have changes in consciousness when the blood sugar is raised or lowered. There are some neurological disorders that are related directly to nutritional/metabolic disorders, e.g. Wernicke's encephalopathy and Wilson's disease.

WERNICKE'S ENCEPHALOPATHY

Wernicke's encephalopathy is due to the deficiency or inability to absorb vitamin B$_1$ (thiamin). This may be the result of poor nutrition or of long-term alcohol misuse that interferes with thiamin absorption and utilization.

Pathophysiology and clinical presentation

Wernicke's encephalopathy is accompanied by loss of neurons, proliferation of glial cells and demyelination. There is also an increase in small blood vessels that may bleed. All these changes occur in several parts of the brain and patients will have ataxia, paralysis of eye muscles and confusion. Dysarthria is also found. Sometimes patients may progress to coma. The hypothalamus can be affected so hypothermia can occur.

Management

The treatment involves giving thiamin. This may be given parenterally if absorption of thiamin is impaired. Many people will improve with treatment, but others will go on to have problems

that require long-term care and support. Korsakoff's syndrome, which is characterized by severe memory impairment, nystagmus (flickering eyeball movement) and gait problems, often follows episodes of Wernicke's encephalopathy and is also treated with thiamin. However, the damage done to the nervous system cannot be reversed and so the care needs to continue over time.

WILSON'S DISEASE

Wilson's disease (hepatolenticular degeneration) is a rare inherited disorder in which there is an inability to deal with dietary copper, causing it to build up in various organs and resulting in liver and brain damage.

Pathophysiology and clinical presentation

The copper, which is present in small amounts in food, cannot be attached to a circulating serum protein. As a result, unbound (metallic) copper is deposited in the brain, kidneys, cornea and liver. The brain damage can be severe. It affects quite specific parts of the brain and results in abnormal movements such as grimacing, writhing, rigidity, dysphagia and dysarthria and unsteady gait. Patients may have seizures and there may be learning difficulties.

Management

Early diagnosis as soon after birth as possible is vital, so that treatment can be started to prevent long-term damage. The treatment of choice is penicillamine, a chelating drug (one that binds metallic ions). Penicillamine will chelate circulating copper and remove excess deposits of tissue copper. The treatment usually needs to be followed for life. A low-copper diet may help. This means restricting seafood, dark red meats and offal, mushrooms, nectarines, chocolate, dried fruit, dried peas and beans. A dietician must be consulted so that the diet provides the necessary nutrients. Cooking should not be done in copper vessels, and in some areas the water supply has a high copper content and should be avoided. Because of liver damage, alcohol is also best avoided.

DEGENERATIVE DISORDERS

There are many types of degenerative disorder of the nervous system, although some are extremely rare with only a handful of occurrences throughout the world. Some are so rare that diagnosis is problematic as there is nothing with which to compare the signs and symptoms. It therefore follows that signs and symptoms are very varied depending on the function of the part of the nervous system affected. Commonly encountered degenerative disorders include Parkinson's disease, Alzheimer's disease and motor neuron disease.

PARKINSON'S DISEASE

Idiopathic Parkinson's disease (paralysis agitans) is a chronic, progressive, degenerative neurological condition resulting from the loss of dopamine-producing (dopaminergic) neurons within an area of the brain known as the substantia nigra. These neurons have connections with the three brain structures, known as the basal nuclei (sometimes called ganglia), that normally control voluntary movement. The loss of the dopamine-producing neurons and hence the neurotransmitter dopamine results in the characteristic signs of the disease, such as tremor. There are numerous effects and, although not generally life-threatening, it can be extremely limiting and distressing for sufferers who have a number of specific nursing needs.

Epidemiology and aetiology

Most new cases of Parkinson's disease occur in people over 65 years of age. However, it is worth noting that 1 in 7 patients are diagnosed under 40 years of age. The prevalence within the general population is approximately 1 in 1000, increasing to 1 in 100 in those over 65 years of age. The prevalence can be expected to increase with the ageing population, but combined evidence from epidemiological studies is insufficient to show if the patterns are changing or if environmental factors are important in the aetiology of the disease (Flaten 1993). It affects men and women equally.

Parkinson's disease is idiopathic (no known cause has been found), and the pathophysiological mechanism is not completely understood. There have, however, been a number of theories expressed regarding possible precipitating factors or causative agents. Parkinson's disease is not principally genetic, although some people may have some hereditary predisposition, which when combined with another precipitating factor may result in the disease.

Considerable interest in recent years has focused on a possible environmental neurotoxic agent, following the production of parkinsonian-like effects in drug misusers after the self-administration of an opiate-like 'designer drug', subsequently found to be contaminated with methyl-phenyl-tetrahydropyridine (MPTP). MPTP is converted within the brain to a more toxic compound that is taken up by and destroys the dopamine-producing neurons. Paraquat, a widely used herbicide, structurally resembles MPTP (Flaten 1993), and hence the hunt for an environmental neurotoxic causative agent.

Many patients display signs and symptoms that resemble those of Parkinson's disease, but the characteristic neuropathological changes within the substantia nigra on postmortem are absent. Possible identifiable causes of this 'parkinsonism' include drugs such phenothiazines, infections of the CNS, chemical neurotoxins (e.g. carbon monoxide), structural brain lesions (e.g. tumours) and metabolic disorders.

Pathophysiology

Normally the inhibitory neurotransmitter dopamine exists in balance with an excitatory neurotransmitter acetylcholine (ACh); it is this balance that results in coordinated voluntary movement. When dopamine is reduced, the balance is lost and excessive excitation of voluntary muscles occurs in the absence of normal inhibition. The signs of Parkinson's disease such as tremor and rigidity do not appear until 50% of the dopamine-producing neurons have been lost and corresponding dopamine production has fallen by 80–85%.

Clinical presentation

Parkinson's disease is typically characterized by tremor, rigidity and bradykinesia (see below). However, patients may present

---

Box 14.7 Effects of rigidity in Parkinson's disease
(Adapted from Lannon et al 1986)

- Facial muscles
  — mask-like expression
- Facial and respiratory muscles
  — speech becomes slurred, slow and monotonous
- Facial and pharyngeal muscles
  — difficulty chewing
  — difficulty swallowing
- Trunk muscles
  — balance problems
  — difficulty sitting, standing from a seated position and turning in bed

---

with non-specific symptoms that include tiredness and aching limbs, mental slowness and, interestingly, small handwriting.

- The characteristic tremor of Parkinson's disease is a coarse resting tremor of distal muscles (i.e. fingers) that disappears during sleep or voluntary movement. It is often exacerbated by stress and is usually one of the first signs of the disease to be noticed.
- Rigidity is resistance to passive movement of an extremity. Patients become unable to relax selectively or contract skeletal muscle for voluntary movement. Rigidity can affect many muscle groups and will cause specific problems depending on the group affected (see Box 14.7).
- Bradykinesia is slowness of movement and difficulty initiating movement and is experienced by almost all patients with Parkinson's disease. Patients also have a shuffling gait, often described as festinating. This makes it difficult voluntarily to stop their body propelling forward once movement has started, which often results in falls. By contrast, patients may experience periods of 'freezing' or akinesia, when they are unable to initiate forward movement altogether. This often occurs when two different actions are attempted simultaneously.

It is now recognized that Parkinson's disease is a more complex syndrome consisting of neurobehavioural disturbances and symptoms occurring outside the CNS (De Keyser 1993) (see Box 14.8, p. 320)

Medical/surgical management

Drug therapy is the mainstay of managing Parkinson's disease and follows one of two approaches. The aim is either to reverse the biochemical deficit by increasing the dopamine concentration or reducing the acetylcholine concentration, or to delay or reverse the underlying process. In addition to drug therapy, patients may need referrals to the appropriate therapists – physiotherapist, OT or SLT.

Drugs

There are no perfect drugs for the treatment of Parkinson's disease; drug effects can control symptoms but cannot offer a cure. The drugs used fall into four main categories: dopaminergics, dopamine receptor agonists, monoamine-oxidase-B inhibitors and antimuscarinics (anticholinergics).

Box 14.8 Neurobehavioural and other manifestations of Parkinson's disease
(Adapted from De Keyser 1993)

- Mental
  - slowness of thought (bradyphrenia)
  - dementia
  - depression
- Ocular
  - reduced blinking
- Respiratory
  - olfactory deficits
  - voice changes
- Cardiovascular
  - postural hypotension
- Gastrointestinal
  - increased salivation and drooling
  - dysphagia
  - delayed gastric emptying
  - constipation
- Urogenital
  - detrusor hyperreflexia, *or*
  - urinary obstruction due to bradykinesia of the urinary sphincter
- Skin
  - seborrhoea with greasy skin
  - pedal oedema
- Somatosensory
  - pain
  - paraesthesia
  - vestibular involvement
- Thermoregulation
  - profuse sweating
- Sleep
  - insomnia
  - daytime somnolence
  - general fatiguability

Dopaminergics

Prior to the introduction of dopaminergics, the prognosis was poor, with patients dying within 7–10 years from the complications of immobility. Dopaminergics such as L-dopa are used to replenish dopamine. Because dopamine does not cross the blood–brain barrier, L-dopa (a dopamine precursor) is administered. Once absorbed from the small bowel, L-dopa passes through the blood–brain barrier, where it is converted to dopamine. Some L-dopa is converted enzymically before it crosses into the brain and it can cause hypotension and nausea. These unwanted effects are avoided by combining L-dopa with an enzyme inhibitor (e.g. carbidopa) that prevents any conversion to dopamine outside the blood–brain barrier, e.g. co-careldopa. After long-term use (3–5 years) patients begin to experience end-of-dose failure and an 'on–off effect'. Over 50% of Parkinson's disease sufferers experience fluctuations in the motor response to L-dopa after 5 years. End-of-dose failure means that patients require their next dose of L-dopa at more frequent intervals and can experience more drug side-effects as

a result. The on–off effect is a rapid fluctuation from mobility to a parkinsonian state of acute and extreme rigidity. Many patients describe being suddenly 'switched off', like an electric light. It is unpredictable, can last from a few minutes to hours and bears no relation to timing of L-dopa doses. It is, however, an effect related to the drug therapy and not the disease process. The incidence of the on–off effect increases with duration of L-dopa therapy and after 10 years most patients are affected. Modified-release L-dopa preparations may be useful in decreasing end-of-dose effects.

Dopamine receptor agonists (dopaminomimetics)

These include bromocriptine, lisuride and pergolide, which mimic the effects of dopamine within the brain, acting directly at the dopamine receptors. When given in a daily dose, combined with L-dopa they have been found to smooth out the troublesome motor fluctuations. They have similar side-effects to L-dopa.

Apomorphine is also a potent dopamine agonist but its peripheral side-effects (e.g. nausea, vomiting, postural hypotension and sedation) must be controlled with the drug domperidone. Apomorphine has been shown to rapidly and consistently reverse the 'off' period motor deficit. Other symptoms associated with the 'off 'period, such as functional bladder outlet obstruction and pain, have also benefited. Administration of apomorphine is usually supervised by a specialist and started in hospital. It is administered subcutaneously either by intermittent injection via a Penject if the patient is able or via continuous infusion using a Graseby syringe pump for patients who require more than 10–12 injections per day. Most patients will be able to discontinue domperidone after 6 months of apomorphine use. Skin nodules that may occur as a side-effect of apomorphine can be reduced by rotating injection sites and maintaining good hygiene. Reduction in daily 'off' periods appears to be maintained by up to 50% on long-term follow-up, i.e. apomorphine does not appear to reduce in efficacy in the same way as L-dopa.

Monoamine-oxidase-B inhibitors

Monoamine-oxidase-B inhibitors, e.g. selegiline, prevent dopamine breakdown by blocking the action of the enzyme monoamine-oxidase B, and therefore extend its action. Additionally they prevent the reuptake of dopamine at the presynaptic dopamine receptors in the neuron. Selegiline is used alone in early Parkinson's disease, and with L-dopa to decrease 'end-of-dose' effects.

Antimuscarinics (anticholinergics)

These drugs redress the dopamine–ACh balance by reducing ACh transmission. Drugs, e.g. benzhexol, partially block ACh receptors terminating in the basal nuclei (ganglia) and also block the uptake of dopamine by the neurons, thereby increasing amounts of free dopamine. Antimuscarinics are used to control symptoms such as tremor in the early stage of Parkinson's disease.

Surgical interventions

Stereotactic surgery using three-dimensional measurements to determine the exact position is sometimes used within specific parts of brain, e.g. pallidus (pallidotomy) or thalamus

(thalamotomy), in patients who do not respond well to drug therapy. The procedures are still offered in a few centres and a new trial is planned to determine whether a specific approach to pallidotomy produces a sustained reversal of bradykinesia, rigidity and L-dopa-induced dyskinesia (involuntary choreic movements) in advanced Parkinson's disease. During the 1980s, experimental procedures were undertaken, in which dopamine-producing cells were transplanted into the substantia nigra. Initially the transplanted cells were taken from the adrenal medulla of the patient (autotransplantation), and once placed within the basal nuclei would hopefully continue to produce dopamine. Initial results appeared promising, but there were also complications and mortality associated with the procedure. Far more controversial was the transplantation of dopamine-producing cells obtained from fetal tissue, with the associated ethical issues (Fletcher 1992).

▶ Nursing management

Parkinson's disease is progressive and even with the best medical/surgical therapies, patients can expect deterioration and increased dependence. People with Parkinson's disease experience particular problems and have specific nursing needs, and some common problems are discussed here. Nurses also play a pivotal role in coordinating the efforts of the multidisciplinary team involved with patient management. Specialist Parkinson's disease nurses and other specialist nurses (e.g. continence, nutrition) can improve quality of life and act as a resource for patients, their families and other nurses. One of the main problems affecting patients is the unpredictable pattern of disease progression or rate of progress, so they need to be prepared and able to adapt to their own changing needs. Optimal management requires both patients and family members to play an active part in adapting to the life changes the condition brings.

Mobility

Some of the main problems relate to mobility. Patients will experience difficulty initiating movement and usually have rigidity and bradykinesia. Particular actions become difficult because of the rigidity, such as turning in bed and rising from a chair. The patient's brain works faster than the muscles and this may lead to frustration. A bed with a firm mattress and a high-backed chair with arms can enhance mobility. Poor posture, a festinating gait and difficulty turning around, coupled with diminished postural responses to correct loss of balance, can often result in falls. Freezing can also become a problem as patients become rooted to the spot.

What these patients need most is time. Nurses and carers need to wait until they are ready to move and allow them time to do things themselves. Patients need time to adapt to their changing abilities and it is important to preserve whatever function they have. A careful assessment, making use of patients' experiences, and early referral to physiotherapy and OT are vital. Specific problems can be approached in the following ways:

- if turning round is problematic, ask the patient to use a wider circle
- using a high-seated chair with arm rests makes rising easier

- if freezing occurs, this can be helped by asking the patient to step over an imaginary line, or count 'one-two' out loud with each step.

Patients may find tasks needing fine movements difficult, e.g. doing up buttons or shoelaces, and self-care tasks such as shaving. Nurses can advise about clothing adaptations such as Velcro fastenings and the OT should be asked to help.

Pain can also be associated with rigidity and an 'off' state, although this is not always recognized. In particular, patients may experience disturbing muscle cramps at night. Off-period pain is often relieved when patients become mobile again and this has been helped by the use of apomorphine, which reverses the 'off' state within 15 minutes.

Communication

Communication problems (verbally and non-verbally) commonly occur for a number of reasons. Voice production very often becomes quieter as the disease progresses and speech can become slurred, monotonous and slow due to rigidity of respiratory and facial muscles. Emotional expression is compromised due to the patient's mask-like facial expression and this can often lead to despondency; such feelings of distress and frustration may exacerbate symptoms. Patients may appear demanding and this can lead to them being labelled as 'difficult' and, coupled with their minimal responses, cause nurses and carers to reduce social interaction with them. Loss of facial expression and absence of body language in this client group have been shown to have a negative effect on health professionals (Pentland 1987).

Patients may appear cold, unfeeling or intellectually dull, and the lack of facial expression may give a false impression of low mood, but this does not mean that patients lack understanding. Written communication is also difficult due to micrographia (small handwriting), which is often illegible. Patients need sufficient time to communicate and successful care requires their involvement in the planning process along with their relatives and carers. Nurses may feel that they do not have the time to wait, but it is important to make that time and listen to what patients have to say in order to help them overcome the loss of confidence and social isolation that they may be experiencing.

Nutrition

As with most activities, eating can be a slow process. Using cutlery may be difficult and the food will become cold before it is finished. The OT should be involved and can provide special cutlery and other modifications. One of the most potentially harmful problems is the possibility of aspiration, often silent (without a cough). Rigidity affects facial and pharyngeal muscles, making chewing and swallowing difficult. Patients may dribble saliva and eating becomes a messy process that leads to embarrassment and reluctance to eat. In order to maintain safety during eating or drinking, it is important that patients sit upright and well forward, and are not rushed. If dysphagia is suspected, early referral to a SLT is vital before patients develop complications following aspiration.

Patients are also at risk of malnutrition due to factors already mentioned, as well as anorexia, reduced sensitivity to taste and smell, depression, increased energy requirements due

321

to muscular rigidity and increased involuntary movements (Beyer et al 1995). Simple nutritional screening and assessment tools can be used to detect risk and it is useful to monitor dietary intake and involve the dietician in patient care (see Ch. 11).

The absorption of L-dopa may be affected by protein in the diet and there is an argument for restricting protein intake in order to improve the effectiveness of drug therapy (Carter et al 1989). However, with the potential risk of malnutrition, this is probably not advisable and it may be better to plan protein intake, e.g. evening main meal, so that any reduction in drug efficacy occurs during sleep (Kempster & Wahlqvist 1994). It may also be useful to time meals to coincide with patients' 'on' periods, when any difficulties may be less pronounced.

Elimination

Patients with Parkinson's disease may experience urinary incontinence and should be referred to a specialist continence nurse (see Ch. 12). In addition the OT can give advice about adaptations to clothing and lavatory facilities.

Patients are at risk of developing chronic constipation for a number of reasons: reduced gut motility, reduced mobility, inadequate dietary fibre and fluid intake and as a side-effect of antimuscarinic drugs. Nurses should monitor bowel action and advise patients regarding fibre and fluid intake. Where constipation does occur, nurses should administer the prescribed laxative.

Nurses' role in medication management

Patient education is a high priority for nurses in order to achieve compliance with drug regimens. Patients will often require drug doses to be adjusted on an individual 'trial and error' basis and this needs careful explanation. Drug doses need to be titrated against effects and side-effects, such as dyskinesia, in order to achieve the right balance for an individual. Dyskinesia may be distressing for the observer, but some patients prefer this to the parkinsonian symptoms they would otherwise experience. Nurses have an important role in dose adjustment through accurate observation and documentation of the drug effects and side-effects. This may be achieved by working with patients in completing a patient diary, or 'on–off' chart as they are sometimes referred to.

It is important to remember that patients who experience 'off' states may change dramatically from one minute to the next and this poses the greatest obstacle to normal living. Carers may find it hard to understand that patients are not being deliberately obstructive when they can no longer perform a movement they could do moments before. Timing of drug doses is of paramount importance. As the 'on–off' effect begins to affect patients, the frequency of L-dopa needs to be increased and often requires administrations at 1.5- to 2-hourly intervals (i.e. outside 'routine' drug round times). It is vital to administer drugs at the times prescribed, as a delay of even 15 minutes can make a difference. Wherever possible, patients should be encouraged to self-medicate, promoting independence and control.

It is also important to remember that commonly used antiemetics and tranquillizers, e.g. prochlorperazine, metoclopramide, chlorpromazine, trifluoperazine, haloperidol and thioridazine, are contraindicated in Parkinson's disease as they exacerbate symptoms by blocking dopamine receptors.

ALZHEIMER'S DISEASE

This condition is seen mainly in older people but it can affect younger adults as well (see Ch. 32). It is characterized by memory loss, behavioural changes such as aggression, or wandering. Mood changes and depression may occur and eventually loss of control over voluntary movement. Dementia occurs in later stages.

Histological changes in the brain include plaques consisting of damaged cells and abnormal proteins such as amyloid precursor protein, which gives rise to beta-amyloid fragments. It is the beta-amyloid fragments that appear to cause most of the loss of neuronal function. Alzheimer's disease is also characterized by neurofibrillary tangles in the neurons. Later there is a marked atrophy of brain tissue.

The aetiology is unknown although genetic links or history of brain injury may be implicated in some cases. Environmental factors and viruses have all been suggested as causes, but no evidence has been found to corroborate this.

▶ Nursing management

The care of Alzheimer's patients depends on the location of the lesions and the stage of the illness. In the early stages, patients are aware of the changes and these can be very frustrating and frightening. In the later stages, they may become dependent on carers for every aspect of care.

Key points are as follows:

- Support patients and family members with information and practical help.
- Try to maintain active participation from both patients and carers.
- Stimulating activities such as games, creative pastimes or reminiscence increase patient confidence and may help to preserve some functions.
- Carers frequently find the behavioural changes very difficult to cope with; support, contact with self-help groups and respite care may help.
- Plan care to minimize confrontation in behavioural challenges; do not argue with or reprimand the patient, but find a distracting activity instead.
- Maintain patient dignity by treating them as adults.
- Plan care to help patients with activities that can no longer be performed, but maximize self-care where possible.

Drugs that may help to maintain function in the earlier stages of Alzheimer's disease include donepezil hydrochloride, rivastigmine and galantamine. They inhibit acetylcholinesterase, the enzyme that breaks down the neurotransmitter acetylcholine (which is depleted in Alzheimer's disease), and in addition galantamine is a nicotinic receptor agonist. They may also increase the amount of acetylcholine in the brain. These drugs are not suitable for all patients with Alzheimer's disease and the National Institute for Clinical Excellence (NICE) recommends that they are normally used for patients with a Mini-Mental State Examination score above 12 points and that certain other conditions are met, e.g. that the diagnosis of Alzheimer's is made in a specialist clinic and the views of the carers are sought (NICE 2001).

MOTOR NEURON DISEASE

Motor neuron disease (MND) is a blanket term that covers several similar degenerative conditions (see Box 14.9) that affect both upper and lower motor neurons, but not sensory neurons. Many people with MND have symptoms from more than one variant. Note that it is often called motor neurone disease but for consistency the spelling neuron is used.

MND occurs most commonly in people over 40 years of age. The cause is unknown in 90% of cases, but in about 10% there is a familial link. Researchers have failed to show any corroborated evidence related to environmental factors. Men are more commonly affected than women in a ratio of 1.5:1. MND is usually fatal within 2–5 years but some people have survived more than 10 years. There are no tests that positively identify MND so a diagnosis is made by a neurologist according to the pattern of signs and symptoms. These vary according to the type and stage of the illness but include:

- weakness progressing to paralysis (the pattern depends on the nerves affected)
- fasciculation – rapid twitching without muscle contraction (seen as muscles lose the nerve supply)
- where MND affects the upper motor neuron, reflexes may persist and muscle wasting does not occur
- where the lower motor neuron is affected, there will be muscle atrophy and loss of reflexes. The neurons controlling continence in the spinal cord are usually spared
- normal sensation, including pain and discomfort due to position.

At present there is no curative treatment available, so patients are treated symptomatically.

▶ Nursing management

Nurses have an important role in supporting patients, families and other carers. Care points include the following:

- Plan care to allow maximum use of residual function.
- Emotional support for patients and carers is vital as this disease has a poor prognosis and the prospect of losing all

Box 14.9 Types of motor neuron disease

- Amyotrophic lateral sclerosis (ALS)
  — upper and lower motor neurons
  — usual type
- Progressive bulbar palsy (PBP)
  — lower motor neurons from the cranial nerves of the medulla (the older name for the medulla was the bulb)
  — PBP affects swallowing and speech muscles
- Primary lateral sclerosis (PLS)
  — upper motor neurons
  — occurs less frequently
- Progressive muscular atrophy (PMA)
  — lower motor neurons
  — occurs less frequently

voluntary activity can make patients extremely fearful. Referral to voluntary MND groups and for expert psychological care is important.

- Provide total care, with emphasis on prevention of pressure ulcers (as patients cannot move), careful positioning to enable eye contact with other people, and prevention of contractures and other problems of immobility such as poor chest expansion. Physiotherapy helps to prevent problems of immobility.
- Swallowing may become a problem, including the swallowing of saliva. Drugs such as tricyclic antidepressants (because of their antimuscarinic action), propantheline and atropine may be used to reduce salivation. Many patients with MND fear drowning in their own saliva. Specialized swallowing techniques taught by the SLT may help in the earlier stages when there is still residual function. Percutaneous endoscopic gastrostomy (PEG) may be used to ensure adequate nutrition (see Ch. 11).
- A stool softener and stimulant laxative may be given to promote a bowel action, but suppositories or a microenema are often necessary for full evacuation due to muscle weakness; peristalsis is unaffected as involuntary muscles are supplied from the ANS so are not affected by MND.
- Urinary incontinence is rare but patients are dependent on carers for all help as the weakness or paralysis prevents normal voiding. Toileting on request is most effective although patients may not be able to speak or summon help so carers needs to be vigilant. In later stages, sheath drainage for men and pads for women may be needed.
- Communication is often affected by either poor chest movement or paralysis of the speech muscles. Word charts, alphabet boards and computer devices such as a speech synthesizer may be used. Language function is unaffected; it is important to remember that patients can still understand speech. If patients have a hearing impairment, carers will need to care for and maintain the hearing aid to avoid patient isolation (see Ch. 16).
- Pain associated with position and spasticity is a common feature and needs to be managed comprehensively.
- Difficulty with breathing (dyspnoea) is common, especially in the later stages, and is often the most feared problem. Depending on assessment, patients should be positioned to maximize air intake, usually sitting up or sitting forward with arms raised and supported on a bed table (orthopnoeic position). Physiotherapy and drug treatment are used to prevent respiratory complications. In the late stages of the disease, patients may need respiratory support with mechanical ventilation.
- Referral should be made to palliative care services and specialist nurses, as appropriate (see Ch. 34).

SPINAL CORD DISORDERS

Patients with spinal cord disorders often require care in a specialist setting such as a spinal injuries unit. Spinal cord compression is mentioned briefly here, but readers are directed to Chapter 33 for a fuller account. Likewise prolapsed intervertebral disc causing pressure on spinal nerve roots is discussed in

Chapter 27. An outline of spinal trauma is provided in this chapter but readers needing more information are advised to consult a specialist text.

SPINAL CORD COMPRESSION

Spinal cord compression (SCC) is extremely serious and can occur over time but may present acutely when metastatic cancer involves the vertebrae and following spinal trauma. Early detection is vital in order to start treatment before irreversible nerve damage occurs. SCC has a number of causes, including:

- vertebral causes (most common), such as metastatic cancers (see Ch. 33), trauma (see below) and prolapsed intervertebral disc (see Ch. 27)
- spinal cord and meningeal causes, e.g. tumour (see below) or infection.

SPINAL TUMOURS

Spinal tumours may also cause neurological signs. There is pain that may be local or radiate along the path of the affected nerves. Spinal tumours are often malignant and can be secondary or primary. They affect all age groups. The main treatments available are surgery, radiotherapy and sometimes chemotherapy (see Ch. 33). The effects of the disease and the long-term results of treatment depend on the area involved. Patients will require rehabilitation, and in the case of inoperable tumours, palliative care and support for patients and their families is vital (see Ch. 34).

▶ Nursing management: spinal surgery

Spinal surgery is undertaken for a variety of conditions apart from tumours, including spinal injuries (see below) and prolapsed intervertebral disc. The exact nature of the surgery, the patient's response and the surgeon's preferences will influence care, but patients will have care that includes:

- pain relief
- observation of vital signs and wound leakage as with any surgery (see Ch. 29)
- checking for bladder problems (such as retention), bowel dysfunction or paralytic ileus where abdominal or sacral nerves are involved. Following cervical or high thoracic spine surgery, patients should be observed for respiratory distress, voice changes due to laryngeal nerve damage and dysphagia, and sensation and movement in the arms
- following surgery below the thoracic level the nurse should check for circulatory and nerve problems in the extremities by making frequent checks of limb colour, warmth, foot pulses and movement
- observation for leakage of CSF and signs of infection, such as headache, wound changes and pyrexia
- maintaining correct spinal alignment, avoiding movements that may twist or strain the spine. Mobilization will depend on type of surgery, correct use of braces or other orthotic devices.

SPINAL TRAUMA

Spinal injury occurs when the spinal cord is damaged or severed. As the main motor and sensory pathways to and from the body use the spinal cord as a communication trunk, any damage will interfere with functions below the level of the damage.

Aetiology

Spinal injuries occur most commonly as a result of accidents, e.g. road traffic accidents and sporting injuries (such as those incurred in a rugby scrum or diving in shallow water). Falling down stairs or off a ladder are also common causes, as landing on the head can flex the neck and damage the spinal cord.

Clinical presentation

A high spinal injury will result in the loss of limb and trunk movement and feeling (quadriplegia/tetraplegia if all four limbs affected). Respiration may also be affected, necessitating respiratory support. A low spinal injury may affect movement and feeling in the legs (paraplegia), loss of bowel and bladder control and, in men, erectile dysfunction (see Ch. 25). Following spinal injury patients are likely to develop spinal shock, which will occur hours or days after spinal injury. There is a period of flaccid paralysis, when muscle tone is lost and the limbs are floppy, and spinal reflexes are absent. When spinal shock subsides, reflexes show a vigorous response and high muscle tone which can lead to spasticity, deformity, loss of function and clonus (rhythmical jerking of the limbs, especially the lower legs).

Management of the spinal injury patient

Patients with spinal injuries are usually transferred to a specialist unit for treatment. They often require emergency surgery to decompress the spinal cord and stabilize bony injury. This is a very delicate procedure as moving and transferring patients with spinal injury can cause further damage to the cord, and currently damage cannot be reversed once it has occurred.

For this reason moving patients before the spine has been stabilized is a very skilled procedure involving several carers, maintaining the spine in supported alignment at all times. The movement is coordinated and careful so that further damage is not caused during the procedure. Once the spine is stable, patients may be mobilized. They may have a plaster jacket applied or wear a brace support that consists of a metal frame supporting the head, neck and torso. Traction is used sometimes if the break is very high in the cervical spine. Following surgery, patients may require many months to recover and undergo rehabilitation. The rehabilitation will cover all aspects of care, but the actual need is based on a holistic assessment involving a multidisciplinary team of nurses, doctors and therapists. For example, patients with low spinal damage may be able to use a wheelchair unaided and return to work, whereas those with a high spinal injury may be unable to breathe unaided and require respiratory support. This will take considerably more rehabilitation input to achieve some independence and autonomy for patients.

▶ Nursing management

The nursing care plan should deal effectively with all the issues described below as well as patient care problems identified by individual assessment. Nurses should ensure that risk of complications is minimized. This will, of course, involve collaborative working with members of the multidisciplinary team.

Common problems

The problems experienced by patients with spinal injuries are those associated with immobility, as described below.

Respiratory infection

This may occur as patients may not be able to expand the chest fully and ventilate effectively. Inability to cough may lead to poor clearance of secretions. Supine position, which is used in many instances, increases the danger of aspiration of food and drink into the respiratory tract. Careful management at mealtimes is necessary if patients are placed in a position that compromises the airway. They may require chest physiotherapy and even suction to keep the chest clear.

Gastrointestinal dysfunction

This can occur because normal mobility is required for effective bowel activity. Patients may need a nasogastric tube and intravenous fluids initially if paralytic ileus is present, which can happen in spinal shock. Faecal incontinence is common following a spinal injury and requires sensitive and effective management (see Ch. 12). The bowel may be atonic resulting in constipation. A bowel programme will be devised based on assessment and may involve regular mealtimes and use of stool softener laxatives complemented by microenemas, suppositories or digital stimulation. Digital stimulation is performed at regular times and involves inserting a finger just inside the anal canal and moving it in a circular motion for 30 seconds to a minute. This stimulation usually produces a reflex emptying of the bowel. In some cases, manual removal of faeces may be necessary. When this is necessary, always observe local or RCN guidelines. Manual removal can trigger dysreflexia (see p. 526) so a skilled carer using local anaesthetic gel as a lubricant must always do it.

Cardiovascular changes

These occur as orthostatic (postural) hypotension. The recumbent position may desensitize the baroreceptors and then the blood pressure will not adjust to compensate for position changes. A tilt table may be used to prevent orthostatic hypotension. This is a table that can be raised to a vertical position with the patient secured. It allows a change of position while patients are still in a 'supine' alignment. Deep vein thrombosis or pulmonary embolus may also occur due to loss of movement in the legs (see Ch. 19).

Musculoskeletal changes

Musculoskeletal changes such as loss of bone density may occur when the bones are not stimulated by weight-bearing. Muscle mass is lost through disuse. Heterotopic ossification occurs when soft tissue, such as muscle and ligament, turns to bone. This is accompanied by pain and swelling and may require surgical treatment. Ossification may occur in the shoulder of a spinal injury patient. Patients may be placed on the tilt table in physiotherapy to increase weight-bearing, which reduces bone loss and may help with muscle mass.

Metabolic changes

The basal metabolic rate increases following trauma such as spinal cord injury, so patients will require increased energy intake to maintain adequate nutrition. Additional protein is not effective in maintaining muscle mass and may even lead to increased urea in the blood. Loss of bone density can cause a rise in serum calcium. Hypoglycaemia can occur as there may be increased secretion of insulin as a result of immobility.

Urinary tract problems

Urinary tract problems include incomplete bladder emptying, infections and urinary tract stones. Continence will be affected in most instances of spinal injury and will require careful management, as severing the spinal cord results in an atonic bladder (see Ch. 12). This happens rapidly after injury and may persist. It may be necessary to use an indwelling catheter in the early stages. In the rehabilitation phase, patients may be suitable for intermittent self-catheterization. Various bladder retraining techniques may be used to re-establish continence. Bladder problems such as infection or distension are a major cause of autonomic dysreflexia (see p. 526).

Communication problems

Communication may be affected if patients cannot move to see other people, cannot write or use a keyboard and cannot speak (which may arise if ventilation is necessary in high cervical spine lesions). The use of mirrors may increase field of vision. Reading devices such as page turners are available. Computerized communication devices such as head pointers and spectacle frames with a small light can be used to give access to a keyboard. Speech is only affected in spinal injuries where loss of respiration occurs, as much of speech is mediated by the cranial nerves.

Sexual difficulties

Sexuality may be challenged with many problems such as body image, erectile dysfunction, performance issues and relationship problems. Counselling and early referral to expert care is necessary. The Spinal Injuries Association produces a selection of information books about spinal injury and sexual function.

Psychosocial challenges

These are substantial, with a huge need for good support and rehabilitation. There may be financial, occupational, relationship and housing issues as well as depression as a reaction to the catastrophic life change. Coping strategies may be many and varied and some may appear dysfunctional. Counsellors, clinical psychologists and social workers will be involved in the resolution of these problems. The family and informal carers need to be involved in care from the outset. If patients are to go home with family carers, they must be consulted and their advice taken so that an appropriate care plan is devised – a care plan that does not consider the needs of all concerned will fail.

Skin problems

Skin will require special attention as most spinal injury patients will be at high risk of developing pressure ulcers. Frequent changes of position are needed and patients can be taught to check pressure areas with a mirror and relieve pressure. Patients may be totally dependent on carers for skin hygiene and personal freshness.

Mobility

This is affected in almost all spinal injuries and patients will need rehabilitation to achieve maximum mobility. Management is required to prevent increasing spasticity of the affected limbs. Unresolved spasticity can lead to contracture of soft tissue around joints such as tendons and ligaments. Physiotherapy and drugs such as baclofen and tizanidine may provide some relief. Sometimes surgery is required to release contractures, but careful planning and care in consultation with the physiotherapy team should prevent this happening.

Sensorimotor losses

With sensory loss there is a danger of further damage from burns (e.g. scalding in the bath or from cigarettes) and pressure ulcers. Patients may be at greater risk of hypothermia as they will not be able to shiver to generate heat. The motor control of sweating, shivering, vasodilatation and constriction can be damaged in a high cervical cord injury and therefore temperature management, such as careful use of clothing, will be necessary.

Sleep disturbance

The patient may have sleep disturbance associated with concerns about the future and spasticity that can be worse at night. Psychological support should be offered and good spasticity management should help with the latter.

Autonomic dysreflexia

Autonomic dysreflexia is a particular problem in spinal injuries and is a serious complication in people with a high spinal lesion anywhere above the sixth thoracic vertebra. Dysreflexia is a syndrome due to uninhibited sympathetic reflexes following noxious stimuli. An understanding of the physiology of dysreflexia is useful to explain the sequence of events that occur during an attack. When a sympathetic sensory receptor is stimulated below the level of the lesion, e.g. a full/distended bladder or bowel, or even a somatic noxious stimulus, such as a pressure ulcer, afferent impulses travel up the spinal cord but are blocked by the lesion. The sympathetic ganglia at and below the level of the lesion respond to the blocked signals by initiating vasoconstriction and arteriolar spasm. The resulting rise in blood pressure is monitored by baroreceptors in the aortic arch, carotid sinus and cerebral vessels, and in an attempt to maintain homeostasis the heart rate falls and blood vessels dilate. Efferent signals dilate the surface vessels causing flushing and sweating where the signals get through, i.e. the part of the body above the lesion. Impulses to the body below the lesion are blocked and this leads to 'gooseflesh' and pallor as a result of the sympathetic stimulation. The blood pressure continues to rise and now the vessels above the level of the lesion dilate in an attempt to restore normal blood pressure. The continuing rise causes increasing pressure in dilated cerebral blood vessels and the patient is now in danger. When assessing patients, the following signs and symptoms may be present:

- hypertension – may be very high with systolic pressure > 200 mmHg
- sweating above the level of the lesion due to the sympathetic response
- bradycardia is most common, as the parasympathetic response is to lower the heart rate to reduce the rising pressure detected by the baroreceptors; however, tachycardia can also occur
- peripheral vasodilatation above the level of the lesion causes flushing, whereas there will be pallor and 'gooseflesh' below the level of the lesion; there is often a clear line of demarcation between the two zones
- patients report a strange feeling that is hard to define
- they will have a pounding headache with nasal congestion due to vasodilatation
- they may report shivery chills and an anxious feeling
- blurred vision
- nausea
- chest pain.

It is important that nurses and carers plan care so as to avoid situations that lead to noxious stimuli, such as bladder and bowel distension, bladder infection and blocked catheters. This means that effective bowel and bladder care is necessary for people with spinal injuries (see p. 325). The use of local anaesthetic lubricant before catheterization and rectal procedures helps to prevent noxious stimuli. In fact, most instances of dysreflexia are due to bladder distension or infection. Normal activities such as sexual activity and childbirth can also act as triggers. Tight clothing, including leg bag straps, may initiate a dysreflexic response.

Apparently minor things such as ingrowing toenails may provide the noxious stimulus, and podiatry may be required for prevention. Pathological conditions including burns and fractures, and dysmenorrhoea can also provide the trigger. Pressure ulcers should be rigorously avoided.

Education of patients and carers is an important part of management of dysreflexia. They should be taught how to recognize signs and symptoms. They must be able to intervene effectively so they need to know the essentials of managing dysreflexia. Many people who are susceptible carry a kit with them at all times consisting of medication, local anaesthetic gel, gloves, a spare catheter, suppositories and instructions and warnings for carers and bystanders.

All those providing care, as well as patients themselves, should be vigilant for signs of autonomic dysreflexia. Early detection and urgent medical attention are vitally important. An outline of care and treatment, should autonomic dysreflexia occur, is given in the Guidelines for Care Priorities box 14.5.

Unresolved dysreflexia may result in retinal haemorrhage, subarachnoid or intracerebral haemorrhage (stroke), seizures, coma and death.

PERIPHERAL NERVE DISORDERS

The function of peripheral nerves can be affected by damage to the cell body, the axon, the myelin sheath or its blood supply. A neuropathy is a pathological process that affects the peripheral nerves and may involve axonal degeneration or demyelination.

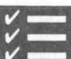

GUIDELINES FOR CARE PRIORITIES

14.5 Autonomic dysreflexia

Urgent medical intervention and treatment are required.

- Explain what is happening and what treatment may be required.
- Offer support and reassurance to all concerned.
- Identify and remove the cause of the noxious stimulus (checking the bladder first).
- Raise the bed head if the client is lying down to use gravity to help to decrease the blood pressure.
- Monitor blood pressure every 5 minutes.
- Loosen tight clothing including anti-embolic stockings and leg bag straps.
- Administer prescribed medication, which includes vasodilator antihypertensive drugs such as nifedipine.

- Treat bladder distension: a bladder washout can be used but no more than 30 mL of blood temperature saline, as an increase in bladder pressure may increase the noxious stimuli.
- If catheterization or recatheterization is necessary, local anaesthetic lubricant must be used and given time to work.
- Treat bowel distension and flatus, and if rectal procedures are needed the use of local anaesthetic gel is required. An enema may be needed but remember that an enema may be the trigger for the dysreflexic event in the first place.
- Review care plan with regard to avoiding noxious stimuli.
- Once the situation has stabilized, take the opportunity to check the patient's/carer's knowledge and identify learning needs.

POLYNEUROPATHY

Polyneuropathy is a diffuse (affecting many nerves), symmetrical disease which may be acute or chronic. It may be progressive, relapsing or transient and can affect motor, sensory or autonomic nerves. Polyneuropathies can be classified according to their cause, distribution or mode of onset and include hereditary neuropathies, inflammatory demyelinating neuropathies (including Guillain–Barré syndrome), neuropathies associated with diabetes, cancer, other systemic diseases, nutritional deficits, drugs and toxins.

GUILLAIN–BARRÉ SYNDROME

Guillain–Barré syndrome (GBS) is a demyelinating disorder.

Epidemiology and aetiology

Guillain–Barré syndrome is a rare neurological condition with an incidence of 1.6 per 100 000 per annum. It has a peak age of onset between 16 and 25 years and affects more males than females. The cause of GBS is unknown, but there are a number of theories as to its aetiology. It is generally agreed that GBS is an autoimmune disorder and it is thought to be due to an abnormal response to a virus. Allergy and hypersensitivity have also been suggested as causes, although there is little evidence to support this.

Pathophysiology

Guillain–Barré syndrome is an acute post-infective disease of the PNS that can cause total skeletal paralysis without affecting consciousness. Fifty per cent of cases follow an upper respiratory tract or gastrointestinal tract infection. In common with MS, the myelin sheath around the neurons is destroyed by the body's own immune system, but in GBS this occurs in PNS, whereas the demyelination of MS occurs in the CNS. This results in slowed conduction velocities along the axons and consequent loss of function. In more severe cases, axons can also be damaged,

but this is a condition that is usually self-limiting and most patients do recover, with axons having the ability to regenerate to some extent.

Clinical presentation

The onset of symptoms can take hours or days. Generally speaking, the more rapid the onset, the quicker the recovery, but most patients will have made a full neurological recovery within 6 months. Symptoms initially worsen and then plateau between 2 and 4 weeks after the onset. Symptoms are varied and unpredictable, with some patients being mildly affected and others being so severely affected that they require respiratory support and admission to intensive care. Symptoms include both sensory and motor dysfunction, with paraesthesia and sensory loss and muscle weakness in the limbs progressing in a glove-and-stocking pattern, upwards from the toes and fingers.

Respiratory difficulty and failure can develop if the peripheral nerves supplying the diaphragm and intercostal muscles become demyelinated. This leads to flaccid paralysis of the respiratory muscles and patients will present with an increased respiratory rate but shallow respirations with increasing dyspnoea and hypoxia.

Cranial nerves can also become involved, predominantly the facial (VII), glossopharyngeal (IX), vagus (X) and hypoglossal (XII) nerves (see Table 14.2, p. 279). Patients can therefore develop facial palsies, dysphagia, cardiac arrhythmias and postural hypotension due to the autonomic involvement.

Most patients recover completely, but some are left with residual disability of varying severity. A small percentage die and some progress to a remitting–relapsing chronic form of the disease (chronic idiopathic demyelinating polyneuropathy) but for most patients GBS is a one-off event.

Specific investigations

Diagnosis is based mainly on the clinical presentation and history given by the patient. Lumbar puncture is performed, which will show an elevated level of protein within the CSF. EMG will demonstrate delayed conduction velocities along the peripheral nerves. Arterial blood gases (see Ch. 9) are measured and respiratory investigations carried out, e.g. vital capacity will be reduced if the respiratory muscles are affected (see Ch. 20).

Medical management

Intravenous immunoglobulin shortens the illness if given soon after onset. Plasma exchange has been tried, but again is not always helpful. Other management is aimed at detecting and treating respiratory failure should it occur and symptomatic relief. Corticosteroids are not effective.

▶ Nursing management

As with most other neurological disorders, patient outcomes are improved by the involvement of a multidisciplinary team, especially the physiotherapist and OT.

Respiratory care

One of the greatest risks with GBS is respiratory failure. If the respiratory muscles become affected, the patient's vital capacity will drop. If this falls below 1.5 litres, medical staff may consider intubation and ventilation, so careful monitoring via spirometry is essential. Oxygen saturation and respiratory rate and depth should also be observed. Patients requiring respiratory support may require ventilation for up to 6 months, and because consciousness is not affected, they can become extremely bored or depressed. When discharged from the intensive care/high-dependency area to a ward, patients and relatives may experience anxiety, as nursing will no longer be on a one-to-one basis, so explanation and reassurance that a nurse can be summoned is required.

Cardiac care

Patients are also at risk of hypertension and postural hypotension, tachycardia or bradycardia and cardiovascular collapse due to autonomic nerve involvement. It is therefore essential that the heart rhythm is monitored, and blood pressure and pulse recorded. Any cardiac arrhythmias should be reported immediately.

Prevention of complications

Patients are at risk of complications caused by immobility, but especially chest infection and DVT (due to the flaccid paralysis of muscles causing deep veins to lack proper support). Anti-embolic stockings should be worn at all times and it is recommended that these be worn until patients are mobile for at least 50% of the time. Patients may also be given subcutaneous heparin or another anticoagulant to reduce the risk of DVT.

Nurses must be alert to the risk of pressure ulcer development and ensure that this is quantified and appropriate preventative measures put in place. Patients may need help with personal care and will soon become fatigued by physical activity. Nurses should plan periods of rest between nursing activity and therapy.

Constipation due to immobility and involvement of nerves supplying the bowel is a particular problem and causes great distress to patients. An adequate fibre and fluid intake is recommended to reduce the risk of constipation and laxatives may be used if this becomes a problem. Retention of urine may occur due to peripheral demyelination affecting the nerve supply to the detrusor muscle, preventing it from contracting. Catheterization may be necessary. Nurses should monitor both bowel action and urinary output.

Foot drop may develop and patients may require an orthotic splint to support the limb. A bed cradle should also be used to keep the weight of bedclothes off the lower limbs and help in preventing this. Contractures may also develop later, so it is important that the physiotherapist and nurses ensure that passive exercises that put joints through a normal range of movement are undertaken. Care should be taken, however, as the muscles affected become flaccid and joints that are usually supported by them can hyperextend. This can be a particular problem for the knee joint when patients are on bed rest and can become particularly painful, so a pillow under the knees is often extremely helpful.

Nutritional management

Patients may experience swallowing difficulties and are at risk of aspiration due to cranial nerve involvement. Swallowing assessment should be undertaken and, if a patient is thought to be at risk, enteral feeding may be used. This would require the involvement of both a dietician and a SLT in the decision-making process.

Patients may experience difficulty eating and drinking due to facial muscle paralysis, making lip closure and chewing difficult. It is the responsibility of the nurse to ensure that patients take in sufficient nutrition. A high-protein diet is often recommended, especially during the rehabilitative phase as muscle mass is lost due to the flaccid paralysis and disuse. Muscle wasting can be one of the biggest barriers to successful rehabilitation.

Pain management

Patients with GBS can experience pain for a number of reasons. Hyperextended joints that have not been supported properly can be extremely painful and become inflamed. Anti-inflammatory drugs and co-proxamol are often used for pain relief in the acute stages. It is important not to administer analgesia that may cause respiratory depression as a side-effect as patients are already at risk of respiratory difficulty.

In the rehabilitative phase, paraesthesiae may occur. This can be a burning sensation or pins and needles, as the axons regenerate, and is persistent. This can be extremely distressing and is treatable with carbamazepine.

Psychological support

Being diagnosed with GBS can be extremely frightening for both patients and families, especially once the risks of respiratory depression and possibility of requiring intensive care are explained. This is a very rare condition and not one that many people will have come across before, so the nurse plays a vital role in explaining the condition and what is likely to happen. It is important to reassure patients that the vast majority of people usually recover fully within 6 months.

SUMMARY: MAIN POINTS

- The structure and function of the nervous system determine the care requirements for patients when there is a pathological change. For instance, the motor cortex is in the frontal lobes; the blood supply to the frontal lobes can be disrupted; if the motor cortex is ischaemic, the patient will display paralysis, weakness and tone changes.

- Patient care is dependent on their needs and these vary widely, because the nervous system affects most physiological functions in some way. Assessment techniques will provide some additional information on which to base care.

- Neurological conditions can affect anyone at any age. Some are very common, such as headache, and some are very rare with only a few known cases worldwide.

- The same pathological processes that affect the rest of the body can affect the nervous system, i.e. congenital and developmental problems such as Huntington's disease; tumours such as glioma; infections such as meningitis and herpes zoster; trauma such as head or spinal injury; ischaemic damage such as stroke; and degenerative disorders such as multiple sclerosis or Parkinson's disease.

- The location of care for patients with neurological disease varies from community to specialist units.

- The nervous system has different healing capabilities from many other body systems and neurological damage cannot always be undone. This underlines the importance of rehabilitation and long-term care.

SELF-TEST: CRITICAL THINKING ACTIVITIES

1 Richard has been admitted to your ward following a stroke. He is paralysed on the right side of his body. Is his speech likely to be affected?

2 He has some problems swallowing and coughs and splutters when you give him water to drink. What action should you take and why?

3 A week after admission he is losing weight. The consultant asks Richard and his wife to consider a percutaneous endoscopic gastrostomy (PEG). After the doctor goes, Richard and his wife ask you to explain what this involves as they did not understand the doctor. What would your answer be?

4 Richard complains constantly of pain in his shoulder.
— How could you assess the effectiveness of your interventions?
— Which other professional discipline may be able to help with shoulder pain?

5 In his fourth week he has a further stroke and becomes unconscious.
— What care will he need?
— How will you support his wife?

 ## FURTHER READING

Davis S, O'Connor S. Rehabilitation nursing: foundations for practice. London: Baillière Tindall; 1999.

Hickey JV. The clinical practice of neurological and neurosurgical nursing, 5th edn. Philadelphia: Lippincott; 2003.

Hinchliff S, Montague S, Watson R. Physiology for nursing practice, 2nd edn. London: Baillière Tindall; 1999.

Lindsay KW, Bone I, Callander R. Neurology and neurosurgery illustrated, 3rd edn. Edinburgh: Churchill Livingstone; 1997.

 ## USEFUL WEBSITES

www.ace.org.uk – Age Concern (England)
www.alzheimers.org.uk – Alzheimer's Society
www.cancerbacup.org.uk – British Association for Cancer United Patients (BACUP)
www.epilepsy.org.uk – Epilepsy Action (British Epilepsy Association)
www.carersonline.org.uk – Carers UK
www.dlf.org.uk – Disabled Living Foundation

www.headway.org.uk – Headway – brain injury association
www.gbs.org.uk – Guillain–Barré Syndrome Society
www.kingsfund.org.uk – The King's Fund
www.meningitis.org.uk – Meningitis Research Foundation
www.migraine.org.uk – Migraine Association
www.mssociety.org.uk – Multiple Sclerosis Society
www.parkinsons.org.uk – Parkinson's Disease
www.stroke.org.uk – Stroke Association

REFERENCES

Barton J, Levene J, Kladakis B, Butterworth C. Stroke: a group learning approach. Nurs Times 2002; 98(7): 34–35.

Beyer PL, Palarino MY, Michalek D, Busenbark K, Koller WC. Weight change and body composition in patients with Parkinson's disease. J Am Diet Assoc 1995; 95: 979–983.

Bonita R. Epidemiology of stroke. Lancet 1992; 339: 342–344.

Branas P, Jordan R, Fry-Smith A, Burls A, Hyde C. Treatments for multiple sclerosis: a rapid and systematic review. Health Technol Assess 2000; 4(27).

Cancer Research UK. Brain cancer. Online. Available: http://www.cancerreasearchuk.org. 2002.

Carter JH, Nutt JG, Woodward WR, Hatcher LF, Trotman TL. Amount and distribution of dietary protein affects clinical response to levodopa in Parkinson's disease. Neurology 1989; 39: 552–556.

Chudley S. The effect of nursing activities on intracranial pressure. Br J Nurs 1994; 3(9): 454–459.

Currie R. Spasticity; a common symptom of multiple sclerosis. Nurs Stand 2001; 15(33): 47–52.

Davies E, Hopkins A. Good practice in the management of adults with malignant cerebral glioma: clinical guidelines. Br J Neurosurg 1997; 11(4): 318–330.

Dean G, Elian M. Age at immigration to England of Asian and Caribbean immigrants and the risk of developing multiple sclerosis. J Neurol Neurosurg Psychiatry 1997; 63: 565–568.

De Keyser J. Non-motor manifestations of Parkinson's disease. Focus Parkinson's Dis 1993; 5(3): 58–63.

DeLisa J (ed). Rehabilitation medicine: principles and practice. Philadelphia: JB Lippincott; 1988.

Department of Health. National service framework for older people. Online. Available: http://www.doh.gov.uk/nsf/olderpeople.htm. 2001.

Dinnes J, Cave C, Huang S, Major K, Milne R. The effectiveness and cost-effectiveness of temozolomide for the treatment of recurrent malignant glioma: a rapid and systematic review. Health Technol Assess 2001; 5(13).

Flaten TP. Time trends in the epidemiology of Parkinson's Disease. Focus Parkinson's Dis 1993; 5(3): 52–57.

Fletcher S. Innovative treatment or ethical headache? Fetal tissue transplantation in Parkinson's disease. Prof Nurse 1992; 7(9): 592–595.

Folstein MF, Folstein SE, McHugh PR. Mini mental state: a practical method for grading the cognitive state of patients for the clinician. J Psychiatr Res 1975; 12(3): 189–198.

Foreman MD. Acute confusional states in the elderly: an algorithm. Dimens Crit Care Nurs 1984; 3(4): 209–211.

Freeman JA, Thompson AJ. Building an evidence-base for multiple sclerosis management: support for physiotherapy. J Neurol Neurosurg Psychiatr 2001; 70(2): 147–148.

Goodkin DE. Interferon beta therapy for multiple sclerosis. Lancet 1998; 352: 1486–1487.

Hickey JV. The clinical practice of neurological and neurosurgical nursing, 4th edn. Philadelphia: Lippincott; 1997.

International League Against Epilepsy Commission on Classification and Terminology. Proposal for revised clinical and electroencephalographic classification of epileptic seizures. Epilepsia 1981; 22: 489–501.

Kempster PA, Wahlqvist ML. Dietary factors in the management of Parkinson's disease. Nutr Rev 1994; 52: 51–58.

Kraft GH. Rehabilitation still the only way to improve function in multiple sclerosis. Lancet 1999; 354: 2016.

Lannon MC, Thomas CA, Bratton M, Jost MG, Lockhart-Pretti P. Comprehensive care of the patient with Parkinson's disease. J Neurosci Nurs 1986; 18(3): 121–131.

Levin V A. Neuro-oncology: an overview. Arch Neurol 1999; 56: 401–404.

Lindsay KW, Bone I, Callander R. Neurology and neurosurgery illustrated, 3rd edn. Edinburgh: Churchill Livingstone; 1997.

Meningitis Research Foundation. About meningitis and septicaemia. Online. Available: http://www.meningitis.org.uk. 2002.

MS Society. Facts on multiple sclerosis available from: http://www.mssociety.org.uk/what_is_ms/index.html. 2001.

National Institute for Clinical Excellence (NICE). Alzheimer's disease – donepezil, rivastigmine and galantamine (No 19). Online. Available: http://www.nice.org.uk. 2001.

North B, Reilly P. Raised intracranial pressure. Oxford: Heinemann Medical; 1990.

Parkin D, Jacoby A, McNamee P, Miller P, Thomas S, Bates D. Treatment of multiple sclerosis with interferon-β: an appraisal of cost-effectiveness and quality of life. J Neurol Neurosurg Psychiatry 2000; 68: 144–149.

Pentland B. The effects of reduced expression in Parkinson's disease on impression formation by health professionals. Clin Rehab 1987; 1: 307–313.

Polman CH. Treatment recommendations for interferon-β in multiple sclerosis. J Neurol Neurosurg Psychiatry 1999; 67: 561–566.

Teasdale G, Jennett B. Assessment of coma and impaired consciousness: a practical scale. Lancet 1974; ii: 81–84.

Teasdale G, Knill-Jones R, van der Sande J. Observer variability in assessing impaired consciousness, coma. J Neurol Neurosurg Psychiatry 1978; 41: 603–610.

Trauma.org. Traumatic brain injury. Online. Available: www.trauma.org/neuro/index.html. 2000.

Williams AC. Patient care in neurology. Oxford: Oxford University Press; 1999.

Woodward S. Impact of neurological problems on urinary continence. Br J Nurs 1996; 5(15): 906–913.

Woodward S. Neurological observations – 1. Glasgow coma scale. Nurs Times 1997a; 93(45): suppl 1–2.

Woodward S. Neurological observations – 2. Pupil response. Nurs Times 1997b; 93(46): suppl 1–2.

Woodward S. Neurological observations – 3. Limb responses. Nurs Times 1997c; 93(47): suppl 1–2.

World Health Organization MONICA Project Investigators. World Health Organization MONICA project: monitoring trends and determinants in cardiovascular disease: a major international collaboration. J Clin Epidemiol 1988; 41: 105–114.

15 Nursing patients with problems of the eye and vision

Mary Shaw

'I was on placement in outpatients and I thought it would be really boring but in fact it's been really interesting. A patient with glaucoma came in today and she was telling me that she had no idea that she had it until she went for her usual eye test. I haven't had my eyes tested for years – maybe I should!'

(Student nurse)

THIS CHAPTER WILL HELP YOU

- Understand eye structures and explain their function
- Make an assessment of the ophthalmic patient
- Describe ophthalmic investigations and tests
- Appreciate the need for health education and health promotion in order to prevent ocular trauma, detect problems early and minimize the complications of eye diseases
- Outline the needs of the adult with visual impairment and blindness
- Describe the care needs and nursing interventions required by patients with a variety of ophthalmic disorders
- Describe the care needs and nursing interventions required by patients undergoing ophthalmic surgery
- Describe the emergency care needed by patients who have sustained trauma to their eyes.

KEYWORDS

Astigmatism	Miotic (myotic)
Cataract	Occulentum (Oc)
Cycloplegic	Ocular
Emmetropia	Ophthalmology
Glaucoma	Refraction
Guttae (G)	Retinopathy
Hypermetropia	Vision
Hyphaema	Vision testing
Hypopyon	Visual acuity
Mydriatic	Visual impairment
Myopia	

INTRODUCTION

Caring for people with eye problems is not every nurse's favourite duty. Some nurses will make an active choice to work in the field of ophthalmology but others will avoid it because they 'don't like eyes or anything to do with them'.

However, it is reasonable to suppose that at any one time, the majority of people with problems of the eye or their vision are within the general community, and not in specialist ophthalmic units. For example, you may be caring for a patient with diabetes mellitus on a renal unit; this patient is likely to have or develop an ocular complication of that condition (see Chs 17 and 24). Working in a care setting with older people (see Ch. 32) you will inevitably have cared for someone with an age-related cataract. Similarly, in the accident and emergency department (see Ch. 30) you could well care for patients who have sustained trauma that is the direct result of their poor vision, e.g. the lady who falls down the stairs because she did not have her spectacles on, and many patients with foreign bodies or eye trauma.

There are as many as 1 million people in the UK who are registered blind or partially sighted (Low Vision Services Consensus Group (LVCG) 1999). It is also known that many people eligible to register blind or partially sighted have not done so (Baker & Winyard 1998).

The World Health Organization (WHO) (1997) estimate that globally there are approximately 38 million people who are blind and some 110 million others who have low vision. In the UK it is thought that there are at least 1.7 million people who have a serious sight problem (Bruce & Hadi 2000).

The trend towards day-case surgery, with many ophthalmic units aiming at 90% day surgery for cataracts, has resulted in a radical rethinking of how ophthalmic patients should be cared for. In addition, because of improvements in surgical technique and anaesthesia, and the use of preoperative assessment clinics, there has been a reduction in the length of time a patient has to stay in hospital (see Ch. 29).

Having seen the benefits of pre-assessment clinics in reducing cancellations on the day, many hospitals plan for the majority of patients requiring routine in-patient operations to be admitted on the day of surgery, and they are likely to be discharged home the next day. There is evidence that patients attending for day surgery make fewer demands on community services than those who are in-patients for surgery (Buckingham et al 1997). There is possibly some need to re-evaluate this in light of the increase in numbers attending for day surgery in recent years.

It is highly probable that you will be caring for patients with an ophthalmic condition that is concurrent with another illness. Hamer & Collinson (1999) recognize that co-morbidity can be a reason for modifying standard care plans to meet the needs of individual patients. For example, patients undergoing heart surgery may also be on long-term treatment for primary open-angle glaucoma (POAG). Without their topical eye medication, such patients are likely to lose their vision.

Population trends show a marked increase in the number of people living into old age (see Ch. 32). It is known that problems associated with vision increase with age (McBride 2000, 2001), e.g. cataract, macular degeneration, glaucoma and diabetic retinopathy (Vaughan et al 1998). Because of this, there is a subsequent demand on ocular services both in hospital and in community settings. Indeed, the UK government is focusing on the modernization of cataract services that will result in 250 000 cataract operations being performed in England in the year 2003 (NHS Executive 2000). It should be noted that this figure does not include the private sector.

In response to the increasing demands on ophthalmic services, many specialist ophthalmic nursing roles have emerged, such as cataract nurse practitioners who undertake most of the patient's care with the exception of the surgery itself but including postoperative examination and discharge. In theatre, some nurses have expanded their role to include the administration of local anaesthetic or acting as first assistant. Some outpatient services and investigations are being run or supported by specialist ophthalmic nurses, including glaucoma, oculoplastic, vitreo-retinal and dry eye clinics. For some time now, nurses have been seeing patients in nurse-led emergency eye centres. Such expanded roles have improved the quality of service offered to patients.

Early in this chapter, the problems encountered by those with impaired vision and the nursing strategies that can improve quality of life are discussed, as is the management of ophthalmic medications. These important issues are covered before the common conditions affecting the eye and sight. The nursing management of patients having day-case cataract surgery is discussed very fully, and many of the principles of care described are applicable to patients having surgery for other eye conditions.

ANATOMY AND PHYSIOLOGY – AN OVERVIEW

The eyeball is the organ of sight and it is situated in the bony orbit and protected by the lids and the eyelashes. The lacrimal system is responsible for the production and drainage of tears and extraocular muscles act to move the eyeball.

EYEBALL

The human eyeball is spherical in shape, with an anterior bulge (see Fig. 15.1).

Layers of the eyeball

There are three distinct layers that contain the intraocular contents: the outer, inner and middle layers.

Outer layer

The outer fibrous layer comprises two distinct structures: the cornea and the sclera (see Fig. 15.1). The cornea is the transparent anterior one-sixth of the eyeball. There are five distinct layers, but not all regenerate when damaged. It is avascular (i.e. it does not have its own blood supply as the presence of blood vessels would interfere with vision), obtaining some of its nourishment from the blood vessels at the corneosclerotic junction or limbus (the point at which the cornea and the sclera meet – seen as an outer dark circle of the iris, though it does become whiter with age), aqueous humour in the anterior chamber and the tear film. The cornea has an excellent sensory nerve supply (just think how it irritates when you get a speck of dust or eyelash in your eye and how your eye waters). The cornea is the main refractive surface of the eye. Refraction is the bending of light rays so that images fall on the part of the retina known as the fovea centralis.

The sclera (the white of the eye) is the tough fibrous outer layer, which is continuous with the cornea anteriorly and the optic nerve posteriorly. It is composed of white fibrous tissue. Its functions include protection of the eyeball contents, prevention of light rays scattering and attachment for the extraocular muscles. Blood vessels and nerves enter and leave through it.

Middle layer

The middle layer is known as the uveal tract and has three distinct parts: the iris, the ciliary body and the choroid (see Fig. 15.1). The iris is the coloured part of the eye, visible through

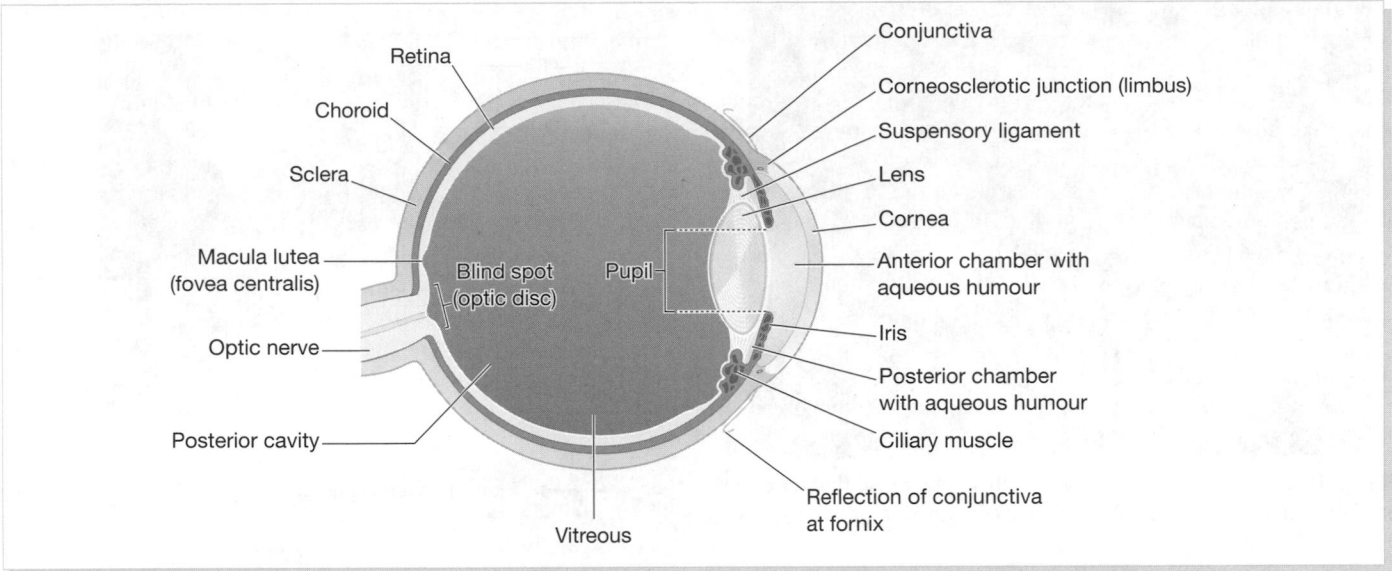

Figure 15.1 Section through the eyeball.

the cornea. It contains circular and radial muscle fibres that control the amount of light entering the eye. The pupil is the space in the centre of the iris. The iris determines pupil size according to light intensity and emotional state. The iris muscle fibres are controlled reflexly by autonomic fibres of the oculomotor or third (III) cranial nerves (see Ch. 14).

Contraction of the pupil (miosis) occurs in bright light and also during accommodation of the lens, e.g. when reading. Dilation of the pupil (mydriasis) happens in dim light but also during arousal, including sensations such as fear and excitement (see Ch. 6). The pupil is normally round, and both pupils work together in synchronization. This means that if you shine a pen-torch onto one eye, that pupil and the fellow pupil will normally constrict briskly at the same time (see Ch. 14).

The ciliary body contains muscle fibres that help to control the shape of the lens in accommodation. Specialized cells of the ciliary body known as the ciliary processes produce aqueous humour (see below). The choroid lies between the sclera and the retina. It is mainly comprised of blood vessels and contains pigment cells. The function of the choroid is to provide a blood supply to the retinal pigment epithelium and the peripheral sensory retina.

Inner layer

The inner layer of the eye is the retina (see Fig. 15.1), which comprises the neural retina containing the photosensitive cells (rods and cones) and other nerve cells, and the pigmented epithelium. The rods and cones are responsible for discriminating between light and dark. The nerve impulses generated by the retinal cells pass along the optic pathways to the visual cortex of the brain where they are interpreted as images. The fibres of the optic nerve leave the retina at a point known as the optic disc or blind spot (which has no light-sensitive receptors). At the side of the optic disc is the macula lutea (the yellow spot); this has a small depression, the fovea centralis.

Like the film of a camera, the retina is smooth and detects images projected onto it by the lens. Images are normally focused onto the macula lutea. The cones are numerous at the macula lutea and so are responsible for fine, central vision. The cones contain visual pigments that allow us to see colour. The rods contain the pigment rhodopsin and are concerned with peripheral vision, vision in dim light and the discrimination of shapes and forms.

The retina obtains its nourishment from the choroid and the central retinal artery. The retinal artery is an end artery, and if it becomes occluded or damaged the retinal cells will be deprived of oxygenated blood, as there are no alternative blood vessels. The retina is nourished from a system of underlying retinal blood vessels. Between the blood vessels and the retina is Bruch's membrane. Normally this membrane allows free flow of nutrients to the sensory retina. In common with the brain (blood–brain barrier), the neural retina is protected by a blood–retina barrier.

The view through the pupil of the structures at the back of the eye using an ophthalmoscope is termed the fundus (see Fig. 15.2, p. 334). This view includes the retina with the optic disc, macula lutea, fovea centralis and the retinal blood vessels. The optic disc can bulge when intracranial pressure is raised (see Ch. 14), a condition called papilloedema.

Structures and cavities inside the eye

Vitreous, a gel-like substance, occupies the large posterior cavity/space behind the lens (see Fig. 15.1). It is formed during embryonic development and it does not have the capacity to regenerate. Vitreous is replaced by aqueous humour when it is lost due to trauma or surgical intervention. It is avascular. The vitreous helps to transmit light to the retina, playing a part in refraction.

The iris divides the anterior cavity of the eye into the anterior and posterior chambers; both are filled with aqueous humour. The anterior chamber is the space behind the cornea and in front of the iris. The posterior chamber is the area behind the iris and in front of the lens.

Aqueous humour is produced constantly and flows from the posterior chamber, through the pupil into the anterior chamber

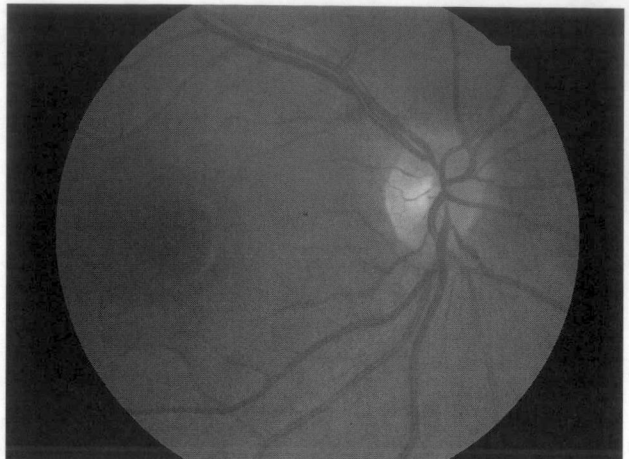

Figure 15.2 Normal fundus showing normal optic disc (lighter circle on right-hand side of picture). (Reproduced with kind permission from Kanski 1999.)

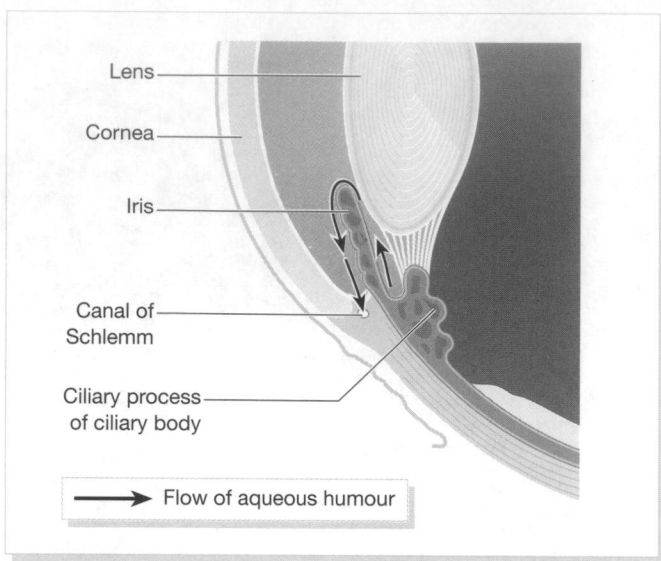

Figure 15.3 Production and drainage of aqueous humour.

(see Fig. 15.3). It drains through the trabecular meshwork, into the canal of Schlemm (a venous sinus encircling the eye at the junction of the cornea and sclera) and on into the venous circulation. The correct volume is maintained by production being equal to the amount draining into the venous system. It provides nourishment to the lens and cornea, removes waste and helps to maintain intraocular pressure (IOP) in the range 10–21 mmHg.

The crystalline lens is located behind the iris and pupil and in front of the vitreous body. The lens is transparent and bi-convex, having a greater posterior curve. The lens is contained within a capsule and its position is maintained by the suspensory ligaments (zonules) (see Fig. 15.1).

The lens changes shape in order to focus near and distant objects on the retina. Accommodation is the term used to describe the focus of the eye from distant to near objects. The lens obtains its nourishment from the aqueous humour.

REFRACTION, ACCOMMODATION AND FOCUSING

Focusing concerns the bringing together of light rays to create an image on the retina. It is the brain that helps us to make sense of these images. We also need to have a memory store to aid understanding of what we see.

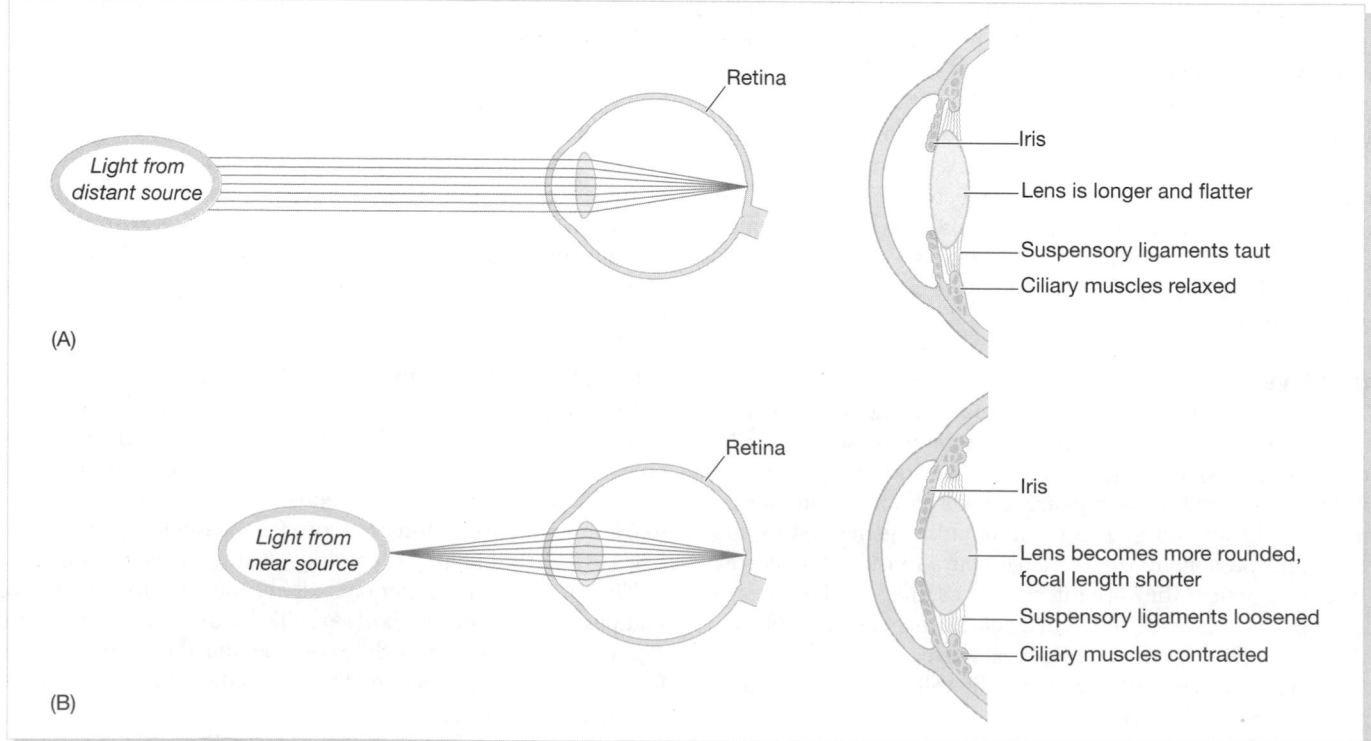

Figure 15.4 Accommodation: (A) for distant objects; (B) for near objects.

Accommodation is the change of refractive (dioptic) power of the eye in response to involuntary stimuli brought about by converging the eyes to focus on a near object. This causes the crystalline lens to change its shape to become thicker and increases its power. Normal vision (emmetropia) means that images are focused sharply on the retina when accommodation is relaxed (see Fig. 15.4). Additionally, when we focus on a near object, the pupils constrict, limiting the amount of light entering the eye.

Refractive errors

When the image falls behind the retina, this is known as hypermetropia (long-sightedness); this is usually caused by the eyeball being short in length. When the image falls short of the retina, this is known as myopia (short-sightedness); the eyeball in such cases is usually long. Astigmatism, a further refractive problem, is caused by defects in the curvature of the cornea. Myopia and hypermetropia are correctable by spectacles, contact lenses or refractive surgery (see Fig. 15.5).

RETINAL PHYSIOLOGY AND THE VISUAL PATHWAY

Sufficient amounts of visual pigments are required before the rods and cones can convert light energy to electrical (nerve) impulses. The four visual pigments are formed from combinations of retinene (retinal), a light-sensitive chemical, and a protein (opsin). Retinene is derived from vitamin A (retinol), lack of which can impair night vision and, in severe cases, cause blindness.

Rods contain the pigment rhodopsin which responds to dull light by changing shape and bleaching; this produces the receptor potential and triggers a nerve impulse, which is transmitted to the optic nerve. Cones have three visual pigments that contain retinene but have different proteins. These three cone types respond to bright light of the green, blue or red wavelengths. Impulses from the cones are also transmitted to the optic nerve. (Normal colour vision is inherited as a dominant gene on the X chromosome.)

The images brought into focus on the retina are translated into electrical impulses that are transmitted via the visual pathway to the visual cortex of the cerebrum where they are interpreted. In order to ensure that the images are seen as one, providing binocular vision, the nerve pathways follow a particular route. Those nerve fibres on the temporal (lateral) side of the retina of each eye continue on the same side, whilst the fibres on the nasal (medial) side cross over at the optic chiasma (see Fig. 15.6). Damage, through disease or trauma, to any part of the visual pathway will result in loss of part or all of the vision, e.g. hemianopia (loss of half the visual field) following a stroke (see Ch. 14).

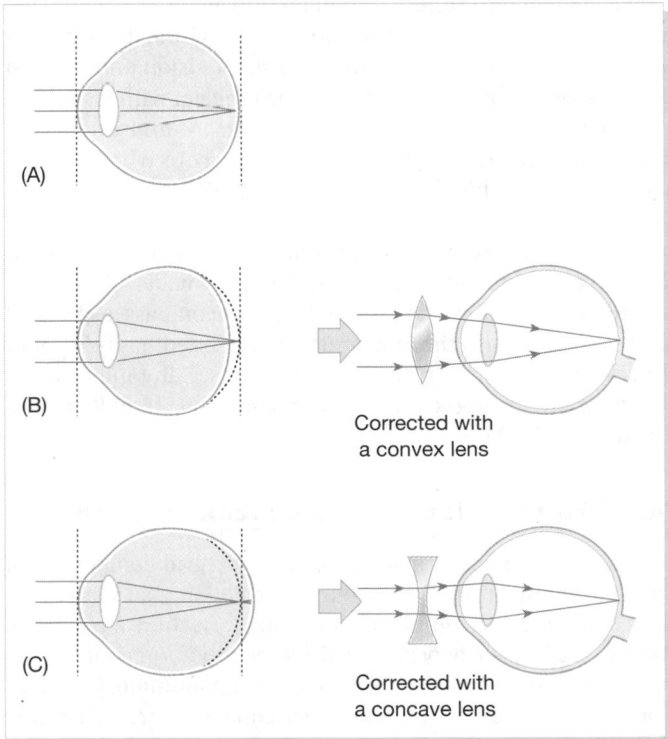

Figure 15.5 (A) Emmetropia; (B) hypermetropia with correction; (C) myopia with correction.

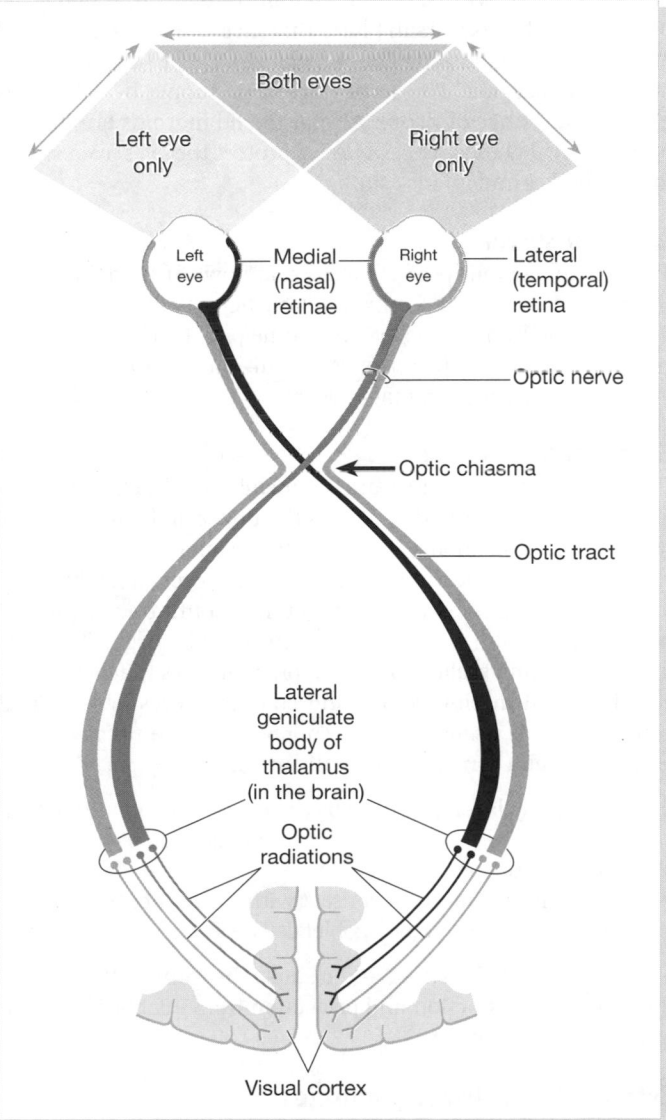

Figure 15.6 Visual pathways and visual fields.

Light and dark adaptation

The eyes adapt to different light intensity in different ways. Dark adaptation is the adjustment the eye makes to darkness. The pupil dilates to ensure that the maximum amount of light can enter the eye and it is the rods of the retina that are stimulated. Sensitivity to light increases as well. As we grow older it takes much longer to adapt to the dark.

Light adaptation relates to the adjustments made by the eye to bright light. The visual pigments bleach and the pupil constricts. Sensitivity to light diminishes.

ACCESSORY STRUCTURES

The orbit and the eyelids provide protection for the eyeball and the orbital contents. The orbital contents comprise the extraocular muscles, blood vessels and nerves, including the optic nerve, and fat.

Eyelids, lashes and eyebrows

The eyelids protect the eyeball from trauma and excess light. The lids are covered with skin and contain muscles that allows lid movement, fibrous (tarsal) plates that give shape and form, and also secretory glands (meibomian glands). Eyelashes are present at the lid margins. The lashes are kept supple by sebaceous glands (the glands of Zeiss). Also at the lid margins are the orifices of tarsal glands. The eyebrows protect the eyes from sweat, foreign bodies and intense sunlight.

Lacrimal system

The lacrimal glands produce tears that flow through ducts into the upper conjunctival fornix. Blinking helps to disperse the tear film over the front of the eye and so helps keep the cornea and conjunctiva moist. The tears drain into the back of the throat via the nasolacrimal drainage system.

Conjunctiva

The conjunctiva is the thin mucous membrane that lines the eyelids (palpebral conjunctiva), forms the upper and lower fornices (topical eye medication is instilled into the inferior fornix), and is reflected to cover the anterior surface of the eyeball (bulbar conjunctiva). The conjunctival epithelium is continuous with that of the cornea, and with the skin at the eyelid margin. The conjunctiva has an excellent blood supply that gives the back of the eyelids a reddish-pink colour and contains accessory lacrimal glands. There is a sensory nerve supply to the conjunctiva.

The tear film comprises three distinct layers:

- an outer oily layer produced by the meibomian glands, which serves to prevent evaporation and spillage of tears
- a middle aqueous layer
- an inner mucin layer (in contact with the corneal surface) produced by conjunctival goblet cells.

Tears not only lubricate and cleanse the front of the eyeball, but also aid in refraction and protection from infection (contain antibacterial enzymes).

Extraocular (extrinsic) muscles

Ocular movement is brought about by six extraocular muscles attached to the eyeball and the bony orbit. The muscles are innervated autonomically by cranial nerves (see Ch. 14) that give the degree of control of eyeball position and movement needed for focusing on distant and near objects. The eyes can also be moved voluntarily.

The extraocular muscles comprise four rectus muscles and two oblique muscles:

- superior rectus – moves eyeball upwards [oculomotor (III) cranial nerve]
- inferior rectus – moves eyeball downwards [oculomotor (III) cranial nerve]
- lateral rectus – moves eyeball outwards [abducens (VI) cranial nerve]
- medial rectus – moves eyeball inwards [oculomotor (III) cranial nerve]
- superior oblique – moves the eye out and downwards [trochlear (IV) cranial nerve]
- inferior oblique – moves the eye out and upwards [occulomotor (III) cranial nerve].

NURSING ASSESSMENT OF OPHTHALMIC PATIENTS

Patients presenting at a hospital A&E department with an ophthalmic condition or ocular trauma will be assessed differently from those attending for a preoperative assessment. By necessity the former will initially be assessed using a triage framework (see Ch. 30) and the latter will be assessed using a recognized model of nursing.

Some problems with vision may not initially appear to be related to the eye. For example, patients who visit their GP with headaches could be suffering from an undiagnosed eye problem such as acute glaucoma. On the other hand, visual disturbances such as diplopia (double vision), blurring of vision and sore red eyes may be obvious indicators of some problem with vision.

Details of any previous ocular disease, trauma or surgery must be accurately recorded, showing clearly to which eye the history relates. This includes whether patients wear contact lenses or spectacles.

The nursing assessment of patients with an ocular condition should be systematic and purposeful. The model of nursing will reflect local need but should also encompass aspects of need associated with the temporary or permanent loss of vision. Nurses need to consider the importance of seeking information about vision during all nursing assessments (see Reflective Practice box 15.1).

PAST MEDICAL HISTORY AND GENERAL HEALTH

Details of past medical history form an integral component of the assessment in order to obtain information that could give clues to the present complaint. For example, is there a history of diabetes mellitus or hypertension? Either condition could cause problems to the eye. A history of systemic inflammatory disease, alongside ocular signs and symptoms, could support a diagnosis of uveitis (see p. 362).

It is important to obtain relevant details of family history of a particular condition or disease. Patients with a close family

15.1 Seeking information about a patient's vision

How often, as part of patient assessment, do you actively seek information about patients' vision or any ocular disease they may have?

Student activities

1. Consider a patient you have admitted recently. During your nursing assessment, how much importance did you place on his or her visual function? What questions did you ask to help you understand the patient's ability to function normally in a visually orientated society? Could he or she see the written information that you provided?

   - Look at the instruction sheets, how big is the print size?
   - Could a patient with poor vision read it?
   - Consider the benefits of assessing ocular health as part of the care planning process
   - Could the patient 'see' the visual cues to good communication you were using, such as a smile or nod of the head?
   - Did the patient wear spectacles or contact lenses? Did these assist the patient or was vision still poor?

2. Consider the ways in which poor vision could affect patients' interaction with health care professionals, their ability to follow recommended treatment plans and possibly their recovery from surgery or illness. You may wish to discuss some of the issues with your colleagues and consider how you might improve communication and outcomes for a person with impaired vision admitted with a non-ophthalmic condition.

15.1 Taking a history of the present complaint

Nurses should obtain information about the following in order to obtain a full history of the present complaint:

- When did the patient become aware of the problem?
- How long has it lasted and is the condition intermittent or constant?
- Is there a history of illness, allergy or trauma?
- What medication is currently being taken?

There is a need to obtain some specific detail in relation to the condition, e.g. about the presence of:

- Vision changes – loss of acuity, blurring, flashes or halos, night blindness or glare from light sources
- Presence of 'floaters'
- Diplopia
- Abnormal eye movement, including paralysis of movement
- Swelling of the eye, conjunctiva or eyelids
- Redness of the eyelids or conjunctiva
- Itching/burning sensation
- Soreness or pain and the location, as it could be of the eye itself or around the eye
- Photophobia
- Tearing (watering)
- Discharge from the eye and the nature of the discharge, e.g. green or yellow pus, mucus
- Pupil changes, shape, size and reaction. Are the pupils the same size and do they react together or not?
- Headache
- Nausea and vomiting.

Details should be recorded appropriately in the nursing record. It is appropriate to obtain specific detail of how the vision deficits impact on the ability to self-care. Sudden loss of vision is potentially more catastrophic than vision that has deteriorated 'silently' over a long period of time. Many people may have begun to adapt to vision loss so it is pertinent to ask about any vision aids used. These include spectacles, magnifying lens and illumination.

---

member (parents and siblings) with primary open-angle glaucoma (POAG) are at increased risk of developing the condition.

Information gathered about a patient's past ocular history (e.g. previous eye injury or surgery) will help guide the ophthalmic nurse towards making a diagnosis but will also support the plan of care drawn up with the patient. For example, in the case of a patient presenting at an A&E department following an accident at work with a corneal foreign body, a history of similar incidents will guide patient education. Similarly, if a patient attends hospital with a recurrent corneal ulcer, this should prompt an enquiry about whether the person is a contact lens wearer.

HISTORY OF PRESENT COMPLAINT

In assessing the present complaint, there is a need to get accurate information of both objective and subjective signs and symptoms (see Guidelines for Care Priorities box 15.1). Nurses will also undertake general observations such as weight, vital signs and urine test. The latter may still be useful in the diagnosis of diabetes mellitus.

EXAMINATION OF THE EYE

An ability to examine the eye thoroughly is a vital skill of the ophthalmic nurse. It provides information on which a diagnosis can be made and appropriate and timely action taken. Many actions involve the ophthalmic nurse working to patient group directions or protocols. These serve to expedite diagnosis and treatment.

Examination of the eye is an essential part of any patient assessment. There are several issues that need to be addressed when doing so, including:

- the age of the patient
- the mental state of the patient
- the degree of pain or discomfort – for example, it would be difficult to test visual acuity on someone in acute pain

15.2 Routine examination of the eye

First of all, look at the eyelids whilst they are closed.

- Do they look healthy?
- Is there any evidence of watering or spasm of the lids?
- Are the eyelids a normal colour and healthy looking? Is bruising present or are they red and inflamed?
- Is there any frank discharge or crusting and, if so, what colour? Note the position of the eyelids; determine whether they are closing properly. Are the lids turning into the eye or away from the eyeball? Are the lashes turning in and rubbing against the cornea or conjunctiva? Can you see any swelling or lump on the lid or lid margin that could indicate that a cyst (meibomian cyst) or sty (hordeolum) is present? The lid should be everted if a foreign body (FB) is suspected.

Ask the patient to open his or her eyes.

- Look at the conjunctiva. Does it appear normal or is there evidence of infection or inflammation? Does the patient complain of itching? Is it pink or injected (red and angry looking)? Is there any discharge present?
- Is the cornea clear or is it cloudy? Look at the iris – is it clear? Is part or all of the view obscured by blood (hyphaema) or pus (hypopyon)?

Pupil reaction

Examination of pupil reaction can give important diagnostic information, especially in relation to the integrity of the iris, retina and optic nerve. It is important to ascertain whether the patient is taking any medication that could affect normal pupillary function; examples include guttae (G) cyclopentolate hydrochloride, a mydriatic and cycloplegic (a drug that dilates the pupil and also paralyses the ciliary muscle), or G. pilocarpine, a miotic (a drug that constricts the pupil).

The pupils should be evaluated as to:

- colour (normally black), shape, size
- whether they are equal in size
- reaction to both dim and bright light stimulus.

Examine the pupil. Is it uniformly round and is it reacting to light in a normal way? Normally, if you shine a light on one eye, that pupil will constrict and so will the other at the same time. Note whether medication that has been instilled is having the desired effect. For example, when G. cyclopentolate hydrochloride has been instilled to dilate the pupil, it should be uniformly round and unreactive to light.

---

caused by a piece of metal lodged on the cornea. It may be necessary to instil local anaesthetic drops providing their use is not contraindicated; these should, of course, be prescribed or be included in a local protocol

- the environment should be conducive. Privacy and quietness are vital
- informing the patient of the procedure and gaining his or her cooperation and informed consent.

Routine examination of the eye requires a good pen-torch. Ask the patient how their eyes are and whether they are in any pain or discomfort. Each eye should be systematically examined and a comparison should be made of each eye in turn (see Guidelines for Care Priorities box 15.2).

Following the nursing assessment, patients will probably require one or more investigations to be undertaken. In many ophthalmic settings, nurses not only undertake these tests and investigations themselves, but are also able to order them as part of locally agreed protocols.

For some time now, ophthalmic nurses have expanded their role to include many routine investigative procedures previously undertaken by technicians or doctors (see below).

GENERAL DIAGNOSTIC TESTS AND MEDICAL INVESTIGATIONS

The doctor will undertake a physical examination of the patient as appropriate. Some conditions will require additional tests and investigations such as X-rays, CT scans, MRI scans and blood tests. Swabs for microscopy to detect viruses or bacteria are ordered where the patient's condition dictates. Use is also made of photography; straight facial photographs or those of surgical or accidental trauma are taken as a record to show progress or regression. A full description of routine eye examination is provided in Guidelines for Care Priorities box 15.2.

Before any investigation, patients are fully informed about the test and test procedure in order to obtain consent and ensure cooperation. In some instances, this consent is in written format; this would be the case for fluorescein angiography, which is an invasive procedure.

Many of the tests and investigations require contact with the eyeball itself. If this is the case, topical local anaesthetic drops will be instilled first, such as guttae (G) (eye drops) oxybuprocaine hydrochloride; one or two drops will have the desired effect in approximately 20 seconds. Patients should be warned that the drops do sting when first instilled. The anaesthetic effect lasts about 20 minutes.

OPHTHALMOSCOPY

An ophthalmoscope is a hand-held instrument that allows the nurse, doctor or optometrist to examine the interior structures of the eye. This instrument is not used very often now but can still be used to aid diagnosis. It is of particular use in the examination of the retina, retinal blood supply and the optic disc (see Fig. 15.2). It can be used to detect retinal haemorrhages or changes to the optic disc, as in glaucoma.

SLIT LAMP EXAMINATION

The slit lamp is basically a table-mounted binocular microscope that provides a three-dimensional view of the ocular structures (see Fig. 15.7). It has an adjustable light source and the magnification can also be changed.

TESTING VISUAL ACUITY

Testing visual acuity (VA) is one of the most important investigations for any patient presenting with reduced vision, ocular disease or trauma, and as a baseline measurement. The test most commonly used is the 'Snellen test type' (see Fig. 15.8A), although there are others available. The test chart should be located in a well-lit space that allows the patient's VA to be measured at 6 metres from the chart.

The Snellen chart has a series of letters, numbers or tumbling Es arranged in lines of diminishing size. The largest single letter, number or E is on the top row and the smallest on the bottom row. All of the letters, numbers or Es are of a particular shape and breadth and are black on a white background. As you can see from Figure 15.8, as the image size reduces on each line, an additional letter, number or E is added. When the adult cannot read standard letters, understand what the letters represent, or say the name of the English letter, a number chart or the E type is used (see Fig. 15.8B). These can be particularly helpful where language or learning disabilities are an issue. Patients look at the chart and show the position of the E with one they hold.

VA is usually expressed as a fraction. The first number, the numerator, represents the distance from the chart in metres. The second number, the denominator, is the distance at which a person who has average normal vision can read a particular line. For example, if a patient can read the second line from 6 metres, vision would be recorded as 6/36.

Vision should normally be tested at a distance of 6 metres, as at this distance accommodation is ruled out. Each eye must be tested separately. If patients normally wear glasses or contact lenses for distance, then vision should be tested both with and without them and recorded as such.

If patients can read all of the letters on the chart at 6 metres, VA would be recorded as 6/4. Some patients can read the letters on a particular line but not all of them; for example, if at 6 metres they can read only four letters on line six, then VA is recorded as 6/9–2. If they can read all the letters on line six but only one off the next line, VA would be recorded as 6/9+1.

Should patients be unable to read the largest letter on the chart, they should move nearer to it, usually in 1-metre stages. The distance is then adjusted when recording the VA. For example, if they can read only the top line at 3 metres, the VA would be recorded as 3/60.

Those unable to read the chart at 0.5 metres are assessed in terms of their ability to count fingers (CF) at a distance of approximately 0.5 metres. If they can, the VA is recorded as CF at 0.5 metres.

In the event that patients' vision is so poor they cannot count fingers, then test whether they can detect any hand movements (HM). If they can, record VA as HM only for that eye. It may be the case that patients cannot detect even HM. They may only be able to perceive light in that eye. If so, record VA as perception of light only (PL) in that eye.

As poor uncorrected distance vision may be due to a refractive error, the need to determine the corrected VA is vital in order to assess ocular health more accurately. An uncorrected VA of 6/9 or less should be re-checked using pinholes. This helps to rule out refractive blur from conditions such as myopia and astigmatism. With these conditions, light would be poorly

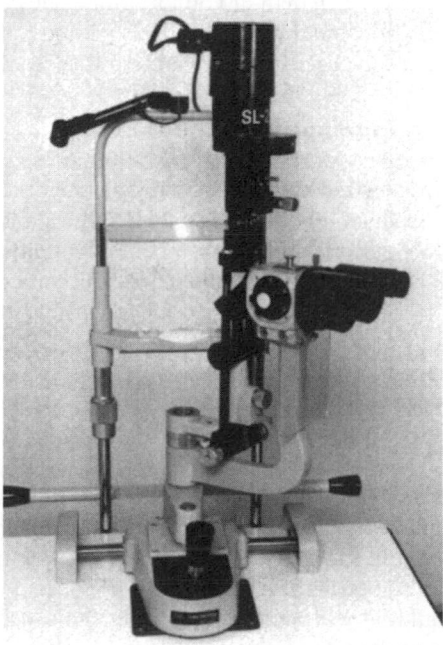

Figure 15.7 Slit lamp. (Reproduced with kind permission from Millodot & Laby 2002.)

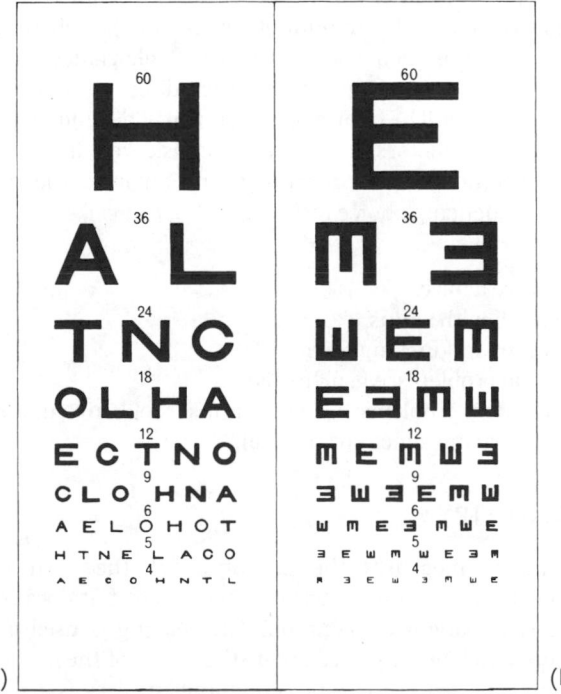

Figure 15.8 Visual acuity testing: (A) Snellen test type; (B) Snellen 'E' chart.

focused on the retina. Viewed through pinholes, only the centrally aligned light rays are focused on the retina, and the image viewed will therefore be clearer. Record the pinhole correction separately.

COLOUR VISION TESTING

Colour vision testing is used to detect defects in the function of the three types of cone cells of the retina that respond to bright light of the green, blue or red wavelengths. It is thought that 7% of the male population suffer from colour blindness, many of whom may be unaware that anything is wrong. Colour sensitivity is reduced in some ocular conditions, e.g. optic neuritis, and some macular disorders.

The usual method of testing is the Ishihara test, which involves patients looking at a series of colour plates with numbers or letters embedded within them. They are asked to say what the letter or number is. People with normal colour vision are able to see the number or letter on every plate, whereas those with defective colour vision may see none of them (monochromatic defect), or may only be able to identify some of them, depending on which type of cone is defective.

GONIOSCOPY

Gonioscopy is a routine assessment tool for any patient suspected of having glaucoma. It is usually performed when the ophthalmologist wants to examine in detail the drainage angle for aqueous humour. This will be examined using a gonioscope to assess the degree to which the drainage angle is open.

VISUAL FIELD TESTING

Visual field (see Fig. 15.6, p. 335) testing (perimetry) is performed to evaluate the amount of central and peripheral vision loss in conditions such as primary open-angle glaucoma. There are several types of machines, including automated and Goldmann types. The choice of machine will depend on clinical need but other factors do need to be considered, as some tests take longer and require more cooperation from the patient. Factors influencing choice include:

- age
- cognitive ability
- mental health status
- communication, language
- physical problems, e.g. arthritis
- some visual problems, e.g. nystagmus (rapid, involuntary oscillatory movement of the eye).

KERATOMETRY

Keratometry measures the curvature of the cornea. The keratometer is a non-contact test instrument but does require a degree of patient cooperation. The reading is used in conjunction with biometry to calculate the power of the intraocular lens implant used at the time of cataract surgery (see p. 349). Some keratometers are automated and provide a more rapid reading.

BIOMETRY

Biometry is a special test that helps to determine the power of the artificial lens that will be implanted at the time of cataract surgery. It is an A-scan of the axial length of the eye. This test does take some time to perform and requires a degree of patient cooperation. It is normally done when patients come to the preassessment clinic and it is usual to do the test on both eyes. This allows comparisons to be made but also means that when the second cataract operation takes place (should this be necessary) the data will be already available. The keratometry reading will be fed into the biometer as part of the detail needed to calculate the intraocular lens power. Patient comfort is essential, as the test can take some time to perform (Stanford 2000), and patients should be positioned in an adjustable chair with a headrest.

The equipment used is a biometer. There is a contact type and this involves placing a probe into contact with the cornea. It is therefore necessary to apply a topical local anaesthetic such as G. oxybuprocaine hydrochloride, or G. proxymethacaine hydrochloride may be used as this does not sting.

Operators need to be mindful of their own position and posture during the test, as there is a risk of repetitive strain injury to the back, wrist and shoulders. There are non-contact biometers on the market, and these are being used more frequently now.

FOCIMETRY

This is a non-invasive test to measure the power of spectacle lenses. The information is also used in calculating the power of the intraocular lens implant.

GOLDMANN APPLANATION TONOMETRY

This is a contact method for measuring the intraocular pressure (normally between 10 and 21 mmHg). The eyes are anaesthetized beforehand to reduce patient discomfort and to aid cooperation. G. lidocaine (lignocaine) hydrochloride drops and G. fluorescein stain are instilled in order to ensure an accurate reading.

CORNEAL TOPOGRAPHY

This is a computerized system for mapping the contour of the cornea and displaying data that is useful to the clinician. It can be used to aid diagnosis and management of conditions such as keratoconus, a condition where the cornea becomes conical in shape, and to obtain clinical data prior to corneal or refractive surgery; it may also assist in contact lens fitting. Pachymetry is the measurement of corneal thickness.

FLUORESCEIN ANGIOGRAPHY

This diagnostic test involves the injection of fluorescein intravenously, usually into a vein in the arm or hand, to highlight the retinal vessels and their condition, the state of the macula and optic disc. It also highlights the presence of choroidal tumours. Patients should be warned that following the procedure their skin will turn yellow for a short time, as will their urine while the dye is excreted. There is also the risk, albeit very small, of an anaphylactic reaction occurring.

Prior to the examination, it is necessary to dilate the pupils with a mydriatic such as G. tropicamide, so that the fundus can be viewed. Colour and black and white photographs are taken and are used to inform diagnosis and treatment. Some patients experience nausea and vomiting. This investigation can lead to patients having an anaphylactic reaction. Nurses should be aware of this risk and ensure that emergency drugs and equipment are available should they be required. If there are no ill effects, patients can usually go straight home.

ORTHOPTIC EXAMINATION

In the orthoptic department, various complex tests will be undertaken, including those to determine how well the eyes are working together (binocular vision).

GENERAL DISEASE PREVENTION AND HEALTH EDUCATION

Nurses have an important role in promoting ocular health and in preventing accidents. It is possible to prevent some eye injuries. Following the manufacturers' instructions when working with machinery or corrosive liquids seems an obvious thing to do, at work and at home, but so often is not. Wearing suitable eye protection can prevent eye injuries. Eye protection should be worn when using a garden strimmer, as debris flies freely in all directions and could easily cause corneal trauma or even penetration of the eyeball. It may also be appropriate for people in the immediate vicinity to protect their eyes as well. When working underneath cars, DIY enthusiasts should protect their eyes from rusty metal or oil by wearing protective goggles.

At work, employers have a duty of care to ensure that safety equipment is available for use and that there are safe systems of working. They should also ensure that staff are trained in their use. Staff trained as first aiders should be available in the workplace, as should emergency equipment such as the correct fluid to irrigate the eye after chemical accidents. Employees also have a duty of care to wear the protective equipment provided. For example, when welding, welding masks or goggles should be worn to protect from welders' flash ('arc-eye').

Nurses, when drawing up cytotoxic drugs, should also protect their eyes, not just their uniforms and skin.

At home or at work, aerosols and cleaning liquids should be directed away from the user's face and those of anyone else in the vicinity.

Some natural phenomena can cause injury to the eye. You should never look directly at the sun during an eclipse but rather use some alternative method or even content yourself to watch it on the television.

Despite links to skin cancer, people still use sunbeds on a regular basis. If they are to be used, it is imperative that the eyes are protected from UV radiation with protective eye shields.

Screening for ocular health is essential for people who are at risk of developing ocular disease. All who have diabetes mellitus should have their eyes examined, not just a sight test every 12 months. Those with a close family history (first-degree relatives) of primary open-angle glaucoma and others at higher risk, such as African and African Caribbean individuals, should have a thorough eye check every year, once over 40 years of age. At the health check, visual acuity, intraocular pressure (IOP), visual fields and the health of the retina and optic nerve should be tested.

Adults over 60 years of age should attend their optometrist annually, because older adults are known to develop problems with their vision, often silently and painlessly. They may have consciously or subconsciously adapted their lifestyle to the visual loss, not aware that they could get treatment or assistance to improve their lifestyle.

VISUAL IMPAIRMENT

Many otherwise healthy adults do not see very well because of refractive errors such as myopia, hypermetropia, presbyopia (long-sightedness caused by a failure of accommodation typically commencing in the late 40s) and astigmatism. These visual anomalies are usually corrected with spectacles or contact lenses. Some people have chosen to correct the error by laser (LASIK) treatment. As we age, the ability of the eye to accommodate to near objects, especially for reading, diminishes. People often compensate for this by holding books or newspapers further away. This condition (presbyopia) is normally corrected with reading glasses.

Visual impairment may be a temporary phenomenon; for example, should you get soap in your eyes, the response is for the eyes to water heavily (tearing) and for vision to become blurred for a few moments. Cataracts, whilst having a major effect on vision, can in most cases be removed with resulting improvement to vision. However, the visual impairment may also be permanent, e.g. with some congenital abnormalities or following severe eye trauma that results in vision loss of that eye. In this latter instance, binocular vision and depth perception will be lost.

The causes of visual impairment include:

- congenital conditions, e.g. genetic abnormalities
- developmental anomalies, e.g. strabismus (squint)
- secondary to systemic disease, e.g. diabetes mellitus (see Ch. 17) and rheumatoid arthritis (see Ch. 27)
- primary disease of the eye itself, e.g. glaucoma, age-related macular degeneration
- trauma to the globe, e.g. penetrating injury
- cerebrovascular conditions, where damage to the visual pathway, e.g. that caused by a stroke (see Ch. 14), can lead to loss of a part of the field of vision (hemianopia)
- trachoma – an infection caused by *Chlamydia trachomatis*
- vitamin A deficiency.

When talking about vision, it must be remembered that it is not simply a question of the ability to see near and distant objects clearly. It is also about the field of vision, the ability to judge depth, discriminate colour and see just one image at a time (Barton 1998).

The RNIB (Baker & Winyard 1998) reported that there were as many as 1 million people aged over 65 with visual impairment. These people experience problems that could be directly or indirectly related to their visual impairment. Four areas of concern were identified:

- Unmet care and daily living needs, including dependence on informal care networks to help with reading letters and bills, the result being a sense of loss of privacy as well as some needs going unmet.
- Mobility problems occurring because of poor and inadequate transport. Losing all or part of one's sight affects confidence in going outdoors to do errands or visit friends.
- Isolation – there is a close relationship between poor mobility and isolation from friends and family. Even when getting out and about, many partially sighted or blind people report that their vision problem leads to their being ignored by those with sight, including health care professionals.
- Poverty and inadequate information about benefits. Of those surveyed, 90% of older blind persons were living in poverty, with an income less than half the national average. Many people with visual impairment do not know about benefits to which they may be entitled.

REGISTRATION AS BLIND OR PARTIALLY SIGHTED

There may reach a point in treatment when the ophthalmic consultant begins to discuss with patients the possibility of their being registered as blind or partially sighted. This is a very traumatic time for patients and their families. The consultant will generally be sure that every treatment option has been tried and that the best course of action is to admit the fact to patients. Whilst the consultant may spend some time discussing this and the reasons, patients may be so devastated at the news as not to 'hear' what is being said and why. They will leave the consultation feeling a variety of emotions. They should be given immediate support from the nursing staff. Patients will need time to make some sort of sense out of what they have been told. There may be a need to let them talk immediately to people from the statutory and voluntary organizations dealing with people with visual problems. These include social workers (most social services departments have groups of staff that specialize in the field of visual impairment) and Henshaws Society for Blind People (Hsbp) or the RNIB (see 'Useful addresses', p. 365). Patients may only want to know about these initially, choosing to think about what has been said, and perhaps discuss the situation with family or friends. Later they may be more receptive to the help and support that can be provided. Even though they may have anticipated the news, they are likely to embark on a grieving process upon hearing it (see Reflective Practice box 15.2).

Registration as blind or partially sighted is a major step for any patient to take. They very often see it as a retrograde step, feeling that it may result in loss of independence or active employment. This need not be the case at all. Registration opens the way for benefits, help and services. The ophthalmic consultant and the patient will discuss the registration category and whilst it is the consultant who undertakes the eye examination and fills in the relevant form for those who are eligible, patients can choose not to register. In England and Wales the form is the BD8, in Northern Ireland the A655, and in Scotland the BP1.

Each local authority has a register of blind or partially sighted people in their area. This helps them to plan services.

15.2 Loss of vision

Imagine that you have just been told that a close friend (about your age) has lost his or her sight and nothing else can be done for that person.

Student activities
- Think about how the person would react to this news.
- What help and support do you think he or she will need from now on to come to terms with that news?
- How do you think you can best help and support the person? What information will you need to be able to do this effectively?

▶ **Nursing management: patients with visual impairment**

The goal of any nursing intervention for patients with an ophthalmic disorder should be to maximize patient well-being, whilst supporting them to be as independent as possible (RCN 2000).

Communication

Ensuring adequate communication for patients with visual impairment calls for well-developed communication skills (see Ch. 3). It is particularly important to follow the usual good practice rules for speaking to patients; for example, maintaining eye contact is just as important as it is when conversing with someone with normal vision. The visually impaired person will pick up on non-verbal cues during conversation as readily as anyone can. If you are talking to a visually impaired person and you smile and nod as appropriate to the conversation, the conversation will have a natural flow and pauses and your voice tone will also reflect the mood.

There are two groups of individuals that require some additional consideration in relation to communication, namely those from minority ethnic groups whose first language is not English and people with learning disabilities. Easy access to, and subsequent use of, health care services is particularly difficult for these individuals. Appropriate treatment depends on accurate diagnosis, and subsequent management of that condition requires patient understanding. If patients are to make informed choices about treatment, difficulties relating to their visual impairment will be compounded if nurses fail to communicate effectively.

Interpreter services can be used to good effect, but such services are not without their problems. For example, patients and health care professionals need to trust that interpreters will give the correct information to both parties and that they will not embellish or censor information, albeit unwittingly. Poor interpretation can result in a delay in timely treatment, isolation and delayed recovery. It is vital that nurses and patients establish a therapeutic relationship (Dias & O'Neil 1998).

Safety and maintaining independence

The goal of any nursing intervention or interaction should be to maintain patient independence as well as ensuring their safety.

Safety issues to consider relate to the environment in which patients are to be cared for, including the access to it. As has already been suggested, the majority of those with visual impairment are older people who are likely to have other problems such as difficulty with mobility. Consideration should be given to how someone arrives at the unit, ward or department. Even if you are not working in an ophthalmic unit, many of your patients and visitors will have some visual problem. Like any other disability, visual impairment must be given some consideration when planning and providing service.

The corridors need to be well lit and well signed and they should not be cluttered with equipment. Direction signs should be readable by someone who has visual problems. It is important that signs are large enough, uncluttered and that there is good contrast between the letters and background.

Stairs should be well lit and contrast provided so that the edge of steps can be seen more clearly. If you are guiding patients, you should let them know that stairs are there. It may be appropriate to offer an alternative to stairs such as a lift.

The clinical environment should be described to patients as they are guided around, in sufficient detail for them to negotiate their way around safely. This should include pointing out specific features and landmarks. If they are sharing accommodation or clinical space, they should be made aware of this and also the presence of visitors. Where appropriate, they should be introduced. Do not expect patients to be able to find their way around the unit after one guided explanation. It may be necessary to guide them each time; on the other hand, some people will rapidly adapt to their new environment.

Nurses must be sensitive to specific patient needs. When caring for people with a visual impairment, it is not enough to place something in front of them; nurses must also provide an explanation so they know what to do with it. As you approach patients, let them know you are there by introducing yourself and making it clear you wish to talk to them. If you are placing items on a locker or table, tell them exactly where they have been placed. It is sometimes necessary to guide their hands to the object in question, warning them if it is hot or sharp. If vision is affected on one side, items should be placed on the opposite side. For example, if patients have a pad and/or bandage over their left eye, place items on a table on their right-hand side, ensuring the better eye can focus on the object. It may be necessary to describe in detail what is in front of patients, such as food on a plate. It is usual to locate things in terms of a clock face. It is helpful to come back to check they have been able to cope with their food and drinks.

Physical contact can help patients to be aware of the presence of other people. Such contact should be made sensitively; for example, as you enter a room and you say hello to patients, touch their hand or arm gently with the palm of your hand. In this way, they will be able to locate where you are. Do be aware that if patients have been dozing, they may initially jump.

Explaining the stages of a nursing intervention will assist patients in understanding what is happening to them. If you are being assisted by other health care staff, avoid situations where you are talking over patients or where both of you are speaking at the same time.

Whilst this is rare, it is worth noting that some people who are blind experience visual hallucinations, a condition called Charles Bonnet syndrome. One lady reported she repeatedly saw a taxi outside her home and people coming into her house. These people do need reassurance that they are not going mad (Harrison 2000).

Services and support

Patients and their family members often require help and support for a long time after they have attended hospital or a clinic. Knox (1998) suggests that nurses consider the use of psychological theory in helping those affected by visual impairment. Services available for patients and families are many and varied. It can be confusing for them as to where they should go for help and support. Social services will undertake an assessment of needs and should be contacted early, with patients' consent. People with visual impairment, like anyone else, can be fiercely independent and offers of help and support need to be dealt with sensitively.

Voluntary organizations such as the RNIB and Hsbp can provide practical advice, detail of visual aids and information leaflets and tapes, as well as counselling services and self-help groups. Some voluntary groups are disease-specific, e.g. the International Glaucoma Association (www.iga.org.uk).

Home adaptations may be necessary and patients should be assessed as to their particular needs. Simple changes can be made at low cost. For example, changing the lighting need not be expensive. Changing to a brighter light bulb can make it easier to see. The provision of a standard lamp or table lamp can improve the lighting for reading or other activities, including hobbies (RNIB 1997).

Low vision aids can improve the quality of patient life. These include spectacles, sunglasses, magnifiers, monoculars, adapting lighting to suit the vision loss and the task, use of contrast such as light on dark, highlighting similar objects using different colours, etc. (Cleary 1995). Ideally, patients should be assessed to determine their specific needs. This service may be offered through social services or voluntary groups, but may also be provided by a high-street optometrist.

Mobility aids are available, e.g. guide canes, but patients will have to be trained in their use. Some people with a visual impairment may benefit from a guide dog (see Special Issues box 15.1, p. 344).

Education and employment training can be vital aspects of a rehabilitation programme for someone who is blind or partially sighted. Local authorities and voluntary organizations provide this, including residential packages.

Some people benefit from learning to read Braille or Moon. Such training is not compulsory and not everyone who is blind can read such texts, but those who do find it enhances their lives. Braille books (fiction and non-fiction) are available from the National Library for the Blind and are delivered directly to the home. Some books are written for sighted people to enable them to read to others who can then follow the Braille text for themselves. Many organizations produce written communications in large print and some will provide Braille communications, e.g. banks and electricity supply companies.

Talking books are an alternative for many people with or without visual problems. Audiotapes of local news can also be arranged. Some consideration needs to be given to the type of tape player and whether headphones are needed. The latter may be essential where patients do not live alone.

SPECIAL ISSUES

15.1 Guide dogs

Patients who might benefit from having a guide dog are assessed on an individual basis, usually by a representative from the Guide Dogs for the Blind (GDB). Not everyone is suited to having a guide dog. Those who are considered suitable are trained in how to care for and get along with their dog. Inevitably, the dog and the handler will develop a close working relationship and a bond of friendship, so when the time comes for the dog to retire, patients will have to learn how to cope with this situation as well as that dog's replacement. There will be times when the patient and the dog will have to be temporarily parted, e.g. whilst the patient is in hospital as an in-patient. At such times if a family member cannot care for the dog, the GDB can be approached to make boarding arrangements.

Student activities
- What might be the impact on patients who have to be separated from their guide dog when admitted to a hospital for planned or emergency treatment?
- Do you think it could influence their recovery?
- How do you think they may behave during the separation?
- What could the nursing staff do to ease the situation for patients, such as obtaining up-to-date news about how the dog has settled in its new surroundings?

 EVIDENCE-BASED PRACTICE

15.1 Getting the correct eye medication

It is obviously vital that patients having regular eye medications have the correct drugs prescribed if they are admitted to hospital for a non-ophthalmic condition. O'Sullivan et al (2001) in a small study of 22 patients identified only seven who were prescribed the correct eye medication.

Student activities
- Read the article by O'Sullivan et al (2001).
- Find out what safeguards exist in your clinical areas to ensure that eye medicines are correctly prescribed.
- Think about a patient who did not receive the correct medication for an existing ophthalmic condition when admitted for an unrelated disorder. Why do you think this happened?
- What interventions by the nurse can ensure that the correct medicine is prescribed?

Reference
O'Sullivan EP, Malhotra R, Migdal C. Prescription of eye drops. Postgrad Med J 2001; 77(912): 654–655.

TV licence concessions are available to people registered blind or partially sighted. Tax and other benefits are available to be claimed for those registered blind. In the UK, the Inland Revenue has a leaflet, IR170, that explains individual entitlements.

▶ Nursing management: ophthalmic medications

Topical medication – drops and ointment
Topical eye medication is just as important as any other prescribed medication. It is imperative that patients, health professionals, family members or carers are mindful that eye drops and ointments are drugs, and that patients' sight may depend on following treatment regimens. When patients with existing eye conditions are admitted to hospital for another reason, such as a heart attack or for surgery, it is vital that the nurse ascertains what eye medication is being used and ensures that the correct regimen is prescribed and administered (see Evidence-based Practice box 15.1). An overview of the common drugs used in ophthalmology is provided in Table 15.1, but readers requiring detailed information should consult an authoritative resource such as the *British National Formulary* (www.bnf.org.uk).

There are many reasons why patients fail to instil their drops or apply their ointment (see below). In addition, it should be

Table 15.1 Drugs used in ophthalmology

Drug group	Examples	Remarks
Mydriatics		
Cycloplegics (antimuscarinics)	Atropine sulphate, tropicamide, cyclopentolate hydrochloride, homatropine hydrobromide	Antimuscarinics act via the parasympathetic nervous system. They paralyse the sphincter muscle of the iris and the ciliary muscle. They dilate the pupil such as for examination
Non-cycloplegics (sympathomimetics)	Phenylephrine hydrochloride 2.5–10%	These act via the sympathetic nervous system. They stimulate the dilator muscle but do not affect the ciliary muscle. They dilate the pupil. Side-effects include raised IOP, sensitivity, hallucinations, psychotic disturbance, contact dermatitis
Miotics	Pilocarpine 1–2%	Constricts the pupil by acting on the parasympathetic nerve endings of the sphincter muscle. Improves drainage of aqueous humour and is used in the treatment of raised IOP. Side-effects include stinging and burning on instillation and blurred vision, headache, sweating, bradycardia, colic and occasionally bronchospasm *(continued)*

Table 15.1 *(cont'd)*

Drug group	Examples	Remarks
Beta-blockers	Betaxolol, levobunolol, timolol maleate	They lower IOP in patients with POAG. They are β_1- and β_2-receptor antagonists (blockers) and so reduce production of aqueous humour. Side-effects include local hypersensitivity, superficial punctate keratitis (corneal inflammation), blurred vision, headache, allergy, reduction of resting heart rate, disorientation, diarrhoea and dizziness. Contraindicated in patients with asthma and/or chronic obstructive airways disease
Sympathomimetic	Brimonidine tartrate	A selective α_2-receptor agonist used to reduce IOP. May be used as alternative or adjunct therapy in POAG, sometimes in conjunction with a beta-blocker
Carbonic anhydrase inhibitors	Acetazolamide, brinzolamide, dorzolamide	They inhibit the production of aqueous humour and so reduce IOP. Side-effects include loss of appetite, tingling of fingertips, acidosis, general malaise and potassium deficiency
Antiprostaglandin analogues	Bimatoprost, latanoprost, travoprost	Increase uveoscleral drainage of aqueous humour. Used to reduce IOP in patients with POAG. Can change iris colour and care should be taken if only one eye is being treated and in patients with a mixed-colour iris
Antibacterials	Broad-spectrum: chloramphenicol 0.5% drops or 1% ointment, neomycin, gentamicin, ciprofloxacin, ofloxacin Antibacterials with specific range of action: fusidic acid, chlortetracycline	Antibiotics are used to treat ocular infections. Usually used topically. May be administered systemically or by subconjunctival, or intraocular injection for some infections Side-effects similar to oral medication including local allergy
Antifungals – fungal infections affecting the eye are rare and advice from a specialist unit should be obtained regarding the use and availability of antifungal drugs		
Antivirals	Aciclovir 3% Fomivirsen sodium	Used to treat herpes simplex infection Used for retinitis caused by cytomegalovirus (CMV).
Anti-inflammatory Corticosteroids	Hydrocortisone acetate 1% drops, 0.5% ointment, prednisolone acetate 0.5%, dexamethasone	Inhibit inflammation, oedema and allergy. Should not be used if virus ulcer of the cornea is suspected or diagnosed. Topical use can result in perforation of the cornea. They should be used with caution
Other inflammatory drugs	Azelastine, levocabastine (antihistamines); sodium cromoglicate (cromoglycate); lodoxamine	Used for allergic conjunctivitis
Local anaesthetics	Amethocaine 0.5% and 1%, oxybuprocaine 0.4%, proxymethacaine, lidocaine (lignocaine)	Short-acting local anaesthesia to surface of the eye Side-effects include one or more of the following: burning sensation on instillation, corneal epithelial toxicity
Diagnostic agents	Fluorescein 2%, rose bengal 1%	Fluorescein highlights damaged tissue. It is also used when fitting contact lenses, applanation tonometry, testing for leaking corneal wound (Siedel's test). i.v. use for fundal photography (fluorescein angiography) Rose bengal is more sensitive than fluorescein. It is rarely used
Lubricants and artificial tears	Liquid paraffin, e.g. Lacri-lube, carbomers, acetylcysteine	Used to treat 'dry eye' conditions, or when normal protective mechanisms are compromised, such as loss of blinking reflex in unconscious patients (see Ch. 14)

recognized that where patients are dependent on a carer to assist with drop installation, concordance with treatment could be compromised if the carer fails to attach importance to the treatment needed. Felinski (1989) and Shaw (2000, unpublished data) both highlight that district nurses may not give the same priority to drop instillation as they would to giving other medication. It has been shown that the outcome of treatment depends heavily upon patients themselves; they need to be informed about their condition and treatment options. Having considered those options they can make an informed choice about their involvement in treatment. They need time to adapt to their circumstances and time and the opportunity to practise drop or ointment instillation, if this is the form of treatment for them (see Fig. 15.9). Nurses need to spend time educating patients and demonstrating drop and ointment technique, allowing them the opportunity to practise (see Health Promotion box 15.1). Drop aids do have their place but are not suited to all patients. Some may need input from the district nurse. Patients need to be educated about safe storage of their eye medication, i.e. stored as per the manufacturers' instructions and out of the reach of children.

If nurses are to transmit clear information about patient education and instruction to others, it needs to be in a format that can be easily understood. Figure 15.10 is an example of a document used to record details of how patients can best instil their drops. It is suggested that such information can help to prevent unnecessary duplication and possible confusion for patients.

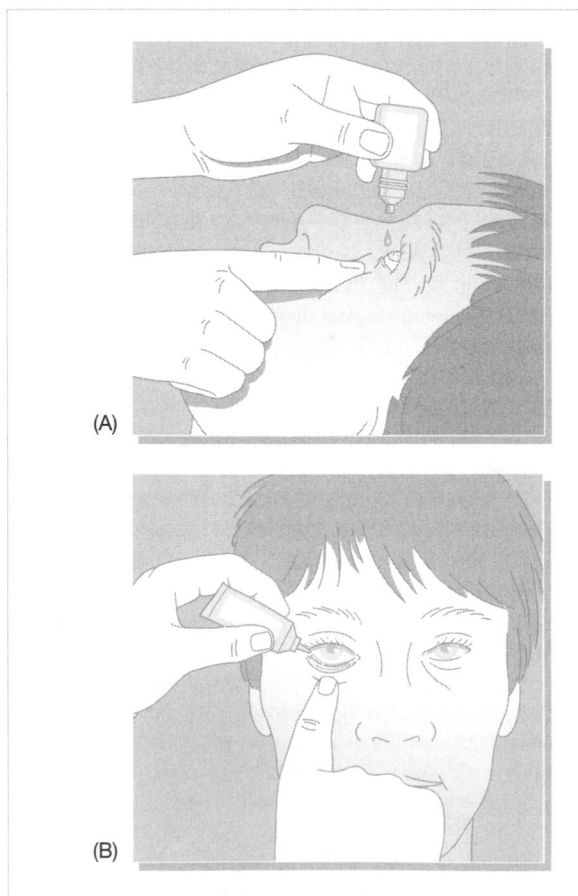

Figure 15.9 Instillation of eye medication: (A) drops; (B) ointment.

Factors influencing medication instillation and associated problems

The factors influencing medication instillation and associated problems may be related to the person's physical condition, level of knowledge and understanding, psychosocial factors, or the treatment regimen.

 HEALTH PROMOTION

15.1 Instilling eye medication (Adapted from Nicol et al 2000)

In order to instil eye medications effectively and safely, patients need information about the procedure from the nurse as well as sufficient opportunities to practise and ask questions. Nurses should reinforce the importance of following eye medication regimens, and the correct care and storage of drops, ointment and any equipment used. Patients should be advised about checking expiry dates on the drugs and reminded that the drug is prescribed only for them. Normally, separate containers for drops or ointment should be used if both eyes are being treated.

Administering eye medication – guidelines for patients
- Check that you are instilling the correct medications into the correct eye at the correct time.
- Wash your hands.
- Remember that the medication may sting and cause blurred vision for a short time, so don't move about or drive until your vision is back to normal.
- Remove the cap from the medication.
- Gently pull down the lower eyelid to form the small pocket (inferior conjunctival fornix). Both eye drops and ointment are instilled into this pocket (see Fig. 15.9).
- Instil the drops or ointment as per prescription, i.e. the number of drops and the order if the treatment involves more than one drug. If you have both drops and ointment, use the drops first, as the greasy ointment may stop the drops working properly. Make sure that the dropper or ointment tube does not touch any part of the eye.
- If you are using ointment, start at the inner part by your nose and squeeze a ribbon of ointment about 1–2 cm in length along the inside edge of the eyelid.
- Shut your eyes gently and count slowly to 60 after instilling your eye medication so that the drug is not absorbed systemically.
- If you need more than one drop per eye, blink normally between drops to disperse the drug.
- Wash your hands.
- Store the medications correctly.
- Check that you have sufficient medications, particularly over weekends and holiday periods.

NB: Seek professional advice if anything unusual happens, such as your eye feeling different after the medication, or if you have any questions about your condition and treatment.

St. Anywhere's Hospital Trust

Patient's name: ....

Hospital record number: ....

Nurse's name: ....

Date: ....

Technique descriptor	No drop aids used	Mirror – static/pivot	Drop aid Add type	Sitting	Lying/ standing
One handed; (bottle clasped between thumb and forefinger and one finger pulling the lid down)					
Bridge of nose used to rest drop bottle					
One hand-finger on cheek					
Moorfields' technique; (knuckle on cheek other hand for dropper)					
Forehead used to rest drop bottle					
Onto closed lids into inner canthus					
Other:					

Figure 15.10 Record of observed drop instillation technique.

Physical

- Lack of dexterity – it is necessary for patients to be able to handle, control and manipulate the dropper or tube of ointment.
- Mobility – problems with movement; neck rigidity; neck or back pain; painful and/or arthritic hands.
- Poor vision – can interfere with patient education. Patients may not be able to read instructions or see well enough to select the correct drops.
- Ocular pain – if patients are in pain, they may find it hard to concentrate on instilling the drops or they may fear

that the drops will cause more discomfort (most drops sting on instillation).
- Level of general health – acute or chronic conditions that are concurrent with the ocular problem as well as how ill or well the patient feels.

Knowledge and understanding

- Level of knowledge of condition, treatment and side-effects of treatment.
- Level of understanding – if patients understand why the drops or ointment are needed and the consequences of not

using them, they can make an active choice to use the prescribed medication. People with learning disabilities may need to be assisted/prompted to instil their medication whilst maintaining their autonomy and independence.

- Poor memory – patients forget to instil the drops, or forget they have already done so.
- Level of motivation/willingness – this can be influenced by health education and promotion.

Psychosocial

- No access to materials/equipment to clean the eye or instil the drops – for example, at work there may only be the public toilets.
- Lack of time – a busy lifestyle can get in the way of drop times.

Treatment regimen

- Multiple drops – simple regimens are preferable to complex ones with multiple drop types.
- The need to use 'Minims' – some drops are provided without preservatives and are intended for single use. They are supplied in small containers. The lids are small and difficult for some to grasp and remove. In addition, the container needs to be squeezed with some force to expel the contents.
- Both eyes requiring treatment – this causes some confusion, especially if each eye requires different treatment. Clear written and verbal instructions should be given. Where possible, the doctor will endeavour to keep the prescription simple.
- Drop bottle design, including breaking seals/opening tops, can be difficult for some people. The carer or pharmacist may have to assist when new bottles or tubes are needed.

PAINLESS VISUAL IMPAIRMENT

CATARACT

A cataract is opacity of the crystalline lens. It is a very common condition and can occur at any age (Forrester et al 1996).

Aetiology and epidemiology

There are several causes of cataract, including:

- congenital
- age-related, as part of the normal ageing process
- drug-induced, e.g. treatment with corticosteroids as eye drops or taken systemically
- trauma
- metabolic diseases such as diabetes mellitus
- radiation.

By far the most common type of cataract is the age-related type.

WHO (1997) estimated that there were 16 million people worldwide whose blindness is due to cataract. In Britain, it is known that there are many thousands of older people who could have improved quality of life if they had their cataracts removed. In England alone it is estimated that as many as 200 000 cataract operations are needed to be performed each

year (Royal College of Ophthalmologists 2001). Despite the numbers with visual impairment or blindness resulting from cataract, cataract extraction and lens implant is a relatively easy operation, but it is not without complications.

Clinical presentation

Cataracts may be very evident in that, when the pupil is examined, it looks white (see Fig. 15.11A) or, in mature cataracts, brown. On the other hand, the cataract may only be seen upon closer examination with an ophthalmoscope or slit lamp.

Effects of cataract on vision include:

- gradual reduction in visual acuity with patchy vision loss in advanced disease (see Fig. 15.11B)
- glare or dazzling lights especially at night
- diplopia.

The impact that age-related cataract has on lifestyle will vary, but the loss of vision is usually very gradual. Indeed, many patients are not aware that they have them. It is not unusual for people visiting their optometrist for a routine vision check, perhaps because they are having problems seeing distant objects clearly, to be advised that they have cataracts.

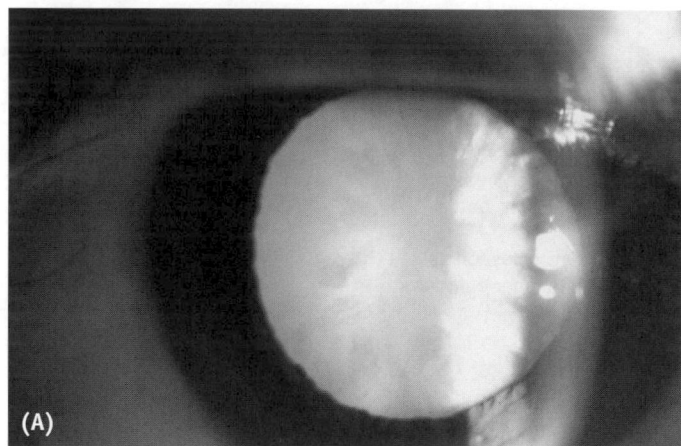

(A)

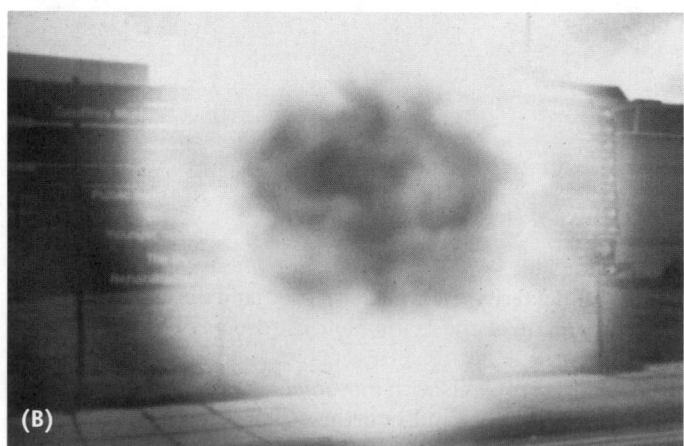

(B)

Figure 15.11 Cataract. (A) Mature cataract seen through the pupil. (Reproduced with kind permission from Kanski 1999.) (B) Simulation of vision associated with advanced cataract. (Reproduced with kind permission from RNIB.)

Surgical management

There are several types of operation to remove cataracts. The most frequently seen are phacoemulsification (phaco) and extracapsular cataract extraction (ECCE). In ECCE, the anterior lens capsule is torn (capsulorrhexis) and the lens (cortex and nucleus) removed with surgical instruments. The posterior capsule remains intact and the replacement intraocular lens (IOL) is placed within it. With phaco, the nucleus and cortex are ultrasonically fragmented and the lens matter aspirated (American Academy of Ophthalmology 1997a).

The choice of the type of anaesthetic is made by the doctor in consultation with the patient at the preoperative assessment. These choices include various types of local anaesthetic and, less commonly, general anaesthetic. Much of ophthalmic surgery is now undertaken using local anaesthetic techniques. Many older patients have other health problems and these must be considered in decisions about anaesthetic. Patients are generally required to lie flat during their operation and this may be difficult for those with other conditions such as chronic respiratory disease. Sedation is not necessarily an option, as drowsy patients could forget where they are during surgery and move their head at a crucial time.

It is becoming increasingly common to manage cataract surgery on a day-case basis; indeed, the target set by the UK government is 80% (see Ethical Issues box 15.1). People who have concurrent health problems, such as insulin-dependent diabetes mellitus or heart disease, will usually be selected for an in-patient stay, although this does not always have to be the case. Patients with learning disabilities should not be excluded from day surgery as this may in fact be far less disruptive to their routine. It is acknowledged that there are other issues that could result in an in-patient stay, including patient choice (Royal College of Ophthalmologists 2001).

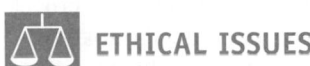

ETHICAL ISSUES

15.1 Day-case cataract surgery

The NHS Executive (2000) recommends cataract surgery should be undertaken as day surgery and that on the day of surgery the time spent in the surgery unit should be 90 minutes.

Student activities

Consider the ethical implications of this recommendation to patients, bearing in mind the following:

- age and mobility of the patient
- ability of the older person to self-care
- ability to comply with postoperative treatment, including instilling drops
- consequences of failing to instil drops
- impact on the relatives/carers/community resources
- amount of time the nurse has for patient education.

Reference

NHS Executive. Action on Cataracts. London: DoH; 2000. (Also online. Available: www.doh.gov.uk/cataracts.htm.)

Consideration will be given as to the type of surgery, and assessment will also be carried out to determine the power of the intraocular lens (IOL) implant needed. Informed consent will also be obtained once the risk of complications, including blindness (albeit a very small risk), has been discussed with patients.

Complications of cataract surgery include:

- Endophthalmitis – a rare complication with inflammation of the whole of the eye, it can lead to blindness. There is intense pain, photophobia, reduced vision and patients feel generally unwell. Treatment involves hospitalization, identification of the microorganism and intensive topical antibiotic therapy plus intravenous antibiotics. Antibiotics may also be given by the intracameral (into the eye) route. Initially the antibiotic drops are usually given every 15 minutes and then every half hour, including overnight.
- Corneal oedema – there is reduced vision and ocular discomfort.
- Raised IOP – patients feel unwell and complain of headache, pain around the eye that is not resolved with usual analgesia, nausea and occasionally vomiting.
- Flat anterior chamber.
- Dislocated or wrong IOL.
- Haemorrhage – this can be seen as red liquid in the anterior chamber (hyphaema).
- Uveitis (see p. 362).
- Infection – discharge from the eye.
- Retinal detachment (see p. 354) – patients may complain of a shadow or curtain in their field of vision and a sensation of flashing light (Okhravi 1997).

Any of these complications must be treated with urgency, and assistance sought from medical staff. The local ophthalmic unit can be contacted for advice when patients present at a non-specialist unit.

▶ Nursing management

Preoperative assessment including discharge planning

Regardless of whether patients are to have surgery as in-patients or as a day-case admission, the preoperative assessment should cover the same aspects. This usually takes place between 1 and 3 months ahead of planned surgery. The majority of the preoperative assessment is usually undertaken by the nurse, the doctor reviewing this and also establishing that patients have a cataract requiring surgery and that they actually want to have the surgery.

The preoperative assessment includes:

- visual acuity measurement
- health review – blood pressure, urinalysis, ECG and blood tests, if indicated
- ocular health – confirmation of diagnosis, history of disease or trauma, intraocular pressure, anterior chamber and fundal check
- keratometry, biometry, applanation tonometry
- nursing history, patient education, understanding of condition and treatment
- discharge planning, including drop technique.

Despite attempts to reduce the amount of time that patients have to wait from diagnosis of cataract and the referral by the optometrist or general practitioner to surgery, many patients will have several weeks before they get an appointment to see a consultant. It is during this time that they may begin to dwell on the implications for them of their condition. They may be uncertain about what a cataract is, although they will recognize the effect on their vision. Fear of loss of independence and concern about how successful the removal of the cataract will be in improving their vision are matters that may cause anxiety. It is known that there is little support for patients during this crucial period of waiting (Rose 1997).

Nurses will need to spend time with patients to ensure there is a clear understanding of the condition, about the pending surgery and the pre- and postoperative management. McBride (2000) found that many patients leave consultations anxious and upset and not fully understanding their condition or the treatment for it. In light of these findings, the consultation should take place in a quiet place and privacy must be assured. Materials to support this health education activity should include models or diagrams, and written (in suitable letter size and appropriate language) or taped information to back up what is said. This is because patients are likely to find the visit to hospital stressful.

Details of social circumstances will assist nurses in determining, along with patients, what (if any) support services will be needed postoperatively. Nurses should ascertain the following:

- availability of transport to and from hospital on the day of surgery and subsequent appointments
- whether there is a telephone at home for use in an emergency
- whether patients can instil their own drops, or if there is someone available to do this if necessary
- whether a district nurse will be needed to assist with drop instillation
- whether a social worker review is required.

Immediate preoperative care and management in the theatre

Patients will usually arrive an hour before their allocated time for surgery, unless they are in-patients and have been admitted the day before surgery. They should be greeted by the nurse and shown to their bed or chair. A name bracelet will be applied, to ensure that they undergo the correct surgery. The consent form will be checked.

The detailed nursing assessment undertaken previously will be confirmed and any changes to health status noted. Vital signs will be taken and recorded.

Patients will have fasted according to local protocols (see Ch. 29). The nurse should check that they have taken their usual medication, bringing any changes to the attention of medical staff.

Also dependent on local practice, patients may be given a theatre gown to wear. Increasingly, in some units, patients wear their own clothing. They will have been asked to wear loose clothing so that staff in theatre can apply monitoring equipment.

Special consideration will be given to patients with diabetes, who will have their blood glucose monitored hourly.

Insulin-dependent diabetics will have been advised about how much insulin they should take on the day of surgery. Patients having anticoagulant therapy should normally have an INR of 2 or below (see Ch. 18).

In order to expedite discharge following surgery, postoperative medication will be prescribed and the prescription sent to pharmacy.

All patients will have the eye to be operated on marked, which is usually done by the medical staff. This is to ensure that the correct eye is operated upon. In addition, the identity of individual patients is also checked against their name band and the notes/prescription.

Pupillary dilation is essential prior to cataract extraction in order to facilitate the surgery. This is usually achieved by the instillation of short-acting mydriatics and cycloplegics such as G. cyclopentolate 1%. Within 1.5 hours, pupil dilation and cycloplegia are obtained. This is sometimes used in conjunction with G. phenylephrine 2.5%, a powerful mydriatic. One drop of each is instilled every 15 minutes, on three occasions. Alternatively, G. tropicamide is instilled. Some units give these drops to patients to begin to use at home before they come to the hospital. Patients should be warned that the drops have the effect of reducing vision whilst increasing sensitivity to light. Like most drops, they sting when they are instilled.

If patients wear glasses or a hearing aid, these should be worn to the operating department so that they can see and hear what is going on. The glasses will, of course, be removed during the surgery, but it may be possible to retain the hearing aid, thus allowing patients to respond to requests during surgery.

In order that they are comfortable during the operation, patients should be given the opportunity to void urine before transfer to the operating department.

During the operative phase and with local anaesthetic, a nurse will stay with patients at all times. Their role is to monitor patients' vital signs and to hold their hand in order to provide both comfort and a means for them to communicate anxieties to the staff. The local anaesthetic will be given in the anaesthetic room (see Special Issues box 15.2).

It is important for patients to know that during ocular surgery, their head and face will be draped with sterile towels, leaving only the eye that is to be operated on exposed. Oxygen or air is circulated under the drapes to help prevent feelings of claustrophobia. It is normal to monitor ECG and oxygen saturation during the operation.

At the end of surgery, a clear cartella shield will be placed over the eye to protect it from accidental injury.

Immediate postoperative care

Nurses will receive a handover report from the theatre nurse outlining the procedure, any complications that may have occurred and giving any specific instructions about postoperative care (although some units operate a system of continuity of care whereby nurses follow patients throughout their hospital visit).

On return to the ward or day-case unit, patients are likely to be feeling tired, fatigued and yet relieved that the operation is over. They need to be allowed to rest, e.g. in bed or in a reclining chair. Some units will only have reclining chairs; this should be a consideration during the preoperative assessment.

SPECIAL ISSUES

15.2 Local anaesthesia for cataract surgery

This is usually given as sub-Tenon's membrane (outer fascia of the eyeball – from the corneoscleral junction to the optic nerve) injection or as a peribulbar injection. The eye will first of all have local anaesthetic drops instilled. The lids will then be cleaned with aqueous povidone-iodine solution (having established that the patient is not allergic to iodine). The anaesthetic will then be introduced through a conjunctival incision via a blunt, angled needle. This will have the effect of numbing and immobilizing the eye as well as rendering it sightless. This effect is only temporary and the patient should be advised that it usually wears off after a few hours.

Many nurses are now becoming involved in expanded roles; sub-Tenon's anaesthetic is one such. Nurses who perform this role feel it provides patients with an improved quality of care, as they are able to spend more time with them. Their medical colleagues who have previously performed this task are usually in a hurry between cases.

Student activities
- Do patients in your area have access to a specialist ophthalmic nurse?
- Find out what other expanded roles are undertaken by specialist ophthalmic nurses.
- Search the literature for research that supports the view that expanded roles for specialist nurses improve the experience of patients.

Patients having general anaesthesia will need longer to recover and will require the standard monitoring of any patient having this type of anaesthetic, including ensuring they have passed urine prior to discharge (see Ch. 29).

Having fasted before and during surgery, patients will welcome a drink and a light snack at this point. Blood pressure and pulse will be recorded and should be within normal limits prior to discharge.

The cartella shield will remain in place for the first 24 hours, after which it should be worn only at night for 2 weeks, to prevent inadvertent injury. If a patient were to rub the eye, it could cause iris prolapse, something that will usually result in further corrective surgery. The shield should be washed in hot soapy water and stored dry between uses. It should be fixed in place with tape.

Pain management is important. As patients return to the unit, the local anaesthetic is likely to still be having some effect but this does not mean that they will not be experiencing some pain or discomfort. For example, immobility during surgery could cause arthritic joints to become sore and stiff; or patients may begin to experience breakthrough pain. In any case, nurses should ask patients whether they are experiencing pain or discomfort. It is helpful to use a verbal analogue scale (see Ch. 7). This is because it does not require vision to see a scale and it also provides an objective means for determining the effectiveness of

medication. As ocular pain, sometimes associated with nausea, could be indicative of raised IOP, it is vital to get accurate information from patients as to the exact nature of the pain and where the pain is coming from, as it may or may not relate to the eye. If nausea and/or vomiting persist, the IOP should be checked. If the IOP is high, oral acetazolamide (a carbonic anhydrase inhibitor – see Table 15.1, p. 345) may be prescribed and it may be necessary to administer a prescribed antiemetic. Paracetamol should be sufficient to relieve the pain and discomfort experienced following cataract surgery, although many patients experience no pain or discomfort postoperatively.

Patients should be encouraged and enabled to mobilize within their own limits as soon as they feel able. Initially, they may require some assistance, especially if their vision in the eye not operated on is poor. The local anaesthetic injection to the operated eye will prevent that eye from seeing. In addition, patients will be in unfamiliar surroundings. For these reasons, patients should be provided with a call bell.

Discharge education and instructions
- Education regarding drop instillation – the importance of following the prescription, to include name, purpose and frequency and duration of administration; storage and side-effects; how to obtain further supplies. Check ability to instil drops, including the use of appropriate drop aids, or the need for assistance of the district nurse.
- Cleaning the eye, and cartella shield wear and storage.
- Return to usual activities, including light work after 24 hours. Driving activity can be resumed when advised by the consultant team.
- Recognizing signs and symptoms of complications. Contact the hospital if vision deteriorates, flashing lights are experienced, there is pain that is not relieved with usual analgesia, discharge from the eye and an allergic reaction to the drops (usually presents as pink irritable eyelids).
- Where appropriate, district nurse referral.
- Follow-up appointment.
- Letter to general practitioner.
- Take home medication. Following cataract extraction this usually includes an anti-inflammatory drop containing an antibiotic, e.g. G. betamethasone (a corticosteroid) combined with the antibiotic neomycin. In addition, a cycloplegic may also be prescribed to prevent ciliary spasm; this is likely to be G. cyclopentolate twice daily and should be stored in a refrigerator between uses. The aim is to prescribe as uncomplicated a drop regimen as possible to improve patient concordance.
- Written discharge instructions, including a contact number to use in an emergency. The instructions should be clear and simple, Ariel font size 16 pt.

Some centres will see patients the following day and perform the first dressing, and examine the eye. Such patients then have a final follow-up at 3 weeks. Others recall the patient at 3 weeks, the first dressing being undertaken by patients themselves or the appointed carer. At 3 weeks, the examination includes determining patient progress, visual acuity measurement, IOP check, and review of anterior chamber activity and the retina. These reviews could be undertaken by a specialist ophthalmic nurse or the ophthalmologist. At this visit, arrangements could be made for the other eye to be operated on. In addition, patients are advised to visit their optometrist to have necessary corrective spectacle lens or lenses prescribed.

Patients should normally expect some improvement with their vision within a few hours of surgery, but it may take a few weeks before the vision settles. This is why they are not encouraged to get new glasses for at least 1 month.

Nursing management in the community
Buckingham et al (1997) suggest that postoperative cataract patients form a small and yet significant part of the district nurse's caseload. District nurse support to the patient at home or in other community settings can be crucial to achieving a satisfactory postoperative outcome. To do this, the district nurse needs to receive adequate information from the referring nurse, including detail of the treatment needed as well as accurate detail about what education and support have already been given.

DIABETIC RETINOPATHY

Diabetes mellitus (see Ch. 17) is a leading cause of blindness in people below the age of 60. Diabetic retinopathy (DR – retinal disease caused by diabetes) occurs more frequently in type 1 diabetics (40%) but it is also seen in patients with type 2 diabetes (20%) (Kanski 1999).

Aetiology
According to Kanski (1999), there are clearly identifiable risk factors for diabetic retinopathy:

- how long the patient has had diabetes
- poor glycaemic diabetic control (see Ch. 17); good glycaemic control can slow the progress of the condition
- other factors adversely affecting the condition include pregnancy, systemic hypertension and renal disease.

Specific investigations and screening
Patients will have their eyes examined and visual acuity tested, and fluorescein angiography will be performed. Those with diabetes will need an annual sight check, including examination of the retina through a dilated pupil.

Pathophysiology and management
It is suggested that there are three stages of DR: background retinopathy, pre-proliferative diabetic retinopathy and proliferative diabetic retinopathy.

Background retinopathy
Background retinopathy occurs about 10 years after the onset of diabetes. This stage is usually asymptomatic. Changes occur in the retinal blood vessels that result in retinal ischaemia and hypoxia. Microaneurysms develop and small dot and blot haemorrhages. In addition, changes occur in the walls of the retinal vessels that allow fluid leakage, leading to retinal oedema. Exudates also leak out of the vessels. Vision is put at risk as the macula (maculopathy) becomes involved (Kanski 1999). Microvascular changes will eventually lead to the formation of new vessels. Fluorescein angiography is used to highlight the extent of the retinal changes. Treatment involves laser photocoagulation, which effectively seals leaky blood vessels and destroys parts of the retina to prevent further changes occurring in those parts.

Laser treatment can be painful for some patients and peribulbar injection may be necessary. They will need to be adequately prepared for the treatment, including giving informed consent. Topical anaesthetics such as G. oxybuprocaine are usually administered in order to gain patient cooperation and facilitate the procedure. Some patients do seem to experience marked discomfort (photophobia) during laser treatment whilst others do not. Some centres use inhaled Entonox as an analgesic agent. This has allowed the laser operator to do a more thorough job and reduce the number of return visits for treatment.

Pre-proliferative diabetic retinopathy
In pre-proliferative retinopathy, the vascular changes become more pronounced. The vessels 'bead' and 'loop'. Infarctions can be seen on the retina as dark blot haemorrhages and cotton-wool spots become visible (Kanski 1999). Such patients require close monitoring and support.

Proliferative diabetic retinopathy (see Fig. 15.12A)
There is growth of new leaky blood vessels (neovascularization) that can cause the vitreous to detach and also haemorrhage into the vitreous. These lead to scar tissue formation, and the traction resulting from the scarring pulls at the retina, causing it to tear or detach.

The new vessels will be treated with laser. Again, analgesia and reassurance are essential features to the success of the treatment. If the haemorrhages are severe enough, surgery may be indicated, requiring a pars plana vitrectomy to remove vitreous gel that is providing the scaffolding on which the new vessels depend. Eventually, the retina itself may become detached, requiring surgery to re-attach it (Kanski 1999).

▶ Nursing management
Nurses will provide explanation and ongoing support for patients having investigations and laser therapies or surgery as outlined above. It is important for nurses to stress the importance of annual sight screening, and the benefits of good glycaemic control in halting the progression of DR. This is the role of the ophthalmic nurse in some centres and usually in collaboration with the diabetic nurse specialists.

The loss of vision is obviously of major importance to patients and their families. The extent of the loss will vary depending upon the structures affected. With maculopathy, for example, central vision becomes gradually worse. This can affect the ability to see faces at a distance, and reading can become problematic, as fine print is difficult to see. In proliferative DR, the bleeding into the vitreous causes patchy blurring of vision (see Fig. 15.12B). Untreated, the eyesight could be lost altogether.

The reduction in visual acuity can affect patients' ability to manage self-blood glucose monitoring and insulin injections. The diabetes specialist nurse should be consulted regarding alternative ways of delivering insulin. The reduced vision and

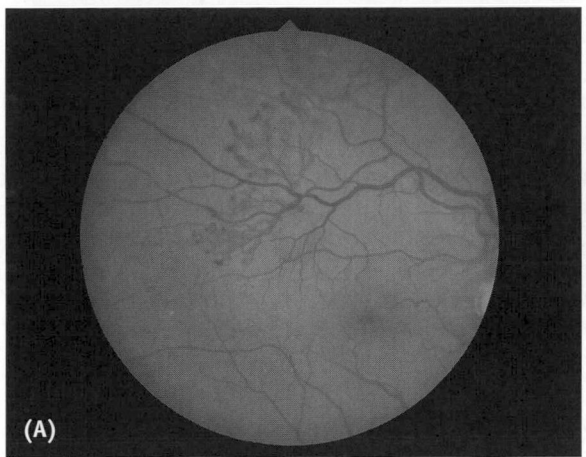

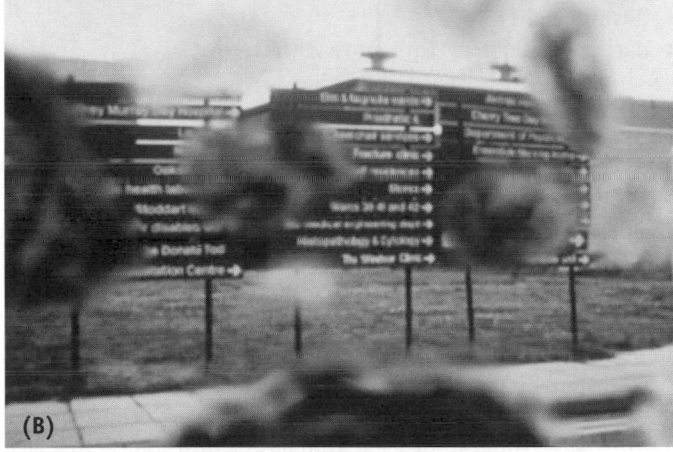

Figure 15.12 Diabetic retinopathy. (A) Proliferative diabetic retinopathy – showing area of new retinal vessels. (Reproduced with kind permission from Kanski 1999.) (B) Simulation of patchy vision loss. (Reproduced with kind permission from RNIB.)

the impact this has on patients and their lifestyle must be considered, e.g.:

- relationships with family and friends
- ease of travelling, whether you drive or use public transport
- the ability to work
- the ability to manage domestic activities in and around the home
- impact on non-verbal communication if unable to see other people's faces
- leisure activities such as visiting the cinema, playing ball games or running.

The nursing support for patients with vision loss is covered in detail in the section on visual impairment (see pp. 342–344).

AGE-RELATED MACULAR DEGENERATION

Age-related macular degeneration (AMD) is a leading cause of blindness in people aged over 50. The aetiology is unknown. A lack of awareness of AMD and its treatment leads to considerable and unnecessary loss of sight (Murphy 2002).

Pathophysiology, presentation and management

Age-related macular degeneration takes two forms: dry (the most common) and wet. AMD affects the macula lutea located at the central posterior part of the retina, an area necessary for reading and seeing fine features such as faces. Unfortunately patients may not be aware of having a problem and may not seek advice until the degeneration is well advanced.

Dry or atrophic AMD

With age, Bruch's membrane (between the underlying retinal blood vessels and the retina) begins to accumulate debris, including some that can be seen on retinal examination, called drusen (yellow deposits). In time the accumulated debris interferes with the transfer of nutrients, which may eventually result in degeneration of retinal macula cells. This causes central vision to deteriorate (see Fig. 15.13, p. 354) and leads, for example, to blurring when reading newsprint; in addition, patients describe photophobia, flashing lights, poor colour vision and visual hallucinations (see p. 342). Whilst the degenerative process occurs over a period of time, it is usually diagnosed in people aged 55–60 (York et al 2000).

Currently there are no laser treatments for dry AMD (RNIB 2002a); however, patients can be helped to maximize residual vision with, for example, low vision aids.

Wet or disciform AMD

Occasionally, the blood vessels grow into Bruch's membrane between the retina and the underlying blood vessels. It is the body's way of reversing the problems with nutrition to the retina. But these new vessels are leaky and allow fluid/blood to leak out causing a 'blister' to develop. This makes the macular uneven which distorts the central vision. The progress of this condition can be fast. Medical treatment is aimed at plugging the leaks and yet conserving the overlying retina (York et al 2000).

There is some treatment available for wet AMD, such as limited thermal laser photocoagulation to seal leaky vessels. However, some treatments, such as photodynamic therapy (PDT) using cold lasers and photosensitive drugs, are expensive and many health providers will not fund this treatment.

> ▶ **Nursing management**

The focus is on education aimed at raising awareness of AMD and early detection in addition to the support of patients during investigations and after diagnosis:

- Education – regular eye tests every 2 years for those over 50, information about AMD and treatments. Encouraging patients to seek help if their vision changes between routine tests.
- Screening and investigations – use of a special Amsler grid; patients who report blurring, wavy or distorted lines or absent areas are referred for examination by an ophthalmologist and sometimes a fluorescein angiography.
- According to Murphy (2002), patients with AMD often give easily missed clues, such as not being able to pour fluids into a glass or cup accurately. This emphasizes the

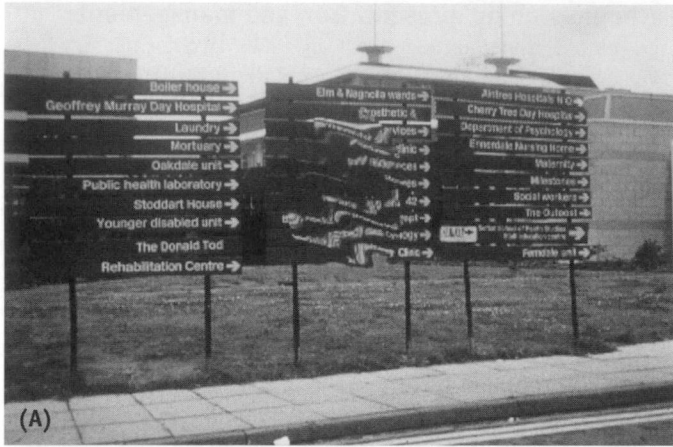

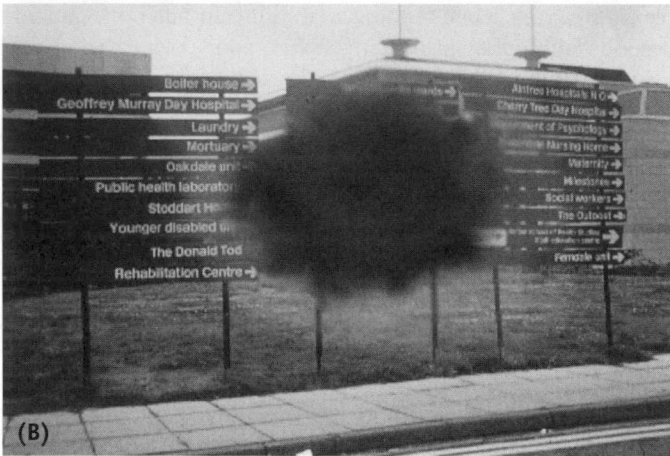

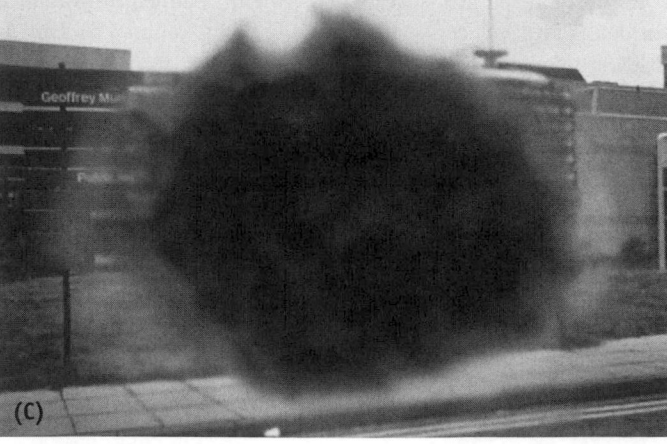

Figure 15.13 Simulation of vision changes in age-related macular degeneration. (A) Early changes including distorted central vision. (B) Later – central vision lost. (C) Typical 'big black blob' in middle of vision. Peripheral vision is retained. (Reproduced with kind permission from RNIB.)

importance of finding out about vision during every nursing assessment.
- Support during diagnosis and treatment.
- Advice about ongoing support and help to maximize residual vision (see section on 'Visual impairment', pp. 342–344).

RETINAL DETACHMENT

This is when the neural retina becomes separated from the retinal pigment epithelium. There are two major classifications relating to whether or not a hole is present in the retina:

- When a hole is present, it is referred to as rhegmatogenous – causes include myopia, after cataract extraction, trauma such as a blow to the head and age-related degeneration of the retina.
- When there is no hole, it is referred to as non-rhegmatogenous – causes include diabetes, tumours and inflammation.

Clinical presentation
Symptoms include:

- a shadow or curtain in the field of vision
- flashing lights
- dark spots (floaters) that move with the eye.

Medical/surgical management
Prompt treatment is essential but if the macula lutea is affected, the central vision could be lost permanently. Retinal detachment involving the area containing the macula lutea is treated as an emergency admission with surgery on the day of admission or the following day. Frequently patients are required to adopt a position or 'posture' of the head postoperatively in order to prevent further damage. Preparation for surgery will include dilation of the pupil so that the interior of the eye can be viewed.

Occasionally gas and/or air are injected into the eye during the operation to ensure that the retinal layers stay together (tamponade). Air is absorbed within days whilst some gases take weeks. Patients should not fly whilst they have a gas bubble in their eye. They must seek advice from their ophthalmologist. Silicone oils are sometimes used for the same reason and this has the effect of distorting vision. The oil will need to be removed at some point in the future.

Some types of surgery for retinal detachment do not require postoperative posturing, e.g. when the detachment is repaired with cryotherapy (intense cold) and an encircling band. Other types of retinal detachment may be less urgent and so admission can be planned.

Some retinal holes can be sealed with an argon laser in the outpatient department. This is usually performed under local anaesthesia.

▶ Nursing management

Patients admitted as an emergency are bound to have fears and anxieties, not just in relation to their visual prognosis, but also about arrangements for home or work.

Depending on the type of surgery, the ophthalmologist will have given patients information about the need for postoperative posturing. If the macula is at risk, for example, the likely posture will be 'face down'. This requires patients to gaze downwards for anything from 50 minutes per hour to the whole time. This does not mean patients will have to stay in bed: they can be shown many variations to relieve the discomfort and boredom. In addition, equipment may be available to relieve discomfort. Nurses have an important part to play in helping patients overcome the complications of this regimen.

Patients need to know that pain and, in some cases, nausea and vomiting are not uncommon postoperatively. They need reassurance that relevant medication will be given in a timely manner.

Patients will normally only be in hospital for two days so it is important to ensure adequate arrangements are made for discharge home.

PRIMARY OPEN-ANGLE GLAUCOMA

There are many types of glaucoma, including primary open-angle glaucoma (POAG) and primary closed-angle glaucoma (see p. 357). POAG is a chronic condition, whereas primary closed-angle glaucoma generally presents as an acute condition. Both can result in loss of vision if they remain untreated, but the diagnosis and treatment of each are quite different.

Aetiology and epidemiology

Glaucoma is said to occur when the intraocular pressure (IOP) is high enough to cause damage to the optic nerve (see Fig. 15.14A) at the point it leaves the eye and subsequently disrupts the visual

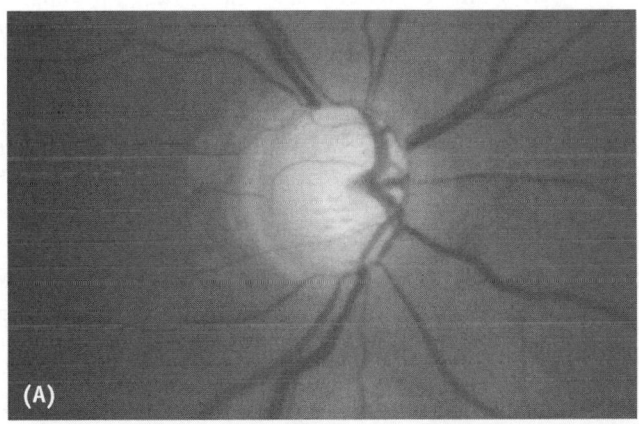

(A)

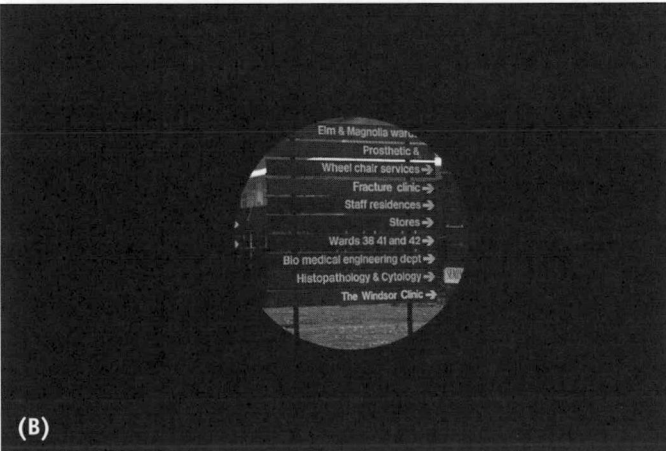

(B)

Figure 15.14 Glaucoma. (A) Retinal changes with cupping in end-stage glaucoma. Note how the blood vessels at the optic disc are displaced. (Reproduced with kind permission from Kanski 1999.) (B) Simulation of 'tunnel vision'. (Reproduced with kind permission from RNIB.)

field (Kanski 1990, Pavan-Langston 1996). It is a major cause of irreversible blindness in the UK and the USA. In the UK, glaucoma affects approximately 2 in every 100 people aged over 40 (Kanski et al 1996).

POAG causes bilateral painless sight loss in middle-aged and older people. It is primarily because the onset is insidious. Very often it is only detected when patients visit their optometrist for a routine sight test. It is estimated that in the UK alone that there are 250 000 cases of POAG but that only half have been detected (IGA 2002).

The exact cause of POAG is not fully understood but there are some recognized risk factors. It is known that people with a close relative who has glaucoma and African Caribbean individuals are at a higher risk of developing the condition.

The risk factors include (American Academy of Ophthalmology 1997b):

- level of increased IOP
- family history of condition
- race
- increasing age.

Associated disorders include (American Academy of Ophthalmology 1997b).

- hypertension
- myopia
- diabetes mellitus
- central retinal vein occlusion.

Clinical presentation

The onset of POAG is insidious, progressing slowly and painlessly. Central vision remains intact and so patients fail to notice the peripheral loss of vision –'tunnel vision' (see Fig. 15.14B). Occasionally patients get involved in scrapes and bumps because of visual field loss, but they fail to act, as they attribute this to 'old age'.

Specific investigations

Investigations that will be undertaken to aid diagnosis are:

- visual acuity
- perimetry
- ophthalmoscopy
- tonometry
- gonioscopy.

Medical/surgical management

Treatment is usually medical and the goal is to reduce the flow of aqueous humour and/or improve its outflow. It depends heavily on the patient. Patients have to agree with the diagnosis, recognize that the condition will progressively worsen if the treatment regimen is not followed, and that the subsequent damage will have a marked impact on lifestyle (see Reflective Practice box 15.3). Surgery is not usually a primary treatment for POAG but may be considered at a later stage if patients do not respond to medical treatment, e.g. trabeculectomy (creating new drainage channels – see p. 356) or the insertion of a drainage valve.

There are several types of drugs in the form of drops used in the treatment of POAG, but they are not without their side-effects.

15.3 Primary open-angle glaucoma (POAG)

Imagine what it may be like to be told you have POAG. You are an active adult who enjoys work and recreational activities. You drive and are enjoying life at the moment. You have not noticed a problem with your eyes but a routine medical resulted in your referral to an ophthalmologist. You have been told that you must now put drops in your eye twice a day for the rest of your life, otherwise you will eventually go blind.

- What is your initial reaction?
- How easy will it be for you to comply with the drop treatment?
- How will you explain things to your family and your employer? Indeed, will you tell them at all?
- Will you find it easy to attend for follow-up appointments?

The goal of medical management is to optimize IOP control and at the same time ensure that side-effects are minimal. As the treatment is very much dependent on patients complying with the therapy, such treatment should have only minimal effect on their lifestyle.

An example of a treatment regimen is G. betaxolol hydrochloride 0.5% twice daily. This is a beta-blocker and it decreases IOP by reducing the flow of aqueous humour. Systemic side-effects are minimized by asking patients to close their eye gently and count slowly to 60 after instilling the drops. The intention is to control the IOP using as few drugs as possible as this will improve patient compliance with treatment. Treatment with eye drops will be for life unless surgery is indicated. Caution should be used if patients have breathing problems such as asthma or obstructive airways disease, as beta-blockers can induce bronchospasm, in which case alternative treatments will be prescribed.

Alternative or adjunct therapies include sympathomimetics such as G. brimonidine tartrate 0.2% twice daily, which may be used in conjunction with a beta-blocker. Carbonic anhydrase inhibitors such as G. brinzolamide or G. dorzolamide may be used. Many of these drops sting on instillation or have unwelcome side-effects, such as changing the colour of the pupil, and foul breath, which could influence patient compliance with treatment. Occasionally patients may be prescribed oral acetazolamide. This is usually prescribed for short-term use. It is a sulphonamide and has the effect of lowering IOP by reducing the production of aqueous humour. There are some unwelcome side-effects, including nausea, taste disturbance, headache and fatigue.

Some patients may be prescribed G. pilocarpine 2% or 4%. This is a miotic and makes the pupil small and not reactive to light and dark stimulus. Such patients should be advised to take care when entering a darkened area as they will need time to adjust to the light conditions. This is because the pupil will not dilate to allow more light to enter the eye. Prostaglandin analogues, e.g. latanoprost, may be prescribed when patients cannot have other drugs.

Further drug information is outlined in Table 15.1 (pp. 344–345). Readers requiring more details about the drugs used in glaucoma are advised to consult a national formulary such as the BNF (www.bnf.org.uk).

Once a diagnosis of POAG has been made, patients will have to make a few adjustments to their lifestyle, not just adapting to the routine of instilling drops. For example, if they drive, the Vehicle Licensing Authority and their insurance company will have to be told. With a particular level of visual field loss, they may no longer be allowed to drive. The consultant ophthalmologist will advise patients on this. They work to specific guidelines relating to the actual visual acuity (wearing glasses) and degree of visual field loss.

Follow-up appointments must be made. Initially, patients may be seen monthly until their condition becomes stable. Then they will be seen every 3 months, but as the condition stabilizes it may be possible to make appointments that are less frequent. Many follow-up clinic appointments may be to see a nurse practitioner who is specially trained to support patients with POAG. This has the effect of freeing up the consultant to see new patients, but also provides continuity for current patients, as they are likely to see the same person on each visit.

In the event that the POAG is not well controlled (reduction in IOP) by medication or laser therapy, and there continues to be progressive changes to the optic disc or visual fields, surgery may be considered. The surgery is likely to be trabeculectomy (new channels are created to improve the drainage of aqueous humour and reduce IOP), combined with phacoemulsification of the lens (see p. 349). This can be undertaken as a day case or, where circumstance dictates, as an in-patient.

▶ Nursing management

Nurses will need to prepare and support patients through the investigations to establish the diagnosis. POAG will result in patients having some degree of visual field loss. This could cause them to knock into furniture or doors, especially in unfamiliar surroundings. They should be supported in finding their way around the unit and yet not have their independence taken from them.

It is known that IOP fluctuates throughout the day (American Academy of Ophthalmology 1997b) so a one-off measurement is to be viewed with some caution. Patients are occasionally requested to attend hospital for several hours so that their IOP can be measured at different times. This is known as 'phasing'. The nurse should give patients an explanation of what will be required of them during the time they are attending the hospital. This is in order to gain their consent and cooperation. In addition, patients may feel at a loose end between tests. Whilst they are attending for 'phasing', facilities should be provided for patients to obtain snacks and drinks. They can usually leave the hospital between tests if they so wish.

Nursing interventions in POAG should be aimed at supporting patients in making appropriate choices with regard to their care, as follows:

- Explanation of the condition, including the nature of the irreversible visual loss and how further loss can be avoided, must be included.

- Nurses have a vital role in educating patients about drug treatment (which will be for life) including drop administration technique (see pp. 344, 346–348). Many drugs used to treat POAG have unwanted side-effects, but the aim is to try to minimize these effects through patient education.
- Education should be supported with appropriate materials such as models and diagrams. Information leaflets/booklets should be provided and in the language and format most accessible for patients.
- Patients should be referred to appropriate agencies, both statutory and voluntary, such as social services and the International Glaucoma Association (IGA).
- The importance of attending for follow-up should be stressed.

Caring for the patient having surgery

When medical treatments have not controlled POAG and surgery is to take place, patients will have a preoperative assessment. This follows a similar path to the cataract assessment but with the inclusion of detail about the trabeculectomy. Routine tests prior to local or general anaesthetic will be undertaken.

Care immediately pre- and postoperatively should be as per post cataract extraction, but dilating drops *must not* be instilled into the eye preoperatively.

The surgery involves the formation of a bleb under the conjunctiva. This is visible to the naked eye as a bulge under the conjunctiva and should be observed at first dressing. The anterior chamber (A/C) should be formed but not flat, which can be checked by shining a torch onto the front of the eye and viewing the eye from the temporal side, noting the depth. A flat A/C is indicative of the bleb draining too freely. A pad and firm bandage should be applied to seal the bleb. Care must be taken to ensure the eyelids are closed under the pad, and patients should be advised to keep them closed and a double pad used in order to prevent accidental damage to the cornea.

Postoperatively, drops will be prescribed for use in the operated eye only, to prevent infection and inflammation and to rest the eye. The other eye should be treated as before. It should be noted that patients could be having as many as five or six different types of drops and this can lead to errors.

A typical example of postoperative medication for the operated eye is as follows:

- G. prednisolone four times daily
- G. chloramphenicol four times daily
- G. atropine twice daily.

Following discharge, patients may need the assistance of a district nurse to ensure the drops are instilled. They will have been using drops previously, but reassessment of need could highlight difficulties. Specific instructions will need to be in a format that patients can use easily.

PAINFUL OCULAR CONDITIONS AND TRAUMA

PRIMARY CLOSED-ANGLE GLAUCOMA

Primary closed-angle glaucoma (PCAG) is an acute condition characterized by an elevated IOP (as high as 70 mmHg). The normal outflow for aqueous humour is blocked because of partial or complete closure of the drainage angle. It is usually unilateral (Kanski et al 1999).

Aetiology

The condition affects middle-aged and older people. The incidence in females is four times greater than that in males. Another factor associated with PCAG is race, it being common in people from South-east Asia and Eskimos, yet rare in Africans. The latter group, it should be noted, may not experience the same level of pain as others and so damage to the optic nerve and blood supply could be more advanced at diagnosis (Kanski et al 1996).

Clinical presentation

Patients present with severe pain around one eye. The eye is typically red and the pupil is oval and semi-dilated. Visual acuity is reduced and patients are intolerant of light (photophobic). They may also complain of seeing halos around lights. This is because of corneal congestion. Occasionally, patients may experience nausea and vomiting. They will be feeling generally unwell (Kanski et al 1996). PCAG is a medical emergency as the raised IOP can cause permanent damage and loss of vision.

Medical management

Management is aimed at urgent reduction of IOP and relief of symptoms. The examination of the eye will include visual acuity and IOP measurement. The drugs used will include:

- slow i.v. infusion of mannitol (osmotic diuretic) to reduce IOP
- i.v. acetazolamide to reduce aqueous humour production
- analgesia and antiemetic, also given i.v.
- G. pilocarpine 2% to the affected eye to open the drainage angle, and G. pilocarpine 1% to the unaffected eye prophylactically
- G. levobunolol hydrochloride or similar beta-blocker twice daily (unless contraindicated, see p. 345) with corticosteroids four times a day (Kanski et al 1996).

Laser iridotomy to both eyes is usually performed the following day when the eye has settled. A laser is used to make a hole in the iris, thereby allowing aqueous humour to flow from the posterior chamber to the anterior chamber, from where it drains through the canal of Schlemm (see Fig. 15.3, p. 334). The pupil is constricted with drugs prior to laser iridotomy, which is performed after the front of the eye has been anaesthetized.

▶ Nursing management

The specific nursing management will focus on providing information and reassurance, relief of symptoms and preparation for laser iridotomy, and will include the following:

- explanations about treatment and care
- a quiet darkened room to aid pain relief
- a vomit bowl for patients; tissues and water to drink, and mouthwashes and facilities to brush their teeth after vomiting
- maintaining a record of fluid balance

- administration of prescribed i.v. drugs or assistance in giving them; observation of the cannula site for signs of inflammation
- administration of prescribed analgesia and antiemetic drugs as required and monitoring of effects
- instillation of prescribed ophthalmic medication
- diet and fluids to be offered as tolerated.

Preparing patients for laser iridotomy will include ensuring that they have fully understood the explanation given by the ophthalmologist. Nurses should check the consent form has been completed. Most importantly, nurses will need to reassure patients that local anaesthetic eye drops such as G. oxybupro-caine will be used, that they will feel very little during the procedure and that a nurse will be with them throughout; this will improve compliance. This is usually done in the outpatient or retinal department.

Complications include bleeding and raised IOP. The IOP will be checked following the procedure to ensure it is not elevated.

Despite patients coming in quite unwell, if they respond to treatment they may be discharged home the day after the laser iridotomy.

Topical anti-inflammatory drops will be prescribed post-procedure, such as G. prednisolone four times daily for 1 week. It is not necessary for patients to continue with their glaucoma medications, as this is an acute condition. An outpatient follow-up appointment will be given for 2 weeks' time, or sooner if symptoms return.

ENUCLEATION

This is the removal from the orbit of the eye and part of the optic nerve. It may be performed for the following:

- severe damage to the eyeball
- to prevent sympathetic endophthalmitis (severe inflammation of the other eye, which can occur weeks or even years after an eye injury)
- painful blind eye
- disfigurement and a painless blind eye
- intraocular tumour (rare in adults; readers requiring more information are advised to consult an ophthalmology text [see 'Further reading', p. 365, Kanski 1999]).

If patients have been in pain for some time, or disfigured, they may welcome the surgery; however, patients with trauma to the eye not only have that incident to contend with, but they also have to think about losing the eye as well. The former will have had time to begin to make adjustments. Likewise, those with an intraocular tumour also have to deal with a diagnosis of cancer (see Ch. 33).

There is little written about the impact of loss of an eye, but issues relating to body image and grieving require some consideration.

Before surgery, patients should be given the opportunity to speak to an ocular prosthetic team. The development of implants to support the artificial eye has meant that good cosmetic results are possible. The problem is that the process takes time, up to 3–6 months.

Patients need to be aware of the complications of this type of surgery:

- haemorrhage
- infection
- ptosis (drooping eyelid, see p. 363) because of loss of orbital volume
- entropion or ectropion (see p. 364), lid laxity
- problems with muscle motility affecting movement of the prosthesis
- conjunctival deficiency that can be rectified with mucous graft
- tear deficiency
- expulsion of the implant
- inflammation of the orbit.

The surgery can be performed under local or general anaesthetic. This is a matter that will be discussed with the surgeon.

▶ Nursing management

Standard preoperative preparation is required and additionally the head of the bed should be inclined at 45°. Patients are given information about the management of postoperative pain, nausea and vomiting (a feature of enucleation surgery with baseball implant of acrylic and hydroxyapatite implants made from coral).

Immediately postoperatively, there will be a pressure dressing of a pad and bandage that will remain untouched for 1 week. Pain should be managed with appropriate analgesia. Nausea and vomiting should also be prevented with appropriate anti-emetics given prophylactically. The dressing should be observed for signs of haemorrhage. It is important to examine the back of the neck/pillows in case bleeding is trickling behind the dressing.

Psychological support is essential in the ensuing days and weeks. Patients may, for example, be introduced to others who have had enucleation surgery previously. They will also need to be taught to control their pain effectively at home. There are some support groups that patients can be put in touch with.

The first dressing will be done on an outpatient basis, usually by a specialist nurse. Patients may or may not want to look at their face straight away. The first dressing can be an uncomfortable experience for patients and it may be necessary for them to be given analgesia first.

A conformer, to maintain the shape of the socket, will sometimes be in place. Patients will be shown how to remove and insert this, and how to keep it clean by using hot soapy water and thoroughly drying it afterwards.

This and subsequent visits will include seeing the prosthetic team. Over the next few weeks the implant will be prepared ready to accept the artificial eye.

When a patient with an artificial eye attends the A&E department or is admitted to hospital with a non-ophthalmic condition, the nurse should ascertain whether the eye needs any specific care and provide facilities or assist as necessary. Where patients are unable to communicate their needs, nurses should seek advice from a specialist nurse.

CORNEAL DISORDERS – AN OVERVIEW

The outer epithelial layer of the cornea can heal without scarring, but damage to the deeper layers can result in permanent scarring. Damage to the inner lining, the endothelium, will lead to corneal oedema. Disorders of the cornea include injury, infection, degeneration, congenital and nutritional disorders. It is worth noting that any corneal disorder has the capacity to cause corneal oedema, ulcers, opacities or perforation.

When the cornea becomes traumatized or diseased, it can result in the following signs and symptoms:

- pain
- photophobia
- excess lacrimation (tearing)
- blepharospasm (eyelid spasm)
- ciliary injection – blood vessels at the corneal margin become inflamed
- miosis (small/constricted pupils associated with iris sphincter muscle spasm), reduced vision
- discharge, e.g. green or yellow pus.

CORNEAL ULCERS

There are many types of corneal ulcer. This section will deal specifically with corneal ulcers severe enough to result in hospital admission. Most patients with a corneal ulcer will have their care and treatment managed in the community independently or with help and support from the practice/community nurse or GP. If patients are at risk of corneal perforation, they will be admitted to hospital for intensive treatment. In addition, if there is a need for intensive drop therapy and patients are not able to instil their own drops, or home support is not available, admission to hospital is indicated.

Aetiology

Corneal ulcers may be caused by bacterial (*Staphylococcus aureus* or *Pseudomonas aeruginosa*), viral (e.g. herpes zoster ophthalmicus) or fungal infection. In addition, they may be the result of allergy. The nature of the ulcer, its shape and the associated medical and ocular history can give clues as to the cause. Overuse of contact lenses is a frequent cause of corneal ulcers.

Specific investigations

It is often necessary to identify the causative organism in order to ensure the correct treatment. One way this is done is by scraping cells off the cornea with a special instrument (by a specialist practitioner), after the instillation of short-acting local anaesthetic drops. The cells are put onto a culture plate and then sent to the laboratory for culture and sensitivity.

Medical management

Whether or not they are admitted to hospital, patients will require some analgesia (e.g. paracetamol or co-codamol) to relieve pain. The intensity of the ocular pain can be quite debilitating for patients; it may even disturb sleep. Topical analgesia is contraindicated because of the effect that such drops have on the corneal epithelium. Topical antibiotic drops such as G. ofloxacin or G. chloramphenicol will be prescribed and may

need to be instilled as often as every half-hour during the day. In addition, a mydriatic drop such as G. cyclopentolate will be prescribed to dilate the pupil, reduce pain and prevent posterior synechia (adhesion between the iris and crystalline lens).

Corneal ulceration and its effects may be so severe as to require a corneal graft to improve vision. The graft is obtained from an eye donated for use after death. Donors must be free from infection and are screened for HIV and hepatitis viruses (RNIB 2002b). Other conditions where corneal grafting may be undertaken include:

- corneal dystrophy – rare inherited disorders that affect corneal transparency
- scarring such as following chemical injury.

The specific care following corneal grafting is beyond the scope of this chapter and readers should consult a specialist textbook for details of aftercare and complications that include rejection.

▶ Nursing management

Patients are unlikely to be prepared for admission to hospital and may have concerns and anxieties that need to be relieved. The hospital social worker can be an excellent source of support in these circumstances.

There is the potential for cross-infection and patients with infections should not be cared for in the same room as surgical cases. Standard (previously referred to as universal) precautions should be followed (see Ch. 13) to prevent the spread of infection. Local policy guidelines should be followed, especially where this involves isolating patients in single room accommodation. Such isolation may be important to prevent the spread of infection, but it can isolate people who are already possibly concerned about the long-term effect of the condition on their vision. Fear of permanent sight loss must not be underestimated. Whilst maintaining integrity of infection control, nurses must make positive approaches to patients to establish a therapeutic relationship. This includes timely patient education.

When first admitted, the priority will be to make patients welcome, calm their initial fears, relieve pain and commence topical treatment. In the first 24–48 hours, intensive drop treatment may need to continue during the night, the goal being to promote healing and prevent further deterioration. There will inevitably be some sleep deprivation. It would be wrong for a nurse to leave patients sleeping at night, or during the day for that matter, mistakenly thinking they need the sleep more than the medication. Adhering to the regimen protects patients from permanent damage and loss of the eye (see Older Adults: Nursing Priorities box 15.1, p. 360).

CORNEAL DAMAGE DUE TO FOREIGN BODY

By far the most frequently seen corneal condition is a foreign body (FB); these are often metallic. They may be the result of work or DIY incidents but could be the result of wind-blown dust. It is important for the nurse to take an accurate history of the incident, including what safety precautions, if any, had been taken prior to the incident. Advice can be given, where this is appropriate, about suitable safety precautions such as wearing

OLDER ADULTS: NURSING PRIORITIES

15.1 Margaret

Margaret (not her real name) is a 74-year-old widow. She lives alone in a detached bungalow. She has severe rheumatoid arthritis that affects her neck, hands and arms. Margaret has one son but he lives and works some distance away. Margaret has been treated previously for right corneal ulcer. The ulcer has now recurred and is severe enough for her to be admitted to hospital. A corneal scrape has been undertaken in the outpatient department. G. chloramphenicol (Minims) has been prescribed for the right eye every half-hour, including overnight G. atropine (Minims) twice daily. In addition, co-codamol is prescribed every 6 hours for pain. Visual acuity in the right eye is hand movement only and in the left is 6/36. She wears glasses for reading. Margaret is worried about security at her home. She is not in receipt of any support services.

Student activities

- How will you address Margaret's immediate care needs?
- How may sleep deprivation affect Margaret? (see Ch. 4)
- What support services may be organized during discharge planning in order to help Margaret maintain independent living in her own home?
- How will you address Margaret's ongoing nursing management to prepare her for discharge home?

protective goggles. Quite often, patients will recall something going into the eye, but it is not unusual for them to attend hospital complaining of having a gritty eye that is watery and photophobic. Where a FB is lodged beneath the lids (subtarsal), patients will complain of a painful gritty sensation on blinking.

▶ Nursing management

Nurses will need a great deal of skill and dexterity to calm patients enough for a full examination to be undertaken. As part of an expanded role, many nurse practitioners work autonomously in clinical settings and have full responsibility for assessing, diagnosing and treating ophthalmic emergencies and, where appropriate, referring cases to ophthalmic medical staff.

It is important to obtain an accurate visual acuity as part of the examination and history-taking. Reduced visual acuity could be indicative of penetrating injury. Because of pain and blepharospasm, it will probably be necessary to instil a drop of topical anaesthetic such as G. oxybuprocaine into the eye to facilitate examination and removal of the FB. Patients should get rapid relief as a result, but they need to be advised that these drops cannot be continued as they can cause damage to the corneal epithelium. Drops can be made accessible for nurses to use without a doctor's prescription if they are made part of patient group directions.

Details of the incident will give vital clues as to the speed at which the FB entered the eye and what type of material it may be. The eye should be examined, preferably under a slit lamp (see p. 339). The upper lid should be everted as the FB could be lodged underneath. The eye should be stained with G. fluorescein to check whether there is an abrasion. The anterior chamber should be examined for any activity that could be indicative of inflammation, e.g. inflammation surrounding the cornea (ciliary injection).

Any FB should be removed with a green needle after instillation of local anaesthetic drops (this procedure should only be undertaken by those specially trained and judged to be competent to do this). Metallic FBs leave a rust ring that will have to be removed if complications are to be avoided. Occulentum (Oc) (eye ointment) chloramphenicol is given for use three to four times per day for 2 weeks. As well as the antibiotic content, the ointment provides some lubrication and relief from discomfort. Any residual pain can be relieved with paracetamol every 6 hours as required.

Patients will need to return after 2 days for removal of the rust ring, which should have softened because of the action of the ointment. Prior to rust ring removal, topical local anaesthetic will be instilled. Following removal with a green needle, a dose of Oc chloramphenicol will be applied.

Nurses should again, where appropriate, promote eye health, including eye protection and preventing accidents (see 'General disease prevention and health education', p. 341).

CORNEAL ABRASIONS

Abrasions result from part or complete removal of a focal area of corneal epithelium. Patients usually complain of intense pain, lacrimation and blepharospasm. It may be the result of a subtarsal FB. The eye is examined after local anaesthetic drops have been instilled, to ensure cooperation and provide short-term pain relief. G. fluorescein stain is used to highlight the damaged or lost epithelial cells. On slit lamp examination using a blue filter, the stained area shows up green.

When the abrasion is large, G. homatropine 2% is instilled at once to give some pain relief by reducing iris spasm. Abrasions heal by about 1 mm per side each day, but this takes longer in older people. Patients are prescribed a topical antibiotic such as chloramphenicol (drops or ointment) or G. fusidic acid. They are advised to rest and not to drive until the abrasion is healed.

Some corneal abrasions result in complications including recurrent erosion syndrome. This is particularly so when the abrasion has been caused by a fingernail (Eke et al 1999). Patients with recurrent abrasions will need to repeat the topical antibiotics and receive advice regarding lid hygiene. However, a course of oral doxycycline may be needed where these measures do not work.

CHEMICAL INJURY

Patients sustaining chemical injury are treated in the A&E department as an emergency. The most frequently seen types of chemicals are:

- alkalis – such as cleaning fluids, mortar or ammonia; they act very rapidly to disrupt the ocular structures
- acids – cause most damage on initial contact. Car battery fluid is often the offending fluid; solvents also cause pain and discomfort.

Health and safety in the home and workplace can help to prevent chemical injury but it is not possible to protect from an attack by someone intent on causing injury.

Management

Immediate irrigation is vital to prevent lasting damage. Normal saline 0.9% is the fluid of choice and this is delivered via a giving set with a controllable nozzle, as follows:

1. Sit the patient in a chair that gives head support.
2. Remove contact lenses if worn.
3. Instil topical anaesthetic such as G. oxybuprocaine to relieve pain and gain cooperation.
4. Protect the patient's clothing and use a receiver to collect the fluid.
5. The whole of the cornea and conjunctiva should be irrigated; it will be necessary to evert the eyelids to do this properly.
6. Large particles can be removed with a cotton bud.
7. The pH of the eye should be checked and irrigation continued until the substance has been neutralized.

Following irrigation, patient assessment should be completed and recorded. Treatment will depend on the nature and extent of the damage.

CONJUNCTIVAL CONDITIONS

The conjunctiva may be affected by disease, infection and trauma. Many conditions respond to treatment, but others can lead to more long-term damage to the eye or the extraocular structures.

CONJUNCTIVITIS

This is inflammation of the conjunctiva, the main causes of which are:

- bacterial infection, usually *Staphylococcus aureus*, *Streptococcus* or *Haemophilus*
- viral infection such as adenovirus
- *Chlamydia*, e.g. *Chlamydia trachomatis*, which causes trachoma; this is a major cause of blindness worldwide, especially in hot dry climates where it is widespread.

Conjunctivitis may also result from allergies to, for example, drops or eye makeup. Overuse of contact lenses can also cause conjunctivitis (see Health Promotion box 15.2). Conjunctivitis can be spread to others, especially where face cloths and towels are shared. This could be the case where people are living in cramped, overcrowded conditions, e.g. rough sleepers, hostels.

Clinical presentation

Clinical features include:

- minor gritty (FB) sensation
- occasionally photophobia
- hyperaemia (red and slightly engorged conjunctiva)
- purulent discharge with bacterial infection, especially on waking
- watery discharge – associated with viral and allergic conjunctivitis.

Visual acuity is not normally affected.

Management

Conjunctival swabbing for microbiological examination is not recommended as a routine, partly because of cost and also because choice of treatment is based on history and clinical presentation.

Management includes the following:

- bacterial infection – a topical broad-spectrum antibiotic is prescribed, e.g. G. chloramphenicol four times daily for 7–10 days
- adenoviral infections – left to run a natural course as there is no treatment, but patients will need an explanation as to why they are having no treatment
- herpes simplex virus – can be treated with Oc aciclovir
- *Chlamydia trachomatis* – G. chlortetracycline four times daily for 6 weeks
- allergic conjunctivitis – responds well to G. sodium cromoglicate (cromoglycate) and advice about avoiding the allergen.

Patients and staff also need advice regarding hygiene to prevent spread of infection or re-infection (see Health Promotion box 15.3, p. 362).

 HEALTH PROMOTION

15.2 Care of contact lenses

Wearers of hard or soft contact lenses may occasionally contract conjunctivitis. There is a trend for young people to wear non-prescription contact lenses to alter the colour of their eyes. They are not always given help and advice on how to care for them. The most frequent cause is the contamination of the contact lens case itself. Contact lens wearers should wash their hands before and after they insert and remove their lenses to help reduce the risk of infection. In addition, the lens case should be washed in hot soapy water and left to air-dry. They do not always do this because they simply forget or the conditions are less than ideal, e.g. when busy at work or in a nightclub rest room.

Manufacturers of lens cleaning solutions are continuing to develop one-step cleaning and soaking solutions. Many of them are also providing lens cases with each new bottle of contact lens solution. Many contact lens prescriptions are available as daily disposable, eliminating the need for cleaning and storage. Some wearers, in an attempt to economize, will occasionally reuse disposable lenses. This is clearly a practice that is not recommended and must be discouraged.

HEALTH PROMOTION

15.3 Preventing the spread of conjunctivitis

Perhaps the most important aspect of management of conjunctivitis is patient and staff education to prevent the spread of infection. Patients and the staff treating them should be aware that thorough handwashing is vital before and after examining, cleaning or treating the eye. At home, patients should be advised to use separate face cloths and flannels to those of other members of the household, otherwise the infection could spread to others. Pillowcases should also be changed and washed daily. Health care staff caring for ophthalmic patients who are diagnosed with adenovirus should be advised to avoid contact with patients and fellow workers. This is to prevent potentially serious outbreaks of infection. Health workers with adenovirus must avoid contact with patients and colleagues. They will normally be required to remain off sick whilst infected. Because the condition can be very easily spread, it is not sufficient to be undertaking non-clinical duties alone.

CONDITIONS OF THE UVEAL TRACT

UVEITIS

Uveitis is inflammation of the uveal tract. It is classified according to the anatomical structures involved: anterior uveitis involves the iris or the ciliary body and occasionally both; posterior uveitis affects the choroid. Panuveitis is inflammation affecting the whole uveal tract.

Aetiology

Anterior uveitis is uncommon and presents either acutely or as a chronic episode that starts gradually, lasting for several weeks. It is usually unilateral (MREH 2000). Frequently the cause is unknown, but it may be associated with:

- trauma
- systemic inflammatory disease such as ankylosing spondylitis (see Ch. 27) and inflammatory bowel disease (see Ch. 22)
- HIV disease (see Ch. 25).

Clinical presentation

- Pain
- Photophobia
- Ciliary injection
- Red eye
- Tearing
- Blurred vision
- Slit-lamp examination – cells and flare are seen in the anterior chamber
- Pus may be present in the anterior chamber (hypopyon)
- Pupil is usually constricted (miosed) when posterior synechiae causes an irregular pupil
- IOP is occasionally raised.

Management

As this is likely to be an acute episode, patients can be very anxious that their vision has deteriorated. In addition, they will be experiencing pain, discomfort and photophobia.

Pain will be managed and a thorough ophthalmic examination will be undertaken, including any relevant history. This needs to be done in a sensitive way as patients' sexual history will have to be discussed. Investigations include blood tests and, where relevant, X-rays.

Treatment involves the administration of corticosteroid drops such as G. prednisolone 1%, one drop every 30 minutes to 2 hours during the acute phase, and for milder attacks, 0.5% once daily may be sufficient. In addition, a cycloplegic may be prescribed to dilate the pupil and help prevent posterior synechiae. Any underlying cause should be treated.

Patients are unlikely to be admitted to hospital so an assessment of their drop technique is essential, as is education about the condition (MREH 2000). This is where nurses can reinforce the importance of persisting with the treatment. If uveitis is neglected, vision may be permanently affected.

CONDITIONS AFFECTING THE EYELIDS

There are several conditions of the eyelids that should be recognized early in order to prevent patient discomfort and, in some cases, loss of sight. The eyelids are normally in close contact with the eyeball. Occasionally, as a result of trauma, disease or ageing, the lids do not function normally.

BLEPHARITIS

Blepharitis is a chronic inflammation of the eyelids and is relatively common. Occasionally, it is associated with conjunctivitis. It is usually bilateral and affects people of any age.

The most frequent cause of blepharitis is bacterial infection. The causative organism is usually *Staphylococcus aureus* or *S. epidermidis*. It is sometimes associated with poor facial hygiene, but there are other factors, including allergy (e.g. chloramphenicol eye drops or eye make up), dandruff, excess production of lipid from the meibomian glands, acne rosacea and occasionally lice infestation (Schwab et al 1997).

Clinical presentation

Patients present with eyelid irritation that may be associated with a burning sensation or itching. The eyelids may be red and the lid margins swollen. It may be possible to see visible scales on the eyelashes. The loss of eyelashes is not unusual. If left untreated, blepharitis can cause complications, including (Parvan-Langston 1996):

- chronic infection
- trichiasis (abnormal growth and position of eyelashes)
- chalazion
- conjunctivitis
- corneal ulceration
- eyelid scarring.

Non-urgent ophthalmic surgery, such as cataract extraction, may be delayed if blepharitis is detected. This is because of the risk of postoperative infection, which could be sight-threatening.

▶ Nursing management

This chronic condition can be treated effectively and nurses have a vital role in its prevention, recognition and subsequent treatment, including patient education, particularly in community settings. Because of the different causes of blepharitis, it is essential to make an individual assessment of patient need.

Hygiene is key to treatment and patient comfort. The face, including the eyelids and eyebrows, should be washed at least twice a day and the hair kept clean and free of dandruff. Antibiotic ointment may also be prescribed and should be applied after cleansing the lids. Individuals should have their own towels and face cloths, and ideally clean ones should be used each day. If eye makeup is worn, it should be removed each day and certainly before going to bed.

Scaly deposits should be removed by 'scrubbing' the lids with cotton buds or flannel wrapped around a finger, dipped in a mixture of warm water and a few drops of baby shampoo (1 teaspoonful of baby shampoo to a mug full of water). If patients are sensitive to baby shampoo, warm water alone may be used. Even when the condition has cleared, the hygiene regimen should be continued twice a week to prevent recurrence.

Relief from soreness and itching can be obtained by applying warm compresses to the eyelids for 5–10 minutes twice a day. Moisten a cloth under a running tap of hot water, repeating as the cloth cools.

CHALAZION

A chalazion is a swelling in the meibomian gland due to a blocked duct. Both the upper and lower lids may be affected. The retained meibomian gland secretions cause a firm, round swelling of the eyelid. It is important to make a clear diagnosis, as there are other causes of lid swelling, including haemangioma (collection of blood vessels) or cancer.

They are likely to resolve spontaneously within a few weeks. Where the swelling fails to subside, incision and curettage may be necessary. This is normally performed under local anaesthesia and as a day case. This type of surgery is now often performed by an ophthalmic nurse practitioner.

There may be pain associated with the chalazion which can be relieved with analgesics such as paracetamol. Some relief can be gained from applying, with great care, a hot compress or steam to the affected eyelid (see Guidelines for Care Priorities box 15.3).

A chalazion is not usually infected, and therefore the routine use of antibiotics is not recommended. However, occasionally they may become infected, e.g. by *Staphylococcus aureus*. As well as analgesia and heat treatment, antibiotic ointment such as Oc chloramphenicol, three or four times per day for 14 days, will be prescribed.

STY OR EXTERNAL HORDEOLUM

This is an acute infection (usually by *Staphylococcus aureus*) of the sebaceous gland at the base of an eyelash follicle. There is abscess formation which frequently has a point associated with an eyelash. It is tender and causes the patient acute pain and discomfort.

Treatment aims to relieve pain and reduce the swelling. Hot bathing, as described previously, may aid drainage of the abscess. The offending lash can be plucked to drain the abscess but this procedure can be very painful for patients. Antibiotic ointment such as Oc chloramphenicol is prescribed to be used on the lid margin four times daily for 7–10 days. Stollery (1997) advises that, where there is recurrence of the condition, patients should be screened for diabetes mellitus.

PTOSIS

Ptosis may be defined as the drooping of the upper lid; sometimes intermittent, it may be unilateral or bilateral. If the droop is sufficient to cover all or part of the pupil, vision can be affected. Ptosis may be congenital or acquired; in the latter case, it may be:

- mechanical – increased lid weight due to tumour, oedema, scar tissue
- involving muscle and nerves – trauma, myasthenia gravis (see Ch. 27), Bell's palsy (see Ch. 14).

Treatment may be correction of the ptosis with surgery to the lid levator (lifts) muscle or tumour removal. Underlying causes are treated.

DRY EYES

A deficiency associated with any aspect of the tear film will result in dry eye, causing discomfort, but if untreated it may lead to loss of vision. Dry eye may also be caused by deficient blinking, e.g. when staring at a computer screen. Dry eye can occur at any age. There may be no obvious signs of tear deficiency; however, dead corneal and conjunctival epithelial cells can be seen when stained with G. rose bengal 1%. Breaks in the tear film can be observed when the tears are stained with G. fluorescein.

Clinical presentation

The presentation may include:

- red eye (occasionally)
- gritty, itchy eye
- burning sensation
- poor tear production
- ache round the eye
- sticky eye (occasionally), usually in the morning.

The treatment is aimed at relieving symptoms, although patients may take some convincing that they have dry eye, particularly when they may be complaining that their eyes are watering. This is because the deficient oil film causes tears to spill over into the cheek. Artificial tears will be prescribed and should be instilled as often as they are needed.

AGE-RELATED DISORDERS

Entropion

This is a condition where the eyelid turns inwards. It usually affects the lower lid. The eyelashes irritate the eye, causing marked discomfort as well as tearing (watering) of the eye. If the condition is allowed to go untreated, the cornea is likely to ulcerate (see p. 359) and could become permanently scarred. Such scarring is likely to interfere with vision and will affect the lifestyle of the individual.

Causes of entropion include:

- spasm of the obicularis oculi muscle (normally closes the eyelids)
- disease or trauma of the eyelids or conjunctiva that results in contraction of the conjunctiva.

Some temporary relief from the discomfort can be obtained by applying tape to the lower lid. Cut a strip of narrow hypoallergenic tape to approximately 1.3–2.5 cm in length. Apply the narrow end close to the lid margin and secure it to the cheek, ensuring that the lid is in close contact with the eyeball. Over-correction will cause ectropion (see below). In addition, offending lashes rubbing against the cornea can be removed.

Treatment will normally be by corrective surgery to evert the eyelid. This is usually performed under local anaesthesia. An alternative to surgery is the use of local injections of botulinum toxin to relieve blepharospasm by paralysing the muscle. This procedure would need to be repeated every 3 months or so.

Ectropion

The eyelid in this case turns outwards, away from the eyeball. The eyelids do not close properly, leaving the eyeball exposed, and the tear film is not evenly distributed. This has an adverse effect on the cornea and conjunctiva. The eye will water because the tears cannot drain into the punctum, and the cheek will become sore owing to frequent wiping away of tears. Patients may feel uncomfortable about their personal appearance.

The causes include:

- relaxation of the obicularis oculi muscle
- trauma to the lids or conjunctiva
- Bell's palsy (see Ch. 14).

The management depends on the cause, but it is usually surgical. However, the quality of the patient's lifestyle can be improved by the use of artificial tears and lubricating ointment to the eye and barrier cream to the cheek to protect the skin.

SUMMARY: MAIN POINTS

- People with eye problems are not only cared for in specialist ophthalmic units. You will, as part of your everyday work, come into contact with people with eye disease and/or problems with their vision.
- Not everyone likes to deal with the eye; your patients must not suffer as a consequence.
- The clinical environment in which you care for patients should also reflect the needs of the visually impaired.
- There are more people eligible for registration as blind or partially sighted than are currently registered.
- Assessment of visual function as part of any nursing assessment should be made to ensure that patients' independence is maintained and, where new or previously unrecognized problems are found, action is taken to provide the necessary management.
- Early detection of eye and vision problems can help prevent unnecessary blindness and the distress this can cause. The nurse can play a vital role in the care and prevention of eye disease and trauma.
- Eye medication that patients bring into hospital or use in the community are drugs and should be treated as such. Failure to assist patients in maintaining their ongoing ocular therapy can result in irreversible blindness.
- Referral to statutory and voluntary services should be done in a timely manner.
- Loss of vision does affect lifestyle and people who have visual problems may grieve for that loss. They need help and support during this time.
- Health education can help prevent disease progress and accidents.

SELF-TEST: CRITICAL THINKING ACTIVITIES

Shiba Choudhury, aged 42 years, has type 1 diabetes mellitus. Her visual acuity is as follows: left – hand movements only, right – 6/36. There is no improvement with glasses or pinholes. Shiba's blood glucose control is poor. At home she has two teenage children. Her husband works long hours as a sales representative and is often required to be away from home for 2 or 3 days at a time. Sheba has no apparent help at home from statutory or voluntary services.

Shiba is admitted to the ward as a planned admission for vitreoretinal surgery. Outline the nursing assessment and plan of care for her management whilst in hospital, including detail of the help and support she will need when she is discharged home.

FURTHER READING

Allen M, Knight C, Falk C, Strang V. Effectiveness of a pre-operative teaching programme for cataract patients. J Adv Nurs 1992; 17: 303–309.

Barnes G. The suitability of cataract patients for day surgery. Prof Nurse 1997; l2(4): 264–268.

Bruce I, McKennell A, Walker E. Blind and partially sighted adults in Britain: the RNIB survey. Vol 1. London: HMSO; 1991.

Chawla HB. Ophthalmology. A symptom based approach, 3rd edn. Oxford: Butterworth-Heinemann; 1999.

Kanski J. Ophthalmology: colour guide, 2nd edn. Edinburgh: Churchill Livingstone; 1997.

Maclean H. The eye in primary care. Oxford: Butterworth-Heinemann; 2002.

 ## USEFUL ADDRESSES

Guide Dogs for the Blind Association
Hillfields
Burghfield Common
Reading
Berkshire RG7 3YG
Tel: 0870 600 2323
(www.gdba.org.uk)

Henshaws Society for Blind People (HSBP)
John Derby House
88–92 Talbot Road
Old Trafford
Manchester M16 0GS
Tel: 0161 872 1234
(www.hsbp.co.uk)

International Glaucoma Association (IGA)
108c Warner Road
London SE5 9HQ
Tel: 0207 737 3265
(www.iga.org.uk)

Macular Disease Society
PO Box 16
Denbigh LL16 5ZA
Helpline 0800 328 2849
(www.maculardisease.org)

National Library for the Blind
Cromwell Road
Bredbury
Stockport SK6 2SG
Tel: 0161 355 2000
(www.nlbuk.org)

The Partially Sighted Society
Queen's Road
Doncaster DN1 2NX
Tel: 01302 323 132
(www.leeder.demon.co.uk)

Royal National Institute for the Blind (RNIB)
105 Judd Street
London WC1H 9NE
Tel: 0207 388 1266
Helpline: 0845 766 9999
(www.rnib.org.uk)

Wales Council for the Blind
Shand House
20 Newport Road
Cardiff CF2 1YB
Tel: 029 2047 3954
(www.wcb-ccd.org.uk)

 ## USEFUL WEBSITES

www.freebooks4doctors.com/fb/spec6.htm#ophth – FreeBooks4Doctors – *internet access to free medical books*

www.wills-glaucoma.org – Glaucoma Service & Foundation at Wills Eye Hospital

www.goodhope.org.uk/Departments/eyedept – Good Hope Hospital NHS Trust – *information for health professionals and patients. Health professionals can download patient information leaflets*

www.concordance.org – Medicines Partnership – a 2-year initiative supported by the Department of Health, aimed at putting the principles of concordance into practice

www.healthcentre.org.uk/hc/pages/eye.htm – UK Health Centre (Eye Conditions and Visual Handicap page) – *an internet health resources library*

REFERENCES

American Academy of Ophthalmology. Lens and cataract. San Francisco: AAO; 1997a.

American Academy of Ophthalmology. Glaucoma. San Francisco: AAO; 1997b.

Baker M, Winyard S. Lost vision. Older visually impaired people in the UK. London: RNIB; 1998.

Barton W. Role of ophthalmic nurses with visually impaired patients. Insight 1998; XXIII(1): 5–10.

Bruce I, Hadi F. RNIB: beyond 2000. Br J Visual Impairment 2000; 18(3): 106–110.

Buckingham K, Campbell SE, Olver LR. Use of community resourses following inpatient and day case surgery for cataract. Br J Commun Health Visiting 1997; 2(10): 495–500.

Cleary ME. Helping the person who is visually impaired: concerns, questions, remedies and resources. J Ophthal Nurs Technol 1995; 14(5): 205–211.

Dias MR, O'Neil E. Examining the role of professional interpreters in culturally sensitive health care. J Multicultur Nurs Health 1998; 4(1): 27–31.

Eke T, Morrison DA, Austin DJ. Recurrent symptoms following corneal abrasion: prevalence, severity and the effects of a simple regimen of prophylaxis. Br J Ophthalmol 1999; 13: 343–347.

Felinski S. Not seeing eye to eye. Nurs Times 1989; 85(20): 57–59.

Forrester JV, Dick AD, McMenamin P, Lee WR. The eye. Basic sciences in practice. London: WB Saunders; 1996.

Hamer S, Collinson G. Evidence-Based Practice. A handbook for practitioners. London: Baillière Tindall (in association with the RCN); 1999.

Harrison MA. Perspective on Charles Bonnet syndrome and age-related macular degeneration. CE Optometry 2000; 3(3): 119–120.

International Glaucoma Association (IGA). Glaucoma fact file. London: IGA; 2002.

Kanski JJ. Synopsis of ophthalmology, 6th edn. London: Wright; 1990.

Kanski JJ. Clinical ophthalmology. A systematic approach, 4th edn. Oxford: Butterworth-Heinemann; 1999.

Kanski JJ, McAllister JA, Salmon JF. Glaucoma. A colour manual of diagnosis and treatment, 2nd edn. Oxford: Butterworth-Heinemann; 1996.

Knox KA. Applying psychological theory to visual impairment: something to consider. Ophthalm Nurs 1998; 2(2): 14–18.

Low Vision Services consensus group. Low vision services recommendations for future service delivery in the UK. London: RNIB; 1999.

Manchester Royal Eye Hospital, Manchester (MREH). Uveitis. Clinic patient information leaflet. Manchester: MREH; 2000.

McBride S. Patients talking. London: RNIB; 2000.

McBride S. Patients talking 2. The eye clinic journey experienced by blind and partially sighted adults: a quantitative study. London: RNIB; 2001.

Millodot M, Laby DM. Dictionary of ophthalmology. Oxford: Butterworth-Heinemann; 2002

Murphy S. Saving sight. Pract Nurse 2002; 23(12): 42–44.

NHS Executive. Action on cataracts. London: DoH; 2000.

Nicol M, Bavin C, Bedford-Turner S, Cronin P, Rawlings-Anderson K. Essential nursing skills. London: Mosby; 2000.

Okhravi N. Manual of primary eye care. Oxford: Butterworth-Heinemann; 1997.

Parvan-Langston D. Manual of ocular diagnosis and therapy, 4th edn. Boston: Little, Brown; 1996.

Rose KE. Caring for patients with cataract. Nurs Stand 1997; 11(2): 49–53.

Royal College of Nursing (RCN). The nature, scope and value of ophthalmic nursing. London: RCN; 2000.

Royal College of Ophthalmologists. Cataract surgery guidelines. London: RCO; 2001.

Royal National Institute for the Blind. Colour and contrast. London: RNIB; 1997.

Royal National Institute for the Blind. Understanding age-related macular degeneration. Royal College of Ophthalmologists. Online. Available: www.rnib.org.uk/macdegen.htm. 2002a.

Royal National Institute for the Blind. Corneal graft factsheet. Online. Available: http://www.rnib.org.uk/info/corneal.htm. 2002b.

Schwab IR, Epstein RJ, Harris DJ et al. External eye disease and cornea. In: Weingeist TA, Liesegang TJ, Slamovitis TL, eds. Basic and clinical science course. San Francisco: AAO; 1997.

Stanford P. A framework of practice for intraocular lens measurement. Int J Ophthalm Nurs 2000; 4(1): 10–11.

Stollery R. Ophthalmic nursing, 2nd edn. Oxford: Blackwell Science; 1997.

Vaughan DR, Astbury T, Riordan E. General ophthalmology, 7th edn. London: Appleton & Laing; 1998.

WHO. Global initiative for the elimination of avoidable blindness. Vision 2020. WHO/PBL/97.61 Rev. 1. Geneva: WHO; 1997.

York J, Glaser B, Murphy R. Understanding macular degeneration. J Ophthalm Nurs Technol 2000; 19(3): 116–119.

16 Nursing patients with problems of the ear and hearing

Hilary Harkin, Francis Vaz

'They said he wasn't really responding but he's OK when I'm there. I wonder if it's because he can't hear what they're saying, I know how to make sure he can hear what I say but maybe they don't. He's got a hearing aid but doesn't like wearing it so I bet he hasn't told them. I think I'll mention it to the nurse next time I go in.'

(Patient's relative)

THIS CHAPTER WILL HELP YOU

- Relate the anatomy and physiology of the ear for health education and disease prevention

- Carry out a nursing assessment on patients with problems of the ear and hearing in the community and in hospital

- Understand common disorders affecting the ear and hearing and the rationale of treatment

- Promote the quality of life of the patient with problems of the ear and hearing

- Understand the nursing management of caring for a patient undergoing surgery on the ear.

KEYWORDS

Aural toilet	Otitis media
Cholesteatoma	Otorrhoea
External auditory canal	Otoscopy
Mastoid cavity	Perforation of tympanic membrane
Mastoiditis	
Otalgia	Tympanic membrane

INTRODUCTION

There are many issues for the nurse to consider when caring for patients with problems of the ear and hearing. With the wide range of medical/surgical conditions that exist, varying from minor to life-threatening, the nurse can develop skills that are appropriate to the specialty. Effective communication skills are essential in nursing patients who are deaf and hard of hearing (Ch. 3), as is knowledge of the anatomy and physiology of the ear. Understanding and promoting ear care provide the nurse with the opportunity to improve the quality of life of the patient. This chapter describes the nursing care of patients with problems of the ear and hearing and provides cross-references to many other chapters, as nurses will come across patients with these problems in every area of their practice:

- Communication skills form an essential part of the nursing of patients who are deaf or hard of hearing (Ch. 3).
- Ear care falls within the nurse's remit and nurse-led clinics are currently providing patients with flexible appointments and knowledgeable, research-based practice (Ch. 1). Nurses managing such clinics need to have the knowledge and ability to prescribe medication for the ear. This raises issues of the organization and management of nursing care, including nurse prescribing.
- The external ear (pinna and external auditory canal) is lined with skin. It can be affected by a range of dermatology and oncology conditions (Ch. 28). The middle ear is lined with mucous membrane and the secretions are affected by disorders such as bronchiectasis and cystic fibrosis (Ch. 20). The smallest bones in the body are the three ossicles located in the middle ear, and they can be affected by osteogenesis imperfecta, osteitis deformans and osteoporosis (Ch. 27).
- Patients with many diverse conditions, e.g. tonsillitis (Ch. 21), cancer of the tongue and of the head and neck, may complain of otalgia (earache). Systemic illness can affect the

hearing and people with diabetes mellitus are more likely to suffer from hearing loss (Ch. 17). Nurses will meet patients with acute ear infections and foreign bodies in the ear in primary care settings and in the accident and emergency department (Ch. 30).

A guidance document in ear care has been developed by the Action on ENT steering group. These are available on the NHS Modernisation Agency website (www.modern.nhs.uk). They provide guidance in the areas of ear irrigation (syringing), aural toilet and microsuction. The Primary Ear Care centre has developed a website that enables practitioners to download guidelines on ear irrigation and health interventions regarding care of the ears (www.earcarecentre.com).

OVERVIEW: ANATOMY AND PHYSIOLOGY OF THE EAR

ANATOMY OF THE EAR

The ear is composed of three parts: the external (outer), middle and inner ear (Fig. 16.1). All three parts, from the outer to the inner ear, are involved in conduction of sound. The inner ear also houses the organ of balance. This is why balance and/or hearing can be affected by certain ear conditions.

External ear

The auricle or pinna is composed of fibrocartilage which is covered by skin, and it is the part the layperson usually refers to as 'the ear'. It is divided into different parts, including the helix, conchae and lobe. The pinna directs sound waves down into the external auditory canal (EAC) or the ear canal. The EAC is lined with skin and is approximately 24 mm long in adults. The outer one-third of the canal is formed by fibrocartilage and the inner two-thirds is bony. The dead skin of the canal, dust and debris mix with the ceruminous secretions from the glands in this region and give rise to cerumen (ear wax). The function of cerumen is to protect and lubricate the ear canal and it has bactericidal properties to protect the canal from infection. Hairs are located in the outer cartilaginous part of the EAC. The hairs help to trap and waft debris out of the EAC. The hairs also protect the thin skin of the canal by holding the wax away from the skin, as cerumen is acidic and would irritate the lining of the canal. At the deep end of the EAC is the tympanic membrane (eardrum). The cylindrical shape of the EAC enables centrifugal migration of the dead skin cells out of the canal.

The nerve supply of the external ear is complex and includes several cranial nerves (V, VII, IX and X) together with supply from the cervical plexus. The Xth cranial nerve (vagus) has an auricular branch in the EAC and stimulation of this nerve can occur during an ear examination, leading to reflex coughing. Referred pain from any of the other cranial nerve distributions or cervical nerves can cause otalgia (earache).

Middle ear

The tympanic membrane is commonly referred to as the eardrum (Fig. 16.2). It separates the external ear from the middle ear and functionally is part of the middle ear. The majority of the tympanic membrane has three layers:

- an epithelial lining continuous with the ear canal
- a middle fibrous layer which gives the drum strength and the ability to vibrate
- a third mucosal layer that is continuous with the mucosa of the middle ear.

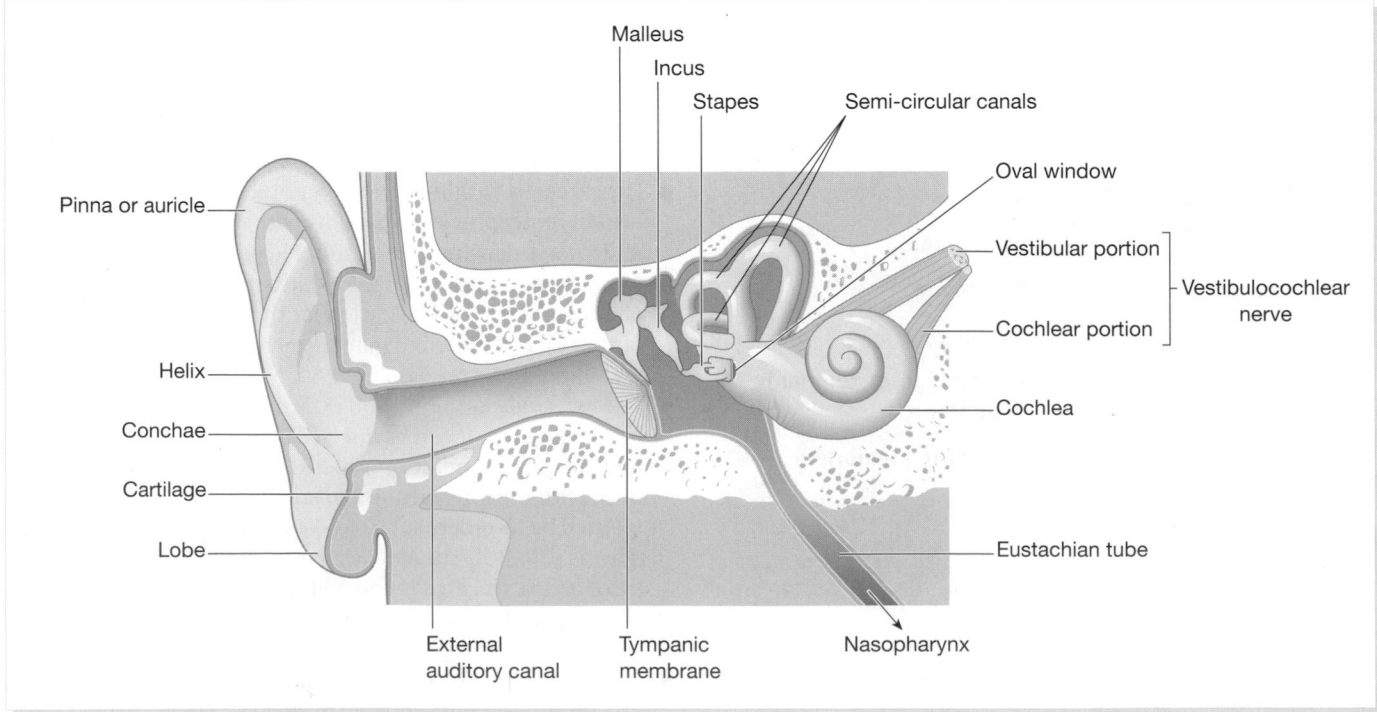

Figure 16.1 Anatomy of the ear.

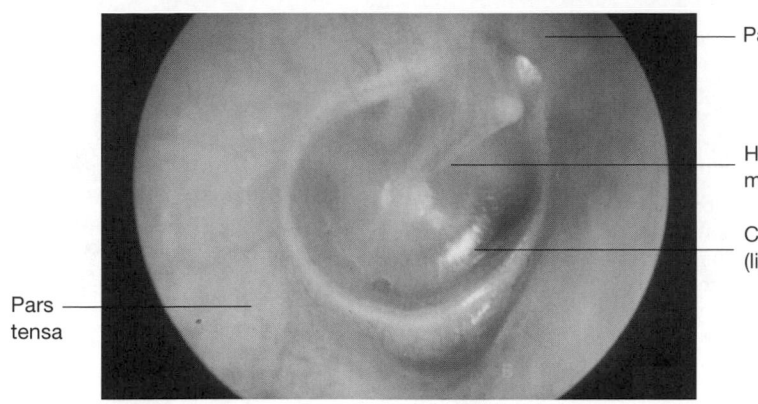

Pars flaccida

Handle of malleus

Cone of light (light reflex)

Pars tensa

Figure 16.2
The right tympanic membrane (eardrum).

These three layers exist in continuity in the lower four-fifths of the tympanic membrane, the pars tensa, which is the main sound-transmitting part of the tympanic membrane. The fibrous layer is absent in the upper tympanic membrane, referred to as the pars flaccida. It is vital to ensure that this area is viewed during ear examination (see p. 371–372) as it is the most vulnerable part of the tympanic membrane and the most prone to serious ear disease.

The middle ear contains three tiny bones or ossicles: the malleus, incus and stapes. The handle of the malleus (hammer), the first of the three ossicles, is embedded in the fibrous part of the tympanic membrane and is the most prominent feature to visualize (Fig. 16.2). The malleus articulates with the incus (anvil), which in turn articulates with the stapes (stirrup). This continuity of the ossicles ensures the transmission of sound waves from the vibrating eardrum across the bones to the cochlea of the inner ear. The stapes is the smallest bone in the body and its footplate is attached to the margins of the oval window of the cochlea with ligaments. The ear is protected from loud sounds as the stapedius muscle, the smallest muscle in the body, dampens the tilting movement of the vibrating stapes. Ligaments fix the stapes to the oval window. This lies above a further opening in the cochlea called the round window. Between the two windows is a swelling referred to as the promontory, which is the basal turn of the cochlea.

As previously mentioned, the middle ear is lined with mucosa. The secreted mucus drains into the nasopharynx via the eustachian tube (or pharyngotympanic tube) which functions to equalize pressure on either side of the tympanic membrane. The opening of the eustachian tube is sited anteriorly in the middle ear. The upper respiratory tract is lined with mucosa and hence the eustachian tube can provide a pathway for infections to travel to the middle ear. In order to reduce the infection risk, the tube normally remains closed and opens on swallowing, sniffing and yawning. This allows for air to pass up the tube which will aerate the middle ear and mucus will drain down to the back of the throat. In adults the tube is about 33 mm long, more vertical and better developed than in children. This allows gravity to assist in the efficient drainage of the middle ear. Problems with drainage of the tube are more likely to occur when the tube is more horizontal and the associated musculature for opening does not function. This situation occurs with poor development of the facial skeleton, as in a person affected with a cleft palate (see Reflective Practice box 16.1).

R|Я REFLECTIVE PRACTICE

16.1 Problems caused by a blocked eustachian tube

Think about the problems a patient may experience if the drainage of the eustachian tube is affected. You may have experienced a sensation of blockage in your ears when you were flying in a plane. Why might this occur? You may also have found that when you swallowed or yawned, the blocked feeling improved along with the sensation of your ears 'popping'. Think about the connection between your ears, nose and throat.

The width of the middle ear is approximately 2 mm across its centre to the basal turn of the cochlea. Since the tympanic membrane has only three thin layers, when viewing the drum the examiner can often see certain features of the middle ear (Fig. 16.2). If there was a central perforation, the basal turn of the cochlea would be viewable through the hole.

The mastoid antrum is contained within the temporal bone and is composed of numerous air cells. It is connected to the attic region of the middle ear by the aditus. The roof of the middle ear is a thin plate of bone which forms a barrier between the middle ear and the meninges and brain (Ch. 14). This plate of bone also separates the mastoid antrum from the brain and can provide a route for infection to travel from the ear to form an extradural abscess and thrombosis in the sigmoid venous sinus. The floor of the middle ear is also composed of thin bone and separates the cavity from the internal jugular vein, which may be exposed if the plate of bone is deficient. The tympanic branch of the glossopharyngeal nerve (IXth cranial nerve) enters the cavity through the floor.

A branch of the facial nerve (VIIth cranial nerve) runs through the middle ear. This is called the chorda tympani and supplies the anterior two-thirds of the tongue with the sensation of taste. Patients who undergo middle ear surgery may complain of a metallic taste in their mouth post-surgery when the chorda tympani has been affected.

Inner ear

The inner ear is responsible for both hearing and balance (Fig. 16.1). It is embedded in the temporal bone and consists of a bony labyrinth filled with a fluid called perilymph. Within this fluid floats a membranous labyrinth filled with another fluid

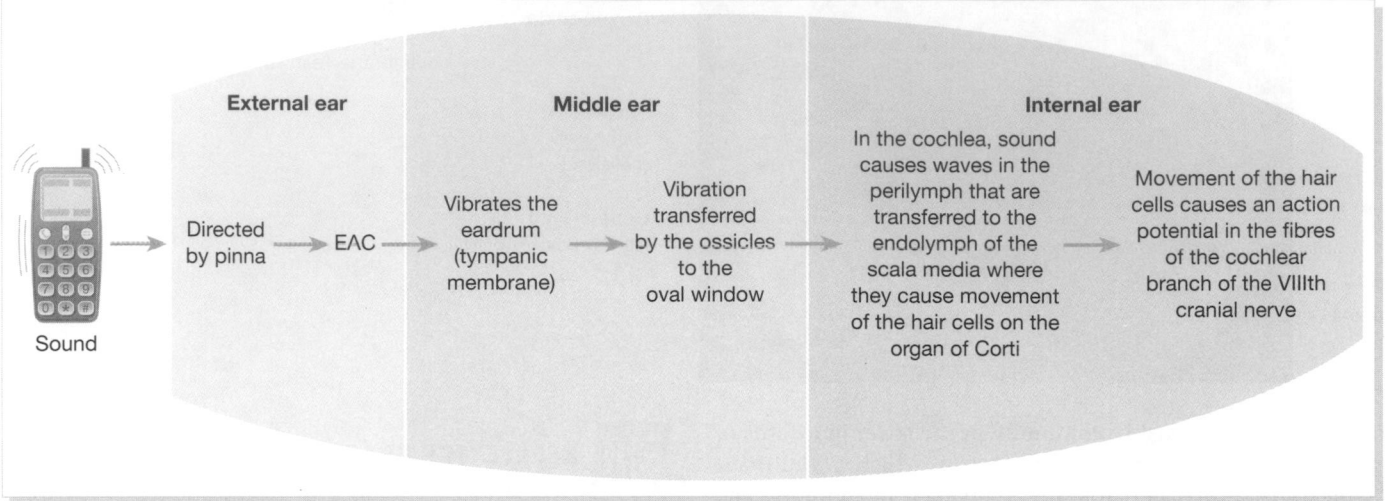

Figure 16.3 The physiology of hearing.

called endolymph. The vestibular part of the labyrinth comprises three semi-circular canals, the utricle and the saccule. It is innervated by the vestibular nerve. The auditory part of the labyrinth comprises the cochlea and is supplied by the cochlear nerve. These two nerves will fuse in the temporal bone to become the single vestibulocochlear nerve (VIIIth cranial nerve).

The cochlea is concerned with hearing. It is approximately 33 mm in length and similar in appearance to a whelk sea shell coiled two and three-quarter times. The continuous coil is divided into three parts: the scala vestbuli, the scala media and the scala tympani. Housed within the cochlea is the organ of Corti, the organ of hearing consisting of a complex arrangement of hair cells. It is the organ of Corti that has the ability to change the transmitted vibrations into nerve impulses.

The three semi-circular canals are concerned with balance of the body and, combined with the other senses, ensure an awareness of our body position in space.

PHYSIOLOGY OF HEARING

Sound travels in the atmosphere as compressions of air, known as waves. The sound wave needs to be channelled from the outside world through the external, middle and inner ear and then sent to the brain where it is integrated with other sensory inputs (Fig. 16.3). Once sound enters the cochlea, it stimulates specific areas depending on the frequency of the sound, i.e. the number of waves per second (measured in hertz, Hz). Low frequencies stimulate the apex of the cochlea and high frequencies the basal turn. The human ear can generally hear frequencies in the range 20–20 000 Hz. Although this varies between individuals, humans tend not to perceive sound waves above and below these limits (but remember that the range encompasses sounds such as a pin dropping and that of a jet engine). Animals, on the other hand, have different audible ranges, and dogs, bats and dolphins can hear sounds produced by special whistles that are not audible to the human ear.

We can distinguish the quality, pitch and loudness of sound and the direction it has originated from by comparing the

impact the sound has on each ear. The loudness of sound is measured in decibels (dB).

▶ Nursing assessment

A thorough nursing assessment that includes an understanding of all the health problems that can have an impact on the ear is essential for providing holistic nursing care to the patient with a problem of the ear and hearing.

Ear care falls within the nurse's remit and nurse-led clinics are providing patients with flexible appointments in a clinic that offers continuity of care and knowledgeable, research-based practice. The nurse assesses the patients, their hearing (see p. 373) and their ear complaints through history-taking and a systematic examination (see p. 371).

Figure 16.4 shows instruments that are frequently used in ear care.

HISTORY-TAKING

There are essential questions that patients should be asked prior to the examination: the reason for them attending, the length of time they have had the complaint and whether it has occurred before. If patients are under the care of the ENT (ear, nose and throat) department or have undergone surgery to the ear, they may be required to return for a review by the ENT surgeon or nurse specialist. The nurse should ask them about:

- pain
- discharge – colour, amount, odour, viscosity, frequency
- hearing loss
- tinnitus (noises in the ear)
- insertion of objects into the ear
- problems with dizziness.

Once the nurse has questioned patients regarding the complaint and documented the results, the examination can commence with both nurse and patient sitting comfortably and at the same level.

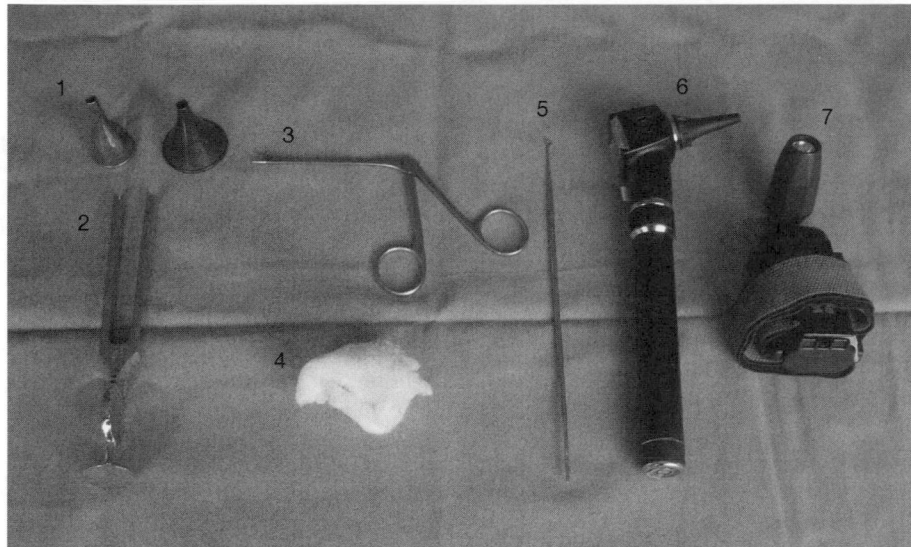

Figure 16.4 Instruments used in ear care (left to right). 1. Choice of aural speculae; 2. 512-Hz tuning fork; 3. crocodile forceps; 4. cotton wool; 5. Jobson Horne probe; 6. otoscope; 7. headlight.

EXAMINATION OF THE EAR

Ear care is often not seen as a priority and there is research suggesting that such care is being carried out by poorly trained personnel (Harkin 2000, Price 1997). Ear examination should only be carried out by practitioners who have been appropriately taught and assessed as competent and who can document their findings. It is necessary to be able to draw the tympanic membrane such that abnormal features, e.g. perforations, can be described in detail.

The rule to follow is to begin the examination with the better hearing ear. It is essential to be able to distinguish the different areas of the drum and to be able to draw the features that are visible when examining a patient's ear. It is important to sit at the same level as the patient to ensure that all of the drum will be visualized and the patient's safety maintained. A headlight is used during the ear examination (Fig. 16.5), and the tympanic membrane is examined using an otoscope (auriscope) (Fig. 16.6). The otoscope has a white light and allows for magnification of the area being viewed (see Guidelines for Care Priorities box 16.1).

Otoscopy – looking for abnormalities
External ear

- Check the condition of the skin around the pinna for:
  - dry skin conditions (Ch. 28)
  - lesions which may be squamous or basal cell carcinomas (Ch. 28) (especially in the sun-exposed regions of the ear)
  - post-auricular scars indicating surgery
  - pre-auricular sinus (congenital sinus that is sited just anterior to the pinna and may connect with the EAC).
- In the presence of local infection, straightening the pinna may prove painful as the lining of the skin is closely adhered to the cartilage underneath. Look at the entrance to the canal with a headlight (Fig. 16.5) and observe for furuncles (infected hair follicles).
- Check if the canal looks oedematous and if there is discharge present. If the discharge is mucoid in origin there must be a perforation as there is no mucous lining in the external ear. A thin liquid may be indicative of otitis externa (an inflammatory condition of the EAC).

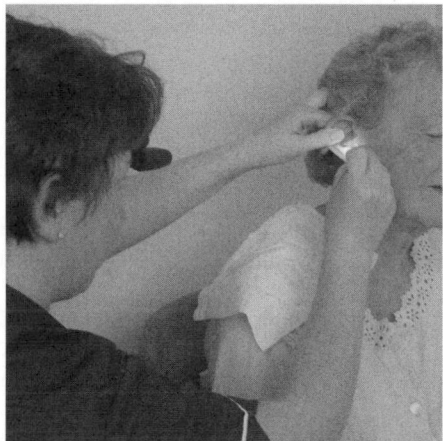

Figure 16.5 Carrying out an ear examination using a headlight.

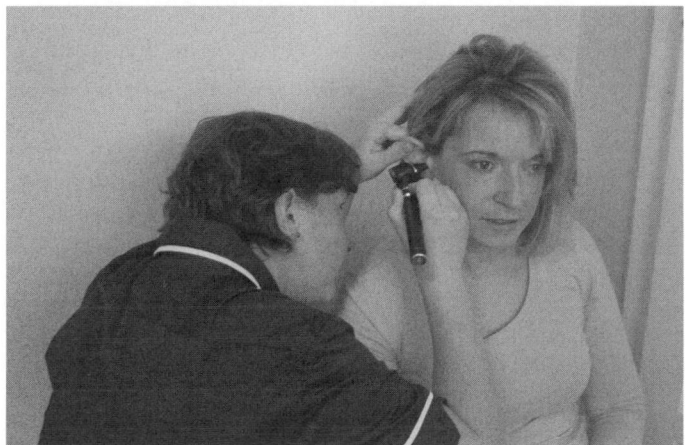

Figure 16.6 Carrying out an otoscopic examination.

GUIDELINES FOR CARE PRIORITIES

16.1 Examination of the ear

- Patients should have the procedure explained to them and informed consent obtained, reassuring them that they can stop the examination at any time if they wish.
- Ensure the instruments are prepared and at hand. If patients are wearing glasses or a hearing aid, they should be requested to remove them.
- Examine around and behind the pinna using a headlight (see Fig. 16.5).
- Straighten the external auditory canal (EAC) by pulling the pinna upwards and backwards (see Fig. 16.5). Check the size of the EAC opening to judge the size of speculum to be used for the examination. It should be large enough to ease the viewing of the drum but be of a comfortable fit for the patient. The speculum is necessary to pass through the hairs that would otherwise hamper a thorough examination; therefore, it should not be necessary to insert it beyond 8 mm in an adult, as this is where the hairs are located.
- Turning on the otoscope, insert the speculum into the patient's EAC (see Fig. 16.6). Observe the condition of the skin of the canal and observe the tympanic membrane, checking that the appearance is normal (see Fig. 16.2). Remove the speculum from the ear and release the pinna. If a patient wears a hearing aid normally, ask for it to be reinserted so that you can discuss the findings. Document the procedure before continuing with further ear care, to ensure that features seen will not be forgotten. If an abnormality is seen on the tympanic membrane, you must have the ability to draw that part, in order to be accountable for the procedure and to provide the person onto whom you are referring the patient with details of your findings.
- Document what was seen in the ears, the treatment and advice given to the patient, and the rationale.

- Using an otoscope, look at the skin of the canal for evidence of implements being inserted in the canal, such as foreign bodies or cotton buds pushing wax down the canal beyond the outer third where the ceruminous glands are located.
- Exostosis (bony overgrowths) in the ear canal are caused by cold water stimulation. They are most commonly found in the ears of cold water swimmers.

Middle ear

- Look for evidence of an abnormal tympanic membrane such as a dull appearance, retraction, perforation or inflammation. Check the light reflex exists (seen as a cone of light in the antero-inferior segment of the tympanic membrane produced by membrane concavity). Next work your eyes up the handle of the malleus to the pars flaccida (Fig. 16.2). Then look around the rim of the drum and to the anterior recess to check for the presence of debris. It is essential to be systematic with the assessment and ensure that all areas of the drum are viewed to be certain that there is no abnormality. The more proficient you become at examining normal tympanic membranes (Fig. 16.2), the easier the recognition of abnormal membranes will be.
- There be may be scarring on the tympanic membrane with the appearance of a white plaque indicating previous middle ear infections. This scarring is called tympanosclerosis.
- A thickened drum such that the malleus cannot be seen may indicate an otitis externa. In this case, the drum would not vibrate as effectively, resulting in impaired hearing.
- Look for a fluid level or bubbles in the middle ear indicating an effusion of fluid in the middle ear or eustachian tube dysfunction. Check the ability of the eustachian tube to open, by asking patients to take a deep breath, pinch their nose and blow out their cheeks, keeping their mouth closed. This should open the eustachian tube with the result that air will rush up to the middle ear and the drum will move quickly in response to this introduction of air. Some patients understand this as 'popping their ears as on an aircraft'. Lack of movement can indicate a tube dysfunction.
- Observe the colour of the tympanic membrane; blue may indicate fluid and yellow may indicate glue ear (thick mucoid fluid behind the tympanic membrane). Is the drum bulging and red indicating acute otitis media (acute inflammation of the middle ear)?
- If the pressure of air inside the middle ear is less than atmospheric pressure (negative pressure), a retraction pocket may develop in the tympanic membrane. If this builds up with migrating keratin debris, a cholesteatoma (squamous debris in the middle ear) may form. Check for a crust or a perforation in the attic.
- Is the tympanic membrane drawn onto the malleus and incus, making the bones more prominent? In severe cases of retraction, the drum can be drawn onto the stapes and the promontory (part of the basal turn of the cochlea).
- A fluid-filled blister on the drum is usually caused by a viral infection and is called bullous myringitis.
- A hole in the tympanic membrane is a perforation. Observe where it is situated and whether there is a margin of the drum remaining at the edge. Also document its size as a percentage.

GENERAL OTOLOGICAL DIAGNOSTIC TESTS AND MEDICAL INVESTIGATIONS

CALORICS

This investigation is useful to test the integrity of the labyrinth and its connections. It stimulates the lateral semi-circular canals by the irrigation of water into the EAC first at 30°C and then at 44°C. This thermal current produces within the intact vestibular system a response of nystagmus (rhythmic oscillatory movements of the eyes), the duration of which can be measured. It is individually performed on each ear using first one temperature then the other. The different temperatures produce nystagmus in opposite directions.

IMAGING

Computed tomography

Computed tomography (CT) is used in the ear to look at cholesteatoma and also at the extent of carcinomas and their involvement in the petrous (stony) temporal bone.

Magnetic resonance imaging

Magnetic resonance imaging (MRI) is most often used in the assessment of lesions such as acoustic neuromas (see p. 389).

ELECTROCOCHLEOGRAPHY

Electrocochleography (ECOG) is an electrical test of the response of the cochlea to sound. It is useful to measure the threshold of hearing and may also demonstrate characteristic changes in Ménière's disease (see 'Further reading' for more information).

HEARING ASSESSMENT AND TESTS

Nurses can assess a patient's hearing without using audiometry. Subjective testing of hearing can be carried out using the voice. Although voice tests are not diagnostic in themselves, they allow nurses to identify patients who are at risk of a hearing loss and they can then be referred quickly and appropriately to the local audiology department for advanced screening.

Voice tests should be carried out frequently in the older adult. They can form part of a routine assessment that will not increase the time of the general assessment or inconvenience the patient. When patients enter the assessment room, they can be questioned while their back is turned, e.g. while they are closing the door. Know the distance across the room from where you are standing. Patients who have difficulty hearing a normal conversational voice, i.e. with a loudness of about 40–50 dB, from 12 feet have some degree of a hearing loss. An ear examination should be carried out to ensure that there is no wax or debris in the EAC which may be impeding the hearing. Speak to patients about their perception of their hearing. Questions can be asked about the hearing loss, which may indicate the nature of the problem, e.g.: 'Is it worse or better in noisy surroundings such as on a busy street or in public places?'; or 'Do people appear to mumble when they are speaking?'.

Hearing loss can be gradual in onset, so patients may not have noticed it. It is often partners or relatives of patients who are complaining that the television volume is turned up too loud, or that the patients are not hearing them in the car when they are not looking at them. Many NHS Trusts have set a standard such that adults over the age of 65 years with a bilateral hearing loss in the absence of other symptoms are eligible for a direct referral to the audiology department.

Tuning fork tests

Nurses can establish the type of hearing loss by using tuning fork tests, which are a reliable method of ascertaining whether a hearing loss is conductive or sensorineural in origin (see p. 374). Their importance as part of a nursing assessment should not be underestimated.

There are two well established tuning fork tests in regular use – Rinne's and Weber's – and they test both air and bone conduction of sound. A 512-Hz tuning fork is used for both tests as a higher frequency tuning fork does not create sound for long enough to test hearing adequately, and a lower frequency fork creates too much vibration for the patient to be able to distinguish sound from vibration.

Rinne's test is performed by striking a tuning fork on your elbow and then placing it a few inches from the entrance of the EAC (air conduction) in the acoustic axis, followed by placing the base of the tuning fork on the mastoid process (bone conduction) located behind the ear. In the normal individual, air conduction (AC) is greater than bone conduction (BC).

Weber's test is performed by striking a tuning fork and placing the base on the forehead. If the sound is heard in the midline, Weber's test is said to be central and normal. Information on Rinne's and Weber's tests can be found in the ENT books in 'Further reading'.

Audiometry

This is the keystone of ear/hearing investigations. It is ideally performed in a soundproof room usually with headphones for air conduction and with an alice band-like instrument abutting the mastoid process for bone conduction.

Different frequencies are tested with varying intensities of sound measured in decibels (dB). Each ear is tested in turn for both air conduction and bone conduction. When hearing aids are to be fitted, the audiologist will test the maximal loudness tolerated by the individual, as the amplification should not exceed this level or it will be uncomfortable for the patient.

The normal range of hearing is accepted, over the frequencies, to be from 0 to 20 dB. A range of hearing below this level, i.e. a hearing loss > 20 dB, is considered to demonstrate a hearing loss. Further information on simple audiometry can be found in 'Further reading' (e.g. Ellis 2002).

Tympanometry

This is a commonly performed, quick and painless procedure. It involves introducing a sound into the EAC, at the same time varying the pressure in the EAC. The amount of sound reflected from the tympanic membrane is measured, allowing its compliance to be calculated. Tympanometry can provide a quick, easy method of discovering whether there is a problem within the middle ear.

Brain stem evoked responses

Brain stem evoked responses (BSERs) measure different electrical potentials from electrodes placed on the head and mastoid prominences in response to varying intensities of sound. A characteristic waveform is produced if the vestibulocochlear nerve is stimulated. This test is used to examine thresholds of hearing and also to investigate for acoustic neuromas.

► **Nursing care of patients undergoing hearing investigations**

Patients undergoing a general anaesthetic for the investigation to be carried out tend to be nursed in a day care setting. The nurse can alleviate anxiety by explaining to patients that audiological investigations do not usually require any large machinery or scans. Most imaging departments have patient information leaflets about the scanning equipment (e.g. CT and MRI), what will happen during the procedure and how long it will take. These information leaflets should be readily available on all units where the patients are nursed.

Hot or cold water stimulus (caloric testing) may cause vertigo (the sensation of movement without the physical stimulus) and an anti-emetic, e.g. prochlorperazine, may be prescribed to help to control dizziness. When patients are feeling dizzy, they often feel nauseous and may neglect to drink fluids. They should be advised to attempt small frequent amounts of liquids and solids 1 hour after taking the anti-emetic medication. The risk of dehydration is increased if vomiting occurs and patients may require admission until the vertigo has resolved.

Electrocochleography (see p. 374) requires the placement of an electrode through the tympanic membrane. The test is carried out in the audiology department and patients are required to be very still. Analgesia should be administered after the procedure. Cotton wool may be placed just outside the external ear canal, as there may be a small amount of blood loss. Patients should be advised to keep the ear dry (with cotton wool soaked in Vaseline or ear plugs) for 1 week and to change the cotton wool as appropriate. After 48 hours, or when the blood loss has stopped, the cotton wool can be removed.

All investigations involving the ear may cause vertigo. It should be ensured that patients have an escort to take them home and that they will not be left alone for 24 hours after the procedure. Patients should be advised to mobilize gently and take slow, steady movements when walking up stairs.

GENERAL DISEASE PREVENTION AND HEALTH EDUCATION

Nurses can have a considerable positive impact on the quality of life of patients with ear and hearing problems. Nursing and medical training in ear care is not standardized nationally and experience often depends on the ENT input during their training. Ear care is an aspect of patient care that nurses can and should carry out to the highest standard. However, at present this is dependent on the personal interest of the nurse rather than on a minimum standard of ear care. Ear care is often seen as a low priority within the realms of health care provision (Harkin & Rodgers 1999) and there is not enough current research to demonstrate whether the ear care that is being practised by nurses is evidence-based.

The holistic care of patients should include a knowledgeable nursing assessment of their ears, as there are a significant number of people who would benefit from such an assessment on admission to hospital or community care. For example, hearing loss is more common in diabetes mellitus (Ch. 17) due to the increased tendency to infections and also neuropathy. When the nurse is carrying out a diabetic clinic, assessment of hearing should be part of the patient's care. Early detection will ensure that the patient is assessed by the audiology department and provided with support in the form of counselling and environmental aids.

Nursing courses on the care of older adults should include ear care in the curriculum, as the improvement in patient comfort when wax is removed as well as the improvement in hearing have a considerable impact on quality of life. The consequent improvement in the ability of patients to understand their treatment also helps to reduce the anxiety associated with hospitalization (see Ch. 3).

Nurses caring for patients who suffer from dermatological conditions should also include ear care in the nursing assessment on admission, because despite the fact that this group of patients is being treated for skin problems, the skin lining the ear canal is often neglected.

The importance of holistic nursing practice cannot be stressed enough and this should include competent, knowledgeable research-based ear care. The nurse will see a direct improvement in a patient's condition if health education about the ear has been heeded. Further information regarding teaching patients to care for their ears can be found in the section on excess ear wax (p. 376).

PREVENTING NOISE DAMAGE

A large part of the role of an occupational health nurse consists of educating patients about noise-induced hearing loss. Noise ranks second, after physical injury, as an occupational health hazard. Workers are entitled to compensation if a company has not taken precautions to reduce noise, or has not advised employees on methods to protect themselves from a noise-induced hearing loss and provided them with the requisite protection. Nurses should be aware that noise damage can cause symptoms of stress (see Ch. 6), raised blood pressure, headaches, nausea and hearing loss. When carrying out an assessment, nurses should question patients about noise in the workplace. Occupational health departments must perform risk assessment and management where noise levels interfere with conversation or irritate workers. This will include measuring noise levels, implementing measures to reduce noise, carrying out hearing tests and providing ear protection for workers. Nurses can carry out subjective hearing tests (see p. 373), but where people are working in noisy environments, e.g. in a factory, they should have frequent hearing tests carried out by an audiologist. It is important for nurses to explain to patients the need to protect their ears and to highlight the danger of the irreversible effects of noise-induced damage. This information should also be given where leisure activities expose people to high levels of noise, e.g. loud music or shooting.

HEARING IMPAIRMENT

Classically, two types of hearing loss are described: sensorineural and conductive hearing loss. However, there can be significant overlap between the two and a mixed hearing loss is not uncommon. A conductive loss is incurred if there is any obstruction to the conduction of sound through the external and middle ear, while a sensorineural hearing loss is incurred if there is disruption of the transmission of sound from the inner ear onwards to the brain.

There are several conditions that affect hearing ability, including excess wax, hereditary conditions and acquired conditions such as noise-induced damage. It is estimated that there are 8.7 million people in the UK who are deaf or hard of hearing (Royal National Institute for the Deaf [RNID] 1999). The RNID maintains that there is a vast communication gap between the health care professions and the hard of hearing and deaf community, with the consequence that the latter receive a relatively poor service. Few health professionals have basic skills such as signing, and many are unaware that there are problems with communication (Robins & Mangan 1999). It is important that nurses work to bridge this gap, to ensure improved care and to reduce feelings of isolation from the health care system experienced by the deaf community.

COMMUNICATING WITH PEOPLE WITH HEARING PROBLEMS

Hospitalization can be a frightening experience for many patients, and those who are hearing-impaired have an added disadvantage, as communication with health care staff is likely to be hampered. There is a shortage of trained interpreters, and nurses need to be aware of the ways in which communication with the hearing-impaired can be facilitated and of their role in doing so (see Ch. 3 and Guidelines for Care Priorities box 16.2). Robins & Mangan (1999) provide numerous examples of poor communication in health care settings, outline technological support and offer practical advice, e.g. making sure that patients who normally lip-read have their glasses.

Nurses should establish how hearing-impaired patients wish to communicate, e.g. by lip-reading, using sign language via an interpreter or family member, using pen and paper or computer. It is also important for nurses to have a knowledge of the facilities, benefits and support available to the hearing-impaired. The RNID provides free leaflets for patients containing information on all aspects of hearing impairment and support groups (see 'Useful addresses', p. 391). The RNID also offers a range of services to deaf and hard of hearing people, their families and professionals who work with them. The Primary Ear Care Agency (see 'Useful addresses') provides nurses and all members of the health professions with training in ear care, including deaf awareness and training in the sympathetic hearing scheme.

HEARING AIDS

There are 5 million people in the UK with a hearing loss such that they would benefit from using a hearing aid, but at most only 2 million people have obtained them (RNID 1999). Hearing aid users tend to be poorly supported and hence the aids tend to be used infrequently by those who have them. A report from the RNID (1999) highlighted inadequate support and guidance for hearing aid users, and noted that there was an average waiting time of 1 year for an assessment appointment. As a result, the NHS Executive is currently reviewing the hearing aid service provided in the UK.

There are around 20 million people in the UK over the age of 50 and, of these, approximately 40% have some degree of hearing impairment. Nurses have a great deal of contact

GUIDELINES FOR CARE PRIORITIES

16.2 Improving communication with people who have hearing problems (Adapted from Robins & Mangan 1999)

- Try to find a quiet location if possible
- Reduce the effects of background noise, such as the television, and remember that hearing aids will amplify all noises
- Make sure that the person can see your face. Sit or stand facing the light and maintain eye contact (taking account of what level is culturally appropriate)
- Sit or stand at the same level as the person, at a distance of 1–2 m
- Speak clearly and slightly slower than usual
- Shouting causes distortion and will make it even more difficult for the person to hear what you are saying
- Make sure that you do not cover your face when talking, e.g. with your hand or papers
- Gestures and other non-verbal communication can be helpful, but excessive use or exaggerated facial expressions are best avoided
- Use the level of language that is appropriate for the person, not the person's level of hearing.

with patients with a hearing loss and are increasingly being called upon to support and advise the hearing aid wearer. It is important for nurses to be able to undertake routine tasks and make minor repairs to hearing aids, such as changing the tubing and batteries, and to understand the different types of hearing aid. Nurses can reinforce the teaching about hearing aids that they receive from the audiology department by helping patients to maintain and fit their aids correctly and manage basic problems.

The NHS supplies certain hearing aids free of charge to patients. A basic NHS hearing aid that is worn behind the ear costs approximately £40; more sophisticated models cost around £150, while digital aids purchased by patients in the private sector can cost considerably more. The basic NHS hearing aid has a small switch with the letters M, T and O on it. When the switch is in the 'M' position the microphone is turned on and the hearing aid will amplify sound. The 'O' position denotes that the aid is turned off and not amplifying sound and the 'T' position allows the person to use the 'loop systems' installed in various venues, such as theatres, and to use an appropriate television set. In the 'T' position, the hearing aid will pick up sounds the user wishes to hear without interference from background noise.

Patients should be given the option of wearing their hearing aid to theatre. It will, of course, be taken out during the operation, but theatre staff should be requested to re-insert the aid before patients wake up in the recovery room, so that they can communicate with the staff. The patient can turn on the aid when they feel ready.

Special doorbells and telephones and other devices are also available for those with hearing impairment. Information about the full range of such devices can be obtained from the RNID.

EXCESS EAR WAX

Normal wax production is discussed above. In most individuals, the action of hair follicles and jaw movement cause wax to migrate into the cartilaginous part of the ear canal, from where it can be easily removed with tissues (Zivic & King 1993). Any inhibition of this normal migration can lead to a build-up of wax. Ceruminous gland activity varies between racial groups and this should be taken into account when examining ear wax. For example, Chinese populations tend to produce small amounts of dry cerumen ('rice bran' wax) which results in dryness of the EAC, whereas Caucasian and African Caribbean populations tend to produce a wet, sticky form of wax. It is important for nurses to have an understanding of the different types of wax produced prior to carrying out ear examination.

As cerumen is exposed to air, it becomes darker in colour and of a drier consistency. Often the darker the wax, the harder the consistency and sometimes softening drops (ceruminolytics) may be required prior to removal (see Health Promotion box 16.1).

Pathophysiology

Anxiety and fear result in increased secretions from the ceruminous glands. People who have frequent ear syringing often say that wax builds up quicker after each procedure. This may be because cleaning of the canal wall encourages secretion from the ceruminous glands. The ageing process also has an effect by reducing sebum secretion, resulting in a drier type of cerumen that is more likely to become impacted in the EAC (see Older Adults: Nursing Priorities box 16.1). People with learning difficulties are also recognized to suffer from wax impaction (Roeser & Ballachanda 1997). The specific reason for this is unknown, but communication difficulties and other factors that cause anxiety can increase ceruminous gland activity and result in an over-production of wax.

Excess wax may cause inflammation, which, if severe, can give rise to otitis externa (see p. 382).

Clinical presentation

A build-up of wax may cause:

- conductive hearing loss
- irritation
- brownish smelly discharge
- tinnitus
- otitis externa.

Specific investigations

Wax can be identified during an otoscopic examination of the EAC. A headlight can be used to enhance the view of the wax, without the use of instruments, by pulling the pinna upwards and outwards to straighten the EAC.

Medical/surgical management

Wax impaction will require some form of medical or nursing intervention. In the community this could take the form of ear irrigation or aural toilet. In the ENT outpatient department a suction machine combined with a microscope is used to remove wax and clean the ear. People with wax impaction who are unable to tolerate removal, e.g. adults with learning difficulties, may be admitted to a day surgery setting where the wax is removed under general anaesthetic.

 OLDER ADULTS: NURSING PRIORITIES

16.1 Ear wax

As people age, the skin becomes drier and the secretion of sebum is reduced. The hairs in the external auditory canal (EAC) become coarser, trapping the wax and thus causing impaction. For these reasons people over the age of 65 years are more likely to suffer from problems related to wax. Ear examination in the older adult should be carried out as a routine assessment and, because wax impaction has a marked effect on the quality of individuals' lives, it should be given priority together with the other vital assessments at the time of admission. Removal of wax will improve hearing and reduce the incidence of problems with hearing aids. The use of cotton buds increases the likelihood of problems with wax and can also cause irritation of the skin of the EAC. Research has found that 32% of subjects aged over 60 years introduced an object into their ears to clean them on a regular basis and 34% were concerned with wax build-up (Ney 1993). Health education should involve explaining to the patient the dangers of inserting objects such as cotton buds, hair grips and pen tops, which cause the wax to be pushed further down into the EAC towards the tympanic membrane. This may cause deafness, otitis externa, tinnitus, pain and itching. When older adults suffer from dry skin around or in the ear, moisturizer should be applied to the outer ear daily and olive oil drops instilled inside EAC on a regular basis (one drop once a week).

Reference

Ney DF. Cerumen impaction, ear hygiene practices and hearing acuity. Geriatr Nurs 1993; 14(2): 70–73.

► Nursing management

Nursing management of excess ear wax can take the form of ear irrigation, aural toilet (cleaning the ear of debris with the use of a headlight and instruments) or microsuction. In the hospital ENT department, wax is generally removed by microsuction and aural toilet and the establishment of nurse-led clinics provides patients with flexible and regular appointments for ear care. Ear irrigation tends to be carried out more commonly in the community. In common with other invasive nursing procedures, ear irrigation has both contraindications and the potential for complications. Prior to undertaking ear irrigation there should be education, training and supervised practice by a recognized expert. As Wilson & Roeser (1997) wrote: 'Practitioners increase their chances of success in these situations by using their knowledge, skill and experience to consider all aspects of the procedure, to perform the procedure with care and to document the procedure accurately'.

A review by the Medical Defence Union of general practice procedure claims over 5 years revealed that ear irrigation accounted for 19% of the total (Price 1997). A metal syringe had been used in 92% of the irrigation cases and poor technique was the underlying problem in 43% of cases. Sharp et al (1990) demonstrated that there is significant water pressure generated

HEALTH PROMOTION

16.1 Choice of eardrops and administration

Patients will often ask the nurse's advice about which drops to take prior to ear irrigation. They may have seen advertisements regarding wax-dissolving drops, but these often cause irritation. Some contain urea hydrogen peroxide, a substance that would not be applied to skin elsewhere on the body and therefore one which should probably not be used for the delicate skin of the external auditory canal (EAC); while others contain traces of peanut oil and so are contraindicated in those with a nut allergy. The drops may well break up wax, as advertised, but the effect on the skin and the irritation they often cause are matters of some concern.

Sodium bicarbonate is alkaline and as such may break up the acidic wax, but again is a substance that would probably not be used on skin elsewhere on the body. Olive oil is a safe method of softening ear wax and lubricating the EAC. There are no contraindications to its use and so it can be instilled in a mastoid cavity or if a perforation is present. The British National Formulary (2002) states that 'the simple remedies are just as effective and less likely to cause irritation'.

How to administer eardrops
Prior to prescribing, it is essential to consider whether patients will be able to administer their own eardrops or whether they will require support from district nurses or a relative. If help is needed, it would be advantageous to prescribe drops that are to be administered twice daily rather than three times daily. If a patient is in a nursing home, a spray dispenser could be prescribed, so the patient would not have to lie down while it was being administered.

An alternative to drops is the insertion of an appropriate ointment into the ear canal with the patient being followed up in a nurse-led clinic (Wilde et al 1995).

To administer eardrops, patients should be advised as follows:

1. Lie on a bed with the affected ear towards the ceiling.
2. With one hand, pull the pinna upwards and outwards to straighten the EAC.
3. Squeeze the dropper until the required number of drops have been instilled. Maintain that position for 5 minutes.
4. Wipe off the excess drops that pool outside the ear when you sit up. Do not insert cotton wool, as this will absorb the drops.
5. Check that the drops will not stain the bed linen or, alternatively, protect the bedding with old material.
6. If the drops are to be inserted into both ears, separate bottles of drops are required (except in the treatment of wax) and repeat steps 1–4. The drops are for single patient use and many prescription drops are to be discarded 1 month after opening.
7. Ensure you keep your ears dry (by the use of cotton wool soaked in petroleum jelly or ear plugs) when bathing and if you have, or are prone to, an ear infection.

References
British National Formulary. Number 44, September. London: British Medical Association and Royal Pharmaceutical Society of Great Britain; 2002. (online www.bnf.org)

Wilde AD, England J, Jones AS. An alternative to regular dressings for otitis externa and chronic suppurative otitis media? J Laryngol Otol 1995; 109: 101–103.

---

using the metal syringe, and unlike an electronic ear syringe, in which a variable pressure control allows the practitioner to control the flow of water, in a metal syringe the water pressure cannot be controlled. Litigation arising out of ear irrigation has often been due to poor maintenance of the equipment and to incorrect attachment of the nozzle of the syringe (Price 1997). The Medical Devices Agency states that metal syringes should not be used.

When a full ear examination has been carried out and it has been ascertained that there is wax to be removed, the nurse must ensure there are no contraindications to the procedure being performed (see Special Issues box 16.1).

Tinnitus and dizziness are potential complications of ear irrigation and nurses should always ask patients whether they suffer from either prior to performing the procedure. This ensures protection from litigation in the event of a complaint. Patients should have the ear irrigation procedure explained and should be made to understand that it can be stopped at any time if they wish. The nurse should then make sure they are sitting comfortably during the procedure. When performing ear irrigation in older adults, nurses must be sure that they can sit still for the 15 minutes or so it takes to carry out the examination and procedure and should ensure that the environment

is warm and the seating comfortable. Patients may prefer a relative or a nursing colleague to be present to reassure and support them. Nurses should also consider the understanding and safety of patients with Parkinson's disease (see Ch. 14), Alzheimer's disease or a learning disability. If patients find it difficult to sit still or tolerate an ear examination then irrigation should not be attempted, as there is a danger that they may jerk their head onto the syringe, causing discomfort; some may even find the noise of the machine frightening (see Guidelines for Care Priorities box 16.3, Reflective Practice box 16.2).

PRESBYCUSIS

Presbycusis is hearing loss caused by age-related degenerative changes of the inner ear.

Pathophysiology

This condition is due to degeneration of the inner and outer hair cells of the inner ear and of the cerebral components of hearing. The commonest explanation for this is progressive decreased blood supply due to small blood vessel disease that often occurs with age. This compromises both cerebral and inner ear blood supply.

SPECIAL ISSUES

16.1 Contraindications to ear irrigation

If the nurse establishes that there is a contraindication to irrigation, the patient will require aural toilet or microsuction, which is cleaning of the ear using a microscope and suction. This is mainly performed within the ENT outpatient department.

Below is a list of reasons why ear irrigation would not be carried out on an individual:

- If the patient has suffered complications with previous ear irrigation

- If the patient has a perforation in the tympanic membrane or a mucoid discharge, which would indicate a perforation
- If the patient has had ear surgery – all forms of ear surgery are contraindications to irrigation, apart from grommets that are no longer in place and have been discharged from the ENT department for 18 months
- If the patient has had a cleft palate, as such patients are more prone to middle ear disease due to poor development of the facial skeleton
- Oedematous canal with pain and tenderness of the pinna

 GUIDELINES FOR CARE PRIORITIES

16.3 Ear irrigation

1. Ensure the equipment for use is within easy reach (see Fig. 16.4).
2. Prepare the electrical syringe.
3. The tap water for use in the ear should be at body temperature (37°C); if it is too hot/cold, the semi-circular canals will be stimulated, causing dizziness.
4. The tip on the syringe should be clicked and secured into place.
5. Patients should be seated comfortably with their back resting against the chair and the nurse should be positioned sideways facing their shoulder.
6. Running the water through the tubing ensures that no air bubbles are trapped and gives patients the opportunity to become accustomed to the noise and water pressure of the machine. A container or kidney dish should be placed below the ear lobe against the skin to collect the water and debris.
7. Water pressure should initially be set to a minimum and increased if necessary and with the patient's permission.
8. A headlight should be focused on the patient's external auditory meatus and the pinna straightened to aid the removal of wax (see Fig. 16.7).
9. Observing the debris, stop irrigating after the wax is removed or after 5 minutes. Examine the ear with an otoscope to check if the tympanic membrane can be visualized and if all the wax has been removed. If the wax has been removed, stop irrigation and dry the canal. If the drum cannot be visualized, and the patient remains comfortable, continue to irrigate for up to 10 minutes. If the wax remaining is too hard, irrigation should be stopped and the patient asked to continue ear-softening drops for 1 week.
10. Excess water should be removed from the external auditory canal to reduce the risk of an external ear infection (otitis externa) post-irrigation.

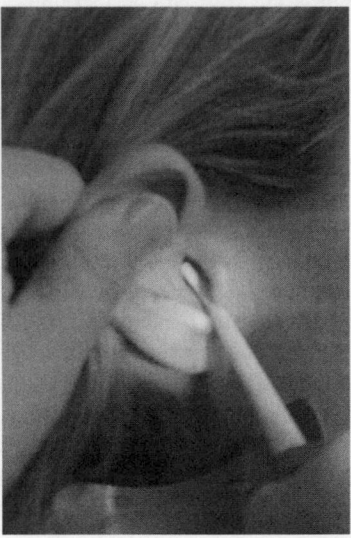

Figure 16.7
Carrying out the ear irrigation procedure.

11. Ensure that you document the procedure as follows:
    — what was seen on examination in the ears
    — the results of the irrigation, e.g. normal wax removed
    — any complications experienced
    — otoscopy results post-irrigation
    — advice given to the patient that is appropriate to the reason for the wax build-up. For example, advise the patient not to insert objects such as cotton buds into the ears.

NB. If it is necessary to proceed to irrigate the second ear after unsuccessful irrigation of the first ear, it is worth re-attempting the procedure after 10 minutes. The instillation of water during the irrigation procedure can often soften wax after it has been left for 10 minutes.

R|Я REFLECTIVE PRACTICE

16.2 Elsa

Elsa has psoriasis (see Ch. 28) and has attended her general practitioner with pain in both ears. She has complained of itchy ears for several months and has always inserted cotton buds after showering. Elsa requires ear irrigation every 6 months due to a build-up of wax. The chemist advised her to use olive oil eardrops for 1 week prior to attending her appointment to have her ears irrigated. On examination, Elsa has normal wax in both ears, but it has been pushed onto the tympanic membrane.

Student activities

- What is the link between Elsa suffering from itchy ears and her psoriasis?
- Why is the wax pushed onto the eardrum and what effect does this have on the skin of the ear canal?
- What advice will you give Elsa before and after irrigating her ears?

Clinical presentation

Presbycusis usually presents in older adults. Sufferers often complain that other people are mumbling when speaking to them and have to have things repeated several times. They tend to find group conversations harder to follow and, having to concentrate harder, tend to tire more easily. They often find it difficult to hear on the telephone and tend to turn the radio and television up so that they are too loud for other listeners. The rest of the otological history is often normal.

Specific investigations

A pure tone audiogram often shows the sensorineural hearing loss that is characteristically high frequency in its nature.

Medical/surgical management

Hearing aids (see p. 375) are of benefit but will require adjustment for the patient.

▶ Nursing management

Where in-patients are thought to suffer from presbycusis, nurses can carry out a holistic assessment which should include questions on how the patients perceive their hearing. The NHS supplies patients with free hearing aids, batteries, repairs, medical examinations and follow-up appointments, but patients are often unaware of this provision. Posters and literature should be available in health centres, GP surgeries and care of the elderly units, etc., to inform people and encourage them to consider whether they or a partner may benefit from a hearing aid.

People often deny that they have problems with their hearing and are reluctant to attend the audiology department because presbycusis is seen as a condition affecting older adults (see Older Adults: Nursing Priorities box 16.2). Patients will require nursing support and reassurance. They can be advised to contact Hearing Concern or the RNID for further information and support. Hearing aid wearers tend to be more prone to wax

65 83 50 71 OLDER ADULTS: NURSING PRIORITIES

16.2 Hearing aids

There is a significant deterioration of hearing with advancing age (presbycusis) that can be improved with the use of hearing aids. Around 50% of hearing impairment occurring in those aged 65 years and over can be corrected with the use of aids, but only 10% are wearers. The poor usage of aids in older adults is partly due to a low referral rate from general practitioners and an acceptance of the hearing loss as a part of growing older. There is a stigma attached to wearing hearing aids that discourages the older adult from seeking a hearing assessment. Nurses can improve the referral rate to the audiology department and support and educate patients regarding their hearing loss and the benefit of hearing aids. The consequences of an unrecognized and unsupported hearing loss in older adults are social isolation and psychiatric morbidity (Herbst 1980). The improvement to the quality of life of older adults who have a hearing aid successfully fitted and maintained should be reiterated to reluctant patients. There tends to be poor audiology follow-up with problems with hearing aids and this is an aspect of care that nurses can be involved in, especially those nurses working within the community environment.

Reference

Herbst K. Hearing impairment and mental state in the elderly living at home. Br Med J 1980; 281: 903–905.

accumulation. Therefore, patients should have their ears examined by the nurse every 6–9 months to maintain the benefit of the aid as well as patient comfort.

OTOSCLEROSIS

Otosclerosis is a hereditary condition that affects the middle ear ossicles, most notably the stapes, causing a conductive deficit in hearing.

Pathophysiology

In otosclerosis the lamellar bone of the ossicles changes to woven bone, leading to fixation of the ossicles, particularly the stapes. Fixation prevents the normal conduction of sound and leads to a conductive hearing loss.

Clinical presentation

Patients may complain of tinnitus and a decrease in hearing that is often better in crowds. Women often complain of the condition worsening during pregnancy, as hormones may influence progression. A tuning fork examination may demonstrate the conductive hearing loss. General examination of the tympanic membrane reveals little, except occasionally the so-called 'flamingo flush' associated with otosclerosis.

Specific investigations

A pure tone audiogram is essential to show the gap between air and bone conduction. A speech audiogram in which words are presented at varying intensities instead of pure tones is often helpful to demonstrate whether the patient would benefit from surgery.

Medical/surgical management

Management must be tailored to the needs of the patient. Hearing aids with audiological input are a simple, safe and non-invasive way of improving hearing loss.

Stapedectomy is the operation of choice, but is not without significant risk (of severe sensorineural hearing loss) even in the hands of an expert. This operation involves removing the immobile part of the stapes and replacing it with an artificial stapes in the form of a piston that allows movement for the conduction of sound.

▶ Nursing management

Care of the patient undergoing stapedectomy is covered in detail in the section on middle ear surgery (see p. 385). Specifically, the nurse should remember that otosclerosis is a hereditary disease, so patients will be concerned about hearing loss in their children. Patients may also be influenced by the standard of care their own parents received while undergoing stapedectomy. Often a sufferer's hearing is better in an environment with background noise, so contrary to general advice, any discussions with the patient may be improved by being within range of a television or radio.

NOISE-INDUCED HEARING LOSS

Hearing loss as a result of excess noise is an increasingly important problem. It has now become a compensatable condition if incurred in the workplace, when an employer has not taken sufficient care to protect the hearing of employees.

Aetiology and epidemiology

In the past, noise-induced hearing loss was seen as a condition that affected people working in heavy industry – hence the name 'boilermaker's disease', as it affected riveters working inside ships' boilers who were continuously exposed to loud noise. In recent years, people have become increasingly aware of the complications of loudness levels in both occupational and recreational situations:

- occupational exposure occurs in people who work with heavy machinery or with aircraft, etc., where noise exposure is continuous
- recreational exposure occurs during leisure activities such as shooting and discos.

Pathophysiology

It is postulated that the hair cells in the inner ear suffer metabolic exhaustion because of an overload of work; then, with further exposure, they are thought to become permanently non-functional.

Clinical presentation

Patients usually complain of tinnitus and a decrease in the hearing in one or both ears depending on the type of exposure.

Specific investigations

A full otological history is essential to exclude other causes of hearing loss. A pure tone audiogram often shows a classical sensorineural hearing loss that is centred at the 4 kHz level and which may be unilateral or bilateral depending on the exposure.

Medical/surgical management

Medical management tends to involve compensation claims. Compensation may be possible for those who have worked in a noise-filled environment and amounts can be calculated according to the degree of hearing loss, the amount of noise above the acceptable limits in the working environment and the percentage disability.

▶ Nursing management

Readers are directed to the earlier discussion regarding hearing impairment, in particular communication with people with hearing problems and hearing aids.

TRAUMA AND FOREIGN BODIES

Trauma to the external and middle ear occurs frequently. It is most often seen in the primary health care setting or in the accident and emergency department. Traumatic injuries to the ear should always be excluded when there is a head injury. Additionally, patients with trauma to one part of the ear must be examined to exclude damage to different parts of the ear.

Foreign bodies in the ear are more common in children, but certainly do occur in adult patients.

HAEMATOMA OF THE PINNA

A haematoma of the pinna is a collection of blood under the skin overlying the pinna.

Aetiology

A haematoma is caused by external physical trauma to the outer ear, e.g. a punch or when rugby players bang their heads together in a scrum.

Pathophysiology

Trauma results in bleeding from just above the cartilage of the pinna. This raises a tense swelling under the skin of the pinna that produces an unsightly swelling.

Clinical presentation

Patients have swelling and tenderness of the pinna that may be red in appearance (erythematous). This is a clinical diagnosis and rarely requires any special investigations unless other pathology exists or is suspected.

Medical/surgical management

Haematoma requires immediate treatment to prevent irreversible damage to the cartilage of the ear. The haematoma is aspirated with a needle or incised and drained, and a pressure dressing is applied. Patients may need nitrous oxide/oxygen inhalation or local anaesthetic while the haematoma is being aspirated or drained. The ear is painful and analgesia will be prescribed, e.g. co-proxamol. Follow-up in the outpatient clinic is essential to observe for return of the haematoma. As a prophylactic measure, it is prudent to prescribe a broad-spectrum antibiotic to prevent infection. Failure to treat the haematoma adequately may lead to complications such as perichondritis (inflammation of the cartilage of the pinna) or ischaemic damage to the cartilage, leading to a deformity of the pinna referred to as a 'cauliflower ear'.

▶ Nursing management

Patients will require a sterile dressing to cover the incision and this will be further covered with a firm crepe bandage applied around the head and affected ear. They should be advised to keep the bandage clean and dry, and not to shower until the wound is healed – a bath will be more appropriate. Repeat dressings may be required for approximately 5 days and patients should be told to return to the ENT department if the dressing becomes soaked with blood or the ear becomes very painful. They should avoid sleeping on the affected ear and should also avoid contact sports for 6 weeks. Patients need to be warned that if they resume contact sports, e.g. boxing or rugby, repeated trauma to the ear may result in cosmetic deformity to the pinna ('cauliflower ear').

TRAUMATIC PERFORATIONS OF THE TYMPANIC MEMBRANE

This is a common injury most often seen in general practice or the A&E department.

Aetiology

Perforation may be caused by a change in air pressure secondary to external direct trauma, such as a blow to the ear, or to a sudden blast or explosion. Solid object trauma is not uncommon during inappropriate ear cleaning. Excessive pressure and poor technique when irrigating ears can perforate the tympanic membrane.

Pathophysiology

A perforation is a hole in the tympanic membrane and is described as being 'safe' or 'unsafe'; this is not to imply safe or unsafe for irrigation, as ear irrigation is always contraindicated when any perforation is suspected. Safe and unsafe are the terms used to describe the position of the perforation. Superior perforations (in the pars flaccida) are more at risk of forming cholesteatoma (squamous debris in the middle ear) compared with safer inferior perforations (in the pars tensa). This is related to the migration of the skin cells when trying to heal over a perforation. When examining a perforation, it is essential to document the type, size and position.

Clinical presentation

People usually present after the traumatic event with a slight decrease in their hearing. They may have complained of pain and slight blood loss at the time of the trauma and perforation occurring. It is essential to confirm that the trauma has not created a sensorineural hearing loss. This is done using tuning fork tests, which may demonstrate a mild conductive loss.

The tympanic membrane may reveal a small amount of haemorrhage or more often a small linear perforation in the pars tensa.

Specific investigations

A pure tone audiogram may be performed if the hearing loss is significant or if the hearing does not return to normal.

Medical/surgical management

The vast majority of traumatic perforations will spontaneously close. Prophylactic antibiotic eardrops should be prescribed where a potentially infected implement or foreign body might have caused the trauma.

Regular review in the outpatient department or the general practice setting is necessary to ensure that the perforation closes and that the hearing returns to normal. This may take up to 3–4 months. An ENT referral is essential if the perforation or the hearing loss persists.

▶ Nursing management

One of the nursing priorities is to reassure patients that there is a strong likelihood that the perforation will heal and hearing will return to normal. Appropriate ear advice is essential and includes:

- keeping the ear dry
- not swimming
- protecting the ear by using cotton wool with Vaseline as an ear plug whilst showering
- not inserting anything into the ear.

People who develop discharge from the ear need to return to the clinic or general practitioner, as this is a sign that the ear is infected and topical antibiotic eardrops should be commenced.

FOREIGN BODIES IN THE EAR

Foreign bodies in the ear are more common in children than in adults, but they do occur in adults who have inserted cotton buds or other objects into their ear canals.

Clinical presentation

Patients usually present early with a decrease in hearing and mild irritation of the canal. Otalgia, otorrhoea (discharge from the ear) and hearing loss are not uncommon where the presentation is late. Nurses need to be aware that some individuals with learning disabilities may have, as a result of a behavioural abnormality, inserted a foreign body and may be unable to explain what has happened.

The presence of a foreign body is usually a clinical diagnosis and no investigations are required.

Medical/surgical management

Unless the foreign body is easy to remove in the emergency department or general practice the majority should be referred to the ENT surgeon or nurse. The first attempt at removal is often the best attempt as patients of all ages become nervous if a second attempt is required. Foreign bodies are either organic or inorganic. The organic type of foreign body tends to be hydroscopic (absorb water readily) and swells with irrigation. The inorganic type if small may be gently irrigated out of the ear. Insects should be killed by instilling olive oil at room temperature prior to their removal. The vast majority of foreign bodies can be removed using a Jobson Horne probe, suction or a pair of crocodile forceps, together with a good light source and microscope.

▶ Nursing management

The nurse, with the relevant skills, can remove foreign bodies from the ear using microsuction, aural toilet or irrigation. Irrigation should not be carried out when the foreign body is suspected to be organic matter (peas, lentils) as it would absorb the water and swell in the external ear canal, causing further trauma and increasing the difficulty of removal. Both ears must be examined and it is essential to ensure a normal tympanic membrane and ear canal are seen and documented on removal of the foreign body. The nurse has to consider the reason why an adult was inserting objects in the ears. It may have been to block out the noises of tinnitus or to stop itching. It is also important to investigate the reason for the insertion of the object in patients who are unable to verbalize pain, tinnitus or problems with their ears. Clients with learning disabilities or dementia (see Ch. 32) who frequently insert foreign bodies should be referred to the ENT department for a thorough assessment of their ears and hearing. A holistic approach to ear care requires that practitioners question the reasons for the occurrence and implement strategies that reduce the risk of repetition.

INFECTIONS AND INFLAMMATORY CONDITIONS OF THE EAR

This is a diverse group of conditions which are frequently seen in both the ENT outpatient clinic and the primary care setting. The majority of infections and inflammatory conditions can be quite painful and therefore it is necessary when treating the actual condition to ensure the patient has effective analgesia.

It is easier to understand the inflammatory or infective conditions affecting the different parts of the ear by starting with the external ear – the pinna and EAC – and the middle ear (otitis media).

PERICHONDRITIS

Perichondritis is an inflammatory condition affecting the cartilage of the pinna.

Aetiology

Perichondritis can follow a haematoma of the pinna, a furuncle in the EAC, infection after piercing to the tragus or helix or even surgery involving an external approach to the middle ear.

Pathophysiology and clinical presentation

The infective microorganism is often *Pseudomonas* species and will cause a localized inflammatory reaction in the pinna. There is swelling, local warmth and discoloration of the pinna. The pinna is exquisitely tender and the patient may be pyrexial. A fluctuant swelling would imply that an abscess has formed.

Medical/surgical management

The treatment for the majority involves the use of analgesia and antibiotics. A swab is taken for microscopy, culture and sensitivity, and an appropriate antibiotic, e.g. penicillin, is given until antibiotic sensitivities are known from swabs. An appropriate dressing for the ear is applied. Where an abscess is present, an incision and drainage are essential with thorough irrigation of the abscess cavity and the commencement of antibiotics.

▶ Nursing management

This is the same nursing care as that required for the patient with haematoma of the pinna (see p. 380).

OTITIS EXTERNA

Otitis externa is inflammation of the EAC. It is extremely common and is often associated with infection. Ten per cent of the population will be affected by otitis externa at some time in their lives.

Aetiology

Several types of otitis externa, with different aetiologies, are recognized:

- Infective – this may be bacterial (*Pseudomonas*, *Staphylococcus aureus*, *Proteus*) or fungal (*Aspergillus* or *Candida*)
- Reactive – secondary to sensitive skin conditions such as eczema, psoriasis or seborrhoeic dermatitis (see Ch. 28)
- Malignant – it is important to mention that this condition is not cancer; it tends to occur in people with diabetes mellitus or in immunocompromised individuals.

Predisposing factors for otitis externa may include:

- irritation of the external canal with cotton buds or other implements
- wet EACs from swimming and humid environments
- narrow EACs.

Pathophysiology

Whatever the predisposing factor associated with otitis externa, the skin of the EAC becomes oedematous. This swelling can affect the normal epithelial migration and an accumulation of debris occurs. Infection can occur in addition to the build-up of debris and oedema. Malignant otitis externa is a severe form that leads to bony exposure in the EAC, and erosion and infection of part of the temporal bone. Additionally it may also be associated with lower cranial nerve palsies (VII–XII; see Ch. 14) as the disease progresses.

Clinical presentation

Otalgia, otorrhoea and a blocked sensation in the ears are common in the acute stage. People with the chronic form frequently complain of pruritus (an itchy sensation). The discharge tends to be thin and of a liquid consistency.

The EAC is often inflamed and covered with debris. Occasionally oedema limits the view in the EAC. The tympanic membrane is often thickened without the feature of the malleus being identified so there may be an accompanying hearing loss. After the acute stage has subsided, it is essential to look at the tympanic membrane to exclude any middle ear pathology that may give rise to similar symptoms.

Specific investigations

A swab is taken for microscopy, culture and sensitivity if the infection does not respond to a first-line treatment with topical antibiotic drops.

Medical/surgical management

The options for treatment include gentle ear irrigation, antibiotic eardrops containing a corticosteroid, aural toilet with the possibility of the insertion of an ear wick.

Malignant otitis externa requires an urgent referral to the ENT surgeon and warrants admission with intravenous antibiotics and debridement of the EAC under general anaesthetic.

▶ Nursing management

It is essential that the debris in the ear canal is removed in order for the eardrops to be absorbed effectively. The nurse (suitably trained and experienced) can carry out gentle ear irrigation for about 2 minutes and this procedure often feels soothing for patients. The nurse must dry mop the length of the external ear canal to ensure that there is no water pooling in the anterior recess that could exacerbate the condition. Patients will need reassurance that their hearing will improve if any hearing loss was caused by a thickened tympanic membrane secondary to the otitis externa. As the infection may have been caused by insertion of implements into the EAC, it is vital that the nurse provides appropriate health education. The ear must be kept clean and dry especially when bathing. This can be achieved by inserting cotton wool covered in Vaseline into the concha of the ear. In situations where patients are unable to self-administer the prescribed eardrops, the nurse could insert an antibiotic-soaked dressing or an ear wick into the canal. This will have to be changed every 48 hours until the condition has improved. The nurse who is trained in ear care in both the community and hospital setting manages otitis externa very successfully.

Malignant otitis externa

A trigger factor for malignant otitis externa may have been ear irrigation and leaving water pooling in the canal for infection to spread. Patients must be advised to return if there is discharge, inflammation or pain post-procedure so that cases similar to this condition can be recognized and treated quickly. If ear irrigation is the trigger, patients should be advised not to have their ears irrigation again and it would be worth offering feedback to the health professional who carried out the procedure. The nurse should ensure that patients are given the intravenous antibiotics as prescribed and that any increase in pain, discharge or temperature is reported to the doctor. As patients can develop cranial nerve palsies, the nurse should examine the facial nerve (VIIth cranial nerve) frequently in the initial stages to ensure deterioration is recognized and treated early. This is done by asking patients to smile, close their eyes, raise their eyebrows and puff out their cheeks to test the branches of the facial nerve and to compare the two sides of the face for symmetry. Holistic care is essential and nurses should be aware of the individuals who tend to be affected by this disease: older people, those with diabetes and immunocompromised individuals.

ACUTE SUPPURATIVE OTITIS MEDIA

Acute suppurative otitis media (ASOM) is an acute infection of the middle ear.

Aetiology

The condition is associated with:

- eustachian tube dysfunction
- adenoidal hypertrophy, upper respiratory tract infections (URTIs) and a narrowed nasopharyngeal airway
- nasopharyngeal carcinoma obstructing the eustachian tube with increased frequency in people of Chinese origin (see Ch. 21).

Pathophysiology

Acute suppurative otitis media is most often due to a bacterial infection that gains entry into the middle ear cavity via the eustachian tube or a perforated tympanic membrane. Once in the middle ear cavity, the infective microorganism causes an inflammatory process that can lead to a thick, mucoid discharge via a perforation in the tympanic membrane.

Clinical presentation

Acute suppurative otitis media usually affects children and follows an URTI, but can occur in adults. Otalgia is common and the pain associated with pressure in the middle ear cavity causes irritability in children. Some individuals may be pyrexial. On otoscopy the tympanic membrane may appear dull and there may be fluid or even pus evident in the middle ear. The blood vessels down the handle of malleus are generally dilated. The fluid will increase until the pressure causes the tympanic membrane to rupture. This provides relief as the pressure in the middle ear is released. Purulent otorrhoea may develop as pus drains from the middle ear cavity.

Specific investigations

A swab of the ear discharge is sent for microscopy, culture and sensitivity. A pure tone audiogram is of use after the acute event to check the state of the hearing; however, during the infective period an audiogram is of little use.

Medical/surgical management

Acute suppurative otitis media can spontaneously resolve on occasions. Early treatment with a short course of oral antibiotics may be of benefit. The majority of the microorganisms causing ASOM are sensitive to simple penicillins.

Where there is ear discharge, it is necessary to dry mop the EAC followed by the instillation of a short course of eardrops.

A cause should be sought for recurrent ASOM, especially if it is unilateral. An examination under anaesthesia of the post-nasal space may be warranted to exclude nasopharyngeal cancer. In childhood ASOM, insertion of a grommet is an excellent treatment option.

▶ Nursing management

The nurse can advise patients to try steam inhalations and decongestants, as they may help to alleviate symptoms by improving eustachian tube function and drainage of fluid from the middle ear. When patients are having grommets inserted, it is important to consider the reason for surgery. Adults with a potential nasopharyngeal cancer preventing middle ear drainage will need information and explanation in an attempt to alleviate their fears and anxieties (see Ch. 3). Extra care should be taken to ensure patients find their stay in hospital as comfortable as possible, as they may be returning for radiotherapy or radical cancer surgery. Children with adenoidal enlargement blocking the opening of the eustachian tube will have adenoid removal in addition to grommet insertion.

Discharge advice

The nurse should show patients what a grommet looks like. Grommets extrude spontaneously from the tympanic membrane some 2–12 months after insertion and are so small that patients may miss them. Swimming can be resumed 2 weeks after surgery, but some surgeons may prefer their patients to avoid swimming until their follow-up in the outpatient department. Patients should prevent shampoo getting into the ear as this will change the water tension and may allow entry into the middle ear via the grommet. Patients should therefore be advised to place cotton wool with Vaseline in the bowl of the ear to prevent this occurring. Patients who develop ear discharge or pain should return to their GP for antibiotic eardrops.

Nurses should reassure patients that the hole remaining in the tympanic membrane after the grommet has fallen out tends to heal in a short period of time. There is a chance of the otitis media recurring when the grommets extrude and this may warrant a further set of grommets. Patients will be reviewed in the ENT department until the disease has resolved.

CHRONIC SUPPURATIVE OTITIS MEDIA

Chronic suppurative otitis media (CSOM) is a chronic inflammatory process in the middle ear cavity. It has a number of classification systems, including the tubotympanic (related to pathology in the pars tensa of the tympanic membrane) and the atticoantral (related to pathology in the pars flaccida of the tympanic membrane).

Tubotympanic

This type is generally referred to as a 'safe' condition, because there is a decreased risk of significant intracranial complications, and involves a perforation with a margin of the tympanic membrane remaining in the pars tensa. Most of the perforations arise as a consequence of ASOM.

Clinical presentation

The condition is often associated with a conductive hearing loss secondary to perforation, erosion of the ossicles or tympanosclerosis (a fibrous scar on the tympanic membrane). There may also be intermittent mucoid discharge.

Otoscopic examination may demonstrate the perforation and this is described with regard to its position and size and also the state of the middle ear mucosa (dry or wet). A swab of the ear discharge is sent for microscopy, culture and sensitivity.

Medical/surgical management

Regular otoscopy to review the state of the tympanic membrane and middle ear may be all that is required in some cases of asymptomatic CSOM. Intermittent eardrops and aural toilet may be necessary for the treatment of episodes of otorrhoea.

For recurrent discharge, repair of the tympanic membrane (myringoplasty) is an option, but the pros and cons should be discussed with the individual before operation. The advantages of the operation are that a dry ear is a definite possibility and thus allows the patient to enjoy a life free of aural discharge. The disadvantages include the chance of failure and also the potential for risk to the hearing and damage to the facial nerve perioperatively, together with the chance of dizziness postoperatively.

Atticoantral

This type is associated with a cholesteatoma (squamous debris in the middle ear) that may be congenital (due to groups of epithelial cells left in the middle ear during development) or acquired. The acquired type arises from negative middle ear pressure, marginal perforations where epithelium grows into the middle ear, metaplasia (change from the normal lining to a skin-like lining of the middle ear) of middle ear mucosa with CSOM, and implantation of epithelium with perforation of the tympanic membrane.

Atticoantral CSOM is generally referred to as an 'unsafe' ear because it can be associated with significant intracranial complications and is usually linked with a retraction pocket or a perforation in the pars flaccida of the tympanic membrane.

Clinical presentation

Patients may be asymptomatic. More often they complain of an offensive discharge, decreased hearing and occasionally vertigo and tinnitus. Examination may reveal a perforation, attic crust (a piece of keratin debris sited over the pars flaccida of the tympanic membrane), a retraction pocket in the pars flaccida, or may show an aural polyp which tends to occur in chronic inflammation.

Specific investigations

A CT scan of the middle ear is performed to assess the extent of the cholesteatoma.

Medical/surgical management

Small retraction pockets in the pars flaccida may be managed medically if they can be completely cleaned of debris in the clinic. If the debris cannot be removed, it will be necessary to examine the patient's ear under anaesthesia. In some cases, surgery on the mastoid bone is needed. This is because most of the cholesteatoma sacs tend to enlarge into the mastoid bone.

COMPLICATIONS OF SUPPURATIVE OTITIS MEDIA

Apart from the problems already discussed, reduced quality of life and time lost from work or study, there are several potentially serious complications of suppurative otitis media.

Intracranial complications

- Abscess formation – extradural (outside the dura of the brain), subdural (under the dura of the brain) or intracerebral (within the brain substance)
- Sigmoid sinus thrombosis – clot formation in the sigmoid venous sinus that drains venous blood from within the skull.

Some information is provided in Chapter 14, but readers are encouraged to consult a specialist neurosurgical textbook, e.g. Lindsay & Bone (1997).

Temporal bone involvement

- Petrositis – infection and inflammation within the petrous (stony) part of the temporal bone
- Mastoiditis – infection and inflammation within the mastoid part of the temporal bone
- Labyrinthitis – inflammation of the organ of balance within the inner ear
- Sensorineural hearing loss.

Middle ear involvement

- Tympanosclerosis – thickened scar tissue affecting the tympanic membrane or middle ear mucosa
- Adhesions
- Perforations
- Ossicle erosion
- Facial nerve palsy.

> ▶ **Nursing management of the patient undergoing ear surgery**

PRE- AND POSTOPERATIVE CARE

General perioperative care is covered in Chapter 29. This section covers specific aspects of caring for patients undergoing ear surgery, many of whom have some hearing impairment. The nurse should take steps to overcome the associated communication problems (see p. 375, Ch. 3). Patients may wish to communicate via sign language with an interpreter, by lip-reading or by computer. Most wards have access to a computer should patients want this type of help. Alternatively, they may want a family member to interpret for them. Nurses will need to have a basic understanding of common ear operations so that they can confirm the information given to the patient by the surgeon (see Table 16.1). Patients will require specific information about the operation, e.g. the site, dressings, packs and whether hair shaving is required. Minor ear operations do not require the hair to be shaved, but for more extensive surgery, the surgeon usually shaves 1 inch of hair from the area behind the pinna. Patients should be reassured that the hair will grow back. Details of pain control and the relief of vertigo and nausea are discussed preoperatively.

Patients often suffer vertigo after ear surgery. Privacy, tissues, mouth care and kindness can never be underestimated.

Prochlorperazine as prescribed should be given to relieve symptoms of vertigo. Intravenous fluids are administered until the nausea settles and the patient can tolerate oral fluids. Water should be attempted first, and then a slow increase to other fluids. Light snacking can then be encouraged.

Patients are offered a bed bath and assistance in removing the surgical gown to increase their comfort. Visitors should be kept to a minimum. A bedside fan may be helpful as a dizzy sensation can cause patients to experience hot flushes. Care should be taken when patients first attempt to mobilize as they may feel dizzy and faint. This may simply be due to the anaesthetic agents but may also be related to surgery performed close to the semicircular canals, which are concerned with maintaining balance. Assistance with putting on slippers or shoes will prevent patients from having to bend down, which will exacerbate the dizziness. Patients should be told to ask the nurse to accompany them to the bathroom or lavatory, to ensure their safety.

The majority of patients who undergo middle ear surgery will have a pack inserted into the EAC or mastoid cavity for up to 2–3 weeks postoperatively. The pack splints the EAC and reduces the risk of infection entering the middle ear. The pack often contains iodine and nurses must ensure that patients are questioned preoperatively about sensitivities and that the surgeon and theatre nurses are aware of any allergies so that an alternative pack can be prepared.

Due to the close proximity of the facial nerve (VIIth cranial nerve) to the operative area, the surgeon may request that facial nerve observations are carried out. These observations are done when the vital signs are monitored and will identify any facial nerve paralysis; patients are asked to:

1. raise their eyebrows
2. close their eyes tightly
3. puff out their cheeks
4. smile.

This tests the branches of the facial nerve that are important on the face. Each exercise is compared to the opposite side and symmetry or weakness is noted. The result of the observations are charted on a specifically designed sheet and documented in the nursing notes. Changes to the facial movement should be documented and reported to the surgeon. The surgeon should be informed immediately if movement deteriorates or suddenly changes.

Patients may have gauze over the affected ear and a crepe bandage firmly placed over the gauze and around the head for the first postoperative night. The dressing needs to be secure to ensure that the blood loss is absorbed by the gauze rather than pooling under the skin and forming a haematoma. If blood loss appears on the outside of the bandage or trickles down the face, the surgeon should be informed. The bandage is removed by the nurse 24 hours postoperatively, and if necessary the area around the ear is cleaned of blood. The pack inside the ear should not be touched, but clean cotton wool is inserted in the concha of the ear and changed as needed. Prior to discharge, the nurse should check if the stitches are dissolvable, or, if they need to be removed, when this should be done and by whom. Patients must understand the advice outlined below and have received both verbal and written instructions. The ward telephone number should be provided in case they wish to seek further advice.

Table 16.1 Commonly performed ear operations

Operation	Condition for which performed	Brief explanation of the surgery involved
Myringoplasty	Perforation (hole) in the tympanic membrane	A graft of temporalis fascia is most often used and placed under the perforation to seal the hole that exists. With time this should be maintained and the perforation cease to exist
Tympanoplasty	Ossicular or tympanic membrane damage secondary to middle ear disease	There are a number of these procedures that are aimed at improving the transmission of sound via the tympanic membrane and ossicular chain. There are varying degrees of ossicular damage with ear disease and these are all treated by a different type of tympanoplasty
Mastoidectomy	Cholesteatoma	An operation involving the drilling of the mastoid bone that would normally be filled with air cells. The drilling out of the bone allows for the removal of the disease (cholesteatoma) in the bone
Cochlear implant	Profound hearing loss	This is an electronic device that is implanted with a wire insertion into the cochlea and secured to the skull. Approximately 2 weeks after the operation an external aid is fitted. This will cause the stimulation of the electrodes within the cochlea and hopefully stimulate any residual neural tissue within the cochlea

DISCHARGE ADVICE FOR THE PATIENT

- Part of the dressing in the ear canal may become dislodged due to jaw movement. Do not push the dressing back into the EAC or pull the dressing out of the EAC; ask an adult to snip the dislodged part of the dressing, using clean scissors. Attend the clinic at your planned appointment. If the whole pack comes out of the EAC, you need to telephone the ward and attend immediately. There is a risk of the canal wall becoming stenosed (narrowed).
- Ensure that the ear is kept dry. Do not wash your hair for at least 5 days. When you shower, keep your ear dry by inserting cotton wool coated in Vaseline in the concha of the ear. Direct all water away from the affected ear, ensuring that the wound is also kept dry.
- If the skin surrounding the stitches becomes painful and inflamed or begins to discharge, attend your GP for advice.
- Do not travel by air, swim or dive until you have attended the outpatient department and discussed the implications with the surgeon.
- There may be a metallic taste in the mouth due to the nature of the surgery and proximity to the chorda tympani.
- Do not blow your nose violently. First gently clear one nostril and then the other. When you sneeze, keep your mouth open to reduce the pressure.
- Avoid sleeping on the side of the surgery until the ear is healed.

If patients complain of feeling dizzy, encourage them to be careful when mobilizing. They should only attempt gentle movement when they have company. Encourage them to take the medication (prochlorperazine) as prescribed, and if the dizziness persists, increases in severity or is accompanied by nausea, they should return to the hospital.

The nurse must stress that patients must never have their ears irrigated.

DISORDERS OF BALANCE

The integration of sensory input from the eyes, the labyrinth of the inner ear and proprioceptors in joints govern balance. It is important to realize that problems with balance will occur if there is an abnormality in any one of the components. The midbrain and cerebrum normally integrate these sensory inputs and relay nerve impulses to the appropriate muscle groups in order to maintain posture and balance.

Vertigo is the sensation of movement without an associated sensory input to the brain, and may occur with many different conditions.

MÉNIÈRE'S DISEASE

Ménière's disease is a condition characterized by episodic vertigo, tinnitus and deafness. It accounts for 10–20% of true vertigo in ENT clinics.

Aetiology

The aetiology is still unknown, but current theories include labyrinthine ischaemia (lack of blood supply) or an auto-immune response in which the body's immune system attacks the labyrinth as though it were a foreign body.

Pathophysiology

The underlying pathology includes a distension of the endo-lymphatic system that leads to distortion of the semi-circular canals and the cochlea, resulting in the symptoms of Ménière's disease.

Clinical presentation

Patients can recognize that they are about to have an attack, the so-called 'aura'. They then experience a combination of symptoms, including a feeling of fullness in the ear, deafness, tinnitus and vertigo. The symptoms are episodic and last a few hours at a time. In the long term, vertigo will improve in 70% of patients, regardless of the treatment. It is, however, the deterioration in hearing that accompanies the condition that is of concern.

Specific investigations

The vast majority of diagnoses are made from the history, but specialist investigations such as electrocochleography and the glycerol dehydration tests (the use of glycerol to mildly dehydrate the patient and also to decrease the swelling in the endolymphatic system, thus increasing the hearing) can be used to aid diagnosis.

The use of pure tone audiogram is essential to trace any changes in hearing with time. Classically a low-frequency sensorineural hearing loss develops.

Medical/surgical management

Drugs may be used to alleviate symptoms. Betahistine (a labyrinthine vasodilator) seems to be of benefit, although the true mechanism is uncertain. Vestibular sedatives, such as prochlorperazine (a phenothiazine) or cinnarizine, used in the acute attack can help to alleviate vertigo and nausea.

Surgical and other treatments include:

- endolymphatic sac decompression to prevent the endolymphatic hydrops
- vestibular nerve section
- destruction of the vestibular labyrinth with surgery or ultrasound, or the instillation of gentamicin (an aminoglycoside antibiotic) where the vestibulotoxic (toxic to the vestibular apparatus) side-effect can be used for treatment.

BENIGN PAROXYSMAL POSITIONAL VERTIGO

Benign paroxysmal positional vertigo (BPPV) is a condition of short-lived vertigo associated with sudden movements of the head. It is common, easily diagnosed and treatable.

Aetiology and pathophysiology

Benign paroxysmal positional vertigo often occurs after a head injury and is thought to be caused by chalk-like particles dislodged into the semi-circular canals. Sudden head movements may cause these particles to stimulate the sensory organ in the semi-circular canals.

Clinical presentation

Patients complain of a rotatory vertigo that occurs shortly after a sudden head movement. It lasts for a few seconds to minutes. Classically the vertigo occurs when patients lie down or get up from the bed.

Specific investigations

The condition is confirmed by performing the Hallpike manoeuvre. This manoeuvre simulates a sudden head movement and precipitates nystagmus and vertigo in the patient.

Medical/surgical management

The condition can generally be improved with specific manoeuvres such as the Epley manoeuvre, which displaces the chalk-like material out of the semi-circular canal. It is effective but may need more than one treatment. Readers requiring more details on the complex Epley manoeuvre are advised to consult an ENT text.

ACUTE LABYRINTHITIS

Acute labyrinthitis is an inflammatory/infective process affecting the labyrinth. It may be bacterial or viral in origin.

Clinical presentation

Classically, patients complain of a preceding upper respiratory tract infection followed by rapid onset of severe vertigo that leads to nausea and vomiting. The vertigo can be very distressing for patients in the most acute stages. Their hearing may or may not be affected. A good history together with spontaneous nystagmus is usually enough to make the diagnosis. It is essential to exclude the diagnosis of meningitis (see Ch. 14).

Medical/surgical management

The best treatment in the acute stages is with vestibular sedatives. These sometimes have to be administered as an intramuscular or sublingual preparation, as oral medications cannot always be retained due to vomiting.

Vestibular rehabilitation overseen by an audiologist with an interest in balance may help an individual recover confidence and improve balance in the more chronic cases.

> ► **Nursing management of patients with disorders of balance**

Psychological support starts in the initial consulting rooms and is an important part of the management of all patients with disorders of balance. It is important to question patients about the medication they take, their smoking habits and alcohol intake. Drugs with an action on the central nervous system (CNS) may cause dizziness if a greater dose than recommended is taken. Antihypertensive drugs, beta-blockers and non-steroidal anti-inflammatories have also been associated with dizziness. Patients should be given a full explanation of why the loss of balance has occurred, which will provide them with assurance and support. Patients can often sense when an attack is about to occur so they should be advised to sit or lie down if possible and ensure they are in a safe environment. They should record when the episodes occur to try to identify the trigger and hence learn to avoid contact with it. Attacks tend to occur in groups, so when patients develop imbalance they should be advised to rest if possible. It is important to explain the nature of the disorder to the family to reduce their anxiety and encourage their support.

It is important to maintain fluid hydration as the episode may occur with nausea and vomiting. If patients are unable to tolerate fluids due to the nausea and vomiting, they may become dehydrated, in which case they will be admitted under the care of a general physician and nursed on a medical ward.

If prochlorperazine given intramuscularly does not control the dizziness, an intravenous infusion of cyclizine can be commenced.

One of the priorities in nursing patients with balance problems is to maintain a safe environment. They should be advised to obtain assistance when they mobilize and not to attempt stairs alone. In the home they should have solid objects placed strategically in parts of the room so they have something to hold onto for stability. Objects that patients will be required to pick up should be placed within easy reach and they will require assistance with footwear as bending down may exacerbate the dizziness. If patients are also suffering from nystagmus, advise them to focus on a fixed object at eye level, such as the handle of a door, and to inhale deeply. The dizziness should subside.

A physiotherapist can teach patients exercises to help control the dizziness, and an occupational therapist can assess patients in their home environment and ensure their safety prior to discharge.

Patients can be referred to a hearing and/or balance therapist for further psychological support and the nurse should provide the telephone numbers of information and support groups and encourage patients to make contact with them (see 'Useful addresses', p. 391).

TINNITUS

Tinnitus is the sensation of sound that does not come from an external source. It is a troublesome and common condition that is not always curable. It can occur in any age group but is more common with increasing age. Persistent tinnitus occurs in about 10% of the population, with one person in six complaining about regular or constant tinnitus (RNID 1999). It is essential to exclude worrying pathology (such as an acoustic neuroma) in the assessment of tinnitus and then to treat and support the sufferer as best one can.

Aetiology
■ Local – any hearing loss presbycusis, Ménière's, acoustic neuromas, noise-induced
■ General – hyperdynamic circulations (as in hypertension or anaemia), carotid bruits (the noise associated with a carotid artery stenosis), caffeine intake from tea, coffee or alcohol.

Pathophysiology
The aetiology is unclear but it has been postulated to arise from 'cross talk' across vestibulocochlear nerve neurons. Whatever the cause of the tinnitus, it is recognized that there is also a central component that may augment the effect tinnitus has on individuals.

Clinical presentation
Tinnitus affects people in different ways. For some, it is a minor irritant which is tolerated fairly easily, while for others, the incessant nature of the problem can cause such severe distress that it can lead to suicide. It is for this reason that the complaint of tinnitus should never be taken lightly. A full otological and general history must be taken to exclude other pathology.

Specific investigations
A pure tone audiogram is of use in establishing the degree of hearing loss that may be attributable to the tinnitus. Other investigations may be of use in looking for specific causes of tinnitus, such as a basic blood screen (full blood count, urea and electrolytes, erythrocyte sedimentation rates), CT scan of the ear and MRI scan of the head and neck.

Medical management
Treatment of any underlying causes is undertaken. Most people find a thorough examination by an ENT specialist reassuring. They will give the patient a clear explanation of the condition, some helpful advice, together with direction towards self-help groups.

▶ Nursing management

As there is generally no medical or surgical care for the relief of tinnitus, patients will rely on the nurse for support. Tinnitus will have an impact on lifestyle, and nurses can empower patients with knowledge on how to control their problem by accessing and passing on information about various management strategies and sources of support available (British Tinnitus Association 2001). The effect that these noises can have on a person should not be underestimated; it is recognized that tinnitus can cause social isolation, aggressive behaviour, anxiety, depression and, in extreme circumstances, suicide. The nurse can help patients come to terms with their diagnosis and reinforce what the ENT surgeon has told them about their condition. Patients should be directed towards specialized help such as that provided by a hearing therapist or self-help groups. Tinnitus counselling provides patients with information and advice on all aspects of the problem and its management. In these sessions, relaxation techniques can be taught and patients offered the use of complementary therapies.

Hearing aids can be of use; they can amplify the hearing and thereby reduce the tinnitus, as straining to hear can focus the subconscious brain to pick up noises more easily.

A combined hearing aid/masker is often used which produces a continuous sound that matches the tinnitus and therefore distracts the patient. Pillow speakers are a useful option; these work on a similar principle to the masking but help to deal with the condition at night, which is often the time when tinnitus sufferers are troubled the most.

Tinnitus is often made worse or triggered by stress. Therefore, if the nurse teaches patients stress management exercises, these may empower them in the control of their tinnitus (see Ch. 6). Tinnitus can cause sufferers to miss bits of conversation, as their ability to concentrate is affected. They are then at risk of becoming depressed and socially isolated. The nurse in the outpatient department can refer patients to a community colleague to ensure that they have continued support.

Tinnitus may be triggered by certain foods/drinks, e.g. chocolate, caffeine and red wine, and patients are encouraged to maintain a food diary in order to try to ascertain what their trigger might be, so as to avoid it in the future. Nurses can encourage patients not to focus on the noises but to attempt distraction therapy. An increase in the number of hobbies they engage in may help to stop patients focusing on the tinnitus. It is an important role for the nurse to ensure that patients believe that members of the health team are listening to their symptoms and are trying to help.

TUMOURS

Tumours of the ear are a diverse group. Benign tumours often only require treatment if they prove to be troublesome. This is because surgery to the canal itself can have important sequelae. Malignant tumours, if treated in their early stages, do very well with minimal cosmetic deformity.

BENIGN TUMOURS OF THE EXTERNAL AND MIDDLE EAR

There are a number of benign tumours of the external ear, but they are relatively rare. Generally they are treated with local excision if they are troublesome or require a diagnosis to exclude malignancy. These tumours include papillomas, adenomas and other rarities such as fibromas and chondromas.

An interesting group of benign tumours include the bony hard exostosis that is seen in people who swim in cold water. These are often bilateral and require treatment only if troublesome. They will require removal if they occlude the view to the tympanic membrane or are obstructing the canal causing the keratin debris to build up behind the exostosis.

MALIGNANT TUMOURS OF THE EXTERNAL AND MIDDLE EAR

The most common malignant tumours of the external and middle ear are squamous cell carcinoma and basal cell carcinoma (see also Ch. 28). This condition is frequently seen in people who have had significant sun exposure, e.g. agricultural workers, sailors and labourers.

Clinical presentation
Patients often complain of a small ulcer or lesion on the pinna. The lesion may not produce any symptoms. Occasionally it bleeds or causes irritation. Clinical examination for signs of regional lymph node enlargement is essential as this is the first site of spread.

Medical/surgical management
Excision of a wedge (including the lesion) from the pinna is acceptable for a small lesion, leaving the patient with minimal cosmetic deformity. If the lesion is of significant size, an assessment of the EAC and temporal bone is essential. Occasionally a radical excision of the ear is necessary which may also be accompanied by an excision of part of the temporal bone. Basal cell tumours are also radiosensitive, which provides the clinician with another treatment option.

▶ Nursing management

Removal of a small lesion is usually performed in a day surgery setting. For details of care required by patients undergoing a more radical removal of a larger tumour, see Chapter 28.

TUMOURS OF THE INNER EAR

Acoustic neuroma
This is a relatively rare tumour that occurs at an area that abuts the apex of the petrous part of the temporal bone (in the skull) and the midbrain, the so-called cerebellopontine angle. The importance of the location of this benign tumour can create serious problems.

Aetiology
Generally the aetiology is unknown except for the rare association with the condition of neurofibromatosis. In this condition there is an association with bilateral acoustic neuromas.

Pathophysiology
This is a benign neoplasm of the Schwann cells of the nerve (see Ch. 14). These are the cells that surround the nerves outside the CNS. The neoplasm is mostly associated with the vestibular part of the vestibulocochlear nerve. It is therefore more accurately referred to as a vestibular schwannoma.

Clinical presentation
Patients are often asymptomatic for a long time; however, the classic complaints are a change in the hearing possibly associated with some tinnitus. Vertigo is a rare symptom. With larger tumours that invade the cerebellopontine angle, other cranial nerve palsies can occur (affecting cranial nerves V, VI, VII, IX and X) and headaches, diplopia and altered levels of consciousness have all been described.

Specific investigations
- A pure tone audiogram is necessary to establish if there is an asymmetric sensorineural hearing loss that warrants further investigation.
- MRI scan of the cerebellopontine angle is now the gold standard investigation for the diagnosis and the follow-up of patients with acoustic neuromas.

Medical/surgical management
The vast majority of acoustic neuromas that are diagnosed in healthy individuals are treated surgically. There are a number of approaches to removing the tumour. Further general information about neurosurgery can be found in Chapter 14 and more specific information in the texts listed in 'Further reading'.

▶ Nursing care

The care of the patient undergoing removal of an acoustic neuroma occurs on a specialist neurosurgical unit (see Ch. 14 and 'Further reading'). However, the specialized nursing care is similar to the nursing care of patients undergoing ear surgery. The surgeon will have informed the patient that surgery will result in hearing loss in the affected ear. Reassurance should be given regarding the type of hearing aids available on the NHS, such as ear canal aids as well as digital hearing aids. If the patient has good hearing in the unaffected ear they may not require a hearing aid.

SUMMARY: MAIN POINTS

- Many people complain of ear irritation that causes discomfort and this often leads to the insertion of objects such as cotton buds into the external auditory canal (EAC). This can lead to a build-up of wax and inflamed skin. Health information on how to care for ears can promote comfort and reduce the frequency of intervention to remove wax.

- Nurses should support and encourage hearing aid wearers and, through practice, reinforce the teaching of the audiology department on how to care for hearing aids and deal with common problems.

- On initial consultation, it is important to question patients about problems they may be having with their ears and hearing. As the patient advocate, the nurse should be the one to communicate with patients and ensure they have the right support from the health sector to maintain their quality of life as best as possible.

- Nurses involved in delivering care to patients with problems relating to the ear and hearing should have good communication skills, a thorough knowledge of the anatomy and physiology, competent skills in performing ear care and an awareness of the appropriate investigations and support network.

SELF-TEST: CRITICAL THINKING ACTIVITIES

1 Within 5 minutes of commencing irrigating a 70-year-old woman's ears, the nurse has to stop as the patient is complaining of water going down the back of her throat. What will you find when you examine the ear with an otoscope? Consider what you would do and your rationale.

2 A 28-year-old pregnant woman complains of a progressive hearing loss and is concerned as her mother became very hard of hearing at a similar age. On examination, both eardrums appear normal. What may be the cause of the hearing loss? Do you feel that the person warrants a referral to the ENT department? What is your rationale for that decision?

3 A patient has had grommets inserted 3 weeks ago. He telephones the ward to ask whether he can fly abroad in 1 week. What advice will you give to the patient? Consider the rationale for this.

4 You are nursing an 85-year-old woman who is having difficulty understanding you. When her son visits, you discover that she usually wears a hearing aid but he has been unable to locate it. Consider what you will include in your nursing care plan and how you will approach having the aid replaced and maintained in your area of nursing.

 FURTHER READING

Burton M (ed). Hall and Colman's diseases of the ear, nose and throat, 15th edn. Edinburgh: Churchill Livingstone; 2000.

Coopey S. Ear syringing – a case for clinical governance. J Commun Nurs 2001; 15(1): 20–22.

Corbridge R. Essential ENT. London: Arnold; 1998.

Ellis P. A companion to ENT for medical students and general practitioners. London: The Medical Defence Union; 2002.

Harkin H, Vaz FM. The provision of ear care by the practice nurse in the primary health care setting. Prim Health Care 2000; 10(10): 30–33.

Harkin H. Review of the literature of ear care. Prim Health Care 2000; 10(9): 37–41.

Harkin H. Evidence based ear care. Prim Health Care 2000; 10(8): 25–30.

Hooper M. Aural hygiene and the use of cotton buds. Nurs Stand 1991; 6(12); 38–39.

Jones AS. Key topics in otolaryngology and head and neck surgery. Oxford: Bios Scientific Publishers Ltd; 1995.

Kaye A. Essential neurosurgery, 2nd edn. Edinburgh: Churchill Livingstone; 1996.

Lewis-Cullinan C, Janken JK. Effect of cerumen removal on the hearing ability of geriatric patients. J Adv Nurs 1990; 15: 595–600.

Lindsay K, Bone I. Neurology and neurosurgery illustrated, 3rd edn. Edinburgh: Churchill Livingstone; 1997.

Liston R, Solomon S, Banerjee AK. Prevalence of hearing problems, and use of hearing aids among a sample of elderly patients. Br J Gen Pract 1995; 45: 369–370.

Robertson DG, Bennett DC. The general practice management of otitis externa. J Roy Army Med Corps 1992; 138: 27–32.

Rodgers R. Hear my plea. Nurs Times 1996; 92(46): 36–37.

Rodgers R. How safe is your syringing? Commun Nurse 1997; June: 28–29.

Rodgers R. Understand the legalities of ear syringing. Pract Nurse 2000; 19: 166–169.

Rodgers R. Continuing education: preventive ear care. Nurse Pract 2002; March: 71–73.

USEFUL ADDRESSES

Royal National Institute for Deaf People (RNID)
19–23 Featherstone Street
London EC1Y 8SL
Tel: 020 7296 8000
Helpline: 0808 808 0123
Fax: 020 7296 8199
Textphone: 020 7296 8001
www.rnid.org.uk

RNID Tinnitus Helpline
2 Pelham Court
Pelham Road
Nottingham NG5 1AP
Tel (voice/textphone, Mon–Fri, 10am–3pm): 0345 090 210

The Primary Ear Care Centre
Kiveton Park Primary Care Centre
Chapel Way, Kiveton Park
Sheffield, South Yorkshire
S26 6QU
Tel: 01909 772746
Fax: 01909 774934
www.earcarecentre.com

Ménière's Society
98 Maybury Road
Woking
Surrey GU21 5HX
Tel: 01483 740 597
Textphone: 01483 771 207

British Society of Hearing Therapists
Hearing Centre
Yardley Green Unit
East Birmingham Hospital
Birmingham B9 5PX

British Tinnitus Association
www.tinnitus.org.uk

Hearing Concern
7–11 Armstrong Road
London W3 7JL
Tel: 020 8743 1110
Textphone : 020 8742 9151
National telephone helpline: 01245 344 600

BT Age and Disability
9th Floor
Burne House
Bell Street
London NW1 5BZ
Tel: 0345 581 456

The Link Centre for Deafened People
19 Hartfield Road
Eastbourne
East Sussex BN21 2AR
Tel: 01323 638 0230
Fax: 01323 642 968
e-mail: linkcntr@dircon.co.uk

REFERENCES

British National Formulary. Number 44, September. London: British Medical Association and Royal Pharmaceutical Society of Great Britain; 2002. (online www.bnf.org)

British Tinnitus Association. Helping patients with tinnitus: guidance for nurses. Nurs Stand 2001; 15(3): 39–42.

Harkin H, Rodgers R. Aural care in the primary setting. Prim Health Care 1999; 9(2): 28–29.

Harkin H. Evidence-based earcare. Primary Health Care Journal 2000; 10(8): 25–30.

Herbst K. Hearing impairment and mental state in the elderly living at home. Br Med J 1980; 281: 903–905.

Ney DF. Cerumen impaction, ear hygiene practices and hearing acuity. Geriatr Nurs 1993; 14(2): 70–73.

Price J. Problems of ear syringing. Pract Nurse 1997; 14: 126–128.

Robins J, Mangan M. Seen and not heard. Nurs Times 1999; 95(37): 30–32.

Roeser RJ, Ballanchanda BB. Physiology, pathophysiology, and anthropology/epidemiology of human ear canal secretions. J Am Acad Audiol 1997; 8(6): 391–400.

Royal National Institute for the Deaf. Waiting to hear. RNID: London; 1999.

Sharp JF, Wilson JA, Ross L et al. Ear wax removal: a survey of current practice. Br Med J 1990; 301: 1251–1252.

Wilson PL, Roeser RJ. Cerumen management: professional issues and techniques. J Am Acad Audiol 1997; 8: 421–430.

Zivic RC, King S. Cerumen impaction management for clients of all ages. Nurse Pract 1993; 18(3): 29, 33–36, 39.

17 Nursing patients with endocrine and metabolic disorders

Maggie Watkinson

'I was looking after a woman with diabetes today. I thought I knew a bit about it 'cos we did it in the last module but I've learnt such a lot from her. She really knew her stuff – I suppose you have to know a lot if you have to live with a chronic condition like that'

(Student nurse)

THIS CHAPTER WILL HELP YOU

- Explain how changes to normal physiology can result in specific diseases of the endocrine system

- Describe the epidemiology of endocrine diseases, where this is known

- Relate the clinical presentation of the specific diseases studied to the underlying pathophysiology

- Discuss current therapies available for specific diseases, indicating any side-effects these may have

- Apply knowledge gained about the specific diseases studied to the clinical setting

- Explore the psychological and social effects the specific diseases may have on the individual

- Assess, plan, implement and evaluate the nursing care required for individuals with the specific diseases

- Critically examine your own attitudes to individuals with endocrine diseases, particularly diabetes mellitus

- Debate the professional, legal and ethical issues associated with the nursing role in the care of people with diabetes mellitus.

KEYWORDS

Addison's disease	Hyperthyroidism
Corticosteroids	Hypoglycaemia
Cushing's syndrome/disease	Hypoparathyroidism
	Hypothyroidism
Diabetic ketoacidosis	Insulin
Endocrine gland/structure	Oral hypoglycaemic agents
Hormone	Thyroidectomy
Hyperglycaemia	Type 1 diabetes mellitus
Hyperparathyroidism	Type 2 diabetes mellitus

INTRODUCTION

Endocrine conditions are generally very uncommon, apart from thyroid diseases, which are usually treated on an outpatient basis, and diabetes, which is discussed below. This means that many nurses will not encounter individuals with the more uncommon conditions, as they are likely to be referred to specialist centres for investigation, diagnosis and treatment. However, the investigations frequently take time to complete, and endocrine conditions very often have lasting effects necessitating lifelong follow-up. Consequently, nurses may encounter people who are undergoing these processes and, although not directly involved, may need to provide information and support.

Some specialist centres benefit from the services of endocrinology specialist nurses; they undertake many of the investigative tests and provide information to patients and their families, and other health care professionals.

Diabetes mellitus is one of the commonest chronic conditions in the world, particularly the Western world, and is becoming more so. It is predicted that the number of people with diabetes mellitus in 2025 will be double that which it was in 1997 (World Health Organization 1997). Although most of this rise will occur in developing countries, westernized societies will still be affected. In the UK, for instance, the estimate is that the number of people with diabetes mellitus will increase to 2.9 million people by 2010 (Amos et al 1997) from today's estimate of 1.3 million. Given that diabetes mellitus costs approximately 9% of hospital budgets alone (Currie et al 1997), the impact of this rise is potentially enormous, in terms of both money and the provision of quality care.

Partly for these reasons, diabetes mellitus has been recognized as an important health care issue. The fourth of the National Service Frameworks (NSFs) (Department of Health 2001) deals with diabetes mellitus; the standards of care (see Special Issues box 17.1) were published in 2001 (Department of Health 2001) and the delivery strategy was published in 2003 (Department of Health 2003). The NSF is likely to have a profound impact on service delivery, albeit over a 10-year period.

As well as being common, diabetes is a serious condition, which affects people physically and also psychologically and sociologically. As a result, quality of life for many people with diabetes is severely reduced.

The long-term complications can affect almost any part of the body; for this reason, nurses working in any setting are likely to encounter individuals with the condition. In the context of this book, the chapters on cardiovascular disorders (Ch. 19), ophthalmology (Ch. 15), neurological problems (Ch. 14) and renal disease (Ch. 24) are of particular relevance. In addition, the theme of health promotion, and the chapters dealing with communication (Ch. 3) and nursing those with a chronic illness (Ch. 35) are also pertinent.

Diabetes specialist nurses, who may be based in secondary or primary care, and often work across both sectors, are invaluable sources of information, education and expert advice about diabetes and the care of those who have it. Indeed, their role not only includes direct care of people with diabetes, but also the continuing education of other health care professionals. Those who wish to know more about nursing people with diabetes and diabetes care should contact their local diabetes nursing team to find out what learning opportunities exist.

ANATOMY AND PHYSIOLOGY – AN OVERVIEW

The overview in this chapter will briefly cover the hypothalamus, pituitary, thyroid, parathyroid and adrenal glands, and the endocrine pancreas. Knowledge of relevant anatomy and physiology provides the base for understanding the conditions, treatments and nursing care needed by people with diabetes mellitus (classified as a metabolic disorder with widespread manifestations) and endocrine problems.

The endocrine structures, which function closely with the nervous system, are vital for the regulation of physiological processes and maintaining homeostasis. These structures (see Fig. 17.1) include:

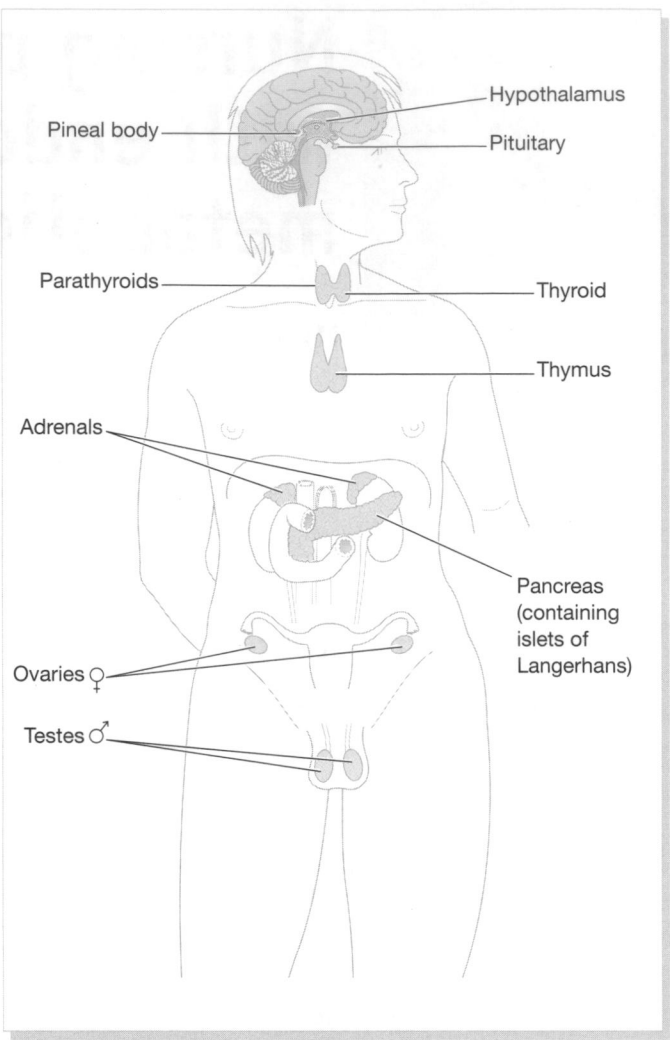

Figure 17.1 Location of major endocrine structures. (NB – Both female and male structures are illustrated.)

- hypothalamus
- pineal body
- thymus gland
- pituitary gland
- thyroid gland
- parathyroid glands (usually four)
- adrenal glands (two)
- gonads – testes or ovaries (two) (see Ch. 25)
- endocrine pancreas (islets of Langerhans).

Please note that a discussion of the pineal gland and the thymus gland is beyond the scope of this chapter.

In addition to the major endocrine structures, hormones are produced by several other tissues, e.g. kidney, heart, gastrointestinal tract, placenta and inappropriately by some cancers.

The endocrine structures produce or release stored chemical hormones directly into the extracellular spaces to enter the blood and lymph for onward transport to target cells in distant organs. Hormones regulate and fine-tune the metabolic activities of most cells, and influence diverse functions, including

SPECIAL ISSUES

17.1 Diabetes National Service Framework

The Diabetes National Service Framework (NSF) is the fourth in a series of NSFs. Unlike the preceding three, it has not been published as one complete document. The first section, the standards, was published in 2001 (Department of Health 2001). The delivery strategy was published in January 2003 (Department of Health 2003). There are 12 standards, as described below.

Standard 1: Prevention of type 2 diabetes
The NHS will develop, implement and monitor strategies to reduce the risk of developing type 2 diabetes in the population as a whole and to reduce the inequalities in the risk of developing type 2 diabetes.

Standard 2: Identification of people with diabetes
The NHS will develop, implement and monitor strategies to identify people who do not know they have diabetes.

Standard 3: Empowering people with diabetes
All children, young people and adults with diabetes will receive a service which encourages partnership in decision-making, supports them in managing their diabetes and helps them to adopt and maintain a healthy lifestyle. This will be reflected in an agreed and shared care plan in an appropriate format and language. Where appropriate, parents and carers should be fully engaged in this process.

Standard 4: Clinical care of adults with diabetes
All adults with diabetes will receive high-quality care throughout their lifetime, including support to optimize the control of their blood glucose, blood pressure and other risk factors for developing the complications of diabetes.

Standard 5: Clinical care of children and young people
All children and young people with diabetes will receive consistently high-quality care and they, with their families and others involved in their day-to-day care, will be supported to optimize the control of their blood glucose and their physical, psychological, intellectual, educational and social development.

Standard 6: Clinical care of children and young people
All young people with diabetes will experience a smooth transition of care from paediatric diabetes services to adult diabetes services, whether hospital or community-based, either directly or via a young people's clinic. The transition will be organized in partnership with each individual and at an age appropriate to and agreed with them.

Standard 7: Management of diabetic emergencies
The NHS will develop, implement and monitor agreed protocols for rapid and effective treatment of diabetic emergencies by appropriately trained health care professionals. Protocols will include the management of acute complications and procedures to minimize the risk of recurrence.

Standard 8: Care of people with diabetes during admission to hospital
All children, young people and adults with diabetes admitted to hospital, for whatever reason, will receive effective care of their diabetes. Wherever possible, they will continue to be involved in decisions concerning the management of their diabetes.

Standard 9: Diabetes and pregnancy
The NHS will develop, implement and monitor policies that seek to empower and support women with pre-existing diabetes and those who develop diabetes during pregnancy to optimize the outcomes of their pregnancy.

Standard 10: Detection and management of long-term complications
All young people and adults with diabetes will receive regular surveillance for the long-term complications of diabetes.

Standard 11: Detection and management of long-term complications
The NHS will develop, implement and monitor agreed protocols and systems of care to ensure that all people who develop long-term complications of diabetes receive timely, appropriate and effective investigation and treatment to reduce their risk of disability and premature death.

Standard 12: Detection and management of long-term complications
All people with diabetes requiring multi-agency support will receive integrated health and social care.

The NSF is an important development in diabetes care; the implementation, over the next 10 years, should ensure people with diabetes receive high-quality care from all sectors of the health service.

References
Department of Health. National Service Framework for Diabetes: Standards. London: Department of Health; 2003.
Department of Health. National Service Framework for Diabetes: Delivery Stratergy. London: Department of Health; 2003.

growth, reproduction, use of energy and nutrients, electrolyte and water balance, and reponses to stress.

The onset of hormone action is usually slower than that of the nervous system, but hormones often control longer-term functions such as metabolism, reproductive cycles, etc. There are, however, exceptions, e.g. blood glucose control or the immediate responses to an intense stressor (see Ch. 6), which are much more rapid.

HORMONES

Hormones are either amino acid-based/protein, e.g. insulin, or steroids derived from cholesterol, which include some hormones from the adrenal glands and the sex hormones. Hormones change the metabolism of specific target cells by binding to receptor proteins that may be on the cell surface (water-soluble hormones) or within the cell (lipid-soluble hormones). Target cell metabolic activity may be changed in a variety of ways, including the following:

- activating or deactivating enzymes
- increased protein production, e.g. enzymes
- changing cell membrane permeability to ions (see Ch. 8)
- production of regulatory molecules
- secretion of substances from cells
- influencing cell division.

Hormones such as thyroxine and some steroid hormones act at gene level (DNA); they enter the cell and bind to receptors to influence protein synthesis. The effects of this type of hormone action usually take a while to become obvious.

Hormones that are unable to enter the target cell act indirectly through regulatory intermediates, special G proteins and 'second messengers'. Second messengers, such as cyclic adenosine monophosphate (cAMP), act in place of the hormone. They cause enzyme cascade amplification, a process where several enzymes are activated, in turn stimulating still more. This type of cascading enzyme action allows some hormone effects to happen rapidly in response to changing homeostatic needs, e.g. glucagon increases blood glucose if levels fall.

Having different modes of hormone action provides the flexibility needed for maintaining homeostasis, allowing, for example, rapid action with immediate effects, e.g. adrenaline (epinephrine), or action over hours or days, e.g. cortisol.

A large group of regulatory lipids (fatty substances), e.g. prostaglandins etc., also have hormone-like effects in the body. They are generally regarded as local hormones because they act over a limited range in local target cells.

Hormone secretion is controlled by:

- other hormones (hormonal)
- concentration of substances such as electrolytes in body fluids (humoral)
- the nervous system (neural).

Some hormones may use more than one control mechanism.

The regulation of most hormone release is through a negative feedback inhibition mechanism, whereby release stops as the hormone level rises (see Fig. 17.2) and commences when the hormone level falls. Mechanisms controlling the hormones that respond to extracellular substances work in a similar way, where high plasma levels of the substance inhibit hormone release and so on. Positive feedback mechanisms, where high levels stimulate even more hormone release, are uncommon and not everyday events, e.g. the release of oxytocin during labour.

After use, hormones are broken down by enzymes in the liver, lungs and kidneys and excreted via bile or urine.

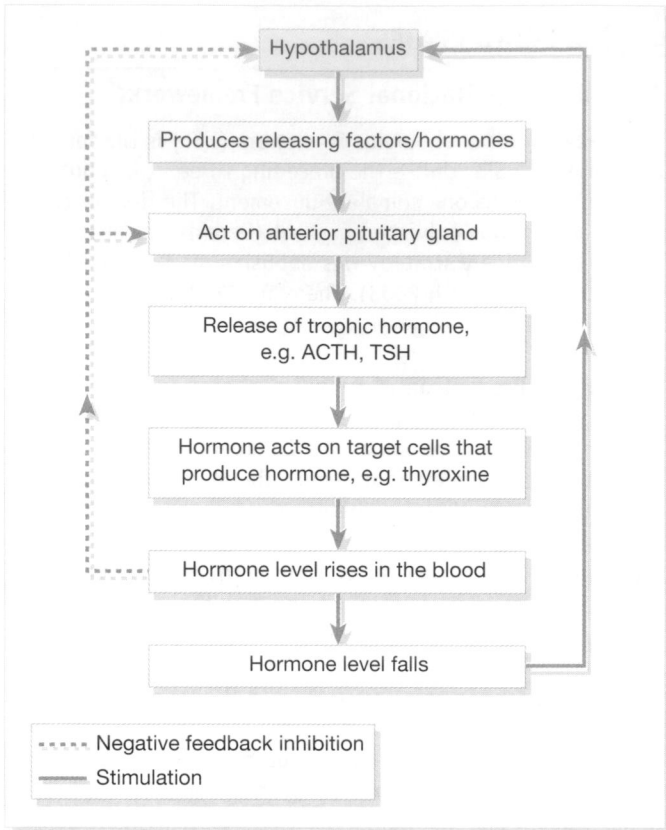

Figure 17.2 Negative feedback inhibition.

HYPOTHALAMUS

The hypothalamus has a central role in maintaining homeostasis. It is situated in the diencephalon of the forebrain (between the cerebrum and the brain stem – see Fig. 17.1 and Ch. 14). It secretes the releasing/inhibiting hormones that control secretion of some anterior pituitary hormones, and makes the two hormones stored and released by the posterior pituitary.

PITUITARY GLAND

The pituitary gland stimulates many other endocrine structures and metabolic processes. It is tiny, weighing only about 0.5 g, and comprises two separate structures: the anterior lobe (adenohypophysis) and the posterior lobe (neurohypophysis). The two lobes hang from the hypothalamus by a stalk containing blood vessels and nerve fibres (see Fig. 17.1). The pituitary gland sits in the pituitary fossa of the sphenoid bone. Its proximity to the optic nerves means that pituitary tumours may cause visual problems if they press on the optic nerves (Ch. 15).

Anterior lobe (adenohypophysis)

Releasing and inhibiting hormones that travel in the portal system of blood vessels from the hypothalamus control the hormones produced by the anterior lobe of the pituitary gland. The six anterior pituitary hormones include four that stimulate other endocrine structures (trophic hormones) (see Fig. 17.3):

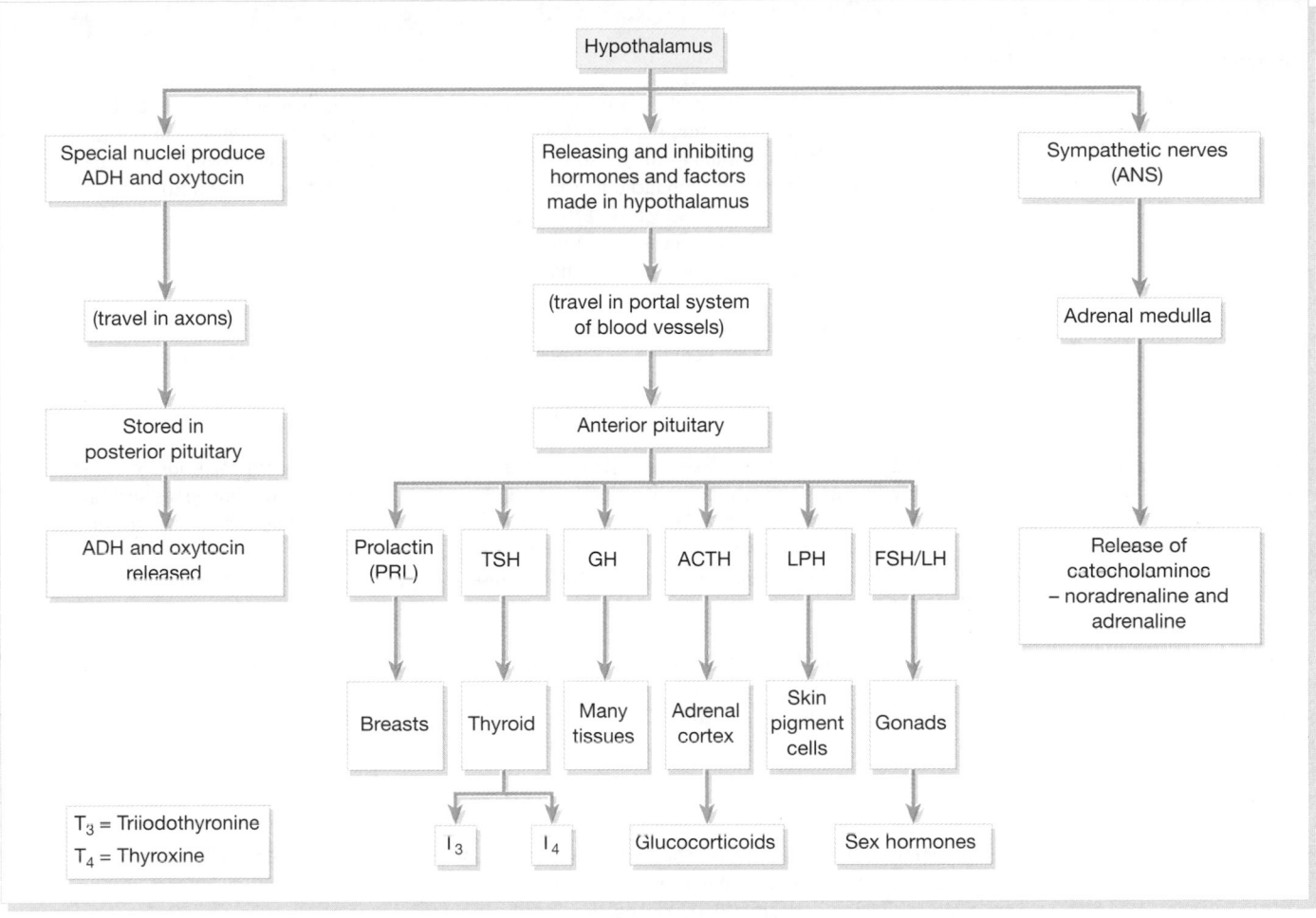

Figure 17.3 Hypothalamus and pituitary gland – hormones secreted and target cells.

- adrenocorticotrophic hormone (ACTH)
- thyroid-stimulating hormone (TSH)
- two gonadotrophins (acting on the ovaries or testes) – follicle-stimulating hormone (FSH) and luteinizing hormone (LH).

The other two act on other tissues:

- growth hormone (GH)
- prolactin (PRL).

In addition, the anterior lobe produces a precursor molecule (prohormone), which forms substances including ACTH and beta-lipotrophin (LPH), which act on melanocytes (skin pigment cells – see Ch. 28). Further details and the effects of the anterior lobe hormones are provided in Table 17.1, page 398.

Posterior lobe (neurohypophysis)

No hormones are produced in the posterior lobe but it stores and secretes two: oxytocin and antidiuretic hormone (ADH – arginine vasopressin [AVP] or vasopressin). These hormones are produced in the hypothalamus and travel in the nerve fibres of the stalk to the posterior lobe. Their release from the posterior pituitary is under neural control from the hypothalamus.

Oxytocin is important in parturition (childbirth) and is also required for the 'let-down' (ejection) of milk during lactation. ADH (arginine vasopressin) reduces diuresis (urine production) in the kidneys (see Ch. 24). ADH is released in response to an increase in plasma osmolality or a decrease in plasma volume. ADH causes some parts of the kidney tubules to become more permeable to water. Hence the kidney reabsorbs more water, less urine is produced, and the plasma osmolality/volume returns to normal.

The release of ADH is regulated by a negative feedback mechanism; as plasma osmolality starts to fall and circulating blood volume is restored, the rate of ADH release is slowed. ADH release is important as part of maintaining fluid balance homeostasis (see Ch. 8). It also increases blood pressure by causing vasoconstriction. This pressor effect accounts for its other name, vasopressin.

THYROID GLAND

The thyroid gland is situated in the front of the neck. There are two lobes that lie on either side of the trachea and below the larynx (see Fig. 17.1). It has an extremely good blood supply and the resultant vascularity increases the need for careful

Table 17.1 Anterior lobe pituitary hormones and effects

Hormone	Details	Effects
Growth hormone (GH)	Protein hormone. Secretion regulated by two hypothalamic hormones: growth hormone-releasing hormone (GHRH) and growth hormone-inhibiting hormone (GHIH), also called somatostatin (small amounts also produced by the pancreas and intestinal cells). GH secretion, which is at its highest during childhood and adolescence, increases during sleep and after exercise and is affected by emotions and nutrition	Widespread effects on body tissues – stimulates the growth of bone, cartilage and muscle, and influences the metabolism of nutrients
Thyroid-stimulating hormone (TSH)	Glycoprotein (protein + carbohydrate) hormone. Secretion is stimulated by the hypothalamic hormone thyrotrophin-releasing hormone (TRH) and inhibited by high levels of thyroid hormones acting on the hypothalamus and pituitary	Stimulates thyroid growth and secretion of two thyroid hormones
Adrenocorticotrophic hormone (ACTH)	ACTH is a polypeptide hormone. Release is stimulated by the hypothalamic factors, corticotrophin-releasing factor (CRF) and arginine vasopressin (AVP). ACTH tends to be highest in the early morning, but stressors (see Ch. 6) override the circadian rhythm. High glucocorticoid levels inhibit release of CRF and ACTH	Stimulates the secretion of glucocorticoid hormones such as cortisol from the adrenal cortex
Gonadotrophins: Follicle-stimulating hormone (FSH); luteinizing hormone (LH) known as interstitial cell stimulating hormone (ICSH) in males	FSH and LH/ICSH are glycoproteins. After puberty, secretion is stimulated by gonadotrophin-releasing hormone (GnRH) from the hypothalamus	FSH stimulates oocyte or spermatozoa production. LH/ICSH functions with FSH to stimulate ovulation in females, and hormone release in both females (oestrogens, progesterone) and males (testosterone)
Prolactin (PRL)	Protein hormone. PRL secretion is increased by prolactin-releasing hormone (PRH) from the hypothalamus, and inhibited by prolactin-inhibiting hormone (PIH) or dopamine, and by high levels of PRL. Levels are increased during sleep. Suckling also increases PRL secretion	PRL stimulates milk production (lactation) following childbirth

haemostasis during surgery and vigilant postoperative observation (see p. 433 and Ch. 29).

The gland is composed of many follicles where thyroglobulin is produced. This colloidal substance forms two of the three thyroid hormones (thyroxine, triiodothyronine). It is stored in the follicles until required. A third hormone (calcitonin) is secreted by cells between the follicles.

Thyroid hormones

The three thyroid hormones are:

- thyroxine (T_4) – regulates metabolism
- triiodothyronine (T_3) – regulates metabolism
- calcitonin – concerned with calcium homeostasis.

Thyroxine and triiodothyronine

Thyroxine and triiodothyronine are formed from the amino acid tyrosine with the addition of either four atoms of iodine (T_4) or three (T_3). The hormones can be stored as colloid for several weeks. They travel in the blood to their target cells bound to a protein, thyroxine-binding globulin (TBG). Thyroid hormones influence many body processes, including:

- the rate at which cells use oxygen (basal metabolic rate – BMR)
- glucose metabolism and use of fats to produce energy
- the synthesis of protein
- maintaining body temperature
- normal development and growth of the skeleton and nervous system
- normal functioning of the nervous system in adults
- reproduction.

Thyroid-stimulating hormone (TSH) from the anterior pituitary controls the production and release of T_3 and T_4 (see Table 17.1) through a negative feedback inhibition mechanism. The release of T_3 and T_4 is also influenced by other hormones, e.g. glucocorticoids (see below), and situations where physiological demands change, such as during pregnancy.

Calcitonin

Calcitonin has a fine-tuning role in calcium and phosphate homeostasis. It opposes the action of the parathyroid hormone and lowers the levels of calcium and phosphate in the plasma. (see below, and Ch. 24). Calcitonin reduces calcium reabsorption from bone and helps its deposition, and increases the amount of calcium and phosphates excreted in the urine. Calcitonin is released if plasma calcium levels rise above normal (2.1–2.6 mmol/L).

PARATHYROID GLANDS

There are usually four parathyroid glands situated on the back of the thyroid gland (see Fig. 17.1). However, there may be extra glands situated elsewhere in the neck or chest. Each parathyroid gland is enclosed in a connective tissue capsule and consists of cords of hormone-secreting cells interspaced with vascular channels. There is only one hormone secreted by these glands, parathyroid hormone (PTH or parathormone).

Parathyroid hormone

Parathyroid hormone is a protein hormone and maintains plasma calcium levels within the normal range of 2.1–2.6 mmol/L. Normal muscle contraction, nerve impulse transmission and blood clotting depend on having the correct level of calcium. PTH maintains calcium and phosphate homeostasis by its effects on the small intestine, bone and kidneys. It raises calcium levels and reduces phosphate levels in the plasma by causing the kidneys to reabsorb calcium and prevent phosphate retention. The kidneys are also stimulated by PTH to convert vitamin D to the active form, 1,25-dihydroxycholecalciferol (see Ch. 11); 1,25-dihydroxycholecalciferol causes the intestinal cells to increase calcium absorption from food. PTH stimulates osteoclasts (see Ch. 27) in bone to reabsorb bone and release calcium and phosphate into the blood.

The release of PTH is stimulated by hypocalcaemia (low level of calcium in the plasma) and inhibited by hypercalcaemia (plasma calcium above normal).

ADRENAL GLANDS

The two triangular adrenal (suprarenal) glands are situated on the upper pole of each kidney (see Fig. 17.1). Each adrenal gland has a middle part or medulla, and a cortex around the outside. The medulla and cortex are really two separate endocrine structures that develop from different embryonic tissues.

Adrenal cortex

The cortex has an outer capsule and three distinct layers that secrete the steroid hormones, made from cholesterol, known collectively as corticosteroids (glucocorticoids, mineralocorticoids and sex hormones). The layers (from the outside working in) are as follows:

- zona glomerulosa – secretes mineralocorticoids, hormones that regulate electrolyte/fluid balance
- zona fasciculata – secretes glucocorticoids which are important metabolic hormones
- zona reticularis – secretes small amounts of glucocorticoids and sex hormones.

The common steroid structure of the corticosteroids means that different hormone groups will have some overlap of function, e.g. glucocorticoids also have some mineralocorticoid effect.

Glucocorticoids

The most important glucocorticoid is cortisol (hydrocortisone). Glucocorticoids have widespread effects in many metabolic processes and in long-term responses to stress (see Ch. 6), including the following:

- Stimulate gluconeogenesis (production of glucose from non-carbohydrate sources, e.g. lactate, alanine and glycerol in the liver), which increases glucose storage, as glycogen, in the liver. Cortisol inhibits the uptake and use of glucose by skeletal muscle. Overall these processes increase blood glucose levels
- Increase protein breakdown for energy use (via gluconeogenesis) and decrease protein synthesis
- Increase the release of fatty acids for energy
- Cause some sodium and water reabsorption by kidney tubules
- Cause vasoconstriction and hence an increase in blood pressure in conjunction with hormones from the adrenal medulla
- Increase calcium excretion by the kidney and block intestinal absorption
- Suppress inflammation, allergy and immune processes
- Delay tissue repair/wound healing
- Stimulate the secretion of gastric acid and enzymes.

Glucocorticoid release is again regulated by a negative feedback mechanism through corticotrophin-releasing factor (CRF) and ACTH (see Table 17.1). Increasing levels of cortisol will inhibit both the hypothalamus and pituitary. Glucocorticoid release follows a circadian rhythm (see Ch. 4) with an early morning peak and dip in the evening. Stressors such as hypoglycaemia (low blood glucose) override the circadian rhythm and extra glucocorticoids are released as part of physiological coping mechanisms (see Ch. 6).

Mineralocorticoids

Aldosterone is the most important mineralocorticoid. It contributes to electrolyte (especially sodium) and fluid homeostasis by causing the distal kidney tubules to reabsorb sodium and water and excrete potassium or hydrogen ions (see Ch. 24) and indirectly helps in the control of arterial blood pressure.

Aldosterone release mostly depends upon the concentration of ions in the blood, plasma osmolality and the blood pressure. Aldosterone is secreted if sodium and chloride levels fall or potassium levels increase in the blood, and when the volume of extracellular fluid (see Ch. 8), and hence the blood pressure, is low. These events trigger the renin–angiotensin response and the release of aldosterone (see Chs 19 and 24).

Sex hormones

The amount of sex hormones secreted by the adrenal cortex is very small, mainly androgens (male hormones) with very small amounts of oestrogens and progesterones (female hormones). Their role is uncertain, but levels are high during fetal life and increase at puberty, and abnormal secretion can lead to virilization (masculinization) in females.

Adrenal medulla

The medulla comprises cells situated around blood vessels and sinusoids. In common with parts of the nervous system, the medulla secretes two catecholamine hormones: adrenaline (epinephrine) and noradrenaline (norepinephrine). These two hormones enhance the action of the sympathetic nervous system in the 'fight or flight' response to stress (see Ch. 6). Noradrenaline is also a neurotransmitter in the autonomic nervous system (sympathetic division).

Both adrenaline and noradrenaline are monoamines (having one amine group) and more adrenaline than noradrenaline is produced. Their metabolic effects are similar; however, adrenaline has most effect on the heart, whereas noradrenaline has most effect on vasoconstriction and blood pressure. The effects include:

- increased heart rate
- vasoconstriction
- increase in blood pressure
- diversion of blood to the vital organs
- rise in blood glucose level
- increase in respiratory rate and bronchodilation
- dilation of the pupil.

The release of medullary hormones is through sympathetic nerve stimulation in response to an immediate stressor (see Ch. 6).

Stress responses and the adrenal glands

Although the physiological responses to stressors have been covered in some depth in Chapter 6, it is worth underlining the important role of both parts of the adrenal gland in helping the body to adapt to a specific stressor and maintain homeostasis. The adrenal medulla along with the autonomic nervous system responds rapidly but usually only for a short time, whereas the response of the adrenal cortex is slower and more prolonged.

THE PANCREAS

The pancreas, a soft tapering gland situated in the left upper abdomen, is around 23 cm in length and is tucked behind the small bowel and the stomach (see Figs 17.1 and 17.4). The pancreas is a mixed gland, having both endocrine and exocrine functions (see Ch. 23). It receives arterial blood from the mesenteric and splenic arteries, and venous blood returns to the general circulation by way of the hepatic portal vein and the liver.

The endocrine part of the pancreas consists of clusters of special cells called islets of Langerhans scattered throughout the pancreas. Within these islets are α cells, which secrete the hormone glucagon, and β cells, which secrete the hormone insulin. Together, insulin and glucagon are the main hormones responsible for the regulation of blood glucose.

In addition, other islet cells produce several substances including somatostatin. Somatostatin is the same substance as growth hormone-inhibiting hormone (GHIH) produced by the hypothalamus (see p. 396). Its secretion from the pancreas inhibits the release of glucagon, insulin and the pancreatic enzymes.

Pancreatic hormones and glucose homeostasis

Both insulin and glucagon are peptides, or chains of amino acids. The precursor to insulin is a long peptide chain called proinsulin, which is joined in a spiral shape by disulphide

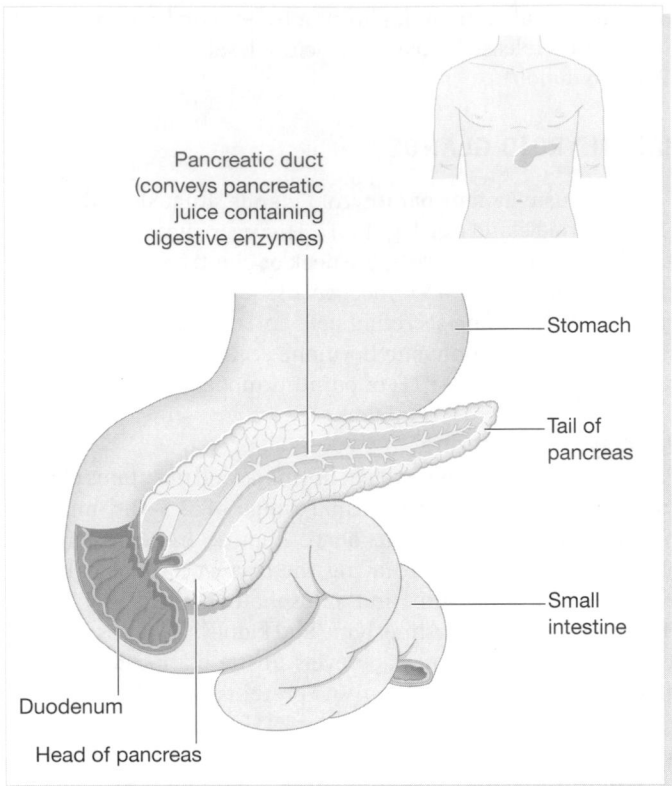

Figure 17.4 Position of the pancreas.

bridges. Just prior to release into the circulation, the connecting peptide, or c-peptide, is broken off, leaving two chains of amino acids still joined together with the bridges. The 'a' chain contains 21 amino acids and the 'b' chain has 30.

When a meal is ingested, only about 40% of the glucose contained in it arrives in the general circulation immediately, from where it enters the cells of the body. Once the glucose is in the cell, it undergoes glycolysis, i.e. it is broken down to provide energy. However, the hormone insulin is required to transport glucose across the cell membrane and is also involved in intracellular glycolysis. Approximately 60% of the glucose in the meal is absorbed from the small intestine and arrives at the liver via the hepatic portal vein. Glucose is stored in the liver, and also in the muscles, as its storage compound glycogen in a process called glycogenesis. Insulin is also required for this process to occur.

When an individual is fasting, overnight and between meals, glucose is still required, however, for normal physiological function. In the fasting state, blood glucose comes from glucose stores through the process of glycogenolysis, or the conversion of glycogen back into glucose, which is released into the circulation, from whence it enters the body's cells. Glycogenolysis is stimulated by glucagon.

As well as glycogenolysis, gluconeogenesis (*gluco* = glucose; *neo* = new; *genesis* = make) also occurs in the fasting state. This is the process whereby glucose is made, in the liver, from lactate, alanine and glycerol. Lactate is converted from glucose in muscle tissue and returned to the liver. Alanine is a breakdown product from protein metabolism and glycerol is a breakdown product from fat metabolism. Thus it can be seen that some breakdown

---

Box 17.1 Functions of insulin

Carbohydrate metabolism
- Promotes glycogen synthesis and storage
- Inhibits glycogen breakdown
- Inhibits gluconeogenesis
- Promotes cellular glucose uptake

Protein metabolism
- Promotes protein synthesis
- Inhibits protein breakdown (proteolysis)

Fat metabolism
- Promotes fat synthesis
- Promotes triglyceride storage
- Inhibits triglyceride breakdown (lipolysis)

---

products from carbohydrate, protein and fat metabolism are 'recycled' to make new glucose. Gluconeogenesis is also stimulated by glucagon.

Glycogenolysis and gluconeogenesis are the methods by which a constant supply of glucose is available to the body, even in the fasting state. They are both stimulated by glucagon release from the Islets of Langerhans.

It can be seen that insulin and glucagon are partners in glucose homeostasis; insulin lowers blood glucose and glucagon raises it. In the normal state, these two hormones work together to ensure that the normal blood glucose level of 4–7 mmol/L is maintained at all times.

In addition to a role in carbohydrate metabolism, insulin is also involved in the metabolism of fats and proteins (see Box 17.1).

NURSING ASSESSMENT

The nursing assessment of people with endocrine conditions will predominantly involve physiological measurements and individuals' knowledge and learning needs in relation to their condition. For instance, many people being investigated for endocrine conditions, or indeed being treated for them, are not physically unwell.

However, accuracy and attention to detail are important. Precise baseline observations of physiological parameters, such as weight, blood pressure and pulse, are essential, as these are frequently abnormal in endocrine conditions.

The investigations that individuals with endocrine conditions undergo are often complex, time-consuming and repetitive. People who have not yet had a diagnosis are likely to be anxious about the implications of the results. It is important for nurses to assess what their fears and anxieties are, as well as their learning needs, to ensure appropriate care is given.

The nursing assessment of people with diabetes mellitus in many circumstances will focus almost entirely on identifying individuals' abilities to effectively manage their own condition and, consequently, their learning needs. This is because people with diabetes mellitus, unlike those with many other conditions, have to manage it themselves on a daily basis. For instance, decisions about activity, eating and the management of medication all require frequent attention. Unusual events, like concurrent illnesses or holidays, often require extra effort.

Because most diabetes mellitus care exists outside the context of nursing, many existing nursing models are not easily adapted for use when an individual's needs are mostly of an educational and psychosocial nature. An alternative is to consider a seminal sociological work that explored chronic illness and quality of life. Strauss et al (1984) undertook a study to explore the social and psychological problems faced by people living with chronic illnesses and devised a framework to consider these problems of daily living. The eight categories in the framework are:

- preventing medical crises and managing them if they occur
- controlling symptoms
- carrying out prescribed regimens
- preventing or living with social isolation caused by reduced contact with others
- adjusting to changes in the course of the disease
- attempting to normalize interaction with others and lifestyle
- funding
- dealing with any psychological, marital or family problems that may occur.

These categories can serve as a useful model for assessing an individual's ability to cope with diabetes mellitus. For example, preventing hypoglycaemia, or treating it effectively, would be included in the 'preventing medical crises' category. Similarly, giving an insulin injection would be included in the 'managing prescribed regimens' category.

Whatever framework is used to assess the nursing needs of people with diabetes mellitus, it must be remembered that, in most circumstances, meeting physical needs is likely to be only a small element of the care required (see Evidence-based Practice box 17.1, p. 402).

DIAGNOSTIC TESTS AND MEDICAL INVESTIGATION – GENERAL

Diagnostic tests and medical investigations are used in conjunction with careful history-taking and physical examination to confirm a diagnosis and to monitor disease progress and the efficacy of management regimens. It is important that nurses have an understanding of common investigations and the need for any special preparation. This knowledge allows them to provide explanation and reassurance for patients and families and to ensure that patients are adequately prepared, and that the test is safe and successful.

The range of investigations used in the diagnosis of endocrine disorders is outlined here, but these and other specific tests of endocrine function are discussed in more detail along with the disorder. The diagnosis of diabetes mellitus, however, is covered in some detail and the ongoing monitoring tests are discussed later in the chapter. The investigations are as follows:

- *A general physical examination* plus, for example, visual field checking
- *Plain X-rays*, e.g. to detect displacement/compression of the trachea by an enlarged thyroid gland, or the characteristic bone changes of parathyroid disease
- *Computed tomography* (CT) and *magnetic resonance imaging* (MRI) may be used, for example, to visualize the pituitary gland, thyroid gland, etc.

EVIDENCE-BASED PRACTICE

17.1 Psychological care: living with diabetes

As with other chronic illnesses, living with diabetes is hard work. Individuals have many social issues to deal with as well as psychological ones (see Ch. 35). At diagnosis there may be feelings of grief for lost health, independence and freedom (Richmond 1998), as well as anger, denial or sadness, some of which do not resolve even when the initial period of shock is over. Indeed, the incidence of depression in people with diabetes is double that of those without it (Lustman et al 2002).

Other losses that may become evident include those of spontaneity and social integration; many people with diabetes feel 'different' and tend to be more socially isolated. Some occupations are not open to people with diabetes, the armed services, for example, and being an airline pilot. Some, such as large goods vehicle drivers treated with insulin, may lose their jobs, thus incurring financial penalties too. Healthy eating is also relatively expensive.

People with diabetes not only have to learn to cope with their treatment regimens and the increased uncertainty of what their futures hold (Callaghan & Williams 1994), but also have to cope with the attitudes of health professionals who are often pejorative and 'blame' the individual for their 'lack of compliance' and poor glycaemic control.

Several studies have explored how many individuals do come to terms with living with diabetes. For example, Callaghan & Williams (1994) undertook a qualitative study to explore the challenges of living with diabetes and people's perceptions of the nursing care they received. Individuals in their study valued person-centred care from accessible, knowledgeable and technically skilled nurses. The study emphasized the importance of nurses understanding 'disease' as not only the biomedical perspectives, but also the experiences of individuals who live with it (Callaghan & Williams 1994).

The study by Paterson et al (1998) concluded that the lived experiences of the people with diabetes they studied focused on learning to balance the management of their disease with the desire for a normal life. Helpful professional care-givers were perceived as those who valued the person with diabetes as an individual.

These investigations emphasize the importance of nurses giving individualized care to those with diabetes, and viewing them as people who are trying to incorporate diabetes into their lives, not as 'diabetics'.

Student activities

- Review the nursing care plan of someone with diabetes in your workplace. Have his or her psychological needs been assessed?
- How would you use the evidence from the studies outlined to improve the provision of individualized care to people living with diabetes?

References

Callaghan D, Williams A. Living with diabetes: issues for nursing practice. J Adv Nurs 1994; 20: 132–139.

Lustman PJ, Singh PK, Clouse RE. Recognizing and managing depression in patients with diabetes. In: Anderson BL, Rubin RR, eds. Practical psychology for diabetes clinicians. Effective techniques for key behavioural issues, 2nd edn. Alexandria, Virginia: American Diabetes Association; 2002.

Paterson BL, Thorne S, Dewis M. Adapting to and managing diabetes. Image J Nurs Scholar 1998; 30: 57–62.

Richmond J. How important are the psychosocial aspects of diabetes? J Diab Nurs 1998; 2(5): 146–149.

- *Radionuclide scanning* such as ^{99m}technetium scans and the uptake of radioactive iodine (^{131}iodine) in the diagnosis of thyroid disease
- *Histological examination* of material obtained, e.g. by fine-needle aspiration of a thyroid nodule
- Blood tests, including basic haematological tests, e.g. haemoglobin and full blood count, and biochemical blood tests, including electrolyte levels, liver function tests, cholesterol and enzymes such as lactate dehydrogenase; blood glucose and glucose tolerance tests (see below); hormone levels in plasma, e.g. prolactin, insulin-like growth factor-I (IGF-I), cortisol, TSH, T_3 and T_4, and PTH, etc.
- *Measuring plasma and urine osmolality*, and water deprivation tests in suspected cases of diabetes insipidus
- *Stimulation tests*, e.g. ACTH stimulation test where tetracosactide (tetracosactrin) is given to stimulate hormone secretion after which blood samples are taken to measure cortisol levels
- *Suppression tests*, e.g. low-dose dexamethasone suppression test for Cushing's syndrome, where plasma and 24-hour urine cortisol is measured following the administration of dexamethasone
- *Electrocardiography* to detect cardiac abnormalities in hypothyroidism (see p. 435)
- *Urine tests* for glycosuria (glucose in the urine), electrolytes such as urinary calcium and hormones or their metabolites, e.g. vanillylmandelic acid.

DIAGNOSIS OF DIABETES MELLITUS

The diagnosis of diabetes mellitus must be made based on symptoms and venous plasma glucose results. Capillary blood glucose results are insufficiently accurate for diagnostic purposes. In the symptomatic individual, a random venous plasma glucose result of 11.1 mmol/L is indicative of diabetes mellitus. In those without symptoms, two fasting venous plasma glucose samples must be taken, on different days; results higher than 7 mmol/L indicate diabetes mellitus.

An oral glucose tolerance test (OGTT) may be performed instead. The individual must be fasted from midnight before the test and cease smoking from this time and for the duration of the test. A venous plasma glucose blood sample is taken prior to the individual taking 75 g of anhydrous glucose powder in water (~ 300 mL). After 2 hours, the venous plasma glucose is measured again. Levels higher than 11.1 mmol/L for the 2-hour post-glucose result again indicate diabetes mellitus (World Health Organization 1999).

Fasting venous plasma glucose results of less than 7 mmol/L and 2-hour results of more than 7.8 mmol/L indicate impaired glucose tolerance (IGT). Many people with this condition develop diabetes mellitus in later years and have an increased risk of cardiovascular events; they should be given healthy living advice and followed up at least annually (World Health Organization 1999).

Impaired fasting glycaemia (IFG) exists when the fasting venous plasma glucose result is between 6.1 and 7 mmol/L, but the 2-hour post-glucose load result (if measured) is less than 7.8 mmol/L (World Health Organization 1999).

Once the diagnosis is made, medical investigations include an assessment of the general health of the individual. In older people with type 2 diabetes mellitus, particular attention is paid to the cardiovascular system as it is estimated that approximately 50% of newly diagnosed individuals have hypertension (UKPDS 1998a).

GENERAL DISEASE PREVENTION AND HEALTH EDUCATION

Until fairly recently, there was no strong evidence that diabetes mellitus could be prevented. Although there are some studies that have investigated the possibility of preventing or at least delaying the onset of type 1 diabetes mellitus, this is not yet possible in clinical practice.

However, type 2 diabetes mellitus can be prevented. Two studies have recently been published with astonishingly similar results. Tuomilehto et al (2001) and The Diabetes Prevention Program Research Group (2002) both achieved a 58% reduction in the risk of developing type 2 diabetes mellitus. The former group achieved this by providing individualized weight reduction, exercise and reduced fat/increased fibre diets to individuals with impaired glucose tolerance. The latter group also provided intense and individualized lifestyle advice to people with impaired glucose tolerance; their subjects also had a 58% reduction in the incidence (the number of new cases) of diabetes mellitus.

The value of healthy eating, regular activity and weight reduction in the overweight or obese in preventing type 2 diabetes mellitus can clearly be seen. However, although many people with impaired glucose tolerance and type 2 diabetes mellitus are aware of these health messages, some have great difficulty in changing their self-care behaviour accordingly. The diabetes mellitus prevention studies demonstrate the importance of ongoing support in achieving these goals. In addition, smoking cessation (see Ch. 20) is an important health promotion strategy for those with diabetes mellitus, due to the increased risk of cardiovascular disease (see Ch. 19). This is particularly pertinent for those with type 2 diabetes mellitus.

There is very little specific health promotion in respect of preventing other endocrine disorders; however, nurses should encourage people to seek early professional advice if they have signs or experience symptoms. In addition, it is important to ensure that all individuals have sufficient information about general lifestyle measures they can take to improve their health, such as healthy eating and maintaining normal weight, exercise, smoking cessation, etc.

DISORDERS OF THE ENDOCRINE PANCREAS

Diabetes mellitus (hereafter referred to as diabetes) is the general term used to describe a group of diseases which are characterized by hyperglycaemia (a high blood glucose level). Diabetes results from defects in insulin secretion or insulin action, or both, which affect the metabolism of carbohydrates, proteins and fats (see Box 17.1, p. 401).

There are several types of diabetes; the two main types – type 1 and type 2 – are discussed below. Other types of diabetes include gestational diabetes. This affects some women in pregnancy and resolves once the baby is born. It may be treated with diet alone or with diet and insulin. Oral hypoglycaemic agents are not given to pregnant women with diabetes because of the potentially damaging effects on the fetus. For the purposes of treatment and care, see the type 1 diabetes section for those treated with insulin and the type 2 diabetes section for those treated through management of diet alone.

Maturity-onset diabetes of the young (MODY) is very uncommon and is caused by genetically inherited defects in pancreatic β-cell function. It is treated most commonly through management of diet alone.

Secondary diabetes occurs as a result of other disease processes or medical treatments. It can occur following pancreatitis, pancreatic carcinoma, pancreatic trauma and partial or total pancreatectomy (see Ch. 23). Diabetes may also occur secondary to other endocrine diseases such as acromegaly, Cushing's syndrome, glucagonoma and phaeochromocytoma (see below). Once these conditions have been treated, the diabetes usually resolves. Diabetes may also be precipitated, in those with insulin resistance, by many drugs. The most common drugs are glucocorticoids (corticosteroids), thiazide diuretics and thyroid hormone.

There are also several genetic disorders associated with an increased incidence of diabetes. These include Down's syndrome, Friedreich's ataxia and Huntington's chorea.

TYPE 1 DIABETES

Type 1 diabetes used to be known as juvenile-onset diabetes or insulin-dependent diabetes mellitus (IDDM).

Aetiology and epidemiology

The underlying cause of type 1 diabetes is an absolute deficiency of insulin. In over 90% of cases, the cause is autoimmune destruction of the insulin-producing cells of the pancreas. It is thought that individuals inherit a genetic predisposition to develop type 1 diabetes. Environmental 'triggers' (currently not identified but which may possibly be viruses), β-cell toxins or, in some cases, certain proteins then stimulate an autoimmune response (Williams & Pickup 1999). β cells in the islets of Langerhans in the pancreas are destroyed, eventually leading to a total insulin deficiency. The process of β-cell destruction can take several years, although it is usually fairly rapid in children and young adults.

Type 1 diabetes accounts for approximately 10–15% of all cases of diabetes in the UK. The incidence of type 1 diabetes is increasing, particularly in young children, and the cause of this is not known. Although type 1 diabetes can occur at any age, most is diagnosed in individuals less than 40 years of age and there are peaks in the incidence rates in preschool children and around puberty.

There are also differences in incidence rates throughout the world. For example, northern Europe has a higher incidence and prevalence of type 1 diabetes than countries in the Far East. This would suggest that genetic or other environmental factors might be relevant.

Less than 10% of type 1 diabetes has no known aetiology and is termed idiopathic. Most of the individuals with this kind of diabetes are of African or Asian descent and their disease is strongly inherited.

Pathophysiology

By the time of diagnosis, most individuals with type 1 diabetes have no, or very little, circulating endogenous insulin as a result of β-cell destruction. As already discussed, insulin is required for the metabolism of all three macronutrients: carbohydrates, proteins and fats. In the absence of insulin blood glucose levels rise rapidly (hyperglycaemia) as ingested carbohydrates cannot be used for energy production. Because of this energy lack from the primary source – carbohydrate, the individual will usually feel tired and lethargic.

A normal blood glucose level is 4–7 mmol/L. Glucose enters the urine (glycosuria) when the blood glucose level reaches approximately 10 mmol/L. This figure is called the renal threshold for glucose. Glycosuria occurs because the amount of glucose entering the filtrate exceeds the amount that can be actively reabsorbed in the kidney tubule. By a process of osmotic diuresis, water in excess amounts is also excreted as urinary glucose rises, which causes excess urination (polyuria). As polyuria leads to dehydration, affected individuals will feel thirsty and massively increase their intake of oral fluids (polydipsia) in an attempt to rectify this; unfortunately, however, the fluid intake cannot match fluid output and dehydration ensues. In extreme circumstances this can be severe.

Because carbohydrates cannot be used as a source for energy, fats are used instead. In the absence of insulin, unrestrained lipolysis occurs (the breaking down of body fat into free fatty acids and triglycerides). This causes a radical and rapid weight loss; some individuals report losing 2–3 stones in weight in as many weeks.

Clinical presentation

The onset of symptoms in type 1 diabetes is usually very rapid, occurring over days or weeks. Individuals usually present with a history of polyuria, polydipsia, lethargy and weight loss. They may have minor infections, such as oral candidiasis (thrush), pruritus vulvae, balanitis (see Ch. 25) or furunculosis (boils). White cell function is compromised when hyperglycaemia exists and people with diabetes are more prone to infections, both bacterial and viral, if their blood glucose levels are high.

Some individuals may present with diabetic ketoacidosis (DKA), although this is becoming less common as primary care health professionals are more adept at recognizing the symptoms of hyperglycaemia.

Specific investigations

A diagnosis of type 1 diabetes can be made based on the symptoms, a random venous plasma glucose level of more than 11.1 mmol/L (see p. 402) and the history of a rapid onset of symptoms and weight loss in a young person.

Urine should be tested for ketones. A negative result or a trace of ketones (0.5 mmol/L) is clinically insignificant but people with newly diagnosed type 1 diabetes are likely to have raised urinary ketone levels. Moderate amounts of urinary ketones (4 mmol/L when tested with Ketostix) or high levels (8 or 16 mmol/L) are indicative of type 1 diabetes. Some units are using a bedside blood ketone meter rather than urine test strips, as the latter only measure acetone and acetoacetic acid, not 3-hydroxybutyrate, which is quantitatively the most important ketone body (Williams & Pickup 1999).

If the individual is unwell, all the investigations for diabetic ketoacidosis should be undertaken (see section on diabetic ketoacidosis, pp. 422–424).

Medical management

Most people with new type 1 diabetes are referred immediately to secondary care diabetes teams for a formal diagnosis, if this has not already occurred, and for initiation of treatment (Fox & MacKinnon 1999). If they are acutely ill, they will be admitted to hospital and the protocol for diabetic ketoacidosis will be commenced. All children with diabetes of whatever type must be referred to paediatric specialist diabetes teams. Most children with newly diagnosed diabetes are currently admitted, although many units are endeavouring to manage the diabetes at home if the child is not unwell.

The medical management of type 1 diabetes is always treatment with dietary therapy and insulin. First aid dietary advice may be given by the physician or by a nurse, if the dietician is not available, although this is unlikely to be the doctor's priority.

Following examination and assessment of the individual's biomedical status, insulin therapy will be initiated immediately. If the individual is not acutely ill, and does not have diabetic ketoacidosis, insulin may be administered subcutaneously. A 'well' adult or young adult with newly diagnosed type 1 diabetes is unlikely to be admitted to hospital unless the diagnosis is made by the primary care team out of office hours, as the specialist diabetes team can commence treatment on an outpatient basis.

▶ Nursing management

The nursing needed by an individual with type 1 diabetes consists mostly of educational (see Guidelines for Care Priorities box 17.1) and psychological care. Specific needs obviously differ at different stages of the illness. For example, educational and psychological care at the time of diagnosis will be intense, whereas care required for someone who has had diabetes for many years may be related only to the concurrent condition. Indeed, one of the goals of nursing is to enable people with diabetes to effectively manage their own condition. Individuals who

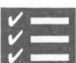

GUIDELINES FOR CARE PRIORITIES

17.1 Diabetes patient education

Despite many studies examining diabetes patient education having been undertaken, there is still a lack of clear evidence about what, where and how it should be done, and by whom. What is clear, however, is that, overall, it is beneficial (NICE 2002).

Several recent documents have given guidelines for the provision of diabetes patient education. Hiscock et al (2001) suggest the following:

- *Information when?*
  - Wait until after post-diagnostic 'adjustment time' before giving large quantities of information
  - Develop an incremental and ongoing approach to the provision of information
  - Provide accessible information quickly in response to patients' needs
- *Information how?*
  - Recognize diversity in preferences for information presentation. Provide information in a number of different formats: personal, one-to-one explanation, written or taped material, telephone helplines
  - Encourage a positive tone to information provision
- *Information and support from whom?*
  - Nurses: recognize and expand the crucially important role played by diabetes nurses
  - Other people with diabetes: establish mechanisms to enable people with diabetes to meet and learn from each other
- *Information and support to whom?*
  - People with diabetes
  - Partners and carers: provide the opportunity for partners/carers to be involved in information sessions
- The wider community: consider ways of informing the wider community about diabetes to help reduce stigma. Establish a systematic process of informing schools about diabetes.

Naqib (2002) recommends that diabetes education should be a planned lifelong process. She also states that the educational outcomes that have achieved the best outcomes are ones that use behavioural models and adult education principles to facilitate improving self-care behaviour. The process of patient education should involve assessment of learning needs, a learning/education plan and evaluation. The framework to support effective education includes up-to-date material, adequate physical resources, such as space in which to teach, and skilled staff. She also gives examples of good practice.

The most recent publication to discuss diabetes patient education (NICE 2002) also recommended that it should be an ongoing process and that different methods should be tried until the best for each individual is identified. The full guidance is available on the NICE website (www.nice.org.uk); the existing evidence for different methods is examined in detail here.

References

Hiscock J, Snape R, Legard D. Listening to diabetes service users: qualitative findings for the Diabetes National Service Framework. London: National Centre for Social Research; 2001.

Naqib, J. Patient education for effective diabetes self-management: report, recommendations and examples of good practice. London: Diabetes UK; 2002.

National Institute for Clinical Excellence. Management of type 2 diabetes: management of blood glucose. London: NICE; 2002.

have achieved mastery are going to know more about diabetes, and in particular their own diabetes, than health care professionals (see Reflective Practice box 17.1, p. 406).

This section will therefore describe the educational and psychological care required by people with type 1 diabetes at different stages of their condition, commencing with care at diagnosis. Although diabetes specialist nurses may deliver much of this care, all nurses will encounter people with diabetes throughout their careers and have an important role to play.

Education at diagnosis

People with newly diagnosed diabetes are likely to be feeling a range of emotions; they may be shocked, frightened or numb. Some, however, may be feeling a sense of relief that their diagnosis is 'only' diabetes rather than the cancer they were thinking they had (Jerreat 1999).

Because of these emotions, initial education should be delivered in small chunks, at a pace that allows individuals to absorb the information. The first step is to answer any questions patients may have, although frequently these do not get asked until the initial impact of the diagnosis has passed. As always, a good assessment of needs is vital. Some people may have previous experience of diabetes, e.g. if a family member has it. Many people will have heard of a person who had to have a leg amputated because of diabetes, or, on a more positive note, of famous individuals with diabetes such as Gary Mabbutt, the football player, or Sir Steve Redgrave who have achieved success despite having diabetes.

Giving insulin injections

The primary concerns of many people relate to insulin injections. It is best to deal with these concerns quickly, on the day of diagnosis if possible, as individuals are unlikely to be able to absorb any more information until these are resolved. Many people ask why insulin cannot be taken by mouth. As insulin is a protein, like many other hormones, it cannot be given orally as it would be digested by the digestive enzymes, and therefore needs to be injected.

The best way to help individuals is for nurses to demonstrate giving an injection by performing a 'dry' injection, i.e. using an empty syringe, on themselves. The insulin should be drawn up by the nurse but the nurse should then ask the person with

R|Я REFLECTIVE PRACTICE

17.1 Self-care of diabetes

Martin (not his real name), who has had type 1 diabetes for 11 years, is admitted to hospital for planned surgery. He has an abdominal hernia. Martin's glucose levels are well controlled with twice-daily insulin. At home, he performs blood glucose monitoring, using a meter, which he has brought with him. He also usually gives his own insulin, using a reusable insulin pen.

Following his operation, which he has recovered from well, Martin states that he would like to manage his own diabetes for the remainder of his hospital stay. He is told that it is the ward's 'policy' that the nursing staff perform all blood glucose tests, and that his insulin pens must be locked in the medicine cupboard when not in use. He is also told that the nurses are responsible for ensuring he gets the correct dose of insulin as prescribed by the doctors, so they must give it.

Following this discussion, Martin's insulin is given only 3 minutes before his evening meal arrives and the blood glucose level is measured after it!

Unfortunately, these situations are not uncommon, particularly when individuals are admitted for non-diabetes-related reasons (Hiscock et al 2001). Current recommendations are that in-patients who are capable of managing their own diabetes should be allowed to do so (Audit Commission 2000, Department of Health 2001).

Student activities
- What might Martin think about the ward's 'policies'?
- What do you think about them?
- What are the background factors that may influence the ward's policy? Are there hospital policies related to the self-administration of medicines, for example? How confident are the nurses on the ward in relation to their diabetes knowledge?
- How might Martin feel about having the responsibility of managing his day-to-day diabetes care removed from him?
- What do you think the impact on Martin's confidence in managing his diabetes may be?
- Think about where you work or, if you are not currently working in an in-patient environment, think about a previous placement. Compare the practices in your workplace with the scenario described above, as well as the recommendations for best practice. What changes, if any, need to occur in your own environment? How could you change your own practice? You might find it helpful to look at the Special Issues box 17.1 (particularly Standards 3 and 8) (p. 395).

References
Audit Commission. Testing times: a review of diabetes services in England and Wales. London: Audit Commission; 2000.
Department of Health. National Service Framework for Diabetes: Standards. London: Department of Health; 2001.
Hiscock J, Snape R, Legard D. Listening to diabetes service users: qualitative findings for the Diabetes National Service Framework. London: National Centre for Social Research; 2001.

---

diabetes to self-inject into either the abdomen or the thigh. Insulin injections are usually completely painless and the relief experienced after having done one's first injection is enormous.

Practising on an orange for days before giving an injection, which is totally unlike injecting into flesh, and 'being kind' to people by doing their injections for them at first are usually counterproductive as anxieties about doing it oneself can be heightened by the delay.

Patients need further information about injection technique and equipment (syringes, needles, etc), as follows:

- Swabbing of the skin with alcohol wipes is contraindicated. Prolonged use of these over time causes the skin to toughen, making injections more difficult. Stinging at the injection site may also occur unless the alcohol is dry (McCarthy et al 1993)
- Needle length – insulin syringes are available in two needle lengths, 8 and 12.7 mm (a shorter needle is supplied for children and very thin people – see p. 408). The shorter needle is less likely to cause anxiety and should be used unless the individual is very overweight, an unlikely occurrence in newly diagnosed type 1 diabetes
- Angle of injection – all subcutaneous injections of insulin should be delivered at 90° to the skin surface, whatever the length of needle. To ensure it is delivered into subcutaneous tissue, rather than muscle, raising a skin fold is necessary for most individuals in most injection sites (apart from the buttocks). In the past, subcutaneous injections were delivered at 45° to the skin; this practice should not occur when using modern insulin needles

- Syringe sizes – syringes are available in three sizes: 0.3, 0.5 and 1 mL. The two smaller sizes are available in both needle lengths: 8 mm and 12.7 mm. The 1 mL syringe is only available with a 12.7 mm needle. The smaller syringes are suitable for individuals using smaller doses of insulin (e.g. children) and are also useful for those whose eyesight precludes them from reading the marks on the larger syringes, which are closer together (see Fig. 17.5). At diagnosis, individuals' vision may be blurred due to osmotic changes in glucose concentration in the lens; this problem resolves after approximately 6 weeks. They may need reassurance that they do not have early visual complications of diabetes.

Once the first injection is over, drawing up insulin, or the use of an insulin 'pen', can be taught. It is preferable to avoid teaching people with diabetes how to mix two insulins together on the first day. All types of insulin are supplied in one strength, 100 units/mL. If only one insulin is to be used, the technique of drawing up insulin is as described in the Health Promotion box 17.1.

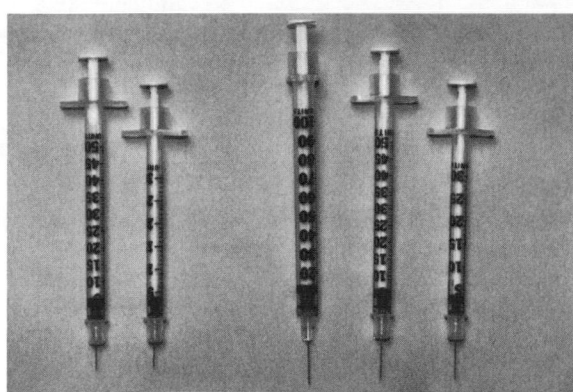

Figure 17.5   Insulin syringes.

Once individuals have mastered drawing up one type of insulin, they may practise drawing up two types of insulin together if their insulin regimen requires this. This may not occur until the following day. If two insulins are to be drawn up the technique is shown in Health Promotion box 17.1.

Many people with diabetes prefer not to use insulin syringes. They often feel there is a stigma attached to using overtly medical devices, particularly syringes, due to the association with illicit drug users. Consequently a variety of insulin delivery devices have been developed which make 'drawing up' easier and which have fewer medical connotations.

Diabetes specialist nurses have an intimate knowledge of insulin delivery devices and should be involved, wherever practicable, in the decision-making process when people with diabetes new to insulin are choosing the device they wish to use. Indeed, they may be the only people who have easy access to the full range of available devices. People with diabetes who are new to insulin treatment should be given the choice, wherever possible, about which insulin delivery device to use.

There are essentially three types of devices available:

- *Preloaded insulin devices or pens* – as their name suggests, these devices contain cartridges of insulin already loaded into them. Once finished, the whole pen is discarded. These pens are the most expensive method of delivering insulin and in some centres they are limited to those who have problems with manual dexterity or visual difficulties, who would consequently find reloading cartridges difficult, but who could maintain independence with a preloaded device (see Fig. 17.6)
- *Reusable insulin pens* – these are loaded with insulin cartridges; once they are used, a fresh cartridge is inserted and only the empty one is disposed of. These pens are currently the most popular method of delivering insulin. Younger individuals have a tendency to choose the most visually appealing pen, whereas older people tend to choose the pen they find easiest to use (see Fig. 17.7)
- *Insulin dosers* – these are a recent development; they use cartridges and similar technology to the pens above but are not pen-shaped (see Fig. 17.8).

 HEALTH PROMOTION

17.1 Technique of drawing up insulin

If only one insulin is to be used
- Draw up into the syringe the equivalent amount of air as the amount of insulin to be given.
- With the vial standing upright, insert the syringe needle into the vial and then push the air into the vial (this is to stop a vacuum developing in the vial).
- Invert the vial, ensuring the tip of the needle is below the level of the insulin and draw up the insulin beyond the mark designating the amount of insulin to be given.
- Tap any air bubbles to the top of the syringe, and then eliminate them back into the vial.
- Move the plunger to the correct mark on the syringe and remove the vial.
- Perform the injection.

As with any new skill, practice will be required. Ensuring the individual has either handwritten or pre-printed instructions to follow is essential, as is a practise syringe and vial.

If two types of insulin are to be used
- Gently agitate the vial of cloudy insulin to ensure the insulin is mixed thoroughly.
- Draw up into the syringe the equivalent amount of air as the amount of cloudy (or longer-acting) insulin to be given.

- With the vial standing upright, insert the syringe needle into the vial of cloudy insulin and then push the air into the vial. Remove the syringe.
- Draw up into the syringe the equivalent amount of air as the amount of clear (or soluble) insulin to be given.
- With the vial standing upright, insert the syringe needle into the vial of clear insulin and then push the air into the vial.
- Invert the vial, ensuring the tip of the needle is below the level of the insulin and draw up the clear insulin beyond the mark designating the amount of insulin to be given.
- Tap any air bubbles to the top of the syringe, and then eliminate them back into the vial.
- Move the plunger to the correct mark on the syringe (the number of units of clear, or soluble, insulin required) and remove the vial.
- Insert the needle into the vial of cloudy insulin.
- Draw up the cloudy insulin, being careful not to go beyond the correct dose (the total number of units of insulin required), and remove the vial.
- Perform the injection.

As before, patients will need to practise the new skill. The nurse should ensure that the individual has either handwritten or pre-printed instructions to follow, as well as a practice syringe and vial.

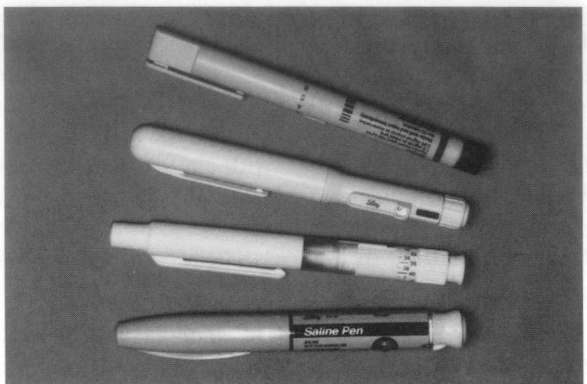

Figure 17.6 Insulin devices (preloaded).

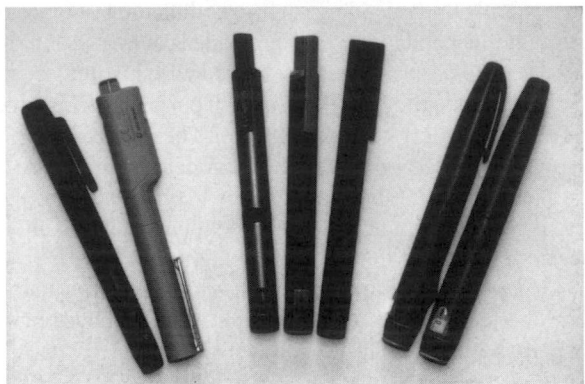

Figure 17.7 Reusable insulin pens.

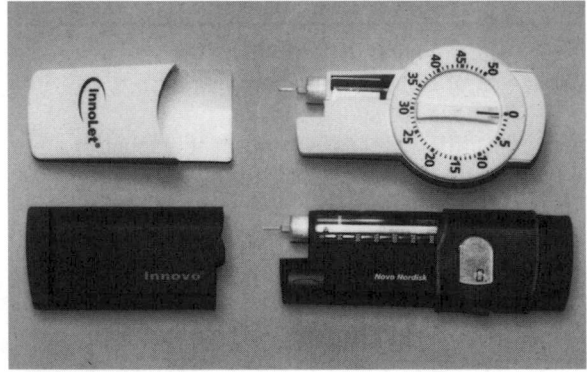

Figure 17.8 Insulin dosers.

Pen needles are available in lengths of 5 or 6 mm (most commonly used for children with diabetes or very thin young men), 8 mm (suitable for most people), or 12.7 mm. The shorter needles are psychologically more acceptable, although it is important that the correct length of needle is used (see Box 17.2). The diabetes specialist nurse, or pharmacy, will provide the needles.

Again, once the decision has been made about which particular device to use, individuals with diabetes will need to practise. The diabetes specialist nursing team can provide sterile water cartridges for this purpose. Written instruction leaflets, with pictures, are available with every insulin delivery device to assist the individual and nursing staff.

Box 17.2 Needle lengths and corresponding usage

12.7 mm
- Obese adults, with a pinch
- Can be used in the buttocks on most people, without a pinch

8 mm
- Normal weight people, with a pinch

5 or 6 mm
- Children
- Very thin adults, particularly men, with a pinch

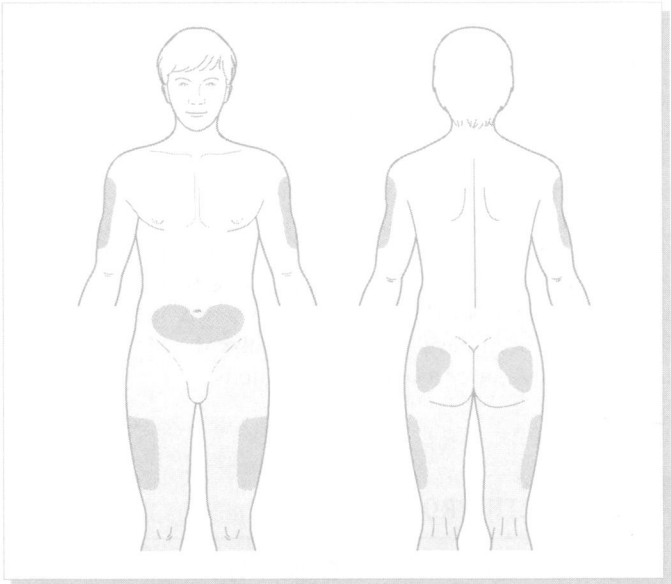

Figure 17.9 Insulin injection sites.

Over the next few days, people with newly diagnosed diabetes will need to learn more about their insulin injections and other aspects of managing their diabetes. The speed at which information is given depends on the speed at which individuals can absorb the information. It is very common to have to repeat information; for this reason providing written guidance, wherever possible, is advised.

Other information about insulin injections is discussed below.

Injection sites. Insulin may be injected into the upper outer arms, the abdomen, the upper outer thighs or the buttocks (see Fig. 17.9). However, insulin is absorbed at different rates from different areas (Bantle et al 1993), so individuals should be advised to inject into the same area at the same time of day. For instance, a man may choose to inject into his thighs in the morning because they are more accessible, and his abdomen in the evening because he can undo a shirt button relatively easily. To avoid lipohypertrophy (see Special Issues box 17.2), however, people with diabetes should be advised to avoid injecting into the same square inch of flesh within these areas for a week. Self-injecting into the upper outer arms is often discouraged because it is not possible to 'take a pinch' and giving an intramuscular

SPECIAL ISSUES

17.2 Lipohypertrophy

Lipohypertrophy is an increase in fatty tissue caused by repeated injections of insulin into the same spot. Insulin has a trophic (growth) action and repeated exposure of fat cells to it encourages enlargement. The resulting 'lump' can be unsightly and also cause erratic absorption of insulin (Jerreat 1999). This may result in very erratic glucose control, with results swinging wildly from the hypoglycaemic range to hyperglycaemia within a few hours.

Reference

Jerreat L. Diabetes for nurses. London: Whurr Publishers; 1999.

---

injection is therefore more likely. A pinch when injecting into the buttock is not necessary as there is sufficient subcutaneous fatty tissue.

People with diabetes need to be informed that exercising a limb that has just been injected with insulin may cause increased insulin absorption and, if the glucose levels are well controlled, subsequent hypoglycaemia because of the increased blood flow in the underlying muscle.

Timing of injections. Most insulins (apart from analogue insulins) should be injected 20–30 minutes before eating, to enable the insulin to be absorbed from the fat under the skin into the bloodstream. This is because the insulin molecule is large and complex, and time for it to become diffused and broken down into small enough particles for absorption into the circulation is required. The exception to this are the insulin analogues. These are 'designer insulins' that have had their molecular structure altered to enable them to start to be absorbed immediately after injection. Readers needing specific information about this should consult an up-to-date formulary such as the British National Formulary or access the information at www.bnf.org.uk.

Sharps disposal. People with diabetes are generally unable to acquire sharps boxes, although some health authorities have made arrangements for this to occur and small sharps boxes have recently become available on prescription. This is such a new initiative that many local authorities have not yet made arrangements for collection and disposal. However, in the absence of any such arrangement, patients should be advised to clip their needles using a Safeclip device, available on prescription, and dispose of the remaining needle hub or syringe in a homemade sharps container. This should be an opaque thick plastic bottle, such as those used for fabric conditioner or bleach, with a screw-top lid. When full, the Safeclip and the closed plastic bottle should be disposed of in the domestic rubbish. Nurses should always discover what local arrangements exist in their area before giving information about sharps disposal to people with diabetes.

Storage of insulin. Insulin not in use should be stored in the domestic refrigerator, in either the salad compartment or the door. It should not be frozen, as this will destroy it. Insulin in use may be stored at the ambient temperature for up to 1 month. If insulin is stored in refrigerators in a clinical area for security

reasons, it should be removed from the fridge for 1 hour prior to injection; cold insulin is uncomfortable!

People with diabetes should be informed about not allowing their insulin to be exposed to extreme temperatures; from 30°C upwards insulin activity progressively deteriorates. Care should be taken, for example, to avoid keeping loaded insulin pens or syringes in direct sunlight or above radiators. Those travelling to hot countries can purchase insulin storage bags to keep their insulin cool. The diabetes specialist nurses will have information about these.

Dietary advice

Immediately type 1 diabetes is diagnosed the person with diabetes should be referred to the dietician, who will undertake a full dietary assessment and provide individualized education within the next few days. However, while the individual is waiting to see the dietician, 'first aid' dietary advice will be necessary. Individuals should be advised to avoid very sugary drinks such as lemonade or other carbonated soft drinks and to avoid adding sugar to hot drinks; 'diet' drinks, however, such as diet cola or low-calorie squash, are good alternatives. They should also be informed about the importance of eating regular meals, i.e. breakfast, midday meal and evening meal, and having a bedtime snack.

Blood glucose monitoring

It is the nurse's role not only to perform accurate bedside capillary blood glucose monitoring but also to teach a newly diagnosed individual with diabetes how to perform his or her own monitoring. Most people with diabetes choose to purchase a blood glucose meter, because they cannot be prescribed for this purpose in the UK, although a visually read blood glucose monitoring system is available on prescription, as are the disposable items for use with meters (test trips and lancets). In some centres, the diabetes specialist nursing team can supply meters free of charge. There are approximately 10 different types of meter available at the time of writing.

As with the supply of insulin delivery devices, it is essential to use the expertise of the specialist nurse team when assisting people with diabetes to choose their blood glucose meter. It is often tempting to recommend the meter used in the hospital or clinical setting but this may not be suitable for the individual's future use at home or in everyday life. The diabetes specialist nurse will also need to demonstrate the meter to the person with diabetes if nursing team members are unfamiliar with it. Whatever the meter used (or not), the underlying principles of blood glucose monitoring are the same (see Guidelines for Care Priorities box 17.2, p. 410)

Blood glucose tests are usually performed four times a day at most (unless an insulin infusion is running, in which case, blood glucose tests are carried out hourly). They should be done just before main meals and at bedtime. When the glucose levels are reasonably well controlled (blood glucose level of 4–9.9 mmol/L), testing frequency may be reduced to twice daily, on one day before breakfast and the evening meal, and the next before the midday meal and at bedtime and so on (see Fig. 17.10A, p. 410).

Once the blood glucose levels are well controlled, i.e. blood glucose 4–7 mmol/L before main meals and 4–8 mmol/L at

GUIDELINES FOR CARE PRIORITIES

17.2 Blood glucose monitoring

- It is essential that blood glucose monitoring (BGM) be performed on clean hands; any contaminants, e.g. orange juice or alcohol, are likely to affect the result obtained.
- The finger should be pricked on the side as it is less painful than pricking the pad.
- Blood should be 'milked' out of the finger, rather than squeezed. Squeezing applies pressure, which prevents blood flow and may also cause interstitial fluid to enter the blood sample, leading to inaccurate results. It is also useful to wait 5 seconds or so prior to 'milking'.
- Washing hands in warm water can help with blood flow as well.
- A finger pricker designed for the purpose must always be used. Using lancets alone may cause damage to the fingers and can be extremely painful. Nurses must ensure the finger pricker they are using is specifically designed for multiple-person use to prevent cross-infection (Douvin et al 1990). The finger prickers supplied with most meters are designed for single-person use only and must never be used for another individual.

- The meter (or visually read system) must be used strictly according to the manufacturer's instructions; most are supplied with helpful leaflets for the basics of BGM as well as more comprehensive instruction manuals for reference purposes.
- It is essential that sufficient blood is obtained to cover the blood glucose-testing strip; insufficient samples will give inaccurate results.
- The results must be recorded; in the hospital situation this should be on the appropriate chart, but people with diabetes should also be encouraged to record their results in a BGM diary, available from the diabetes specialist nursing team. Many meters have a memory function, recording the result and the date and time of day the test was performed, but it is not easy to detect patterns in results using this function.

Reference

Douvin C, Simon D, Zinelabidine H, Wirquin V, Perlemuter C, Dhumeaux D. An outbreak of hepatitis B in an endocrinology unit traced to a capillary-blood-sampling device. N Engl J Med 1990; 322(1): 322–357.

Date	Before breakfast	Before midday meal	Before evening meal	Bedtime	Notes
	x		x		
		x		x	
	x		x		

(A)

Date	Before breakfast	Before midday meal	Before evening meal	Bedtime	Notes
	x				
		x			
			x		
				x	
	x			x	**To gym**
		x			
			x		

(B)

Figure 17.10 Blood glucose monitoring profile. (A) Twice daily; (B) four times (various) a day.

bedtime, testing may be reduced to once daily at various times with extra tests if there are any concerns (see Fig. 17.10B).

Most blood glucose meters are supplied with quality control solutions. As all blood glucose meters should be subjected to regular quality control checks in the clinical setting, so too should people with diabetes be shown how to check their own meters on a regular basis, at least once a week, or according to local protocols.

The 'honeymoon' period

People with newly diagnosed type 1 diabetes need to be informed that they may experience the 'honeymoon' period shortly after they develop diabetes. There are often a few β cells still left in the islets of Langerhans at the time of diagnosis; these can recover following the administration of exogenous insulin so that they produce insulin again. This may occur to such an extent that insulin injections are not required, although this is uncommon.

Some individuals notice nothing and some have a relatively short period of reduced insulin doses. Others may have a honeymoon period lasting up to a year. However long it lasts, individuals who experience it will always need insulin in larger doses in the future. Unless they are warned that this event is possible, people with type 1 diabetes may think the diagnosis is a mistake or that they have been cured.

Goals for blood glucose control

It is vitally important that people with diabetes are informed about recommended targets for glucose control and that negotiation with regard to their personal goals is undertaken. Achieving perfect glucose control in the immediate post-diagnosis period is unlikely to occur. A reasonable target in this phase would be to reduce blood glucose levels to those at which symptoms of hyperglycaemia (lethargy, polyuria and polydipsia) are not apparent. This is generally less than 15 mmol/L.

Driving

In the UK people with newly diagnosed diabetes must be informed that they have a legal responsibility to inform the Drivers and Vehicle Licensing Authority (DVLA) in Swansea that they have type 1 diabetes; their doctor will be sent a questionnaire regarding their fitness to drive. Licenses will be issued for a

3-year period, although on some occasions these are only for 1 or 2 years. They must also inform their insurance company or their insurance will not be valid.

Unfortunately people with type 1 diabetes are unable to hold large goods vehicle (LGV) or passenger service vehicle (PSV) licences. For those affected, this has an obvious implication for employment prospects.

Hypoglycaemia

Although hypoglycaemia, or a hypo, is unlikely to occur in the first week after diagnosis, the person with diabetes should be taught to recognize the signs and symptoms of mild, moderate and severe hypoglycaemia, the causes of 'hypos', how to prevent them occurring and how to treat them if they do occur (see section on hypoglycaemia, pp. 421–422).

Testing for ketones

People with diabetes should be shown how to test their urine for ketones and a brief explanation of the reasons for doing so given. Ketostix are used for the estimation of ketones in urine. The strip is dipped in urine, removed and the excess urine shaken off. Fifteen seconds afterwards, the strip is read by comparing the colour on the reagent pad to those on the side of the container. The results may be negative, trace (0.5 mmol/L), small (1.5 mmol/L), moderate (4 mmol/L) or large (8 or 16 mmol/L). Immediately after diagnosis, ketones are likely to present in the urine in moderate or large quantities, but the amount tends to reduce rapidly. Following the period immediately after diagnosis there should be no ketones in the urine.

A brief explanation of the purpose of testing urine for ketones is required. Due to the lack of insulin, the body is unable to use carbohydrates to produce energy. Fats will be used instead. If these are metabolized, or 'burned', in large amounts, the body is unable to use the breakdown products of fat metabolism, ketones. These are then excreted via the kidneys into the urine (ketonuria). (Further information on ketonuria may be found in the section on 'Diabetic ketoacidosis', pp. 422–424.)

Education required over the next 3 months

A member of the diabetes specialist nursing team will deliver, on an outpatient basis, most of the educational care required over the next 3 months. However, nurses may encounter people with diabetes during this period and should contribute to the educational process in this situation.

As one of the goals of diabetes education is to equip people with diabetes with the information they need to effectively manage their own diabetes on a day-to-day basis, they should be taught how their insulin regimen works and also how to adjust their own insulin doses according to prevailing patterns of blood glucose results and what activities they undertake. The initial step is to discuss the types of insulin they are using. Full information is given below. However, the amount of information given to each person with diabetes must be specifically tailored to individual needs; factors to take into account when teaching include intellectual capacity, emotional status and physical status. Therefore, not all of the information given below will be required for all people with diabetes. Give the essential pieces of knowledge to enable understanding and supply the rest of the information if the individual indicates a wish to know more. The

information about these rather 'dry' topic areas should be given in small chunks and people must be given the opportunity to practise using the information between sessions to enable effective learning.

Types of insulin

Short-acting insulins. Soluble insulin is, as the name suggests, insulin in solution. As such it has a clear appearance. The pH of these insulins is 7.0 and they are often referred to as the neutral insulins. All soluble insulins have a short duration; they start being absorbed 20–30 minutes after injection and peak between 1.5 and 4 hours after injection (see Fig. 17.11A). The duration of these insulins is approximately 6–8 hours post-injection, although this can differ in individuals.

Analogue insulins. These are a new development and are also known as 'designer' insulins. The structure of the insulin molecule has been altered to enable immediate absorption following injection. For this reason they are very popular with those needing a flexible insulin regimen as it enables them to inject immediately before eating, or indeed up to 15 minutes afterwards.

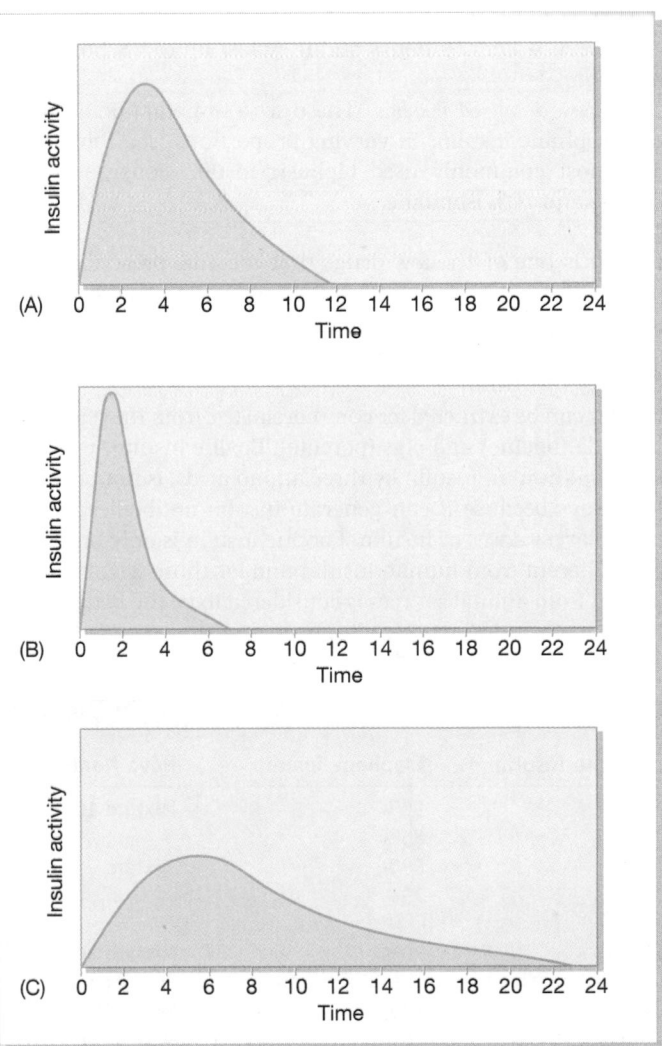

Figure 17.11 Time action profiles for insulin. (A) Short-acting insulin; (B) analogue insulins; (C) isophane insulins.

The peak absorption is 0.5–2 hours post-injection and the duration is about 5 hours (see Fig. 17.11B, p. 411).

Intermediate-acting insulins. Isophane insulins are insoluble suspensions of insulin combined with protamine, a protein which delays the absorption of the insulin. They may alternatively be designated as NPH (Neutral Protamine Hagedorn) after the laboratories in which they were developed. Isophane insulins start to be absorbed about 1 hour after injection; their peak is between approximately 2 and 12 hours, depending on the specific insulin used, and the duration is between 18 and 24 hours, again depending on the specific insulin (see Fig.17.11C, p. 411).

Lente insulins are made by adding excess zinc ions to insulin. They tend to start being absorbed later than the isophane insulins, at about 2 hours after injection, but peak at similar times and have approximately the same duration. Any insulin with excess zinc ions cannot, theoretically, be mixed with soluble insulin as the excess zinc 'blunts' the effect of the quick-acting insulin, by combining with it to make more lente insulin. However, in practice this is often done by people who have had type 1 diabetes for many years. If diabetes control is good, they should not be discouraged from mixing their insulins.

Long-acting insulins. Ultralente insulins are very long-acting; they start to be absorbed 2–4 hours after injection, their peak is between 4 and 24 hours and they last up to 28 hours after injection.

Biphasic or 'mixed' insulins. These are a combination of soluble and isophane insulins in varying proportions (see Table 17.2). The most commonly used biphasic insulin consists of 30% soluble and 70% isophane.

Insulin is one of the few drugs that must be prescribed by its proprietary or 'trade name' rather than the generic term, as each insulin has a different time action profile.

Sources of insulin

Insulin can be extracted for commercial use from the pancreases of cattle (bovine) and pigs (porcine). Bovine insulin, which differs from human insulin by three amino acids, is not often used nowadays because it can generate insulin antibodies, necessitating larger doses of insulin. Porcine insulin is only one amino acid different from human insulin and for those wishing to use insulin from animal sources is considered to be the better option because of a reduced antigenic effect.

Human insulin is bioengineered. Enzymatically modified porcine insulin (emp) is made by cleaving the different amino acid and replacing it with the correct amino acid to make human insulin.

Most 'human' insulin, however, is produced by recombinant DNA technology. The genetic material of either the bacterium *Escherichia coli* or yeast cells is altered. These reprogrammed organisms then 'grow' insulin rather than more of themselves. The source of the insulin can be identified; prb (proinsulin recombinant bacteria) insulin is produced from *E. coli* and pyr (proinsulin yeast recombinant) from yeast. In both these cases, the precursor to insulin, proinsulin, is produced, which is then converted to insulin and purified.

It is important that individuals using insulin from one source are not changed arbitrarily to another species, as glucose control may be compromised. Admission to hospital is one possible cause of such an event! Religious beliefs can often preclude individuals from using insulin from animal sources. For example, those of the Jewish or Muslim faiths are unlikely to use porcine insulin, and Hindus are not likely to wish to use bovine insulin. Individuals who follow a strict vegetarian or vegan diet are also likely to refuse insulin from animal sources on ethical grounds.

Insulin regimens

There are almost as many insulin regimens as there are insulins themselves. However, the following two are the ones most likely to be used long term for those with newly diagnosed type 1 diabetes. Whatever regimen is used, the goal is to try and achieve as normal an insulin profile as possible, given the individual's lifestyle (see Fig. 17.12). Different centres do have different policies in relation to commencing insulin therapy so it is best to check local policies.

The basal bolus regimen. This regimen necessitates four injections a day. The longer-acting dose, which serves as a baseline or 'basal' dose, is given at bedtime. An injection of short-acting insulin, the bolus, is given before each main meal (see Fig. 17.13A). If this is a 'normal' insulin, such as Actrapid, Velosulin or Humulin S, it should be given 20–30 minutes before eating to ensure it is being absorbed at the same time as food.

However, the advent of 'designer' insulins has enabled those using them to give the short-acting insulin with, and even up to 15 minutes after, a meal. Novorapid is one such insulin, and the other is Humalog. It should be noted that the time action curve

Table 17.2 Biphasic or 'mixed' insulins

Soluble insulin	Isophane insulin	Novo Nordisk	Lilly	CP Pharm	Aventis
10%	90%	Mixtard 10			
15%	85%				Insulin Comb 15
20%	80%	Mixtard 20	Humulin M2		
25%	75%		Humalog Mix 25		Insulin Comb 25
30%	70%	Mixtard 30 Pork Mixtard 30	Humulin M3	Hypurin Porcine 30/70	
40%	60%	Mixtard 40			
50%	50%	Mixtard 50	Humulin M5 Humalog Mix 50		Insulin Comb 50

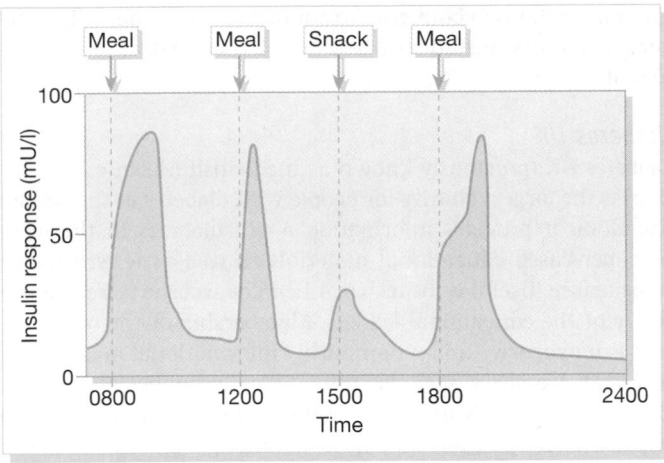

Figure 17.12 The physiological insulin profile.

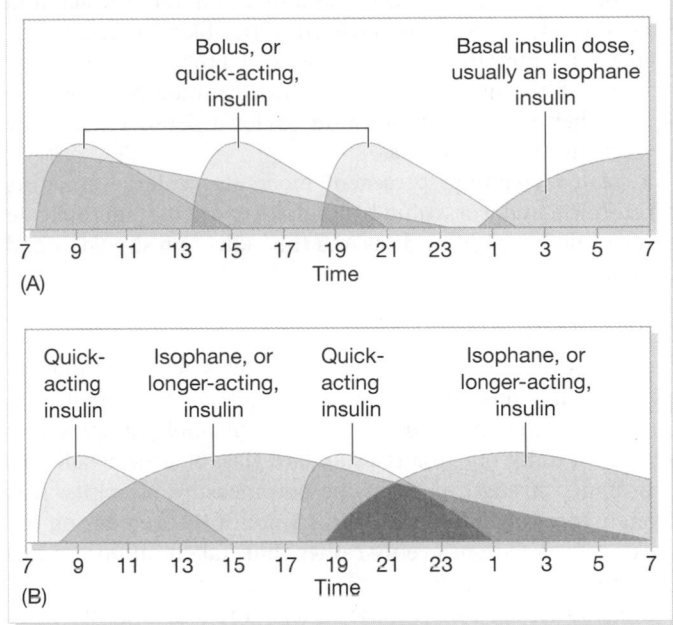

Figure 17.13 Insulin profiles. (A) The basal bolus insulin regimen; (B) the twice-daily regimen.

for these 'designer' insulins is much shorter than that shown in Fig. 17.13A.

The basal bolus regimen is suitable for people who have flexible lifestyles, e.g. younger people, those working shifts and people who travel a lot. The disadvantage of more injections is outweighed by the flexibility of this regimen, as meals do not have to be eaten at the same time every day.

The twice-daily regimen. This regimen requires two injections a day. With each injection, a mixture of a longer-acting insulin, such as Insulatard or Humulin I, is given in conjunction with a shorter-acting soluble insulin such as Actrapid or Humulin S (see Fig. 17.13B). The insulins may either be administered as a 'fixed mixture', or drawn up from separate vials and mixed in a syringe – free mixing.

Fixed mixtures may be advantageous for individuals who have manipulative difficulties, as it is only necessary to draw up one lot of insulin. These insulins may also be used in insulin pens, which are useful particularly for those who have visual problems. The fixed-mixture insulins are available in 10/90, 15/85, 20/80, 25/75, 30/70, 40/60 and 50/50 proportions, where the first figure refers to the amount of soluble insulin in the preparation. Each individual may require two different mixtures to achieve good glycaemic control.

Because these insulins contain 'normal' soluble insulin, they must be injected 20–30 minutes before a meal. However, there are three 'designer' mixtures available, which may be injected immediately before eating; these are Humalog Mix 25, Humalog Mix 50 and Novomix 30.

Free mixing enables the relative proportions of each insulin to be adjusted precisely without requiring a change in prescription.

The twice-daily regimen tends to be more suitable for those who eat their meals at set times, or who wish only two injections a day. On occasions the twice-daily regimen may be initiated with twice-daily isophane insulin only; the short-acting component is added later, once the individual has become confident with the mechanics of insulin delivery.

Prescription exemption

People with diabetes treated with insulin or oral hypoglycaemic agents are exempt from paying prescription charges. This includes any future prescriptions for items not related to their diabetes. Certificates are available from the general practitioner (GP); they will need to be shown to the pharmacist whenever prescriptions are presented. The hospital pharmacy and the diabetes nursing team should provide initial supplies of equipment and insulin.

Sick day rules

The most important thing people with type 1 diabetes should be taught is that they should *never* stop taking their insulin, even if they do not feel like eating because of a concurrent illness (Fox and MacKinnon 1999). The reason for this is that when the body is stressed, the stress (or counter-regulatory) hormones, adrenaline (epinephrine) and cortisol, are secreted in larger amounts than normal, to provide the body with extra energy to assist in combating the illness (see pp. 399–400 and Ch. 6). Counter-regulatory hormones stimulate the production of glucose in the liver and increase the conversion of stored glucose, glycogen, back into glucose. In someone without diabetes, increased amounts of insulin are secreted to utilize the extra glucose. A person with type 1 diabetes is obviously unable to do this. Counter-regulatory hormones are also insulin antagonists, i.e. they reduce the physiological effects of insulin. The net effect of all this hormone activity is an increased blood glucose level. This can occur during a cold or 'flu', and in more serious illnesses. In the latter case, people with type 1 diabetes can require as much as three times their normal insulin dose, even if they are not eating.

If eating is problematic during an intercurrent illness, people with type 1 diabetes should be informed that they could replace their normal meals with liquid carbohydrate, such as milk, Lucozade or other sugary drinks. It is also advisable to increase their intake of non-carbohydrate fluids.

Blood glucose levels should be tested four times a day and urine should be tested for ketones if the blood glucose level is above 15 mmol/L. Insulin doses will probably need to be increased, although the newly diagnosed should be advised to contact their diabetes specialist nurses for assistance until they have learned how to do this.

Repeated vomiting, persistent moderate or large amounts of ketonuria and worsening hyperglycaemic symptoms indicate incipient diabetic ketoacidosis and the individual should attend hospital urgently.

Alcohol intake

The advice given to people with diabetes about alcohol is essentially the same as that given to the general population. Men may have a maximum of 21 units of alcohol per week and women 14 units; one unit is a standard glass of wine, a half-pint of ordinary strength beer or one pub measure of spirits. It is strongly recommended that, if this amount is taken during the week, it is spread out evenly rather than taken on one or two days only.

Mixers should be low-calorie or 'diet', to avoid large increases in blood glucose levels. Where possible, wines should be dry rather than sweet. Low-alcohol beers tend to have a lot of sugar in them and should therefore be avoided. So, too, should strong beers where most of the sugar has been converted to alcohol. Excess alcohol increases the risks of severe hypoglycaemia (see section on hypoglycaemia, pp. 421–422).

Those people with diabetes who are concerned with their weight need to be informed that alcohol has many calories and a reduction in alcohol intake can help with weight control.

Work

There are some jobs that people with diabetes are excluded from doing; these include jobs in the armed forces (although in some circumstances people may be moved to posts which are 'behind the scenes' and not related to active service), airline pilots and offshore work. Although there have been blanket bans in the past, such as in the fire and police services, attitudes are slowly changing; for example, there is one instance of a man with type 1 diabetes successfully continuing his career in the fire service on active duty.

Any job that requires a large goods vehicle (LGV) or passenger carrying vehicle (PCV) driving licence may also mean the individual becomes unemployed or has limited career options, although those with type 2 diabetes treated with diet alone or diet and oral hypoglycaemic agents may still retain these licences.

Shift work may cause problems for some individuals in relation to the timing of meals and snacks and also insulin doses. In these situations, individuals should be referred to the diabetes specialist nursing team for assistance in working out how to manage their diabetes in the context of work.

Smoking

People with diabetes should ideally not smoke, as it is an added risk factor for the development of cardiovascular complications of diabetes. However, expecting someone with newly diagnosed type 1 diabetes to give up smoking immediately is somewhat unrealistic. People should be informed of the increased risks and given information about who to contact (usually their GP's surgery in the first instance) when and if they make the decision to quit.

Diabetes UK

Diabetes UK (previously known as the British Diabetic Association) is the largest charity for people with diabetes in the United Kingdom. It provides information about diabetes in the form of paper-based educational materials as well as a very useful website (see 'Useful websites', p. 442). The website is free, as are many of the educational leaflets. Membership of the organization is inexpensive and a bi-monthly informational magazine is provided. Members may also attend local branches of Diabetes UK, which generally meet four or more times a year and provide opportunities to obtain support from other people with diabetes. The diabetes specialist nursing team will be able to provide information about joining Diabetes UK, the free educational materials as well as a catalogue, and the local branches.

Diabetes complications

Discussing diabetes complications can be a difficult topic. However, unless people with diabetes have an understanding of the potential risks of long-term high blood glucose levels, they have inadequate information upon which to base their decisions about their own glucose control.

One way to begin is to ask them whether they know of any people with diabetes and whether those individuals have any long-term health problems, or whether they have heard any 'horror stories' related to diabetes. Giving up-to-date and correct information in relation to these issues is a priority. For example, it is now known, as a result of a landmark study, the Diabetes Control and Complications Trial (DCCT 1993), that maintaining blood glucose levels as near normal as possible reduces the risks of developing long-term complications of type 1 diabetes. Also, diabetes care has improved radically over the last two decades; for example, home blood glucose monitoring has only been available since the early 1980s and the strips and lancets available on prescription since 1988. In the early 1980s, there were relatively few diabetes specialist nurses and education about diabetes was somewhat scarce. In these circumstances it was difficult to maintain 'good' diabetes control, and consequently reduce the risks of complications.

Screening for complications has also improved as well as the treatments for them. The recommendation for people with diabetes is that they receive an annual review that includes:

- eye screening to ascertain whether any diabetic retinopathy (disease of the retina) is present (see Ch. 17)
- check on the blood and nerve supply to the feet
- blood tests to determine renal function (see Ch. 24)
- blood lipid status and blood pressure measurement (see Ch. 19).

Early detection of complications is vital to enable treatment to commence; this may prevent complications worsening or reduce the severity of them. Further information is available about specific diabetes complications in the relevant section.

Once the discussion about complications has occurred, negotiations about the individual targets for blood glucose control (glycaemic control) can occur. The 'textbook' targets are to have capillary blood glucose levels of 4–7 mmol/L before main meals, 10 mmol/L or lower 2 hours after meals, and 5–8 mmol/L at bedtime.

Longer-term glycaemic control can be assessed by measuring the percentage of glycosylated (glycated) haemoglobin ((HbA_1, HbA_{1c}). This is the fraction of haemoglobin that binds glucose. The assay provides a measure of average blood glucose levels, and hence the degree of glycaemic control, over about 8 weeks. Most centres nowadays use 'DCCT aligned results' – HbA_{1c}; this enables results measured in different laboratories to be compared where necessary.

The target HbA_{1c} for people with type 1 diabetes is 7% or lower. Recent guidance on type 2 diabetes from the National Institute for Clinical Excellence (NICE 2002) advises that 'For each individual, a target HbA_{1c} (DCCT aligned) should be set between 6.5% and 7.5%, based on the risk of macrovascular and microvascular complications'.

Foot care

Newly diagnosed people with type 1 diabetes are unlikely to have any foot complications in the near future, if at all. However, it is wise to ensure they know how to look after their feet to reduce the likelihood of problems occurring in the future (see Health Promotion box 17.2).

Holidays and travel

Holidays require forward planning, particularly if they are abroad. Prior to the trip, the relevant vaccinations must be acquired and sufficient supplies of insulin and blood glucose testing equipment need to be acquired to last for the duration of the holiday as well as spares in case they get lost. Food for the journey also needs to be taken in case of hypoglycaemia ('hypos').

HEALTH PROMOTION

17.2 Foot care for people with diabetes

People with diabetes are encouraged to adopt the following foot care tasks:

- Wash feet regularly, preferably daily
- Dry carefully, patting dry rather than rubbing
- Apply moisturizer to dry skin, but avoid using it between the toes
- Check feet daily for abrasions or discoloration
- Do not use proprietary corn plasters or hard skin remover (they contain acids which can burn away healthy as well as hard skin)
- Avoid extremes of temperature
- Avoid walking barefoot out of doors
- Ensure footwear fits correctly
- If there is some sensory deprivation (numbness in the feet), check shoes for foreign objects by eye and feeling inside with the hand
- Use a state-registered podiatrist/chiropodist only and visit when necessary
- Cut toenails following the line of the toe, never into the corners.

If travelling by air, insulin and blood glucose testing strips must be packed in hand luggage; they will get frozen in the hold of the aircraft, which will destroy the insulin. A letter explaining the person has diabetes is necessary for customs; it can avoid lengthy explanations of why syringes are needed, for example. Identification when travelling abroad is crucial, as is adequate insurance cover in case of serious illness. It is wise to take a supply of over-the-counter medicines, such as travel sickness pills and oral rehydration salts in case of diarrhoea and vomiting.

Long flights involve lengthened or shortened days, which can cause havoc with usual insulin regimens. Specific advice from the diabetes specialist nursing team is required in this instance. Diabetes UK also provides extremely useful information about holidays and travel; the diabetes specialist nursing team should have information about how this may be acquired.

Ongoing diabetes education

Ongoing diabetes education should occur throughout the life of people with diabetes and should occur in a planned fashion during outpatient visits and also opportunistically. Any individual admitted to hospital at any time, for example, should have his or her diabetes learning needs assessed. Many will have had their diabetes for a long time and may assume, along with the health care professionals caring for them, they know all that is necessary. However, needs can change, e.g. in relation to insulin delivery as eyesight deteriorates with age, and people's knowledge may become out of date fairly quickly. Some information may have been forgotten and need to be given again, or people may be unaware of new recommendations for diabetes care as a result of research. An example of the latter is the change in targets for glycaemic control.

TYPE 2 DIABETES MELLITUS

Type 2 diabetes was previously known as maturity-onset diabetes or non-insulin-dependent diabetes mellitus (NIDDM).

Aetiology and epidemiology

The underlying causes of type 2 diabetes are less well understood than those of type 1 diabetes. However, there are undoubtedly environmental factors involved as the incidence rises dramatically in those who are obese. Those who have gained 10 kg in weight in adulthood are three times more likely to have diabetes than those who have not, for example. Other risk factors include a family history of type 2 diabetes, ethnic origin, a sedentary lifestyle, previous gestational diabetes and increasing age.

It is known that the body's sensitivity to insulin decreases with weight increase; approximately 80% of people with type 2 diabetes are overweight or obese. Truncal, or central, obesity is associated with a greater risk of type 2 diabetes. These people are often described as being 'apple-shaped', whereas people with a more peripheral spread of weight might be described as 'pear-shaped'. Central obesity, as well as increasing the risks of developing diabetes by as much as four times, is also more likely to increase the risks of developing cardiovascular disease.

Type 2 diabetes tends to 'run' in families. People with a strong family history are more likely to develop it themselves in later life, particularly if they have a first-degree relative with the condition (a parent or sibling). If both parents have type 2 diabetes, as many as three out of four children could develop the condition.

The genetic components of type 2 diabetes are not clear. However, as well as a strong association with family history, type 2 diabetes is also more prevalent in some ethnic groups. For example, people of south Asian or African Caribbean descent living in the UK have an increased prevalence of type 2 diabetes (Williams & Pickup 1999). In the Asian population, the incidence of diabetes is increased sixfold compared with Caucasian populations and in the African Caribbean population it is increased threefold. The prevalence of diabetes is also increased in people of Chinese descent and other non-white groups.

It is known that low activity levels increase the risk of developing type 2 diabetes, particularly in those who are overweight or obese. Exercise and activity increase the body's sensitivity to insulin and can help to prevent obesity.

Gestational diabetes is that which occurs in pregnancy and resolves following the birth of the baby. Unfortunately, approximately 50% of these women will develop type 2 diabetes in later life.

The prevalence of type 2 diabetes increases steeply with age; approximately 5–20% of people over the age of 65 years have diabetes, although as many as half of these may be undiagnosed. Most people with type 2 diabetes are diagnosed after the age of 40, although the number of children and young adults with type 2 diabetes is rapidly increasing; this is probably because the number of children and young adults with sedentary lifestyles and who are overweight or obese is also increasing in Westernized societies.

Overall, type 2 diabetes accounts for approximately 85–90% of all cases. In the UK, it is estimated that 1.3 million people have diabetes, most of which is type 2. It has also been estimated that there are about 1 million people who have as yet undiagnosed type 2 diabetes.

Partly because of the increasing prevalence of obesity and physical inactivity, it is projected that a diabetes epidemic is occurring. The World Health Organization predicts that by 2025 the world population of people with diabetes will be double that which it was in 1997. Although most of this rise will occur in developing countries there will be some increase in first world societies. In the UK, the population is ageing; this, as well as increasing rates of obesity, means that the number of people with type 2 diabetes is projected to rise dramatically.

Pathophysiology

The two main pathophysiological defects in type 2 diabetes are impaired insulin secretion and insulin resistance. In type 2 diabetes there is a failure of the β cells to produce insulin appropriately in response to glucose from meals – the first phase response. Although some insulin is secreted, there are inadequate amounts and the secretion is delayed. This means that blood glucose levels rise above normal and stay raised after eating. In type 2 diabetes of long duration there is also a reduced second-phase insulin secretion, meaning that blood glucose levels in the fasting state will also be raised.

As well as insulin secretion defects, the problem of insulin resistance occurs in type 2 diabetes. This occurs when the body does not respond to available insulin effectively. It has been noted that in obese people the number of insulin receptors on cell surfaces is reduced. The pancreas responds by producing more insulin to activate the available receptors more frequently, thereby allowing glucose to cross the cell membrane. Hyperinsulinaemia (high level of insulin in the blood) is often, therefore, a feature of obesity. However, not all obese people have diabetes. It is suggested that people with type 2 diabetes may also have a post-receptor defect within the cells themselves. Insulin has a role to play in the intracellular metabolism of glucose and it is mooted that there are as yet unclear defects in this intracellular function.

It is also not certain whether insulin resistance precedes a deficiency in insulin secretion although this is probable. The likely scenario is as follows. In those who are insulin-resistant, insulin secretion is increased in an effort to normalize blood glucose levels. Hyperinsulinaemia ensues. Eventually, in some individuals, the β cells in the islets of Langerhans are unable to produce sufficient insulin to control blood glucose levels and hyperglycaemia is the result. The diagnosis of type 2 diabetes occurs after this point.

Clinical presentation

The symptoms of type 2 diabetes are the same as in type 1 diabetes, although the onset is slow in comparison. However, people with type 2 diabetes are resistant to ketosis because they have sufficient insulin secretion to avoid unrestrained breakdown of fat (lipolysis). Weight loss can be a feature of type 2 diabetes but it is not extreme, and indeed may go unnoticed by the individual.

Most people with newly diagnosed type 2 diabetes are overweight. They may be aware of symptoms of hyperglycaemia (lethargy, polyuria and polydipsia) but many deny these or have attributed them in the past to increasing age. For example, men may expect nocturia 'at my time of life'. Unfortunately primary care staff may also miss the symptoms and many people with type 2 diabetes are identified via opportunistic screening.

Because prevailing blood glucose levels are frequently high for long periods of time, people with type 2 diabetes may be diagnosed with existing long-term complications of diabetes; i is thought that this occurs in at least 25% of cases.

Very occasionally people with newly diagnosed type 2 diabetes may present with hyperosmolar non-ketotic hyperglycaemia (HONKH). This condition is similar to diabetic ketoacidosis, but without significant amounts of ketones present. Blood glucose levels are extremely high (usually > 50 mmol/L), the patient is severely dehydrated and the risk of death is high, at approximately 30% (see the section on 'Diabetic ketoacidosis', pp. 422–424).

Specific investigations

A diagnosis of type 2 diabetes can be made based on symptoms and a random venous plasma glucose level of greater than 11.1 mmol/L in those who are more than 40 years of age and are overweight. However, in the absence of symptoms, the diagnosis must be made based on the results of two fasting plasma glucose levels on two different days; results of 7.0 mmol/L or above are diagnostic. If, however, the results of this are uncertain, i.e. a fasting plasma glucose below 5.5 mmol/L and a random result between 5.5 and 11.1 mmol/L, a glucose tolerance test should be performed (see p. 402).

For a glucose tolerance test, the individual should be tested in the morning after 3 days of an unrestricted diet and usual physical activity.

Medical management

Many people with type 2 diabetes are managed in primary care by their GP and practice nurse. Type 2 diabetes may be treated with:

- diet alone (see p. 419)
- diet and oral hypoglycaemic agents (OHAs, see below)
- diet and insulin (see pp. 411–413)
- a combination of all three regimens, although this is not very common.

Most GPs and practice nurses are confident in managing type 2 diabetes when it is treated with diet, or diet plus oral therapy, but tend to refer those requiring insulin treatment to secondary care services. As political initiatives are changing the ways in which chronic illness care is managed, however, many more people with type 2 diabetes requiring insulin therapy will have all their needs met by primary health care professionals in the future.

As well as having a role to play in the management of glycaemic control, the medical management of type 2 diabetes involves regular review to ensure the early diagnosis and treatment of diabetic complications should these occur.

Oral therapy for diabetes

As many as 50% of people with type 2 diabetes need to take oral therapy to help control their blood glucose levels. Oral hypoglycaemic agents (OHAs) can be used to treat type 2 diabetes, although they should not be initiated until 3 months 'trial of diet' has occurred. Nurses should be familiar with the different types of OHAs and their action, side-effects and contraindications, etc.

An overview of examples, action and some side-effects is provided but readers are advised to consult their latest national formulary, e.g. BNF, for full details of doses, side-effects and contraindications. There are several types of OHA that are used in different circumstances and these are discussed below.

Sulphonylureas

Sulphonylureas, e.g. glibenclamide, gliclazide (see Table 17.3), are the most common type of OHA currently in use. These drugs were initially produced during the 1950s. It was noted that sulphonamides, used to treat tuberculosis, tended to cause hypoglycaemia, and the sulphonylureas were developed from these. They work by stimulating the pancreas to produce insulin and consequently must be used for those with residual β cell function. Sulphonylureas reduce fasting blood glucose levels but cannot target postprandial (after meals) blood glucose rises. They cause hyperinsulinaemia, which unfortunately leads to weight gain. Sulphonylureas should not be used in the presence of ketoacidosis.

The side-effects of the sulphonylureas are uncommon and usually mild. They include:

- transient hypersensitivity reactions, which manifest as allergic skin reactions and usually resolve approximately 6–8 weeks after initiation of therapy
- gastrointestinal disturbances such as nausea, vomiting, diarrhoea and constipation
- rarely, blood disorders such as leucopenia or thrombocytopenia, among others, and liver function disturbances can occur.

Chlorpropamide has more side-effects than most of the other sulphonylureas, and for this reason is generally no longer used. It has an extremely long duration of action and can cause severe and prolonged hypoglycaemia. It can also cause facial

Table 17.3 Sulphonylureas

Generic name	Length of action	Timing of dose	Comments
Chlorpropamide	24–72 h	Daily before breakfast	Not generally used due to long duration and risk of hypos
Glibenclamide	18–24 h	Daily before breakfast (occasionally dose divided and given b.d.)	Care needs to be taken in older people because of the long duration and risk of hypos
Gliclazide	10–15 h	Up to 160 mg as a single dose; higher doses divided and taken before breakfast and evening meal	Very commonly used
Glimepiride	24 h (half-life 5–8 h)	Taken before breakfast	4 mg is usually the maximum dose
Glipizide	16–24 h	Up to 15 mg may be given before breakfast; higher doses divided	
Gliquidone		Before breakfast; maximum single dose 60 mg; maximum daily dose 180 mg in two or three divided doses	Rarely used
Tolbutamide	6–12 h	Before breakfast or in two or three divided doses. Maximum dose 2 g	Can be useful for older people as the duration of action is so short, but they may also have difficulties remembering to take it!

flushing following consumption of alcohol. Glibenclamide can also cause severe and prolonged hypoglycaemia because of its length of action and should be avoided in older people. Its use is declining.

People with diabetes should be informed that sulphonylureas work best if they are taken approximately half an hour before they eat, rather than with food. Larger doses should be divided equally and taken before breakfast and the evening meal if the dose is prescribed twice daily (b.d.), and before breakfast, the midday meal and evening meal if prescribed three times a day (t.d.s.).

Biguanides

Metformin is the only biguanide available in the UK. The biguanides work by decreasing gluconeogenesis, by increasing the peripheral uptake of glucose and, possibly, by reducing some carbohydrate absorption from the gut. As with the sulphonylureas, it is only effective if there is some residual β-cell function and so is only used for individuals with type 2 diabetes. Because metformin does not increase pancreatic insulin secretion, it does not cause hypoglycaemia. It is not associated with weight gain and consequently is the therapy of choice for people with type 2 diabetes who are overweight. Metformin should be withdrawn prior to surgery, in which case insulin therapy should be instigated.

However, metformin can have unpleasant gastrointestinal side-effects. Nausea, vomiting and diarrhoea are all common, as well as a metallic taste in the mouth. The diarrhoea can be particularly distressing and some people are unable to tolerate even a small dose. The side-effects may persist and metformin therapy cannot be used in this instance. Vitamin B_{12} absorption can also be affected. Metformin can have an anorexic effect. Lactic acidosis is a very rare side-effect of metformin treatment; it is not seen in practice very often as its use is avoided in high-risk individuals.

Metformin must be taken with food in order to reduce the incidence of side-effects. It can be taken with the first mouthful of food, or in the middle of the meal.

Alpha glucosidase inhibitors

Alpha glucosidase inhibitors became available in the 1990s. Acarbose is the only example currently available in the UK. It works by delaying the digestion and absorption of sucrose and starches in the gut, thus reducing blood glucose levels. Unlike the sulphonylureas, it has a postprandial effect. Acarbose can be used alone, with metformin or with one of the sulphonylureas.

Unfortunately the marked gastrointestinal side-effects have limited its use. The more common side-effects of acarbose are flatulence, which can be extreme, soft stools, diarrhoea, abdominal distension and pain. Rare side-effects are abnormal liver function tests and skin reactions.

Acarbose should be swallowed whole with liquid immediately before meals, or chewed with the first mouthful of food. Dose increments should be gradual to reduce the risk of side-effects.

Thiazolidinediones

Thiazolidinediones, e.g. rosiglitazone and pioglitazone, are a new type of oral therapy for diabetes developed in the 1990s. They work by reducing insulin resistance in the adipose tissue, the skeletal muscle and the liver. Glucose uptake is consequently improved. They are sometimes called insulin sensitizers. The thiazolidinediones (or 'glitazones') are currently only licensed for use in conjunction with either a sulphonylurea or metformin and should be initiated in those people with type 2 diabetes who have not achieved glycaemic control despite maximal doses of oral monotherapy.

The thiazolidinediones can cause gastrointestinal disturbances, weight gain (although this is not usually as much as that gained with sulphonylurea use), oedema, anaemia, fatigue, hypoglycaemia, headache, visual disturbances, dizziness, arthralgia, haematuria and erectile dysfunction. More uncommon side-effects are sweating, alopecia, dyspnoea, altered blood lipids and proteinuria. Each of the two thiazolidinediones currently available has slightly different side-effect profiles. Hepatic toxicity is rare but liver function tests must be performed before initiation and at 2-monthly intervals for the first year, and thereafter annually. They must not be prescribed if hepatic impairment is present or a history of heart failure, or in combination with insulin due to the risk of heart failure.

Meglitinides (non-sulphonylurea prandial glucose regulators)

The only meglitinide currently available is repaglinide. This is a new class of oral agent developed in the 1990s. Repaglinide works in a similar way to the sulphonylureas by stimulating insulin secretion from the β cells in the islets of Langerhans, but it has a rapid onset of action, a short duration of action and also a postprandial effect, minimizing postprandial glucose rises. Consequently, it is taken with meals – usually immediately before a meal, but can be taken up to 30 minutes before. If the meal is omitted, so is the drug. It may also be used in conjunction with metformin. Repaglinide should not be given in diabetic ketoacidosis.

The side-effects associated with repaglinide include abdominal pain, diarrhoea, constipation, nausea, vomiting, hypersensitivity reactions, including rashes and urticaria, and elevated liver enzymes.

Amino acid derivatives (non-sulphonylurea prandial glucose regulators)

Nateglinide is the only available amino acid derivative. It, too, stimulates the secretion of insulin from the pancreas; early phase insulin release in response to a meal is restored and postprandial glucose spikes are reduced. There is no prolonged hyperinsulinaemia as with the sulphonylureas. It should ideally be taken 1 minute before meals but can be taken up to 30 minutes before eating. Nateglinide should not be used in type 1 diabetes or diabetic ketoacidosis.

The side-effects of nateglinide include hypoglycaemia and, rarely, hypersensitivity reactions such as rashes, raised liver enzymes, gastrointestinal complaints, headache and respiratory infections.

▶ Nursing management

As in type 1 diabetes, the primary nursing role is to enable people with diabetes to manage their own condition wherever possible (see Reflective Practice box 17.1). The main nursing functions, therefore, are to provide education and psychological support to people with type 2 diabetes (see Guidelines for Care Priorities box 17.1 and Evidence-based Practice box 17.1).

Many people with newly diagnosed type 2 diabetes are shocked at the news of the diagnosis but others, who may have had a suspicion they have the condition because of past experiences with other family members, may be less surprised. Similarly, the range of education needs is likely to be wide.

The most important educational need for people with type 2 diabetes is related to diet, given that most of them will be overweight at diagnosis. All people with newly diagnosed type 2 diabetes should be referred to a dietician for individual assessment and advice about their eating; this assessment should ideally occur within 4 weeks after diagnosis. Unfortunately, however, due to a shortage of dieticians in many areas, this sometimes does not occur. It is the nurse's responsibility in this instance to provide the individual with information about healthy eating with diabetes. It is also the role of nurses, working in all contexts, to reiterate information about healthy eating when necessary. However, it must be remembered that 'nagging' is not an effective means of education (see Ch. 1).

As well as educating people with diabetes about healthy eating, they need information about their other treatments for diabetes such as oral hypoglycaemic agents (see above). This education should occur at the time the therapy is commenced and should be updated at periodic intervals.

Dietary management of diabetes

Dietary management of diabetes is the 'cornerstone of treatment'; both oral hypoglycaemic therapy and insulin treatment supplement effective healthy eating on the part of the individual with diabetes. The goals of dietary management of diabetes are to maintain health and quality of life for as long as possible, and avoid the vascular complications of diabetes (Ha & Lean 1998).

Before the early 1990s, people with diabetes were taught to count carbohydrates, usually in 10 g 'exchanges' or 'portions'. Some people who have had diabetes for many years still tend to use the system of dietary management they were originally taught and carefully organize their meals around the amount of carbohydrate they need.

However, nowadays, newly diagnosed people with diabetes are taught the principles of healthy eating (see Health Promotion box 17.3 and Ch. 11). Some individuals may need to make radical changes to achieve a healthy eating pattern. It is best not to try and change everything immediately as this task is too difficult for most people. Small incremental changes in eating patterns, which become permanently integrated into the lifestyle, are more likely to be successful in the long term. It is worth pointing out, however, that the principles of healthy eating apply to the whole family; this may help to remove the stigma of a 'special diet', and it is so much easier if everyone in the household is having similar food. Furthermore, there are health benefits for everybody.

 HEALTH PROMOTION

17.3 The principles of healthy eating

The principles of healthy eating are the same for all of us. However, for people with diabetes, healthy eating is the 'cornerstone' of their treatment.

- Eating regularly is important for glucose control. This does not mean that meals have to be eaten at exactly the same time each day, but that it is important to have breakfast, lunch and dinner every day.
- High carbohydrate (40–60%) – starchy foods, such as bread, potatoes, pasta, rice, chapattis, etc., should be taken at every meal. Carbohydrates fill people up, reducing hunger, and also have only 3.75–4.2 kcal/g compared with fats with 9 kcal/g. Carbohydrate is the best source of energy for the body.
- High fibre slows the absorption of carbohydrates from the gut and reduces the risks of intestinal problems, including constipation.
- Low fat (30%), particularly low in saturated fats – reducing the intake of fats helps those who are overweight to lose it. Crash diets are not recommended; instead a slow steady weight loss, if necessary, is healthier. Even if the target weight is not achieved, any reduction in weight is beneficial to health. A diet that contains high amounts of saturated, or animal, fats is linked to an increased risk of heart disease. Examples of foods that contain saturated fats include butter, cheese, milk and fatty meats.

- Monounsaturated fats such as olive oil or rapeseed oil are better alternatives as they can reduce the risks of heart disease. Cooking methods can also have an impact on fat intake. People should be advised to grill or steam their food, for example, rather than frying or roasting it.
- Five portions a day of fruit and vegetables – as for us all, the recommendation is that people with diabetes eat five helpings a day of fruit and vegetables. This helps maintain an adequate intake of vitamins and minerals and aids in intestinal health. One portion is a serving of vegetables, or one average size piece of fruit.
- Avoiding sugary drinks – contrary to popular belief, people with diabetes are not prohibited from taking sugar in their diet. However, adding sugar to hot drinks or drinking 'regular' soft drinks such as cola or lemonade is not advisable as blood glucose levels can rise rapidly. Low-calorie fruit squashes or 'diet' carbonated drinks are alternatives.
- Less salt – although only about 20% of total salt intake is accounted for by adding it in cooking or at the table, reducing this amount can help with lowering blood pressure. Cooking fresh foods, rather than relying on processed or convenience foods can also aid in salt reduction.
- Alcohol as for the rest of the population (maximum of 21 units per week for men and 14 for women). It is best not to 'save up' the units for a weekend, but to even out consumption during the week.

Oral medication – the nursing role

People with diabetes often do not take their tablet therapy correctly. A common reason for this is lack of knowledge about how the tablets work, when they should be taken in relation to meals and what the potential side-effects are. The obvious implications of this lack of knowledge are uncontrolled blood glucose levels and the potential worsening of side-effects.

The nurse's role is to ensure that people with type 2 diabetes using oral therapy have an adequate knowledge to take their tablets in the correct amounts and at the correct times and to be aware of the possible side-effects and consequences of incorrect administration of oral therapy. All possible opportunities to assess knowledge should be taken. For example, nurses should include this aspect in their assessments of patients' needs on admission to hospital. Browne et al (2000) also suggest that practice nurses assess knowledge base during a patient's annual diabetes review, usually undertaken in primary care for people with type 2 diabetes. They also recommend that people with diabetes be provided with both oral and written information about their diabetes tablets (see Health Promotion box 17.4).

Another issue that is pertinent for nurses working in hospitals is that of ensuring that in-patients receive their tablets at the correct time. If it is not possible to ensure that patients receive their therapy appropriately, it may be worthwhile considering self-administration of medication, particularly if patients' knowledge base is good and they have been doing this in the community.

Monitoring diabetes

Like individuals with type 1 diabetes, those with type 2 diabetes also need to engage in self-monitoring of their glucose control.

They may choose to perform capillary blood glucose monitoring (discussed on pages 409–410), particularly if their diabetes is not controlled on maximum oral agents. Blood glucose monitoring provides 'here and now' results, i.e. the result obtained gives information about the blood glucose level at a particular point in time. However, not everyone feels the need for such specific information and may feel that urinalysis for glucose is adequate.

Glucose in urine is measured by dipping a test strip into a fresh sample of urine, shaking any excess urine off the strip and, after waiting the requisite time, comparing the colour on the test pad to the colours on the side of the test strip container, and then recording the result. Results range from 0.1 to 5% depending on the brand of test strips used. The desirable result is a negative glucose reading. The renal threshold (see p. 404 and Ch. 24) for glucose is approximately 10 mmol/L (this rises with age), so a negative result means that there has been a blood glucose level of less than 10 mmol/L since the individual last passed urine. However, urinalysis cannot detect hypoglycaemia or the blood glucose level at a given point in time. In addition, a negative urinalysis result for glucose means that the blood glucose could be low, normal or even higher than normal. For these reasons, urine glucose testing is not recommended for use by individuals who are actively trying to improve their blood glucose control.

Where blood glucose monitoring is performed, the nurse should educate the person with diabetes in the way described in the section on type 1 diabetes (pp. 409–410 and also HbA_{1c} on p. 415). However, well controlled individuals (blood glucose levels 4–7 mmol/L before meals and at bedtime) may do fewer tests, perhaps only two a week and occasional 'extras'.

 HEALTH PROMOTION

17.4 Example of an information sheet for sulphonylureas

The following is patient information about taking one of the oral hypoglycaemic agents. It is designed to be completed by the nurse and then given to the person with diabetes for use when at home. How else might you use this information sheet? (For example, it could serve as an assessment of patients' knowledge about their OHAs; the nurse could pose the questions asked in the handout.)

Sulphonylureas
The name of the sulphonylurea is:

How does it work?
All the sulphonylureas work by stimulating, or 'telling', the pancreas to produce more insulin.

What are the side-effects?
If your dose is too high, you can have a hypo (low blood sugar). Other side-effects are usually mild and do not often

happen. They include rashes, which usually go away after 6 weeks, an upset digestive system and headaches.

When should I take it?
Sulphonylureas should be taken about half an hour before food.

My dose is:
… tablet(s) … times a day before: breakfast ☐, midday meal ☐, evening meal ☐.

Student activities
Prepare similar patient information material for the other oral hypoglycaemic agents. Use the information provided in the text as your source material.

Points to remember:
● Avoid the use of jargon
● Keep sentences short – less than 10 words, if possible
● Do not use words of more than two syllables where possible – more syllables are acceptable if they are suffixes such as 'ing', 'ation' or 'itis'.

ACUTE COMPLICATIONS OF DIABETES

HYPOGLYCAEMIA

Hypoglycaemia (a low blood glucose level) occurs in people with diabetes treated with insulin or sulphonylureas. It is not, however, a feature of type 2 diabetes treated with diet alone.

Aetiology and epidemiology

Hypoglycaemia, or 'hypos', are due to a relative excess of insulin circulating in the bloodstream. In people without diabetes, or those with diabetes not treated with insulin or sulphonylureas, insulin production in the pancreas is reduced as blood glucose levels drop.

Hypoglycaemia, therefore, is a result of the treatment of diabetes. People with type 1 diabetes who have 'tight' glycaemic control are more likely to have a threefold increase in the number of severe hypoglycaemic episodes than their less well controlled counterparts (Diabetes Control and Complications Trial [DCCT] Study Group 1993). Approximately 25–30% of people treated with insulin experience at least one episode requiring assistance from another person every year. People with type 2 diabetes well controlled on sulphonylureas may also experience hypoglycaemia needing assistance from others.

The underlying causes of hypoglycaemia are usually:

- unexpected activity, e.g. spring cleaning or gardening
- missed or delayed meals
- excessive alcohol intake
- excess insulin
- long duration of diabetes.

Pathophysiology

Symptoms of hypoglycaemia can be classified in several ways. The most helpful way to categorize them for people with diabetes is to label symptoms as mild, moderate or severe (see Box 17.3). Mild hypos are defined as those which individuals are able to identify and treat themselves. Moderate hypos occur when individuals have not lost consciousness, but require assistance from another, and severe hypos are classed as those in which unconsciousness occurs.

Most of the mild symptoms are caused by a release of adrenaline (epinephrine) and noradrenaline (norepinephrine) following activation of the autonomic nervous system. These two hormones act on the liver and stimulate the conversion of stored glycogen back into glucose (glycogenolysis) to raise the blood glucose level.

Most of the moderate symptoms are caused by neuroglycopenia, wherein the brain is deprived of sufficient glucose. The neuroglycopenic symptoms occur when there is insufficient glucose in the brain for neurons to connect properly. Glucose is the fuel the brain utilizes for energy; once there is a deficit, brain function is compromised. Some of these symptoms are non-specific, in as much as there is no known cause, e.g. headache.

The autonomic symptoms (sometimes referred to as the adrenergic symptoms) serve as an 'early warning' system. They occur when the brain first recognizes that the blood glucose level is dropping below normal and before there is insufficient glucose

> **Box 17.3 Signs and symptoms of mild, moderate and severe hypoglycaemia**
>
> *Mild hypoglycaemia*
> - Sweating
> - Tremor
> - Pallor
> - Tachycardia/palpitations
> - Hunger
> - Tingling in tongue or fingertips
> - Anxiety
> - Double or blurred vision
> - Headache
>
> *Moderate hypoglycaemia*
> - Unsteady gait
> - Slurred speech
> - Confusion
> - Unusual behaviour
> - Drowsiness
> - Incoordination
>
> *Severe hypoglycaemia*
> - Seizures
> - Unconsciousness

available for proper brain function. Unfortunately a long duration of diabetes can mean that some individuals lose this early warning mechanism. In this instance, blood glucose monitoring is vital.

Clinical presentation

Those having a mild hypoglycaemic episode most commonly appear pale and sweaty and may have a fine tremor. There is commonly a 'glassy-eyed' appearance too. Each individual is likely to experience the same symptoms with each episode of hypoglycaemia, although these may change over a period of years.

Individuals experiencing a moderate hypo may appear as if they are drunk. They often have slurred speech, an uncoordinated gait and may be verbally and physically aggressive. Those experiencing a severe hypo will be unconscious and may be having a seizure.

Specific investigations

People experiencing mild hypos may wish to confirm this by performing a capillary blood glucose measurement, although it may be difficult to perform well if tremor is experienced.

If there is any doubt of hypoglycaemia being the cause of strange behaviour in an individual having a moderately severe hypo, a capillary blood glucose test must be performed. However, this can be difficult if the individual does not believe this is the case and in this instance treatment should be instigated anyway; that a hypoglycaemic episode has occurred is confirmed by the individual's recovery.

Hypoglycaemia resulting in unconsciousness must be confirmed with a venous blood glucose sample wherever possible. Capillary blood glucose measurement systems (near patient testing) have a greater range of inaccuracy at hypoglycaemic levels.

Medical management

Mild hypos should initially be treated with 10 g of oral glucose. This may be given in the form of glucose tablets, e.g. Dextrosol or Lucozade, powder or liquids, e.g. Lucozade (see Box 17.4). Individuals should begin to recover within 10 minutes. If they do not feel better, the 10 g dose should be repeated. If glucose is not available, anything containing sucrose may be used as an alternative. Sugar should not be put in hot drinks; it takes too long to cool the drink for safe consumption. Orange juice is a palatable alternative. Chocolate may be used, but it must be noted that using any foodstuffs containing fat to treat hypoglycaemia is likely to result in a delayed response; the fat delays the absorption of glucose from the digestive tract.

If the hypo occurs before a meal, the meal should then be eaten to provide 'longer-acting' carbohydrates to prevent the blood glucose level falling again. If, however, the episode occurs between meals, a snack containing starchy carbohydrate should be taken for this purpose. Examples include biscuits or a sandwich.

Moderately severe hypos may be treated in the same way if the individual is able to swallow. Some individuals carry Hypostop with them to use in such situations. This is a clear gel, which contains glucose; it is packaged in a tube which is easily transportable and opened. However, it is very sweet and some individuals find it induces nausea.

Oral glucose of any kind must not be given to people with severe hypoglycaemia until they have regained consciousness. Glucagon may be given. It must be given by injection; this could be subcutaneous, intramuscular or even intravenous although it is not frequently given in this way. Non-professional carers of people with diabetes usually give it via the subcutaneous route, but health care professionals should give it intramuscularly if possible as it will work more quickly. Glucagon takes approximately 10 minutes to work.

Individuals must always be given a meal following glucagon administration as the hormone stimulates the release of all the glycogen stored in the liver. Consequently, there is no glycogen left should the individual experience another hypo. Feeding replaces the store of glycogen. Glucagon can also induce nausea. For this reason, it is frequently only given in a 0.5 unit dose rather than the full 1 unit dose, especially for children.

Severe hypoglycaemia may also be treated with intravenous glucose; 50 mL of 50% dextrose may be given by a physician. However, this can damage veins and should be given slowly. The advantage is that it is virtually instantaneous in its effect.

▶ Nursing management

Although the treatment of hypoglycaemia is described above as medical management, it is in reality usually the individual with diabetes or a relative or friend who treats it. Nurses, too, tend to see more hypoglycaemic episodes than doctors.

Once the hypo has been treated and the individual has recovered, it is important to try and elicit why it occurred. For instance, it may be that the person has done more gardening than had been anticipated. Discovering the cause and discussing it can serve as a useful opportunity for education; the individual may be able to work out ways of preventing hypos in future similar circumstances. For the gardening example, it would be

> ### Box 17.4 Foods/fluids containing 10 g carbohydrate
> **Solids**
> - 3 Dextrosol or Lucozade tablets
> - 2 teaspoons table sugar
> - 1 digestive biscuit
>
> **Liquids**
> - 50 mL Lucozade
> - 100 mL milk

advisable to take a break every couple of hours to have a snack, for instance. It is helpful to allow people to work out their own solutions to problems rather than giving them the 'answers'.

If the hypo was self-treated, it may be useful to review how it was treated. Many people with diabetes do not know that foods containing fat delay the absorption of glucose. Hypos can be seen as an opportunity to eat foods that would not normally be eaten, chocolate being a popular choice. However, if people with diabetes have been treating their hypos successfully in this way for years they may decide to continue their practice. As long as their choices are made following access to all the relevant information, they must be allowed to decide what will be best for them as individuals.

Hypoglycaemia is an unpleasant experience, which is feared by many people with diabetes (Jerreat 1999). Some even purposefully manage their diabetes to avoid hypos altogether with the consequent risks of high blood glucose levels. The fear may be related to potentially being embarrassed in public, a fear of dying during a hypo or an intense dislike of feeling out of control.

Once the specific reasons for fear of hypos have been identified, the nurse needs to decide whether further education is appropriate. For instance, some people with diabetes may assume that having a severe hypo will lead to death if they are not found. They are often unaware of the 'back-up' systems of the body – glycogenolysis and gluconeogenesis – which in most instances correct the hypoglycaemia within a few hours. Giving this information in an appropriate way may resolve this fear for individuals. However, many fears are not amenable to more information. In this instance, the nurse must listen carefully and sensitively, acknowledging the difficulties of living with diabetes and hypos.

DIABETIC KETOACIDOSIS

Diabetic ketoacidosis (DKA) is an uncommon acute complication of diabetes, usually involving people with type 1 diabetes. It occasionally affects people with type 2 diabetes at times of acute physiological stress, during serious intercurrent illnesses such as myocardial infarction or cerebrovascular events.

Aetiology and epidemiology

Diabetic ketoacidosis is caused by an absolute or relative insulin deficiency. It may arise at diagnosis of type 1 diabetes, although this is becoming less common as early diagnosis rates are improving. For those with established diabetes, an episode of intercurrent infection or another acute illness such as a myocardial infarction is frequently the cause of DKA. It can also occur as a result of missed insulin or mismanaged diabetes, either by people with diabetes themselves or by health professionals. Occasionally there is no obvious cause.

DKA is the main cause of diabetes-related deaths in children and young people. Overall mortality rates are between 0.65 and 3.3%, and rise in older people.

Pathophysiology

Because of the role of insulin in the metabolism of carbohydrates, proteins and fats, there are biochemical disturbances consequent to the total or relative insulin lack observed in DKA. In the absence of insulin, carbohydrates cannot be metabolized and glycogen stores in the liver are converted back into glucose. Gluconeogenesis is also increased. Proteins are broken down into amino acids and, following hepatic gluconeogenesis, add to the hyperglycaemia. Fats are mobilized to provide energy. Lipolysis (the breakdown of fats) occurs in an unrestrained way and ketone bodies are generated as by-products of fat metabolism.

The result is hyperglycaemia, which can be extreme. This is followed by an osmotic diuresis as glucose is excreted in the urine in an attempt to correct blood glucose levels. Polyuria and glycosuria ensue. Despite polydipsia (excessive drinking) occurring in an attempt to rectify the dehydration, it is likely to become progressively more severe. As the dehydration worsens, so does the loss of the electrolytes sodium and potassium. Vomiting, if it occurs, is likely to aggravate the dehydration and electrolyte imbalance (see Ch. 8). Hypovolaemia caused by the dehydration can give rise to shock (see Ch. 9) and also reduced renal perfusion and glomerular filtration in the kidneys, which in turn increases the blood glucose level as glucose is not excreted in the usual amounts.

As ketones (3-hydroxybutyrate, acetoacetate and acetone) are weak acids, an excess amount causes metabolic acidosis. If death occurs due to DKA, it is likely to be due either to the metabolic dysfunction or cardiac arrhythmias subsequent to the potassium imbalance.

Clinical presentation

Individuals with DKA are likely to have extreme hyperglycaemia. Blood glucose levels will be higher than 13 mmol/L; they can often be very much higher than this and levels of 80 mmol/L, although uncommon, have been known. Individuals are also likely to have lost weight due to dehydration and the reduction of both fat and muscle. They are likely to look 'dry' and there will be signs of dehydration.

Kussmaul breathing is likely to occur. This is deep, rapid and laboured and is caused by acidosis. Ketones can be excreted by the lungs and the breath will smell of them. The smell is said to resemble nail-varnish remover, pear drop sweets or even newly mown hay, but unfortunately not all health care professionals can smell ketones.

Patients will complain of extreme thirst and will have polyuria. The urine will be very dilute and strongly positive for both glucose and ketones when tested. In the very late stages of the development of DKA, urine output may be decreased due to the hypovolaemia (see Ch. 9). Individuals will have tachycardia and may be hypotensive as a result of dehydration.

Initially, individuals may be hypothermic, probably due to peripheral vasodilatation caused by the acidosis. However, once the biochemical abnormalities have been resolved, pyrexia may be evident several hours later, if the underlying cause is due to infection.

People with DKA may complain of muscle aches and pains or cramps, particularly in the legs. This may be due to dehydration and electrolyte imbalance or to loss of muscle bulk. They may also have visual problems, complaining of blurred vision. This is caused by osmotic changes in the lens of the eye. Individuals may also complain of abdominal pain; on occasion people have undergone surgical procedures for this. However, it must not be forgotten that an acute abdominal event can precipitate DKA.

Nausea and vomiting usually occur relatively late in the development of DKA, unless this has been precipitated by a concurrent illness involving these symptoms. In the extreme state, individuals may be unconscious, but this only occurs in 10% of cases. These individuals should be cared for in an intensive care unit (see Ch. 31).

Cerebral oedema (see Ch. 14) is a rare complication of DKA in adults and the pathophysiology is not well understood. It is more common in children and has a high mortality rate. Adult respiratory distress syndrome (ARDS, see Ch. 9) is also a complication of DKA, particularly in older people. Thromboembolism is another potential problem (see Ch. 19).

Specific investigations

Specific investigations include bedside tests for the blood glucose level and urinalysis for glucose, ketones and indications of infection. A midstream or catheter sample of urine should be sent for culture to explore the possibility of a urinary tract infection as the precipitating cause (see Ch. 24).

Venous blood samples for laboratory analysis of glucose, electrolytes, urea, creatinine, osmolality, a full blood count, cardiac enzymes and culture should be sent. Arterial blood pH and gas tension samples should be analysed.

An electrocardiograph (ECG) and a chest X-ray should be performed.

Medical management

The priority in managing DKA is to rectify the fluid and electrolyte losses (see Ch. 8) and to treat the insulin deficiency. Intravenous infusions to deliver normal saline initially, followed by 5% dextrose when the blood glucose level has fallen to 15 mmol/L, and continuous insulin are initiated. Potassium is added to the saline to replace the deficit after the first litre of fluid, following the return of blood results. Potassium levels are assessed regularly and the dose for each litre of intravenous fluid adjusted accordingly. Care needs to be taken with fluid replacement in older people and those with ischaemic cardiac disease, as they may develop fluid overload. Soluble insulin is infused, using a syringe-driver pump, at 5–10 units/hour depending on capillary blood glucose results, which are measured hourly. Once the patient is eating and drinking normally, and there is no ketonuria, the infusions may be discontinued 1 hour following the administration of a dose of subcutaneous insulin. Local protocols may differ slightly and these should always be checked.

If there are problems with renal perfusion and output, a urinary catheter will be inserted to monitor fluid output.

A nasogastric tube should be passed in any unconscious person or in those who are vomiting profusely or continuously.

The cause of the DKA is thoroughly investigated and treatment for any underlying pathology commenced.

▶ Nursing management

The first priority in nursing a person with DKA is usually physical care, although psychological needs may be met at the same time. The family will also need information and ongoing support.

The individual will need to be carefully observed, as follows:

- Measurements of blood pressure, pulse and respirations will be made, initially at half-hourly intervals and then reducing as the physical condition improves.
- Temperature must be measured hourly for the first few hours even if it is initially normal; pyrexia due to an underlying infection may not be evident until the fluid deprivation is rectified.
- All fluid intake and output must also be carefully measured and recorded.
- Capillary blood glucose levels should be recorded hourly while the insulin pump is running. As with all blood glucose readings, it is essential that these results are accurate, as insulin doses will be based on them. If blood glucose levels do not fall as expected, the insulin pump should be checked to ensure it is working correctly.
- The insertion site of the intravenous lines should be carefully observed for signs of extravasation and infection. Ideally, the two infusions should run through the same cannula, using a 'y' connector or octopus, and non-return valves.

Mouth care is vitally important for people with DKA. Because of the dehydration and increased respiratory rate, they are likely to have a very dry mouth. Mouthwashes and a toothbrush and paste should be made available, and if necessary the individual helped to use them.

The nurse may need to administer analgesia to relieve the general aches associated with DKA. These, however, tend to resolve fairly rapidly once treatment commences.

Positioning is important. Because of hyperventilation (caused by acidosis) most people feel more comfortable in an upright position, well supported with pillows. It is also important to encourage regular movement because of the increased risks of deep vein thrombosis (DVT) following dehydration and immobility, particularly in older people.

Many people with DKA are physically recovered within about 24 hours. However, as well as providing physical care, the nurse should give psychological support. Many people with already diagnosed type 1 diabetes are surprised and scared about how ill they can become over a very short space of time. Active listening and empathetic support can mitigate feelings of loss of control over the situation.

Nurses should also try to identify if the episode of DKA was caused by an error in insulin administration or not following 'sick day rules'. When the individual is ready, education to rectify any knowledge deficits in relation to problems identified will be required to try to ensure that similar situations do not recur.

LONG-TERM DIABETES COMPLICATIONS

In general the long-term, or chronic, complications of diabetes are categorized into micro- and macrovascular categories. Microvascular complications, as the name suggests, affect small blood vessels and nerves. Retinopathy (see Ch. 15), which affects the retina in the eye, nephropathy which affects renal function (see Ch. 24) and neuropathy – sensory, motor, or autonomic nerve damage – are included in this category. Macrovascular complications affect large blood vessels and include ischaemic heart disease, cerebrovascular events and peripheral vascular disease (see Chs 14 and 19).

Aetiology and epidemiology

It was not until 1993 that there was strong evidence that the cause of microvascular complications of diabetes was chronic hyperglycaemia. In the Diabetes Control and Complications Trial (DCCT Study Group 1993), a cohort of people with type 1 diabetes was studied. There were two distinct groups: one had strict glucose control over a 9-year period and the other had less strict control. The group with strict control showed a reduction in the incidence of clinically important retinopathy, nephropathy and neuropathy. The incidence of retinopathy, for example, was reduced by 76%, and in those who had early retinopathy on entering the trial, the average risk of progression was reduced by 54%.

The evidence to support the theory that chronic hyperglycaemia is also responsible for the aetiology of long-term complications in type 2 diabetes was provided by the United Kingdom Prospective Diabetes Study, the results of which were published in 1998. Intensive therapy in one group of people with type 2 diabetes was associated with a 25% reduction in microvascular complications.

However, the risks of developing macrovascular complications were not significantly reduced by strict glycaemic control in either the DCCT (1993) or the UKPDS (1998b). A separate study within the UKPDS (1998a) showed that good blood pressure control did reduce the risk of macrovascular complications. Other studies have demonstrated that lipid levels and smoking are both contributors to macrovascular disease.

Therefore the aetiology of diabetes complications is both hyperglycaemia and hypertension, in conjunction with dyslipidaemia (abnormal blood lipids) and lifestyle issues such as smoking habits, activity levels, eating habits and body mass index (BMI).

In the Western world, diabetic retinopathy is a leading cause of blindness in the working population. Approximately 2% of the population of people with diabetes in the UK become blind as a result of retinopathy, although this figure should reduce as screening and treatment improve. Unfortunately, the incidence and prevalence of diabetic retinopathy in the UK are not known; 80–100% of people with diabetes will develop some form of diabetic eye disease after 20 years' duration of their condition, but this may not be sight-threatening.

Approximately 30% of people with type 1 diabetes will have proteinuria after 20 years' duration of diabetes. Once this is persistent, renal function gradually deteriorates towards end-stage renal failure. In type 2 diabetes the prevalence differs according to ethnic origin. About 25% of those of European descent develop nephropathy and as many as 50% of those of Asian, African Caribbean or Japanese origin will develop it to some degree. However, not all individuals will reach end-stage renal failure. Neuropathy is the most common of the microvascular complications. However, because there are many manifestations of neuropathy, the prevalence is difficult to determine.

Diabetes-related macrovascular (large blood vessel) disease includes cerebrovascular events (CVEs) such as stroke (see Ch. 14), cardiovascular disease (CVD) and peripheral vascular disease (PVD) (see Ch. 19). Estimates of the prevalence of macrovascular complications vary between countries but people with type 2 diabetes, in particular, are nearly twice as likely to have a non-fatal myocardial infarction (MI) as those without diabetes and between two and three times more likely to have a fatal MI. The risks of stroke are increased two- to threefold. Estimates of the increased risk of amputation due to PVD range between five and 16 times that of the normal population, although neuropathy will be a contributing factor in many of these instances.

Overall, cardiovascular mortality is increased three- to fourfold, compared with those without diabetes. Cardiovascular disease is the commonest cause of death in those with type 2 diabetes.

Pathophysiology

The pathology of diabetes complications is not entirely clear; although research in this area has answered many questions, there are many more still unanswered. However, it is now clear that chronic hyperglycaemia damages a variety of tissues. This has been demonstrated by the landmark DCCT and UKPDS studies already referred to. It is also known that genetic susceptibilities are a factor. For example, some people with relatively poor glucose control do not develop many complications and others, with 'tight' control, develop them at an earlier stage and more severely.

Excess glucose seems to cause tissue damage through repeated episodes of acute changes in cellular metabolism. For example, sorbitol (sugar alcohol) is formed from glucose within cells. Sorbitol does not easily cross cell membranes and accumulates. It is thought that excess amounts in certain cells may cause damage. For instance, it may contribute to decreased nerve conduction because it impairs the normal transport of electrolytes across nerve cell membranes.

In other tissues, hyperglycaemia is thought to increase the synthesis of basement cell membranes and increase the permeability of capillaries (Williams & Pickup 1999). Proteins which have become glycated (i.e. they have glucose attached to them) can damage blood vessel walls, causing thickening. In small blood vessel disease (microangiopathy), there are also disturbances in capillary blood flow and pressure, blood viscosity and red cell aggregation.

Other factors, such as hypertension and hyperlipidaemia, also have a role to play in the development of macrovascular disease.

It is known that the pathogenesis of large blood vessel disease is identical to that in people without diabetes, but chronic hyperglycaemia increases the risk of these events occurring in those with diabetes, possibly because of increased platelet aggregation, or 'stickiness'. Macrovascular disease in people with diabetes is often more severe than in those without diabetes, and more

extensive. Hyperinsulinaemia and insulin resistance are thought to be possible factors in the increased incidence of cardiovascular disease. It has been shown, for instance, that insulin could possibly promote atherogenesis (formation of atheroma). However, the mechanisms for this process are unclear.

Clinical presentation

Retinopathy (see Ch. 15)

Background retinopathy does not usually cause symptoms, so individuals with this condition are unaware of it. It can only be detected by visualization of the retina using an ophthalmoscope. Background retinopathy is the term used to describe a variety of features, including microaneurysms (dots), haemorrhages (blots), hard exudates and small areas of retinal ischaemia (cotton wool spots). Preproliferative retinopathy occurs if the retinal ischaemia worsens. Proliferative retinopathy refers to the development of new blood vessels in the retina (neovascularization). These changes and the growth of fibrous tissue may lead to vitreous haemorrhages and detachment of the retina. Retinal oedema and thickening close to the macula can cause loss of central vision. Unless individuals with diabetes have an annual visual check, retinopathy may develop to the stage at which it becomes threatening to vision.

Nephropathy (see Ch. 24)

Early renal damage does not cause any symptoms. However, the detection of urinary microalbuminuria indicates that early nephropathy is occurring. As the disease progresses, proteinuria develops. This stage can last for many years, and in some cases the proteinuria is intermittent. However, once it becomes persistent, it is an indication that renal function will progressively decline towards end-stage renal failure; people with diabetes will experience the same signs and symptoms as those without.

Neuropathy

The commonest diabetic neuropathy is a sensorimotor neuropathy, which affects the lower limbs. It is usually symmetrical, diffuse and affects the feet and legs in a 'stocking' distribution. There are usually no symptoms. Pain sensation is lost, which can give rise to injuries which initially go unnoticed. For example, it has been known for an individual to present with a drawing pin in the sole of the foot. However, in later stages, people may feel numbness, tingling sensations, cold feet or burning. Occasionally, peripheral diabetic neuropathy can be extremely painful and some individuals develop hypersensitivity to touch. Hands may be affected although this is not common.

People with diabetic neuropathy may present with a neuropathic foot ulcer (see Chs 10 and 19). These are typically fairly small on the surface of the foot and have a 'punched-out' appearance. They are often very deep, however, and can also track sideways. If infection ensues, bony structures can be affected, resulting in osteomyelitis and subsequent amputation (see Ch. 27).

Mononeuropathies, those affecting a single nerve, are relatively uncommon and usually resolve over time. The femoral nerve can be affected, causing diabetic amyotrophy. The third and sixth cranial nerves can also be affected.

People with diabetes can also develop problems with nerve compression. Examples include carpal tunnel syndrome wherein the median nerve is involved, ulnar nerve compression and foot drop (see Ch. 27).

Autonomic neuropathy is a relatively common complication of diabetes, the incidence of which increases with duration of diabetes. Any organ served by the autonomic nerves may be affected. One of the more common problems is erectile dysfunction and it is estimated that 50% of men with diabetes experience this (Drucquer & McNally 1998) (see Ch. 25).

Gustatory sweating, which is induced by eating, can occur. Other sweating abnormalities are often evident, particularly in relation to the foot. In this instance, there is often reduced sweating which contributes to the development of hyperkeratosis (development of hard, dry skin or callus – see Ch. 28). This is prone to cracking, which can lead to the introduction of infection and consequent foot ulcers.

Gastrointestinal complications include gastroparesis (delayed gastric emptying, which can cause vomiting or regurgitation of food), constipation and diabetic diarrhoea. Diabetic diarrhoea can be very severe but is relatively uncommon. It tends to be intermittent, with episodes of normal bowel function or constipation in between bouts of diarrhoea. All these problems are caused by damage to the nerves that innervate the gut; motility is either slowed or increased depending on whether the sympathetic or parasympathetic nerve fibres are damaged.

Cardiovascular autonomic complications include postural hypotension; on standing, individuals may experience a range of symptoms from dizziness to loss of consciousness. Cardiac innervation may also be affected but this is usually symptomless. It may be detected by electrocardiograph changes during the Valsalva manoeuvre (see Ch. 19). 'Silent' or painless myocardial infarcts may also occur in people with diabetes. It is thought that the lack of pain may be due to autonomic nerve damage.

The bladder may be affected by autonomic damage, but this is rare. It does not empty completely, leading to an increased risk of urinary tract infections.

Other autonomic complications include an increased peripheral blood flow (arteriovenous shunts between capillaries do not function correctly), abnormal pupil reactions, oesophageal dysfunction and impaired counter-regulatory hormone responses to hypoglycaemia.

Cardiovascular complications

Those individuals presenting with cardiovascular complications of diabetes, i.e. CVE, CVD or PVD, will display the same signs and symptoms as the general population. As with the general population, hypertension is generally asymptomatic.

Specific investigations

The investigations undertaken to detect complications include an annual review (see p. 414), including:

- examination of the retina, via an ophthalmoscope
- measurement of the blood pressure, both lying and standing (stand for 2 minutes)
- urinalysis for protein and/or microalbuminuria
- foot examination to test for neuropathy and circulation (dorsalis pedis and posterior tibial pulses – see Ch. 19)
- blood tests for renal function, lipid profile and glucose control.

If probable complications are detected, further relevant investigations may be undertaken depending on the specific signs and symptoms under investigation. For example, a person with a history of possible gastroparesis may require an endoscopy to exclude other diagnoses and to confirm the diagnosis; an individual with a neuropathic foot ulcer will require X-ray studies to assess whether osteomyelitis is present.

Medical management

The progression of diabetes complications can be slowed with 'tight' control of blood glucose levels and, in the instance of cardiovascular disease, control of hypertension. It is therefore important that the individual receives the appropriate treatment in order to achieve this. In some cases, this may necessitate an individual with type 2 diabetes commencing insulin therapy.

Retinopathy can be very effectively managed with laser treatment; blindness can be prevented in approximately 90% of patients with proliferative retinopathy following appropriate laser therapy. Those who have suffered a vitreous haemorrhage may benefit from a vitrectomy, wherein the vitreous gel is removed.

Nephropathy is managed by treating hypertension, encouraging good glycaemic control and the correction of cardiovascular risk factors. Angiotensin-converting enzyme (ACE) inhibitors are the drugs of choice for blood pressure control as they have some renal protective properties. Unfortunately, about one-third of people with renal damage die of cardiovascular events before they develop renal failure. As renal function deteriorates, dietary protein restriction will be required. Those treated with oral hypoglycaemic agents (OHAs) will need to be treated with insulin when their serum creatinine levels reach 200 μmol/L, as the kidneys clear many OHAs.

Neuropathy is difficult to treat. Improved glycaemic control, correction of any vitamin B_{12} deficiency, avoidance of excess alcohol and treatment of uraemia need to be dealt with initially.

Peripheral neuropathy that results in burning pain may be treated with tricyclic antidepressants; amitriptyline is the most commonly used of these. If these agents prove to be ineffectual, gabapentine may be prescribed. Capsaicin cream is occasionally used. This is derived from hot peppers and is applied to the affected areas. Care must be taken to avoid accidental application to mucous membranes such as in the mouth or genital area, as a severe burning sensation in these sensitive places is likely to be the result!

Stabbing or lancing pain may be treated with anticonvulsants, such as carbamazepine or phenytoin, tricyclic antidepressants or capsaicin. Symptoms of painful cramp generally respond well to quinine sulphate. Contact discomfort (allodynia) may be treated with Opsite film and 'restless legs' may respond to clonazepam.

Following the taking of a thorough medical/sexual history to determine the contribution of psychological factors to erectile dysfunction, there are a range of treatment methods, including improved glycaemic control, removal of causative drugs, reduced alcohol intake, intraurethral prostaglandins, e.g. MUSE, sildenafil, the use of vacuum tumescence devices and surgical penile implants (see Ch. 25).

The treatment of other autonomic neuropathies is mostly limited to symptom control, although glycaemic control is important. Those with gastroparesis may be prescribed pro-kinetic drugs (which increase gut motility), such as meto-clopramide, and given advice about eating small regular meals. Constipation and diarrhoea are generally treated symptomatically. Stimulant laxatives are used, if required, to treat constipation, and opioid derivatives such as codeine or loperamide are used to treat diarrhoea. Broad-spectrum antibiotics may also be prescribed if there are concerns about bacterial overgrowth in a hypomotile bowel.

There are no current pharmacological treatments for a hypotonic bladder. Some individuals are taught how to manually express their bladders and, in severe circumstances, intermittent self-catheterization. Antibiotics are required to treat urinary tract infections.

The treatment of cardiovascular complications is also complex (see Chs 14 and 19). The factors that contribute to the risks of heart attacks and strokes are hypertension, hyperlipidaemia and hyperglycaemia as well as the lifestyle issues of smoking, activity levels and weight. Drug treatments for cardiovascular complications may therefore be required in conjunction with non-pharmacological strategies.

Those with known coronary heart disease should be taking 75 mg aspirin daily (a 'baby' aspirin tablet). Hypertension needs to be controlled; the target blood pressure is a maximum of 140/80 mmHg. Blood pressure control is important for the management and prevention of both macro- and microvascular complications of diabetes. To achieve this blood pressure target may necessitate the person with diabetes taking several drugs of different types. For example, an individual may be taking ramipril (an ACE inhibitor), bendrofluazide (a diuretic) and atenolol (a beta-blocker).

Dyslipidaemia is also controlled. The serum cholesterol target is less than 5 mmol/L, the LDL (low-density lipoproteins) target is less than 3 mmol/L and the HDL (high-density lipoproteins) target is more than 1.1 mmol/L. In simple terms, LDL cholesterol is 'bad' and HDL is 'good'. Triglyceride levels should be less than 2 mmol/L. Many people with diabetes, particularly those with type 2 DM, have high LDL and low HDL cholesterol levels and high overall cholesterol levels; this increases the risk of cardiovascular disease.

Drug therapies to achieve the lipid targets include the HMG-CoA reductase inhibitors (statins) such as simvastatin, which reduce cholesterol, and possibly fibrates, e.g. bezafibrate, to reduce triglycerides, if hypertriglyceridaemia is evident.

The treatment of diabetic foot ulcers depends on the underlying pathophysiology. Neuropathic foot ulcers frequently take many months to heal; it is important to prevent infection during this time. Existing infection may require long-term treatment with broad-spectrum antibiotics. Long-term expert podiatry care is also required to deal with removal of callus and dress the ulcers with the most appropriate wound care products. The relief of pressure to the wound is also vital. This is achieved with the use of pressure-relieving footwear supplied by an orthotist, such as Scotchcast boots, or total contact plaster casts.

Those with exclusively ischaemic ulcers, which are rare, or ulcers with an ischaemic component may require angioplasty or bypass surgery to improve blood flow. Gangrene necessitates amputation.

▶ Nursing management

People with the complications of diabetes are, like others with chronic conditions, largely seen as outpatients or are cared for in a community setting. However, the most likely reason for an individual with diabetes to be admitted to hospital is for treatment of complications.

Wherever the individual is seen, the nurse's role in relation to diabetic complications is likely to involve predominantly education and psychological care, although there will be some elements of physical care, e.g. in relation to foot ulcers.

With regard to nursing assessment there are consequently some physical assessments to be made. For example, individuals may have bowel problems as a result of autonomic neuropathy or a diabetic foot ulcer. Most of these physical problems should be elicited following a nursing assessment using a recognized theoretical framework and from the medical notes.

The nursing assessment should also include patients' understanding and knowledge of their diabetes complications. For example, they may understand that they have hypertension and hyperglycaemia but be unaware that in conjunction these are two risk factors which increase the likelihood of a cardiovascular event in the future. Similarly, people with diabetic foot ulcers may be aware that they have some diabetic nerve damage but have no knowledge of the importance of well-fitting shoes in preventing further ulcers.

As well as knowledge, patients' attitudes towards their complications need to be explored. Someone with a firm belief that long-term complications are an inevitable consequence of having diabetes may not change that belief easily. In cases like this, further exploration of the issue is required, possibly by nurses experienced in discussing these difficult areas. People with firm beliefs in their own abilities to cope with adversity, however, tend to be more receptive to immediate education about ways in which they can influence their own health.

The emotional state of patients will need to be explored. For example, a person who has recently developed a complication of diabetes may find that feelings of loss and grief that were felt at the time of the original diagnosis of diabetes are experienced again, and time to 'come to terms' with these may be required. Others may blame themselves for their complications and some may be angry that, despite taking good care of their diabetes, they have developed them anyway.

The self-care skills of people with diabetes complications need to be assessed. As well as general diabetes management issues such as healthy eating, blood glucose monitoring and injection skills, where relevant, the specific skills in relation to self-management of diabetes complications need to be assessed. For instance, individuals with diabetic neuropathy will need to have their practical foot care skills assessed.

As with general diabetes-specific nursing care, the role of the nurse in caring for people with diabetes complications is mostly that of a patient educator, as well as providing psychological support. Any knowledge or skill deficits should be addressed where possible.

Those with diabetic retinopathy may experience deterioration in visual acuity, which can affect their ability to maintain independence in performing self-blood glucose monitoring and insulin injections. The nurse may need to involve the diabetes specialist nurse in finding alternative insulin delivery devices and blood glucose testing equipment.

Individuals with diabetic nephropathy may require support and education about achieving optimal glucose control and also, if they are taking a protein-restricted diet, help with meal choices. Referral to a dietician may be necessary. Those with renal failure may be treated with continuous ambulatory peritoneal dialysis (CAPD) or haemodialysis and will need specific care in this instance (see Ch. 24). Glucose control is often difficult to achieve with CAPD and the services of the diabetes specialist nursing team may also be required.

Those who experience postural hypotension can be encouraged to sit on the edge of the bed for several minutes before attempting to stand, to reduce the risk of 'dizzy spells' or loss of consciousness. Similarly, when rising out of a chair, individuals may find it beneficial to stand still for a few minutes before walking off. In some instances, compression stockings may be beneficial, although some people have great difficulty in applying them correctly.

People with gastroparesis should be taught to eat small meals frequently. In the hospital environment, nurses should ensure that suitable meals are available and given to patients at appropriate intervals. People with constipation will need information about minimizing this: encouragement to drink at least 1.5 litres of water a day, to eat the recommended five portions a day of fruit and vegetables and, if necessary, to take appropriate aperients. Referral to a dietician is also desirable.

Those with neuropathic or ischaemic foot problems need to have the principles of good foot care reiterated, if they have any knowledge deficits. They may also need assistance with alternative ways of carrying out self-care when at home. For example, some older people are unable to examine the bottom of their feet well because of limited mobility or poor eyesight. Showing them how to use a mirror for this purpose may help to maintain independence. People with diabetic foot ulcers need to be referred to a podiatrist, preferably a diabetes specialist podiatrist with advanced skills in the management of diabetic foot ulcers.

Those with hypertension should be taught about non-pharmacological ways of reducing blood pressure. These include a low-fat, low-salt diet, reduced alcohol intake, increased activity, weight reduction in the overweight and cessation of smoking. As well as giving information about these aspects of self-care, nurses should explore barriers to behaviour change in those who find it difficult to actually carry out such changes. For instance, individuals may be aware that half an hour a day of brisk walking, enough to make them slightly warm and increase the pulse rate, is recommended. They may, however, find it difficult to fit this activity into a busy life. Discussing options, such as walking to work or getting off the bus a few stops earlier, may help them to solve the problem.

People who have an atonic bladder may need information about an adequate fluid intake and may need to be taught how to express their bladders manually. In extreme circumstances, they may need to be taught how to catheterize themselves intermittently and the services of a specialist nurse may be required for this (see Ch. 12).

Because people with diabetes complications are usually taking several medicines, another educative role of nurses is to ensure that they know what all their medicines do, when to take them, particularly in relation to food, and what the potential side-effects may be. Some individuals, particularly older people, may need help in remembering to take their medicines at the correct times. Devising individualized charts, which can be ticked as each medicine is taken, or providing tablet dosing boxes may be helpful. As many older people with diabetes will have complications, nurses must also ensure that they can open the packaging.

As well as educative care, nurses need to provide psychological care. Diabetes complications can have a huge negative impact on individuals' quality of life (Glasgow et al 2001). Enabling people to talk about their feelings can be helpful, as well as involving family members in providing support. Other support groups may be useful, such as those organized by local branches of Diabetes UK. The diabetes specialist nursing team can usually provide information on these.

The importance of individualized nursing care for those with diabetes complications is paramount. Although the physical effects may be similar in different people, their abilities to cope with them can differ widely. Nurses, in conjunction with other members of the diabetes team, have an important role in educating and supporting these patients.

DISORDERS AFFECTING THE PITUITARY GLAND

PITUITARY TUMOURS

Most pituitary tumours are adenomas (benign tumours of glandular epithelium). The majority of them are small, being less than 10 mm across (microadenomas). Those that are more than 10 mm in diameter are known as macroadenomas. Pituitary adenomas are benign in the sense that they do not spread to other parts of the body. However, many cause hypersecretion of anterior pituitary hormones (see p. 398). Those which produce excess amounts of thyroid-stimulating hormone (TSH) and adrenocorticotrophic hormone (ACTH) are discussed in the sections dealing with thyroid and adrenal problems, respectively (pp. 431 and 437).

Other tumours which occur less commonly are craniopharyngiomas, meningiomas, and primary and metastatic malignant tumours (see Ch. 14).

ACROMEGALY AND GIGANTISM

Acromegaly and gigantism are caused by excessive growth hormone (GH) secretion. If the GH excess occurs before the epiphyses of the long bones have fused, gigantism results and this extremely rare condition is therefore seen in children and adolescents. Some individuals with gigantism can grow to heights in excess of 7 feet.

Excess secretion following fusion of the epiphyses occurs in adults and results in acromegaly.

Aetiology and epidemiology

Acromegaly is usually caused by persistent oversecretion of growth hormone from an anterior pituitary adenoma; these tumours account for 99% of acromegaly cases. Other, very rare, causes include excess secretion of growth hormone-releasing hormone (GHRH) from hypothalamic tumours and ectopic secretion of GH or GHRH from non-endocrine tumours such as small-cell lung tumours.

The incidence is three to four per million people per year.

Pathophysiology and clinical presentation

The signs and symptoms of acromegaly are the result of high levels of circulating GH and insulin-like growth factor-I (IGF-I), which are secreted from the pituitary adenoma. These hormones have somatic, or growth, effects and metabolic effects. The tumour itself may cause visual disturbances and other local problems such as cranial nerve palsies (see Box 17.5).

The development of acromegaly is very slow, over many years. The average age at presentation is between 40 and 45 years. Because of the insidious onset of the condition, it may pass unnoticed until individuals find themselves changing shoe size or needing to enlarge rings. Relatives and friends may comment on a changed appearance, provoking a visit to the doctor. Cardiovascular problems or back pain or joint symptoms may also be reasons for seeking help, as may headaches or visual changes, although the latter are less common.

Specific investigations

Blood samples for serum IGF-I and GH will be taken. A raised IGF-I will be diagnostic. An oral glucose tolerance test (see

---

Box 17.5 The signs and symptoms of acromegaly

Somatic (or growth) signs and symptoms
- Enlarged hands and feet
- Enlarged or prognathous jaw
- Coarse facial features (enlargement of the nose and frontal bones)
- Teeth become spread (interdental separation)
- Soft tissue enlargement (e.g. deeper voice, carpal tunnel syndrome)
- Hyperhydrosis (increased sweating)
- Skin and hair thickens
- Cartilage and synovial enlargement – arthropathy
- Osteoporosis
- Cardiovascular disease – hypertension, left ventricular hypertrophy, cardiomyopathy
- Organ enlargement

Metabolic signs and symptoms
- Insulin resistance – secondary diabetes mellitus (see p. 403)
- Lipogenesis and weight gain
- Nitrogen retention

'Local signs' and symptoms
- Headache
- Visual field defects (due to upward growth of tumour to the optic chiasm)
- Cranial nerve palsies
- Enlarged pituitary fossa
- Menstrual dysfunction (decreased secretion of other pituitary hormones due to a compression)
- Erectile dysfunction
- Hypogonadism

'Diagnosis of diabetes mellitus', pp. 402–403) may be performed with GH being measured 2 hours post-glucose load. In acromegaly, this value is usually raised, whereas in normal individuals it falls. Other pituitary function tests may be performed if there is a suspicion that the adenoma is secreting other hormones as well.

A magnetic resonance imaging (MRI) scan of the pituitary can show tumours as small as 2 mm in diameter. Although not used for diagnostic purposes, skull X-rays may show an enlarged pituitary fossa (sella turcica) or erosion of the fossa floor. Other bony changes of the skull may also be identified. If the MRI scan is normal, radiological studies to identify the locality of tumours elsewhere will be undertaken.

Medical/surgical management

The best treatment is surgical removal of the tumour using the trans-sphenoidal route (via the sphenoid sinus). Trans-sphenoidal adenomectomy (removal of the adenoma) is generally successful in treating about 80% of microadenomas, but the figure is lower for macroadenomas. However, patients must be informed of potential complications following surgery, e.g. diabetes insipidus (see p. 431).

Octreotide is an analogue of growth hormone-inhibitory hormone (GHIH) or somatostatin and is used when surgery is not possible or has failed. It is also used in patients receiving radiotherapy (to shrink the tumour) or to treat severe symptoms such as sleep apnoea or headaches prior to surgical intervention. Octreotide is given by subcutaneous (short-acting) or intramuscular (depot) injection. Lanreotide is a recently introduced alternative.

Radiotherapy can be used in patients who are unable to have surgery or in whom surgery has failed, as well as those who are not controlled with medication. Unfortunately, the reduction in excess GH and IGF-I hormones takes a long time to achieve and approximately 50% of patients experience a reduction in other pituitary hormones within 10 years.

Patients will require long-term follow-up for many years to assess the effectiveness of therapy.

▶ Nursing management

People with acromegaly may be anxious following diagnosis of their condition. Providing clear explanations of the investigations to be undertaken is important and patients should be given the opportunity to ask questions about these. Giving appropriate leaflets or website addresses may also be useful (see p. 442).

Some patients may be anxious about their appearance and explanations of the causes for these changes are necessary. For some, body image will have been severely affected; reassurance that successful treatment can reverse many of the changes can be encouraging, e.g. informing people that, in some cases, there have been improvements (such as reduced skin thickness) within days of surgery.

Other individuals may be anxious about the treatment itself, particularly when faced with the prospect of neurosurgery, albeit via the sphenoid sinus. Again, clear explanations of what to expect should be given (see Ch. 14 for further details about neurosurgery). Most individuals are discharged within a few days post-surgery.

PROLACTINOMAS

Prolactinomas are anterior pituitary tumours which secrete excess amounts of the hormone prolactin, and can affect both sexes.

Aetiology and epidemiology

Prolactinomas, like other pituitary adenomas, are caused by a mutation of the hormone-producing cells, in this case prolactin. They account for approximately 30–40% of all pituitary adenomas. More women than men are diagnosed because of the effects on menstruation; however, the tumours in men are frequently larger due to the delay in presentation.

Pathophysiology and clinical presentation

Hyperprolactinaemia inhibits gonadotrophin secretion and the resultant signs and symptoms are mostly related to this. In women, hypogonadism (deficiency of gonad function, in this case the ovaries) can cause infertility and menstrual problems (amenorrhoea or oligomenorrhoea – see Ch. 25). The degree of symptoms, e.g. whether premenopausal women have oligo-menorrhoea or amenorrhoea, is related to the levels of prolactin secreted. Women may also experience galactorrhoea (inappropriate milk secretion). Eventually they may develop osteoporosis due to reduced oestrogen levels. Women usually present with menstrual problems or infertility. Postmenopausal women have reduced gonadotrophin secretion anyway and prolactinomas in this instance are usually identified only if the tumour is sufficiently large to cause neurological symptoms such as headaches or impaired vision.

In men, hypogonadism can result in reduced libido, infertility, hair loss, decreased muscle mass and osteoporosis. Men may develop gynaecomastia (abnormal enlargement of the breast) but galactorrhoea is less common than in women. They may also experience erectile dysfunction.

Specific investigations

Hyperprolactinaemia can occur for reasons other than the presence of a prolactinoma, e.g. some medications. MRI scans are therefore essential for accurate diagnosis. Visual field studies may also be useful, particularly if there is a history of headaches or field defects.

Medical/surgical management

Initial treatment of prolactinomas is the administration of a dopamine-receptor stimulant to reduce the size and secretion of the tumour. Current medications are bromocriptine, cabergoline and quinagolide.

If drug therapy is ineffective or not tolerated, trans-sphenoidal adenomectomy is a treatment option. Radiotherapy is reserved for the prevention of regrowth of residual tumour tissue following surgery to remove a large macroadenoma.

▶ Nursing management

Those individuals with prolactinomas may be experiencing distress relating to infertility or concern about their future chances of having children. Men may also be distressed by the physical changes associated with a prolactinoma, such as erectile dysfunction and loss of muscle mass, and have body image problems. Nurses should ensure that patients have sufficient information and are referred to appropriate specialist services (e.g. a specialist nurse in erectile dysfunction, counselling or infertility services), and provide psychological support for patients and family members.

ANTERIOR PITUITARY HYPOSECRETION

Hyposecretion of the anterior pituitary hormones can occur with any of the hormones, or all six. In the latter case, this is referred to as panhypopituitarism.

Aetiology and epidemiology

Anterior pituitary hyposecretion, total or selective, can occur in patients with pituitary adenomas, other pituitary tumours, following pituitary surgery or irradiation or following head injury (Thorner 1996). The most common effect is the cessation of gonad function due to a deficiency of gonadotrophins (LH or FSH) or suppression of these hormones by hyperprolactinaemia.

GH deficiency is the next most likely scenario, followed by deficient amounts of TSH and ACTH. A prolactin deficiency is uncommon.

Pathophysiology and clinical presentation

The signs and symptoms of anterior pituitary hyposecretion will be related to each individual hormone deficit (see Table 17.4). Patients with pituitary tumours may present with signs and symptoms of local compression. Those whose hypopituitarism follows trauma etc. will present with symptoms and signs of their particular hormone deficiency.

Specific investigations

The investigations performed are determined by the presenting symptoms and signs. However, radiological studies of the

Table 17.4 Signs and symptoms of anterior pituitary hyposecretion

Deficiency	Symptoms and signs
Gonadotrophins (LH and FSH)	Men — Poor libido — Infertility — Erectile dysfunction Women — Infertility — Menstrual disorders — Amenorrhoea
Growth hormone (GH)	Adiposity (weight gain) Reduced strength Thin, dry skin and cool peripheries Cold intolerance Impaired psychological well-being
Thyroid-stimulating hormone (TSH)	Hypothyroidism (see p. 435)
Adrenocorticotrophic hormone (ACTH)	Adrenal cortex insufficiency (secondary)

pituitary gland, visual field testing and measurement of plasma hormone levels are all possible.

Medical and surgical management

The underlying cause of the hypopituitarism also determines the treatment. Surgery for pituitary tumours is indicated and radiotherapy may be necessary. Hormone replacement therapy is required in those instances where the cause of the problem is hyposecretion following previous surgery, irradiation or trauma. A relatively new treatment is growth hormone replacement therapy for adults, which is given by subcutaneous injection.

▶ Nursing management

People with hypopituitarism need explanations of their condition and psychological support to help them to cope with the body image difficulties they may be experiencing. Thorough explanations of investigations and surgical or radiation therapies will be required if these are performed.

The nurse will need to teach people about their hormone replacement therapy, which can be complex in panhypopituitarism. Those taking GH will need to be taught how to give subcutaneous injections using a pen injection device.

The importance of regular attendance at outpatient appointments for monitoring of pituitary function needs to be discussed.

DIABETES INSIPIDUS

Diabetes insipidus (DI) is a condition in which excessive amounts of very dilute urine are passed. In most cases, there is a consequent increased intake in oral fluids – polydipsia – to compensate for the increased urine output.

Differential diagnoses include primary polydipsia, whereby the polyuria is caused by excessive drinking, and nephrogenic diabetes insipidus, which is caused by an inability of the kidneys to respond to antidiuretic hormone (ADH).

Aetiology and epidemiology

Diabetes insipidus is caused by an inadequate release of ADH. Approximately 30–50% of cases are idiopathic. Other causes include neurosurgical trauma, mainly following trans-sphenoidal resection of pituitary tumours, other cerebral trauma involving the hypothalamus and posterior pituitary gland, primary and secondary tumours, and infiltrative diseases such as sarcoidosis.

An autoimmune process probably causes the destruction of ADH-secreting cells in the hypothalamus in idiopathic DI. In relation to neurosurgery, approximately 10–20% of individuals develop DI following the trans-sphenoidal removal of microadenomas, whereas 60–80% develop the condition following macroadenoma removal. It may only be temporary.

Diabetes insipidus is an uncommon condition; however, specific epidemiological data are unavailable.

Pathophysiology and clinical presentation

The lack of ADH causes the kidneys to excrete excess amounts of water, leading to polyuria and very dilute urine. This also occurs at night, giving rise to nocturia. The water loss can be severe, with amounts of 10–15 litres not being uncommon.

Individuals will drink large amounts of fluids to compensate, leading to polydipsia.

Individuals with idiopathic DI will usually present with a history of a rapid onset of symptoms (over a couple of days). Following surgery or trauma, the symptoms are usually evident within 24 hours.

Specific investigations

Urine and plasma osmolality samples are taken at the same time. Dilute urine with a concentrated plasma osmolality would be expected in DI. Plasma sodium levels are measured; the result to be expected in DI is high-normal.

It is common to perform a water deprivation test. Patients are deprived of any fluids and urine volume and osmolality are measured hourly. Two-hourly plasma osmolality and sodium are also measured (local procedures may differ slightly). In normal individuals, as the plasma osmolality rises (due to water deprivation), the urine osmolality would also rise as the kidneys respond to ADH release to conserve water. In those with DI, the urine does not become more concentrated and plasma osmolality rises above normal. At this point exogenous ADH is given (2 µg intramuscularly or 20 µg intranasally). If the urine becomes more concentrated, the diagnosis of DI is confirmed.

Medical management

The treatment of DI is with desmopressin, the analogue of ADH. This can be taken intranasally, by subcutaneous or intramuscular injection or by mouth.

▶ Nursing management

During the diagnosis phase of care, nurses are responsible for the measurement of patients' fluid intake and output. It is extremely important that these measurements are accurate to the nearest 10 mL of fluid. Accurate body weight measurement and collection of urine samples for osmolality are important, too, especially during the water deprivation test. A clear explanation of what will occur during the test is necessary and reminders to collect all urine samples may be required. A sufficient supply of containers is essential, as is easy access to toilet facilities.

Those with DI can find the water deprivation test distressing, as their thirst can be very acute. It has been known for some individuals to succumb to drinking water straight from the tap in desperation. For this reason they will often need considerable psychological support and encouragement to complete the test.

Following diagnosis, individuals require explanation of their condition and education about the management of their desmopressin therapy, including self-administration of the drug. They will also need information about who to contact should their treatment regimen need revising.

DISORDERS AFFECTING THE THYROID GLAND

These include hyperthyroidism or thyrotoxicosis (overactivity of the thyroid gland), which may be caused by a variety of disorders, and hypothyroidism or myxoedema (underactivity of the thyroid gland), which is often due to an autoimmune disorder.

The terms thyrotoxicosis and hyperthyroidism are frequently used interchangeably. Thyrotoxicosis occurs when the body is exposed to excess amounts of circulating thyroid hormone. Usually this is due to hyperactivity of the thyroid gland – hyperthyroidism. The most common conditions causing hyperthyroidism are Graves' disease, thyroiditis, toxic multinodular goitre and toxic solitary adenoma. Uncommon causes include pituitary tumours producing TSH (very rare), iodine-induced hyperthyroidism and metastatic thyroid carcinoma.

GRAVES' DISEASE

Graves' disease is the most common cause of hyperthyroidism and accounts for approximately 75% of all cases in the UK.

Aetiology and epidemiology
The exact aetiology of Graves' disease is unknown, but it is an autoimmune disease of the thyroid gland and tends to run in families. It is possible that an environmental 'trigger', probably an infection, leads to autoimmune destruction of thyroid cells in genetically susceptible individuals. More females than males develop the disease; the prevalence is approximately 20 per 1000 in females and 2 per 1000 in males. Individuals tend to be between 20 and 40 years of age at diagnosis.

Pathophysiology and clinical presentation
The majority of signs and symptoms of Graves' disease are caused by the increase in metabolic rate due to the excess thyroid hormone. They include a diffusely enlarged thyroid gland (goitre), features of hyperthyroidism (see Box 17.6), ophthalmological features and, occasionally, pretibial myxoedema, a skin condition associated with Graves' disease (raised pink/purple plaques on the front of the legs).

The ophthalmological features can range from lid lag (stare) and lid retraction to proptosis (protrusion of the eyeball) or exophthalmia, periorbital and conjunctival oedema, extraocular muscle involvement, corneal abrasions caused by failure to close the eyelid, and sight loss due to optic nerve involvement (see Ch. 15). All of these, apart from the lid lag and lid retraction, are peculiar to Graves' disease.

Graves' disease usually develops gradually, and individuals present to their doctor with a variety of symptoms, most commonly increased irritability, decreased weight despite an increased appetite, and heat intolerance. However, occasionally the presentation is acute.

Special investigations
The diagnosis is confirmed by laboratory measurements of thyroid hormones. Free or total T_4 (thyroxine) and T_3 (triiodothyronine) levels will be raised and TSH (thyroid-stimulating hormone) will be undetectable. Thyroid antibodies in conjunction with raised T_4 and T_3 levels confirm the diagnosis as Graves' disease. An isotope scan (radioactive iodine) of the thyroid gland may also be performed.

Medical and surgical management
The treatment of Graves' disease is to control the excess amounts of hormone, using drugs that inhibit the synthesis of thyroid hormone (thionamides), treatment with radioactive iodine to reduce the bulk of thyroid tissue, or surgical removal of part of the thyroid gland.

Carbimazole is the most commonly used drug, although propylthiouracil may be used for those sensitive to the former. Carbimazole may suppress bone marrow function, causing pancytopenia or agranulocytosis, and should be stopped if patients develop infections, particularly sore throats (see Ch. 18); however,

---

Box 17.6 General and specific signs and symptoms of hyperthyroidism (McGregor 1996)

General
- Heat intolerance, sweating
- Fatigue, apathy
- Tremor

Cardiovascular (see Ch. 19)
- Palpitations, tachycardia
- Dyspnoea
- Angina
- Atrial fibrillation
- Heart failure

Gastrointestinal (see Ch. 22)
- Weight loss despite increased appetite
- Diarrhoea, steatorrhoea
- Vomiting

Genitourinary (see Chs 24 and 25)
- Polyuria and polydipsia
- Amenorrhoea
- Infertility

Neuromuscular (see Chs 14 and 27)
- Fatiguability
- Restlessness
- Proximal muscle weakness
- Choreoathetosis (irregular involuntary movements)
- Hypokalaemic periodic paralysis
- Myasthenia gravis

Psychiatric
- Irritability, nervousness
- Agitation, emotional lability
- Psychosis

Dermatological (see Ch. 28)
- Pruritus
- Palmar erythema
- Pretibial myxoedema
- Vitiligo
- Hair thinning
- Onycholysis

Ocular
- Lid lag (stare)/lid retraction, proptosis or exophthalmia

this occurs in fewer than 1% of patients. Initial doses are relatively high, but once the patient is clinically euthyroid (having normal thyroid function) after approximately 4–8 weeks, maintenance doses are then given for 6–12 months.

A blocking and replacement regimen may also occur. High doses of carbimazole are given to suppress the production of thyroid hormones and replacement thyroxine is also given for a period of 6–12 months. Between one-third and one-half of patients achieve a long-term remission. Carbimazole is weakly immunosuppressive and it is thought that the autoimmune destructive process may be stopped in this way.

Those with severe cardiovascular symptoms may initially be treated with beta-blockers, such as propranolol, to reduce the symptoms, until the thionamides have been effective.

A very rare complication of hyperthyroidism is hyperthyroid or thyrotoxic crisis ('thyroid storm') caused by a sudden increase in the signs and symptoms of hyperthyroidism. It is a life-threatening medical emergency characterized by pyrexia, tachycardia, other arrhythmias such as atrial fibrillation, and confusion and agitation. Hyperthyroid crisis may be associated with infection, or may occur soon after thyroid surgery or treatment with radioactive iodine. The management includes rehydration with i.v. fluids, propranolol, hydrocortisone, antibiotics as appropriate, and carbimazole and oral iodine.

If drug treatment is not successful, partial thyroidectomy may be performed. Treatment with thionamides prior to surgery is given to make the patient euthyroid. It is particularly important that patients are euthyroid prior to surgery in order to reduce the risk, albeit very slight, of a hyperthyroid crisis occurring postoperatively. Oral potassium iodide (Lugol's solution) may occasionally be prescribed, with carbimazole, for 10–14 days prior to partial thyroidectomy to improve control and decrease thyroid size and vascularity. Post-surgery, approximately 80% of patients are euthyroid, 15% develop hypothyroidism and 5% relapse (McGregor 1996).

Radioactive sodium iodide (radio-iodine) may be used to treat hyperthyroidism. The thyroid follicular cells are destroyed by the isotope, which is given orally. Most patients develop hypothyroidism as a consequence of this treatment, requiring replacement therapy. However, this can take 2 or 3 months, so treatment with thionamides or beta-blockers is necessary for this period. Radioactive iodine may also be used following a relapse after thyroid surgery and is increasingly being used for those with cardiac disease.

▶ Nursing management

If hyperthyroidism is treated medically, or with thionamides prior to surgery, the nurse's role is to educate patients about their medications. Those taking oral potassium iodide should be advised always to take the drug solution well diluted in milk or water. As individuals may be anxious or restless, this is best done by giving small 'chunks' of information at any one time.

As individuals' metabolic rates are increased, they may not be able to maintain body weight; ensuring adequate nutrition, particularly preoperatively, is also important. Those who are heat-intolerant may find a fan beneficial. However, the goal of medical treatment prior to surgery is to make the patient euthyroid, so these problems should not be manifest at the time of admission.

Other preoperative nursing care includes explanations of what to expect postoperatively. The nursing team should ensure patients have sufficient information about the procedure itself, if required, and that they have sufficiently understood medical explanations. Patients must also be shown how to perform deep breathing exercises and should be encouraged to practise these, as well as the postoperative positioning required to prevent strain on the suture line.

Postoperatively, patients will need careful nursing because of the risk of complications. They should be nursed in an upright position, with the head and neck well supported with pillows. This should be comfortable for patients and also ensure the least strain on the suture line.

As the thyroid gland is highly vascular, there is a risk of haemorrhage which can compress the trachea, although this event is very uncommon. Clip or suture removers should therefore be kept at the bedside for at least 24 hours to enable rapid removal should haemorrhage occur. An increase in pulse rate and a decrease in blood pressure could indicate haemorrhage. For this reason, half-hourly observations of blood pressure, pulse and respiration rate should be performed; the frequency of measurements may be reduced as patients recover and if the observations are stable.

A pulse oximeter may be used to monitor pulse rate. Irregular or laboured breathing, or any stridor (harsh sound during breathing) should also alert the nursing team to the possibility of haemorrhage. The wound should be observed for any signs of swelling, every half hour initially. It is also vital that nurses observe for signs of obvious bleeding, which must include checking the pillow behind the patient's head as blood may be leaking from under a dressing pad. Any change in vital signs, breathing problem or wound swelling should be reported to the medical staff immediately. If clips do need to be removed to allow blood compressing the trachea to escape, the wound should be covered in saline-soaked gauze. The patient will then return to theatre for treatment to the offending blood vessel and resuturing.

Breathing difficulties, particularly noisy breathing or stridor, a hoarse voice and swallowing difficulties may indicate damage to the recurrent laryngeal nerves, resulting in vocal cord spasm and paralysis of the larynx. If both nerves are affected, patients will require a tracheostomy. This, however, is an uncommon complication, which is more likely to occur if a total thyroidectomy has been performed.

Nurses should also be aware of the remote possibly of a hyperthyroid crisis (see above) occurring shortly after surgery. They should monitor pulse, blood pressure and temperature and inform the medical staff immediately of changes in vital signs, if patients become confused or agitated, or there is an alteration in conscious level.

An intravenous infusion will be in situ; this will usually be discontinued on the first postoperative day. Oral fluids may be taken when patients are able. A soft diet may be given on the evening of surgery, as patients are able. A fluid balance chart must be maintained.

As there is a small risk of postoperative hypoparathyroidism (see p. 436) due to inadvertent removal of the parathyroid glands, patients should be observed for signs of tetany (muscle spasms) and asked if they have any tingling in their fingers or toes. Any such signs should be reported to the medical staff. If this occurs, an i.v. infusion of calcium gluconate will be commenced.

Postoperative analgesia and antiemetics need to be given as required and prescribed. Although chest infections and deep vein thrombosis are uncommon after thyroid surgery, the nursing team should provide care aimed at preventing these occurrences.

If clips have been used for wound closure, alternate ones are removed on the second postoperative day, with the remaining clips being removed on the fourth day. If a continuous suture had been used, this is removed on the fourth postoperative day.

Many patients are discharged from hospital on the day after surgery, depending on their condition.

THYROIDITIS

Most cases of thyroiditis are due to an infection of the thyroid gland; in this instance it is usually referred to as subacute thyroiditis, but is also known as granulomatous giant cell or de Quervain's thyroiditis. 'Silent' (painless) thyroiditis can also cause hyperthyroidism.

Aetiology and epidemiology
Subacute thyroiditis is an uncommon condition caused by a viral infection of the thyroid, usually following an upper respiratory tract infection. Silent thyroiditis is an autoimmune condition and is also uncommon.

Pathophysiology and clinical presentation
Destruction of the follicles leads to release of thyroid hormone in large quantities, leading to signs and symptoms of hyperthyroidism. The ability to make new thyroid hormone is impaired and a period of hypothyroidism then ensues. Eventually, thyroid function returns to normal.

In 'silent' thyroiditis, the disease process is a lymphocytic infiltration of the gland. As in subacute thyroiditis, thyroid hormones are released from damaged cells in large amounts. The cells are temporarily unable to produce thyroid hormones, leading to a subsequent period of hypothyroidism. This eventually resolves and normal function is resumed.

Individuals with subacute thyroiditis usually present with pain in the thyroid and sometimes an accompanying fever. The pain may be severe. However, in some cases there is no pain at all. Those with 'silent' thyroiditis may have an enlarged thyroid gland, but it is not painful.

Special investigations
If iodine isotope scans are performed, the uptake is low in thyroiditis. There may be biochemical evidence of hyperthyroidism if tests are performed during the initial stages of the disease.

▶ Nursing and medical management

Aspirin may be sufficient to control the symptoms of subacute thyroiditis, and occasionally glucocorticoids may be used. If the hyperthyroid phase causes marked clinical disease then carbimazole may be used, but this is uncommon.

The nursing needs of people with thyroiditis are generally educational. Patients need to be informed about their condition and given information about pain control or other medications, where used. Patients are unlikely to be admitted to hospital.

TOXIC MULTINODULAR GOITRE AND TOXIC SINGLE ADENOMA

As the name suggests, in a multinodular goitre the thyroid gland is enlarged but with distinct nodules palpable. This is in contrast to Graves' disease in which the enlargement is diffuse. Single adenomas appear in younger patients, about 30–40 years of age.

Aetiology and epidemiology
The toxic multinodular goitre tends to give rise to hyperthyroidism in an older age group than in Graves' disease.

A single palpable nodule is the cause of single toxic adenoma. It accounts for approximately 2% of all cases of hyperthyroidism.

Pathophysiology and clinical presentation
The overproduction of thyroid hormone for both toxic multinodular goitre and toxic solitary adenoma is usually less than in Graves' disease and the signs and symptoms are therefore less severe (see Box 17.6, p. 432).

The presentation of hyperthyroidism in both of these conditions is usually less dramatic than that of Graves' disease. Indeed, initially the only abnormality evident with toxic single adenoma is a borderline suppression of TSH.

Special investigations
Blood tests reveal excess amounts of the thyroid hormones T_3 and T_4. A radioisotope scan will indicate the presence of both multinodular and single nodule disease.

Medical/surgical management
The treatment of choice is radioactive iodine. Larger doses than that for Graves' disease may be required in the case of toxic multinodular goitre, although they are similar for a single nodule. Those who have large goitres, or nodules, may require surgery.

▶ Nursing management

Patients receiving oral radioactive iodine treatment need information about how to reduce radiation exposure to their family members and friends. Individuals should be advised to sleep alone and to avoid kissing and sexual intercourse. Long periods of physical contact are also to be avoided, particularly with children and pregnant women.

A high fluid intake is advised to avoid constipation and to increase urinary output, thus reducing the amount of iodine in the body. Using separate eating utensils for the first few days after treatment reduces the chance of contaminating others with radioactive saliva.

Hygiene is essential. Handwashing after going to the lavatory is imperative, and the sink should be cleaned afterwards. Flushing the lavatory several times after each use is also advised. A daily shower, and cleaning the bath or shower thoroughly after each use will reduce the risk of contamination from sweat. These precautions need to be observed for 2–5 days after the treatment. Specific instructions should be acquired from the local medical staff.

Patients may be very apprehensive about radioactive iodine treatment and need opportunities to discuss these fears. They also need reassurance that the treatment will be effective. All patients should be advised to attend follow-up appointments regularly, as they will eventually become hypothyroid and will need monitoring and replacement therapy.

HYPOTHYROIDISM

Hypothyroidism, or myxoedema, occurs when there is an insufficient amount of circulating thyroid hormones. Primary hypothyroidism results from thyroid disease and secondary hypothyroidism from pituitary or hypothalamic disease or damage.

Aetiology and epidemiology

Most hypothyroidism, like Graves' disease, is autoimmune in nature. Autoimmune hypothyroidism is called Hashimoto's disease or Hashimoto's thyroiditis. The autoimmune process results in extensive infiltration of the gland by lymphocytes; it is this, as well as hyperplasia of remaining thyroid tissue in response to TSH stimulation, which gives rise to the characteristic goitre. Other disorders causing hypothyroidism include primary thyroid atrophy, which is probably end-stage Hashimoto's disease and is characterized by the lack of a thyroid goitre; post-radioactive iodine therapy and post-surgery. Between them, these causes account for about 95% of all hypothyroidism.

The specific aetiology of the autoimmune process is unknown in Hashimoto's disease. It is more common in women than in men and most usually affects those between the ages of 30 and 50. Approximately 3% of women and about 0.3% of men (Nussey & Whitehead 2001) have the condition. A family history is relatively common.

Secondary hypothyroidism results from damage to the pituitary or hypothalamus associated with tumours, radiotherapy, surgery or trauma. Thyroid-stimulating hormone (TSH) synthesis becomes impaired in these circumstances.

Individuals can develop hypothyroidism if there is an insufficient intake of dietary iodine. This cause is virtually unseen in Western countries, although it is common in iodine-deficient areas of the world.

Pathophysiology and clinical presentation

The signs and symptoms of hypothyroidism are shown in Box 17.7. There are many of these, owing to the fact that lack of thyroid hormone has an effect on every system in the body.

The onset of hypothyroidism is generally slow. Patients may present with any of the signs and symptoms listed, or, if they have Hashimoto's disease, with a goitre.

Special investigations

The diagnosis of Hashimoto's disease is suspected if a goitre is present. It is confirmed following low thyroid hormone levels, with thyroid antibodies and high TSH levels.

▶ Nursing and medical management

Most patients with hypothyroidism are managed on an outpatient basis. The treatment for hypothyroidism is with thyroxine, i.e. replacement therapy. The dose is adjusted to individual needs.

Box 17.7 Signs and symptoms of hypothyroidism

Signs
- Weight gain
- Dry, coarse, scaly skin – pale or yellow
- Coarse, brittle hair
- Bradycardia
- Hair loss
- Anaemia
- Puffy eyes and sometimes hands
- Oedema*
- Cerebellar signs*
- Deafness*
- Psychiatric signs ('myxoedema madness')*

Symptoms
- Lethargy
- Fatigue
- Cold intolerance
- Depression
- Poor concentration
- Aches and pains, paraesthesia
- Carpal tunnel syndrome
- Constipation*
- Hoarse voice*
- Menorrhagia*

*Less common signs and symptoms.

The nurse's role is to educate individuals about their condition, stressing the importance of taking thyroxine as prescribed. Individuals also need to be aware that regular blood tests to check the appropriateness of the dose will be required. In the initial stages, patients may require psychological support, as some of the signs and symptoms relating to an altered physical appearance may be distressing. Reassurance that these should resolve following the commencement of treatment is often required.

SIMPLE GOITRE

A simple goitre may also be called a non-toxic goitre. A thyroid enlargement occurs but there is no altered function. The cause of the condition is unknown. Women are affected more than men, particularly at puberty and during pregnancy. Surgery may be required if there are symptoms associated with tracheal obstruction. If this occurs, replacement thyroid hormone therapy is necessary (McGregor 1996).

THYROID CANCER

Thyroid cancer can be primary, i.e. arising from cells in the thyroid gland, or secondary to other cancers.

Aetiology and epidemiology

Although thyroid cancer is the most common of the endocrine cancers, it is rare, with only about 30 people in a million in the UK being diagnosed annually. The death rate is even lower (Nussey & Whitehead 2001).

There are two main types of thyroid carcinomas – papillary and follicular. Eighty per cent of all tumours are papillary, 10% are follicular and the remainder are Hurthle cell, medullary or anaplastic carcinomas.

More thyroid cancers are diagnosed in women than in men (it is two to four times more common) and the women tend to be between the ages of 45 and 50 years.

Pathophysiology and clinical presentation

Thyroid cancers do not generally give rise to hypo- or hyperthyroidism, although both are possible. The most likely sign is a thyroid nodule which is relatively fast-growing. Occasionally local symptoms, such as dysphagia, dyspnoea or a hoarse voice, may be apparent, indicating disease spread to other structures in the neck. Patients generally present with an asymptomatic thyroid nodule.

Specific investigations

Distinguishing malignant from benign thyroid nodules is difficult using imaging tests. The best investigation to do this is a fine-needle aspiration for histological examination. Thyroid function is also assessed.

Medical/surgical management

The management of thyroid cancer is to surgically remove either some or all of the thyroid gland with the tumour. Thyroid hormone therapy will be required postoperatively, partly to suppress any remaining tumour and to replace hormones lost following gland removal. Postoperative radioactive iodine treatment may be given to those with residual disease or metastases.

▶ Nursing management

The nursing care of individuals undergoing surgery or radioactive iodine treatment is as described on pages 433–434. However, the diagnosis of cancer is usually very frightening and individuals and families will need reassurance that the outcome of treatment for thyroid cancer is usually very good.

DISORDERS AFFECTING THE PARATHYROID GLANDS

HYPOPARATHYROIDISM

Hypoparathyroidism is the most common cause of chronic hypocalcaemia (reduced serum calcium level) and is due to a lack of parathyroid hormone (PTH). Pseudohypoparathyroidism refers to the condition in which the body is resistant to the action of PTH. In this case, PTH concentrations are high.

Aetiology and epidemiology

Hypoparathyroidism can be congenital. However, the most likely cause in adults is damage following thyroid or laryngeal surgery (see p. 433 and Ch. 21). The incidence of hypoparathyroidism after thyroidectomy varies greatly (Kanis 1996). Rarely, it may be due to polyendocrine autoimmune disease.

Clinical presentation

The symptoms and signs of hypoparathyroidism are due to hypocalcaemia and hyperphosphataemia (increased serum phosphate level). Insufficient calcium causes neuromuscular irritability, giving rise to spasms (tetany) in the hands and feet (carpopedal spasm), paraesthesia in the face, fingers and toes and, occasionally, abdominal cramps. It may also cause irritability, emotional lability, memory impairment, lethargy and sometimes seizures in extreme cases (Kanis 1996).

In adults, symptoms and signs of hypoparathyroidism are most likely to be detected during routine appointments following thyroid surgery. Occasionally hypoparathyroidism may become manifest when there is a greater demand for calcium, e.g. during lactation.

Specific investigations

Serum calcium and phosphate levels are measured. If pseudo-hypoparathyroidism is suspected, PTH and responses to exogenous PTH may be measured.

Medical management

The treatment of hypoparathyroidism is with calcium and vitamin D supplementation, to restore normal calcium and phosphate levels. Ergocalciferol, alfacalcidol or calcitriol tablets may be used. Measurements of plasma calcium levels are initially performed weekly to avoid hypercalcaemia due to excess doses. Plasma calcium levels should be measured 6-monthly thereafter.

▶ Nursing management

Hypoparathyroidism is usually managed on an outpatient basis. The nurse's role is to provide explanations of the condition and its treatment. Information about the importance of regular blood tests to check calcium levels should also be given.

HYPERPARATHYROIDISM

Hyperparathyroidism occurs when there is an excess of parathyroid hormone (PTH). PTH is the hormone responsible for calcium balance in the body, so most of the manifestations of hyperparathyroidism are related to an elevated serum calcium level.

Aetiology and epidemiology

Primary hyperparathyroidism usually occurs as a result of a single adenoma on one of the four parathyroid glands. The annual incidence is estimated at 45 per 100 000 of the population (Nussey & Whitehead 2001). Women are 2.5 times more likely than men to have the condition and the incidence rises with age.

Hyperplasia of the parathyroid glands or multiple adenomas are less common causes of primary hyperparathyroidism. Even more rare causes are parathyroid cancers (< 1%) or familial hyperparathyroidism.

Clinical presentation

Most individuals with hyperparathyroidism have no symptoms or signs of hypercalcaemia. Those who do may have hypertension, malaise and fatigue, depression, constipation, anorexia, polydipsia, polyuria, renal colic, joint and bone pains. There are other, rare, ophthalmological, neurological, rheumatological and gastrointestinal signs.

Between 50 and 70% of all cases of primary hyperparathyroidism present with hypercalcaemia. This is asymptomatic, so most cases are identified incidentally following blood analyses. Most of the remaining individuals present with renal calculi.

Specific investigations

Blood samples for calcium and PTH levels are taken. Twenty-four-hour urine samples may also show high calcium levels. X-ray studies may be undertaken to ascertain whether there are skeletal signs. Visualization of the parathyroid glands themselves, to ascertain whether an adenoma or general hyperplasia of the glands is present, is difficult regardless of the radiological technique used and is not always performed.

Medical and surgical management

Surgery is the treatment of choice for primary hyperparathyroidism. The treatment of a single parathyroid adenoma is removal of the adenoma, leaving normal parathyroid tissue in the other three glands. If hyperplasia is the cause of the hyperparathyroidism, three and a half glands are removed. Parathyroid surgery can be difficult as the glands are usually the size of a lentil, although experienced surgeons have a success rate of approximately 95% (Nussey & Whitehead 2001).

Those who have only mild hypercalcaemia and no symptoms may not require surgery; a high fluid intake is recommended to reduce the risk of developing renal calculi.

Bisphosphonates (pamidronate or alendronate), which inhibit bone resorption, may be given to the approximately 15% of those with bone involvement, although the effects are not long-term. Surgery is usually performed following symptom improvement,

▶ Nursing management

Apart from explanations about the nature of their condition, most of the nursing care of patients with hyperparathyroidism involves that required around the time of surgery.

Preoperatively, patients should be given explanations of what to expect following surgery and, if they wish, details of the surgery itself. Although this is most likely to be given by the medical staff, the nursing team may need to repeat the information.

Postoperative care following parathyroidectomy is similar to that given following thyroid surgery. As for thyroid surgery, patients must be observed for bleeding and airway obstruction due to compression of the trachea. In addition, they must be observed for signs of tetany (muscular spasms), which is common postoperatively in those with significant bone disease. Intravenous calcium is given in these circumstances, as well as vitamin D. Postoperative hypocalcaemia may persist for several days. Once hypocalcaemia is corrected, the tetany resolves.

An intravenous infusion will be in situ on return from surgery. Intravenous fluids are usually given for at least 24 hours. Fluid intake and output should be measured until patients are eating and drinking normally; the latter should be encouraged when they are fully conscious.

Postoperative observations of blood pressure, pulse, respiration rate and temperature should be performed and gradually reduced in frequency as patients recover. Analgesia should be given as necessary, and as prescribed.

Once patients have recovered from surgery, information about their medication needs to be given. Calcium and vitamin D may be required for some time. Discharge from hospital usually occurs 1–2 days postoperatively.

DISORDERS AFFECTING THE ADRENAL GLANDS

ADRENAL CORTEX INSUFFICIENCY

Primary adrenal insufficiency is known as Addison's disease. The adrenal cortex is destroyed, resulting in a lack of cortisol production and mineralocorticoids. It is usually easily diagnosed and treated but can be fatal if not recognized.

Secondary adrenal insufficiency is due to lack of stimulation of the adrenal glands as a result of pituitary or hypothalamic disease. The most common cause is trauma to the area following neurosurgery or resection of an ACTH producing tumour. Less commonly, the pituitary gland fails to produce ACTH, following infection, radiotherapy or haemorrhage. However, the most common cause of secondary adrenal insufficiency is sudden cessation of glucocorticoid treatment.

Aetiology and epidemiology

Autoimmune destruction of the adrenal cortex accounts for approximately 80% of Addison's disease; tuberculosis is responsible for between 7 and 20% of cases, with other infectious diseases, adrenal infarction or haemorrhage, drugs and metastatic cancer or lymphoma causing the rest. The prevalence of Addison's disease is approximately 35–60 cases per million people.

Clinical presentation

The signs and symptoms (see Box 17.8) of Addison's disease usually have a very slow onset, unless illness or other stress causes adrenal crisis. Those with an insidious onset of Addison's disease are likely to present with general fatigue and weakness and are likely to have noticed skin discoloration if it has

---

Box 17.8 Signs and symptoms of primary adrenal insufficiency

- Weakness, tiredness and fatigue
- Weight loss
- Anorexia
- Hyperpigmentation
- Vitiligo (patches of skin with complete loss of pigmentation)
- Hypotension
- Postural dizziness
- Hypoglycaemia
- Gastrointestinal symptoms – nausea, vomiting, constipation, abdominal pain, diarrhoea
- Salt craving
- Muscle or joint pains

occurred. Adrenal crisis usually presents as shock in previously undiagnosed Addison's disease, or in an individual who has not taken sufficiently increased amounts of replacement therapy during a concurrent illness. Other common symptoms of adrenal crisis are abdominal tenderness and fever.

Specific investigations

In patients who present with mild and chronic signs and symptoms, the basal serum cortisol and plasma ACTH levels are measured. An individual with primary adrenal insufficiency will have a low cortisol level and a high ACTH result. However, there is often a period of several weeks before the latter result is available.

Those presenting with adrenal crisis obviously need more urgent diagnosis. In this situation, the basal serum cortisol is measured and a short tetracosactide [tetracosactrin (Synacthen)] test is performed. Synthetic ACTH is administered intravenously or intramuscularly; plasma cortisol levels are measured after 30 and 60 minutes. In primary adrenal insufficiency, there would be no response, as endogenous ACTH levels are already high. A basal plasma ACTH measurement can also be performed but the result will not be immediately available.

Radiological investigations to determine the cause of the Addison's disease should be performed. For example, an abdominal CT scan can detect calcified adrenal glands, which suggests a non-autoimmune cause.

Medical management

The treatment of chronic primary adrenal insufficiency is replacement therapy with glucocorticoids. Hydrocortisone, prednisolone or dexamethasone may be used. Mineralocorticoids (fludrocortisone) also need to be replaced.

Adrenal crisis is managed by treating the shock with intravenous fluids, giving normal saline with dextrose if blood glucose levels are low (see Ch. 9). Intravenous hydrocortisone is given (after the short tetracosactide test if necessary) to replace glucocorticoids. The underlying illness also needs to be treated. Once stable, the glucocorticoids will be administered orally and mineralocorticoids introduced.

▶ Nursing management

Individuals with primary adrenal insufficiency require education about their disease and why they need replacement therapy. They also need to know how to manage minor illnesses in the context of increasing their corticosteroid doses and how to manage major illnesses. They should be advised to carry identification, such as a Medic-Alert card or bracelet, in the event of an emergency (see Health Promotion box 17.5). Patients are reminded about the importance of having an adequate supply of their medication, particularly over weekends and public holidays, and during periods spent away from home on business or holiday.

ADRENAL CORTEX HYPERSECRETION – CUSHING'S SYNDROME

Cushing's syndrome is a collection of signs and symptoms caused by excess cortisol. There are various causes of Cushing's

 HEALTH PROMOTION

17.5 Information for people undergoing corticosteroid ('steroids') treatment

To avoid acute adrenal insufficiency, individuals who have been taking steroid treatment (for any condition) for 3 weeks must be advised as follows:

- Never stop taking the medicine suddenly. The dose should be reduced gradually.
- Read the patient information leaflet that comes with your medicine.
- Carry a steroid treatment card at all times. Show it to anyone who treats you.
- Wear a Medic-Alert bracelet (or similar).
- Contact the GP urgently if you develop an illness or if you come into contact with a person with an infectious illness. If you have never had chickenpox, contact with people who have it, or shingles, should be avoided. If contact does occur, you should contact your doctor immediately.

(See the text for further information.)

syndrome but they fall into two broad categories: those that are ACTH-dependent and those that are ACTH-independent, i.e. excess cortisol is evident without raised ACTH levels.

Aetiology and epidemiology

Around 66–70% of all cases of ACTH-dependent Cushing's syndrome arise from Cushing's disease, which is caused by a pituitary tumour releasing excess ACTH. The other causes of ACTH-dependent Cushing's syndrome are ectopic tumours secreting ACTH and ectopic tumours which release excess amounts of corticotrophin-releasing hormone (CRH), the hormone normally produced in the hypothalamus that stimulates the pituitary gland to secrete ACTH.

ACTH-independent Cushing's syndrome is most commonly caused by exogenous administration of glucocorticoids (or 'steroids'), followed by adrenocortical adenomas and carcinomas, which account for 18–20% of Cushing's syndrome. Another, rarer, cause is bilateral micronodular dysplasia of the adrenal glands.

Apart from iatrogenic causes (due to treatment with glucocorticoids), the incidence of Cushing's syndrome is rare; however, precise figures are unavailable.

Pathophysiology and clinical presentation

The signs and symptoms of Cushing's syndrome are the result of chronic exposure to excess cortisol (see Box 17.9). Long-term excess cortisol gives rise to altered fat and carbohydrate metabolism, a compromised immune system and osteoporosis following decreased intestinal calcium absorption and bone formation. The causes of hypertension in Cushing's syndrome are uncertain.

Because there are so many signs and symptoms of Cushing's syndrome, people may present with any of these. However,

Box 17.9 Signs and symptoms of Cushing's syndrome

- Central obesity (with relatively thin arms and legs)
- 'Moon' face
- A 'buffalo hump' due to fat deposition at the back of the neck
- Thin hair
- Glucose intolerance
- Weakness, proximal myopathy or muscle weakness
- Hypertension
- Psychiatric changes – two-thirds have depression but psychosis may occur
- Easy bruising
- Abdominal striae (stretch marks)
- Thin skin – once damaged this is prone to infection and heals slowly
- Hyperpigmentation (excess ACTH production)
- Fungal infections of the skin
- Oligomenorrhoea or amenorrhoea
- Erectile dysfunction
- Ankle oedema
- Backache, vertebral collapse, loss of height, fractures (caused by osteoporosis)
- Exophthalmia (due to fat being deposited behind the eyes)
- Peptic ulcer
- Cataracts
- Hirsutism (excess androgen production)*
- Acne (excess androgen production)*

*In women the adrenal glands are the major source of androgens, so those with adrenal carcinomas may also be producing excess amounts of these hormones, giving rise to hirsutism and acne. Men with Cushing's syndrome do not show signs of androgen excess because their major source is in the testes.

they frequently present with skin problems, such as bruising, stretch marks and discoloration, which are not as attributable to other causes.

Specific investigations

Diagnosing the fundamental cause of Cushing's syndrome is extremely complex. Once exclusion of exogenous glucocorticoids intake has occurred, investigations to determine whether hyper-cortisolaemia is present take place. Twenty-four-hour urine samples are analysed for the presence of cortisol. Blood samples are taken at 9.00am and again at midnight to establish whether the normal diurnal rhythm of cortisol is present. A low-dose dexamethasone suppression test may be performed. In normal circumstances, cortisol secretion is suppressed by dexamethasone; in Cushing's syndrome this does not occur.

The diagnosis must differentiate between pseudo-Cushing's syndrome and true Cushing's syndrome. High cortisol levels in the blood can occur in patients who are physiologically stressed (e.g. by a severe bacterial infection), the severely obese, depressed patients and, rarely, those with chronic alcoholism. The last two are referred to as pseudo-Cushing's syndrome.

Once Cushing's syndrome has been confirmed, investigations are carried out to determine whether it is ACTH-dependent or not. The initial step is to measure plasma ACTH. Low ACTH levels in a patient with high cortisol levels indicates the ACTH-independent disease. The next diagnostic step is to undertake a scan (MRI or CT) of the adrenal glands to ascertain an adrenal tumour.

Those who have high ACTH levels should undergo a high-dose dexamethasone suppression test. If urinary cortisol excretion is suppressed, the diagnosis is Cushing's disease, i.e. a pituitary tumour. Investigations continue as for other pituitary tumours.

If cortisol excretion is not suppressed, further radiological investigations to find the ectopic tumour producing ACTH must be undertaken.

Medical and surgical management

Cushing's syndrome caused by exogenous glucocorticoid therapy is treated by withdrawal of the medication. However, this must be done gradually and under medical direction.

The treatment for Cushing's disease is trans-sphenoidal adenomectomy to remove the pituitary tumour (see treatment of pituitary tumours, p. 428). For those in whom pituitary surgery or irradiation has failed, bilateral adrenalectomy and replacement glucocorticoid and mineralocorticoid therapy are required.

Most tumours that secrete ACTH or CRH are not resectable. However, where this is possible, removal usually results in a cure. In inoperable cases, the excess cortisol can be controlled with adrenal enzyme inhibitors, such as metyrapone.

Those who have adrenal adenomas are cured following a unilateral adrenalectomy. However, carcinomas usually recur following surgery and the tumours do not generally respond to radiotherapy or chemotherapy.

The prognosis following treatment for Cushing's syndrome is generally good, unless the tumours are cancerous.

▶ Nursing management

Individuals with Cushing's syndrome require careful nursing, as they may be extremely unwell before treatment. A thorough assessment of the person's needs is essential prior to planning nursing care. The most common problems are discussed below.

The muscle weakness that is often evident frequently results in an inability to rise from a crouching position or mobilize for long periods. Some individuals may also need help in transferring from the bed to a chair. Providing assistance with positioning, mobilization and personal hygiene is likely to be necessary, as individuals will probably tire easily.

Some may also have suffered spontaneous fractures due to osteoporosis; careful positioning and handling are required as well as adequate pain relief prior to any period of sustained movement such as washing. Those with rib fractures may need encouragement to breathe deeply in order to reduce the risks of infection, which are unfortunately raised due to the compromised immune system. A physiotherapy referral may be required. When sitting, the legs should be elevated to reduce ankle oedema.

Four-hourly observations of temperature, pulse and respiration rate are therefore required, and any abnormalities should be reported to the medical staff immediately. The person is likely to be hypertensive; blood pressure should also be recorded 4-hourly.

The skin of a person with Cushing's syndrome is likely to be thin and fragile. Such people are very prone to wounds caused by skin 'shearing', making care of pressure areas essential, as well as extremely careful handling when being moved in bed. Additionally there is a risk of injury from the nails, watches and rings of carers. Any wounds present are prone to becoming infected and need to be dressed using an aseptic technique. The choice of adhesive dressings or tape is important in these circumstances, as they may damage the very thin skin when being removed. Where possible, light bandages are preferable.

Those with secondary diabetes should have their blood glucose levels measured 6-hourly and treatment given as prescribed. Bruising at injection sites is probable and the finest and shortest needles are required to reduce this.

The psychological effects of Cushing's syndrome may be profound; many people have depression and most will experience difficulties arising from the change in their body image. The hirsutism, acne, the 'buffalo' hump, abdominal striae and obesity all contribute to this. Reassurance that most of these features will resolve following treatment is required. Individuals also need time to talk about their feelings, as well as clear explanations of the investigations being carried out. Prior to surgery, explanations of the procedures, to reiterate those given by the medical staff, and information about what to expect postoperatively are necessary.

Care following adrenalectomy

Traditionally, adrenalectomy was performed using the open abdominal technique, necessitating a large incision close to the ribs. Breathing is painful after this procedure and there are subsequent risks of developing a chest infection postoperatively as well as the other complications associated with abdominal surgery (see Chs 22 and 29). Nowadays adrenalectomy is increasingly being performed using laparoscopic surgery. This is obviously less invasive surgery and patients consequently experience less stress and postoperative pain and may be discharged after 2–3 days in hospital (see Ch. 29 for more detailed information about postoperative care). Nurses should ensure that patients fully understand the importance of any replacement therapy with glucocorticoids and mineralocorticoids (see 'Adrenal cortex insufficiency', pp. 437–438).

PRIMARY ALDOSTERONISM

Primary aldosteronism is a condition in which excess amounts of aldosterone, a mineralocorticoid, are produced.

Aetiology and epidemiology

Primary aldosteronism is due to an aldosterone-producing adrenal adenoma (APA), otherwise known as Conn's syndrome (60%), an angiotensin II-responsive APA, primary adrenal hyperplasia, an aldosterone-producing adrenal carcinoma (3–5%) or glucocorticoid-suppressible hyperaldosteronism.

These conditions are all rare (Brook & Marshall 2001).

Pathophysiology and clinical presentation

Primary aldosteronism is generally asymptomatic, although some individuals have symptoms of hypokalaemia (low serum potassium level), such as muscle weakness, polyuria and polydipsia, and paraesthesia. Hypokalaemia is usually present and most patients are hypertensive.

The hypokalaemia is caused by aldosterone-induced retention of sodium by the kidney; it is exchanged for potassium, which is excreted in the urine. Most diagnoses of primary hyperaldosteronism are incidental.

Specific investigations

Plasma renin activity is measured; in primary aldosteronism it is low or undetectable. Twenty-four-hour urine samples may be tested for levels. Radiological tests may be performed to try to identify whether an adrenal adenoma is present.

Medical and surgical management

Medical therapy includes treatment with the aldosterone receptor agonist spironolactone or angiotensin II agonists such as losartan. Angiotensin-converting enzyme (ACE) inhibitors may also be used.

Surgical removal of adrenal tumours is a therapeutic option.

▶ Nursing management

The nurse's role in relation to medical therapy is to teach patients about their condition and how to take their treatment (in tablet form) appropriately. For the care required following adrenal surgery, see the section on Cushing's syndrome (above).

PHAEOCHROMOCYTOMA

A phaeochromocytoma is a tumour of the adrenal medulla that produces excess amounts of the catecholamine hormones, adrenaline (epinephrine) and noradrenaline (norepinephrine).

Aetiology and epidemiology

The aetiology of phaeochromocytomas is unknown; 80% of them are undiagnosed and discovered at postmortem (Nussey & Whitehead 2001). They are extremely rare, with an incidence of approximately 1 per million per year, and are usually benign. There is no gender difference in incidence. They can occur at any age, although the majority are diagnosed between the ages of 20 and 50 years.

Pathophysiology and clinical presentation

The symptoms and signs of a phaeochromocytoma all relate to the function of catecholamines. As these are released periodically, symptoms and signs tend to be paroxysmal and also rather non-specific. Cardiovascular problems include hypertension. Sudden postural drops may also occur. Headache, sweating and palpitations are often present. Episodes of pallor and paraesthesia may also occur. The individual may be anxious and suffer palpitations and panic attacks. About 90% of phaeochromocytomas are located in the adrenal glands; however, the remaining 10% occur outside the adrenal gland, in the sympathetic chain.

Patients usually present with hypertension and a history of unusual symptoms, as above. Most individuals investigated for a phaeochromocytoma do not have the disease.

Specific investigations

Three 24-hour urine collections are measured for vanillylmandelic acid (a breakdown product of catecholamine metabolism). A glucagon stimulation test may also be performed (catecholamine secretion from a phaeochromocytoma is increased by glucagon). Once the diagnosis is confirmed, radiological studies to ascertain the location of the tumour are performed.

Medical/surgical management

The only cure for phaeochromocytoma is surgery. However, initial medical treatment is designed to reduce the risks of acute catecholamine release during the operative procedure. This treatment is usually α-adrenergic blockade, e.g. phenoxybenzamine, followed by combined α- and β-adrenergic blockade, e.g. labetalol.

▶ Nursing management

As with other endocrine diseases, patients need clear explanations of their condition and symptoms. People with phaeochromocytomas may be anxious, and relieving this where at all possible is desirable.

For care required during the perioperative phase, see the section on Cushing's syndrome (above).

ADRENAL SEXUAL DISORDERS: CONGENITAL ADRENAL HYPERPLASIA

Congenital adrenal hyperplasia (CAH) refers to a group of disorders characterized by excessive secretion of adrenal androgens.

Aetiology and epidemiology

Due to a deficiency in one of the enzymes involved in their synthesis, cortisol and aldosterone are unable to be metabolized correctly in the adrenal glands. The precursors to these hormones are used for androgen production instead. Due to stimulation of ACTH, the adrenal glands enlarge. The condition, which has various forms, is inherited and affects approximately 1 in 10 000 people in the UK.

Pathophysiology and clinical presentation

The effects of excess androgen synthesis result in virilization. In males it may not be noticed, but in severe forms females develop external male sexual characteristics. Clitoral hypertrophy may occur, as well as fusion of the labial folds. In some instances, the child may be identified incorrectly as a male. Problems that may occur in later life are primary amenorrhoea, precocious puberty, and short stature from early fusing of the epiphyses of the long bones.

The lack of glucocorticoids may lead to adrenal crisis.

In severe cases, the condition is usually evident at birth. Late-onset forms of the condition may result in precocious sexual development in boys, or virilization in females.

Specific investigations

Blood tests to ascertain ACTH levels (which will be high) and the precursors of corticosteroid production will be performed. An ACTH stimulation test may be carried out.

Medical/surgical management

Treatment is with glucocorticoids and mineralocorticoids. These hormones suppress the production of androgens. Some female babies may need plastic surgery to correct the labial fusion.

▶ Nursing management

People with CAH need information about taking their medicines correctly (see Health Promotion box 17.5, p. 438). They may also need psychological support and specialist counselling, especially if the diagnosis was not made in infancy. Possible difficulties, particularly for young women, include body image problems and fears about sexual activity.

SUMMARY: MAIN POINTS

- Although many 'pure' endocrine disorders are not often encountered by nurses, it is important for them to have some knowledge about these conditions in case they come across individuals who live with them. It can also be intellectually stimulating; endocrinology knowledge is increasing rapidly and it is a fascinating area of health care.

- Diabetes, however, is extremely common and is becoming more so. Nurses are likely to meet more and more people with it.

- Nurses have a vital health promotion role in the prevention of type 2 diabetes.

- It is incumbent upon all nurses, not just those who specialize in diabetes care, to deliver high-quality care and endeavour to remain up to date with their diabetes knowledge.

- The prevention of diabetes complications and screening that aims to detect complications at an early stage are important elements of holistic individualized nursing care.

- Keeping up to date means staying abreast of not only the 'scientific' aspects of care, but also the issues surrounding quality of care and new ways of working in partnership with people with diabetes in order to help them to manage and live effectively with it.

- Diabetes care is undergoing great change; this, and the fact that diabetes nursing can encompass physical care of every system of the body, as well as educational activities and psychological care in all clinical settings, makes it an exciting and rewarding area to work in.

SELF-TEST: CRITICAL THINKING ACTIVITIES

1 Look at a nursing care plan for a person with diabetes in your clinical setting. Using a model or framework for guided reflection (Gibbs 1988, Johns 1996) consider the following questions in relation to diabetes issues:
   — Does the care plan address physical, social, psychological and educational needs?
   — Has existing knowledge and practice of diabetes self-management been evaluated?
   — Have the goals been negotiated?
   — Has the rationale for each nursing action been included?
   — Have the diabetes specialist nursing team been involved in the patient's care?
   — Do they need to be?
   — How different would your care plan look? Why?

2 Thelma (not her real name) has just been diagnosed as having hypothyroidism. She is 45 years of age and is married with two children. Her youngest child is 13 years old and

the oldest is 19. He has recently left home. Thelma works as a care assistant in a local nursing home. She tells you that she is worried she may lose her job; she keeps forgetting things lately and can tell the nursing home manager is getting fed up with her. She also says that she is slower than she used to be and can't get her work done as quickly as she used to. Thelma suddenly bursts into tears. She is somewhat incoherent, but you gather that she is feeling unattractive because she has put on weight and has dry skin. She tells you that she was a size 10 and her husband used to tell her that her hair was her crowning glory (it is now very dry and coarse). She also says her sex life is non-existent because she is 'too tired to bother'.

Using a recognized model of nursing, e.g. the Roper et al (1996) Activities of Daily Living model, or Orem's (1995) self-care model, devise a nursing care plan for Thelma, giving a rationale for all your nursing actions.

 FURTHER READING

Anderson BL, Rubin RR. Practical psychology for diabetes clinicians. Effective techniques for key behavioural issues, 2nd edn. Alexandria, Virginia: American Diabetes Association; 2000.

Anderson B, Funnell M. The art of empowerment: stories and strategies for diabetes educators. Alexandria, Virginia: American Diabetes Association; 2000.

Audit Commission. Testing times: a review of the diabetes services in England and Wales. London: Audit Commission; 2000.

Hiscock J, Snape R, Legard D. Listening to diabetes service users: qualitative findings for the Diabetes National Service Framework. London: National Centre for Social Research; 2001.

Krentz AJ, Bailey CJ. Type 2 diabetes in practice. London: Royal Society of Medicine Press; 2001.

Naqib J. Patient education for effective diabetes self-management: report, recommendations and examples of good practice. London: Diabetes UK; 2002.

Sinclair AJ, Finucane P. Diabetes in old age, 2nd edn. Chichester: John Wiley; 2002.

Williams G, Pickup JC. Handbook of diabetes, 2nd edn. Oxford: Blackwell Science; 1999.

Useful journals

Diabetes Digest. London: SB Communications Group.
Diabetes and Primary Care. London: SB Communications Group.
Journal of Diabetes Nursing. London: SB Communications Group.
Practical Diabetes International. Chichester: John Wiley.

 USEFUL WEBSITES

www.diabetes.audit-commission.gov.uk – Audit Commission (diabetes)
www.desg.org – Diabetes Education Study Group (DESG) of the European Association for the Study of Diabetes (EASD)
www.doh.gov.uk/nsf/diabetes – Diabetes National Service Framework

www.diabetes.org.uk – Diabetes UK
www.nelh.nhs.uk – National Electronic Branch Library for Diabetes
www.nice.org.uk – National Institute for Clinical Excellence
www.pituitary.org.uk/resources/di.shtml – The Pituitary Foundation

REFERENCES

Amos AF, McCarty DJ, Zimmet P. The rising global burden of diabetes and its complications. Diabetic Med 1997; 14: S7–S85.

Bantle JP, Neal L, Frankamp LM. Effects of the anatomical region used for insulin injections on glycaemia in type 1 diabetes. Diabetes Care 1993; 16: 1592–1597.

Brook CGD, Marshall NJ. Essential endocrinology. Oxford: Blackwell Science; 2001.

Browne DL, Avery, L, Turner BC, Kerr D, Cavan DA. What do patients with diabetes know about their tablets? Diabetic Med 2000; 17: 528–531.

Currie CJ, Kraus D, Morgan CLI, Gill L, Stott NCH, Peters JR. NHS acute sector expenditure for diabetes: the present, future and excess in-patient cost of care. Diabetic Med 1997; 14(8): 686–692.

Department of Health. National Service Framework for Diabetes: Standards. London: DoH; 2001.

Department of Health. National Service Framework for Diabetes: Delivery Stategy. London: DoH; 2003. OnLine. Available: www.doh.gov.uk/nsf/diabetes/delivery.

Diabetes Control and Complications Trial Research Group (DCCT). The effect of intensive treatment of diabetes on the development and progression of long-term complications in insulin-dependent diabetes mellitus. N Engl J Med 1993; 329(14): 977–986.

Diabetes Prevention Program Research Group. Reduction in the incidence of type 2 diabetes with lifestyle intervention or metformin. N Engl J Med 2002; 346(6): 393–403.

Drucquer MH, McNally PG. Diabetes management: step by step. Oxford: Blackwell Science; 1998.

Fox C, MacKinnon M. Vital diabetes. London: Class Publishing; 1999.

Gibbs G. Learning by doing: a guide to teaching and learning methods. Oxford: Further Education Unit, Oxford Brooks University; 1988.

Glasgow RE, Toobert DJ, Gillette CD. Psychosocial barriers to diabetes self-management and quality of life. Diabetes Spectrum 2001; 14(1): 33–41.

Ha TKK, Lean MEJ. Technical review: recommendations for the nutritional management of patients with diabetes mellitus. Eur J Clin Nutr 1998; 52: 467–481.

Jerreat L. Diabetes for nurses. London: Whurr Publishers; 1999.

Johns C. Using a reflective model of nursing and guided reflection. Nurs Stand 1996; 11(2): 34–38.

Kanis JA. Disorders of calcium metabolism. In: Weatherall DJ, Ledingham JGG, Warrell DA, eds. Oxford textbook of medicine, 3rd edn. Oxford: Oxford University Press; 1996.

McCarthy JA, Covarrubias B, Sink P. Is the traditional alcohol wipe necessary before an insulin injection? Diabetes Care 1993; 16(1): 402.

McGregor AM. The thyroid gland and disorders of the thyroid. In: Weatherall DJ, Ledingham JGG, Warrell DA, eds. Oxford textbook of medicine, 3rd edn. Oxford: Oxford University Press; 1996.

National Institute for Clinical Excellence. Management of type 2 diabetes: management of blood glucose. London: NICE; 2002 (Also online. Available: at www.nice.org.uk).

Nussey SS, Whitehead SA. Endocrinology: an integrated approach. Oxford: BIOS Scientific Publishers; 2001.

Orem DE. Nursing: concepts and practice, 5th edn. St Louis: Mosby; 1995.

Roper N, Logan W, Tierney A. The elements of nursing, 4th edn. Edinburgh: Churchill Livingstone; 1996.

Strauss AL, Corbin J, Fagerhaugh S et al. Chronic illness and the quality of life, 2nd edn. St Louis; CV Mosby; 1984.

Thorner MO. Anterior pituitary disorders. In: Weatherall DJ, Ledingham JGG, Warrell DA, eds. Oxford textbook of medicine, 3rd edn. Oxford: Oxford University Press; 1996.

Tuomilehto J, Lindstrom J, Eriksson JG et al (for the Finnish Diabetes Prevention Study). Prevention of type 2 diabetes mellitus by changes in lifestyle among subjects with impaired glucose tolerance. N Engl J Med 2001; 344(18): 1343–1350.

UK Prospective Diabetes Study (UKPDS) Group. Tight blood pressure control and risk of macrovascular and microvascular complications in type 2 diabetes: UKPDS 38. Br Med J 1998a; 317: 703–726.

UK Prospective Diabetes Study (UKPDS) Group. Intensive blood-glucose control with sulphonylureas or insulin compared with conventional treatment and risk of complications in patients with type 2 diabetes. (UKPDS 33). Lancet 1998b; 352(9131): 837–853.

Williams G, Pickup JC. Handbook of diabetes, 2nd edn. Oxford: Blackwell Science; 1999.

World Health Organization. World health report 1997. Geneva: WHO; 1997.

World Health Organization. Department of Noncommunicable Disease Surveillance. Definition, diagnosis and classification of diabetes mellitus and its complications. Geneva: WHO; 1999.

18 Nursing patients with blood disorders

Linda Bywater, Elizabeth Rawlings

> 'I was really worried about having a blood transfusion – well you read such a lot of scare stories about catching things or getting the wrong blood or something. When I mentioned this to the nurse he was really nice and said that the risks of catching anything were very low. He also explained what they do to make sure you get the right blood. He even offered to get the haematologist to come and see me if I was still worried.'
>
> *(Patient)*

THIS CHAPTER WILL HELP YOU

- Understand the structure and function of the haematological system
- Carry out a general assessment of a haematology patient
- Describe the national guidelines for the safe administration of blood products
- Understand the management of the main transfusion reactions
- Plan nursing care for patients with a range of haematological conditions
- Describe the side-effects of haematological treatments and identify care priorities.

KEYWORDS

Anaemia	Haemostasis
Apheresis	Leukaemia
Bone marrow biopsy	Lymphoma
Central venous catheters	Monoclonal antibody
Differentiation	Mucositis
Haemoglobinopathy	Myeloma
Haemolysis	Neutropenia
Haemopoiesis	Pancytopenia
Haemopoietic growth factors	Stem cell
Haemopoietic stem cell transplantation	Thrombocytopenia
	Tumour lysis syndrome

INTRODUCTION

Nursing patients with blood disorders is a highly specialised and extremely challenging field of practice. Patient-centred care and support from nurses working alongside other members of the multidisciplinary team are essential in this varied specialty. Patients may present with acute and potentially life-threatening disorders such as acute leukaemia, or lifelong conditions such as sickle cell disease that can seriously affect daily living. As a result, patients and their families often face huge physical, psychological and social challenges. In such circumstances, there are many opportunities for nurses to provide truly holistic care. This may clearly be of great value to patients and their families. It can also be highly satisfying for the nurse.

OVERVIEW: ANATOMY AND PHYSIOLOGY

The haematological system consists of the blood and the bone marrow. Blood is a thick, red fluid that circulates within the vascular system. It consists of blood cells suspended in a fluid called plasma. Normal blood volume is around 5 L. The functions of blood are summarized below:

- Transportation
  - oxygen from the lungs to the tissues for cellular respiration
  - nutrients from the gut to the tissues
  - waste products of metabolism from the tissues for excretion by the lungs, kidneys and liver
  - hormones from the endocrine glands to target organs, other chemicals and drugs
- Regulation
  - body temperature
  - normal pH
  - fluid volume
- Defence
  - against infection
  - coagulation to prevent excessive blood loss.

PLASMA

Plasma accounts for 45% of the blood volume. It is a straw-coloured fluid composed of water and dissolved substances, including plasma proteins, clotting factors, hormones, electrolytes, gases, nutrients and cellular waste products. Albumin, the most abundant plasma protein, plays an important role in maintaining the circulating plasma volume. Plasma that has had the clotting factors removed is called serum.

BLOOD CELLS

There are three main types of blood cell: red cells (erythrocytes), white cells (leucocytes) and platelets (thrombocytes). All have distinctive roles and functions.

Red cells

Red cells are the most numerous of the blood cells ($3.8–6.5 \times 10^{12}$/L) and give blood its characteristic colour. The main function of red cells is to transport oxygen and some carbon dioxide. Red cells are biconcave, non-nucleated discs; this shape provides the maximum surface area for gas absorption and exchange. They are also very flexible, which enables them to pass through blood vessels with a diameter half that of a red cell. Red cells contain the molecule haemoglobin, which consists of four globin chains (two alpha chains and two beta chains), each surrounding an iron-containing haem group. Haemoglobin readily binds with oxygen when it is in an oxygen-rich environment such as the lungs. Conversely, haemoglobin releases oxygen in an oxygen-poor environment, such as the body tissues. By this mechanism, oxygen is transported from the lungs to the tissues for cellular respiration. As body tissues take up oxygen, they release carbon dioxide. This is transported to the lungs for excretion either as bicarbonate ions in the plasma or combined with the haemoglobin. The haemoglobin molecule also helps to prevent changes in pH by acting as a buffer.

Iron is an essential component of haemoglobin. In fact, haemoglobin contains most of the body's iron – approximately 3 g in total. A small quantity of iron is also stored within the muscles, liver and spleen. Iron is efficiently recycled by the body when red cells reach the end of their normal life span of around 120 days. However, some iron is lost as a result of normal growth and development, during menstruation in females, and in faeces. This can generally be replaced by eating iron-rich foods such as red meat, offal and green vegetables. Other nutrients that are essential for the production of healthy red cells include vitamin B_{12}, folic acid, protein and copper (Ch. 11).

White cells

The normal white cell count is around $4.0–11.0 \times 10^9$/L. White cells function as a defence against infection and in surveillance for abnormal cells such as cancer. White cells are nucleated and may be classified as myeloid cells or lymphocytes.

Myeloid cells

Myeloid white cells can be further subdivided into neutrophils, eosinophils, basophils and monocytes. All except monocytes may also be classified as granulocytes, due to the presence of granules in the cytoplasm. Neutrophils, eosinophils and basophils are sometimes known collectively as polymorphonuclear white cells.

Neutrophils are the most numerous, contributing about 40–70% of the total number of white cells ($2.5–7.5 \times 10^9$/L). Neutrophils provide a first line of defence in many infections but are relatively short-lived. Neutrophils help to control infection by ingesting and destroying pathogens, a process known as phagocytosis. They are attracted to a site of an infection by substances released by infected or damaged cells. Huge numbers of neutrophils can congregate at a site of infection forming pus.

Eosinophils account for less than 5% of the total white cell count ($0.04–0.4 \times 10^9$/L). They are activated in response to allergic disorders, such as asthma (Ch. 20), eczema (Ch. 28) and hay fever, or parasitic diseases.

Basophils make up less than 1% of the white cell count ($0.01–0.1 \times 10^9$/L) and play a role in hypersensitivity reactions.

Monocytes form 2–10% of white cells. As they mature, they move out of the bloodstream and into body tissues where they become macrophages. Macrophages can destroy pathogens by phagocytosis and can enhance the immune response. They also remove and break down ageing or damaged blood cells (mononuclear–macrophage system).

Lymphocytes

Lymphocytes form around 30–40% of the total white cell count in the peripheral bloodstream ($1.5–3.0 \times 10^9$/L). Large numbers are also found within the lymph nodes. Lymphocytes can be subdivided into T cells and B cells.

T cells mature in the thymus gland where they are 'educated' to react with foreign antigens rather than body cells (Mehta & Hoffbrand 2000). They play an important role in cell-mediated immunity.

B cells mature in the bone marrow. Some B cells differentiate into plasma cells that produce immunoglobulins and play an important role in humoral immunity.

Platelets

Platelets are small fragments of much larger cells called megakaryocytes. They are formed in the bone marrow and play a vital role in the clotting process (see p. 448). The normal platelet count is around $150–400 \times 10^9$/L.

BLOOD GROUPS

An individual's blood group is determined by the presence or absence of specific proteins, or antigens, on the surface of red cells. The two major blood group classifications are the ABO system and the rhesus system. Many other blood groups have been identified but they are less clinically significant.

ABO system

There are four main blood groups: A, B, AB and O. The ABO system is based on two antigens, A and B, which are carried on the surface of red cells. An individual's blood group is determined by the inheritance of these antigens. People with antigen A are blood group A and those with antigen B are group B. Those who have both A and B antigens are group AB. Individuals who have neither antigen are group O. Certain blood groups can predominate in different racial populations (Table 18.1).

Table 18.1 ABO blood groups in the UK (Caucasians)

Blood group	Percentage
O	47
A	42
B	8
AB	3

Individuals who are blood group A will have anti-B antibodies in their plasma. Conversely, those who are group B will have anti-A antibodies. Those with blood group O will possess both anti-A and anti-B. People with group AB will possess neither antibody. Antibodies (immunoglobulins) are special proteins that circulate in plasma as part of the body's immune system. They target and bind to foreign antigens, which initiates an immune reaction and leads to the destruction of the targeted cell. Consequently, if a person with blood group A is transfused with group B blood, an incompatibility reaction will occur, causing haemolysis (breakdown of red cells). This can be life-threatening so it is essential that transfused blood is compatible with that of the recipient (see Table 18.2 and p. 452).

Table 18.2 ABO blood group compatibility

Recipient	Donor			
	A	B	AB	O
A	Yes	No	No	Yes
B	No	Yes	No	Yes
AB	Yes	Yes	Yes	Yes
O	No	No	No	Yes

Rhesus system

Rhesus antigens may also be found on the surface of red blood cells. Those who have rhesus antigens are termed Rh(D)-positive and those without are Rh(D)-negative. People who are Rh(D)-negative do not naturally produce anti-rhesus (anti-D) antibodies. Anti-D will be formed if the Rh(D)-negative person is transfused with Rh(D)-positive blood. A second transfusion could therefore cause an incompatibility reaction. In a similar way, an Rh(D)-negative woman who carries an Rh(D)-positive fetus may develop anti-D. During a second or subsequent pregnancy with an Rh(D)-positive fetus, the anti-D antibodies may cause haemolysis of fetal blood cells, leading to haemolytic disease of the newborn, which can cause intrauterine death. Anti-D can be given to Rh(D)-negative women to prevent sensitization of the immune system. This is usually administered within 72 hours of sensitizing events such as labour, miscarriage or bleeding during pregnancy.

HAEMOPOIESIS

In the fetus, blood cell formation, or haemopoiesis, commences in the yolk sac, liver and spleen. Towards the end of pregnancy, the bone marrow becomes the primary site for haemopoiesis and blood cell formation occurs in all bones. During childhood much of this active red marrow is replaced by fat; it is then termed yellow marrow. By adulthood, the red haemopoietic marrow is confined to the pelvis, vertebrae, sternum and the ends of the long bones.

Red marrow consists of a mesh of bony strands containing a thick, red, jelly-like substance. It comprises fat cells, small blood vessels and immature blood cells. Pluripotent stem cells are found within the red marrow. Stem cells have the ability to self-replicate but they can also differentiate into mature blood cells. A single stem cell can differentiate through several stages to become any type of blood cell (Fig. 18.1).

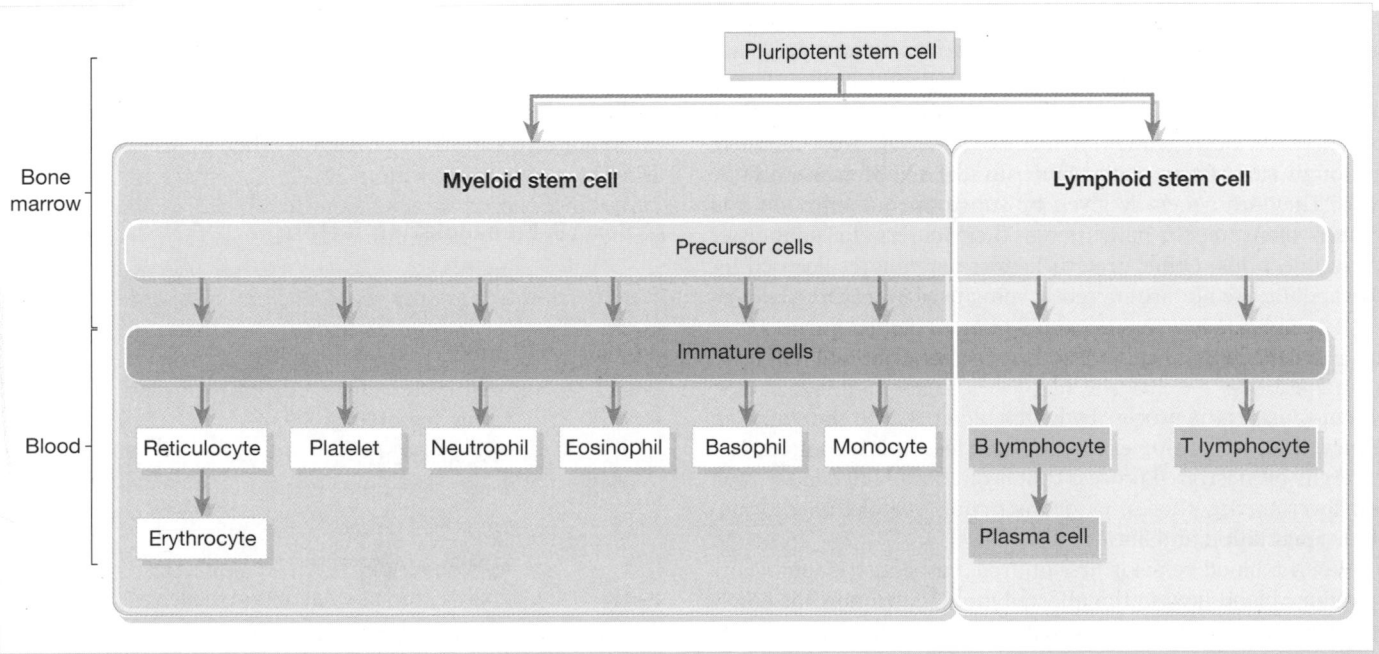

Figure 18.1 Haemopoiesis.

Table 18.3 Haemopoietic growth factors

Growth factor	Target cell
Erythropoietin	Red cell precursors
Thrombopoietin	Platelet precursors
Granulocyte colony-stimulating factor (G-CSF)	Granulocyte precursors
Granulocyte-macrophage colony stimulating factor (GM-CSF)	Myeloid and macrophage precursors
Stem cell factor (SCF)	Stem cells
Interleukin-3	Myeloid and platelet precursors
Interleukin-6	Platelet and B-cell precursors

The bone marrow is a highly active organ producing about 3 000 000 cells every second. Normal haemopoiesis requires sufficient supplies of energy, protein, vitamins and minerals. It is regulated by a series of growth factors that act upon the stem cells and cause them to differentiate into specific cell types. Growth factors can also speed up the maturation process. Many growth factors have been isolated and some are used therapeutically to enhance specific blood cell production (Table 18.3).

Erythropoietin (EPO) stimulates red cell production; it is produced in the kidneys and levels are regulated by oxygen concentrations in the blood. Recombinant (genetically engineered) forms are now available to treat patients with chronic anaemia secondary to bone marrow dysfunction or cytotoxic therapy (Ch. 33). It is also used for patients with chronic renal failure (Ch. 24).

Granulocyte colony-stimulating factor (G-CSF) and granulocyte-macrophage colony stimulating factor (GM-CSF) stimulate the production of white blood cells and can be used therapeutically to accelerate white blood cell regeneration following haemopoietic stem cell transplantation (bone marrow transplantation) (see p. 474). They can also limit the period of neutropenia (reduced neutrophil count) following cytotoxic chemotherapy (see p. 470). Both growth factors are generally well tolerated, although side-effects can include flu-like symptoms and bone pain. They are generally given by subcutaneous injection and nurses often teach patients or their carers to administer these injections. Other growth factors are not yet licensed for therapeutic use but are currently being used in research.

HAEMOSTASIS

Haemostasis is the process by which blood clots at the site of an injury, thus preventing excessive blood loss. It is a complex and carefully orchestrated process that is often explained in terms of four overlapping phases: vasoconstriction, platelet plug formation, coagulation and fibrinolysis.

When a blood vessel is first injured, vasoconstriction occurs to reduce blood flow to the affected area. Platelets immediately begin to adhere to the damaged endothelium, and swell and aggregate around the site of injury. This creates a primary haemostatic plug and temporarily halts blood loss. The intrinsic

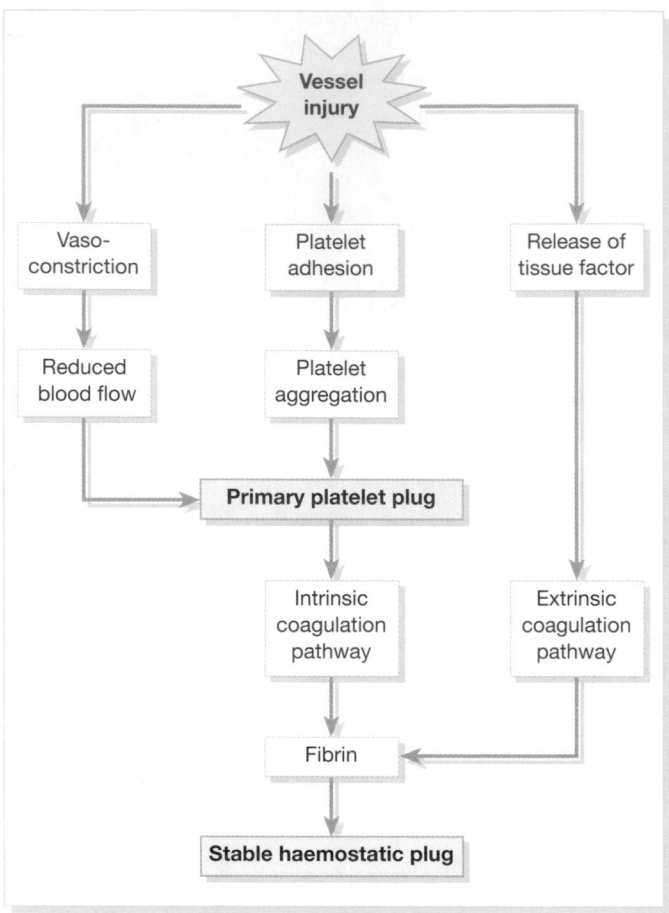

Figure 18.2 The coagulation process.

coagulation pathway is initiated when granules within the platelets break down and release chemical substances into the bloodstream, while substances released by the damaged endothelium initiate the extrinsic coagulation pathway. These pathways interconnect within the coagulation cascade (Fig. 18.2).

During the coagulation cascade, coagulation factors (Box 18.1) in the blood act sequentially to convert the plasma protein prothrombin into thrombin. Thrombin then converts the plasma

Box 18.1 Coagulation factors

I	Fibrinogen
II	Prothrombin
III	Tissue factor
IV	Calcium
V	Labile factor
VII	Proconvertin
VIII	Anti-haemophilic factor
IX	Christmas factor
X	Stuart–Prower factor
XI	Plasma thromboplastin antecedent
XII	Hageman factor
XIII	Fibrin stabilizing factor

protein fibrinogen into fibrin, a durable substance that reinforces the primary platelet plug to form a more stable haemostatic plug. A feedback mechanism exists to limit clot formation to the area of damage after coagulation has been established. Once formed, fibrin absorbs thrombin to halt the coagulation process. As tissue damage is repaired, the fibrinolytic system is activated to dissolve the clot.

Blood clots or thrombi can form inappropriately within blood vessels when no vascular injury has occurred. Thrombus formation can be triggered by various factors, including blood stasis due to poor venous return from lower extremities and the build-up of atheromatous plaques within vessels. Haematological disorders associated with very high blood viscosity, e.g. polycythaemia (see p. 459), can also predispose to thrombus formation. Thrombi can restrict blood flow to a body area or cause complete occlusion of a vessel. Part of a thrombus can break off and circulate in the bloodstream; this is termed an embolus. Emboli can become lodged in small blood vessels of the lungs (Ch. 20), heart or brain and cause tissue ischaemia and infarction (Chs 19 and 14).

GENERAL NURSING ASSESSMENT

Haematology disorders are highly varied so a basic understanding of the patient's underlying condition is a necessary prerequisite for skilled nursing assessment. Nurses should also be aware of recent blood tests or laboratory results and should understand their significance. This will help them to ascertain whether patients are anaemic or at particular risk of infection or bleeding. The monitoring of vital signs is also necessary, as people with haematological disorders can be at increased risk of serious complications such as haemorrhage or septic shock (Ch. 9). Medical advice should always be sought if patients are hypotensive, tachycardic or pyrexial. Other problems that are often associated with haematological disorders include anxiety, fatigue, anorexia and pain. Before considering how these factors might be assessed, it is worth pointing out that in clinical haematology, as in many other disciplines, patient care and assessment are often combined as a joint undertaking involving many members of the multidisciplinary team. For this reason, nurses should appreciate the roles of other team members and be able to enlist their input wherever appropriate.

ANXIETY

When assessing a patient's level of anxiety, nurses should aim to create an environment that will maximize the exchange of information (Ch. 3). Privacy and comfort are clearly important in this context, as is a respectful approach. Because it is vital to gain an understanding of patients' own perspectives, the use of open questioning is particularly appropriate. This can elicit valuable information about the effects of illness upon the daily lives of patients and those around them. It can also provide insight into patients' coping strategies and their existing support networks. It should be remembered, however, that gathering such information can take time – patients may not reveal their main anxieties at a first meeting. Much may depend upon the gradual development of the nurse–patient relationship.

Moreover, difficult and intense issues may come to light, particularly if patients are facing life-threatening illnesses. Nurses must therefore be both sensitive to patients' needs and aware of their own limitations. It is often preferable for the inexperienced nurse to draw things to a close and enlist the help of more experienced team members than to persist with an assessment if patients appear distressed. Occasionally, patients may also be referred to a trained nurse-counsellor or psycho-oncologist for further assessment.

FATIGUE

Fatigue can dramatically affect physical activity and mental function. Fatigue may result from physical factors, such as loss of appetite, nausea, anaemia, pain and malignancy, or psychological causes, e.g. anxiety and depression. It can also be a persistent side-effect of certain treatments, e.g. chemotherapy or radiotherapy. Assessing the underlying cause is therefore important. A baseline assessment of the extent of the fatigue and the person's ability to maintain normal activities should also be made. This can assist the joint planning and evaluation of care and support interventions and the setting of achievable goals.

SKIN AND MUCOSA

An observation of skin condition is another important part of any nursing assessment (Ch. 28). This can provide information regarding patients' nutritional state (Ch. 11), the presence of infection and haemorrhagic tendencies – particularly if there are signs such as dryness, pallor, flushing, inflammation, jaundice, bruising or petechiae (small red spots caused by bleeding under the skin or mucous membranes). The presence of more generalized rashes may indicate infection or drug reactions. Infected skin lesions can be a serious complication in people who are severely immunocompromised as a result of disease or its treatment (Ch. 33). The skin around indwelling central venous catheters should also be observed for signs of infection or bleeding.

Similarly, the patient's mouth should be assessed for inflammation, ulceration or bleeding (Ch. 22). Inflammation of the oral or gastrointestinal mucosa (mucositis) can be a significant problem for haematological patients who have impaired immunity. Mucositis can cause severe pain, loss of appetite and can increase the risk of systemic infection. A number of oral assessment tools are available to help with this type of assessment. Patients should also be asked about any changes in bowel habit, as both diarrhoea and constipation are common treatment side-effects that can produce considerable knock-on effects in terms of anorexia, discomfort, anxiety and fatigue.

APPETITE

It can be useful to ask patients about their nutritional intake and any recent weight loss. Anorexia or loss of appetite can be a side-effect of haematological treatments or psychological distress. Unexplained weight loss may be associated with certain haematological malignancies, e.g. lymphoma (see p. 469). In some circumstances it may be helpful to refer the patient to a dietician or specialist nutrition nurse who can provide more detailed nutritional assessment and advice (Ch. 11).

PAIN

Pain can accompany many haematological disorders and may be acute or chronic, depending on the underlying condition. The characteristics, site and intensity of pain should be assessed and then regularly monitored in order to evaluate the efficacy of treatment. Pain assessment tools can be helpful in this context as they provide a patient-centred approach to pain management (Ch. 7). Pain assessment and control require a multidisciplinary approach. Medical staff may clearly assess the need for analgesia – although monitoring the effects of this and ensuring that the most effective analgesia is prescribed may require joint assessment and input from medical staff, nurses and patients. In some instances it can be useful to enlist the help of specialist pain relief teams or palliative care teams (Ch. 34) who possess particular expertise in symptom control. Other professionals, such as physiotherapists or occupational therapists, may provide assessment and care interventions to enable patients to cope with chronic pain such as that associated with haemophilia or myeloma.

DIAGNOSTIC TESTS

Patient assessment and treatment decisions must clearly be informed by accurate diagnosis of the underlying condition. In haematology, blood testing and bone marrow sampling often guide the process of diagnosis.

BLOOD TESTS

Most haematological tests are carried out on venous blood samples. Nurses using simple venepuncture techniques frequently obtain samples.

Full blood count
A full blood count (FBC) provides the following information:

- haemoglobin and red cell count
- haematocrit or packed cell volume (PCV) – the percentage blood volume comprising red cells
- mean cell volume (MCV) or size of red cells
- white cell count
- differential counts for neutrophils, eosinophils, basophils, lymphocytes, monocytes
- platelet count
- reticulocyte count.

Reticulocytes are immature, nucleated red cells; they normally account for 1% of red cells in the peripheral blood. The reticulocyte count can give an indication of bone marrow activity in anaemic patients. Reticulocytes increase at times of rapid red cell production.

Blood film
Blood films are used in the diagnosis and monitoring of a wide range of haematological conditions. A blood sample is spread on a slide and viewed under a microscope. This allows assessment of the size and shape (morphology) of blood cells.

Erythrocyte sedimentation rate
Erythrocyte sedimentation rate (ESR) measures the rate at which columns of red cells fall in a capillary tube. The rate is determined by the concentration of proteins dissolved in the plasma. A raised ESR can indicate an inflammatory disorder, infection, anaemia or malignancy.

Coagulation screen
The coagulation screen measures:

- prothrombin time (PT) – assesses the extrinsic coagulation pathway. It is prolonged in people having warfarin therapy, in those with liver disease where the normal production of coagulation factors is inhibited, and in disseminated intravascular coagulation (DIC) (Ch. 9)
- activated partial thromboplastin time (APTT) – assesses the intrinsic coagulation pathway. It is prolonged in heparin therapy, haemophilia A, liver disease and DIC
- international normalized ratio (INR) – measures the PT of the patient compared with a standard.

Coombs' test or direct antiglobulin test
A positive Coombs' test or direct antiglobulin test (DAT) indicates the presence of red cell antibodies. It is used to diagnose red cell haemolysis.

BONE MARROW SAMPLING

Bone marrow sampling or biopsy is a diagnostic procedure that is increasingly being carried out by specialist haematology nurses. Sampling of the bone marrow can take two forms: bone marrow aspirate and trephine (Fig. 18.3A). Samples are usually taken from the posterior iliac crest (Fig. 18.3B). This procedure is very quick but it can be uncomfortable and some patients may prefer to be sedated with short-acting benzodiazepines such as midazolam or to inhale nitrous oxide and oxygen.

Prior to sampling, nurses should ensure that patients both understand and are fully prepared for the procedure. For both types of sampling, the surrounding skin area is cleaned and a local anaesthetic, usually lidocaine (lignocaine), is injected. The bone marrow needle is inserted through the skin into the cortex of the bone, the stylet is removed and a syringe attached to the hub of the needle. Approximately 0.5–1 mL of marrow is then aspirated into the syringe, which can cause a sharp pain for a few seconds. A bone marrow trephine uses a similar technique, but a core of bone and marrow is removed.

Patients who are sedated with short-acting benzodiazepines should be closely observed until they are fully recovered. Their respiratory rate and oxygen saturation levels (Chs 9, 20 and 31) should be monitored, as respiratory depression can occur. The puncture site should be observed for bleeding or inflammation, particularly if the patient has a low platelet count or white cell count, although bleeding is generally minimal. Following a bone marrow test, the patient may feel some discomfort. This can normally be relieved with a mild analgesic such as paracetamol.

A variety of tests can be performed on bone marrow. Aspirated marrow can be spread on a slide for analysis under a microscope. This enables an assessment to be made of the number and type of cells present. More sophisticated tests can

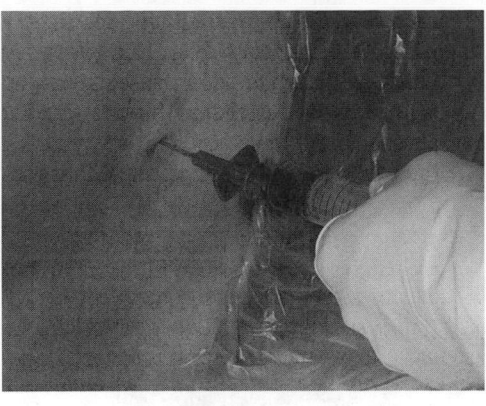

(A)

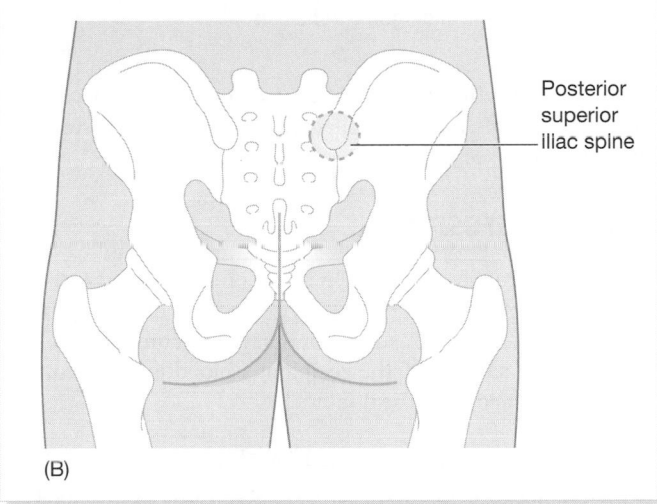

Posterior superior iliac spine

(B)

Figure 18.3 (A) Patient undergoing bone marrow sampling (biopsy). (B) Usual site for bone marrow sampling.

be used to identify specific malignant cells and abnormalities of the chromosomes or DNA.

BLOOD DONATION AND TRANSFUSION

In the UK, the National Blood Service manages all blood donations.

BLOOD DONATION

Donors must be healthy volunteers aged between 18 and 70 years, and prospective donors are screened through a detailed health questionnaire. The fitness to donate and the risk of transmitting an infection to the recipient are assessed. Donors' haemoglobin levels are also checked to ensure they are not anaemic. Additional factors that would preclude blood donation are:

- donation in the last 12 weeks
- weight less than 50 kg
- history of viral hepatitis
- visit to a malaria region within 12 months
- history of drug misuse
- membership of a high-risk group for HIV infection

- recent history of hypersensitivity
- pregnancy within 12 months
- tattoo or body piercing within 12 months
- recent immunization
- previous treatment with human pituitary extract (some growth hormone or fertility treatments before 1985)
- family member has had Creutzfeldt–Jakob disease (CJD)
- recent or current illness
- recent or planned major surgery.

Once screened, donors can proceed to give blood. Blood donation takes approximately 15 minutes. About 450 mL of blood is taken from a vein in the arm. Giving blood is very safe, although donors are advised not to give blood more than three times a year. The main complications of blood donation are bleeding from the puncture site, bruising or fainting due to the loss of blood volume or psychological factors. After donation, nurses should advise donors to rest for a short period, have a drink or light snack, and maintain a good fluid intake for the rest of the day. Smoking and alcohol are best avoided for a few hours after donation as they can increase the risk of fainting.

Donated blood and blood components are routinely screened for hepatitis B and C, HIV and syphilis. In the UK, blood is also leucocyte-depleted, i.e. most of the white cells are removed. This measure was instigated due to the theoretical risk of transmitting variant Creutzfeldt–Jakob disease (vCJD) through transfused white cells. An additional benefit is that leucocyte depletion reduces the risk of febrile reactions. It has, however, substantially increased the cost of blood transfusions.

TYPES OF BLOOD PRODUCT TRANSFUSION

Whole blood may be used to treat acute massive haemorrhage. However, it is more usual to use components of whole blood. In this way, patients receive only the components that they need and donor blood can be used more efficiently.

Packed red cells

Units of packed red cells, or volume-reduced blood, have had much of the plasma removed. This increases the relative concentration of red cells. Packed red cells are given to correct anaemia or to replace blood lost during surgery or haemorrhage. The aim is to produce the greatest benefit to the patient while reducing the risk of fluid overload or allergic reactions to plasma factors (see p. 452).

Platelets

Platelet transfusions are generally only used when the recipient's own platelet count falls below 10×10^9/L, or below 50×10^9/L if invasive treatment is required. Ideally, donor platelets should be of the same blood group as the recipient, but in practice this is not usually essential. However, those with specific platelet antibodies may require donated platelets from human leucocyte antigen (HLA)-compatible donors.

Granulocytes

Granulocytes are occasionally given to patients who are severely neutropenic (see p. 456) and have an overwhelming infection that is not responding to antibiotics. However, the benefit of granulocyte transfusions has yet to be fully established and transfusions can be quite hazardous. Transfusion reactions are more likely to occur and pulmonary infiltration of transfused white cells can lead to severe respiratory distress. Apheresis is the process used to collect granulocytes (see below).

Fresh frozen plasma
Fresh frozen plasma (FFP) is a rich source of coagulation factors. It is used to treat those whose own coagulation factors have become depleted due to liver disease, DIC or major blood loss. FFP can be stored for up to a year if frozen. It is defrosted immediately prior to use.

Albumin
Albumin may be used to treat hypovolaemia (decreased blood volume), particularly in severe burns or shock. It can also be used to treat resistant oedema. Albumin exerts an osmotic pressure that encourages fluid to move into the circulation from the tissues. However, synthetic plasma expanders can be equally effective and in recent years there has been some evidence to suggest that the use of crystalloid solutions is safer and more effective in the treatment of hypovolaemic shock (Cochrane Injuries Group 1998).

Factor VIII and factor IX
Factors VIII and IX are coagulation factors that are used in the treatment of haemophilia. In the past, these factors were solely derived from human sources and some products became contaminated with HIV and hepatitis C, leading to high rates of infection among those with haemophilia (see p. 477). The use of heat treatments and the development of recombinant or genetically engineered products have now largely eliminated this risk.

Cryoprecipitate
Cryoprecipitate is obtained from FFP and contains concentrated fibrinogen and factor VIII. It may be used in the treatment of liver disease, DIC and acute massive haemorrhage.

APHERESIS

Apheresis is a technique whereby a single blood component is removed from a patient or donor. During apheresis, the patient's or donor's blood is gradually passed through an automated cell separator. The desired blood component is drawn off and the remainder is returned to the patient. The person undergoing apheresis will require two peripheral venous access devices, or a central venous catheter with two lumens, to enable blood to be removed and returned (Fig. 18.4). Apheresis can be used to collect or remove platelets, plasma (plasmapheresis), white cells (leucopheresis) or stem cells.

Apheresis can have certain advantages over whole blood donation insofar as there is no depletion of red cells and the volunteer can donate more frequently. Apheresis is most commonly used to obtain platelets and plasma from healthy donors. Plasmapheresis is also used to remove plasma from people with disorders affecting plasma proteins and to remove toxic substances from the blood. Fresh plasma can then be transfused (plasma exchange). Leucopheresis can be used to treat patients

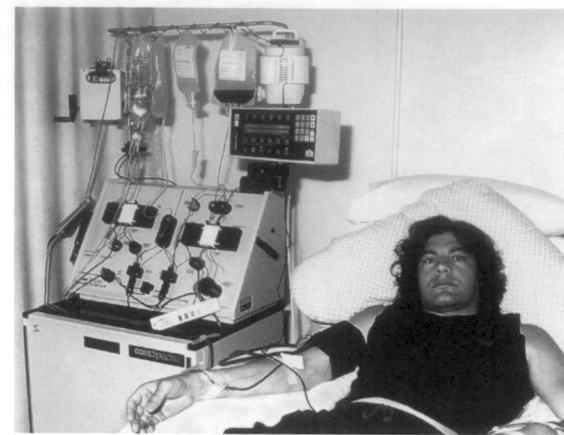

Figure 18.4 Patient undergoing apheresis.

with very high white cell counts, such as those with chronic leukaemia. Stem cells can be collected for haemopoietic stem cell transplantation (see p. 474).

BLOOD TRANSFUSION

During blood transfusion, whole blood or packed red cells are administered to a patient whose own supply is depleted due to blood loss or disease. To ensure patients receive compatible blood transfusions, a sample of the recipient's blood is first grouped and cross-matched with the donor's blood.

Pre-transfusion compatibility testing
The recipient's ABO grouping and rhesus status are first established. The recipient's blood is also screened for a range of red cell antibodies by adding drops of the blood to solutions containing known antigens. The presence of antibodies can be determined because the mixing of incompatible blood causes clumping of the red cells (agglutination). A donated unit of the same group is then selected for cross-matching. Red cells taken from the donor unit are mixed with the recipient's plasma. If agglutination does not occur, compatibility is confirmed.

Safe administration of blood
A blood transfusion can be a life-saving intervention but it is also potentially hazardous. Care must be taken when administering any blood product. Nurses have a central role in preventing and managing the complications of transfusion (see Reflective Practice box 18.1). National guidelines have been produced that outline the principles of safe transfusion (British Committee for Standards in Haematology 1999; summarized in Guidelines for Care Priorities box 18.1).

COMPLICATIONS OF TRANSFUSION

Complications of transfusion may range from relatively minor febrile reactions to extremely serious incompatibility reactions that may be fatal. Nurses should always be alert to the possibility of a reaction, and should stop the transfusion and take other appropriate action immediately a reaction is suspected. The most common types of transfusion reaction and appropriate actions to take are discussed below.

REFLECTIVE PRACTICE

18.1 Preventing and managing the complications of blood transfusion

William has a haemoglobin level of 8.0 g/dL and is prescribed a 3-unit blood transfusion.

Student activities

- William expresses fear about the risk of transfusion-related infection. What information could you give him about the risk of infection? Reflect on how you might communicate the risks and benefits of transfusion.

- List the short-term complications of blood transfusion.
- Considering the whole process of blood transfusion from blood donation, compatibility testing and administration, what nursing interventions can be made to reduce the risks of transfusion-related complications?
- Plan the nursing care for William undergoing a blood transfusion, taking account of both his physical and psychological needs.

GUIDELINES FOR CARE PRIORITIES

18.1 Principles for safe blood transfusion

A summary based on national guidelines that outline the principles of safe transfusion (British Committee for Standards in Haematology 1999) is as follows:

- Patients do not need to give written consent for blood transfusion. However, the risk of transfusion should be fully explained and nurses should ensure that patients have all the information they require. The National Blood Service produces a useful patient information sheet for this purpose; this is available through hospital transfusion laboratories.
- Before commencing a blood transfusion the nurse should record the patient's temperature, pulse, blood pressure and respiratory rate to establish baseline values.
- To ensure that the correct blood is administered a registered nurse or midwife should check the patient's details against the information on the prescription, the blood bag and the cross-match form. Some hospital policies may stipulate that two nurses participate in this checking procedure. The check should be carried out at the bedside and should include the patient's name, date of birth, hospital number and the blood unit number and expiry date. It should also confirm that the blood group of the donor unit is compatible with that of the patient.
- Blood should not be used after midnight on the expiry date.
- To reduce the risk of bacterial proliferation within blood, transfusions should be initiated within 30 minutes of

the blood leaving storage. Blood should never be temporarily stored in drug refrigerators. No drugs should be added to blood.

- Blood should be administered through a blood giving set, which incorporates a filter above the drip chamber (Nicol et al 2000), into a peripheral venous cannula or central venous line. A unit of blood is normally transfused over 3–4 hours. The duration of each unit of blood should not exceed 6 hours. Blood remaining in the bag after this period should be discarded in a clinical waste bin.
- Serious transfusion reactions usually become evident within 30 minutes of commencing a unit. The patient's temperature, pulse and respiratory rate should therefore be recorded 15 minutes after the start of each unit. Any significant changes from baseline should be reported to the medical team at once. These checks represent a minimum standard and local policies may require more frequent checks of vital signs. As a general principle, all patients should be closely observed throughout the transfusion.
- Once the transfusion is complete, blood bags can be disposed of in clinical waste bins.

References

British Committee for Standards in Haematology. The administration of blood and blood components and the management of transfused patients. Transfus Med 1999; 9: 227–238.

Nicol M, Bavin C, Bedford-Turner S, Cronin P, Rawlings-Anderson K. Essential nursing skills. London: Mosby; 2000.

Blood incompatibility

The transfusion of an incorrect or incompatible blood component is an extremely serious hazard of blood transfusion. It is most frequently due to a failure in the bedside checking procedure or a sampling error (SHOT Steering Group 2000). A reaction will usually be evident within the first few minutes of the transfusion. Signs and symptoms are:

- agitation
- flushing
- pain at the venepuncture site, and in the abdomen, flank or chest

- fever
- hypotension
- bleeding
- oliguria.

If such a reaction is suspected, the transfusion should be stopped immediately and venous access maintained with normal saline. Medical assistance should be requested urgently as this is a potentially life-threatening complication. Meanwhile the nurse should monitor the patient's vital signs, including oxygen saturation and urine output. Throughout this, the patient will require support and reassurance, and it is important to maintain a calm and controlled environment. The blood transfusion laboratory must be informed of the incident and blood samples obtained for a full blood count, cross-match, coagulation screen, biochemical analysis and blood cultures. The blood bag should be retained and returned to the blood laboratory for further investigation. A hospital incident form should be completed once the patient's condition has been stabilized.

Circulatory overload

During blood transfusion, an increase in the circulating volume may lead to hypertension and pulmonary oedema (Ch. 8). Patients most at risk are those with underlying cardiac conditions (Ch. 19). The rate of transfusion should be reduced for these patients and some may require prophylactic diuretics, e.g. furosemide (frusemide). Patients should be closely observed for signs of respiratory distress (dyspnoea, increased respiratory rate, restlessness, agitation). If symptoms occur, the transfusion should be stopped, medical advice sought and vital signs recorded.

Febrile reactions

Febrile reactions occur in 1–2% of blood transfusions but are more common with platelet concentrates and in patients who have had previous transfusions. Antibodies within the patient's plasma are activated in response to leucocytes within the donated blood. Patients become pyrexial and may complain of shivering. Symptoms often commence 30–60 minutes after the start of the transfusion. In severe reactions, the transfusion should be stopped and medical staff and the blood transfusion laboratory informed. Mild reactions can be treated with an antipyretic, such as paracetamol. The patient should be kept warm and the transfusion slowed. The transfusion can be completed if symptoms do not progress. The incidence of such reactions should decrease now that blood is routinely leucocyte-depleted.

Allergic reactions

Some patients develop sensitivity to components of the donated plasma and may experience allergic reactions such as urticaria (wheals or hives), wheezing, facial oedema and fever. These reactions usually respond to treatment with an antihistamine such as chlorphenamine (chlorpheniramine). The transfusion should be stopped if a reaction occurs, but can be recommenced after 30 minutes if the symptoms subside.

Anaphylactic reactions are a much more severe, but fortunately rare, form of allergic reaction that can lead to widespread oedema, bronchial constriction, heart failure and circulatory collapse. If an anaphylactic reaction occurs, it is an urgent and potentially life-threatening complication. The procedure outlined under incompatibility reactions should be followed. The patient's airway should be maintained – this may require the insertion of a laryngeal airway or endotracheal intubation in some instances – and oxygen should be administered. Adrenaline (epinephrine) and chlorphenamine (chlorpheniramine) are given to counteract this type of reaction.

Acute bacterial reactions

Acute bacterial reactions occur when contaminated blood or blood components are transfused. In such circumstances, the patient can rapidly develop septic shock (Ch. 9). The procedure outlined under incompatibility reactions should be followed.

Delayed complications of transfusion

- *Delayed haemolysis* 1–2 weeks after the transfusion, often after the patient has been discharged. It is characterized by anaemia and jaundice.
- *Iron overload.* A blood transfusion contains a quantity of iron. However, the body is not able to excrete large amounts of iron, and patients who are transfused regularly over a long period of time can become iron-overloaded, e.g. patients with thalassaemia (see p. 461). As iron is deposited around the body, progressive organ damage can occur. Patients at risk of iron overload may require daily subcutaneous infusions of the chelating drug desferrioxamine to aid iron excretion. Desferrioxamine binds to iron and enables it to be excreted in urine.
- *Transmission of viral infections.* The risk of viral contamination is now very small given modern screening techniques. However, the risk of acquiring hepatitis B or C is estimated at 1 in 200 000 transfusions, and of acquiring HIV as 1 in 2 million.
- *Transfusion-associated graft-versus-host disease* (TA-GVHD) is a rare complication of transfusion. It occurs when T cells in the donated blood react with the recipient's cells. This typically occurs in the bone marrow, although cells in the gastrointestinal tract, skin and liver may also be targeted. Reactions can be severe. Death may result from infection or haemorrhage if blood cell counts are lowered due to bone marrow depression. TA-GVHD is most likely to occur in people whose immune systems are already compromised as a result of disease or treatment. Those at particular risk should receive irradiated blood products.

ALTERNATIVES TO BLOOD TRANSFUSION

Blood is an expensive resource and supply relies on the goodwill of donors. As has been demonstrated, there is also a risk associated with transfusion. For this reason, alternatives to conventional blood transfusion are being sought. Patients may ask for information about these alternatives, some of which are listed below:

- Steps should be taken to prevent excessive blood loss during surgery due to pre-existing factors. Where appropriate, antiplatelet and anticoagulant therapies should be discontinued several days prior to surgery and causes of anaemia should be investigated and treated if practicable.
- It may be possible for patients to store their own blood prior to elective surgery. This blood can be transfused into the patient during the post-surgical period if required. This type of autologous transfusion is available in some centres. However, it can be logistically difficult and expensive to manage. Moreover, the shelf-life of autologous blood can expire if surgery is delayed.
- New surgical techniques that limit blood loss, or salvage blood and recycle it back into the patient, are being developed. Such developments may limit the need for postoperative blood transfusion in the future.
- Red cell and platelet substitutes are also being developed, but at present these are less effective and far more expensive than conventional blood transfusions.

⚖ ETHICAL ISSUES

18.1 The treatment of Jehovah's Witnesses with blood disorders

The religious doctrine of Jehovah's Witnesses advocates that Witnesses should abstain from blood. Traditionally, this has precluded Witnesses from accepting whole blood or any of its four main components, namely red cells, white cells, platelets or plasma. Witnesses who do not comply with this doctrine risk exclusion from the Jehovah's Witness community.

This teaching has effectively reduced the number of therapeutic options available to Witnesses with blood disorders, and on occasion Witnesses have died rather than undergo blood transfusion. However, in 2000 the Jehovah's Witnesses' Watchtower Society issued two important directives:

- The first placed the onus on members who accept blood to disassociate themselves from congregations. Previously, there was an onus on the congregation to actively investigate and expel those they suspected of not following the teaching (Muramoto 2001).
- The second stated that Witnesses may, if their consciences permit, receive products derived from the four major blood components (although not the components themselves). In effect, Witnesses can now receive haemoglobin-based blood substitutes and drugs such as interferon that were previously prohibited.

While the tenet to abstain from blood still stands, these developments place a much greater emphasis upon individual conscience. Nursing implications are that:

- Nurses should be aware of the ethical dilemmas that Jehovah's Witnesses may face when having treatment for blood disorders.
- Jehovah's Witnesses should be given adequate time and support when making their own decision about whether or not to accept blood products. It is important to note that individuals may not have previously needed to think about their position on this issue.
- If a Witness does feel that blood transfusion is acceptable (and some Witnesses interpret the teaching to mean not eating rather than not transfusing blood), it is up to him or her to disclose it to other congregation members. Nurses should therefore do all that they can to ensure that patient confidentiality is respected.

Reference
Muramoto O. Bioethical aspects of the recent changes in the policy of refusal of blood by Jehovah's Witnesses. Br Med J 2001; 322: 37–39.

- Haemopoietic growth factors (see p. 448) such as erythropoietin, the growth factor that stimulates red cell production, are increasingly being used to treat people with chronic anaemia. Erythropoietin can help to maintain haemoglobin at an acceptable level, reducing the need for regular transfusions. As erythropoietin takes approximately 7–14 days to produce a response, it is not suitable for use in acute situations.

The provision of alternatives to blood transfusion is an extremely important issue for Jehovah's Witnesses, who will often refuse a transfusion of any blood product (see Ethical Issues box 18.1). Advice on how to manage the care of Jehovah's Witnesses in these circumstances can be sought from the local Jehovah's Witness Hospital Liaison Committee.

DISEASE PREVENTION AND HEALTH EDUCATION

Haematological disorders may affect one or more elements of the haematological system. They can be broadly classified in terms of red cell, white cell and bone marrow disorders, and disorders affecting haemostasis. Blood and bone marrow disorders are extremely varied in their aetiology. Some result from an autoimmune response, some are inherited congenital disorders, while others develop due to an acquired genetic abnormality. Many of these disorders cannot be prevented at present, although patients may still try to identify the cause of their illness in order

to rationalize it in some way. These patients require support and reassurance as they come to terms with their diagnosis (Chs 3 and 6). People with a diagnosis or family history of inherited haematology disorders, such as haemophilia, thalassaemia and sickle cell disease, may also benefit from genetic and prenatal counselling and information from specialist nurses.

While disease prevention is not always possible in the haematology setting, health education is a major responsibility for nurses. Patients should be given information regarding their disease, its treatment and the prevention of complications. Health advice given to any patient should be individualized to that patient's needs, lifestyle and cultural background. It is also important to offer advice in a sensitive way that respects the patient's autonomy. A diagnosis of a haematological disease can be devastating and, when offering health advice, nurses must balance the need to maintain the individual's safety alongside his or her need to preserve a sense of control and normality.

GENERAL HEALTH EDUCATION

Health education issues related to specific disorders are discussed throughout the rest of the chapter. However, the following general guidance is relevant to many haematology patients.

Diet

Patients should be advised that a balanced diet is essential to support healthy blood cell production. This requires a sufficient supply of iron, vitamins, protein and calories. A diet containing fruit and vegetables, cereals and protein foods such as meat and dairy products will supply all the necessary nutrients (Ch. 11). Strict vegans should be encouraged to maintain an adequate intake of vitamin B_{12}, as this vitamin is not found in plants. Patients who are at risk of infection should be advised on how to maintain a low microbial diet in order to reduce the risk of gastrointestinal infections (see p. 466).

Smoking

Tobacco smoking is contraindicated in most blood disorders. Smoking has been associated with an increased risk of haematological malignancies, such as acute leukaemia. Smoking reduces the oxygen-carrying capacity of red cells and should be discouraged in those with anaemia, polycythaemia or sickle cell disease (see below). Smoking also predisposes people to chest infections, which is of particular concern for people who are immunocompromised. At the same time, it must be recognized that smoking may act as an important method of stress management (Ch. 6) for patients with serious blood disorders. Advice should therefore be offered with tact and understanding.

Activity and exercise

Tiredness and fatigue are common features of many haematological disorders and treatments. If patients are experiencing fatigue, nurses should assist them to plan their daily activities and set realistic goals. Promoting gentle exercise is important as this can enhance the patient's sense of well-being and improve the quality of sleep. However, periods of rest should be planned around periods of activity. The charity BACUP produces a useful booklet on advice for managing fatigue (see 'Useful Addresses'). Nurses can also teach relaxation techniques to enhance rest (Ch. 6).

Further information

Haematological patients should be taught how to monitor their own condition and should be given details of who to contact should problems or complications arise. Neutropenic patients with a high risk of infection are generally taught to monitor their own temperature and are provided with 24-hour emergency contact details should they develop pyrexia. Verbal information should be backed up with other forms, e.g. written or multimedia (National Cancer Directory 2000). Patients should also be made aware of additional sources of information, including local or national support groups. Remember, newly diagnosed or anxious patients may find it hard to assimilate all that is being presented to them. Nurses may therefore need to sensitively reinforce information on a number of occasions.

Educating other professionals

In specialized areas such as clinical haematology, the nurse's educational remit often extends beyond patients and their families. Other health care professionals may also require education and advice to assist them in caring appropriately for haematology patients in other hospital and community settings. The importance of sharing knowledge and expertise across care pathways and professional boundaries is now well recognized (Calman & Hine 1995, Department of Health 1997). It can lead to greater consistency and equity, and can improve patients' experiences of care.

RED CELL DISORDERS

Red cell disorders are very varied. Some may arise due to insufficient red cell production or excessive red cell loss. Others are caused by red cell dysfunction. This section describes some of the most common red cell disorders and how the nurse can play a crucial role in caring for people with these disorders.

ANAEMIA – GENERAL POINTS

Anaemia is a term used to describe the insufficient oxygen-carrying capacity of blood. Anaemia is said to be present if the haemoglobin concentration of blood falls below 13.5 g/dL in males or 11.5 g/dL in females (normal ranges are 13.5–18.0 g/dL in males, 11.5–16.5 g/dL in females).

Aetiology

There are many potential causes of anaemia, including traumatic haemorrhage, surgery, disease or its treatment, chronic blood loss, nutritional deficiencies and hereditary factors.

General investigations

Diagnosis and classification may be determined by blood tests, the microscopic examination of blood films and, where indicated, bone marrow biopsy.

Clinical presentation

Signs and symptoms of anaemia most commonly appear when the haemoglobin concentration falls below 9–10 g/dL. That said, some people with considerably lower haemoglobin levels could be asymptomatic, whereas others with relatively mild anaemia may experience marked symptoms. A number of factors may contribute to this discrepancy, such as cause of anaemia, speed of onset, age and general health, including the presence of cardiac and respiratory disease (see Older Adults: Nursing Priorities box 18.1).

65 83 50 71 OLDER ADULTS: NURSING PRIORITIES

18.1 Anaemia in older adults

Anaemia is a common haematological condition in older adults and may arise due to dietary deficiencies or underlying disease. Older adults with coexisting atherosclerotic or cardiorespiratory disorders may be particularly symptomatic, as their body systems are less able to compensate for lowered haemoglobin levels.

Care priorities

- A careful assessment should be undertaken so that the underlying cause of anaemia can be promptly identified and treated.
- Where appropriate, nurses should advise older patients on how best to maintain an adequate diet and manage symptoms such as weakness and fatigue.
- If necessary, a suitable home care package should also be initiated in consultation with the patient and other care professionals.

Table 18.4 General signs and symptoms of anaemia

Signs and symptoms	Reasons and rationale
Weakness and fatigue	Reduced oxygen for muscle contraction causes fatigue
Breathlessness	The respiratory rate increases. This is particularly evident on exertion, as the body attempts to increase oxygen supply to active tissues
Dizziness	Caused by a lack of oxygen reaching the brain
Tachycardia and palpitations	Heart rate increases and the person becomes aware of the heart beating, as the demand for oxygen increases and the cardiovascular system tries to supply more oxygenated blood to the tissues
Angina pectoris and congestive cardiac failure, particularly in older adults (see Ch. 19)	Anginal pain may occur if the myocardium is deprived of oxygenated blood. Cardiac failure may be precipitated in people with existing heart disease
Pallor of the skin and mucosa, particularly the conjunctival membranes	The skin and mucosa are paler than normal because haemoglobin, which normally produces the 'pinkish' coloration, is reduced. Skin pallor will be evident in people with light skin, but it may only be detected in the mucosa of individuals with darker skin.

General signs and symptoms of anaemia are related to reduced oxygen delivery to body tissues and impaired normal metabolism, as well as the increased demands placed upon body systems (Table 18.4). Other general effects and signs and symptoms associated with specific types of anaemia are discussed in the following sections.

HAEMORRHAGIC ANAEMIA

Haemorrhagic anaemia results from excessive blood loss.

Aetiology
Blood loss may arise from acute haemorrhage, e.g. after severe trauma or surgery. It can also result from smaller scale but persistent haemorrhage, especially from the gastrointestinal tract (e.g. peptic ulcer), the genitourinary tract (e.g. menorrhagia) or malignancy (Chs 22, 24 and 25). Over time, this may also lead to iron deficiency anaemia.

Clinical presentation
It is worth noting that individuals may lose up to 20% (1.0 L) of their blood volume without any outward signs of anaemia. Beyond this, peripheral vasoconstriction, tachycardia and hypotension develop. If blood volume depletion exceeds 30–40% (1.5–2.0 L), symptoms of hypovolaemic shock appear (Ch. 9). A rapid blood loss of more than 40% requires immediate intervention to prevent fatality.

Medical/surgical management
In haemorrhagic anaemia, the main treatment priorities are to arrest any bleeding and restore the circulating plasma volume. The former may require surgical intervention. The latter may initially be achieved using crystalloid infusions (see Ch. 9 for further discussion). Colloid infusions that contain albumin may also be used for volume replacement; however, these should be administered in accordance with clear protocols or guidelines. This is because studies have suggested that there may be a higher mortality rate among those receiving colloid than among those receiving crystalloid solutions (Cochrane Injuries Group 1998).

Blood (packed red cells) transfusion may be required if the haemoglobin level falls below 10 g/dL. It is almost always required if the haemoglobin level falls below 8 g/dL, or if there is a rapid loss of more than 30% of the total blood volume. As platelets and clotting factors are also depleted in major haemorrhage, platelets may be transfused if the platelet count falls below 50×10^9/L, or 100×10^9/L if there is multiple trauma or head injury with a high risk of further bleeding. Fresh frozen plasma (FFP), and occasionally cryoprecipitate, may be needed to correct coagulation factor deficiencies.

▶ Nursing management
Patients suffering from acute haemorrhage require close observation. This may involve identifying the site of bleeding and providing first aid treatment, such as applying pressure to a bleeding wound. Respiratory rate, heart rate, blood pressure and oxygen saturation level should be closely monitored and any deterioration reported urgently to the medical team. Nurses should ensure that patients maintain an adequate fluid input and urine output, and should administer prescribed blood products in line with local guidelines (see p. 453). Any acute event will be a frightening experience for patients and their families. Nurses should therefore help to maintain a controlled and calm environment, keeping patients informed of what is happening to them.

IRON DEFICIENCY ANAEMIA

This refers to anaemia caused by a deficiency of iron.

Aetiology
Iron deficiency anaemia can result from inadequate dietary intake, although in developed countries this is rarely the sole cause, as iron is found in many readily available foods, especially red meat, offal, green leafy vegetables, dairy products and some fortified cereal products. Instead, iron deficiency anaemia is more likely to occur when extra demands are placed on body iron reserves, which can be a result of normal growth and development or pathological disorders.

Females tend to be more susceptible to iron deficiency anaemia than males. This is because menstruation, especially if it is abnormally heavy (menorrhagia), pregnancy and lactation lead to increased iron loss. In pregnancy, the woman expands her own blood volume while also accommodating fetal demands for iron. Blood loss during labour may further deplete iron stores. Iron is also passed to the infant during breast-feeding.

Iron deficiency anaemia can also stem from many pathological conditions that cause chronic bleeding or malabsorption. Chronic bleeding commonly results from gastrointestinal disorders such as gastritis, peptic ulcers, oesophageal varices and haemorrhoids, or uterine disorders such as fibroids and malignant tumours. Malabsorption can occur as a result of gastric resection or inflammatory bowel conditions such as ulcerative colitis.

Special investigations

In iron deficiency anaemia, blood tests typically reveal a reduction in the haemoglobin and iron content of blood. The platelet count may also be slightly elevated if the person is actively bleeding. Blood film examination reveals pale (hypochromic), abnormally small (microcytic) red cells. Pencil-shaped red cells (poikilocytes) may also be observed.

Identification and treatment of the underlying causes of iron deficiency anaemia are clearly important. When more straightforward causes, such as undernutrition, pregnancy or menorrhagia, seem unlikely, further investigations are undertaken to determine the source of the anaemia, including faecal occult blood tests, physical and rectal examination, endoscopy, sigmoidoscopy or colonoscopy, and X-ray and ultrasound investigations, where indicated.

Clinical presentation

As well as general symptoms of anaemia, people with severe iron deficiency anaemia may complain of headache, a burning sensation in the mouth or tongue, difficulty or discomfort when swallowing (dysphagia) and a craving for unusual or non-nutritious foods (pica). They may exhibit a smooth, reddened tongue, stomatitis and brittle, ridged or 'spoon-shaped' fingernails.

Medical management

Iron replacement to correct the anaemia and replenish the body's iron stores should be instituted. As a general rule, oral iron preparations are as effective as parenteral preparations. Oral preparations, such as ferrous sulphate, have the added advantage of being easy to administer and relatively cheap. Oral iron preparations may be offered prophylactically to pregnant women in combination with folic acid.

▶ Nursing management

Nurses should stress the importance of compliance to people taking oral iron preparations. This is because treatment may need to continue for up to 6 months after the haemoglobin has returned to normal, and symptoms have subsided, in order to replenish body iron stores. People should be advised that it is best to take oral iron preparations before food, as an acid environment enhances iron absorption. Nurses should also inform patients of the side-effects of iron supplements, which may

include nausea, epigastric pain, diarrhoea or constipation. Patients need to be made aware that ferrous sulphate can also cause blackening of the stools and discoloration of the urine. Additional support may focus upon managing symptoms such as fatigue (see above) and giving dietary information to try to prevent recurrence.

MEGALOBLASTIC ANAEMIAS – GENERAL

Megaloblastic anaemias are characterized by the presence of large, abnormal immature red cells (megaloblasts) in the bone marrow.

Pathophysiology and aetiology

Red cell production is ineffective and many red cells are destroyed in the marrow. Consequently, fewer mature red cells enter the bloodstream. Those that do tend to be enlarged (macrocytic) and misshapen. The life span of these cells may also be reduced by up to 50% (50–60 days).

Acute megaloblastic anaemia may be induced by certain therapies, including prolonged inhalation of nitrous oxide and medications, such as zidovudine (azidothymidine, AZT) and the cytotoxic drug hydroxycarbamide (hydroxyurea). Excessive alcohol intake can also predispose to megaloblastic anaemia. However, megaloblastic anaemias are most commonly due to vitamin B_{12} or folic acid deficiencies, both substances that play a role in DNA synthesis. A deficiency in either substance may therefore slow or impair cell development. All body cells may be affected to some degree. Rapidly proliferating cells, such as those found in the bone marrow, are most affected.

MEGALOBLASTIC ANAEMIA DUE TO VITAMIN B_{12} DEFICIENCY AND PERNICIOUS ANAEMIA

Vitamin B_{12} is found in meat and dairy products but not in plants (Ch. 11). While herbivores obtain B_{12} from bacterial activity in the gut, humans cannot synthesize B_{12} in this way. Vitamin B_{12} is commonly added to fortified cereal products. Nevertheless, people who adhere to a strict vegan diet or those who are generally malnourished may still be at risk of deficiency.

During digestion, B_{12} is released from foodstuffs by the action of hydrochloric acid and pepsin in the stomach. It then binds to intrinsic factor, a substance produced by gastric parietal cells. This facilitates the eventual absorption of B_{12} in the ileum. Some B_{12} is stored in the liver. The rest is transported to the bone marrow and other tissues.

Aetiology and pathophysiology

Megaloblastic anaemia can therefore result from reduced gastric secretion of intrinsic factor or malabsorption. This can follow gastric surgery or small bowel resection (Ch. 22). Megaloblastic anaemia may be slow to manifest. It has been estimated that anaemia due to B_{12} deficiency may take 2–10 years to develop, even after total gastrectomy, due to the presence of B_{12} stores (Hugh-Jones & Wickramasinghe 1996). Inflammatory bowel disorders such as Crohn's disease may impair B_{12} absorption. However, the classic cause of megaloblastic anaemia in vitamin B_{12} deficiency is the inadequate production of intrinsic factor, a condition known as pernicious anaemia.

Pernicious anaemia is an autoimmune disease in which the body's antibodies become targeted against gastric parietal cells and intrinsic factor. Although the exact mechanisms are not completely understood, the parietal cells and the stomach lining become atrophied, thus impairing the production of intrinsic factor and other gastric secretions. Pernicious anaemia has been linked with other autoimmune disorders, including autoimmune thyroid disorders and vitiligo (Chs 17 and 28). Hereditary factors are also thought to play a role, as the disease tends to occur in families and is associated with blood group A. Pernicious anaemia predominately affects middle-aged, Caucasian females.

Clinical presentation

The general signs and symptoms of anaemia develop as B_{12} stores are diminished. In addition, people with megaloblastic anaemia may appear mildly jaundiced, or lemon yellow, due to the increased breakdown of abnormal, immature erythrocytes in the bone marrow. What particularly characterizes severe B_{12} deficiency is the presence of progressive, degenerative changes in the central and peripheral nervous systems (Ch. 14). Vitamin B_{12} is important for the maintenance of myelin, a protective substance that surrounds some nerves and helps to speed the transmission of nerve impulses. As a result, people may complain of tingling (paraesthesiae) and weakness or numbness (neuropathy) in the extremities. This often begins in the feet and legs, progressing to ataxia, or unsteady gait. Poor vision, loss of balance, impotence, loss of bladder and bowel control, and paralysis can develop over time. If untreated, damage can be irreversible and the condition is potentially fatal.

▶ Nursing management

For those people who have an inadequate intake of vitamin B_{12}, care may focus on giving dietary advice; it may be appropriate to refer them to a dietician. For those suffering neurological symptoms, assistance may be required with activities of daily living. This may involve input from primary care nurses, social services and occupational therapy.

In cases of malabsorption, vitamin B_{12} stores are replenished by a series of intramuscular injections of hydroxocobalamin, followed by 3-monthly booster injections, usually for life. Injections are given prophylactically for those undergoing total gastrectomy. Once the diagnosis is made and treatment initiated, the patient will usually be followed up by primary care practitioners. Hydroxocobalamin injections can cause an anaphylactic reaction so patients should remain in the surgery for at least 30 minutes after administration. Patients should be encouraged to continue treatment even when their symptoms have resolved. As with all chronic conditions, patients require clear information regarding their condition in addition to understanding and support.

MEGALOBLASTIC ANAEMIA DUE TO FOLIC ACID DEFICIENCY

Good sources of folic acid are meat, green vegetables and wholegrain or fortified cereal products (Ch. 11). Folic acid is absorbed in the small intestine and is stored in the body as folate.

Aetiology

Folic acid deficiency can arise from insufficient intake, increased requirements or malabsorption. Reserves are small and deficiencies can arise, particularly in those who overcook their food and consume only small amounts of fresh or uncooked vegetables. People drinking large amounts of alcohol may also become deficient.

Increased body requirements predominantly occur during pregnancy and lactation. The prevention of folate deficiency around conception and in early pregnancy is extremely important, as it has been positively associated with an increase in fetal neural tube defects, such as spina bifida.

Poor absorption may be secondary to small bowel surgery or inflammation. Treatment with certain drugs, particularly sulphonamides, trimethoprim and methotrexate, can also impair folic acid metabolism.

Clinical presentation

Clinical features of folic acid deficiency are similar to B_{12} deficiency, except that neurological impairment is not a feature.

Medical management

The focus is on prevention, and prophylactic folic acid supplements are therefore advisable for pregnant women and those planning to conceive. Simple oral supplements can also be used to treat an established deficiency. However, folic acid should never be prescribed alone unless B_{12} deficiency has been firmly excluded as a cause of megaloblastic anaemia, as this can precipitate a degeneration of the spinal cord (Hugh-Jones & Wickramasinghe 1996).

ANAEMIA OF CHRONIC DISEASE

Anaemia of chronic disease may occur in conjunction with a wide range of inflammatory, infective or malignant conditions, including rheumatoid arthritis, inflammatory bowel disorders, tuberculosis, AIDS, lymphoma and metastatic cancers. The exact mechanisms of this disorder are not completely understood, but they appear to involve the body's immune response to the underlying disease.

This type of anaemia is usually mild to moderate, and the symptoms of anaemia can often be overshadowed by the symptoms of the underlying disease. Haemoglobin levels rarely fall below 9 g/dL.

Mild anaemia may not require any therapy. In more severe anaemia, blood transfusion can facilitate symptom control. Modern treatment regimens may include the use of erythropoietin to relieve patients' symptoms and improve their quality of life (see Ethical Issues box 18.2 and p. 455). Nurses can provide physical assistance to patients suffering fatigue and can help them adapt their lifestyles to their functional ability.

POLYCYTHAEMIA

Polycythaemia may be primary or secondary and can be defined as a rise in haemoglobin levels beyond the normal upper limits of 16.5 g/dL in females and 18.0 g/dL in males. The haematocrit and packed cell volume are also elevated. In primary proliferative polycythaemia (PPP), the amount of urate in the blood is

⚖️ ETHICAL ISSUES

18.2 High cost of drugs used in symptom control

- Erythropoietin is one of a growing number of non-curative high-cost drugs that may be used to alleviate patient symptoms.
- Running alongside the development of new treatments is a clear requirement for health professionals and managers to allocate the resources that are available to them in ways that are both cost-effective and equitable.

Student activities

- Think about how members of the public might feel about NHS resources being used to fund high-cost drugs for symptom control, rather than treatments that offer a cure.
- List the points you would make in support of using erythropoietin for symptom control.
- What sort of information about the use of erythropoietin would you need for completing the previous activity?

increased and there is often an increase in the number of neutrophils and platelets. PPP is a disorder that most commonly arises in people over the age of 50. It is caused by the mutation of a stem cell that produces excessive numbers of red cells. Secondary polycythaemia can be due to hypoxia, such as in lung disease or at high altitude, increased secretion of erythropoietin by the kidneys or tumours, or the misuse of the drug erythropoietin to enhance athletic performance.

Clinical presentation

People with polycythaemia often have a ruddy appearance due to the increased number of red cells in the circulation. Physical examination may reveal splenomegaly (enlargement of spleen). Symptoms of polycythaemia tend to be related to an increase in blood volume and blood viscosity and include headaches, fatigue, dizziness, breathlessness, visual disturbances, sweating, pruritus and gout. However, the most serious complication is thrombosis. Thrombi can lead to vascular occlusion, peripheral gangrene, deep vein thrombosis (DVT), embolus formation, stroke and heart attack (Chs 14, 19 and 20).

Medical management

In primary polycythaemia, the aim of treatment is to maintain the haematocrit within normal limits. This helps to control symptoms and reduces the risk of thrombosis. In the short term, this is usually accomplished by venesection. During venesection, around 500 mL of blood is removed from the venous circulation via a needle into an arm. The procedure is normally carried out in the outpatient setting by a doctor or specialist nurse on a regular basis. In more severe cases, drugs such as hydroxycarbamide (hydroxyurea) or interferon may also be given to suppress bone marrow function. Aspirin may be prescribed to reduce platelet activity and inhibit clot formation. In older people, radioactive phosphorus may be used to reduce marrow activity; unfortunately this form of treatment can cause acute leukaemia after some years.

HAEMOLYTIC ANAEMIAS – GENERAL

The haemolytic anaemias encompass a diverse range of inherited or acquired disorders.

Pathophysiology

They are characterized by the premature destruction, or haemolysis, of red cells. There is usually a compensatory increase in red cell production. If an adequate level of functioning red cells is maintained, the person is said to be in a compensated haemolytic state.

Clinical presentation

Symptoms can occur, however, if the rate of red cell manufacture falls below the rate of destruction or if the red cells produced are abnormal, such as in those with sickle cell disease (see p. 461).

In addition to the general signs and symptoms of anaemia, people with haemolytic anaemia often appear mildly jaundiced. Enlargement of the spleen (splenomegaly) and liver (hepatomegaly) can result from increased organ activity in the breakdown of red cells. Gallstones may be precipitated by the accumulation of red cell breakdown products in the gallbladder. If haemolytic anaemia has been present since childhood, a compensatory expansion of the bone marrow may lead to skeletal abnormalities.

AUTOIMMUNE HAEMOLYTIC ANAEMIA

In autoimmune haemolytic anaemia (AIHA) the patient's antibodies are targeted against antigens found on the surface of their red cells.

Aetiology

Underlying causes can include other autoimmune diseases, infection, the use of some drugs and disorders such as lymphoma or chronic lymphocytic leukaemia (see pp. 468–469). However, in many cases no cause can be determined, and the condition is thus said to be idiopathic.

Medical/surgical management

Autoimmune haemolytic anaemia is usually treated with corticosteroids such as prednisolone. If this proves ineffective, second-line treatments include splenectomy (removal of the spleen) or the use of immunosuppressive drugs such as azathioprine, ciclosporin, and cytotoxic drugs such as chlorambucil and cyclophosphamide. If the anaemia in AIHA is severe enough, blood transfusion may be required. A form of AIHA is exacerbated in low temperatures, and people with this condition should therefore be advised to keep warm, and any transfused blood they receive should be given through a blood warmer.

HAEMOGLOBINOPATHIES

The haemoglobinopathies are inherited disorders that affect haemoglobin production. They are commonly divided into two groups: disorders resulting from reduced haemoglobin synthesis, e.g. the thalassaemias; and those that produce abnormal haemoglobin, such as sickle cell disease. Both are associated with considerable long-term health problems, including chronic haemolytic anaemia.

THALASSAEMIA

Thalassaemia is a haemoglobinopathy that results from a reduced synthesis of haemoglobin components.

Aetiology and pathophysiology

Thalassaemia can occur in people of all ethnic backgrounds but is most commonly found in people with Mediterranean ancestry. It occurs when the gene responsible for globin production is faulty. People who inherit the faulty gene from both parents are said to have thalassaemia major, whereas those who inherit a faulty gene from only one parent have thalassaemia trait. In thalassaemia, the synthesis of alpha- or beta-globin chains, essential for haemoglobin production, is reduced because of a genetic abnormality. This leads to red cell fragility, with impaired oxygen-carrying abilities that are more rapidly destroyed by the spleen.

Clinical presentation

People with thalassaemia trait are usually asymptomatic or have very mild anaemia. However, those with thalassaemia major develop severe anaemia from infancy or early childhood. Consequently, they may fail to thrive, experience recurrent infections and developmental delays. Both the liver and spleen become enlarged due to excessive haemolysis, while expansion of the bone marrow leads to alterations in the bone structure. Thus, children with thalassaemia major who receive inadequate treatment can develop bony deformities, osteoporosis and pathological fractures (Ch. 27).

Medical/surgical management

Thalassaemia is managed by giving regular blood transfusions to maintain the haemoglobin level at around $11-12$ g/dL; this reduces the symptoms of anaemia and suppresses the production of the abnormal red cells (Howard & Hamilton 1997). Splenectomy may help to reduce red cell destruction and reduce transfusion requirements. Currently the only curative option for thalassaemia is haemopoietic stem cell transplantation (see p. 474). However, this is a high-risk procedure and is only recommended for children who have a suitable sibling donor. It is hoped that new advances in gene therapy will bring safer curative options.

There are a number of risks associated with frequent blood transfusion. People who are regularly transfused can develop antibodies against donor blood. This increases the risk of transfusion-related reactions, so that over time it can become difficult to select compatible units of blood. Frequent blood transfusion can also lead to the excessive accumulation of iron in vital organs, particularly the heart, liver and endocrine organs. This can precipitate secondary conditions such as diabetes mellitus and congestive heart failure due to progressive organ damage (Chs 17 and 19). The risk of these complications can be minimized by the long-term administration of iron-chelating drugs such as desferrioxamine, which binds to iron and enables it to be excreted in urine. To prevent the adverse complications of iron overload, iron chelation should begin in childhood. Treatment is given by subcutaneous infusion over 8–12 hours. As infusions may need to be repeated three to seven times a week, they are usually given overnight.

▶ Nursing management

The nursing care of patients with thalassaemia can have an impact throughout the individual's life. Nurses should ensure the safe administration of blood products and be aware of the increased risk of transfusion reactions. Patients normally receive 3 units of blood every 3–4 weeks. This can cause enormous lifestyle disruptions, with major implications for schooling and employment. In such circumstances it is important to educate teachers and employers, as well as patients, about thalassaemia so that they understand the importance of regular treatment.

The risk of transmitting viral infections through blood products has been reduced but can be a source of great anxiety to people who will have to rely on transfusions for the rest of their lives. Nurses need to be sensitive to these fears. Venous access can become a problem as peripheral veins become damaged through frequent venepuncture and cannulation. Consequently, many patients will require long-term venous access devices. These may adversely affect body image and serve as a constant reminder of their disease.

Similarly, iron chelation therapy can also have a major impact on a patient's lifestyle and body image. Nurses can teach patients to administer their drugs safely and provide the necessary support to encourage compliance. They can also refer patients to self-help groups where they can share their experiences and gain further support from others with the same or similar conditions.

People with thalassaemia, or those with a family history of the disorder, may require a great deal of information and sensitive counselling, including genetic, preconceptual and antenatal counselling. Although people with thalassaemia can have children, all will carry thalassaemia trait. Women may also need to consider any personal health risks, particularly if they already have some degree of organ damage due to iron overload. People with thalassaemia trait should be informed of the risks of thalassaemia for their offspring if their partners also carry the trait.

Nursing people with thalassaemia requires a range of skills and knowledge. Clinical nurse specialists can have a dramatic impact in this context by providing long-term care and support for patients and their families. They can also serve as a point of contact for local self-help groups and other health care professionals.

SICKLE CELL DISEASE

Sickle cell anaemia is an inherited haemoglobin disorder that is caused by an abnormality in the beta-globin gene.

Aetiology and pathophysiology

If a person inherits a gene for normal adult haemoglobin (HbA) from one parent and a gene for sickle haemoglobin (HbS) from the other, he or she is said to have sickle cell trait. People with sickle cell trait are carriers of sickle cell anaemia but have no clinical problems and have normal blood counts. The inheritance of an HbS gene from both parents, on the other hand, results in sickle cell disease (HbSS).

Sickle cell anaemia is most commonly found in people of African, African Caribbean or African-American descent, but can also be found in those with Indian, Middle Eastern, Far Eastern and southern European ancestry. The high prevalence of the abnormal gene in people of African ancestry appears to be due to the protection that sickle cell trait offers against falciparum malaria in childhood.

When HbS becomes deoxygenated, crystals are formed within the red cells. The cells become distorted and take on the characteristic sickle shape (Fig. 18.5). When red cells are oxygenated they can return to their normal shape. However, with time, affected cells become increasingly rigid and inflexible and are destroyed prematurely by the cells of the mononuclear-macrophage system in the spleen and liver. The life span of an HbSS cell is around 5–30 days, compared with 120 days for a normal red cell.

Clinical presentation

Sickle cell disease is characterized by chronic haemolytic anaemia and intermittent painful crises. Patients with sickle cell disease will often have a haemoglobin level of between 6 and 10 g/dL. Many people function relatively normally at these levels, as the body adjusts to a low Hb and also because HbS is a more efficient transporter of oxygen than HbA. As with other haemolytic anaemias, patients will usually be mildly jaundiced and have splenomegaly.

Sickle cell crises are precipitated when large numbers of cells become sickle-shaped; the rigidity of these cells prevents them passing through small blood vessels, the blood vessels become occluded and tissue ischaemia and infarction can result. These crises are associated with excruciating pain in the affected area of the body. Crises are unpredictable and can occur very suddenly; they can last for a matter of hours or persist for several weeks. While the exact mechanisms are unclear, crises appear to be triggered by a range of factors including:

- reduced tissue oxygenation
- infection
- dehydration
- temperature extremes
- high altitude
- excessive alcohol consumption
- strenuous exercise
- general anaesthesia
- emotional stress
- pregnancy.

The frequency and severity of sickle cell crises vary from one individual to another. Severe crises can have life-threatening consequences, particularly when vaso-occlusion occurs in the brain or lungs.

Other problems faced by people with sickle cell disease include an increased risk of infection, tissue necrosis due to repeated tissue infarction, renal insufficiency (Ch. 24) and retinal disease (Ch. 15).

Medical/surgical management

At present, there is no cure for sickle cell disease apart from haemopoietic stem cell transplantation from a sibling donor (see p. 474). Unfortunately this procedure is only suitable for a small minority of patients. Sickle cell disease is not usually treated with transfusions, as patients are able to tolerate quite low haemoglobin levels. The treatment of sickle cell crises will depend on the severity. Mild crises may be managed at home with simple analgesics such as paracetamol, bed rest and oral fluids. Severe crises will require hospital admission for strong analgesics, fluid replacement, oxygen therapy and close observation.

On admission to hospital, the pain experienced by those in sickle cell crisis is often excruciating, and strong analgesics, such as morphine or diamorphine, should be offered prior to examination and detailed assessment. Nitrous oxide and oxygen may provide some short-term pain relief in the interim. Intravenous fluids are normally commenced if the person is dehydrated and unable to maintain an adequate oral intake. Oxygen therapy is given to counteract hypoxia and prevent further sickling of the red cells. Antibiotics are prescribed if there are signs of infection. Particularly close attention should be given to the patient with chest pain, as a sickling crisis affecting the lungs, sometimes called chest crisis, carries a significant risk of mortality. This type of crisis may justify an exchange transfusion whereby some of the patient's own blood is removed and donated blood is transfused by apheresis (see p. 452).

The cytotoxic drug hydroxycarbamide (hydroxyurea) is being given to some people with sickle cell disease; it is not curative but may reduce the frequency and severity of crises. This drug suppresses bone marrow function so patients should have their blood counts monitored frequently to ensure that they do not fall below safe levels. The long-term effects of hydroxycarbamide (hydroxyurea) are, as yet, unknown.

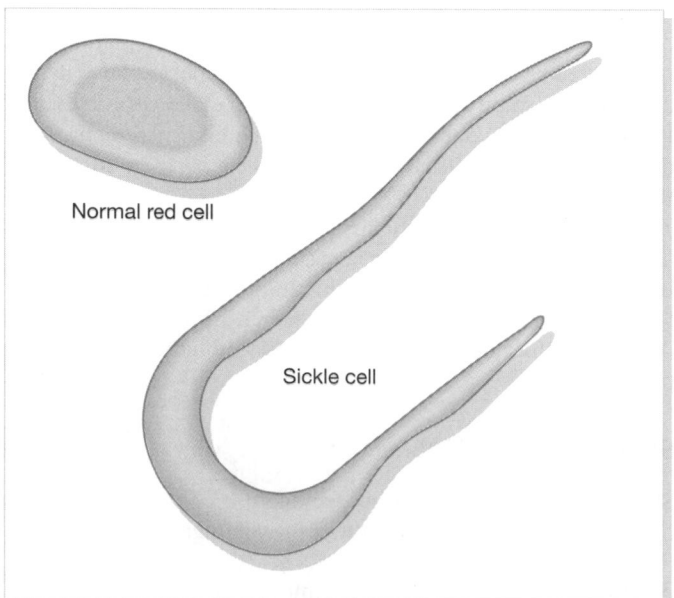

Normal red cell

Sickle cell

Figure 18.5 A sickle cell.

▶ Nursing management

Pain relief is a major priority when nursing patients in sickle cell crisis and should always be managed in close partnership with patients. People with sickle cell disease are often very knowledgeable about their condition and will know what analgesics are most effective for them. They are also best able to judge their own level of pain. Empathy and trust are important in this context. Problems can arise if nurses or other health care professionals underestimate the degree of pain that people with sickle cell crisis are enduring, or mislabel them as drug addicts if they urgently demand opioid analgesics (Oni 1998). Here, it is worth remembering that the provision of inadequate levels of pain relief can lead to a worsening of the crisis.

One way in which patients can play a positive role in their own pain management is through the use of patient-controlled analgesia (PCA) devices. These deliver a regular dose of parenteral analgesia that is titrated to the needs of the individual with a bolus function that the patient can control independently. Regular monitoring to ensure that pain relief remains appropriate should be carried out. The use of pain charts, whereby patients subjectively score their pain levels over time, can prove extremely useful for this (Ch. 7). The side-effects of opioid drugs such as nausea and constipation should be monitored and treated as necessary.

Dehydration can precipitate a crisis or make it worse as the blood becomes more viscous and flow is reduced. It is important that patients have a fluid intake of at least 3 L daily. If they are unable to drink adequately, this should be supplemented intravenously. A fluid balance chart can be used during the acute phase of the crisis to monitor intake and urine output.

Hypoxia can also cause or aggravate a crisis. Oxygen saturation levels should therefore be monitored along with the respiratory rate, and nurses should be mindful of the fact that high-dose opiates can suppress respiratory function. Oxygen therapy is often required, particularly for chest crises.

Nurses should observe for signs of infection, such as a raised temperature, cough or skin lesions. The presence of chest pain should be immediately reported to the medical team as this may indicate a chest crisis. Patients should be encouraged to rest as much as possible in order to reduce their oxygen demand. Nurses should ensure that patients can easily access everything they need.

As the crisis subsides, people with sickle cell anaemia may benefit from teaching about progressive relaxation and visualization. These techniques may help people to manage the psychological and emotional aspects of pain, and cope day to day with this unpredictable and potentially life-threatening disease (Thomas et al 1998).

In the absence of cure, nurses should advise sufferers on how to manage their condition while maintaining as normal a lifestyle as possible (see Health Promotion box 18.1). As with thalassaemia, people with sickle cell disease may also benefit from skilled counselling from specialist haemoglobinopathy nurses. They need advice and support to balance their lifestyle with the disease. Specialist nurses also offer genetic counselling for carriers of sickle cell disease wanting children.

An important role is to educate others about sickle cell disease; there remains much ignorance surrounding this disorder

 HEALTH PROMOTION

18.1 Managing sickle cell disease and maintaining as normal a lifestyle as possible

Some general recommendations of the UK Sickle Cell Society (www.sicklecell.co.uk) include the following:

- Maintain general health and nutrition.
- Avoid situations that may trigger a crisis, including exposure to cold, dehydration and sports such as scuba diving and skydiving.
- Treat infections early.
- Consider taking prophylactic penicillin and having pneumococcal vaccination.
- Consider taking folic acid supplements.
- Undergo regular blood tests.
- Carry a haemoglobinopathy card or letter that gives details of the condition.

among health care professionals, schools and employers, which can have a detrimental effect on sufferers.

DISORDERS OF THE BONE MARROW

APLASTIC ANAEMIA

Aplastic anaemia is a very rare but serious disorder that can be fatal if left untreated.

Aetiology and pathophysiology

Aplastic anaemia can result from exposure to certain chemicals, cytotoxic drugs, radiation and some viruses, including Epstein–Barr, HIV and parvovirus. In approximately 50% of cases, it results from an idiopathic, autoimmune reaction whereby the patients' antibodies target and destroy their own stem cells. There is a congenital form of aplastic anaemia, Fanconi's anaemia, that occurs in children.

Aplastic anaemia arises because of a reduction in the number of stem cells in the bone marrow. This leads to a marked decrease in all types of blood cell production.

Special investigations and clinical presentation

The reduction in all blood cells (pancytopenia) means that patients may present with signs and symptoms of anaemia, bleeding and bruising and persistent infections. A full blood count will reveal a low haemoglobin, low white cell count (leucopenia) and low platelet count (thrombocytopenia). A bone marrow aspirate will demonstrate a hypoplastic (few cells) marrow.

Medical management

- Elimination, where possible, of any identifiable underlying cause and giving supportive treatments.
- Autoimmune aplastic anaemia may respond to treatment with antilymphocyte globulins (ALGs).
- Corticosteroids or immunosuppressants such as ciclosporin.

- In resistant cases – haemopoietic stem cell transplantation may be the only means of re-populating the bone marrow (see p. 474).
- Supportive treatments aimed at maintaining adequate blood counts – blood or platelet transfusions.
- Growth factors, e.g. G-CSF, to stimulate neutrophil production and reduce the risk of infection.

► Nursing management

Nursing support should include the management of anaemia, thrombocytopenia and neutropenia (see p. 465).

Nurses should inform patients of the side-effects of corticosteroids, such as weight gain, hypertension, sleeplessness, mood swings, diabetes, increased infection risk, increase in appetite and gastric irritation. Changes in weight should be monitored. Patients should have their blood pressure measured at regular intervals. Wherever possible, corticosteroids should be given early in the day to improve sleep at night. Oral preparations should be taken with food to help prevent gastric irritation. Daily urinalysis should be performed to detect the presence of glucose. If glucose is present on urinalysis, a blood glucose test should be carried out. Insulin treatment may be required for secondary diabetes mellitus. Where appropriate, relatives should also be informed of the changes in mood that can accompany corticosteroid treatment, as this will allow them to support the patient more effectively.

Major infection poses a serious risk to people with aplastic anaemia, and any signs of infection should be reported promptly to the medical team. It should be remembered that patients taking corticosteroids might not present with pyrexia, even in the case of serious sepsis. In such circumstances a significant tachycardia may be the first sign of infection that can be observed.

Patients with severe aplastic anaemia have a life-threatening condition and may require a great deal of psychological support from nursing staff. If they are candidates for a haemopoietic stem cell transplant (see p. 474), they will also require clear and accurate information about the procedure and its likely outcomes. If a family member is to act as a donor, he or she will also require information and support from health care professionals.

MYELODYSPLASIA

Myelodysplasia, or myelodysplastic syndrome (MDS), describes a group of disorders of the bone marrow that are characterized by the presence of abnormal stem cells and progressive bone marrow failure.

Aetiology and pathophysiology

Blood cell formation is undermined, leading to lower peripheral blood counts. Those blood cells that are produced may not function normally. MDS is mainly a disease of older adults, although children and younger adults can be affected. In severe cases, MDS can evolve into acute leukaemia.

Medical management

- Haemopoietic stem cell transplantation – a curative option for younger people

- Supportive treatment for older adults – regular blood or platelet transfusion for anaemia and thrombocytopenia; associated iron overload is treated with chelating drugs (see p. 461)
- Growth factors, such as G-CSF and erythropoietin, to enhance marrow function
- Low-dose cytotoxic chemotherapy, using drugs such as cytarabine, may help slow the progression of MDS.

► Nursing management

Myelodysplastic syndrome is a debilitating disorder that can persist for years. Lowered blood cell counts may lead to symptoms such as anaemia, thrombocytopenia and recurrent infection; the nursing care for these conditions is described elsewhere in this chapter. Advice can be given on how to manage fatigue, the prevention of infection and maximizing nutritional input.

Regular hospital visits for blood transfusion or other treatments can place a considerable strain on the personal resources and family relationships of people with MDS, many of whom are older adults. Careful nursing assessment, to elicit whether extra resources such as home care or transport are necessary, should therefore be undertaken. Individualized care is important in this as in other areas.

Most patients will experience progressive marrow failure and will die of infection. Psychological support is essential to help patients through the progress of their disease and early referral to palliative care teams is advisable (Ch. 34).

MYELOMA

Myeloma is a malignant disorder affecting bone marrow.

Aetiology and pathophysiology

The aetiology is unknown. It results from an uncontrolled proliferation of plasma cells that are derived from B lymphocytes and produce immunoglobulins. The incidence of myeloma increases with age. The mean age of diagnosis is around 60 years; less than 5% of patients are aged below 40.

Clinical presentation

The onset of myeloma is insidious and the disease can be quite advanced when a diagnosis is reached. Patients may present with backache or symptoms of anaemia. However, the proliferation of abnormal plasma cells within the bone marrow can result in a wide range of clinical features. Normal bone marrow function can be inhibited, leading to low blood cell counts and eventual bone marrow failure. Bone damage is also characteristic. This can be seen on X-ray as holes in the bone, known as lytic lesions. Disintegration of bone can result in abnormally high serum calcium levels (hypercalcaemia), severe pain, pathological fractures and spinal cord compression (Chs 33 and 34). Malignant plasma cells secrete large quantities of abnormal immunoglobulins that may increase blood viscosity. This can cause renal failure and damage to other major organs.

Medical management

- Cytotoxic drugs and corticosteroids – not curative and average survival is about 3 years

- Cure may be achieved for younger patients through the use of haemopoietic stem cell transplantation
- High-dose chemotherapy with autologous peripheral blood stem cell rescue (see p. 474) may improve life expectancy for some older adults
- Bisphosphonates, e.g. pamidronate, to control bone destruction
- Local radiotherapy for pain control
- Plasmapheresis to reduce blood viscosity.

▶ Nursing care

The focus is mainly on symptom control, the identification of emergency situations such as hypercalcaemia and spinal cord compression (Chs 33 and 34) and psychosocial support.

Pain is often the major problem (Ch. 7). Bone pain can be very intense and can restrict mobility and severely undermine the patient's quality of life. Opioid drugs provide the mainstay of pain control; other analgesics can be useful but most anti-inflammatory drugs are contraindicated if the patient has thrombocytopenia. Local radiotherapy and long-term epidural medication are also important methods of pain control. Progressive relaxation and visualization techniques may be useful. However, complete pain relief in myeloma patients can be difficult to achieve. Nurses working with these patients should therefore help them to set realistic goals in terms of both pain management and activities of daily living. It may be helpful to administer analgesics prior to periods of activity. Here, it should be remembered that prolonged inactivity could exacerbate problems such as osteoporosis or bone destruction. Home support may be necessary for some patients. Referral to the palliative care team (Ch. 34) or specialist pain relief team can provide additional support.

Increased pain should always be investigated, as it can be a sign of pathological fractures. Increased back pain may indicate vertebral collapse or spinal cord compression, particularly if the patient experiences sensory loss or changes in bowel or bladder control. Spinal cord compression is a serious complication of myeloma and should be viewed as an emergency. It can produce permanent loss of function or paralysis if it is not promptly treated (Ch. 14).

Symptoms such as anorexia, nausea, vomiting, constipation, lethargy and confusion may be associated with hypercalcaemia due to increased bone destruction. If these symptoms are unresolved, they may lead to a downward spiral as patients become more and more reluctant to eat and drink. The maintenance of a good fluid intake and a healthy, fibre-rich diet should be encouraged. The judicious use of antiemetics may assist patients in maintaining an adequate intake. Laxative medications may be necessary to prevent constipation, particularly for those taking opioid drugs.

Renal failure is a frequent complication of myeloma, and urine output should be monitored in patients who become acutely unwell.

As with other bone marrow disorders, patients with myeloma may also have symptoms arising from lowered or dysfunctional blood cell production. These should be managed appropriately according to individual need. Nurses should be aware of the patient's full blood count to assess the risk of infection and bleeding and symptoms of anaemia. Patients receiving chemotherapy may display side-effects related to their treatment (see p. 471).

In most cases, this is an incurable disease that results in increasing levels of pain and incapacity. Palliative care teams provide vital assistance with symptom relief and psychological support. Family members can find it very distressing to witness the progression of this disease and the provision of counselling and bereavement care is often crucial (Ch. 34).

WHITE CELL DISORDERS

The nursing care of patients with white cell disorders is extremely challenging. Patients frequently require an enormous amount of psychological support and education, whilst their medical condition can fluctuate rapidly. Not infrequently, patients will die as a result of their disease or its treatment. This can exact an emotional toll on nurses working in the field. Burnout is a recognized problem in haematology units and therefore part of the nurse's responsibility is to offer support to colleagues as well as patients. A strong and cohesive team approach can be crucial in mitigating the effects of such stress (Ch. 6).

NEUTROPENIA

Neutropenia is usually defined as a neutrophil count of $< 1.0 \times 10^9$/L, but some centres define it as a neutrophil count of $< 0.5 \times 10^9$/L (Ch. 33).

Aetiology

Neutropenia can often result from bone marrow failure due to an underlying disease such as leukaemia, or exposure to substances that are toxic to the bone marrow such as cytotoxic drugs, radiation and chemical exposure.

Medical management

Patients who are neutropenic have a vastly increased risk of infection. Once an infection develops, the lack of body defences means that the patient's condition can very rapidly deteriorate, leading to septic shock. An infection in a neutropenic patient is a medical emergency and requires urgent treatment with antimicrobial drugs and supportive measures as appropriate. Infections can result from cross-infection and some may be hospital-acquired (nosocomial) (Ch. 13). Many are caused by organisms already present on the patient's body and are harmless in normal circumstances. The majority of infections are bacterial, although viral infections, e.g. cytomegalovirus (CMV) and herpes simplex, and fungal infections, e.g. *Aspergillus* and *Candida*, can also pose serious risks for patients.

▶ Nursing management

The focus of nursing care for neutropenic patients is to:

- minimize the risk of infection
- monitor closely for early signs of infection
- act promptly should an infection be suspected
- provide patient education and support.

Minimizing infection risk

It is impossible to completely eliminate the risk of infection for neutropenic patients, but various strategies may reduce this risk. In the past, neutropenic patients were often nursed in strict protective isolation. However, such measures are not always necessary and may have a detrimental psychological impact. Nowadays, people tend to be nursed in less stringent isolation, or may remain at home, depending on the intensity of the treatment and the duration of the neutropenia.

Most centres now adopt a common-sense approach to infection control, whereby normality is preserved as far as possible whilst minimizing risk. The general principles are that:

- Neutropenic patients should be nursed away from infected patients – clean single room, or in some centres a sterile laminar air flow environment where positive pressure filters sterile air through the room (Ch. 33).
- Strict handwashing should be observed by all personnel entering the patient's room and before any care episode.
- Staff or visitors with an obvious infection, or those who have been in contact with an infectious illness, should avoid contact with the patient.
- Special care should be taken during any invasive procedures.

The general environment should be kept meticulously clean and patients should also be encouraged to maintain high standards of personal hygiene and mouth care. Good general hygiene with regard to food preparation should also be maintained. Thus, food should be stored correctly and should be consumed well within its expiry date. Foods should be thoroughly cooked as the process of cooking destroys most microorganisms. Raw vegetables, salads and nuts are best avoided. Fruit is only recommended if it has been peeled. Soft cheeses, raw eggs and unpasteurized dairy products should not be eaten when patients are neutropenic. That said, a degree of common sense should be used when advising patients about diet. The risk of infection from food is relatively small in comparison to the patients' need for good nutrition. It is also psychologically important for patients to eat foods that they desire and feel able to tolerate.

Observing for signs of infection

Neutropenic patients require close observation for signs of infection:

- Vital signs monitored 4-hourly, or more frequently if infection is present or suspected.
- Observation for any obvious signs and symptoms such as pyrexia, tachycardia, hypotension, altered respiratory rate, skin inflammation, cough, sore throat or diarrhoea.
- Central venous access devices and peripheral cannulae should also be monitored for signs of redness or inflammation.

It is important to note that normal signs of infection, such as pus formation, do not occur in people with neutropenia due to their low white cell count. Pyrexia may also be masked by corticosteroid therapy, and tachycardia may be the first sign of significant sepsis.

Management of infection

The medical team should be informed immediately whenever an infection is suspected. A temperature of 38°C or above is usually an indication for intravenous antibiotic treatment. Antibiotics should not be delayed and should be administered as soon as blood cultures (peripheral and central) have been taken. Most units have a written policy for the treatment of neutropenic sepsis (Ch. 33). Nurses should be familiar with this.

Nurses caring for the patient with neutropenic sepsis must ensure that:

- Vital signs and oxygen saturation level are frequently checked until the patient's condition stabilizes.
- An adequate fluid intake is maintained to prevent dehydration and reduce the risk of shock – rapid intravenous fluids are often indicated.
- An accurate fluid balance chart is kept to monitor renal function.
- The patient is kept comfortable and well informed about what is happening.

In most cases, patients will respond to treatment with intravenous antibiotics and will recover within a few days. However, for some, overwhelming infection results in a rapid deterioration of the patient's condition with a significant associated mortality.

Patient education and support

Increasingly, patients remain at home when they are neutropenic. This is partly to maximize their time at home between treatment cycles, and partly because the risk of infection can be lower in their own environment. Education and support of this group of patients are essential parts of the nurse's role. Nurses should ensure that patients and their families are able to take adequate precautions to prevent infection and are clear about what to do if the patient becomes unwell. At the same time, nurses should try to prevent patients or their relatives becoming unduly anxious. Patients should be taught to record their own temperature and should be provided with a 24-hour contact number for the haematology unit. The nurse should emphasize that contact should be made at the first sign of infection, as neutropenic patients can become extremely ill very quickly. Advice about maintaining a low-microbial diet and central line care should be given as appropriate. Caring for a neutropenic patient at home can place an enormous strain on family members and they need reassurance that they can contact nurses at the hospital at any time for advice.

ACUTE LEUKAEMIA

Acute leukaemia is a life-threatening, malignant disorder that results from the uncontrolled proliferation of abnormal immature blood cells (blast cells) within the bone marrow. It can be divided into two broad categories: acute myeloid leukaemia (AML) and acute lymphoblastic leukaemia (ALL). This distinction depends on whether the malignancy has occurred in the lymphoid or myeloid cell lines. The leukaemic cells crowd the marrow and prevent normal blood cell formation. Leukaemic cells eventually spill out into the peripheral blood and can go on to infiltrate other organs.

A diagnosis of acute leukaemia requires urgent medical attention as the rapidly deteriorating bone marrow function can lead to life-threatening complications, primarily infection. Without treatment, death would occur within weeks or months.

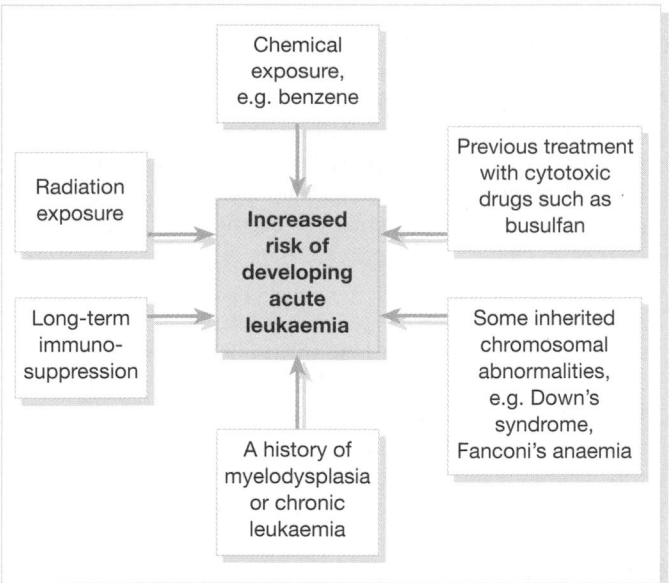

Figure 18.6 Factors associated with an increased risk of developing acute leukaemia.

Aetiology

In most cases the cause of leukaemia is unknown, but some factors appear to increase the risk of developing the disease, e.g. exposure to radiation (Fig. 18.6).

Clinical features and investigations

Acute leukaemia has a rapid onset. Patients will usually present with a short history of weight loss, bruising, bleeding, pallor, fatigue and repeated infection. A full blood count will often reveal anaemia and thrombocytopenia. White cell counts can be elevated or very low. Leukaemic blast cells are visible on the blood film. A definitive diagnosis is usually made from bone marrow biopsy.

Acute myeloid leukaemia

Acute myeloid leukaemia can be classified into eight subtypes depending on the characteristics of the leukaemic blast cells. AML is rare in childhood and the incidence increases with age. Secondary AML is sometimes seen in people who have previously been treated with cytotoxic chemotherapy or radiotherapy.

Medical management

Treatment for AML involves intensive chemotherapy that is given in a number of courses or cycles. Patients generally receive four or five courses of chemotherapy over a period of about 6 months. Each course of chemotherapy consists of a combination of cytotoxic agents given over several days and requires hospital admission. These intensive blocks of chemotherapy cause profound bone marrow suppression, leaving patients severely pancytopenic for about 3 weeks until normal bone marrow function recovers. Frequent blood and platelet transfusion is often required after chemotherapy. However, infection can be the most serious complication of treatment. Neutropenic sepsis (see p. 466) and septic shock can be major causes of mortality in patients undergoing treatment for AML.

The aim of treatment is to induce and consolidate a durable disease remission. About 75% of adults treated for AML have a positive response to first-line chemotherapy treatments and achieve a complete remission. Complete remission is defined as less than 5% of blast cells remaining in the marrow. Around 30% of adult patients will be cured with conventional chemotherapy. Haemopoietic stem cell transplant (see p. 474) can increase the rate of cure to about 50%, but it is a highly toxic procedure with a range of long-term side-effects.

Patients who fail to respond to chemotherapy or those who experience a relapse of their disease have a relatively poor prognosis with standard chemotherapy treatments. However, if a remission is achieved by the use of second-line chemotherapy regimens, further treatment involving haemopoietic stem cell transplantation will improve the prospect of long-term survival.

Acute lymphoblastic leukaemia

Acute lymphoblastic leukaemia (ALL) is the most common form of haematological malignancy in children. ALL does, however, occur in adults, with the incidence increasing with age. It is more common in males than in females. In children, long-term survival can be expected in 70% of cases; for adults the figure is around 35–40%.

Many of the signs and symptoms of ALL are similar to those of AML and result largely from bone marrow failure. There are, however, some specific manifestations associated with ALL, including enlarged lymph nodes (lymphadenopathy), enlarged liver and spleen (hepatosplenomegaly) and infiltration into the central nervous system (CNS).

Medical management

Acute lymphoblastic leukaemia is treated with a very complex drug regimen that includes both cytotoxic and immunosuppressant drugs. Some of the cytotoxic drugs are given intravenously, some by intramuscular injection, and some intrathecally via the spinal canal to treat CNS disease. Treatment for ALL can take up to 2 years to complete. Fortunately, a large proportion of the treatment can be given on an outpatient basis, as patients tend not to be rendered so profoundly neutropenic as those having treatment for AML. Patients do, however, remain immunocompromised for long periods and remain at risk of serious infection.

As with AML, those who have a poor response to first-line treatments or those with poor prognostic indicators may be suitable candidates for haemopoietic stem cell transplantation.

▶ **Nursing management: acute leukaemia**

A diagnosis of acute leukaemia is clearly devastating for both patients and their families. The situation can be compounded by the fact that, once the diagnosis is confirmed, treatment should commence as soon as possible, usually within 24 hours. Skilled nursing is required to support patients and their relatives in coming to terms with the diagnosis. At the same time, nurses must provide them with a great deal of complex information about the disease and its treatment (see Reflective Practice box 18.2). Patients should be made aware of the short-term and long-term effects of treatment prior to its commencement. These effects are outlined in the section covering the treatment of malignant blood disorders.

R|R REFLECTIVE PRACTICE

18.2 A diagnosis of acute leukaemia

John is 32 years old and has been admitted to the haematology unit. His wife Jill accompanies him. They have been told that John has acute leukaemia and should commence chemotherapy within 24 hours.

Student activities
The couple will require information regarding his disease, its treatment, the side-effects, prognosis, central line care and dietary advice.

- How would you structure the information?
- What factors may hinder the exchange of information?
- What methods of information-giving would you employ?

Patients may remain pancytopenic throughout much of their treatment. Nurses should therefore be aware of patients' recent blood and laboratory results. This will enable them to appropriately assess their level of anaemia, potential for bleeding and risk of infection. Patients with diminished platelet counts should be observed and monitored for signs of bleeding. These can include tachycardia, restlessness, confusion, spontaneous bruising, petechiae, nose or gum bleeds, oozing from around central line sites, abdominal pain, haematuria and melaena.

Anaemia is generally corrected by blood transfusion. Platelet transfusions are indicated if the platelet count falls below $10 \times 10^9/L$ or there are signs of bleeding. General principles of infection control for this group of patients are outlined in the section on neutropenia. However, it must be stressed that infection is a major cause of morbidity and mortality; the nursing care of these patients should therefore be meticulous.

It has already been noted that some patients will not recover from this disease and may die as a result of leukaemia itself or from complications of treatment. Once it becomes clear that curative treatment is no longer appropriate, the management of symptoms becomes a priority to facilitate a peaceful death for the patient. The role of nurses in this process is pivotal as they seek to maintain the comfort and dignity of the patient whilst offering emotional support to them and their family. These situations can put enormous strain on the personal resources of nurses and a strong team approach is vital to managing stress (Ch. 6). The involvement of palliative care teams should be facilitated at the earliest opportunity, they can offer expertise in symptom control and bereavement care for relatives as well as support for ward staff.

CHRONIC LEUKAEMIA

Chronic myeloid leukaemia

Chronic myeloid leukaemia (CML) is a stem cell disorder that results in the unregulated production of myeloid white cells.

Aetiology and pathophysiology

The aetiology is unknown but it is generally associated with a specific, acquired chromosome abnormality, the Philadelphia (Ph) chromosome (a shortened chromosome 22 occurring from a reciprocal translocation of material with chromosome 9). CML can affect any age group but mainly affects people between the ages of 40 and 60 years. For a small proportion of people, CML will remit spontaneously. More commonly, the disease will become progressively unresponsive to treatment. Eventually it will move from a chronic to an accelerated phase when it transforms into an acute leukaemia. On average, survival is about 3–7 years.

Clinical presentation

Chronic myeloid leukaemia has an insidious onset and is frequently diagnosed by a routine blood test. The usual clinical features include anorexia, weight loss, anaemia and hepatosplenomegaly. A full blood count will reveal a high white cell count. This can increase blood viscosity and result in such symptoms as headache, blurred vision and breathlessness.

Medical management

The initial treatment involves lowering the white cell count. Apheresis (see p. 452) and the use of oral cytotoxic drugs such as hydroxycarbamide (hydroxyurea) or busulfan can help to achieve this. Treatment with subcutaneous interferon-alpha can help to correct any chromosomal abnormality and prolong survival, but it is not curative.

Allogeneic (obtained from a compatible donor) stem cell transplantation is the main curative option for those with CML and is best performed during the chronic phase of the disease. The decision to undergo the high-risk process of transplantation can be very difficult at this stage, as people may feel relatively well and may still be coming to terms with the implications of their disease. Support from health care professionals, including specialist nurses, can be very important at this time (see p. 469).

A new drug treatment that is currently under investigation for the treatment of CML is imatinib. This targets Philadelphia chromosome positive cells in order to prevent abnormal cell proliferation. If imatinib does prove to be effective, it could provide a more acceptable alternative to transplantation in the future.

Chronic lymphocytic leukaemia

Chronic lymphocytic leukaemia (CLL) is a proliferative disorder of the lymphocytes. These cells then accumulate in the blood, bone marrow, lymph nodes and spleen. CLL is the most common form of leukaemia and usually occurs in later life; 95% of cases are seen in people over the age of 50 years.

Clinical features

In the early stages, the symptoms of CLL are mild and include fatigue, weight loss and some enlargement of lymph nodes, liver and spleen. However, the disease is marked by a slow but progressive bone marrow failure. The mean survival of patients with CLL is about 10 years. As CLL is essentially a disease of older people, patients will often die from unrelated causes.

Medical management

Treatment is generally delayed until symptoms become troublesome, often for a period of years. If symptoms do progress, oral cytotoxic agents such as chlorambucil can help to control the disease and reduce symptoms. Eventually, the disease is likely to progress and require more aggressive treatments. The cytotoxic drug fludarabine is often the treatment of choice. Combination chemotherapy regimens such as CHOP (cyclophosphamide, hydroxydaunorubicin, vincristine [oncovin] and prednisolone) may also be used for second-line treatment but they are not curative. Haemopoietic stem cell transplantation may be offered to some relatively young patients in the hope of effecting a cure, but this is not routine at present.

▶ Nursing management: chronic leukaemia

Many patients with chronic leukaemia receive all of their treatment in busy outpatient clinics. In the past, this meant that many received very little nursing input. In order to rectify this, haematology units are increasingly employing clinical nurse specialists. These nurses can offer support, patient education and advice about symptom management. They can also play a role in coordinating patient care, educating other professionals, and helping patients to access additional forms of care and support, including community and palliative care support, should this become necessary.

THE LYMPHOMAS

The lymphomas are a diverse group of tumours that originate in lymphoid tissue. Lymphomas can primarily be divided into two groups: Hodgkin's lymphoma (Hodgkin's disease) and non-Hodgkin's lymphoma (NHL).

Lymphomas can arise in any age group but predominantly affect adults. The incidence of Hodgkin's lymphoma tends to peak in young adults between the ages of 20 and 30, making it one of the most common malignancies in this age group. It peaks again after the age of 50 years. More males than females are affected by Hodgkin's lymphoma. Non-Hodgkin's lymphoma usually occurs at around 50 years of age, and incidence is more evenly distributed between the sexes.

Aetiology and pathophysiology

The aetiology is largely unknown, although genetic and environmental factors may be implicated. Certain viruses, particularly Epstein–Barr virus (EBV) and human T-cell leukaemia virus (HTLV-1), may also be a factor. People who are immunocompromised appear to be more susceptible to NHL. Predisposing factors may therefore include long-term corticosteroid therapy, immunosuppressant therapy following organ or stem cell transplant, and pre-existing autoimmune disease (Mehta & Hoffbrand 2000). People who are HIV-positive and those with AIDS have an increased risk of developing aggressive lymphomas, such as Burkitt's lymphoma.

Lymphomas can spread throughout the lymphatic system and into the surrounding organs, CNS, lung, skin and bone marrow. Patterns of spread vary according to lymphoma type and site of origin. Hodgkin's lymphomas tend to spread in a contiguous manner to neighbouring lymph nodes. The spread of NHL tends to be more diffuse. Prognosis varies with the subtype and stage of the disease.

Clinical presentation

People with lymphoma commonly present with a non-painful swelling of one or more lymph nodes. In Hodgkin's lymphoma, this typically affects the cervical lymph nodes at the side of the neck. People with NHL tend to present with more generalized lymphadenopathy. If abdominal or thoracic nodes are primarily affected, individuals can present with very large, bulky tumours. When other organs are involved at presentation, it can initially prove difficult to distinguish between lymphoma and other forms of solid tumour. A patient history may reveal the presence of systemic symptoms, namely fever, night sweats and unexplained weight loss. Other common symptoms are pruritus, particularly in Hodgkin's lymphoma, and fatigue. Those with Hodgkin's lymphoma may also report alcohol-induced pain at tumour sites. Additional signs and symptoms may be due to the involvement of a particular organ or body area.

Special investigations

A definitive diagnosis of lymphoma is generally obtained from lymph node or tissue biopsy followed by histological examination and chromosomal (cytogenetic) analysis. The stage of lymphoma is determined by a combination of blood tests, X-ray, computed tomography (CT) or magnetic resonance imaging (MRI), and bone marrow biopsy. Blood cell counts and biochemistry may appear normal in early stage disease. Indicators of more advanced disease include anaemia, pancytopenia, a raised ESR and abnormal liver function tests.

HODGKIN'S LYMPHOMA

In Hodgkin's lymphoma, stage of disease is an important prognostic indicator that strongly influences treatment selection. Staging of Hodgkin's lymphoma is generally based upon the widely accepted Ann Arbor system (Box 18.2). Staging criteria include the extent and distribution of lymphadenopathy, the involvement of other organs and the presence or absence of systemic symptoms (see above).

For early-stage Hodgkin's lymphoma without systemic symptoms, localized radiotherapy to the affected lymph node regions can be curative. More advanced disease is treated with cytotoxic chemotherapy. A standard regimen for this is ABVD (adriamycin, bleomycin, vinblastine and dacarbazine) given on an outpatient basis.

Box 18.2 Ann Arbor staging of Hodgkin's lymphoma

I   Node involvement in one lymph node area

II   Two or more lymph node areas affected, but on the same side of the diaphragm

III   Lymph nodes involved above and below the diaphragm

IV   Involvement in extranodal sites, such as the bone marrow, liver and testes
    a   Absence of systemic symptoms
    b   Presence of systemic symptoms such as fever, night sweats and weight loss

---

General considerations for the nursing care of patients having cytotoxic chemotherapy are outlined below in the section on the 'Management of malignant blood disorders'.

NON-HODGKIN'S LYMPHOMA

In NHL, disease classification and rate of tumour cell division tend to have more prognostic significance than does the stage. In terms of general treatment principles, major distinctions can be made between indolent (low-grade) NHL and aggressive or highly aggressive (high-grade) NHL. Indolent NHL may require no specific treatment initially. Indeed, a conservative 'watch and wait' policy may be reasonably adopted for months, or even years, if patients are asymptomatic. If treatment is given, the options include localized radiotherapy or chemotherapy. Such treatments are rarely curative. Consequently, the immediate benefits of treatment interventions should always be carefully weighed against possible toxicities. Premature intervention can reduce the scope for further treatment at a later stage.

The ineffectiveness of current treatments for indolent NHL seems to be linked to the slow rate of cell division in low-grade tumours, which limits the action of many cytotoxic agents. However, newer agents are now being assessed. These include fludarabine, interferon-alpha and monoclonal antibodies (see p. 475).

Conversely, people with more aggressive, rapidly multiplying tumours may respond well to chemotherapy. An effective and widely used regimen for aggressive lymphoma is CHOP (cyclophosphamide, hydroxydaunorubicin, vincristine [oncovin] and prednisolone). Repeated cycles are given over a period of up to 6 months, usually as an outpatient procedure.

BURKITT'S LYMPHOMA

Highly aggressive lymphomas, such as Burkitt's lymphoma, generally require more intensive chemotherapy regimens. Until recently, Burkitt's lymphoma was a very rare disease that was associated with EBV infection and was predominately found in children of African origin. These children typically presented with localized tumours to the jaw and responded well to relatively simple chemotherapy regimens. There is an increasing incidence of Burkitt's lymphoma among adults in both Europe and North America; this is often associated with HIV infection. People with this form of Burkitt's lymphoma tend to present with widespread, rapidly progressing, abdominal or mediastinal tumours. CNS disease and bone marrow involvement are often present. Treatments for Burkitt's lymphoma include complex and intensive chemotherapy regimens, which comprise chemotherapy with CNS treatment and haemopoietic growth factor support. Chemotherapy for CNS disease (methotrexate and cytarabine) is given intrathecally in order to bypass the blood–brain barrier. Haemopoietic growth factors (G-CSF) are given to reduce the duration of chemotherapy-induced neutropenia. This can be particularly important for people who are already immunocompromised due to HIV infection.

People undergoing such intensive treatments require hospitalization and very close monitoring. Those presenting with very bulky disease need particularly close observation in the early stages of treatment due to the risk of tumour lysis syndrome (see p. 473).

RELAPSED LYMPHOMA

Approximately 10% of people with early stage Hodgkin's lymphoma will fail to achieve remission or will relapse after initial therapy. For people with stage IV Hodgkin's lymphoma (Box 18.2) or those with NHL, the overall relapse rate is nearer 50%. Those who relapse may achieve a complete or further remission following second-line chemotherapy regimens. Nowadays, people may also opt for further high-dose chemotherapy followed by autologous peripheral blood stem cell rescue or allogeneic stem cell transplantation (see p. 474).

A promising new treatment that is licensed for selected forms of lymphoma is anti-CD20 monoclonal antibody therapy. These monoclonal antibodies target antigens on the surface of lymphoma cells and lead to their destruction. The advantage of this is that other cell types are unaffected. This is not the case for cytotoxic chemotherapy (see below).

NURSING AND MEDICAL MANAGEMENT OF MALIGNANT BLOOD DISORDERS

Three forms of treatment for malignant haematological conditions are outlined:

- cytotoxic chemotherapy
- haemopoietic stem cell transplantation
- monoclonal antibodies.

CYTOTOXIC CHEMOTHERAPY

Cytotoxic drugs are antiproliferative agents that are used in the treatment of many malignant haematological and non-haematological conditions (further detail can be found in Ch. 33). Most of these agents exert an effect during cell replication. Cytotoxic drugs can potentially affect all cells in the body. Abnormal tumour cells or rapidly dividing cells (bone marrow, gastrointestinal mucosa, skin, hair follicles, sperm and oocytes) are most vulnerable. Chemotherapy regimens often combine drugs from different groups, which can maximize treatment efficacy as drugs will act upon cells at different stages of the cell cycle in different ways (Ch. 33) or work synergistically. Some cytotoxic drugs can be taken orally. More intensive regimens are normally given intravenously.

Long-term central venous catheters

Long-term central venous catheters, such as Hickman lines, are often used to facilitate the safe administration of cytotoxic drugs. They also provide a route for giving intravenous fluids, blood products and other intravenous medications, and permit frequent blood sampling without the discomfort associated with venepuncture (Ch. 11).

These lines are tunnelled under the skin and exit from the chest. A Dacron cuff anchors the line within the tunnel. Risks associated with the use central venous catheters include infection and thrombus formation. The line site should therefore be regularly inspected for signs of infection such as soreness or inflammation (see Evidence-based Practice box 18.1). Thrombi can occur at the tips of central venous catheters. If a line is

EVIDENCE-BASED PRACTICE

18.1 Prevention of infection at the site of tunnelled central venous catheters

The site of a tunnelled central line acts as a potential port of entry for pathological microorganisms into the patient's bloodstream. Care of this site is critical for minimizing this risk. The following principles can guide practice:

- Dressing of the site is recommended for the first 21 days after a line is inserted.
- The site should be cleaned with chlorhexidine-based solutions (Harrison 1997). This should be allowed to dry before a dressing is applied (Terry et al 1995).
- The exit site of a tunnelled central line can be covered with a semi-permeable transparent dressing or a dry dressing; research indicates that neither is superior to the other (Brandt et al 1996).
- Wet or soiled dressing should be changed immediately as they provide an optimal environment for bacterial proliferation (Cornock 1996).
- After 21 days, fibroblasts form around the cuff of the catheter. This anchors the line and creates a natural barrier to microorganisms. At this time the sutures may be removed from the line site and it requires no dressing (BCSH 1997).

- All central line sites should be observed daily for signs of infection, which should be reported to the medical team promptly.

References

Brandt B, De Palma J, Irwin M, Shogun J, Lucke JF. Comparison of CVC dressings in bone marrow transplant patients. Oncol Nurs Forum 1996; 23(5): 829–836.

British Committee for Standards in Haematology (BCSH). Guidelines on the insertion and management of central venous lines. Br J Haematol 1997; 98: 1041–1047.

Cornock M. Making sense of central venous catheters. Nurs Times 1996; 92(49): 30–31.

Harrison M. CVCs: a review of the literature. Nurs Stand 1997; 11(27): 43–45.

Terry J, Baranowski L, Lonsway RA, Hedrick C (eds). Intravenous – clinical principles and practice. Philadelphia: WB Saunders; 1995.

Further reading

Dougherty L, Lamb J. Intravenous therapy in nursing practice. Edinburgh: Churchill Livingstone; 1999.

---

blocked it should be reported to the medical team for prompt action. Blocked lines should never be forced. Fibrinolytic drugs may be used to dissolve clots in situ, while the prophylactic use of warfarin can lower the risk of thrombus formation.

The presence of a central venous catheter is a constant symbol of illness and can adversely affect the patient's body image. Nurses should therefore be sensitive to the possible impact of this on patients.

Most patients will go home with their lines in situ and must be shown how to care for them. Many patients become skilled in flushing their lines and can self-administer intravenous antibiotics. However, some patients are not able to participate in the care of their lines due to poor technique or squeamishness; nurses should assess a patient's ability to self-care before discharge.

Administration of cytotoxic drugs

Nurses who have undertaken suitable post-registration training frequently administer cytotoxic drugs. Because these are, by definition, potentially harmful to body tissues, great care should be taken to prevent accidental spillage or contamination during administration (Ch. 33) and hospital policies concerning these drugs should be strictly adhered to. Universal precautions should also be taken when handling the body fluids of patients undergoing treatment (Ch. 13).

Side-effects of cytotoxic drugs

Cytotoxic treatments produce a wide range of side-effects and can have a dramatic impact on quality of life. Most side-effects result from damage to normal rapidly dividing tissues such as the bone marrow, gastrointestinal mucosa and hair follicles. They include pancytopenia, nausea and vomiting, mucositis, diarrhoea, constipation, alopecia and fatigue. Psychological effects can include anxiety and depression and altered body image. Longer-term effects can include infertility. The very intensive regimens used to treat haematological malignancies can also result in particularly severe and even life-threatening complications such as neutropenic sepsis (see p. 466), tumour lysis syndrome (see p. 473), major organ damage and secondary malignancies.

Pancytopenia

One of the most significant problems associated with cytotoxic treatments for haematological malignancies is bone marrow depression leading to pancytopenia. Bone marrow function can be suppressed for several weeks after treatment. Chemotherapy is usually given in intermittent cycles to minimize the effects of marrow depression and to enable the marrow to recover. Here, a balance often needs to be achieved between maximizing bone marrow recovery and minimizing the chance of disease recurrence. Haemopoietic growth factors can be given therapeutically to increase the rate of marrow recovery so that treatment intensity and efficacy can be maintained.

Blood product support is often required and patients remain neutropenic for prolonged periods. The nursing care for anaemia, neutropenia and thrombocytopenia is discussed in the relevant sections of this chapter. Nurses should be aware of the blood counts of their patients in order to assess their condition.

Nausea and vomiting

Nausea and vomiting are distressing symptoms that can produce a range of additional effects such as anxiety, fatigue, anorexia and fluid and electrolyte imbalance (Ch. 8). Anxiety can exacerbate symptoms and may precipitate anticipatory nausea that is very difficult to control. Frequent retching can cause discomfort and potentiate bleeding in patients with thrombocytopenia or mucositis. Nurses should therefore ensure that all patients undergoing cytotoxic chemotherapy receive effective antiemetic cover. A variety of antiemetics may be prescribed depending on the chemotherapy regimen and its potential to cause emesis. In regimens where there is a relatively low risk of emesis, symptoms may be well controlled by the use of antiemetics such as metoclopramide. Regimens with a higher risk of emesis may require the use of $5HT_3$ antagonists, such as ondansetron or tropesitron, in combination with the corticosteroid dexamethasone (Ch. 34). Patients who are nauseated should be encouraged to maintain a good oral fluid intake. Food may be better tolerated if the principle of 'little and often' is adhered to. Distraction and relaxation therapies may also be helpful.

Mucositis

The mucous membranes of the gastrointestinal tract are composed of rapidly dividing cells that are particularly susceptible to the effects of cytotoxic drugs. Such treatments can give rise to mucositis throughout the gastrointestinal tract where it causes ulceration, bleeding and pain. Because the integrity of the mucosa is undermined, there is also an increased risk of infection. This is of particular concern when patients are neutropenic, and prophylactic antibiotics or antifungal medications may be prescribed.

Oral mucositis is termed stomatitis. The mouth can become extremely dry (xerostomia) and the saliva can become thick and stringy or absent. Regular oral assessment, including a baseline assessment prior to treatment, should be undertaken. A number of oral assessment tools are available, and unit policies should be adhered to.

Criteria for oral assessment may include:

- dryness (mouth and lips)
- colour
- ulceration
- bleeding
- pain
- ability to speak
- ability to maintain an oral intake or perform oral care.

Good oral care regimens can help to reduce the chances of infection (Chs 33 and 34). Wherever possible, patients should visit their dentist and rectify dental problems before commencing treatment. To minimize trauma to oral mucosa, patients should be encouraged to clean their teeth twice daily with a soft toothbrush. Chlorhexidine-based mouthwashes can be used to help control the spread of some oral bacteria and other microorganisms. Keeping the mouth moist is important and patients should be encouraged to drink if they can tolerate it. If this is not possible, artificial saliva can sometimes be helpful. Eating can be very difficult, and can be compounded by anorexia, nausea and taste changes. Patients should be encouraged to eat whatever they feel able to tolerate (Ch. 11). Spicy foods are usually best avoided. A light diet or dietary supplements such as fortified milkshakes or sip feeds may be better tolerated. Advice from a dietician can be extremely useful in this context. Benzydamine mouthwashes, soluble paracetamol and topical cocaine preparations can provide effective first-line analgesia for mucositis. Pain relief is usually most efficacious if given before meals.

Mucositis can be extremely severe when intensive, high-dose treatments are administered. Severe pain from mucositis may require treatment with intravenous opioids such as morphine. The use of patient-controlled analgesia (PCA) pumps is particularly appropriate as they can enable patients to exert greater control over their circumstances (Ch. 7). Patients with very severe mucositis may be completely unable to tolerate oral food or fluids and may need to be supported with intravenous fluids and nasogastric feeding or total parenteral nutrition (Ch. 11).

Bowel disturbances

Diarrhoea and constipation are common side-effects of chemotherapy. As with other side-effects, prevention is better than cure. Hence, patients should be informed of the potential for these symptoms to occur and should be encouraged, wherever possible (but see above), to maintain an adequate oral fluid intake. Patients should also be encouraged to report any changes in bowel habit so that treatments such as anti-diarrhoeal drugs or laxatives can be prescribed at an early stage as appropriate. In the case of diarrhoea, stool samples should be obtained for culture to rule out any infective cause.

Hair loss

Many of the cytotoxic regimens used to treat acute haematological malignancies will cause temporary hair loss (alopecia). This can have an enormous psychological impact on patients and can undermine their body image. Hair loss usually occurs around 2 weeks after chemotherapy commences. Nurses should make sure that patients are aware of this side-effect and have an opportunity to work through their concerns and prepare for hair loss. Grants for wigs are available on the NHS, and nurses may advise patients on suitable styles. Wigs should be ordered as soon as possible so that they are available when the hair loss occurs. Scarves and hats can provide acceptable and stylish alternatives and can be used to express individuality. Patients should be advised to keep their heads covered in strong sunlight to protect them from sunburn. Heat loss can be a problem in winter. The hair will usually start to grow back about 6 weeks after treatment is completed, but it may be a different shade or texture.

Fatigue

Fatigue can have an enormous impact on quality of life. It can make accomplishing simple everyday activities and maintaining normal social relationships extremely difficult. Fatigue can persist after treatment is completed and may be heightened by depression. Managing fatigue can be challenging and nurses should offer support and understanding to patients and their relatives. Patients should be informed that fatigue is a normal side-effect and that they are not alone in experiencing it. The effects of fatigue upon the individual and whether it occurs at certain times of the day or after particular activities should be assessed. This can highlight ways in which patients might usefully adapt their routines to minimize the effects. Patients should be advised to punctuate periods of activity with periods of rest. Light exercise can decrease fatigue and improve the quality of sleep. Relaxation techniques can be used to enhance rest periods.

Infertility and sexuality (Ch. 25)

Sperm and oocyte production is often affected by cytotoxic therapy. However, conception can still occur and patients should be advised to use appropriate contraception throughout their treatment due to the potentially adverse effects of cytotoxic drugs upon the fetus. Fertility can be permanently reduced after treatment. The recovery of fertility is rare for people undergoing high-dose chemotherapy (Apperley et al 2000).

Patients should always be informed of the possibility of infertility prior to commencing treatment. Male patients should also be given the option of storing sperm. For females, the storage of oocytes is still relatively experimental and can be difficult to achieve in the short time span between diagnosis and treatment. Embryo storage may be possible prior to planned high-dose treatments. Assisted conception using in vitro techniques may increase the chances of pregnancy after treatment. Other alternatives include surrogacy or adoption.

The psychological impact of infertility can have long-term consequences and can adversely affect an individual's perception of their sexuality. This can be compounded by factors such as weight loss, alopecia and fatigue. Loss of libido is common both during and after treatment. Males may experience temporary or long-term erectile dysfunction. Women may experience menopausal symptoms such as flushing or vaginal dryness and itching – although hormone replacement therapy may help to relieve this in the longer term. Women having treatment for haematological malignancies may be given drugs such as norethisterone to suppress normal menstruation and reduce the potential for blood loss.

Nurses should offer patients and their partners the opportunity to discuss sexual issues if they so wish (see Reflective Practice box 18.3). Sensitivity is clearly important in this, as in many other areas. Referral to specialist counsellors may sometimes be appropriate.

Tumour lysis syndrome

Cytotoxic drugs can have a very rapid effect on tumour cells, which can cause problems in patients with large, bulky tumours. As the cells die, they release substances into the bloodstream that can be highly toxic and lead to elevated levels of urate, potassium and phosphate with a corresponding fall in calcium. This condition is called tumour lysis syndrome (TLS). TLS tends to occur during the first few days of treatment and can result in renal failure due to the crystallization of uric acid in the renal tubules, acidosis, cardiac failure and death. It can be prevented by the administration of allopurinol before and during cytotoxic treatment and by maintaining a good diuresis. Patients should therefore be encouraged to drink 2–3 L of fluid daily. People with bulky tumours or a high tumour burden will require intravenous fluids prior to and during treatment. Sodium bicarbonate may also be given to reduce acidosis. An accurate measure of fluid balance is essential to monitor renal function and to assess adequate fluid intake.

R|Я REFLECTIVE PRACTICE

18.3 Sexuality and patients undergoing cytotoxic chemotherapy

In 1975 the World Health Organization emphasized sexuality as an aspect of health. Sexuality affects our identity, social relationships, feelings of well-being and emotions in addition to sexual activity itself. Lamb (1996) estimated that 90% of cancer patients experience some problems associated with sexuality, and yet nurses rarely discuss sexual issues with patients.

Student activities
- What factors could adversely affect patients' perceptions of their sexuality when undergoing treatment for a haematological malignancy?
- How can nurses address some of these issues?
- What inhibits nurses from addressing these issues?

The BACUP booklet 'Sexuality and Cancer' is a useful resource (www.cancerbacup.org.uk).

References
Lamb M. Sexuality and the cancer patient. Gynaecol Oncol Nurs 1996; 6(3): 38–45.
World Health Organization (WHO). Education and treatment in human sexuality: the training of health professionals. Technical Report Series 572. Geneva: WHO; 1975.

Late effects

The long-term side-effects of cytotoxic treatment can include permanent organ damage. All major organs can be affected and damage is often dose-related. Those having high-dose chemotherapy prior to haemopoietic stem cell transplantation are therefore particularly vulnerable. Close monitoring of the patient is essential to enable problems to be detected and treated as early as possible. Ironically, the drugs used to treat malignant illnesses can cause the genetic mutations that lead to secondary malignancies. The immediate benefits of treatment can clearly make this an acceptable risk for patients.

New and improved treatment regimens that limit the adverse effects of cytotoxic treatments are constantly being sought. Many haematology patients are treated in accordance with national or international research studies. The aim of these studies is to maximize the effectiveness of treatment regimens while reducing their overall toxicity.

In spite of the dramatic array of side-effects, many patients tolerate intensive chemotherapy remarkably well and manage to maintain some degree of normality in their lives. The role of nurses in supporting patients and their families throughout their treatment cannot be underestimated. Skilled nursing is essential for the management of symptoms, treatment of complications, patient education and psychological support. This is what makes haematology nursing so challenging.

HAEMOPOIETIC STEM CELL TRANSPLANTATION (HSCT)

Haemopoietic stem cell transplantation (bone marrow transplantation) enables normal blood cell production to be re-established in patients whose bone marrow function is inadequate or has failed as a result of disease or its treatment. It is used to treat a range of haematological conditions, including leukaemia, lymphoma, myeloma, aplastic anaemia, thalassaemia and sickle cell disease. Research studies are being conducted to assess its efficacy in some solid tumours, including breast, ovarian and germ cell tumours.

There are two main types of haemopoietic stem cell transplant: autologous and allogeneic. In autologous transplants, the patient's own stem cells are collected and later re-infused following very high-dose chemotherapy and/or radiotherapy treatments. This procedure is sometimes called stem cell rescue. When the bone marrow is the primary site of disease or in cases where there is pre-existing bone marrow failure, allogeneic transplantation may be indicated. In allogeneic transplants, stem cells are obtained from a HLA-compatible donor. These are infused into the recipient and serve to repopulate the bone marrow with healthy stem cells.

Human leucocyte antigens (HLAs) are carried on the surface of cells. They form part of the immune system and determine tissue type compatibility. The best chance of finding a good match is from a sibling donor, as both the donor and recipient share the same gene pool. If no compatible sibling is available, a matched unrelated donor (MUD) transplant may be considered. Unrelated donors are located via national and international donor registers. Finding a suitable matched unrelated donor is a complex process (see Special Issues box 18.1). Moreover, some HLA incompatibilities are not detected by routine matching techniques. This can increase the risk of complications such as graft-versus-host disease (see p. 475).

The decision to undergo a high-risk procedure such as stem cell rescue or allogeneic transplantation requires very careful consideration. It is important that candidates are given sufficient information to enable them to come to a decision that is right for them. Transplant candidates must take in a great deal of complex treatment information; the giving of this usually takes place over a period of weeks or even months. During the decision-making period, ongoing support from health care professionals can be vital (see Reflective Practice box 18.4). Nurses should ensure that transplant candidates have ample opportunity to discuss the implications of treatment and voice any concerns they may have. It should be remembered that many candidates are already coping with life-threatening illness and confronting their own mortality. Creating a sympathetic environment, and the use of techniques such as open questioning to facilitate discussion, and careful listening, is very important in this context (Ch. 3).

 SPECIAL ISSUES

18.1 Bone marrow donation

There is a 1 in 4 chance of any sibling having compatible bone marrow cells to a patient. For those who do not have a suitable donor within the family, an unrelated donor can be sought from the bone marrow donor register. Males are preferred for bone marrow donation because:

- They are generally larger and can provide a higher yield of bone marrow cells.
- They are less likely to suffer from anaemia, which prohibits donation.
- They tend to be more available than females as it is not possible to donate during and for 1 year after pregnancy.
- Women who have had a pregnancy will often have antibodies in their blood; this makes them less suitable as donors.

However, on the Anthony Nolan Bone Marrow register, only 30% of volunteers are male.

Student activities
- What measures could bone marrow registers take to encourage male volunteers?
- What factors may inhibit potential donors from joining the register?

For more information visit the Anthony Nolan Bone Marrow Trust website: www.anthonynolan.org.uk

---

R│Я REFLECTIVE PRACTICE

18.4 Decision support for haemopoietic stem cell transplantation (HSCT)

Patients must assimilate a large amount of complex information when deciding whether to undergo HSCT. The giving of appropriate support prior to transplant has been linked to patients' psychological adjustment afterwards (Molassiotis 1997). Because transplant candidates may already be coping with the physical and psychological demands of life-threatening illness, the need to maintain hope and a positive outlook is often very important.

Student activities
- How would you ensure that candidates for HSCT have adequate information on which to base their decisions without overloading them?
- What sources of information might candidates use when making a decision?
- How would you check that candidates understand and appreciate any adverse implications of treatment without undermining their coping mechanisms or their ability to maintain hope for the future?
- What sort of environment might enhance this type of disclosure?

Reference
Molassiotis A. A conceptual model of adaptation to illness and quality of life for cancer patients treated with bone marrow transplant. J Adv Nurs 1997; 26: 572–579.

When a decision to proceed with transplant has been made, stem cells are collected (harvested) from the patient or donor either directly from the bone marrow or via the peripheral blood using apheresis (see p. 452). It is common for specialist nurses to perform both harvesting procedures.

Bone marrow harvesting is carried out in theatre. The patient is anaesthetized and multiple punctures are made in the posterior iliac crests. Marrow is then aspirated until the desired yield is obtained. Usually around 500–1000 mL of bone marrow is aspirated, depending on the size of the recipient. The harvested marrow is then infused into the patient via a central venous catheter; the marrow cells will circulate in the blood to the bone marrow spaces and then start to proliferate.

Although stem cells are mainly found in bone marrow, they can be made to spill out into the peripheral bloodstream by the controlled use of chemotherapy and/or haemopoietic growth factors such as G-CSF. Once stem cells enter the circulation in sufficient quantities, the patient or donor is able to undergo peripheral blood stem cell harvest by apheresis. This procedure can be repeated for up to three consecutive days in order to obtain an adequate number of stem cells. Stem cells collected in this way are infused into the recipient in the same way as bone marrow or they can be frozen and stored for future use.

People generally undergo stem cell transplantation during a period of disease remission following standard treatment for haematological malignancies. In preparation for transplantation, patients receive conditioning treatments that are designed to eradicate any remaining disease. Conditioning regimens are selected in accordance with disease type. Some combine cytotoxic chemotherapy with total body irradiation (TBI). These treatments can be extremely arduous. However, the aim is always to maximize treatment effectiveness while minimizing toxicity.

Stem cell administration is a relatively simple technique. Stem cells are infused into the recipient in a similar way to blood transfusion. Nurses administering stem cells should closely monitor patients' vital signs (temperature, pulse, respiration rate), oxygen saturation levels, weight and fluid balance. Patients receiving a large volume of marrow are at risk of fluid overload. Patients may occasionally react to donor cells during the infusion, although this is relatively rare as they are already immunocompromised by conditioning regimens. The prophylactic use of antihistamines such as chlorphenamine (chlorpheniramine) can help to prevent this.

The side-effects and complications of stem cell transplantation are primarily related to the cytotoxic and immunosuppressive effects of conditioning regimens. The immune system is severely compromised and patients are rendered profoundly neutropenic. In these circumstances, even minor everyday infections can prove life-threatening. Consequently, patients are nursed in conditions of protective isolation for around 2–4 weeks after transplantation, depending on transplant type. Protective isolation means that the external environment is manipulated in order to reduce the risk of infection. The degree of isolation can vary with transplant type and local policies. However, the overall aim is to maintain the safety of patients while balancing their needs for continuing human contact and emotional support throughout the period of stem cell engraftment.

During the post-transplant period, red blood cell and platelet production is also inhibited and most patients require blood transfusion and blood product support. Other side-effects of cytotoxic chemotherapy such as nausea and vomiting, mucositis, diarrhoea, fatigue and alopecia are common and can be severe. High-dose chemotherapy or radiotherapy can also precipitate a range of additional and potentially serious complications, including organ failure and haemorrhage (Apperley et al 2000).

Graft-versus-host disease

An additional risk associated with allogeneic transplantation is the development of graft-versus-host disease (GVHD). This is an immune reaction whereby T cells in the transplanted marrow, or graft, attack the recipient's cells. The risk of GVHD increases in transplants from unrelated donors and in older people. GVHD most commonly affects the cells of the skin, gut or liver. GVHD may simply manifest as a minor skin rash, but in extreme cases it can cause severe cell destruction leading to widespread ulceration of the skin or gut, profuse diarrhoea, bleeding, infection and liver failure. Severe GVHD will often prove fatal.

In the past, T-cell depletion of the donor marrow was seen as a means of reducing the incidence and severity of GVHD. However, this was also found to be associated with a higher rate of disease relapse after transplantation. The reason for this appears to be that T cells within the graft can also exert some form of graft-versus-tumour effect. This effect is now being exploited in the development of non-myeloablative or 'mini' allografts.

Non-myeloablative stem cell transplants

The toxic effects of conventional allogeneic stem cell transplantation mean that these very arduous treatments are only suitable for people who are relatively young and fit. There is, however, a growing move to develop better-tolerated conditioning regimens to enable a wider range of recipients to benefit from stem cell transplantation. The resulting non-myeloablative transplants are designed to suppress the recipient's immune system sufficiently to allow engraftment of the donated marrow. The aim is for the grafted T cells to then destroy any remaining malignant cells. However, the longer-term effectiveness of these transplants has still to be evaluated.

MONOCLONAL ANTIBODIES

Monoclonal antibodies are a fairly recent addition to the range of treatment options for haematological malignancies. Monoclonal antibodies harness the body's natural immune system to destroy malignant cells. Different types of cell have specific antigens on their surface. The theory behind monoclonal antibody therapy is that, if the antigens on the surface of tumour cells can be identified, genetically engineered antibodies can be generated to target and destroy the tumour cells. Monoclonal antibodies are an exciting development in cancer care and are increasingly being used alongside standard treatments.

▶ Nursing care

Monoclonal antibodies are specifically targeted; therefore they do not cause the same array of side-effects as conventional chemotherapy. These drugs are given by intravenous infusion.

The most common complications of treatment are infusion-related reactions. Patients receiving monoclonal antibodies should be closely observed for signs of adverse reaction such as shivering, fever or dyspnoea. Patients' vital signs should be monitored throughout the infusion. Reactions can usually be treated with paracetamol, antihistamines such as chlorphenamine (chlorpheniramine), or bronchodilators such as salbutamol. As the first dose of a monoclonal antibody can sometimes cause tumour lysis syndrome (see p. 473), patients should have a fluid input of 3 L in 24 hours and their urine output should be monitored.

DISORDERS OF HAEMOSTASIS

Disorders of haemostasis may be due to reduced or abnormal platelet production or abnormalities in the coagulation process. There are several disorders arising from these factors:

- thrombocytopenia
- disseminated intravascular coagulation (DIC)
- haemophilia.

THROMBOCYTOPENIA

The term thrombocytopenia is used to describe an abnormally low platelet count below the normal range of $150–400 \times 10^9/L$. It is worth noting, however, that many people function normally with far lower platelet counts. Spontaneous bleeding tends to occur when the platelet count falls below $10 \times 10^9/L$.

Aetiology

Platelet counts can be temporarily reduced as a result of infection, alcohol consumption and the use of common medications such as penicillin, heparin and quinine, while non-steroidal anti-inflammatory drugs (NSAIDs) and aspirin can inhibit platelet aggregation and extend bleeding time. This effect can be beneficial in people with a tendency to thrombus formation, but harmful in those with thrombocytopenia or other bleeding disorders.

In the longer term, thrombocytopenia is most often due to inadequate platelet production or increased platelet destruction. Inadequate platelet production may be secondary to conditions such as myelodysplasia or aplastic anaemia. It can also result from bone marrow infiltration by malignant cells as in acute leukaemia, lymphoma and myeloma. Treatments for these conditions can also inhibit platelet production by suppressing bone marrow activity. All of these factors are considered elsewhere in the chapter.

Increased platelet destruction is often immunological in nature and may be secondary to autoimmune conditions such as systemic lupus erythematosus (Ch. 27) or HIV infection (Ch. 25). There may, however, be no obvious underlying cause, as in chronic idiopathic thrombocytopenic purpura (ITP).

In ITP, antibodies in the bloodstream target antigens on the surface of platelets and mark them for destruction in the mononuclear–macrophage system. As a result, the life span of platelets may be reduced from an average of 5–9 days to 1–2 days or, in some cases, a few hours. This condition is most prevalent in adults, particularly females, and is characterized by periods of remission.

Clinical presentation

On diagnosis, the platelet count is often below $20 \times 10^9/L$, while other blood cell counts are normal. Bone marrow biopsy may demonstrate a normal or elevated number of megakaryocytes. This helps to distinguish ITP from disorders arising from inadequate platelet production. Physical examination may reveal petechiae. Other symptoms can include spontaneous bruising, nosebleeds and bleeding gums. Women may complain of menorrhagia.

Medical management

The aim of treatment is to preserve platelets by reducing the number of circulating antibodies. In the short term, intravenous immunoglobulin therapies can bring about a rapid but temporary increase in the platelet count. High-dose prednisolone given over a period of 4–6 weeks can induce longer-term remission, although side-effects may occur (see p. 464). For those who do not respond to corticosteroid therapy, splenectomy may be a reasonable option, as approximately 60% of people who undergo splenectomy achieve a long-term response (Hugh-Jones & Wickramasinghe 1996). For those who relapse after splenectomy, other immunosuppressant medications such as azathioprine, ciclosporin and cyclophosphamide may be prescribed.

▶ Nursing care

The nursing care of patients with thrombocytopenia includes assessing risk, detecting signs of bleeding, administering drug treatments and platelet transfusions, and providing patient education and support.

The nurse caring for a patient should always be aware of the current platelet count and understand that a serious bleeding risk exists if it is below $10 \times 10^9/L$ (normal range $150–400 \times 10^9/L$). Nurses should also be aware of any additional factors that may enhance the risk of bleeding, such as hypertension, menstruation, trauma or a history of peptic ulceration. Severe sepsis can dramatically increase the risk of bleeding in vulnerable patients.

Careful observation is necessary to detect any bleeding process that may be occurring. Patients should be encouraged to report bleeding gums, nosebleeds or the presence of bruising or petechiae. Urinalysis and testing for faecal occult blood can also indicate the presence of bleeding. Severe haemorrhage can happen spontaneously and may be life-threatening if it occurs in sites such as the brain or gastrointestinal tract. An intracranial bleed may be suspected if a patient experiences a rapid change in conscious level, becomes agitated or confused, or collapses (Ch. 14). In such instances, urgent medical attention is required.

Any thrombocytopenic patient who is actively bleeding must have vital signs checked frequently to detect early signs of hypovolaemic shock (Ch. 9). Intravenous fluid and blood or platelet transfusion may be indicated.

Outpatients at risk of bleeding should be advised to report any bleeding promptly to the haematology unit. Women may benefit from hormone treatment to suppress menstruation. Patients should be aware of the risks of taking over-the-counter medications that can reduce platelet activity such as aspirin or ibuprofen. Fortunately, dramatic bleeding events are rare and patients should be encouraged to enjoy their usual activities within common-sense guidelines, although high-impact activities may be best avoided to reduce the risk of trauma.

DISSEMINATED INTRAVASCULAR COAGULATION

Disseminated intravascular coagulation (DIC) results from the simultaneous overactivation of both the coagulation and fibrinolytic pathways, leading to widespread clotting and thrombus formation throughout the body. As clotting factors become exhausted, generalized bleeding can also occur.

Aetiology

The conditions associated with the development of DIC include inadequate organ perfusion, such as hypovolaemia and/or sepsis, liver disease, trauma, burns and malignancy. DIC often precedes multiple organ dysfunction syndrome (MODS) (Ch. 9). Primary haematological causes can include blood transfusion incompatibility reactions and acute myeloid leukaemia, particularly of the acute promyelocytic subtype. The latter occurs because substances released during the breakdown of the abnormal promyelocytes can precipitate coagulation. This can lead to a rapidly progressing DIC, particularly in the early stages of cytotoxic treatment when the number of leukaemic cells is likely to be high.

Medical management

Disseminated intravascular coagulation is a serious disorder requiring immediate medical attention (Ch. 9). The condition is primarily rectified by treating the underlying cause and by giving supportive therapies such as platelet transfusion. Fresh frozen plasma and cryoprecipitate may also be given to correct deficiencies. Low-dose heparin infusion may be used to prevent further coagulation problems, although this can be a dilemma in the haematological setting where patients are at increased risk of bleeding. Patients with promyelocytic leukaemia may also be prescribed all-trans retinoic acid (ATRA) before beginning cytotoxic treatment to help reduce the number of circulating promyelocytes.

> ▶ **Nursing management**

Patients with DIC need to be closely monitored for signs of bleeding or shock (see p. 476). It can be a very frightening experience for both patients and their relatives, who may require a considerable amount of support and education.

HAEMOPHILIA

Haemophilia is an inherited disorder that results in a lifelong deficiency of one of two essential coagulation factors: factor VIII (haemophilia A) or factor IX (haemophilia B or Christmas disease). The severity of haemophilia is in direct proportion to the level of factor deficiency. The genes for both factor VIII and

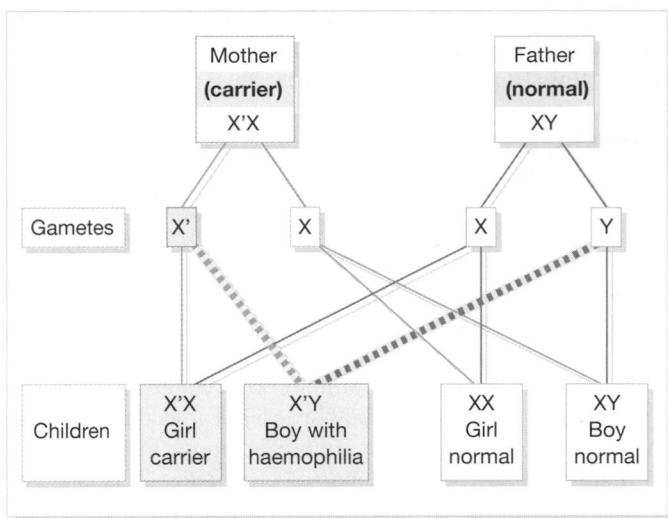

Figure 18.7 The inheritance of haemophilia (adapted from Brooker 1998).

factor IX are found on the X chromosome. This means that inheritance is sex-linked and the vast majority of people with haemophilia are males, while females are carriers (Fig. 18.7). Haemophilia A is more common than haemophilia B, although the clinical features of both types of haemophilia are similar.

Pathophysiology and clinical presentation

In haemophilia, the activated partial prothrombin time (APTT) is prolonged. This means that people bleed for longer after trauma or surgery, including relatively minor procedures such as dental extraction. In severe cases, spontaneous bleeding may also occur. The effects of this can be serious. Repeated bleeds into muscles or joints can cause severe pain, swelling and deformity, as well as long-term arthritic changes and mobility problems. However, with careful management and the use of modern therapies, many of the more severe complications of haemophilia can now be prevented.

Multiprofessional management

The management of haemophilia is a complex process that requires close collaboration and partnership between patients, their families and the multiprofessional team of nurses, doctors, dentists, physiotherapists, social workers, counsellors and laboratory staff. Haemophilia Comprehensive Care Centres and Haemophilia Centres have been set up around the UK to provide the necessary level of expertise (NHS Management Executive 1993). Comprehensive Care Centres provide a 24-hour point of access as well as a forum for teaching and education. Staff within these centres also run home therapy programmes. These enable people with haemophilia to administer their own treatments if they so wish, the benefits of which include the following:

- Bleeding episodes can be treated promptly.
- People with haemophilia and their families can exert more control.
- There is minimal disruption to normal daily routines.

Prompt action is vital when bleeding occurs, and many people with haemophilia become adept at recognizing bleeds and initiating treatment at a very early stage.

Treatment

Bleeding is usually treated by intravenous injection of the deficient factor. Dosage is dependent on the severity of the bleed and the degree of factor deficiency. People with severe haemophilia, those undergoing surgery and children may also use coagulation factors prophylactically.

Highly purified concentrates of human factor VIII and factor IX are available for replacement therapy. However, the past use of non-heat-treated human products has been linked to the spread of serious blood-borne viral infections such as HIV and hepatitis C. An important breakthrough in recent years has therefore been the development of genetically engineered recombinant clotting factors. Because these are not derived from human sources, the chances of viral contamination are negligible. Consequently, there has been considerable pressure to make these products available for all people with haemophilia in the UK (see Ethical Issues box 18.3).

A proportion of those having regular replacement therapy develop antibodies (inhibitors) to factors. These people may respond to treatment with higher doses of factor. Alternatively, they may be offered treatment with porcine (derived from pigs) factor VIII or factor VIII inhibitor bypassing agent (FEIBA).

Milder forms of haemophilia A may respond to treatment with desmopressin (DDAVP). Desmopressin can be given by intravenous injection or nasal spray, temporarily boosting plasma levels of factor VIII, while antifibrinolytic agents such as tranexamic acid may be used to promote clot stability, e.g. following dental surgery.

▶ Nursing care

Pain management is an important aspect of nursing care. Giving education and advice on how to bring about the early resolution of bleeds can help to prevent pain to a large extent. Rest, relaxation, distraction, warm baths and mild analgesics such as paracetamol may provide sufficient pain control in small bleeds. It is important that patients avoid the use of aspirin or NSAIDs as these can prolong the clotting times and exacerbate the problem.

More severe bleeds may clearly require the administration of stronger analgesics, such as opioids, but it should be noted that intramuscular injections are generally contraindicated for people with haemophilia.

Chronic pain due to joint deformity or arthritis can be difficult to control and may require some degree of trial and error. The long-term use of narcotic analgesics is usually avoided wherever possible as, in the past, some people with haemophilia became dependent on these medications. The development of modern Cox 2 inhibitors, such as rofecoxib, has been a major breakthrough in the treatment of chronic pain in haemophilia. These drugs work in a similar but more selective way to NSAIDs but do not significantly interfere with platelet function. The use of orthopaedic aids such as splints, crutches and walking sticks can also be helpful in some cases by shifting body weight away from joints that are particularly painful (Ch. 27).

There is no cure for haemophilia, although advances in gene therapy may offer hope for the future. In the meantime, an extremely important aspect of nursing care is to help people with haemophilia and their families to live with the condition. This may take the form of education, support and counselling, including genetic, preconceptual and antenatal counselling.

For parents who are adjusting to the birth of a child with haemophilia, the outlook can be very positive. With modern therapies, most people with haemophilia can now lead normal lives and, while aggressive contact sports are probably best avoided, children with haemophilia need not be overprotected. Indeed, participating in normal social and physical activities is an important part of their overall physical and mental development. People with haemophilia should, however, be advised to carry a Medi-Alert card.

 ETHICAL ISSUES

18.3 The availability of recombinant products for people with haemophilia

Prior to the mid-1980s, over 1200 haemophiliacs in the UK contracted HIV from contaminated products, and over 3000 contracted hepatitis C (Cowe & Fuller 1999). As a result, many face the possibility, or the reality, of AIDS or severe liver disease. The provision of effective support for those affected by these conditions is clearly important. Access to specialist nurses and counsellors is usually provided within Comprehensive Care Centres. Referring people to support groups, such as The Haemophilia Society, can provide them with an additional source of help and support.

Ethical implications
- The risk of viral transmission from blood products derived from human sources cannot be completely eliminated.
- For this reason, all haemophiliacs in Scotland are now offered treatment with recombinant clotting factors.
- However, in England, only haemophiliacs under 16 years of age or those who screen negative for viruses such as HIV and hepatitis receive these relatively expensive products.

Student activities
- What might be the pros and cons of either stance?

NB: Difficulties within the manufacturing process may sometimes limit the worldwide availability of recombinant products.

Reference
Cowe A, Fuller S. Introduction to haemophilia (on-line version: www.haemophilia.org.uk). London: Haemophilia Society.

SUMMARY: MAIN POINTS

- Nursing haematology patients is a challenging and varied area of practice. The delivery of effective care requires many clinical and psychosocial skills.

- The nurse is pivotal in providing information to patients/families regarding their disease and treatment.

- A sound knowledge of the haematology system and the functions of blood are essential for planning appropriate nursing care.

- The most common complication of blood transfusion is administration of the wrong product. Nurses have a central role in ensuring the safe administration of blood components.

- Media coverage of the infection risks of blood transfusions has led to high levels of anxiety. Patients require accurate and sensitive information about the risks and benefits of transfusion.

- Haematology patients commonly have chronic fatigue. Its effect on quality of life is often underestimated.

- Acute leukaemia requires urgent treatment, leaving little time for patients and families to adjust to the diagnosis before treatment is initiated. Skilled nursing can help by providing ongoing support and appropriate information.

- Cytotoxic drugs produce many side-effects. Nurses need an awareness of these problems and their solutions.

- Infection is the major risk to patients undergoing treatment for malignant blood disorders. Nurses should understand effective infection control measures and communicate these to patients. They need to be able to identify early signs of infection and facilitate prompt treatment should infection occur.

- Bone marrow transplantation is a highly toxic procedure but is often the only curative treatment option for aggressive haematological malignancies.

- There is a shortage of bone marrow donors, particularly from minority ethnic groups.

- Long-term issues following treatment for haematological malignancies include infertility and disease relapse, and psychological morbidity often occurs after treatment.

- Inherited blood disorders pose many difficulties; generally incurable they will adversely affect a patient throughout life. There are also implications for a patient's offspring and wider family. Specialist nurses provide a vital service to these patients.

- Haematology is a highly dynamic field of practice – research is changing the ways that patients are treated and strives to improve patient outcomes.

- Many patients will not recover from serious blood disorders, and palliative care skills are very relevant for nurses in this specialty.

- Working with haematology patients can cause emotional strain for health care professionals. A strong team approach to care is vital for providing staff support.

SELF-TEST: CRITICAL THINKING ACTIVITIES

1 Why do people with sickle cell disease experience pain? What role do nurses have in managing this pain?

2 What factors contribute to the increased risk of infection for many haematology patients? How can nurses reduce the risk of infection?

3 What factors may contribute to the development of fatigue in haematology patients and what advice would you give to patients?

 FURTHER READING

Cook N. Central venous catheters: preventing infection and occlusion. Br J Nurs 1999; 8(15): 980–989.

Drewett SR. Complications of central venous catheters: nursing care. Br J Nurs 2000; 9(8): 466–478.

Groenwald S, Frogge M, Goodman M, Yarbro C. Cancer symptom management. Boston: Jones and Bartlett; 1996.

McClellend B. Handbook of transfusion medicine. London: HMSO; 1996.

McKay J, Hirano N. The chemotherapy survival guide. Oakland, CA: New Harbinger Publications; 1995.

Mehta A, Hoffbrand V. Haematology at a glance. Oxford: Blackwell Science; 2000.

Department of Health. Better blood transfusion: The appropriate use of blood (HSC 2002/009). London: DoH; 2002

Salter M. Altered body image: the nurse's role. London: Baillière Tindall; 1997.

Twycross R. Symptom management in advanced cancer. Oxford: Radcliffe Medical Press; 1995.

USEFUL WEBSITES

www.cancerbacup.org.uk
www.depressionalliance.org
www.haemophilia.org.uk
www.anthonynolan.org.uk
www.leukaemiacare.org

www.sicklecell.co.uk
www.ukts.org – thalassaemia
www.bloodnet.nbs.nhs.uk
www.shot.demon.co.uk

REFERENCES

Apperley JF, Gluckman E, Gratwohl A. The EBMT handbook: blood and marrow transplantation. France: European School of Haematology; 2000.

British Committee for Standards in Haematology. Guidelines on the insertion and management of central venous lines. Br J Haematol 1997; 98: 1041–1047.

British Committee for Standards in Haematology. The administration of blood and blood components and the management of transfused patients. Transfus Med 1999; 9: 227–238.

Brooker C. Human structure and function. Nursing applications in clinical practice, 2nd edn. London: Mosby; 1998.

Calman K, Hine D. A policy framework for commissioning cancer services. London: HMSO; 1995.

Cochrane Injuries Group. Human albumin administration in critically ill patients: systematic review of randomised controlled trials. Br Med J 1998; 317: 235–240.

Department of Health. The new NHS. London: HMSO; 1997.

Howard MR, Hamilton PJ. Haematology. New York: Churchill Livingstone; 1997.

Hugh-Jones NC, Wickramasinghe SN. Lecture notes on haematology, 6th edn. Oxford: Blackwell Science; 1996.

Mehta A, Hoffbrand V. Haematology at a glance. Oxford: Blackwell Science; 2000.

National Cancer Directory. Towards a cancer information strategy: overview. March 2000. Winchester: NHS Information Authority; 2000.

NHS Management Executive. Provision of haemophilia treatment and care. London: HMSO; 1993.

Oni L. Sickle cell disease and the carer-client relationship. Nurs Times 1998; 94: 26.

SHOT Steering Group. Serious hazards of transfusion annual report 1998–1999. Manchester: SHOT Steering Group; 2000.

Thomas VN, Wilson-Barnett J, Goodhart F. The role of cognitive behavioural therapy in the management of pain in patients with sickle cell disease. J Adv Nurs 1998; 27: 1002–1009.

19 Nursing patients with cardiovascular disorders

Jillian Riley

'It's not indigestion, they said, it's angina. I know I've put on a bit of weight and don't get much exercise these days, and I do enjoy the odd pint and a cigarette but I never thought I'd get heart disease. The Practice Nurse says she will help me to look at what I eat and think of ways to get more exercise – it's hard when you drive a lorry all day. I'm determined to give up smoking now – she has really made me think.'

(Patient)

THIS CHAPTER WILL HELP YOU

- Understand the rationale for caring for a patient with some of the more common cardiovascular disorders

- Describe specific cardiovascular investigations and understand how to prepare the patient for them

- Understand the nurse's role in the assessment of the cardiovascular system and how this can contribute towards planning care

- Contribute to the health promotion needs of the population with regard to cardiovascular health.

KEYWORDS

Angina	Coronary heart disease
Arrhythmia	Haemodynamic instability
Atheroma	
Cardiac output	Palpitations
Cardiac rehabilitation	Stroke volume
Chest pain	Syncope
	Venous return

INTRODUCTION

Nursing patients with disorders of the cardiovascular system takes place in many diverse settings, ranging from the community to the acute hospital arena. Cardiovascular disorders may lead to many of the conditions discussed in the other chapters of this book, such as stroke (see Ch. 14), and nurses will encounter the sequelae of these disorders in every area of practice.

Immense changes have occurred over the past decade, through advances in both technology and pharmacology, and these have led to many changes in the care delivered by nurses.

As is well known, coronary heart disease (CHD; atheroma of the coronary arteries which may lead eventually to angina, myocardial infarction or heart failure) is considered a preventable cause of premature death affecting more than 120 000 people in the UK (ONS 1998). The role of preventative care within this field poses an additional challenge to the nurse.

Another important topic covered in some detail in this chapter is cardiopulmonary resuscitation, which has implications for nurses in every area of practice.

ANATOMY AND PHYSIOLOGY: AN OVERVIEW

For the body to receive adequate nutrition, a constant supply of oxygen (O_2) and nutrients must be delivered to the cells and the waste products of cellular metabolism removed. Fundamental to this process are an efficiently working pump system, the heart, and a circulatory system able to carry the nutrients around the body. This circulatory system consists of both a systemic and pulmonary circulation. The systemic circulation pumps blood to the body organs and tissues providing O_2 and nutrients while removing the waste products of metabolism. The pulmonary system takes the blood to the lungs where it is oxygenated and carbon dioxide (CO_2) removed. An effective pump (the heart) will ensure the circulatory system provides blood to the body organs and tissues. Any reduction in cardiovascular function will lead to disorders of cellular metabolism and organ dysfunction.

481

THE HEART

The adult heart weighs around 300 g and is about the size of an adult fist. It is situated between the lungs in the mediastinal area of the thoracic cavity and extends from the second to the fifth intercostal (between the ribs) spaces (see Fig. 19.1). It is bounded anteriorly by the sternum, and the vertebral column posteriorly.

The heart wall

The wall of the heart comprises three layers: the outer pericardium, the myocardium (or major muscle mass) and the endocardium (see Fig. 19.2A).

The pericardium

The heart is enclosed within the pericardium. It is composed of several layers: the fibrous pericardium forms the outer layer of connective tissue that anchors the heart in place and a double serous layer. The inner serous layer is called the epicardium. Between the serous layers is the pericardial cavity, containing serous fluid. As with any serous fluid, it functions to lubricate the movement of the heart within the pericardial sac and reduce friction.

The myocardium

The myocardium is made up of specialized striated cardiac muscle fibres, joined together in bands and spirals, and is responsible for the heart contracting and relaxing. If the muscle cells are damaged in any way, the force of the contraction of the heart is reduced. Each cardiac cell is very small, and a vast number of these cells are needed to make up the myocardium (Cheitlin et al 1993). They are designed to work together to create the forceful contraction needed to pump blood into the circulatory system.

The endocardium

The endocardium is the innermost layer of the heart wall, composed of a layer of endothelial cells. These line the heart chambers and cover the valves. The endocardium creates a smooth surface that helps to prevent blood sticking and clotting together.

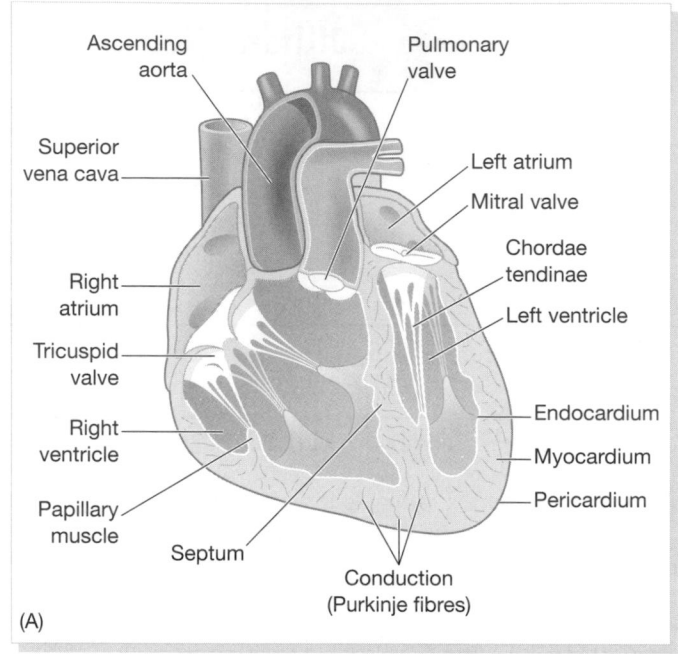

(A)

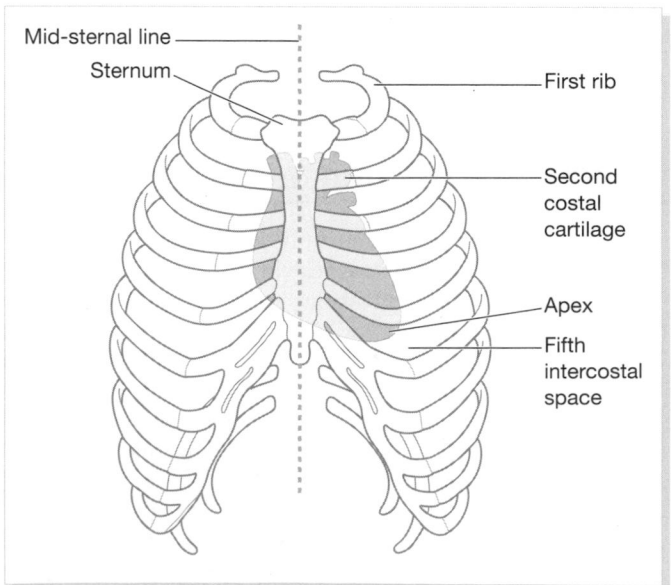

Figure 19.1 Position of the heart in the thoracic cavity.

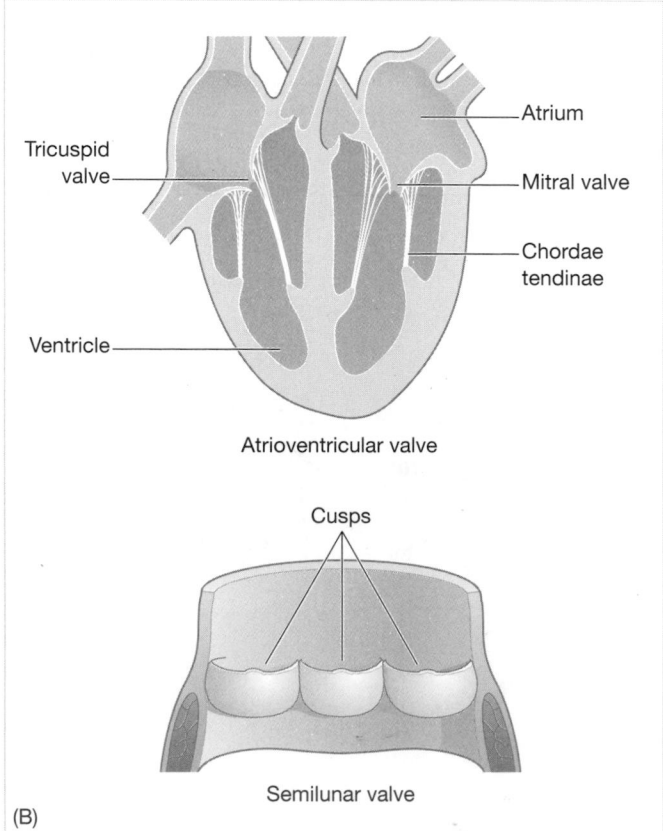

(B)

Figure 19.2 (A) The heart – showing the wall, chambers and position of valves. (B) Atrioventricular and semilunar valves.

The heart chambers and valves

The heart has four chambers; two upper receiving chambers called atria and two lower pumping chambers the ventricles (see Fig. 19.2A). These are divided into the right and left sides by the septum that lies longitudinally in the heart (see Fig. 19.2A).

The atria are separated from the ventricles by the atrio-ventricular valves (AV valves) and semilunar valves are situated between the ventricles and the aorta and pulmonary artery (see Fig. 19.2B). The valves are important in ensuring that blood flows in one direction only through the heart.

The mitral valve is the left AV valve while the tricuspid valve lies between the right atrium and right ventricle. As the mitral valve is close to the aortic valve, disease of this valve frequently affects the function of the aortic valve.

At the opening of the ventricles lie the semilunar valves: the pulmonary valve at the junction of the right ventricle and the pulmonary artery and the aortic valve at the point where the aorta leaves the left ventricle. The coronary arteries originate from an opening 1–2 cm above the aortic valve.

The AV valves are stabilized by the chordae tendineae. These are fan-like structures located between the AV valves and the papillary muscle on the heart wall (see Figs 19.2A and B). These are necessary to prevent the valve bulging into the atria when the ventricles contract.

Coronary circulation

The coronary vasculature traverses the heart and is composed of coronary arteries (which branch from the aorta), coronary veins and the capillary network. These supply the myocardium with O_2 and nutrients, and remove the waste products of metabolism. Three major coronary arteries supply the myocardium with O_2: the right coronary artery, the left anterior descending and the circumflex arteries (see Fig. 19.3). These latter two

divide from the left main stem artery. The arteries form a dense network of arterioles and capillaries that traverse the external surface of the heart and penetrate the myocardium. Once the muscle has been supplied with O_2, the blood returns to the right atrium of the heart via the coronary sinus. The lungs then reoxygenate the blood. As the myocardium works continuously, the muscle requires a large supply of O_2 and extracts about 70% of the available O_2 from the blood. Other tissues extract in the region of only 30% of the available O_2. When the heart muscle has to work harder, as in exercise, obesity or when the heart is beating fast (tachycardia), the requirement for O_2 increases. The heart is able to adapt to this by increasing the diameter of the arteries, thus increasing the supply of blood and O_2. It is when the arteries are damaged, e.g. by atheroma (a proliferation of smooth muscle cells and accumulation of lipid within the intima of the large arteries), that they are unable to dilate sufficiently to meet an increase in O_2 demand. This explains why people may experience ischaemic chest pain (angina) when exercising.

The coronary arteries primarily fill with blood during diastole when the heart muscle is relaxed – an important point to remember when considering the effects of cardiac disorders that cause a shortening of diastole (see pp. 484–485).

THE ELECTRICAL CONDUCTION SYSTEM

The electrical conduction system comprises four main structures (see Fig. 19.4):

- the sinus or sinoatrial (SA) node, on the posterior surface of the right atrium
- the atrioventricular (AV) node, at the junction of the right atrium and right ventricle
- the atrioventricular bundle (bundle of His) and branch bundles, which lie in the septum between the two ventricles
- the Purkinje fibres, which spread out through the ventricular muscle mass.

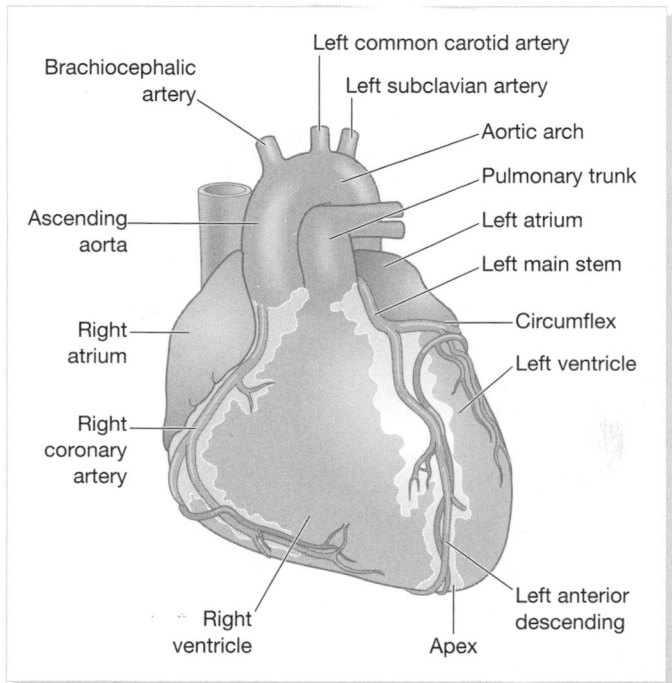

Figure 19.3 The coronary circulation.

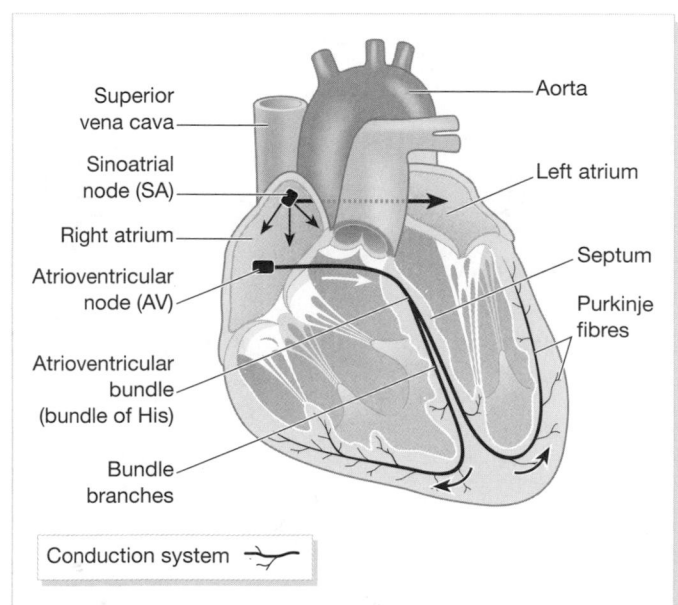

Figure 19.4 Conduction through the heart.

The sinus node is the pacemaker of the heart and beats at its own intrinsic rate of 60–100 beats/min (bpm). This is the fastest rate within the conduction system and so the sinus node initiates each heartbeat. From the sinus node, the impulse passes to the AV node and results in atrial systole. The impulse then passes to the bundle of His, the right and left bundle branches and the Purkinje fibres. This causes the ventricular muscle fibres to contract and expel the blood.

THE CARDIAC CYCLE

The cardiac cycle comprises the events occurring during one heartbeat, the rhythmic contraction and relaxation of the heart as it pumps blood around the body and to the lungs. It can be divided into stages (see Fig. 19.5):

- The first stage is called *ventricular filling*. Here the AV valves are open and blood flows from the atria to the ventricles.

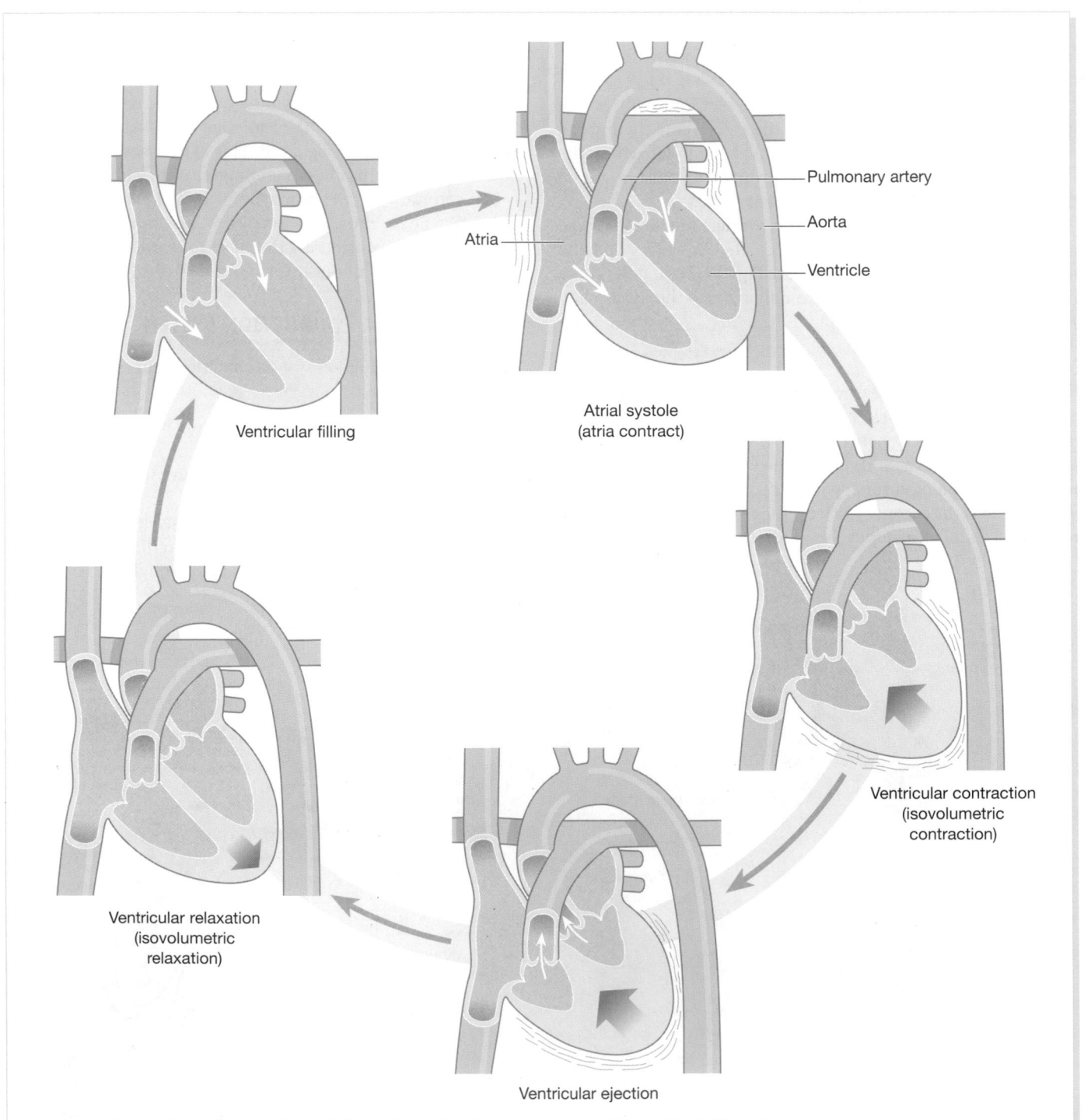

Figure 19.5 The cardiac cycle.

- The second stage is *atrial systole*. The heart starts to contract and blood is squeezed out of the atria and into the ventricles. This completes ventricular filling.
- The third stage occurs when the ventricles start to contract (*ventricular contraction*). The increase in pressure in the ventricles forces the AV valves to shut, preventing any further movement of blood into the ventricles.
- The ventricles continue to contract and become closed chambers (all the heart valves are shut); this is called the *isovolumetric contraction* stage. Pressure builds up within the ventricles until it exceeds the pressure of the pulmonary or systemic circulation and the semilunar valves are forced open. It is during this stage that the heart utilizes the most energy and O_2.
- In the next stage of the cardiac cycle, *ventricular ejection*, blood is ejected into the circulation.
- The last stage of the cardiac cycle is when the ventricles start to relax (*ventricular relaxation*). Eventually ventricular pressure falls and back pressure in the great vessels closes the semilunar valves and again the ventricles are closed chambers (*isovolumetric relaxation*).

Meanwhile the atria have been filling with blood and the rising pressure soon opens the AV valves. Once this cycle of events is completed, the cardiac cycle repeats itself. Normally the whole cycle takes less than 1 second to complete.

The purpose of the cardiac cycle is to create a cardiac output (CO). This is defined as the volume of blood pumped out of the heart in 1 minute and is expressed in litres per minute (L/min). The average adult heartbeat pumps out about 70 mL of blood. This is referred to as the stroke volume (SV). As the average heart rate is around 70 bpm, the cardiac output will be 70 mL × 70 = 4900 mL or just under 5 L/min.

Cardiac output, then, is dependent upon myocardial contractility and the volume of blood in the heart (the venous return).

THE VASCULAR SYSTEM

Blood is supplied to body tissues through arteries, arterioles and capillaries and returns to the heart via the venules and veins. Arteries and veins are composed of three layers:

- The outer *tunica adventitia* is a layer of connective tissue and a fibrous matrix. This gives structure to the vessel.
- The *tunica media*, or middle layer, is composed of muscle cells which give the vessel elasticity. The large arteries need to be more elastic than the smaller ones as they have to contend with higher pressures. They therefore have a thicker tunica media.
- The *tunica intima* is a layer of endothelial cells that line the vessel lumen. These cells secrete vasoactive substances such as endothelium-derived relaxing factor (EDRF) and endothelin. These substances lead to vasodilatation and vasoconstriction, respectively, and prevent platelet aggregation. It is now thought that the endothelial cells play an important part in the development of atheroma.

The arteries

Blood is pumped forcibly out of the heart into the aorta by the left ventricle. The elastic wall of the aorta distends and then recoils, forcing blood along the smaller arteries or arterioles. The arterioles also have a muscular wall, although it is less developed than that of the larger arteries, which contracts and relaxes to encourage the movement of the blood. These end in capillaries, thin-walled vessels comprising a single layer of endothelial cells that enable the easy exchange of O_2 and nutrients between the cells and the blood and the removal of the waste products of metabolism.

The veins

Blood travels back to the heart and lungs through venules, which drain the capillaries and pass the blood on to the veins. The walls of the veins are less muscular than those of the arteries, as less pressure is generated within the venous system. Without the structure of the well-developed arteries, they are easily compressed by muscle contraction around them. This creates a 'milking' effect that aids venous return. You may hear this referred to as the 'calf pump'. Many of the veins also have valves within them, which help blood return to the heart. If these valves become damaged, blood may return to the heart more slowly. This will allow platelets to clump together and form clots. When these form in the deep veins of the legs or pelvic veins, the condition is referred to as deep vein thrombosis (see p. 525).

Blood pressure

Blood pressure is the pressure exerted upon the blood vessel walls. Clearly it will vary throughout the vessels and should be greatest in the large arteries closest to the heart.

Blood pressure is affected by the force of contraction of the heart, the amount of circulating blood, blood viscosity, venous return to the heart and the elasticity of the vessel walls that creates the resistance to the flow of blood (systemic vascular resistance). The following equation may help you to understand this:

$$\text{Blood pressure (BP)} = \text{cardiac output (CO)} \times \text{systemic vascular resistance (SVR)}$$

Blood pressure is recorded as a systolic pressure when the heart contracts and a diastolic pressure when the heart is relaxed:

- As the heart contracts, blood is ejected from the left ventricle into the systemic arteries. This is recorded as the systolic blood pressure.
- Following ventricular ejection, blood moves along the arteries, and the elastic vessel walls start to recoil. This is then recorded as the diastolic blood pressure.

In health, the adult blood pressure is around 120 mmHg (mercury) systolic pressure and 70 mmHg diastolic pressure. This is recorded as 120/70. Clearly, certain factors may alter the blood pressure, such as age, position, exercise and emotional state. Otherwise it is kept at a fairly constant level through the body's own regulatory system.

Blood pressure is regulated by neural, chemical and renal responses. Any change in the blood O_2 level or pH (e.g. through exercise) will stimulate chemoreceptors in the aortic arch and the carotid artery to pass messages to the vasomotor centre of the brain. The body responds by reflex vasoconstriction, which raises the blood pressure. Blood pressure is also regulated by pressor receptors. These lie close to the chemoreceptors in the aortic arch and carotid bodies and respond to changes in pressure or stretch. When arterial blood pressure rises, the pressor receptors are stretched and impulses are passed to the vasomotor centre. These impulses cause blood vessel walls to dilate and the blood pressure will fall. Impulses from these pressor receptors also pass to the cardio-inhibitory centre, causing a reduction in heart rate and force of contraction. As blood pressure is related to cardiac output, a reduction in both the rate and force of contraction will reduce cardiac output and hence blood pressure.

The body also compensates for a low blood pressure through the renin–angiotensin–aldosterone system (RAAS). Here, a decrease in the renal blood flow promotes the release of renin by the juxtaglomerular cells in the kidney, which in turn leads to a production of angiotensin II and aldosterone (see Ch. 24). Aldosterone causes the retention of sodium and water, increasing the circulating blood volume, while angiotensin II is a powerful vasoconstrictor. Thus blood pressure rises.

NURSING ASSESSMENT

It is important for the nurse to collect and analyse patient data, and to assist in decision-making regarding nursing problems, goal setting and care planning. This forms an important part of the nurse's work. It is vital to remember that undertaking a comprehensive cardiovascular assessment is necessary in all nursing situations.

NURSING HISTORY

This section will focus on the specific requirements for a nursing history of the patient with commonly identified cardiovascular disorders.

A general health history should include an assessment of the patient's primary problem, past history, family history and details of social activities and lifestyle that may have an impact upon cardiovascular status. These include factors such as diet, smoking, alcohol intake, exercise and any family history of cardiovascular disorders.

It is important for the nurse to determine the detail of health history to be taken and to vary this according to the patient's presenting symptoms. For example, if patients are breathless, a short health history should be obtained until the breathlessness has been treated sufficiently to enable them to talk more freely.

Commonly identified problems related to cardiovascular illness include breathlessness, chest pain (any form of chest pain and not necessarily angina), syncope (a sudden loss of consciousness, frequently caused by a sudden drop in blood pressure or a cardiac arrhythmia) and palpitations (a fluttering sensation that is felt in the chest, usually caused by a fast or irregular heartbeat) and the nurse should include questions to ascertain if the patient has experienced any of these.

PHYSICAL ASSESSMENT

Physical assessment should include an assessment of the skin, arterial pulses and chest pain.

Skin
Skin colour
Cyanosis in the patient with cardiovascular disease may indicate pulmonary congestion or a reduced cardiac output where insufficient O_2 reaches the tissues. Assessment is through inspecting the colour of the skin (which can be more difficult in patients with darker skins) and mucous membranes. The mucous membranes of the mouth, lips and eyes should be inspected; a bluish hue may indicate central cyanosis. Peripheral cyanosis may be indicated by a bluish hue of the toes and fingers. Clearly cyanosis may also occur due to poor oxygenation in the lungs in a patient with a respiratory disorder (see Ch. 20).

Capillary refill
Pressure can be applied to the nail beds and then released. If colour returns to the nail bed quickly, then cardiac function is adequate.

Skin temperature
Skin that feels warm to the touch has a good blood supply and the cardiac output can be presumed adequate. However, fever or infection must be eliminated (see Ch. 5). Skin that is cold may indicate vasoconstriction, possibly due to poor cardiac function.

Skin turgor
When a fold of the skin is lifted, it will quickly return to its position if the patient is well hydrated. This is useful to assess the hydration status in a patient on diuretic therapy (see Ch. 8). It is important to remember that, with ageing, the skin becomes less elastic and will not return to its original position so quickly.

Oedema
Both the presence and severity of oedema can be used as an indicator of cardiovascular function. Oedema is more likely to be seen in the dependent parts of the body such as the ankles, feet and legs. If a person spends long periods of time sitting, then the dependent area for oedema to accumulate is the sacral area. When oedema is visible the patient has retained at least 4 kg (4 L) of fluid. This could again indicate inadequate cardiac function and is often seen in patients with heart failure (see p. 516). An assessment tool to measure and record oedema consistently should be used. One such tool is to press three fingers into the area to be assessed for 5 seconds, and then release. The depth of indentation is then used to record oedema (Talbot & Meyers-Marquardt 1997):

+1	0–0.5 cm
+2	0.5–1.0 cm
+3	1.0–2.5 cm
+4	> 2.5 cm.

Arterial pulses
A great deal of information can be gained from feeling pulses and detecting the flow of blood. Pulse rate and rhythm are commonly and conveniently assessed using the radial artery. However, there are situations when alternative pulses should be examined to complete the patient assessment (see Fig. 19.6).

Radial artery pulse. If the radial pulse is irregular, such as in atrial fibrillation (see p. 499), additional information may be

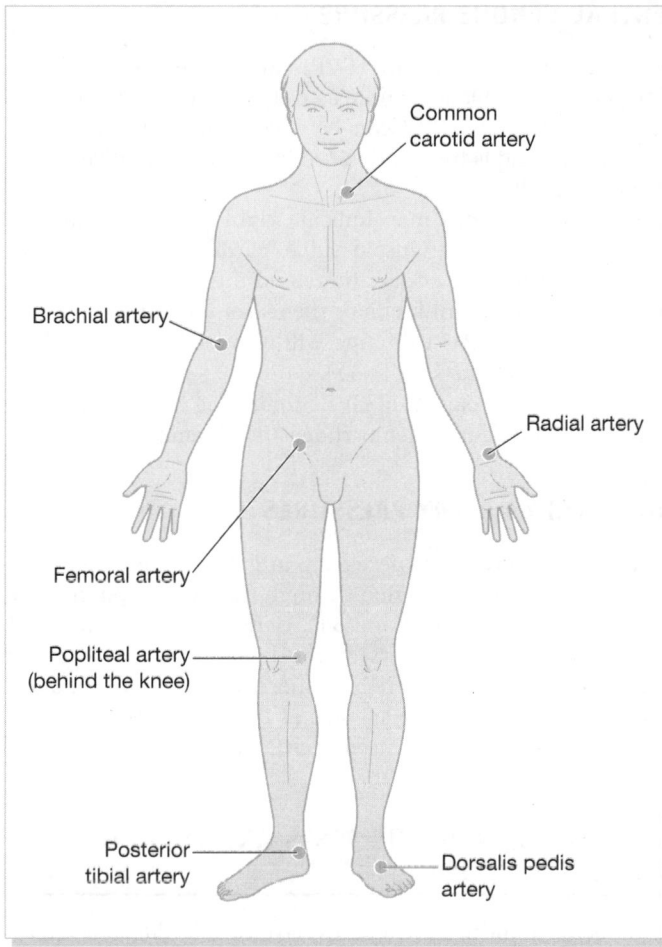

Common
carotid artery

Brachial artery

Radial artery

Femoral artery

Popliteal artery
(behind the knee)

Posterior
tibial artery

Dorsalis pedis
artery

Figure 19.6 Arterial pulses.

gained from listening to the heartbeat. A simultaneous apex and radial beat may then be counted. This is when two nurses assess the rate simultaneously; one counts the radial pulse rate while the other counts the heart rate by placing a stethoscope over the apex of the heart. This can be found in the midclavicular line at the fifth intercostal space. If a few heartbeats appear early and weak, you may need to consider premature ventricular contractions (see p. 502). In this instance, the frequency of abnormal beats should be assessed over a full minute. If more then six are counted, consider undertaking a 12-lead ECG (see pp. 488–490).

Carotid artery pulse. A patient who is shocked (see Ch. 9) or who has suffered a cardiopulmonary arrest (see p. 495) is likely to be peripherally vasoconstricted and the radial pulse will be difficult to palpate. In these circumstances the carotid pulse should be used. This can be found either side of the mid-neck and is a measure of the central circulation.

Pulses in the legs can be used to assess the peripheral circulation. The femoral, popliteal, dorsalis pedis and posterior tibial artery pulses can be used to detect the flow of blood in the legs. Assessment of these pulses forms an important part of the patient evaluation following cannulation of the limbs, e.g. as occurs during a cardiac catheterization, or when peripheral arterial disease (see p. 523) is present or suspected.

Chest pain

Chest pain can result from various conditions, which may be non-cardiac or cardiac in origin. A careful history of the pain is important. The following points should be considered in the assessment of chest pain:

- precipitating factors – e.g. exercise or strong winds and cold weather
- location of pain – cardiac pain is frequently central and may radiate to the back, arms and jaw
- description of pain (see Evidence-based Practice box 19.1) – cardiac chest pain may be variously described as a heavy sensation, aching or crushing (Hofgren et al 1994)
- intensity of pain – here it is useful to use a Likert scale and ask the patient to grade the pain (see Ch. 7). Remember that non-verbal communication (see Ch. 3) such as facial expressions can be used to determine the severity of pain (Albarran et al 2000)
- factors that relieve the pain – e.g. it may subside on resting or stopping a particular activity.

 EVIDENCE-BASED PRACTICE

19.1 The use of chest pain assessment tools

The use of chest pain assessment tools is widespread in cardiac care. Through the use of these tools, it is possible to determine if an intervention to relieve pain has been successful. A visual analogue scale rating pain from 0 (no pain) to 100 (worst pain possible) is easy for both the patient and the nurse to use (Thompson et al 1994).

Word descriptors have also been used to assess pain. Patients are asked to use sensory or affective pain descriptors to describe their pain. Sensory descriptors may include 'pressing', 'aching', 'cramping' or 'gnawing'. Affective word descriptors may include 'worrying', 'annoying', 'frightening' or 'suffocating'; (Gaston-Johansson & Gustafsson 1985).

More complex tools for the assessment of pain such as descriptive scales (Hofgren et al 1994) or the McGill Pain Questionnaire may be too complex for the assessment of acute pain.

References

Gaston-Johansson F, Gustafsson M. A baseline study for the development of an instrument for the assessment of pain. J Adv Nurs 1985; 10: 539–546.

Hofgren C, Karlson B, Herlitz J. Word descriptors in suspected acute myocardial infarction: a comparison between patients with and without confirmed myocardial infarction. Heart Lung 1994; 23(5): 397–403.

Thompson D, Webster R, Sutton T. Coronary care unit patients' and nurses' ratings of intensity of ischaemic chest pain. Intensiv Crit Care Nurs 1994; 10: 83–88.

Common causes of chest pain

Not all chest pain is cardiac in origin and accurate assessment is an important skill to learn. Some common causes in both the cardiac and non-cardiac categories are summarized below.

Cardiac in origin
- Angina – caused by CHD or severe anaemia
- Myocardial infarction (MI)
- Aortic stenosis
- Dressler's syndrome
- Aortic aneurysm/dissection.

Non-cardiac in origin
- Oesophagitis (see Ch. 22)
- Peptic ulcer (see Ch. 22)
- Musculoskeletal injury or disease (see Ch. 27)
- Pleurisy (see Ch. 20).

BLOOD PRESSURE

Arterial blood pressure is an important component of assessment and must be measured accurately (Nicol et al 2000). This takes skill, patience, practice and the correct equipment in working order. Treatment often depends upon the patient's blood pressure reading, and therefore measurements must be standardized to provide reliability. The blood pressure can be monitored indirectly using a cuff and either a sphygmomanometer and stethoscope or an electronic measuring device.

The normal adult blood pressure reading is in the range 100–120 mmHg (systolic) and 60–80 mmHg (diastolic). Blood pressure should be routinely measured with the person sitting down because the influences of gravity will result in a lower blood pressure on standing.

The pressor receptors are able to respond rapidly to changes in pressure and normally the blood pressure remains fairly constant regardless of posture. However, a patient who is dehydrated or one who has been in bed for a period of time may feel dizzy or faint on standing. It would then be necessary to record the blood pressure in different positions: sitting, standing and lying.

The systolic blood pressure reading depends upon the cardiac output. A low systolic pressure may indicate poor cardiac function, or a decrease in the circulating blood volume. The diastolic pressure represents the resistance of the arteries. A high reading may indicate an increase in vascular tone, e.g. because the person is cold.

The 30–50 mmHg difference between systolic and diastolic pressures is termed the pulse pressure. Abnormalities may indicate certain disorders, such as an increase in pulse pressure in hyperthyroidism (see Ch. 17).

Blood pressure may also be monitored using an intra-arterial line when a cannula is inserted into a small artery, usually the radial artery, and connected to an oscilloscope. Invasive monitoring lines are considered to be very accurate. However, there are disadvantages associated with their use, such as the need to cannulate an artery, the risk of haemorrhage, occlusion of the artery, peripheral ischaemia and infection. For these reasons, direct arterial blood pressure monitoring is generally used only in patients in a high-dependency unit (see Chs 9 and 33).

CENTRAL VENOUS PRESSURE

The central venous pressure (CVP) can be used as a measure of the circulating blood volume as well as cardiac function (see Chs 9 and 31). The CVP can be easily measured in a ward environment and is frequently used in the postoperative period (Nicol et al 2000).

High CVP readings may indicate right ventricular failure, incompetence of the tricuspid valve, cardiac tamponade (see below) and volume overload. Increased intrathoracic pressure caused by artificial ventilation or the use of continuous positive airway pressure (CPAP) therapy will also lead to higher than normal CVP readings (see Ch. 31).

The risks to the patient of CVP monitoring include infection of the intravenous site, haemorrhage and air embolism.

PULMONARY ARTERY PRESSURES

In certain situations it is necessary to gather additional information about cardiac function through the use of a pulmonary artery catheter (see Chs 9 and 31). Here a catheter is inserted through the right chambers of the heart until it sits in the pulmonary artery. This enables more accurate information about the workings of the left side of the heart to be gathered and it is a procedure that is used in critically ill patients.

GENERAL DIAGNOSTIC TESTS AND MEDICAL INVESTIGATIONS

A number of non-invasive and invasive cardiac diagnostic tests can be used to provide additional information to assist in the diagnosis and monitoring of cardiovascular function. Although staff with the required skills and experience will undertake these investigations, the nurse caring for a patient with a cardiovascular disorder requires some knowledge and understanding of these procedures in order to prepare the patient and family adequately.

THE ELECTROCARDIOGRAM

The electrocardiogram (ECG) depicts the electrical activity of the heart. By placing electrodes at various sites on the surface of the body, the depolarization (the inside of the cell membrane becomes electrically positive with respect to the outside) and repolarization (the cell membrane potential returns to the polarized negative resting state) of the myocardial cells can be detected. These are termed leads and make up the ECG. Depolarization and repolarization occur when changes to the electrical charge of the myocardial cell membrane lead to contraction and relaxation. As the myocardial cell becomes positively charged during depolarization, electrical activity will move towards one of these leads, resulting in a positive or upright deflection on the ECG. As the cell repolarizes, the deflection will return to the baseline. The resulting normal pattern, known as sinus rhythm (see Fig. 19.7), depicts the electrical activity through the atria and ventricles and can provide information on the activity of the cells in a particular part of the heart and the conduction pathways.

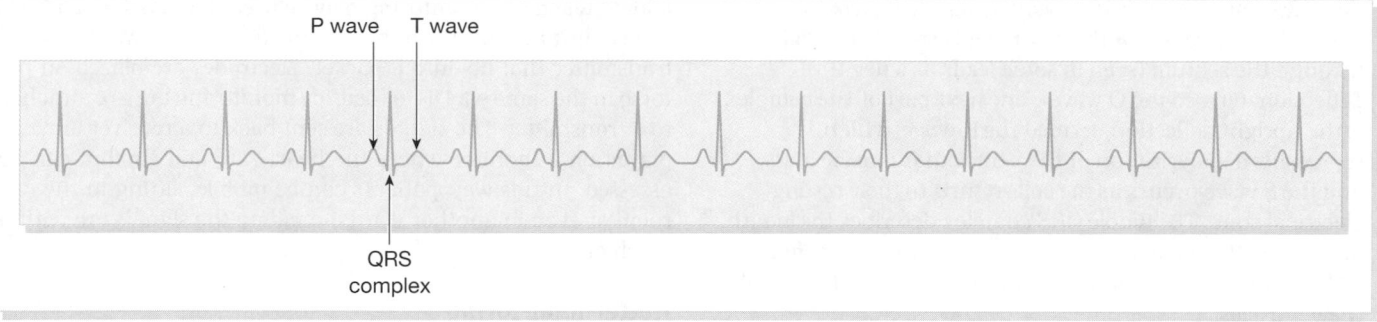

Figure 19.7 Sinus rhythm.

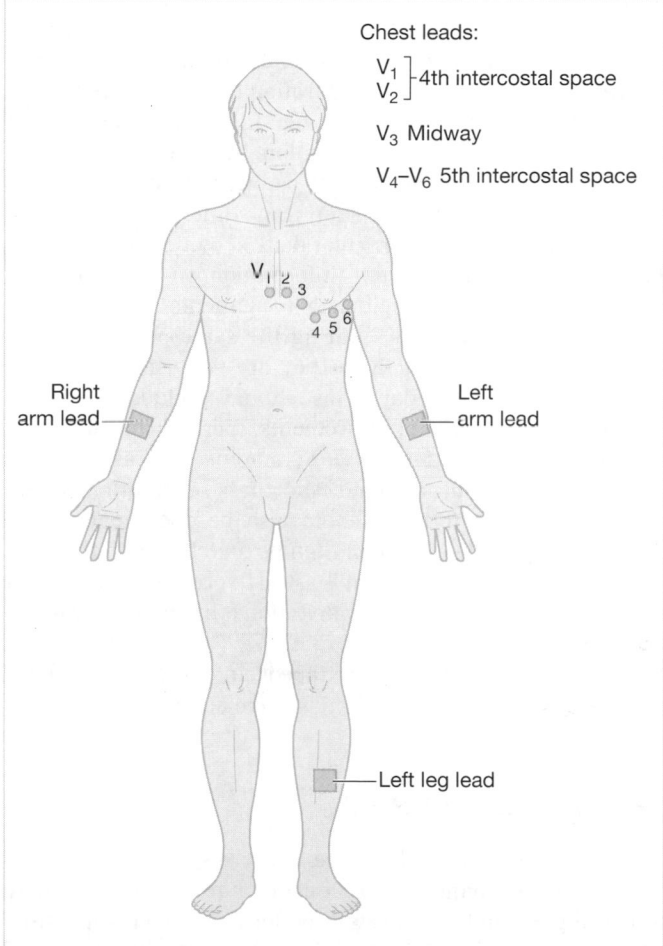

Figure 19.8 Position of ECG leads.

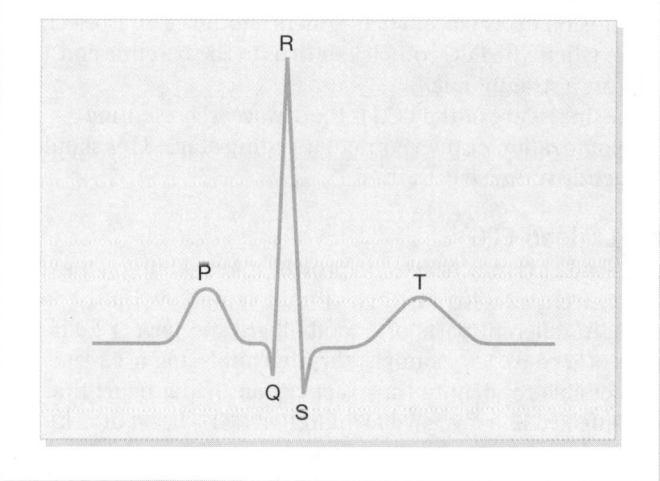

Figure 19.9 P-QRS-T complex.

electrode jelly, to enhance contact with the skin and impulse transfer. Substances that may prevent adhesiveness of the electrode or create impedance, such as dressings, should be removed, and it may be necessary to remove rough skin cells by gentle abrasion. Poor contact may result in the baseline wandering, making ECG interpretation difficult and possibly inaccurate.

The ECG is recorded on special squared paper. This enables the pattern to be examined and compared with previous recordings. For fuller detail on the ECG, you should refer to a more specialized text (see 'Further reading').

The deflections occurring during the cardiac cycle are referred to as the P-QRS-T complex, with each part of the complex representing electrical activity at a different part of the heart (see Fig. 19.9):

- The P wave is usually a rounded dome-shaped deflection. It occurs as the wave of depolarization passes through the atria to the AV node. Following the P wave, the atria contract (atrial systole).
- The interval between the P wave and ventricular contraction is termed the PR interval and is measured from the beginning of the P wave to the beginning of the QRS complex. It must be long enough to allow complete ventricular filling before the ventricles start to contract. A reduced PR interval will therefore lead to a decrease in cardiac output.

The ECG is recorded using 12 leads: six standard limb leads and six precordial or chest leads. The precordial leads are termed V_1–V_6 and are positioned around the chest wall, while the six standard limb leads (I, II, III and aVR, aVL and aVF) are obtained by placing electrodes on the right and left arms and on the left leg (see Fig. 19.8). The best position for limb leads is on the distal portion of the arms and legs. To reduce muscle tremor, the 12-lead recording should be made with the patient in the supine position, whenever this can be tolerated. Skin is a poor conductor of electricity and so careful preparation is required. Pre-prepared adhesive electrodes are used, which contain an

- The QRS complex represents ventricular depolarization. Initial depolarization of the ventricles is from left to right through the septum (seen in some leads as a negative deflection, termed the Q wave). The next part of the complex is the upright deflection, termed the R wave, which represents depolarization of the ventricular muscle mass, and the S wave occurs as the cells return to their resting electrical state. The whole QRS complex describes the length of time for electrical activity to depolarize the ventricular cells. If wide, it may indicate abnormal conduction through the ventricles.

- The ST segment follows the QRS complex and represents the end of ventricular depolarization and the start of repolarization. It is during this period that coronary artery perfusion takes place. This segment should be an isoelectric line where the ECG complex returns to the baseline and forms a straight line.

- The final wave of the ECG is the T wave, representing repolarization or the ventricular resting stage. This should be a gently rounded deflection.

The 12-lead ECG

A 12-lead ECG may be used to provide information on the heart activity from 12 different angles (in the same way that 12 people sitting in different parts of a football ground have 12 different views of a goal). For example, through analysing a 12-lead ECG it is possible to identify the exact region of the heart that has been affected in a myocardial infarction (MI – heart attack).

Prior to this procedure patients should be encouraged to wear loose-fitting clothes and to lie down on a bed or couch. If they are unable to lie down, e.g. due to breathlessness, they may be more comfortable at a 45° angle. It is more important that they lie as still as possible to ensure a good tracing. The procedure should not cause discomfort and usually only takes about 5 minutes to complete. Nurses are often responsible for taking the 12-lead ECG recording and should have some understanding of its interpretation.

For more information about how to perform a 12-lead ECG and how to interpret the recording, you should refer to a more detailed text (see 'Further reading').

Bedside monitoring

At times it is important to obtain a continuous tracing of the heartbeat. This would normally occur in a high-dependency, intensive care or coronary care unit where the prompt identification of arrhythmias (disturbances in the rate, rhythm or conduction of the heart) enables rapid treatment. Most ECG bedside monitors can record only one view of the heart at any one time and require patients to have at least three leads positioned on their arms and legs. Although the best position for limb leads is on the distal part of the limbs, for continuous tracings this position produces too much artefact through muscle movement and the leads are therefore placed on the torso. Three leads are positioned on the right and left upper chest wall and one on the left lower chest wall. Frequently the lead II position is chosen for bedside monitoring as it records a positive R wave and a clear view of the P wave.

Bedside ECG monitoring requires patients to be relatively immobile either in bed or sitting in a chair. When the condition allows, telemetry monitoring may be used. This enables patients to get up and move around the hospital. They wear a small transmitter that fits into a pocket. Electrodes are placed on the torso in the same way as for bedside monitoring but are attached to a transmitter. The signals are sent back to a receiver and displayed on a monitor where the heart rate and rhythm can be assessed. In this way, patients can be mobile, sitting in the day room or even in another ward, providing the signals are within reach of the receiver.

Holter monitoring

This is used when a continuous tracing of cardiac electrical activity over a 24-hour period is needed. The Holter tape is a miniature electrocardiograph worn by the patient. The ECG electrodes are placed on the torso sufficiently securely to obtain a good tracing for the 24 hours. This usually requires more extensive skin preparation than is required for an ECG. The chest is often shaved in men to enable better contact and the electrodes taped into position. As these are to be in place for 24 hours, patients must be aware that they cannot shower, bathe or swim during that time. However, they should continue with their regular daily activities, as the Holter tape test is designed to obtain information on the heart rate and rhythm during normal activity. Patients will be asked to keep a diary of activities during the same period, making accurate entries of the activity they are performing, and the time, throughout the day. This should include strenuous exercise, smoking, bowel movements, periods of anger or emotion and sexual intercourse. Symptoms such as dizziness, chest, neck, jaw and arm pain, shortness of breath, nausea, weakness and palpitations should also be documented. The information from the diary can then be matched with the ECG. With certain devices the patient is asked to press a record button if they feel symptoms such as palpitations that may indicate an arrhythmia.

Once the test is complete, the tape is analysed and the diary inspected to see if any arrhythmias correlate with a particular activity.

EXERCISE TEST TREADMILL

This test is used to see how the heart responds to exercise. During the test, patients exercise on a treadmill. This may induce angina and so must be performed under supervised conditions. Both the ECG and blood pressure are recorded frequently throughout.

Often this test can be reassuring to patients, confirming that they are able to undertake exercise without chest pain. This is especially important to some patients following an MI. However, for others, the test may cause concern about their inability to exercise, and early consultation with their cardiologist is important.

ECHOCARDIOGRAM

This test is used to assess the structure, function and blood flow through the heart. High-frequency sound waves are aimed at the heart and the echo of these waves is picked up by a transducer and viewed on a screen.

A Doppler echocardiogram may sometimes be carried out. Here a probe is placed on the chest wall. A conductive jelly is applied to this so that any sound waves from the heart can be transmitted to a screen.

A transoesophageal echocardiogram (TOE) may also be performed. Here a probe is passed down the oesophagus. This particular form of echocardiogram is useful to assess the function of the aortic and mitral valves and the left ventricle. As the probe is passed down the oesophagus, it is usual to use a local anaesthetic, such as a lidocaine (lignocaine) spray on the throat, and a light sedative. For these reasons, patients should be advised not to eat or drink for 6 hours before the test and should not be allowed home until they have woken fully and are able to take fluids. As they will have been given a sedative, they should be encouraged to have a friend or member of the family collect them from the hospital, and should not drive or ride a motor vehicle for at least 12 hours.

MAGNETIC RESONANCE SCANNING (MRI)

This technique is used to obtain three-dimensional images of the heart – the chambers, vessels, function and size. For this test, patients are expected to lie flat, enclosed within a scanner, for around 30 minutes. It is not an uncomfortable procedure but some patients may find it difficult to lie like this for the required time period, while others may find the scanner claustrophobic. Nurses can reduce patient anxiety by answering questions, describing the equipment and procedure, and reinforcing the information with written material.

CHEST X-RAY

The chest X-ray is useful to determine the size of the heart. An enlarged heart may indicate heart failure or cardiomyopathy. The size of the aorta can also be evaluated and may be used to diagnose and assess an aortic aneurysm.

The chest X-ray also provides a view of the lungs. The presence of pulmonary oedema, for example, may indicate heart failure.

BLOOD TESTS

These include both general tests and very specific tests.

Cardiac enzymes

During illness causing cell damage, the cell membrane may be disrupted and chemical substances not normally found in the blood will leak from the cell into the bloodstream. When cardiac muscle cells are damaged, possibly from ischaemia or actual damage to the cells as occurs in MI, certain enzymes (not all are cardiac-specific) will leak from the cell and be detected in the blood. These are referred to as cardiac enzymes and provide important information which can be used to plan care. For example, if there is severe damage to the cardiac muscle, large amounts of cardiac enzymes are released into the blood. Cardiac enzymes are also released according to the time since the injury and it is important to draw blood samples at clearly defined intervals. The date and time of the blood sampling must be clearly identified on the blood tubes and the laboratory

request form. The enzymes routinely measured in the blood are outlined below:

- Creatinine phosphokinase (CPK) is present in skeletal, cardiac and brain tissue where it is involved in the production of energy for cellular contraction. The isoenzyme (an enzyme which has several forms – found in diverse sites but catalyses the same reaction) CPK MB has been found predominately in the myocardium and therefore this test is used to diagnose MI. Levels of CPK MB should be measured every 6 hours following a suspected MI. Levels will rise at 4–6 hours, peaking at 12–24 hours. If there is no further damage to the myocardium, the levels should start to fall, returning to the baseline after 3–4 days. CPK MB levels will also rise following percutaneous transluminal coronary angioplasty (PTCA), cardiac surgery or unstable angina. Increases may also be seen with pericarditis or myocarditis.
- Other enzymes may include aspartate aminotransferase (AST). Following cellular injury, levels will rise sharply over 8–12 hours, peaking at 24–48 hours. The levels will return to normal by day 5. However, AST is found in the liver as well as the heart and so raised AST levels cannot be used as a reliable indicator of damage to the heart muscle.
- Lactate dehydrogenase (LDH), another enzyme involved in the production of energy in the cell, is released following injury to the cell. It is released over 2–10 days, peaking at 3 days, and so may be used to detect myocardial damage that has possibly occurred a few days before.
- More recently troponin I has been used as a blood test to detect the presence of myocardial injury. Troponin is a protein found exclusively in cardiac cells where it is involved in the process of cellular contraction. Troponin I can now successfully identify patients who have myocardial damage. Troponin I will be found in the blood between 3 and 4 hours following an MI.

Full blood count and erythrocyte sedimentation rate

A full blood count can provide useful information to inform the care of the person with cardiovascular disease. A low red blood cell count or reduced haemoglobin level indicates anaemia. For the person with cardiovascular disease, anaemia may precipitate angina or exacerbate heart failure and should be treated.

The white blood cell (WBC) count will be raised in the presence of an inflammatory process and, in a person with cardiovascular disease, may indicate an acute MI or infective endocarditis (IE). Four days following an MI, the WBC count may rise as white blood cells invade the necrotic tissue as a natural part of the healing process. As a raised WBC count is indicative of infection, other causes, such as a concomitant infection, should be ruled out. Some drugs used for the person with cardiovascular disease (such as digoxin, aspirin, heparin and procainamide) may also lead to a raised WBC count.

The erythrocyte sedimentation rate (ESR) is a non-specific indicator of the inflammatory process and again may be elevated following MI or IE.

If an infection is suspected then blood cultures should be taken to identify the exact pathogen. Blood must be drawn from a clean venous site and placed into special culture bottles. These blood cultures must be taken at specific times and a particular number of days apart and local policy should be observed. The blood must be put into the bottle carefully, avoiding any outside contamination that may affect the results of the culture. Preliminary results should be available on the blood culture within 24 hours and appropriate antibiotics commenced if the results are positive.

Coagulation studies

Some patients with cardiovascular disease are maintained on an anticoagulant such as warfarin. In these cases, it will be important to obtain regular results of their clotting time. In the UK the international standardized ratio (INR) is referred to. Blood is drawn at regular intervals and the dose of warfarin titrated against the result. The INR is kept at different levels, dependent on the reason for the anticoagulation. For example, a person on warfarin therapy for atrial fibrillation should have the INR maintained around 2.0–3.0, while following prosthetic valve replacement the INR should be higher, at 2.5–4.0 (Woods et al 2000).

Blood lipid profile

Blood lipid levels are used to determine risk for CHD. The lipid profile includes low-density lipoproteins (LDLs), high-density lipoproteins (HDLs) and triglycerides.

CORONARY ANGIOGRAPHY

Coronary angiography enables the physician to assess the coronary vessels, cardiac function and intracardiac pressures. It is performed under sterile conditions in the cardiac catheter laboratory.

Prior to the procedure, the groin area should be shaved. Patients are advised not to eat or drink for 4 hours before the procedure in case an emergency operation is required. A local anaesthetic is injected into the area where the catheter will be inserted, e.g. the groin area for the femoral artery approach, and intravenous sedatives may be given during the angiography as the procedure and equipment may be frightening. A catheter is inserted through either the femoral or brachial artery and radio-opaque contrast medium is injected into the heart and coronary arteries. The contrast media used may make the patient experience a warm flushing sensation when first injected and patients should be warned of this before it occurs. Very occasionally a patient may be allergic to the dye, feeling nauseous, vomiting and perhaps developing hypertension or respiratory distress.

Once the contrast is injected, pictures are recorded on film or digitally and can be reviewed at a later date. Coronary angiography is usually performed to assess the severity of CHD. The disease is usually defined as single-vessel, two-vessel, three-vessel or left main stem disease. The diseased coronary artery should be noted, along with the exact location of the atheroma and the extent to which the atheroma obstructs the lumen (see Fig. 19.10).

Following the procedure, the femoral catheter should be removed prior to the patient returning to the ward. Firm pressure must be applied to the area and a pressure dressing placed over the puncture site. The patient should remain on bed rest for

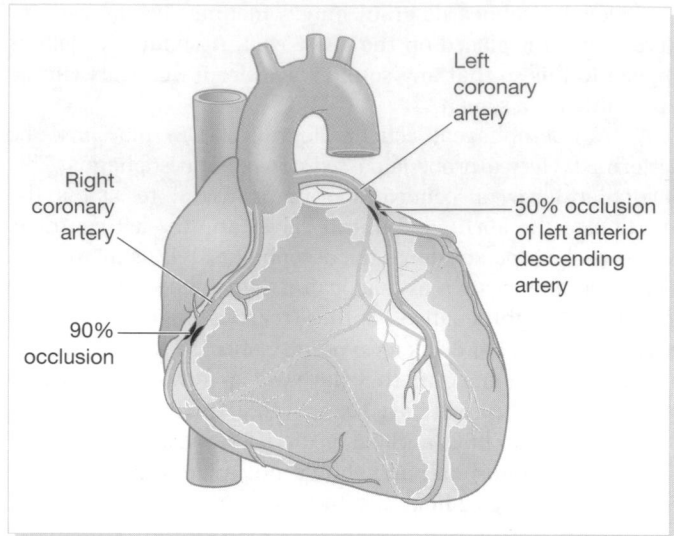

Figure 19.10 Diagram showing severe calcification of the right coronary artery and a smaller obstruction of the left anterior descending artery. This patient will require a percutaneous transluminal coronary angioplasty and stent to the right coronary artery.

approximately 4 hours, lying flat or at a maximum angle of 45° head up. The cannulated leg must be kept straight. Initially, on return to the ward, the limb should be observed for bleeding, pedal pulses, colour, warmth and sensation every 15 minutes. This can be gradually reduced if the condition is stable. Patients should be advised that bleeding from the site may occur if extra strain or pressure is applied to the area. They should be told to apply digital pressure to the puncture site when they cough or laugh for the first day, and to avoid stooping or heavy lifting that would expose the site to additional strain.

Patients should also be encouraged to drink plenty of fluids to flush the contrast from the system, as again, very occasionally, it may lead to renal failure.

The whole experience of coronary angiography can be worrying; not only the procedure itself and the equipment used, but also the potential diagnosis that may follow the test. For some patients, their employment may be affected by the results. It is important that before they leave the hospital they have a chance to discuss the test results and have an early appointment to discuss this further with a cardiologist.

ELECTROPHYSIOLOGY STUDIES (EPS)

These are more specific investigations for arrhythmias undertaken in the cardiac catheter laboratory. A small wire is inserted into the femoral vein and passed into the heart. A map of electrical impulses from the heart is sent to a screen to provide more exact information on the site and nature of the arrhythmia (see section on disorders of electrical conduction later). During the study the cardiologist may provoke arrhythmias to see how the heart reacts. If abnormal pathways responsible for an arrhythmia are detected, they are ablated (removed) by radiofrequency waves sent down the catheter.

GENERAL DISEASE PREVENTION AND HEALTH EDUCATION

The focus here will be CHD, which is the largest cause of morbidity and mortality amongst the cardiovascular disorders. Additionally, as is clear from this chapter, many other cardiovascular disorders may be traced back to CHD.

Despite the declining incidence of CHD, it remains a major cause of premature death in the UK and accounts for a high cost to the NHS. The UK government aims to reduce death from CHD and stroke by at least 40% by the year 2010 (Department of Health 1999). In other words, these two diseases currently account for the death of around 200 000 people each year in the UK (ONS 1998) and the government aims to reduce this figure to 120 000 over the next 10 years. Although the incidence of CHD is declining among the higher social classes, the worst off in our society have not really benefited. It is this inequality in health, highlighted in the late 1970s (Department of Health 1978), that the government has pledged to address through the National Service Framework for Coronary Heart Disease (Department of Health 2000); for example, reducing the prevalence of smoking is one of the standards for reducing heart disease in the population. Nurses, especially those working in primary care, have an important role in smoking cessation programmes.

The major reduction in CHD seen in recent years may be attributed to the improvements in social and economic conditions. However, there is a long way to go to improve the conditions of the UK population to encourage a more healthy approach to living. Consider, for example, the current situation regarding the perceived safety of the streets and the controls on food pricing. Streets that are perceived as unsafe to walk in will encourage the use of cars, and the high prices of fruit, vegetables, lean meat and fish will encourage a poorer diet. A population-focused approach to health, then, is essential to reduce the risk of CHD. Yet it has proved difficult for governments to achieve, and currently the UK has a higher mortality from CHD in the under-65 age group than any other European country (Department of Health 1999).

An individual approach to health is more tangible and the nurse can make a major contribution towards this. It aims to identify patients at risk and then to target them for reduction in their risk.

Many risk factors for CHD have been identified and can be subdivided into factors that are non-modifiable and those that are modifiable. The non-modifiable risk factors such as increasing age, gender (being male) and familial risk are not addressed here and readers are advised to consult the 'Further Reading' suggestions.

Important modifiable risk factors for CHD have been identified: hypercholesterolaemia (high cholesterol level in the blood), hypertension (high blood pressure), physical inactivity and smoking. Other modifiable factors include poor nutrition with high fat intake, obesity and diabetes. It is easy to see how all these factors are interrelated. For example, someone who eats a poor diet may well become obese and, consequently, physically inactive. It is this multifactorial approach to identifying risk factors and offering appropriate advice that is the cornerstone of treatment today (see Health Promotion box 19.1).

 HEALTH PROMOTION

19.1 Prevention of coronary heart disease

Coronary heart disease is the leading cause of premature death and the UK government has pledged to reduce this high incidence. Identifying people at risk and providing health promoting activities are some of the main target areas identified within the national service frameworks for coronary heart disease (Department of Health 2000).

Key points for health promoting activities include:

- healthy eating (see Ch. 11)
- smoking cessation (see Ch. 20)
- physical activity.

Student activities

Make a diary entry of your own food intake, smoking habits and physical activity over a 7-day period.

- Did you meet the current recommendations of eating five portions of fruit or vegetables a day, not smoking and exercising for 30 minutes five times a week?
- List the barriers that may have prevented you meeting these recommendations such as shift work, fruit too expensive, etc.
- List the barriers that you overcame to achieve these recommendations.
- Reflect on these activities and think how you can use the experience to help patients make changes in their lifestyle.

Reference

DoH. National service framework for coronary heart disease. London: DoH; 2000.

HYPERCHOLESTEROLAEMIA

Cholesterol, a fatty substance, is made by the body in the gut and liver and is also found in our diet. It is essential to the body for the growth and development of cell membranes and steroid hormones. Cholesterol in the body binds with proteins to create lipoproteins. These lipoproteins can be divided into different groups. The two major groups are high-density lipoproteins (HDLs), which have a protective effect for CHD risk, and low-density lipoproteins (LDLs), which lead to the development of atheroma. High levels of LDL and low levels of HDL are associated with CHD risk.

High blood cholesterol levels can be reduced through diet modification, physical activity or drugs. There is a vast amount of information in the literature on healthy eating (see Ch. 11); yet it is sometimes difficult for the patient to find the right message. A diet low in fat will lower the blood cholesterol level, yet cholesterol is essential to the body and it is important to remember that it is the ratio of HDL to LDL that is important.

Other measures that may be considered to improve cholesterol levels include stopping smoking, increasing exercise and drinking one unit of alcohol a day (a small glass of wine or half a pint of beer). For more information, see the section on lifestyle changes and exercise below.

To maintain a healthy ratio of LDL to HDL does not only require attention to diet. Exercise, considered beneficial in the reduction of CHD, is thought to increase HDL levels, while smoking may reduce them. Attention to these factors may assist in maintaining a healthy cholesterol level. For more information, see the section on lifestyle changes and exercise below.

Drug therapy

For some patients, high cholesterol levels may be caused by genetic factors (familial hypercholesterolaemia) that lead to raised levels of LDLs. In these patients, cholesterol-lowering drugs (resins) should be used. These drugs prevent the absorption of cholesterol from the gastrointestinal tract and so reduce serum cholesterol levels. They have a good safety record and can reliably be used for familial hypercholesterolaemia where therapy may be required for several years. In all other patients with CHD and high cholesterol levels (> 5 mmol/L), the HMG-CoA reductase inhibitors (statins) such as simvastatin can be chosen.

HYPERTENSION

Hypertension is a particular risk factor for CHD, but again cannot be viewed in isolation. It is associated with a three- to four-fold increase in risk of MI and stroke (Jensen et al 1991). High salt intake in the diet, a high alcohol intake, poor physical activity and obesity may all contribute to hypertension and the associated risk of CHD.

SMOKING

Smoking is a significant risk factor for CHD and possibly the most preventable. The CHD risk among smokers increases with the number of cigarettes smoked, the number of years of smoking and the younger the age at which smoking started (Jensen et al 1991). This is especially true for women. Before the climacteric, oestrogen increases the level of HDL (protective factor for CHD) in the blood. However, smoking will reduce HDL levels. For women who take an oral contraceptive and smoke, the risk of CHD is even higher. Additionally, smoking reduces the supply of O_2 to the myocardium, increases the viscosity of the blood, making it more likely to clot, and injures the endothelial lining of the arteries, leaving them more susceptible to atheroma development.

Patients should be given professional advice and help to stop smoking. This may be through the use of cognitive therapy and nicotine replacement. The UK government has pledged to reduce smoking within the general population by means of more widely available smoking cessation classes (Department of Health 2000). Patients should be made aware of this help and encouraged to accept it. Some patients may benefit from a drug specifically used to support smoking cessation. Bupropion (amfebutamone) may be used, but should only be prescribed after a consultation when it is clear that the person has decided to cease smoking and has set a date for this. The complete course should be taken despite some of the side-effects of insomnia, headache and a dry mouth (MacConnachie 2000).

LIFESTYLE CHANGES AND EXERCISE

A diet high in fat and sodium or one with too little non-starch polysaccharide (fibre) such as fruit and vegetables is important in the aetiology of CHD. Many snack and convenience foods are high in fat, sugar and sodium, which are used to improve the flavour of bought meals. However, none of this helps to create the 'heart healthy diet'.

A heart healthy diet should include at least five pieces of fruit or vegetables a day, lean meat or fish (avoiding too much red meat), grains and cereals for the vitamin B group and a reduction in fat intake. Food should be baked, grilled or steamed and any skin removed from meat prior to cooking. Oils high in monounsaturated fats should be used, such as some margarine and olive oil.

Patients may need help to understand a heart healthy diet from either a dietician or a nurse specially trained in dietary advice. Weight reduction and lowering of blood pressure, blood cholesterol and blood glucose can all be achieved through a healthy diet and will contribute to reducing the risk of CHD.

Social class and income influence diet. Yet the food we eat not only influences the risk of developing CHD but also affects how we feel, how much energy we have and body weight. All these factors may influence the amount of physical activity undertaken by an individual.

Physical activity protects against CHD by reducing obesity and blood pressure. Aerobic exercise such as a brisk walk, jogging or cycling should be undertaken at least three times a week for a period of 30 minutes. It is not always easy to maintain regular exercise and this may be a particular problem for older people (see Special Issues box 19.1). Not only does exercise reduce weight and blood pressure, but it may also have a direct effect on reducing CHD by increasing HDL levels.

 SPECIAL ISSUES

19.1 Encouraging physical activity in older people

As the older population of the UK is increasing in number, the importance of addressing strategies to encourage physical activity in this group must be considered.

Keeping fit when growing older may be difficult. Older people may have co-morbidities such as osteoarthritis or osteoporosis, both of which may make exercising difficult. Perhaps they live alone and have no-one to go for a walk with or perhaps they are frightened of getting chest pain while out.

In North America, shopping malls are frequently used by older people as a safe environment for them to walk. They can also be used regardless of the weather. Some shopping malls even open before shop opening times to encourage this. In the UK, sports centres are now holding exercise or swimming classes for older people and short walks may be advertised in the local sports facilities, health centres or libraries.

Student activities

Find out what facilities are available in your local area to encourage safe exercise by older people.

CARDIOPULMONARY ARREST AND RESUSCITATION

In cardiopulmonary arrest, there is a sudden cessation of cardiac output or breathing. This results in a loss of consciousness, myocardial ischaemia and eventually to death. Fast and efficient resuscitation is therefore essential to save lives and reduce morbidity in survivors of a cardiopulmonary arrest.

Aetiology
Possible reasons for a cardiopulmonary arrest include:

- myocardial ischaemia
- cardiomyopathy
- respiratory insufficiency
- severe forms of heart block
- electric shock
- anaphylactic reactions to certain drugs and other substances
- electrolyte imbalance
- hypovolaemia.

It is important to remember that there may be no pre-existing disease and that a cardiopulmonary arrest may be the first sign of a serious cardiovascular disorder.

Pathophysiology and clinical presentation
Cessation of either cardiac or respiratory activity will rapidly lead to a cardiopulmonary arrest if treatment is not initiated as soon as possible. A cardiac arrest may result from pulseless ventricular tachycardia, ventricular fibrillation or asystole (see pp. 500–501). When the initial cause is respiratory, the arrhythmia is caused by tissue ischaemia due to respiratory insufficiency.

The cardiac output is reduced and the body is unable to obtain sufficient O_2 to meet metabolic requirements. This results in a rapid loss of consciousness. The person suffering a cardiopulmonary arrest will be unresponsive, not breathing and have no palpable pulse. There is cyanosis or pallor, and the pupils dilate.

The clinical presentation is discussed further below.

▶ Nursing management

The outcome of a cardiopulmonary arrest is dependent upon the speed of action. The supply of O_2 to the brain must be restored within 4 minutes if irreversible damage is to be avoided.

Assessment of the patient's Airway, Breathing and Circulation – the ABC of resuscitation – must be accurate and fast, and must take place prior to the initiation of cardiopulmonary resuscitation (CPR). All nurses should understand the ABC of cardiopulmonary resuscitation and practise their basic life support (BLS) skills of resuscitation regularly (Resuscitation Council (UK) 2000a and Fig. 19.11). Most hospitals in the UK employ resuscitation training officers and encourage nurses to obtain regular simulation practice. This section is only intended as an introduction to CPR and should not be used as a replacement for attendance at resuscitation training days.

Assessment and resuscitation of the airway and breathing
When initially faced with a situation of suspected cardiopulmonary arrest, the following procedure should be carried out:

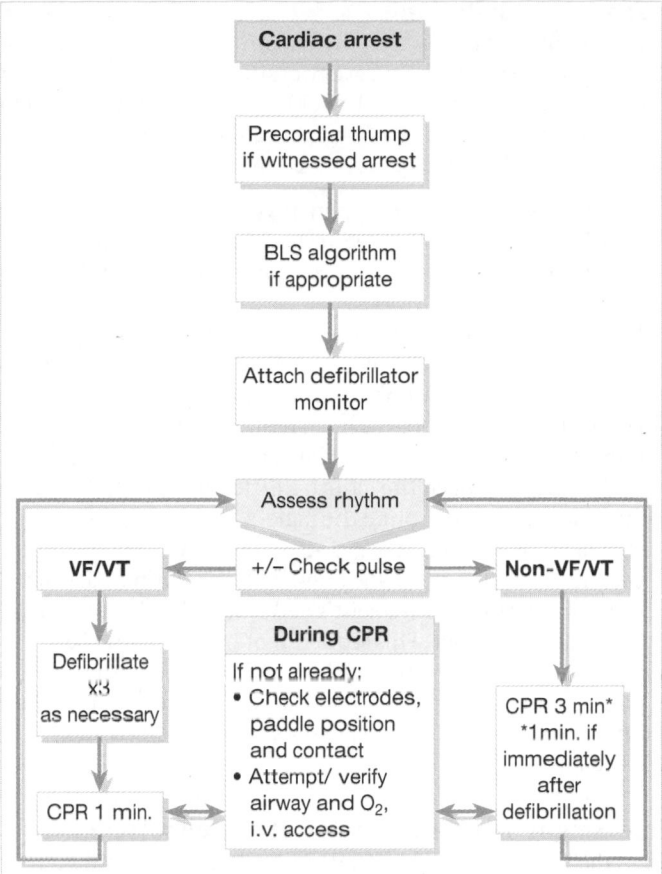

Figure 19.11 Algorithm – advanced life support (ALS). (Adapted from Resuscitation Council UK 2000b.)

- Level of consciousness should be assessed. If the patient responds to gentle shaking of the shoulders or to loud speaking, then he or she should be left in the same position and help sought if needed. You should be familiar with the process for obtaining help from the cardiac arrest team in your place of work and location of emergency equipment. If the patient is unresponsive, you should call for help.

- The airway should be opened. Placing a hand on the forehead and gently tilting the head back can achieve this. Placing fingertips under the patient's chin should lift the chin. The patient's position should only be altered if it is not possible to open the airway using this action. In this case, the patient should be moved onto the back. This should be avoided if there appears to be either head or neck injury.

- Any visible obstruction should be removed from the airway.

- It should now be possible to check for any signs of breathing by:
  — looking at the chest wall for movement
  — placing your ear close to the patient's mouth and listening for breath sounds
  — placing your cheek close to the patient's mouth to feel any movement of air. (NB. No more than 10 seconds should be used in assessing for movement of air.)

Steps in resuscitation

If there is any indication that the patient is breathing, he or she should be turned into the recovery position (readers are advised to consult a current first aid book) and monitored until help arrives. If there is no sign of breathing then pulmonary resuscitation should be commenced, as follows:

- The airway should be kept open. If you are in a hospital you may have access to an oropharyngeal airway that you can insert until the cardiac arrest team arrive and the patient can be intubated.
- You should prepare to give the patient two effective breaths. Again, in a hospital you may be able to use an Ambu-bag connected to an O₂ supply to deliver these breaths. Otherwise you will need to ensure the head remains tilted and the chin lifted. Pinch the soft tissue of the nose with the index finger and thumb and open the mouth a little. Take a deep breath and place your lips around the patient's own and blow steadily into the mouth over 1–2 seconds. While doing this, you should watch to see the chest wall rise. Then take your mouth away from the patient's and watch the chest wall fall as the air comes out. This sequence of events should be repeated so that two effective breaths are given to the patient. Small plastic pocket shields are now available for use and should be used if at all possible to prevent the risk of infection to the rescuer.

Assessment and resuscitation of the circulation

Once the two breaths have been performed, the patient's circulation must be assessed. The carotid pulse in the neck (see Fig. 19.6) should be palpated, as this is easily accessible.

If a pulse is not palpable, external cardiac massage should be started immediately: the fingers of both hands should be locked together and placed over the xiphoid sternum. Firm pressure is then applied with the heels of the hands. The elbows should be kept straight so that the pressure is exerted downwards. This will increase the intrathoracic pressure and provide effective compression of the heart to push blood into the arteries. The pressure should be sufficient to depress the sternum by about 2 cm in an adult to create an effective cardiac output while reducing the risk of fracture to the ribs.

Cardiopulmonary resuscitation

If there is only one person present, the chest should be compressed 15 times before two repeat breaths are given. When two people are present, the same ratio of 15:2 should be used, with one rescuer undertaking chest compression while the other cares for the airway.

As soon as possible the patient should be attached to a cardiac monitor so that the presence of a heart rate and rhythm may be detected. It is unlikely that, following a cardiac arrest, the heart will spontaneously regain normal activity. The aim should be to maintain oxygenation of the brain and heart until the cardiopulmonary arrest team arrives and advanced life support (ALS) can be started (see Fig. 19.11).

An intravenous line should be inserted as soon as possible so that emergency intravenous drug therapy can be given. If the patient is found to be in ventricular fibrillation, a defibrillator should be used.

Defibrillation is used to treat pulseless ventricular tachycardia or ventricular fibrillation. Two paddles are placed on the chest wall, one on each side of the heart – one in the right upper sternum, mid-clavicular region and the other at the fifth intercostal space, mid-axilla region. An electrical current of between 200 and 360 joules is delivered through the paddles. This causes all the myocardial cells to contract so that the sinus node can fire and the heart return to a sinus rhythm. As an electrical current is being used, strict safety precautions should be taken. The paddles should only be charged once they are in position on the chest wall and all personnel should stand well clear of the patient or bed when the electric shock is delivered. Clearly, it is also important to ensure that there is no spillage of water in the vicinity that could conduct the electric current.

Defibrillation is an important part of ALS and nurses should undertake specific training prior to using a defibrillator. This training should form part of all hospital personnel training and be regularly updated.

During resuscitation from a cardiac arrest, it is important that a team leader directs the procedure (see Ch. 30). This will normally be an experienced nurse or doctor. All treatment should be accurately recorded during a cardiac arrest and hospitals have their own policies regarding the roles of the cardiac arrest team members. The Resuscitation Council for the UK regularly updates the guidelines for practice to ensure the best possible results are achieved (Resuscitation Council 2000). All hospital personnel and health care professionals should be familiar with the most recent recommendations.

In England, only around 1 in 50 people will survive an out-of-hospital arrest (Department of Health 2000). In response to this, the government intends to place defibrillators in public places and, through the 'Health Skills' programme, teach the public how to use them. The defibrillators will be automated, so that if someone collapses, the paddles will detect the heart rhythm and only deliver a shock if the rhythm is ventricular tachycardia or fibrillation. This feature means that the devices will be safe for all members of the public to use, as they will not deliver an electric shock inappropriately.

Following successful CPR, patients are generally transferred to a high-dependency area for monitoring. If they remember losing consciousness they may be very frightened and will require careful support. People may describe the whole event as a 'near death experience' and they may fear recurrent cardiac arrests, which can reduce their quality of life and make them fearful of leaving the house.

Relatives who witnessed the arrest and resuscitation may also require support and possibly counselling (see Ch. 30). Sometimes the family will want to learn BLS so that they can use it if the person suffers a further cardiopulmonary arrest. However, despite prompt and effective resuscitation, the patient will not always survive.

For severely ill patients with a terminal illness such as heart failure or cancer (see Ch. 34), it is important for the team, the patient and their family to consider, in advance, if they wish to be resuscitated in the event of a cardiopulmonary arrest (see Ethical Issues box 19.1). No decision should be made not to resuscitate until it has been discussed with the patient and the family. This requires considerable skill and should be undertaken only by an experienced nurse or physician.

ETHICAL ISSUES

19.1 When not to resuscitate?

The decision not to resuscitate is arguably one of the most difficult that the medical team has to make. In the person who is mortally ill, such as when terminally ill with cancer or a severe cardiac or respiratory disorder, the aim of care is to preserve the dignity of the patient and enable a peaceful death. It would then not be morally correct to undertake resuscitation. However, both the patient and relatives should be aware of this decision and have an opportunity to discuss it with the medical staff.

This communication between hospital personnel, patients and their relatives is difficult and is not always easy to initiate. Yet it is essential for all staff to be involved in, and aware of, any decision made. It is also important that people are reassured that neither they nor their relatives will be left to die if there is a chance of prolonging life in an acceptable way to achieve a reasonable quality of life.

The Resuscitation Council (UK) (2001) suggest that the following are considered prior to making a decision not to resuscitate:

- the patient's own wishes – possibly indicated in an advance directive
- the patient's wish to be resuscitated should be respected where possible
- the view of relatives who may be aware of the patient's wishes
- the patient's prognosis – both intermediate and longer term
- the previous quality of life
- the views of all medical and nursing staff involved in the patient's management
- the patient's human rights – the right to life and the right not to be subjected to degrading treatment
- probability of successful resuscitation
- the perceived ability of the patient to cope with a possible disability.

NB. Resuscitation must not be carried out against the recorded and sustained wishes of a mentally competent adult patient.

Reference

Resuscitation Council (UK). Decisions relating to cardiopulmonary resuscitation. A joint statement from the British Medical Association, the Resuscitation Council (UK) and the Royal College of Nursing. Resuscitation Council (UK). Online. Available: www.resus.org.uk 2001.

CARDIOVASCULAR DISORDERS

The groups of disorders covered in this chapter include:

- disorders of electrical conduction
- CHD

- heart failure – acute and chronic
- valvular heart disease
- infective endocarditis
- disorders of the myocardium
- disorders of the pericardium
- disorders of the vascular system
- congenital heart disease.

Readers requiring more detailed information about particular disorders and the care needed are directed to the suggestions in 'Further reading'.

DISORDERS OF THE ELECTRICAL CONDUCTION SYSTEM – ATRIAL ARRHYTHMIAS

SINUS BRADYCARDIA

A normal rhythm is termed sinus rhythm (see Fig. 19.7) and bears all the hallmarks of normal conduction. However, when the heart beats at a rate below 60 bpm, the term bradycardia is used.

Aetiology

Sinus bradycardia may be a sign of ill health, and causes such as disease of the sinus node or hypothyroidism (see Ch. 17) should be considered. It may also be associated with increased stimulation of the vagus nerve. This may occur during excessive vomiting or, for example, on removal of a femoral cardiac catheter sheath. Sinus bradycardia may be common in healthy, young adults such as athletes where it is generally well tolerated.

Clinical presentation

Cardiac output is determined by the heart rate multiplied by stroke volume; hence a sinus bradycardia may lead to a decreased cardiac output. Although generally well tolerated, for some the reduced cardiac output may cause a feeling of dizziness and light-headedness and may even cause syncope attacks.

Medical management

It is only necessary to treat sinus bradycardia if the patient is symptomatic. In these situations, it may be necessary to increase the heart rate with intravenous atropine or even a pacemaker.

A cardiac pacemaker provides artificial electrical stimulation to the heart and is used when there are serious conduction defects affecting the patient's normal level of functioning. Pacemakers consist of electrodes, a battery unit, a pulse generator and a lead system. Older pacemakers tended to be set at a predetermined rate, whereas externally programmable pacemakers are now used, which can alter rate in response to physical activity and greatly improve the person's quality of life.

Pacemakers may be used on a temporary or permanent basis depending on why they are needed.

▶ **Nursing management**

The nursing management is dependent on the type of pacemaker used and the information and educational needs of the patient.

Temporary pacemaker

If a temporary pacing system is used, it is inserted under local anaesthetic in a clinical room off the main ward. Aseptic technique is used and the pacing system is inserted via the subclavian vein. The leads exit the vein and are attached to a pacing box.

Once connected to a temporary pacing system, patients will need to be relatively immobile as the pulse generator is outside the body and should not become disconnected. They should have their cardiac rhythm continuously monitored either by bedside ECG recording or through telemetry. When the pacemaker fires, a pacing spike will precede the ECG complex of the paced chamber (see Fig. 19.12). Having undergone an invasive procedure, patients should also be monitored for signs of infection (e.g. pyrexia) and the temperature recorded 4-hourly for the first 2 days.

Permanent pacemaker

A permanent system is also generally inserted under local anaesthetic under aseptic conditions. However, it is usually inserted in a cardiac catheterization laboratory or the operating theatres. A pocket is made under the skin in the left pectoral region and the pacemaker is inserted. The leads are then inserted directly into the subclavian vein. Again, following insertion, the patient should be attached to a cardiac monitor until it is known that the pacemaker is working correctly.

Various complications may occur at the time of the pacemaker insertion:

- Pneumothorax may develop soon after insertion and the patient will rapidly become short of breath. A chest X-ray should be ordered following the insertion of the system to detect the presence of air that may have entered the pleural space.
- Infection may occur. If left untreated this may lead to infective endocarditis (see p. 516). The insertion site should be observed for inflammation, indicating infection, and following the insertion a course of antibiotics should be given.
- Bleeding may occur from the site of insertion and often there is significant bruising that may become very painful and limit the mobility of the arm. The insertion site must be regularly observed for haematoma.

Caring for patients with a cardiac pacemaker requires the nurse to monitor and record the ECG and to determine if the pacemaker is working correctly. When the pacemaker fires, a large spike (pacing spike) is seen on the ECG (see Fig. 19.12). This should immediately precede contraction of the chamber. If the ventricles are paced, the pacing spike is seen just prior to the QRS complex (see Fig. 19.9). If the atria are paced, the pacing spike should be seen just prior to the P wave. If the pacemaker is not functioning correctly, the pacing spikes will be unrelated to the ECG waveform and patients are likely to complain of feeling dizzy or faint with a reduced cardiac output. Occasionally the pacing wires are displaced and stimulate the diaphragm, in which case patients are likely to experience hiccupping. The pacemaker leads may become displaced if patients are too active in the early stages of recovery, e.g. lifting their arms over their heads.

Certain types of machinery and electrical devices may affect the pacemaker system. Correctly 'earthed' home appliances should not cause any problems, but certain larger pieces of electrical equipment or electromagnetic fields may interfere with the functioning of the pacemaker. Equipment that may cause problems include arc welding sets, airport security detectors and some types of electrical dental equipment. Conversely, pacemakers may trigger anti-theft devices in shops. Patients should be made aware of these possibilities and should be given an identification card to carry with them.

Following pacemaker insertion, patients should not drive until they have attended their first pacemaker check. Additionally, persons with a pacemaker are not allowed to hold a heavy goods vehicle (HGV) licence. For these reasons it is important to discuss patients' employment and some may need to consider alternatives. Patients are also advised to avoid direct contact sports where a blow to the area of the pacemaker may be sustained.

Some patients become very anxious when a pacemaker system is first inserted. The fact that they are now relying on an electrical device to make their heart work can lead to great anxiety about the consequences of it failing to work correctly. Both patients and their families will need someone to talk to regarding such concerns. It is useful to give them contact details for the cardiology nurse specialist so that they may discuss any concerns and questions as they arise.

Regular follow-up is required. It is important to ensure that the pacemaker is functioning correctly, and at these times patients should have an opportunity to discuss any questions that have arisen. It is also important to teach patients and their families how to count the pulse rate. Patients should be encouraged to do this on a monthly basis and should be aware of

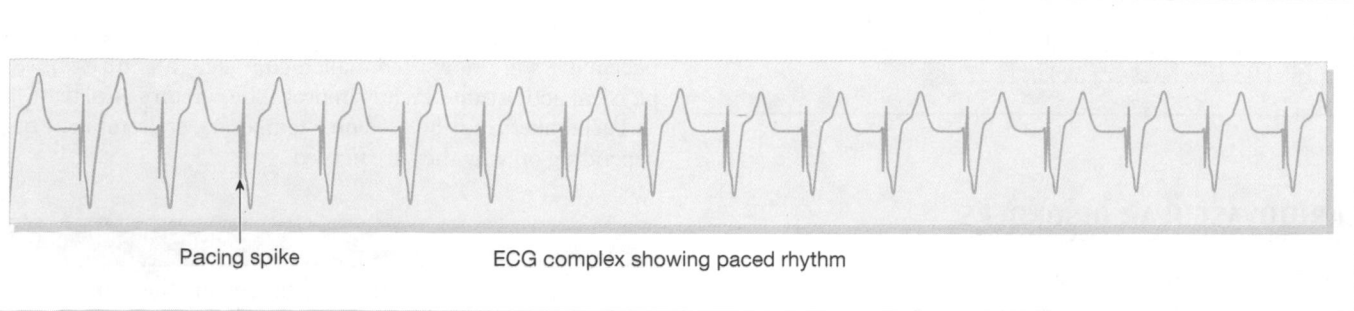

Pacing spike

ECG complex showing paced rhythm

Figure 19.12 Electrocardiogram with pacing spike.

when to report changes to their doctor. Every opportunity should be used to assess these skills, and they should be reinforced at every clinic visit. It may be useful to provide a personalized booklet stating the pacemaker mode, pulse rate parameters and contact phone numbers. Patients can then record their pulse rates in this booklet, taking it to any follow-up clinic appointment.

SINUS TACHYCARDIA

When the heart beats at a rate greater than 100 bpm, but again bears all the hallmarks of normal conduction, it is referred to as a sinus tachycardia. However, the rate rarely exceeds 150 bpm in adults. The significance of sinus tachycardia is twofold. During the cardiac cycle (see p. 484), ventricular filling and coronary artery perfusion take place during diastole. With a heart rate above 130 bpm, diastole is shortened and therefore cardiac output and coronary artery perfusion are compromised.

Clinical presentation

Sinus tachycardia may lead to a fall in cardiac output, together with reduced myocardial blood supply. The heart muscle needs more O_2 when it beats fast; hence in patients with angina, tachycardia may precipitate an anginal attack, while for those with heart failure it may lead to chest pain or a worsening of their symptoms (see p. 510). Some patients may feel palpitations when their heart beats quickly.

Medical management

Sinus tachycardia may be a sign of ill health, occurring when the patient is pyrexial, anaemic (see Ch. 18), or has hyperthyroidism (see Ch. 17) or poor cardiac function. However, in a healthy adult, sinus tachycardia will be found during exercise or in response to emotional stress and will not need treating. Treatment is usually directed at the underlying cause.

ATRIAL FIBRILLATION

Atrial arrhythmias originate in the atrium, and atrial fibrillation (AF) is probably one of the more commonly recognized arrhythmias. In AF, the electrical activity in the atria is completely disorganized.

Pathophysiology

The heartbeat does not originate in the sinus node but in cells throughout the atria. This leads to a disorganized pattern of impulses reaching the AV node, which are then conducted sporadically to the ventricles. Ventricular contraction is irregular and frequently fast. Atrial systole is ineffective and the atria are never completely full of blood or empty, which may lead to a decreased cardiac output.

Clinical presentation

Some patients only notice symptoms on exercising when they are more susceptible to the reduced cardiac output. Others may have cold fingers and toes, feel dizzy or notice palpitations.

As the atria are not contracting forcibly, blood may become stagnant in the atria and thrombi may form on the atrial wall. When the heart returns to a normal sinus rhythm and the atria contract forcibly, emboli may break off and travel in the circulation. There is then a significant risk of cerebrovascular accident (CVA) and, unfortunately, AF is sometimes only diagnosed once a patient has suffered a CVA, stroke (see Ch. 14).

Atrial fibrillation may also be found more commonly amongst older people, in patients with valvular heart disease, CHD or following cardiac surgery (Kern 1998). Other causes of AF include hyperthyroidism, hypertension, pulmonary embolus (PE) and congenital heart defects (see p. 528).

Medical management

Underlying causes of AF, such as hyperthyroidism, are treated where possible. The treatment of AF is primarily through drug therapy or synchronized direct current (DC) cardioversion. Drugs such as digoxin, beta-adrenoceptor antagonists (beta-blockers) such as atenolol, or amiodarone are frequently used to slow the heart rate and control the irritable focus.

Synchronized DC cardioversion may be used to halt the abnormal foci and allow the sinus node to take over as the heart's pacemaker. Here a controlled electric shock momentarily stops the heart, allowing the natural pacemaker of the heart (the sinus node) to initiate the heartbeat and thereby allowing sinus rhythm to be restored.

▶ Nursing management

Nurses have an important role in monitoring patients with AF and ensuring that information needs regarding medication and other treatments are met. AF may be anticipated if the radial pulse rate is weak and irregular. The apex/radial heart rate is counted simultaneously by two nurses (see p. 487). The ECG will show an irregular heart rate with no definable P wave. Instead, fibrillatory waves (a wavy base line) are seen (see Fig. 19.13).

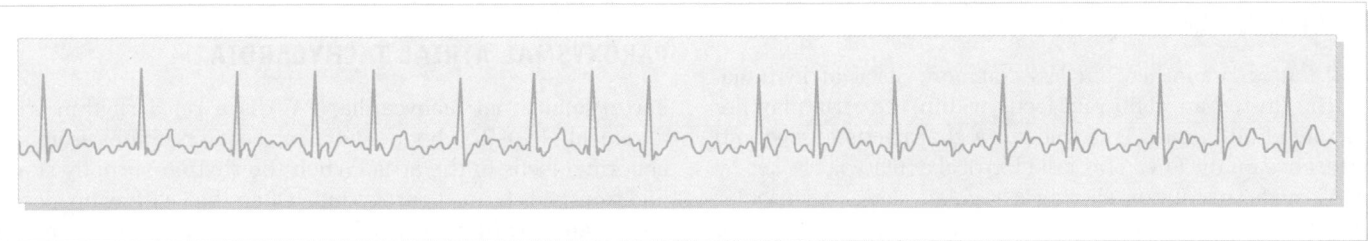

Figure 19.13 Atrial fibrillation. Note the wavy baseline of fibrillating waves.

Patients prescribed amiodarone should be warned that it may cause a bluish-grey discoloration of the skin on exposure to sunlight. They should therefore be advised to avoid direct sunlight when on this medication.

Nurses should be aware of potential side-effects associated with the use of digoxin. The drug has a long half-life (the time taken for plasma levels of the drug to fall to half of the initial level) and it is possible for plasma levels to reach toxic levels (see below). This may happen if maintenance doses are given too frequently, and toxicity is particularly likely to occur in older people. Digoxin may cause gastrointestinal side-effects, including anorexia, nausea, pain and diarrhoea. Other side-effects include confusion and delirium, which are easily attributable to another cause in older patients. The heart rate may fall and nurses should monitor the pulse and report bradycardia of < 60 bpm.

Nursing patients having synchronized DC cardioversion

Nurses are well placed to minimize anxiety by providing patients with information about what will be happening to them. Patients will require a general anaesthetic and should have no food or fluids by mouth for at least 4 hours. They will be attached to an electrocardiograph and the lead identified where the characteristics of the arrhythmia are clearest. This is normally lead II. Two paddles are placed on the chest wall, one on each side of the heart: one towards the apex, and the other towards the base. The paddles are charged to between 100 and 150 joules. The current will pass through the chest wall and affect the heart muscle more readily if any impedance is removed. Transfer of the electrical current is enhanced if electrode jelly is applied to the paddles, which should then be held firmly against the chest wall.

As an electrical current is being used, strict safety measures should be applied (see p. 496). The electric shock may lead to some redness and burning of the skin, and flamazine cream may be applied to the area.

If sinus rhythm is not restored, further shocks may be required. When sinus rhythm is restored or, alternatively, when the cardiologist considers that further shocks will not be effective, patients are woken from the anaesthetic. Nurses should observe their condition and ensure their safety during the recovery period (see Ch. 29). Unfortunately sinus rhythm is not always sustained, and future elective cardioversions may need to be considered.

Some patients may be admitted to the hospital as a day case for the procedure, which should take no more than 15 minutes. They should be allowed to go home once they are fully awake, but should not drive due to the sedative action of the drugs.

ATRIAL FLUTTER

Atrial flutter is another, but less common, atrial arrhythmia. In atrial flutter, an abnormal focus within the atria may fire at a rate of 300 bpm. This leads to a characteristic sawtooth appearance on the ECG. This fast electrical activity is blocked by the AV node, usually producing a regular, slower ventricular rate. This results in fast flutter waves which are blocked in a regular pattern. Consequently, there may be four flutter waves to every ventricular beat. This would be termed a 4:1 block.

Aetiology

Causes of atrial flutter include CHD, heart failure and chronic pulmonary disease (see Ch. 20). Atrial flutter may also be a precursor of atrial fibrillation.

Clinical presentation and medical management

The patient is likely to have palpitations or episodes of syncope. As the atria do not contract well, thrombi may form within them, and although this is less common than in AF, some patients may present following a CVA.

Atrial flutter is also treated with digoxin, beta-adrenoceptor antagonists (e.g. atenolol) and amiodarone or cardioversion (see above, atrial fibrillation).

▶ Nursing management

For details of nursing management, see the section on atrial fibrillation (p. 499).

PREMATURE ATRIAL CONTRACTION, ATRIAL EXTRASYSTOLES OR ATRIAL ECTOPIC BEATS

Premature atrial contraction (PAC) may precede the onset of AF or supraventricular tachycardia. Irritable cells in the atria initiate the stimulus and the beat is conducted along an abnormal pathway. On the ECG this is seen as an early and abnormally shaped P wave.

Clinical presentation

As PACs may be rapid, it is important that the AV node slows conduction to the ventricles. If the fast, premature beats are not inhibited, a tachycardia will develop. This will dramatically reduce the cardiac output, leading to dizziness and syncope.

Medical management

Treatment is not usually required unless the cardiac output is affected. If treatment is required, drugs such as digoxin or amiodarone will be used.

▶ Nursing management

Premature atrial contractions are often benign and may be associated with stress, smoking and high caffeine intake. If they become problematic, the patient should be given information about how to avoid the cause. This may involve the development of coping strategies to reduce stress (see Ch. 6), help with smoking cessation, and alternatives to high caffeine drinks and medication containing caffeine.

PAROXYSMAL ATRIAL TACHYCARDIA

Paroxysmal atrial tachycardia (PAT) is a rapid rhythm with a rate of 150–200 bpm. The heartbeat originates from an abnormal focus in the atria. When the rhythm abruptly starts and stops, it is termed paroxysmal. Often the PAT has no identifiable cause. Otherwise it may be associated with congenital heart abnormalities, valvular heart disease and cardiomyopathy. In such patients, it may lead to a low cardiac output.

Clinical presentation

The rhythm is regular with coordinated atrial and ventricular activity, and therefore the effect upon cardiac output is generally less severe than in AF, although patients are more likely to feel palpitations as the fast rhythm starts and then stops. If the patient already has a risk of thrombus formation within the heart chambers, PAT may lead to emboli breaking off and, hence, to a CVA.

Medical management

Again treatment is only required if cardiac output is reduced, when digoxin, amiodarone or synchronized cardioversion may be used (see p. 499).

▶ Nursing management

For patients with existing heart disease and PAT who have a reduced cardiac output, it is important that the heart rate is slowed and measures to reduce stimulation of the heart are taken. Patients should be advised to rest, reduce their intake of alcohol, caffeine and nicotine, and where possible either reduce their exposure to stressful situations or learn relaxation strategies (see Ch. 6). Patients who have repeated and frequent episodes of PAT should be encouraged to make lifestyle changes to reduce stimulation of the heart.

SUPRAVENTRICULAR TACHYCARDIA OR NARROW COMPLEX TACHYCARDIA

Supraventricular tachycardia (SVT) is the term used for any tachycardia that originates from a focus above the ventricles but where the exact origin is uncertain. Therefore it may be seen as an umbrella term for atrial flutter, atrial tachycardia or junctional tachycardia (where the foci are situated within the junctional tissue of the AV node). The heart rate is greater than 100 bpm and may be as fast as 280 bpm. The P wave is unclear or not present. The QRS complex may be normal if the ventricular cells can conduct the rhythm or, as is more commonly seen, narrow (see Fig. 19.14).

Aetiology and clinical presentation

Many of the causes for SVT are benign, such as excessive caffeine intake, alcohol, smoking and stress. It can, however, warn of CHD.

As the rate is fast without a good atrial systole, the cardiac output will be reduced and patients may complain of cool fingers and palpitations. For others, the fatigue and dizziness associated with a low cardiac output may prevent them from going to work during episodes of SVT.

Medical management

Treatment is aimed at the cause. It may be necessary to use drug therapy such as adenosine or verapamil. Alternatively the heart rate may be slowed by gentle massage of the carotid sinus. This stimulates the parasympathetic vagus nerve and slows the heart rate. It should, however, only be performed by a physician as it may lead to asystole. Alternatively the heart rate may be slowed by using the Valsalva manoeuvre to stimulate the vagus nerve. Here the patient breathes in and then slowly exhales against a closed glottis.

Radiofrequency ablation of the abnormal pathways may be used for symptomatic supraventricular tachycardia, or where abnormal atrial tissue is responsible for the abnormal pathway as in Wolff-Parkinson-White syndrome.

▶ Nursing management

Again, if a cause can be identified, patients should be advised of any lifestyle changes that may reduce the likelihood of these arrhythmias developing. Some patients may have to change their employment to one that is less stressful, while others may even have to give up their work.

DISORDERS OF THE ELECTRICAL CONDUCTION SYSTEM: VENTRICULAR ARRHYTHMIAS

These arrhythmias originate from cells in the ventricular muscle mass or the Purkinje fibres and are considered the most dangerous and potentially life-threatening type. As they affect ventricular contraction they can severely reduce cardiac output.

PREMATURE VENTRICULAR CONTRACTION, VENTRICULAR EXTRASYSTOLES OR VENTRICULAR ECTOPIC BEATS

Premature ventricular contraction (PVC) arises from an abnormal focus in the ventricles that depolarizes early and the impulse is conducted abnormally through the ventricles.

Aetiology and pathophysiology

On the ECG this is seen as a QRS complex with a broad and bizarre shape, which is not preceded by a P wave. It is only when they become more frequent than around 10/min, if they

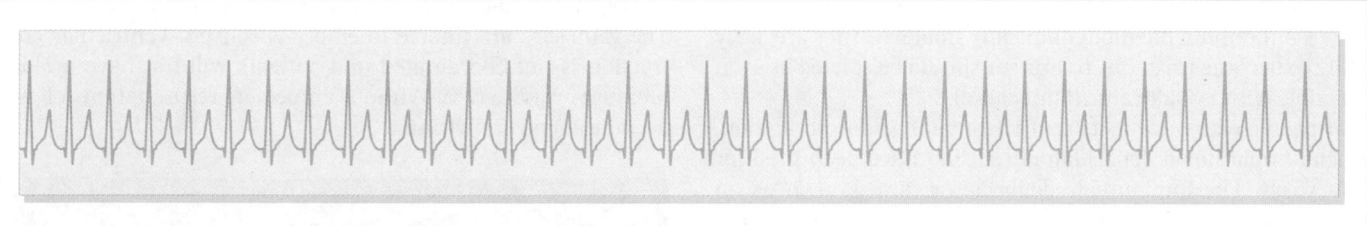

Figure 19.14 Supraventricular tachycardia (SVT). Note the narrow QRS complex.

originate from multiple sites (multifocal) or they occur in salvoes (runs of three or more), that they are considered dangerous.

Premature ventricular contractions are probably one of the most common arrhythmias, but in the absence of CHD, they are usually benign and may result from exposure to stress, excessive caffeine, alcohol or nicotine intake. However, they may also indicate myocardial ischaemia or heart failure. It is when an ectopic beat occurs close to the preceding T wave that it may precipitate ventricular tachycardia or ventricular fibrillation and signal danger.

Clinical presentation

Premature ventricular contractions frequently pass unnoticed and only occasionally will the person complain of palpitations. Healthy people tend to notice the palpitations more often when at rest.

Medical management

Treatment is required if they appear dangerous, in which case a bolus dose of intravenous lidocaine (lignocaine) is given, followed by an intravenous infusion.

> ► Nursing management

Patients who are symptomatic should be monitored and the rhythm observed for the frequency of PVCs. If frequent, it may be necessary to undertake a 12-lead ECG or a Holter tape.

VENTRICULAR TACHYCARDIA

Ventricular tachycardia (VT) may occur in certain conditions such as cardiomyopathy or CHD where the myocardium is diseased and the person may readily develop a fast ventricular heart rate. These people are at risk of sudden death from the arrhythmia (Schilling & Kaye 1998). VT is a serious arrhythmia and is usually associated with heart disease.

Pathophysiology

Ventricular tachycardia is caused by rapid firing from ectopic foci in the ventricles and results in a rapid ventricular rate (see Fig. 19.15A).

Clinical presentation

Due to the speed of the rhythm, the reduction in cardiac output is severe and may rapidly lead to unconsciousness. The pulse rate may not be palpable (pulseless VT) or it may be fast and thready. The blood pressure is likely to fall rapidly.

Medical management

Where cardiac arrest occurs, resuscitation must be started immediately (see section on CPR, p. 495). At times, patients may be in VT but remain haemodynamically stable. As they are likely rapidly to become unstable, treatment should be started as soon as possible with i.v. lidocaine (lignocaine).

For people who have recurrent VT or ventricular fibrillation, artificial implantable defibrillators (AICDs) have been used for many years. The implantable defibrillator (also known as an internal cardioverter) is inserted into the clavicular region and the electrodes are placed on the ventricular muscle tissue. The device can sense the heartbeat. If VT or ventricular fibrillation is

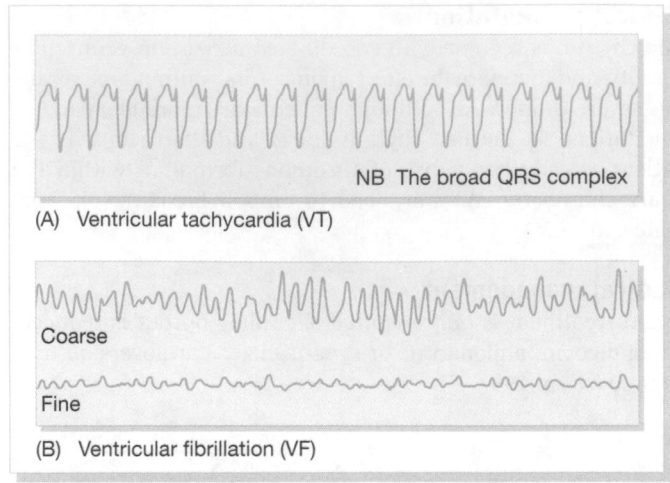

Figure 19.15 Ventricular arrhythmias. (A) Ventricular tachycardia (VT) – note the broad QRS complex. (B) Ventricular fibrillation (VF) – coarse and fine.

detected, the device will fire a small electric shock to the heart cells to restore sinus rhythm (Schilling & Kaye 1998). Radio-frequency ablation of the abnormal pathways may be used for ventricular tachycardia not treatable in other ways.

> ► Nursing management

Treatment must be started as soon as possible. If the patient has no discernible pulse, defibrillation should be used and ALS measures commenced (see pp. 495–496). When an implantable defibrillator has been inserted, patients will often feel this shock as a sudden jolt through their chest. For some, the shock may lead to a momentary loss of consciousness and they may fall to the ground. This may cause some patients extreme embarrassment and make them reluctant to leave their homes. However, for others, who may previously have had a restricted quality of life due to the fear of sudden death, the AICD will restore them to normal functioning (Porterfield et al 1999).

VENTRICULAR FIBRILLATION

In ventricular fibrillation (VF) the ventricles are no longer contracting. Instead, there is a characteristic fast quiver of the ventricles, which fails to produce any cardiac output.

Pathophysiology

Ventricular fibrillation results from several abnormal foci within the ventricles that fire in an abnormal and chaotic fashion. There are rapid, fibrillatory waves seen on the ECG (see Fig. 19.15B). The ventricles are unable to empty effectively. Ventricular contraction is not coordinated and patients will not have a blood pressure or pulse rate. Without immediate resuscitation, VF will become a fatal arrhythmia.

> ► Nursing management

Treatment is commenced as soon as possible with defibrillation and advanced resuscitation (see pp. 495–496).

CORONARY HEART DISEASE

Coronary heart disease is caused by atheroma affecting the coronary arteries, which eventually may lead to angina, myocardial infarction or heart failure.

Aetiology and epidemiology

It must be remembered that the risks for CHD are mutifactorial, although there are major risk factors, e.g. hypercholesterolaemia, hypertension, physical inactivity and smoking (see section on general disease prevention and health education, above).

Deaths from CHD show marked regional differences in the UK, the highest levels being in the north of England, Northern Ireland and Scotland (Petersen et al 2000). The premature death rate from CHD shows socioeconomic variation, with higher rates in manual workers, and it is also higher in South Asians living in the UK (Petersen et al 2000).

Pathophysiology

Coronary heart disease starts as an atheromatous plaque within the coronary arteries (see Fig. 19.16). The exact mechanisms that lead to this are uncertain. Lipid accumulates under the intimal lining of the coronary artery, possibly where this layer has been damaged by hypertension, chemicals in tobacco smoke or other noxious chemical irritants (Woods et al 2000). As the lipid infiltrate is foreign matter in the intima, macrophages attempt to engulf it, and this creates what are known as foam cells. The thin lipid layer now becomes a larger obstruction within the coronary artery. Smooth muscle cells start to invade the area and undergo mitosis and the whole area enlarges. As the wall of the coronary artery is now damaged and irregular in shape, platelets will clump around the obstruction, leading to thrombus formation. This further reduces the lumen size.

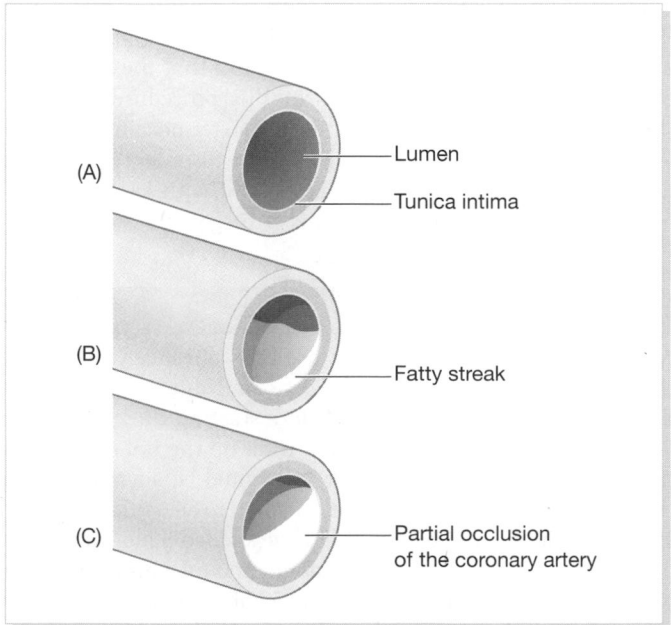

Figure 19.16 Atheroma formation. (A) Normal artery. (B) Early atheroma development. (C) Severe atheroma.

The obstruction to the coronary artery can severely narrow the lumen and affect blood supply to the myocardium. If the blood supply is reduced to such an extent that it does not meet myocardial demand for O_2, supply and demand become unbalanced. At this point the myocardial cells will stop functioning properly in that region of the myocardium normally supplied by the affected artery.

ANGINA PECTORIS

When an atheromatous plaque obstructs more than 50% of the lumen of the coronary artery, the flow of blood to the myocardium is only adequate for the heart at rest. This means that when the demand for blood increases, such as during exercise or emotional episodes, the narrowed coronary artery cannot increase the blood supply sufficiently to meet myocardial needs and the patient will experience chest pain. This is referred to as angina. In the UK more than 1.5 million suffer from this condition (Peterson et al 2000).

Usually angina is caused by atheroma. However, when the supply of O_2 to the myocardium is reduced by severe anaemia or aortic stenosis, or when the myocardium needs more O_2 than can be supplied (as in hypertrophic cardiomyopathy or hyperthyroidism – see Ch. 17), the patient will experience angina which is not caused by atheroma.

Occasionally the coronary artery will go into spasm, which will also reduce the blood supply to the myocardium and lead to angina. Although coronary artery spasm may be associated with atheroma, it may also be found in people with normal coronary arteries, particularly women.

Clinical presentation

The classic symptoms of angina are retrosternal chest pain that is frequently described as burning, squeezing or pressing. Sometimes patients do not describe pain but experience a sensation of breathlessness, or tingling in the jaw, arm, back or epigastrium. The pain is likely to start when activities are undertaken that require an increase in myocardial blood supply. This could involve running for a bus, doing the gardening or shopping, lifting heavy items, or expressing emotions such as anger. Previously healthy adults may first notice these symptoms when they are at the gym or out jogging. Remember that angina does not just affect older people.

Angina is more often experienced in cold weather when the coronary vessels may go into spasm. It is also possible that during cold weather, platelets become sticky, which increases the likelihood of platelet aggregation on the damaged endothelium with further occlusion of the coronary artery.

In patients with diabetes mellitus (see Ch. 17) the nervous system has often been damaged, resulting in an altered perception of pain. These patients are more likely to have myocardial ischaemia that does not display the typical pattern of chest pain and may make the diagnosis more difficult.

When the chest pain is experienced, the person will usually stop the activity that brought it on. The pain may last for several minutes once this trigger is removed, but it rarely lasts longer than 15 minutes.

Other symptoms may develop when the myocardium is starved of O_2. These include arrhythmias such as PVCs or even VT (see p. 502).

Specific investigations

The primary health care team usually manages patients with angina. A history of the pain and its precipitating factors will be taken. Blood lipid levels will be measured. Additionally an electrocardiogram should be recorded to assess the heart rate and rhythm. If the angina is severely limiting the person's daily activities or becomes more frequent, then an exercise treadmill test should be undertaken. Recommendations from the National Services Framework for CHD in England suggest that coronary angiography should then be used to assess the degree of stenosis of the coronary arteries (Department of Health 2000).

Medical and surgical management

Initial treatment is likely to consist of drug therapy and advice about positive lifestyle changes. A drug commonly used in the treatment of angina is sublingual glyceryl trinitrate (GTN), or another nitrate such as isosorbide dinitrate. Other drugs frequently used include diltiazem and verapamil, both of which dilate the coronary arteries. Beta-adrenoceptor antagonists (beta-blockers) such as atenolol may be useful to reduce the heart rate, contractility and blood pressure and so decrease the myocardial O_2 demand.

Patients should also be prescribed low-dose aspirin. This will reduce the risk of further platelet aggregation and of the atheroma developing further.

Individuals found to have high blood cholesterol levels (> 5.0 mmol/L) should be prescribed an HMG-CoA reductase inhibitor (statin), e.g. simvastatin. This category of drug is used to lower blood cholesterol levels. However, it should never be used instead of encouraging lifestyle changes to reduce blood cholesterol levels.

In situations where angina severely affects activity and quality of life, angioplasty and stent insertion, myocardial revascularization or surgical treatment will be considered.

Percutaneous transluminal coronary angioplasty stent

Percutaneous transluminal coronary angioplasty (PTCA) and stent is increasingly being used in the UK, as it can be carried out in the cardiac catheter laboratory and only requires a short hospital stay.

Although the concept of PTCA was introduced in the 1960s, the first clinical case was performed in the late 1970s by Gruentzig (Apple & Lindsay 2000). Since then it has become widely used in the treatment of CHD (Windecker et al 1998). A catheter with a small balloon on the end is inserted into the femoral artery and passed into the coronary arteries. When the catheter is sitting in the stenosed portion of the artery, the balloon is inflated. The arterial muscle wall is stretched and the lumen widened. This allows a greater blood supply to flow down the coronary artery and reduces the angina (Meluch & Mitchell 1997). This procedure has been further developed and an intra-coronary stent is now used alongside PTCA. The intracoronary stent is a wire mesh tube that is placed in the coronary artery following successful balloon inflation of the stenosed portion of artery. It is used to keep the artery open once it has been stretched by the PTCA (Bevans & McLimore 1992).

The potential problem of vessel occlusion by thrombus aggregating to the arterial wall or the stent requires the administration of glycoprotein IIb/IIIa inhibitors, such as abciximab (NICE 2000), or platelet inhibitors such as ticlopidine or clopidogrel prior to, during and following the procedure.

Percutaneous myocardial revascularization

This is a newer form of treatment carried out in only a few centres in the UK. Using the same process as angiography, a catheter is passed through the femoral artery and into the left ventricle. A laser energy source on the tip of the catheter is placed directly against the myocardium. Channels through the myocardium are created from the endothelium to the subepicardial surface (below the epicardium or visceral pericardium). Blood can then use these channels to supply the myocardium with O_2 and nutrients.

Cardiac surgery

For some patients, PTCA is not possible and cardiac surgery may be of benefit. Traditional cardiac surgery involves bypassing the diseased coronary arteries with a graft, a portion of the saphenous vein from the leg; this is known as a coronary artery bypass graft (CABG). Approximately 50% of saphenous vein grafts are occluded within 5–10 years following surgery and alternative vessels are now being used such as the internal mammary artery (IMA).

For traditional coronary artery bypass surgery, a median sternotomy approach is employed, the heart is stopped and a cardiopulmonary bypass machine is used to maintain the circulation and gaseous exchange. Cardiopulmonary bypass (CPB) temporarily acts as the heart and lung. Blood is pumped around the body and gaseous exchange takes place through an oxygenator. This operation therefore leaves the patient with a large sternal wound, severe pain and the possibility of CVA from the cardiopulmonary bypass machine. Alternative methods of cardiac surgery are now being used.

Minimally invasive cardiac surgery (MICS) avoids the median sternotomy and CPB and is used in selected patients. A thoracotomy incision (opening into the thoracic cavity) is made and the heart is stabilized using a small device that minimizes the movement of that part of the myocardium that the surgeon is operating upon. The advantages of this procedure are that, through avoiding CPB, there can be a shorter hospital stay and less risk of CVA, renal failure or respiratory disorders (Maglish et al 1999). As a result it may be associated with less morbidity and mortality than traditional forms of surgery.

▶ **Nursing management**

Nurses are able to help patients use GTN effectively by asking them to note the activities that cause an angina attack and advising them to take the GTN before starting these activities. For example, if a man is unable to walk up the hill outside his house without an angina attack, he should be advised to take the GTN before leaving the house and then to climb the hill more slowly. He should also be told that if he suddenly has an angina attack, he should stop what he is doing and take his GTN. If the chest pain has not resolved within 5 minutes, a further dose should be taken. Patients should, however, be told that if the pain is not relieved within 15 minutes of using the GTN, they should call for an emergency ambulance.

GTN can be given in various forms – as a sublingual tablet or spray, or transdermally as an ointment or patches. Nurses should explain that when administered by the sublingual or transdermal routes the drug enters the systemic circulation, thus avoiding the first-pass metabolism in the liver that would render GTN ineffective if taken orally. GTN loses potency during storage and should only be used as a fresh preparation; patient supplies should be kept in an airtight container and replenished every 6 months.

Sublingual GTN tablets may cause a burning sensation on the tongue, flushing or headaches. The vasodilator effects of the drug cause all of these. However, the side-effects may be uncomfortable for the patient, who should be warned that they are normal. If patients are unable to tolerate these side-effects, they may prefer to use GTN in a spray form, when the effects are sometimes reduced. More severe angina will be treated with a longer-acting preparation of a nitrate such as a GTN patch. This should be placed on a hairless part of skin such as the forearm where it is slowly absorbed into the bloodstream. It should not be placed over skin that is broken as the drug will be rapidly absorbed and the patient may develop hypotension (low blood pressure). It should be effective for 6 hours, but if a slow-release form of the ointment is used, the effect will last for 12 hours. Sometimes patients develop a tolerance to the drug and, if this occurs, the patch should be removed for 4–6 hours every day. The best time for this must be tailored to the individual patient's lifestyle, so that the period without the nitrate is that period when the person is less active (possibly in the early evening).

Patients should be given advice about lifestyle. This is particularly important for those found to have a high cholesterol level and may include advice regarding smoking cessation clinics in the area, physical activity, meticulous control of blood glucose levels in diabetic patients (see Ch. 17) and how to eat a 'heart healthy diet' (see Ch. 11). The role of the nurse in promoting health in the patient diagnosed with angina is clear.

Chest pain is very frightening and, following its onset, people may start to lead sedentary lives, giving up activities they enjoy, and they may even become frightened to go out with friends. Sometimes patients' families will start to limit their activities, and this is likely to contribute to depression and a reduced quality of life. Helping patients to assess their lifestyle and activities and to use GTN to enable them to continue with those activities they wish to will limit the inactivity that often follows the onset of angina. If, despite good advice on lifestyle modifications and drug therapy, the angina severely limits the person's activities, PTCA stent or surgery will be considered.

Readers requiring more information about nursing patients who are having cardiac surgery are advised to consult a specialist book (see 'Further reading').

Nursing patients following PTCA

The care following a PTCA will be similar to that following coronary angiography. However, patients having PTCA are treated with substances to prevent the formation of thrombi and vessel occlusion (see p. 504), and haemostasis therefore poses a particular challenge following removal of the femoral sheath. This is achieved through a variety of techniques, including manual pressure, femostops or angioseals (Barbiere 1995, Apple & Lindsay 2000). It is particularly important that patients

are given clear instructions about the care of the femoral area. Retroperitoneal haemorrhage, haematoma formation, severe bruising and CVA are all complications associated with the procedure (Meluch & Mitchell 1997). PTCA is increasingly performed as a day-case procedure and the nurse's contact with patients in hospital is reducing. It is important that nurses take the opportunity to encourage patients to attend cardiac rehabilitation classes and initiate discussion about the secondary prevention of CHD.

UNSTABLE ANGINA

Unstable angina may occur in a patient with known angina, or may itself be the initial sign of CHD. In unstable angina, chest pain develops without exertion, often while the patient is either resting or sleeping.

Pathophysiology

Unstable angina is associated with an atheromatous plaque that is beginning to rupture. The central part of the atheroma is made up of dead tissue that the macrophages have slowly destroyed. This portion, then, is like a volcano waiting to erupt. The top of the atheroma will eventually blow off, platelets will clump around the rupture and thrombus will form on top. The obstruction to the vessel wall is further increased and myocardial O_2 supply is severely reduced. It is therefore clear how unstable angina develops at rest, may become progressively worse over a few days, and is associated with a worse prognosis than stable angina.

Clinical presentation

Patients who previously suffered from stable angina will often describe the pain of unstable angina as being different: it lasts for a longer period of time, is not relieved by the normal methods (e.g. rest or GTN) and may well radiate differently over the chest wall (Cheitlin et al 1993). The angina will also often get progressively worse over a few days.

Specific investigations

Patients with unstable angina will require a 12-lead ECG to assess for myocardial ischaemia. This will show up as depression of the ST segment in leads that are looking at the ischaemic heart muscle. Continuous bedside electrocardiography should be used for at least 24 hours following the onset of chest pain, or for longer if the pain has not subsided.

An exercise treadmill test is useful once the angina has subsided and prior to discharge. This will help both the patient and the physician to understand the extent of the myocardial ischaemia. If positive changes of ST-segment depression or ventricular arrhythmias are observed during the test, the patient may be referred for a cardiac catheter for further diagnosis and treatment of the CHD.

Medical management

Treatment should aim at increasing myocardial blood flow and achieving pain relief. To disperse the platelets that have collected around the ruptured atheroma, which may completely occlude the artery, the patient with unstable angina should be given aspirin on admission and this should be continued daily afterwards. Heparin should also be prescribed, either as an intravenous infusion for between 2 and 5 days or subcutaneously in low-molecular-weight form (Department of Health 2000).

Intravenous glyceryl trinitrate (nitroglycerine) should be given to dilate the coronary arteries and improve the myocardial blood supply. This should be increased gradually until the pain subsides or a maximum dose is established. Once a therapeutic dose has been achieved, the infusion should be maintained for a further 24 hours.

Diamorphine should be prescribed intravenously to rapidly relieve the chest pain. This occurs through its analgesic properties and its effect on dilating the coronary arteries (Jowett & Thompson 1996).

It is only when pain has not subsided over a period of 48 hours with maximum treatment that more aggressive forms of management should be considered. The intra-aortic balloon pump (IABP) is increasingly in use for unstable angina. This aims to improve coronary blood flow while reducing the work of the heart. Alternatively, the patient may be referred for emergency PTCA or cardiac surgery.

▶ Nursing management

Unstable angina may be a precursor to myocardial infarction or may precipitate ventricular arrhythmias, and patients should be admitted to hospital for observation and rest. They should be connected to an electrocardiograph for constant ECG monitoring, started on a pain chart and preferably cared for on a coronary care unit (CCU) for at least 12 hours (Department of Health 2000). Diamorphine should be given as repeated intravenous bolus doses until the chest pain has subsided.

The intravenous infusion of GTN should be increased incrementally at 2- to 5-minute intervals until the pain subsides or a maximum dose is established. The patient's blood pressure must be recorded at 15-minute intervals. If the systolic pressure falls by more than 20 mmHg from the baseline, or the systolic pressure falls below 100 mmHg, the GTN should not be increased further.

Patients should be encouraged to rest in bed or undertake minimal exertion to reduce the myocardial O_2 demand. They should be allowed to sit up in a chair if they wish, use a commode and care for their personal hygiene at the bedside. To encourage rest, visiting may be kept to a minimum. However, if the absence of family increases patient anxiety, they should be present but asked to help the patients to relax as much as possible.

Heparin should be maintained for between 2 and 5 days, by which time the chest pain should have resolved and patients will be starting to mobilize. However, they may find that the infusion limits their mobility and independence, while subcutaneous heparin may be painful and lead to bruising. They may consequently be reluctant to continue with this therapy. It is essential that nurses are aware of the importance of this medication in preventing the risk of further unstable angina or myocardial infarction and that they encourage patients to continue with their vital treatment.

With rest, to reduce the myocardial O_2 demand, and nitrates and heparin to increase the myocardial O_2 supply, the chest pain should start to subside. It must be remembered that if patients are in pain, the increased sympathetic nervous system stimulation will cause them to be tachycardic and vasoconstricted, thereby increasing the myocardial O_2 demand still further.

Once the pain has subsided, patients should be kept in hospital and encouraged to gradually increase their exercise. This period of nurse–patient contact should be used to discuss CHD and any specific lifestyle changes that should be considered to reduce the risk of worsening disease.

MYOCARDIAL INFARCTION

Myocardial infarction (MI) occurs when there is an abrupt cessation to blood flow within the coronary arteries leading to an area of infarction in the myocardium.

Epidemiology

Myocardial infarction is a common cause of death in Western countries. There are over 270 000 MIs each year in the UK, and about 50% are fatal (Peterson et al 2000). However, where the MI is fatal, possibly 30% of these deaths occur before the patient reaches a hospital. It is also interesting to note that only about 25% of patients aged less than 70 have previously documented angina.

Pathophysiology

Myocardial infarction is frequently caused by the rupture of an atheromatous plaque. Thrombus forms on top of this rupture and results in complete occlusion of the affected coronary artery. Oxygenated blood will not reach the myocardial cells and, if this lasts longer than 20–30 minutes, the cells will die, leaving an area of necrosed tissue (infarct) (Jowett & Thompson 1996).

Myocardial infarctions can be divided into two major groups:

- transmural – the infarcted area extends through the full thickness of the myocardium
- subendocardial – only the inner layer of the myocardium is affected. A subendocardial infarct will not reduce the cardiac output as significantly as a transmural infarction.

Clinical presentation

The classical presentation of an acute MI is with severe chest pain that is not resolved by rest and lasting longer than 30 minutes. Frequently the pain comes on in the resting state and this may distinguish it from stable angina; patients may even be woken from sleep with severe chest pain. They may describe the pain as the worst they have ever experienced and it is often accompanied by light-headedness, nausea and vomiting. Prior to this, patients may well have an overwhelming sense of tiredness, although this can only be associated with the MI retrospectively. Unfortunately for some, the first sign of an MI is sudden death, presumed to be caused by VF, while others may not experience pain and have what is termed a silent infarction. The latter is more common amongst the older person or in those with an altered pain perception, such as occurs with diabetic neuropathy (see Ch. 17). Some individuals report extreme anxiety with feelings of impending death.

Other presenting signs may result from the reduced cardiac output. Patients are likely to appear grey and sweaty, and may be peripherally cool. If the MI is severe, they may have dyspnoea caused by pulmonary oedema, hypotension and confusion due to reduced cerebral blood supply.

The complications of an MI can rapidly lead to death. These include ventricular septal defect, aneurysm or rupture of the papillary muscle leading to mitral regurgitation. Other severe life-threatening complications may arise from damage to the electrical conduction system, leading to ventricular arrhythmias (Forbess & Bashore 1996).

Specific investigations

A 12-lead ECG

If patients are in the acute stage of an MI, changes to the ST segment will be seen. By analysing each of the 12 leads for ST-segment elevation (>1 mm or 2 small squares), it is possible to determine if the myocardium has infarcted and identify the area of damage. The ECG may also show inversion of the T wave and Q wave formation in affected leads. These may indicate that an MI has occurred at some time in the past, but probably too long ago for thrombolytic therapy (see below) to be effective. Increasingly the nurse is responsible, through the use of protocols and a nurse-led service, for the initiation of thrombolytic therapy and so must be skilled in ECG interpretation.

Blood tests

Blood is tested for various cardiac enzymes (see above, cardiac enzymes). Additionally urea and electrolytes should be checked for possible abnormalities, the blood glucose level should be measured to identify diabetes, although it may be raised in response to the stress of pain and illness, and the lipid profile should be assessed.

Medical management – immediate care

When patients are suspected of having an MI, arrangements should be made for immediate admission to hospital. A properly equipped emergency ambulance should be called to facilitate this transfer with appropriately trained paramedic staff.

Aspirin should be given as soon as possible, either by paramedic staff or self-administered. Aspirin works by inhibiting the aggregation of platelets and adherence to the thrombus. O_2 should be given to help reduce the pain from ischaemic heart tissues and redress the myocardial O_2 supply and demand imbalance.

Once in hospital, pain should be relieved through rapid administration of intravenous (i.v.) diamorphine in conjunction with an antiemetic such as metoclopramide and GTN.

Reperfusion of the myocardium should be attempted as soon as possible through the administration of thrombolytics. Ideally they should be given within 1 hour of the onset of pain (Department of Health 2000) but may be of benefit within 12 hours. Thrombolysis is started either as pre-hospital delivery with reteplase or tenecteplase, or in hospital where an appropriate choice is made from streptokinase, alteplase, reteplase or tenecteplase (NICE 2002). Streptokinase is the most widely used thrombolytic in the UK. The prescribed dose should be given intravenously over 1 hour. Streptokinase is a protein extracted from streptococcal strains and antibody production will occur. Repeat use within 1 year is therefore contraindicated. Streptokinase is used to lyse (break down) the clot, which has formed over the atheromatous plaque and so is associated with a risk of haemorrhage. Tissue plasminogen activator (tPA)

Box 19.1 Criteria for thrombolytic therapy

Inclusion criteria for thrombolytic therapy
ST elevation of 1 mm in leads II, III and aVF; 1 mm in leads I and aVL; and 2 mm in leads V_1–V_6
Clinical presentation of cardiac chest pain
Onset of chest pain < 12 h

Exclusion criteria for thrombolytic therapy
Spinal or intracranial surgery within the past 2 months
Uncontrolled, severe hypertension
Active internal bleeding or known bleeding disorder
Haemorrhagic CVA within the past 6 months
Retinal laser surgery within 1 week
Aortic dissection

is an alternative thrombolytic agent and should ideally be given over 90 minutes and accompanied by an i.v. infusion of heparin. A newer thrombolytic drug, reteplase, can be administered over a much shorter period (two bolus doses, 30 minutes apart). This enables more rapid myocardial reperfusion and it is also associated with a reduced risk of CVA (Albarran & Kapeluch 2000).

Contraindications to thrombolytic agents do exist and unfortunately not all patients will benefit from thrombolysis (see Box 19.1).

PTCA may be used to open the occluded artery and reduce the possible complications of acute MI. However, for the procedure to be effective, it must be performed as quickly as possible and therefore requires a cardiac catheter laboratory and staff to be constantly available. Within the UK, this form of treatment is not always a practical option.

▶ Nursing management

Initial stage

Patients should be encouraged to seek help at the earliest possible opportunity in order to achieve the goals of care. It is important that the general public is aware of the signs and symptoms of an MI (or 'heart attack') and that seeking medical help should be a priority (Alonzo & Reynolds 1997).

The need for the rapid treatment of life-threatening arrhythmias has led the UK government to place automated defibrillators in many public places (Department of Health 1999). When the defibrillator paddles are placed against the chest wall, they will detect the heart rhythm, delivering a shock only as required. They can now be found at railway stations, on aeroplanes and in shopping malls and the public is increasingly being trained in their use.

On admission to hospital, it is essential that a rapid diagnosis be made so that myocardial reperfusion can be initiated as soon as possible. The UK government, in an attempt to reduce the morbidity and mortality associated with MI, have the stated aim that by the year 2003 reperfusion will be started within 20 minutes of arriving in hospital (Department of Health 2000). This requires skilled staff to assess patients as quickly and accurately as possible. In the A&E department, nurses should be able to accurately assess patients with a possible MI and, through the triage system, enable them to receive prompt treatment (Quinn 1995, Caunt 1996) (see Ch. 30).

With the onset of chest pain comes extreme anxiety for both patient and family. A quiet waiting room should be offered to the family, equipped with a telephone, and they should be informed of the diagnosis and treatment given to their relative. Alternatively, they may wish to stay with the patient during the assessment, and should be allowed to do so providing this does not increase anxiety.

Nursing assessment of a patient after suspected MI

The nursing assessment for a patient with a suspected MI should include:

- Assessment of pain (see chest pain assessment, p. 487). Pain should be measured using a pain scale devised for cardiac chest pain, and GTN and prescribed analgesia administered intravenously until the pain subsides. If the chest pain returns or worsens, this may indicate further ischaemia or injury and a 12-lead ECG should be performed.
- Recording of and analysis of the ECG. It is important to determine which part of the heart is damaged and therefore which coronary arteries are likely to be involved. It is then possible to be aware of potential complications.

Common complications after MI

The most common complication occurring within the first 6 hours following an MI is ventricular arrhythmia (Quinn & Thompson 1995), which may occur as the myocardium is being reperfused with blood (reperfusion arrhythmia). Throughout the administration of the thrombolytic, the heart rate, blood pressure and respiration rates should be recorded at 15-minute intervals with continuous ECG monitoring. The ECG should continue to be monitored for arrhythmias, and ideally thrombolytics should be given where experienced staff are available to treat any complications. This may be on a CCU, in the A&E department or by appropriately trained paramedical staff.

Complications of thrombolytic therapy should be observed for and include:

- haemorrhage
- hypotension
- bradycardia
- allergic reaction
- reperfusion arrhythmias.

Later care in hospital

As lack of independence increases feelings of stress (Jowett & Thompson 1996), early mobilization is now encouraged following an MI. However, patients should be encouraged to rest for the first 2 days, sitting in a chair and using a commode by the bedside. By the third day they should be slowly mobilizing, taking short walks around the bed space. Although encouraged to use bathroom facilities, they should be wheeled to the lavatory and bathroom, unless their bed is next door. By the fourth day they should be helped to walk up a flight of stairs and by the fifth day they should be fairly independent in their activities of daily living, preparing for discharge home. Clearly activity must

be planned for each individual and any shortness of breath, palpitations or chest pain recorded and the activity then stopped.

Throughout their hospital stay, patients should be encouraged to inform staff as soon as they have any chest pain, and note any particular activities they were undertaking at the time. Relief of pain is important. Initially i.v. opioids should be given and i.v. nitrates titrated until the pain is relieved. As the condition allows, the i.v. drugs should be withdrawn and oral analgesia and nitrates given when required. Patients should be taught how to use GTN in a spray or sublingual form during their hospital stay.

Nutrition is important and the hospital stay, albeit quite short, provides a useful forum for discussion on diet. Patients should be assisted in the choice of appropriate food. A low-fat diet should be encouraged in hospital, and time should be spent discussing strategies to continue a 'heart healthy' diet at home. Nurses should organize additional input from a specialist nutrition nurse or dietician as appropriate. High-fibre diets should also be encouraged, especially in the immediate post-MI phase when immobility and opioid use may lead to constipation.

Although patients are likely to experience both nausea and vomiting, fluid replacement should be given cautiously. Following an MI, the myocardium becomes stiff and any increases in fluid volume may rapidly lead to pulmonary oedema if left ventricular function is impaired.

One of the aims of nursing care for patients following an MI is to reduce the workload of the heart. This can be assisted through nursing them in a quiet environment, with the provision of reassurance and support. By reducing anxiety and therefore catecholamine secretion, myocardial workload is reduced. To address the imbalance between myocardial O_2 supply and demand, prescribed O_2 is frequently administered via a face mask. Occasionally, a mask may seem claustrophobic to the patient, in which case O_2 may be delivered via nasal cannulae. To measure O_2 levels, pulse oximetry (see Chs 8, 9 and 31) should be used.

Discharge planning

Discharge planning, which involves the patient, the family and the health care team, should start as soon as possible after admission. By knowing patients and their domestic and work situation, the nurse can develop a discharge plan that is both culturally sensitive and meets the needs of individual patients.

Cardiac rehabilitation

Patients should be encouraged to attend cardiac rehabilitation and discuss all the modifications to lifestyle that may be necessary. The current trend for shorter length of hospital stay leaves less time for nursing staff to talk about CHD risk and lifestyle, and this is a potential disadvantage of this trend.

Cardiac rehabilitation aims to improve quality of life and reduce morbidity and mortality. For some, the diagnosis of CHD will lead to dramatic changes in their lifestyle, while others may need help to adjust to the diagnosis and to gain confidence in carrying on as normal a life as possible. A formal rehabilitation programme should be offered to all patients with a diagnosis of CHD and may be held in the hospital, GP surgery, health centre or other community setting such as the local school or church hall.

For those living in isolated rural communities poorly served by public transport, or where attendance at a formal programme is difficult, the 'heart manual' (Lewin et al 1992) with exercise and relaxation tapes, books and a diary for patients to work through may be useful.

Cardiac rehabilitation is divided into four phases that are clearly explained in the National Service Framework for Coronary Heart Disease (Department of Health 2000).

Phase 1 cardiac rehabilitation

Phase 1 is the stage when the diagnosis is first made. This usually occurs in hospital following an MI or revascularization through PTCA or cardiac surgery. During this phase, patients and their family members should be given time to talk to a specialist nurse about CHD and its management. Verbal information, supplemented with written material, is a useful strategy. Discharge planning should include a discussion on when patients should return to work, to driving, and to any forms of exercise. This information should be tailored to the needs of the individual patient and so should be given by a specialist nurse working in cardiac rehabilitation (see Guidelines for Care Priorities box 19.1).

Phase 2 cardiac rehabilitation

Phase 2 is the early period, usually following discharge from hospital. At this time, patients and their families are beginning to adjust to the diagnosis and to understand some of the lifestyle changes it may require. Many patients feel quite isolated during this period. A telephone helpline and a nurse-initiated telephone follow-up are useful to enable questions to be asked and answered, for information to be reinforced and so that patients may be encouraged to attend the formal exercise programme of phase 3 cardiac rehabilitation.

 GUIDELINES FOR CARE PRIORITIES

19.1 Discharge home following a myocardial infarction

- Assessment of physical, psychological and social needs
- Smoking – advice on smoking cessation, clinics, nicotine replacement patches
- Dietary advice – promoting healthy eating and reducing obesity. Refer to a dietician if necessary
- Alcohol consumption – limit consumption to 2 units of alcohol/day
- Employment issues – may need to consider strategies to reduce stress or a change in employment
- Physical activity – may need to consider strategies to increase physical activity
- Sexual activity – advice regarding the resumption of sexual activity
- Education about medication
- Rehabilitation – referral to a programme of cardiac rehabilitation and details of this
- Telephone helpline number
- Information on cardiac support groups

Phase 3 cardiac rehabilitation

Phase 3 is the formal rehabilitation phase. This is an easily recognized phase when patients undergo a structured programme of exercise, stress management and dietary advice. Patients should attend the programme for at least three sessions each week for between 6–12 weeks. This phase requires considerable time commitment by patients and their families, and for some there will be practical difficulties to overcome (e.g. lack of transport, child care issues and low income). Health care professionals should ensure that formal programmes are useful to patients, and where practical difficulties exist, staff should assist patients in finding imaginative solutions.

Phase 4 cardiac rehabilitation

Phase 4 is the final phase and refers to the long-term maintenance of any lifestyle changes. This may include such areas as referral to smoking cessation clinics (Coats et al 1995) (see Older Adults: Nursing Priorities box 19.1).

65 83 50 71 OLDER ADULTS: NURSING PRIORITIES

19.1 Cardiac rehabilitation in older people

Rehabilitation for people with heart disease consists of exercise, advice regarding modification to diet and education and assistance with smoking cessation. The goals are to reduce morbidity and mortality and improve the quality of life of the sufferer. Programmes of cardiac rehabilitation are now well established in the UK and are of proven benefit. However, it would appear that many older people either fail to attend these programmes or do not complete the course.

An individual exercise programme tailored to the specific needs of the older person, alongside lifestyle advice and stress management, may well be of greater benefit to the person living alone.

One obvious problem may well be the venue of the cardiac rehabilitation programme. Many are hospital-based and require the person to attend the hospital at least twice a week for the 8- to 10-week period. This may lead to a greater urgency to place more cardiac rehabilitation programmes in community or primary care settings but with close cooperation between primary and secondary care.

Another issue is whether older people are referred to cardiac rehabilitation programmes less often than younger patients.

Student activities (see Further reading, e.g. Halm et al 1999)

- Do you think that there are any differences (e.g. based on age or gender) in referral rates to cardiac rehabilitation?
- If the answer is yes – why do you think health professionals may be reluctant to refer older people or other groups to cardiac rehabilitation programmes?
- Older people who are referred to programmes might not attend or may fail to complete the course. Why do you think this happens?

HEART FAILURE

Heart failure can be categorized as either acute heart failure, such as that caused by cardiogenic shock after MI, or chronic heart failure where deteriorating cardiac function occurs over a longer period of time.

CARDIOGENIC SHOCK

Cardiogenic shock describes a situation in which impaired tissue perfusion associated with shock has been caused by the inability of the heart to maintain a cardiac output sufficient to ensure that cellular requirements are met (see Ch. 9).

Aetiology

The causes of cardiogenic shock include:

- an acute MI, when the contraction of the heart is reduced
- arrhythmias – fast atrial fibrillation or one of the ventricular arrhythmias
- cardiac tamponade – the presence of blood or fluid in the pericardial sac inhibiting cardiac contraction
- severe chronic heart failure
- pulmonary embolus
- mitral and aortic valve disease (see p. 515)
- dissection of the aorta (see p. 522).

Clinical presentation

The patient with cardiogenic shock will present with symptoms due to the inadequate perfusion of organs (see Ch. 9):

- Hypotension – a diagnosis of cardiogenic shock is made if, along with the other presenting signs or symptoms, the blood pressure is below 80 mmHg systolic
- There will be tachycardia as physiological compensatory mechanisms are initiated in response to the reduction in cardiac output and the pulse is likely to be weak and thready
- Ventricular arrhythmias will result from myocardial ischaemia
- There will be oliguria (reduced urine output) due to poor renal perfusion
- The patient will feel cool and clammy to touch.

Medical management

Treatment aims to restore tissue perfusion through improving the cardiac output:

- The cardiac output should be maximized through the use of drugs. Drugs that increase the force of the cardiac contraction are termed positive inotropes and include dopamine, dobutamine and adrenaline (epinephrine).
- Cardiac output may be assisted with the IABP (see p. 506).
- O_2 therapy, possibly even through intermittent positive pressure ventilation (IPPV), may be required (see Chs 20 and 31)
- If a coronary artery is occluded, PTCA or cardiac surgery may be considered.
- Cardiac output can be maximized through controlling any arrhythmias (see pp. 497–502).

- The patient with cardiogenic shock will frequently have pulmonary oedema and a fast-acting loop diuretic such as furosemide (frusemide) is usually given intravenously.

▶ Nursing management

The goals of nursing for these acutely ill patients must parallel those of the medical management. They should be nursed in a HDU or CCU where regular observation of their haemodynamic status can be made (see Chs 9 and 31). This should include the assessment of the heart rate and rhythm through continuous electrocardiography, blood pressure recordings, central venous pressure monitoring, pulmonary artery occlusion pressure and cardiac output measurements and urine output. Regular assessment of the respiratory status and cerebral perfusion should also be made. If the brain is underperfused with blood, patients will become restless, agitated and confused. They must then be protected from harm and their level of consciousness recorded (see Ch. 14). Medical staff should be alerted if this appears to deteriorate.

Patients with a poor cardiac output will also have poor tissue perfusion and be susceptible to pressure ulcers (see Ch. 10). Regular turning may not be possible as it may induce hypertension. They should therefore be nursed on a pressure-relieving mattress.

During this phase of an acute illness, special support for family members is necessary. They are likely to be extremely anxious and will need regular communication with the nurses caring for their relative as well as from the medical staff.

CHRONIC HEART FAILURE

Chronic heart failure affects a large proportion of the population, with an enormous cost to the NHS, patients and their families (Hobbs 1999). Following a diagnosis of heart failure, many patients will not survive more than 5 years and during this time are likely to have repeated hospital admissions. It is important for health care professionals to gain a good grasp of the condition, and for this reason the topic is given some prominence and is covered in some depth.

Aetiology

Possible reasons for the increasing number of patients with heart failure in the UK are that people are living longer and more are surviving a myocardial infarction (MI). Other causes of heart failure include coronary heart disease, hypertension, valvular heart disease, cardiomyopathy, congenital heart disease and alcohol or drug misuse.

Pathophysiology

The heart is unable to maintain a cardiac output sufficient to perfuse the tissues and cells. Blood pressure is low and the body compensates for this through the action of the sympathetic nervous system and the RAAS. Activation of these mechanisms results in vasoconstriction and sodium and water retention. In the short term, these mechanisms maintain blood pressure and cardiac output, but in the longer term they directly damage the myocardial cells.

The pulse rate is likely to be raised as a result of the sympathetic nerve stimulation and may well be irregular, possibly atrial fibrillation (see p. 499). Patients may be aware of an irregular heartbeat or palpitations.

Most cases of heart failure result from left-sided failure. If the left side of the heart is not pumping well, the left ventricle will start to dilate to accommodate the increased blood volume. In time, this leads to back pressure in the lungs and fluid accumulates in the alveoli (pulmonary oedema).

Right-sided heart failure existing in isolation is likely to be associated with a chronic lung condition that has placed excessive strain upon the right ventricle. Such conditions may include cystic fibrosis or chronic obstructive pulmonary disease (COPD) (see Ch. 20). Additionally most forms of congenital heart disease place a strain on the right side of the heart and may result in right-sided heart failure.

A combination of both right- and left-sided heart failure is termed congestive heart failure or congestive cardiac failure.

Clinical presentation

Signs and symptoms of *left-sided heart failure* include (see also Reflective Practice box 19.1):

- pulmonary congestion
- persistent coughing (pink-tinged, frothy secretions in extreme cases)
- breathlessness (dyspnoea) is a common symptom and is more likely to occur during exercise or when the person is lying down
- nocturnal breathlessness and coughing
- a strong, bounding pulse, alternating with a weak thready one – this commonly occurs in severe left ventricular failure and is termed pulsus alternans.
- blood pressure may be normal due to the action of compensatory mechanisms. Ultimately the blood pressure will fall as heart failure progresses and compensatory mechanisms become inadequate
- atrial fibrillation – a common arrhythmia in heart failure
- activation of the RAAS leads to the retention of fluid; this may result in the patient experiencing nocturia.

Signs and symptoms of *right-sided heart failure* include:

- oedema of the feet, ankles, sacrum or any other dependent part of the body
- ascites (accumulation of fluid in the peritoneal cavity)
- the reduction in cardiac output is likely to leave the person with cool peripheries and he or she may complain of cold fingers and toes
- in moderate to severe heart failure, patients may also have anorexia, possibly due to venous congestion of the gastrointestinal tract, or shortness of breath
- when the liver is congested with venous blood, patients may appear jaundiced.

Specific investigations

- ECG – to detect arrhythmia frequently seen in the patient with heart failure: atrial fibrillation, atrial flutter and premature ventricular beats. Evidence of myocardial ischaemia from an imbalance of O_2 supply and demand may also be seen

R|Я REFLECTIVE PRACTICE

19.1 The physical problems of heart failure

Tom, aged 70 years, was diagnosed with heart failure 2 years ago. Over the past week, he has woken during the night feeling very breathless and frightened.

Student activities
- Why do you think Tom becomes breathless during the night?
- Why does he feel less breathless when he gets up and spends the rest of the night sleeping in a chair?
- What advice could you give Tom to help prevent these attacks of paroxysmal nocturnal dyspnoea (PND)?
- Think about a patient you have cared for with heart failure.
- Other than attacks of PND, what other symptoms did your patient experience because of breathlessness?
- What actions may reduce these symptoms?

- Chest X-ray – this is a useful tool to assess the size of the heart and to visualize any evidence of pulmonary oedema
- Serum electrolytes – these are measured as an imbalance may occur. Hyponatraemia may be found in patients who are on a strict low-sodium diet. Hyperkalaemia may be secondary to renal failure from prolonged heart failure, while diuretic therapy may lead to reduced potassium, sodium and magnesium levels (see Ch. 8)
- Regular measurements of urea and creatinine levels – used to assess renal function. Patients with heart failure may show early signs of deteriorating renal function
- Echocardiogram – provides information about the function of the valves, the cardiac chambers, the presence of pleural effusion (excess fluid collection between the layers of the pleura), chamber enlargement and ventricular hypertrophy. This evidence can be used to make a diagnosis of heart failure, and also informs clinicians of the degree of severity of the condition.

Medical/surgical management

Medical treatment includes loop diuretics, angiotensin-converting enzyme (ACE) inhibitors, digoxin and beta-adrenoceptor antagonists (beta-blockers). As this drug therapy has many implications for nursing care, a fuller explanation of these drugs is given.

Loop diuretics, such as furosemide (frusemide), or the potassium-sparing diuretic spironolactone, an aldosterone antagonist, are useful in heart failure as they promote the excretion of the accumulating sodium and water. They reduce both the intravascular volume and the extracellular fluid, thereby reducing the symptoms of pulmonary congestion and the discomfort of peripheral oedema (Bradley 2000).

ACE inhibitors, such as captopril or enalapril, inhibit the RAAS. The effects include a decrease in sodium and water retention, potassium excretion is decreased and vasoconstriction is reduced.

Digoxin (a positive inotrope) is given to improve myocardial contractility and increase cardiac output. It will therefore reduce the pulmonary congestion. However, it has a narrow therapeutic index, an indicator of the difference between a therapeutic dose and one that causes toxicity. Regular serum digoxin levels should be assessed and if a patient presents with symptoms of digoxin toxicity, the drug should be discontinued. Digoxin may also correct arrhythmias such as atrial fibrillation and therefore ensures patients have coordinated and effective contraction of the atria and ventricles.

Beta-blockers (negative inotropes), such as carvedilol or bisoprolol, play an important part in the pharmacological management. Used in conjunction with ACE inhibitors, they have been found to improve left ventricular ejection, improve exercise tolerance, reduce arrhythmias, reduce myocardial ischaemia and enhance coronary artery blood flow. Patients receiving beta-blockers are therefore likely to have fewer hospital admissions and a better quality of life (McMurray 1999).

Although vasoconstriction is a compensatory mechanism for a low cardiac output, the increase in afterload (i.e. the back pressure of blood in the aorta and pulmonary artery that creates the resistance that ventricular contraction must overcome to pump blood into the circulation; a high afterload increases the work required by the myocardium) and preload (the degree of stretch present in the myocardial muscle cells at the end of diastole; it depends on the end-diastolic volume) that results will adversely affect cardiac function. Vasodilators, such as nitrates, can therefore be used to improve cardiac output. Arterial dilation may be used to reduce the work of the heart. Hydralazine (vasodilator) and amlodipine (calcium-channel blocker) are the more commonly used drugs for this purpose.

Revascularization of the myocardium through PTCA or CABG may be considered. Additionally, some patients may be offered other treatment options, e.g. the left ventricular assist device or heart transplantation (see pp. 518–520).

▶ Nursing management

Nurses have an important role in the management of patients with heart failure, particularly in helping them to achieve a level of symptom control through self-management that reduces admissions to hospital and improves quality of life.

Advice on drug regimens

The pharmacological interventions for heart failure can reduce symptoms, increase exercise tolerance and enhance the quality of life. It is important for nurses to ensure that patients have a full understanding of their medication and use their guidelines to adjust or even withhold their medication as their condition dictates.

Non-adherence to drug regimens has been associated with increased hospital admissions among patients with heart failure (Michalsen et al 1998). Adherence to medical regimens is too extensive a subject to consider here, although it is worth noting that the complexity and number of drugs may be important factors to consider.

According to the health belief models (see Ch. 1), patients will be more inclined to take their medication if they are aware of the positive effects. The symptom control, increased exercise tolerance and improved quality of life may outweigh some of the disadvantages and provide positive feedback to encourage the continuation of the drug regimen.

Diuretics usually result in a rapid feeling of improvement in patients, as they allow them to exercise and breathe more easily. However, these drugs may lead to a significant diuresis and care should be taken that patients do not become dehydrated. This is of particular importance if they become ill, pyrexial or are subject to hot and/or humid environmental conditions, when they will be more susceptible to dehydration.

The fact that these drugs promote diuresis may make patients reluctant to take them. A plan for the dose regimen should be prepared with patients and they should be familiar with ways to accommodate their lifestyle. For most patients, a diuretic should be taken in the morning and/or early evening to reduce nocturia and encourage adherence to the medication.

ACE inhibitors should reduce both the pulmonary congestion and peripheral oedema. Consequently patients should be less breathless, have an increased exercise tolerance and experience fewer exacerbations of heart failure. This should improve their quality of life, making it easier for them to mobilize, breathe, eat and sleep. To encourage compliance with these medications, these important benefits should be stressed. Some patients develop a dry cough when taking ACE inhibitors. This is a troublesome side-effect but it is rare. Others notice a rash and alterations in taste when prescribed captopril. This particular side-effect has not been found when enalapril is used instead. The most common side-effects of ACE inhibitors are hypotension, headache and dizziness.

Some of the drugs used in heart failure [e.g. furosemide (frusemide)] may lead to potassium depletion. For a patient taking digoxin, this could lead to digoxin toxicity. Patients should therefore be informed of the symptoms that may indicate a low serum potassium level, muscle weakness and cramps (see Ch. 8), and should be encouraged to eat potassium-rich foods such as bananas, tomatoes and citrus fruit if they experience these symptoms (see Ch. 11).

Digoxin toxicity may lead to bradycardia, gastrointestinal side-effects, visual disturbances and cardiac arrhythmias, and again, patients taking digoxin should be encouraged to contact their GP or heart failure clinic if they experience these.

When beta-blockers are prescribed, they should be titrated against symptoms over a period of weeks, increasing the dose until the desired therapeutic effect is achieved. This will require patients to return to the GP practice or heart failure clinic on a regular basis. The importance of regular review should be stressed, otherwise the dose of drug may be inadequate to provide symptom relief. Throughout this slow titration period, patients require regular assessment of their blood pressure as well as assessment for worsening signs of heart failure or symptomatic bradycardia or heart block, all side-effects of the drugs. Beta-blockers may be associated initially with unpleasant side-effects such as sleep disturbances (see Ch. 4), nightmares (more common with lipid-soluble beta-blockers), depression and fatigue and also with initial exacerbation of the patient's symptoms. Other side-effects of beta-blockers include transient hypotension, light-headedness and dizziness, and patients may even faint when the drug is commenced or the dose is altered. These are not indications to either reduce or stop the drug and they should disappear after a few days.

Nitrates are frequently used to treat patients with heart failure. Side-effects include flushing, headaches and postural hypotension. Unfortunately these are found more commonly amongst older people. Severe headaches may require a change in dose or even discontinuation of the nitrate.

To prevent severe postural hypotension (which may occur with nitrates, ACE inhibitors or beta-blockers), patients should be advised about avoiding dehydration where possible. Again, it may be necessary to warn them of dehydration caused by hot and humid environmental conditions and to avoid alcoholic beverages. Additionally, they should be encouraged to get out of bed slowly and avoid any abrupt changes in posture.

The effective pharmacological treatment of the symptoms of heart failure should lead to an improving quality of life for these patients, albeit a gradual process. Oedema makes it difficult for some patients to wear shoes and walk, and frequently leads to a heavy feeling of the legs that limits mobility. Breathlessness compounds the immobility, fatigue and decreased quality of life. The drugs described above should reduce these symptoms.

Self-monitoring and self-management

The development of self-monitoring and self-management skills is important for patients with heart failure and the nurse has a substantial role in assisting patients in this area. Patients in heart failure should be encouraged to weigh themselves daily. An increase of 1–2 kg may mean that they need to alter their diuretic therapy and they should be taught how to manage this to maintain their ideal weight. Through diuretic management patients may be able to alter their sodium intake at times and the heart failure clinic nurse should provide them with this information. Oedema is unlikely to become apparent until about 5 L of fluid has been retained, which is equivalent to around a 5 kg gain in weight (1 L of pure water = 1 kg in weight).

As a high intravascular sodium level leads to water retention, limiting salt (sodium chloride) intake in food or cooking can also reduce oedema. Salt intake should be reduced to about 2–3 g/day and patients with heart failure should be referred to a dietician. Additionally the nurse can encourage a low-salt diet through advice on how to shop and cook. For example, many convenience and sweet foods contain high levels of salt and are best avoided. Adding salt at the table or during cooking should also be avoided. In situations where partners shop and cook for the household, they should also be given information on how to avoid a high salt intake. Low-salt diets can be very bland and spices and herbs can be used to flavour food in the absence of salt (see Ch. 11).

Traditional medical views held that exercise should be restricted in patients with heart failure. Currently, however, supervised exercise, in the form of rehabilitation classes (Taylor 2000) designed for patients with heart failure, is recommended. It is thought that exercise increases peak exercise capacity and enhances quality of life. Other benefits include the prevention of problems such as constipation (see Special Issues box 19.2).

Patients with mild heart failure may not demonstrate any symptoms while at rest; these may only become apparent when they increase their level of activity, e.g. breathlessness on exertion. Patients with more severe heart failure are likely to be breathless even at rest. The person who is breathless is likely to look anxious and possibly flushed or cyanosed.

People with heart failure will experience severe fatigue, even when undertaking only small amounts of activity. This tiredness can be so overwhelming that they find it difficult to maintain their normal activities, such as going to work or even washing and dressing.

Overall, the tiredness, breathlessness and oedema associated with heart failure may make it difficult for patients to continue their normal functioning, with a consequent decrease in quality of life.

Some patients with heart failure learn to control fluid retention by altering the dose of diuretics. Increasing self-management and symptom control allows these patients to adjust their drug dosages themselves; for example, patients may make an adjustment in the diuretic dose to deal with a worsening of symptoms such as breathlessness. These areas of

 SPECIAL ISSUES

19.2 Constipation affecting the person with heart failure

Constipation is a state in which an individual experiences difficulty with defaecation. This frequently leads to discomfort and an increase in straining during attempts to pass hard faeces. Causes of constipation in the person with heart failure are as follows:

- Fluid restriction of 1500–2000 mL/24 h
- Reduced fibre intake due to abdominal bloating and discomfort
- Inactivity due to oedema, fatigue and breathlessness
- Dehydration from mouth breathing when breathless and fluid restriction
- As part of the pathology of heart failure where the gastrointestinal tract is not receiving sufficient oxygen or is congested with venous blood.

Nursing assessment

- Identify the cause of constipation in each person
- Ascertain the person's normal bowel pattern
- Identify self-management measures used to cope with constipation.

Nursing management

- Ensure the person is not dehydrated
- Encourage small, frequent meals to reduce bloating
- Encourage patients to eat a piece of fruit as a snack
- Encourage gentle mobilization. More active mobilization is useful for selected persons with heart failure following an assessment by a specialist
- Consider the use of pharmacological interventions, stool softeners and stimulants.

self-management should be discussed by the patient and the heart failure nurse, GP or dietician. Nurses in primary care have a central role in the education and management of these patients. Increasingly, they are running clinics to assist patients in understanding their disease and the titration of medication.

The symptoms of heart failure can be relieved, but the disease itself cannot be cured and there will be a steady decline in patient ability to function normally. It is therefore appropriate to consider when patients and their families require palliative care from a specialist nurse. Macmillan nurses are now using their specific skills to care for patients with heart failure and hospice care is provided (see Ch. 34 and 'Further reading').

VALVULAR HEART DISEASE

Valvular heart disease may be congenital or acquired and causes either valve stenosis or valve regurgitation (incompetence).

ACUTE RHEUMATIC FEVER

Acute rheumatic fever is a systemic inflammatory disease that damages the endothelial lining of the heart as well as the skin and connective tissue. It mainly occurs in children and young adults.

Aetiology and epidemiology

The aetiology of acute rheumatic fever is infection with certain strains of group A beta-haemolytic *Streptococcus* that cause upper respiratory tract infections. It is thought that the lymphatic channels from the tonsils carry the *Streptococcus* from the throat to the heart (Woods et al 2000).

The incidence of acute rheumatic fever and the consequent rheumatic heart disease is declining in the UK, but it still accounts for most acquired heart disease in children and is still more prevalent in developing countries.

One possible reason for the decline in acute rheumatic fever in the UK, despite the still relatively common streptococcal throat infection, is the widespread use of antibiotics.

Pathophysiology

The disease causes carditis (inflammation of the heart) which may involve individual layers, i.e. pericarditis, myocarditis and endocarditis. It is the involvement of the endothelium lining the heart chambers and valves that leads to rheumatic heart disease. There is also joint inflammation with arthritis, and skin involvement. Sometimes late involvement of the central nervous system leads to chorea.

Clinical presentation

In the acute illness, the patient will demonstrate:

- fever (see Ch. 5)
- a history of a sore throat
- anorexia
- lethargy
- arthralgia (joint pains) – 'flitting arthritis' with the inflammation moving from joint to joint

- a macular skin rash (see Ch. 28) known as erythema marginatum and subcutaneous nodules, especially over the joints
- specific signs of carditis may be present, such as breathlessness, heart murmurs, or oedema if there is heart failure
- chorea – evidenced by involuntary movements.

Specific investigations

- Investigations to diagnose the cause of the fever and systemic disease – these will include a throat swab to isolate the microorganism, WBC and ESR
- Blood samples – to test for rising levels of antistreptolysin O antibodies (ASO)
- ECG – may show a prolonged PR interval or heart block as the conduction pathways of the heart become inflamed and conduction slows
- Chest X-ray – to show pulmonary congestion or cardiac enlargement
- Echocardiogram – to show if pericarditis has resulted in a pericardial effusion (collection of fluid between the layers of the pericardium).

Medical management

Antibiotics such as penicillin should be used to treat any streptococcal throat infections as a prophylactic measure. However, to ensure that antibiotic resistance does not develop, it is important that viral throat infections are not treated in the same way. Once rheumatic fever has been diagnosed, antibiotics should be prescribed alongside drugs to reduce pain and inflammation such as aspirin. Corticosteroids may be prescribed where carditis is present, or if the joint inflammation is severe.

Any signs of cardiac involvement should be treated (see below for pericarditis and myocarditis). Appropriate supportive treatment is given for arrhythmias and heart failure.

▶ Nursing management

Patients should be made as comfortable as possible and treated for their fever, by maintaining fluid intake, attention to hygiene and cooling measures if appropriate (see Ch. 5). Patients are confined to bed during the acute phase of rheumatic fever, which may be for a period of some weeks in patients who have had carditis. This presents a challenge for nurses in terms of preventing and managing the complications of immobility, e.g. muscle wastage, constipation and boredom. The nurse should work with other health professionals, such as physiotherapists and occupational therapists, to minimize the effects of prolonged bed rest.

Effective pain relief is important and nurses should monitor patients for symptoms of aspirin toxicity such as tinnitus (see Ch. 16) and nausea.

Observations of vital signs (temperature, pulse, respiration and blood pressure) are recorded as frequently as the condition dictates and abnormalities such as an irregular pulse rate should be reported to the medical staff. Additionally the nurse should be alert to the signs of complications such as breathlessness and oedema present in heart failure.

Table 19.1 Valvular heart disease

	Mitral stenosis	Mitral regurgitation	Aortic stenosis	Aortic regurgitation
Aetiology	• Rheumatic heart disease • Increasing age • Calcification of the valve • More common in women	• Rheumatic heart disease • Infective endocarditis • Complications of myocardial infarction	• Calcification of the valve • Congenital heart disease • Rheumatic heart disease	• Increasing age • Marfan's syndrome
Pathophysiology	• Valve leaflets thicken and valve is unable to open fully • Blood flow is reduced into the left ventricle • Left atrium enlarges • Pulmonary congestion occurs • Low cardiac output	• Valve closes but does not remain shut when the ventricle starts to contract • Blood regurgitates into the left atrium during ventricular contraction • Low cardiac output • Pulmonary congestion	• Valve leaflets thicken and valve is unable to open fully • Reduced blood flow into the systemic circulation • Blood flow into the coronary arteries decreases	• Valve closes but does not remain shut when the ventricle starts to contract • Blood regurgitates into the left ventricle • Ventricular hypertrophy (enlargement)
Clinical presentation	• Shortness of breath • Paroxysmal nocturnal dyspnoea • Fatigue • Heart failure • Atrial fibrillation	• Shortness of breath • Paroxysmal nocturnal dyspnoea • Fatigue • Heart failure • Atrial fibrillation	• Shortness of breath • Syncope • Fatigue • Angina	• Fatigue • Shortness of breath • Palpitations • Heart failure
Specific investigations	• Auscultation – may detect heart murmur • Echocardiography – size of opening of valve • Cardiac catheterization – measure heart pressures • ECG – to detect atrial fibrillation • Chest X-ray – heart size and lung fields	• Auscultation – may detect heart murmur • Echocardiography – degree of regurgitation • Cardiac catheterization – measure heart pressures • ECG – to detect atrial fibrillation • Chest X-ray – heart size and lung fields	• Auscultation – may detect heart murmur • Echocardiography – size of opening of valve • Cardiac catheterization – measure heart pressures	• Auscultation – may detect heart murmur • Echocardiography – degree of regurgitation • Cardiac catheterization – measure heart pressures • ECG – left ventricular hypertrophy
Medical/ surgical management	Medical • Nitrates • Treat heart failure • Treat atrial fibrillation Surgical • Valvuloplasty • Valve replacement	Medical • Treat heart failure • Treat atrial fibrillation Surgical • Valvuloplasty • Valve replacement	Surgical • Aortic valve replacement	Medical • Nitrates Surgical • Aortic valve replacement

VALVULAR HEART DISEASE

Valvular heart disease (VHD) is often divided into categories depending upon whether the valve is stenosed or regurgitant. These categories are further divided to describe the affected valve. More commonly these will include mitral stenosis, mitral regurgitation, aortic stenosis and aortic regurgitation (see Table 19.1).

Valves that are unable to open fully restrict the flow of blood and are referred to as stenosed. Valve stenosis increases the pressure required to maintain the flow of blood and leads to enlargement of the heart chambers.

If the heart valves are unable to close competently, they are referred to as regurgitant (incompetent). This results in a situation where blood flows backwards, there is enlargement of the heart chamber subject to the back flow of blood, and the forward flow of blood is reduced.

Occasionally the valve is diseased in such a way that it is both stenosed and regurgitant. In this case it will neither open fully nor close completely.

The aetiology, pathophysiology, clinical presentation, investigation and medical/surgical management of VHD are outlined in Table 19.1, and some information about valve replacement is provided on page 516. However, detailed coverage of valve surgery is beyond the scope of this book and readers requiring more specific information are directed to the suggestions in 'Further reading'.

▶ Nursing management

Patients will need to be given all the care required for someone with heart failure (see pp. 512–514). Patients with diseased valves and those who have undergone surgical valve replacement are at risk of infective endocarditis. Advice regarding the prevention of this potentially serious condition must be stressed (see p. 516).

For patients who have developed mitral regurgitation over a period of time, and have developed left ventricular failure, the risk of valve replacement may outweigh the perceived benefits of the operation and they may not be considered suitable to undergo such a procedure. The nursing management of their heart failure to provide symptom relief is therefore paramount. However, if they do undergo surgery, it is likely to be complicated. Both the patients and their families should be prepared for this longer postoperative course.

Valve replacement – surgical management

Over recent years there has been a profusion of replacement valves available on the market. These may be mechanical (metal) or biological (tissue). Biological valves may be made from pig tissues (xenograft – tissue from another species) or the pericardium, or may be taken from a cadaver heart (homografts). The choice of valve may depend upon the age of the patient, religion (e.g. some religions will not allow the use of a pig valve), the patient's views on animal welfare and the long-term need for anticoagulation required with some mechanical valves.

A valve replacement requires that patients will have to undergo open-heart surgery. As valvular heart disease occurs more frequently in older people, it must be remembered that the operative risk rises with age.

Although the surgeon makes the choice of valve, it is useful for the nurse to have some knowledge of the factors that influence this choice and so be able to answer any questions that patients or their family members may have. The mechanical valve has the advantage of lasting for several years, but having a mechanical prosthesis implanted means that patients will need to take anticoagulation for life. Mechanical valves should not be used in women of child-bearing age or patients with a contraindication to anticoagulation, such as a previous CVA (see Ch. 14), gastrointestinal bleed (see Ch. 22), alcohol misuse, or someone who is known to be reluctant to take the required drugs. Bioprosthetic valves may not require anticoagulation, but may only last for 8–10 years, after which they degenerate and require replacement. They may be useful when anticoagulation is not advisable or in patients whose life expectancy is limited (e.g. those with another illness, such as certain cancers). Homografts do not require anticoagulation, and although initially they were thought to last for a long time, it is now thought that they too will need replacement after about 8–10 years.

Contraceptive advice is necessary when valvular heart disease is present in women of child-bearing age. If the disease is asymptomatic or the symptoms minor, then pregnancy will normally be safe, although the mothers-to-be will require careful monitoring throughout. However, if the women already have symptoms of heart failure, it may be necessary to perform a valve replacement prior to them planning a family. The choice of valve is then important to avoid anticoagulation, and a tissue valve or homograft will be used.

INFECTIVE ENDOCARDITIS

Infective endocarditis (IE) was previously referred to as acute, subacute or chronic bacterial endocarditis, but the term IE is now used to describe all of these categories. IE results from a microbial infection of a heart valve or the endocardial lining of the heart.

Aetiology and epidemiology

The infection is usually bacterial, and the organisms responsible include *Staphylococcus aureus*, *Staphylococcus epidermidis*, *Streptococcus faecalis* and *Streptococcus viridans*. More rarely the infection may be due to a fungus, *Rickettsia* or *Chlamydia* (see Ch. 13).

Over the past 50 years, the pattern of IE in the UK has changed, largely due to the reduced incidence of rheumatic heart disease. The population at risk includes:

- people with diseased valves (such as mitral or aortic stenosis or regurgitation)
- following prosthetic valve replacement
- following cardiac surgery
- congenital heart disease
- i.v. drug misusers
- patients with an i.v. or central line in situ
- IE may develop on normal heart valves when an infection elsewhere in the body (frequently from periodontal disease) travels to the endocardium.

In the UK, only about 4000 cases occur each year; consequently it is rare for a GP to see IE and the symptoms may be missed. Mortality may be as high as 50% in patients with a prosthetic valve (British Cardiac Society 1996), while in the older population it may carry a mortality rate of 70% (Woods et al 2000). Prompt diagnosis and treatment are therefore essential.

Pathophysiology

Vegetation (fibrin, microorganisms and platelets) grows on the leaflet of the heart valve or on the endocardium itself. This can be a single or multiple lesion and may be several centimetres in size. As the endocardium is normally a smooth, continuous layer of cells it should be resistant to the growth of vegetation. However, in areas where the blood flow is turbulent, as through a narrowed or diseased valve, endothelial damage may occur and vegetation may adhere to the surface. When microorganisms stick to this vegetation, the process of IE commences, which ultimately leads to erosion of the valve tissue. Part of the vegetation may break off and form emboli, which may travel to the brain or other systemic sites.

Clinical presentation

Symptoms of IE are often non-specific, resulting in diagnostic delay, and may include:

- low-grade fever and night sweats, chills and rigors
- splenomegaly (enlargement of the spleen)
- petechiae (small, red lesions caused by an effusion of blood) on the skin and mucous membranes
- splinter haemorrhages (long black streaks under the nail bed)
- cardiac murmurs may be heard if the vegetation damages the heart valves
- clubbing of fingers in long-term disease
- subconjunctival haemorrhages
- haematuria
- signs of heart failure.

Box 19.2 Prophylactic use of antibiotics

High risk
Prosthetic valves
Previous infective endocarditis
Immunosuppression

Average risk
Rheumatic/acquired valvular heart disease
Congenital heart disease
Cardiomyopathy

Specific investigations

Prior to treatment it is necessary to establish the exact microorganism responsible for the infection and at least three sets of blood cultures should be taken from different puncture sites (British Cardiac Society 1996).

Echocardiography may be used to see if any vegetation affects the valve action. Commonly, valves fail to close effectively and regurgitant flow will be present. During the acute period of IE, patients are likely to have weekly echocardiograms to assess valve function.

Medical management

The use of antibiotics has improved the treatment of IE, and the prophylactic use of antibiotics for those at risk has reduced the incidence (see Box 19.2).

Once a diagnosis of IE has been made and the organism responsible is isolated, i.v. antibiotics are commenced. The course of treatment is usually continued for at least 6 weeks and patients may require the insertion of a central or Hickman line. Antibiotics, frequently penicillin and gentamicin, must be given until the blood cultures are negative. Oral antibiotics are then prescribed and must be continued for 4–6 weeks to ensure the infection has cleared.

Surgery is indicated only when patients develop heart failure, have many relapses of the condition or develop an abscess on the valve. Ideally, surgery should be delayed until it is clear that there is no active infection, which could infect the replacement valve.

▶ Nursing management

The prophylactic use of antibiotics for those at risk of IE should be encouraged whenever they undergo a procedure where the mucous membranes may be breached. Such procedures would include dental care, body piercing and body tattoos. As many of these patients are feeling fit and well, they may not be aware of the need to take antibiotics and nurses will need to stress the importance of both taking and completing the prescriptions (see Health Promotion box 19.2).

Those at risk of IE should also be advised to prevent dental disease through good oral care and regular treatment by dental hygienists. Ulcers from ill-fitting dentures or teeth braces should be avoided, as these are other potential causes of mucosal damage.

When patients are diagnosed with IE, they will need all the care required for someone with a fever and infection

 HEALTH PROMOTION

19.2 Preventing infective endocarditis

Infective endocarditis (IE) is an infection of the endocardium or inner lining of the heart and valves. The infection can be life-threatening, leading to dysfunction of the heart valves and ultimately heart failure. Patients at risk of IE should limit their exposure to infection that might enter the systemic circulation. When this is not possible, they should be prescribed and encouraged to complete a course of antibiotics. Prophylactic antibiotics should therefore be prescribed when they undergo body piercing, dental work, investigations that require instrumentation (such as uroscopy) or any invasive procedures or surgery.

Student activities

Think about the information you would include in a handout or website for patients who are at risk of IE (e.g. following a heart valve replacement) who are being discharged from your care in hospital.

(see p. 514). Additionally they will need specific assessment of their haemodynamic status. The infection may lead to the heart valves becoming regurgitant and patients will have signs similar to those outlined in Table 19.1. Regular assessment of the heart rate and rhythm and blood pressure may provide early warning signs that they are beginning to develop heart failure.

Nurses should be alert to the possibility of an embolus breaking off from vegetations. If emboli originate in the left side of the heart, they may lodge in the brain where they could cause a cerebral abscess. Any changes in the level of consciousness of the patient should be reported. Sometimes the emboli are very small and cause only transient obstruction to the cerebral blood flow and patients may only exhibit a brief change in level of consciousness or show signs of inappropriate behaviour. Again these should be reported.

Occasionally, the endocarditis will develop around the tricuspid valve, something that is more commonly found amongst i.v. drug misusers. Any emboli that break off will travel from the right side of the heart to the lungs and may lead to a pulmonary abscess. Patients will develop worsening fever, general malaise and may start to expectorate blood-specked sputum. Again these signs and symptoms should be reported.

Once blood cultures are negative, and if patients are haemodynamically stable, antibiotics should be continued for a further 4–6 weeks. It is often difficult to encourage patients to continue with antibiotic therapy once they begin to feel well and this poses a challenge to the nurse.

DISORDERS OF THE MYOCARDIUM

Disorders affecting the myocardium include myocarditis and the cardiomyopathies.

MYOCARDITIS

Myocarditis refers to inflammation of the myocardium. It is usually diagnosed once there is considerable cardiovascular dysfunction.

Aetiology

Causes of myocarditis include:

- infections – commonly viral infections (Coxsackie virus), but bacterial infections may also occur (staphylococcal and pneumococcal)
- autoimmune disease such as systemic lupus erythematosus (SLE) (see Ch. 27)
- endocrine disorders such as thyroid disease and diabetes (see Ch. 17).

Pathophysiology

The inflammatory process develops in the myocardium in response to the particular causative agent and this ultimately leads to death of the myocardial cells and poor cardiac function. Additionally there is interstitial fibrosis, which may contribute to arrhythmias seen in the patient with myocarditis.

Clinical presentation

Patients will present with a history of a flu-like or viral illness. As a result of poor cardiac function, they will have signs and symptoms of heart failure, such as fatigue, shortness of breath and palpitations.

Specific investigations

- ECG – this is likely to show small QRS complexes indicative of low voltage. Heart blocks may also be seen as the interstitial fibrosis interrupts the conduction pathway
- Echocardiogram – this is likely to confirm poor ventricular function
- Cardiac biopsy – this will be taken to enable a definitive diagnosis. It may be undertaken via echocardiogram; patients will be prepared in the same way.

Medical management

Patients will be treated for their heart failure (see p. 510) and, if their condition deteriorates, they should be considered for a heart transplantation or left ventricular assist device (see p. 519).

► Nursing management

Patients with myocarditis will be severely ill and, along with their families, will require considerable psychological support. The deterioration in their condition is likely to have been very fast, possibly over a few days.

They will require the same care as a person with heart failure.

CARDIOMYOPATHY

Cardiomyopathy describes a disease of heart muscle that results in both structural and functional abnormalities. There are three main forms of cardiomyopathy: dilated, hypertrophic and restrictive. The aetiology, pathophysiology, clinical presentation, investigations and medical management are outlined in Table 19.2. Readers requiring more specific information are directed to the suggestions in 'Further reading'.

► Nursing management

Patients with cardiomyopathy should be advised to reduce their alcohol intake, even where this is not thought to be the cause. Alcohol may depress the cardiac muscle and, as this is already weak, may reduce cardiac output further. The nurse will need to advise patients on the suggested number of units of alcohol each week and to spread these out evenly (see Ch. 23). A discussion on alternative drinks such as alcohol-free wine or lagers, which are now freely available, may be included.

Patients should be encouraged to follow a healthy diet (see Ch. 11). People who are overweight or obese will need help to reduce weight and may need the help of a dietician or specialist nurse to reach their ideal weight. Any excess body weight will place additional strain upon the heart. Moderate physical exercise should be encouraged unless it precipitates symptoms; however, competitive sports should be avoided.

As patients with cardiomyopathy develop heart failure, nursing management should include all the care given to patients in that group (see p. 510).

Patients with cardiomyopathy who are considering becoming pregnant should be offered advice regarding the familial risk of the disease, the particular risks associated with pregnancy and the specific management required as pregnancy progresses. Pregnancy increases fluid volume and, consequently, cardiac output. This may precipitate heart failure, and prescribed drugs such as warfarin or antiarrhythmics may complicate the pregnancy.

The familial risk of cardiomyopathy poses other dilemmas for patients and their families. The risks to future children must be considered and first-degree relatives should be offered screening. However, this will require the skills of specialist counsellors and support services (see below).

Cardiomyopathy cannot be cured and all forms of treatment are palliative. If heart failure progressively worsens, patients may be considered for assessment for heart transplantation or a left ventricular assist device. For these forms of treatment, very careful assessment of both the physiological and psychological condition of the patient is required.

Patients with cardiomyopathy and their families often need help to adjust to the illness and it may be useful to refer them to a support group. The Cardiomyopathy Association is a voluntary organization able to provide support and can put patients and their relatives in touch with a local support group.

Heart transplantation

Heart transplantation has developed both in surgical technique and immunological therapy and is now associated with a survival of 80% at 1 year, and just under 60% at 4 years. However, the demand for transplant organs exceeds the supply. The allocation of these organs requires careful medical, ethical and societal considerations, which have led to a national organ procurement and distribution network. Patients with severe

Table 19.2 Cardiomyopathy

Type of cardiomyopathy	Dilated cardiomyopathy	Hypertrophic cardiomyopathy	Restrictive cardiomyopathy
Aetiology	• Unknown • Coxsackie virus • Alcohol misuse • Postpartum • Familial	• Genetic	• Unknown • Sarcoidosis • Amyloidosis
Pathophysiology	• Dilation of both ventricles • Mitral valve regurgitation	• Ventricular walls thicken • Septum enlarges and obstructs the flow of blood into the systemic circulation • Left atrium enlarges	• Ventricular walls fibrose and stiffen
Clinical presentation	• Heart failure • Shortness of breath • Paroxysmal nocturnal dyspnoea • Oedema • Fatigue • Dizziness • Palpitations – atrial fibrillation, supraventricular tachycardia, ventricular tachycardia	• Angina • Atrial fibrillation • Ventricular arrhythmias • See dilated cardiomyopathy	• See dilated cardiomyopathy
Specific investigations	• Echocardiography • 12-lead ECG • Holter tape • Exercise test • Chest X-ray	• See dilated cardiomyopathy • Myocardial biopsy	• See dilated cardiomyopathy • Myocardial biopsy
Medical/surgical management	Medical • Treat heart failure • Treat arrhythmias Surgical • Pacemaker • Implantable defibrillator • Left ventricular assist device • Heart transplant	Medical • Treat heart failure • Treat arrhythmias Surgical • Alcohol ablation of the septal artery • Implantable defibrillator • Heart transplant	• Treat heart failure • Treat arrhythmias
Special considerations	• Risk of sudden death – an AICD (also known as an internal cardioverter) may be considered	• See dilated cardiomyopathy	

heart failure are carefully assessed, both physically and psychologically. Once considered suitable for heart transplantation, their names are added to a list of potential recipients and kept on a national database. The allocation of the donor heart is based upon severity of illness, ABO blood type compatibility and an assessment of the match between the body sizes of the donor and the recipient.

▶ Nursing management

Donor organs are not freely available and patients must be warned that they may have a long wait and that their condition may deteriorate in the meantime. The waiting time can be very difficult for both patients and their families, and the former frequently worry that they have been forgotten. It is useful to give them a contact name so that they may discuss any concerns or anxieties they have. Hospitals offering a transplant service normally have a specially trained nurse to liaise with patients and families during this time. This nurse can allay any fears or anxieties, by telephone, at clinic visits and sometimes by e-mail. This contact also allows the nurse to become aware of any changes in a patient's physical or mental condition, which may affect the outcome of transplantation.

Left ventricular assist devices

During a long wait for heart transplantation, a patient's condition may deteriorate and it is increasingly common to support the failing left ventricle with a left ventricular assist device (LVAD) (see Fig. 19.17). In some cases, the patient's own heart function improves with the rest provided by an assist device. The mechanical LVAD can then be removed, as the patient's own heart is functioning adequately. A patient in this position will no longer require a heart transplant and his or her name can be removed from the transplant register. Clearly these patients

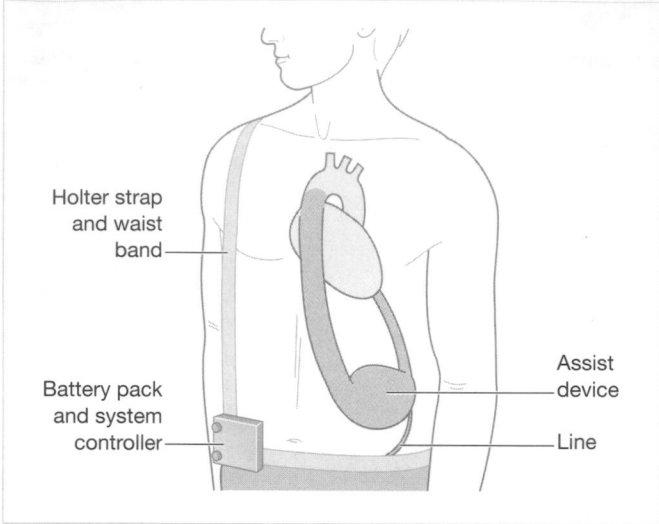

Figure 19.17 Left ventricular assist device.

would then be followed up closely and should be reassured that if their heart starts to fail again they would be reconsidered for transplantation.

The LVAD is now a totally implantable device. It is implanted into the peritoneal cavity. One tube is attached to the apex of the left ventricle, while the other is joined to the ascending aorta (Chilcott et al 1998). A small driveline exits through the abdominal wall and connects to an external power source. This is a battery worn either as a belt or a Holter, depending upon the manufacturer of the device.

▶ Nursing management

These totally implantable systems mean that patients can move around freely and even take gentle exercise. They are asked to avoid high-impact jumping, such as using a jogging machine, as the device may move within the body. As the battery source is external, patients must avoid getting the driveline wet. They are therefore unable to exercise in water, such as swimming or water aerobics. Additional advice is to avoid taking a bath and ensure the driveline of the device is covered when they shower. Patients with a LVAD can be discharged home and some will return to work. The improvement in quality of life and psychosocial functioning for these patients is tremendous and should ensure that they are in the best possible condition both medically and psychologically when a transplant organ becomes available.

DISORDERS OF THE PERICARDIUM

PERICARDITIS

Pericarditis is inflammation of the pericardium.

Aetiology

About 15% of patients will develop pericarditis following a myocardial infarction (see p. 506). When it develops after

3 weeks, it is referred to as Dressler's syndrome. Other causes include:

- infection – viral (Coxsackie virus, influenza or herpes zoster), bacterial (*Pneumococcus*) or fungal (aspergillosis) infections
- cancers such as those of the breast (see Ch. 26) or lung (see Ch. 20)
- injury to the chest wall or migration of pacing wires from their position in the endocardium
- renal failure, which may cause uraemic pericarditis to develop (see Ch. 24).

Pathophysiology

The inflammatory process leads to a pericardial effusion (accumulation of fluid in the pericardial sac) as the pericardium secretes more fluid into the enclosed space around the heart. In severe situations, this may lead to cardiac tamponade (see p. 521), which restricts the normal stretching of the heart as it fills with blood.

In constrictive pericarditis, the inflammation occurs slowly and the pericardium is thickened. Although this may also constrict the function of the heart, the slow process leads to more subtle symptoms.

Clinical presentation

Inflammation of the pericardium leads to fever, general malaise and pain. Frequently the inflammation leads to chest pain, which is felt particularly on inspiration or when lying down. It may radiate to the shoulder in a similar way to angina, which may confuse the diagnosis. Patients will often have to sit forward or kneel on all fours to obtain relief. On auscultation, a pericardial rub will be heard; this is a high-pitched, scratchy sound caused by friction between the pericardial layers.

Once a pericardial effusion develops, the pain often subsides or disappears altogether. If the pericardial effusion is severe, it may create pressure around the heart that prevents the normal stretching required for filling during diastole, which results in a fall in cardiac output.

Specific investigations

An ECG may show ST-segment elevation. However, on careful analysis this should not be confused with the ST-segment changes of an MI; there are no Q wave changes and the T waves are not inverted.

Medical management

Treatment for pericarditis includes relief of the pain. Aspirin also reduces pyrexia but non-steroidal anti-inflammatory drugs (NSAIDs) such as indomethacin may be needed to control pain. If the pericarditis does not resolve, a pericardial tap will be performed and the fluid sent for microbiological examination (for identification of microorganism and antibiotic sensitivities), thus allowing the appropriate choice of antibiotic.

▶ Nursing management

During the time of acute fever, patients should be encouraged to rest and maintain an adequate oral intake of fluids (see Ch. 5). Usually the prognosis is good.

Patients should be continuously monitored for arrhythmias and their blood pressure recorded every 4 hours. Any indication that cardiac tamponade may be developing (low blood pressure and raised jugular venous pressure) must be noted and medical aid sought immediately.

CARDIAC TAMPONADE

Cardiac tamponade refers to fluid in the pericardium, usually blood or serous fluid. This fluid compresses the heart and does not allow it to stretch during diastole. Ventricular filling is reduced, as is the cardiac output.

Aetiology

Any disease that may lead to pericarditis may ultimately result in cardiac tamponade. Chest trauma or surgical intervention that may cause the heart or aorta to bleed can cause acute tamponade. Tamponade is also a complication of elective cardiac surgery.

Pathophysiology

Cardiac tamponade causes the heart to be constricted by high pressure from outside. The right atrium and right ventricle are compressed, filling is compromised and the CVP will start to rise (see p. 488). Left ventricular filling is also compromised, resulting in low cardiac output and a fall in blood pressure.

Clinical presentation

If cardiac tamponade develops rapidly, patients may become haemodynamically unstable, which constitutes a medical emergency. In acute cardiac tamponade, patients are anxious, sweating, dyspnoeic and dizzy with a high CVP, hypotension and tachycardia.

Specific investigations

A chest X-ray may detect an enlarged heart indicative of tamponade. ECG may be helpful in determining the underlying cause. Echocardiography can be used to confirm the diagnosis and ascertain the best site for withdrawing fluid by pericardial tap.

Medical management

As this is an emergency situation, medical assistance should be summoned immediately and excess fluid removed from the pericardium, a procedure known as a pericardial tap. If tamponade is recurrent (as may occur with some forms of malignancy), a small window may be made in the pericardium. This will prevent further collections of fluid compromising cardiac function.

Patients who develop cardiac tamponade following cardiac surgery should be returned to the operating theatre so that the bleeding can be arrested.

▶ Nursing management

The nursing management of a patient with cardiac tamponade depends upon the cause. Clearly if it constitutes a medical emergency, the nursing priority will be the maintenance of cardiac output until medical assistance arrives. Subsequently the nurse should assist with the removal of the fluid.

DISORDERS OF THE VASCULAR SYSTEM

HYPERTENSION

Hypertension refers to systolic blood pressure > 140 mmHg and a diastolic blood pressure > 85 mmHg (Curzio & Kennedy 1996). It is considered a major risk factor for the development of atheroma, although the mechanisms for this are unclear. Possibly the high pressure in the coronary arteries damages the endothelium, thus allowing lipid deposition in the arterial wall.

Aetiology — study of causes of disease

Transient elevations of blood pressure are normal under conditions of anxiety or excitement and during exercise.

The underlying cause of secondary hypertension is unknown in the vast majority of patients (over 95%) and is called essential hypertension. Hypertension has a multifactorial aetiology and the factors associated with it include obesity, diabetes, high salt intake, alcohol misuse and smoking. Genetic factors are also important and about 30% of cases are thought to be familial (Hanson 1997). Certain racial groups have a higher prevalence of hypertension, e.g. African-Americans and the Japanese.

Blood pressure rises with age and hypertension is rarely seen in the under-25 age group unless they have a primary illness, such as renal failure.

The known causes of secondary hypertension include:

- pregnancy (pre-eclampsia)
- coarctation of the aorta (see p. 528)
- renal artery stenosis
- parenchymal renal diseases such as glomerulonephritis (see Ch. 24)
- certain drugs – corticosteroids and the oestrogen-containing oral contraceptives
- endocrine disorders (see Ch. 17) such as Cushing's disease, acromegaly and phaeochromocytoma.

Clinical presentation

Frequently hypertension is diagnosed from a routine medical examination, as the person does not demonstrate any symptoms. However, if symptoms do occur, they include headaches, dizziness or burst blood vessels in the eyes. An elevation of blood pressure over a prolonged period of time may lead to what is referred to as end-organ damage, i.e. damage to the kidneys (renal failure), eyes (cataracts and conjunctival haemorrhage – see Ch. 15), central nervous system (papilloedema, transient ischaemic attacks and cerebrovascular accident – see Ch. 14), heart (left ventricular failure and atheroma) and blood vessels (aneurysm).

Medical management

Medication is only used in the treatment of hypertension where nursing management involving lifestyle changes is unsuccessful. Diuretics such as bendroflumethiazide (bendrofluazide) or furosemide (frusemide) and ACE inhibitors such as captopril are frequently prescribed to remove excess salt and water and cause arterial vasodilatation. Other antihypertensive drugs include beta-adrenoceptor antagonists (beta-blockers) such as atenolol that block the sympathetic nervous system response and cause vasodilatation. Calcium channel blockers (amlodipine or nifedipine) may be prescribed.

Other drugs that may be used include alpha$_1$-adrenoceptor antagonists (prazosin), drugs that act directly to cause vasodilatation (such as hydralazine), or drugs that act centrally (such as clonidine).

▶ Nursing management

Accurate blood pressure monitoring is essential to diagnose hypertension and then to decide upon the treatment options. The correct cuff bladder size is vital for accurate measurement of blood pressure and is especially important in overweight individuals where unreliably high recordings may occur with a cuff that is too small. All those involved in the management of hypertensive patients should be aware that Korotkoff phase V diastolic blood pressure is used in the diagnosis and management of hypertension.

It may be difficult to obtain reliable blood pressure values in the general practice surgery or outpatient clinics, where patients may well be anxious. Repeat blood pressure recordings should be obtained before a diagnosis of hypertension is made and sometimes ambulatory blood pressure recording is necessary to remove the anxiety created in general practice, the so-called 'white coat' factor. Patients are taught how to use a small portable device that measures blood pressure. They will then be able to record their blood pressure over a period of 24 hours, away from the surgery environment.

As hypertension is often asymptomatic, opportunities should be taken to check an individual's blood pressure. This may be on every visit to a medical professional such as a GP or practice nurse. Drop-in clinics where a regular assessment of blood pressure can be made may contribute to an early diagnosis. Although the risk factors for CHD are multiple, it is still important to detect hypertension as early as possible and initiate treatment as a means of reducing CHD. However, a word of caution: nurses must consider the ethical implications of taking a person's blood pressure when that person has clearly chosen to consult for an unrelated condition or problem.

Once hypertension is diagnosed, the main aim of treatment must be to reduce the risk of end-organ damage by reducing blood pressure. Guidelines for treatment have been provided by the British Hypertension Society (Ramsey et al 1999). Patients should be encouraged to eat a low-salt and low-fat diet. They may need advice about losing weight and starting a regular exercise programme. Smoking cessation should be encouraged. Relaxation techniques and the use of biofeedback have been found to combat hypertension associated with lifestyle stresses (see Ch. 6). Primary prevention is important, especially amongst those with a family history.

Patients should be taught to record their blood pressure at home, usually while sitting, as blood pressure values will vary with posture (see p. 488). They should also become familiar with any symptoms or signs that may indicate a worsening of their condition, including deteriorating eyesight, burst blood vessels in the eyes or a cerebrovascular incident. Patients encouraged with self-monitoring may adapt to their chronic illness in a more positive way.

AORTIC ANEURYSM AND DISSECTION

An aortic aneurysm occurs when there is a weakness in the aorta that allows a portion of the vessel wall to protrude. Sometimes this bulge may rupture, with potentially devastating results. The aneurysm is classified according to the site in the aorta, and the severity of the condition depends on how close it is to the heart. For example, if an aneurysm in the ascending aorta ruptures, there would be a rapid and dramatic reduction in circulating blood volume and cardiac output from which the patient would be unlikely to survive.

Aortic dissection occurs when the intima of the aorta starts to tear. This may take place anywhere from the ascending aorta to more distal parts. Again the severity depends upon the proximity of the area of dissection to the heart.

Aetiology

People at risk of developing an aneurysm/dissection include those with atheromatous disease, inherited conditions where the arterial walls are diseased (e.g. Marfan's syndrome) or aortitis. Hypertension may also lead to aortic aneurysm/dissection, as the aorta is exposed to high pressures for a prolonged period of time.

Clinical presentation

The signs of aortic aneurysm may be insidious and include shortness of breath, backache and hoarseness; these vary depending upon the site of the aneurysm. If the aneurysm affects the abdominal aorta, patients may experience central abdominal tenderness, loss of appetite and nausea. Abdominal aortic aneurysms (AAAs) are more commonly associated with older men and those who are hypertensive.

Aortic dissection is frequently acute. Patients will suddenly complain of chest, jaw, back and abdominal pain. Beyond the site of the dissection, they are unlikely to have any pulses and a rapid diagnosis can be made. For example, dissection of the abdominal aorta will lead to absent pulses from the femoral region and below.

Specific investigations

When an aortic aneurysm is suspected, patients should be prepared for various investigations. X-ray, ultrasound or MRI scan of the abdomen or chest will be used to provide information on the size and location of the aneurysm. This is important to guide the decision on treatment.

Screening of the group aged over 65 years (at risk of hypertension) through ultrasound has been suggested for the early detection of an aortic aneurysm. If present, repeat ultrasounds should be offered every 9 months (Herbert 1997).

Medical management

Once a diagnosis of aneurysm is made, it is very important to try to reduce the blood pressure and reduce the risk of the aneurysm rupturing. Patients should be followed up regularly and referred for surgery when the aneurysm starts to enlarge or if they develop pain. If the aneurysm is found in the ascending aorta, surgical ligation will be undertaken as soon as possible as the risk of rupture is great, with devastating consequences. Small aneurysms are now treated with aortic stents inserted through a small femoral incision, in a similar manner to an intracoronary stent (Herbert 1997). Aneurysms that form distal to the heart may be monitored, as they often grow more slowly.

With aortic dissection, the blood pressure must be lowered rapidly and a fast-acting vasodilator such as sodium nitroprusside is frequently given intravenously. Patients usually should be rapidly prepared for surgery, as without prompt treatment aortic dissection has a very poor prognosis. For surgical repair of an aortic dissection, a Dacron graft is sutured to the dissecting aorta.

▶ Nursing management

When aortic aneurysm is diagnosed it is important that strategies are used to reduce the blood pressure. This should include pharmacological and non-pharmacological methods (see above). If the aneurysm is already rupturing the situation is treated as an emergency. The blood pressure must be lowered immediately and preparation should be made to prepare the patient and their family for surgical ligation or stent insertion.

PERIPHERAL ARTERIAL DISEASE

Peripheral arterial disease (PAD) is usually caused by atheroma and affects the arteries of the legs more often than those of the arms. Similar atheromatous disease may occur in the arteries of the pelvis, abdomen, or the carotid arteries.

Aetiology

Risk factors for PAD include:

- age over 50 years
- gender (more commonly found in men; Doughty et al 2000)
- family history
- diabetes
- smoking
- hyperlipidaemia
- obesity
- physical inactivity
- hypertension.

Pathophysiology

Peripheral arterial disease (PAD) results from atheromatous plaque accumulating within an artery, where it will reduce or even obstruct the flow of blood. The process of atheroma development is the same as that affecting the coronary arteries (see p. 500). Most frequently this is seen where the arteries branch, such as the iliac or femoral arteries. In diabetic patients the disease more commonly affects the distal tibial arteries.

Specific investigations

The diagnosis is usually made from the history and the presence or absence of pulses. The assessment must include a description of the pain and factors that both precipitate and alleviate it.

A physical assessment should include observation of the leg and blood flow. Pulses should be palpated, starting with the dorsalis pedis. If this is not palpable, the posterior tibia should be palpated (see Fig. 19.6). If pulses are not palpable, then a hand-held Doppler probe should be used. Conductive jelly should be applied to the area and the Doppler moved slowly until a pulse is heard. If a pulse cannot be detected, complete arterial occlusion should be suspected.

Angiography can detect the exact location and extent of the atheroma and is used if the condition is very severe. The procedure is carried out in a similar way to coronary angiography.

Clinical presentation

The peripheral pulses are absent or very difficult to palpate. The main symptom is that of intermittent claudication when patients experience discomfort or cramp in the lower limbs and buttocks which is associated with exercise and relieved after resting for 1 or 2 minutes. Slowly, the distance patients are able to walk without experiencing pain becomes less (Apple & Lindsay 2000). The pain occurs because the flow of blood down the narrowed artery is insufficient to meet the oxygen demands of tissues with a high metabolic rate. The site of discomfort is usually distal to the diseased area and it is therefore possible to localize the site of the occlusion. Patients who develop discomfort in their calf are likely to have atheromatous changes affecting the femoral artery, whereas discomfort in the buttocks or thigh may be due to disease of the iliac artery. These symptoms should not, however, be confused with the pain of osteoarthritis (see Ch. 27), sciatica or muscle strain.

Only when the disease is severe will patients experience pain at rest. This is described as a constant, dull ache. Classically this pain is in the toes and feet, and is worse at night, keeping patients awake. It is also worse in cold temperatures.

Observation of the leg will show that it is cold and blanched. Frequently the skin is shiny and hairless from the poor supply of nutrients and the calf muscles and toenails may atrophy. In extreme cases, there is obvious gangrene affecting the toes.

Chronic ischaemia leads to loss of skin integrity and arterial ulcers may be present. Unlike venous ulcers, they are extremely painful and more likely to occur on the foot or heel (see Ch. 10).

Medical and surgical management

Once a diagnosis of PAD is made, risk factor modification (e.g. smoking cessation) is an important aspect of management. The treatment of patients with hypertension or diabetes should aim to improve the control of these conditions. Opioid analgesia may be required for the severe pain of advanced PAD. Aspirin or clopidogrel is used to reduce platelet aggregation. Exercise will encourage the development of a collateral circulation. When symptoms persist, the skin condition deteriorates or acute ischaemia occurs, revascularization is required. This may require bypass surgery, embolectomy or percutaneous transluminal angioplasty.

If surgery is undertaken, an incision is made close to the affected artery and either a portion of vein or an artificial graft is used to bypass the blockage. As blood flows down the graft, warmth and sensation will slowly return to the limb, reducing the ischaemia.

Angioplasty (similar to PTCA) and stent is a simpler, less invasive method of restoring blood flow, but is not an option for widespread disease, or small vessels. When the disease is severe and arterial ulcers have developed, amputation may be the only option to reduce the pain, limited lifestyle and risk of acute infection.

▶ Nursing management

The cornerstone of treatment for PAD is risk factor stratification and lifestyle modification. Smoking cessation is vitally important as continued tobacco consumption leads to progressive arterial occlusion and limb ischaemia (Apple & Lindsay 2000). Meticulous control of blood glucose levels is important for the diabetic patient with PAD (see Ch. 17).

A walking programme may help to relieve the pain of intermittent claudication, increase the distance patients can walk without experiencing pain, and increase their sense of well-being. A typical walking pattern includes walking 30–60 minutes, 4–5 days each week. Patients should be encouraged to walk at a speed of 2 miles per hour (Doughty et al 2000). Telling them the distance to their local shops, for example, will help them to identify how far and how quickly they should be walking.

Patients with nocturnal rest pain often find that allowing the foot to hang off the side of the bed at night offers some relief.

Patients undergoing revascularization (angioplasty and stent, arterial graft or embolectomy) procedures are prepared physically and psychologically for anaesthetic and surgery as appropriate (see Ch. 29). Following revascularization procedures, it is important for the nurse to observe the circulation distal to the original obstruction. This should include palpation of distal pulses (e.g. dorsalis pedis, posterior tibial), skin colour and temperature, sensation and pain. Additionally blood pressure, pulse, temperature, respiration and colour are monitored. Pain assessment and the provision of effective pain relief are important. Nurses should note that the pain relief needs of individual patients might be influenced by the degree and type of pain they experienced with PAD prior to surgery (see Ch. 7).

Arterial ulcers may develop on the feet or pressure points and further damage should be prevented by ensuring that patients have well-fitting shoes and avoid trauma and tight-fitting socks and stockings. Podiatry services may be required for some patients, particularly those with diabetes. Once an arterial ulcer has developed, healing is unlikely unless tissue oxygenation is corrected through arterial grafting. Infection and gangrene are caused by poor tissue perfusion and collection of waste products in the tissues. Ultimately this will lead to amputation.

Amputation

Amputation will be considered if, through removing the cause of the pain and increasing mobility, a patient's quality of life can be improved. However, the loss of a limb is both disfiguring and extremely worrying, and patients are likely to have concerns over their ability to cope with normal daily activities following the operation. It is important that patients and their families are prepared physically and psychologically for the operation and given sufficient time to discuss any concerns. During the preoperative period, they should be made aware of the available services and aids that may assist them in the postoperative period.

The care throughout the pre- and postoperative period must be multidisciplinary; the occupational therapist, physiotherapist, social worker and dietician all have vital roles to play. A home assessment may be planned so the occupational therapist can prepare the home with aids that may be needed, e.g. bath aids, wheelchair ramps or stair lifts. The physiotherapist can teach exercises to strengthen the limbs that will have to work differently, e.g. the arm muscles to manipulate crutches. Wound healing is encouraged by good nutrition and the dietician may be able to provide useful advice for patients and their families. It may also be important to carefully review dietary requirements postoperatively. Initially patients may be less active and utilize fewer calories. However, when fitted with an artificial limb, energy consumption and caloric requirement may increase.

Postoperatively phantom limb pain may occur, when patients can still feel pain in the amputated part of their body. This may exist for up to 2 years following the amputation, but does become less severe (Herbert 1997). Otherwise pain from the amputated area may be caused by osteomyelitis, where the bone becomes infected. As the arterial blood supply is poor, healing will be delayed and the wound may break down. This will lead to pain from further infection of the area (see Ch. 27 for further discussion of stump care). Adequate pain control in the postoperative period is important. Movement is difficult and passive leg exercises should be encouraged to reduce the risk of thrombus formation. Flexion contraction can be avoided through exercising the limb and ensuring that it is not held in a flexed position. If flexion contraction occurs, it will be more difficult to fit the prosthesis (see Ch. 27).

The limited mobility and poor arterial perfusion mean that these patients are at risk of pressure ulcer formation. They should be encouraged to mobilize from the first day postoperatively as this will not only reduce postoperative complications but will also increase their self-confidence.

RAYNAUD'S PHENOMENON AND DISEASE

Raynaud's phenomenon is caused by spasm of the peripheral arteries. The spasm occurs on exposure to cold and usually affects the fingers. It is associated with connective tissue disorders such as SLE or scleroderma, certain drugs (ergotamine, beta-adrenoceptor antagonists) and exposure to vibration and cold. It may also be associated with occupational trauma from a constant tapping of the fingertips (piano playing or typing), compression of the nerves (carpal tunnel syndrome) or PAD. The condition is termed Raynaud's disease when it occurs in the absence of an obvious cause. This is more common in women.

Clinical presentation

Raynaud's phenomenon/disease may present with a history of numbness or extreme pain of the fingertips. In cold conditions or stress, severe arterial vasoconstriction occurs. Patients will have numbness and tingling of their fingers and toes, which are very pale or have a bluish hue when the condition is exacerbated. As blood flow returns, the digits become dark red and painful, and patients experience a burning sensation. The nails often appear disfigured due to the reduced blood supply. Smoking clearly contributes to vasoconstriction and will exacerbate the condition. In extreme situations gangrene of the fingertips may occur (Herbert 1997).

Medical management

Treatment is aimed at reducing exposure to factors that trigger the arterial spasm: keeping the fingers and toes warm and reducing stress. Those affected should stop smoking. Calcium channel blockers such as nifedipine may be prescribed to reduce the arterial spasm.

The fingers should be protected from trauma and kept warm by wearing gloves (thermal if needed). Smoking cessation is important and patients may need to be referred to a special smoking cessation clinic. If they are prescribed a calcium channel blocker, such as nifedipine, they should be warned that the vasodilatory effects might lead to flushing, headaches, nausea and palpitations.

If stress is a trigger, relaxation strategies should be taught and encouraged (see Ch. 6).

VARICOSE VEINS

Varicose veins are veins that have tortuous dilations. They are usually found in the superficial veins of the legs. They are present in approximately 10–20% of the population, and in about 3% will lead to venous leg ulcers (Morison & Moffat 1994).

Aetiology
- Trauma
- Deep vein thrombosis (see below)
- Pregnancy (hormone effects and increased pressure within the abdomen)
- Abdominal tumours causing increased abdominal pressure
- Occupations that involve long periods of standing
- Ageing process
- Familial.

Pathophysiology
When the valves in the veins become damaged, venous return is impaired. The blood is slowed and the veins dilate. Collateral blood vessels develop and become superficial and tortuous.

Clinical presentation
As blood accumulates in the veins, the superficial veins bulge and appear as tortuous, purple vessels with 'spider veins' visible under the skin. The legs become unsightly and patients may complain of a dull ache after a period of standing.

Medical management
Treatment includes injecting a sclerosing agent into the veins or surgical removal of the varicose veins (vein stripping). This has a cosmetic advantage and also removes the aching and risk of venous ulcers developing. The blood will then find new collateral vessels for venous return.

Following the injection or surgery support hosiery should be worn for about 6 weeks. Patients should be advised to walk for 30 minutes twice daily, elevate the legs when sitting and avoid too much standing.

DEEP VEIN THROMBOSIS

Deep vein thrombosis (DVT) is a thrombus that has formed in a deep vein, usually in the legs or pelvis. It is often a precursor of pulmonary embolus (PE), a potentially fatal condition.

Aetiology
The predisposing factors of DVT are venous stasis (slow blood flow), changes to blood coagulation and trauma affecting the veins. These three factors are known as Virchow's triad and any factor may act in isolation to cause DVT, or alternatively they may act together:

- *Venous stasis.* Blood flowing through the leg veins is slowed by the effects of gravity and this is exacerbated by physical inactivity. Slow blood flow provides conditions for intravascular coagulation. Patients at risk are those who are immobile for any reason. This includes patients confined to bed or chair, older people who may be frail, obese people, following surgery (particularly longer than 30 minutes and involving abdominal, pelvic or lower limb surgery), those with pre-existing cardiovascular disorders such as heart failure that also slow blood flow, and those travelling on long-haul flights (see p. 526) (Wallis & Autar 2001).
- *Blood coagulation changes.* Blood becomes more liable to coagulate in certain situations – blood disorders such as polycythaemia (see Ch. 18), the presence of certain factors (e.g. factor V Leiden), hormone therapy, (e.g. oral contraceptives), cancers and dehydration (see Ch. 8).
- *Trauma.* Vein trauma may damage the endothelial lining, which provides conditions for thrombus formation. Damage may be caused during surgery (e.g. the pelvic veins during gynaecological procedures) or during the administration of i.v. drugs.

Several other factors are associated with DVT and certain groups of people are at high risk, including:

- increasing age (> 40 years)
- obesity
- pregnancy (when the abdomen is compressed by pregnancy, the risk of thrombus formation in the leg veins is increased) and during the puerperium
- smoking
- previous DVT
- venous insufficiency/varicose veins.

Specific investigations
- Doppler ultrasonography – measures blood flow
- Venography – opaque contrast medium is injected into a vein in the foot. Pictures are taken as the dye travels through the ankle, calf and thigh
- Venometer – a device that measures venous drainage can be used to confirm diagnosis. It has the advantages of being portable and quick to use, thus reducing the time taken to make a definite diagnosis (Wallis & Autar 2001)
- Impedance plethysmography (IPG) – a non-invasive technique that utilizes an inflatable cuff around the thigh to impede venous return. Electrodes placed on the calf measure the time taken for venous blood flow to recommence as the cuff is deflated (Geraghty et al 2001)

■ Other investigations:
— screening blood for D-dimer (a fibrin breakdown product – see Ch. 18)
— scanning tests using radioactive fibrin may be used to locate the thrombus
— MRI scanning.

The selection of investigations is based on the particular clinical presentation, and a combination of tests is often used.

Clinical presentation

Making a diagnosis from physical signs and symptoms is not always easy, as many patients have only minimal changes or no physical changes can be detected.

The signs and symptoms of DVT include:

■ localized pain or tenderness in the leg or calf; Homans' sign is positive where calf pain is experienced when the foot is dorsiflexed
■ swelling of the ankle, calf or thigh
■ warmth and redness around the affected area
■ pallor of the leg
■ dilated distal veins.

Medical management

The immediate treatment for DVT is anticoagulation using heparin. Standard (unfractionated) heparin may be administered by i.v. infusion, but increasingly a daily, subcutaneous injection of low-molecular-weight heparin (LMWH) is used for DVT. A major benefit of using LMWH is the reduction in hospital stay. Some form of heparin is likely to be prescribed for 5–7 days and an oral anticoagulant such as warfarin, or more rarely phenindione, is commenced at the same time. The activated partial prothrombin time (APPT) is used to monitor the level of anticoagulation when standard heparin is used and for making adjustments to the dose of warfarin, the aim being to maintain the international normalized ratio (INR) at 2.5 when warfarin is prescribed for DVT; the target INR is increased to 3.5 for recurrent DVT. Warfarin will be continued for 3–6 months to dissolve the clot and help prevent recurrence. Usually this is sufficient to dissolve the clot (Herbert 1997).

Prophylaxis for DVT is indicated for patients who are assessed as being at increased risk by virtue of having one of the three predisposing factors, or other factors (see p. 525). This usually involves the use of graduated compression stockings and subcutaneous heparin (see Ch. 29), but the benefits of physiotherapy and early mobilization should be stressed.

▶ Nursing management

Nurses have an important preventative role through the assessment of patients at risk of DVT and implementation of the measures discussed above. Several risk scales are available, such as the Autar DVT risk assessment scale (Autar 1996).

Evidence is growing with respect to the link between DVT risk and long-haul flights. The associated immobility, venous stasis, dehydration and reduced air pressure all contribute to the formation of a DVT. People contemplating long flights should consider these risks, and those with a history of thromboembolic conditions should be encouraged to seek medical advice. Passengers undertaking long flights should be advised to avoid dehydration by drinking plenty of non-alcoholic fluids, to take regular exercise around the plane and perform foot and ankle exercises while sitting. Some experts suggest that compression stockings should be worn during long flights but this has yet to be tested in large-scale randomized controlled trials.

Nurses are also important members of the multiprofessional team managing the care of patients with an established DVT. The appointment of specialist nurse practitioners has led to the establishment of many nurse-led services that cater for patients with DVT and others requiring anticoagulation.

Patients should be reminded to take their medication as prescribed, observing themselves for bruising, swelling, gum bleeding, nose bleeds or any evidence of gastrointestinal bleeding. They should be encouraged to attend the anticoagulation clinic and alter the dose of warfarin only as prescribed. Many nurse-led anticoagulation services offer telephone helplines and will give advice about medication to individual patients. Nurses should stress the importance of taking warfarin at the same time each day.

Graduated compression stockings should only be used when patients are fully anticoagulated. It is vital that patients are accurately measured for stockings (Geraghty et al 2001), which are then fitted correctly, and nurses should ensure that patients are competent in using them. The circulation should be observed daily for ischaemia and again nurses should make sure that patients understand how to make these checks.

Patients with chronic venous insufficiency should be referred to a specialist tissue viability nurse before graduated compression stockings are used, because there may be situations in which they should be avoided.

The leg area should not be rubbed or massaged as this may encourage the movement of the clot and increase the risk of PE. Encouraging patients not to sit or lie with their legs crossed and to mobilize as much as possible will also reduce this risk. Nurses should work in collaboration with physiotherapists to implement a suitable programme of leg exercises, mobilization and activity. Brisk walking, swimming and jogging (if appropriate) once discharged home will help reduce venous stasis and any risk of a future DVT.

Early discharge after a diagnosis of DVT makes it more difficult for nurses to provide comprehensive patient education, especially where the patient and their family are still coming to terms with the implications of such a diagnosis. The nurse can reinforce verbal information with specially prepared written material and, where available, the telephone helpline provides a vital back-up after discharge.

PULMONARY EMBOLUS (see also Ch. 20)

A DVT may break off and travel in the veins and through the right side of the heart into the pulmonary circulation where it will cause a PE that leads to infarction of lung tissue. DVT is the commonest cause of PE. Preventing PE obviously depends on the prophylactic measures put in place to prevent DVT (see above). Pulmonary emboli may be massive, acute, small/ medium-sized or chronic multiple microemboli and are estimated to cause some 30 000 deaths every year in the UK.

Nurses involved in the management of patients with DVT should be alert to the possibility of the patient having a PE. Vital signs of heart rate, blood pressure, temperature and respiration should be recorded every 4 hours to detect early signs of PE. Dependent on the type of PE, patients develop chest pain (often pleuritic), shortness of breath, pyrexia and haemoptysis (coughing up blood). A massive PE leads to sudden and severe dyspnoea and chest pain, cyanosis, tachycardia, hypotension, syncope and oliguria.

Treatment includes urgent resuscitation as appropriate (such as CPR), oxygen, pain relief, anticoagulation or thrombolytic drugs. Surgical intervention may occasionally be indicated; this may be an embolectomy or a procedure that modifies the venous system to prevent recurrent emboli reaching the pulmonary circulation.

THROMBOPHLEBITIS

Phlebitis is inflammation of a vein and usually affects the superficial veins. When thrombus forms around the area of inflammation, it leads to the development of thrombophlebitis.

Aetiology

Thrombophlebitis in a superficial vein may be caused by the presence of an i.v. cannula or catheter used to administer drugs or the infusion of fluids. Where thrombophlebitis occurs in a deep vein, it will be due to the presence of a DVT.

Clinical presentation

The inflamed area will be warm to touch and mottling of the affected area is often present. If an i.v. cannula has been inserted, the site is likely to be painful and a firm red streak will be seen along the vein. In severe instances, when the clot has obstructed the blood flow, the area will be cold and cyanosed.

▶ Nursing management

Immediate action requires the removal of the cannula. The limb should be elevated to reduce oedema and pain relief should be given. Further information about the prevention of phlebitis can be found in Chapter 8.

There is a significant risk that emboli may break off a clot in one of the deep veins and travel to the lungs where it will cause a PE. Patients should be assessed for this and any warning signs such as shortness of breath or coughing up of bloodstained fluid should be reported immediately (see above and Ch. 20).

CHRONIC VENOUS INSUFFICIENCY

This condition is caused when the valves of the veins become incompetent and leaky, leading to venous hypertension.

Aetiology

Venous insufficiency is usually present in both legs. The causes include:

- DVT
- after removal of the saphenous vein for use in CABG
- obstruction to the deep veins such as from a tumour of the pelvis or abdomen

- familial valve incompetence
- infection.

It is associated with obesity.

Pathophysiology

As chronic venous insufficiency develops, venous return will be inhibited and venous congestion will develop. The leaky valves allow back-flow of high-pressure blood from the deep veins to the low-pressure system of superficial veins, which leads to venous hypertension. The increase in venous pressure causes the capillary hydrostatic pressure to rise and the transudation of fluid and fibrinogen (coagulation factor) into the extracellular spaces leading to oedema.

Clinical presentation

Patients may have a dull ache and heaviness in their legs when standing. This is often relieved when they sit down or elevate the legs.

Often they will have oedema of the legs that worsens over the day. The fluid in the extracellular spaces contains substances that may cause pigmentation, itchy skin and venous eczema. This may progress to induration, fibrosis and eventually the formation of a venous ulcer. This type of ulcer accounts for approximately 70–90% of all leg ulcers (Doughty et al 2000) (see Ch. 10).

▶ Nursing management

Important aspects of management include measures taken to improve venous return, protect the legs from injury and prevent the development of venous ulcers. When the saphenous vein has been harvested for cardiac surgery, patients are more at risk of developing a venous leg ulcer.

Muscle movement aids venous return and patients with chronic venous insufficiency should be encouraged to operate the 'calf pump' by walking and performing exercises involving the foot, ankle and leg. However, they should be encouraged to sit with their legs elevated, whenever this is possible, to improve venous return. Patients should not stand for long periods of time without operating the 'calf pump'. Sometimes this is difficult to achieve for patients whose work involves driving, sitting at a desk or standing. Patients should be advised to raise their legs above heart level when lying down. It may be useful to arrange for the foot of the bed to be elevated. This strategy should not be used, however, if patients have any degree of cardiac dysfunction as it may precipitate pulmonary oedema.

Improving venous return should be encouraged to assist the removal of waste products and reduce oedema. This will also reduce the toxic damage to tissues that may increase the risk of venous ulceration.

Patients prone to leg injuries should wear support hosiery to encourage venous return and prevent further damage to the area. However, support hosiery can be hot, needs to be fitted correctly by a specialist and should be replaced every 3–6 months as it loses its elasticity. Some patients may lack the manual dexterity, strength or cognitive ability to use hosiery correctly.

Increasing awareness about the effects of apparently minor trauma is important. Patients may already know about potential hazards in their environment, but nurses who practise in the community, the workplace, minor accident units and emergency departments are well placed to advise on the prevention of minor trauma. Other measures may include strategies to reduce falls in older people (see Ch. 32) and lifestyle changes such as wearing trousers or thick tights to increase leg protection.

Although compression bandaging is the most effective form of treatment for venous ulcers, it must not be used if there is any evidence of arterial insufficiency. In order to apply compression bandages safely, staff should be correctly trained in their use (see Ch. 10 for a detailed coverage of venous ulceration).

CONGENITAL HEART DISEASE

Only the more common congenital heart defects will be discussed here. If the condition is diagnosed, most children will now undergo corrective surgery in childhood and consequently many live into adulthood. A brief understanding of some of these defects is therefore useful for the nurse working with adult patients and clients.

Congenital heart disease affects about six to eight children in every 1000 live births, although clearly the extent and severity of these defects vary. Approximately 50% of these children will require treatment. It is rare to be able to identify the exact cause of congenital heart disease, although genetic predisposition and environmental causes are often implicated. Factors affecting the

development of the heart within the first 10 weeks of gestation may lead to these defects; 5–8% are thought to be due to a chromosome abnormality, as in Down's syndrome, while about 1% may be due to toxic causes such as maternal heroin or alcohol misuse, or maternal toxoplasmosis (a protozoan infection transmitted in the faeces of cats), rubella during pregnancy, maternal HIV infection or diabetes.

The most common congenital heart defects are septal defects, absence of (or abnormality affecting) the heart valves, abnormalities to the flow of blood inside the heart and to the main arteries, and abnormalities that impede the flow of blood through the vessels. Clearly more than one abnormality may be present at any one time.

The pathophysiology, clinical presentation and surgical management are outlined in Table 19.3. Readers requiring more specific information are directed to the suggestions in 'Further reading'.

▶ Nursing management

Surgical and pharmacological advances mean that more babies born with a congenital heart defect are surviving into adolescence and even adulthood. Unfortunately, many will have undergone negative experiences involving repeated hospital admissions and surgery during childhood. This may affect their perceptions of their current health and consequently recovery from any further surgery or other illness. Nowadays, more procedures are undertaken using invasive cardiology techniques that are not associated with surgical scarring and disfigurement, and length of hospital stay can be shorter.

Table 19.3 Congenital heart defects

Defect	Atrial septal defect	Coarctation of the aorta	Tetralogy of Fallot
Pathophysiology	• Opening between the two atria • Blood shunts from the left to the right side • Increased blood volume, right ventricle • The right atrium dilates • Pulmonary blood flow increased	• Narrowed portion of aortic arch – the aorta is narrowed • Increased pressure in the aorta before the narrowing • Decreased pressure in the aorta distal to the narrowing	• Ventricular septal defect • The aorta overrides the septal defect • Right ventricular hypertrophy • Stenosed pulmonary valve
Clinical presentation	• In early life, the pulmonary vessels are able to cope with this increased flow, but as the patient grows older, pulmonary hypertension and dyspnoea develop • Right ventricular failure	• Differences in blood pressure between the right and left arms • Frequent headaches • Epistaxis • Leg cramps • Fatigue • Heart failure if undiagnosed	• Central cyanosis • Clubbing of the fingers and toes • Pulmonary stenosis • Moderate hypoxaemia • Limited exercise tolerance • Right ventricular failure
Surgical management	• Dacron patch is sutured over the hole • Small umbrella-like device may be inserted into the defect	• The narrowed portion is dilated • Open heart surgery where the narrowed portion is removed and replaced with a graft	• Closure of ventricular septal defect • Repair of stenosed pulmonary valve

SUMMARY: MAIN POINTS

- Coronary heart disease remains a major cause of premature death in the UK and accounts for a high cost to the NHS.

- Important modifiable risk factors to CHD have been identified, such as hypercholesterolaemia, hypertension, physical inactivity and smoking.

- Nurses have a vital role in the prevention of cardiovascular disease.

- Nurse-led initiatives in the care and management of patients with cardiovascular diseases are increasingly common.

- Symptomatic angina may be relieved by PTCA and stent, or cardiac surgery.

- All health care staff should be familiar with the use of an automated external defibrillator.

- Cardiac rehabilitation has proven benefits for people with cardiac disease, who should be encouraged to attend a cardiac rehabilitation programme.

- The number of people with heart failure in the UK is increasing. People must be empowered with the skills of self-monitoring and self-management in order to enhance their quality of life.

- Hypertension is a major risk factor for the development of cardiovascular disease such as CHD and stroke.

- Following the diagnosis of PAD, cessation of smoking is vitally important as continued tobacco consumption leads to progressive arterial occlusion and limb ischaemia, while meticulous control of blood glucose levels is important in the diabetic patient.

- Varicose veins are usually found in the superficial veins of the legs. In about 3% of cases, they will lead to venous leg ulcers.

- DVT, a preventable condition, forms when there is venous stasis, blood coagulation changes or trauma to veins. It may lead to PE, a potentially fatal condition.

- Through successful treatment and palliation of symptoms, people with a congenital heart disease are now presenting in adult wards and nursing and medical staff should be familiar with some of the more common problems they encounter.

SELF-TEST: CRITICAL THINKING ACTIVITIES

Anwar, aged 50 years, is admitted to your ward for repair of an inguinal hernia. His medical history indicates that he suffers with mild angina and takes GTN on an occasional basis to relieve his chest pain. Preoperative blood tests have revealed that his serum cholesterol level is 8.0 mmol/L.

1 How would you plan secondary prevention advice for Anwar and what topics do you think should be included?

2 After returning to the ward, Anwar complains of tightness in his chest. He is very anxious. The registered nurse responsible for Anwar's care decides to record an ECG, which shows ST-segment elevation in two leads (II and aVf):
— What observations do you think would be appropriate?
— List the priorities of Anwar's care.
— What do you think might be causing the tightness in Anwar's chest?
— What measures might be used to relieve the tightness in his chest?

 FURTHER READING

Broekman B. Discussing resuscitation with patients, why not? Resuscitation 1998; 37(2): 62.

Coats A, McGee H, Stokes H, Thompson D. BACR. Guidelines for cardiac rehabilitation. Oxford: Blackwell Science; 1995.

Dracup K, Moser D. Beyond socio-demographics; factors influencing the decision to seek treatment for symptoms of acute myocardial infarction. Heart Lung 1997; 26(4): 253–262.

Gavin M, Bethall H, Turner S. The acute mood effects of a single exercise session on cardiac patients. Coronary Health Care 2000; 4(2): 71–75.

Halm M, Penque S, Doll N, Beahrs M. Women and cardiac rehabilitation: referral and compliance patterns. J Cardiovasc Nurs 1999; 13(3): 83–92.

Hampton J. The ECG made easy, 5th edn. Edinburgh: Churchill Livingstone; 1997.

Hatchett R, Thompson D. Cardiac nursing: a comprehensive guide. Edinburgh: Churchill Livingstone; 2002.

Jevon P. A matter of life and death. Nurs Times 2001; 97(37): 32–34.

Julian D, Campbell Cowan J, McLenachan J. Cardiology, 7th edn. London: WB Saunders; 1998.

Lavie C, Milani R. Benefits of cardiac rehabilitation and exercise training in elderly women. Am J Cardiol 1997; 79(5): 664–666.

Linden B. Evaluation of a home based rehabilitation programme for patients recovering from acute myocardial infarction. Intensiv Crit Care Nurs 1995; 11: 10–19.

Lindsay G, Gaw A. Coronary heart disease prevention. A handbook for the health care team. Edinburgh: Churchill Livingstone; 1996.

Manelli A, Moodie D. Adult congenital heart disease. In: Topol E, ed. Comprehensive cardiovascular medicine. Philadelphia: Lippincott; 1998.

Normington K, Goodwin S. A personalised approach to cardiac rehabilitation. Prof Nurse 2000; 15(7): 432–436.

Quinn, T. Thrombolysis in accident and emergency: the exception not the rule. Are we denying patients lifesaving treatment? Accid Emerg Nurs 1999; 7(1): 39–41.

Quinn T, MacDermott A, Caunt J. Determining patients' suitability for thrombolysis: coronary care nurses'

agreement with an expert cardiological 'gold-standard' as assessed by clinical and electrocardiographic 'vignettes'. Intensiv Crit Care Nurs 1998; 14(5): 219–224.

Riley J. The ECG: its role and practical application. In: Hatchett R, Thompson D, eds. Cardiac nursing. A comprehensive guide. Churchill Livingstone: Edinburgh; 2002.

Stokes H. Education and training towards competency for cardiac rehabilitation nursing in the UK. J Clin Nurs 2000; 1(3): 411–419.

Thow M, Isoud P, White M, Robertson I, Keith E, Armstrong G. Uptake and adherence of women post myocardial infarction to phase III cardiac rehabilitation: are things changing? Coronary Health Care 2000; 4(4): 174–178.

USEFUL ADDRESSES AND WEBSITES

Action on Smoking and Health (ASH)
109 Gloucester Place
London W1H 4EJ

British Association for Nursing in Cardiac Care
9 Fitzroy Square
London W1T 5HW
www.bcs.com/bancc

British Heart Foundation
14 Fitzhardinge Street
London W1H 4DH
www.bhf.org.uk

British Organ Donor Society
Balsham
Cambridge CB1 6DL
www.argonet.co.uk/body/

Cardiomyopathy Association
40 The Metro Centre
Tolpits Lane
Watford
Herts WD1 8SB

Coronary Prevention Group (CPG)
2 Taviton Street
London
WC1H 0BT
www.healthnet.org.uk

Health Development Agency
Trevelyan House
30 Great Peter Street
London SW1P 2HW
www.hda-online.org.uk

REFERENCES

Albarran J, Durham B, Chappel G, Dwight J, Owens J. Are manual gestures, verbal descriptors and pain radiation as reported by patients reliable indicators of myocardial infarction? Preliminary findings and implications. Intensiv Crit Care Nurs 2000; 16: 98–110.

Albarran J, Kapeluch H. Role of the nurse in thrombolytic therapy – expanding the clinical horizons. In: Cruickshank J, Bradbury M, Ashurst S, eds. Aspects of cardiovascular nursing. Dinton: Quay; 2000.

Alonzo A, Reynolds N. Responding to symptoms and signs of acute myocardial infarction – how do you educate the public? A social-psychological approach to intervention. Heart Lung 1997; 26(4): 263–272.

Apple S, Lindsay J. Principles and practice of interventional cardiology. Maryland: Lipincott Williams and Wilkins; 2000.

Autar R. Nursing assessment of clients at risk of deep vein thrombosis. The Autar DVT scale. J Adv Nurs 1996; 23(4): 763–770.

Barbiere C. Control of bleeding after transfemoral catheterisation. Crit Care Nurse 1995; 15: 51–53.

Bevans M, McLimore E. Intracoronary stents: a new approach to coronary artery dilation. J Cardiovasc Nurs 1992; 7(1): 34–49.

Bradley C. Drug therapy review: spironolactone in heart failure – new role for an old drug. Intensiv Crit Care Nurs 2000; 16(6): 403–404.

British Cardiac Society. Valvular heart disease: investigation and management. Recommendations. J Roy Coll Phys 1996; 30(4): 309–315.

Caunt J. The advanced nurse practitioner in CCU. Care Crit Ill 1996; 12(4): 136–139.

Cheitlin M, Sokolow M, Mcilroy M. Clinical cardiology. East Norwalk: Appleton Lange; 1993.

Chilcott S, Atkins P, Adamson R. Left ventricular assist as a viable alternative for cardiac transplantation. Crit Care Nurs Quart 1998; 20(4): 64–79.

Coats A, McGee H, Stokes H, Thompson D. BACR. Guidelines for cardiac rehabilitation. Oxford: Blackwell Science; 1995.

Curzio J, Kennedy S. Hypertension. In: Lindsay G, Gaw A, eds. Coronary heart disease prevention. A handbook for the health care team. Edinburgh: Churchill Livingstone; 1996.

Department of Health. Black report. A report of a Royal Commission on Health Inequalities. London: HMSO; 1978.

Department of Health. Saving lives: our healthier nation. London: The Stationery Office; 1999.

Department of Health. National service framework for coronary heart disease. Modern standards and service models. London: Department of Health; 2000.

Doughty D, Waldrop J, Ramundo J. Lower-extremity ulcers of vascular etiology. In: Bryant R. Acute and chronic wounds, 2nd edn. St Louis: Mosby; 2000.

Forbess L, Bashore T. Mechanical complications of myocardial infarction. Emerg Med 1996; 28: 26–46.

Geraghty S, Russell J, Gilbourne S, Young J. Deep vein thrombosis – aetiology and prevention. Nurs Times 2001; 97(17): 34–36.

Hanson L. Hypertension and concomitant disorders. London: Science Press; 1997.

Herbert L. Caring for the vascular patient. Edinburgh: Churchill Livingstone; 1997.

Hobbs F. The scale of heart failure: diagnosis and management issues for primary care. Heart 1999; 82(Suppl. IV): 8–10.

Hofgren C, Karlson B, Gaston-Johaansson F, Herltiz J. Word descriptors in suspected acute myocardial infarction: A comparison between patients with and without confirmed myocardial infarction. Heart Lung 1994; 23(5): 397–403.

Jensen G, Nyboe J, Appleyard M et al. Risk factors for acute myocardial infarction in Copenhagen II: smoking, alcohol intake, physical activity, obesity, oral contraception, diabetes, lipids, and blood pressure. Eur Heart J 1991; 12: 298–308.

Jowett N, Thompson D. Comprehensive coronary care, 2nd edn. London: Baillière Tindall; 1996.

Kern L. Management of postoperative atrial fibrillation. J Cardiovasc Nurs 1998; 12(3): 57–77.

Lewin B, Robertson I, Cay E, Irving J, Campbell M. Effects of self-help post myocardial infarction rehabilitation on psychological adjustment and use of health services. Lancet 1992; 389: 1036–1040.

MacConnachie A. Drug therapy review. Bupropion (Zyban) for smoking cessation. Intensiv Crit Care Nurs 2000; 16: 266.

McMurray J. Major beta blocker mortality trials in chronic heart failure: a critical review. Heart 1999; 82(Suppl. IV): 14–22.

Maglish B, Schwartz L, Matheny R. Outcomes improvement following minimally invasive direct coronary artery bypass surgery. Crit Care Clin North Am 1999; 11: 177–187.

Meluch F, Mitchell S. Decreasing intracoronary stent complications. Dimens Crit Care Nurs 1997; 16(13): 114–121.

Michalsen A, Konig G, Thimmes W. Preventable causative factors leading to hospital admission with decompensated heart failure. Heart 1998; 80: 437–441.

Morison M, Moffat C. A colour guide to the assessment and management of leg ulcers, 2nd edn. London: Mosby; 1994.

NICE. Angina (unstable) and coronary syndromes – glycoprotein IIb/IIIa inhibitors (No 12). National Institute for Excellence. Online. Available: www.nice.org.uk 2000.

NICE. Full guidance on the use of drugs for early thrombolysis in the treatment of acute myocardial infarction. (Guidance No 52). National Institute for Excellence. Online. Available: www.nice.org.uk 2002.

Nicol M, Bavin C, Bedford-Turner S, Cronin P, Rawlings-Anderson K. Essential nursing skills. London: Mosby; 2000.

Office for National Statistics (ONS). Mortality statistics: cause. Series DH2 no 25. London: HMSO; 1998.

Peterson S, Rayner M, Press V. Coronary heart disease statistics. British Heart Foundation Statistics Database 2000. London: British Heart Foundation; 2000.

Porterfield L, Morton P, Butze F. The evolution of internal defibrillators. Crit Care Clin North Am 1999; 11(3): 303–310.

Quinn T. Can nurses safely assess suitability for thrombolytic therapy? Intensiv Crit Care Nurs 1995; 11: 126–129.

Quinn T, Thompson D. Administration of thrombolytic therapy to patients with acute myocardial infarction. Accid Emerg Nurs 1995; 3(4): 208–214.

Ramsey L, Williams B, Johnston G et al. British Hypertension Society guidelines for hypertension management 1999: summary. Br Med J 1999; 319: 630–635.

Resuscitation Council (UK). Basic life support. Resuscitation guidelines. London: Resuscitation Council. Online. Available: www.resus.org.uk 2000a.

Resuscitation Council (UK). ALS manual, 4th edn. London: Resuscitation Council; 2000b.

Schilling R, Kaye G. Epidemiology and management of failed sudden cardiac death. Hosp Med 1998; 59(2): 116–119.

Talbot L, Meyers-Marquardt M. Pocket guide to critical care assessment, 3rd edn. St Louis: Mosby; 1997.

Taylor A. The effects of exercise training on patients with chronic heart failure. Coron Health Care 2000; 4(1): 10–16.

Wallis M, Autar R. Deep vein thrombosis: clinical nursing management. Nurs Stand 2001; 15(18): 47–54.

Windecker S, Meyer BJ, Bonzel T et al. Interventional cardiology in Europe 1994. Working group coronary circulation of the European Society of Cardiology. Eur Heart J 1998; 19(1): 40–54.

Woods S, Froelicher E, Underhill-Motzer S. Cardiac nursing, 4th edn. Philadelphia: Lippincott; 2000.

20 Nursing patients with respiratory disorders

Glenda Esmond

'We did oxygen therapy in the skills lab today and she told us to see what it feels like to have an oxygen mask on. I was surprised how quickly my mouth became dry and I couldn't hear very well because of the hissing noise. I was glad I only had to wear the thing for a few minutes. Now I have some idea what it feels like – and I'm not even breathless!'

(Student nurse)

THIS CHAPTER WILL HELP YOU

- Review the anatomy and physiology of the respiratory system
- Apply knowledge of disordered pathophysiology in clinical decision-making
- Understand the assessment skills required to plan respiratory care
- Understand the nursing care required for patients with respiratory disorders
- Identify and evaluate the psychological and social impact of chronic respiratory illness upon individuals, their family members and significant others
- Identify and evaluate strategies to promote respiratory treatment adherence
- Identify the function of specialist nurses and the interprofessional team in providing holistic respiratory care.

KEYWORDS

Bronchoconstriction	Hypoxia
Cor pulmonale	Hypoxic respiratory drive
Cyanosis	
Dyspnoea	Hypercapnia
Haemoptysis	Respiratory failure
Hypoxaemia	Ventilation

INTRODUCTION

Respiratory disease is a major cause of acute and chronic ill health, affecting approximately 8 million people and resulting in tens of thousands of deaths every year in the UK (British Lung Foundation 2000). The burden of respiratory disease on the National Health Service (NHS) is steadily increasing. It is the single most common reason why people consult their general practitioner (GP) and accounts for about 20% of all hospital admissions. The impact on the individual is more difficult to measure, although it has been recognized that disability is a frequent consequence of respiratory impairment.

ANATOMY AND PHYSIOLOGY – AN OVERVIEW

The respiratory system comprises the upper and lower airways and the thoracic cage (Fig. 20.1). The upper airway includes the nose, mouth, nasopharynx, oropharynx, laryngopharynx and larynx and has a protective role. The nasopharynx filters, warms and moistens the air before it enters the lungs, protecting the lung from exposure to microorganisms, toxic gases and particulates larger than 10 microns (μm) in diameter. Any particles that are deposited in the airways are propelled upwards towards the oropharynx by the mucociliary system. The mucus traps the particles and the cilia (microscopic hair-like projections) sweep the mucus upwards so that it can be expectorated. Ciliary movement can be impaired by tobacco smoke, pollution and excessive mucus production. The larynx protects the lower airways by closing during swallowing to prevent food entering the lower airways. It is also responsible for initiating the cough reflex, as it is sensitive to particles that cause irritation.

The lower airways include the trachea, bronchi, lungs, bronchioles (conducting air passages) and alveoli, which are small grape-like sacs that extend from alveolar ducts, responsible for the passage of gases between the lungs and the bloodstream. These structures work in combination with the thoracic cage, which includes the ribs, sternum and vertebrae, in affecting the exchange of oxygen and carbon dioxide in the lungs.

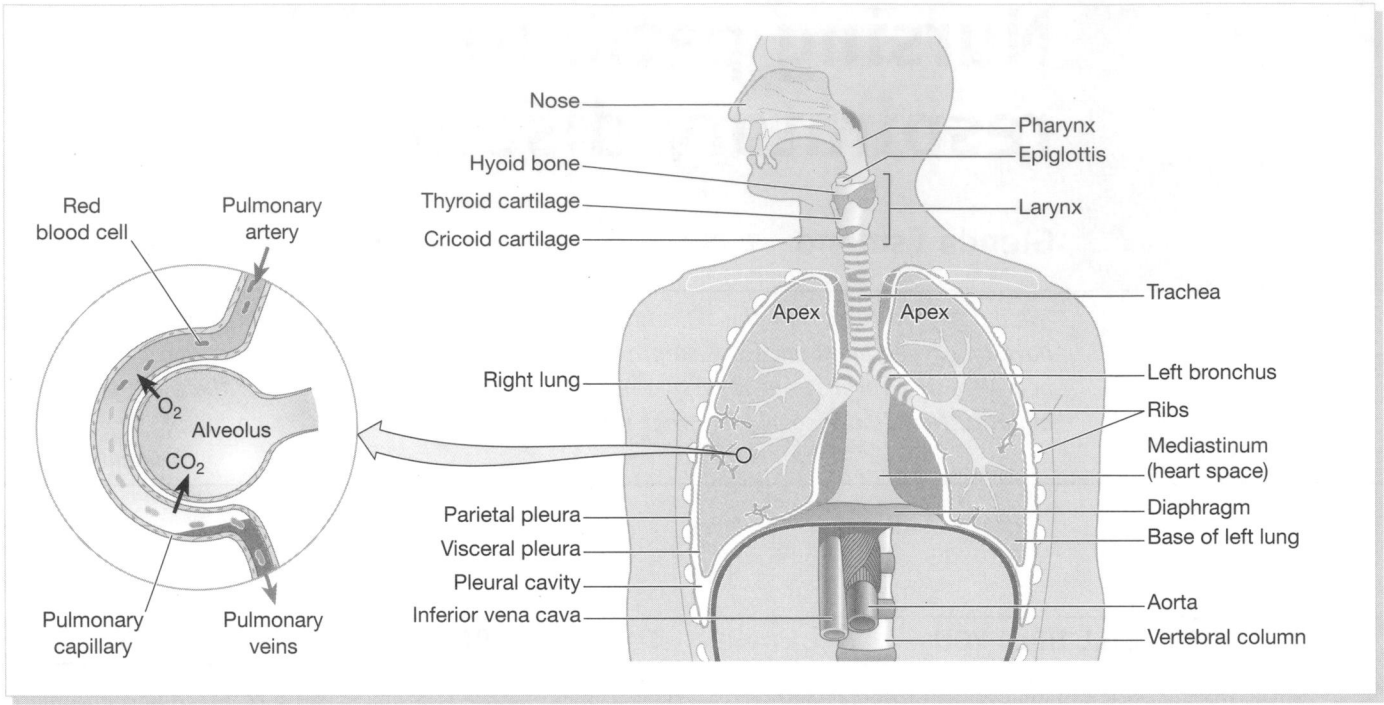

Figure 20.1 The respiratory system.

CONTROL OF BREATHING

The rate and depth of breathing, both mostly involuntary, are controlled by complex interactions between many physiological processes to allow an adequate exchange of oxygen and carbon dioxide.

Respiratory centre

The medullary respiratory centre, situated in the medulla oblongata, primarily controls breathing through stimulating the contraction of the diaphragm and the external intercostal muscles, which expand and contract the thoracic cavity. During inspiration, the diaphragm contracts and flattens, causing the thoracic cavity to lengthen, whilst the external intercostal muscles contract to expand the chest. This creates a negative intrapulmonary pressure. During expiration the diaphragm rises and the intercostal muscles relax, resulting in a positive intrapulmonary pressure. Air pressure differences allow the movement of air in and out of the lungs. All gases move from an area of higher pressure to one of lower pressure. During inspiration, air is drawn into the lungs, which then flows through the bronchi and into the bronchioles, alveolar ducts and alveolar sacs until it reaches the alveolar capillary membrane. The lungs are able to expand and move easily because the visceral pleura that lines the lungs and the parietal pleura that lines the mediastinum and chest wall create a potential space, known as the pleural cavity. It contains a small amount of lubricating fluid that allows easy movement between the pleura when the lungs expand.

Pulmonary stretch receptors

Pulmonary stretch receptors are located in the smooth muscle of the bronchi and bronchioles which respond to inspiration by sending impulses through the vagus nerve to the medullary respiratory centre when the lungs are filled with air, inhibiting further inflation of the lungs. This is known as the Hering–Breuer reflex and prevents over-inflation of the lungs.

Chemoreceptors

Peripheral chemoreceptors located in the aorta at the aortic arch (aortic body) and at the carotid bifurcation (carotid body) send impulses by sensory nerves to the medullary respiratory centre in response to a decrease in oxygen and pH, and an increase in carbon dioxide in the blood. The chemoreceptors in the carotid bodies are the main oxygen sensors and are stimulated to increase the breathing rate when there is a significant decrease in oxygen levels, i.e. below 90% or 8 kPa.

The normal stimulus to breathe is the rising level of carbon dioxide that easily crosses the blood–brain barrier into cerebrospinal fluid where it hydrates to form carbonic acid and then dissociates into bicarbonate and hydrogen ions. The hydrogen ions stimulate the central chemoreceptors in the medulla oblongata to send impulses to the medullary respiratory centre to increase the respiratory rate, thereby eliminating excess carbon dioxide.

GAS TRANSPORT

The main function of the respiratory system is the transfer of gases, principally oxygen and carbon dioxide. Gas transfer occurs by diffusion and includes the movement of oxygen from the alveolar capillary membrane to the mitochondria within the cells, and the movement of carbon dioxide from tissue capillaries to the alveolar capillary membrane. There are millions of alveoli, each surrounded by pulmonary capillaries and lined by a single layer of epithelium. This allows maximum gas exchange because the barrier between the gas in the alveoli and the blood in the capillaries is very thin (0.5 μm thick).

Oxygen transport

During inspiration, oxygen is taken into the lungs and passes down the trachea and bronchi and into the alveoli, where it comes into contact with the pulmonary circulation. Once the oxygen diffuses across the alveolar capillary membrane, it is carried in arterial blood to the heart and pumped around the body in two ways. Approximately 3% dissolves in the plasma, with the remaining 97% being carried in the red cells, bound to haemoglobin. Each haemoglobin molecule can reversibly bind (i.e. it can give it up again) four molecules of oxygen to form oxyhaemoglobin. The maximum amount of oxygen that can chemically combine with haemoglobin is called the oxygen capacity. The oxygen capacity plus the oxygen carried as dissolved oxygen is termed the oxygen content.

Carbon dioxide transport

Carbon dioxide, the waste product of metabolism, is transported in the blood in three forms: as dissolved carbon dioxide, as bicarbonate ions and as carbamino compounds (carbamino-haemoglobin). The carbon dioxide diffuses from the blood capillaries across the alveolar capillary membrane to the alveoli to be exhaled. Because of the properties of haemoglobin, the unloading of oxygen and the loading of carbon dioxide are reciprocal events. When the carbon dioxide levels rise, the affinity of haemoglobin for oxygen decreases.

Ventilation and perfusion

Adequate alveolar ventilation and perfusion are required for normal gas exchange. Alveolar ventilation ($\dot{V}$) is the volume of gas (approximately 4 litres) that reaches the alveoli per minute, while perfusion ($\dot{Q}$) is the amount of blood that flows through the pulmonary capillaries per minute (approximately 5 litres). The normal $\dot{V}/\dot{Q}$ ratio is 0.8, although this will change in various parts of the lung due to gravitational forces. In a healthy individual, these gravitational differences do not affect adequate gaseous exchange; however, in lung disease, the mismatch is wider and is the most common cause of low oxygen levels in arterial blood (hypoxaemia). With effective ventilation and perfusion, oxygen is able to diffuse from the alveoli into the blood to achieve a partial pressure (PaO_2) of between 10 and 13 kPa.

ACID–BASE BALANCE

The respiratory system also has an important role in maintaining acid–base balance. The regulation of acid–base balance is expressed as pH, which measures acidity and alkalinity, or hydrogen ion concentration (H^+) in the body. The normal pH of arterial blood is 7.35–7.45. A fall in pH (< 7.35) indicates an increase in hydrogen ions causing an acidosis. In respiratory disease this is due to raised carbon dioxide levels, caused by alveolar hypoventilation. This situation can be corrected through increasing ventilation, but if the respiratory acidosis continues, the action of buffers and the renal system will be activated to maintain homeostasis. Buffers (bicarbonate, proteins and phosphate) combine with the acid to prevent excessive

changes in hydrogen ion concentration. The kidneys contribute to the regulation of acid–base balance by increasing or decreasing the bicarbonate concentration. This is the most efficient mechanism, but it takes several hours or even days for the renal system to change the plasma bicarbonate level.

CAUSES AND PREDISPOSING FACTORS OF RESPIRATORY DISEASE

The most common causes of respiratory disease are:

- smoking
- allergens and trigger factors
- genetics
- microorganisms
- poverty.

SMOKING

Currently 28% of adult males and 26% of adult females in the UK are smokers, with a higher prevalence among teenagers, those in their early 20s and those in lower socioeconomic groups (Office of National Statistics 1998). The majority of smokers take up the habit as teenagers when there is often peer group pressure to smoke, and a third of teenage smokers go on to become lifelong smokers.

Tobacco smoke, which contains nicotine, tar, carbon monoxide and 4000 chemicals, is currently the leading cause of respiratory ill health and premature death. In susceptible individuals, smoking may affect the respiratory system and cause:

- lung cancer
- chronic bronchitis
- emphysema
- recurrent infections in the airways
- damage and loss of efficiency in the lungs.

Fletcher & Peto (1977) demonstrated that smoking accelerates the normal decline in lung function due to the ageing process from about 30 to 45 mL/year (Fig. 20.2). Disability can

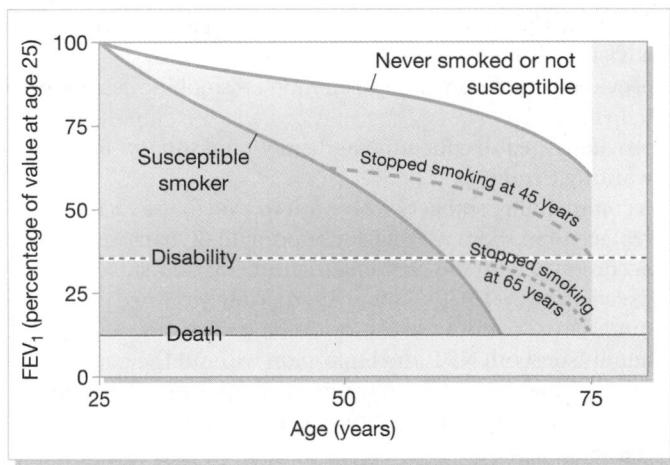

Figure 20.2 The effects of smoking on the decline in lung function. (Adapted with kind permission from Fletcher & Peto 1977.)

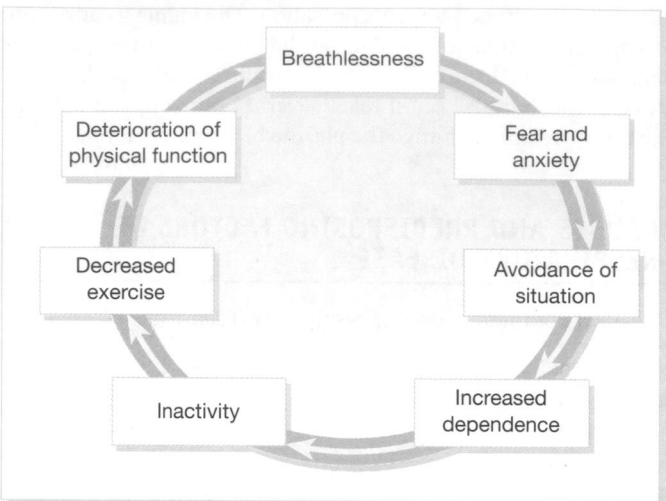

Figure 20.3 Vicious cycle of breathlessness.

be a consequence of this increased loss of lung function, as functional impairment can result in fatigue and breathlessness which impacts on the individual's ability to perform normal activities of daily living (ADL). Increased dependency on others often ensues, as there is a tendency to avoid activities that may provoke breathlessness. Williams (1990) describes this as the vicious cycle of breathlessness (Fig. 20.3), which, if not alleviated, will result in social isolation. Smoking cessation activities are aimed at preventing this accelerated decline in functional ability.

Smoking cessation

To reduce the incidence of respiratory disease it is necessary to discourage teenagers from starting smoking, and established smokers need to be encouraged, motivated and enabled to stop smoking. Evidence-based smoking cessation guidelines have been developed to assist health care professionals to develop smoking cessation strategies that fit in with the overall tobacco control (West et al 2000).

Nurses are in an ideal position to encourage and enable smokers to quit the habit through:

- assessing the smoking status of patients at every opportunity
- advising all smokers to stop smoking
- providing smokers with information on smoking cessation help lines
- providing health education and emotional support to those wanting to quit
- recommending smokers who want to stop to use nicotine replacement therapy (NRT) or bupropion (Zyban) in accordance with the National Institute for Clinical Excellence (2002) guidance. Appropriately trained nurses involved in smoking cessation clinics can administer both NRT and bupropion without the need for a doctor's prescription using a patient group direction (Department of Health 1999a). For NRT, nurse prescribing is also an option
- referring to specialist smoking cessation services if necessary.

Nicotine

Nicotine is absorbed into the bloodstream when tobacco smoke is inhaled, creating a physical dependence upon the drug. There can also be a psychological dependence, as smoking may be used as a means of coping with stress, boredom and anxiety. There are two aspects to smoking cessation: firstly, dealing with the nicotine addiction that causes withdrawal symptoms, consisting of agitation, insomnia, irritability, anger, anxiety, difficulty concentrating, restlessness and increased appetite; and secondly, dealing with the behavioural aspects of smoking, as it is a personal habit which may be linked to psychological stresses or social behaviour.

Nicotine replacement therapy

Nicotine replacement therapy has been shown to double the chances of success of smokers wishing to quit (West et al 2000), and provided that it is used in sufficient quantity and for a long enough period of time, it reduces the withdrawal symptoms. The dose needs to vary according to the number of cigarettes smoked, with heavy smokers requiring high doses of NRT initially. Manufacturer's instructions must be followed carefully to ensure that the correct dose is achieved. NRT is available as:

- nicotine skin patches
- nicotine gum
- Nicorette nasal spray
- Nicorette inhalator.

The delivery method of NRT is usually a matter of individual preference and should be discussed with the person intending to quit smoking.

Bupropion (Zyban)

Bupropion is an antidepressant that has been shown to reduce the nicotine withdrawal symptoms through desensitizing the brain's nicotine receptors (Jorenby et al 1999). There have been reports of side-effects that include seizures (estimated at less than 1 in 1000 risk), dry mouth, gastrointestinal problems, insomnia, tremor and headaches and therefore may not be suitable for some individuals. The National Institute of Clinical Excellence (2002) recommend bupropion as an alternative to NRT in adults, although careful history-taking to exclude contraindications (i.e. history of seizures or pregnancy) is required. There is insufficient evidence to support the use of a combination of bupropion and NRT.

Behavioural change

Smoking is a complex habit and dealing with the nicotine withdrawal alone may not be sufficient to quit. Emphasis needs to be placed on the psychological and social aspects of the habit as well as the management of the nicotine withdrawal symptoms if smoking cessation is to be achieved. The most commonly used approach to behavioural change for smoking cessation is based on the Prochaska & DiClemente (1984) change model, which assumes that the individual attempting to change behaviour will follow a series of stages:

- Pre-contemplation – is not interested in considering a change in behaviour

HEALTH PROMOTION

20.1 Quitting smoking

Percival (2001) identified that individuals are likely to succeed in stopping smoking if they are motivated and suggested that nurses can assist the smokers by:

- Finding out what the patient already knows and believes about lifestyle and health
- Developing a partnership with the patient in which the nurse acts as an expert who can help, whilst the patient remains in control of the choices concerning health
- Recognizing that not all patients are ready for change and many may need help to understand the impact their chosen lifestyle is having before overcoming their barriers to change
- Letting the patient decide what, when and how to change, and eliciting a commitment to change
- Tackling one aspect of behaviour at a time; this is usually more successful than trying to remove several risk factors simultaneously

- Facilitating the patient to develop an action plan with specific, achievable goals
- Building up patients' belief in their ability to succeed in achieving the goals they have set for themselves and providing support during the process.

Student activities

- Discuss with a smoker the reasons he or she smokes and identify what barriers there are for stopping smoking.
- Using the Prochaska & DiClemente (1984) change model, think of things that might help someone stop smoking for each of the stages and identify the skills required by the nurse to implement these strategies.

References

Percival J. Smoking and smoking cessation. In: Esmond G, ed. Respiratory nursing. Edinburgh: Baillière Tindall; 2001, ch 3.

Prochaska JO, DiClemente C. The transtheoretical approach: crossing traditional foundations of change. Homewood, IL: Don Jones/Irwin; 1984.

- Contemplation – is considering a change in behaviour but has not yet made the decision
- Preparation – has made a commitment to change behaviour but has not planned to do so
- Making a change – is implementing a plan that will change behaviour
- Maintenance – is continuing to make changes to behaviour and maintaining the healthier lifestyle.

Being able to assess a person's stage of change will allow the nurse to use appropriate strategies to help (see Health Promotion box 20.1).

GENETICS

There are a relatively small number of respiratory diseases that are a result of abnormal gene mutations:

- cystic fibrosis (see p. 550)
- chronic obstructive pulmonary disease caused by alpha-1-antitrypsin (1% of cases)
- bronchiectasis resulting from immunodeficiencies (see p. 552).

The other area of interest in genetics in relation to respiratory disease is in identifying the genetic factors that make some individuals more susceptible (see Ethical Issues box 20.1).

MICROORGANISMS

Microorganisms have two roles in respiratory disorders: they may cause the respiratory disease (e.g. pneumonia and tuberculosis); or they may exacerbate an underlying respiratory disease (e.g. asthma and COPD). These are discussed later in the chapter.

 ETHICAL ISSUES

20.1 Genetic screening

In the future, the ability to identify the genes that make individuals susceptible to respiratory ill health could be of benefit in preventative therapy, although some people may not wish to know of the possibility that illness may befall them.

- How much information would you like to be given about susceptibility to diseases that may not affect you for 10–20 years?
- How can the public be protected from discrimination (i.e. being unable to get life assurance) if a gene was found that makes them susceptible to a life-threatening condition in the future?

POVERTY

The prevalence of respiratory disease, particularly COPD, is higher amongst the lower socioeconomic groups. The main causative factor is the higher smoking rates amongst manual workers (Office of National Statistics 1997), but the association of low birthweight and reduced lung function is also an important factor. Maternal smoking, which is higher in lower socioeconomic groups, has been linked with low birthweight and recurrent respiratory infections in childhood. Poor housing and social deprivation have also been shown to be causative factors of respiratory illness.

Table 20.1 Allergen and trigger avoidance

Allergen/irritant	Avoidance management measures
House dust mite	Vacuuming regularly Wooden flooring better than carpet Open windows Mattresses and pillows should have a protective cover
Animals (i.e. cats, dogs)	Daily hoovering Keep pets from living areas and bedrooms Wash pets frequently Complete avoidance wherever possible
Outdoor (i.e. pollution, pollen)	Reduce exposure Stay indoors when there are high levels of allergens (e.g. pollen) reported and close windows Self-management of asthma medication
Viral infections	Flu vaccination Difficult to avoid but attempt to avoid visiting people if they have a 'cold' or 'flu'
Exercise	Include a warm-up and cool-down in routine Wear scarf over nose and mouth in cold weather Improve general fitness – helps exercise-induced bronchospasm Use bronchodilator inhaler prior to exercise
Tobacco smoke	Reduce smoking environments (e.g. pubs) Reduce exposure to passive smoking (e.g. ask people not to smoke in the house) Smoking cessation

ALLERGENS AND TRIGGER FACTORS

Allergens are the cause of extrinsic asthma, i.e. where an environmental cause can be identified, and tends to be associated with atopy (allergic reactions). Atopic individuals have high levels of immunoglobulins (IgE) and often suffer from related diseases such as eczema (see Ch. 28) and rhinitis (see Ch. 16). When there is a history of atopy, it is possible to determine the responsible allergen through skin prick or patch testing. Unlike allergens, trigger factors do not cause respiratory disease, but can exacerbate existing respiratory diseases such as asthma and chronic obstructive pulmonary disease (COPD).

Wherever possible, the offending allergen or trigger factor should be avoided; however, this is not always possible and in these cases exposure should be reduced and symptoms controlled using medication to treat bronchoconstriction (narrowing of the airways). Table 20.1 identifies common allergens and trigger avoidance measures.

NURSING ASSESSMENT OF RESPIRATORY STATUS

The assessment of respiratory status is important in determining the severity of the respiratory problem in order to prioritize care. During the acute phase of respiratory illness (i.e. acute asthma 'attack' or acute infective exacerbation of COPD), the emphasis is placed on physiological assessment in order to detect life-threatening situations that require immediate treatment. However, the impact of the respiratory problem on the activities of daily living as a consequence of breathlessness, and the psychosocial aspects are equally important if the patient and family are to cope with the consequences of chronic respiratory illness. Respiratory assessment requires observation,

communication and clinical skills and should include assessment of physiological factors, mental state, causative factors, symptoms, impact on ADLs and psychosocial factors (see Guidelines for Care Priorities box 20.1).

PHYSIOLOGICAL ASSESSMENT

Physiological assessment should include assessment of the following.

Respiratory rate, rhythm and depth

Normal breathing should be regular and appear effortless with a respiratory rate in adults between 12 and 20 breaths/min. The majority of patients with underlying respiratory disease will have an elevated respiratory rate (> 20 breaths/min) to facilitate adequate oxygenation and ventilation. Respiratory depression (< 12 breaths/min) may occur due to exhaustion and fatigued respiratory muscles caused by the work of breathing. The use of sedatives and opioid analgesics may also cause respiratory depression. Observation of the rhythm and depth of breathing should be assessed, as this will indicate the quality of each breath. Slow, shallow breathing is a sign of respiratory depression and indicates that there is an insufficient number and quality of breaths to sustain adequate ventilation. Equally, a rapid, irregular breathing pattern that does not allow expansion of the lower lobes of the lungs will also result in ventilatory failure.

Chest movement

The chest movement should be symmetrical and is best observed by standing in front of the patient rather than to one side. If one side of the chest is not expanding as well as the other, this may indicate a collapsed lung due to pneumothorax (air in the pleural space) or the presence of bronchial obstruction. The

GUIDELINES FOR CARE PRIORITIES

20.1 Respiratory assessment

This involves assessment of the following:

Physiological
- Respiratory rate (normal adult 12–20/min)
- Breathing rhythm and depth
- Are accessory muscles being used?
- Skin colour – is there cyanosis?
- Oxygen saturation (normal 95%+)
- Smoking history
- Triggers
- Peak expiratory flow rate (peak flow)
- Cough (productive/dry)
- Chest tightness/wheeze
- Chest pain/ache/soreness
- Is the patient disorientated/confused?
- Sputum colour, viscosity and volume
- Fluid retention/presence of oedema
- Temperature, blood pressure and pulse

Impact of breathlessness on activities of living
- Identify deficits
- Mobility
- Nutrition

Psychosocial
- The patient's perception/concerns
- Housing
- Community support

patient's use of accessory muscles in the neck and shoulders (the sternocleidomastoid and trapezius muscles) should also be observed as this indicates that the patient is unable to use the diaphragm and external intercostal muscles sufficiently to maintain ventilation.

Oxygen levels

Observation of skin colour and pulse oximetry will indicate whether the patient is receiving adequate oxygenation. The patient's skin should be observed for blueness of the lips, tongue and oral mucosa, as this indicates the presence of central cyanosis caused by hypoxaemia (low oxygen levels in arterial blood). In patients with dark skin, it may not be possible to see changes in lip colour and therefore the oral mucosa and tongue should always be examined. Hypoxaemia will also be detected through performing pulse oximetry as this will detect oxygen saturation levels outside the normal limits of 95–100%. When examining the skin, the presence of peripheral oedema should be noted as this may indicate cor pulmonale (right ventricular hypertrophy and failure) due to vasoconstriction of the pulmonary circulation as a result of local hypoxia in the lungs. Another sign of chronic tissue hypoxia is finger clubbing, which is where the terminal phalanges of the fingers become enlarged and the base of the nail feels spongy.

MENTAL STATE

Respiratory assessment should include assessment of mental state, because confusion and disorientation may be a sign of severe hypoxia resulting in a reduced supply of oxygen to the brain. Asking relatives and friends if they have noticed a change in mental state may be helpful when the nurse has not previously known the patient. The patient's level of alertness also needs to be assessed as drowsiness may indicate hypercapnia (raised levels of carbon dioxide in arterial blood).

CAUSATIVE FACTORS

Causative factors that influence the patient's respiratory health status, such as allergens, the environment and smoking, should be identified so that potential health education strategies can be implemented. As smoking is a major cause of respiratory illness, a thorough smoking history should include current and past smoking habits, with the total pack-years of smoking being estimated. One pack of 20 cigarettes smoked per day for 1 year is equal to one pack-year. Assessing the patient's present and past occupations may indicate exposure to toxic substances, such as asbestos and industrial chemicals. Through identifying exposure as the causative factor of respiratory disease, the patient and their family may be eligible for compensation.

SYMPTOMS

The most common symptom associated with respiratory disease is breathlessness, although cough and wheeze, often described by patients as chest tightness and muscular chest pain, can be equally troublesome. Through assessing symptoms at regular intervals, it is possible to monitor treatment effectiveness. Assessment for the presence of infection is important as it causes much respiratory disease, such as pneumonia and tuberculosis. A raised temperature and pulse rate, a raised white blood cell count, positive blood cultures and a productive cough with yellow or green sputum (see p. 553) indicate the presence of infection.

IMPACT ON ACTIVITIES OF DAILY LIVING

Assessing the impact of breathlessness on all the activities of daily living (ADL) will allow the nurse to plan care more effectively, identifying the need for referral to occupational therapy, physiotherapy, dietetics and social services as appropriate. Particular attention to mobility and nutritional status is essential, as breathlessness has been shown to cause immobility as well as malnutrition due to increased energy requirements and poor appetite (Margereson & Esmond 1997). Patients with underlying respiratory disease should be observed for increasing breathlessness and oxygen desaturation (lowering of oxygen levels) on exertion, as this may indicate the need for supplemental oxygen to prevent complications of immobility. Assessment of the patient's nutritional status should include body mass index (BMI, see Ch. 11), identification of recent significant weight loss, eating habits and changes in appetite. Patients found to have a BMI less than 20 or a recent weight loss greater than 10% should be referred to a dietician.

PSYCHOSOCIAL FACTORS

The chronic nature of much respiratory disease can affect a patient's psychological state and relationships with family and friends. Through assessing the patient's perceptions and concerns, coping strategies, such as relaxation techniques to alleviate fear and anxiety or activity pacing to allow greater mobility, can be identified to assist with adaptation to chronic respiratory illness. The introduction of nurse-led clinics, usually run by practice nurses or respiratory nurse specialists, has assisted those suffering from chronic respiratory illness to feel at ease discussing psychosocial issues. This is usually achieved through the nurse building a therapeutic trusting relationship with patients over a period of time so that a profile of perceptions and concerns can be developed. Consideration of current social issues and need for referral to social services or community nursing should be continually assessed so that interventions can be identified at the earliest opportunity.

RESPIRATORY INVESTIGATIONS

The symptoms of breathlessness, wheeze, chest tightness and cough can be associated with many different respiratory conditions. Respiratory investigations are used to determine the cause of respiratory symptoms, allowing appropriate treatment to be commenced, to monitor disease progression, and assess treatment effectiveness. The most commonly used respiratory investigations are respiratory function tests, pulse oximetry, chest X-ray, sputum microscopy, culture and sensitivity, and bronchoscopy.

RESPIRATORY FUNCTION TESTS

Respiratory function tests assess the functioning of the lungs through measuring flow rates and lung volumes. Although there are many different tests available to diagnose and monitor treatment and lung disease, the most commonly used respiratory function tests are peak expiratory flow rate (PEFR), forced expiratory volume in 1 second (FEV_1) and forced vital capacity (FVC).

Peak expiratory flow rate

Peak expiratory flow rate (commonly referred to as 'peak flow') is measured in litres per minute (L/min) and is an objective measure that detects airflow obstruction in the larger airways. If the airways are narrowed then the rate of expiration is limited and the PEFR will be lower than the predicted normal value for the person's age, height and sex. Measurement of PEFR is an integral part of the self-management of asthma; it is also used in acute asthma to monitor response to treatment, through comparing the PEFR before and after bronchodilator therapy. An increase in PEFR after bronchodilator therapy will indicate that opening of airways (bronchodilation) has occurred. PEFR is simple to measure using a Wright peak flow or mini-Wright peak flow meter. To ensure the measurement is accurate, patients must be taught how to perform the test (Fig. 20.4). Patients must be standing or sitting in an upright position and are required to make a seal with their lips around

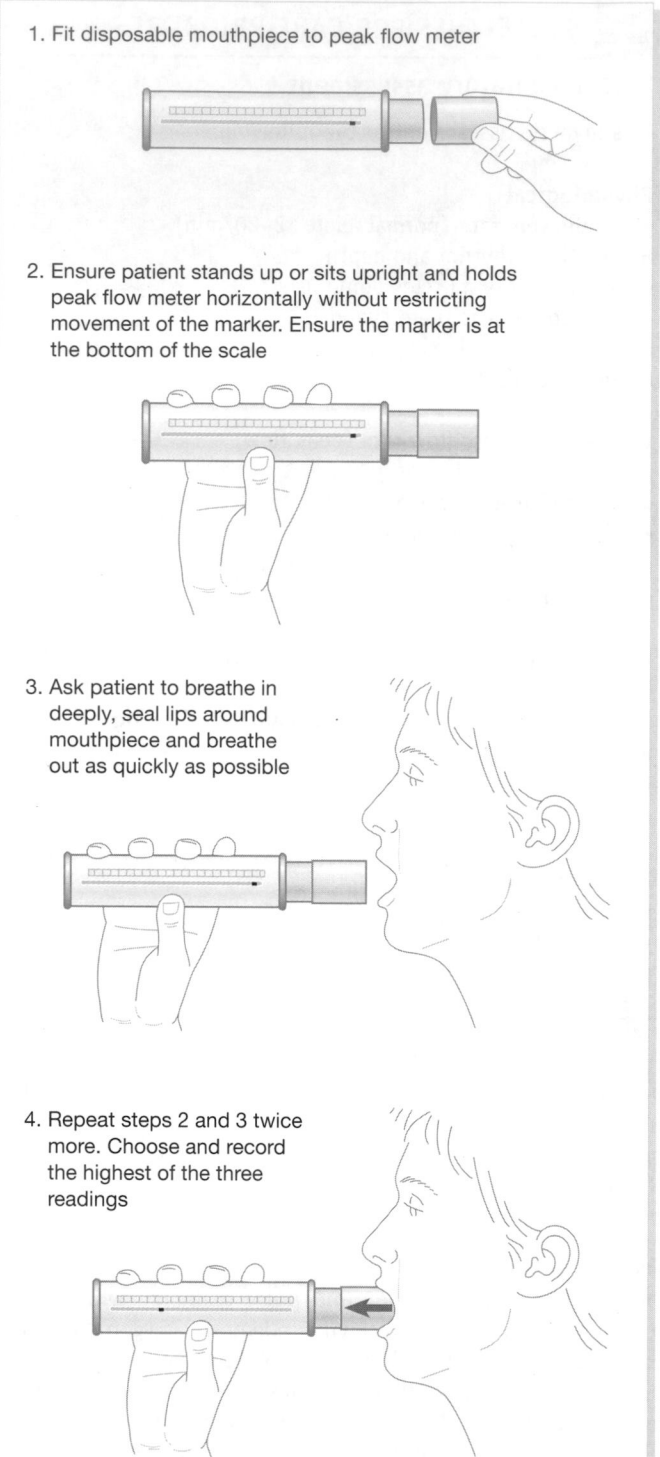

1. Fit disposable mouthpiece to peak flow meter

2. Ensure patient stands up or sits upright and holds peak flow meter horizontally without restricting movement of the marker. Ensure the marker is at the bottom of the scale

3. Ask patient to breathe in deeply, seal lips around mouthpiece and breathe out as quickly as possible

4. Repeat steps 2 and 3 twice more. Choose and record the highest of the three readings

Figure 20.4 Measuring peak expiratory flow rate (PEFR) using a peak flow meter.

the mouthpiece before exhaling forcibly. The test is repeated three times and the highest result recorded.

FEV_1 and FVC

The forced expiratory volume in 1 second determines the amount of air that is exhaled in the first second of a forced expiration. FVC is the total amount of air exhaled from maximal inspiration to maximal expiration. A spirometer is the instrument used to measure FEV_1 and FVC and can detect obstructive patterns of breathing which occur in asthma, COPD, cystic fibrosis and bronchiectasis; and restrictive patterns of breathing due to fibrosing alveolitis, sarcoidosis, asbestosis, kyphoscoliosis and muscular dystrophies.

Reversibility testing

Respiratory function tests can also be used to determine the extent to which airflow obstruction can be reversed with bronchodilators. The respiratory function test is performed before and fifteen minutes after administration of a bronchodilator, and the two results compared. An increase in FEV_1 or PEFR of greater than 15% is representative of a positive response and indicates the presence of asthma. This is not the case in COPD where the airflow is fixed and the respiratory function test will either show limited (< 15%) or no reversibility following bronchodilators.

NURSING ROLE IN RESPIRATORY FUNCTION TESTS

The nurse is in an ideal position to prepare patients for and support them during and after respiratory function tests by ensuring that:

- the procedure is explained to patients and any concerns addressed
- patients are not wearing restrictive clothing
- patients are made aware that the test is performed in an upright sitting position
- patients have not recently had a meal as abdominal distension may restrict diaphragmatic movement
- loose dentures or chewing gum are removed
- patients have emptied their bladder and are comfortable before the test is performed
- pain is controlled as this can inhibit patients taking a deep breath.

PULSE OXIMETRY

Pulse oximetry is a simple, non-invasive way of measuring peripheral oxygen saturation of arterial blood (SaO_2) to determine whether the values are within the normal range (95–100%). A probe consisting of a small light-emitting diode on one side and a light detector on the other is placed on the patient's finger. The technique works because of the light-absorbing characteristics of haemoglobin (see Ch. 9). In hypoxaemia, the 'blueness' of the blood will be measured by the pulse oximeter. Although clearly useful, pulse oximetry has its limitations. It is unable to detect changes in carbon dioxide levels (Bateman & Leach 1998) and produces inaccurate readings at saturation levels below 82% (Carter 1998), so may not be reliable in severe respiratory disease. Inaccurate readings may also be due to a number of other factors. These include:

- peripheral vasoconstriction
- anaemia

- high bilirubin blood levels
- movement (i.e. shivering or fitting)
- nail varnish/false nails
- blockage of the light detector
- dark skin pigment
- intravenous dyes
- severe hypoxaemia
- high levels of carboxyhaemoglobin due to smoking
- exposure to carbon monoxide.

CHEST X-RAY

Chest X-ray is a valuable aid to diagnosis of respiratory disease and will show the lung fields, pleura, rib cage, diaphragm shape and size of the heart. Chest X-ray is usually performed when patients present with persistent cough, chest pain, unexplained breathlessness, haemoptysis (coughing up blood), weight loss and pyrexia. Respiratory abnormalities found using chest X-rays include:

- over-inflated lung field – may be found in people with severe asthma or COPD
- consolidation or shadowing indicating infection
- specific shadowing that may indicate a primary or secondary tumour
- cavities that may indicate active tuberculosis (TB)
- calcification that may indicate that patients have previously suffered TB although it is not presently active
- pneumothorax (air in the pleural cavity)
- pleural effusion (fluid in the pleural cavity).

SPUTUM

The diagnosis of respiratory infections can be achieved through microbiological analysis of sputum. A specimen of muco-purulent or purulent sputum, not saliva, should be collected in a sterile container, to prevent contamination, prior to antibiotic therapy being commenced. Sputum should never be left for long periods before being transferred to a laboratory, otherwise an overgrowth with Gram-negative organisms may occur. Patients should be asked to rinse their mouth before the specimen is obtained to prevent contamination of the sputum with food, which renders it unusable by the laboratory. The laboratory will perform microscopy, culture and sensitivity to antibiotics. Sputum will contain causative microorganisms in patients with:

- pneumonia
- tuberculosis
- infective exacerbation of chronic bronchitis
- cystic fibrosis and bronchiectasis.

Observation of sputum

The observation of sputum colour, viscosity, odour and amount is vital in order to monitor the effectiveness of antibiotic treatment. Patients who are producing sputum require:

- a sputum pot with a lid, as swallowing the sputum may cause nausea. Expectorating into a tissue can increase the risk of cross-infection as tissues are often re-used and left lying around

- tissues to allow patients to wipe excess secretions from their mouth and nose
- mouthwash/mouth care as sputum is often foul tasting
- encouragement with fluid intake as dehydration will increase the viscosity of the sputum.

BRONCHOSCOPY

Flexible fibreoptic bronchoscopy is an invasive procedure that is commonly used to diagnose:

- lung cancer
- tuberculosis
- pneumonia and other respiratory infections.

Bronchoscopy and related procedures (lung biopsy, brushing and lavage) are usually performed under sedation and local anaesthetic to the throat. Sedatives, such as midazolam, may cause respiratory depression, hypoventilation and hypotension, and local anaesthetics applied to the throat may lead to laryngospasm and bronchospasm Therefore, patients need careful monitoring during the procedure and for 6–8 hours afterwards as bronchoscopy can cause bronchospasm, hypoxaemia, fever, pneumonia, pneumothorax and haemorrhage. On discharge, patients should be given information (usually a post-bronchoscopy leaflet) explaining how they should feel during the first 12 hours and detailing what to do if prevailing symptoms worsen or new symptoms develop. The proven safety of bronchoscopy must not lead to complacency when caring for these patients. It is not usually necessary to admit patients to hospital following bronchoscopy unless significant post-bronchoscopic bleeding, pneumothorax and/or respiratory distress occur.

COMMON RESPIRATORY DISORDERS

ASTHMA

Asthma is a chronic inflammatory condition that results in narrowing of the airways caused by inflammation and bronchoconstriction.

Epidemiology

Asthma is one of the most common respiratory conditions, affecting aproximately 1 in 13 adults in the UK (National Asthma Campaign 2001). The prevalence of asthma has steadily increased over the last 25 years and accounts for aprroximately 40 000 hospital admissions each year. It is estimated that asthma prescriptions account for 10% of the total NHS spending on drugs and that around 17 million working days are lost due to asthma (British Lung Foundation 1996). Although death rates from asthma are slowly declining, there are still 1 500 people who die from asthma, a third of whom are people under the age of 65 years.

Pathophysiology

The narrowing of the airways (Fig. 20.5) is usually reversible, although in some patients with chronic asthma, the inflammatory process can result in damage to the protective endothelial layer, smooth muscle hypertrophy and mucus plugging, leading to irreversible air flow obstruction.

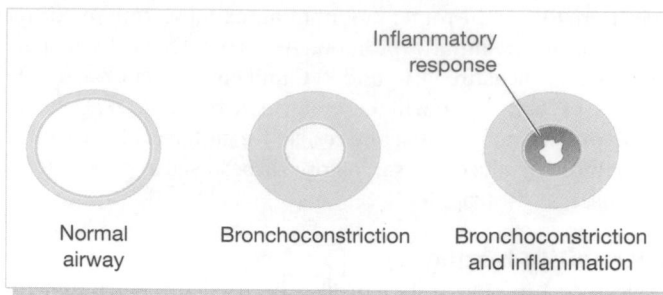

Figure 20.5 Changes in the airways as a result of asthma.

The symptoms produced in response to the narrowing of the airways are:

- inspiratory wheeze
- dry non-productive cough
- dyspnoea
- chest tightness.

Treatment options for asthma

The aim of treatment is to control symptoms and prevent asthma 'attacks', and it therefore needs to be targeted at prevention and control of inflammation and bronchoconstriction. The *British Guidelines on Asthma Management* (British Thoracic Society/SIGN 2003) recommend a stepwise approach that corresponds to the severity of asthma based on symptoms and peak flow measurements (see Guidelines for Care Priorities box 20.2). The main treatments used to control asthma are bronchodilators and corticosteroids.

GUIDELINES FOR CARE PRIORITIES

20.2 Stepwise asthma management

The British Thoracic Society/SIGN (2003) guidelines on asthma use a stepwise approach to asthma management. Patients are started at the step most appropriate to the severity of their condition and treatment should be stepped up as necessary to achieve asthma control. Stepping down should also be considered if treatment has been stepped up to alleviate symptoms during an exacerbation (e.g. respiratory infection or allergen exposure).

- *Step 1* – inhaled short-acting β_2 agonist (e.g. salbutamol) as required
- *Step 2* – add inhaled corticosteroid < 800 µg/day for adults (e.g. beclomethasone)
- *Step 3* – add long-acting β_2 agonist (e.g. salmeterol)
- *Step 4* – add any or all of the following to control asthma:
  — increase inhaled corticosteroids to < 2000 µg/day
  — long-acting β_2 agonist
  — leukotriene receptor antagonist (e.g. montelukast or zafirlukast)
  — methylxanthine (e.g. theophylline)
- *Step 5* – daily oral corticosteroid (e.g. prednisolone) or regular booster courses of oral steroids

Bronchodilators

Beta-2 agonists or sympathomimetic bronchodilators exert their effect on the beta-receptors and, by mimicking the actions of adrenaline (epinephrine), relax the smooth muscle of the airways. The most commonly used bronchodilators are the short-acting β_2 agonists, such as salbutamol and terbutaline. These act as 'relievers' and provide quick relief of symptoms, with the peak bronchodilator effect being reached within 15 minutes and a duration of action of approximately 6 hours. If symptoms persist, particularly at night, a long-acting β_2 agonist, such as salmeterol, may be introduced as the duration of action is 12 hours. Other classes of bronchodilator are also used, namely methylxanthines (theophylline) and muscarinic antagonists (ipratropium bromide and oxitropium bromide). These work by opposing the effects of acetylcholine neurotransmitters and blocking the cholinergic reflex of the vagus nerve that causes bronchospasm in some asthmatic patients.

Corticosteroids

Corticosteroids such as beclomethasone, budesonide and fluticasone can be given by the inhaled route, orally or intravenously to treat asthma. They act as a 'preventer' by reducing the inflammatory response of the airways provided they are taken continuously. The inhaled route is the preferred route of delivery as the systemic effect is minimal and there are fewer side-effects (e.g. osteoporosis, diabetes, weight gain and increased body hair) that can occur with prolonged use of oral steroids (2 months or more).

During episodes of acute asthma, inhaled corticosteroids may be insufficient to control the symptoms as only 10–25% of the drug reaches the respiratory tract. In these circumstances, oral prednisolone or intravenous hydrocortisone may be needed. Although the side-effects of inhaled corticosteroids are less severe (hoarseness and oral candidiasis), it is important to remember that if the powder is deposited on the back of the throat and then swallowed, systemic side-effects will occur. This can be reduced by using a large-volume spacer (Fig. 20.6A), a dry powder device, such as the turbohaler (Fig. 20.6B), or a breath-actuated device, such as the Easi-breathe (Fig. 20.6C), to deliver the corticosteroid. In addition, patients should be advised to rinse their mouth after inhalation.

Leukotriene antagonists

Cells involved in the pathogenesis of airway inflammation produce cysteinyl leukotrienes that can cause an inflammatory response in bronchial asthma. Leukotriene antagonists (montelukast and zafirlukast) represent a new class of drugs for the treatment of mild to moderate asthma. They are used to block the effects of the released cysteinyl leukotrienes that cause bronchoconstriction, plasma exudation, mucous secretion and possibly inflammation in bronchial asthma. A major advantage of leukotriene antagonists is that the drugs are available in oral form which may improve adherence to treatment.

ACUTE SEVERE ASTHMA

It is important that patients and nurses are able to detect acute severe asthma (previously called status asthmaticus), as delay in recognizing deterioration may be fatal. Box 20.1 outlines the symptoms of acute asthma and classifies them into acute severe asthma, life-threatening asthma and near fatal asthma.

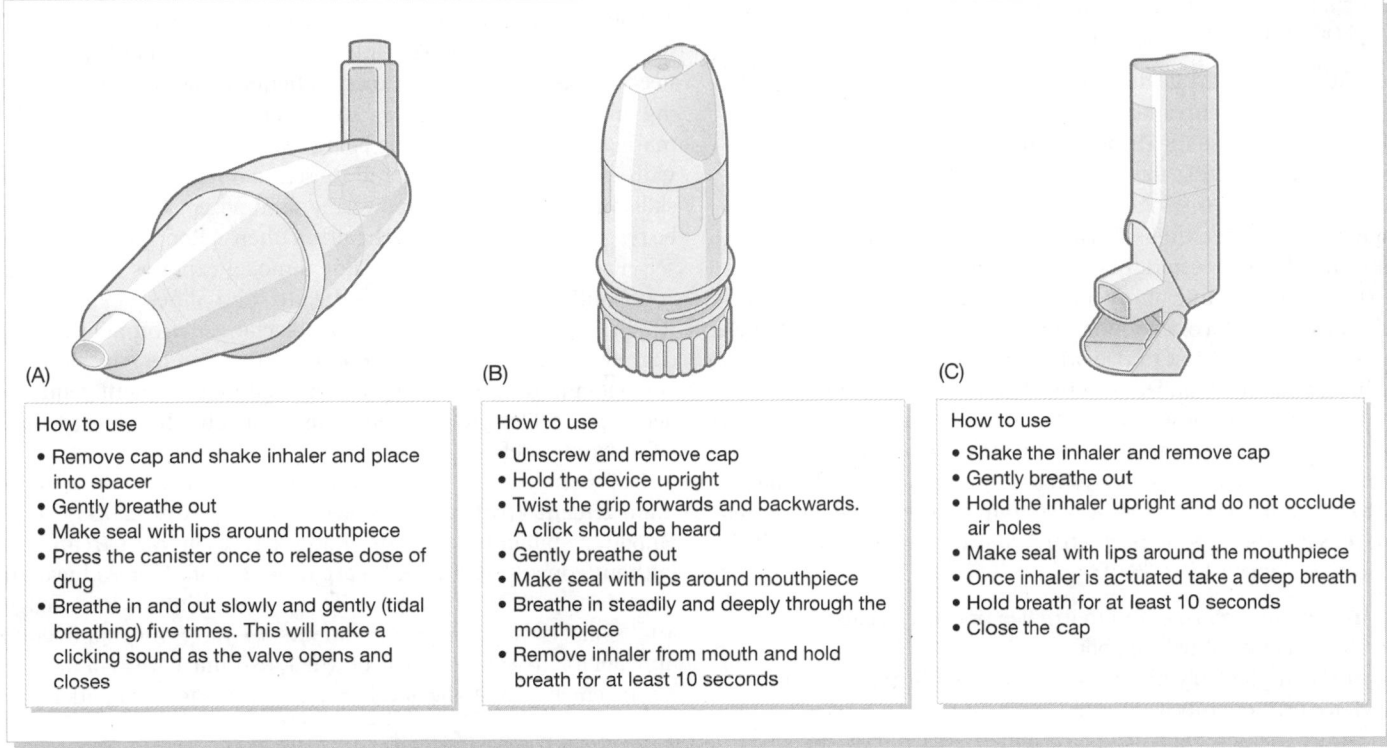

(A)

How to use
- Remove cap and shake inhaler and place into spacer
- Gently breathe out
- Make seal with lips around mouthpiece
- Press the canister once to release dose of drug
- Breathe in and out slowly and gently (tidal breathing) five times. This will make a clicking sound as the valve opens and closes

(B)

How to use
- Unscrew and remove cap
- Hold the device upright
- Twist the grip forwards and backwards. A click should be heard
- Gently breathe out
- Make seal with lips around mouthpiece
- Breathe in steadily and deeply through the mouthpiece
- Remove inhaler from mouth and hold breath for at least 10 seconds

(C)

How to use
- Shake the inhaler and remove cap
- Gently breathe out
- Hold the inhaler upright and do not occlude air holes
- Make seal with lips around the mouthpiece
- Once inhaler is actuated take a deep breath
- Hold breath for at least 10 seconds
- Close the cap

Figure 20.6 Inhaler delivery devices. (A) Metered dose inhaler (MDI) with spacer. (B) Dry powder device – Turbohaler. (C) Breath-actuated devices – Easi-breathe.

Box 20.1 Levels of severity of acute asthma

Moderate asthma exacerbation
- Increasing symptoms
- PEFR > 50% best or predicted
- No features of acute severe asthma

Acute severe asthma
- PEFR 33–50% best or predicted
- Respiratory rate > 25/min
- Heart rate > 110/min
- Severe dyspnoea
- Inability to complete sentences in one breath

Life-threatening asthma
- PEFR < 33% best or predicted – bradycardia
- SaO_2 < 92%, PaO_2 < 8 kPa – dysrhythmia and hypotension
- Chest silent – exhaustion
- Cyanosis – confusion
- Feeble respiratory rate – coma

Near fatal asthma
- Symptoms of life-threatening asthma
- Raised $PaCO_2$ and/or requiring ventilation

The aim of treatment is to prevent hypoxia and to reduce bronchoconstriction and inflammation of the airway and therefore patients will immediately require:

- high-flow oxygen (40–60%)
- nebulized bronchodilators delivered via an oxygen supply (6–8 L/min)
- oral prednisolone (40–60 mg) or intravenous hydrocortisone (100 mg) (British Thoracic Society/SIGN 2003).

Patients with an acute exacerbation of their asthma *must* be given high concentrations of oxygen (40–60%) using a high-flow mask, such as the Hudson or non-rebreathing mask. Unlike patients with COPD there is little risk of precipitating hypercapnia ($PaCO_2$ > 6.0 kPa) with high-flow oxygen. Hypercapnia may occur due to exhaustion and fatigue of respiratory muscles, and may lead to respiratory arrest if not reversed. Beta-2 agonists and muscarinic antagonists in high doses will be administered to ensure bronchoconstriction is alleviated as quickly as possible. The decision to use oral or intravenous corticosteroids will depend on the patients' clinical state.

Unfortunately, despite the introduction of asthma guidelines and increased awareness of treatment of acute asthma, 1500 people die in the UK each year (National Asthma Campaign 2001). There are several factors that have been identified as increasing the risk of premature death from asthma (British Thoracic Society/SIGN 2003):

- inadequate treatment with inhaled or oral steroids – as asthma control will be poor
- non-compliance with treatment and monitoring – as signs of deterioration may be ignored
- failure to attend appointments and self-discharge – may indicate denial about the life-threatening consequences of uncontrolled asthma

- mental health problems, including psychiatric illness, current or recent tranquillizer use, deliberate self-harm and alcohol or drug abuse
- learning disabilities – because symptoms are often under-reported.

It is important, when assessing patients with acute asthma, to consider whether there are any additional risk factors so that discharge planning can be as effective as possible. For example, early discharge would not be appropriate for high-risk patients as they are unlikely to complete the course of treatment.

▶ Nursing management: asthma

The role of the nurse in asthma care will depend on the severity of the patient's symptoms. The majority of people with asthma are cared for by practice nurses in the community who provide preventative asthma care. This is achieved by monitoring peak flow rates, checking inhaler technique, providing allergy avoidance advice and developing patient self-management plans. Acute asthma care, which is discussed later in this chapter, usually requires care from accident and emergency nurses, medical/respiratory ward nurses and, in some cases, critical care nurses. Asthma/respiratory nurse specialists should be involved with discharge planning as they provide liaison between primary and secondary carers to ensure that continuity of care is achieved. They will also follow up severe asthmatic patients in nurse-led asthma clinics where they provide education and support in developing individualized self-management plans.

Self-management plans

The UK government's white paper, *Saving Lives: Our Healthier Nation* (Department of Health 1999b), outlines a self-management strategy for people with chronic illness, identifying the need for them to become 'expert patients' by actively participating in the management of their care. The concept of self-management is increasingly being used to help patients to cope with their chronic illness, and therefore nurses need to develop skills in enabling and empowering, and accept that people can be responsible for their own health. Cohen & Rodriguez's (1995) self-management of chronic illness model explores dimensions contributing to the patient's health and illness experience, which include the physiological, social, environmental and cognitive (i.e. beliefs, perceptions and attitudes) influences. For patients to make choices about self-management requires decisions on lifestyle preferences, informed by their knowledge, values and beliefs.

Self-management has become an integral part of asthma management (British Thoracic Society/SIGN 2003) and empowers patients to make changes to their own treatment without consulting a health care professional. Nurses have an important patient education role, as acquisition of knowledge and skills is necessary for patients to have the confidence and ability to take control of their asthma care. For a self-management plan to be developed it is necessary that patients:

- have knowledge of the disease process
- are able to perform and interpret peak flow measurements
- are able to recognize symptoms

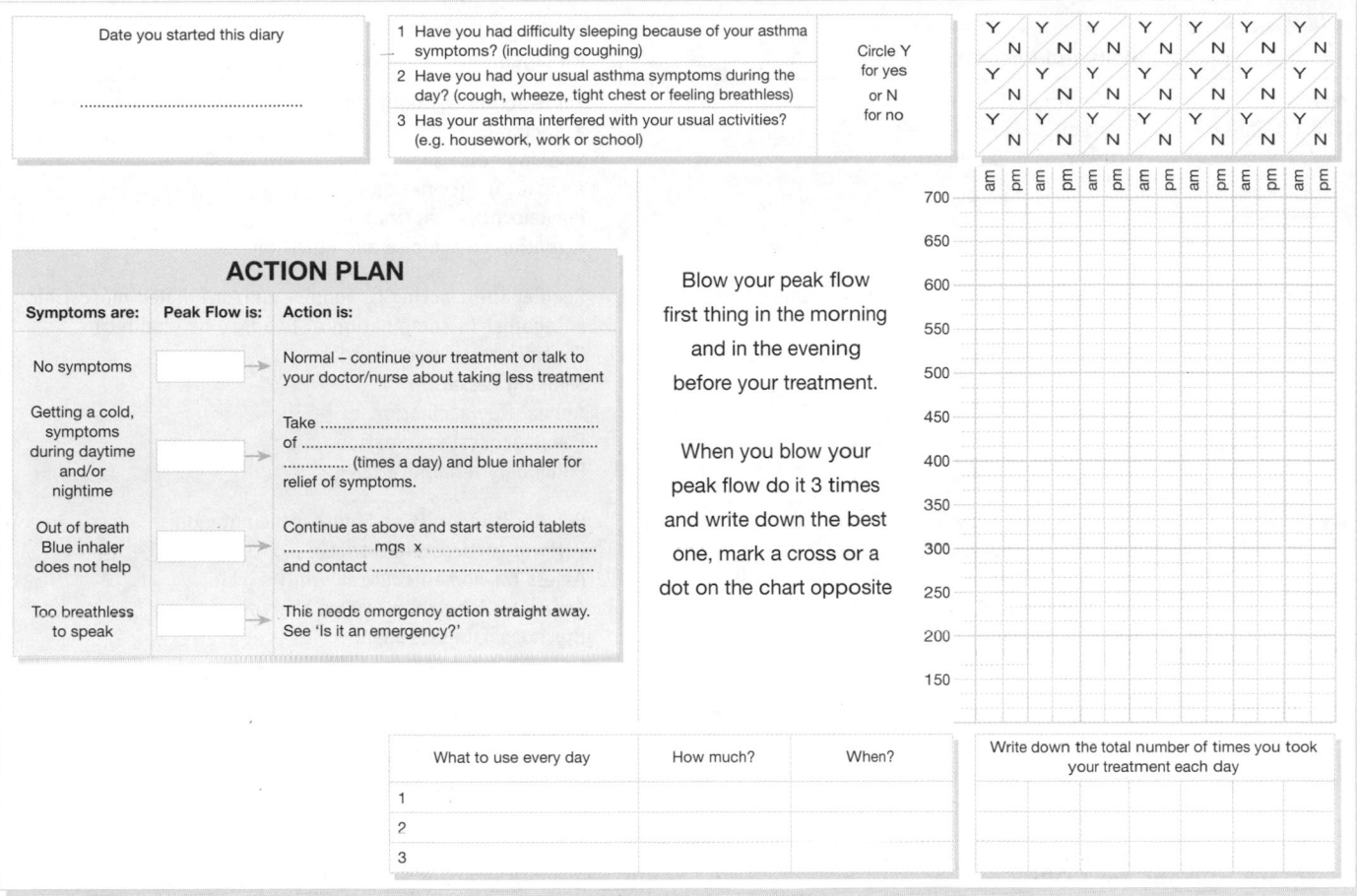

Figure 20.7 Self-management plan.

- have the confidence to adjust medication
- have sufficient insight to know when professional advice is required.

The National Asthma Campaign produces pre-printed self-management plans (Fig. 20.7) that can be individualized for patients, but they will only be successful if combined with education, support and agreement between the health care professional and the patient.

CHRONIC OBSTRUCTIVE PULMONARY DISEASE

The World Health Organization's (WHO 2002) *Global Initiative for Obstructive Lung Disease* (GOLD) defines COPD as 'a disease state characterised by air flow limitation that is not fully reversible'. The air flow limitation is usually both progressive and associated with an abnormal inflammatory response of the lungs to noxious particles and gases. Unlike previous definitions, GOLD emphasizes how COPD is caused by inhaled irritants. Tobacco smoke is the most important risk factor for the development of COPD, although other noxious particles and gases may result from occupational exposure, such as coal mining and welding.

Epidemiology

There are over 600 000 people in the UK with COPD, representing a prevalence of around 1% of the population (British Thoracic Society 1997a), and the disease is responsible for about 26 000 deaths each year. The majority of patients with COPD are over the age of 65 years, and it affects 7% of men over the age of 75. The inherited deficiency of α_1-antitrypsin, a protective enzyme that counteracts the action of proteolytic enzymes in the lungs, predisposes smokers to COPD. Alpha-1-antitrypsin deficiency accounts for 1–2% of COPD cases and is usually associated with the early development of emphysema, affecting people under the age of 40 years.

Pathophysiology

Chronic obstructive pulmonary disease is a term used to describe a number of overlapping conditions:

- chronic bronchitis – chronic inflammation of the membranes of the trachea and bronchi resulting in a productive cough on most days for at least 3 months in at least two consecutive years
- emphysema – abnormal, permanent enlargement of the terminal air spaces due to destruction of the alveolar wall
- chronic asthma that has become unresponsive to treatment.

The underlying feature of COPD is that it is a chronic, slowly progressive disorder characterized by airway obstruction which does not change markedly over several months and the impairment of lung function is largely fixed (British Thoracic Society 1997a).

Table 20.2 Chronic obstructive pulmonary disease severity and management

	Signs and symptoms	Management
Mild (FEV$_1$ 60–80%)	No abnormal signs 'Smoker's cough' Little or no breathlessness	Short-acting β$_2$ agonist or inhaled muscarinic antagonist as required Smoking cessation Annual flu vaccination Pneumococcal vaccination Attention to exercise and nutrition
Moderate (FEV$_1$ 40–60%)	Breathlessness (+/– wheeze) on moderate exertion Cough (+/– sputum) Reduction in breath sounds and presence of wheeze	Regular short-acting β$_2$ agonist and/or inhaled muscarinic antagonist (a combination of two may be required) Consider corticosteroid trial Smoking cessation Annual flu vaccination Pneumococcal vaccination Pulmonary rehabilitation
Severe (FEV$_1$ < 40%)	Breathlessness on any exertion/at rest Wheeze and cough often prominent Lung overinflation usual Cyanosis Peripheral oedema	Regular β$_2$ agonist and muscarinic antagonist Perform corticosteroid trial Assess for home nebulizer Assess for long-term oxygen therapy Psychosocial assessment Smoking cessation Annual flu vaccination Pneumococcal vaccination Pulmonary rehabilitation

Treatment options for COPD

The management of COPD is dependent on the severity of the disease process and the associated symptoms. Table 20.2 outlines the types of symptoms and the treatments used to manage each stage, based on the British Thoracic Society (1997) guidelines on the management of COPD.

The aim of treatment is to prevent further deterioration in lung function, control unpleasant symptoms, increase physical activity and improve the individual's quality of life. The treatments outlined in Table 20.2 are for those patients who have stable COPD and therefore the majority of treatment will take place in the community or outpatient setting. It is during acute exacerbations, usually as a consequence of respiratory infection, that patients will require hospital intervention or admission. It is for this reason that patients with COPD are advised to have flu vaccine every year.

Some of the treatments for COPD are similar to those used in asthma as both have an obstructive airway component requiring bronchodilator treatment to alleviate bronchoconstriction and corticosteroids for treatment of inflammation of the airway. Although there are similarities in treatment for asthma and COPD, it is necessary to understand that there are differences between the two diseases. COPD shows little or no day-to-day variability in symptoms or reversibility, whereas asthma is variable and reversible; thus the expectation is that treatment can have a greater impact.

Due to the chronic nature of COPD, the nurse has an important role in supporting and advising patients on how best to cope with the consequences of breathlessness on everyday activities and how to manage their treatment at home. The respiratory nurse specialist caring for COPD patients often has a primary and secondary care remit and is in the ideal position to provide pulmonary rehabilitation programmes and community and/or outpatient follow-up for patients recently commenced on long-term oxygen or nebulizer therapy. The mainstay treatments for severe COPD are:

- long-term oxygen therapy
- home nebulizer therapy
- pulmonary rehabilitation.

Long-term oxygen therapy

The use of long-term oxygen therapy in patients with chronic hypoxaemia (PaO$_2$ < 7.3 kPa) due to COPD has shown an increase in survival by approximately 5 years when 28% oxygen was administered for 15–16 hours/day (Nocturnal Oxygen Therapy Trial Group 1980, Medical Research Council Working Party 1981). The reason for low concentrations of oxygen being administered to COPD patients is that they develop sensitivity to falling oxygen levels in the blood rather than raised levels of carbon dioxide. If a higher percentage of oxygen is administered, this may reduce the stimulus to breathe and lead to carbon dioxide retention.

Long-term oxygen therapy is often delivered by an oxygen concentrator rather than oxygen cylinders. This frees patients from relying on the delivery of the cylinders, allows them to be more mobile around the home and eliminates the need for storage of numerous cylinders. The oxygen concentrator is powered by electricity and draws in room air, which is then passed through bacterial filters and molecular sieve beds that remove nitrogen and carbon dioxide and concentrate the oxygen. This is then delivered to the patient through a flow meter. Oxygen concentrators have been found to be well accepted and tolerated by the majority of patients (Restrick et al 1993).

According to the domiciliary oxygen guidelines (Royal College of Physicians 1999), patients newly started on long-term oxygen therapy should have written instructions and outpatient or community follow-up so that the following aspects of care can be addressed:

- monitoring of oxygen saturation (SaO$_2$) to ensure that oxygen therapy is correcting hypoxaemia (SaO$_2$ > 92%)
- psychological and social concerns and issues that may prevent the patient complying with the oxygen therapy
- monitoring of the patient's condition and observation for signs of deterioration (e.g. peripheral oedema)
- assessing whether continued domiciliary oxygen is required.

Respiratory nurse specialists are often the most appropriate people to provide the education, support and follow-up required for patients recently commenced on long-term oxygen therapy as they work alongside the respiratory physicians and liaise with GPs and community nurses (see Health Promotion box 20.2).

Nebulizer therapy

The use of nebulized β$_2$ agonists and muscarinic antagonists are indicated for acute exacerbations of COPD and in severe disease when high-dose bronchodilator treatment is indicated (British Thoracic Society 1997b).

The jet nebulizer is the most widely used device (Fig. 20.8). Compressed gas (oxygen or air) is forced through a narrow opening in the base of the nebulizer unit, creating the negative pressure required to draw up the drug solution from its reservoir. When the liquid collides with the jet of gas, it fragments into droplets that then impact on a baffle. The smallest particles form a therapeutic mist for the patient to inhale, while larger particles return to the reservoir and are recycled until the prescribed

dose has been given, usually about 10 minutes. A flow rate of 6–8 L/min produces 50% of the particles at a diameter of less than 5 μm, which allows deposition of the drug in the lungs.

Compressed air is the most common source for driving a nebulizer unless a high rate of inspired oxygen (i.e. for asthmatic patients) is indicated and prescribed. To prevent worsening of carbon dioxide retention, patients with type II respiratory failure, whose stimulus to breathe is driven by low levels of oxygen rather than high levels of carbon dioxide, should always use compressed air to drive the nebulizer. The use of a nasal cannula to deliver the prescribed flow rate of oxygen during nebulization will prevent hypoxaemia (Esmond 1998).

The decision as to whether masks or mouthpieces are used should be made with consideration of patient ability and the prescribed medication. Very breathless patients may find a face

HEALTH PROMOTION

20.2 Domiciliary oxygen therapy

The nurse has an important role in patient education in relation to:

- Oxygen safety issues
- Positioning of the machine within the home to prevent noise disturbance
- Planning the patient's day to accommodate the use of oxygen for 15–16 hours/day
- Positioning the oxygen outlets to maximize mobility so patients are able to walk around the house using their oxygen
- Preventing nasal and ear discomfort from use of a nasal cannula or mask
- Dealing with embarrassment and altered body image due to wearing a mask or nasal cannula.

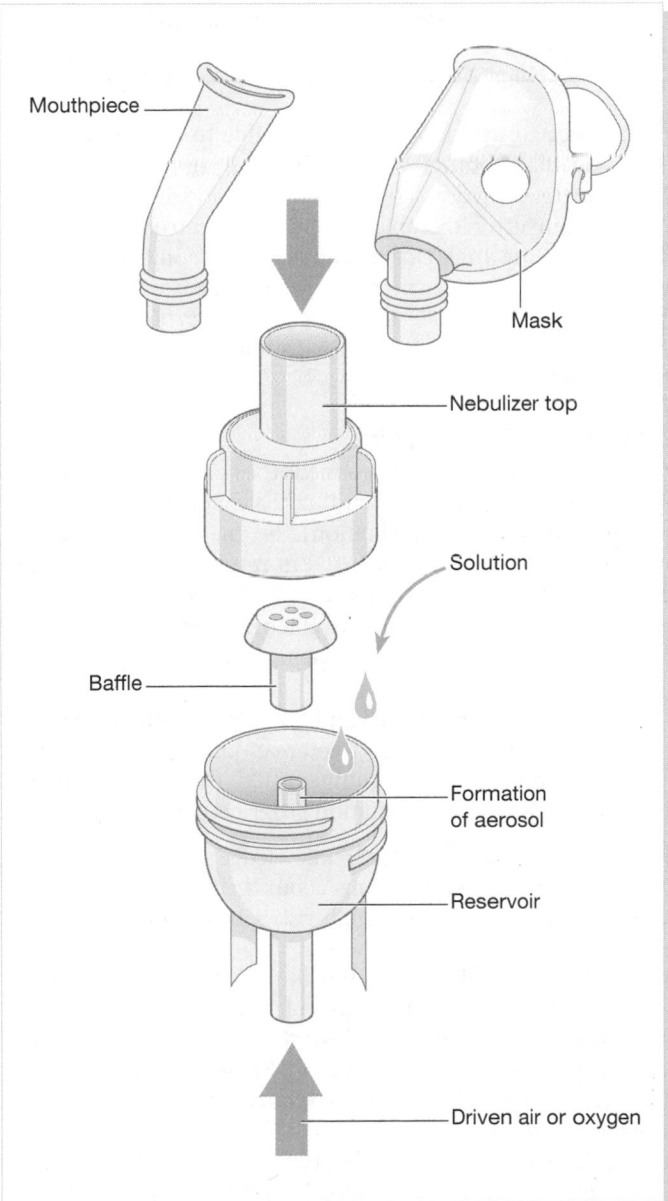

Figure 20.8 Jet nebulizer. (Adapted with kind permission from Medic-Aid.)

HEALTH PROMOTION

20.3 Nebulizer therapy

When self-administering nebulizer therapy, patients should be advised to sit comfortably in an upright position with the back supported, lips sealed around the mouthpiece or mask applied closely to the face and asked to breathe at a normal comfortable rate. Nebulization of the drug is complete when the nebulizer 'spits' intermittently or when no further aerosol mist is emitted.

Effective cleaning of the nebulizer is important for both infection control and performance. Washing in warm soapy water is recommended after every use. After washing, the nebulizer should be rinsed and stored dry in a plastic bag to prevent contamination by dust or airborne organisms. The majority of nebulizers are for single patient use and should be changed in accordance with the manufacturer's instructions.

---

mask easier to use and some are unable to use mouthpieces effectively. If a mouthpiece can be used, it should be chosen as there is better drug deposition in the lungs and fewer side-effects from certain drug therapies. Nebulized ipratropium bromide may cause acute angle closure glaucoma if it comes into contact with the eye and this is more likely to occur if a mask is used. Patients should be made aware of possible problems and told to report any eyesight changes (Esmond 1998) (see Health Promotion box 20.3).

Pulmonary rehabilitation

Pulmonary rehabilitation has a focus that is different from rehabilitation offered to patients with other conditions (e.g. cardiac or musculoskeletal rehabilitation), as there is no cure and patients do not have the potential to return to the pre-disease state, as the lung damage is not reversible. It is all about patients achieving their own maximum potential within the limits of their disease and being able to live and cope with a respiratory disability.

The aim of pulmonary rehabilitation is to reduce respiratory symptoms, increase exercise tolerance, improve psychological coping and improve overall quality of life. The common components of pulmonary rehabilitation programmes include:

- *Education* – increase patients' knowledge so that they are empowered to make decisions about their health needs, including modification of high-risk behaviours such as smoking
- *Exercise* – the majority of rehabilitation programmes use interval training which consists of 2–3 minutes of high-intensity training (e.g. bicycle or step-ups) alternating with equal periods of rest (Ries 1997). This allows patients to exercise safely and learn how to control their breathlessness whilst exercising
- *Breathing control* – patients are taught breathing techniques using their diaphragm, designed to slow respiratory rate while increasing their tidal volume
- *Psychosocial intervention* – patients with COPD have a high incidence of depression and anxiety and therefore need to be

able to develop coping strategies to deal with the impact of respiratory disability on their lives
- *Nutritional intervention* – patients with COPD require nutritional advice and support as they are at high risk of malnutrition. Both the practical aspect of preparing meals as well as the physiological barriers, such as breathlessness and reduced appetite due to infection, need to be addressed. Usually small, regular high-calorie meals or snacks are better tolerated than two large main meals per day (see Ch. 11).

For pulmonary rehabilitation to be successful, a multiprofessional approach is essential. The team should include a respiratory nurse, a physiotherapist, a dietician, a psychologist, an occupational therapist and a respiratory doctor. Organization of the programme is usually undertaken by the respiratory nurse and/or the respiratory physiotherapist, with input from the other disciplines as appropriate.

Management of an acute respiratory exacerbation of COPD

Patients with an acute exacerbation of COPD present with worsening symptoms of a previously stable condition, which will include:

- increased inspiratory wheeze and presence of chest tightness
- increased breathlessness at rest and/or on exertion
- increased sputum volume
- increased sputum purulence and change in colour (e.g. white/yellow to green)
- fluid retention (e.g. ankle oedema) due to hypoxaemia resulting in cor pulmonale.

As the underlying cause of the acute exacerbation is usually infection, patients are likely to be commenced on corticosteroids and antibiotic therapy, and given increased doses of bronchodilators. Diuretic therapy will be added if fluid retention has occurred. During an acute exacerbation COPD, patients are likely to develop type I respiratory failure (low oxygen levels in arterial blood) or, if already in type I respiratory failure, to develop type II respiratory failure (low oxygen and high carbon dioxide levels in arterial blood). It is therefore necessary to monitor arterial blood gases and treat with oxygen therapy and, if necessary, non-invasive ventilation or respiratory stimulants. These will be discussed later in this chapter.

Most patients with an acute exacerbation will need hospitalization but there are some nurse-led initiatives such as the Acute Respiratory Assessment Service (ARAS) (Flanagan et al 1999) and the Acute Chest Triage Rapid Intervention Team (ACTRIT) (Callaghan 1999) that have been established to support patients at home during acute respiratory exacerbations. The nurses base their assessment of whether patients are suitable to remain at home and their management on the British Thoracic Society (1997a) guidelines for the management of COPD (see Guidelines for Care Priorities box 20.3). Patients assessed as suitable for home treatment will be provided with an oxygen concentrator, nebulizer and home visits from the respiratory nurses, who will monitor progress and provide advice and support. Another important role is liaison between primary and secondary care. Once recovered from their acute exacerbation, patients will be discharged back into the care of the GP and community nursing service.

GUIDELINES FOR CARE PRIORITIES

20.3 Chronic obstructive pulmonary disease

The British Thoracic Society (1997a) guidelines on the management of COPD suggest that the following questions will help to guide the decision on where the patient is likely to be most effectively cared for during an acute respiratory exacerbation of COPD (i.e. at home or in hospital):

- Is the patient able to cope at home?
- Is there a normal level of consciousness?
- Is the patient able to perform activities of daily living despite being breathless?
- Is the patient in good general condition?
- Is the patient's SaO_2 above 90% when breathing air or is the patient receiving long-term oxygen therapy?
- Has the patient got a good level of activity?
- Has the patient got good social circumstances?

Using these questions when assessing a patient with an acute exacerbation of COPD will identify what support is required if the patient is to be cared for at home, as questions answered 'no' will indicate that intervention is required.

LUNG CANCER

Lung cancer describes any tumour that originates in the airways or lung and tobacco smoke is the most significant factor in its causation.

Epidemiology

Lung cancer is the most common cancer in the UK with around 40 000 cases diagnosed each year. Tobacco smoking is still overwhelmingly the most common cause of lung cancer and more than 90% of patients diagnosed with the disease die from it.

Pathophysiology

Lung cancer is classified according to histological cell types. Over 95% of lung cancers can be separated into small cell lung cancer (SCLC), accounting for approximately 20% of all lung cancers, and non-small cell lung cancer (NSCLC), consisting of squamous cell, adenocarcinoma and large cell carcinoma. Another rare form of lung cancer is mesothelioma, a type of cancer of the lining of the lung (pleura), caused by the inhalation of asbestos dust; it is classified as an occupational lung disease.

Clinical presentation

A patient with suspected lung cancer is likely to present with:

- breathlessness
- cough
- pleuritic chest pain
- haemoptysis (blood in sputum)
- loss of appetite and weight loss
- hoarseness of voice.

It is important to diagnose the type and to determine the stage of a lung cancer at presentation as this has an influence

Box 20.2 Treatment options for different types of lung cancer

Non-small cell lung cancer (squamous cell carcinoma, adenocarcinoma, large cell carcinoma)
- Thoracic surgery (20% of patients suitable)
  — lobectomy (removal of lobe of lung)
  — pneumonectomy (removal of lung)
- Radical radiotherapy
- Chemotherapy – offered as part of a clinical research trial as not of proven benefit

Small cell lung cancer
- Chemotherapy
- Radiotherapy (often used post-chemotherapy)

Mesothelioma
- Palliation of symptoms (see Ch. 32)

on the prognosis and the choice of treatment. Investigations (chest X-ray, bronchoscopy, cytology, histology, CT scan and bone scan) will be carried out to identify the type of lung cancer, the extent of the cancer and whether there is spread to other organs. The results are then used in staging the cancer so that a treatment plan can be determined (see Box 20.2).

▶ Nursing management

Nurses have an important role in caring for patients with lung cancer through:

- Assessment of social, emotional, physical, financial and spiritual needs.
- Emotional support of patient and family in coming to terms with the diagnosis and coping with the treatments that may have unpleasant side-effects (e.g. chemotherapy causing nausea and hair to fall out).
- Education and information about lung cancer and the treatments that have been offered so that informed choices can be made.
- Good symptom control, particularly in relation to breathlessness and pain (see Ch. 34).
- Discharge planning, which may include referral to a palliative care team, social services and community nurses.

The role of lung cancer nurse specialists is important as they are usually present at the time of diagnosis and help patients to make informed choices about treatment options and provide support for patients and family members during treatment. As one of the most unpleasant symptoms is breathlessness, there is a move towards nurse-led breathlessness clinics (Corner et al 1995). These clinics use an integrated approach that emphasizes the importance of not separating the physical and psychological aspects of breathlessness. Bredin et al (1999) describe how the integrated approach attempts to promote a therapeutic relationship where patients are able to talk about their breathlessness and be heard. The principles of this approach are as follows:

- The mind and body are considered inseparable.
- The meaning of breathlessness is explored as part of therapy.

20.1 Breathlessness

James is a 69-year-old who has been a life-long smoker and has been recently diagnosed with non-small cell lung cancer. He has had radical radiotherapy, as he is not suitable for surgery. Breathlessness is causing him distress, as he is unable to get out to visit his family because he is too frightened.

- Suggest medical treatment that may help James' breathlessness.
- Identify the benefits that James may get from attending a breathlessness clinic run by the lung cancer nurse specialist.

- Symptoms are redefined as problems in relation to their effect on the person's life.
- A therapeutic relationship with the patient is developed.
- There is mutual inquiry, where the patient and nurse work together as equals to discover and develop ways of managing breathlessness.

Interventions adopted to alleviate breathlessness tend to involve (see also Reflective Practice box 20.1):

- cognitive strategies – addressing fears and anxieties and explaining how anxiety can lead to panic and hyperventilation which can exacerbate breathlessness
- behavioural modification – the teaching of techniques to help patients cope with breathlessness may include goal-setting, diaphragmatic breathing control, relaxation techniques and activity pacing
- counselling strategies – listening to fears around dying and acknowledging the psychological distress that breathlessness can evoke
- pharmacological agents – the use of oxygen therapy, opioids and bronchodilators can be of some benefit in alleviating breathlessness, although are best used in conjunction with cognitive, behavioural and counselling strategies.

CYSTIC FIBROSIS

Cystic fibrosis (CF) is the most common life-threatening genetic disease, affecting approximately 1 in 2500 live births in the UK. One in 25 Caucasians in the UK are carriers of the CF gene. As it is a recessive genetic disorder, when both parents are carriers of the abnormal gene there is a 1 in 4 chance of each pregnancy producing a child with CF.

Epidemiology

There are approximately 7500 people with CF in the UK, which is a relatively small number of people, considering that it affects 1 in 2500 live births. This is because, despite increasing survival, the median age of death is only 31 years, although babies born in the 21st century are expected to have a mean survival of over 40 years. With the majority of patients with CF now reaching adulthood, it is no longer exclusively a childhood disease.

Pathophysiology

Cystic fibrosis involves a basic dysfunction of the exocrine gland ducts due to altered sodium and chloride channel function at the epithelial cell surface. This results in the production of abnormally concentrated secretions that tend to block exocrine ducts. CF is a multisystem disorder that primarily affects the respiratory and digestive systems, although there are often associated problems of liver disease, cystic fibrosis-related diabetes (CFRD), arthropathy and male infertility.

The main cause of morbidity and mortality in CF is bacterial lung infections (Davis et al 1996). A background of chronic lung sepsis, usually due to *Staphylococcus aureus*, *Haemophilus influenzae* or *Pseudomonas aeruginosa*, is punctuated at increasingly frequent intervals by acute infective exacerbations. In response to persistent inflammation, pulmonary fibrosis and bronchiectasis (collection of necrotic material and bronchial secretions in dilated bronchi) progress, culminating in respiratory failure and death.

Treatment

Treatment is aimed at delaying progression of the disease through maintaining lung function by preventing and controlling lung infections. This involves:

- lifelong physiotherapy to assist mucus clearance from the lungs
- administration of a combination of oral, nebulized and intravenous antibiotics to control infection
- nebulized bronchodilators (e.g. salbutamol)
- anti-inflammatory medication (i.e. oral or inhaled steroids)
- nutritional support consisting of pancreatic enzyme supplementation, fat-soluble vitamin supplementation and 20–50% increased calorie intake
- monitoring disease progression (FEV_1, FVC, SaO_2 and weight).

Lifelong physiotherapy

Physiotherapy is initiated from the time of diagnosis and becomes part of the daily routine (Pryor & Prasad 2002); the patient and family are taught how to clear bronchopulmonary secretions. Types and frequency of treatment will vary with age and severity of disease, but usually involves breathing control, percussion to mobilize secretions, postural drainage to assist with movement and huffing (a forced expiration technique) to expectorate sputum. Exercise is also encouraged as it can assist with mobilization of secretions.

Antibiotic therapy

Antibiotic therapy will vary and depends on the most recent sputum culture result, the previous clinical response to agents already used and allergies. High doses of antibiotics over a longer duration are required if treatment is to be successful since they must penetrate pus-filled cavities and areas of poor perfusion.

The quinolones (e.g. ciprofloxacin) may be the best first-line oral antibiotic therapy, although the response is unlikely to be of benefit if the patient has recently received ciprofloxacin. Some other broad-spectrum oral agents (i.e. doxycycline, erythromycin) should be considered as these may improve lung function (probably by treating other pathogens and reducing exoenzyme production by *Pseudomonas aeruginosa*). Anti-staphylococcal agents (i.e. flucloxacillin) are frequently given indefinitely following the isolation of *Staphylococcus aureus*.

For intravenous anti-pseudomonal therapy, the most common first-line approach is a combination of a beta-lactam antibiotic or penicillin (i.e. ceftazidime, aztreonam or tazocin) and an aminoglycoside (i.e. gentamicin, tobramycin, amikacin). Single agents are not recommended as there is increased probability that resistance will develop.

Anti-pseudomonal agents may be given via the nebulized route on initial isolation of *Pseudomonas aeruginosa* in combination with ciprofloxacin orally to eradicate it and delay colonization. Once colonized with *Pseudomonas aeruginosa*, nebulized antibiotics (e.g. colistin, tobramycin (TOBI), gentamicin) may be administered indefinitely. The use of bronchodilators before nebulized antibiotics can prevent bronchospasm. In general, patients are asked to take bronchodilators (usually nebulized) before physiotherapy, which is itself performed before nebulized antibiotics (UK Cystic Fibrosis Trust's Antibiotic Group 2000).

Anti-inflammatory medication

The inflammatory response to infection is treated with anti-inflammatory medication, such as corticosteroids. The inhaled route is the preferred route of delivery as the systematic effect is minimal and there are fewer side-effects, particularly as CF patients have an increased risk of developing osteoporosis and diabetes, which can occur with prolonged use of oral steroids (2 months or more).

Nutritional requirements

Patients with CF have an increased requirement for energy and protein due to a high resting energy expenditure, poor appetite and malabsorption. The aim is to achieve 20–50% more energy than is usually required for their age and sex. Patients find achieving their energy requirements difficult, particularly during chest infections when a poor appetite due to breathlessness, foul-tasting sputum and coughing (which often results in vomiting) may contribute to a reduced food intake. Use of home-made or commercial liquid supplements during this time can be helpful in providing the increased energy requirements.

Over 90% of patients with CF suffer pancreatic enzyme insufficiency requiring pancreatic enzyme supplements to digest their food. Steatorrhoea (fatty stools) and weight loss indicate uncontrolled malabsorption. The importance of taking enzyme supplements just before and throughout eating all meals and snacks is stressed. It is necessary to increase the dose with higher fat foods. CF patients are at risk of deficiencies of the fat-soluble vitamins A, D, E & K. However, routine daily supplementation of a water miscible form of the fat soluble vitamins and adequate enzyme replacement therapy should prevent vitamin deficiency.

Acute respiratory exacerbations of CF

The aim of treating acute respiratory exacerbations is to prevent loss of lung function as a consequence of lung tissue damage from infection. Acute exacerbations are characterized by some or all of the following symptoms:

- increased breathlessness
- change in sputum volume, colour and viscosity
- tiredness
- loss of appetite
- increased coughing.

These symptoms rely on the patient reporting them, and therefore monitoring lung function (FEV_1 and FVC), oxygen saturation (SaO_2) and nutritional status (weight and BMI) allows a more objective assessment of deterioration in clinical status. Because early detection of acute respiratory exacerbations is necessary to initiate early treatment and thereby prevent permanent loss of lung function, monitoring of disease progression is necessary so that changes from the patient's baseline can be detected and acted upon.

During acute respiratory exacerbations there is an increased risk of other respiratory complications which include:

- increased incidence of asthma and bronchial hyperreactivity
- pneumothorax
- haemoptysis
- allergic bronchopulmonary aspergillosis (ABPA)
- cor pulmonale.

These complications are not unique to CF patients and are discussed later in this chapter.

Some exacerbations may be managed at home from the outset, with a combination of oral, nebulized and intravenous (i.v.) antibiotics. More severe infections or patients who cannot self-administer i.v. antibiotics may require hospitalization, during which time i.v. therapy is initiated and controlled oxygen therapy can be administered. Many patients may also require more intensive assistance from the CF team, which includes physiotherapy, nutritional support, psychological support and rest.

Home intravenous therapy

There are a number of advantages and disadvantages for patients self-administering intravenous (i.v.) antibiotics at home. It should not be seen as an 'easy option', but it can offer a degree of choice and flexibility. Patients can either continue a course of antibiotics initiated in hospital or perform the entire course at home. Selection and training of patients to self-administer i.v. medication must be done on an individual basis. Motivation, home stability and family support as well as practical ability need to be assessed. Teaching programmes need to be tailored for individuals at their own pace. It is essential that patients and/or carers are both competent and confident before home i.v. therapy is undertaken.

▶ Nursing management

Cystic fibrosis places many demands on individuals and their families. The treatment regimen can be demanding, symptoms unpleasant, and coping with emotions associated with a life-threatening chronic illness is often stressful. The CF nurse has an important role in supporting patients and families and is often the person they contact for support and advice. They usually become involved in the care during transition from the paediatric to adult team which can be quite a traumatic time, as the person with CF is having to deal with issues of adolescence as well as getting to know a new team. All nurses caring for CF patients need to be aware of the developmental needs of adolescents and young adults and the burden that a life-threatening illness can present. Strategies to assist patients and family members to cope include:

- reduction of anxiety by giving information and explanations
- providing encouragement and practical suggestions for coping (e.g. how to fit treatment around a busy lifestyle)
- helping patients cope with 'loss', of physical function, changes in body image, and death of other CF patients whom they have got to know due to frequent spells in hospital and attendance at the same outpatient clinics
- a supportive relationship to reduce stress of coping alone
- counselling to cope with emotional stressors such as denial, guilt, anger and fear
- information about support groups (e.g. Cystic Fibrosis Trust).

End-stage management

As the mean age of death is currently 31 years, the majority of people with CF now die in adulthood. There are many challenges in caring for CF patients as they enter the terminal stages of their disease. An important option to consider at this time is lung transplantation.

Transplantation

Patients with end-stage CF are young, well motivated, used to attending hospitals and performing treatments and take an active interest in the management of their disease. This makes them good candidates for transplantation. Heart–lung transplantation is the technique of choice, as it is technically an easier procedure. This usually includes 'domino' heart transplantation, where the CF transplant patient donates his or her heart to a patient requiring a heart transplant. Double-lung transplantation is technically more difficult to perform but is now possible due to the development of direct revascularization of the bronchial arteries.

The timing of surgery is vital. It should not be performed too early because approximately 25–30% of patients die within the first postoperative year from complications associated with transplantation (e.g. organ rejection or haemorrhage), and therefore the risk is too great. However, neither must it be too late because suitable donor organs may not be found in time or the patients may become too ill to successfully undergo transplantation. Transplantation is not the most appropriate option for all patients who have end-stage CF, nor is it a type of treatment that all patients wish to consider. Dying is often discussed more openly when transplantation is no longer an issue.

Management principles

Whether or not patients are on the transplant waiting list, the principles of end-stage management remain the same. The aim is to control unpleasant symptoms that arise from respiratory infection and loss of lung function. The most troublesome symptom is breathlessness, although muscular chest pain can also cause distress. A combination of treatments will be used in the terminal phase of CF to control symptoms as follows:

- oxygen therapy
- non-invasive ventilation (NIV)
- positioning to alleviate breathlessness

- opioids to control pain and breathlessness
- analgesics to control muscular chest pain (e.g. non-steroidals)
- complementary therapy (e.g. massage or aromatherapy)
- relaxation techniques (e.g. tapes).

Anxiety, depression and panic can cause distress and increase breathlessness; therefore emotional support to the patient and family are essential if symptoms are to be controlled. As patients with CF are aware that they are likely to have a shortened life, their own involvement and that of their family in the decisions being made to control symptoms may help all concerned to cope with death more easily.

Gene therapy

The aim of gene therapy is to correct the underlying basic genetic defect in the lungs as this is the major cause of mortality. Gene therapy trials in CF have been ongoing for several years but there are problems associated with safety (viral vector gene therapy) and efficacy (liposomal gene therapy). Despite great efforts, gene therapy is still considered to be several years away from being an effective therapy (Geddes & Alton 1999).

BRONCHIECTASIS

Bronchiectasis is a chronic dilation of the bronchi caused by inflammation as a result of:

- childhood infections (i.e. bronchiolitis)
- immunodeficiency syndromes (i.e. hypogammaglobulinaemia)
- allergic bronchopulmonary aspergillus (a fungus) (ABPA)
- pneumonia
- cystic fibrosis
- tuberculosis
- alpha-1-antitrypsin deficiency.

Epidemiology

The incidence of bronchiectasis has decreased over the past 50 years due to the widespread introduction of immunization against childhood infections and with antibiotic treatment. Unfortunately the incidence is unknown as it is often as a consequence of a disease (e.g. cystic fibrosis or tuberculosis).

Pathophysiology

Collections of necrotic material and bronchial secretions in the dilated bronchi result in inflammation that causes secondary bacterial infection and fibrosis in the lung. This will result in recurrent and persistent lower respiratory tract infections, causing production of large amounts of purulent sputum, bronchoconstriction, cough and haemoptysis.

Treatment

The principles of treatment are the same as the respiratory management for cystic fibrosis.

RESPIRATORY TRACT INFECTIONS

Respiratory infections can be divided into upper respiratory tract infections (URTIs) involving the nose and pharynx, and lower respiratory tract infections (LRTIs) involving the trachea, bronchi and lungs. URTIs are usually minor and are mainly due to viral infections, such as rhinovirus and influenza. In patients with underlying respiratory disease, URTIs can be more serious as they often develop secondary LRTIs which can be life-threatening, especially when a pneumonia develops. According to the *Lung Report II* (British Lung Foundation 2000) between 5 and 15% of patients admitted to hospital with pneumonia will die despite apparently appropriate antibiotic treatment.

PNEUMONIA

Pneumonia is the term used when the infection affects the parts of the lungs responsible for transferring oxygen to the blood and therefore radiological changes on chest X-ray can be observed (Fig. 20.9).

Classic symptoms of pneumonia include:

- cough – often non-productive with bacterial pneumonia, but with subsequently increased production of mucopurulent yellow/green sputum
- pleuritic chest pain
- pyrexia
- loss of appetite
- low oxygen levels.

Epidemiology

Pneumonia is a leading cause of illness and is associated with significant mortality and utilization of health service resources. More than 66 000 people die of pneumonia in the UK each year, with an increased prevalence amongst the elderly, aged 75 and over (British Thoracic Society 2001).

Pathophysiology

Pneumonia may be acquired in the community or in hospital, when it is known as a nosocomial infection as it has been acquired from other patients, the environment or health care workers. The type of pneumonia is determined by the causative organism, e.g. *Pneumococcus* pneumonia, *Streptococcus* pneumonia and *Pneumocystis carinii* pneumonia (PCP).

Pneumonia can occur in previously healthy people although there is a higher incidence amongst people where there are predisposing factors including:

- impaired respiratory defences (e.g. reduced cough reflex or tracheostomy)

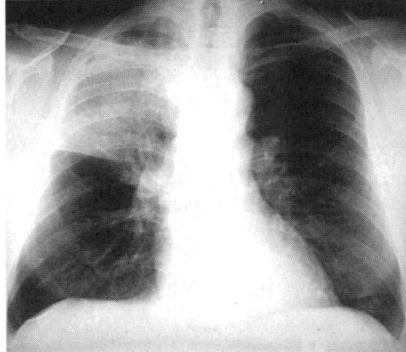

Figure 20.9 Chest X-ray showing a patient with pneumonia.

- old age, because of a less efficient immune system
- underlying respiratory disease (e.g. asthma, COPD, cystic fibrosis or tuberculosis)
- secondary to influenza
- immunodeficiency diseases (e.g. HIV/AIDS or on chemotherapy)
- aspiration of vomit (aspiration pneumonia) or associated with chronic diseases such as alcoholism, hepatic and renal disease.

Complications of pneumonia include meningitis, empyema (pus in the pleural space), lung abscess and septicaemias. Death occurs most often in the elderly and in those with debilitating chronic conditions, especially when it is secondary to recent influenza.

Specific investigations

Patients will have investigations that include chest X-ray, sputum microscopy, culture and sensitivity, blood cultures, white cell count (WBC), pleural fluid microscopy, culture and sensitivity, pneumococcal antigen tests and serological tests.

Treatment

The aim of treatment is to identify the cause of the pneumonia, deliver appropriate treatment and rule out other causes of disease. The treatment of pneumonia will require antibiotic therapy active against the causative organism. Initially a broad-spectrum antibiotic such as amoxycillin, ampicillin or erythromycin will be used until sputum microbiological results are available. The choice of the oral or intravenous route will depend on the severity of presenting features. For example, a patient with a decreased oxygen saturation (< 95%) would be admitted to hospital and given intravenous antibiotics initially and then changed to oral once there is clinical improvement.

Prevention of pneumonia

A pneumococcal vaccine is available (Salisbury & Begg 1996) and is recommended for high-risk groups, such as older people and those with underlying respiratory disease. The polyvalent vaccine is a single 'one-off' injection, although in immuno-compromised patients and those who have undergone splenectomy, a booster is recommended every 5 years. Vaccination against influenza ('flu' vaccine) is also recommended and needs to be administered annually between late September and early November. In addition, causative risk factors, which include poverty, poor housing, malnutrition, environmental exposure to pollutants, smoking (both active and passive) and excessive alcohol consumption, need to be addressed if mortality rates are to be reduced (see Older Adults: Nursing Priorities box 20.1).

▶ Nursing management

The needs of the patient with pneumonia will be determined by the causative factors and symptoms. To assist with sputum clearance, the patient needs to be encouraged to expectorate the sputum through coughing and therefore will need sputum pots, tissue and frequent mouthwashes. Chest physiotherapy will also

OLDER ADULTS: NURSING PRIORITIES

20.1 Flu vaccination

The Department of Health provides information on influenza ('flu') and flu immunization (http://www.doh.gov.uk/flu.htm) which states:

- For most people, flu is an unpleasant but self-limiting illness, the main symptoms lasting up to about a week. Treatment is symptomatic and those affected are advised to stay at home, rest and drink plenty of fluids.
- For people in certain 'high-risk' groups, such as those with underlying respiratory, heart or renal disease or who are elderly, flu is a significant cause of serious illness and death. Complications such as bronchitis and pneumonia are more common in those in high-risk groups (those with underlying respiratory, heart or renal disease) especially if they are also elderly, and mortality is almost entirely in these groups.
- Flu-like illness may be due to viruses other than flu. Even during a flu epidemic, a proportion of so-called 'flu' is due to other viruses.

Flu immunization

- Flu vaccine should be offered to all people aged 65 years and over.
- Vaccination is also recommended for people of any age with underlying conditions that put them at higher risk of serious illness from flu and for those in long-stay residential accommodation.
- The aim is to increase the uptake each year until a 70% uptake in people aged 65 years and over is achieved (the uptake in 2001 was 60%).
- Strategic health authorities are being asked to work with their local general practitioners and primary care trusts to contact all people aged 65 years and over, and to achieve the target uptake.

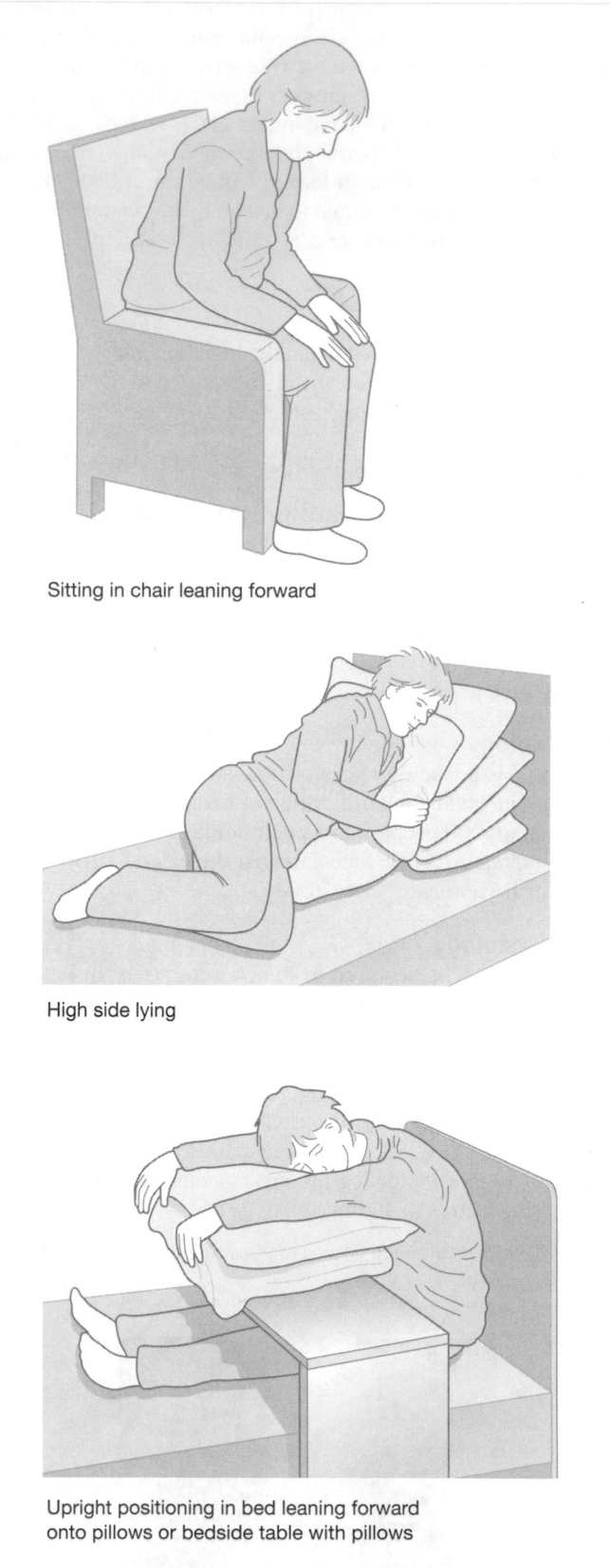

Sitting in chair leaning forward

High side lying

Upright positioning in bed leaning forward onto pillows or bedside table with pillows

Figure 20.10 Positioning the breathless patient.

be initiated to assist with airway clearance and usually consists of postural drainage, percussion and breathing control.

Positioning the patient in an upright position supported by pillows or leaning against a bed table will alleviate breathlessness by allowing effective lung expansion (Fig. 20.10). The cause of breathlessness in pneumonia is usually associated with hypoxaemia and therefore administration of oxygen is required. The dryness of oxygen will restrict the expectoration of sputum so it is advisable to use humidified oxygen therapy and offer frequent drinks or mouthwashes.

The patient with pyrexia requires sufficient fluid intake to replace fluid lost in sweat, which will assist with excretion of toxins from the body. An antipyretic, such as paracetamol, may be used to control body temperature and make the patient more comfortable (see Ch. 5). Additional analgesia may be required, as paracetamol alone may be insufficient to control pleuritic chest pain. Both pyrexia and pain may have an adverse effect on nutrition and therefore nutritional supplementation, using high-protein supplements such as Ensure Plus, Fresubin or Fortisip, may be necessary during the acute phase.

Having pneumonia can be a very frightening experience and therefore psychological support of the patient and family is required. Listening to fears and anxieties can be very supportive and during severe breathless episodes the patient may be reassured by the presence of the nurse or a family member.

TUBERCULOSIS

Tuberculosis (TB) is a notifiable disease which, in accordance with the Public Health Act (Department of Health 1984), requires individuals diagnosed to be notified to the Consultant in Community Diseases Control (CCDC) or Director of Public Health who is responsible for TB surveillance and control of the spread of TB within the local community.

Epidemiology

In 1993, the World Health Organization (WHO) declared TB a global emergency as it is estimated that a third of the world's population is infected (World Health Organization 1994). More than three million people worldwide die each year from a disease that can and ought to be cured (British Lung Foundation 2000).

Pathophysiology

Tuberculosis is a chronic infectious disease caused by the tubercle bacillus, *Mycobacterium tuberculosis*. It mainly affects the lungs as it is transmitted by inhalation of infected droplets of sputum coughed up by someone with active TB. However, other parts of the body (extrapulmonary) can be affected, with the bacterium entering the bloodstream through the lymphatic system. The commonest forms of extrapulmonary disease are lymphadenopathy, pleural effusion, pericardial TB, miliary TB and TB meningitis.

Most people infected with *Mycobacterium tuberculosis* never develop active disease as the body's immune system makes the bacterium dormant. Soon after the primary infection enters the lung, the inflammatory response occurs and a calcified lesion is left. The primary infection remains dormant but may be reactivated (post-primary infection) if the immune system is weakened, resulting in active tuberculosis.

The risk factors for developing active TB are associated with the immune system weakening and exposure to infectious TB and include:

- immunodeficiency (i.e. HIV and AIDS)
- immunosuppression (i.e. steroids, chemotherapy)
- close contact with someone newly diagnosed with infectious TB
- homelessness, particularly those with a history of alcohol misuse and malnutrition
- older adults, particularly those resident in long-term care facilities
- those with chronic respiratory disease (e.g. bronchiectasis and cystic fibrosis).

Clinical presentation

Tuberculosis is caused by bacteria and therefore the symptoms are associated with infection, including:

- chronic cough
- pyrexia
- weight loss
- night sweats
- general malaise
- haemoptysis (blood in the sputum).

Specific investigations

A strong medical history as well as a combination of investigations lead to the diagnosis of pulmonary tuberculosis.

- A chest X-ray may identify the presence of cavities that may indicate active TB or calcification, demonstrating that the patient has a primary infection that is not presently active.
- Three sputum samples, obtained on separate days wherever possible, should be sent for microbiological analysis. The presence of acid fast bacillus (AFB) in sputum indicates that the patient has active (smear-positive) TB. A smear-negative result cannot exclude the presence of TB until the sputum culture, which takes approximately 8 weeks, also proves negative.
- Tuberculin skin test (e.g. Heaf test) is used to detect past or present tuberculosis infection. A positive Heaf test when there has been no Bacillie-Calmette-Guérin (BCG) vaccination, or a grade 3 or 4 Heaf when BCG vaccination has taken place, would give rise to suspicion of active TB, although this alone would not be sufficient to diagnose the disease.

Treatment of pulmonary tuberculosis

The British Thoracic Society (1998) has produced guidelines on the type of antibiotics to be used in the management of TB in the UK. Currently, first-line treatment for tuberculosis consists of a 6-month treatment regimen of rifampicin, isoniazid, pyrazinamide and ethambutol or streptomycin for 2 months and then rifampicin and isoniazid for a further 4 months. The fourth drug, ethambutol or streptomycin, can be omitted when patients have a low risk of developing resistance to isoniazid.

Multi-drug resistant tuberculosis

Pulmonary tuberculosis is a treatable condition but if initial therapy is inadequate or the course of treatment is not completed, multi-drug resistant tuberculosis (MDR-TB) can develop. The reasons for this occurring are:

- inadequate treatment (single drug therapy or low dose)
- failure to complete course of antibiotics because of poor adherence to treatment
- asymptomatic after 2–4 weeks of treatment and so patients believe they no longer need the medication
- lack of knowledge and understanding of TB and its treatment
- inability to access health care, which is prevalent amongst the homeless and minority ethnic groups if there are language problems.

Role of the nurse in prevention and treatment of tuberculosis

With the increasing incidence of drug resistance in reported cases of TB, the nurse has an important role in developing strategies to prevent MDR-TB occurring. Treatment of TB usually takes place at home, with only those with severe illness, secondary complications (e.g. pleural effusion or adverse drug reactions) or social problems being admitted to hospital. If admitted to hospital, patients with, or suspected of having, active pulmonary TB should be nursed in a single room so that isolation precautions for airborne infections can be implemented. Once patients have commenced TB treatment and had three consecutive smear-negative sputum results, they can be nursed on an open ward. Patients with, or suspected of having, MDR-TB should be cared for in a negative pressure room, and because of the serious consequences of contracting MDR-TB, staff caring for them should wear dust mist-fume masks as these provide greater protection (see Ch. 13).

The TB nurse specialist and/or health visitors work in collaboration with public health officials, respiratory physicians and microbiologists and are responsible for contact tracing, screening and treatment supervision. The role of the TB nurse is essential in providing education and support to patients during treatment and thereby improving adherence and completion of therapy. The nurse must be aware of the psychosocial impact that TB can have on individuals and communities. There still remains a great deal of stigma associated with TB, partly because of the high incidence in minority ethnic groups, homeless people and those with HIV. In addition, the majority of patients are in the lower socioeconomic groups, often living in poverty with poor access to health care.

Contact tracing

Contact tracing means tracing associated cases, people who have been in contact with the person diagnosed with TB (index or source case), who may be infected but have no evidence of active disease. Contact screening is usually carried out by the TB nurse specialist who will screen close contacts (people living in same house and very close associates such as boyfriend/ girlfriend) of the index case. The British Thoracic Society's (2000) guidelines on control and prevention of TB recommend that contact screening includes inquiry into symptoms of TB, BCG vaccination status, tuberculin testing (e.g. Heaf test), chest X-ray and sputum. Contacts who have symptoms and/or radiological changes are likely to be smear positive and therefore urgent referral to the respiratory physician is necessary so that treatment can be initiated if TB is diagnosed.

Treatment supervision of tuberculosis

Adherence to therapy is essential if TB is to be controlled and MDR-TB is to be prevented. Baker (2001) suggests that placing the emphasis on supporting rather than monitoring patients is likely to improve treatment completion rates, as it allows exploration of factors that may lead to patients not adhering to treatment. These may include lack of knowledge, social problems, health beliefs, cultural beliefs and chaotic lifestyle. Through the nurse working in partnership with the patient, strategies to improve adherence can be individualized.

 HEALTH PROMOTION

20.4 Tuberculosis

Peter has been living in a hostel and sleeping rough for the last 15 years and has an alcohol problem. He is not registered with a GP as he does not have a permanent address. Through the tuberculosis nurse specialist contact tracing another index case, Peter has been identified as a close contact of a person with smear-positive infective tuberculosis. He attends for screening where he has a physical examination, chest X-ray, Heaf test, sputum specimen sent for AFBs. He is diagnosed with smear-positive tuberculosis and commenced on rifampicin, izoniazid, pyrazinamide and ethambutol.

Student activities
- Why was Peter at risk of being infected with tuberculosis?
- What strategies could be adopted to increase Peter's adherence to treatment?
- If Peter does not complete his 6 months of treatment, what might be the consequences?

The WHO advocates directly observed therapy (DOT) for all people with TB, which is where patients are observed taking their therapy by a health care professional. This strategy is labour-intensive and often difficult to achieve and in the UK is only implemented if patients are assessed to be at high risk of non-adherence. Homeless people are a group at such a risk as they have difficulty accessing health care and obtaining medication. Incentives such as provision of meals and taxis have been used in association with DOT to encourage homeless people to attend appointments. A move towards the medication being provided by the hospital free of charge to patients is being advocated, as they often stop their medication because either they presume that they have completed the course or they do not have access to a GP (see Health Promotion box 20.4).

Tuberculosis remains a major cause of concern as it is steadily increasing throughout the world. The treatment of the disease alone will not solve the problem as many of the factors are linked to social deprivation and lack of health care facilities. As well as addressing the issues of disease control, those formulating social policy need to look at the causative factors because, without tackling these, it is likely that tuberculosis will remain a problem.

INTERSTITIAL LUNG DISEASES

Interstitial lung diseases are a group of rare conditions characterized by cellular and extracellular infiltrates in the spaces between the pulmonary capillary endothelial cells and the pulmonary alveolar epithelium. The most common of these rare diseases are:

- cryptogenic fibrosing alveolitis
- sarcoidosis
- vasculitis
- neurofibromatosis.

With these diseases, inflammation invades the alveoli resulting in fibrosis (scarring) and causes the lungs to become stiff. The effect is that transfer of gas between the pulmonary capillaries and alveoli is reduced, and the work of breathing increased. Treatment consists of corticosteroids (prednisolone) and immunosuppressants (cyclophosphamide and azathioprine) to control the inflammatory process and prevent further lung damage. The most disabling feature of interstitial lung disease is breathlessness, and in the later stages oxygen therapy is required to control this.

RESPIRATORY FAILURE

As a result of respiratory disease, the mechanics of breathing can be impaired, leading to respiratory failure, i.e. the inability to maintain adequate oxygenation and adequate carbon dioxide elimination. There are two types of respiratory failure: type I respiratory failure, when there is only an oxygenation problem resulting in hypoxaemia (low oxygen level in arterial blood); and type II respiratory failure, when there is a ventilatory problem, resulting in hypoxaemia and hypercapnia (high carbon dioxide level in arterial blood). Effective ventilation is required to eliminate or 'blow off' carbon dioxide, the waste gas of respiration. In addition, chemical reactions in the body are dependent on a balance of acids and bases to maintain a normal pH. If the body has had insufficient time to compensate for raised levels of carbon dioxide then the pH in the blood becomes abnormally low (< 7.35) indicating a respiratory acidosis, which is a life-threatening situation. Table 20.3 identifies the normal levels of oxygen, carbon dioxide and pH in arterial blood and the changes in these values in patients with type I or type II respiratory failure.

Treatment

The aim of treatment for respiratory failure is to provide additional oxygenation for those in type I respiratory failure, and additional ventilation to provide oxygenation and elimination of carbon dioxide for those in type II respiratory failure. The treatment options are as follows:

- *type I respiratory failure*
  — oxygen therapy
  — continuous positive airway pressure (CPAP) (see Ch. 31)
- *type II respiratory failure*
  — oxygen therapy
  — respiratory stimulants (e.g. doxapram)
  — non-invasive ventilation (NIV)
  — endotracheal intermittent positive pressure ventilation (IPPV) (see Ch. 31).

Oxygen therapy

The aim of oxygen therapy is to increase the fractional inspired oxygen (FiO_2) above 21% (air) to ensure adequate saturation of haemoglobin.

In the presence of type I respiratory failure, oxygen therapy must be prescribed at a level which will correct hypoxaemia, and patients with severe asthma or pulmonary embolism may require 60–100% oxygen initially to prevent hypoxia, until specific disease management is initiated.

In the presence of type II respiratory failure, the low levels of oxygen are providing the respiratory drive, i.e. the stimulus to the respiratory centre in the medulla. High percentages of oxygen can reduce the hypoxic respiratory drive, causing carbon dioxide retention and a respiratory acidosis (see Ch. 8). This is because patients with underlying respiratory disease such as COPD develop sensitivity to falling oxygen levels in the blood rather than raised levels of carbon dioxide. If a higher percentage of oxygen is administered, this may reduce their stimulus to breathe and lead to carbon dioxide retention. If the rising levels of carbon dioxide remain untreated, narcosis, disorientation and ultimately death due to respiratory acidosis will occur. These patients require low percentage oxygen (24–28%) initially. The oxygen can be gradually increased on the basis of repeated arterial blood gases so that carbon dioxide levels can be monitored. Patients with COPD can receive more than 28% oxygen, provided arterial blood gases indicate that there is no evidence of carbon dioxide retention, as only 10–15% of COPD patients are at risk of hypercapnia (Bateman & Leach 1998). However, it is unusual to administer more than 35% oxygen to patients with type II respiratory failure.

Monitoring patients receiving oxygen therapy

- Arterial blood gases should be performed before oxygen therapy is commenced wherever possible.
- Arterial blood gases for patients in type II respiratory failure, or pulse oximetry for patients in type I respiratory failure, should be measured within 2 hours of commencing oxygen therapy and oxygen adjusted accordingly.
- In patients at risk of type II respiratory failure, arterial blood gases should be measured if there is a change in the patient's condition or if the percentage of supplemental oxygen is changed.

Problems associated with oxygen therapy

- Retention of carbon dioxide because high percentages of oxygen can reduce the hypoxic respiratory drive in patients with type II respiratory failure.
- Mucosal drying that can cause pain and discomfort and mucociliary dysfunction, which prevents warming and filtering of the air breathed into the lungs.
- Dehydration of respiratory secretions and subsequent sputum retention.
- Fire is a risk as oxygen is a combustible gas, therefore patients need to be given advice on the dangers of smoking and exposure to naked flames (i.e. gas fires and cookers). Facial burns and death of patients who smoke when using oxygen has occurred.

Table 20.3 Arterial blood gases			
	Normal	Type I respiratory failure	Type II respiratory failure
pH	7.35–7.45	7.35–7.45	< 7.35
$PaCO_2$	4.5–6.0 kPa	4.5–6.0 kPa	> 6.0 kPa
PaO_2	10–13 kPa	< 8.0 kPa	< 8.0 kPa
SaO_2	95%+	< 90%	< 90%

■ Oxygen toxicity can occur if high concentrations of oxygen (> 60%) are given for more than 48 hours. Alveolar membrane damage occurs, progressing to acute respiratory distress syndrome.

Oxygen delivery devices

There is a variety of oxygen devices available but they can be categorized into two types:

Variable performance, i.e. nasal cannula, Hudson mask and any system that does not incorporate a 'Venturi' mechanism. These deliver a percentage of oxygen that depends on the rate and depth of the patient's respirations. These oxygen devices are suitable for patients who are stable and whose respiratory rate does not vary to any great extent. These are generally used for patients on long-term oxygen therapy (LTOT). The use of a nasal cannula allows patients to eat and communicate while receiving oxygen therapy.

Fixed performance. Fixed performance devices include in the delivery circuit a 'Venturi' coloured adaptor or the use of the Venturi principle incorporated into the humidification delivery device (e.g. Respiflow humidification system). The Venturi supplies oxygen to the patient at a precise flow rate that causes mixing of the oxygen with air drawn into the system through holes in the adaptor (Fig. 20.11). The large number of wide holes in the mask will also allow removal of carbon dioxide. This system is more accurate and is not dependent on the patient's rate and depth of respirations. During acute respiratory episodes, these are the masks of choice as they provide accurate concentrations of oxygen and prevent patients re-breathing their own carbon dioxide.

Oxygen flow rates

The flow rates of the different oxygen delivery systems are not interchangeable; for example, 2 litres of oxygen delivered from nasal cannula will not give the same percentage of oxygen as 2 litres through a Venturi system. To prevent confusion, oxygen should be prescribed as a percentage or, when a flow rate in litres per minute (L/min) is prescribed, the type of device to be used also needs stating on the prescription. It is important to follow

R|Я REFLECTIVE PRACTICE

20.2 Oxygen therapy

Think of patients that you have nursed who were receiving oxygen therapy in your clinical area.

● What types of oxygen devices were used? Classify them into variable and fixed performance devices.
● Identify which types of patients require each of the different oxygen devices and why.

the manufacturer's instructions to ensure accurate flow rates are achieved (see Reflective Practice box 20.2).

Humidification of oxygen

When oxygen is delivered at low flow rates (e.g. 1–2 L/min) and in the absence of respiratory tract infections, the oropharynx or nasopharynx may be able to provide adequate humidification. However, oxygen is very drying and therefore humidification should be considered for patients with:

■ flow rates above 2 L/min
■ respiratory infections
■ tracheostomy
■ nasal discomfort/dryness.

Fell & Boehm (1998) identified that lack of humidification can lead to secondary respiratory complications. The drying of secretions can cause pain and increase the risk of respiratory infections, as expectoration of sputum may be inhibited, with the consequence of lung collapse in the small airways (atelectasis), reducing lung expansion.

Humidification systems must provide a mist of the correct particle size in order to deliver a therapeutic aerosol. The particles should be less than 5 μm in order to reach the peripheral airways of the lungs. The most commonly used humidification system is the large volume nebulizer (e.g. Respiflow), which will provide adequate levels of humidification for the majority of patients (see Fig. 20.12).

Patients with tracheostomy require humidified gases because air does not pass through the nose and pharynx, which normally filters and warms it. Lack of humidification in a patient with a tracheostomy can have dire consequences, as secretions that are too viscous to pass through the suction catheter will accumulate and block the inner lumen of the tube (see Ch. 21). The most effective mode of humidification is a heated water system (e.g. Fisher Paykel) delivering 100% relative humidity and this should be used for patients receiving oxygen therapy via a tracheostomy.

▶ Nursing management: patients receiving oxygen therapy

As well as ensuring patients are receiving the prescribed percentage of oxygen using an appropriate oxygen device, the nurse needs to consider their comfort. As oxygen can cause mucosal drying, the development of mouth ulcers is not

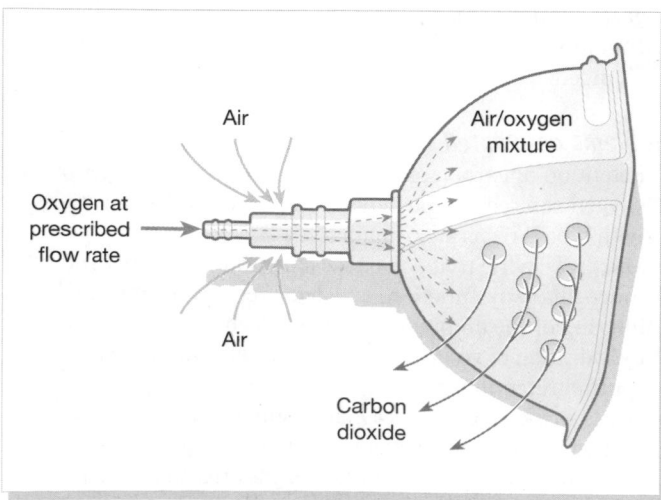

Figure 20.11 Venturi fixed performance oxygen mask.

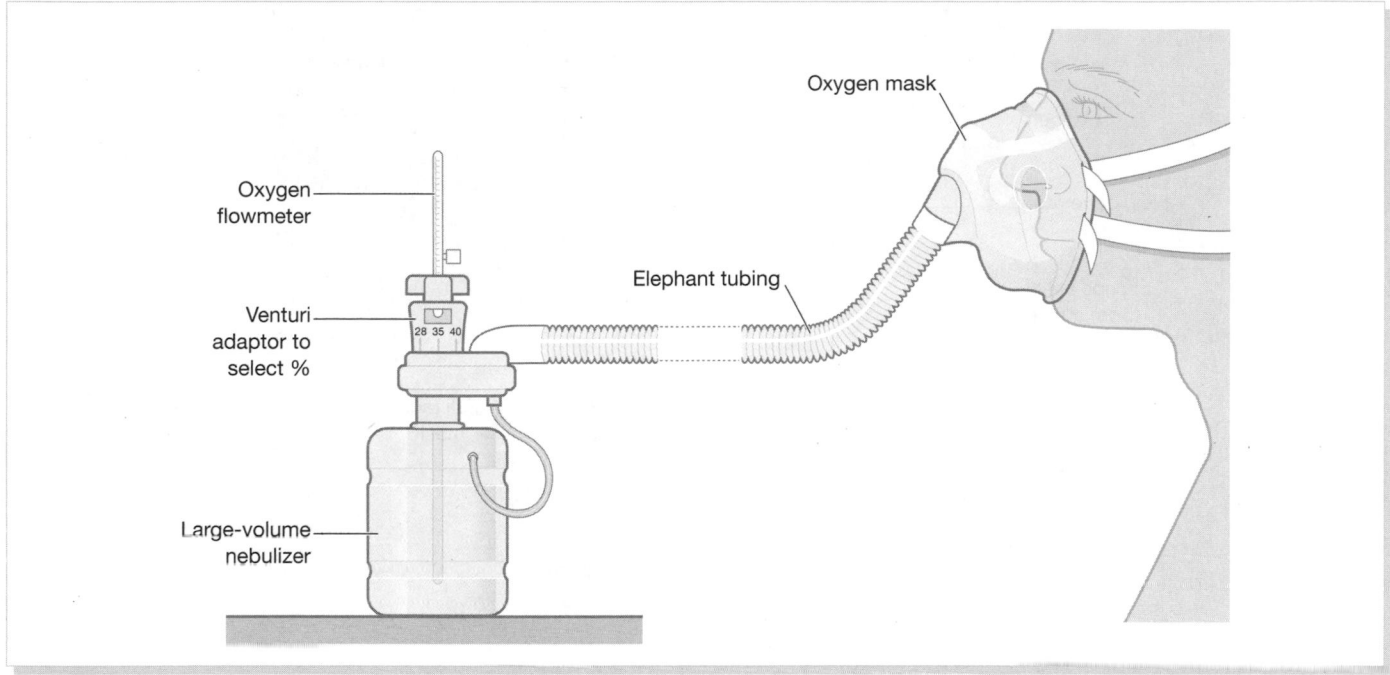

Figure 20.12 Humidification of oxygen.

uncommon in patients receiving continuous oxygen therapy. The nurse needs to perform regular mouth care to prevent the development of mouth ulcers as the consequence of pain and difficulty with eating and drinking can have a significant adverse effect on recovery. The use of humidification may counteract the drying effect, and is indicated if patients complain of discomfort or if there are signs of mouth ulceration. Some patients may have difficulty with communication as the oxygen mask creates a barrier when speaking and the noise of the oxygen may interfere with their ability to hear. Facing patients, taking time and speaking clearly can improve communication, prevent isolation and enable them to express concerns and care needs. The nurse also needs to be aware that pressure ulcers can occur under the oxygen mask straps, and therefore inspection behind the ears for redness and ulceration is necessary. If the straps are causing pressure and/or discomfort, padding behind the ears may help.

Continuous positive airway pressure

Oxygenation can be enhanced by using continuous positive airway pressure (CPAP), which increases lung volume and keeps the alveoli open at the end of each breath to allow more time for gaseous exchange. A full-face mask is strapped in position and needs to be tight fitting, as any leaks will reduce the effectiveness of the positive pressure (see Fig. 20.13). The aim of treatment is to increase functional lung capacity and compliance, decrease the work of breathing, improve ventilation and perfusion, increase oxygen saturations, mobilize secretions, and re-expand collapsed alveoli. CPAP relies on the patient's own respiratory effort and therefore is indicated for treatment of type I respiratory failure when there is:

- restrictive patterns of breathing (e.g. fractured ribs, pain)
- atelectasis, often secondary to pneumonia

- increased work of breathing due to the respiratory effort required to maintain adequate oxygen levels
- difficulty with clearing secretions, particularly when the cough reflex is reduced due to fatigue.

Continuous positive airway pressure needs to be used with caution and by experienced practitioners as it is contraindicated in patients with pneumothorax, bullae (air cysts inside the lung), lung abscess, haemoptysis and hypotension. The majority of patients receiving CPAP will be cared for in a critical care environment, such as a HDU or an ICU (see Ch. 31).

Respiratory stimulants

Doxapram is an intravenous preparation used to reduce carbon dioxide levels through stimulation of the central nervous system to increase the respiratory rate. It is the only respiratory stimulant that should be considered in the treatment of type II respiratory failure where the patient has become drowsy due to carbon dioxide retention. Monitoring of oxygen, carbon dioxide and pH levels is vital. Patients may develop marked anxiety and sometimes hallucinations due to the stimulation of the central nervous system and it is usually only tolerated for 24–48 hours. The patient and family need to be aware that doxapram may produce agitation and hallucinations, as these are distressing side-effects.

Non-invasive ventilation

Non-invasive ventilation (NIV) is a form of ventilation using a well-fitting nasal or full-face mask, and unlike CPAP does not rely on the ability of the patient to breathe spontaneously as the machine has both inspiratory and expiratory phases. It is used to treat patients in type II respiratory failure and has the advantages of being non-invasive, being able to provide adequate oxygen levels with carbon dioxide clearance, decreasing

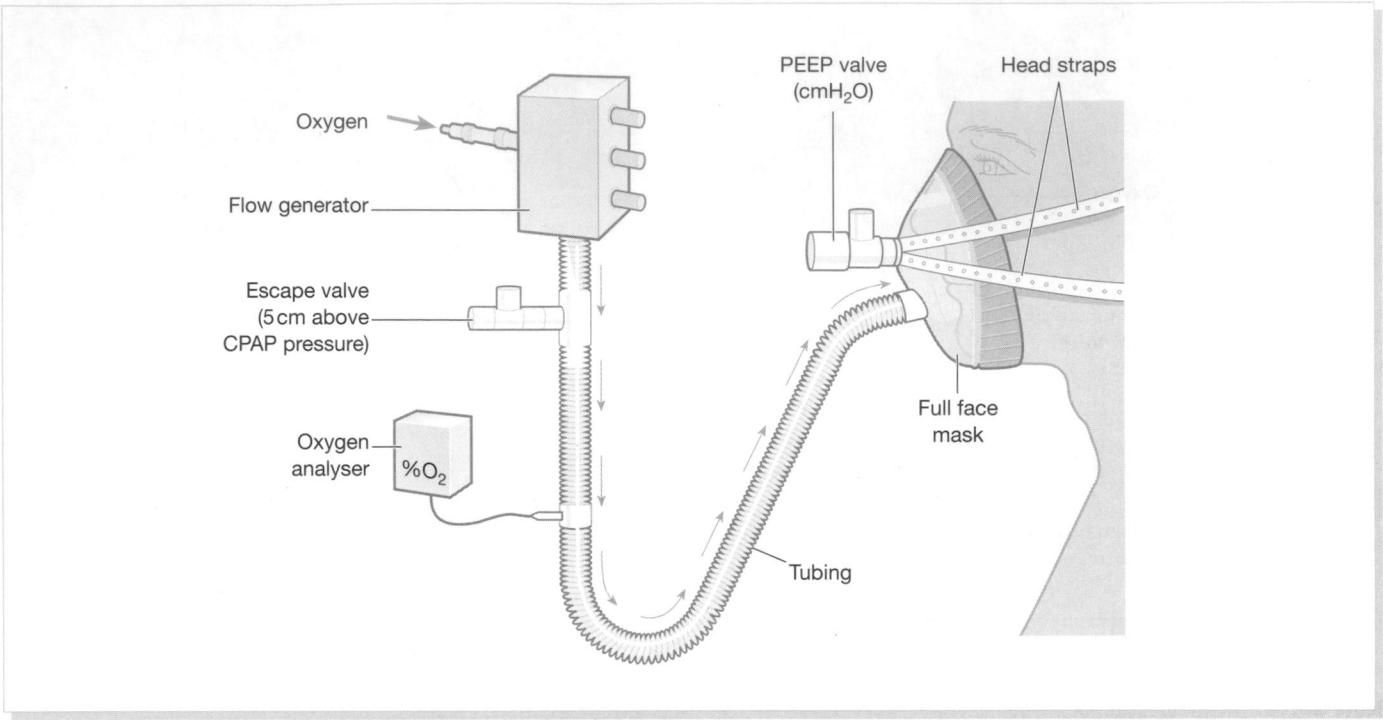

Figure 20.13 Continuous positive airway pressure (CPAP).

the work of breathing and improving the quality of sleep. For it to be successful, the patient must be able to cooperate with treatment, have normal swallowing reflexes, haemodynamic stability and the ability to clear bronchial secretions. The nurse caring for patients receiving this treatment needs to be skilled so that they are able to troubleshoot problems, such as mask problems, dry nose, air leaks, eye irritation and gastric distension. Patients will require psychological support to deal with the effects of altered body image from wearing a facial mask.

PNEUMOTHORAX

A pneumothorax occurs when the integrity of either layer of the pleura is breached allowing air to enter the pleural cavity and leading to lung collapse. There are three types (Gallon 1998), as described below.

Spontaneous pneumothorax

This occurs as a result of the rupture of small blebs, cysts or bullae (air cysts inside the lung). This type of pneumothorax can occur in healthy people, although those with underlying respiratory disease have an increased risk, particularly those with emphysema.

Traumatic pneumothorax

This is caused by blunt chest trauma, a penetrating injury (e.g. stab wound or fractured rib) or secondary to insertion of a sub-clavian cannula or during bronchoscopy. High pressures during mechanical ventilation or CPAP can also cause a pneumothorax as the visceral pleura can be breached. Trauma, particularly with penetrating injuries, can also cause blood to enter the pleural cavity, which is known as a haemothorax.

Tension pneumothorax

Both spontaneous and traumatic pneumothorax can develop into a tension pneumothorax. This is a life-threatening event because air enters the pleural space on inspiration but cannot leave on expiration; the increased pressure causes the mediastinum to shift, which moves the heart towards the opposite side.

Signs and symptoms

The first sign of pneumothorax is the sudden onset of dyspnoea with unilateral chest pain that may radiate to the shoulder or arm and becomes worse on inspiration. On physical examination there is hyperresonance and decreased breath sounds on the affected side and asymmetrical chest movement. Severe dyspnoea, cyanosis, hypotension and tachycardia signify a tension pneumothorax, requiring immediate treatment.

A chest X-ray will confirm the presence and the amount of air in the pleural cavity and, unless there is a tension pneumothorax, will be performed before initiation of treatment. The chest X-ray along with the signs and symptoms will determine the management of the pneumothorax.

Treatment

Treatment options for pneumothorax include the following:

Thoracocentesis. A needle is inserted into the second intercostal space anteriorly to allow the air to escape. This is used in an emergency to relieve a tension pneumothorax. A chest drain (see below) will then be required.

Conservative medical management. Allows the air in the pleura to be absorbed by the body and is used when the pneumothorax is small (< 15% of lung collapsed) and the patient is asymptomatic.

Needle aspiration. Aspiration of the air using a fine needle attached to a 50 mL syringe with a three-way tap is used for

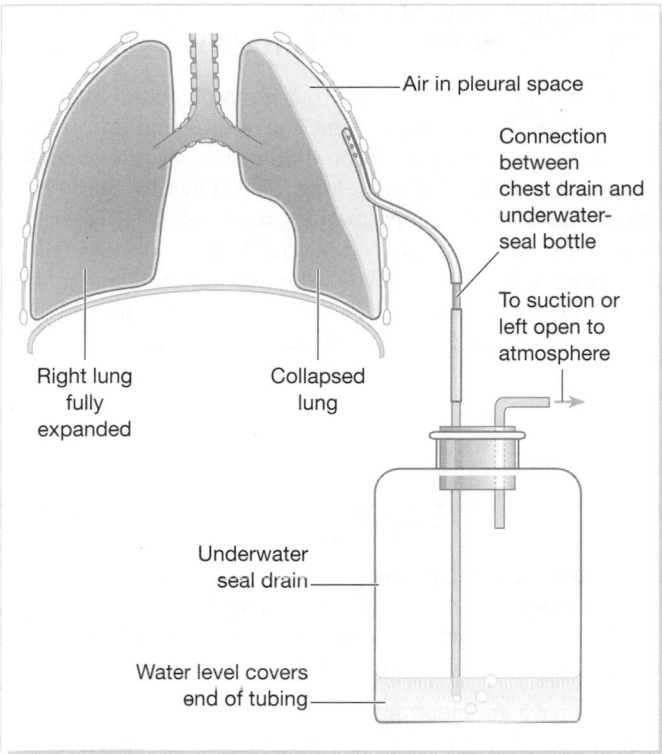

Figure 20.14 Underwater-seal chest drainage system.

patients with a pneumothorax where < 20% of the lung is collapsed and they are symptomatic.

Intercostal chest drain. Under local anaesthetic, a drain is inserted into the fifth intercostal space in the anterior axillary line and is then attached to an underwater sealed drain. The aim of the underwater-seal drain is to allow air to escape from the pleural space but not to re-enter.

Pleurodesis or pleurectomy. Failure to re-expand the lung with intercostal chest drainage or two or more recurrences may require referral to a thoracic surgeon for an abrasive pleurodesis (adhesion of the two pleural membranes so that no space exists) or pleurectomy (stripping of parietal pleura to obliterate pleural space).

▶ Nursing management: underwater-seal drains

The nurse has an important role in caring for patients' chest drains, as many of the potential complications can be prevented if the principles of chest drain management are understood and implemented.

Maintenance of the underwater seal
The underwater sealed drainage system (Fig. 20.14) acts as a one-way valve, allowing air to bubble out through the water during expiration, but because the end of the tube is covered by water, air is prevented from being drawn back into the pleural cavity during inspiration (Avery 2000). If at any point the seal is broken, air can enter the pleural cavity causing the lung to collapse again. The nurse needs to ensure that the water level in the chest drain bottle covers the end of the tube and that the drain and connections are secure and not leaking. The nurse

needs to check that the chest drain bottle is kept below the chest level to prevent fluid entering the pleural cavity.

Maintaining drain patency
The level of water in the tube will 'swing' and 'bubble' as the patient breathes, indicating that the tube is patent and draining. As the lung re-expands, the bubbling will stop and the swing will decrease. Any rapid decrease in the swing may indicate the tube is blocked or kinked and, if not corrected, the lung will collapse. Clamping of the tube is not recommended, unless the connection becomes disconnected, because this mimics the removal or blocking of the tube and may lead to lung collapse.

Prevention of infection
The chest drain is held in place by a purse-string suture which will prevent air leak; therefore, an air-tight dressing should not be used as this increases the risk of infection. A small dry key-hole dressing with an adhesive border should be used and checked daily. If clean and dry, it only needs to be changed every 48–72 hours. If the site becomes infected, this can track up the tube and cause an empyema (pus in the pleural cavity). Infection can also occur during insertion of the chest drain or when the bottle is changed, and therefore an aseptic technique is important.

Pain management
Adequate analgesia is important because if pain is not controlled, patients will restrict their breathing and coughing, which could lead to a lower respiratory tract infection.

Removal of chest drain
Once the lung has re-expanded and there is no further leakage of air or fluid, the drain can be removed. Prescribed analgesia should be administered prior to chest drain removal, as it can be a painful procedure. The main complication associated with chest drain removal is air re-entering the pleural cavity. To prevent this, patients should avoid breathing in during removal; to this end they are asked to hold their breath while the drain is pulled out and the purse-string suture tied to seal the wound.

PLEURAL EFFUSION

Pleural effusion is an accumulation of fluid in the pleural space and is usually secondary to respiratory infections, such as pneumonia and tuberculosis, or malignancy due to lymphatic obstruction or metastasis to the pleura. To determine the cause, pleural fluid is aspirated using a fine needle and sent in a sterile container to the laboratory for analysis. The treatment of pleural effusion consists of treating the underlying cause (e.g. antibiotics for infection) and drainage of the fluid. This can be achieved by pleural aspiration or through the insertion of a chest drain. If left untreated, empyema (pus in the pleural cavity) can develop.

HAEMOPTYSIS

Haemoptysis is the coughing up of blood and occurs when the pulmonary blood vessels rupture. The main reasons for haemoptysis are infection and scarring in the lung, which weakens the walls of the blood vessels, and lung cancer because the tumour can erode into the blood vessels. Blood loss can range from a few flecks to a massive bleed of 200 mL or more.

Coughing up blood, even in small quantities, can be distressing to the patient and family, but a massive haemoptysis (> 200 mL) can be life-threatening and cause panic. The nurse needs to remain calm as this will be supportive and can alleviate anxiety. The initial treatment is to correct hypovolaemic shock and treat any associated clotting disturbances. Oxygen and intravenous sedation are usually prescribed and should be administered without delay. If bleeding continues, a bronchoscopy will be performed to identify the bleeding point so that bronchial artery embolization can be used to stop it.

ASPERGILLUS AND ALLERGIC BRONCHOPULMONARY ASPERGILLOSIS

Aspergillus fumigatus is a fungus that is mainly found in animal manure and rotting vegetation. The spores can be inhaled into the lungs causing chronic infection or disseminated aspergillosis where invasive lung infections by *Aspergillus* occurs. Allergic bronchopulmonary aspergillosis (ABPA) can develop in people who have an allergic response to *Aspergillus*. Patients who develop APBA develop asthma and are treated with prednisolone to treat the wheeze, and antifungals, such as itraconazole and amphotericin, to treat the infection.

SUMMARY: MAIN POINTS

- Lung disease affects around 8 million people in the UK and results in tens of thousands of deaths annually, with a higher incidence of respiratory disease in the lower socioeconomic groups.

- The main cause of respiratory disease is overwhelmingly tobacco smoking.

- Breathlessness is the main cause of distress associated with respiratory disease which impacts on the individual's ability to perform activities of daily living.

- Due to the chronic nature of much respiratory disease, self-management skills need to be taught so that individuals are empowered to manage their condition and make decisions about their health.

- Nurses have an important role in improving the quality of life of people with respiratory disease through holistic care.

- The development of respiratory nurse specialist roles provides continuity of care across primary and secondary care and a focal point for patients to seek advice and support.

SELF-TEST: CRITICAL THINKING ACTIVITIES

1 What are the main predisposing factors to respiratory disease?

2 When assessing a patient with respiratory disease, what clinical skills and tools are required?

3 What impact does breathlessness have on the individual and what strategies can be adopted to alleviate the effects of breathlessness?

4 Who are the key members of the interprofessional team in respiratory care, and what are their roles?

 FURTHER READING

Esmond G (ed). Respiratory nursing. Edinburgh: Baillière Tindall; 2001.

Pryor JA, Prasad A (eds). Physiotherapy for respiratory and cardiac problems, 3rd edn. Edinburgh: Churchill Livingstone; 2002.

Simonds A (ed). Non-invasive respiratory support. London: Arnold; 2001.

 USEFUL WEBSITES

www.lunguk.org – British Lung Foundation
www.brit-thoracic.org.uk – British Thoracic Society
www.cftrust.org.uk/ – Cystic Fibrosis Trust
www.goldcopd.com/ – Global initiative for obstructive pulmonary disease

www.asthma.org.uk – National Asthma Campaign
www.nice.org.uk – National Institute of Clinical Effectiveness
www.thorajnl.com – Thorax (The journal of the British Thoracic Society)

REFERENCES

Avery S. Insertion and management of chest drains. Nurs Times 2000; 96: 3–6.

Baker T. Tuberculosis returns. Nurs Times 2001; 97: 56–57.

Bateman NT, Leach RM. ABC of oxygen: acute oxygen therapy. Br Med J 1998; 317: 798–801.

Bredin M, Corner J, Krishnasamy M et al. Multicentre randomised controlled trial of nursing intervention for breathlessness in patients with lung cancer. Br Med J 1999; 318: 901–904.

British Lung Foundation. Lung disease: a shadow over the nation's health, lung report. London: British Lung Foundation; 1996.

British Lung Foundation. Lung disease: a shadow over the nation's health, lung report II. London: British Lung Foundation; 2000.

British Thoracic Society/SIGN. The British guidelines on asthma management. Online. Available: www.brit-thoracic.org.uk. 2003.

British Thoracic Society. The burden of lung disease. Online. Available: www.brit-thoracic.org.uk . 2001.

British Thoracic Society. Guidelines for the management of chronic obstructive pulmonary disease. Thorax 1997a; 52(Suppl 5): S1–28.

British Thoracic Society. Current best practice for nebuliser treatment. Thorax 1997b; 52(Suppl 2): S1–106.

British Thoracic Society. Chemotherapy and management of tuberculosis in the United Kingdom: recommendations. Thorax 1998; 53: 536–548.

British Thoracic Society. Control and prevention of tuberculosis in the United Kingdom: code of practice 2000. Thorax 2000; 55: 887–901.

Callaghan S. ACTRITE: acute chest triage rapid intervention team. Acc Emerg Nurs 1999; 7: 42–46.

Carter BG. Accuracy of two pulse oximeters at low arterial haemoglobin oxygen saturation. Crit Care Med 1998; 26: 1128–1133.

Cohen S, Rodriguez M. Pathways linking affective disturbances and physical disorders. Health Psychol 1995; 14(5): 374–380.

Corner J, Plant H, Warner L. Developing a nursing approach to managing dyspnoea in lung cancer. Int J Palliat Nurs 1995; 1: 5–11.

Department of Health. Public Health (Control of Disease) Act. London: The Stationery Office; 1984.

Department of Health. Review of the prescribing, supply and administration of medication (2nd Crown Report). London: The Stationery Office; 1999a.

Department of Health. Saving lives – our healthier nation. London: The Stationery Office; 1999b.

Esmond G. Nebuliser therapy update. Prof Nurse 1998; 14(1): 39–43.

Flanagan UM, Irwin A, Dagg K. An acute respiratory assessment service. Prof Nurse 1999; 14: 839–842.

Fletcher CM, Peto R. The natural history of chronic airflow obstruction. Br Med J 1997; 1: 1645–1648.

Gallon A. Pneumothorax. Nurs Stand 1998; 13: 35–39.

Geddes DM, Alton E. The CF gene: 10 years on. Thorax 1999; 54: 1052–1053.

Jorenby DE, Leischow SJ, Nides MA et al. A controlled trial of sustained release bupropion, a nicotine patch, or both for smoking cessation. New England Journal of Medicine 1999; 340: 685–691.

Margereson C, Esmond G. Chronic obstructive pulmonary disease: The role of the nurse. Nurs Times 1997; 93, 20: 5–8.

Medical Research Council Working Party. Long term domiciliary oxygen therapy in chronic hypoxic cor pulmonale complicating chronic bronchitis and emphysema. Lancet 1981; i: 681–686.

National Asthma Campaign. Asthma Audit 2001. Online. Available: www.asthma.org.uk. 2001.

National Institute of Clinical Effectiveness. Guidelines on the use of nicotine replacement therapy and bupropion for smoking cessation. London: National Institute of Clinical Effectiveness; 2002.

Nocturnal Oxygen Therapy Trial Group. Continuous or nocturnal oxygen therapy in hypoxaemic chronic obstructive lung disease. Ann Intern Med 1980; 93: 391–398.

Office of National Statistics. Prevalence of cigarette smoking by sex and socio-economic group. London: National Statistics; 1997.

Office of National Statistics. Prevalence of cigarette smoking by sex and age: 1974 to 1998, living in Britain. London: National Statistics; 1998.

Prochaska JO, DiClemente C. The transtheoretical approach: crossing traditional foundations of change. Homewood, IL: Don Jones/Irwin; 1984.

Pryor JA, Prasad A (eds). Physiotherapy for respiratory and cardiac problems, 3rd edn. Edinburgh: Churchill Livingstone; 2002.

Restrick LJ, Paul WA, Braid GM, Cullinan P et al. Assessment and follow up of patients prescribed long term oxygen treatment. Thorax 1993; 48: 708–713 .

Ries AL. Pulmonary rehabilitation. Joint ACCP/AACVPR evidence based guidelines. Chest 1997; 112: 1363–1396.

Royal College of Physicians. Domiciliary oxygen therapy services: clinical guidelines and advice for prescribers. London: Royal College of Physicians; 1999.

Salisbury D, Begg N. Immunisation against infectious disease. London: HMSO; 1996.

UK Cystic Fibrosis Trust's Antibiotic Group. Report of the UK CF Trust's Antibiotic Group. Bromley: Cystic Fibrosis Trust; 2000.

West R, McNeill A, Raw M. Smoking cessation guidelines for healthcare professionals. Thorax 2000; 55(12): 987–999.

Williams SJ. Chronic respiratory illness and disability: a critical review of the psychosocial literature. Social Sci Med 1990; 28: 79–80.

World Health Organization. Tuberculosis: a global emergency: WHO report on the tuberculosis epidemic. Geneva: WHO; 1994.

World Health Organization. Global initiative for obstructive pulmonary disease (GOLD). Online. Available: www.goldcopd.com. 2002

21 Nursing patients with nose and throat disorders

Sue Stringer

> 'He had a special opening in his neck for his breathing and it scared me to death when he coughed – I thought the whole tube would come out. Luckily the nurses were never far away. They cleared the tube with a special tube and explained why he coughed. They also showed me how it was tied round his neck so it couldn't come out.'
>
> *(Patient's relative)*

THIS CHAPTER WILL HELP YOU

- Understand the specific needs of patients with common disorders of the nose and throat and the nursing care required

- Develop an awareness of the medical and surgical management of nose and throat disorders in a variety of settings

- Develop an awareness of common nose and throat emergencies that may be encountered and the appropriate nursing care for each

- Plan for discharge and give specific advice.

KEYWORDS

Anosmia	Rhinorrhoea
Cilia	Rhinosinusitis
Epistaxis	Stridor
Hyposmia	Tracheostomy
Olfaction	

INTRODUCTION

Nursing patients with nose and throat problems is often much more involved than simply caring for someone who has undergone minor surgery such as tonsillectomy. With the rapid advances in technology, there is now a wide choice of treatment options available for patients with nose and throat disorders, such as microsurgery and endoscopy. Treatment advances have transformed care delivery in the speciality. The length of postoperative hospital stay has also been reduced, so that patients previously hospitalized for a week or more now spend an average of 1.5 days in hospital or have day surgery. However, patients undergoing the more extensive or radical surgery that is now available will be in hospital for 12–14 days and require very intensive nursing care. Thus caring for patients with nose and throat disorders can be a very challenging and rewarding experience, as this chapter will demonstrate.

Nose and throat emergencies are frequently encountered and nurses must be able to recognize these and give appropriate care. Conditions affecting the nose, throat and ears are often interconnected and therefore Chapter 16 (Nursing patients with problems of the ear and hearing) should be read in conjunction with this one. A knowledge of the other systems that may be involved is also essential (see Chs 18, 19 and 20), as is a knowledge of the mechanisms of hypovolaemic shock (Ch. 9). Readers will also need a working knowledge of perioperative care (Ch. 29), and the care of older adults (Ch. 32) and patients with cancer (Ch. 33). Communication is another area that is vitally important (Ch. 3), as patients suffering from throat disorders often have problems in this area, e.g. after removal of the larynx. Patients with nose and particularly throat disorders may be nutritionally compromised and Chapter 11 provides information on dealing with this eventuality, while pain management (see Ch. 7) is an area that is always of relevance where surgical procedures are involved.

OVERVIEW OF ANATOMY AND PHYSIOLOGY

THE NOSE

The nose is part of the respiratory tract; it contains the receptors for smell (olfaction) and helps to produce speech. It consists of bone, cartilage and other connective tissue and is divided into two halves by the nasal septum (Fig. 21.1A). The lateral wall of the nose comprises three ridges of bone, called turbinates, which increase the surface area of the nasal cavity (Fig. 21.1B). The nasal cavity is lined with respiratory mucosa which enables the nose to moisten, warm and filter inspired air. Filtered particles are trapped in the mucus (0.5–1 L/day), which is moved by cilia to be swallowed or expectorated. The other important function of the nose is olfaction, and the area concerned with this is located at the roof of the nasal cavity.

The nose and sinuses receive a good blood supply via branches of the carotid arteries. Little's area, situated at the front of the nasal septum, has a particularly rich blood supply and is the site of many nosebleeds.

THE PARANASAL SINUSES

The paranasal sinuses – maxillary, frontal, ethmoid and sphenoid – are hollow cavities located in the skull (Fig. 21.1B). They are lined with respiratory mucosa. Functions of the sinuses include lightening the skull, reducing the impact of facial trauma and giving the voice resonance. The latter is confirmed by the dull, nasal sounding voice in a person with a cold.

THE PHARYNX

The pharynx is a muscular tube, extending from the back of the mouth into the throat. It is divided into three compartments anatomically, described according to their position – the nasopharynx, oropharynx and hypopharynx (Fig. 21.1B). The

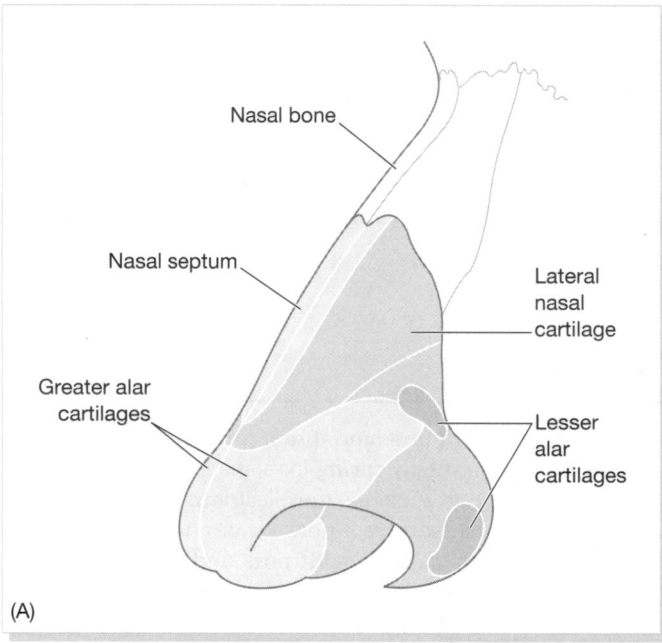

(A)

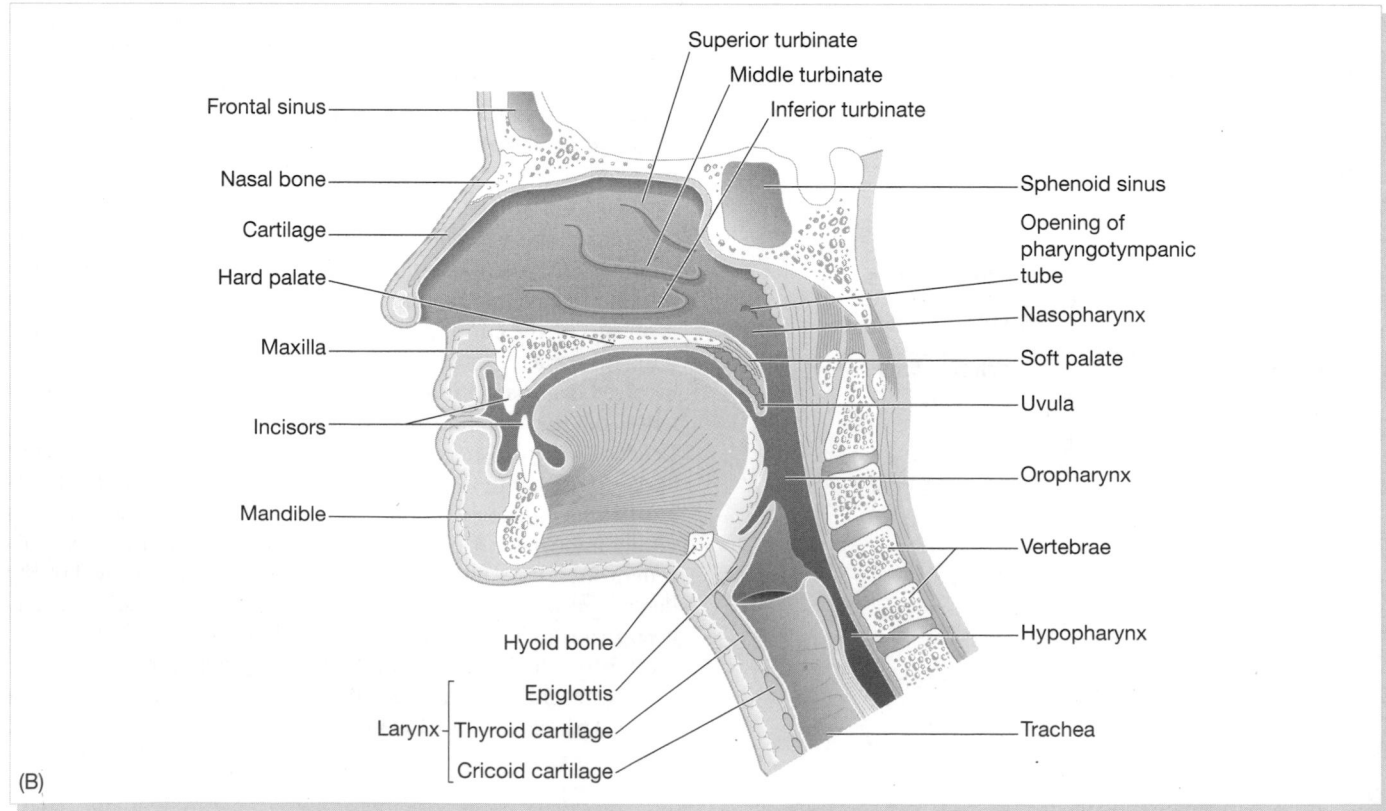

(B)

Figure 21.1 (A) The structure of the nose, showing the bones and cartilage. (B) Sagittal section through the head and neck.

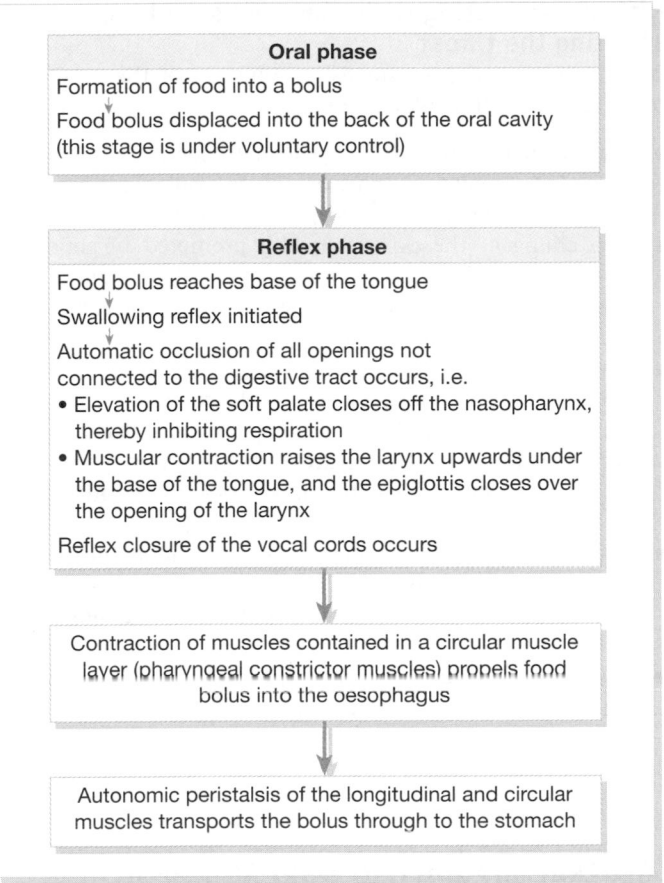

Oral phase
Formation of food into a bolus
Food bolus displaced into the back of the oral cavity (this stage is under voluntary control)

Reflex phase
Food bolus reaches base of the tongue
Swallowing reflex initiated
Automatic occlusion of all openings not connected to the digestive tract occurs, i.e.
• Elevation of the soft palate closes off the nasopharynx, thereby inhibiting respiration
• Muscular contraction raises the larynx upwards under the base of the tongue, and the epiglottis closes over the opening of the larynx
Reflex closure of the vocal cords occurs

Contraction of muscles contained in a circular muscle layer (pharyngeal constrictor muscles) propels food bolus into the oesophagus

Autonomic peristalsis of the longitudinal and circular muscles transports the bolus through to the stomach

Figure 21.2 The physiology of swallowing (adapted from O'Donoghue et al 1992, Becker et al 1994).

tonsils, a ring of lymphoid tissue (Waldeyer's ring) situated in the pharynx at the entrance to the food and air passages, help to protect the body from infection. The nasopharynx is exclusively respiratory, but the other two parts provide a route for food and fluids as well as air. Swallowing has both voluntary and involuntary stages (Fig. 21.2).

The pharynx is a resonating chamber contributing to the pitch and melody of the voice and helping to turn sounds produced by the vocal cords into intelligible words. Other structures are also involved in this process, including the lips, tongue and soft palate.

THE LARYNX

The larynx is located at the top of the trachea and is responsible for producing sound. It is a specialized section of the trachea and is formed by the hyoid bone and the thyroid, cricoid and arytenoid cartilages (Fig. 21.3A). During swallowing the airway is protected as the epiglottis covers the larynx.

The larynx contains the true vocal cords or folds. Each vocal cord comprises a delicate vocal ligament and the vocalis muscle and is covered with mucosa. Their length varies, which is why men, with longer cords, have deeper voices than women. At the front of the larynx, the vocal cords are joined together at approximately the level of the Adam's apple (thyroid prominence) and

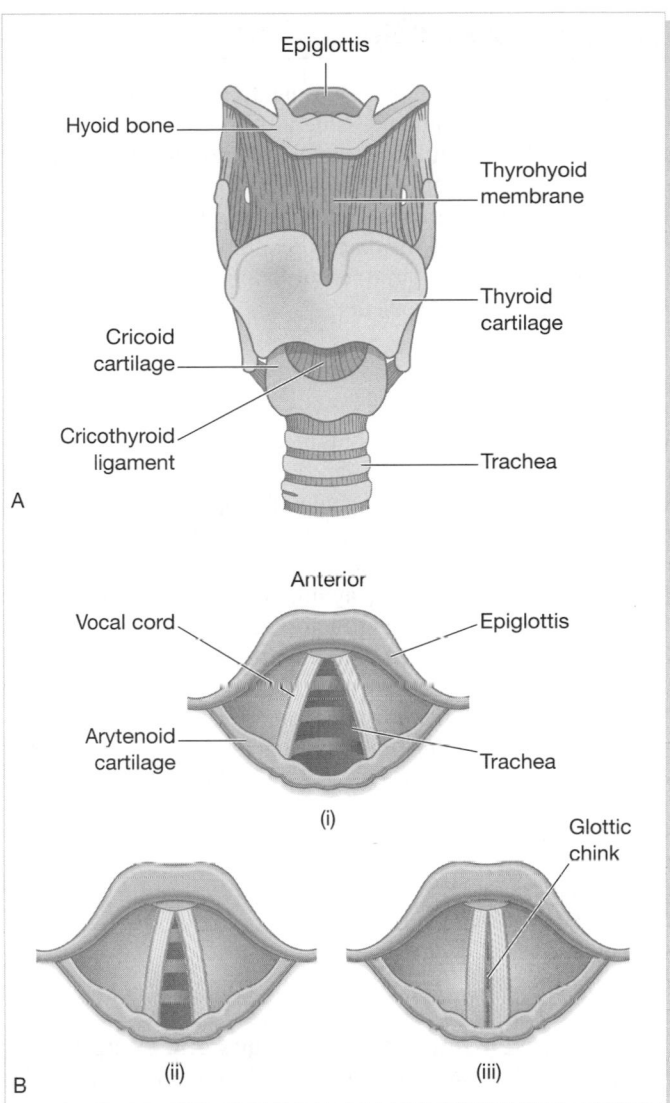

Figure 21.3 (A) Anterior view of the larynx. (B) Positions of the vocal cords. (i) Respiratory or lateral position: when the muscles relax, the arytenoid cartilages rotate laterally and abduct, separating the vocal cords, and no sound is produced. (ii) Paramedian position: tension of the vocal cords – seen in recurrent laryngeal nerve paralysis. (iii) Phonatory or median position: when the muscles of the arytenoid cartilages contract, the cartilages adduct and rotate medially. This pulls the vocal cords together, narrowing the gap between them. As air is forced through this 'chink', vibration of the cords occurs, producing sound.

are firmly anchored to the thyroid cartilage. Posteriorly, the vocal cords are attached to moveable cartilages, allowing their position to be altered depending on the function of the larynx (Fig. 21.3B). An opening (the glottis) between the true vocal cords allows air movement through the larynx.

THE TRACHEA

The trachea extends from the lower end of the larynx to its bifurcation into the two main bronchi. It is composed of 16–20 horseshoe-shaped rings of cartilage.

NURSING ASSESSMENT

In order to provide patients with individualized and appropriate nursing care, a thorough assessment of their general condition is required, which should include, in addition to the presenting condition, an assessment of their general health. This is accomplished by collecting information from or about the patient, by physical observation of the current condition and by reviewing the information, identifying actual or potential problems and then prioritizing these problems.

NURSING HISTORY

A nursing history should be obtained at an early stage so that a nursing care plan can be developed to meet the patient's needs. Important elements include biographical details, family dynamics, anxieties and previous medical history.

Vital signs (blood pressure, pulse and temperature) are recorded to obtain a baseline against which to compare subsequent recordings and to identify any abnormalities. Body mass index is calculated (Ch. 11). This ensures that appropriate drug doses are prescribed and that weight change can be monitored. Urine is tested to identify any abnormalities, e.g. glycosuria.

A nursing history regarding the current symptoms and the progression of the presenting complaint should be established. Other factors include:

- smoking
- alcohol intake
- previous surgery
- medications and allergies
- family history.

Patients presenting with nasal signs and symptoms

Patients are asked about specific nasal symptoms, which helps to establish the diagnosis, allowing the subsequent treatment and nursing care plan to be formulated. The questions should include information about:

- Nasal obstruction – permanent or intermittent, unilateral or bilateral, or variable
- Precipitating factors – such as dust, pollen, alcohol, pets or medications
- Other factors – environmental temperature or humidity and body position, e.g. worse when lying down; history of nasal trauma or surgery
- Nasal discharge – extent and colour (clear, yellow, green or bloodstained), site of origin (front or back of the nose) and whether unilateral or bilateral
- Bleeding – unilateral or bilateral, bloodstained secretions or frank blood
- Visible deformity
- Sense of smell – can range from normal to hyposmia (reduced sense of smell) and complete anosmia (absent sense of smell).
- Pain – ranging from generalized dull headaches and facial aches, to well-localized pain; similarly, pain can be intermittent or persistent, may radiate to other sites, and may be aggravated by bending forwards or straining.

Patients presenting with signs and symptoms affecting the throat

Again, it is essential to establish the history of the presenting complaint, including information about:

- Pain – ranging from a dull ache to acute soreness. It may be persistent or may occur on speaking or swallowing; some patients may complain of referred otalgia (earache)
- Voice changes – these are often what prompted the patient to seek medical help. Changes range from mild hoarseness to total loss of voice and can occur suddenly or gradually; they can be intermittent or constant
- Dyspnoea (difficulty breathing) or stridor (a harsh, vibrating sound produced by a partial airway obstruction) – often late signs of laryngeal or pharyngeal pathology, these can be extremely alarming. The nature of the stridor or dyspnoea should be established, whether it occurs at rest or during exercise
- Dysphagia (difficulty swallowing) – the duration and what causes problems (fluids, solids or semi-solids), and any evidence of coughing or choking during eating or drinking
- Palpable neck lumps – it is important to establish how long the lump(s) have been present, as well as the site, size, mobility, consistency, skin temperature and colour, and tenderness.

GENERAL DIAGNOSTIC TESTS AND MEDICAL INVESTIGATIONS

Some investigations may be carried out by nurses, enabling an early diagnosis to be made. These include examination of the nose and throat, palpation of the neck, skin tests and bacteriological tests.

EXAMINATION OF THE NOSE

The external nose
Nurses should observe:

- the skin
- deformities
- masses
- mobility of nasal bones.

The internal nose
Anterior rhinoscopy allows visualization of the anterior septum, inferior turbinate and middle turbinate. It involves use of a nasal speculum, a good light source and a head mirror. It allows observation of the mucosa, secretions, crusts, perforations and septal deviation.

Posterior rhinoscopy can be carried out indirectly using a nasopharyngeal mirror, allowing visualization of the posterior nasal cavity (Fig. 21.4). Alternatively, a nasendoscope can be used to examine the same areas under direct vision. This method is particularly useful for patients who are unable to tolerate indirect posterior rhinoscopy. Both methods can be used to observe for nasal polyps, enlarged adenoids or nasopharyngeal tumours.

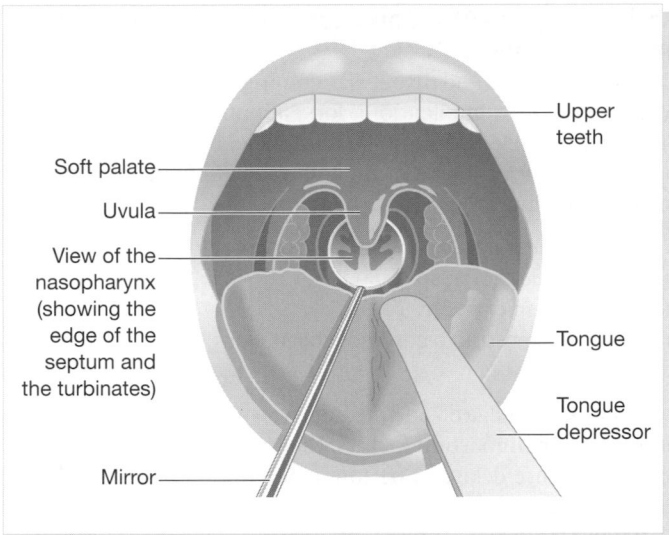

Figure 21.4 Posterior rhinoscopy. This involves depression of the base of the tongue, whilst introducing a small warmed mirror into the space between the soft palate and the posterior pharyngeal wall. This allows examination of the posterior end of the turbinates, posterior end of the septum and the roof of the nasopharynx, including the openings of the pharyngotympanic tubes.

EXAMINATION OF THE THROAT

Palpation of the neck

The neck should be exposed and inspected from the front. Palpation is carried out from behind, with the head slightly flexed to ensure soft tissue relaxation. The neck is palpated systematically with the pads of the fingers and both sides compared. Palpable abnormalities include lymph nodes, tumours, cysts and abscesses.

Internal examination

Indirect laryngoscopy allows inspection of the throat using a laryngeal mirror. Any abnormal masses or ulcerated areas can be identified, and vocal cord mobility assessed.

Endoscopic laryngoscopy involves examination of the throat with a flexible fibreoptic endoscope or rigid endoscope passed along the floor of the nose, allowing a good view of the nasopharynx and larynx. Areas that may be hidden during indirect laryngoscopy may be examined. Direct laryngoscopy allows excellent illumination and examination of the throat under direct vision and is carried out under general anaesthesia with a rigid laryngoscope.

Microlaryngoscopy involves addition of an operating microscope to improve illumination and magnification of the hypopharynx, larynx and upper trachea.

GENERAL INVESTIGATIONS

Blood tests

Blood tests such as a full blood count, urea and electrolytes, liver function, thyroid function and coagulation studies can reveal underlying disorders.

Radiology and scanning

Plain X-rays can demonstrate nasal fractures, intranasal foreign bodies, fluid levels in the sinuses and sinus disease. Plain X-rays of the sinuses are of limited value as they fail to demonstrate precise detail.

Computed tomography (CT) scans are valuable for imaging bony structures and can show normal structures in fine detail and subtle pathological changes.

Magnetic resonance imaging (MRI) provides assessment of the head and neck without exposing the patient to ionizing radiation. Soft tissue is demonstrated well, but because bone appears as a 'void', MRI is of little value in diagnosing nasal and sinus pathology.

Ultrasound scanning can be used to differentiate between solid lesions (e.g. malignant lymph nodes) and cystic lesions (e.g. branchial cysts). This technique may also be used to facilitate fine-needle aspiration of lesions, where cells are obtained for analysis.

Angiography may be used to demonstrate intracranial complications and the blood supply of vascular tumours. It may also be used in conjunction with embolization to control epistaxis and to reduce the vascularity of tumours.

SPECIFIC INVESTIGATION OF NASAL FUNCTION AND PATHOLOGY

Rhinomanometry

Rhinomanometry assesses the patency of the nasal airway and measures the nasal airflow and pressure at the nostrils during respiration. This is carried out using a face mask and a piece of pressure tubing that is inserted into the nasal cavity. During spontaneous respiration, information regarding nasal patency is recorded by a manometer.

A cruder method involves holding a polished metal plate beneath the nose during respiration, and comparing the resulting 'fogging'.

Immunological investigations

Skin tests. These are relatively inexpensive, quick to perform and carry a low risk of anaphylaxis (a severe reaction to injection of a foreign substance). They are frequently used to identify a specific allergen. Sensitivity to common allergens such as pollen, house-dust mite, and animal fur, can be identified. This allows for subsequent allergen avoidance or desensitization.

Radio-allergosorbent test (RAST). This involves combining a sample of the patient's serum with known isolated antigens and measuring the subsequent reaction.

Microbiological investigations

Nasal swabs. These may be of little value diagnostically, as many microorganisms which cause sinus infection are nasal commensals (normally found in the nose without causing harm).

Proof puncture of the maxillary antrum. This allows a sample of pus to be obtained for microscopy and culture to identify the causative organism. The area beneath the inferior turbinate is prepared by application of a topical anaesthetic agent. The bone is then punctured with a pointed trocar contained in a hollow cannula. The trocar is then removed allowing the contents of the sinus to be aspirated via the cannula.

Investigation of olfaction

Olfactometry involves a variety of tests. Olfactory substances such as cinnamon, vanilla, menthol and coffee are presented to the patient, and the ability to distinguish between them is noted.

Investigation of mucociliary clearance

The saccharin test. This test aims to investigate the efficiency of the cleaning system of the nose. This is achieved by placing a fragment of saccharin on the anterior end of the inferior turbinate, using a nasal speculum and forceps, and noting the time taken for the cilia to waft the saccharin into the pharynx, i.e. when the saccharin can be tasted. This occurs within 10–20 minutes if the mucociliary transport mechanism is normal.

Brush biopsy. This involves obtaining a specimen of mucosa from the turbinate via the nostril using a bronchoscopy brush and subsequent examination of ciliary action using a microscope.

SPECIFIC INVESTIGATION OF THE THROAT

Swallowing analysis

A contrast swallow with contrast medium such as barium sulphate may be used to demonstrate the upper digestive tract. This method is useful for patients with dysphagia.

Videofluoroscopy and high-speed cine recordings facilitate the detailed assessment of swallowing using fluorescent fluid and can be useful in the evaluation of neurological disorders (Ch. 14).

Manometry involves measurement of pressure in the lumen of the oesophagus at various points and can be combined with radiography such as fluoroscopy.

Voice analysis

Electrolaryngography and electromyography of the laryngeal muscles are just two of the several methods described for measurement of the voice. They involve recording the electrical currents generated by the active muscles of the larynx during speech.

Video stroboscopy. This allows assessment of the mucosal waveform of the vocal cords and involves examination of the larynx with a nasendoscope linked to a video camera and a stroboscopic light. This light flashes at the same speed as the object being viewed with the effect of 'freezing' the image. This can then be viewed on a television screen.

GENERAL DISEASE PREVENTION AND HEALTH EDUCATION

Many disorders of the nose and throat are preventable and certain predisposing factors are known, e.g. working in a dusty environment. Some conditions may be successfully treated in the community, either following consultation with a GP or simply by seeking advice from a nurse or pharmacist (removing the need to use secondary services). Therefore a proactive approach can only be beneficial, making disease prevention and health education invaluable.

Education of patients ranges from giving information on the prevention of life-threatening conditions like cancer (e.g. cessation of smoking) to information on less serious nose and throat problems such as rhinitis (e.g. to avoid known allergens) or guidelines on the management of sore throats.

Aetiology, prevention and early detection of nose and throat cancer

Cancer of the nose and throat is becoming increasingly common, with devastating implications for patients and their families. Some cancers are known to be influenced by lifestyle, personal habits and risk factors within the environment. Preventative measures include:

- alerting the public to the dangers of smoking
- reducing alcohol misuse
- reducing sun exposure
- avoiding exposure to carcinogens at work, e.g. asbestos and nickel.

Public knowledge of, and attitudes towards, cancer of the nose and throat are important factors. Diagnosis and management of many cases are delayed due to a combination of fear and lack of knowledge.

It is vital to increase awareness of the significance of common symptoms such as hoarseness, oral ulceration and dysphagia, and of the fact that early diagnosis and treatment offer the best chance of cure.

NOSE AND THROAT DISORDERS – GENERAL CONSIDERATION

Disorders of the nose and throat can have profound effects on the everyday life of patients, from nasal obstruction and rhinorrhoea (nasal discharge) associated with sinusitis, to cosmetic deformities of the head and neck, and problems with swallowing, breathing and talking caused by throat cancer. Therefore, although the particular condition may seem routine and commonplace to health professionals, the impact on the person could be considerable and must be considered.

INFECTION AND INFLAMMATION OF THE NOSE AND SINUSES

RHINITIS

Rhinitis is inflammation of the nasal mucosa.

Aetiology and pathophysiology

The aetiology of rhinitis may be allergic (see Special Issues box 21.1), infective, atrophic and vasomotor. Rhinitis is characterized by mucosal inflammation, swelling and increased secretions.

Clinical presentation

Presentation includes:

- nasal obstruction due to mucosal oedema
- rhinorrhoea
- hyposmia or anosmia
- 'irritation' of the entire head
- excessive sneezing
- conjunctivitis
- fever and general malaise.

Secondary bacterial infection is characterized by mucopurulent (mucus and pus) nasal secretions.

SPECIAL ISSUES

21.1 Allergic rhinitis: 'hay fever'

Hay fever is a common condition characterized by sneezing, watery nasal discharge and sore and watering eyes. It causes distress and misery to many people every summer although it may be perennial.

Student activities

- Discuss the effects of this condition and treatment on the quality of life of those affected. In particular, consider how it might impact on everyday activities, such as working, studying, driving, sleeping, taking exams, leisure activities and sport.
- What self-help measures are available? Ask someone with hay fever or, if you suffer, think about what measures help you.

In the case of atrophic rhinitis, wasting (atrophy) of the nasal tissues occurs and the nasal cavity becomes filled with offensive-smelling crusts. Removal of these crusts reveals an abnormally wide nasal cavity and atrophy of the inferior turbinate.

Specific investigations

Investigations should involve establishing the history of the condition, skin testing and possibly radio-allergosorbent testing. In the case of atrophic rhinitis removal of the crusts confirms the diagnosis.

Medical/surgical management

Management of allergic rhinitis is based on allergen avoidance and symptomatic treatment with local corticosteroid preparations for use in the nose (Table 21.1). Antibiotics may be necessary if bacterial infection is present.

Surgical procedures include electrocautery or trimming of the inferior turbinates. In vasomotor rhinitis, all possible mechanical points of irritation are removed, such as septal deviations. Division of the parasympathetic nasal fibres may be indicated, as vasomotor rhinitis is an autonomic nervous system disorder, with attacks sometimes linked to mechanical and chemical stimuli.

Management of atrophic rhinitis ranges from simple conservative measures to operative procedures designed to prevent drying out of the nose by narrowing of the nasal cavity.

▶ Nursing management

Patients with rhinitis will be managed at home. Therefore much of the nursing management involves advice and education.

Advice is given on eliminating or avoiding known irritants, e.g. pollen, animal fur, the house dust mite. Information regarding products available to help with this, such as mattress covers, is offered. Patients should be taught about steam inhalations and administration of corticosteroids, decongestants and sedatives, e.g. in the form of nasal drops and sprays (Fig. 21.5).

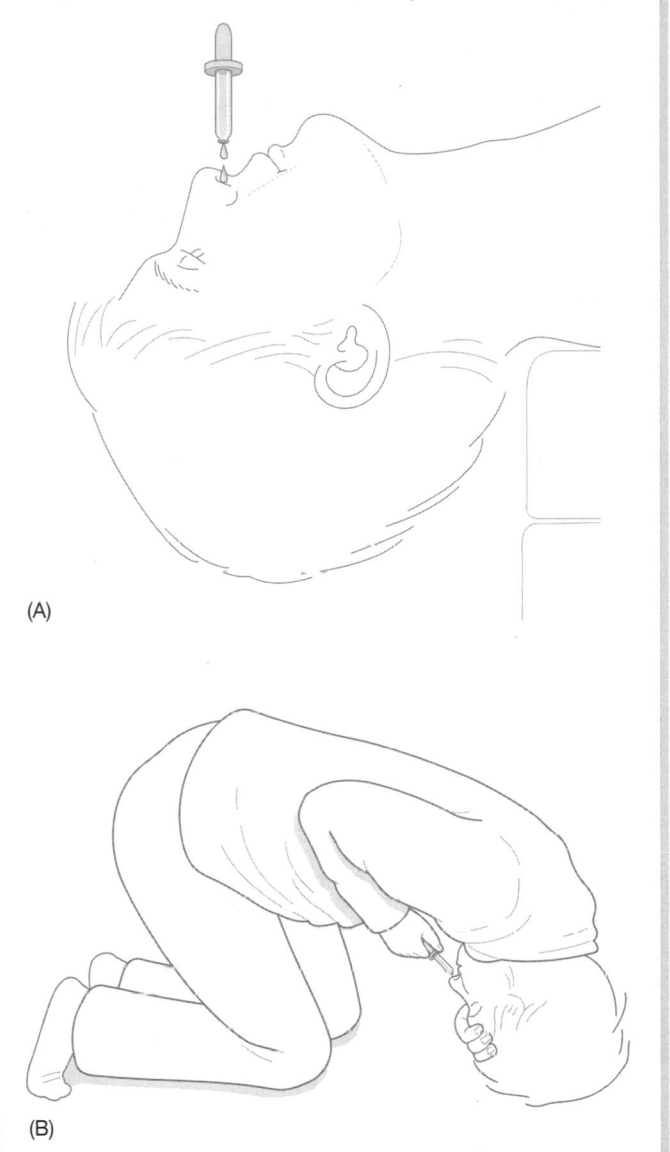

(A)

(B)

Figure 21.5 Methods of administration of nasal drops. (A) With the head tipped backwards (best achieved by lying on a bed with the head hanging over the edge). (B) With the head tipped forwards (technically more difficult!).

Patients with atrophic rhinitis often have very low self-esteem, due to the foul-smelling nasal discharge, and so reassurance and psychological support are essential. In order to reduce the impact of the odour, advice may be given on cleaning, douching and the application of oily emulsions to the nose to prevent the accumulation of crusts. Use of perfumes and air fresheners or deodorizers around the home may also be suggested. It should also be emphasized to the patient that the odour may not be obvious to others.

Vasomotor rhinitis can be associated with stress, and therefore advice regarding stress management and relaxation techniques may be appropriate (see Ch. 6). Coping strategies may be needed and support is given to help patients manage the condition and make lifestyle changes (see Health Promotion box 21.1).

Table 21.1 Drugs used on the nose (adapted from *British National Formulary* 1999)

Name of preparation	Mode of action	Indications	Side-effects
Antihistamine Azelastine hydrochloride	Inhibits the effects of histamine (histamine is released when the allergen is encountered) – used in nasal allergy. Less effective than topical corticosteroids, but more effective than cromoglycates	Allergic rhinitis	Irritation of the nasal mucosa; taste disturbances
Topical corticosteroids Betamethasone sodium phosphate Flunisolide Budesonide	Synthetic corticosteroids used for their anti-inflammatory effect to treat many kinds of inflammation, especially those caused by allergic disorders	Allergic and vasomotor rhinitis	Sneezing after administration, dryness and irritation of nose, epistaxis
Sodium cromoglycate	Mode of action is not fully understood, but it is thought to prevent the release of inflammatory mediators. Less effective than topical corticosteroids	Prophylaxis of allergic rhinitis (should be started 2–3 weeks before the hay fever season commences)	Local irritation, transient bronchospasm (rarely)
Sympathomimetic drugs Ephedrine hydrochloride	Topical decongestant. Acts as a vasoconstrictor	Nasal congestion	Changes in heart rate and blood pressure, anxiety, restlessness, tremor, insomnia. Prolonged or excessive use can result in local irritation, a diminished effect (due to tolerance), and rebound congestion
Antimuscarinic Ipratropium bromide	Inhibits the release of acetylcholine, relaxing smooth muscle and reducing the production of secretions	Watery rhinorrhoea associated with perennial rhinitis	Dry mouth, urine retention (rarely) and constipation
Cocaine hydrochloride	Vasoconstrictor	Used in the examination and treatment of epistaxis, and during nasal surgery (reduces bleeding)	May cause cardiac arrhythmias, especially when used in conjunction with adrenaline (epinephrine)
Dexamethasone and neomycin	Anti-infective preparation	Nasal infections	Prolonged or widespread topical application may lead to sensitivity reactions and/or the development of resistant strains of bacteria
Chlorhexidine and neomycin	Anti-infective preparation	For prevention or eradication of nasal staphylococci. Often used following nasal cautery	Nil recorded
Mupirocin	Anti-infective preparation	As for chlorhexidine and neomycin, but should be reserved for resistant cases, including methicillin-resistant *Staphylococcus aureus* (MRSA)	Nil recorded

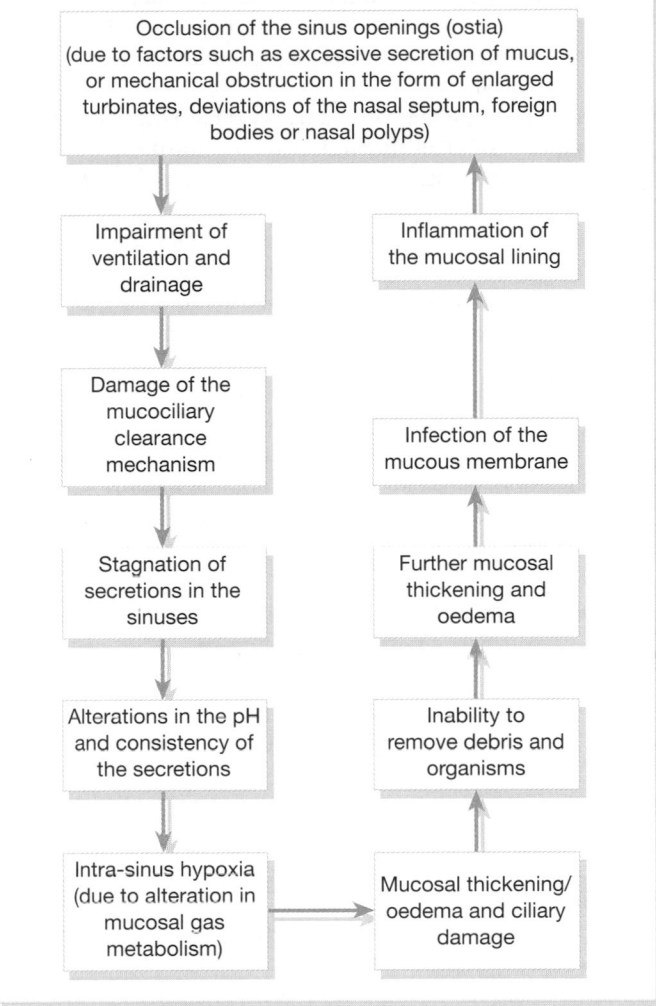

Figure 21.6 Mucociliary clearance and sinusitis (O'Donoghue et al 1992, Becker et al 1994, Evans 1994).

21.1 Self-help for patients with chronic rhinosinusitis

Chronic rhinosinusitis can be a very debilitating and problematic disorder. Although it can be treated surgically, there are several conservative self-help measures that patients can undertake in their home environment in order to ease their symptoms. Such measures include:

- allergen avoidance
- steam inhalations
- administration of nasal sprays/drops.

Student activities
- Using the measures outlined above as a guide, think about what advice you would offer to a patient with chronic rhinosinusitis.

SINUSITIS

Sinusitis is inflammation of the paranasal sinuses and may be acute or chronic.

Aetiology
Acute sinusitis is often a sequela to upper respiratory infections, such as the common cold, but can occur secondary to dental problems. Chronic sinusitis may occur due to inadequate ventilation of the sinuses due to nasal obstruction, or may follow acute sinusitis.

Pathophysiology
Sinusitis often occurs as the inflamed nasal mucosa becomes oedematous and eventually obstructs the opening of the sinuses and pus forms in the sinus (Fig. 21.6).

Clinical presentation
Characteristics of sinusitis include:

- Frontal headaches and facial pains, exacerbated by activities such as bending forwards. Acute sinusitis may cause severe pain, whereas chronic sinusitis may be characterized by a dull ache. Such symptoms can cause great misery, with adverse effects on every aspect of life. In some cases there may be aggravation of chest problems such as asthma (Pearce 1998)
- Nasal obstruction
- Diminished sense of smell
- Pyrexia may accompany acute sinusitis
- Rhinorrhoea (yellowish-green or bloodstained) or postnasal drip.

Various complications may occur, including osteomyelitis, complications affecting the eyes and orbits (such as orbital cellulitis) and spread of infection to the brain, e.g. intracerebral abscesses and venous sinus thrombosis (Ch. 14).

Specific investigations
- Anterior and posterior rhinoscopy or fibreoptic nasendoscopy
- Plain sinus X-rays
- CT scan
- Nasal swabs and/or proof puncture
- Blood cultures.

Medical/surgical management
This may consist of conservative management: antibiotics, analgesia, steam inhalations, topical corticosteroids and decongestants, and systemic decongestants (Evans 1994). Short-term (maximum 7 days) administration of vasoconstrictor sprays may be useful to open the sinus opening (ostia).

If conservative measures fail, there are a number of surgical procedures:

- Sinus washout may be carried out under local or general anaesthesia and involves puncturing the maxillary sinus underneath the inferior turbinate. Saline is introduced into the cavity, displacing debris or pus out through the ostia.

- Antrostomy increases drainage of the maxillary sinus.
- Septal or turbinate surgery improves the airflow to the nose and sinuses and facilitates access for administration of topical medications.
- Functional endoscopic sinus surgery (FESS) involves direct examination of all of the sinuses with a fine nasal endoscope. The sinus openings can be enlarged, improving ventilation and drainage. Diseased tissue within the sinuses is also removed. This restores the mucociliary transport mechanism and usually relieves the patient's symptoms. The main advantage of FESS is that it is minimally invasive. CT scanning prior to endoscopic sinus surgery is essential, creating a 'map' to enable the surgeon to visualize and comprehend the layout of the sinuses during the procedure (Evans 1994). However, potentially serious complications may still occur, such as bleeding, black eyes, adhesions, double vision, partial or complete blindness, injuries to the carotid arteries, and even intracranial injuries (Petroff 1997).

▶ Nursing management

Most patients with sinusitis will be managed in the community by the primary care team. However, patients with severe acute sinusitis may need hospital admission.

Acute sinusitis

In acute sinusitis, nursing care aims to assist patients physically and psychologically during investigations and to relieve symptoms.

Pain is relieved and nasal decongestant drops, e.g. ephedrine hydrochloride, can be administered to decongest the sinus ostia. Antibiotics should be used to treat infection; the choice of drug should, where possible, be dictated by culture and sensitivity results. In severe cases, intravenous antibiotics may be indicated, and thus care of the intravenous cannula will be necessary. Steam inhalations and nasal drops should be administered as prescribed and the patient encouraged to take an active part in such management.

If patients feel generally unwell and debilitated, bed rest should be encouraged and assistance with daily living activities may be appropriate. Oral fluids should be encouraged to prevent dehydration; however, intravenous fluids may be required initially. Fan therapy may help to reduce pyrexia and maintain patient comfort (Ch. 5) and regular mouth care will be essential due to mouth breathing.

Patients must be observed closely for evidence of complications:

- extension of infection to the soft tissues, characterized by skin redness, 'boggy' swelling of the face (around the cheeks and eyes) and tenderness to touch
- orbital complications – glazed, swollen eyelids, pain on pressure, eyeball displacement or protrusion, double vision (diplopia), visual deterioration or limited eye movement
- intracranial complications – headache and sensation of pressure in the head, irritability, restlessness, convulsions, increasing fever, bradycardia, general deterioration, altered consciousness or inappropriate behaviour (Becker et al 1994).

Preoperative nursing – sinus surgery

Surgery may be considered where there is no response to conservative treatment. Prior to this, CT scanning is needed to assess the extent of the disease. All procedures relating to pre- and postoperative care must be fully explained and any questions answered to allay anxiety and allow patients to make informed choices.

Postoperative care – endoscopic sinus surgery

In addition to routine postoperative care (Ch. 29) and specific care following nasal surgery, other important observations must be made:

- visual acuity (focusing ability) or alteration in eye movement
- presence of eye pain
- sudden rise in temperature
- bruising or swelling around the eyes
- severe headaches
- abnormal neurological signs – fits, altered consciousness.

Any abnormalities are reported immediately to the surgeon as they could signify postoperative complications. The airway should also be observed and respirations monitored, as the patient will usually have a nasal pack in situ, which could potentially become displaced into the pharynx. Pain levels are assessed (Ch. 7) and appropriate analgesia is given as prescribed.

Several weeks may elapse before the mucosa of the nose and sinuses is fully healed and measures to prevent infection should be implemented. Prophylactic oral antibiotics are commenced on the day of surgery.

Steam inhalations help to reduce the nasal congestion which inevitably follows nasal surgery. Care must be taken to minimize the risk of scalding. The addition of substances to the inhalation, e.g. menthol crystals, is not advisable, as they may irritate the mucosa.

Topical corticosteroid drops are commenced 3 days postoperatively to reduce mucosal inflammation. Prior to administration of the nasal drops, patients should be encouraged to blow their noses gently. After ensuring that the nozzle or dropper is clean and intact, they are asked to lie down with the head tilted back (Fig. 21.5A). Following instillation, patients breathe via the mouth and remain in position for several minutes to allow the drops to reach the ethmoid sinuses. Alternatively, they could adopt a kneeling position (Fig. 21.5B) to allow the nasal drops to reach the ethmoid sinuses. However, this manoeuvre will not be suitable for all patients.

Discharge advice and follow-up care

On discharge the patient should be advised to continue with the topical corticosteroids, steam inhalations and antibiotics until their outpatient appointment (7–10 days later), when their nose is usually decrusted by the surgeon and healing assessed using nasendoscopy.

EPISTAXIS AND SEPTAL DEVIATION

EPISTAXIS

Epistaxis (nosebleed) is a common emergency in ENT and A&E departments and can generally be controlled fairly easily. Some bleeding, however, is extremely difficult to control and can result in significant morbidity and distress for the patient and may be life-threatening.

Aetiology and pathophysiology

The causes of epistaxis are varied and may be local or general:

Local causes include trauma, tumours, hereditary haemorrhagic telangiectasia, nasal infections and sudden environmental or atmospheric pressure changes, e.g. during flying. Vascular degeneration (common in older adults) has also been implicated.

General causes may include coagulation defects, e.g. thrombocytopenia and haemophilia, cardiovascular conditions, such as hypertension, mitral stenosis and arteriosclerosis, and chronic hepatic and renal disease and anticoagulant drugs.

Clinical presentation

Epistaxis may range from a minor trickle to a torrential haemorrhage. Bleeding may originate from the anterior or posterior portion of the nose. Each patient presents with individual problems and needs. Some are calm, relaxed and haemodynamically stable, whereas others are anxious, fearful and nauseous. Where bleeding is severe, they may present with hypovolaemic shock (Ch. 9).

Specific investigations

- *A full blood count* – haemoglobin, red cell count and parameters, white cell count, platelet count and haematocrit; blood group is ascertained and blood cross-matched if transfusion is required
- *Coagulation screen* – to eliminate bleeding disorders
- *Anterior rhinoscopy* (see p. 573).

Medical/surgical management

Depending on the amount of bleeding, first aid (see p. 576) and stabilization with intravenous fluids or plasma may be needed. Management of profuse epistaxis must take priority over finding the cause. However, certain significant facts must be ascertained (Phillips 1997a).

Intravenous access should be established and fluids or blood administered as appropriate. Anterior rhinoscopy is performed to locate the origin of the bleeding. Any examination or treatment to the nose can be facilitated using a topical anaesthetic and vasoconstricting solution applied either as a spray or on cotton wool pledgets placed inside the nose.

Once the patient is stabilized, the aim is to stop the bleeding. Methods of haemostasis include the following:

- Nasal cautery – if a bleeding point can be located, it may be cauterized with either silver nitrate or electrocautery
- Nasal packing and balloons – where the bleeding point cannot be identified, or is inaccessible, nasal packing may be required. A variety of packing materials are now commercially available, e.g. bismuth iodoform paraffin paste or nasal tampons (Fig. 21.7).

If the nose is bleeding posteriorly or cannot be controlled by cautery or anterior packs alone, it will be necessary to insert anterior packs in conjunction with either a postnasal pack or balloon. Hospital admission is strongly advised after anterior packing because the pack may be dislodged into the throat

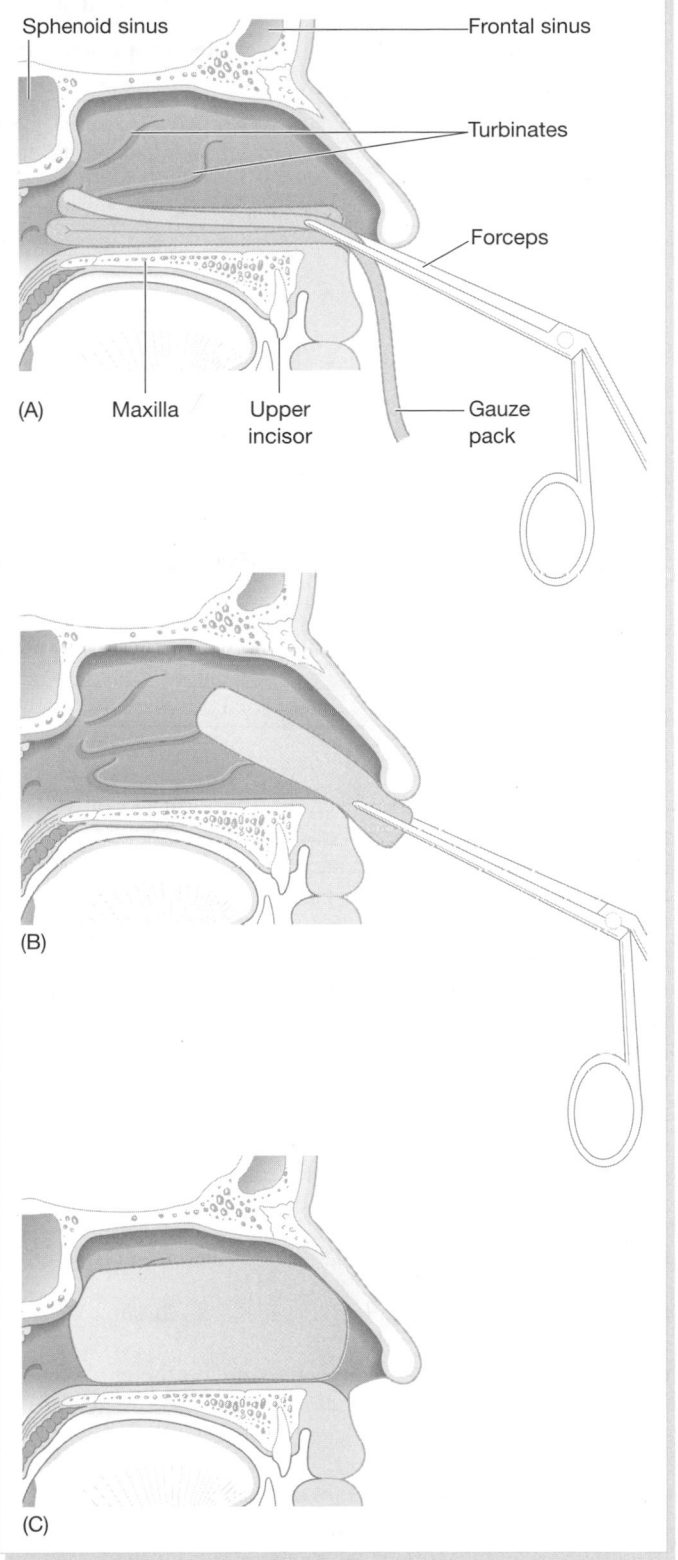

Figure 21.7 Nasal packing. (A) The gauze pack is introduced into the nose in horizontal layers from the floor of the nose upwards. (B) The nasal tampon is introduced into the nose using forceps (following preparation with a suitable lubricant). (C) As the pack absorbs exudate or blood from the nose, it swells in size, thereby applying pressure to any bleeding vessels.

Table 21.2 Complications of nasal packing (adapted from von Schoenberg et al 1993, Murthy & McKerrow 1995)

Associated with pack insertion	Associated with maintenance of the pack	Associated with pack removal	Late complications
Pain	Hypoxia and hypoxaemia – may lead to myocardial infarction and stroke	Pain or discomfort	Secondary haemorrhage
Vasovagal attack	Obstructive sleep apnoea	Trauma	Adhesions
Cardiovascular collapse (due to hypovolaemic shock, vasovagal reflex, reactions to local anaesthesia/ vasoconstricting drugs)	Infection – local, e.g. sinusitis, or general, e.g. bacteraemia or toxic shock syndrome Fever Abscess	Haemorrhage	Septal perforation
Trauma to soft palate, nares, mucosa	Pharyngotympanic tube obstruction – may lead to otitis media with effusion, acute otitis media, haemotympanum Bleeding or haematoma		Nasal infection
	Accidental pack displacement which compromises the airway Unusual chronic inflammatory response induced by petrolatum and lanolin-based ointments used in postoperative packs		Pharyngeal incompetence and stenosis Paraffin granulomata (rare)

(potential for asphyxia). However, if posterior packs or balloons are used, hospital admission is essential, as the risk of pack displacement, and hence asphyxia, is greater. Most patients with nasal packs in situ will receive light sedation, e.g. diazepam, to relieve anxiety and promote bed rest. Oral antibiotics will be prescribed for patients with posterior packs or balloons.

The complications of nasal packing include pain, trauma, pack displacement, hypoxia, infection, toxic shock syndrome and otitis media (Table 21.2).

In addition to haemostasis, patients with untreated hypertension may require antihypertensive drugs. Other underlying conditions are treated or an appropriate referral is made. Where cautery or packing fail to control bleeding, other methods are available, including:

- septal surgery – improves access and makes nasal packing easier
- arterial ligation – generally reserved for life-threatening epistaxis (Bent et al 1999)
- arterial embolization – involves passing a catheter via the femoral artery into the offending artery and obstructing it with polyvinyl alcohol particles (Phillips 1997a).

▶ Nursing management

Examination and treatment for epistaxis can be distressing and alarming for patients and nurses should provide physical and psychological support. Patient cooperation can make the difference between a successful procedure and an unsuccessful one.

Initial care (First aid)

When a patient initially presents with an epistaxis, first aid measures are employed, regardless of the location, be it in the A&E department, the ward, the GP's surgery, or at home. These measures are as follows:

- Maintain a calm atmosphere and reassure by explaining all procedures and care.
- Sit the patient down.
- Provide a receptacle to catch the blood, and also in case of vomiting.
- Encourage the patient to lean forwards over the receptacle.
- Encourage the patient to breathe gently through the mouth and to spit out blood, rather than swallowing it.
- Apply pressure to the soft part of the nose (Little's area) for approximately 10 minutes.
- Apply ice packs to the nose and forehead to ease bleeding through reflex vasoconstriction of the blood vessels.
- Evaluate the extent of blood loss and record the amount.

In a health care setting, ensure that oxygen and suction equipment are accessible. Monitor blood pressure and pulse as required (every 15–30 minutes initially) to observe for hypotension and tachycardia resulting from blood loss, or hypertension which could be contributing to the epistaxis. Ensure that intravenous access is patent and administer intravenous fluids as prescribed.

Ongoing nursing measures (see also Older Adults box 21.1) Careful monitoring of vital signs and general condition is important not only in the acute phase but also in the period following, in order to detect the development of complications. For example, choking indicates pack displacement; pyrexia could signify infection; and irritability, restlessness and disorientation could indicate toxic shock syndrome or hypoxia.

Oxygen should be administered if prescribed, as should antibiotics and sedatives. Most patients with nasal packing in

65 83
50 71 **OLDER ADULTS–NURSING PRIORITIES**

21.1 Epistaxis

- Older adults may have age-related changes and disorders that contribute to epistaxis and the severity of bleeding, such as hypertension and other cardiovascular diseases.
- They may be less able to cope with physiological stresses, such as severe blood loss.
- They may have other age-related changes, e.g. poor mobility, that must be considered in their nursing management.
- Discharge planning should take account of the factors likely to affect the patient's ability to self-care at home, e.g. the manual dexterity and cognitive ability to administer nasal drops and antihypertensive drugs. In addition, it may be necessary to address other health and social care issues, such as housing, assistance needed with activities of daily living, help available from family or neighbours, finances, lifestyle and risk assessment and a patient who is normally a carer. Referrals to social services, physiotherapists, occupational therapists and community nurses may be necessary.

situ (particularly posterior packs or balloons) will require regular analgesia, e.g. paracetamol or weak opioid.

Due to the inevitable mouth-breathing and dried blood inside the mouth, oral hygiene is essential and should be carried out as required. Bed rest is necessary to prevent further haemorrhage and patients will need help with daily living activities (although independence should be encouraged where possible). This will include assistance with hygiene and elimination and, because even walking to the lavatory should be discouraged, provision of urinals or bed pans may be necessary or use of a wheelchair to the lavatory.

Patients with nasal packs in situ (particularly posterior packs) may find eating and drinking difficult. Regular cool fluids should be encouraged, but hot fluids that may cause vasodilatation and further bleeding should be avoided. Straws should be provided to keep the nasal dressing dry.

Blood may continue to ooze through the nasal packs and the soiled nasal dressing should be replaced in order to preserve patient comfort and dignity.

Discharge advice

Patients should be given discharge advice as follows:

- Avoid nose blowing for at least 2–3 days. Then only do so very gently one nostril at a time, to allow the fragile nasal mucosa time to heal.
- Avoid strenuous activities, such as heavy lifting or exercise, for 2–3 weeks.
- Avoid contact sports for at least 4–6 weeks.
- Avoid bending down with the head forwards which can raise blood pressure, leading to further bleeding.
- Avoid straining during defaecation for 4–6 weeks, which also increases blood pressure. Prevent constipation by having a high-fibre diet and taking adequate fluids. A laxative may be necessary.

- On no account remove scabs which may form in the nose as this will lead to further bleeding. Such scabbing can be particularly problematic following nasal cauterization. In order to avoid scab formation and prevent infection, petroleum jelly or an ointment containing chlorhexidine and neomycin may be applied to the nostrils twice daily.

DEVIATED NASAL SEPTUM

Aetiology

The nasal septum usually has some degree of bending and, in fact, a septum that is perfectly straight and in the midline is rare. Causes of deviation include genetic factors, fractures or birth injury.

Pathophysiology

Anatomical deformities include dislocation of the caudal or lower end of the septum into one of the nostrils or deviation of the posterior part of the septum further back in the nose. Displacement of the nasal septum causes altered airflow through the nose and sinuses which results in impaired ventilation of the sinuses and hypertrophy of the middle turbinate bone.

Clinical presentation

The most common complaint is nasal obstruction, unilateral or bilateral. Some patients may present with a cosmetic deformity of the external nose. Recurrent sinus infections or epistaxis may also be encountered.

Specific investigations

Rhinomanometry may be carried out (more objective than patient testimony). Sinus X-rays or CT scan may be performed to exclude sinus involvement.

Medical/surgical management

No intervention is required where deviation and symptoms are minor. In severe cases, however, correction of the nasal septum may be undertaken.

Submucosal resection of the nasal septum

This operation is generally performed for deformities of the middle part of the septum.

Septoplasty

This is a more conservative procedure and is usually performed for septal (caudal end) dislocation. It involves minimal removal of cartilage, and cautious repositioning of the septum in the midline (see Evidence-based Practice box 21.1).

▶ **Nursing management**

Preoperative nursing – septal surgery

Patients require information about what to expect postoperatively. For example, they should be told that they may have a nasal pack initially and normal nasal breathing will be impossible. Reassurance should be given that they will automatically breathe through the mouth instead. Prior warning should also be given regarding postoperative bleeding and the need for

EVIDENCE-BASED PRACTICE

21.1 Septal surgery as day-case procedures

In 1996, Benson-Mitchell et al conducted a study into septal surgery as a day-case procedure. They hypothesized that many procedures that have traditionally been considered to require an overnight stay may be carried out on a day care basis. The outcome of their study supported this hypothesis, concluding that providing strict selection criteria are followed, day-case septoplasty is a safe and acceptable procedure and is associated with a low complication rate.

Student activities
- Find out if this type of surgery is undertaken as a day-case procedure in your area and, if not, what are the reasons.
- If day-case septal surgery is undertaken in your area, what selection criteria are used?
- In the light of this literature, consider the pros and cons of day-case septal surgery.

References
Benson-Mitchell R, Kenyon G, Gatland D. Septoplasty as a day-case procedure – a two centre study. J Laryngol Otol 1996; 110(2):129–131.

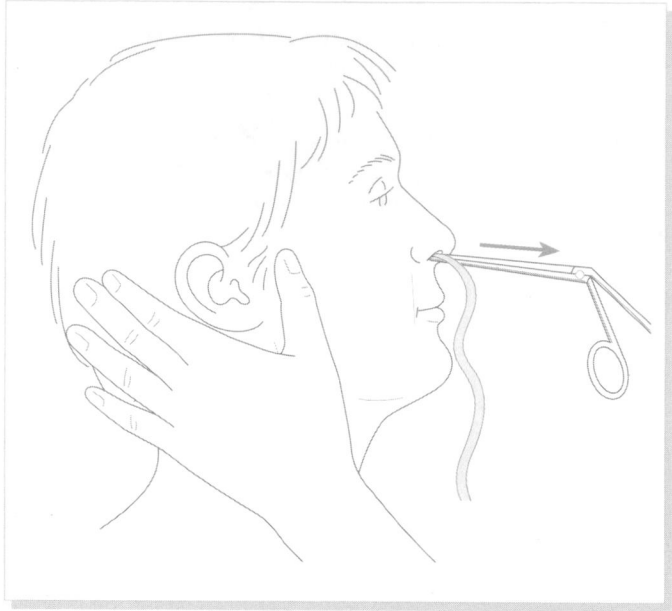

Figure 21.8 Removal of nasal packing. Using a pair of forceps, the end of the pack is grasped tightly and gentle traction applied. The direction in which the pack is eased from the nose should follow the same horizontal plane that was used to insert the pack. The patient's head may be supported with the other hand if necessary.

regular dressing changes. Both of these can cause distress and anxiety in unprepared patients.

Postoperative nursing – septal surgery

Specific care required following septal surgery includes observation of the airway, as nasal packs could be dislodged into the throat. This includes physical observation of the rate, depth and rhythm of respirations. Examination of the patient's throat using a tongue depressor and light may be necessary if pack displacement is suspected. Pulse oximetry or observation of the patient for cyanosis may also be carried out. Observation for bleeding is also required, as haemorrhage is the most common complication following this type of surgery.

Blood pressure and pulse are monitored until stable to detect haemodynamic problems resulting from blood loss or anaesthesia. The temperature should be monitored to detect signs of infection, i.e. pyrexia. A pain assessment should be undertaken and any pain managed appropriately and effectively.

Most patients will have a nasal dressing consisting of a piece of gauze taped underneath the nose or a bolster underneath the nose secured with ties around the back of the head. As blood will leak through the pack onto the dressing, it will require changing several times a day.

Nausea and vomiting may be a problem (swallowed blood irritates the stomach) and prescribed antiemetics should be administered. Food and fluids should be withheld for 1–2 hours postoperatively in case of nausea or significant haemorrhage necessitating a return to theatre for haemostasis.

Mouth care should be offered at least 2- to 4-hourly and should consist of gentle cleaning or rinsing of the mouth. When patients are sufficiently recovered, they can be encouraged to perform their own mouth care. Drinking straws should be provided to prevent contamination of the nasal dressing.

Nasal packs are generally removed the day after surgery, something that is often distressing for patients, who will need explanation and reassurance (Fig. 21.8). Analgesia may also be given prior to the procedure to reduce the discomfort. Following removal of the packs, the nose and surrounding area should be gently cleaned to remove any dried blood.

Discharge advice and follow-up

On discharge, patients are advised to avoid nose blowing for 2–3 days, to avoid strenuous activity or heavy lifting for 2–3 weeks and to avoid straining (see p. 577). Crowded places should be avoided for 1–2 weeks, where contact with upper respiratory infections is likely, and individuals known to be infected should also be avoided. Smoking and smoky areas should similarly be avoided for 1–2 weeks as smoke irritates the nasal mucosa.

The patient should be told that swelling will block the nasal airway for 1–2 weeks after the operation and that a certain amount of oozing and bloodstained discharge is likely for approximately 1 week postoperatively.

Contact numbers should be provided and patients told to seek medical advice if the discharge becomes alarmingly bloodstained or smelly, if they become generally unwell with a fever, if the nose becomes red and sore or if any other problems are experienced.

A review appointment is generally arranged for 4–6 weeks postoperatively, where other potential complications of septal surgery may be recognized, such as septal perforation, septal haematoma, adhesions between the septum and the lateral nasal wall, nasal deformity due to excessive removal of cartilage and anosmia (rarely).

NASAL INJURIES

NASAL FRACTURES

Nasal fractures may be either closed or open. They can occur in isolation or be part of more extensive facial injuries.

Aetiology
Facial trauma sustained during sport, assaults, fights or traffic accidents often results in fractures of the nasal bones. These can occur from the front or the side.

Clinical presentation
Visible signs such as nasal deformity, bleeding, bruising and swelling of the surrounding tissues usually occur. Other symptoms may include pain and nasal obstruction. The nasal bones may also be mobile on palpation (but it is not recommended that this is tried!).

Specific investigation
Although X-rays can be useful where multiple nasal fractures are suspected, their value in the management of isolated nasal fractures is debatable.

Medical/surgical management
Management depends on the severity and when the patient presents. For patients presenting immediately after injury, urgent reduction under local or general anaesthesia must be considered, before swelling makes a satisfactory reduction unlikely. Patients presenting at a later stage, i.e. 24–48 hours after the injury, are generally asked to return after 7 days. Manipulation under general anaesthetic should then be possible when the swelling has subsided.

Depending on the type of injury, the bones may be lifted using an elevator inside the nose or pushed back into place by digital pressure on the side of the nose. Nasal packing may be required to hold the fragments in position. A plaster of Paris or thermoplastic splint will be required in the event of very unstable nasal bones.

For injuries left longer than 10–14 days, reduction becomes impossible and formal rhinoplasty (reshaping of the nose) may be required.

▶ Nursing management

Preoperative nursing management
Nursing management will depend on the stage of presentation. Thus, it may include assisting the patient during control of epistaxis secondary to fracture, pain relief, cleaning lacerations and applying ice packs to reduce oedema and bleeding. The preoperative care for those requiring reduction under anaesthetic is as for septal surgery (see p. 577).

Postoperative nursing management
The nursing management depends on the chosen treatment option. Postoperative care, however, is similar to that required following septal surgery.

If external splinting is required, nursing management will include provision of advice about splint care. For example, as it is essential that the splint remains in position for 7–10 days, care must be taken to ensure that the tape holding it in position does not become wet. Situations where further injury may occur, such as contact sports, must be avoided for 6 weeks postoperatively.

SEPTAL HAEMATOMA

This is a collection of blood between the septal cartilage and the covering mucosa (mucoperichondrium).

Aetiology and pathophysiology
Septal haematomas usually result from nasal trauma and are often bilateral. The septal cartilage derives its blood supply from the perichondrium and necrosis may occur if a septal haematoma is left untreated. This results in collapse of the nasal bridge. Subsequent infection of the haematoma results in septal abscess and possible intracranial sepsis.

Clinical presentation
On examination of the nasal cavities, a bluish, 'boggy', fluctuant swelling will be evident in one or both sides. The patient usually complains of increasing nasal obstruction, pain and tenderness.

Specific investigations
Anterior rhinoscopy and palpation of the swelling with a probe confirm the diagnosis (as the swelling will feel 'boggy').

Medical/surgical management
The risks of necrosis and infection make haematoma evacuation an immediate priority. This is achieved by making a large incision in the mucoperichondrium inside the nasal cavity and draining the haematoma, usually under general anaesthesia. Nasal packing is inserted to encourage healing of the mucoperichondrium and cartilage. Where the haematoma is infected a wound drain may be required.

▶ Nursing management

Patients may experience a significant amount of pain and appropriate analgesia will be required. Antibiotics should also be administered as prescribed to avoid a septal abscess. Care relating to the nasal packs will also be required (as for septal surgery and epistaxis).

SEPTAL PERFORATION

This refers to a hole in the nasal septum, usually in the cartilaginous part.

Aetiology and pathophysiology
Septal perforations result from a variety of causes, including trauma (e.g. habitual nose-picking). Perforation may have iatrogenic causes, such as pressure from nasal packs and balloons, following septal surgery or cauterization. Other causes include syphilis and tuberculosis, malignant conditions such as melanomas or lymphomas, or chemical trauma, e.g. cocaine sniffing or industrial exposure to chrome salts.

Clinical presentation

Patients may present with epistaxis and crusting. Small perforations may cause whistling during respiration. Some patients, however, may be asymptomatic. Fibrosis and collapse of the nasal dorsum may be a late presenting feature. This condition is characterized by saddling or depression of the nasal pyramid.

Specific investigations

Where the cause is unknown, the following tests are performed:

- blood tests, e.g. full blood count, erythrocyte sedimentation rate and serology to exclude syphilis
- biopsy
- chest X-ray to exclude uncommon causes, e.g. Wegener's granulomatosis (autoimmune disease).

Medical/surgical management

No specific treatment is required for asymptomatic perforation. Whistling may be remedied by enlargement of the perforation or the insertion of a silastic button. Rarely, the perforation is closed surgically, using mucosal flaps. Coexisting diseases are managed appropriately, e.g. patients with Wegener's granulomatosis will require corticosteroids, immunosuppression and possibly chemotherapy or radiotherapy.

▶ Nursing management

Saline douches and application of petroleum jelly to the edges of the perforation are useful to combat crusting, and long-term use of antibiotic cream may be necessary to prevent infection. Patients with coexisting diseases, e.g. Wegener's granulomatosis, are often seriously ill and require intensive nursing care, including assistance with all activities of daily living.

Patients having surgery need clear information about the likely postoperative course, including the possibility that the surgery could fail. Postoperative care should include airway observation (may have packs in situ), monitoring of blood pressure and pulse, and monitoring for evidence of infection.

NASAL OBSTRUCTION

Nasal obstruction, although often regarded as trivial, may reduce quality of life for some sufferers. Obstruction leads to mouth-breathing, dry mouth and halitosis. Disturbances of smell and taste can occur and may affect the enjoyment of food. The inability to breathe properly makes physical activity and sport difficult.

NASAL POLYPS

Nasal polyps are pendunculated tumours arising from the mucosa of the sinuses or nose.

Aetiology

The aetiology of nasal polyps is not fully understood, but they may have an allergic origin. Other factors include various drugs, e.g. aspirin, and temperature changes may also have a role.

Nasal polyposis is a chronic condition and recurrence is common. Coexisting asthma and aspirin sensitivity may also

occur. Antrochoanal polyps are single polyps arising from the maxillary sinus and occur much more rarely.

Clinical presentation

Signs and symptoms include severe nasal obstruction, rhinorrhoea, sneezing and reduced or absent sense of smell. Examination reveals pale, grey, glistening sacks of mucosa hanging into the nasal cavity.

Specific investigations

- Anterior rhinoscopy
- Skin tests for allergies
- Possible CT scan to determine the extent of the disease.

Medical/surgical management

Some polyps regress spontaneously but most will require some intervention. Management may include topical corticosteroids. A 3-month course is usually given and approximately 50% will have a good response. Systemic corticosteroids may be given as a short course in severe cases, but are not routinely used because the long-term side-effects outweigh the benefits.

A nasal polypectomy (polyp removal) may be carried out under local or general anaesthesia. Ethmoidectomy involves removal of the ethmoid cells from which the polyps originate. It is used in the management of recurrent polyps. Antrochoanal polyps are excised from their narrow pedicle and removed via the mouth (under general anaesthetic).

▶ Nursing management

Patients being managed conservatively are instructed how to instil nasal drops or sprays. For patients undergoing surgery, pre- and postoperative care is as for any other nasal surgery. Patients with coexisting asthma require close observation of the airway and breathing and the administration of bronchodilators and other asthma drugs as prescribed.

NASAL FOREIGN BODIES

Nasal foreign bodies, e.g. beads, are common in children, but they may also be encountered in adults with learning disabilities.

Clinical presentation

Foreign bodies present with a unilateral foul-smelling nasal discharge.

Medical/surgical management

Due to the patient group commonly affected, removal of foreign bodies often requires a short general anaesthetic (although one attempt at removal under local anaesthesia is usual). A hooked instrument is passed behind the object and it is carefully manipulated out of the nose.

▶ Nursing management

Pre- and postoperative nursing care should be tailored to meet the individual needs of the patient, especially where understanding may be limited. If removal under local anaesthesia is attempted, a great deal of psychological support or distraction may be required. Minor epistaxis often accompanies foreign body removal and reassurance should be given that this will soon stop.

INFECTIONS AND INFLAMMATION OF THE THROAT

Throat infections range from a minor inconvenience to severe life-threatening situations. Examples of such infections include tonsillitis, peritonsillar abscess, pharyngitis and retropharyngeal abscess.

TONSILLITIS

This is acute infection of the tonsils.

Aetiology and pathophysiology

Tonsillitis is usually due to bacterial infection, which may be secondary to a viral infection. Bacteria are normally present in the mouth and pharynx, but these sometimes become pathogenic if the environment changes. Causative organisms include *Streptococcus pyogenes* and *Haemophilus influenzae*. The palatine tonsils have crypts which drain into the oral cavity. If these become occluded, ideal conditions for microorganisms are produced. The formation of pus in the crypts leads to chronic tonsillitis, which can develop regardless of tonsil size.

Clinical presentation

Modes of presentation include sore throat, dysphagia, pyrexia, earache and general malaise. The tonsils are enlarged and red bilaterally, sometimes with pus discharging from the tonsillar crypts. Cervical lymph nodes may be enlarged and tender.

Medical/surgical management

Management consists of analgesia and antibiotics, and possibly a tonsillectomy later if recurrent tonsillitis is troublesome. Severe tonsillitis with dehydration may require admission to hospital for intravenous fluids and antibiotics.

Tonsillectomy

Tonsillectomy involves removal of the entire tonsillar tissue bilaterally. The main indication for tonsillectomy is recurrent tonsillitis (four or more attacks per year for at least 18 months) causing disruption to work or study. Other indications include chronic tonsillitis, unilateral enlargement (which may indicate a malignancy), peritonsillar abscess and very large tonsils, causing sleep apnoea (Phillips 1997b; Ch. 4) or difficulty with swallowing. Patients generally remain in hospital overnight following tonsillectomy, but day-case surgery is now becoming acceptable (Fenton & O'Dwyer 1994).

▶ Nursing management

Pre- and postoperative care – tonsillectomy

Preoperatively the patient should be given an explanation of what to expect postoperatively: soreness and risk of bleeding.

Airway management is a priority following tonsillectomy, and patients should be nursed on their side or semi-prone until fully awake to allow blood and saliva to drain from the mouth. Patients' colour and respirations should be observed and a pulse oximeter used if available.

The main risk following tonsillectomy is haemorrhage, either reactionary (within the initial 24 hours postoperatively) or secondary (up to 14 days postoperatively). Various methods have been used to prevent haemorrhage, with varying degrees of success, e.g. application of fibrin glue (Stoeckli et al 1999) and surgical techniques, such as diathermy and ligation of bleeding vessels.

Close observation of the patient for evidence of haemorrhage, leakage, spitting blood from the mouth or excessive swallowing is essential. Blood pressure and pulse should be monitored regularly (hypotension and/or tachycardia could indicate hypovolaemia). If haemorrhage occurs, hydrogen peroxide mouthwashes are given as prescribed to remove clots from the tonsil beds. If this fails to stop the bleeding, pressure can be applied to the tonsil bed with a gauze swab. If this fails, a return to theatre is usually necessary.

As a severe sore throat and otalgia are known to be significant features of tonsillectomy (Molony et al 1998, Warnock & Lander 1998), many methods of management have been considered. These include topical or injected local anaesthetics and nerve blocks. The most common method of management is oral analgesia, preferably in a soluble or liquid form.

Pain may make many patients reluctant to eat and drink. As eating is important as part of the healing process, some encouragement may be necessary. Analgesia given 30 minutes prior to meals may help. The traditional soft diet postoperatively was later replaced with the recommendation of a rough diet. However, trials have demonstrated no differences in pain, secondary haemorrhage and healing rates between patients instructed to eat a soft diet, those told to eat a rough diet, or those given no dietary advice. Therefore the general consensus today appears to be simply to eat regularly (Bhaskar 1998; see also Evidence-based Practice box 21.2).

 EVIDENCE-BASED PRACTICE

21.2 Diet after tonsillectomy

'Traditionally, soft cold foods have been recommended after tonsillectomy to aid comfort and haemostasis but, more recently, rougher foods have been advocated to promote physiologically normal deglutition' (Cook et al 1992).

A trial was conducted to discover whether post-tonsillectomy dietary advice has any influence on recovery. Cook et al (1992) concluded that as there were no significant differences between the diets regarding postoperative pain, analgesic required, healing rates or secondary haemorrhage, specific post-tonsillectomy dietary advice is unnecessary, other than to encourage regular eating.

Student activities

- Is any particular dietary advice advocated in your area, and if so, what are the reasons given for this?

References

Cook JA, Murrant NJ, Evans KL, Lavelle RJ. A randomised comparison of three post-tonsillectomy diets. Clin Otolaryngol 1992; 17(1): 28–31.

Chewing gum has also been cited as reducing postoperative pain and bringing about a speedier return to normal dietary intake as it may reduce muscular spasm in the throat and jaw. However, Hanif & Frosh (1999) found increased pain and delay in eating and concluded that this practice should not be routinely advocated.

PERITONSILLAR ABSCESS

Peritonsillar abscess or quinsy is a collection of pus around the tonsillar capsule.

Aetiology and pathophysiology

Peritonsillar abscess may follow tonsillitis as inflammation spreads from the tonsil to the surrounding tissue and forms an abscess.

Clinical presentation

Symptoms include severe sore throat, pyrexia, dysphagia, referred otalgia and possibly trismus (difficulty opening the mouth). A characteristic 'hot potato' voice (i.e. thick, indistinct speech) is usually present.

Examination reveals tonsillar enlargement and inflammation, gross asymmetry of the soft palate and displacement of the tonsil towards the midline (Fig. 21.9).

Medical/surgical management

A blood test is performed to exclude infectious mononucleosis. First-line treatment is aspiration or incision and drainage of the abscess to relieve pressure and pain and reduce the risk to the airway. This is achieved by aspiration of the pus or drainage via a small stab incision under local anaesthesia.

High doses of antibiotics are then administered (usually intravenously) and intravenous fluids are often necessary as many patients present are dehydrated due to pain and dysphagia.

Some centres advocate 'hot' tonsillectomy, i.e. removal of the acutely infected tonsils. However, this is generally regarded as technically difficult, with the theoretical risk of abscess rupture during intubation.

▶ Nursing management

Treatment of a peritonsillar abscess can be extremely frightening and patients require immense psychological support. The

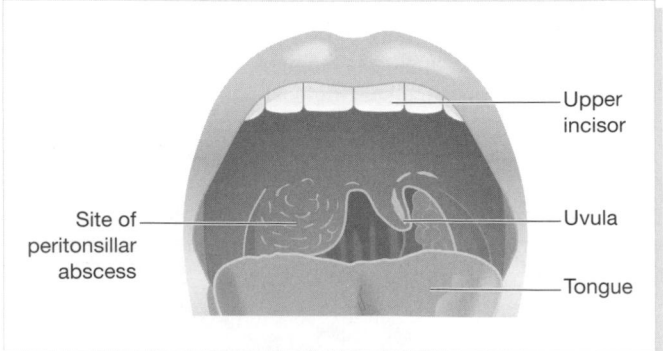

Figure 21.9 A peritonsillar abscess (or 'quinsy'). Note the grossly asymmetric soft palate, with the uvula pushed away from the side of the abscess.

procedure should be fully explained and the fact that it provides immediate relief from severe pain should be emphasized.

Airway observation is essential, as oedema could lead to airway obstruction. This is important both prior to drainage of the abscess and afterwards, as swelling may persist for several days.

Analgesia should be administered as prescribed. Soluble preparations are usually necessary due to dysphagia, but parenteral administration, e.g. intramuscular injection, may be required where dysphagia is severe. High-dose intravenous antibiotics should be administered as prescribed and the cannula site monitored for evidence of inflammation or infection. The temperature should be recorded regularly and pyrexia managed as appropriate (Ch. 5).

Regular mouth care and mouthwashes will be necessary as oral dryness and halitosis frequently occur due to mouth-breathing. Oral fluids should be encouraged to prevent dehydration and supplementary intravenous fluids should be given as prescribed. Dietary advice should be offered; cool, soft foods are more likely to be tolerated.

Assistance with all other activities of daily living, such as personal hygiene, may be required by patients who are dehydrated, lethargic and generally unwell.

DEEP NECK ABSCESSES

These include retropharyngeal and parapharyngeal abscesses.

Aetiology and pathophysiology

These are rare occurrences. Retropharyngeal abscesses are generally related to tuberculosis of the cervical vertebrae, whereas parapharyngeal abscesses may follow tonsillitis or dental infections of the lower jaw.

Clinical presentation

Symptoms are similar to those of a peritonsillar abscess but with neck stiffness. Airway obstruction may also occur due to pressure on the pharynx and larynx. Parapharyngeal abscesses may cause swelling below and behind the angle of the jaw and of the upper neck.

Specific investigations

An X-ray of the neck may reveal an increased soft tissue space in front of the vertebrae.

Medical/surgical management

- High doses of intravenous antibiotics
- Possible surgical drainage
- Tracheostomy (see p. 584) may be necessary to maintain the airway.

▶ Nursing management

This is as for peritonsillar abscess, with particular regard to airway observation.

LUDWIG'S ANGINA

This is cellulitis (inflammation of the soft tissues) affecting the oral floor. It should not be confused with angina pectoris (Ch. 19).

Aetiology and pathophysiology

Ludwig's angina has a variety of causes, including dental infections, lacerations or infections, salivary calculi, and mandibular fractures. Microorganisms gain access and an abscess forms in the loose musculature of the tongue and the connective tissue spaces.

Clinical presentation

Presents with pain and swelling in the floor of the mouth, pyrexia and displacement of the tongue. Dysphagia and excess salivation also occur due to immobility of the tongue. Voice changes and airway obstruction may also occur.

Specific investigations

Soft tissue neck X-rays and possibly MRI scanning are appropriate investigations.

Medical/surgical management

High-dose antibiotics are indicated. Drainage and exploration may be necessary and endotracheal intubation or tracheostomy (see p. 584) may be required to secure the airway in severe cases.

▶ Nursing management

This is as for peritonsillar abscess, but with very close observation of the airway. The risk of airway obstruction is high and patients are best nursed in a high-dependency unit (Ch. 31).

PHARYNGITIS

Pharyngitis is inflammation of the pharynx. It is generally managed in the community. Pharyngitis is usually caused by a virus but secondary bacterial infection may also occur. Oral antibiotics are generally only given for severe bacterial infections.

Symptomatic relief is offered for sore throat, oral analgesia, mouthwashes, local anaesthetic lozenges and steam inhalations. Bed rest may be appropriate for severe pharyngitis with fever.

LARYNGITIS

Laryngitis is inflammation of the larynx.

Aetiology and pathophysiology

Acute laryngitis often occurs following an acute upper respiratory tract infection and generally resolves fairly promptly. Chronic laryngitis is more common in the winter and often follows a cold or influenza. Other precipitating factors include smoking, drinking alcohol and over-using the voice.

Clinical presentation

Hoarseness, dysphonia (difficulty speaking) or aphonia (complete voice loss) and a sore throat may also occur. The larynx looks red and dry and often there is stringy mucus between the vocal cords.

Specific investigations

An indirect laryngoscopy should be performed, followed by direct laryngoscopy or microlaryngoscopy in chronic cases. This may be done under local or general anaesthesia.

Medical/surgical management

Predisposing factors should be eliminated, such as smoke, infections, chronic sinusitis and postnasal drip. Periodic stripping of affected mucosa may be required using microsurgery or laser.

▶ Nursing management following direct laryngoscopy

The priority following direct laryngoscopy is airway observation, as oedema can obstruct the airway.

Local anaesthetic spray is generally applied to the vocal cords during the procedure which could impair the protective reflexes that normally ensure that food or fluids entering the larynx are expelled with a cough. Patients remain nil orally for 2–6 hours postoperatively until the protective reflexes return.

Perforation of the pharynx or oesophagus can occur and is characterized by dyspnoea, back or chest pain and pyrexia. For this reason, diet and fluids are introduced gradually, beginning with sterile water only for the first 6 hours. Nurses should observe for signs of perforation and record the temperature hourly for 6 hours postoperatively.

Analgesia should be administered as prescribed by a parenteral route initially.

If a biopsy is taken, voice rest is necessary to allow the true vocal cords (folds) to recover and patients are advised not to speak for 48 hours and to carry a pen and paper for communication (Ch. 3). Many patients find this very difficult and it is the reason why voice rest must be stressed. After 48 hours, speaking may usually resume, although shouting or whispering must be discouraged to avoid straining the vocal cords. Talking in noisy environments, noisy public houses, discos or in a moving car, where it may be necessary to raise the voice, should also be discouraged.

Patients are advised to reduce alcohol and coffee intake, as both can have detrimental effects by dilating the surface capillaries of the vocal cords. Frequent cool drinks help to prevent a dry throat, as may steam inhalations and humidifiers.

Throat clearing and coughing should also be avoided, and patients should be encouraged to pause for breath more frequently when speaking, to reduce demands on the voice. Support and education regarding cessation of smoking may also be applicable.

Referral to a speech and language therapist may be appropriate where direct laryngoscopy is normal and it is thought that patients are using their voices incorrectly.

LARYNGEAL OBSTRUCTION

Laryngeal obstruction presents an absolute emergency as death can quickly result.

Aetiology and pathophysiology

The causes of laryngeal obstruction include tumours, acute infection or inhaled foreign bodies.

Clinical presentation

The most striking sign of laryngeal obstruction is stridor (a hard, high-pitched respiratory sound). Patients may be restless and anxious. Dyspnoea and cyanosis may be present.

Specific investigations

These will depend on the patient's condition and the nature of the emergency.

- Neck and chest X-ray may show a foreign body and a contrast barium swallow will outline the oesophagus and may reveal tracheal compression.
- Examination under anaesthetic with emergency tracheostomy (see below) may be required to secure the airway.

Indirect laryngoscopy should be avoided as it could cause complete airway obstruction.

Medical/surgical management

The airway is secured with endotracheal intubation or tracheostomy as required. Intravenous corticosteroids to reduce inflammation and antibiotics (if infective) are usually given.

▶ Nursing management

This will depend on cause and treatment but close monitoring of airway will be required in all cases. These needs may be best met in a high-dependency setting. The rate, depth and rhythm of respirations should be monitored and pulse oximetry is essential to monitor for hypoxia (Ch. 31). Humidified oxygen should be administered as prescribed to moisten the respiratory tract, making breathing easier.

Laryngeal obstruction is extremely terrifying for patients and their relatives. Support, explanation and psychological care are imperative. A calming atmosphere should be preserved at all times.

TRACHEOSTOMY

A tracheostomy is an opening into the trachea via the neck (Fig. 21.10A). It may be temporary or permanent (following laryngectomy). Tracheostomy can be performed surgically or percutaneously by inserting a guide wire into the trachea and dilating the tract until it is wide enough for the tracheostomy tube.

Reasons for performing a temporary tracheostomy include the following:

- to bypass upper airway obstruction
- to enable long-term mechanical ventilation
- to facilitate tracheobronchial suction
- to prevent aspiration of secretions.

Tracheostomy tubes

There are many types of tube and choice will depend on such factors as the reason for the tracheostomy, the procedure performed and the ability to tolerate the tube in question (Fig. 21.11). Where the tracheostomy is permanent and self-care is anticipated, the manual dexterity and ability of the patient must be considered; some patients may be unable to remove and clean the inner tube of certain devices. Tubes are generally constructed from metal or flexible synthetic materials. Most synthetic tubes have an inflatable cuff which creates an air-tight seal between tube and trachea. This arrangement prevents the aspiration of secretions into the lungs and facilitates mechanical ventilation.

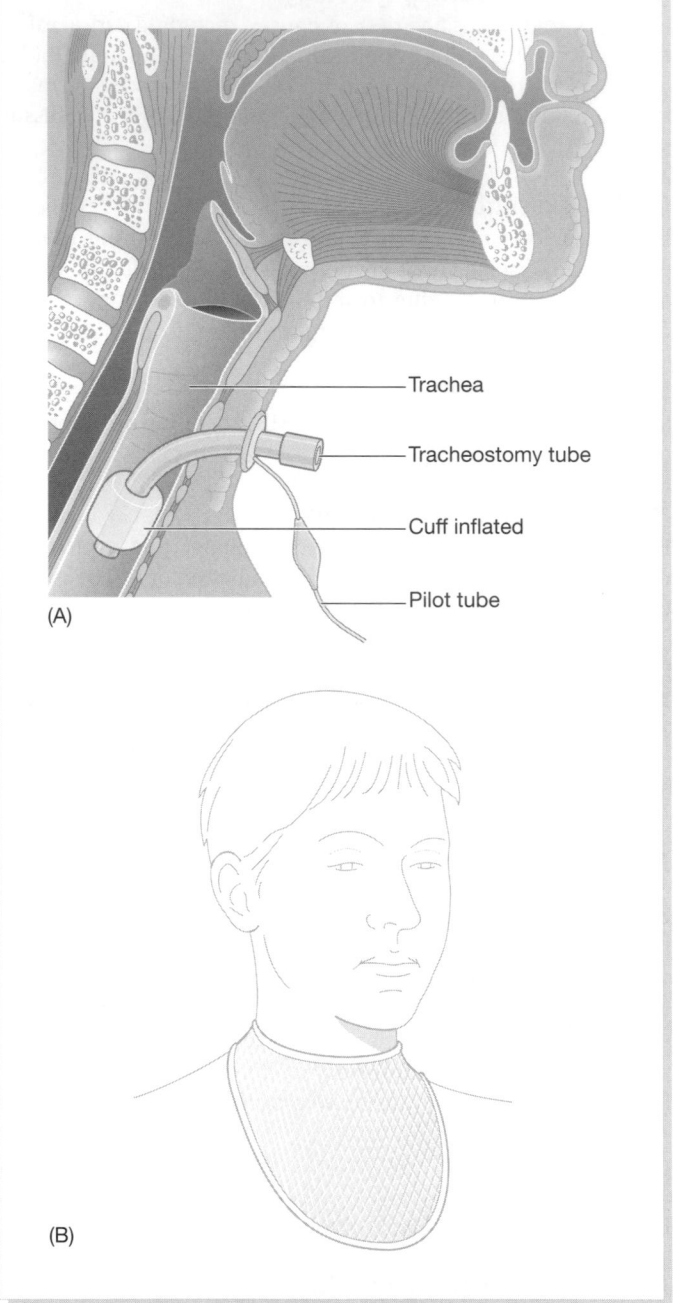

Trachea

Tracheostomy tube

Cuff inflated

Pilot tube

(A)

(B)

Figure 21.10 (A) A cuffed tracheostomy tube in place (tapes not shown). (B) A patient wearing a laryngectomy protector (or 'Buchanan bib'). The bib consists of a layer of foam sandwiched between two layers of cotton mesh. It removes dirt and dust particles from, and warms and moistens, inspired air. The bib may be worn under normal clothing and so is barely visible.

▶ Nursing management

Where possible, nurses must provide information for patients about what to expect after the tracheostomy; this will include tracheal suction and communication problems. In some emergency situations, there is little opportunity for preoperative explanations.

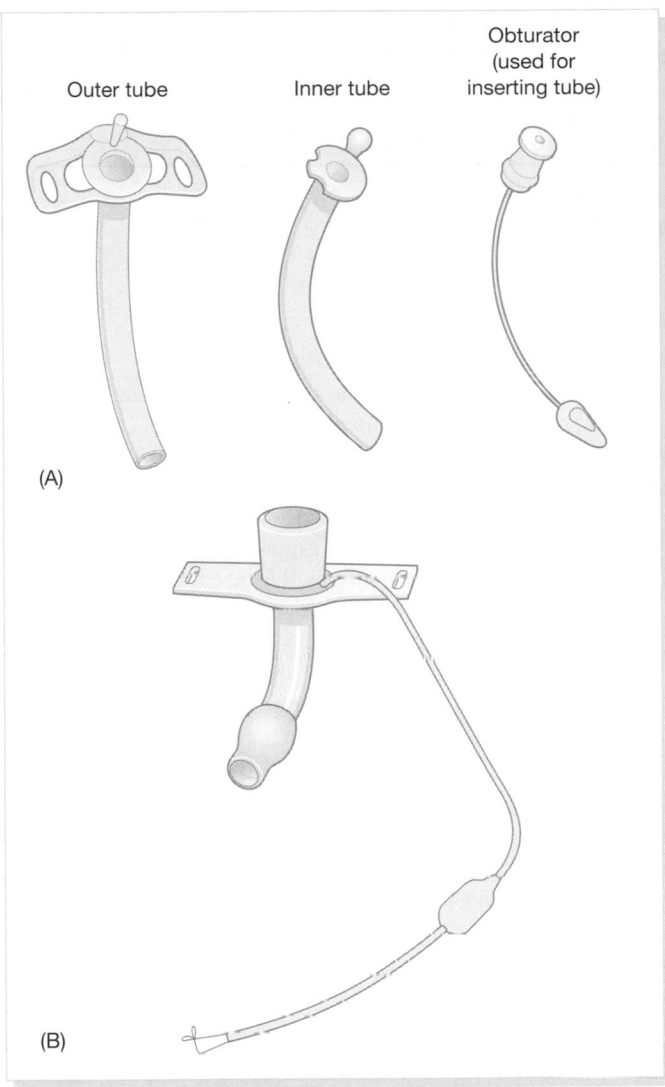

Outer tube   Inner tube   Obturator
(used for
inserting tube)

(A)

(B)

Figure 21.11   Tracheostomy tubes: (A) metal tube; (B) synthetic (polyethylene) cuffed tube.

Postoperative care

General postoperative care is required, which includes observation for haemorrhage, pulse, blood pressure and wound leakage (remembering to check behind the neck). As with any surgery, appropriate pain relief is a priority.

Airway management and preventing chest infection

There is a potential for airway obstruction by secretions or tube displacement. Therefore careful observation of the airway is vital – respiratory rate, depth and rhythm, assessment of respiratory adequacy (indicated by the skin and nail bed colour) and blood oxygen saturation with pulse oximetry. A physical check of airway patency involves placing a hand 2.5 cm away from the end of the tube to assess the amount of air being exhaled.

Deep breathing should be encouraged if possible and supplemental humidification (see below) will be required to prevent drying of the secretions, which makes them difficult to remove.

Tracheal suction is undertaken to remove secretions as necessary. Expectoration of secretions is encouraged to maintain airway patency and prevent infection. If the patient is able to clear secretions by coughing, this reduces the need for tracheal suction (with its associated complications). A sterile tracheal dilator should always be available in case the tube becomes dislodged through coughing or poorly tied tapes.

An adequate fluid intake is required to help keep pulmonary secretions liquid and easily removed. Initially fluids are given intravenously, but oral fluids are introduced gradually where there are no contraindications.

Chest infection is a potential complication following tracheostomy and patients should be observed for signs of infection, pyrexia, yellow/green sputum and 'rattly breathing'. Preventing chest infection involves working with the physiotherapist to encourage expectoration, effective suctioning, pain relief and mobilization as appropriate. Regular mouth care (2-hourly) is also important in preventing infection and promoting comfort, especially where the patient is unable to eat.

Tracheal suction

Tracheal suction is carried out to clear secretions from the airway and remove crusts. Initially it is a sterile procedure and readers are directed to Nicol et al (2000) for a detailed description. It involves the careful introduction of a suction catheter (with suction control apparatus) to about one-third of its length into the tracheostomy. Suction is then applied by occluding the suction control apparatus (but only) as the catheter is withdrawn (using a rotating motion). Suction should only be applied for up to 15 seconds at a time. Complications of tracheal suction include infection, cardiac arrhythmias and tracheobronchial trauma (Clarke 1995). Trauma caused by suctioning can, in extreme cases, cause tracheal necrosis and stenosis. Suction may become a clean procedure for self-care of a permanent tracheostomy.

Loss of upper airway humidification

The normal humidification process in the nose, warming, moistening and filtering inspired air, is bypassed and must be replaced by other means (Hooper 1996, Harkin 1998). Humidification aims to prevent the formation of crusts and this is achieved by several methods (see Guidelines for Care Priorities box 21.1).

Care of the tube and wound

The tapes securing the tracheostomy tube in position are changed whenever they become soiled. Whilst one person holds the tube in position, the old tapes are cut and removed one at a time. If the tube has an inflatable cuff, care must be taken to avoid cutting the pilot tube when cutting the tapes. Two nurses are required to ensure that the tube is not dislodged. New tape is threaded through the hole in the flange and tied securely onto the flange. The tapes are then tied securely around the patient's neck, but the nurse should check that the tapes are not too tight or causing skin soreness. The tapes may be threaded through a foam tube to improve comfort.

Depending on the type of tube used, the inner tube should be removed and cleaned according to local protocols.

The area around the tracheostome may be left exposed or dressed with an absorbent 'keyhole' dressing which is changed

GUIDELINES FOR CARE PRIORITIES

21.1 Humidification after tracheostomy

The upper respiratory tract normally warms, filters and adds moisture to inspired air, a process known as humidification, but this protective system is bypassed in a patient who has a tracheostomy. The main points are as follows:

- The risk of chest infection is increased by inhalation of dry unfiltered air or oxygen.
- The tracheostomy tube may become blocked with crusted tracheal secretions and so adequate hydration is essential to keep secretions moist.
- Initially humidified oxygen or air will be administered via a tracheostomy mask, which is like an oxygen mask but is designed to fit over the tracheostomy.
- Heat and moisture exchangers may be attached to the end of the tracheostomy tube in order to simulate the function of the nose.
- Nebulized saline via corrugated tubing and a tracheostomy mask or with an atomizer spray containing saline can be used.
- Portable humidifiers are available for use in the community.
- Buchanan bibs (Fig. 21.10B) may be worn. This is the preferred option for many patients with a permanent tracheostomy.
- Strict adherence to handwashing and cleaning, emptying and replacing equipment according to local protocols helps to reduce the risk of infection.

whenever soiling occurs. The area must be cleaned with sterile saline as required and any crusts should be carefully removed.

Communication problems

Patients will be unable to speak and the nurse must ensure that the call bell is available for alerting staff to patient needs, such as tracheal suction or analgesia. Patients may be very anxious about the tube blocking and not being able to breathe, and so they must feel confident that they can summon help if the nurse is not at the bedside. Paper and pen should be available and nurses should be alert to non-verbal communication. A system of simple hand signals may be developed where appropriate. Loss of speech can result in patients becoming very isolated. This can be overcome by allowing adequate time for communication, providing a pen and paper and encouraging family involvement in the patient's care. Speaking valves that open on inspiration and close on expiration to produce speech may also be used (if the larynx has not been removed). Referral to a speech and language therapist may be appropriate.

Altered body image

Altered body image may cause distress and nurses should provide support and explanation, but counselling may be required to enable patients with a permanent tracheostomy to accept their new body image and lifestyle. Advice on cosmetic measures, such as covering the tracheostome with specially made scarves, may

also be given. Talking to other patients helps and information about support groups should be provided (see p. 588).

VOCAL CORD PROBLEMS

PARALYSIS

Paralysis can affect either one or both vocal cords, with the former being the most common.

Aetiology and pathophysiology

One of the most common causes is paralysis of the recurrent laryngeal nerve by tumours involving the left lung. Other causes include tumours of the oesophagus, nasopharynx and thyroid gland.

Bilateral vocal cord paralysis is uncommon, but may occur following thyroid surgery or head injuries. The cords are often in the midline position and the airway will be compromised.

Clinical presentation

Unilateral paralysis causes voice changes such as a weak, breathy voice and an ineffective cough. Paralysis affecting both cords causes inspiratory stridor, but a good voice.

Specific investigations

- Laryngoscopy with a rigid or fibreoptic endoscope
- Chest X-ray to exclude lung cancer
- CT scan of the neck.

Medical/surgical management

Bilateral paralysis

A tracheostomy may be necessary if the airway is compromised. Other procedures to increase the airway include arytenoidectomy (arytenoid cartilage removal) and fixing the vocal cord in the lateral position (Becker et al 1994).

Unilateral paralysis

Speech and language therapy may be effective, but surgical procedures may be required. A conservative surgical procedure involves injecting substances, e.g. bovine collagen, into the vocal cord to 'plump it up' and move it closer to the midline. Surgery to the laryngeal framework, such as thyroplasty, may also be performed, where a silastic implant is inserted to move the vocal cord into the midline.

▶ Nursing management

Preoperatively patients will need a thorough explanation of all aspects of care. Voice rest should be mentioned preoperatively and emphasized postoperatively as this is vital following any surgery to the vocal cords.

Postoperative airway observation is essential because of the risk of oedema. Following thyroplasty, the external wound is observed for evidence of infection, redness, heat, tenderness, swelling and discharge. Sutures are usually removed by a practice nurse after 7 days.

TUMOURS OF THE NOSE AND THROAT

SINUSES

Aetiology and pathophysiology

Benign tumours affecting the nose and sinuses include granulomas, osteomas and papillomas but are relatively uncommon. Malignant tumours include squamous cell carcinomas, adenoid carcinomas and malignant melanomas. Adenoid carcinomas are linked to inhalation of hard wood dust, but the aetiology of other tumours is unknown.

Clinical presentation

The large air-filled sinuses may conceal a large tumour for a long time without symptoms. For this reason, the prognosis is often poor. The most common features are epistaxis, pain and nasal obstruction. Visual symptoms and swelling of the palate may occur. Enlarged cervical lymph nodes may be palpable.

Specific investigations

- Sinus X-rays
- CT scan
- MRI scan
- Biopsy via the nose.

Medical/surgical management

A combination of radiotherapy and surgery is generally used. Surgical approaches include intranasal, endoscopic or via an external incision.

▶ Nursing management

This will include pre- and postoperative care and considerable support and explanation in relation to altered body image (Cronan 1993, Burt 1995, Celinski 1996), care of dental prosthesis, helping with coping strategies, adjustment and social reintegration. Further details are provided in Chapter 33.

THE EXTERNAL NOSE

Malignant tumours include basal cell carcinomas, squamous cell carcinomas, malignant melanomas and malignant lymphomas. Management usually involves wide excision, combined with radiotherapy. Readers are directed to Chapter 28 for more information.

BENIGN LARYNGEAL TUMOURS

Benign tumours include vocal cord polyps (inflammatory), nodules (resulting from voice abuse) and papillomata (viral). Hoarseness is the main presenting feature. Some of these lesions respond to speech and language therapy, papillomata may be treated with antivirals, e.g. interferon, but others require surgical removal. Due to the risk of oedema and airway obstruction, an overnight stay in hospital is recommended following vocal cord surgery.

MALIGNANT LARYNGEAL TUMOURS

Aetiology, epidemiology and pathophysiology

These are generally squamous cell carcinomas, often affecting males aged 55–65 with a history of heavy smoking. The stage reached at presentation ranges from mildly abnormal cell changes to invasive carcinoma. Malignancy can affect various sites within the larynx. The most common site is the vocal cords, followed by the area above the cords. Cancers occurring below the vocal cords (subglottic) are relatively rare.

Clinical presentation

Presentation depends on the tumour site. Hoarseness is common. Dyspnoea, dysphagia and referred otalgia may also occur. Cervical lymph nodes may be enlarged.

Specific investigations

Investigations will include:

- indirect laryngoscopy
- microlaryngoscopy and biopsy
- X-rays to exclude lung cancer
- CT/MRI scan.

Medical/surgical management

Management depends on the extent of the disease. Radiotherapy may be indicated; however, where this fails or the cancer recurs, radical surgery may be the only option. Surgery involves laryngectomy (removal of the larynx) in most cases, with part or all of the thyroid gland. The tracheal 'stump' is then sutured to the skin of the neck and the patient breathes via this stoma. If all of the thyroid gland is removed, thyroxine replacement will be necessary (Ch. 17). Where the parathyroid glands are removed with the thyroid, the serum calcium should be monitored and calcium given as required.

▶ Nursing management

This is as for a patient with a tracheostomy. In addition to this, the patient will be nil orally for approximately 14 days postoperatively, allowing the pharynx to heal. Therefore, during this period, enteral feeding (Ch. 11) via a nasogastric or tracheo-oesophageal tube will be necessary. Tracheo-oesophageal feeding occurs through a tube passed into the stomach via a tract (tracheo-oesophageal fistula) running from the trachea to the oesophagus (formed at the time of the laryngectomy). Patients undergoing enteral feeding will require specific care, which includes:

- checking the site of the tube for soreness or excoriation
- checking the position of the tube, according to local protocols, prior to commencement of each feed
- administering feeds according to the prescribed regimen
- accurate recording of fluid balance.

Enormous support and assistance will also be required, to enable the patient to maintain self-esteem and to adjust socially to altered body image and functioning. Adequate time must be given both pre- and postoperatively to enable the patient to ask questions and discuss fears and anxieties. Arranging a preoperative meeting between the patient and someone who is

R|Я REFLECTIVE PRACTICE

21.1 Problems with communication

Patients with throat disease or following surgery may have temporary or permanent loss of speech and problems with communication.

Student activities

Think about a person who is unable to speak because of a throat problem:

- What emotions do you think they might feel?
- How would you explain the loss of voice to the family of a patient who has a tracheostomy?
- How might you help the patient to communicate his or her needs?
- Which other health professionals will be involved in solving the communication problem?

SUMMARY: MAIN POINTS

- Nurses will encounter a wide variety of disorders affecting the nose and throat.
- Disorders range from minor to life-threatening. Some may affect quality of life.
- Emergency situations are often encountered.
- Many patients are managed in the community and time in hospital is minimal.
- Many disorders will require medical and/or surgical treatment (elective and emergency).
- Nurses caring for patients with nose and throat disorders can gain knowledge and experience if learning opportunities are grasped as they arise.
- Caring for patients with nose and throat disorders is both challenging and rewarding.

coping well after a laryngectomy is an invaluable source of support. Such meetings give encouragement to the patient and the opportunity for support both in the immediate postoperative period and in the long term.

Assistance and encouragement with communication will also be vital, as speech is lost (see Reflective Practice box 21.1). Rudimentary measures such as providing pen and paper may be of most help in the initial stages and a nurse call bell should be available at all times. Voice rehabilitation will be necessary and considerable input from the speech and language therapist is essential. Measures available to enable speech following a total laryngectomy include oesophageal speech, use of an artificial larynx or tracheo-oesophageal speech using a voice prosthesis.

Family and partners should be involved in all aspects of care from the diagnosis. Such collaboration reduces isolation for the patient, reduces the fear involved in caring for a patient with a tracheostome and encourages acceptance of altered body image and functioning for all concerned.

SELF-TEST: CRITICAL THINKING ACTIVITIES

1 What advice should be given to a patient going home following treatment (nasal packing) for epistaxis? Think about and explain the rationale for each point.

2 You notice that a patient who had a tonsillectomy earlier in the day is swallowing a great deal whilst asleep. What do you think might be happening? What observations should be performed and why?

3 Find out what discharge advice is given to patients with a tracheostomy or laryngectomy with regard to:
 — preventing respiratory infection
 — keeping the tube (if present) clean and open
 — bathing and swimming.

FURTHER READING

Becker W, Naumann HH, Pfaltz CR. Ear, nose and throat diseases. Stuttgart: Thieme Medical Publishers; 1994.
O'Donoghue GM, Bates GJ, Narula AA. Clinical ENT – an illustrated textbook. Oxford: Oxford University Press; 1992.

Mellor D. Altered body image. Prof Nurse 1996; 11(5): 296–297.
Nicol M, Bavin C, Bedford-Turner S, Cronin P, Rawlings-Anderson K. Essential nursing skills. London: Mosby; 2000.

USEFUL ADDRESSES

The National Association of Laryngectomy Clubs
Ground Floor
6 Rickett Street
London SW6 1RU

Changing Faces
1&2 Junction Mews
London W2 1PN

Let's Face It
(a support group for people with facial disfigurements)
10 Wood End
Crowthorne
Berkshire RG11 6DQ

REFERENCES

Becker W, Naumann HH, Pfaltz CR. Ear, nose and throat diseases. Stuttgart: Thieme Medical Publishers; 1994.

Bent JP, Brennan P, Wood BS. Complications resulting from treatment of severe posterior epistaxis. Laryngol Otol 1999; 113: 252–254.

Bhaskar K. Diet following tonsillectomy. Paediatr Nurs 1998; 10(9): 25–27.

British Medical Association and the Royal Pharmaceutical Society of Great Britain. Bristish National Formulary (BNF). London; 1999.

Burt K. The effects of cancer on body image and sexuality. Nurs Times 1995; 91(7): 36–37.

Celinski M. The reluctant patient: a patient with facial cancer. Nurs Times 1996; 92(20): 26–28.

Clarke L. A critical event in tracheostomy care. Br J Nurs 1995; 4(12): 676–681.

Cronan L. Management of the patient with altered body image. Br J Nurs 1993; 2(5): 257–261.

Evans K. Diagnosis and management of sinusitis. Br Med J 1994; 309: 1415–1422.

Fenton JE, O'Dwyer TP. Adult day-case tonsillectomy: a safe and viable option. Clin Otolaryngol 1994; 19(6): 470–472.

Hanif J, Frosh A. Effect of chewing gum on recovery after tonsillectomy. Auris Nasus Larynx 1999; 26(1): 65–68.

Harkin H. Tracheostomy management. Nurs Times 1998; 94(21): 56–58.

Hooper M. Nursing care of the patient with a tracheostomy. Nurs Stand 1996; 10(34): 40–43.

Molony NC, Santana-Hernandez D, Wardrop PJ, Armstrong M, Moralee SJ. On which day is pain worst following adult tonsillectomy? Int J Clin Pract 1998; 52(6): 372–373.

Murthy P, McKerrow W. Nasal septal surgery: is routine follow-up necessary. J Laryngol Otol 1995; 109: 320–323.

Nicol M, Bavin C, Bedford-Turner S, Cronin P, Rawlings-Anderson K. Essential nursing skills. London: Mosby; 2000.

O'Donoghue GM, Bates GJ, Narula AA. Clinical ENT – an illustrated textbook. Oxford: Oxford University Press; 1992.

Pearce L. Rhinitis: diagnosis and treatment. Nurs Times 1998; 94(39): 46–47.

Petroff PF. Computer assisted endoscopic sinus surgery. AORN J 1997; 66(3): 416–425.

Phillips S. Epistaxis. Prof Nurs 1997a; 12(4): 292–295.

Phillips S. Obstructive sleep apnoea: diagnosis and management. Nurs Stand 1997b; 11(17): 43–46.

Stoeckli SJ, Moe KS, Huber A, Schmid S. A prospective randomized double-blind trial of fibrin glue for pain and bleeding after tonsillectomy. Laryngoscope 1999; 109(4): 652–655.

von Schoenberg M, Robinson P, Ryan P. Nasal packing after nasal surgery – is it justified? J Laryngol Otol 1993; 107: 902–905.

Warnock FF, Lander J. Pain progression, intensity and outcomes following tonsillectomy. Pain 1998; 75: 37–45.

22 Nursing patients with gastrointestinal disorders

Anthony McGrath

'I knew as soon as I was stuck in bed I'd get constipated, I always do. I didn't like to say anything to the nurses, well everyone can hear what you're saying can't they. Luckily they realised how embarrassed I was and instead of a commode by the bed, they said they could wheel me out to the lavatory – what a relief!'

(Patient)

THIS CHAPTER WILL HELP YOU

- Understand the anatomy and physiology of the gastrointestinal tract

- Describe the main pathological conditions affecting the gastrointestinal tract

- Understand the physiological, pathological, psychological, sociological and cultural aspects that influence the care of patients with gastrointestinal disease or disorders

- Describe the nursing management of patients with disorders of the gastrointestinal tract

- Consider the impact of gastrointestinal disease on patients and their families, identify individual needs and take appropriate action to enable them to adjust to changes in their lifestyle

- Understand the rationale for, and nursing care of, patients undergoing diagnostic and therapeutic gastrointestinal endoscopic procedures

- Understand the physical and psychological care required for patients with stoma.

KEYWORDS

Anorexia	Inflammatory bowel disease (IBD)
Dysphagia	
Dyspepsia	Haematemesis
Endoscopy	Melaena
Helicobacter pylori	Peptic ulceration
Hiatus hernia	Pyloric stenosis
Irritable bowel syndrome (IBS)	Stomatitis

INTRODUCTION

Gastrointestinal problems account for approximately 9% of all consultations in general practice (Hungin and Rubin 2000). This chapter will explore the anatomy and physiology of the GI tract and examine the conditions that affect this system. It will explore the nursing assessment and nursing care required for patients with these conditions and the investigations that may be required. It will also look at the role of some of the nurse specialists who work in this wide field of care. Readers should also refer to Chapter 11 (nutrition), as this will be an important aspect of care when dealing with patients with GI problems, and Chapter 23, which addresses the liver and biliary problems. Many of the problems experienced by patients with a GI disorder may in fact be linked to the hepatic system.

OVERVIEW OF THE GASTROINTESTINAL TRACT

The GI tract is a muscular tube approximately 9 metres in length consisting of the mouth, pharynx, oesophagus, stomach, duodenum, jejunum, small and large intestines, the rectum and anal canal (see Fig. 22.1). The GI tract is controlled by the autonomic nervous system. It is responsible for the breakdown, digestion and absorption of food and the removal of solid waste in the form of faeces from the body. It does this by allowing foods to pass through each section and subjecting them to the action of various digestive fluids and enzymes. The fluids and enzymes are secreted by a variety of glands and organs such as the salivary glands, the stomach, small intestine, the pancreas and the liver. It is this secretion of fluids that helps to maintain the function of the tract.

LINING OF THE GI TRACT

The GI tract is lined throughout with mucous membrane and it is constructed in such a way that its various parts can act independently of each other. The walls of the GI tract are made up of four layers of tissues:

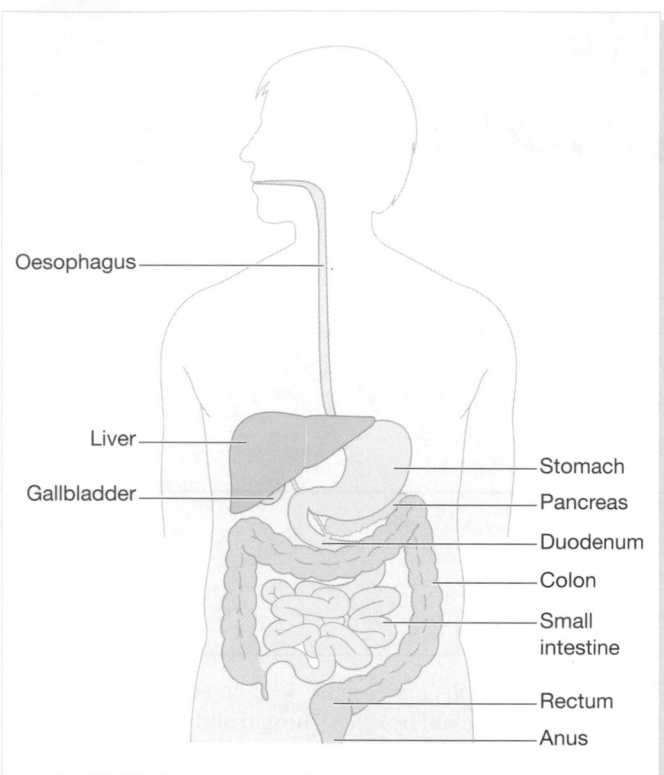

Figure 22.1 The gastrointestinal tract.

- adventitia
- muscularis
- submucosa
- mucosa.

Adventitia

The adventitia or outer layer consists of a serous membrane composed of connective tissue and epithelium. In the abdomen it is called the visceral peritoneum and forms a portion of the peritoneum where it is the largest serous membrane of the body.

The peritoneum

The peritoneum is a serous membrane that lines the abdominal and pelvic cavities, and covers most abdominal viscera. It is a large closed sac of thin membrane that has two layers:

- the visceral layer, the parietal peritoneum, which lines the abdominal and pelvic cavities
- The visceral peritoneum which covers the external surfaces of most abdominal organs, including the intestinal tract.

The serous membrane is composed of a simple squamous epithelium and a supporting layer of connective tissue. The potential space between the visceral and parietal layers is known as the peritoneal cavity and contains serous fluid. In some diseases (e.g. liver disease), the peritoneal cavity fills with serous fluid; this is known as ascites. Some organs protrude into the abdominal cavity, but are not encased in visceral peritoneum. The kidneys lie in this type of position and are said to be retroperitoneal.

The folds of the peritoneum bind the organs to the cavity walls and to each other. The folds include the mesentery, the lesser omentum, the greater omentum and the falciform ligament. The peritoneum also contains the nerve, blood and lymph supplies to the abdominal organs. The mesentery is attached to the posterior abdominal wall and this binds the small intestine to the abdominal wall. The lesser omentum arises from the lesser curvature of the stomach and extends to the liver. The greater omentum is given off from the greater curvature of the stomach, forms a large sheet that lies over the intestines, and then converges into parietal peritoneum. The falciform ligament attaches the liver to the anterior abdominal wall and to the diaphragm.

Muscularis

The muscularis mostly consists of two layers of smooth muscle, which contract in a wave-like motion. The exceptions can be found in the mouth, pharynx and upper oesophagus, which are made of skeletal muscle that aids swallowing. The two smooth layers of muscle contain longitudinal fibres on the outer layer and circular fibres on the inner layer. It is the contraction of theses two layers that assists in breaking down food, mixing it with the digestive secretions and propelling it forward, an action known as peristalsis. Peristaltic action looks like an ocean wave moving through the muscle.

Between the two muscle layers are found the blood vessels, lymph vessels and the major nerve supply to the GI tract. The nerve supply is called the mesenteric or Auerbach's plexus and it consists of both sympathetic and parasympathetic nerves and is mostly responsible for GI motility, which is the ability of the GI tract to move spontaneously.

Submucosa

The submucosa, or submucous layer, consists of connective tissue and elastic fibres and is highly vascular as it houses plexuses of blood vessels, nerves and lymph vessels and tissue. It contains the submucosal or Meissner's plexus, which is important in controlling the secretions in the GI tract.

Mucosa

The mucosa is a layer of mucous membrane that forms the inner lining of the GI tract. It is made up of three layers:

- a lining layer of epithelium which acts as a protective layer in the mouth and oesophagus and has secretory and absorption function throughout the rest of the tract
- the lamina propria, the second layer, supports the epithelium by binding it to the muscularis mucosa and is made up of loose connective tissue that contains blood and lymph vessels
- the muscularis mucosae layer, which contains smooth muscle fibres.

THE MOUTH

In order for solid food to get into the body, it must be first liquefied to enable the digestive enzymes to work. When food enters the mouth, the teeth and tongue work together to reduce the food to small particles.

The tongue

The tongue is a voluntary muscular structure that occupies the floor of the mouth. It is composed of skeletal muscles covered by a mucous membrane and is divided into two halves, each of which consists of both intrinsic and extrinsic muscles. The extrinsic muscles originate outside the tongue and insert into it and these include the hypoglossus, styloglossus and the geniglossus. The intrinsic muscles originate from within the tongue and include the transverses linguae, longitudinalis superior, the longitudinalis inferior and the verticalis linguae. The extrinsic muscles are responsible for moving the tongue from side to side and in and out, whilst the intrinsic are concerned with the size and shape of the tongue. The underside of the tongue is divided in the midline by the lingual frenulum, which limits the movement of the tongue posteriorly. At the base of the tongue it is attached to the hyoid bone. The superior surface and sides of the tongue consist of papillae, which are small projections that contain the nerve endings. As they are concerned with taste, they are often referred to as taste buds.

When food enters the mouth, it becomes moistened with saliva. Saliva is secreted continuously by the glands in the mouth, but more is produced when food is chewed. Saliva is mostly water and contains lingual lipase, bicarbonate and lysozyme, which destroys bacteria, and the enzyme salivary amylase which initiates starch digestion. The nerve endings in the mouth relay information to the brain via the glossopharyngeal and vagus nerves, which control swallowing. The moistened and reduced food is then passed into the oesophagus.

OESOPHAGUS

The moistened and reduced food is passed down the oesophagus by peristaltic motion (see p. 595) into the stomach. However, if for some reason this process is affected, the person will not be able to swallow effectively, and in some cases (e.g. a malignant growth causing obstruction) not at all. The oesophagus is a muscular tube measuring approximately 25 centimetres (cm), which lies behind the trachea. At the lower end of the oesophagus it narrows and forms into the gastro-oesophageal or cardiac sphincter at the opening to the stomach, which relaxes during swallowing to allow food to pass into the stomach and then closes to prevent regurgitation of gastric contents into the oesophagus.

STOMACH

The stomach is a J-shaped distensible pouch with four separate areas: the cardia, the fundus, the body and the pylorus (see Fig. 22.2). The cardia, which surrounds the lower oesophageal sphincter, can be found at the top of the stomach where the oesophagus opens into the stomach. The fundus is the rounded portion found above and to the left of the cardia. The body is the main part of the stomach and the pylorus is the lower segment. The stomach is described as having two curvatures, the lesser and greater curvatures. The lesser curvature lies on the medial (near the midline of the body) border of the stomach and is a continuation downwards from the medial border of the oesophagus; it forms the characteristic J shape as it curves upwards just before the pylorus. The greater curvature forms the lateral

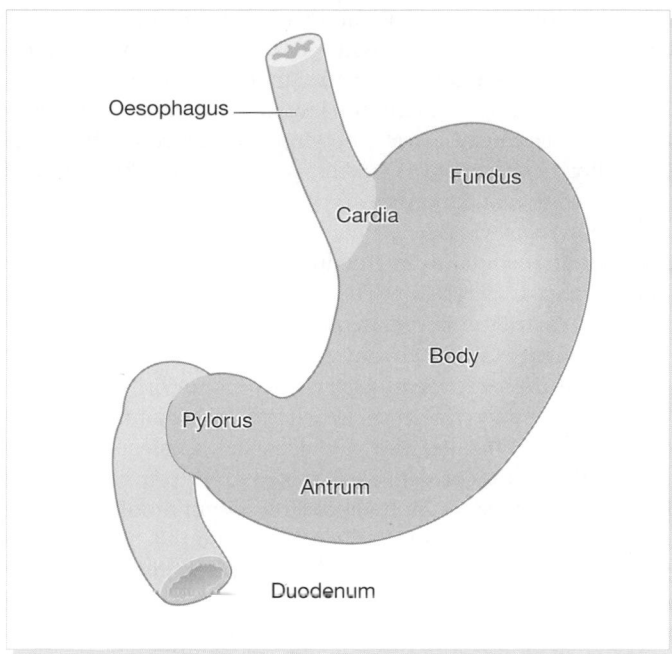

Figure 22.2 The stomach.

border. The stomach is composed of the same four layers found elsewhere in the GI tract; however, there are some modifications. When the stomach is empty, the mucosa lies in longitudinal folds called rugae; when it is full the folds are flattened and the surface appears smooth. The mucus layer is made up of simple columnar epithelium that contains the gastric glands. These glands secrete gastric juice into the stomach in response to the presence of food.

Functions of the stomach

The principal function of the stomach is to begin the digestion of proteins and to macerate food and mix it with the gastric juices, turning it into a liquid called chyme. Waves of peristalsis occur every 15–25 seconds and these aid the mixing process. The gastric mucosa secretes a colourless liquid that contains hydrochloric acid, pepsin and, in infants, renin, which is important in the digestion of milk. Hydrochloric acid is necessary for the conversion of pepsinogen (an inactive form of pepsin) to active pepsin. The cells that produce pepsinogen would themselves be digested by pepsin if it were active. Thus pepsinogen only becomes active pepsin when it comes into contact with hydrochloric acid. Pepsin is responsible for the digestion of proteins by breaking down amino acids into peptides. Whilst in the stomach, the food is churned and mixed with the gastric secretions and turned into chyme before moving into the duodenum.

Gastric emptying

The rate of gastric emptying is strongly influenced by both the volume and composition of gastric contents. For example, when drinking water, the stomach distends, which triggers nerves to commence the digestive process, but as water contains no solids to liquefy, the rate of gastric emptying is very fast. However, when a large meal that contains fats and amino acids enters the stomach, the rate of gastric emptying will be slowed. This is because the presence of fat in chyme will inhibit gastric emptying. The amount of chyme passing into the duodenum is controlled by the amount that the small intestine can process. This is achieved by reducing the level and intensity of the peristaltic contractions. Gastric emptying is inhibited by the secretion of hormones and by the enterogastric reflex, which inhibits gastric secretion and motility.

The enterogastric reflex is controlled by nerve impulses that travel to the medulla from the duodenum, telling it to stop or slow down gastric secretion. The hormones secretin, cholecystokinin and gastric-inhibiting peptide are released in response to various contents in the chyme. Secretin decreases gut motility and inhibits the secretion of gastric juice along with stimulating the release of pancreatic juice, which is rich in sodium bicarbonate ions that neutralize the stomach acid. Cholecystokinin is stimulated by the presence of fats and proteins in chyme that enter the duodenum. It also decreases gut motility, inhibits gastric juice secretion and causes the ejection of bile from the gallbladder. It is also responsible for the secretion of pancreatic juice which is rich in digestive enzymes. The gastric-inhibiting peptide (GIP) is stimulated by the presence of fats and is also responsible for decreasing gut motility and gastric juice secretion. GIP also stimulates the release of insulin.

Portal circulation

This is made up of veins that drain blood from the stomach, spleen, pancreas and gallbladder. Venous blood from the gastrointestinal organs flows to the liver before returning to the heart, allowing blood rich in nutrients and other substances to be processed by the liver before releasing them into the general circulation. In the case of toxic substances, the liver can attempt to detoxify them, rendering them harmless to the body (see Ch. 23 for a more detailed description). Obstruction of blood flow to the liver (e.g. from cirrhosis of the liver) causes the veins in the portal system to become overfilled and engorged. This leads to increased pressure and distension in the portal veins (portal hypertension). In the oesophagus, this gives rise to oesophageal varices, which, if they rupture, cause massive haemorrhage. Patients will vomit large amounts of blood and require emergency treatment (see Ch. 23).

Vomiting

Vomiting is the forceful expulsion of contents of the stomach and sometimes the duodenum. The vomiting centre lies in the brain in the medulla, stimulation of which induces vomiting. The vomiting centre receives signals from the GI tract via the vagus or sympathetic nerves, which inform the medulla when the stomach is overdistended (most common cause of vomiting) or when there is mucosal irritation (e.g. food poisoning). However, signals from outside the GI tract can also cause vomiting, including signals from the bile ducts, peritoneum and a variety of other organs. This can be seen in patients who have calculi (stones) in their common bile duct. Signals from outside the medulla but from within the brain can also stimulate vomiting, e.g. dizziness. Vomiting can also occur when the brain stem is affected, which commonly occurs in hospitals following the administration of analgesic drugs, especially morphine. Unpleasant smells can also induce nausea and vomiting. Prolonged vomiting must never be ignored, especially

in hospitalized patients or those undergoing treatment in the community, as it can have serious consequences, including acid–base imbalance, fluid volume and electrolyte depletion, malnutrition and aspiration pneumonia.

Projectile vomiting is usually caused by a blockage at the pylorus. This can be due to narrowing of the pylorus or as a result of ingestion of a foreign body (e.g. a coin), which blocks the opening. It is important to X-ray all patients who have swallowed a foreign body to ensure that the object has passed through into the small intestine. Once through, most people will then safely pass the object in their stool.

THE SMALL INTESTINE

The small intestine begins at the pyloric sphincter and coils its way through the abdominal cavity and opens at the ileocaecal valve into the colon (see Fig. 22.3). It is approximately 6.5 metres long and has a diameter of approximately 2.5 cm. It comprises three segments:

- the duodenum – approximately 25 cm in length and curves around the head of the pancreas. In the mid-section of the duodenum there is an opening from both the pancreas and the common bile duct. The sphincter of Oddi controls this opening
- the jejunum – approximately 2.5 metres in length and extends to the ileum
- the ileum – the terminal part of the small intestine, which measures about 3.5 metres in length and terminates at the ileocaecal valve. The ileum will usually empty approximately 1.5 litres of fluid into the colon each day.

The walls of the small intestine consist of the same four layers as the rest of the gastrointestinal system (see p. 592); however, the mucosal and submucosal layers are modified. The mucosal

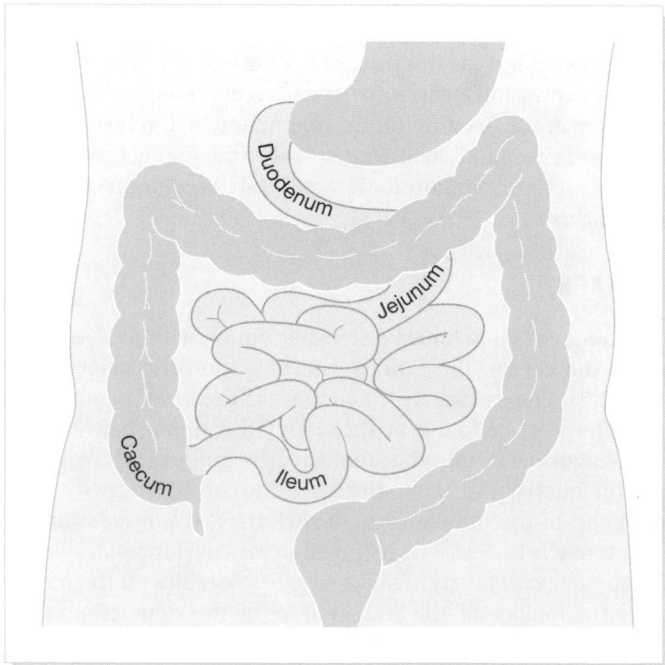

Figure 22.3 The small intestine.

layer consists of a great many glands called intestinal glands, which are lined with glanular epithelium and secrete intestinal juice. The submucosa in the duodenum contains glands that secrete mucus, which is alkaline and designed to protect the small intestine walls from the acid in chyme and to prevent the enzymes from acting on the intestinal wall.

The small intestine is further modified in that, throughout its length, the epithelium that covers the lining and the mucosa is simple, columnar and contains both absorptive and goblet cells. Microscopic examination reveals that the absorptive cells contain finger-like projections known as microvilli. These allow the small intestine to deal with larger amounts of digested nutrients, as they increase the surface area available for digestion. Nutrients pass via the blood capillaries and lymphatic capillaries into the cardiovascular and lymphatic systems. The nerve supply to the small intestine is both sympathetic and parasympathetic.

The surface area of the small intestine is further increased by the presence of circular folds that cause the chyme to twist around as it moves through. This assists the digestive and absorptive processes. Throughout the mucous membrane in the small intestine, there are numerous lymph nodes that occur at irregular intervals.

Functions of the small intestine

The main function of the small intestine is digestion and absorption. Its structure allows the chyme to be broken into small molecules that can be transported across the epithelium and into the bloodstream. This occurs in the presence of pancreatic enzymes and bile, both of which are important in the digestive process. The small intestine absorbs most of the water and electrolytes (sodium, chloride, potassium), glucose, amino acids and fatty acids from the chyme. The small intestine not only provides nutrients to the body, but also plays a critical role in water and acid–base balance.

The chyme from the stomach moves along at approximately 1 cm/min, and as the small intestine is approximately 6.4 metres in length, chyme can remain there for up to 8 hours. The chyme is moved by peristalsis, which is controlled by the autonomic nervous system. Digestion is completed in the small intestine with the aid of juices from the liver and pancreas. Waste is then transported to the large intestine for excretion. The superior mesenteric artery supplies the whole of the small intestine and venous blood is drained into the superior mesenteric vein, which links with other veins to form the hepatic portal vein.

THE PANCREAS

Attached to the duodenum lying posterior to the greater curvature of the stomach is the pancreas. When chyme enters the duodenum, the hormone secretin is released, which stimulates the pancreas to secrete its juices. The pancreatic juices then pass through the pancreatic ducts into the duodenum to aid digestion by neutralizing the acid to continue the digestive process (see Ch. 23).

THE LIVER AND GALLBLADDER

The liver is situated in the right hypochondrium and extends into the epigastric region. Bile that is produced in the liver passes from the hepatic ducts into the cystic duct prior to entering the gallbladder for storage. When fatty foods are detected in the duodenum, the hormone cholecystokinin is secreted. This causes the gallbladder to contract and excrete bile into the duodenum to emulsify the fatty food (see Ch. 23).

LARGE INTESTINE

The large intestine is so called because of its ability to distend. It forms a three-sided frame around the small intestine, leaving its inferior area open to the pelvis, and has four sections: the caecum, colon, rectum and anal canal. The colon is further divided into four sections: the ascending colon, transverse colon, descending colon and sigmoid colon (see Fig. 22.1). Its main function is to absorb water from the contents of the small intestine that pass into it. Whilst the small intestine will absorb some water, this process is intensified in the large intestine until the familiar semi-solid consistency of faeces is achieved.

The large intestine is approximately 1.5 metres in length and extends from the ileum to the anus. Its size decreases gradually from the caecum, where it is approximately 7 cm in diameter, to the sigmoid colon, where it is approximately 2.5 cm in diameter. The large intestine houses a variety of bacteria, known as commensals, that play an important part in digestion. The commensals ferment carbohydrates to release hydrogen, carbon dioxide and methane gas, and synthesize a number of vitamins such as vitamin K and some of the B vitamins. They are also responsible for breaking down the bilirubin into urobilinogen, which gives faeces its characteristic brown colour. Although harmless within the intestine, those bacteria can cause illness, even death, if they leak from the bowel into surrounding tissues, e.g. following perforation of the bowel.

The blood supply to the large intestine is mainly via the superior and inferior mesenteric arteries. The internal iliac arteries supply the rectum and anus. Venous drainage from the large intestine is mainly via the superior and inferior mesenteric veins, and via the internal iliac veins from the rectum and anus. Nerve supply to the large intestine is via the sympathetic and parasympathetic nerves. The external anal sphincter is under voluntary control and is supplied by motor nerves from the spinal cord.

Caecum

The small intestine terminates at the caecum. At the opening to the caecum, there is a fold of mucous membrane known as the ileocaecal valve, which allows the passage of materials from the small intestine into the large intestine and prevents the reflux of contents from the colon back into the ileum. This is important because the contents of the colon are heavily colonized by bacteria, whereas the small intestine is relatively microbe-free. The caecum is a dilated portion approximately 6 cm in width and 8 cm in length. It is continuous with the ascending colon superiorly and has a blind end inferiorly. Attached to the caecum is the vermiform appendix. It is usually 8–13 cm in length but can vary from 2.5 to 23 cm. It has the same structure as the walls of the colon but contains more lymphatic tissue.

Ascending colon

The ascending colon is approximately 15 cm long and joins the caecum at the ileocaecal junction. The ascending colon is covered with peritoneum anteriorly and on both sides; however, its posterior surface is devoid of peritoneum as it ascends on the right side of the abdomen to the level of the liver where it bends acutely to the left. It is at this point that it forms the right colic or hepatic flexure to become the transverse colon.

Transverse colon

This is a loop of colon approximately 45 cm long that continues from the left hepatic flexure across to the left side of the abdomen to the left colic flexure. It passes in front of the stomach and duodenum and then curves beneath the lower part of the spleen on the left side as the left colic or splenic flexure, and then passes acutely downward as the descending colon.

Descending colon

This section of the colon passes downward on the left side of the abdomen to the level of the iliac crest. It is approximately 25 cm in length. The descending colon is narrower and more dorsally situated than the ascending colon (see Fig. 22.1).

Sigmoid colon

The sigmoid colon is approximately 36 cm long. It begins near the iliac crest and ends at the centre of the mid-sacrum, where it becomes the rectum at about the level of the third sacral vertebra. It is mobile and is completely covered by peritoneum and attached to the pelvic walls in an inverted V shape.

Rectum

The rectum is approximately 13 cm in length and lies in the posterior aspect of the pelvis. It ends 2–3 cm in front of and just below the tip of the coccyx where it curves downwards to form the anal canal.

Anal canal

This is the terminal segment of the large intestine and is approximately 4 cm in length, opening to the exterior as the anus. The mucous membrane of the anal canal is arranged in longitudinal folds that contain a network of arteries and veins. The anus remains closed at rest. The anal canal corresponds anteriorly to the bulb of the penis in men and with the lower vagina in the female. Posteriorly it is related to the coccyx. The internal anal sphincter is 2.5 cm long and composed of smooth muscle and can be felt during rectal examination. It controls the upper two-thirds of the canal. The external sphincter is made up of skeletal muscle and is normally closed except during elimination of faeces. The nerve supply is from the perineal branch of the fourth sacral nerve and the inferior rectal nerves.

NURSING ASSESSMENT

The nursing interview is an extremely valuable way of obtaining information which will allow nurses to plan the care of patients, and requires great care and attention. A good nursing assessment will allow nurses to determine patients' problems, formulate a plan of care, and implement and evaluate it. Assessment is a continuous process and evaluation is important to determine the effectiveness of the nursing approach in meeting patients' needs.

ASSESSMENT INTERVIEW

The initial contact and interview is an important milestone in a patient's hospital or clinical experience and should be seen as a time to get to know patients and for them to get to know you. It is therefore important that you introduce yourself and explain your role on the ward or clinical area, and allow time to carry out the interview successfully. An accurate history is one of the most important steps in enabling a nursing diagnosis to be made and will indicate whether further investigations and observations are necessary and facilitate care planning. Whilst it may be seen as friendly and less formal to use patients' first or pet names, many patients and their relatives feel more comfortable with a more formal introduction. Patients will invite you to be less formal and use their first name if that is what they would prefer.

The nursing interview should address two areas: the patient's functional ability and physical assessment. Assessment of functional ability includes issues such as whether patients can feed, wash or mobilize by themselves, e.g. whether they can walk to the toilet unaided, while the physical assessment involves inspection, palpation, percussion and auscultation and is carried out by a doctor or senior nurse. Nurses assess a patient's physical condition by noting temperature, skin condition, pulses, BP and, if skilled, cardiac sounds and lung fields.

As patients will undoubtedly be sharing some very confidential information, it is important to carry out the interview in a quiet area of the ward or a side room to ensure privacy. Patients may feel less inhibited when talking about personal issues and sharing their problems.

Nursing history

When taking a nursing history, it is important to focus on the current complaint and check that patients understand their diagnosis and what will be happening to them. It is also important to check that they know what they can and cannot do and make sure they are aware of what is required of them and what they can expect from the health care team. Patients' past medical history is important as this may alert the nurse to potential problems and the need for further observation. For example, patients who have diabetes will need to have blood sugar levels checked regularly and, possibly, daily urinalysis. They will also need special care regarding their medication if undergoing surgery (see Ch. 29). Older adults also need special consideration (see Older Adults: Nursing Priorities box 22.1).

Questions about patients' employment history can alert nurses to financial problems, which can be referred to the hospital social worker, or the possibility of exposure to an occupational hazard, such as rat-infested water, e.g. in the case of dock and sewer workers. Rats can harbour and excrete an organism via their urine called *Leptospira icterohaemorrhagiae*. This organism enters the body via the skin through either a bite or an abrasion that has come into contact with infected water. This causes a condition known as Weil's disease and can result in jaundice, haemorrhages into mucous membranes and renal damage.

Information about current medication and any over-the-counter medicines may reveal problems. For example, a patient taking aspirin or ibuprofen may suffer from indigestion or

OLDER ADULTS: NURSING PRIORITIES

22.1 Gastrointestinal changes in older adults

As people age, their metabolic rate decreases along with a loss of teeth, which may impair their ability to chew food. Swallowing may be impaired because saliva excretion decreases with age and food is not digested as efficiently as gastric and enzyme secretions are diminished. As the bowel slows, owing to a loss of muscle tone in the intestines, elderly patients are prone to developing constipation.

With older patients, it is important to assess bowel habit, nutritional intake and body mass index (BMI), as well as the presence of dentures, as poorly fitting dentures can cause ulceration and prevent proper chewing. Note any muscle wasting, clothes or rings that are too big, and note patients' colour to detect whether they are anaemic.

abdominal pain. Many patients think that health care professionals are only interested in the medication that they have been prescribed by a doctor. Questions about alcohol and tobacco consumption will provide the opportunity for health education about the effects of these drugs. Another area to explore is foreign travel, as patients may be exposed to a wide variety of conditions and illnesses (e.g. tapeworm infestations and typhoid) that may not be suspected if recent trips abroad are not known about. Such illnesses may have implications for the care required or even require isolation. Questions about family and home circumstances will enable individualized discharge planning to include any need for home care and support.

ORAL ASSESSMENT

Examination of the mouth is important, as the symptoms noted there may be a sign of serious problems. Patients may complain of pain, soreness, dryness, difficulty in swallowing or chewing, difficulty with speech, over-salivation or loss or disorder of taste. Pain can arise from a variety of areas – the teeth, the gums, the tongue or the glands. Check whether patients' lips are cracked or dry and whether there is any evidence of angular stomatitis (inflammation of the corners of the mouth), which appears as reddish-brown cracks or fissures that are moist and superficial in the corners of the mouth. Note the presence of mouth ulcers, especially if they are flat and shallow, as this may indicate carcinoma epithelioma. Note the presence of multiple small black or brown spots on the skin surrounding the mouth, as this may indicate Peutz–Jeghers syndrome, an inherited condition signifying underlying small bowel polyposis.

In some patients, the gums, lips and mouth may appear reddish/orange brown, due to chewing of the betel nut, which turns saliva a brick red colour. Examine the mucous surface of patients' lips, as this will enable you to detect the presence of aphthous ulcers, which are small, painful lesions with a white or yellow base. Note the colour of patients' teeth as they can become discoloured due to tartar deposits from smoking, or reddish-brown due to the chewing of betel nuts.

Clinical presentation

Patients may present with a wide variety of signs and symptoms.

Abdominal pain

Abdominal pain is probably the most important symptom of abdominal disease (Barkauskas et al 1994). Pain can result from smooth muscle spasm, peritoneal irritation, mucosal irritation or direct nerve irritation. The description of the nature of the pain given by patients can be crucial in reaching a diagnosis. Pain caused by a perforated gastric ulcer is often described as 'burning', a dissecting aortic aneurysm as 'tearing', intestinal obstruction as 'gripping', pyelonephritis as 'dull aching', and biliary or renal colic as 'crampy constricting' (Swartz 1995). Patients suffering from generalized peritonitis lie almost motionless with knees flexed, whereas marked restlessness may indicate biliary colic or intraperitoneal haemorrhage (Barkauskas et al 1994).

Anorexia and weight loss

Anorexia means loss of appetite or decreased appetite and can occur for a variety of reasons. Any illness can adversely affect a previously hearty appetite and in most cases the appetite returns when the condition is treated or the course of treatment has stopped. Appetite can be affected by the following: anxiety, emotional upset, nervousness, loneliness, boredom, bereavement and depression. It may also be affected by infections, pregnancy (especially the first trimester), cancer and some cancer treatments, and antibiotics as well as numerous other drugs. Loss of appetite can lead to unintentional weight loss and, in severe cases, malnutrition. Nutritional supplements such as fortified drinks may help, but in severe cases intravenous nutritional support may be required.

Nausea and vomiting

Nausea and vomiting are symptoms of a variety of conditions, such as food poisoning, motion sickness, over-eating and intestinal obstruction. Nausea and vomiting can also be symptoms of diseases such as a myocardial infarction, central nervous system disorders, cancer and renal and liver disorders. Nausea is described as a feeling of uneasiness that often accompanies the urge to vomit; however, it does not always lead to vomiting.

Flatulence

Gas is formed in the bowel as a result of the action of bacteria on undigested food. Even though it can cause discomfort, excessive gas is usually not a serious symptom. Common causes of excessive gas include swallowing air while eating and eating high-fibre foods.

Hiccups

This is caused by an unintentional movement of the diaphragm followed by rapid closure of the vocal cords, which produces the characteristic sound of a hiccup. In most cases, they occur spontaneously and usually disappear after a few minutes. However, in some cases they can persist for days, weeks or even months and will require treatment. In many cases, the cause is unknown; however, they can be brought on by eating hot and spicy foods and by disorders that irritate the nerves controlling the diaphragm (e.g. pneumonia). Holding one's breath and drinking a glass of cold water can help to stop them.

Abnormal stools

Diarrhoea

Diarrhoea is defined as the passage of three or more unformed or excessively watery stools per day. Most diarrhoea will stop in a few days without treatment. Certain drugs, such as antibiotics, can cause or worsen diarrhoea by allowing overgrowth of toxin-producing bacteria, giving rise to diarrhoea. In some cases they can cause a type of colitis (inflamed bowel) leading to severe diarrhoea. Chronic diarrhoea occurs when loose or more frequent stools persist for longer than 2 weeks. The majority of diarrhoeal diseases are caused by infections such as *Cryptosporidium*, *Microsporidium*, *Giardia*, *Salmonella* and *Shigella*. In children, the most common causative organism is a rotavirus.

Constipation

Constipation refers to infrequent passage of stools. The stool becomes hard and difficult to pass. It is also used to describe a lack of bowel movements for more than 3 days; however, the term constipation is a relative term as there is a wide variability in what is considered a normal pattern of bowel elimination. Some people may have consistently soft or near liquid stools, while others may have consistently hard firm stools, but no difficulty in passing them. However, if there is difficulty in passing a hard stool, the mucosal membrane of the anus may become torn, causing bleeding, pain and the possibility of an anal fissure. Constipation in hospitals is a common complication and can be caused by a variety of problems (see p. 609).

Tenesmus

Tenesmus describes the constant feeling that the bowel is not completely emptied and it may be accompanied by pain. It is usually associated with inflammation of the bowel.

Melaena

Melaena is the passage of black, tarry and foul-smelling stools. Black stools usually indicate bleeding from the upper GI tract.

Haematemesis

Haematemesis is the vomiting or regurgitation of blood as a result of bleeding in the upper GI tract, which includes the mouth, pharynx, oesophagus, stomach and small intestine.

Rectal bleeding

Blood in the stool can originate anywhere in the intestinal tract. A bright red colour usually indicates that the blood is coming from large bowel or rectum. Bleeding may occur as a result of anal fissures, haemorrhoids or diverticular disease, but it can also be a sign of malignant disease and so should always be investigated.

Abdominal distension

The abdomen may become distended for a number of reasons, which may be summarized as the 'six Fs' of distension: fat, flatus, fluid, faeces, fibroids and fetus. In patients who have fluid in the bowel, it is important to discover the cause, and women with fibroids will require surgery to have them removed.

Jaundice

This is a yellow discolouring of the skin, eyes and mucous membranes caused by too much bilirubin in the blood. Bilirubin is normally excreted via the bowel, but if for some reason it is unable to do this, due to an obstructed common bile duct, the body excretes it onto the skin and via the urine, which will become dark in colour (see Ch. 23).

ABDOMINAL EXAMINATION

During abdominal examination, the patient will need to lie flat on the bed with his or her head on a pillow and the arms lying loosely at the side. If the patient is tense, flex the knees slightly towards the chest thus relaxing the abdominal muscles. The patient should not be exposed more than necessary but as the liver and spleen lie under the ribs, the lower half of the chest must be exposed in order to undertake examination.

GENERAL DIAGNOSTIC TESTS AND MEDICAL INVESTIGATIONS

There are a number of tests that can be performed to diagnose conditions of the GI tract.

GASTRIC ACID STUDIES

The purpose of gastric acid studies is to determine gastric function by passing a nasogastric (NG) tube and measuring the amount of acid in the stomach. The complete gastric acid study includes a basal gastric secretion test, which measures the level of acid secretion while the patient is in a fasting state. This test is followed by a gastric acid stimulation test, which measures the secretion of gastric acid for 1 hour after injection of a drug that stimulates its output.

In healthy individuals, the basal acid output is just a few millilitres per hour, containing approximately 10 mmol of hydrogen ions per litre, and the maximal acid output following stimulation can reach 27 mmol/L per hour. In patients with gastrinomas that secret large amounts of gastrin (a hormone secreted by the walls of the stomach), a very high basal output may be noted, whereas in patients suffering from duodenal ulcers, a high maximal output is noted.

UREA BREATH TEST

Helicobacter pylori is a bacterium that lives in the mucous lining of the stomach of some people. It has been linked with the development of gastric and intestinal ulceration and stomach cancer. As it is very rich in urease, a good way to detect it is to give urea to patients to take orally. Their expired air is then monitored for carbon dioxide (CO_2), which indicates the breakdown or hydrolysis of the ingested urea. This confirms the presence of a urease-producing organism in the stomach. The test is usually carried out after fasting patients for 6 hours, and three baseline samples are collected. A straw is inserted into a test tube and patients are asked to blow through it until condensation appears on the test tube wall. They are then given 100 ml of a fatty meal, which delays gastric emptying. After a period of 10 minutes, the labelled urea isotope is given to patients and breath samples are collected 30 minutes after that. By finding out whether patients have *H. pylori*, doctors are then in a position to treat it with antibiotics to eradicate it, thus reducing the risk of further problems.

ENDOSCOPY

Although developed in the 1950s, it was not until the 1970s that the flexible fibreoptic endoscope became widely available (see Fig. 22.4) and the greatest developments in this field have been seen in the last 10–15 years. The fibreoptic endoscope, along with video imaging, has revolutionized the inspection of the GI tract. The endoscope provides a direct view of the mucosa and enables biopsies to be taken. It is also used to rectify problems such as strictures and bleeding oesophageal varices. In the upper GI tract, the endoscope can be used to visualize the pharynx (pharyngoscopy), oesophagus (oesophagoscopy), stomach (gastroscopy) and duodenum (duodenoscopy).

Endoscopy of the upper GI tract is used to investigate symptoms such as heartburn, difficulty in swallowing, vomiting and abdominal pain, especially when linked with eating or hunger. Patients undergoing this investigation usually only require light sedation and local anaesthesia to the pharynx. When investigating the lower GI tract, the endoscope allows visualization of the rectum (proctoscopy), the colon (colonoscopy) and sigmoid colon (sigmoidoscopy). One of the most exciting aspects to occur in the world of endoscopy has been the development of nurse endoscopists, who have added a nursing dimension to this role.

BIOPSY

Histological studies can be carried out on tissue taken from suspected mucosal disorders and lesions during endoscopy.

RADIOGRAPHY

There are a number of radiographical investigations that may be carried out, as described below.

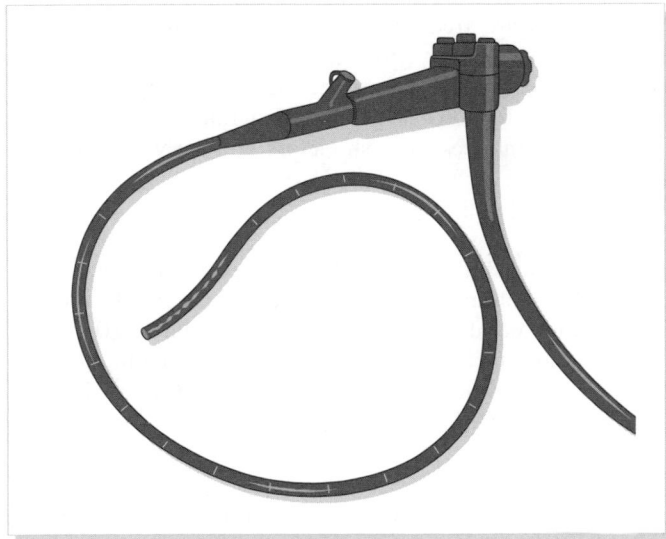

Figure 22.4 A flexible fibreoptic endoscope.

Imaging techniques

Ultrasound, CT scanning and MRI have been found to be extremely helpful in demonstrating abscess, carcinoma and the presence of stones; however, they are not considered effective when demonstrating the outline of the bowel.

Plain X-rays

X-rays of the abdomen and chest are important as they can highlight a number of problems associated with GI disease. The presence of gas under the diaphragm or in the peritoneal cavity can be detected, which may be the result of a perforated bowel along with the presence of a pleural effusion which may be linked to liver disease (covered in more detail in Ch. 23). A plain X-ray can also highlight bowel disorders, such as bowel distension and obstruction. Mechanical bowel obstruction can be seen as air- and fluid-filled loops of bowel before the obstruction and flattened-out, decompressed bowel after the obstruction. Air noted in the small intestine may suggest a paralytic ileus (paralysis of the intestinal muscle).

Radioisotope studies

A scan of white blood cells labelled with indium-111 can be used to locate and measure the activity of inflammatory bowel disease (IBD) as they have been shown to be an accurate means of detecting intestinal inflammation (Tibble et al 1999).

Barium studies

Barium studies are used to investigate the upper GI tract and small intestine. A barium meal (swallow) and follow-through are useful in outlining GI anatomy and can be very helpful in discovering the presence of problems in the oesophagus and small bowel. A barium swallow can reveal abnormalities such as strictures, ulcers, hiatus hernia and problems with the passage of food through the oesophagus. In order to obtain clearer views of the distal small bowel, a small bowel enema is performed. This involves the passing of a tube through the nose and stomach into the jejunum to allow the passage of a contrast medium.

When examining the large bowel, a double-contrast enema with air and barium is administered rectally in order to outline the bowel mucosa. This technique is useful in demonstrating colonic lesions, such as inflammatory bowel disease, polyps and carcinomas. A small amount of barium is introduced into the bowel to provide a thin coating of the mucosal surface, and then air is used to stretch the mucosa, which enables the fine detail of the bowel to be seen. Patients who are to undergo a barium enema will require preparation.

Patient preparation

Two days before the procedure, patients are required to eat a low residue diet, which means they should not eat any fruit, nuts, peas, beans, coarse cereals or fried foods. On the day before the procedure, they should drink only clear liquids, such as clear soup, apple or cranberry juice and ginger ale, and no milk or milk products. Bowel preparation commences the day before the procedure. Once the bowel preparation is taken (e.g. Picolax), patients should not eat or drink anything after midnight the night before the test. Medications should be taken as normal when fasting prior to the test. Patients should not undergo a barium enema study for at least a week following a rectal biopsy, as there is a risk of bowel perforation. They should be advised to drink plenty of fluids following the procedure and for up to a week afterwards to prevent constipation.

BLOOD TESTS

A variety of blood tests may be required.

Iron and folate levels

Iron and folate are both absorbed from the upper section of the small intestine. If the levels are low, this may indicate a wide variety of disorders, such as megaloblastic anaemia, pernicious anaemia (see Ch. 18) and malabsorption syndromes.

Haemoglobin

Anaemia may be due to chronic blood loss, intestinal malabsorption, dietary insufficiency, or reduced or impaired gastric secretion. In patients with Crohn's disease, there may be malabsorption of vitamin B_{12}.

Erythrocyte sedimentation rate (ESR)

A raised ESR is associated with acute and chronic infection and inflammation. C-reactive protein (CRP) is released by the body in response to acute injury or infection and may indicate the acute phase of the disease such as inflammatory bowel disease.

Liver function tests

When the liver is damaged or diseased, liver enzymes, which are normally contained within the liver, escape into the blood. Liver function tests are performed to detect the levels of liver enzymes in the blood.

A low level of albumin in the blood (hypoalbuminaemia) may occur due to the leaking of protein into the gut and is often seen in patients with bowel disease, although it may also indicate poor dietary intake or malabsorption.

An increased number of leucocytes (leucocytosis) and platelets (thrombocytosis) may occur in active inflammatory bowel disease; however, electrolytes can also be deranged in patients with diarrhoea as they lose potassium and in patients with pyloric stenosis (see p. 607).

Faecal occult blood (FOB)

Faecal occult blood refers to blood in the stool that is not visible to the naked eye; it can only be detected in laboratory tests. It is important to check for its presence, as it may indicate the possibility of rectal cancer.

GENERAL DISEASE PREVENTION AND HEALTH EDUCATION

Many of the problems and disorders discussed in this chapter are linked to diet, alcohol intake and smoking. Nurses are thus in a very strong position to offer advice and guidance that may help to reduce the problems faced by patients in their care. However, it is important to recognize that many patients will find it difficult to change their behaviour, and by recognizing this, nurses are in a position to motivate them and offer support. Nurses can provide information and teaching that allow patients to make their own choices. However, it is important also to be able to judge when and what it is appropriate to teach, as some patients may just disregard what is said if the timing is not right.

It is important to begin by building a therapeutic relationship, to gain the patients' trust and demonstrate that you are there, not to judge or to preach to them, but to give them the information that allows them to make choices. On the whole, patients are interested in their own welfare and in getting well. Many will see the benefits and try to change. Again, by offering them support, they are more likely to succeed. By gaining a greater perspective and insight, many patients feel better able to cope. Offering advice on dietary changes and helping patients to cut down or cease smoking and drinking alcohol can have profound effects on the GI tract. For example, encouraging a patient with a hiatus hernia to give up smoking can remove one of the precipitating factors; while encouraging patients to exercise and to drink more water can reduce constipation. Providing advice about diet and encouraging a high-fibre diet can have a positive impact on colorectal cancer and haemorrhoids.

DISORDERS OF THE GASTROINTESTINAL TRACT

DISORDERS AFFECTING THE MOUTH

The mouth is used in speech, respiration and digestion and can be affected in a variety of ways. Nursing assessment and care are aimed at ensuring that the mouth is clean, moist and free from infection. The oral cavity is lined by a layer of rapidly dividing mucosal cells that regenerate every 7–10 days. Problems in the mouth are common and poor oral care is the primary causative factor.

Carcinoma of the mouth

Malignant tumours of the mouth account for 1% of malignant tumours in the UK (Kumar & Clark 2002). They usually develop on the lateral borders of the tongue and the floor of the mouth. They are usually painless in the early stages but may become painful as the tumour advances. They are linked with heavy alcohol consumption, tobacco use and chewing of the betel nut. Oral tumours are treated by surgical excision and/or radiotherapy. Nurses are in a prime position to educate patients about the risks and help them to reduce high-risk behaviours. Early detection is key to increasing the survival rate for these cancers. Box 22.1 summarizes the risk factors and early signs of oral cancer.

Stomatitis

Stomatitis means inflammation in the mouth. Angular stomatitis refers to inflammation in the corners of the mouth and is a common mucosal disorder, affecting approximately 10–25% of the population in the UK. Its aetiology is unknown, although stress and autoimmune factors have been postulated. Patients with IBD are often affected.

Xerostomia

Saliva production is important to the oral cavity and patients with a dry mouth (xerostomia) may have difficulties in swallowing. A dry mouth is common when people are anxious or afraid,

Box 22.1 Oral cancer: risk factors and early warning signs

Risk factors
- Excessive intake of alcohol
- Use of tobacco products
- Ill-fitting dentures
- Lip-biting and cheek-chewing
- Exposure to excessive levels of sunlight

Oral cancer: early warning signs
- Sores on the face, neck or mouth that do not heal within 2 weeks
- Swellings, lumps or bumps on the lips, gums or other areas inside the mouth
- White, red or dark patches in the mouth
- Repeated bleeding in the mouth
- Numbness or pain in any area of the face, mouth or neck

 EVIDENCE-BASED PRACTICE

22.1 Oral care

The aim of oral care is ensure that the patient's mouth is moist, comfortable and free from infection. Oral problems can reduce a patient's quality of life and cause misery and pain. Poor oral care can result in dental decay, halitosis, gingivitis, stomatitis, parotitis, candidiasis, ulceration, tonsillitis and pneumonia.

The use of foam sticks are not as effective as using a soft toothbrush and paste and this should be your first choice.

Care should commence with a full and comprehensive assessment of the patient's mouth and level of hydration, as adequate fluid intake will help to maintain a moist mouth. Note the presence of ulcers and whether the patient has dentures, which will require a thorough cleaning at least once a day. It is known that fluoride protects teeth and in some cases this is added to the water. Fluoride is also an ingredient of many toothpastes and therefore a 3-minute brushing at least once a day is recommended (Miller & Kearney 2001).

Reference
Miller M, Kearney N. Oral care for patients with cancer: a review of the literature. Cancer Nurs 2001; 24(4): 241–245.

or when they are mouth breathing due to a nasal obstruction. However, a variety of diseases can affect saliva production, including fungal infections, mumps and salivary calculi formed from calcium deposits and carbonates. A lack of saliva can predispose patients to the development of salivary gland infection (sialadenitis), especially of the parotid glands (parotitis). Therefore it is important for nurses to include regular oral care in all patients suffering from xerostomia.

White patches in the mouth

White patches in the mouth may be of a transient nature or they may persist. The condition is commonly due to *Candida* (thrush, see below) but is occasionally seen in systemic lupus erythematosus (SLE). Leucoplakia refers to the occurrence of white patches when no local cause is found. Unlike candidiasis, the patches cannot be removed by rubbing the mucosal surface. Leucoplakia is often linked with heavy alcohol consumption and smoking; it is a premalignant condition. However, hairy leucoplakia (a shaggy white patch on the side of the tongue) is associated with HIV and is not premalignant.

Oral candidiasis

Oral candidiasis, also known as thrush, is a fungal infection caused by the *Candida* fungus. It affects the mouth (oral candidiasis) and/or the throat (oesophageal candidiasis). Some medications (e.g. antibiotics and steroids) alter the natural organisms in the mouth, allowing growth of *Candida*. Symptoms include discomfort, a burning feeling and an altered sense of taste. Inspection of the mouth reveals creamy white or yellowish spots on the mouth and throat. These may be accompanied by cracking, redness, soreness and swelling at the corners of the mouth. Patients will be prescribed locally acting medication to suck, such as nystatin pastilles or amphotericin lozenges. In systemic disease, intravenous amphotericin is required.

Ulceration

Ulceration in the mouth can occur for a variety of reasons; however, the most common is idiopathic aphthous ulceration, which refers to painful white ulcers that can occur singly or in crops.

These ulcers can affect the lips, cheeks or tongue and usually heal within 7–10 days. The aetiology is unknown, although there may be a possible link to hormonal factors as they appear more frequently in women and appear to improve during pregnancy. In some cases, there appears to be a strong link with Crohn's disease, especially if there is colonic involvement. Patients are advised to rinse their mouths with an appropriate mouthwash (e.g. chlorhexidine or tetracycline) to prevent the development of secondary infections. In more severe cases, patients may be prescribed corticosteroid (e.g. hydrocortisone) lozenges.

Gingivitis

Gingivitis describes the condition in which the gums become inflamed and swollen due to bacteria in the plaque. The bacteria penetrate the gum tissue, triggering an immune response, which causes the gums to become swollen and tender. Patients may complain of pain when brushing but it is often painless and so goes undetected. The first sign may be bleeding when using dental floss. This is usually accompanied by puffiness in the gums. If left untreated, the gums begin to recede and this can lead to periodontitis, a condition in which the supporting membrane of the teeth and bone are eroded. Regular oral hygiene and visits to the dentist can reverse the effects of gingivitis (see Evidence-based Practice box 22.1).

Disorders of the tongue

There are a number of disorders that can affect the tongue:

- glossitis – inflammation of the tongue causing it to look red, smooth and sore. This is seen in patients with iron deficiency

- stomatitis – the presence of small ulcers
- furring or coating of the tongue – a common condition, often seen in smokers
- a black hairy tongue – due to an alteration in the normal flora of the mouth because of a proliferation of microorganisms that cause a brown staining of the elongated filiform papillae (the tiny projections that give the tongue its velvety appearance). The causes of a black hairy tongue are unknown, although it is seen in patients who have been prescribed with broad-spectrum antibiotics or who have used antiseptic mouthwashes containing chlorhexidine. It is also seen in patients with a history of heavy smoking.

Vincent's angina

This is a pharyngeal infection accompanied by an ulcerative gingivitis (ulcerated gums). It mostly affects young male smokers with poor oral hygiene. Patients complain of painful gums, often with bleeding, halitosis (bad breath), fever and cervical lymphadenopathy (enlarged nodes in the neck).

▶ Nursing management

The mouth can be affected by a wide variety of conditions, and effective mouth care requires nurses to utilize their assessment skills. To facilitate effective assessment, a variety of tools have been developed to act as a guide and prompt when assessing the mouth (Eilers et al 1988, Beck & Yasko 1993). One of the most important aspects of care is to keep the mouth moist. Regular mouth care with a soft toothbrush and paste, rather than foam brushes, can help in reducing problems such as dental caries, gingivitis and halitosis. The prophylactic use of nystatin or amphotericin lozenges can significantly reduce the incidence of candidiasis.

Ulcers that change appearance or become more painful should always be referred to the medical team for further investigation. The use of petroleum jelly on the lips will prevent cracking and retain moisture. Patients should be encouraged to drink to prevent dehydration, which will lead to drying of the mucosa of the mouth (buccal mucosa). Ill-fitting dentures should be removed and, if possible, a new set fitted. On removing dentures it is important to label them and clean them, as they can become clogged with food and debris and can act as a source of infection. Good oral care is a mark of high nursing standards and is considered by the government to be an essential aspect of patient care (Department of Health 2001).

DISORDERS AFFECTING THE OESOPHAGUS

The major symptoms associated with oesophageal disorders are dysphagia (difficulty swallowing), heartburn and painful swallowing. As the lumen of the oesophagus is narrow, it can become blocked and prevent the passage of food. This section will look at some of the conditions that can cause these symptoms.

Oesophageal diverticulum

Diverticulae (small pockets in the lining of the oesophagus) can occur in the mid-oesophagus due to inflammation of the mediastinal lymph nodes, which pull on the oesophagus (traction diverticulum). They can also occur just above the lower oesophageal sphincter (epiphrenic diverticulum). They can cause the regurgitation of food and sometimes cause dysphagia. Diagnosis is by barium swallow and treatment usually requires surgery (diverticulectomy).

Hiatus hernia

The diaphragm separates the stomach from the chest. Hiatus hernia refers to herniation of the stomach through the opening where the oesophagus passes through the diaphragm (called the oesophageal hiatus) into the thorax (see Fig. 22.5). Hiatus hernia may be congenital when a portion of the fundus of the stomach lies anterior to the oesophagus and this is known as para-oesophageal type. In a sliding hiatus hernia, the gastro-oesophageal junction 'slides' through the hiatus so that it lies above the diaphragm. Patients with a sliding hernia may be asymptomatic or they may suffer with reflux. Patients with hiatus hernia may require surgery but there are things that they can do themselves to alleviate their symptoms (see Health Promotion box 22.1).

Achalasia

Achalasia is a disease characterized by an absence of peristalsis (aperistalsis) in the body of the oesophagus. The lower oesophagus fails to relax when food is swallowed, causing the oesophagus to become dilated and the muscle wall to hypertrophy. It results from a degeneration of the nerve cells of Auerbach's plexus (see p. 592). Patients complain of difficulty in swallowing (dysphagia), regurgitation of undigested food and precordial pain, i.e. oesophageal pain over the heart region that is hard to distinguish from cardiac pain. Regurgitation often occurs spontaneously at night and patients are at risk of aspiration pneumonia.

Diffuse oesophageal spasm

This is characterized by dysphagia and abnormal oesophageal motility that can sometimes produce retrosternal chest pain. It can occur as a primary disorder or secondary to achalasia, cancer of the oesophagus or in a neuromuscular disorder. Swallowing is accompanied by abnormal contractions of the oesophagus

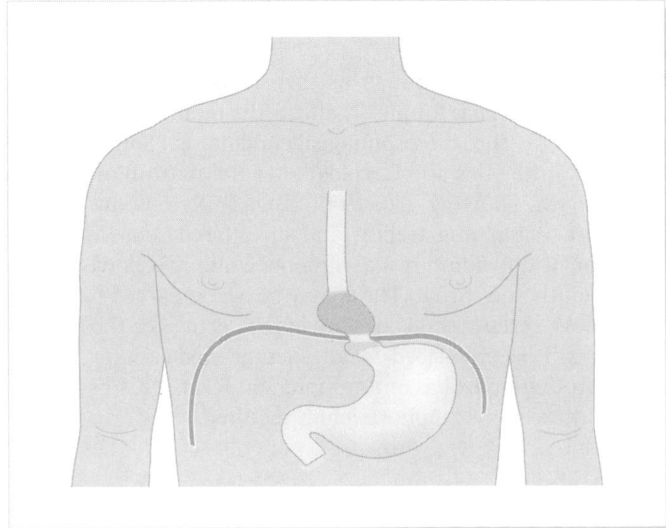

Figure 22.5 Hiatus hernia.

HEALTH PROMOTION

22.1 Avoiding gastro-oesophageal reflux

Reflux can be reduced by considering the following:

- *Diet* – heartburn can occur after large, spicy or fatty meals. Many people find that specific foods provoke symptoms, e.g. hot curries or fish and chips. Therefore try to avoid such foods once identified
- *Smoking* – give up or reduce smoking, as this can make the problem worse
- *Eating habits* – avoid eating just before bedtime or just before exercising
- *Alcohol* – reduce alcohol intake as it can aggravate the symptoms
- *Weight* – lose weight if overweight
- *Raise bed* – if symptoms occur at night, try raising the head of the bed by 10 cm.

Patients should be advised to consult their GP without delay if:

- they get pain when they swallow
- their food 'sticks' on the way down
- they have choking attacks
- they vomit blood.

---

without progression of the waves. Barium study appearances on X-ray are characteristic: the image is described as being like a corkscrew due to the uncoordinated contraction of the oesophageal muscles.

Oesophageal rings and webs

Oesophageal ring, also known as the Schatzki ring, is a narrowing of the oesophagus due to a membranous ridge of mucosa projecting into the lumen of the lower oesophagus. Patients may be asymptomatic, but some complain of dysphagia after eating, especially if the meal has been hurried. Patients are advised to eat slowly and to chew food well. Many patients will only require reassurance.

Oesophageal webs may occur throughout the oesophagus, but mainly in the post-cricoid region near the cricopharyngeal muscle. On X-ray it looks like a web. Patients may be asymptomatic or present with dysphagia and anaemia. In a rare and poorly understood syndrome known as Plummer–Vinson syndrome or Paterson–Brown–Kelly syndrome, which mainly affects middle-aged women, the web is associated with iron deficiency anaemia, koilonychias (spoon-shaped nails), glossitis and angular stomatitis.

Foreign bodies in the oesophagus

Some people, especially children, may be seen in the A&E departments because they have swallowed an object such as a coin or glass or food that is not chewed thoroughly, causing a blockage in the oesophagus. Patients may complain of dysphagia or pain and, if the object is sharp, may present with a haemorrhage. A plain X-ray will confirm the presence of a solid object, but if the object is food, a barium swallow may be necessary to locate the blockage. This is also useful in detecting the presence of strictures or growths that may be impeding the passage of food. Once the object has been identified, it can usually be removed by endoscopy (see p. 599).

EMERGENCY SITUATIONS – THE ACUTE ABDOMEN

This is a surgical emergency and accounts for about 1% of all hospital admissions in the UK (Sweetland & Cook 1999). Patients usually present with severe abdominal pain and may also present with nausea, vomiting, anorexia and possible sepsis. The site of the pain is important and the patient should be asked to indicate the most painful site. In patients complaining of both back pain and abdominal pain, an abdominal aortic aneurysm may be suspected (see Ch. 19). Pain in the upper abdomen may be due to perforation of a gastric ulcer; pain in the mid-abdomen may indicate small bowel disease; pain in the right iliac fossa is commonly due to appendicitis; and pain in the left iliac fossa may be due to diverticulitis. In women with low abdominal pain, ectopic pregnancy must be considered.

Acute abdominal problems may be due to intestinal obstruction, inflammation, ischaemic disorders, systemic disorders and peritoneal disease. The aim of care is to determine whether patients require a medical or surgical referral and to resuscitate the critically ill patient with intravenous fluids and oxygen therapy. The presenting history, the clinical examination and subsequent investigations are critical in determining a diagnosis and immediate treatment.

ACUTE PERITONITIS

Acute peritonitis may be either primary or secondary. In primary peritonitis the peritoneum is infected via the bloodstream, but this is very rare. Secondary peritonitis can be caused by a wide variety of problems, the most common of which is perforation of the GI tract. This can occur when the stomach, gallbladder, bowel or bladder perforates into the peritoneal cavity. Perforation of the colon (large intestine) may due to obstruction, diverticulitis, inflammatory bowel disease or toxic megacolon. A perforated diverticulum of the sigmoid colon is a common cause of peritonitis. Other diseases that are linked to perforation are ulcerative colitis and Crohn's disease. The colon will require resection if the peritonitis is caused by any of these diseases.

Patients will usually present with a sudden onset of abdominal pain, which is made worse by coughing. They will usually lie very still and rigid, afraid to move. In severe cases, tenderness occurs over the entire abdomen, accompanied by vomiting and pyrexia. Patients will usually have no bowel sounds, as peristalsis is absent. If this is the case, time is of the essence and they will require surgery (laparotomy) as soon as possible. There is a risk of multi-organ failure in that the kidneys and liver may fail. Fluids are lost as they leak into the peritoneal cavity, which in turn will lead to dehydration and electrolyte disturbances. Patients will require a series of abdominal X-rays; gas collected under the diaphragm will indicate that the GI tract has been perforated. A nasogastric tube should be passed and attached to suction. Fluids should be replaced intravenously and antibiotic therapy commenced.

INTESTINAL OBSTRUCTION

Patients usually complain of colicky abdominal pain, which is often preceded by vomiting. If the vomit contains faecal matter, this usually indicates that the small bowel is obstructed. Large bowel obstruction may be due to inflammatory or neoplastic pathology. The cause is usually age-dependent, as bowel cancers are rare in younger patients. Unless the obstruction is removed, there is a risk that it will perforate and leak faecal material into the abdomen. Colonic obstruction can occur if the caecum or sigmoid colon twists in on itself. This causes an abrupt onset of symptoms.

Sigmoid volvulus is the twisting of a loop of bowel around its mesentery, causing ischaemia and infarction, and usually occurs in older individuals with a history of straining at stool. Caecal volvulus usually occurs if the caecum is mobile and the mesentery is abnormally long. This is usually a cogenital abnormality. Patients present with abdominal distension, nausea, vomiting and colicky/cramp-like abdominal pain.

INTESTINAL ISCHAEMIA

The formation of thrombus and emboli may cause a blockage to the superior mesenteric artery or vein and is associated with artherosclerosis. Patients usually present with a sudden onset of severe abdominal pain and abdominal tenderness. They will have an elevated white cell count and, in about 50% of cases, a metabolic acidosis. If the bowel has infarcted, surgery is required to remove the infarcted area and the ends are brought onto the skin to form a stoma.

▶ Nursing management

Until a diagnosis is reached, the nursing role will focus on pain relief and close observation of the vital signs to enable any deterioration in the patient's condition to be detected and reported and to enable preparation for surgery if appropriate. Patients are likely to require pain relief and they will need information and reassurance. Vital signs (temperature, pulse, respiration, blood pressure) should be checked and blood samples obtained for full blood count (FBC), urea and electrolytes (U&E), blood sugar and amylase. If there is any possibility of haemorrhage, patients' blood should be cross-matched so that blood will be available for transfusion if necessary. Intravenous (i.v.) fluids may be required. In some cases, the insertion of a central venous pressure (CVP) line should be considered (see Ch. 31). Patients may require a plain abdominal X-ray, and if there is any indication of ileus or obstruction, a nasogastric tube should be passed and the gastric contents aspirated. Nurses will need to document care given and ensure appropriate interventions are recorded, such as fluid balance.

DISORDERS OF THE UPPER GI TRACT

HAEMORRHAGE

Haematemesis is the term used to describe blood that is vomited after bleeding in the upper GI tract. This may be bright red, which indicates recent bleeding, or a brown colour described as 'coffee grounds', which indicates that the blood is old and has been mixed with the acids in the stomach, which has altered the haemoglobin. Patients will require prompt treatment to stop the bleeding and a blood transfusion may be required to replace blood loss.

Haemorrhage in the upper GI tract is a common medical emergency and has an annual prevalence of about 50 cases per 100 000 population. It can occur for a variety of reasons:

- oesophageal varices
- oesophagitis
- acute gastric erosion
- carcinoma
- peptic ulceration
- Mallory–Weiss tears.

OESOPHAGEAL VARICES

There is a high mortality rate associated with oesophageal varices, which develop as a result of portal hypertension (see p. 594). The raised pressure, which is commonly due to alcoholic cirrhosis of the liver, causes the veins to dilate and rupture, leading to serious haemorrhage. Oesophageal varices are found in 50% of patients with cirrhosis of the liver (Odelowo et al 2002). The aim of treatment is to stop the haemorrhage and restore blood volume.

Medical/surgical management

Treatment will depend on the severity of the bleeding and will involve one of the following (see also Ch. 23):

- i.v. vasopressin which causes vasoconstriction, thus restricting portal blood flow
- insertion of an inflatable Sengstaken–Blakemore triple-lumen oesophageal tube, which has a long balloon that is filled with air, in order to apply compression to the varices to stop the bleeding
- direct injection of the varices (via an endoscope) with a sclerosing agent, an irritant solution that causes inflammatory obliteration of the veins
- transluminal intrahepatic portasystemic stent shunt (TIPSS – for patients who do not respond to endoscopic management), which reduces portal pressure by connecting the portal and systemic veins.

OESOPHAGITIS

Oesophagitis refers to inflammation of the oesophagus, which can be due to infection (infective oesophagitis), the ingestion of corrosive agents (corrosive oesophagitis), or the reflux of acid gastric contents into the oesophagus (reflux oesophagitis).

Infective oesophagitis

The most common oesophageal infections are *Candidia* and herpes simplex. Patients may complain of difficulty in swallowing (dysphagia) or painful swallowing (odynophagia). Candidiasis can occur in patients who are on a course of antibiotics, because antibiotics also affect normal flora and reduce resistance to fungal infections. Both candidiasis and herpes simplex occur in patients who are immunosuppressed. Patients on corticosteroids and cytotoxic drugs and those with AIDS may also suffer from these problems.

Medical/surgical management

Candida infections are usually treated with nystatin and/or amphotericin, although in patients who are severely immuno-suppressed, ketoconazole or fluconazole appear to be more effective. Patients with herpes simplex may find that drinks containing a local anaesthetic may be useful or that a course of aciclovir can reduce the symptoms.

Corrosive oesophagitis

The ingestion of a caustic solution (e.g. bleach) causes pain, severe inflammation, haemorrhage and, in some instances, stricture formation. The patient's mouth will be burnt and the patient may be in a state of shock.

Medical/surgical management

Treatment is aimed at reducing and controlling shock and preventing the formation of strictures. On no account should ipecacuanha or any other agent to induce vomiting (emesis) be given because this will bring the caustic solution back into the oesophagus and mouth, causing further damage. Patients who develop strictures will require surgical intervention.

Reflux oesophagitis

This is an inflammatory response secondary to the reflux of gastric contents into the lower oesophagus. It is associated with reduced pressure in the lower oesophageal sphincter and is seen in pregnancy, obesity, hiatus hernia and raised intra-abdominal pressure. Patients complain of heartburn, retrosternal chest pain and a sour or bitter taste in the mouth, especially when stooping or bending down.

Medical/surgical management

Patients should be advised to lose weight if obese, to avoid large meals prior to bedtime and, if a problem at night, to raise the bed head. Some patients find that an antacid reduces the problem, whereas others will require the administration of H_2-receptor antagonists as they reduce gastric acid secretion. In patients with severe problems, a proton-pump inhibitor (e.g. omeprazole), which reduces gastric acid production by blocking the proton-pump mechanism in the stomach, may be more effective.

GASTRITIS

Gastritis may be either acute or chronic. Acute gastritis is usually due to an irritant such as food poisoning or to excessive alcohol intake, which damages the gastric mucosal barrier and can lead to upper gastrointestinal bleeding.

Pathophysiology

In acute gastritis, there is an acute inflammatory infiltrate in the superficial gastric mucosa, predominantly with neutrophils, which can sometimes be accompanied by mucosal erosions. The mucous membrane of the stomach becomes thickened and its rugae are prominent. Chronic gastritis is subdivided into two types: chronic superficial, which is usually as a result of *H. pylori*

colonization; and chronic atrophic, which is linked to vitamin B_{12} malabsorption.

Clinical presentation

Patients with acute gastritis complain of abdominal pain or discomfort, nausea and vomiting and a loss of appetite. Some patients may present with haematemesis due to gastric erosion following the ingestion of aspirin or other forms of non-steroidal anti-inflammatory drugs (NSAIDs). Patients with chronic gastritis may have no symptoms, although some will present with dyspepsia (indigestion). Patients with chronic alcohol misuse may complain of a loss of appetite and nausea and they will frequently vomit mucus that has collected in the stomach overnight (Reflective Practice box 22.1).

Medical/surgical management

In patients who develop GI bleeding, an endoscopy is necessary to confirm the presence of acute ulcers or erosions. However, apart from altering diet and removing the causes, no specific therapy is required.

CARCINOMA OF THE UPPER GI TRACT

Carcinoma of the upper GI tract may occur in the mouth and pharynx, oesophagus and stomach. In many cases, the problem is only discovered when patients present with another problem, such as dysphagia or pain, or it may be detected during a routine dental visit.

Carcinoma of the oesophagus

Patients with carcinoma of the oesophagus are usually aged between 50 and 70 years. It is linked with chronic alcohol and tobacco use. Patients usually present with progressive dysphagia, inability to swallow their saliva, pain and regurgitation of food. Patients will lose a great deal of weight in a short period of time. The tumour can occur in any part of the oesophagus; approximately half of all cases occur in the distal third of the oesophagus and the other half in the proximal two-thirds.

R|Я REFLECTIVE PRACTICE

22.1 Gastritis and alcohol

John has gastritis and suffers from dyspepsia and heartburn. He drinks 4–5 units of alcohol each day, smokes 20 cigarettes daily and is overweight (BMI = 31 kg/m²). John's diet is high in saturated fat and he admits to liking Indian and Chinese food. He takes aspirin and ibuprofen for headaches and pain relief.

Student activities

- Why do you think that John suffers from gastritis?
- What nursing actions could be used to reduce the problems experienced by John?
- Would you recommend John to take alternative medication for his headaches? If so, why?
- What other advice would John need?

Carcinoma of the stomach

Patients with carcinoma of the stomach often present with symptoms which suggest an ulcer, but the symptoms do not get any better and the patients do not have any periods of remission. There appears to be a very strong link with *H. pylori* infection, as this leads to gastritis with atrophy (wasting) and intestinal metaplasia (replacement of one type of cell for another). Most tumours are found in the gastric antrum and are almost invariably adenocarcinoma. Patients develop anorexia and lose a great deal of weight. Chances of survival are improved with early diagnosis and treatment, but gastric cancer has a very poor prognosis. Diagnosis is reached by undertaking radiological studies, endoscopy and biopsy of the gastric mucosa. Patients who present with signs of advanced disease, such as a hard fixed mass in the epigastrium and evidence of secondary deposits in the liver or malignant nodes in the left supraclavicular fossae (Virchow's node), have a very poor outcome.

Medical/surgical management

Surgical intervention (total or partial gastrectomy) appears to offer the best form of treatment, although radiotherapy for squamous cell carcinoma has proved beneficial, as has treatment with chemotherapy. In patients with no infiltration outside the oesophageal wall, the 5-year survival rate is 80%; however, many patients will only present in the advanced stages of the disease and their chances of survival are very poor. In patients with gastric cancer, the 5-year survival rate is approximately 10%. Therefore nurses will need to ensure terminal patients receive palliative treatment, adequate pain relief and emotional support (see Chs 33 and 34).

> ▶ **Nursing management: patients undergoing gastric surgery**

Patients who require surgical intervention are at risk of haemorrhage and pulmonary complications (e.g. chest infection and pulmonary embolus) in the immediate postoperative period. The nurse should arrange for the physiotherapist to see patients prior to the surgery. The physiotherapist will then teach patients breathing exercises that can minimize problems postoperatively. The nurse also needs to ensure adequate pain relief so that patients are able to mobilize as their condition allows. The nurse should also measure patients for graduated compression stockings, as they will reduce the risk of deep vein thrombosis (DVT) and pulmonary embolus (PE). Patients may arrive back on the ward with i.v. fluids in progress to prevent dehydration, and should only be given fluids by mouth when bowel sounds have been heard in all four quadrants of the abdomen. It is important to note that some high-pitched tinkling sounds may be a sign of impending bowel paralysis and are caused by an accumulation of fluid and gas. Patients may also have a nasogastric tube in situ, as this allows for free drainage of gastric contents. If large amounts of fluid are drained, this may indicate paralytic ileus, the absence of peristalsis in the bowel.

Nurses need to be alert to the development of other possible complications that may occur at a later stage, such as dumping syndrome in which patients may faint, experience abdominal pain and show signs of shock. This is due to the osmotic effects of the rapid transit of food from the stomach to the small intestine.

Dumping syndrome can occur after gastrectomy, because large amounts of food may pass suddenly into the intestine, causing a rapid fluid shift and a temporary reduction in circulating volume. Patients should be advised to lie down for up to 30 minutes after meals. Nursing staff will need to ensure that nutritional needs are being met, and regular monitoring of patients' weight and body mass index (BMI) is important (see Ch. 11).

Patients who have had a part of their stomach (partial gastrectomy) removed may develop 'short stomach syndrome' in that they feel full even after a small meal. They may also have an impaired appetite. Nurses will need to liaise with the dietician to ensure that patients receive adequate calorific intake.

Following total gastrectomy, patients will require regular injections of vitamin B_{12}. This is because they are no longer able to produce intrinsic factor (the enzyme necessary for absorption of vitamin B_{12}) due to the lack of gastric acid (the acid required for production of intrinsic factor).

PEPTIC ULCERATION

Peptic ulceration occurs when the inner lining (mucous membrane) becomes ulcerated as a result of the corrosive effects of hydrochloric acid and pepsin, leading to erosion of the mucosal wall. It is one of the most common gastrointestinal disorders and can affect approximately 15% of the population at any one time, although it is more common in men. It is mainly due to *H. pylori* infection, but factors such as smoking, stress, alcohol, NSAIDs and acid hypersecretory states (e.g. Zollinger–Ellison syndrome, which usually affects the jejunum) have also been linked to its development.

Ulceration can occur in the oesophagus, stomach and duodenum, although the majority of ulcers are in the stomach or proximal duodenum. Ulcers extend through the muscularis mucosae and are usually over 5 cm in diameter. Oesophageal ulcers arise in patients with hiatus hernia and gastrooesophageal reflux. Signs and symptoms include epigastric pain radiating to the back, nausea, waterbrash (saliva filling the mouth), heartburn, anorexia and weight loss. The main complications are GI bleeding and perforation leading to peritonitis.

Specific investigations

Endoscopy and barium studies are the most effective, and biopsies may be obtained during endoscopy.

Medical/surgical management

This involves removing the exacerbating factors, and the use of H_2-receptor antagonists, antacids or proton-pump inhibitors. If the ulcer perforates, patients will require immediate surgery. As many patients relapse following the cessation of the H_2-receptor antagonists and because of the clear link with *H. pylori*, many gastroenterologists favour the use of 'triple therapy' as the first line of defence. Triple therapy (e.g. amoxicillin or clarithromycin, metronidazole and omeprazole) can be used for 1 or 2 weeks; however, there are often problems with compliance as some patients find it hard to take so many tablets. Furthermore, when metronidazole is used, patients must abstain from alcohol as they can develop severe reactions to it (see Ethical Issues box 22.1). They may also experience side-effects such as nausea and vomiting, which can sometimes be quite severe.

ETHICAL ISSUES

22.1 Managing a disruptive patient

Mr Jones has been admitted to your ward with a peptic ulcer. He has a long history of alcohol abuse. He has been commenced on metronidazole, which will make him violently sick if he continues to drink, but he is refusing to stay on the ward and you suspect he is drinking in the toilets and disregarding his tablets. He is now causing problems on the ward and disrupting other patients. The doctor has suggested that he should be discharged, as he will not comply with medical instructions; however, the nurses feel that he should be referred for counselling and support. The doctors feel that this would be a waste of resources.

● What ethical issues do you feel that this situation raises?

PYLORIC STENOSIS

This occurs when the area around the pyloric sphincter becomes scarred and oedematous, and in adults it is usually a complication of peptic ulceration. The main feature of this problem is vomiting, which can be projectile, and abdominal discomfort. In the initial stages, when muscle tone is good, patients may vomit soon after meals and at frequent intervals. However, as it progresses, muscle tone decreases and patients vomit the contents 3–4 hours after their meal. Food pools in the stomach and can remain undigested. Patients may also present with anorexia and weight loss. When examining a patient, a distended stomach may be noted, and when listening with a stethoscope over the stomach, a fluid splash may be heard when gently rolling the patient from side to side.

Specific investigations

Barium studies will demonstrate a delay in gastric emptying and a narrowing of the pyloric canal.

Medical/surgical management

The initial treatment of pyloric stenosis is to correct any fluid and electrolyte imbalance and patients will usually require surgical intervention to correct the problem. This commonly involves one of the following:

■ pyloroplasty – surgery to the pylorus to enlarge the outlet
■ truncal vagotomy – the main trunks of the vagal nerves are divided to decrease gastric acid secretion
■ gastroenterostomy – surgical anastomosis between stomach and small intestine to bypass the pyloric obstruction if the duodenum is involved.

MALLORY–WEISS SYNDROME

This is a rare cause of haematemesis in which persistent retching and vomiting leads to small lacerations at the gastro-oesophageal junction. Fresh blood at the conclusion of forceful vomiting suggests a traumatic tear.

▶ Nursing management: patients with acute GI haemorrhage

Patients presenting with an upper GI bleed will require a rapid assessment and treatment. The treatment will depend on the cause and the extent of the blood loss. Management includes the restoration and maintenance of circulating volume. Patients may require the insertion of a CVP line to monitor venous pressures and a low reading may indicate that bleeding is still taking place. Patients will require oxygen therapy to assist with tissue perfusion, a blood transfusion to replace blood loss and to maintain circulating volume. If there is any suspicion of variceal bleeding, they will need immediate endoscopy and possible sclerotherapy (artificial production of fibrosis by injecting a sclerosing agent). Patients with other causes will also require an endoscopy, although nurses will have more time to prepare them to undergo this procedure. Patients who have received more than 6 units of blood and continue to bleed will need to be prepared for surgery.

Patients who do not fall into the above categories will require conservative treatment. Nurses will need to provide support and information to ensure that patients understand the need to remain nil by mouth and the need for bed rest. Patients will also need to have blood cross-matched for at least 6 units, and intravenous fluids will be prescribed. It is important to ensure that the fluid input and output are recorded and that patients are monitored for signs of fluid overload. The volume of any vomit should also be recorded and whether it contains blood or is bloodstained. Faeces should be observed for the presence of melaena (black, tarry faeces due to the presence of blood).

By closely monitoring patients' vital signs, nurses may gain an early warning of shock, a repeat bleed or fluid overload. Patients who require a blood transfusion will need more frequent observations (see Ch. 19). Those who stabilize will need support and encouragement to give up smoking and reduce alcohol intake.

DISORDERS OF THE LOWER GI TRACT

Disorders of the lower GI tract include appendicitis, irritable bowel syndrome, Crohn's disease and constipation.

APPENDICITIS

The appendix is a worm-like tube with a blind end, which projects from the caecum in the right iliac fossa. It contains a large amount of lymphoid tissue and is covered in peritoneum. Acute appendicitis is the most common surgical emergency in the developed world (Sweetland & Cook 1999) and occurs when the lumen of the appendix becomes obstructed. This may be due to swollen lymphoid follicles following an infection, hard faecal material, or the presence of threadworms or tapeworms. Following blockage, organisms from the gut invade, causing an inflammatory response to occur. It can affect any age group but is most common in 8 to 15-year-olds. As there is a risk of perforation, this condition should be treated as an emergency and patients will need to be prepared for surgery as quickly as possible.

Clinical presentation

Patients may present initially with pyrexia, a furred tongue, foetor (unpleasant smelling breath), constipation and central abdominal colic. However, when the peritoneum becomes inflamed, the pain will centre in the right iliac fossa and become more constant. When examining such patients, the surgeon will note that there is usually tenderness and guarding (tensing of abdominal muscles). There may also be tenderness on the right side when a rectal examination is performed. When palpating the abdomen, the surgeon may also note the presence of Rovsing's sign, which refers to pain in the right inguinal fossa when the left inguinal fossa is pressed.

Medical/surgical management

As there is a risk of perforation and peritonitis, the surgeon may wish to operate to remove the appendix (appendicectomy) as soon as possible.

▶ Nursing management

As appendicitis is seen as a surgical emergency, it is important to prepare patients for theatre as quickly as possible. Patients and their family members are likely to be very anxious and so good communication skills are paramount. Explain to them what is happening and what patients are likely to experience when they wake up from the procedure. They should have nothing orally and a nasogastric tube may be passed to empty the stomach of its contents as this will help to prevent regurgitation and possible inhalation of stomach contents into the lungs during induction of anaesthesia. Box 22.2 summarizes the preparation for surgery (see Ch. 29 for further discussion).

In most cases, recovery will be uneventful but it is important that patients are observed closely on their return from theatre. As there will be an abdominal wound, there is a potential for bleeding to occur and therefore it is important to monitor blood pressure and pulse rate. A rapid, weak pulse accompanied by a drop in blood pressure may indicate that a patient is bleeding or becoming shocked. There is also a risk of peritonitis.

PERITONITIS

Peritonitis occurs when the peritoneum becomes inflamed and a reaction is triggered. Serous fluid is produced in response to the inflammation and this becomes infected by the bacteria in the bowel. Therefore, it is vital that nurses monitor the wound site to detect any distension, and noting the presence of unusual levels of pain. The abdominal pain that accompanies peritonitis is intense and agonizing. The abdomen will appear rigid, with little or no movement with respiration, and the abdominal muscles will appear board-like and rigid. The patient may vomit. Patients who develop peritonitis will require further surgery to drain the abdominal cavity, a nasogastric tube to reduce the distension, and intravenous antibiotics to treat the infection. Nurses will then need to ensure that fluid balance is maintained and that patients receive adequate analgesia.

IRRITABLE BOWEL SYNDROME

Irritable bowel syndrome (IBS) is probably the most common GI problem seen by doctors in GI clinics and it affects about 1 in 4 people in the Western world. It is known as a condition of negatives as there is no structural pathology, no known cause, there is no test to diagnose it and in most cases no cure (Hope et al 1999). It is characterized by abdominal pain and discomfort, bloating and a disordered bowel habit, which alters between constipation and diarrhoea and a sensation of incomplete evacuation. Possible causes include psychological factors such as stress and depression, food intolerance, and previous episodes of gastroenteritis. Alcohol, antibiotics and some foods can exacerbate the symptoms.

Investigations and management

As the condition mimics other bowel conditions, it is important to exclude other possible causes. A sigmoidoscopy is useful, especially in patients over the age of 40 who present with a recent change in bowel habit, in order to exclude the possibility of colon cancer. A barium enema and colonoscopy should be performed.

Box 22.2 Preparation for surgery

- Ask the patient to empty the bladder to promote comfort and reduce the possibility of damage during surgery
- If requested by the surgeon, remove or shorten hair around the site with clippers or with a depilatory cream. This is to reduce the risk of wound infection
- Remove all makeup, nail varnish and lipstick to ensure that lips and nail beds can be seen in order to detect cyanosis
- Clean the skin with chlorhexidine to reduce bacterial count
- Remove any prostheses, contact lenses, hearing aids, glasses and dentures and place in a safe place
- Check for the presence of any dental caps or crowns to alert the anaesthetist to prevent damage
- Apply name bands with patient's details to one upper and one lower limb to ensure correct identification

- Ensure the patient has been nil by mouth for at least 4 hours or empty stomach contents with a nasogastric tube to reduce the possibility of regurgitation of stomach contents
- Remove all jewellery and hair pins to reduce the risk of diathermy burns and store in a safe place
- Place the patient in a theatre gown which allows for easy access to the operation site
- Measure and apply graduated compression stockings to prevent deep vein thrombosis
- Give premedication as prescribed to relax the patient
- Ensure all medical and nursing notes and X-rays are collated so that all relevant information is available
- Ensure that the patient understands what is about to happen, that consent has been given and that the consent form has been signed

If patients present with diarrhoea, stool samples should be obtained for culture and sensitivity (to rule out infection) and for faecal fat studies to exclude malabsorption. Biopsies taken during sigmoidoscopy/colonoscopy can exclude the presence of irritable bowel disease (IBD, see below). Once a diagnosis of IBS is made, it is important to reassure patients that there is no underlying malignancy.

Treatment is aimed at controlling the symptoms, and if food intolerance is suspected, an exclusion diet may be helpful. Patients with diarrhoea may find that medication, such as an antimotility drug (e.g. loperamide), is useful in controlling it. When they are constipated, a drug that retains fluid in the bowel, such as an osmotic laxative (e.g. lactulose), is useful. Bulking agents such as bran or ispaghula husk are also useful as they increase faecal mass and stimulate peristalsis. Patients should also be advised to have a balanced diet that includes fibre and sufficient fluid, as this too will prevent constipation. However, it is important to note that the use of fibre can exacerbate the problems in some patients, leaving them feeling bloated and in pain. It has been suggested that hypnotherapy may be useful in controlling the symptoms (Galovski & Blanchard 2002).

CONSTIPATION

This is defined as the incomplete or infrequent action of the bowels or difficulty in defecation. There are a variety of causes and it is important to treat these in order to gain a satisfactory outcome. However, in patients over the age of 40, it is important that the more sinister causes are ruled out, e.g. colorectal cancer. The common causes can be grouped into the following categories:

- diet and fluid intake
- bowel disorders, including tumours and diverticular disease
- local rectal problems causing pain
- faulty bowel habits
- immobility and exercise
- socioeconomic factors
- medication.

Diet and fluid intake

Food in the small bowel is in liquid form, but as it passes through the large bowel, fluid is absorbed, resulting in the semi-solid appearance of faeces. However, if insufficient fluids are taken, the stool will become hard, as its bulk will be reduced. This causes the normal peristaltic movement to slow down and more fluid to be absorbed. Diet is also important, because a diet low in fibre and bulk will slow down peristaltic movement and allow more fluid to be absorbed. Therefore, it is important to ensure patients are drinking sufficient fluid (at least 2 litres a day) and are encouraged to eat fruit and vegetables, wholemeal bread and bran-based cereals.

Bowel habits

Some people put off going to the toilet for a variety of reasons. This may be because they are busy, they are not at home or they are embarrassed about going to the toilet in a strange place, and so they ignore their body and hold onto the stool (see Special Issues box 22.1). This causes fluid absorption, resulting in constipation, and it also alters the gastrocolic reflex. Conditions such as anal fissures and haemorrhoids (see p. 617) can cause

SPECIAL ISSUES

22.1 Preventing constipation in hospital patients

Constipation is not an inevitable consequence of hospitalization. There are a number of things that nurses can do to reduce the risk:

- Ensure that patients have sufficient fluid intake and are drinking at least 2 litres a day. If unable to take oral fluids, make sure that sufficient intravenous fluids have been prescribed and are running to time
- Encourage patients to drink fruit juice, eat fruit and vegetables and other high-fibre foods
- Check each day whether patients have had their bowels open. This will allow potential problems to be identified early and addressed before becoming more severe and more difficult to resolve
- Provide privacy for patients using the bed pan or commode. Imagine what it is like for patients using a bed pan or commode at the bedside to open their bowels. Ask yourself: 'Would I sit in a crowded room with a curtain around me and open my bowels?'. 'Not if I can help it' will probably be your answer! Wherever possible, taking patients to the toilet rather than the other way round is preferable as it provides more privacy. If patients are unable to leave the bedside, make sure the curtains are tightly closed and prevent other staff entering before they have finished.

pain with the result that the patient becomes reluctant to pass stool, the stool remains in the colon longer, more fluid is absorbed and constipation occurs. Patients need to be educated about the dangers of ignoring the call to stool and should be encouraged to open their bowels in the mornings. A hot drink will stimulate peristalsis.

Immobility and exercise

Exercising increases the muscle tone in the abdominal wall and in the bowel and thus aids peristalsis. However, in patients who do not exercise or who are immobile, peristalsis is slowed, resulting in fluid absorption and constipation.

Socioeconomic factors

Income can play a part in the development of constipation. Individuals and families on low incomes may not have the money to buy fresh fruit and vegetables and may not have transport to enable them to shop at the big supermarkets. They are then forced to buy their shopping at the more expensive local shops and thus may be tempted to buy more convenience and processed food, instead of fresh fruit and vegetables. For older people with mobility problems, this is also a factor if they cannot get out to the shops.

Medication

A variety of drugs, e.g atropine, morphine and tricyclic drugs (antidepressants), can cause constipation because they reduce intestinal motility.

▶ Nursing management

Unless patients have a bowel obstruction, the mainstay of treatment will be the use of a fibre-rich diet, a 2- to 3-litre daily fluid intake, mobilization and as much exercise as possible. Medication should only be used as a last resort and only for a short period (see also Ch. 12). The importance of emptying the bowel and not ignoring the call to stool should be emphasized by the nurse. Medication that may prove useful includes bulking agents (e.g. fibrogel), laxatives (e.g. bisacodyl) and osmotic agents (e.g. lactulose). In patients who present with a hard faecal mass, arachis oil, phosphate enemas and glycerine suppositories may be useful (see Box 22.3). In patients whose constipation is caused by reluctance to defecate because of pain (e.g. due to anal fissures, haemorrhoids or diverticulosis), it is important to treat the condition in order to rectify the constipation.

BOWEL DISORDERS INCLUDING TUMOURS AND DIVERTICULAR DISEASE

Disorders of the large bowel can cause pain and restrict the passage of stool. It is important that the underlying condition is treated and this may involve surgical intervention.

HERNIA

A hernia occurs when an organ pushes through the structures (membrane or cavity) that enclose it. The most common types are described below.

Hiatus hernia

The stomach, lower oesophagus and intestine are usually contained within the abdominal cavity as the diaphragm forms a tight seal around the oesophagus. However, in some cases, the diaphragmatic opening becomes enlarged and loose, thus allowing the stomach, lower oesophagus or intestine to push through the oesophageal opening into the thoracic cavity. This is known as a diaphragmatic or hiatus hernia (see p. 602).

Inguinal hernia

This occurs when a portion of the bowel protrudes through the inguinal canal. This can often move freely backwards and forwards, but if it becomes trapped (strangulated), the bowel may become ischaemic, requiring urgent surgery.

Incisional hernia

This refers to the protrusion of a portion of the bowel through an abdominal wound or incision.

Umbilical hernia

This is the protrusion of intestine through the umbilicus.

DIVERTICULAR DISEASE

A diverticulum is a small pouch or pocket protruding from the bowel wall (see Fig. 22.6). They can occur in any part of the gut but appear predominantly in the sigmoid colon. The presence of diverticulae that are asymptomatic is known as diverticulosis and many patients are unaware that they have this condition. When the diverticulae become inflamed, this is known as diverticulitis. Women appear to be affected more than men and it is estimated that by the age of 60, one-third of the population of the Western world will have diverticulosis (Schoetz 1993), as a result of diet. Lack of dietary fibre is thought to lead to the development of the disease, as studies have shown that patients with diverticulitis typically have a low intake of fruit, vegetables and bran and a high intake of meat. It is thought that the lack of fibre leads to high intraluminal pressure, causing the gut mucosa to herniate through the muscle wall.

Faeces can collect in the 'pouches' and this may lead to inflammation, abscess formation, perforation and fistula formulation between the colon and the bladder, vagina or small bowel. Other symptoms of diverticulitis include pain, haemorrhage and stricture formation. However, diverticulitis rarely presents with bleeding (Sher et al 1999).

Box 22.3 Treatment for constipation and bowel cleansing

- Faecal softeners – enemas containing arachis oil lubricate and soften the stool, as well as promoting bowel movement
- Osmotic laxatives – act by retaining fluid in the bowel by osmosis (e.g. lactulose)
- Bulk-forming laxatives – stimulate peristalsis by increasing faecal mass (e.g. ispaghula husk, bran)
- Stimulant laxatives – these increase intestinal motility; prolonged use can cause an atonic, non-functioning colon
- Bowel cleaning solutions – used prior to surgery or examination and should not be used to treat constipation (e.g. Picolax, Kleenprep)

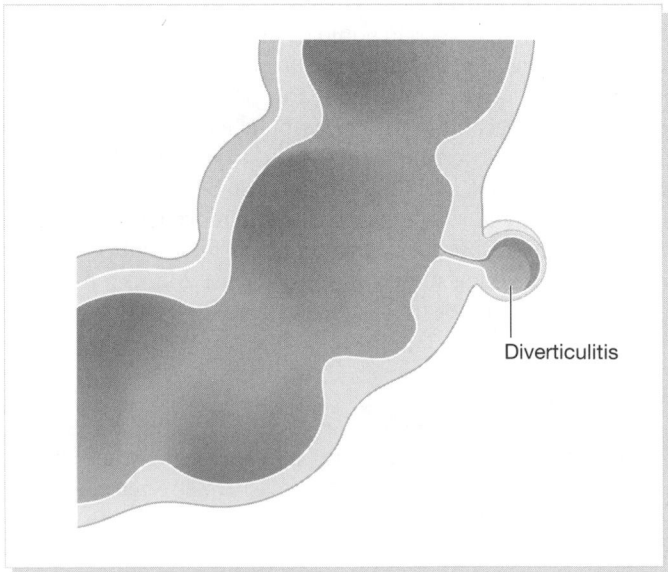

Figure 22.6 A diverticulum.

Clinical presentation

Patients with diverticulitis usually present with pyrexia, altered bowel habit, flatulence, nausea and colicky type pain, which is usually in the left iliac fossa and relieved by defecation. In severe cases, they can present with paralytic ileus, shock and peritonitis, and urgent surgical intervention as an 'acute abdomen' case will be required (see p. 603).

Medical/surgical management

The main treatment for diverticulosis is dietary and nurses should promote the importance of a high-fibre diet along with increased intake of water. It is important that nurses emphasize water, as coffee and tea have a diuretic effect. Patients may be referred for further investigation and will need to be prepared for a barium enema and flexible sigmoidoscopy. It is important that the bowel is empty, as the endoscopist and radiologist cannot visualize it well if faeces is present. Both of these tests can help to rule out the presence of cancer and confirm the diagnosis of diverticular disease. Patients with inflammation will be treated with antibiotics; however, in the event of perforation of the bowel, they will require admission and surgery.

The procedure of choice in the UK is Hartman's procedure, which involves a partial colectomy and the formation of a temporary colostomy. This involves the resection of the sigmoid colon, with closure of the rectal stump. The surgeon then forms an end colostomy in the left iliac fossae. This procedure gives the option of restoring bowel continuity at a later date.

FAMILIAL POLYPOSIS

This is a hereditary disease that usually occurs in the teens and early 20s. Large numbers of adenomatous polyps grow in the colon. These polyps are known to be premalignant and will require removal because, if left untreated, they are almost certain to develop into a colonic cancer. As this is an inherited disease, it is important that patients' family members are also followed up and investigated. Patients will require regular follow-up to remove any polyps that have grown. These can be effectively removed during endoscopy.

COLORECTAL CANCER

This is the second most common cause of cancer deaths in the UK. It affects all age groups, but is more common in those individuals aged 50–70+. Patients older than 70 make up 56% of all presentations (Hope et al 1999).

Aetiology

Colorectal cancer can affect any part of the large bowel, although it is more common in the sigmoid colon and the rectum. It is a disorder of cell growth arising in epithelial disease. The cause of colorectal cancer is still unclear, although diet, IBD and a family history appear to be linked. Benign polyps can grow in the bowel, but there is always a possibility that a benign polyp will become malignant. As discussed above, in patients with familial polyposis, it is essential that the polyps are removed. As the tumour grows, it spreads circumferentially or into the lumen of the bowel, eventually causing obstruction. The tumour spreads by infiltrating the bowel wall and organs via the peritoneal cavity. It is also spread to the liver via the lymphatic system and the blood.

Clinical presentation

Symptoms may only become apparent when the cancer is at an advanced stage. Patients may complain of a variety of symptoms depending on the site affected. Those with a tumour on the left side may present with an altered bowel habit, rectal bleeding and tenesmus (a feeling that the bowel is not emptied). A mass may also be felt when rectal examination is performed. With a tumour on the right side, patients may present with abdominal pain and weight loss. Blood tests may reveal a low haemoglobin level, indicating blood loss. Patients with either left- or right-sided tumours can also present with a fistula, an abdominal mass, bowel obstruction, perforation and haemorrhage.

Investigations and management

Following the initial examination and history, a series of investigations will need to be performed to enable the medical staff to reach a diagnosis and to determine not only the site but also the extent of the problem. Blood samples will need to be taken for haemoglobin levels and liver function tests (LFTs) may indicate possible liver involvement. Other tests include a liver ultrasound to detect any spread of the cancer, a proctoscopy, a sigmoidoscopy, a colonoscopy, barium studies and a chest X-ray. CT scanning will be carried out in most centres as this can help to detect any metastatic disease, especially in the liver. It is more sensitive than ultrasound and can image liver lesions at a resolution of about 1 cm. However, positron emission tomography (PET) scanning, a metabolic imaging examination, can detect and stage most cancers, often before they are evident through other tests.

The cancer will be staged using the modified Dukes' or TNM classification (Porrett & Daniel 1999), as follows:

Grade A   Confined to mucosa
Grade B1   Involves part of the muscle wall
Grade B2   Reaches the serosa
Grade C1   Involves wall, but not completely, and local
           lymph nodes
Grade C1   Involves serosa and lymph nodes.

Depending upon the grade, radiotherapy, chemotherapy and/or surgery (curative or palliative) will be carried out. If it is felt that the cancer cannot be totally removed, or if there are metastases, palliative surgery may be performed to relieve the symptoms and prevent bowel obstruction, improving the patient's quality of life. The type and extent of the surgery undertaken will depend upon the site of the cancer and patients may require a temporary or permanent stoma.

Bowel preparation

Prior to colorectal surgery, a clean bowel is vital if complications are to be minimized. An unprepared bowel places patients at risk of spillage of faecal material into the abdominal cavity. Ideally they should be admitted at least 3 days prior to the surgery and food should be restricted to a low-residue diet. Patients are given

22.1 Bowel preparation using Fleet phospha-soda

- On the morning of the day before surgery, the patient is asked to drink 45 ml of the solution diluted with 120 ml of water, followed by 240 ml of water.
- At midday, 750 mL of water is taken.
- In the evening prior to the surgery, the patient is again asked to drink 45 mL of the solution diluted with 120 mL of water, followed by 240 mL of water.
- The patient should not eat any solid foods the day before and should have nothing by mouth for 4–6 hours prior to the surgery.

medications such as Fleet phospho-soda, Kleen prep or Picolax to clear the bowel (see Guidelines for Care Priorities box 22.1).

Surgical management

Surgical management focuses on resection of the tumour, which may or may not require the formation of a stoma. If the tumour can be surgically removed, this increases the chances of patient survival. The main surgical approaches are described below.

Local excision

Local excision of the tumour involves removing the rectal wall in which the tumour is growing. This procedure is usually only considered if the tumour is lying within easy reach of the anus. Following removal of the tumour, it will be examined by a pathologist to ensure that complete removal has been achieved. If this is not the case, there is a risk of regrowth and the patient will require further surgical intervention.

Anterior resection

Anterior resection is performed for high rectal or low sigmoid cancers. This involves radical removal of the tumour, the segment of bowel to which it is attached, as well as the tissues that contain its lymphatic drainage, and anastomosis (joining together) of the left side of the colon to the distal bowel end. The surgeon may create a colonic pouch which allows patients to have a 'normal' bowel function, or a temporary colostomy or ileostomy, which allows the anastomosis time to heal and to prevent complications.

Abdominoperineal (AP) resection

This involves extensive surgery in which the sigmoid colon is brought out as a colostomy and the rectum and anus are removed. A permanent colostomy is usually performed, although some specialist centres are offering patients total anorectal reconstruction as an alternative to a colostomy.

Hemicolectomy

Right hemicolectomy is performed for cancer in the caecum, ascending and proximal transverse colon. Left hemicolectomy is performed for tumours in the distal transverse colon and the descending colon.

▶ **Nursing management**

Preoperative care

Patients will require the usual preoperative care (see p. 608 and Ch. 29) to ensure that they are safely prepared for surgery and will need to see the specialist stoma nurse if they are to have a stoma formed. The specialist stoma nurse will be able to explain some of the issues around stoma formation and ensure that the stoma is sited correctly. He or she will also be available postoperatively, in the hospital and at home, to offer ongoing support and practical help for patients and their families. The stoma nurse will be able to show patients the various appliances and skin products and explain how they work. Patients will have the opportunity to discuss any issues they are worried about and the stoma nurse can provide information about the various voluntary and patient organizations available to provide support.

Postoperative care

On the patient's return from theatre, the nurse should observe the wound site and monitor the condition of the stoma and whether it is functioning. The colour of the stoma must be closely monitored to ensure it is healthy. It should be reddish-pink in colour and if it appears a purple colour or dark it is imperative that the medical staff are informed as this may indicate that there is a lack of blood supply. The patient's vital signs require frequent monitoring to detect any problems. Pain relief should be administered and any signs of infection or shock should be noted and appropriate action taken. An appliance that allows observation of the stoma without removing the bag should have been applied to the patient whilst in theatre. This must be checked regularly to ensure that it fits well, is not constricting the blood supply, there is no leakage and that the patient feels comfortable. Note the presence of flatus in the bag as this indicates that bowel function is returning.

Patients with a diagnosis of cancer are likely to be frightened, stressed, anxious, depressed or angry, especially if they are worried that the cancer has not been removed. They may be worried that it has spread, that they are going to die, that they will be in pain and also about what will happen to their family or loved ones. They may also be worried about dealing with a stoma and how their partner will react to it. It is important that a senior member of the medical team is available to discuss with them the outcome of the surgery and their prognosis.

If a stoma has been formed, patients will need to come to terms with it if they are going to be able to care for themselves following discharge. They now have their bowel opening onto their skin (see Fig. 22.7) and have to go to the toilet in a different way. They may no longer see themselves as normal and may live with the constant worry that they smell. They have to learn how to change and drain their appliances and how to care for their stoma and the surrounding skin. They will need to learn about how their diet can affect the stoma and its contents. Some patients will find this hard to deal with, so it is important that nurses recognize this and offer good psychological support and approach them in a sensitive and tactful way to build a therapeutic relationship. Whilst it may be hard to deal with the emotional distress of patients and their family members, by being supportive, nurses can help patients come to terms with the situation and help to prepare them for the future. By being there for

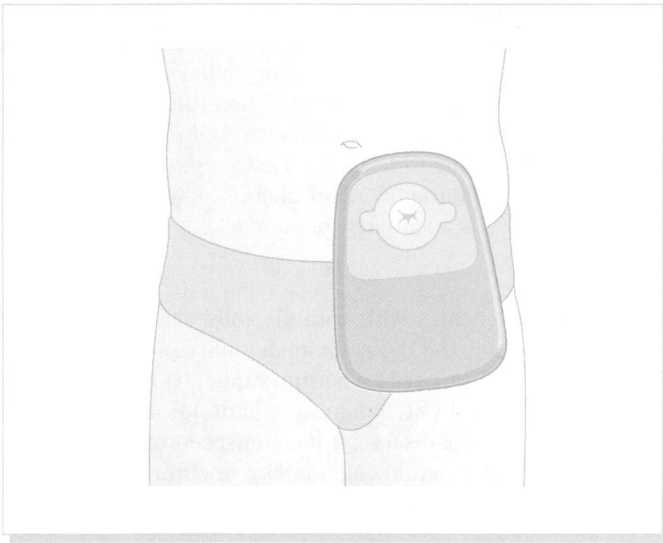

Figure 22.7 Patient with a stoma bag.

patients, listening to and acknowledging their fears, offering good clear explanations and building up trust, and simply by showing they care, nurses can clearly make a difference to the patient experience.

Discharge preparation

By discharge, patients should be able to:

- prepare the equipment required prior to an appliance change
- remove and attach the clip at the bottom of a bag or other mechanism for emptying the bag
- empty a bag safely and into an appropriate receptacle
- remove a bag/wafer from the skin
- clean and dry the stoma and surrounding skin
- measure the stoma to ensure the correct size of appliance is used
- correctly fit a new appliance
- dispose of soiled bags safely
- use accessories confidently
- observe the stoma for complications.

INFLAMMATORY BOWEL DISEASE

Inflammatory bowel disease comprises two major chronic conditions: ulcerative colitis and Crohn's disease. Despite extensive research, the aetiology remains obscure, although various theories have been proposed. The peak age of onset of both diseases occurs in the 20–40 year age group. Women appear to be affected more than men (Lam & Lombard 1999). There appears to be a genetic link to these disorders and, in the UK, both occur at a higher rate in the Jewish community than in the indigenous population. Initially, Crohn's disease affected mainly the white population, but it is becoming more common in Asian immigrants to the UK. The incidence in the Europe and the USA is as follows (Kamm 1996):

- ulcerative colitis – 1 in 1000
- Crohn's disease – 1 in 1500.

The prevalence of both disorders (i.e. the number of people affected in a population at any given time) is as follows:

- ulcerative colitis – 160 per 100 000
- Crohn's disease – 50 per 100 000.

Ulcerative colitis

Ulcerative colitis is a chronic inflammatory disorder that mainly affects the large bowel, although in some cases the distal part of the terminal ileum can be affected (backwash ileitis). Ulcerative colitis is characterized by widespread superficial ulceration and usually extends proximally from the rectum in a continuous fashion. It is a disease characterized by relapses and remissions.

Crohn's disease

Crohn's disease is a chronic, progressive, granulomatous inflammatory disorder. Unlike ulcerative colitis, Crohn's disease can affect any part of the GI tract from the mouth to the anus. There is no pattern to diseased areas and they are generally not continuous. The inflammation may involve the entire thickness of the bowel wall, leading to severe ulceration and the formation of fistulae.

Aetiology

The causes of ulcerative colitis and Crohn's disease are unknown, but there are several theories, which can be linked to both disorders.

Infective causes

Infective causes have been suspected as some patients present with IBD after an episode of gastroenteritis. Hydrogen sulphide, a product of sulphate-reducing bacteria, has been implicated in the development of ulcerative colitis (Forbes 2002). The measles virus has also been linked with the development of Crohn's disease (Thompson 1995). Mycobacteria (microorganisms resembling the tuberculosis bacillus) have also been considered as a cause, as this organism is known to cause a similar disease in animals (Johne's disease). However, whilst bacterial and viral infections have been linked to ulcerative colitis, the link is as yet unproven (Farthing 1993).

Smoking

This is known to provide some protection against ulcerative colitis (Forbes 2002), but increases the incidence of Crohn's disease (Pullan 1996).

Genetic predisposition

In patients with ulcerative colitis, the chances of a sibling, parent or child also having the condition is between 1 in 15 and 1 in 10, which is about 50 times the risk of the general population. Identical twins of a patient with Crohn's disease have a 50% chance of developing the disease themselves.

Diet

Some patients have had success with dietary changes, such as the exclusion of dairy products in ulcerative colitis. In Crohn's disease, elemental feeds (liquid feed with all the nutrients needed in a 'pre-digested' form and thus absorbed through the small intestine) may be used. An elemental diet has been shown to bring about symptomatic relief while simultaneously addressing the often compromised nutritional state of many patients (Wight & Scott 1997).

Clinical presentation

Ulcerative colitis

This is an idiopathic recurrent inflammatory disease that affects the mucosa of the large bowel and rectum. It affects women more than men and is most common between the ages of 20 and 40, although it can occur at any age. It manifests as swelling, inflammation and ulceration of the mucosa, which leads to diarrhoea with the presence of mucus and blood and associated urgency. Outside the tropics it is the commonest cause of bloody diarrhoea (Hope et al 1999). The ulceration usually starts in the rectum and extends proximally toward the small intestine in a continuous fashion. However, in approximately 50% of patients, the disease will remain in the rectum (Brian & Ferguson 1993). On endoscopic examination (sigmoidoscopy), the bowel is red, the mucosa raw and inflammatory pseudo-polyps may be seen.

Systemic problems associated with ulcerative colitis include arthritis, ankylosing spondylitis (stiffness and loss of spinal movement), erythema nodosum (painful swellings, particularly on the shins) and pyoderma gangrenosum (painful ulcers). In the long term, patients may experience problems with liver abnormalities and sclerosing cholangitis (fibrosing inflammation of bile ducts). There is also an increased risk of developing colonic cancer after 8–10 years as ulcerative colitis is premalignant and approximately 2% of patients will develop colorectal cancer.

Crohn's disease

Crohn's disease occurs most commonly in the ileocaecal region, but can occur anywhere from the mouth to the anus. It is transmural inflammation (i.e. affects the full thickness of the intestinal wall), causing thickening and narrowing of the lumen, which can have an adverse effect on the passage of chyme along the gastrointestinal tract. Unlike ulcerative colitis, the progression of Crohn's disease is not uniform along the bowel; instead it skips from place to place, giving rise to so-called 'skip lesions', areas of diseased bowel with healthy areas in between. The clinical features of Crohn's disease can be non-specific and vary according to the area of bowel affected; however, the following symptoms are common:

■ diarrhoea and bleeding, although bleeding is less common than in ulcerative colitis
■ cramping abdominal pain
■ subacute GI obstruction
■ anorexia and weight loss
■ fever
■ anal and perianal lesions (skin tags, abscesses and fistulas)
■ slowed growth in children.

Specific investigations

Blood tests

Serum albumin is low in severe disease because of the lack of good nutrition. Erythrocyte sedimentation rate (ESR) is raised when inflammation is present and is indicative of active disease. However, the C-reactive protein (CRP) test is probably a better test, as CRP is an acute-phase protein and correlates with inflammatory activity. A full blood count may show a low haemoglobin, which can result from either a large or chronic blood loss.

Endoscopic investigations

A rigid or flexible sigmoidoscopy allows visualization of the rectum and sigmoid colon. A colonoscopy allows visualization of the whole colon and terminal ileum. The other benefit of this form of investigation is that it allows the endoscopist to obtain biopsies, which can aid in reaching a diagnosis. To enable effective visualization and the taking of biopsies, it is important that the patient's bowel is adequately prepared.

X-ray

Double-contrast enemas with both air and barium are used to assess the extent of the disease. Good-quality plain abdominal X-rays may reduce the need for barium studies (Hope et al 1999). Computed tomography (CT) scanning is useful in determining the progression of the disease; it has now been used with computers to generate a virtual colonoscopy, and in the future may reduce the need for colonoscopy.

Microbiology

The collection of stool samples can help rule out the presence of an intestinal infection and they can also rule out antibiotic-associated colitis (pseudomembranous colitis), which is caused by colonization of the colon by *Clostridium difficile* bacteria.

Medical/surgical management

As the aetiology of IBD is unknown, treatment is centred on symptom control and is dependent on the severity of the episode. The aim is to bring about a remission in the disease and to maintain this as long as possible. Corticosteroids (prednisolone) form the backbone of treatment in acute episodes, as they help control the inflammation in the bowel. They provide rapid and effective relief in acute exacerbations but are ineffective in maintaining remission and have long-term side-effects such as adrenal suppression, osteoporosis and Cushing's syndrome. Corticosteroids can be given intravenously, orally or rectally. When patients achieve remission, they can be maintained on medications such as the 5-ASA drugs (sulphasalazine, mesalazine), which are drugs from the aminosalicylates group. Aminosalicylates have been in use since the 1950s and have been effective in reducing the relapse rate in ulcerative colitis from 70 to around 25% (Forbes 2002). However, there is a risk of renal toxicity when taking these drugs, which can lead to renal failure; patients should have their renal function checked at least every 6 months. Immunosuppressant drugs (e.g. azathioprine) have been found to be useful in patients with chronic symptoms and allow the use of steroids to be reduced. However, azathioprine can cause bone marrow suppression and it is therefore important that patients' white blood cell count is monitored every 4–6 weeks.

Mild to moderate exacerbations of ulcerative colitis can be treated with oral medication without hospital admission. With severe attacks, hospital admission is usually required for the administration of intravenous fluids and corticosteroids. This allows the close observation of patients, because of the risk of toxic megacolon (extreme dilation of the large intestine) and perforation in severe illness; a blood transfusion may also be needed if patients are anaemic. Local disease of the rectum and sigmoid colon can often be managed by topical therapy of 5-ASA drugs and steroids in the form of suppositories or foam enemas.

Crohn's disease is treated with the same medications as ulcerative colitis, but it is more difficult to control due to the diversity of symptoms. Patients with acute episodes of Crohn's will require a full nutritional assessment (see Ch. 11), as they are prone to weight loss because of poor appetite and reduced food intake. Dietary supplements such as elemental diet, nasogastric feeding or total parenteral nutrition may be the most appropriate way of ensuring adequate nutrition.

If patients do not respond well to medical management or if complications develop, surgery will need to be considered. Approximately 20–30% of patients with ulcerative colitis will require surgery within the first 5 years of diagnosis. A panproctocolectomy, which involves the removal of the anus, rectum and colon with the formation of an ileostomy, is performed. However, there is a risk that patients will develop bladder and sexual difficulties due to nerve damage. Alternatively the terminal ileum can be used to create an ileal pouch, which is then joined to the rectum. At least half of all patients with Crohn's will need surgical intervention during the first 10 years of the disease; however, due to the nature of Crohn's, a panproctocolectomy will not cure the problem.

▶ Nursing management

Despite the symptoms, relapses and remissions, most patients with ulcerative colitis and Crohn's disease will lead a full and active life. Patients will only be admitted to hospital when either long-term medical management has not been successful or an acute exacerbation has not settled down following a course of treatment. There is little doubt that chronic conditions such as IBD have deep and long-term implications for sufferers. However, sound nursing intervention is key to reducing its impact and coordinating care. Nurses are ideally placed to pre-empt and address the multitude of physical and psychological issues that form such a large part of these conditions. Nursing management needs to address the following areas.

Bowel function

Because of the nature of ulcerative colitis and Crohn's disease, patients experience frequent, loose bowel movements, often with the presence of blood and mucus, up to 20 times a day. This is often accompanied by abdominal pain and cramp, and is exacerbated by eating and drinking. Therefore patients may avoid eating as they feel this causes more problems. Patients in hospital should be given a bed near a toilet, ideally in a side room or quiet area of the ward as this will afford them some privacy. By being aware of what patients are experiencing, nurses can promote the benefit of rest to them in order to maximize their recovery. Observation of patients is important and a stool chart should be used to note the amount and frequency of bowel actions. Note the consistency and the presence of blood or mucus as this provides an indication of the extent of inflammation, and whether it is worsening or improving. A stool sample should be obtained to eliminate the possibility of infection.

Patients should be advised on good perianal care. The perianal area is prone to excoriation which can lead to skin breakdown and infection because mucus can leak from the bowel onto the skin, causing severe itching and scratching. Patients should be advised to clean the area with soap and water and to pat it dry to avoid damaging the skin. Some patients find moist toilet tissue or baby wipes useful. In patients who develop sore bottoms, the use of a barrier cream may prove helpful. Patients may need to go to the toilet several times a day and some may worry that they will not get there in time and soil themselves. These patients may prefer to wear an incontinence pad as a precaution against accidents. However, patients who decide to wear pads may also worry about the possibility of odour and whilst it is easy to provide air fresheners and open windows, by providing reassurance you can enhance their self-worth.

Another major bowel problem is abdominal pain and cramps. Antispasmodic medication [e.g. dicyclomine hydrochloride or hyoscine butylbromide (Buscopan)] should be administered as prescribed and patients observed for complications and side-effects such as palpitations, tachycardia and arrhythmias. Patients should not be given anti-diarrhoeal medication during an acute exacerbation, as worsening symptoms or complications may be masked.

Nursing observation

Both ulcerative colitis and Crohn's disease may lead to complications, and therefore observation of patients is important. By observing their temperature, pulse and blood pressure, as well as assessing the level of abdominal tenderness, nurses will be in a good position to recognize the first signs of colonic dilatation, perforation and toxic megacolon. Diarrhoea can result in fluid and electrolyte loss, causing patients to become dehydrated, and an accurately maintained fluid balance chart will assist in determining the need for replacement fluids. Alongside this, it is important to observe for the signs and symptoms of electrolyte imbalance, including hypokalaemia, characterized by muscle weakness and cramp, and hypernatraemia, which presents as a tachycardia and pyrexia. With both conditions, there is a risk of bleeding, although this may be worse in ulcerative colitis. Blood samples should be taken regularly to check the full blood count and nurses should observe for signs of prolonged bleeding – lethargy, tiredness, breathlessness and pale mucosa – which all indicate a drop in iron levels.

Nutritional support

During an acute exacerbation, patients may be disinclined to eat, due to a loss of appetite (anorexia) and/or a fear that to do so may precipitate unwanted bowel movements. Assessment is the key when managing patients with nutritional problems. This should embrace subjective, objective and biochemical methods. Visual observation of patients will reveal whether their clothes fit, whether they look tired, pale or thin. Other methods and tests, such as skin fold thickness and body mass index (BMI), can also prove useful (see Ch. 11). Weight should be monitored at least twice weekly.

Patients should be questioned about their normal diet, and friends and relatives may also provide information. They should be encouraged to eat small, regular meals; nutritional supplements are very useful (milk-based ones should always be served cold). In some cases patients may require nasogastric feeding, which should be performed in consultation with a dietician and the medical team. In patients who require complete rest of the GI tract, total parenteral nutrition may be the best option to improve their nutritional status (see Ch. 11).

Body image and self-esteem

As a nation we in the UK do not talk about our bowels. We do not talk about going to the toilet and tend to keep our bowels private. We also spend a great deal of money trying to make ourselves smell and look nice, as well as having an ideal image of ourselves. When faced with problems that result in us losing our privacy, or problems that affect the way we look, such as a loss of weight along with the indignity of diarrhoea, our self-esteem and body image can suffer an almighty blow. Patients with IBD have to face not only the effects of the illness but also the effects of the medications they are required to take. The corticosteroids can cause weight gain and the characteristic 'moon face' of Cushing's syndrome and this can have an adverse effect on self-esteem. Patients also face the possibility of surgery and stoma formation. This has major implications for body image. Patients may no longer see themselves as 'normal' and they face the prospect of caring for their stoma site for the rest of their lives (see Reflective Practice box 22.2).

By its very nature, IBD can affect people's working lives and may require a person to give up work. This has implications not only financially but also for a person's self-worth. By listening, providing support and allowing patients time to express their fears and anxieties, nurses can help them to adjust to these changes in their lifestyle. Nurses are also in a very good position to refer patients for further help and support. When caring for a sick person, there is a tendency to focus on that person alone; however, these diseases also affect families and it is important to consider them as well. Relationships can be affected and some people become depressed. No two people will react in the same way and responses range from full acceptance to actively avoiding people, even those who were once very close. Although having IBD is not a direct reason to avoid an active sex life, patients often have trouble starting or continuing relationships. The prospect of faecal soiling, urgency, noise and odour can frighten so many people that they avoid close sexual contact. Good care and recognizing the importance of other heath care professionals (sexual counsellors, stoma care nurses) should address these issues, by offering practical advice that is appropriate to the situation.

Work and social implications of IBD

A person's ability to hold down a job may be reduced due to the fact that the illness may require frequent time off for outpatient appointments or hospital admissions. For those still in school or university, there is a risk that they will fall behind. Some patients confine themselves to their home and are afraid to leave the house in case they need the toilet. This can have terrible effects on their ability to work or socialize. Normal social activities such as going to dinner can be fraught with problems and patients often need to cancel at short notice, which can lead to them being considered unreliable.

PSEUDOMEMBRANOUS COLITIS

This is an infectious colitis that occurs as a side-effect to the use of antibiotics. If patients receive prolonged courses of antibiotics, there is a risk that the normal bacteria that colonize the bowel can be wiped out, allowing the overgrowth of *Clostridium difficile*. This Gram-positive anaerobic bacterium causes a severe colitis, producing diarrhoea, abdominal pain, cramps, tenderness and fever. Stools may contain blood, mucus and pus, and if left untreated, toxic megacolon and death can occur. Generally found in hospitalized patients and passed on by poor hand hygiene, pseudomembranous colitis is treated by intravenous antibiotics, such as metronidazole or vancomycin, and source isolation. As a result of this, inflammation will usually abate within 3–5 days.

ANORECTAL DISORDERS

Anorectal problems include pruritus ani, anal fissures, haemorrhoids, fistulae, pilonidal sinuses, abscesses, rectal prolapse, rectal ulcers, skin tags and anal cancer. These are distressing for patients because they cause pain and embarrassment, and in some cases patients are reluctant to seek professional help. However, many of these conditions are ultimately treatable and so it is important that patients are investigated in order to determine the cause and extent of the problem.

PRURITUS ANI

This is an itching sensation felt around the anus. It can be caused by a worm infestation, e.g. threadworm, or anxiety. It can also be caused by poor hygiene or wearing tight underwear. Sometimes it is caused by mucus from the bowel, which acts as an irritant when it comes into contact with the skin. The presence of anal fissures, incontinence, IBD, fistulae, dermatoses, lichen sclerosis and contact dermatitis (see Ch. 28) will also cause this embarrassing problem.

R|Я REFLECTIVE PRACTICE

22.2 Coming to terms with a stoma

Joan is a 28-year-old woman who has had ulcerative colitis for 18 months. She has recently undergone an emergency colectomy with formation of an ileostomy, as she had developed toxic megacolon. You have been asked by the nurse in charge to keep a close eye on her as Joan is very upset to find that she now has a stoma.

Student activities

- What reactions would you expect in a patient who had undergone surgery that had implications for their body image?
- Why is it important to provide psychological support for patients with stomas?
- If Joan did become depressed or agitated, what do you think might help her?
- Think back to other patients that you may have nursed with a stoma – what interventions did they receive?

Medical/surgical management

Patients should be advised to clean themselves thoroughly after going to the toilet; moist wipes have proved very useful in some cases. They should also be advised to avoid spicy foods and to wear loose clothing. If the problem persists, anaesthetic cream may be helpful. If the itching is caused by a specific problem, it is important to treat the cause.

ANAL FISSURE

This is also referred to as 'fissure in ano', which is a tear in the squamous lining of the lower anal canal which causes the patient pain on defecation. In chronic problems, a mucosal tag, known as a sentinel pile, may be noted at the external aspect of the anus. Fissures are usually caused by the passage of hard stool but they can also be caused by syphilis, Crohn's disease, trauma and anal cancer. Patients usually present with a history of pain and rectal bleeding on defecation.

Medical/surgical management

Dietary changes are helpful; patients should be advised to eat a diet high in fibre. The application of local anaesthetic ointment can reduce pain.

HAEMORRHOIDS

Haemorrhoids are anal cushions of vascular tissue that drain into the superior rectal vein. They become dilated and congested because of straining during defecation. They can also occur in pregnancy due to the fact that venous return is delayed because of the pressure exerted by the uterus. Patients usually complain of bleeding from the rectum after opening their bowels, or blood may be seen on the toilet paper after wiping.

ANAL FISTULAE

An anal fistula is an abnormal link between two epithelial surfaces. The cause is still unclear, but there is a strong link to infection of the anal glands, which in turn causes an abscess (cavity containing pus) to form. In Crohn's disease, abscess formation is thought to be due to leakage in the bowel wall, which forms an inflammatory mass. The abscess then causes a track to develop between the two surfaces. The formation of fistulae is linked to the diseases IBD and HIV. Patients will usually present with rectal discharge and skin excoriation and will complain of pain.

Medical/surgical management

It is important to replace any fluid and electrolytes lost. Parenteral nutrition has been found to be helpful, and if surgical intervention is considered, the tract is laid open to allow healing by granulation. Healing usually occurs within 2 weeks.

PILONIDAL SINUS

A pilonidal sinus is a blind ending tract that occurs in the nasal cleft. It is caused by hair at the base of the spine that curls and punctures the skin, causing a foreign body reaction to occur. The opening becomes invaded by bacteria, which cause an abscess to form. Patients will usually complain of pain and they usually note the presence of a foul-smelling discharge.

Medical/surgical management

If infection is present, patients are treated with intravenous antibiotics and the sinus is laid open to allow healing to occur.

PERIANAL ABSCESS

An abscess is a cavity that contains pus and occurs when organisms invade the mucosal wall following a breach or tear. The abscess can then track inferiorly to the perianal region or laterally to the ischiorectal fossae. This causes a great deal of discomfort. Patients will have a fever and complain of throbbing pain and swelling. On inspection, the anal region will appear red, tender and inflamed.

Medical/surgical management

The abscess will be incised and drained and swabs are taken to determine whether the organisms are from the skin or from the bowel. Bacteria from the bowel usually indicate the presence of a fistula, whereas skin flora indicates a skin infection.

RECTAL PROLAPSE

In people with a lax anal sphincter or those who constantly strain during defecation, there is a risk that the rectum may descend through the anus. This is caused by chronic constipation and multiparity (multiple births) in women, as childbirth can damage the pudendal nerves, causing weakness in the sphincters. Patients complain of discomfort, rectal bleeding, incontinence and mucus discharge.

Medical/surgical management

Surgery is the preferred treatment. If patients are fit enough, a laparotomy is performed and the rectum is lifted and secured to the hollow of the sacrum with mesh.

SKIN TAGS

These small growths of skin are also called sentinel piles and occur due to oedema of the skin and fibrosis. They seldom cause trouble and are easily excised. They are associated with anal fissures, and multiple skin tags are associated with Crohn's disease. Treatment is by surgical excision.

ANAL CANCER

This is a rare carcinoma that usually occurs in the elderly, but it is also known to affect young homosexuals as the risk increases in the presence of syphilis and anal warts (human papilloma virus). It is usually a squamous cell carcinoma and originates in the mucosa of the lower anal canal. Patients may present with bleeding, pain, change in bowel habit, discharge, pruritus ani, stricture formation and inguinal lymphadenopathy (lymph nodes in the groin that are hard and knotty).

Medical/surgical management

A biopsy is taken to confirm diagnosis. Patients require radiotherapy and chemotherapy, and in some cases an anorectal excision is performed with the formation of a colostomy.

SUMMARY: MAIN POINTS

- Patients with GI disease face physiological, pathological, psychological, sociological and cultural problems that need to be addressed by good nursing care.

- Gastrointestinal disease can have a major impact on patients and their families.

- Anyone who complains of an altered bowel habit or rectal bleeding should be investigated, as this might be a sign of colorectal cancer.

- Colorectal cancer is the second most common cause of cancer deaths in the UK.

- Constipation in hospital can largely be prevented by good nursing care.

- A stoma specialist nurse provides support for patients and specialist advice for nurses on the care of patients with stomas.

- Crohn's disease and ulcerative colitis can have a significant impact on a person's lifestyle.

SELF-TEST: CRITICAL THINKING ACTIVITIES

1 What can you do to prevent constipation in hospital?

2 What observations are needed for patients with acute abdominal pain, and why?

3 Why is it important to care for a patient's mouth if he or she is taking nothing orally?

 FURTHER READING

Cheshire E. Gastrointestinal system – Mosby's crash course. London: Mosby; 1998.

Haslett C, Chilvers ER, Boon NA, Colledge NR, Hunter JAA. Davidson's principles and practice of medicine, 19th edn. Edinburgh: Churchill Livingstone; 2002.

Middleton SJ, Hunter JO. Therapeutic aspects of nutrition in Crohn's disease. J Irish Coll Phys Surg 1995; 24(1).

Williams J (ed). The essentials of pouch care nursing. London: Whurr; 2002.

Rose JDR, Roberts GM, Williams G, Mayberry JF, Rhodes J. Cardiff Crohn's disease jubilee: the incidence over 50 years. Gut 1988: 29: 346–351.

 USEFUL ADDRESSES

National Association for Colitis and Crohn's Disease (NACC)
98A London Road
St Albans
Hertfordshire AL1 1NY
Tel: 01727 844296
www.nacc.org.uk

British Colostomy Association
15 Station Road
Reading
Berkshire RG11 1LG
Tel: 0118 939 1537
www.bcass.org.uk

Ileostomy Association
Amblehurst
Blackscotch lane
Mansfield
Notts NG18 4PF

Macmillan Cancer Relief
Anchor House
15/19 Britten Street
London SW3 3TZ

Colon Cancer Concern
4 Rickett Street
London SW6 1RU
Tel: 020 7381 4711
www.coloncancer.org.uk

British Digestive Foundation
3 St Andrews Place
London NW1 4LB

USEFUL WEBSITE

www. nice.org.uk – National Institute for Clinical Excellence

REFERENCES

Barkauskas V, Stoltenberg-Allen K, Baumann L, Darling-Fisher C. Health and physical assessment. St Louis: CV Mosby; 1994.

Beck S, Yasko JM. Guidelines for oral care. Crystal Lake: Sago; 1993.

Brian H, Ferguson A. Inflammatory bowel disease. Pract Nurs 1993; 15: 11–12.

Department of Health. The essence of care patient-focused benchmarking for health care practitioners. London: DoH; 2001.

Eilers J, Berger AM, Petersen MC. Development, testing and application of the oral assessment guide. Oncol Nurs Forum 1988; 15: 325–330.

Farthing M. Medical management of Crohn's disease and ulcerative colitis. In: Myers C, ed. Stoma care nursing: a patient centred approach. London: Arnold; 1993, pp. 42–62.

Forbes A. Medical aspects of ulcerative colitis. In: Williams J, ed. The essentials of pouch care nursing. London: Whurr; 2002.

Galovski TE, Blanchard EB. Hypnotherapy and refractory irritable bowel syndrome: a single case study. Am J Clin Hypnosis 2002; 45(1): 31–37.

Hope RA, Longmore JM, Hodgetts TJ, Ramrakha PS. Oxford handbook of clinical medicine, 4th edn. Oxford: Oxford University Press; 1999.

Hungin P, Rubin G (eds). Gastroenterology in primary care: an evidence-based guide to management. Oxford: Blackwell Science; 2000.

Kamm M. Inflammatory bowel disease. London: Martin Dunitz; 1996.

Kumar P, Clark M. Clinical medicine, 4th edn. Edinburgh: Saunders; 2002.

Lam E, Lombard M. Gastroenterology. London: CV Mosby; 1999.

Odelowo OO, Smoot DT, Kim K. Upper gastrointestinal bleeding in patients with liver cirrhosis. J Natl Med Assoc 2002; 94(8): 712–715.

Porrett T, Daniel N (eds). Essential coloproctology. London: Whurr; 1999.

Pullan R. Colonic mucus, smoking and ulcerative colitis. Ann Roy Coll Surg England 1996; 78: 85–91.

Schoetz DJ. Uncomplicated diverticulitis. In: Wolf BG, ed. Surgical clinics of North America. Philadelphia: WB Saunders; 1993.

Sher ME, Cheney L, Ricciardi J. Diverticular disease. In: Porrett T, Daniel N, eds. Essential coloproctology for nurses. London: Whurr; 1999.

Swartz M. Textbook of physical diagnosis, history and examination, 2nd edn. Philadelphia: WB Saunders; 1995.

Sweetland H, Cook J. Surgery: Mosby's crash course. London: Mosby; 1999.

Thompson NP. Is measles a risk for inflammatory bowel disease? Lancet 1995; 345: 1071–1073.

Tibble JA, Sigthorsson G, Bjarnason I. Prediction of relapse in IBD using faecal calprotectin and small intestinal permeability. Gut 1999; 44(suppl 1): A35.

Wight N, Scott BB. Dietary treatment of active Crohn's disease. Br Med J 1997; 314.

23 Nursing patients with hepatic, biliary and pancreatic disorders

Liz Williamson

'Deep down I knew I was drinking too much. Now they tell me they think my liver is in trouble and I have to have some investigations. I almost didn't tell them the truth about how much I drink – I thought they'd say it was all my own fault. But when I did tell them, they were really understanding and supportive and said they can put me in touch with people who can help that sort of thing.'

(Patient)

THIS CHAPTER WILL HELP YOU

- Describe the anatomy, physiology and functions of the liver, gallbladder and pancreas and their role in metabolism, digestion and energy balance of the body in health

- Explain the basis for the nursing assessment information which must be collected to identify patient problems

- Describe in simple terms the various diagnostic tests that patients may undergo

- Describe the pathophysiological basis for the clinical presentations seen

- Identify the opportunities for health promotion with regard to liver, gallbladder and pancreatic function

- Anticipate the nursing care needs for patients with disorders of the liver, gallbladder and pancreas

- Assist patients in understanding their illness and the long-term/lifestyle adaptations they may need to make.

KEYWORDS

Abdominal ascites	ERCP
Acute liver failure (ALF)	Gallstones
Bile	Hepatitis
Biliary colic	Jaundice
Bilirubin	Oesophageal varices
Biliverdin	Laparoscopic cholecystectomy
Cholangiography	
Cholecystectomy	Liver function tests
Cholecystitis	Pancreatitis
Cholecystogram	Paracentesis
Cholelithiasis	Portal hypertension
Cirrhosis	Pruritus
Encephalopathy	Whipple's procedure

INTRODUCTION

The liver, gallbladder and pancreas (see Fig. 23.1) are considered the accessory organs of digestion. When an alteration occurs with the normal function of any of these organs, not only is digestion affected but many other systems too. The impact on patients can range from relatively mild (e.g. hepatitis A) to life-threatening (e.g. liver failure, acute pancreatitis). Many of the conditions are chronic and may require patients to make

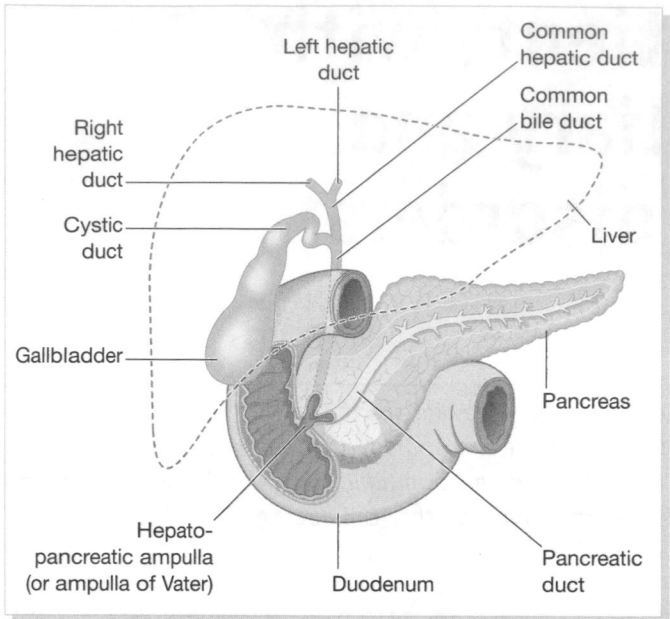

Figure 23.1 Anatomy of the liver, gallbladder and pancreas.

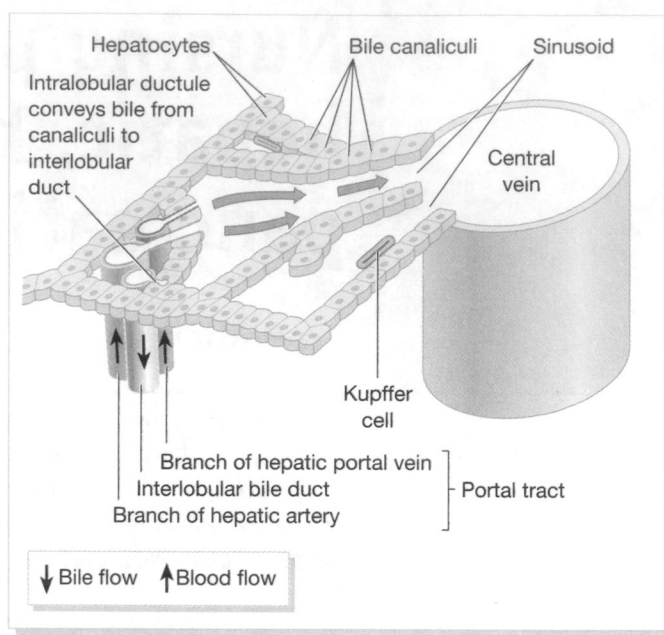

Figure 23.2 Cellular structure of the liver with blood and bile flow.

modifications to their lifestyle over many years. Many public and individual health issues are raised, such as alcohol misuse, blood-borne infections and environmental pollution. The nurse working in the hospital or community setting needs to be able to explain investigations, treatments, diagnoses and prognoses, and to follow up any information given by medical colleagues. The nursing care required can range from the simple, such as teaching a client about a special diet, to the highly complex, such as intensive care monitoring.

ANATOMY AND PHYSIOLOGY OF THE LIVER

The liver is a remarkable organ, playing a vital role in the body's metabolism through the synthesis, processing and/or storage of many of the substances that are essential for normal body functioning. It is the largest gland and solid organ in the body and is situated within the ribcage in the right upper quadrant of the abdomen (see Fig. 23.1). Functionally, it is divided into two parts (left and right) and then subdivided into eight sectors, each with its own blood supply.

The liver is a highly vascular organ, receiving approximately 28% of the body's total blood flow. It receives its blood supply from two sources: the hepatic artery, which delivers oxygenated arterial blood from the aorta; and the hepatic portal vein, carrying partly deoxygenated blood from the stomach, intestines, spleen and pancreas. Blood leaves the liver via the hepatic vein. This dual blood flow ensures that the liver is able to play its key role in metabolism and synthesis of vital substances (see below). The pressure in the hepatic portal vein is normally low (5–10 mmHg), but if there is an obstruction in the liver, portal pressure rises, leading to portal hypertension.

Each sector is subdivided into lobules which are microscopic hexagonal units made up of columns of liver cells called hepatocytes. These are separated by numerous blood vessels and fibrous strands. Each lobule contains a central venule, surrounded by branches of the hepatic artery, hepatic portal vein and bile duct (together known as the 'portal triad') (see Fig. 23.2).

Surrounding the hepatocytes (within the cell membrane) is a network of minute tubules called bile canaliculi, which secrete bile. The lobular bile ducts unite to form the hepatic duct, which joins the cystic duct to form the common bile duct. The blood vessels between the cells are lined with phagocytic cells called Kupffer cells that play a vital role in phagocytosis and antibody production.

FUNCTIONS OF THE LIVER

The liver has a unique spectrum of functions and any abnormality has a great impact on every other system of the body.

Bile production

One of the main functions of the liver is the production of bile, an alkaline fluid, yellow-green or brown in colour. Its main role is in the emulsification of fats and absorption of lipids and fat-soluble vitamins (such as vitamin K) and iron. Bile also has a deodorizing effect on faeces. Without bile salts, around 25–50% of ingested fat would be lost, resulting in a bulky, greasy and offensive stool (steatorrhoea).

Bile pigments are formed as a result of the breakdown of red blood cells and food. These pigments (bilirubin and biliverdin), which give bile its characteristic colour, are reduced to urobilinogen in the intestine through the action of bacteria. Some is excreted in the faeces (as stercobilinogen), giving it the characteristic brown colour. The remainder is absorbed by the terminal ileum, passes to the liver and is re-excreted into the bile.

Metabolic functions

The liver plays a vital role in the metabolism of carbohydrates, proteins and fats and is central to blood glucose homeostasis (see

Ch. 11). During periods of fasting, the liver is able to synthesize glucose from amino acids and lactate, and from fructose and galactose. It also breaks down fatty acids into ketones and acetates. Cholesterol is synthesized by the liver and used for the synthesis of several hormones and in the production of bile. Proteins are deaminated so that the amino acids can be used for energy production and the excess ammonia produced is converted to urea and excreted by the kidneys.

Storage of energy
The liver stores energy (mostly in the form of glycogen) and small amounts of proteins, fats, cholesterol, copper and iron, as well as vitamins A, B_{12}, D, E, K and folic acid. Amino acids derived from digestion are stored and reconstructed into body proteins.

Synthesis of blood components
Plasma proteins, mostly albumin, are synthesized by the liver and serve as part of osmotic regulation. All the clotting factors, apart from factor VIII, are synthesized in the liver, some of which require vitamin K for their synthesis (see Ch. 18). The liver is also able to make red blood cells when demand exceeds supply (a function usually only carried out in the fetal liver).

Destruction of erythrocytes
The Kupffer cells break down worn-out erythrocytes by splitting the iron and globin and releasing the haem. One of the by-products is bilirubin, which is then excreted in bile.

Detoxification
Many drugs and chemicals are metabolized by the liver, to render them harmless before being excreted by the kidneys. For example, the enzyme glutathione binds to paracetamol, converting it from a potentially harmful, fat-soluble substance to a water-soluble substance which can be excreted by the kidneys. It also detoxifies alcohol into energy, carbon dioxide and water. The liver is the principal site of hormone deactivation, including insulin, glucagon, cortisol, progesterone, testosterone and antidiuretic hormone (ADH) which is vital for the body's self-regulation system.

Heat production
Under resting conditions, the liver is responsible for producing most of the body heat; only the muscles produce more.

THE BILIARY SYSTEM
The gallbladder is a pear-shaped sac situated on the underside of the liver (see Fig. 23.1). It is 9–10 cm in length, has musculo-elastic walls and a capacity of approximately 50 mL. The internal surface consists of rugae, folds of tissue which greatly increase the surface area to promote the absorption of water.

The cystic duct arises from the neck of the gallbladder and joins the hepatic duct to form the common bile duct. This unites with the pancreatic duct to form the hepatopancreatic ampulla (or ampulla of Vater), which opens into the duodenum through the hepatopancreatic sphincter (sphincter of Oddi).

Bile concentration and storage
Bile secreted by the liver accumulates in the gallbladder where it is concentrated by absorption of water and electrolytes.

Following a meal, duodenal cells secrete a hormone called cholecystokinin-pancreazymin (CCK). CCK stimulates the smooth muscle within the wall of the gallbladder to contract and relaxes the hepatopancreatic sphincter, allowing bile to flow into the duodenum.

THE PANCREAS
The pancreas is a soft, yellowish, 'fish-shaped' gland, 12–15 cm long, which lies under the greater curvature of the stomach. It is divided into three sections: the head, body and tail. The main pancreatic duct joins with the common bile duct at the hepatopancreatic ampulla. For a full discussion of the endocrine function of the pancreas, see Chapter 17 – this chapter focuses on the exocrine function.

Exocrine cells secrete large amounts of digestive enzymes, water and electrolytes into a system of small ducts which run throughout the pancreas and drain into the main pancreatic duct. The main purpose of the pancreatic fluid is to continue the digestive process started in the stomach. The high bicarbonate level in the fluid (secreted by cells lining the pancreatic ducts) produces a pH of around 8 and this raises the pH of the stomach contents as they enter the duodenum to a level that will not damage the duodenal mucosa.

The enzymes produced are:

- lipases – to digest fats
- amylase – for carbohydrate digestion
- proteases – to reduce proteins to amino acids.

Amylase and lipase are both secreted in the active form; the proteases are released in inactive form as proenzymes, which are not activated until they reach the duodenum. This mechanism protects the pancreas from autodigestion which causes pancreatitis.

NURSING ASSESSMENT
Disorders affecting the liver, gallbladder and pancreas can have a significant effect on body function, and patient assessment needs to take into account a variety of factors, such as dietary habits and lifestyle, as well as changes to the physiological functions of many body systems. Many of the signs and symptoms of liver, gallbladder and pancreatic disorders are distressing and frightening. For example, jaundice (yellowing of the skin and sclera) is highly visible and may cause the patient great anxiety and embarrassment. It is vital during assessment to establish the impact the disorder is having on that particular patient. Also, a great number of diagnostic tests and examinations may be employed and the nurse should be able to explain these and their implications to the patient.

PATIENT HISTORY
During assessment, a wide range of information should be collected from patients and/or their carers, establishing where possible the time-frame of the development of signs and symptoms, to aid diagnosis and prognosis. Information should be gathered in the following areas.

Nutrition

Assessment should include the following:

- daily food intake, eating habits and any factors which affect eating
- specific likes and dislikes, food allergies or intolerances, especially to fats, as this may indicate a problem with bile production or flow
- cultural, religious and social factors that influence dietary intake and habits
- related symptoms, such as anorexia, nausea, vomiting, indigestion and recent changes in body weight
- food intake of nutrients, vitamins and calories
- fluid intake.

Elimination pattern

Determine the patient's usual bowel habits and any recent changes. Note the frequency, nature, form, colour and odour of the stool. Observe for the presence of steatorrhoea (bulky, offensive stools due to inability to digest fats) or clay-coloured stools (lack of urobilinogen). Also establish the volume, colour and frequency of urine and the pattern of voiding, including any nocturia.

Pain or discomfort

Establish with the patient:

- location, type and duration of pain
- any activities which worsen or relieve it
- prescribed or over-the-counter medications being used
- any non-pharmacological measures that help (e.g. sitting upright, curling up, etc.).

Reactions to pain are highly individual and influenced by cultural background. It is essential to understand a patient's pattern of pain expression for effective pain management.

Personal and social history

Determining patients' perception of their own health and the impact a condition is having on their life and work is a vital part of the nursing assessment. Ask patients and/or carers if there have been any episodes of irritability, depression or changes in mental status. Other aspects to consider are marital status, support systems, religious preferences, home conditions and socioeconomic background. This last factor is known to influence health and health promotion activities, with those of lower socioeconomic status engaging in fewer health promotion activities and under-utilizing all types of health care services. For example, there is a marked social class gradient for obesity, a known risk factor for gallbladder disease (Acheson 1998).

Culture and ethnicity

There are many indications of poorer health among the ethnic minority groups in the UK. For example, black people (Caribbean, African and other) and Indians have higher rates of illness than white people and those of Pakistani and Bangladeshi origin have the highest rates. In contrast, Chinese and other Asians have lower rates than the white population (Acheson 1998). Minority ethnic groups in the UK may include migrants from countries where the prevalence of hepatitis B virus carriers is high. When advising about diet and dietary adjustments, ethnic and cultural background must be considered, as food preferences may have emotional and cultural significance.

Activity and lifestyle

Ask the patient about:

- the type and extent of daily activities and any recent adaptations
- leisure time
- usual pattern and amount of sleep
- activities which may increase the risk of hepatitis, such as tattooing, i.v. drug use, ear piercing and recent overseas travel, particularly to developing countries
- alcohol consumption and substance/drug use (through careful questioning).

A great deal of tact and sensitivity is required when enquiring about alcohol consumption and/or drug use. A four-point system with the acronym CAGE has been developed to help assess alcohol intake (Bateson & Bouchier 1997). Affirmative answers to all four questions are strongly indicative of problem drinking; answering yes to two or three is suspicious:

- Have you ever tried to **C**ut down on your alcohol intake?
- Have you ever been **A**nnoyed at criticism of your drinking?
- Have you ever felt **G**uilty about the amount you drink?
- Do you ever have an **E**ye-opener drink to start the day?

Occupational and environmental history

This should include the identification of any factors at home or work which may be toxic to the individual, such as heavy metals (lead, mercury), pesticides and certain chemicals (e.g. carbon tetrachloride, previously used in the dry cleaning industry).

Past medical history and illnesses

Establish whether the patient has had any previous illnesses such as jaundice, gallstones, etc., surgery or trauma to the liver, gallbladder or pancreas, or a blood (or blood product) transfusion. It may be helpful to establish whether there is any family history of relevant illnesses or conditions.

PHYSICAL EXAMINATION

General appearance

Assess whether the patient appears distressed, in pain, tired and agitated or, alternatively, calm, comfortable, etc. Observe for any changes in posture or weight distribution (e.g. due to abdominal ascites) as well as observing the general condition and colour of the skin and sclera of the eyes.

Vital signs

Temperature, pulse, blood pressure and respiration rate should be recorded. Temperature may be affected by liver function and metabolism, as well as being a sign of infection. Respiratory rate may be affected by pain, as well as physiological disturbances associated with pancreatic disorders.

Height and weight

These should be recorded, including any recent changes in body weight, for future comparisons and drug and fluid calculations. The patient's body type should be assessed; obesity may accompany gallbladder disease and malnutrition may exist in patients with substance misuse or cirrhosis.

Skin

Note the temperature, colour and integrity of the skin. Record the presence of any non-healed lesions, tattoos or bruising, which may indicate a problem with blood coagulation. Decreased skin turgor (elasticity) may indicate impaired fluid balance as a result of nausea and vomiting (see Ch. 8), and yellowing of the skin may indicate jaundice. Observe for the presence of any rashes, scratch marks and itching, especially in the absence of any visible rashes.

Physical signs of disease of the liver, gallbladder or pancreas

These may include:

- pitting oedema (due to low albumin levels) – press your thumb over the dorsum of the foot for 5 seconds; when released, the indentation will remain

- abdominal ascites (a collection of fluid in the peritoneal cavity caused by portal hypertension) – there will be distension and asymmetry of the abdomen and umbilical protrusion
- discoloration around the umbilicus or flank, indicating pancreatic haemorrhage.

DIAGNOSTIC TESTS AND MEDICAL INVESTIGATIONS

LABORATORY TESTS

Blood tests

A great number of blood tests may be used in the diagnosis of liver, gallbladder and pancreatic disorders and Table 23.1 summarizes those commonly used. As there are no international standards for some tests, values vary between individual laboratories and it is vital to become familiar with locally agreed values.

Table 23.1 Common blood tests for disorders of the liver, gallbladder and pancreas

Blood test	Normal range	Interpretation
Bilirubin	2–17 μmol/L	Conjugated bilirubin increases with biliary obstruction Non-conjugated bilirubin increases with excessive erythrocyte haemolysis
Cholesterol	3.5–6.5 mmol/L	Elevate when secretion blocked by bile duct obstruction Reduced in severe liver damage
Amylase	< 220 U/L	Released from pancreatic acinar cells during autodigestion Raised 2–3 h after onset of acute pancreatitis but may return to normal after 48 h
Albumin	36–53 g/L	Decreased in chronic liver disease due to impaired protein synthesis
Ammonia	< 1 mg/L	Elevated when severe hepatocellular damage reduces the synthesis of urea from ammonia
Aspartate aminotransferase (AST) Alanine aminotransferase (ALT)	7–40 U/L 10–40 U/L	Released from damaged liver cells, heart, kidney and muscle cells; prolonged elevation in liver disease may be first indicator of chronic active hepatitis
Alkaline phosphatase (ALP)	25–115 U/L	Increased in biliary obstruction and liver disease (cirrhosis, metastases)
γ-glutamyl transferase (GGT)	Male 11–50 U/L Female 7–33 U/L	Elevation of GGT and ALP is a significant indication of liver disorders and bile duct disease; alcohol ingestion causes a rise in GGT
Blood glucose (fasting)	3.6–5.8 mmol/L	Increased following damage to islets of Langerhans and subsequent decrease in insulin production
Hepatitis viral studies	Negative	Used to identify known antigens and antibodies associated with the hepatitis viruses
Calcium	2.2–2.67 mmol/L	Raised in severe acute pancreatitis
Platelets	$150–400 \times 10^9$/L	May fall when spleen is enlarged by portal hypertension
Prothrombin time (PT)	12–15 seconds	Prolonged in acute liver damage and cirrhosis
International normalized ratio (INR) (of clotting time)	1	Prolonged with (i) decreased synthesis of prothrombin due to liver cell damage or (ii) decreased vitamin K absorption due to bile duct obstruction
White cell count	$4–11 \times 10^9$/L	Raised in pancreatitis
α-fetoprotein (AFP)	< 10 μg/L	Usually only synthesized by fetus – raised AFP levels in adults usually indicate hepatocellular carcinoma

Urine tests

Bilirubin is not normally present in urine, but may be present in obstructive jaundice. An increased level of urinary urobilinogen (normally present in small amounts) is a sign of liver damage. Decreased levels of urinary urobilinogen may indicate either obstructive jaundice, when bile is not reaching the intestine, or that the patient is taking oral antibiotics. This reduces the number of intestinal bacteria, whose action is vital in the process of converting bilirubin to urobilinogen. This information should be included on the laboratory form.

Tests on faeces

The failure of pancreatic lipase or bile salts to reach the intestine will result in a stool with high fat content (steatorrhoea) which appears bulky and greasy and has an offensive odour.

ENDOSCOPIC INVESTIGATIONS

Endoscopy allows direct visualization of the gastrointestinal tract and can be used for both diagnosis and treatment.

Endoscopic retrograde cholangiopancreatography

Endoscopic retrograde cholangiopancreatography (ERCP) utilizes a combination of endoscopic and radiological techniques to allow detailed examination of the pancreatic ducts and hepatobiliary system. ERCP is performed to determine the causes of biliary problems, as well as to remove gallstones obstructing the common bile duct. An endoscope is passed via the mouth and stomach into the duodenum, and a catheter is introduced into the biliary system via the hepatopancreatic ampulla. Both the pancreatic and bile ducts can be visualized and explored. Stones in the common bile duct can be removed, stents inserted to keep ducts patent, or biopsies taken. The care of a patient undergoing an ERCP is discussed on pages 642–643.

RADIOLOGICAL INVESTIGATIONS

Plain and contrast X-rays

Plain X-rays rarely provide useful information specifically about liver, gallbladder and pancreatic disorders. Contrast X-rays (cholangiography) using an intravenous dye have now been largely replaced by other tests, especially ultrasound and ERCP.

Scintigraphy (nuclear imaging)

Scintigraphy involves the i.v. injection of a harmless radioactive isotope that is taken up by the Kupffer cells and excreted in bile and is thus useful in the assessment of biliary excretory function and the detection of diffuse liver disease, such as cirrhosis and tumours. Any lesions within the liver appear as a 'cold' area on the scan.

Cholecystogram

Patients swallow a radio-opaque iodine compound to allow imaging of the gallbladder. They eat a fat-free meal the evening before the investigation and then clear fluids only until the investigation takes place the following day. Although once common, this procedure has increasingly been replaced by ERCP.

Computed tomography

Computed tomography (CT scan) gives greater resolution than conventional imaging and is particularly useful for the detection of abscesses and masses. Although usually pain-free, it does require patients to lie still in an enclosed machine. A full explanation of the procedure and the equipment beforehand will allay some of the fears patients may have and ensure their cooperation during the procedure, which takes 25–40 minutes.

ULTRASONOGRAPHY

Ultrasound is quick, safe and non-invasive. It can provide detailed anatomical information, as well as evaluating blood flow using a Doppler probe. It can also detect gallstones, bile duct dilatation, abscesses and tumours.

MAGNETIC RESONANCE IMAGING

Magnetic resonance imaging (MRI) is used to produce cross-sectional images of the liver and is useful for soft focal lesions. It is less useful for imaging the gallbladder and pancreas.

PERCUTANEOUS BIOPSY

Histological examination can provide useful information for both diagnosis and prognosis of liver disease, using a percutaneous approach with a liver biopsy needle. The procedure is performed in the X-ray department by specialist radiologists. Patients should have a clotting screen and a 'group and save' (see Ch. 18) performed beforehand because of the risk of haemorrhage. Baseline measurements of vital signs should be recorded for future comparison.

Patients are placed in the supine position, close to the right side of the bed or trolley. Local anaesthetic is injected and oral sedation may also be given. A biopsy needle is quickly introduced whilst patients hold their breath, and a sample of liver tissue is taken. Because of the risk of haemorrhage, patients are usually on bed rest until the following morning (or at least 4 hours). Observation of vital signs, puncture site, colour and pain levels should be monitored every 15 minutes for the first 2 hours, every 30 minutes for next 2 hours, and then hourly thereafter. Other complications include lung puncture (breathlessness), colon puncture (severe pain), and abdominal pain, rigidity and tenderness (due to peritoneal irritation and inflammation).

DISEASE PREVENTION AND HEALTH EDUCATION

The Department of Health (DoH) document, *Saving Lives – Our Healthier Nation* (DoH 1999a), recognizes the potential of all nurses, health visitors and midwives to play a major part in promoting health and preventing illness. The contact that nurses have with people at critical points in their lives offers a significant opportunity to promote health. During acute illnesses associated with the liver, gallbladder and pancreas, patients may be particularly receptive to advice and support about healthy lifestyle choices. If chronic illnesses develop, such as cirrhosis or chronic pancreatitis, there are important opportunities to help people manage and take control of their condition, minimizing dependence and maximizing well-being. *Making a Difference* (DoH 1999b), which specifically looks at strengthening the nursing contribution to health and health care, identifies the unique opportunities that nurses have to identify patterns and causes of ill health and to join with others to tackle them.

NUTRITION

Obesity has been shown to be a predisposing factor to the development of gallstones, especially in women (Everhart 1993). Opportunities should be taken to encourage and assist patients to maintain a well-balanced diet, reduce fat intake and avoid obesity (see Ch. 11). Patients who are obese should be given encouragement, advice and assistance to reduce their weight. Weight loss should be steady. Rapid weight loss in obese women has been shown to be a significant risk factor for the development of gallstones (Everhart 1993) and is thought to be due to a relative rise in bile concentration; 10–25% of obese people develop gallstones within a few months of starting a very low-calorie diet. The risk is much lower in men but is highest in women with the greatest body mass index and most rapid weight loss.

Food preparation hygiene is vital to reduce the risk of hepatitis A. If hepatitis A is endemic or sanitation levels are poor, it may be best to avoid drinking tap water or eating ice cubes, salads, fresh (unpeeled) fruit and vegetables, shellfish and raw oysters.

ENVIRONMENT

Occupations such as farming, dry cleaning and the chemical industry, that bring people into contact with chemicals such as carbon tetrachloride, arsenic, chloroform, phosphorus or vinyl chloride, potentially increase the risk of toxic hepatitis. Instructions contained in the *Control of Substances Hazardous to Health (COSHH) Regulations* (Health and Safety Executive 1999) require employers to ensure that employees suffer no harm as a result of contact with hepatotoxic substances. Certain household products and cleaning agents contain hepatotoxic chemicals. Occupational health advisors and practice nurses should encourage clients to follow the COSHH regulations and the instructions given on labels.

LIFESTYLE

Smoking

A link with cigarette smoking and pancreatic cancer was identified in a 40-year study of 34 000 male doctors in the UK, which found a threefold increase in incidence amongst heavy smokers (Doll et al 1994).

Alcohol

Alcohol consumption and misuse are closely associated with liver and pancreatic diseases. With an estimated 800 000 problem drinkers in the UK, half of them alcohol-dependent (Paton 1994), alcohol consumption forms a major part of disease prevention. It is not just the 'alcoholic' patient who is at risk. Moderate regular drinking and occasional 'heavy binges' can also lead to health problems. Damage (especially to the liver) from excess drinking, however, is much more common in those

individuals who have been drinking regularly and heavily for more than 5 years (Sherlock & Dooley 1997). Women appear to suffer more damage to their liver, thought to be due in part to a lower percentage of body water so that the alcohol consumed is less diluted. Older people are also particularly susceptible to the effects of alcohol (see Older Adults: Nursing Priorities box 23.1) and nurses in most practice areas can expect to meet older patients who have alcohol-related problems (Mudd et al 1994).

Alcohol misuse is a complex problem. Scare tactics have been found to be ineffective in dealing with alcoholism in the UK; however, government programmes in both France and the USA have led to a small but steady decline in alcohol consumption (Sherlock & Dooley 1997). Early identification and treatment of alcohol dependency improves recovery rates to 68–85% and is much more effective than waiting for the patient to hit 'rock bottom' (Tweed 1989). This approach also improves the likelihood of patients keeping their jobs, their family and their self-esteem. Although alcohol misuse is a global phenomenon, it may be controlled or restricted by religion, especially within the Muslim and Buddhist communities. This may make people from these communities reluctant to seek help or admit to a problem. Mortality from cirrhosis and liver tumours amongst men born in South Asia is nearly twice that of the white male population in the UK (Oyefeso & Ghodse 1998). Nurses in both the hospital and the community can fulfil an important role in giving information about the early identification and impact of problem drinking (see Health Promotion box 23.1). It is vital to remember that family members and significant others may require considerable support. Groups such as Alcoholics Anonymous also provide essential support and information for families as well as treatment programmes.

Sexual practices

The hepatitis B and D viruses are both known to be transmitted in vaginal secretions and semen, as well as blood. Therefore, sexual contact with a person with hepatitis B and D carries a risk of infection. Certain groups of people are known to be at increased risk, e.g. sex workers and homosexual men, and anyone who has unprotected sex with multiple partners (DoH 1998). Every opportunity should be taken to stress the importance of 'safer sex', particularly through the use of condoms and other barrier methods. People from high-risk groups should be offered vaccinations to offer further protection.

Drug users

Sharing needles and having unprotected sex are the major causes of hepatitis C, B and D viruses as all are blood-borne. The hepatitis B vaccine and needle exchange programmes have the potential to reduce the incidence of hepatitis B.

CLINICAL CHARACTERISTICS

Disorders affecting the liver, gallbladder and pancreas have the ability to affect many of the body's systems and can be devastating in their consequences. However, both the liver and the pancreas have the ability to maintain relatively normal function if only part of the organ is affected. Disorders may be chronic or acute and the severity of the condition dictates the

OLDER ADULTS: NURSING PRIORITIES

23.1 Alcohol misuse and the older patient

Depression, loneliness and lack of social support are the most frequently cited reasons by older people for alcohol misuse (Gambert 1997); it is often associated with psychiatric disorders such as depression and anxiety. Clinically, the same amount of alcohol once consumed during younger years with impunity may cause clinical symptoms in later years. Physiological changes associated with ageing (see Ch. 33) make older patients particularly susceptible to problems of acute alcohol toxicity, giving rise to a range of complications such as:

- increased cardiac rate and output; increased blood pressure
- hypothermia from vasodilatation and loss of body heat
- acute gastritis and pancreatitis
- falls and accidents
- alcohol-induced hypoglycaemia
- inhibition of antidiuretic hormone, leading to volume depletion, electrolyte disturbance and dehydration
- cognitive impairment and confusion, even with moderate intake.

Chronic alcoholism can affect almost every system and organ within the body and cause even more problems for the older patient. The decline in extracellular and intracellular fluid and the higher proportion of body fat to muscle means that the alcohol load from a drink reaching the central nervous system is increased with age. Nurses should be aware when assessing a confused older patient that confusion and disorientation may be due to alcohol misuse or withdrawal symptoms, rather than dementia. The cognitive deficits resulting from alcohol misuse also magnify other age-related changes or diseases. Alcohol misuse should also be considered in older patients admitted with hypoglycaemia or malnutrition.

Alcohol is often used (even advised by health professionals) as an appetite stimulant or sleep aid. Although effective in both areas in the short term, long-term use may lead to tolerance and increased use and become a substitute for well-balanced meals and so lead to malnutrition. It may also reduce the amount of REM sleep and thus cause somnolence and irritability during the day. Many older patients do not realize the effect that their alcohol consumption is having, or could have, on their well-being. Nurses are ideally placed to assist patients through education and information.

A thorough nursing assessment is required, paying particular attention to patients' mental state and the nutritional content of their diet; they may require nutritional and vitamin supplements.

Reference
Gambert SR. Alcohol abuse: medical effects of heavy drinking in late life. Geriatrics 1997; 52(6): 30–37.

HEALTH PROMOTION

23.1 Sensible drinking

In 1997, the Department of Health published revised guidelines for alcohol consumption. Most men can safely drink 3–4 units of alcohol a day without significant risks to their health. The maximum health benefit (e.g. protection against coronary heart disease and gallstone formation) for men over 40 lies between 1 and 2 units/day.

For women, the guidelines indicate 2–3 units/day, with the maximum health benefit for postmenopausal women lying between 1 and 2 units/day. Advice for pre-conception or pregnant women is to limit intake to 1–2 units/week; however, some doctors recommend no alcohol as the only completely safe limit.

The guidelines also recommend avoiding binge drinking and also having one or two alcohol-free days per week, particularly following an episode of heavy drinking. To enable patients to stay within these limits, it is vital they understand exactly what a unit is, in terms they can relate to. Broadly, half a pint of standard strength beer, lager or cider, a small glass of wine (note that wine varies in strength between 9 and 13.5% alcohol – therefore some small glasses of wine may be 1.5 units) or a single measure of spirit is equal to one unit of alcohol. Keeping track at home is much more difficult than in a pub, where all the measures are of a standard size.

---

intensity of signs and symptoms. The clinical characteristics of the patient with disorders of the liver, gallbladder and pancreas are summarized in Table 23.2.

Jaundice

Jaundice is a common and distressing sign. The patient will have yellow skin, mucous membranes and sclera, caused by increased amounts of bilirubin in the blood. The discoloration is usually seen first in the sclera and is often accompanied by pruritus (itching). For people with darker skin colour, the palms of the hands and the soles of the feet will be yellow. The primary cause of jaundice may vary (see Table 23.3) but any failure of the bilirubin excretory pathway will result in an accumulation of bile pigment in the blood.

Table 23.2 Disorders of the liver, gallbladder and pancreas – associated clinical characteristics and possible causes

Clinical characteristic	Possible causes
Jaundice – see Table 23.3	
Pruritus – severe itching of the skin, with no rash	Irritation of the subcutaneous sensory nerves by retained bile salts
Pain – dull ache to extremely severe	Impacted stone, peritonitis, inflammation, nerve ending irritation, biliary colic
Digestive disturbances – flatulence, nausea, vomiting, 'fullness', fatty food intolerance	Impaired bile transportation, ascites, biliary colic or obstruction
General constitutional symptoms – anorexia, weight loss, lassitude, weakness	Impaired storage of carbohydrates and protein metabolism
Ascites – soft, distended abdomen, non-specific abdominal discomfort, increased girth	Portal hypertension – increase in blood pressure in the portal vein allows fluid to escape into the peritoneal cavity
Oedema – swelling of the legs and ankles, sacral area, scrotum	Less albumin and other plasma proteins produced – loss of osmotic pressure
Bleeding, e.g. purpura, epistaxis, melaena	Inadequate production of prothrombin and other blood clotting factors by the liver
Varicosities – painless, explosive, massive bleeding from the mouth or rectum	Portal hypertension causing the veins that drain into the portal vein to become grossly dilated and rupture
Fever – may be low grade or chills and a high temperature may be noted	Infection or inflammation of biliary system, pancreas or ascitic fluid
Neurological disturbances – irritability, lethargy and amnesia, tremors, confusion, aggression, stupor and even coma	Ammonia toxicity – liver's inability to convert ammonia (from amino acid metabolism) to urea; ammonia is a CNS toxin
Skin changes – palmar erythema, 'spider naevi', loss of axillary and pubic hair and slow growth of (male) facial hair	Capillary dilatation High oestrogen levels in the blood – hormones are not being degraded by the liver

Table 23.3 Types and causes of jaundice

Type of jaundice	Possible causes	Urinalysis			Faeces	Degree of jaundice
		Colour	Bilirubin	Urobilinogen		
Pre-hepatic or haemolytic	Blood transfusion reactions Haemolytic anaemia	Normal	Slight	++++	Normal to dark in colour	Mild jaundice – 'lemon' colour to skin
Hepatic or hepatocellular	Carcinoma of the liver, excessive drug use, alcoholic cirrhosis or hepatitis, poisons	Dark	Slight	Normal	May be paler and fatty	Variable
Post-hepatic or obstructive	Cancer of the head of pancreas, gallstones, strictures or inflammation of the biliary system	Very dark	+++	Nil	Pale, fatty and offensive	Severe – green tinge to skin

Jaundice is classified as:

- pre-hepatic or haemolytic – caused before the bilirubin reaches the liver; excessive amounts of bilirubin are released from red blood cells
- hepatic or hepatocellular – the pathology is in the liver itself
- post-hepatic or obstructive – bile flow is obstructed after it has left the liver.

Pruritus

Pruritus, caused by an accumulation of bile salts in the skin, is often the most distressing symptom of jaundice for the patient. The patient's skin should be kept clean and dry, and the use of perfumed toiletries avoided. Encourage the patient to keep the nails short and not to scratch. Observe the skin for areas of redness, bruising, or breakdown – moisturizers can be used if the patient has dry skin (see Reflective Practice box 23.1).

23.1 Caring for a patient with jaundice

Mr Patel is a 45-year-old man who has severe jaundice. He is awaiting the results of a number of blood tests to investigate the cause of his condition and is withdrawn and sleeps much of the time. Think about the care a patient with jaundice like Mr Patel may require.

- Why do you think Mr Patel is so withdrawn? What visible signs of jaundice will there be and how might he feel about this?
- Why does Mr Patel feel itchy all the time, and what measures could you take to help alleviate this distressing symptom?
- What fears might he have about his blood tests and how could you allay them?
- What written information is available in your workplace for the patient with jaundice?

DISORDERS AFFECTING THE LIVER

Liver disease may be acute or chronic in nature. Acute liver dysfunction may occur as a complication of hepatitis B or C, as a reaction to hepatotoxic drugs such as paracetamol or halothane, or exposure to toxic chemicals. More often, however, liver dysfunction or failure is chronic. Conditions associated with chronic liver failure include viral hepatitis, medication overdoses, biliary obstruction, and alcoholic cirrhosis.

HEPATITIS

Inflammation of the liver is known as hepatitis, a disease which can range from subclinical to life-threatening. The most common cause is viral, but other causes include excessive use of alcohol, drugs or other types of infectious diseases. Hepatitis may be acute or chronic.

Acute hepatitis. Any condition which causes inflammation within the hepatocytes and which lasts for less than 6 months

Chronic hepatitis. Inflammation lasting for more than 6 months. The term is used to define a range of inflammatory liver diseases ranging from mild chronic persistent hepatitis to severe chronic active hepatitis. Forms of chronic hepatitis are associated with viral infections, such as hepatitis A, B and D, cytomegalovirus, excessive alcohol consumption, inflammatory bowel disease and autoimmune diseases.

VIRAL HEPATITIS

Viral hepatitis (see Table 23.4) is usually caused by a unique group of viruses that only attack the liver, and the types currently known are classified alphabetically from A to G. The hepatitis A and E (HAV and HEV) viruses tend to cause acute hepatitis, rarely lasting more than 6 months. The hepatitis B, C, D and G (HBV, HCV, HDV, HGV) viruses can cause both acute and chronic hepatitis. Other viruses which can cause hepatitis include Epstein–Barr and cytomegalovirus (CMV).

Hepatitis A

The least serious of the five, HAV accounts for the greatest number of hepatitis cases and is prevalent in areas with suboptimal hygiene of water supply and food production. The virus is eliminated in the faeces and therefore stools constitute an infection risk.

Hepatitis B

HBV has been isolated in sputum, urine and faeces, as well as blood and serum. Contaminated surfaces have been implicated in transfer of infective material, but there is no evidence of airborne spread. The disease may become chronic or produce a carrier state, where the individual may be asymptomatic but carry the virus, and thus be able to infect others. Because of the

Table 23.4 Viral hepatitis: comparison of the five most common types (adapted from Hicks Keen 1999)

	HAV	HBV	HCV	HDV	HEV
Likely mode of transmission	Faecal-oral; food-borne most common	Blood or serum; sexual contact; mother to baby (perinatal) transmission	Blood or serum; perinatal transmission rare (unless mother is HIV positive); often transmitted by chronic carriers	Similar to HBV; can cause infection only if individual already has HBV	Faecal-oral; food-borne; water-borne
Population most affected	Children; areas of poor sanitation	i.v. drug users; health care workers; homosexual men; men and women with multiple sexual partners; young children of infected mothers; recipients of certain blood products; patients on haemodialysis	i.v. drug users; patients who received blood products in UK prior to 1991; potential risk to health care workers	i.v. drug users; haemophiliacs; recipients of multiple blood transfusions	Parts of Asia, Africa and Mexico where sanitation is poor
Incubation	2–6 weeks	6 weeks to 6 months	18–180 days	Varies; not well established	

transmission routes, health care workers have an occupational exposure risk to HBV (see Guidelines for Care Priorities box 23.1). HBV carries a significantly higher mortality rate than other hepatitis viruses – up to 30%, compared with 0.2% for HAV (Rogers et al 1998). The World Health Organization estimates that 350 million people are infected worldwide, with around a million deaths a year (Smales 1998). Around 600 acute cases are reported to the Public Health Laboratory Services (PHLS) every year in the UK and there are thought to be around 50 000 chronic carriers.

Hepatitis C

HCV has around a million carriers worldwide. Sexual transmission is rare (Ahmed & Elias 1996). Between 0.5 and 2% of the population of Europe are estimated to have hepatitis C, but its true prevalence is unknown because most people are asymptomatic. It is estimated to be around 300 000–600 000 in the UK (Rogers et al 1998); the number of cases reported to the PHLS

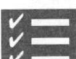

GUIDELINES FOR CARE PRIORITIES

23.1 Hepatitis B: protecting staff and patients

- Handwashing – the single most effective way of reducing cross-infection, this should be carried out before and after all care
- Treat all body fluids as potentially infected
- Wear protective clothing (disposable gloves and aprons) whenever contact with blood, faeces, urine or other body fluids is likely. Masks are not advocated unless there is a risk of being splashed in the face; glasses/goggles will afford additional protection in this situation
- Specimens – bottled samples of blood, urine, sputum or faeces must be enclosed in a sealed plastic bag with the request form kept separately, and be clearly labelled as a biohazard, in order to alert and protect laboratory staff
- Contaminated linen – should be double-bagged and clearly labelled, as should bloodstained clinical waste
- Disposal of any clinical waste should always be as close to the point of use as possible
- Spillages of blood, urine and faeces – should be cleaned wearing plastic gloves and apron. Disinfect the area with paper towels soaked in 1% hypochlorite solution and, if possible, left for 30 minutes (Rogers et al 1998)
- Reporting – any untoward incidents involving patients with hepatitis should be reported, no matter how minor
- Immunization should be offered to all health care workers – offers protection for up to 90% of recipients (Department of Health 1998). It is not a substitute for good infection control practices

References

Department of Health. Guidance for clinical health care workers: protection against blood-borne viruses. London: Department of Health; 1998.

Rogers R, Salvage J, Cowell R. Nurses at risk: a guide to health and safety at work, 2nd edn. London: Macmillan Press; 1998.

has increased 10-fold between 1991 and 1997 (Smales 1998). Its prevalence in health care workers is no greater than that of the average population (Rogers et al 1998).

Hepatitis D and E

HDV is only able to replicate in the presence of HBV. Hepatitis E (HEV) is an RNA virus and is transmitted via the faecal-oral route. Young adults appear to be most at risk and infected pregnant women have a 20% mortality rate. High-risk areas for HEV are Mexico, China and India; the prevalence of both HDV and HEV is very low in northern Europe.

Hepatitis G

HGV has only recently been recognized (RCN 1998) and its exact history and significance remain unknown (DoH 1998).

Pathophysiology

Viral hepatitis can cause considerable liver pathology. Inflammation and necrosis cause swelling and congestion of the liver cells. This causes bile formation and flow to be disrupted, leading to obstructive jaundice and elevated bilirubin levels. Necrosis also causes the levels of serum enzymes [alanine aminotransferase (ALT) and aspartate aminotransferase (AST)] to rise sharply (see Table 23.1). In most cases, the liver is able to regenerate, with only minimal scarring and fibrous tissue formation, and only a few patients are left with residual impairment of liver function. However, recent studies of patients with HCV indicated an increased rate of cirrhosis and liver-related mortality in future years (Ahmed & Elias 1996).

Clinical presentation

The onset of hepatitis usually manifests as vague symptoms such as malaise, irritability, anorexia, nausea and vomiting, muscle or joint aches, pyrexia and headache. As the disease progresses, pain and abdominal tenderness over the right upper quadrant worsen and the urine becomes darker. The patient may have either constipation or diarrhoea and, as jaundice develops, light-coloured stools.

Investigations and diagnostic procedures

Blood analysis reveals that the serum bilirubin levels are elevated, as well as ALT and AST. Prothrombin times may be prolonged. Urinalysis may show high levels of urobilinogen during the early stages of the disease. Serotological tests to identify specific antigen and antibody markers will confirm the diagnosis, the causative virus and the stage of the disease.

Medical management

Medical management tends to centre around symptom control and supportive therapy. The patient's medications should be reviewed and reduced wherever possible. Drugs which are deactivated by the liver, e.g. barbiturates, oral contraceptives and morphine, should be avoided. Patients should also avoid alcohol in order to reduce the workload of the liver. In recent years, specific therapies such as interferon-alpha have been licensed in the UK for the treatment of chronic HBV and HCV patients in order to improve disease progression by reducing the incidence of liver failure (Kowdley 1996). End-stage liver disease due to HCV is a common indication for liver transplantation (see

Ch. 28). If the patient's blood coagulation has been affected by the impaired absorption of vitamin K, it may be prescribed and administered parenterally.

During the recovery stage, physical examinations and blood tests will be carried out to determine the progression of the disease or possible residual liver dysfunction, usually on an outpatient basis. Monitoring may continue for up to 1 year, or longer if necessary.

▶ Nursing management

Following a physical examination of the patient, a nursing care plan can be devised. The physical examination will include:

- measurement of vital signs
- observation of skin, mucous membranes and sclera for signs of jaundice
- observation of urine, faeces and gums for signs of bleeding.

Following a thorough assessment, during which the patient's likely exposure to the virus is tactfully explored, the clinical symptoms which the patient is experiencing are established.

Nutrition and fluids

During the acute phase, patients may suffer from anorexia, nausea and vomiting and maintaining an adequate fluid and nutritional intake may be difficult. Patients require a higher than usual fluid intake (around 3000 mL/day) to compensate for insensible losses due to fever and to facilitate the elimination of urobilinogen in the urine. Intravenous administration of fluids may be necessary until patients are able to tolerate oral fluids. Fluid intake and output should be monitored and there should be close observation for signs of dehydration and fluid overload (see Ch. 8).

Antiemetics (e.g. metoclopramide, dimenhydrinate) should be administered where required to control nausea and vomiting. As soon as patients are able, high-calorie foods in the form of small meals should be offered frequently. Initially, the diet should consist of protein and carbohydrates, with dairy produce introduced slowly, as tolerated (when jaundice has subsided). Fried, fatty and rich foods should be avoided for weeks, even months, after recovery. Alcohol should be avoided for at least 6 months.

Patients should be weighed regularly to monitor their intake and to ensure that any weight loss during the acute phase has been regained.

Rest and sleep

Adequate rest and sleep are vital during the acute and recovery stages. Both in hospital and at home, patients should be encouraged and helped to get periods of uninterrupted rest and sleep, including during the day. Strenuous activities should be avoided during this period, and usual activities only resumed slowly, as patients can tolerate.

Skin care

If patients have a fever, frequent bathing should be encouraged or assisted, with frequent changes of bed linen and personal clothing. Emollients can be added to bathwater or the skin to help relieve itching associated with jaundice. Patients should keep their fingernails short to minimize the effects of scratching,

especially when asleep. A cool environment and loose cotton clothing may also help.

Prevention of spread of infection

Universal precautions (see Ch. 13) to prevent the spread of infection should be used when caring for any patient with viral hepatitis. Isolation is not necessary, unless the patient is bleeding, vomiting or has diarrhoea. The main risk of infection arises from contact with blood or blood products; the main risk to health care workers comes from needlestick injuries (see Guidelines for Care Priorities box 23.2).

☑ GUIDELINES FOR CARE PRIORITIES

23.2 Needlestick injuries and the safe handling and disposal of sharps

Most injuries are preventable. The risks of needlestick injuries should be minimized by implementing procedures for the safe handling and disposal of sharps.

- Place all sharps in an approved, rigid sharps container immediately after use
- Never overfill a sharps container and close securely after use
- Never re-sheathe needles. Where possible, dispose of needle and syringe as a single unit. If re-sheathing is necessary, use either a device or a single-handed 'scoop' method
- Removing needles from syringes increases the risk of needlestick injury. Remove only when essential, e.g. to transfer blood to a container
- Other 'sharps' – including cannulae, administration sets, stitch cutters, razors, broken ampoules, glass, scalpels – should be disposed of with equal care into an approved sharps container
- Training and education – should include the possible risks, the procedures for safe handling and in the event of a sharps injury
- Risk assessments should be undertaken wherever 'sharps' are in use, in conjunction with regular clinical audits to identify where practices could be improved
- In the event of an injury:
  — wash the site liberally with soap and water
  — do not scrub or suck the area
  — irrigate mucous membranes with copious amounts of water
  — encourage free bleeding of puncture wounds
  — report incident promptly and seek urgent advice.

For further information see the recommendations of the Expert Advisory Group on AIDS and the Advisory Group on Hepatitis (Department of Health 1998).

Reference

Department of Health. Guidance for clinical health care workers: protection against blood-borne viruses. London: Department of Health; 1998.

Health education

Patients and their families should be given advice and information about the spread of the virus, especially when being cared for at home. The importance of thorough handwashing, especially after going to the toilet, should be stressed. Barrier methods of contraception should be discussed, as well as other issues relating to safer sexual practices, such as abstinence or reducing the number of sexual partners, and avoiding direct contact with blood, semen or urine. The importance of rest and adequate nutrition should be emphasized. Patients should be advised against taking any drugs not prescribed by their GP and to avoid alcohol for at least 6 months. Known contacts of HAV and HBV are advised to consult a doctor as soon as possible to determine their hepatitis status and the need for treatment. It is important that patients understand the importance of informing any health care workers with whom they have contact of their hepatitis status.

ALCOHOL-INDUCED HEPATITIS

This form of inflammation (acute or chronic) occurs as a result of tissue necrosis caused by alcohol misuse. Symptoms usually develop following a bout of heavy drinking and patients may complain of anorexia, nausea, abdominal pain, jaundice, ascites, fever and changes in mental status (lassitude, mood swings). Some features of malnutrition, such as recent weight loss, are common. Laboratory tests may reveal that patients are anaemic, with an elevated serum bilirubin level and white cell count. A liver biopsy reveals a typically fatty-looking liver.

Nursing care includes offering a diet high in carbohydrate, protein and vitamins and high-calorie drinks. Corticosteroids have been shown to have a beneficial effect in some studies (Bircher et al 1999), but their use remains controversial. The most important factor of long-term care is total abstinence from alcohol.

DRUG-INDUCED HEPATITIS

Many prescription drugs can cause inflammation of the liver, even in small therapeutic doses. These drugs include allopurinol, amiodarone, androgenic steroids, carbamazepine, halothane, chlorpromazine, diazepam and oral contraceptives. Many hepatotoxic drugs, such as paracetamol, NSAIDs, aspirin and vitamin A, can be bought without a prescription. The liver is particularly concerned with the metabolism of drugs administered orally (known as the 'first pass' effect), and with some drugs (e.g. GTN) the oral route is avoided because of this effect.

Paracetamol overdose is one of the most common causes of drug-induced hepatitis. Its use in self-harming incidents has risen with increasing ease of access over the past 20 years. It is now the most commonly used substance in self-poisoning (around 70 000 cases in the UK annually) and is the most common cause of acute liver failure in the UK (Bridger et al 1998). There have also been cases of inadvertent overdose, with patients taking a number of different over-the-counter preparations, all containing paracetamol. Manufacturers are now required to limit pack size and include a warning on all paracetamol-containing preparations of the dangers of inadvertent overdose.

In therapeutic doses, paracetamol is inactivated in the liver by reduction with glutathione into soluble metabolites which are excreted via the kidneys. In higher doses, glutathione is depleted, and toxic substances form which cause cell damage. Hepatitis usually begins 24–48 hours after the overdose, and the levels of liver enzymes rise. Production of clotting factors falls (prothrombin time is a useful prognostic indicator) and there is a drop in the mobilization of glucose, leading to hypoglycaemia. During days 3–5, the patient's symptoms may worsen and if there is no sign of improvement, liver failure and even death may ensue.

Management depends on the interval between overdose and treatment and the plasma levels of paracetamol. Within 4 hours of the overdose, options include:

- gastric lavage
- charcoal to reduce absorption
- ipecacuanha-induced emesis
- methionine administered orally to restore glutathione levels or, if the patient is vomiting, intravenous acetylcysteine.

Nursing care of a patient with drug-induced hepatitis focuses on preventing complications such as bleeding, infection and malnutrition, and monitoring the progress of the disease and the effects of the medical treatment.

TOXIC HEPATITIS

Certain chemicals are known to cause inflammation and degenerative changes in the liver. Chemicals such as carbon tetrachloride, arsenic, chloroform, phosphorus and sulphonamides have all been known to cause toxic hepatitis. Treatment consists of prompt identification and removal of the causative agent, rest and symptomatic care.

CIRRHOSIS

Cirrhosis is a serious liver disease characterized by the destruction of hepatocytes and the formation of dense fibrous scar tissue. Although symptoms may not occur for many years, structural changes gradually lead to total liver dysfunction.

Aetiology and epidemiology

The most common cause of cirrhosis is alcohol misuse. The healthy liver detoxifies small amounts of alcohol to non-toxic compounds which the body can use for energy. If the frequency and/or amount of alcohol consumption increases, acetaldehyde causes hepatocyte damage and chronic liver enlargement, related to the accumulation of fatty acids. If patients stop drinking alcohol at this stage, the prognosis and chances of a full recovery are good. However, if patients continue to drink, the fat deposition process worsens and fatty acids accumulate in hepatocytes.

Worldwide, mortality and morbidity from cirrhosis is increasing. In the USA, it is the leading cause of death amongst men between the ages of 35 and 45.

There are several other types of cirrhosis, the details of which are beyond the scope of this book. Readers are referred to 'Further reading' for more information.

Pathophysiology

Fatty deposits within the liver cause cellular degeneration and the development of non-functioning fibrotic nodules to replace the necrotic cells (which give the liver a roughened 'hobnail' feel on palpation). Liver function becomes increasingly compromised, through decreased cellular blood supply and congestion in the portal system; these changes are irreversible. The congestion can lead to the development of a number of serious effects (see Table 23.5).

Clinical presentation

The early signs of cirrhotic changes often go unnoticed, because the liver has a large reserve capacity. Impaired liver function may gradually appear over a long period of time, sometimes even years. Symptoms may include the following:

- *Initial stages* – lethargy and fatigue, vague digestive disturbances (anorexia, flatulence, nausea), weight loss
- *Later stages* – jaundice, dependent oedema (i.e. swelling of the legs and ankles which is increased by gravity), anaemia, ascites and increased girth, spider naevii (dilated branching cutaneous arteries), bleeding, epistaxis, melaena and haematemesis. Endocrine abnormalities such as gynaecomastia (breast development) and impotence in males, amenorrhoea and infertility in females may develop
- *Advanced stages* – splenomegaly (enlarged spleen), hepatic coma, haemorrhage from oesophageal varices (enlarged tortuous veins in the lower oesophagus).

Investigations

Liver function tests will be carried out to determine the stage and severity of the disease, as well as a full blood count and a clotting screen. Abdominal palpation will be performed to assess the size and nature of the liver and spleen – both may be enlarged due to portal hypertension (causing increased vascular pressure within the organs), and on palpation the liver will be roughened and firm. Patients may also undergo a liver biopsy in the radiology department. Ultrasound, CT scan or ERCP may be performed to identify the cause of the cirrhosis (if alcohol misuse is not suspected).

Medical management

The care patients receive will depend largely on the cause and severity of the disease and the presence of any complications. The first priority is to treat the underlying cause, e.g. exposure to toxins, use of alcohol, biliary obstruction, etc. Complications of cirrhosis are usually inevitable and, for many patients, the only chance of a full recovery lies with a liver transplant. The management of the effects of cirrhosis is detailed in Table 23.5.

▶ Nursing management

Many patients with cirrhosis are seriously ill and require thorough assessment and intensive nursing care, especially during the acute phase of the illness.

Immediate/on admission

Many patients are admitted acutely ill, often bleeding from oesophageal varices and in a state of hypovolaemic shock. During this phase, the aim of nursing care is to detect any worsening of the patient's condition through the close monitoring of vital signs and the maintenance of an adequate circulating volume (see Chs 9 and 31). If the patient is actively bleeding from oesophageal varices, vital signs and level of consciousness should be recorded every 15 minutes. A balloon tamponade tube may be passed nasogastrically to control the bleeding (see Fig. 23.3). The balloon should be maintained at a pressure of around 25–30 mmHg – medical staff will give precise instructions. Inadequate pressure may fail to control the bleeding, while excessive pressure may cause ulceration. The stomach

Table 23.5 Cirrhosis – effects, causes and medical management

Effect	Cause	Medical management
Portal hypertension	Increased vascular resistance leading to the development of an inefficient collateral system with back-flow into the vessels of the spleen, stomach, oesophagus and intestines	Beta-blockers (e.g. propranolol) – reduced hepatic portal blood flow and thus risk of re-bleeding
Ascites	Increased resistance to blood flow and decreased lymphatic protein filtration – force protein into the peritoneal space. Dehydration – causes adrenal glands to secrete aldosterone, causing water and sodium retention	• Restrict sodium and water • Diuretics: — loop [furosemide (frusemide)] — aldosterone antagonist (spironolactone) • Paracentesis • Replace albumin • Peritoneovenous shunt
Oesophageal varices	Portal hypertension causes distension and rupture of vessels in oesophagus – the excessive blood loss is life-threatening. Compounded by disruption to the liver's normal role in the blood clotting process	• Vasoconstrictive agents • Balloon tamponade • Sclerotherapy • Vitamin K
Encephalopathy	Failure by the liver to metabolize and detoxify nitrogenous substances, especially ammonia	• Lactulose • Neomycin

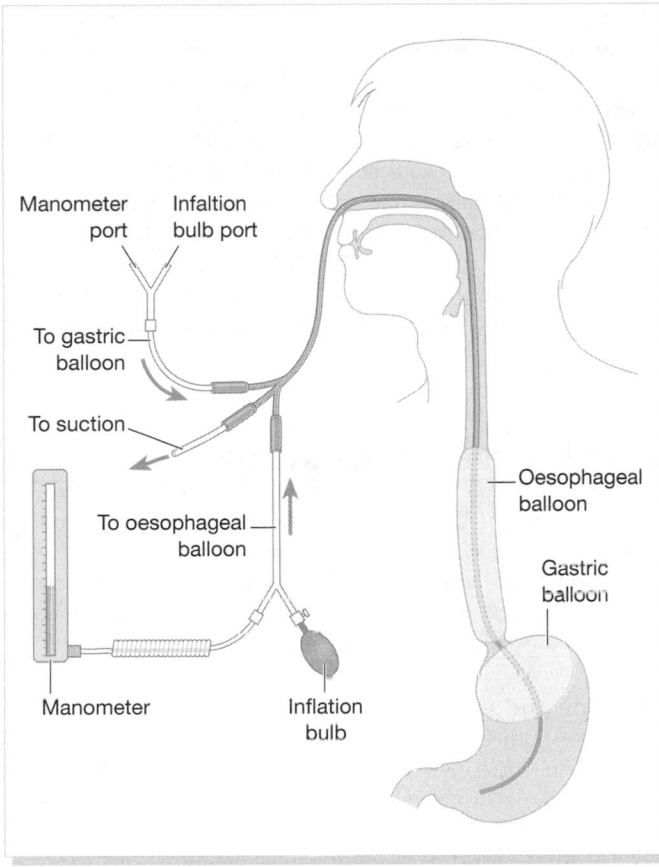

Figure 23.3 A patient with oesophageal varices – balloon tamponade tube in situ.

contents should be aspirated at regular intervals and be closely observed for blood content. If the correct pressure is maintained, the amount of blood should decline.

Patients will not be able to swallow saliva and so a receiver and suction should be available. Conscious patients are likely to be extremely anxious during tube insertion and may experience projectile vomiting and/or deterioration in their general condition. All staff should be skilled in cardiopulmonary resuscitation techniques. Balloon tamponade is usually maintained for 24–48 hours once the bleeding has been controlled; re-bleeding is common, however, when the tube is removed.

During this acute phase, patients' fluid balance should be closely monitored. Intravenous access is vital and i.v. fluids and blood will be administered to correct any hypovolaemia.

Considerable psychological support through explanations and reassurance will be vital for both patients and their carers during this initial stage of care. Some patients may be sedated when the tube is passed, to allay severe anxiety and to ensure they keep still (to avoid inadvertent removal of the tube) and rest.

Once the condition has begun to stabilize, a more thorough assessment of patient needs can be undertaken. Information should be obtained about patients' recent symptoms:

- any recent changes in girth, weight and appetite
- nausea, vomiting or anorexia
- skin and eye colour and itching

- changes in bowel habits and colour of urine
- changes in mental state
- levels of energy, tiredness and general feelings of malaise.

Regular mouth care is vital if patients vomit blood.

Ongoing care

Once the immediate nursing care needs have been met, a more long-term plan of care should be drawn up, in conjunction with patients and relatives, as appropriate.

Monitoring

Ongoing nursing care will involve close monitoring of the vital signs and fluid balance, as well as patients' nutritional intake. Any alteration in consciousness level should be noted as well as any signs of confusion and lethargy. Signs of ascites and changes in body weight should be monitored through daily weight and/or girth measurements. Signs of peripheral oedema, bleeding and bruising should be noted, as well as any other skin changes associated with jaundice.

Ascites

If patients have or develop ascites, this will be one of the priorities of care. A large collection of fluid in the peritoneal cavity can cause discomfort, anorexia, respiratory distress, hernias and aspiration of stomach contents into the lungs (due to an increase in intra-abdominal pressure), and, if the fluid becomes infected, peritonitis.

To relieve the ascites, paracentesis may be performed by medical staff. A cannula is passed into the peritoneal cavity and fluid is gradually drained off into a sterile receptacle. Removal of a large amount of ascitic fluid (more than 2 litres) may predispose patients to hypovolaemia and even circulatory collapse and shock. This is due to the sudden reduction of intra-abdominal pressure, leading to a dilation of blood vessels and pooling of a large volume of blood.

Nursing care of patients involves:

- closely monitoring their vital signs and skin colour during and after the procedure
- administration of prescribed intravenous fluids, which may include blood or albumin
- frequent mouth care and ice chips to minimize discomfort from a dry mouth
- assistance with positioning – patients may be more comfortable in a sitting position, to relieve respiratory distress
- care of the abdominal puncture site.

If the ascitic fluid re-accumulates, a peritoneovenous shunt may be indicated. This is a tube that is implanted to drain ascitic fluid from the peritoneal cavity to the superior vena cava or right atrium.

Pain and discomfort

Patients with cirrhosis may experience varying degrees of pain and discomfort. Analgesic drugs should be used with great caution, because of the risk of further liver damage, and should be discussed with a pharmacist. Diversion therapy and other non-pharmacological measures should be tried.

Skin care

Skin care should include the following:

- assist patients to keep the skin clean and dry
- avoid the use of perfumed toiletries
- encourage patients to keep their nails short and not to scratch
- observe for areas of redness, bruising or breakdown – moisturizers can be used if patients have dry skin.

Infection risk

Patients with cirrhosis are at increased risk of infection because of reduced resistance (related to altered protein metabolism and loss of normal phagocytic function) – hence their temperature should be taken regularly. Precautions should be taken when carrying out procedures or care which may increase the risk of infection, especially if the skin is compromised or broken.

Mobility

If patients have ascites or reduced mobility, deep breathing and coughing should be encouraged (to prevent pneumonia) as well as active/passive leg exercises, to prevent the development of a deep vein thrombosis (see Ch. 19).

Nutrition

As soon as patients are able to drink, oral fluids should be reintroduced. The diet should be high in carbohydrates and vitamins, to compensate for the liver's inability to store them, and low or free of sodium, to reduce ascites. The severity of the disease will dictate how much protein should be taken; if the disease is serious and ammonia levels are high, it should be avoided altogether, as protein may precipitate hepatic encephalopathy. Fats should be kept to a level which makes the diet palatable but reduces the risk of exacerbation of symptoms. A dietician should be consulted for assistance and advice.

Long-term/discharge

Patient teaching is vital to ensure that both patient and family members understand the nature of the illness and the necessary adjustments during the recovery period. This may include:

- advice (preferably written) about diet and the importance of complying with this advice
- the importance of not drinking alcohol or taking any over-the-counter medications which may worsen the condition
- advice and assistance with combating alcohol misuse. Information about self-help groups, such as Alcoholics Anonymous (see 'Useful addresses', p. 650), should be provided for patients and significant others
- avoiding physical strain and unnecessary fatigue during recovery and the need for periods of rest
- avoiding any activities which may cause skin injuries or abrasions (e.g. gardening) or contact with infectious individuals – they are at an increased risk of bleeding and infections
- the symptoms of cirrhosis and the importance of patients reporting them immediately to their doctor or nurse.

Ongoing support and supervision from the primary health care team will be vital during this period.

Prognosis

Patients with cirrhosis of the liver have a variable prognosis. If the disease is diagnosed and treated during the early phase, and patients are sufficiently motivated to comply with the suggested care, then the prognosis may be reasonable. However, if patients have developed complications, especially portal hypertension with oesophageal varices and ascites, then the prognosis may be very poor and a liver transplant may offer the only hope. Visits from community nurses are helpful in monitoring patients' progress, in dealing with any questions patients and family members may have, and in providing physical and emotional support.

LIVER FAILURE AND HEPATIC COMA

Acute liver failure (ALF), also known as fulminant liver failure, is a highly complex syndrome, caused by the breakdown of vital hepatic functions within a few days or weeks. Hepatic coma is the main manifestation of the syndrome and cerebral oedema the major cause of death (Randolph & Jonas 1998).

Aetiology and epidemiology

Acute liver failure is a rare condition with around 150 cases a year in the UK (Lee & Williams 1997). This fact, along with the complex nature of the disease, means that diagnosis is often delayed. The main cause is acute viral hepatitis (around 60–70% of cases); other causes include hepatotoxic drugs (especially paracetamol), underlying chronic liver disease and (more rarely) heat stroke and pregnancy.

Pathophysiology

In ALF, the patient suffers extensive damage to the liver, resulting in multi-organ failure (see Ch. 9). Hepatocytes are destroyed and the liver parenchyma collapses. The course of the disease is a balance of three factors: the ability of the liver to regenerate, the metabolic effects of a non-functioning liver, and the effects of the toxic substances released from the necrotic liver.

The causes of encephalopathy in ALF are not fully understood but may be related to the liver's inability to remove toxic, mainly nitrogenous, substances from the circulation. Raised levels of serum ammonia (a central nervous system toxin), the by-product of bacterial breakdown of protein, are commonly seen, as the liver is no longer able to convert it to urea.

Clinical features

On initial presentation, patients' vital signs and level of consciousness may be stable, with only rather non-specific symptoms (nausea, vomiting); however, patients are at high risk of rapid and unexpected deterioration (Randolph & Jonas 1998). Patients with ALF invariably develop hepatic encephalopathy (coma), metabolic disorders, such as hypoglycaemia (due to the failure of glycogenesis), blood clotting disorders and jaundice. Cerebral oedema, renal impairment, infection and multi-organ failure may also develop. Patients may have fetor hepaticus (a sweetish, slightly faecal smell of the breath), caused by abnormal amino acid metabolites being excreted by the lungs. This is often a sign of imminent coma.

Medical and surgical management

Because of the risk of sudden deterioration and multi-organ failure, caring for patients with acute liver failure is complex – early referral to a specialist liver unit has been shown to improve survival rates (Lee & Williams 1997). The major goal is to provide adequate supportive care to the failing liver and to prevent and treat extrahepatic complications. Intensive care is required and patients' haemodynamic status will be closely observed and maintained (see Ch. 31). Adequate cerebral perfusion is a priority; patients should be nursed flat or no higher than 10–20° of tilt in a quiet room. Patients in a severe coma are likely to need to be artificially ventilated. Laxatives may be given to reduce intestinal ammonia levels by cleansing the gastrointestinal tract. As infection is a major risk, frequent cultures of blood, urine and sputum may be taken. Intracranial pressure may need to be monitored using direct monitoring devices.

For many patients, the only chance for recovery is a liver transplant. The survival rates for patients with severe ALF and hepatic encephalopathy without transplantation is less than 20% – with transplantation it is 60–80% (Sherlock & Dooley 1997). However, only about 1 in 10 patients who might benefit from a transplant ultimately receive one because of the limited availability of livers for transplantation (Lee & Williams 1997).

> ▶ **Nursing management: liver failure**

Nursing care should ideally be carried out in a liver unit or intensive care unit. Frequent observations and recording of vital signs, fluid intake and output, blood glucose levels and signs of complications are vital. Regular and comprehensive neurological assessments (see Ch. 14) are required to detect any worsening neurological symptoms. Patients will usually have a nasogastric tube inserted and oxygen saturation levels should be monitored and oxygen delivered via a mask. If patients are comatose, then full nursing care of a patient in a coma should be instigated.

LIVER TUMOURS

The liver is affected by both benign and malignant tumours. This section will concentrate on primary tumours only (see Ch. 33 for secondary tumours).

Benign tumours. These are usually single and small; patients are usually asymptomatic and the tumour is often discovered accidentally. They can be detected using MRI or ultrasound scans. Surgical removal is not usually necessary for benign liver tumours, unless patients are experiencing pain.

Malignant tumours. These may be primary or (more commonly) secondary. The liver is the most frequent site of blood-borne metastases – it is involved in about a third of all cancers (Sherlock & Dooley 1997). They occur throughout the liver, usually in multiple deposits.

Aetiology and epidemiology

Every year, there are an estimated 1.25 million deaths worldwide from primary liver cancers. Most primary tumours are, in fact, associated with an already diseased liver – the highest frequency is amongst African and Oriental races (due to underlying cirrhosis). The condition is increasing in the West, related to the prevalence of HBV and HCV infections. Alcohol misuse also carries a fourfold increase in the risk of primary cancer of the liver. Men are affected more frequently than women (4–6:1), probably due to their higher alcohol consumption.

Pathophysiology

Primary tumours are highly vascular. Large veins within the liver are often thrombosed and contain a tumour which causes an obstruction and portal hypertension. The tumour cells may mimic some of the usual functions of liver cells – they may secrete bile and contain glycogen. However, as the tumour enlarges and spreads, liver function is compromised, but often not until the tumour has replaced as much as 90% of normal tissue.

Clinical presentation

The clinical picture is often very variable. Early symptoms of liver cancer may be vague (anorexia, weight loss, fatigue) or patients may be admitted with severe liver failure. Most patients complain of pain, but it is rarely severe. The liver is enlarged and may be felt as a hard, irregular lump in the right upper quadrant. About 50% of patients have ascites and some will be jaundiced but rarely deeply.

Investigations

A very high serum alpha-fetoprotein level (AFP > 20 µg/mL) is diagnostic of a primary tumour (AFP is usually only produced by the fetal liver). For all tumours, an ultrasound-guided needle biopsy will confirm the diagnosis through histology.

Medical and surgical management

Surgery is often impossible because too much of the liver tissue is involved or spread to other organs has already occurred. Large liver resections carry high mortality and morbidity rates. However, if the tumour is small and localized within the liver, less radical surgery, with a better outcome, is possible. Chemotherapy may be used, usually 5-fluorouracil and fluorodeoxyridine, and some centres use surgically placed hepatic artery catheters to administer cytotoxic drugs directly into the liver and avoid systemic side-effects (Ellender 1999).

For the majority of patients, however, treatment is restricted to symptom control and the prognosis is bleak.

> ▶ **Nursing management**

Nursing care will focus on symptom control and providing emotional and practical support to the patient who is facing a terminal illness. Patients should be given sufficient time to express fears, anxieties and concerns. Information should be given about the disease, the liver and, if patients want it, their prognosis. Because the prognosis is often so poor, patients do not have a great deal of time to come to terms with the disease and prepare themselves and loved ones, or to put their affairs in order. Consequently, patients, family members and friends will require a great deal of support. Where available, referral should be made to the primary care team, hospice and/or Macmillan nurse, for practical and emotional support (see Chs 33 and 34).

Patients will become increasingly dependent on others and repeated admissions to the hospital or hospice may be necessary for abdominal paracentesis. As they lose more and more weight, care should be directed at maintaining intact pressure areas and preventing moniliasis through regular oral hygiene.

LIVER TRAUMA

Liver trauma usually results from either a penetrating injury (such as laparoscopic surgery, knife wound or gunshot) or blunt trauma (from a steering wheel or fall). Spontaneous rupture can complicate the third trimester of pregnancy and cardio-pulmonary resuscitation. Any injury which disrupts the capsule surrounding the liver carries the potential for severe internal haemorrhage. This may be fatal if efforts at resuscitation and surgical intervention are not timely. Patients need very careful monitoring of vital signs to detect any changes quickly, usually in an ITU. If the liver is leaking bile into the surrounding tissues, then peritonitis may develop. The damaged area may be drained, sutured, packed or resected. Liver cells may be destroyed following injury, resulting in long-term impairment of liver function and serious clotting disorders.

DISEASES AFFECTING THE BILIARY SYSTEM

Disorders of the gallbladder and the bile ducts are extremely common; gallstone disease is known to affect 10–20% of the world's population. Disorders include gallstones, inflammatory conditions, infections and tumours. The vast majority of patients with a gallbladder disorder have gallstones.

CHOLELITHIASIS

Cholelithiasis is the term used for gallstones or calculi in the gallbladder. Gallstones may be one of the following:

- cholesterol stones – pure cholesterol stones (usually solitary) or mixed (cholesterol in a matrix of calcium and protein)
- pigment stones – either brown stones (soft, friable) made up of calcium bilirubinate, calcium soaps and cholesterol, or black stones (hard and brittle) made up of calcium carbonate and phosphate.

Aetiology and epidemiology
The causes of gallstones are not well understood. There are a number of theories about stone formation, which are described below.

Change in bile composition
In cholesterol stones, bile may undergo a change in composition – it becomes saturated with cholesterol, but deficient in bile salts.

Impaired gallbladder function
If the gallbladder doesn't empty completely (bile stasis), gallstones may form. The incidence of gallstones in patients on long-term parenteral nutrition and in women during pregnancy (both conditions where there is gallbladder stasis and incomplete emptying) suggests that gallbladder stasis has a role in the formation of gallstones.

Biliary infections
The majority of brown pigment stones contain Gram-negative bacteria. Bacterial action on bilirubin causes precipitation, and inflammatory debris can form a nidus (point of origin) for stone growth.

Increased enzyme activity
The effect of β-glucuronidase on bilirubin in the gallbladder appears to be connected to black pigment stone formation.

Other predisposing factors
Age
There is a steady increase with age; by age 75, 20% of men and 35% of women will have gallstones (Ransohoff & Gracie 1993).

Dietary links
- Obesity – this is a particular risk factor for women under 50 years of age, associated with increased cholesterol synthesis and excretion, and decreased gallbladder emptying
- Rapid weight loss
- Lack of fibre (longer intestinal transit time)
- Diets low in cholesterol but high in unsaturated fats – there is no evidence that directly links cholesterol intake to gallstones
- Moderate alcohol consumption and a vegetarian diet seem to protect against gallstones (Sherlock & Dooley 1997).

Gender
Gallstones are twice as common in women than in men, particularly under the age of 50 and especially during the postpartum period. Women who take the combined contraceptive pill or HRT have a higher incidence of gallstones. Oestrogen appears to increase biliary cholesterol saturation, which then decreases gallbladder motility.

Other
- Hereditary – relatives of patients with gallbladder disease have an increased frequency of gallstones
- Genetics – e.g. Native American Indians have a genetic predisposition
- Cirrhosis of the liver – 30% of patients have gallstones
- Diabetes
- Bowel resections.

In the West, the incidence is around 10%. It is lowest amongst black Africans and people from the Far East, and highest amongst American Indians. However, prevalence is changing as lifestyles and dietary habits change, especially with higher energy intakes.

Pathophysiology
Stones in the gallbladder are asymptomatic unless they migrate to the gallbladder neck where they become impacted, resulting in the transient blockage of the gallbladder and severe pain (biliary colic). Small stones tend to cause more acute problems, as they are more likely to migrate. Local pressure from gallstones can lead to tissue necrosis in the wall of the gallbladder, allowing bile to leak into the peritoneal cavity, causing peritonitis. Abscesses may form around or near a gallstone and the gallbladder may become acutely or chronically inflamed (cholecystitis).

Clinical presentation

Fewer than half the people with gallstones report any symptoms. For the others, they may experience digestive disturbances such as intolerance of fatty foods, or the most characteristic symptom of the severe pain of biliary colic (in the right upper quadrant, radiating into the back), associated with nausea and vomiting. If the stone lodges in the common bile duct, patients may be jaundiced.

Investigations

Most gallstones can be detected with ultrasound; oral cholecystograms are now only rarely used. Blood tests are not helpful and patients may not be pyrexial.

Medical and surgical management

Many patients with asymptomatic gallstones (i.e. those found incidentally) require no treatment and only a small proportion develop symptoms. However, some centres do offer prophylactic cholecystectomies, depending on the patient's preference and the analysis of risk factors. For patients with symptomatic cholelithiasis, treatment is dictated by the type, frequency and severity of the symptoms. There are two main methods of medical management:

- Physical methods, e.g. ERCP (most common form of treatment) and sphincterotomy (see p. 642) and, less commonly, lithotripsy in which shockwaves are used to disintegrate stones
- Chemical agents – oral bile acid therapy, e.g. ursodeoxycholic acid (UDCA), which dissolves cholesterol gallstones.

In the latter case, however, the recurrence rate is quite high, the therapy is slow to work and many patients are not suitable for this form of treatment (stones must be smaller than 15 mm). Side-effects include diarrhoea, skin rashes, headaches and fatigue.

For many patients with gallstones, surgeons will advise removal, either by laparoscopy or by an open procedure. Although surgery itself may carry higher risks than medical management, the risk of gallstones re-forming is non-existent. Every year in the UK, around 40 000 people undergo cholecystectomy (removal of the gallbladder) (Bryan 1998).

During the 1990s, minimal access surgical techniques ('keyhole' surgery) were rapidly developed and increasingly replaced traditional 'open' procedures. In laparoscopic cholecystectomy, three to four small incisions are made in the abdominal wall and the peritoneal cavity is inflated with carbon dioxide to allow the gallbladder to be visualized and removed via one of the small incisions.

The number of keyhole procedures carried out is continuing to rise as surgeons improve their techniques. In 1994, 80% of cholecystectomies were performed laparoscopically, compared with 30% in 1990–91 (Bryan 1998). The complication rates are usually lower than for open surgery; however, there is concern about the higher risk of biliary duct injury and bile leakage, due mostly to the surgeons' more restricted view (Down et al 1996).

Open cholecystectomies are still performed, when keyhole surgery fails or is contraindicated, because of infection or severe obesity. It is a safe and effective treatment for gallstones, especially when performed electively. The gallbladder is removed via a right subcostal incision and a closed drainage system is usually used to drain blood, serum and bile away from the gallbladder bed.

For older patients requiring sphincterotomy, research has shown that open surgery is preferable to endoscopy. More patients experience recurrent biliary symptoms following endoscopic procedures than following open surgery (Targarona et al 1996).

▶ Nursing management

Patients with gallstones

Nursing care should reflect the patient's symptoms. Patients with mild symptoms will not require hospitalization, but for those experiencing pain, and other distressing symptoms, more active management will be necessary. Patients may need to be fasted and, if nauseous and vomiting, have a nasogastric tube passed. This should be aspirated regularly and antiemetics administered. Intravenous fluids may be prescribed. Patients should be observed for signs of jaundice and the colour of stools should be checked. If there is jaundice, a daily dose of vitamin K may be administered parenterally to counteract any coagulation problems. As the symptoms improve, the nasogastric tube can be removed and clear fluids and then diet reintroduced.

Patients undergoing laparoscopic cholecystectomy

Preparation for laparoscopic surgery is similar to any other abdominal surgery, as is the immediate postoperative care (see Chs 22 and 29). Patients can commence fluids as soon as they are recovered from the anaesthetic, and diet can be started the following day.

Although often less painful than open procedures, patients should still be carefully observed for signs of complications, particularly bile leaks and obstructive jaundice. Pain should be regularly assessed using a pain assessment tool (see Ch. 7), and any sudden increases in pain should be reported to medical staff. Around 30% of patients experience distressing pain in the shoulder. This is referred pain due to nerve irritation from carbon dioxide and abdominal distension (Cason et al 1996) and a large proportion will still require strong analgesia in the form of opiates for the first 2–3 days. Only a very few patients experience vomiting or nausea.

The small incisions heal by primary intention and are rarely sutured, just covered with adhesive plasters – patients can carry out their usual hygiene routine the day after surgery. Many patients are discharged 1 or 2 days after surgery; some are carried out as day cases. Research has shown that patients return to their usual activities after 7–14 days (Cason et al 1996) (see Evidence-based Practice box 23.1). Given the early discharge, it is vital that patients are given clear information about how to identify possible complications such as jaundice, severe pain, the need for analgesia, as well as how to contact community nurses.

Patients undergoing open cholecystectomy

As with any surgery, patients should have a clear understanding of what to expect postoperatively. It is especially important that they know to expect an intravenous infusion, a closed system drain (e.g. Redivac type) and a subcostal incision around

EVIDENCE-BASED PRACTICE

23.1 Laparoscopic cholecystectomy: preoperative information and preparation and postoperative recovery

To enhance recovery and to enable a patient to make an informed decision, preoperative preparation for laparoscopic surgery must reflect postoperative events accurately. The media and many patient information leaflets depict recovery from laparoscopic cholecystectomy as relatively pain-free with minimal disruption to usual daily activities. Cason et al (1996) reviewed the available literature on patient expectations and experiences following laparoscopic cholecystectomy and found that, for many of them, recovery was more difficult, more painful and slower than they had been led to expect.

The studies identified the need for realistic, written information for patients about to undergo 'keyhole' surgery, highlighting the need for discharge analgesia and a slightly longer postoperative recovery period than previously indicated. Most patients resume their normal activities by 7–11 days postoperatively, and the majority return to work between 11 and 14 days.

It is vital that nurses establish what knowledge patients have about laparoscopic surgery and what their expectations are for the postoperative period. Useful and accurate information can then be tailored to the individual patient's needs.

Reference

Cason CL, Seidel SL, Bushmiaer M. Recovery from laparoscopic cholecystectomy procedures. AORN J 1996; 63(6): 1099–1116.

10–15 cm long. Immediate postoperative care is similar to any abdominal surgery (see Chs 22 and 29). Intravenous fluids should be administered until patients are able to tolerate fluids. They are often able to tolerate small amounts of clear fluids as soon as they have recovered from the anaesthetic, although in some, bowel sounds may not return for 1–2 days. They are usually able to drink normally the following day and start eating on day 2–3.

Pain management is vital for patients with an abdominal wound, to enable coughing and deep breathing and to avoid the risks of atelectasis and pneumonia (see Ch. 7). Patients will often have a patient-controlled analgesia (PCA) pump, to enable them to manage their own pain, to avoid the need for frequent intramuscular injections and to allow early mobilization. The wound and drain should be observed regularly and the nature and amount of any drainage noted and reported if excessive, especially if fresh blood or pus. The drain is usually removed after 2 or 3 days and the sutures at around days 5–7 (depending on the patient's age and healing capacity). Patients should be observed for signs of jaundice which may indicate that a gallstone is left in the bile duct.

Patients are usually discharged around 4–7 days postoperatively, depending on their age and fitness. They should be instructed to take regular periods of rest and avoid heavy lifting and strenuous activity for at least 4–6 weeks. They should also be encouraged to eat a normal diet, avoiding fats only if not tolerated. With an uncomplicated recovery, patients should be able to resume usual activities and work after 4–6 weeks.

ACUTE CHOLECYSTITIS

Acute cholecystitis is inflammation of the mucous membrane of the gallbladder wall.

Aetiology and epidemiology

The cause is usually a gallstone in the cystic duct – bile in the gallbladder irritates the gallbladder wall, causing inflammation. Other causes are bacterial infection and pancreatic enzymes. Because gallstones are more common in women, more women than men will present with cholecystitis.

Pathophysiology

Obstruction of the cystic duct by a gallstone causes the gallbladder to become distended. Bacteria proliferate and the wall of the gallbladder becomes first inflamed and then oedematous and thickened, even gangrenous. Empyema (pus in the gallbladder) may develop and cause severe sepsis. Complications include adhesions, abscess, fistula formation, perforation and peritonitis.

Clinical presentation

This can vary from mild tenderness over the right upper quadrant to fulminant gangrene of the gallbladder wall and septicaemia. Pain and tenderness are the most common features, and palpation of the right upper quadrant of the abdomen will cause severe pain and a sudden stop in inspiration (Murphy's sign). Unlike biliary colic, the pain lasts 30–40 minutes without relief, comes on suddenly and may be precipitated by late night eating or fatty foods. Patients may also get referred pain in the right scapula. Flatulence and nausea are common, but vomiting is unusual. Many patients will be pyrexial.

In older adults, gallstones may not cause pain or fever; mental confusion and an elevated alkaline phosphatase may be the only manifestations.

Investigations

The signs and symptoms of acute cholecystitis can be confused with other conditions, such as perforated peptic ulcer, acute pancreatitis, liver abscess or even myocardial infarction or pleurisy. An ultrasound will usually reveal gallstones. Blood tests may reveal a raised white cell count, as well as raised serum bilirubin, alkaline phosphatase and amylase levels.

Medical and surgical management

Initial treatment may involve intravenous fluids and antibiotics, analgesia and rest. The majority of patients will require a cholecystectomy. Surgeons are much more likely to operate during an acute attack than was previously the case, when it was common practice to delay surgery for 6 weeks following an attack. However, many patients suffered relapses during this period and, with antibiotic cover, the benefits of early surgery have been realized (Sherlock & Dooley 1997).

▶ Nursing management

The patient admitted with acute cholecystitis may be severely ill. The main nursing care priorities prior to surgery include:

- pain control, using an opiate such as pethidine – morphine can be effective, but should be used with caution, as it can cause spasm of the hepatopancreatic sphincter and so worsen the pain if there is a stone present
- hourly observations of vital signs until the condition stabilizes
- fasting patients and administration of i.v. fluids and a broad-spectrum antibiotic
- monitoring of patients' fluid balance
- if patients are vomiting, a nasogastric tube should be passed and aspirated and antiemetics given
- comfort measures, such as fresh bed linen, a cooling face cloth or assistance with hygiene, a dark, quiet room, etc.

Oral fluids can be reintroduced and i.v. fluids discontinued once the acute phase has passed. Antibiotics are usually given for 5 days. Patients may be very anxious about the suddenness and severity of their symptoms, and will have many questions about their diagnosis and likely treatment. Involving patients in the planning and delivery of care is vital.

CHRONIC CHOLECYSTITIS

Chronic cholecystitis is caused by the presence of gallstones but progresses more slowly than the acute disease. The gallbladder wall becomes thickened and fibrosed due to chronic irritation.

Clinical presentation
Patients will often have a long history of vague digestive disturbances such as mild abdominal discomfort and flatulence, especially after a heavy or fatty meal, and have a dull, aching pain in the epigastric or right upper quadrant area. Many patients tolerate their symptoms for many years, until their frequency and intensity increase and cause them to seek medical advice.

Management
Once the diagnosis has been confirmed and if the extent and nature of the patient's symptoms are severe, removal of the gallstones or the gallbladder itself is indicated. However, many patients require no treatment apart from education and information about the condition, particularly the need to report worsening symptoms (see Evidence-based Practice box 23.2).

ACALCULOUS CHOLECYSTITIS

Acute acalculous cholecystitis (inflammation of the gallbladder in the absence of stones) is much rarer than gallstone disease but also more serious. It is more difficult to diagnose accurately and mortality is much higher than that of gallstone disease (Chung 1995). The cause is unclear but is probably related to bile stasis and bacterial infection. Ultrasound will reveal a thickened gallbladder wall and treatment will involve a broad-spectrum antibiotic and cholecystectomy.

 EVIDENCE-BASED PRACTICE

23.2 The role of low-fat diets for patients with gallstones

Many people with, or suspected of having, gallstones modify their diet in an effort to prevent recurrence of symptoms or to relieve associated pain. The modifications may be initiated by the patient (following advice from friends, the media) or advised by a health professional. The majority of the modifications involve a low-fat diet. Madden (1992) looked at the advice given to patients by dieticians, and the research available to support that advice. Most dieticians said that they would advise a low-fat diet to avoid pain and other symptoms but there was little consensus over what amount of fat constituted a low-fat diet.

However, a meta-analysis (combining the results of many studies to produce an overview) of available studies found that patients with gallstones were no more likely to report intolerance to fatty food than people without gallstones. Studies have also found that the gallbladder contracts just as much following protein, elemental (e.g. amino acids, peptides, glucose – substances which are readily absorbed and leave a minimal residue in the intestine) or fat-free meals, as well as in response to the mere smell of a tasty meal.

The available evidence indicates that a low-fat diet is not necessary in the treatment of gallbladder disease, except when the bile ducts are obstructed. Patients with specific food intolerances will avoid those substances anyway, regardless of the advice they receive. A healthy diet, with high fibre, small amounts of refined carbohydrates, with a moderate energy restriction for the obese, seems to be much more useful advice for patients with gallbladder disease.

Reference
Madden A. The role of low fat diets in the management of gallbladder disease. J Hum Nutr Dietet 1992; 5: 267–273.

CHOLEDOCHOLITHIASIS AND CHOLANGITIS

Choledocholithiasis refers to gallstones in the common bile duct, and cholangitis is inflammation of the duct. Many people with bile duct stones are asymptomatic for long periods of time, as small stones can pass through the hepatopancreatic sphincter without complications. However, stones can cause cholangitis, or impact in the duct and cause biliary colic and obstructive jaundice. Complications include pancreatitis, liver abscess, biliary-enteric fistula (openings between the gallbladder and duodenum caused by pressure from a stone) and bile duct stricture, caused by inflammation, which can lead to biliary colic and obstructive jaundice.

Aetiology and epidemiology
Most bile duct stones arise in the gallbladder, but they can occur in the absence of a gallbladder (primary duct stones). Around

15% of patients with cholelithiasis have common bile duct stones and this proportion increases with age to around 50% for older patients.

Clinical presentation

The patient with bile duct stones classically presents with right upper quadrant pain, vomiting, fever and shivering (indicating cholangitis) and jaundice. Jaundice may be constant or intermittent as bile builds up and then forces past the stone. Patients characteristically report intermittent, intense pain which causes restlessness and vomiting.

In older patients, symptoms may be confined to sudden and unexplained mental and physical debility, thus making diagnosis more difficult.

Investigations

Ultrasound may detect gallstones in the gallbladder and dilated ducts. An ERCP may confirm the presence of stones in the ducts and remove them. Liver function tests (raised serum bilirubin, alkaline phosphatase) should reveal the extent of any obstruction.

Medical and surgical management

Unlike asymptomatic gallbladder stones, patients found to have bile duct stones will generally require removal because of the long-term risks of biliary obstruction. If patients have obstructive jaundice, drainage of the biliary system is needed.

Choledochostomy with T-tube

The duct is incised and the stones removed and this is often performed in conjunction with a cholecystectomy. Surgery or exploration of the bile duct may result in oedema of the walls of the ducts which can lead to obstruction. A T-shaped tube may be inserted into the duct to maintain patency (see Fig. 23.4). The stem part of the tube is brought out onto the abdominal surface and attached to a drainage bag.

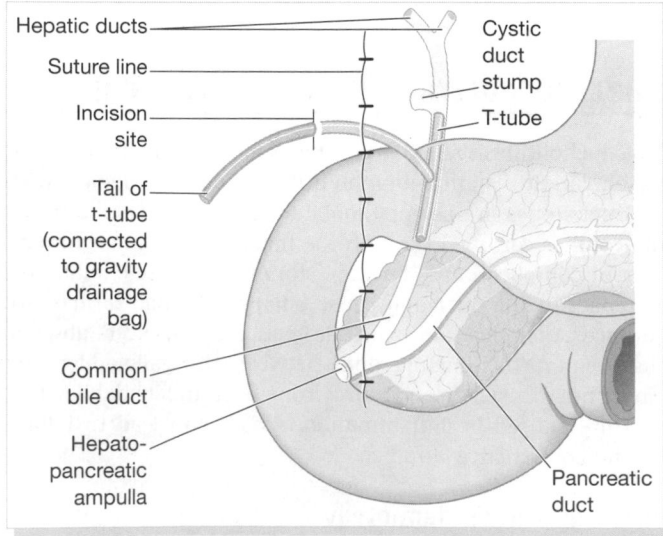

Figure 23.4 Position of a T-tube.

Endoscopic retrograde cholangiopancreatography (ERCP)

This treatment has rapidly become the method of choice for most bile duct stones, especially for sicker patients who might not survive a major surgical procedure. A sphincterotomy is performed by enlarging the hepatopancreatic sphincter using diathermy. Stones can then be extracted using either a balloon (to pull the stone) or a basket (to 'grab' the stone). The success rate for the procedure is extremely high for small stones (almost 100%) and up to 80% for larger stones (more than 15 mm in diameter).

Stenting and lithotripsy

For 10–20% of patients, bile duct stones cannot be extracted through a standard sphincterotomy and so mechanical lithotripsy and/or stenting (insertion of a small tube into the duct) is attempted. If an ERCP has been unsuccessful, a stent will be inserted to keep the duct patent and reduce the risks of complications and morbidity. With large stones (more than 15 mm in diameter), a mechanical lithotripsy technique using a basket to 'crush' the stones has become increasingly successful. A few patients may have laser or 'shock wave' lithotripsy to break up the stones.

▶ Nursing management: bile duct stones

Because of the possibility of a number of different causes for the symptoms, nurses have a vital role to play in assessing patients and providing information to aid an accurate diagnosis. Following admission and the initial management of the most pressing symptoms (e.g. pain, vomiting), a fuller assessment should be undertaken. Particular attention should be paid to any factors that worsen the symptoms (such as a rich or fatty meal) or help to alleviate them. The pattern, severity and type of pain experienced will provide useful information for diagnosis. A thorough assessment of the patient's past history relating to gastrointestinal function is important, looking for signs and symptoms of gallstones.

Patients may be fasted to prevent further vomiting, and intravenous fluids and antibiotics given as prescribed. Mouthwashes should be provided and assistance given if required. Vital signs should be recorded and patients observed for signs of fever and rigor. Pain management is vital (see p. 641). Urinalysis should be carried out, any signs of jaundice reported and fluid intake and output recorded.

The patient undergoing ERCP

Prior to undergoing an ERCP, it is vital that patients are given information about the procedure and what to expect; many are surprised and even horrified to hear that they won't be anaesthetized. A careful explanation of the procedure and the risks and benefits is usually sufficient to allay such fears.

Pre-procedure care includes:

- fasting for 6 hours to reduce the risk of gastric aspiration and to maximize the view through the endoscope
- an intravenous cannula for sedation and to provide i.v. access if required
- cross-matching and clotting screen obtained – haemorrhage is a potential complication of the procedure

- antibiotic cover, especially if a sphincterotomy is to be performed.

Patients usually receive intravenous sedation (e.g. diazemuls) prior to the procedure and this may be supplemented by a short-acting opioid analgesic such as fentanyl. Once the procedure is completed, vital signs should be monitored regularly until patients are stable and awake; any signs of worsening pain should be reported as they may indicate obstruction. Patients should be able to start drinking once they have recovered from the sedation. Ongoing nursing care involves observing for signs of complications such as haemorrhage, jaundice and infection.

The patient with a T-tube

If patients undergo choledochostomy or other bile duct surgery, a T-tube may be inserted to maintain patency of the duct (see Fig. 23.4). The tube will be attached to a drainage bag. In the first 24 hours, there may be 300–500 mL of bile drainage; this should decrease to less than 200 mL after 2–3 days. There may be a small amount of blood on the first day, but persistent bleeding or excessive drainage of bile should be reported to medical staff. To minimize loss of bile, the drainage bag should be positioned at the level of the abdomen. The tube should be well supported to reduce tension on it, to prevent inadvertent removal and prevent kinks in the drainage tube. The entry site should be covered with a sterile dressing and be observed regularly. Any bile spillage on the skin should be quickly cleaned with soap and water.

The T-tube can be clamped during meals to aid digestion and to assess duct patency – any increase in pain should be reported and the tube unclamped. The tube usually remains in place for around 10 days and will be removed following a T-tube cholangiogram to assess duct patency. Some patients may be discharged with a T-tube; they will usually require community nursing to check the drainage and the condition of the skin around the insertion site. T-tube removal is usually straightforward and quick but it may be quite painful, because the tube may adhere to the duct wall and require some effort to free it. A short-acting analgesia (such as fentanyl) or Entonox gas may help patients during the removal. Following removal, the entry site should be closely observed for bile leaks and a sterile dressing applied until it has healed. If skin excoriation occurs because of bile leaks, a hydrocolloid wafer should be applied to the skin to protect it and encourage healing.

TUMOURS OF THE BILIARY TRACT AND GALLBLADDER

Benign tumours of the gallbladder and ducts are rare. In the gallbladder they are usually only detected coincidentally, but in the duct they may cause obstruction. These tumours can be removed and surgery has a high curative rate.

Malignant tumours of the gallbladder (cholangiocarcinomas) are also rare. They are four times more common in women than in men, and there is a frequent association with gallstones and chronic cholecystitis, although there is no evidence of a causal link. Prognosis is poor, as many patients already have metastases,

and the 1-year survival rate is only around 15%. Treatment is usually palliative and consists of biliary stenting to prevent/relieve bile duct obstruction and jaundice.

The incidence of carcinoma of the bile duct seems to be rising (Sherlock & Dooley 1997) and affects slightly more men than women. There is an association with gallstones and ulcerative colitis but again no causative link. The most common feature is progressive jaundice. Prognosis is better than with gallbladder tumours. Surgery involves resection of the tumour and anastomosis of the duct to the duodenum (choledochoduodenostomy) or jejunum (choledochojejunostomy). Alternatively, a stent may be placed in the duct to maintain patency and relieve jaundice and itching. Radiotherapy and chemotherapy have not yet proven effective against cholangiocarcinomas. Death is usually caused by liver failure and/or sepsis rather than due to the tumour itself.

DISORDERS AFFECTING THE PANCREAS

The conditions affecting the pancreas are usually either inflammatory or neoplastic in nature although a small number may be traumatic or due to genetic disorders such as cystic fibrosis (see Ch. 20).

ACUTE PANCREATITIS

Acute pancreatitis refers to acute inflammation of the pancreas, characterized by upper abdominal pain, with raised serum levels of pancreatic enzymes. This is a potentially serious and even life-threatening disorder, depending on the degree of inflammation of the gland. With mild inflammation, patients are able to recover quickly following treatment. If the inflammation is severe and persistent, the damage to the pancreas becomes irreversible and the prognosis is much more serious.

Aetiology and epidemiology

Most cases of acute pancreatitis occur in association with gallstones or alcohol misuse; other causes include trauma (which may be postoperative or following ERCP), certain drugs (e.g. steroids), traumatic injuries and viral infections (mumps, Coxsackie B). However, in 20–30% of cases, an identifiable cause cannot be found.

Acute pancreatitis is becoming more common in the UK. The overall incidence in Scotland is higher than that in England and Wales, which may reflect a greater incidence of alcohol-related disease. Sex and age both influence the incidence of the disease. Where the disease is associated with gallstones, the female:male ratio is around 1.5:1, but where alcohol is the primary cause, this ratio is reversed. Because gallstone pancreatitis is more common than alcohol-related disease, rather more women than men suffer from acute pancreatitis.

Pathophysiology

Acute pancreatitis is an inflammatory response within the pancreatic tissue caused by premature activation of the digestive enzymes. The protective mechanism fails and the pancreatic enzymes begin to digest their own tissue, resulting in necrosis and haemorrhage and a vicious circle of more enzyme activation. The precise causes are still largely unknown and may be dependent on the aetiology:

- gallstone-induced pancreatitis – gallstones impact at the hepatopancreatic ampulla causing biliary (or duodenal) reflux
- alcoholic pancreatitis – ethanol may have a generalized effect on cell physiology or a specific effect on pancreatic secretions.

The risk of multiple organ failure (see Ch. 9) is high during the initial stages of severe disease and is a consequence of the inflammatory process and systemic effects of the activated enzymes. Heart action may be affected because of a fall in serum calcium, causing tetany and prolonged diastole. Later (after 1–2 weeks), systemic septic complications become more prevalent and account for around 80% of the deaths.

Complications of acute pancreatitis include fistula and abscess formation, ascites, duct strictures, diabetes mellitus and pseudocysts (thick-walled capsules within the pancreas which contain exudate, liquefied necrotic tissue and secretions).

Clinical presentation

Because of the vital role of the pancreas in digestion and endocrine function, many body systems can be affected. Table 23.6 summarizes the common presenting symptoms and treatment/ care of the patient with acute pancreatitis.

Other signs and symptoms include:

- tenderness and guarding over the epigastric and hypochondrial areas
- absent or diminished bowel sounds
- jaundice
- grey-blue discoloration of the flank (Grey Turner's sign) or around the umbilicus (Cullen's sign)
- hyperglycaemia and ketoacidosis.

Older adults may present with collapse and hyperglycaemia but without any pain.

Investigations

Acute pancreatitis is associated with many abnormal laboratory tests related to pancreatic, renal, hepatic and pulmonary function and clotting disorders:

Table 23.6 Acute pancreatitis – clinical presentation, possible causes and treatment/care

Clinical presentation	Possible causes	Treatment/care
Pain – constant and severe, becoming more diffuse. Degree of pain correlates with the extent of disease	• Pancreatic oedema • Irritation of the peritoneum • Biliary system obstruction • Chemical irritation of local nerves • Necrosis and inflammation	• Pain assessment • Regular i.m./i.v. pethidine • Reassurance and information
Respiratory problems including shallow breathing	• Anxiety • Pain on inspiration • Increased metabolic demands • Pleural effusions • Elevation of diaphragm • Surfactant production may be affected	• High flow rate humidified oxygen • Oxygen saturation levels • Blood gas analysis • Respiratory observations
Nausea, vomiting – persistent	• Paralytic ileus • Gastric irritation • Severe pain (may stimulate vomiting centre)	• Nasogastric tube • Antiemetic i.m./i.v.
Pyrexia (usually < 38.5°C)	• Initially due to inflammation • Other possibilities include peritonitis, cholecystitis, cholangitis or abscess • Systemic or pulmonary sepsis if prolonged	• Prophylactic antibiotic therapy • Regular temperature recordings
Anuria	• Hypovolaemia • Sodium and water retention (due to release of ADH) • Impaired renal perfusion (due to hypercoagulation)	• Prompt i.v. fluid replacement • Regular blood chemistry monitoring • Urinary catheter
Shock – hypotension, tachycardia	• Peripheral vasodilatation (caused by the release of trypsin) and loss of protein-rich fluid into the retroperitoneal space • Possible haemorrhage from necrosed blood vessels • Constant, severe pain	• Central venous access • Prompt i.v. fluid replacement (blood and plasma) • Regular vital signs and CVP measurement • Fluid balance chart • Regular strong analgesia

- serum amylase – five times the upper limit of normal is a strong indication of acute pancreatitis and reflects the degree of necrotic damage
- serum calcium – low calcium levels usually occur following a severe attack and are at their lowest around 5 days after onset
- clotting studies – to detect any coagulopathy
- oxygen saturation – should be monitored to detect the onset of pulmonary insufficiency.

Other abnormal tests include increased haematocrit, leucocytosis, raised serum urea and glucose and a fall in plasma phosphate and albumin.

The following radiological tests may be used:

- ultrasound for suspected gallstone-related disease
- contrast CT scan for pancreatic fluid collections (abscess or pseudocyst)
- ERCP (with sphincterotomy) to examine the pancreas and gallbladder, and remove stones (once the condition has stabilized).

Medical and surgical management

Early diagnosis and treatment are crucial in improving the outcome of an attack. The severity of the disease has been shown to correlate with the level of abnormality of laboratory test results and various prognostic systems, e.g. Ranson's signs (Misiewicz et al 1994) have been developed to aid diagnosis. These systems take into account various clinical signs and symptoms and enable clinicians to score the severity of the disease and decide on the most appropriate course of treatment.

For many patients, acute pancreatitis is a mild disease which subsides spontaneously in a short time. With bed rest, fasting, a nasogastric tube and analgesia, patients will recover without serious complications and further difficulties. However, 10–15% of patients with acute pancreatitis are extremely ill and require intensive care, directed towards:

- reduction of pancreatic secretions
- relief of pain
- correction or prevention of shock
- management of fluid, electrolyte and glucose imbalance
- prevention of infection.

At present, there is no pharmacological treatment known to be effective in treating pancreatitis.

Patients with gallstone-related disease may undergo a cholecystectomy or ERCP to reduce the risk of further attacks. If a patient develops a pseudocyst, this will be surgically drained (into the stomach) after approximately 6 weeks, when the cyst has developed a toughened wall.

▶ Nursing management

The nursing care required is dependent on the severity of the disease. A thorough and speedy assessment of overall condition is vital in the early stages of the admission.

Immediate assessment and care

A comprehensive nursing assessment will assist in the confirmation of both the diagnosis and severity of the disease. The patient's condition can deteriorate rapidly and so regular and frequent observations of vital signs and general appearance should be carried out, including central venous pressure (CVP) readings, respiratory rate, rhythm and depth, as well as signs of peripheral cyanosis. Patients may be in shock (see Ch. 9) and require i.v. fluid replacement. A urinary catheter should be inserted to facilitate accurate monitoring of fluid balance. Pain relief should be administered to reduce (often very severe) pain. Oxygen should administered at the prescribed rate and saturation levels monitored (see Ch. 9 for more information about shock and multisystem failure and Ch. 31 for caring for critically ill patients).

Patients and significant others will need a great deal of support throughout their illness but the early stages are likely to be particularly traumatic. Clear, simple and short explanations should be made of all the procedures and care – patients with acute anxiety are likely to have short attention spans.

Intermediate care

The patient with acute pancreatitis is likely to experience pain in the abdomen and back, often severe in nature. The location, intensity and nature of the pain should be noted and recorded, as well as any precipitating and relieving factors. Analgesia should be given regularly. Pethidine is usually prescribed; morphine should be used only with care as it may stimulate spasm of the biliary and pancreatic ducts, thereby increasing the pain. PCA may be used as it has been shown to be more successful in achieving pain control than nurse-initiated intramuscular analgesia (McConnell & Lewis 1991). Patients should be kept strictly nil by mouth to decrease pancreatic stimulation and diminish the pain. Even ice chips may aggravate the pain by stimulating pancreatic enzymes. Positioning patients correctly may also help to relieve the discomfort – either lying on the side in a knee-chest position or upright with the trunk flexed. Pain management is discussed in more detail in Chapter 7.

Patients' fluid balance needs careful, ongoing assessment. Their response to fluid and blood replacement should be monitored, through observations of vital signs, signs of peripheral and pulmonary oedema, and the condition of skin and mucous membranes. Any signs of hypocalcaemia, hypokalaemia and hyperglycaemia (see Ch. 8) should be reported to medical staff. Blood glucose levels should be monitored every 1–4 hours. Insulin may be prescribed and is usually administered intravenously.

Patients are also likely to experience nausea and vomiting and a nasogastric tube should be passed to assist in the relief of these distressing symptoms. Regular aspiration will decrease pancreatic secretions and gastric distension, thus promoting comfort. Antiemetics should also be administered. Patients will need frequent nasal and mouth care to minimize discomfort whilst they are nil by mouth and the nasogastric tube is in situ. Petroleum jelly or other moisturizing cream can be used on the lips to prevent painful cracking.

Continuing care

Respiratory difficulties are a common problem for patients with acute pancreatitis, due to acid–base abnormalities, a distended abdomen or pain on inspiration, as well as immobility. If possible, patients should be nursed in a semi-upright position to promote lung expansion. They should be referred to a physiotherapist and taught the importance of deep breathing and coughing exercises, and their pain should be sufficiently well controlled to enable them to carry these out regularly. If patients need continuous oxygen, this should be warmed and humidified to prevent drying of the respiratory tract and secretions.

Patients are kept nil by mouth until abdominal pain and tenderness have subsided. Small amounts of oral fluids are introduced slowly and increased as patients are able to tolerate. Diet is introduced only when patients are able to take oral fluids without any increase in pain or tenderness. Initially, the diet should be primarily carbohydrates, and small, regular meals should be provided. Some patients may need pancreatic enzyme replacement, such as pancreatin. These must be taken with food (and sometimes anticholinergics and antacids) to reduce the effect of gastric acid on the pancreatic enzyme preparation. If patients are unable to eat for a long period, total parenteral nutrition may be required (see Ch. 11).

The convalescent period from acute pancreatitis can be prolonged. Patients should rest and only resume normal activities slowly. It is important that patients understand the nature and likely cause of their disease, and the part they can play in their recovery. A good understanding of their nutritional needs and the impact of alcohol is vital. There is no clinical proof of the need for a low-fat diet or other dietary restrictions during the recovery phase, except for abstinence from alcohol (Forsmark & Toskes 1995). However, patients may have become undernourished and they should be given clear verbal and written instructions about how to achieve a high-protein, high-carbohydrate diet and to avoid any foods which they can no longer easily tolerate, e.g. spicy or fatty foods (see Reflective Practice box 23.2).

CHRONIC PANCREATITIS

Chronic pancreatitis is a progressive, inflammatory, destructive disease which is characterized by varying degrees of pancreatic

---

R|Я **REFLECTIVE PRACTICE**

23.2 Nursing a patient with acute pancreatitis

Mrs Chung is a 52-year-old woman, admitted to a general surgical ward as an emergency. She is in severe pain and appears shocked. The provisional diagnosis is acute pancreatitis.

- Why do you think Mrs Chung is experiencing such severe pain?
- What nursing actions, both drug- and non-drug-related, could you use to provide some relief?
- How will you evaluate the effectiveness of the actions you have taken?
- What is the analgesia of choice, and why, for patients with suspected gallstone-related pancreatitis?

---

insufficiency that persist even after the primary cause or factors have been removed. This results in decreased production of enzymes and bicarbonate and malabsorption of fats and proteins.

Aetiology and epidemiology

Chronic alcoholism is the most frequent cause of the disease. Other causes include hyperparathyroidism (see Ch. 17), congenital abnormalities and pancreatic trauma. The disease is uncommon but increasing, particularly in the Western world where an increasing proportion is related to alcohol misuse. Chronic pancreatitis usually begins in adult life (35–50 years), and in Europe 80% of the cases occur in men (Lendrum 1994).

Pathophysiology

The pancreas is progressively destroyed by repeated attacks of (usually mild) acute pancreatitis. This process results in scarring and calcification of the pancreatic tissue and the damage is irreversible, affecting both endocrine and exocrine functions. The degree of damage and the intensity of the attack are proportional to the amount of continuing inflammation or the frequency of the attacks. The digestion of fat is affected most severely and consequently a high-fat diet stimulates water and electrolyte secretion, which produces diarrhoea and calorie malnutrition. The action of bacteria on faecal fat produces flatus, fatty stools (steatorrhoea) and abdominal cramps. Patients may develop diabetes mellitus because of damage to the insulin-producing cells.

Clinical presentation

Pain is the most prominent feature of chronic pancreatitis – dull to severe, usually in the epigastric region, and often radiating into the back. The frequent passage of foul fatty stools is also common. The presence of obvious oil in the stools (due to the presence of unabsorbed triglycerides) is very indicative of pancreatic malabsorption. Anorexia, vomiting and malabsorption means that most patients will report weight loss. Between 10 and 30% of patients develop overt diabetes mellitus, and jaundice may develop due to inflammation or duct blockage.

Investigations

Chronic pancreatitis should be suspected whenever epigastric pain, steatorrhoea and weight loss occur together. If a plain abdominal X-ray shows calcification of the pancreas, further tests should be unnecessary. Ultrasound and ERCP may be used to determine the size and nature/damage of the pancreas and ducts and to detect the presence of any cysts.

Medical and surgical management

Management centres on the alleviation of symptoms. Non-narcotic analgesia should be tried first but opiate analgesia may be needed as the disease progresses. Enzyme supplements may also help, as well as anticholinergics and antacids (to decrease gastric acid stimulus). Pancreatic stones and strictures may be treated by endoscopy, extraction or stenting.

The role of surgery in the treatment of chronic pancreatitis remains controversial. Some physicians maintain that surgery has no place in treatment, believing that avoidance of alcohol and adequate medical therapy will suffice without the risk of an operation. In contrast, some surgeons believe that only very radical surgery offers adequate pain control (Venables 1994).

▶ Nursing management

As with acute pancreatitis, management of a patient's symptoms is central to nursing care. Pain management is complicated as patients are likely to require analgesia over a long period, even for the rest of their lifetime. Therefore, the lowest effective dose of analgesia should be used, in conjunction with a pain assessment tool, to ensure that patients are pain-free. As the disease progresses, pain levels may increase; this is complicated by the fact that patients will develop a tolerance to a drug, which will necessitate larger doses and increasing strengths of analgesia.

A thorough nutritional assessment is vital to ensure that nutritional needs are being met and to identify strategies to address any deficiencies. This should usually be in conjunction with specialist advice from a dietician or nutrition nurse specialist. Patients are likely to need to take pancreatic enzyme supplements long-term, as well as vitamin supplements (A, B_{12}, D, K and folic acid). Malabsorption and weight loss are addressed through a gradual increase in dietary fat; whilst this serves to increase steatorrhoea moderately, it greatly increases the fat absorption and consequently patients' calorific intake (Lendrum 1994).

In the long term, the key for patient care is total abstinence from alcohol (see Ethical Issues box 23.1). It is also vital that patients fully understand the disease, the possible complications, especially the signs and symptoms of diabetes mellitus, and the importance of monitoring the adequacy of their diet, through regular weight checks.

TUMOURS OF THE PANCREAS

Patients are only usually aware of the disease once it has reached an advanced stage and prognosis is very poor; average survival time is 5–6 months, and of those with resectable lesions, around 7% are alive at 5 years. However, advances are being made in understanding and potential treatments that may offer a better quality of life and potentially better survival rates.

Aetiology and epidemiology

The only proven aetiological factor is the link with cigarette smoking. A 40-year study of 34 000 male doctors (Doll et al 1994) in the UK found a threefold increase in incidence amongst heavy smokers. Patients who have chronic pancreatitis have also been found to have a higher rate of pancreatic cancer (Imrie 1996). Although diabetes is present in a proportion of patients with pancreatic adenocarcinoma, there is little clear evidence that diabetes itself predisposes to pancreatic cancer.

In the UK, 3% of cancers are pancreatic, mostly in the head of the pancreas (Imrie 1996). There has been a slow and steady rise in the incidence of the disease during the 20th century, which is largely due to an ageing population. The average age for patients with cancer of the head of pancreas is the late 60s. It is very rare in those under 25 and uncommon under the age of 45.

Pathophysiology

In 75–80% of cases, the adenocarcinoma is a duct cell cancer which spreads by local peripancreatic invasion or by lymphatic or venous channels. There is a high degree of metastatic spread and, at the time of diagnosis, only 20% of patients will have disease confined to the pancreas.

Clinical presentation

The common presenting features are:

- weight loss, anorexia and jaundice
- pain (poorly localized)
- nausea and vomiting
- diarrhoea, weakness, fatigue or epigastric bloating
- smaller numbers may present with acute pancreatitis or diabetes.

Investigations

- *Blood tests* – patients typically have a raised serum bilirubin and alkaline phosphatase (see Table 23.1). If the degree of bile duct obstruction is high, the alkaline phosphatase may be more than 2000 IU/L and the increase in bilirubin may be very high (around 44 μmol/L)
- *Ultrasound or CT scan* will assist with the diagnosis and staging of the tumour

---

 ### ETHICAL ISSUES

23.1 An alcoholic patient with chronic pancreatitis – a 'lifestyle disease'?

Chronic pancreatitis can be a very debilitating disease and require many hospital visits and treatment. Many patients who have chronic pancreatitis have misused alcohol for many years and the majority are cared for by health care workers who are not experts in substance misuse. Many 'lay' people may think that such patients 'deserve' their ill fortune; that they have brought it on themselves. Even for health care workers, it may be difficult to understand how a person can

destroy their own pancreas through years of alcohol misuse. It is easy to judge these patients harshly.

Student activities

- What are your views on patients with so-called 'lifestyle' diseases?
- In this age of scarce health care resources, what access should patients have to treatment and care, especially if they continue to drink alcohol?
- What local facilities exist to help and support patients who are attempting to stop drinking?

- *ERCP with biopsy* – to assess the level of duct involvement
- *Laparoscopic assessment* – to predict the level of resectability
- *Magnetic resonance imaging* – to outline bile and pancreatic ducts; technical improvements may reduce the need for ERCP in future.

Medical and surgical management

For many patients with advanced disease and distant metastases, the prognosis is very poor and management revolves around relief of symptoms rather than curative therapy. Some centres offer chemotherapy to increase survival times; others advocate radiotherapy plus chemotherapy. However, the overall survival rate is still poor (Imrie 1996). Since most of the patients have obstructive jaundice, endoscopic placement of stents to relieve jaundice and pain is an important part of symptom management. This procedure has a lower complication and mortality rate than bypass surgery and the patients spend less time in hospital. However, many patients require repeat stenting because of blockage.

For patients with intractable pain, a chemical or surgical procedure may be performed to block the nerve pathways (splanchnicectomy) and so reduce the pain (see Ch. 7).

The use of chemotherapy and radiotherapy for pancreatic cancers remains controversial. However, there are early indications that combined therapy, in the form of intraoperative or post-resection radiotherapy and chemotherapy (with 5-fluorouracil), is the way forward for both management and treatment (Uzer & Lehman 1998).

Studies have identified oestrogen-binding proteins in pancreatic carcinoma tissue and low serum testosterone levels. Consequently, the use of anti-androgen drugs is a recent addition to the range of drug therapies for pancreatic cancer (similar to the use of tamoxifen for breast cancer). The use of flutamide has been shown to double average survival times, from 6 months to 12, is well tolerated by patients and has minimal side-effects (Greenway 1998).

For some patients, surgery is an option. A variety of procedures are possible, depending on the stage, location and size of the tumour. The surgery has a high morbidity and this has to be balanced against the possible outcomes. For many patients, surgery is purely palliative, to relieve jaundice or intestinal obstruction.

Surgical procedures

Choledochoduodenostomy

This involves joining the bile duct directly to the duodenum (anastomosis). The tumour is left intact. This is the preferred palliative procedure to relieve jaundice and/or duodenal obstruction, as it is relatively straightforward and confers the most advantages.

Whipple's procedure (pancreatoduodenectomy – see Fig. 23.5)

This procedure is indicated if the tumour is confined to the head of the pancreas. It involves a wide resection of the head of the pancreas and adjacent duodenum, including local lymph tissue, and usually includes a partial gastrectomy. Mortality has fallen dramatically during the last two decades but is still around 10% (Bircher et al 1999).

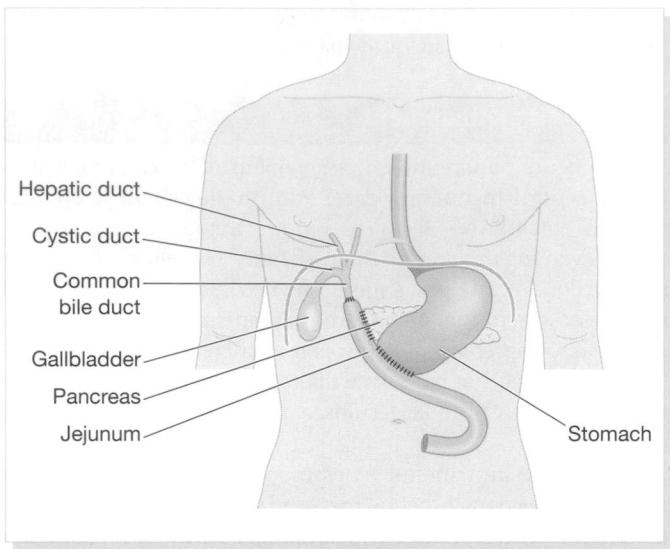

Figure 23.5 Whipple's procedure for cancer of the head of the pancreas.

► Nursing management

Cancer of the head of the pancreas

Nursing care focuses on treatment of symptoms to enhance patients' quality of life. Pain is the main problem for patients with pancreatic tumours. As the disease progresses, pain may become severe and non-opiate analgesia will be inadequate. Specialist advice from pharmacists, anaesthetists and pain management specialists at this stage is vital (for the care of jaundiced patients, see p. 628). As the disease progresses, other complications may develop, such as diabetes, sepsis and pancreatic insufficiency. New enzyme preparations (pellets and micro-capsules), which increase the availability of enzymes in the intestine, allow patients to maintain a normal dietary fat intake, and thus the calorific content and palatability, whilst preventing diarrhoea and steatorrhoea and increasing quality of life. The calorific content and appeal of the patients' diet is vital, as anorexia and weight loss are common. Small, regular meals should be offered, and patients' personal likes and dislikes should be discussed and taken into consideration. Advice from a dietician will assist in the provision of adequate nutrients.

Patients and their families will need considerable support, information and practical assistance (see Chs 7, 33 and 34 for further information).

The patient undergoing a Whipple's procedure

As well as the usual care for any major abdominal surgical procedure (see Chs 22 and 29), patients need particularly thorough preoperative preparation, as many will be over 65 and in a poor state of health. This preparation includes:

- comprehensive information about the nature of the operation, the benefits and risks and any alternatives, as well as the intended outcome (i.e. curative or palliative)
- nutritional status should be as optimal as is possible, through a high-calorie diet prior to the operation

- good hydration, through intravenous fluid administration if necessary
- parenteral vitamin K and a blood transfusion (if jaundiced).

Many postoperative complications would be expected in this age group (cardiovascular, septic or embolic complications), but these patients are also susceptible to hepatorenal syndrome, especially if they are jaundiced. This is a poorly understood condition characterized by sudden renal failure as a result of intrarenal vasoconstriction. Therefore, intravenous fluids will be administered (usually 5% dextrose) and hourly urine measurements should be recorded. Jaundiced patients may experience delayed wound healing, so frequent wound assessments should be carried out.

Referral to a Macmillan nurse specialist (see Ch. 34) will give patients additional support information and practical help, especially following discharge from hospital. Once at home, patients are likely to need ongoing practical and psychological support from community nurses.

TUMOURS OF THE ISLETS CELLS

These rare tumours may be gastrin-secreting (gastrinoma) or insulin-secreting (insulinoma) and arise in the islets of Langerhans.

GASTRINOMA

A gastrinoma is a tumour of the delta cells of the islets of Langerhans which secretes gastrin. This causes gastric hypersecretion and intractable peptic ulceration, a condition known as Zollinger–Ellison syndrome. They can occur in both adults and children and affect both sexes equally. The majority of patients complain of ulcer-type abdominal pain and/or diarrhoea. The most effective treatment is excision of the gastrinoma before it has metastasized. In the past, gastrectomy was the only curative option but the advent of new drugs, such as omeprazole, has negated the need for such radical surgery.

INSULINOMAS

Insulinomas arise from the beta cells of the islets of Langerhans and are found equally in both sexes and at any age, although most are first diagnosed in middle age.

Symptoms are related to hypoglycaemia, which develops after fasting or strenuous exercise. Hypoglycaemia usually develops gradually and the effect is mainly on brain cells which are very sensitive to glucose deficiencies. Initially, patients will be apprehensive, restless and hungry; the symptoms develop into weakness, loss of coordination, disorientation and tremors. Some patients become comatose or suffer epileptic fits. Prolonged or repeated attacks can lead to dementia, permanent brain damage, or even death. Mistaken diagnosis of a psychiatric or neurological problem is not uncommon.

Prompt treatment of the hypoglycaemic attack is necessary. The tumour may be treated with chemotherapy or, preferably, with surgical resection. Surgery has a high curative rate. Without treatment, death is usually inevitable, due to untreated hypoglycaemia.

SUMMARY: MAIN POINTS

- Alcohol misuse often plays a key role in the development of liver and pancreatic disorders and presents a complex issue for individuals, their family and nurses to deal with.

- There are five main types of hepatitis virus – measures to control the spread of HAV and HEV focus on handwashing, while the other three types (B, C, D) are spread through contact with blood and body fluids.

- Cirrhosis is most commonly the result of chronic alcohol misuse. Portal hypertension and bleeding oesophageal varices are two life-threatening complications.

- Patient education is a major part of nursing care for most patients with liver disease because of the long-term nature of the liver problems.

- Paracetamol overdose is a major cause of acute liver failure and requires prompt treatment.

- Risk factors for gallstone formation include obesity, female gender, multiparity and advancing age.

- Acute cholecystitis may cause pain, nausea, vomiting and fluid and electrolyte problems.

- Laparoscopic cholecystectomy (minimal access surgery) is commonly performed to remove inflamed and diseased gallbladders.

- Biliary colic (severe, visceral pain) is caused by the passage of a calculus through the bile duct.

- Acute pancreatitis can result in severe pain, fluid and electrolyte problems, and metabolic disruptions. It may resolve spontaneously, but mortality is high for severe forms.

- Care for the patient with acute pancreatitis focuses on pain management, i.v. fluid administration to prevent or treat shock, and resting the pancreas by fasting.

- Chronic pancreatitis is progressive and is commonly caused by alcohol misuse or gallstones. It results in pain, malabsorption, steatorrhoea and possibly diabetes mellitus.

- Cancer of the pancreas is insidious and has a poor prognosis. Surgery may be possible with adjuvant drug or radiotherapy.

SELF-TEST: CRITICAL THINKING ACTIVITIES

1 What are the priorities of care for a patient with alcohol-induced cirrhosis, and why? How were they achieved? What discharge education should the patient receive and why?

2 A female patient in her 50s asks you for advice about living with gallstones – what advice will you give her?

3 A young woman tells you that her boyfriend (with whom she has a sexual relationship) has been diagnosed with hepatitis B. She is worried about him and the risks to her own health. What advice and information will you give her?

4 A patient you are caring for is going to be discharged with a T-tube in situ, following bile duct surgery.

— What information and instructions will you give to the patient, and why?

— What specific signs and symptoms should the patient look out for, and what action should the patient take if any of these arise?

5 Mr Ahmed, a 66-year-old married man, has been discharged from hospital following palliative surgery for tumour of the head of the pancreas.

— If you were the district nurse, what would you have in mind when visiting Mr Ahmed for the first time?

— What long-term care might Mr Ahmed need from you and your colleagues?

 FURTHER READING

Bassett C. Medical investigations 2: ERCP. Br J Nurs 1997; 6(8): 460–461.

Brodrick RL. Preventing complications in acute pancreatitis. Dim Crit Care Nurs 1991; 10(5): 262–270.

Budden L, Vink R. Paracetamol overdose: pathophysiology and nursing management. Br J Nurs 1996; 5(3): 145–152.

Farthing MJG (ed). Clinical challenges in gastroenterology. London: Martin Dunitz; 1996.

Karnik A, Freeman JW. Acute liver failure. Care Crit Ill 1998; 14(5): 148–154.

Marx JF. Understanding the varieties of viral hepatitis. Nursing 1998; 28(7): 43–50.

O'Shea D, Wynne HA. Disorders of the liver, gallbladder and pancreas. Rev Clin Gerontol 1996; 6: 231–240.

Rutishauser S. Physiology and anatomy: a basis for nursing and healthcare. Edinburgh: Churchill Livingstone; 1997

Williamson L. Self-destruction in the pancreas. Nurs Times 1998; 94(29): 22–28.

Worman HJ. Common laboratory tests in liver diseases. Online. Available: http://cpmcnet.columbia.edu/dept/gi/labtests.html. 20 Aug 2002.

 USEFUL ADDRESSES

Addaction
Tel: 020 7251 5860
Offers community-based services to people who are addicted to alcohol or drugs, offers health information on safe sex and the risks of multiple needle use and HIV/AIDS infection

Alcoholics Anonymous
PO Box 1
Stonebow House
York YO1 2NJ
Tel: 01904 644026
Helpline: 020 7352 3001 (10am–10pm, 7 days)
Provides information through publications and support for people through self-help groups

British Association of Cancer Patients and their Families and Friends (BACUP)
BACUP
3 Bath Place
Rivington Street
London EC2A 3DR
Tel: 0171 696 9003
Helpline: 0808800 1234
Charity consisting of a team of oncology nurses offering emotional support, advice and information by post or phone

British Liver Trust
Ransomes Europark
Ipswich
Suffolk IP3 9QG
Tel: 01473 276326
Helpline: 0808 800 1000
Website: www.british-liver-trust.org.uk/home.asp
Works to help adult liver patients, their families and carers, by providing information and support services, and fostering medical research

Digestive Disorders Foundation
2 Andrew's Place
London MW1 4LB
Tel: 020 7486 0341
Website: www.digestivedisorders.org.uk/leaflets
Produces a range of leaflets for patients on digestive disorders which can be bought by professionals

Drinkline
Tel: 0800 917 8282 (9am–11pm, Mon–Fri; 6pm–11pm Sat–Sun)
Telephone helpline offering support, advice and information to drinkers and their family and friends. Not a counselling line

USEFUL WEBSITES

www.cancer.gov/cancer_information/ – cancer information supplied by the National Cancer Institute; contains information on cancer of the liver, gallbladder and pancreas

www.cdc.gov/ncidod/diseases/hepatitis/ – information on viral hepatitis supplied by the National Center for Infectious Diseases

REFERENCES

Acheson D (chair). Independent inquiry into inequalities in health report. Online. Available: http://www.archive.official-documents.co.uk/document/doh/ih/ih.htm. 1998.

Ahmed M, Elias E. Treatment for hepatitis C. In: Farthing MJG, ed. Clinical challenges in gastroenterology. London: Martin Dunitz; 1996: 188–210.

Bateson MC, Bouchier I A. Clinical investigations in gastroenterology. Dortrecht: Kluwer Academic; 1997.

Bircher J, Benhamou J-P, McIntyre N et al. Oxford textbook of clinical hepatology, 2nd edn. Oxford: Oxford University Press; 1999.

Bridger S, Henderson K, Glucksman E, Ellis A, Henry J, Williams R. Deaths from low dose paracetamol poisoning. Br Med J 1998; 361: 1724–1725.

Bryan J. Cut above the others. Health Service J 1998; 108: 12–13.

Cason CL, Seidel SL, Bushmiaer M. Recovery from laparoscopic cholecystectomy procedures. AORN J 1996; 63(6): 1099–1116.

Chung SC. Acute acalculous cholecystitis. Postgrad Med 1995; 98(3): 199–204.

Department of Health. The health of the nation. London: HMSO; 1992.

Department of Health. Guidance for clinical health care workers: protection against infection with blood-borne viruses. London: Department of Health; 1998.

Department of Health. Saving lives: our healthier nation. London: Department of Health; 1999a.

Department of Health. Making a difference. London: Department of Health; 1999b.

Doll R, Peto R, Wheatley K, Gray R, Sutherland I. Mortality in relation to smoking: 40 years' observation on male British doctors. Br Med J 1994; 309(6959): 901–911.

Down SH et al. A systematic review of the effectiveness and safety of laparoscopic cholecystectomy. Ann R Coll Surg England 1996; 78(3.II): 241–323.

Ellender R. Hepatic arterial perfusion scintography. Prof Nurse 1999; 14(10): 695–699.

Everhart JE. Contributions of obesity and weight loss to gallstone disease. Ann Intern Med 1993; 119(10): 1029–1035.

Forsmark CE, Toskes PP. Acute pancreatitis – medical management. Crit Care Clin North Am 1995; 11(2): 295–306.

Gambert SR. Alcohol abuse: medical effects of heavy drinking in late life. Geriatrics 1997; 52(6): 30–37.

Greenway BA. Effects of flutamide on survival in patients with pancreatic cancer: results of a prospective, randomised, double-blind, placebo controlled trial. Br Med J 1998; 316: 1935–1938.

Health and Safety Executive. Control of substances hazardous to health regulations (COSSH). London: HMSO; 1999.

Hicks Keen J. Hepatic and biliary disorders and pancreatic disorders. In: Swearingen PL, Ross GR. Manual of medical-surgical nursing care, 4th edn. St Louis: Mosby; 1999.

Imrie CW. Pancreatic cancer. In: Farthing MJG, ed. Clinical challenges in gastroenterology. London: Martin Dunitz; 1996: 152–165.

Kowdley KV. Update on therapy for hepatobiliary diseases. Nurse Pract 1996; 21(7): 78–86.

Lee WM, Williams R. Acute liver failure. Cambridge: Cambridge University Press; 1997.

Lendrum R. Chronic pancreatitis. In: Misiewicz JJ, Pounder RE, Venables CW, eds. Diseases of the gut and pancreas, 2nd edn. Oxford: Blackwell Science Publications; 1994: 441–453.

McConnell E, Lewis LW. Managing the patient with pancreatitis. Nursing 1991; 21(11): 98–102.

Misiewicz JJ, Pounder RE, Venables CW. Diseases of the gut and pancreas, 2nd edn. Oxford: Blackwell Science Publications; 1994.

Mudd S, Boyd C, Brower K et al. Alcohol withdrawal and related nursing care in older adults. J Gerontol Nurs 1994; 20(10): 17–27.

Oyefeso A, Ghodse H. Addictive behaviours. In: Rawaf S, Bahl V, eds. Assessing health needs of people from minority ethnic groups. London: Royal College of Physicians; 1998: 141–162.

Paton A. ABC of alcohol. London: British Medical Journal Publishing; 1994.

Randolph A, Jonas M. Fulminant hepatic failure. Online. Available: http://medicina.ub.es/All-Net/english/gipage/liver/. 1998.

Ransohoff DF, Gracie WA. Treatment of gallstones. Ann Intern Med 1993; 119: 606–611.

Rogers R, Salvage J, Cowell R. Nurses at risk: a guide to health and safety at work, 2nd edn. London: Macmillan Press; 1998.

Royal College of Nursing (RCN). Hepatitis: guidelines from the Royal College of Nursing. London: RCN; 1998.

Sherlock S, Dooley J. Diseases of the liver and biliary system, 10th edn. Oxford: Blackwell Scientific Publications; 1997.

Smales C. Hepatitis: symptoms, treatment and prevention. Nurs Times 1998; 94(44): 58–60.

Targarona EM, Ayuso RMP, Bordas JM. Randomised trial of endoscopic sphincterotomy with gallbladder left in situ versus open surgery for common bile duct calculi in high risk patients. Lancet 1996; 347: 926–929.

Tweed SH. Identifying the alcoholic client. Nurs Clin North Am 1989; 24(1): 13–32.

Uzer V, Lehman M. Pancreatic cancer. In: Bone RC, ed. Current practice of medicine. New York: Churchill Livingstone; 1998: vol 4, ch 22.

Venables CW. Surgery for gallstones. In: Misiewicz JJ, Pounder RE, Venables CW. Diseases of the gut and pancreas, 2nd edn. Oxford: Blackwell Science Publications; 1994: ch 38.

24 Nursing patients with urinary disorders

Hilary Fanning

> 'I was on placement with a practice nurse and we had to test a patient's urine. When I found it had protein in it the nurse explained that this might indicate early renal disease. I must look up what all the tests mean, I've never really understood it.'
>
> (Student nurse)

THIS CHAPTER WILL HELP YOU

- Describe the normal structure and function of the urinary system

- Understand the effects that structural or functional derangements have on normal urinary system function

- Describe the common investigations of the urinary tract and the care needed by patients

- Justify nursing interventions pertinent to the management of patients with disordered function of the urinary system

- Identify deficits in your knowledge base and plan strategies to address these

- Describe the role of the renal nurse specialist.

KEYWORDS

Albuminuria	Micturition
Anuria	Nocturia
Catheterization	Oliguria
Compliance	Renal
Dialysis	Renal failure
Diuretics	Suprapubic catheterization
Dysuria	
Glomerular filtration rate	Uraemia
	Uraemic syndrome
Haematuria	Urinalysis
Homeostasis	Urinary tract/system

INTRODUCTION

Nursing care for those with disorders of the urinary tract may be broadly differentiated into the care of patients who have disorders of renal function and those who have functional derangements of the urinary tract. In either case, there is a need for the nurse to be familiar with the anatomy and physiology of the urinary system in order both to understand and to anticipate the likely pathway of medical and nursing care progression. For this reason, some coverage of renal (relating to the kidney) physiology is included; however, readers requiring more detail should consult a more specialized physiology text. There is also a requirement that nurses understand the ways in which disordered function may affect patients' lives, and their ability to perform self-defined roles. Patients who present with a disordered renal and/or urinary tract function may have conditions that are highly amenable to treatment and that will resolve completely. Conversely, they may present with conditions that are persistent and for which no cure is available. The particular skills required from nurses who care for these individuals thus involve the ability to provide both critical care in the short term and care that supports patients' attempts to redefine the nature of their existence in the long term.

For nurses who choose to work within the renal specialty, the scope of practice is extensive. The current drive to increase the availability of haemodialysis facilities in locations close to patients' homes (satellite dialysis units) has led to the evolution of dialysis provision as a nurse-led service. Similarly, with peritoneal dialysis, nurses have responsibility for patient education, monitoring and audit of response to treatment. Like other contexts of care where patients have a chronic condition, such as diabetes, the renal nurse is pivotal to an effective multidisciplinary approach.

For nurses working within the urology specialty, advances in medical treatment and surgical techniques, greater understanding of the aetiology of diseases, and the positive impact of disease surveillance have all led to an extension of nursing roles.

A number of issues raised in this chapter are discussed in greater detail in other chapters. Thus additional information on the multisystem effects of diabetes can be found in Chapter 17, shock and its physiological impact in Chapter 9, gynaecological causes of urinary system dysfunction in Chapter 25, and renal function in the setting of critical care in Chapter 31. Loss of continence is a feature of some conditions discussed in this chapter and the reader is directed to Chapter 12 for a comprehensive discussion of this.

Throughout this chapter, examples of relevance to clinical practice are offered. Readers are asked to further add to this by examining situations encountered in their own practice related to the contents of this chapter and applying the following analysis checks:

- Is this what I have seen in practice?
- How is it the same or different?
- Do I have all the information I need on this subject or are there some deficits?

ANATOMY AND PHYSIOLOGY – AN OVERVIEW

The normal urinary tract/system comprises two kidneys, two ureters, a bladder and a urethra (see Fig. 24.1). Essentially, the functions of the kidney are to preserve fluid and solute homeostasis (the ability of cells to maintain a number of chemical and physical properties within a relatively narrow range). This is achieved through the production of urine by three processes

in the kidney: filtration, reabsorption and secretion. The lower urinary tract provides a conduit for the urine to pass from the body. In addition to fluid and solute balance, the kidneys normally make important contributions to homeostasis in other physiological systems within the body. These are summarized below and discussed in further detail in subsequent sections of this chapter.

Water balance (see Ch. 8)
- Preservation of internal environment of cells
- Preservation of extracellular fluid (ECF) volume
- Contribution to short- and long-term control of blood pressure.

Solute balance (see Ch. 8)
- Preservation of intracellular and extracellular solute concentrations.

Excretion of end products of metabolism
- Maintenance of the internal environment
- Elimination of toxic substances.

Acid–base balance (see Ch. 8)
- Preservation and maintenance of physicochemical buffers, e.g. sodium bicarbonate
- Excretion of 'fixed' acids that cannot be converted to carbon dioxide for excretion by the lungs.

Production of erythropoietin (see Ch. 18)
- Maintenance of red blood cell count and thus oxygen-carrying capacity.

Calcium and phosphate balance (see Ch. 8)
- Maintenance of ionized calcium balance in the ECF
- Preservation of compounded calcium balance in the ECF
- Preservation of calcium and phosphate balance in the skeleton.

Prior to reading the following sections, the reader is asked to keep in mind that in physiological terms, structure reflects function. It thus follows that alterations to structure will impact on function. The importance of understanding the basic functioning of any organ system cannot be overemphasized, and is as important as understanding the impact that disordered function has on the lives of patients, their families and the wider community. In clinical nursing, such knowledge will allow you to integrate what you see in practice with what you know theoretically.

DEVELOPMENT AND MATURATION OF THE KIDNEYS AND URINARY TRACT

The embryonic development of the kidneys and urinary tract begins early in the first trimester of pregnancy, and by the beginning of the second trimester urine is being formed and excreted into the amniotic fluid. Following birth, both the kidneys and the urinary tract undergo additional growth and development. The adult glomerular filtration rate (GFR – the volume of plasma filtered by the kidneys in 1 minute) is usually achieved between

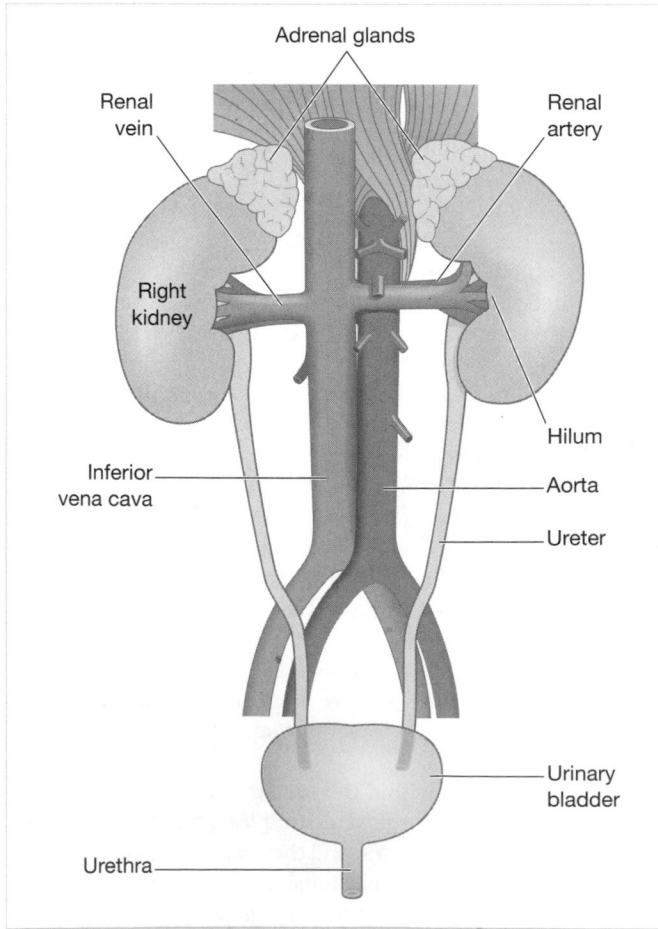

Figure 24.1 Urinary tract.

Table 24.1 Congenital abnormalities of the kidneys and urinary tract

Abnormality	Numbers affected	Consequence
Unilateral renal agenesis – failure to develop one of the two kidneys	1 in 1000 births	Usually asymptomatic, as the other kidney compensates
Bilateral renal agenesis – failure to develop two kidneys	0.3 in 1000 births	Not compatible with extrauterine life
Horseshoe kidney – two kidneys formed but these are fused across the midline, usually at the lower aspect	1 in 600	Usually asymptomatic, but may be symptomatic if urine outflow via the ureters is obstructed
Multiple renal blood vessels	Anomalies in the number of renal arteries and veins are relatively common	Usually asymptomatic
Autosomal recessive polycystic kidney disease	Incidence estimated to be around 1 in 40 000	In neonates, the associated mortality is very high. For those surviving the neonatal period with this condition, morbidity and mortality remain significant
Exstrophy of the bladder	1 in 50 000 births	Exposure and protrusion of the bladder. Surgical intervention with creation of urinary diversion. This may need revision as the child grows
Primary vesicoureteric reflux (VUR)	Estimations of incidence vary (between 0.4–1.8% of infants and young children and up to 9%)	Associated with persistent urinary tract infections in early life. The consequence may be end-stage renal failure secondary to the development of reflux nephropathy

1 and 2 years of age. The ability to produce concentrated urine is limited in babies, but increases rapidly during the first 18 months.

Abnormal intrauterine growth and development may result in anomalies of structure, and thereby functional alterations, of either the kidneys or the urinary tract, or both. The incidence of congenital abnormalities in the urinary system is low, at around 3–4% of the population, but they have important consequences for life (see Table 24.1).

Renal function declines with normal ageing (see Ch. 32). However, despite an age-related decrease in GFR, plasma creatinine (a clinical marker of renal function) does not rise proportionately. This is because GFR is a function of total body mass, and with age, muscle mass, and thus creatinine production, declines.

Other homeostatic mechanisms related to control of volume are altered in older people. Among those reported include blunting of the thirst response and an increase in abnormal serum sodium concentrations (see Ch. 8). In view of the latter, particular care needs to be taken when nursing older patients to ensure that they are adequately hydrated, and that attention is paid to drug dosage (see Ch. 32).

KIDNEYS – MACROSCOPIC STRUCTURE

The kidneys are sited one on either side of the vertebral column. The right kidney is slightly lower than the left, as a consequence of lying under the liver. Both kidneys are retroperitoneal and are protected by an outer layer of renal fascia, a middle layer of fat, and an inner layer of fibrous tissue that adheres closely to the kidney.

The adult kidney is approximately 9.5–12.5 cm in length. This measurement is important since a diminution of renal

mass as measured on ultrasound provides a clinically useful indication of chronic renal damage.

Macroscopically, the kidney has three distinct regions: the outer, dark brown cortex, the medulla and the renal pelvis (see Fig. 24.2). The inner zone of the cortex forms the corticomedullary junction with the medulla. The medulla consists of between eight and 18 triangular wedges that have a striated appearance, the renal pyramids. The medulla is also subdivided into zones: outer, middle and the deepest zone forming the apex of the renal pyramids, the renal papilla. The renal pelvis is

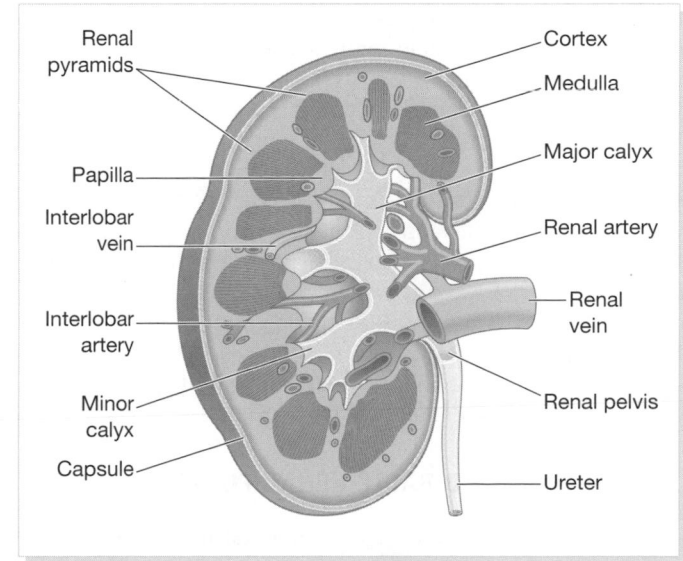

Figure 24.2 Macrostructure of the kidney.

funnel-shaped and opens out from the top of the ureter to divide into two or three major calyces. Each of these is subdivided into between eight and 18 minor calyces. These minor calyces cup the apices of the renal pyramids.

Blood supply to the kidneys

Blood supply to the kidneys is via the renal arteries that arise directly from the abdominal aorta. Prior to entering the kidney, the renal arteries divide into five segmental arteries. These enter the kidney and undergo further subdivision to form lobar arteries, which supply a specific region, or lobe, of the kidney. Lobar arteries subdivide to form interlobar arteries. At the corticomedullary junction, branches arise from the interlobar arteries to form arcuate arteries, and these in turn subdivide to form interlobular arteries. It is from these latter arteries that the afferent arterioles, glomerular capillary knot and efferent arterioles arise.

The kidneys receive about 25% of cardiac output (see Ch. 19). This is approximately 400 mL/min per 100 g of renal tissue at rest, or 1200 mL/min (Valtin & Schaeffer 1995). Such a volume of blood flow appears at first to be disproportionate to the combined mass of renal tissue. For example, the heart receives approximately 250 mL/min per 100 g of cardiac mass at rest. This difference is easily explained if one considers that the bulk of blood supply to the kidneys is not to supply renal tissue *per se*, but rather the blood is to be processed by the functional unit of the kidney, the nephron. A high volume of blood supply to the kidneys is thus required to maintain high GFRs and to provide the oxygen required by active cell transport mechanisms.

The majority of blood supplied, some 90%, perfuses the cortex. The medulla receives only 10% of the total blood supply (outer medulla, 8%; and inner medulla, 1–2%). Clinically this has important consequences for renal function, since even under conditions of normal blood flow, the innermost medulla is short of oxygen (borderline hypoxia). Physiologically, the relatively slow flow of blood through the inner medulla is necessary to enable efficient concentration and dilution of urine (see section on 'Countercurrent exchange', p. 658). However, when normal blood flow to the kidneys is disrupted, hypoxic damage to this region is inevitable, with consequent derangement of normal renal function.

Venous drainage from the kidneys is via the renal veins into the inferior vena cava.

Nerve supply to the kidneys

Nervous supply to the kidneys is mainly from the renal sympathetic plexus. Sympathetic nerves supply the smooth muscle layer of the arterioles and juxtaglomerular apparatus (see p. 658), and stimulation contributes to the regulation of blood flow through the kidneys.

There are also some afferent nerve fibres that are responsible for the transmission of pain.

THE NEPHRON AND BASIC RENAL FUNCTION

The nephron is the microscopic functional unit of the kidney and consists of a renal tubule and a glomerulus, a tight knot of capillaries that lies within the invaginated blind end of the tubule (the glomerular capsule). The renal tubule comprises a proximal convoluted tubule (PCT), loop of Henle, distal convoluted tubule (DCT) and a collecting duct (see Fig. 24.3).

Each kidney has around 1 million nephrons; of these, approximately 85% are cortical, and the other 15% juxtamedullary. The cortical nephrons lie almost entirely within the cortex of the kidney. Cortical nephrons have a short loop of Henle that extends only to or slightly below the corticomedullary junction. In contrast, juxtamedullary nephrons have a very long loop of Henle, which traverses the entire depth of the renal medulla as far as the minor calyces (see Fig. 24.4).

Blood flow through the knot of glomerular capillary loops is delivered via the wide-bore afferent arteriole, a branch of the interlobular artery. Blood leaves the capillary knot through the efferent arteriole. The majority of efferent arterioles in the kidney then subdivide to form a peritubular capillary network that supplies blood to other regions of the nephrons within the renal cortex. A smaller number of efferent arterioles, principally those associated with juxtamedullary nephrons, form a specialized capillary network called the vasa recta. The vasa recta closely follows the long loops of Henle of juxtamedullary nephrons deep in the renal medulla.

Glomerulus and glomerular capsule: glomerular filtration barrier

The first stage in the production of urine, filtration, occurs in the glomerulus and glomerular capsule (see Fig. 24.3). The term GFR refers to the rate at which this occurs. Filtration is the passive transport of fluid and solute, and as such requires no expenditure of energy. Fluid and solute are forced across a filtration barrier, to form an ultrafiltrate of the plasma. That force is supplied by hydrostatic pressure.

Functionally, the glomerulus and the glomerular capsule may be considered as a single entity (Valtin & Schaefer 1995). Its principal function is to provide a filtration barrier between the blood being carried through it and the lumen of the renal tubule. This filtration barrier has the following components and can be thought of as a sieve that has layers of progressively smaller openings:

- a layer of capillary endothelium, with pores of between 70 and 100 nanometres in width
- a basement membrane
- a layer of epithelium, which consists of specialized cells called podocytes. It has filtration slits of between 25 and 60 nanometres in width.

Molecules (glycosialoproteins) with a negative electrical charge are also attached to the cells, forming the filtration barrier. The structure of this physiological sieve thus allows for a high degree of discrimination about what is allowed to filter from the blood to the renal tubule. The filtration barrier discriminates by:

- molecular size
- molecular shape
- electrical charge (negatively charged molecules are repelled by the negative electrostatic barrier).

Detection of albumin in the urine (albuminuria, see below) on urinalysis is regarded as abnormal. However, albumin is a relatively small molecule and theoretically small enough to cross

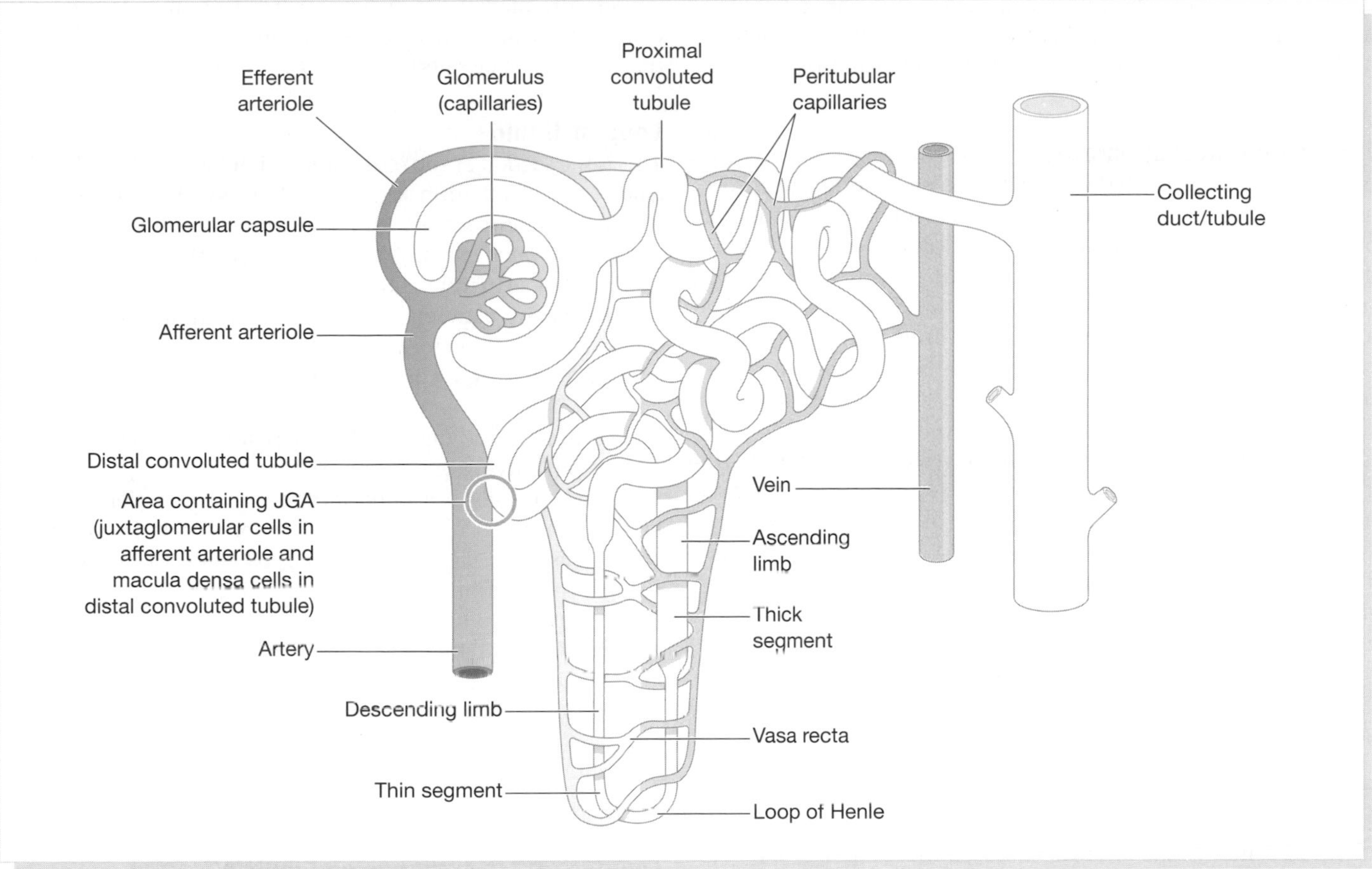

Proximal
convoluted
tubule

Efferent
arteriole

Glomerulus
(capillaries)

Peritubular
capillaries

Collecting
duct/tubule

Glomerular capsule

Afferent arteriole

Distal convoluted tubule

Area containing JGA
(juxtaglomerular cells in
afferent arteriole and
macula densa cells in
distal convoluted tubule)

Artery

Vein

Ascending
limb

Thick
segment

Descending limb

Vasa recta

Thin segment

Loop of Henle

Figure 24.3 A nephron (diagrammatic).

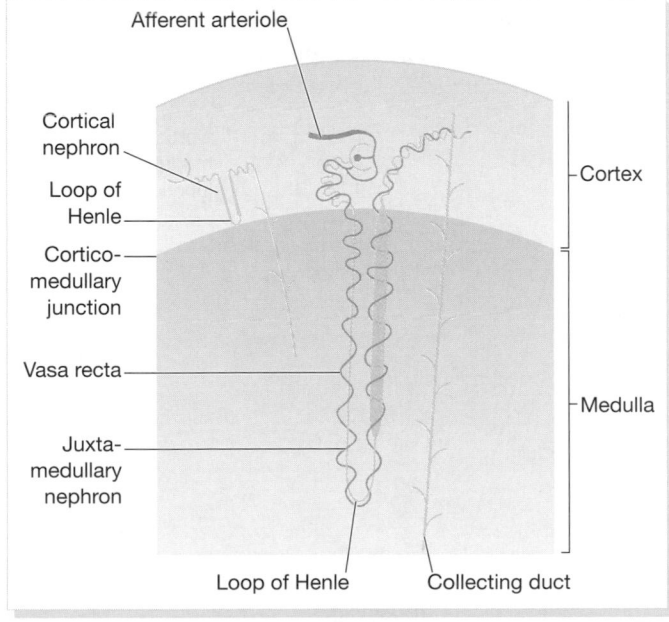

Afferent arteriole

Cortical
nephron

Loop of
Henle

Cortico-
medullary
junction

Vasa recta

Juxta-
medullary
nephron

Cortex

Medulla

Loop of Henle   Collecting duct

Figure 24.4 Cortical and juxtamedullary nephrons.

the glomerular filtration barrier in quantities equal to its concentration in the blood. Under normal conditions, small amounts of albumin do indeed cross the glomerular filtration barrier to enter the PCT, where most is reabsorbed. The remainder (< 150 mg/ 24 hours in adults) is excreted in the urine and, at this level, is not detectable using a commercial dipstick for urinalysis.

So why is it that only small amounts of albumin cross the barrier when molecular size is not a hindrance? The answer to this lies in the fact that the passage of albumin (negatively charged) through the glomerular filtration barrier is inhibited by the negatively charged glycosialoproteins present on the cells in this area. It therefore follows that conditions in which there is structural damage to the filtration barrier or functional disruption of glycosialoproteins, or both, will result in clinically detectable albuminuria. Disorders causing albuminuria include diabetic nephropathy and autoimmune disease damage to the kidney (see p. 682–683).

In addition to the discriminating glomerular filtration barrier, a number of other factors (e.g. hydrostatic pressure) influence filtration of fluid and solute from the blood and into the tubule, and hence determine the GFR. These can perhaps be most easily described using the following equation:

$$GFR = P_{uf} \times k \times S$$

where P_{uf} is the net ultrafiltration pressure, i.e. the force applied by hydrostatic pressure that acts to push fluid and solute across the glomerular filtration barrier; k is the permeability of the capillary wall; and S is the available filtering surface area.

Each of the above factors can change, and thereby influence the GFR; for example, if hydrostatic pressure decreases (i.e. the mean arterial blood pressure falls), then there will be a fall in net ultrafiltration pressure. Clinically, measurement of GFR is important in the assessment of renal function (see pp. 667 and 680).

Juxtaglomerular apparatus

Additional structures associated with this region of the nephron are the macula densa (specialized cells that monitor the amount of sodium chloride in the filtrate in the tubule) and the juxtaglomerular cells (which secrete renin). Together they are referred to as the juxtaglomerular apparatus (JGA). Renin is the substance that initiates the renin–angiotensinogen–angiotensin–aldosterone cascade. It is released into the blood when renal perfusion is reduced or sodium chloride level in the filtrate is reduced. Renin converts angiotensinogen (plasma protein) into angiotensin I, which is subsequently converted to angiotensin II. This is a powerful vasoconstrictor and also stimulates release of aldosterone, a hormone, from the adrenal cortex. Aldosterone causes increased reabsorption of sodium (Na^+) in the nephron. This physiological activity makes a major contribution to both short- and long-term control of blood pressure.

Angiotensin-converting enzyme (ACE) inhibitor drugs, such as enalapril, are used to control hypertension. As their name implies, they inhibit the conversion of inactive angiotensin I into angiotensin II (see Ch. 19 and p. 682).

PCT

The PCT is the hollow extension from the glomerular capsule to the descending limb of the loop of Henle (see Fig. 24.3). It has a significant role in the reabsorption and secretion of solute. The PCT has cells with microvilli (finger-like projections) that increase surface area, and numerous mitochondria generate energy for active transport.

Of the filtrate that enters the PCT, up to 99% is reabsorbed. Individual solutes are reabsorbed in varying degrees. For example, almost all the glucose that filters across is reabsorbed. Reabsorption in the PCT may be passive, down concentration gradients, or active, requiring energy and the use of carrier proteins.

In addition to this, the reabsorption of some solutes from the PCT is transport maximum (T_m) limited. We can use the example of glucose to explain what this means. Glucose is a small molecule and is filtered freely from the blood across the glomerular filtration barrier into the PCT. Reabsorption of glucose requires active transport with a carrier protein. At normal plasma concentrations of glucose, the amount filtered is equivalent to that reabsorbed in the PCT. In this case, no glucose is excreted in the urine. However, when plasma glucose concentration is high, e.g. in diabetes mellitus (see Ch. 17), the amount of glucose entering the filtrate exceeds the carrying capacity of the active transport mechanism. In this case, the glucose that the PCT is unable to reabsorb is excreted in the urine in clinically detectable amounts (glycosuria).

Reabsorption describes the movement of solute from the lumen of the tubule to the circulation, whereas secretion signifies the movement of a solute from the capillaries surrounding the PCT into the lumen of the tubule. The two transport processes are the same, except that they occur in different directions. Examples of substances that are secreted in the PCT

include the diuretic drug furosemide (frusemide – a diuretic drug is one that increases the secretion of urine by the kidneys), morphine and bile salts (see Ch. 23).

Loop of Henle

This is the section of the renal tubule that follows the PCT. It has a descending limb (thin segment), a loop and an ascending limb (thick segment) (see Fig. 24.3). The descending limb is freely permeable to water, but not solute, whereas the ascending limb is impermeable to water, but permeable to solute. The differences in permeability between these two is important in determining the kidneys' ability to form dilute (hypo-osmotic/low solute concentration) and concentrated (hyperosmotic/high solute concentration) urine.

The juxtaglomerular nephrons (with long loop of Henle and accompanying vasa recta) that penetrate the full depth of the renal medulla are important in the production of dilute and concentrated urine. Before describing how hypo-osmotic or hyperosmotic urine is produced, one other related feature requires highlighting. The medullary interstitium (the tissue spaces) surrounding the loop of Henle and the vasa recta becomes increasingly hyperosmotic from the corticomedullary junction to the renal papillae (see Fig. 24.5).

The kidney forms hypo-osmotic or hyperosmotic urine, and generates and maintains the medullary interstitial osmotic gradient, through a process called countercurrent exchange and multiplication.

Countercurrent exchange and multiplication

- *Step 1* (see Fig. 24.6) – filtrate entering the descending limb of the loop of Henle has an osmolality approximately equivalent to that of plasma (285 mOsm/kg H_2O). As the filtrate descends the loop, water moves out into the interstitium because the descending limb of the loop is

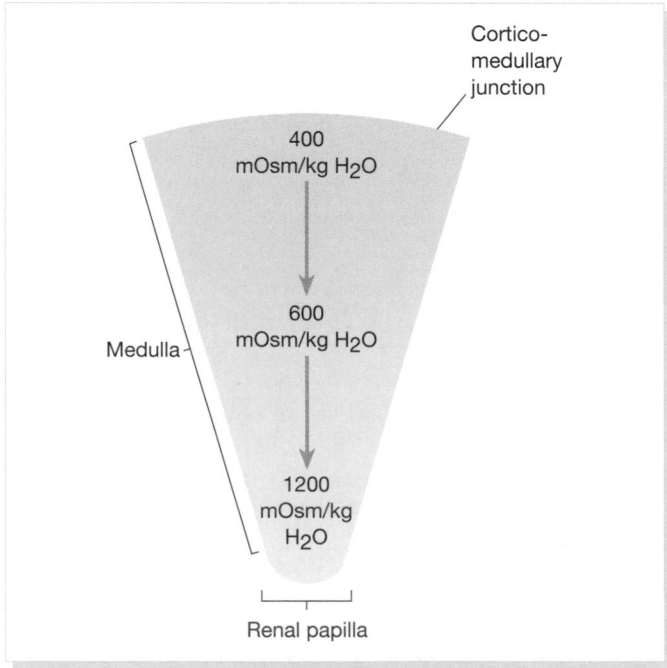

Figure 24.5 Osmotic gradient in the medullary interstitium.

relatively impermeable to solute, but freely permeable to water. The outward water movement is facilitated by the difference in osmolality between the filtrate and the medullary interstitium in the outer medulla (osmotic gradient). The outward movement of water results in the filtrate becoming increasingly concentrated. When the filtrate enters the loop, its osmolality is about the same as that in the medullary interstitium in this region (approximately 1200 mOsm/kg H_2O).

■ *Step 2* (see Fig. 24.6) – as filtrate moves up the ascending limb of the loop of Henle, its osmolality begins to change again (remember that the ascending limb is relatively impermeable to water, but permeable to solute). Thus, in this region, solute moves out of the tubular lumen and into the medullary interstitium (both passive and active transport). When the filtrate reaches the corticomedullary junction again, and begins its passage into the DCT, the osmolality is approximately 100 mOsm/kg H_2O.

While steps 1 and 2 are taking place, an additional process maintains overall balance of water and solute in the medullary interstitium. The relatively slow blood flow in the capillaries of the vasa recta allows for the exchange of water and solute, in a type of recycling, between the blood and the medullary interstitium (see Fig. 24.7, p. 660). This prevents too rapid a removal of solute from this area and serves to maintain the medullary interstitial gradient.

DCT and collecting duct

The DCT consists of four segments with one or more distinct cell types. Hormones that work on specific cell types influence the activity of each segment. Essentially, the function of the DCT is to fine-tune the urine produced by the earlier sections of the nephron (Rose 1994). The collecting duct is continuous with the DCT and opens into the pelvis of the kidney through the renal papillae.

Achieving maximal urinary concentration

A primary function of the kidneys is to conserve overall fluid homeostasis. Normally, changes to the concentration of the filtrate will be relatively small as it passes through the DCT and collecting duct. However, in hypovolaemia (see Ch. 9), the requirement to conserve water increases. Conservation of water by the kidney results in the production of increasingly concentrated urine, with a decrease in excreted volume.

This occurs in the DCT and the collecting ducts under the influence of antidiuretic hormone (ADH, also known as arginine vasopressin). The principal stimulus for ADH release, from the posterior pituitary, is increasing plasma osmolality. A secondary stimulus is a fall in plasma volume. ADH increases permeability to water in the late segments of the DCT and the collecting duct. This allows water to pass from the tubule into the interstitium and thence to the circulation. Release of ADH is controlled by a negative feedback mechanism when plasma

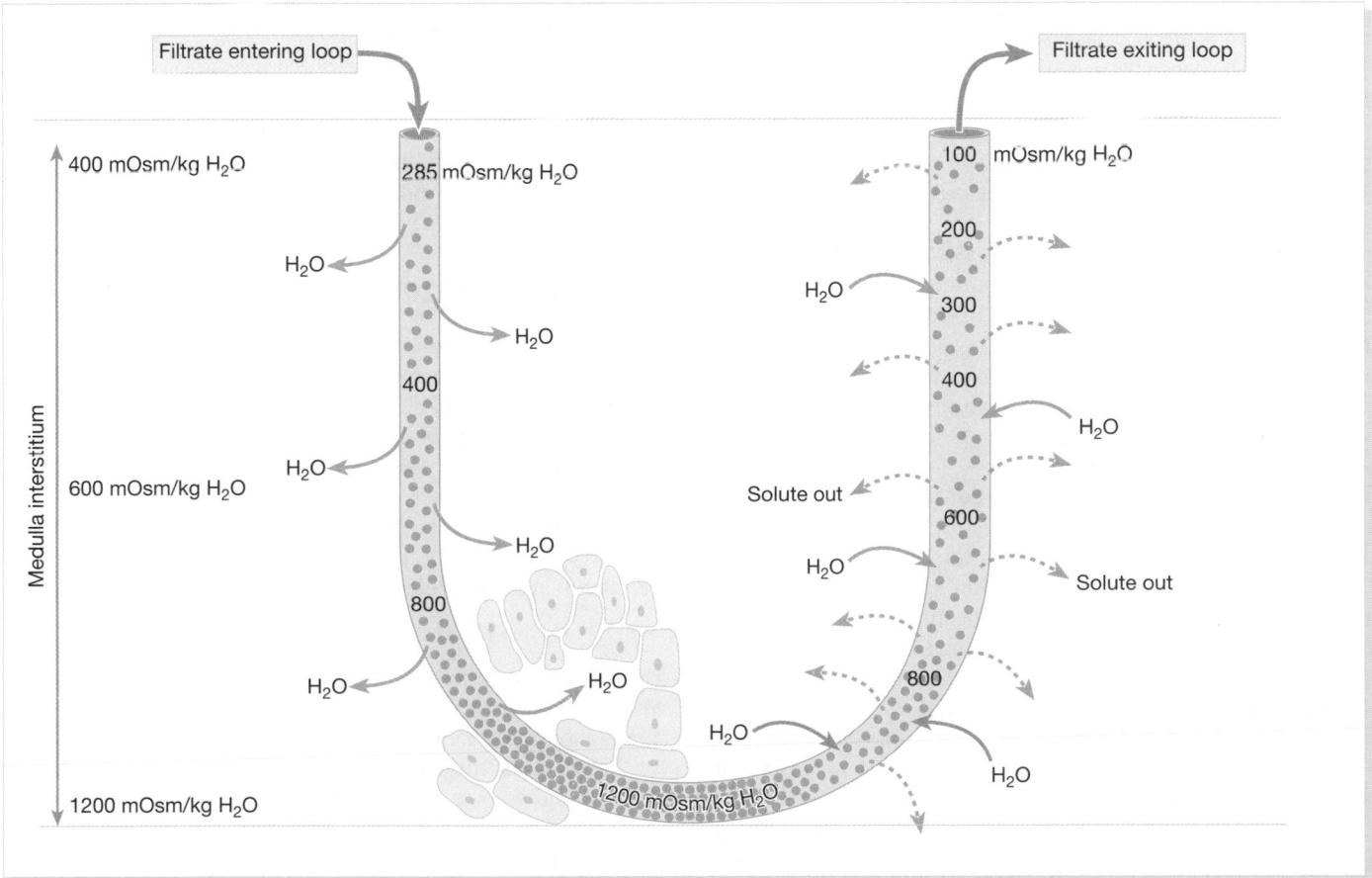

Figure 24.6 Countercurrent exchange and multiplication in the loop of Henle.

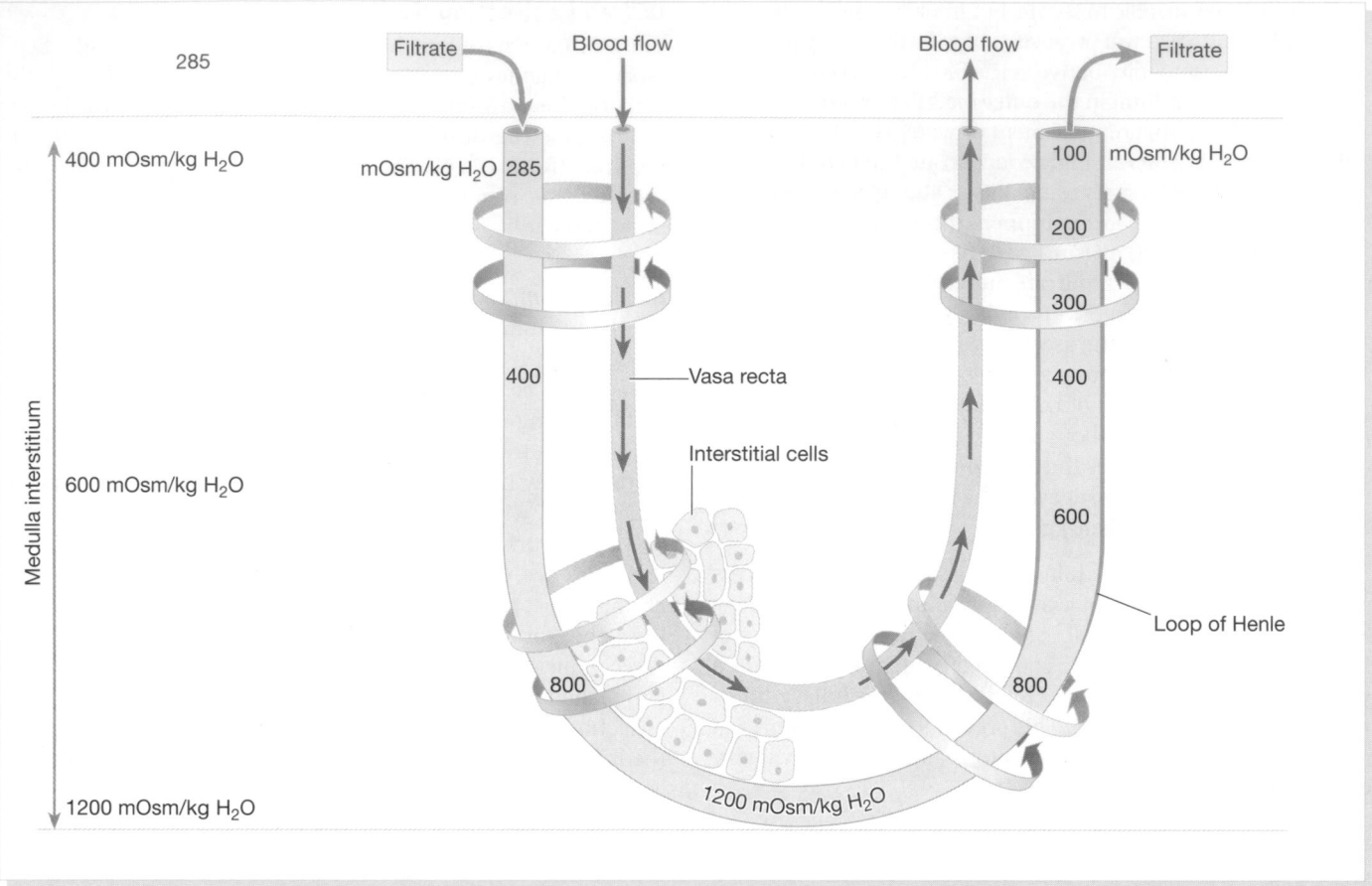

285

400 mOsm/kg H₂O

Filtrate   Blood flow

mOsm/kg H₂O 285

400

Vasa recta

Interstitial cells

600 mOsm/kg H₂O

Medulla interstitium

800

1200 mOsm/kg H₂O

Blood flow   Filtrate

100 mOsm/kg H₂O

200

300

400

600

Loop of Henle

800

1200 mOsm/kg H₂O

Figure 24.7 Exchange between the loop and the vasa recta.

osmolality begins to fall with restoration of circulating blood volume, the rate at which ADH is released is slowed.

Maintaining homeostasis of potassium in the DCT

Secretion of potassium (K^+) into the lumen of the DCT accounts for the majority of K^+ excreted in the urine. A number of active transport mechanisms exist to perform this function. While the primary function is to secrete K^+ for excretion, in hypokalaemia (reduced K^+ level in the plasma), reabsorption of K^+ can also occur in this region.

Summary: fluid and solute homeostasis

The kidneys contribute to fluid and solute homeostasis, and the removal of toxic substances through the production of urine. The processes of filtration, reabsorption and secretion produce urine. Filtration of water and solute occurs at the level of the glomerulus. Most solute reabsorption and some secretion occur in the PCT. For solutes that are not completely reabsorbed or secreted in the PCT, additional regulation of their final concentration in the urine occurs elsewhere in the tubule. Reabsorption and secretion activities in the DCT are regulated by a number of hormones, including ADH and parathyroid hormone (PTH) (see below and Ch. 17). This regulation allows for fine-tuning of final urinary solute concentration such that it adequately reflects homeostatic requirements. The last touches to overall water reabsorption or excretion also occur in the DCT, under the influence of ADH. The urine thus formed then moves down the collecting ducts to enter the renal pelvis and onwards to the lower urinary tract (see below).

RENAL CONTRIBUTION TO ACID–BASE BALANCE

The renal contribution to overall acid–base balance in the body is important. Normally, blood pH is maintained within a relatively narrow, and slightly alkaline, range (pH 7.35–7.45) (see Chs 8 and 9). The body's daily challenge in terms of changes to pH is derived from two sources: endogenous production of acid and diet.

Metabolism in the body produces carbon dioxide (CO_2) and water (H_2O). These combine to form carbonic acid ($H_2CO_3^-$, a weak acid) in a reversible reaction:

$$CO_2 + H_2O \rightarrow H_2CO_3^- \rightarrow CO_2 + H_2O$$

The carbonic acid formed from CO_2 is termed a 'volatile acid', which is normally excreted by the lungs (see Ch. 20).

Metabolism also gives rise to the production of non-volatile (or 'fixed') acids; these must be excreted via the kidneys. Under certain conditions, e.g. anaerobic exercise and highly catabolic states (see Ch. 11), endogenous production of non-volatile acid can rise considerably.

Dietary intake constitutes an additional challenge to maintenance of body pH. Diets that derive protein from meat or wheat products produce an acid load, whereas vegetarian diets produce an alkaline load. Acid production related to dietary intake produces non-volatile acids.

The body counteracts the effects of acid production on pH in three ways (see Ch. 8): chemical buffers, respiratory compensation and via the renal contribution to acid–base balance. The renal contribution to acid–base balance provides for three things:

- conservation of bicarbonate (HCO_3^-) – this is achieved through avid reabsorption of HCO_3^- in the PCT
- regeneration of HCO_3^- – tubular cells generate HCO_3^- and, in doing so, replenish body stores
- secretion of hydrogen (H^+) ions derived from non-volatile acids into the tubule, and thence excretion via the urine. The kidney produces urine of variable pH in a range 4.5–8 in response to homeostatic requirements.

While buffering and respiratory alterations will adjust changes in pH towards normal, it is the renal component that restores the pH to normal. This is noteworthy, as abnormal renal function has a profound effect on the body's ability to maintain acid–base homeostasis.

RENAL CONTRIBUTION TO CALCIUM AND PHOSPHATE HOMEOSTASIS (see Ch. 8)

The kidneys have an important role in calcium and phosphate homeostasis. Approximately 99% of body calcium is stored in the skeleton, where it combines with phosphate. Of the remaining 1%, approximately half exists in its ionized state (Ca^{2+}), while the other half is bound to plasma proteins, primarily albumin. Ionized calcium levels in the body are maintained within a narrow range (2.1–2.6 mmol/L).

Plasma pH exerts an influence on the ratio of ionized to protein-bound calcium in the blood. Acidaemic states increase plasma ionized calcium levels. Alkalotic states have the opposite effect, thus reducing ionized calcium levels. Another factor that influences this ratio is the serum albumin level. If this is low, then the proportion of ionized calcium increases.

PTH, a hormone produced by the parathyroid glands (see Ch. 17), regulates ionized calcium levels by exerting an effect at three main sites in the body:

- bone – the effects of PTH result in the release of calcium and phosphate from the bone into the blood
- small intestine – this is the primary site of calcium absorption from the diet. Calcium absorption by active transport needs physiologically active vitamin D (1,25 dihydroxycholecalciferol). Cells in the kidney contain an enzyme that converts inactive vitamin D to the active form
- the kidneys – PTH stimulates active renal tubular reabsorption of Ca^{2+}, while simultaneously inhibiting phosphate retention.

THE LOWER URINARY TRACT

This comprises the ureters, bladder and the urethra (see Fig. 24.1).

Ureters

The ureters are hollow tubes extending from the pelvis of each kidney to the posterior aspect of the bladder. They convey urine from the kidneys to the bladder. Each ureter has three layers of tissue:

- a lining mucosa of transitional epithelium (urothelium) continuous with the renal pelvis and the bladder
- a smooth muscle layer
- an outer layer of fibrous connective tissue.

The ureters enter the muscular wall of the bladder obliquely. This feature is important for the following reason. When the bladder contracts to expel urine, the muscle layers compress the distal part of the ureters and prevent urine being forced back up the ureters.

The ureters have both sympathetic and parasympathetic nerve supplies. However, local responses to stretch as urine enters from the renal pelvis appear to be the main signal to generate ureteric peristalsis that moves urine to the bladder.

Bladder

The bladder is a hollow muscular sac that lies retroperitoneally on the floor of the pelvis behind the symphysis pubis. In the female, the bladder lies in front of the uterus and vagina. In males, it lies in front of the rectum. The bladder is a receptacle for urine, and in the adult has a maximum capacity of approximately 500 mL. The empty bladder is pyramidal in shape. The neck of the bladder lies inferiorly, and in the male rests on the upper surface of the prostate gland. When full, the bladder becomes ovoid in shape and projects up into the abdomen above the symphysis pubis. It can be easily palpated through the anterior abdominal wall in this position.

Like the ureters, the bladder has three layers. An inner mucosal layer of transitional epithelium, which when the bladder is empty is mostly thrown into folds called rugae. The remainder, which covers the base of the bladder in an area called the trigone, remains smooth. The trigone is demarcated by the openings of the right and left ureters above, and the internal urethral orifice below. The middle muscular layer of the bladder is smooth muscle and is arranged in three layers of interwoven bundles – inner and outer longitudinal layers and a circular layer. This is the detrusor muscle. At the bladder neck, the circular layer of the detrusor muscle thickens to form the involuntary internal urethral sphincter. The bladder also has an external sphincter composed of striated muscle that is under voluntary control (see Ch. 12).

The bladder has both sympathetic and parasympathetic nerve supplies. Sympathetic fibres originate from the first and second lumbar ganglia, and descend to supply the bladder via the hypogastric plexuses. Parasympathetic fibres arise from the sacral nerves and, like the sympathetic fibres, pass through the hypogastric plexuses to the bladder wall.

Urethra

The urethra conveys urine from the bladder to the outside. In females, it is 4 cm long and lies anterior to, and closely associated with, the vagina. The male urethra is approximately 20 cm long and has three parts: prostatic (containing openings for the prostatic and ejaculatory ducts), membranous (traverses the external urethral sphincter) and spongy (traverses the corpus spongiosum of the penis).

With the exception of its termination, which is lined with squamous epithelium, the urethra is lined with transitional epithelium (urothelium) in common with other sections of the lower urinary tract.

Micturition

Micturition (passing urine) is essentially a reflex action. This is demonstrated clearly in the child who is not toilet-trained and in some patients who have sustained damage to the spinal cord (see Ch. 14). Here, once the bladder begins to fill and distend, a simple stretch reflex action is initiated, the detrusor contracts, and micturition occurs. In the continent adult, this simple reflex action is overridden by activity within the cerebral cortex and micturition is inhibited until convenient. The inhibitory fibres which facilitate this pass downward from the cortex in the corticospinal tracts to the second, third and fourth sacral segments of the spinal cord.

The stimulus to void the bladder arises from a combination of increases in urine volume (approximately 300–400 mL of urine), the internal bladder pressure that this generates, and the sensation of bladder wall stretch that is sensed by stretch receptors.

Prostate

In the male, an additional structure associated with the lower urinary tract is the prostate. This triangular structure lies immediately below the bladder neck and completely encircles the upper section of the male urethra (prostatic urethra). The prostate is a fibromuscular glandular organ that normally has two capsules, an outer layer of fibrous tissue and a thin inner fibrous sheath. Both encapsulate the prostatic glandular tissue. Prostatic secretion, which forms part of semen, is mildly acidic and contains enzymes (e.g. acid phosphatase), citrate and calcium. It may be involved in reducing the acidic environment of the vagina, coagulating the secretion from other accessory sex glands (see Ch. 25) and influencing the motility of spermatozoa.

NURSING ASSESSMENT – URINARY SYSTEM FUNCTION

Nursing assessment of the urinary system centres on assessment of function and the individual's ability to contribute to this. Age, level of consciousness, clinical condition, and the presence or absence of physical and neurological deficits will have significant impacts.

Acquiring a history of what is or has been 'normal' for the patient is an indispensable part of overall nursing assessment. It provides a basis for anticipation and planning of care needs and subsequent discharge planning. In this context, eliciting 'normal' refers to the acquisition of an understanding not just of physical and functional characteristics, but also of the nature of the person's existence. The latter assumes even greater importance within the context of establishment and maintenance of a therapeutic relationship with individuals requiring long-term care for renal chronic disease.

Physical assessment will include the following:

■ Micturition
— usual volume and noted changes
— usual flow characteristics: ask about how easy/difficult it

is to start and stop micturition. Is the stream forceful and continuous, or intermittent? Is there dribbling of urine?
— is there pain associated with micturition?
— what colour is the urine and what does it smell of?
— is the urine clear, cloudy, does it contain blood (see 'Urinalysis' below)?
■ Associated symptoms
— loin pain
— nausea
— oedema: periorbital (around the eyes) and dependent, e.g. ankle or sacral oedema. Patient may have noticed weight gain
— headache: check blood pressure (see below)
— alteration in vision: check blood pressure and blood sugar levels
■ Lifestyle
— smoking
— work: exposure to heavy metals or carcinogens, or hot environment and dehydration
— pattern of sexual activity.

A critical approach to the performance of nursing assessment is also an invaluable learning tool for the nurse. An example of how you might use this approach is provided in Box 24.1.

Box 24.1 Developing a knowledge base through patient assessment

Assessment identifies
● Change in pattern of urine excretion, specifically frequency and nocturia

What do I know about this?
● Bacteriuria and urinary tract infection
● In men an early symptom of benign prostatic hyperplasia

How do I think this will be investigated?
● Urine culture, renal ultrasound, plain abdominal X-ray
● Assessment of renal function
● Abdominal and rectal examination
● Micturating cystogram
● Cystoscopy

What are the probable outcomes?
● Treatment for urinary tract infection
● Benign prostatic hyperplasia – possibly transurethral resection (TURP)
● Permanent indwelling urethral or suprapubic catheter
● Changes in body image
● Changes in perception of ability to perform personal roles

Additional knowledge checks
● Do I know enough about these to safely plan holistic patient care?
● What are my care priorities?
● Are these different from those of my nursing and medical colleagues? If so, why?
● Where will I get additional information?

ASSESSMENT OF FLUID AND ELECTROLYTE BALANCE

Although accurate assessment of fluid and electrolyte balance is important in many settings, it is particularly so when nursing patients with renal or urological problems (see Ch. 8).

Fluid balance charts

One of the principal means by which fluid and electrolyte balance is assessed and monitored by nurses is through the accurate maintenance of a fluid balance chart. The literature suggests that maintaining accuracy of these is not entirely unproblematic, and it appears that even nurses doubt their accuracy (Daffern et al 1994). Fluid balance charts should measure all inputs, whether these are ingested or given parenterally. Outputs include urine volumes in addition to drainage from other sites (e.g. nasogastric tubes).

The volume of urine produced from hour to hour varies and is a reflection of hydration and the level of activity of the hypothalamic–pituitary axis, which influences urine osmolality. When required to conserve water, the minimum amount of urine that the kidneys can produce per hour is 0.5 mL/kg. This represents maximal urinary concentration and is equivalent to a urine output of 35 mL/h in a 70 kg adult. The significance of the volume of urine excreted must be interpreted for individual patients.

Daily weight

Daily weighing of patients is a useful adjunct to maintenance of fluid balance charts, and ideally they should be weighed at the same time of day wearing similar clothing. Fluid accounts for around 60% of total body weight in the 70 kg adult (see Ch. 8 for a fuller discussion of age/gender variation). Thus, body weight is a useful indicator of overall fluid balance in the body. Over a 24-hour period, changes in body weight which cannot be accounted for by loss or gain of flesh weight will be due to fluid loss or gain (Valtin & Schaeffer 1995).

Skin turgor and mucous membranes

Turgor is the term used to describe the elastic property of the skin and it is a reflection of interstitial fluid volume. Assessment of turgor can be performed by gently pinching the skin over the back of the hand. In the euvolaemic (adequately hydrated) person, the skin flattens quickly once the pinch is released. Interpretation of this assessment must take into account the age of the patient (skin elasticity declines with age) and the presence of obesity, since the latter may mask changes in skin turgor. Observation of the tongue and mucous membrane hydration also provides an indication of overall fluid balance status (Rose 1994).

Arterial blood pressure

The factors affecting blood pressure include the circulating blood volume (see Ch. 19). The relationship between blood pressure and circulating vascular volume can be summarized using the following formula:

$$\text{Blood pressure} = \text{cardiac output} \times \text{systemic vascular resistance (peripheral resistance).}$$

From this formula, we can see that if cardiac output or peripheral resistance changes, this will have an effect on the blood pressure.

Assessment of blood pressure provides information about overall cardiac function in addition to circulating blood volume and resistance to blood flow in the arterial tree, thereby providing information that is useful in determining fluid status.

Lying (supine) and standing observations of blood pressure may additionally be used to determine overall fluid status. In this instance, the blood pressure is measured initially in the supine position. Patients are then asked to stand and the blood pressure measured again. A rise in the systolic blood pressure of 10–20 mmHg should be observed between these two readings. This is a normal physiological response to positional change. If the systolic pressure is lower in the standing position than in the supine, the patient has postural hypotension. This may be an indication of hypovolaemia (see Chs 8 and 9). However, it may also be an indication that the normal physiological response has been blunted. Peripheral neuropathy associated with diabetes mellitus (see Ch. 17) and loss of vascular tone following a prolonged period of bed rest are two examples of the latter.

Skin temperature

Skin temperature at the extremities can also provide additional qualitative information about overall fluid balance. A decrease in circulatory volume stimulates a sympathetic nervous system response that results in peripheral vasoconstriction and a cool skin. This is an early physiological response to decreases in circulatory volume and may be observed prior to a fall in blood pressure. Skin temperature at the periphery is monitored in tandem with core body temperature (see Ch. 5) and the gradient between the two is noted. Greater differences between skin and core temperature are an indication of increasing peripheral vasoconstriction, and thus of a decrease in circulatory volume. There are many factors that influence skin temperature and results should always be used in conjunction with other assessment tools.

Central venous pressure

Central venous pressure (CVP) monitoring is a useful adjunct in the assessment of vascular volume (see Chs 8, 9 and 31). CVP measurements may be used to guide decisions about oral or parenteral fluid requirements in patients with altered renal function. During dialysis (see p. 689) CVP measurements may be used to inform decisions about the requirements for fluid volume removal.

ASSESSMENT OF URINE – URINALYSIS

Urinalysis is a simple non-invasive test. Despite its simplicity, it should never be regarded as 'routine' (Cook 1995), since it plays a role not just in diagnosis of renal dysfunction, but also in discovery and monitoring of functional alterations. There are a number of commercially available reagent strips on the market (dipstick) that provide information about a number of parameters (see Table 24.2). All of these provide clear directions for use and storage, which should be adhered to in order to minimize the risk of obtaining a false reading. Urinalysis should always begin with simple observation of the colour, clarity and odour of the fresh urine sample. Normal fresh urine is clear, pale yellow in colour (although colour will be affected by concentration), and smells slightly aromatic. It is important to record and report the findings of both observation and dipstick test (see Table 24.2).

Specific gravity

Measurement of specific gravity gives a numerical indication of the solute concentration of the urine. The specific gravity range is 1.002–1.035 (1.0 is the specific gravity of distilled water, i.e. negligible solute concentration; thus the higher the number, the more solute is contained in the urine sample). Dilute urine will have a specific gravity on the lower limit of this range, and concentrated urine will have a specific gravity on the higher limit. Specific gravity estimation provides information about the kidneys' ability to concentrate and dilute urine, and can be used as additional information during investigation into a range of disorders that impact on normal renal function, e.g. diabetes insipidus (see Ch. 17). A fixed specific gravity of 1.010 is common in chronic renal dysfunction because of reduced ability to vary the concentration of urine.

Blood

The presence of blood in the urine is called haematuria. Frank haematuria is obviously abnormal and does not require the use of a dipstick to confirm its presence, since this is visible to the naked eye. Frank haematuria may be traumatic in origin, but it is also associated with malignancy and renal tuberculosis (see pp. 674 and 675). Microscopic haematuria can be detected by dipstick and is also an abnormal finding. In some circumstances, this may be an early indication of damage to the kidneys as a result of some disease processes, e.g. autoimmune diseases.

Glucose

Normally, glucose is not detectable in the urine. Generally, the presence of glucose (glycosuria) indicates that the plasma concentration of glucose (as in diabetes mellitus, as a physiological stress response, and in people taking corticosteroids – see Chs 6, 9 and 17) is greater than the kidneys' ability to reabsorb glucose (see discussion of T_m, p. 658).

Protein

A positive result for protein/albumin (proteinuria/albuminuria) on dipstick is indicative of kidney damage and is a manifestation of glomerular or tubular damage. Persistent protein loss is a sequel to a number of diseases, including nephrotic syndrome, diabetic nephropathy (see pp. 682 and 684) and vasculitis, and its appearance is a significant risk factor for further deterioration of renal function. In the latter examples, protein loss can be

Table 24.2 Normal characteristics of urine and the significance of abnormal findings

Physical/chemical characteristics	Normal findings – observation and dipstick	Significance of abnormal findings
Colour	Pale straw colour to deep amber	Abnormal colour may indicate presence of red blood cells, drug or food residue excretion, presence of abnormal substances, e.g. bilirubin (see Ch. 23)
Clarity/deposits	Clear with possibly slight turbidity caused by mucus	Opacity may indicate presence of white cells/pus/protein
Odour	Freshly voided urine has a faint aromatic odour. An odour of ammonia develops on standing caused by bacterial action on urea. Some foods produce characteristic odours	Abnormal 'fishy' odour may indicate infection. The presence of abnormal substances, such as ketones, may affect the odour
Specific gravity	1.002–1.035	Inability to concentrate or dilute urine, or the presence of abnormal substances, e.g. glucose
pH	4.5–8.0	Inability to produce acid or alkaline urine, UTI, prolonged vomiting
Protein	Negative	Protein in the urine is an indication of glomerular and/or tubular damage, viral illness and UTI
Glucose	Negative	Glucose loss associated with inadequately controlled diabetes; may appear in pregnancy
Ketones	Negative	Ketonuria is an indication of inadequately controlled diabetes, starvation, excessive or prolonged vomiting
Blood	Negative dipstick Red cells – none to 3	Microscopic haematuria is associated with a number of autoimmune-related diseases that damage the nephron and surrounding structures. Urinary causes of frank haematuria include UTI, renal calculi, tumours and trauma
Leucocytes (white cells)	None to 4	Presence may indicate infection or acute interstitial nephritis

NB. Tests for bilirubin and urobilinogen are discussed in Chapter 23.

considerable, and sending a 24-hour urine collection for protein estimation provides more accurate measurement. Protein loss may also be detected where there is concurrent urinary tract infection (UTI), or in association with a number of viral illnesses. In the latter cases, this tends to be transient and ceases when the person recovers from the infection.

pH

The kidney's role in acid–base homeostasis is outlined above. The normal range of urinary pH is between 4.5 and 8.0. When renal function is normal, there is a correlation between dietary intake and urinary pH (high meat protein diets produce acid urine whereas vegetarian diets produce alkaline urine).

Ketones

Ketones in urine (ketonuria) are associated with a physiological state in which body fat, rather than the carbohydrate store in the body, is metabolized for energy such as fasting, vomiting and diabetic ketoacidosis (see Ch. 17).

Leucocytes and nitrites

Dipsticks may also be used to test for the presence of leucocytes (white blood cells) and nitrites. The presence of leucocytes in urine is associated with UTI. However, high leucocyte counts are also associated with acute interstitial nephritis (see p. 684), an inflammatory disorder, and care must be taken to ensure that the presence of leucocytes is not assumed to be an absolute indication of infection.

A positive dipstick for nitrite is associated with bacteriuria (the presence of 100 000 or more bacteria per mL of urine).

GENERAL DIAGNOSTIC TESTS AND MEDICAL INVESTIGATIONS

The purpose of medical investigation is to acquire information about the extent to which an organ is performing in relation to the norm. The results of investigations are like pieces of a puzzle; they fill in some gaps but they can only provide a partial view of the whole picture. Thus, the results of investigations contribute, along with other information, to confirm or reject a diagnosis. It is important that nurses understand common investigations and any requirement for specific physical preparation. This allows them to provide explanation and reassurance for patients and to ensure that patients are adequately prepared, and the investigation is safe and successful. Common investigations are discussed in this section, while others are discussed in sections relating to specific disorders.

PHYSICAL EXAMINATION

A physical examination will be undertaken to assess functioning of the urinary system (see Box 24.2).

ULTRASONOGRAPHY

Ultrasound is relatively simple, painless and non-invasive and is used to investigate both the kidney and the bladder.

Box 24.2 Physical examination to assess functioning of the urinary system

Appearance of patient
- Able/unable to lie flat and breathless
- Periorbital or sacral oedema
- Change in skin colour
- Skin rash (e.g. purpuric)
- Nail beds (any splinter haemorrhages?)
- Evidence of weight loss
- Evidence of pain

Vascular tree
- All pulses present?
- Evidence of bruit over renal or carotid arteries?
- Jugular vein pressure (JVP) – raised/lowered/normal

Cardiac
- Pulse volume, rate
- Heart sounds – normal/abnormal, murmurs, evidence of pericardial rub

Pulmonary
- Breath sounds, pattern of air entry and exit (equal/unequal air entry)
- Trachea central

Abdominal palpation
- Abnormal masses
- Areas of tenderness, 'guarding' or pain
- Palpation of kidney

Rectal examination (men)
- Prostate, smooth with regular outline or hard and enlarged

Eyes (ophthalmoscopy)
- Optic disc (any oedema)
- Small retinal blood vessels

Renal ultrasound

Renal ultrasound provides information about the following parameters (Parsons 2000):

- kidney size – smaller than normal is indicative of chronic renal damage
- obstruction of the collecting system (includes the renal calyces, renal pelvis and the ureters) – dilatation of the collecting system is seen where there is obstruction to outflow of urine (e.g. a calculus in the renal pelvis, or where a ureter is compressed or obstructed)
- echo pattern of the kidneys – e.g. some echo patterns may signify the presence of cysts
- presence or absence of renal calculi.

More recently, the introduction of colour Doppler imaging has allowed for the visualization of renal perfusion.

Preparation for renal ultrasound

Preparation of patients focuses on ensuring that they are given an explanation of the procedure and an opportunity to voice any concerns or queries they may have. There is no specific after-care required, other than making sure that patients are comfortable and receive an indication of when the findings of this investigation will be available.

Bladder ultrasound

Bladder ultrasound provides information about the echoic pattern of the bladder wall. In addition, colour flow Doppler ultrasound can be used to identify urethral obstruction.

Preparation for bladder ultrasound

Preparation will generally include encouraging patients to drink fluids (if appropriate) and desist from voiding urine, so that the bladder is full. This is obviously not achievable in those who have no urine output.

ANGIOGRAPHY

Angiography is a radiographic technique used to demonstrate the arterial system after injection of an opaque contrast medium.

Renal angiography

A renal angiogram is an invasive procedure that is undertaken to assess blood flow through the kidney and the presence or absence of renal artery stenosis. Arterial cannulation is performed via the right or left femoral artery, and a small catheter is passed up through the aorta to the junction between the aorta and renal arteries. The catheter is then passed into the right or left renal artery, or both. Blood flow pressures in the renal artery may be measured at this point. Following cannulation of the renal artery, opaque contrast medium is injected via the catheter. This is carried in by the blood flow through the renal vasculature.

Care of the patient undergoing renal angiogram

There is likely to be some variation in care procedures, both prior to and following renal angiogram, between different hospitals. However, the following is offered as an indication of what is generally included.

Patients must be given information about the procedure such that they can make an informed choice to consent to the procedure. This is not a pain-free procedure and like all invasive procedures carries a risk of complications (e.g. haemorrhage, arterial embolism). Premedication with an anxiolytic drug may be offered to patients. Any history of allergy to opaque contrast or its specific components must be determined prior to this procedure. If there is a patient history of allergy, there must be an unequivocal record to this effect made in the hospital notes and other patient assessment documentation.

A period of fasting may be required prior to renal angiography. Nursing observation prior to the procedure must include maintaining a check on the period of time during which patients are fasting. It is not appropriate to starve individuals for prolonged periods of time (see Ch. 29). In addition, a state of dehydration will increase the nephrotoxic effect of opaque contrast medium, and if abstinence from fluid is prolonged, it may be necessary to maintain hydration with intravenous (i.v.) fluids.

Blood samples will be drawn to record a baseline measurement of urea, electrolytes (specifically, Na$^+$, K$^+$) and serum creatinine, haemoglobin and clotting times. It is important that the results of these tests are known and available prior to the procedure. Abnormal findings dictate the need for correction prior to the procedure. In addition, if there is a decline in renal function following the angiogram, the magnitude of decline is most easily assessed against pre-procedure results. In the event of procedural complications, this set of blood sampling will be repeated.

A period of complete bed rest is always required following renal angiogram, usually for a period of no less than 2 hours. Observations of vital signs are commonly undertaken, particularly pulse, respiratory rate and blood pressure. Haemorrhage is a known complication of renal angiography, and close observation is required following this procedure. The reader is advised here to keep in mind that a fall in blood pressure is a late sign of blood loss and occurs when other compensatory mechanisms have been overwhelmed. The arterial puncture site is observed for bleeding (covert or overt). Covert blood loss may be observed as swelling of the groin in the region of the puncture site, with the subsequent development of bruising beneath the skin. Internal loss of blood from the vessel puncture site into the layers of the artery wall can result in the formation of a pseudo-aneurysm. Ultrasound of the groin will show this if it is suspected.

Bilateral palpation of pedal and/or post-tibial pulses is performed (see Ch. 19). The site of palpation of these pulses should ideally be marked prior to the procedure, along with a description of their presence/absence, and pulse pressure should be recorded as a baseline observation. Bilateral pulses are monitored because it is possible that passing a catheter up the aorta and into the renal artery may dislodge a fatty plaque or other debris within the aorta. If this occurs, then that embolus will be carried downward in aortic blood flow towards the bifurcation of the aorta, whence it can enter either the left or right common iliac artery and be carried in the blood supply to the lower limb (see Ch. 19).

Monitoring of urine output is also necessary. The use of opaque contrast medium carries the risk of precipitating acute deterioration of renal function.

COMPUTED TOMOGRAPHY

Computed tomography (CT) may be undertaken to visualize the urinary system, investigate renal and extrarenal masses, or identify abscesses or calculi. CT scans can be enhanced with opaque contrast medium (see above).

MAGNETIC RESONANCE ANGIOGRAPHY

As a means by which to visualize the renal vasculature, magnetic resonance angiography (MRA) has a distinct advantage over renal angiography (see above), since it may be performed as a non-invasive procedure. Therefore, for certain groups of high-risk patients, e.g. those with renal artery stenosis or diabetes, it may be used in preference. However, this procedure requires patients to lie on a hard surface within the close confines of what is, to all intents and purposes, a metal tunnel. It may therefore be perceived as an unpleasant and claustrophobic experience. Care should be taken to ensure that patients are prepared for this and that, if necessary, and medically appropriate, they receive anxiolytic premedication (Parsons 2000).

Magnetic resonance angiography may also be enhanced with opaque contrast medium. In this case, it is invasive, since arterial cannulation is performed, and the same cautions and observations outlined above (renal angiography) apply.

RADIONUCLIDE SCANNING

Radionuclide scanning of the kidney involves the use of substances, normally cleared from the body by the kidney, that have been labelled with a radioactive isotope, e.g. diethylenetriamine (DTPA) and mercaptoacetyl triglycine (MAG3) labelled with the isotope ^{99}technetium (^{99}Tm). Both these agents are cleared from the blood by the glomerulus and can be used to measure GFR, and thus blood flow through the kidney. The scan involves the i.v. administration of a small volume of either ^{99}Tm-labelled DTPA or ^{99}Tm-labelled MAG3. After a period of about 45 minutes following administration, a gamma-ray camera is used to capture the photons generated by radio decay of the substance used, and in the process generates an image.

UROGRAPHY (PYELOGRAPHY)

This is the radiographic visualization of the renal pelvis and ureter by the introduction of a contrast medium. The medium may be injected into the bloodstream to be excreted by the kidney (intravenous urography) or it may be injected directly into the renal pelvis by percutaneous injection (antegrade urography) or into the ureter by way of a catheter introduced through a cystoscope (retrograde or ascending urography).

Intravenous urography (IVU)

Contrast medium is administered by i.v. injection and a series of X-rays are taken as the kidney excretes the contrast. IVU has been mostly replaced by ultrasound but is still useful for certain conditions, e.g. detection of some urinary cancers. In common with renal angiography (see above), there is a risk of nephrotoxicity, caused by the i.v. iodine-based contrast medium, and dehydration.

Retrograde urography (pyelography)

Retrograde urography may be undertaken to provide a radiographic evaluation of the ureters or renal pelvis, or to obtain samples of urine for cytology or culture from one or both kidneys. Under cystoscopic guidance (see p. 668), a ureteric catheter is advanced into the ureteric orifice and then upwards into the renal pelvis. The catheter is then withdrawn and, as this is being done, opaque contrast medium is injected. A series of X-ray exposures is taken to visualize the passage of the contrast downwards through the ureter(s) and into the bladder. If urine sampling is required, this is performed prior to injection of contrast medium.

Antegrade urography (pyelography)

Contrast medium is injected into the renal pelvis using a fine needle passed through the skin under X-ray or ultrasound guidance. The technique may be used to locate obstruction and insert nephrostomy drainage tubes (see p. 666).

CYSTOGRAPHY

A cystogram (or cystourethrogram) provides a detailed radiographic evaluation of bladder and urethral function. This procedure involves passing a Foley catheter into the bladder. The bladder is then drained of urine and filled with opaque contrast medium under fluoroscopic guidance. From the point at which bladder filling with contrast medium begins, to the point at which the bladder is full, a series of X-ray exposures is taken. If a micturating (voiding) cystogram is required, the Foley catheter is removed and the patient asked to void. Additional X-ray exposures are taken during voiding and when voiding is complete.

RENAL BIOPSY

Renal biopsy involves the removal of a small piece of renal tissue that is usually subjected to electron microscopy, histology and immunofluorescence tests. The procedure may be uncomfortable and anxiety-provoking for patients. For this reason, some renal centres choose to offer premedication with anxiolytics prior to its performance.

Patients are usually placed in the prone position with one pillow (see Fig. 24.8). The kidney to be biopsied is identified by ultrasound, with note taken of its position and depth. The area through which the biopsy needle will be inserted is then marked. Skin overlying the kidney is cleaned with an appropriate bactericidal/bacteriostatic solution. A local anaesthetic, e.g. lidocaine (lignocaine), is then used to infiltrate the skin (see Ch. 29). Following this, a small incision is made in the skin with a scalpel blade. A special renal biopsy needle is inserted, usually under ultrasound guidance, and advanced to the kidney. Patients are asked to hold their breath and the kidney is biopsied. The piece of tissue obtained is immediately viewed under a microscope to ensure that a sufficient sample of the renal cortex has been obtained. Usually this is a sample of not less than 5 mm in length that is subsequently divided into three. One of the samples will be sent for histology, and the other two for electron microscopy and immunofluorescence. If insufficient tissue has

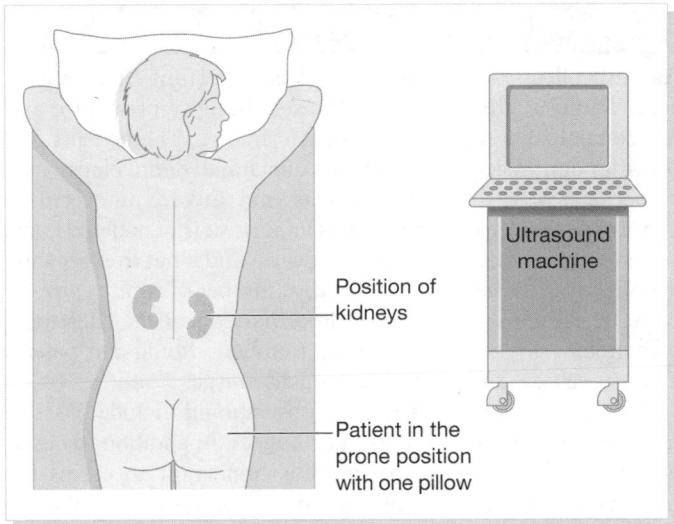

Figure 24.8 Position used for renal biopsy.

been obtained, a subsequent attempt at biopsy will be made. Once the biopsy has been completed, a pressure dressing is applied to the insertion site and patients are asked to remain lying flat in bed.

When a transplanted kidney is biopsied, patients are supine for the procedure and the approach is via the anterior abdominal wall, in the region directly overlying the transplanted kidney. This approach is required because transplanted kidneys are placed in the iliac fossa (see p. 694).

Generally, renal biopsies are performed on the ward area. However, they may also be performed in the ultrasound department under ultrasound guidance. This option is preferred where there is significant additional risk to patients, or where access to the kidney is difficult, as, for example, in an obese patient.

Renal biopsy facilitates accurate description of damage to the renal tissue. However, like other invasive procedures it carries risk, the most significant of these being haemorrhage. The sequelae to haemorrhagic complications following renal biopsy range from the formation of a perirenal haematoma through to bleeding severe enough to warrant surgical intervention, with the attendant risk of emergency nephrectomy (removal of kidney) for uncontrollable blood loss.

Medical care

Part of the medical work-up for renal biopsy involves establishing the nature of risk to the patient, and the extent to which the risks associated with biopsy are justified. As a general rule, patients who are to undergo renal biopsy should have sterile urine (to avoid introducing infection), normal coagulation and blood pressure within the normal range. It is also necessary to establish the number of kidneys and their size and shape prior to biopsy.

Blood samples will be taken for biochemistry, haematology and clotting screen. In addition, it is usual practice to draw a sample for blood group and save. These blood tests provide necessary information that informs the medical assessment of risk. In the case of blood group and save, it is always prudent to anticipate a requirement for blood transfusion, rather than begin the process in an emergency due to active bleeding.

▶ Nursing management

As with all other investigations, it is important that patients receive information regarding the renal biopsy procedure and are competent to consent to its performance. The benefits and the attendant risks must be clearly explained. Renal biopsy may be performed on a day-case basis or may involve an overnight stay in hospital. In either case, it is important that patients know what to expect on admission to the ward, and what to expect and do following discharge. To this end, a number of centres provide patients with pre- and post-care information leaflets. These usually include a contact telephone number, should the patient experience any difficulties following discharge.

Nursing assessment prior to biopsy should include baseline measurement of vital signs and urinalysis. In addition to observation of physical parameters, it is important to assess the patients' expectations of this procedure. For many patients who undergo renal biopsy, the results of this investigation may be the final piece of information required for diagnosis of chronic renal

R|R REFLECTIVE PRACTICE

24.1 Breaking bad news: a diagnosis of end-stage renal failure

Consider the following scenario: you have recently had a renal biopsy and are now attending an outpatient clinic where you are expecting to hear the result of this investigation. The previous conversations that you have had with your consultant, the research you have conducted on the internet, and the way that you seem to feel tired and sick all the time have made you suspect that the news won't be good.

- Would anything make this situation easier for you?
- What help or assistance do you think that the health care professionals could offer you?
- What is your greatest fear and how do you think you will confront and deal with this?

Further reading

Faulkner A. When the news is bad: a guide for health professionals on breaking bad news. Cheltenham: Stanley Thornes; 1998.

Kralik D, Brown M, Koch T. Women's experience of 'being diagnosed' with a long term illness. J Adv Nurs 2001; 33(5): 594–602.

disease. Thus, the outcome of renal biopsy may have a significant impact on the patient's life (see Reflective Practice box 24.1). On the nephrology ward, the point at which renal biopsy is performed may be the point at which nurses are introduced to individuals for whom they will subsequently provide care for a considerable period of time.

Nursing care specific to the post-biopsy procedure will include the following:

- Ensure that patients remain resting comfortably in bed following the procedure.
- Since the risk of haemorrhage is significant, it is important that the frequency of observations of pulse and blood pressure, and of the biopsy puncture site, reflect this risk. As a general rule, observations are performed at 15-minute intervals at least for the first hour, then half-hourly for 2 hours, then hourly for 4 hours.
- Patients may require the administration of an oral analgesic, e.g. paracetamol, following the biopsy. Severe pain and discomfort are not normal sequelae to renal biopsy and warrant prompt attention and investigation if they are reported.
- Urinary output and observation of the presence or absence of blood should be recorded.

CYSTOSCOPY

An internal inspection of the bladder and its three openings is achieved by cystoscopy (see Fig. 24.9). Flexible cystoscopy using a fibreoptic cystoscope with a video display unit attachment

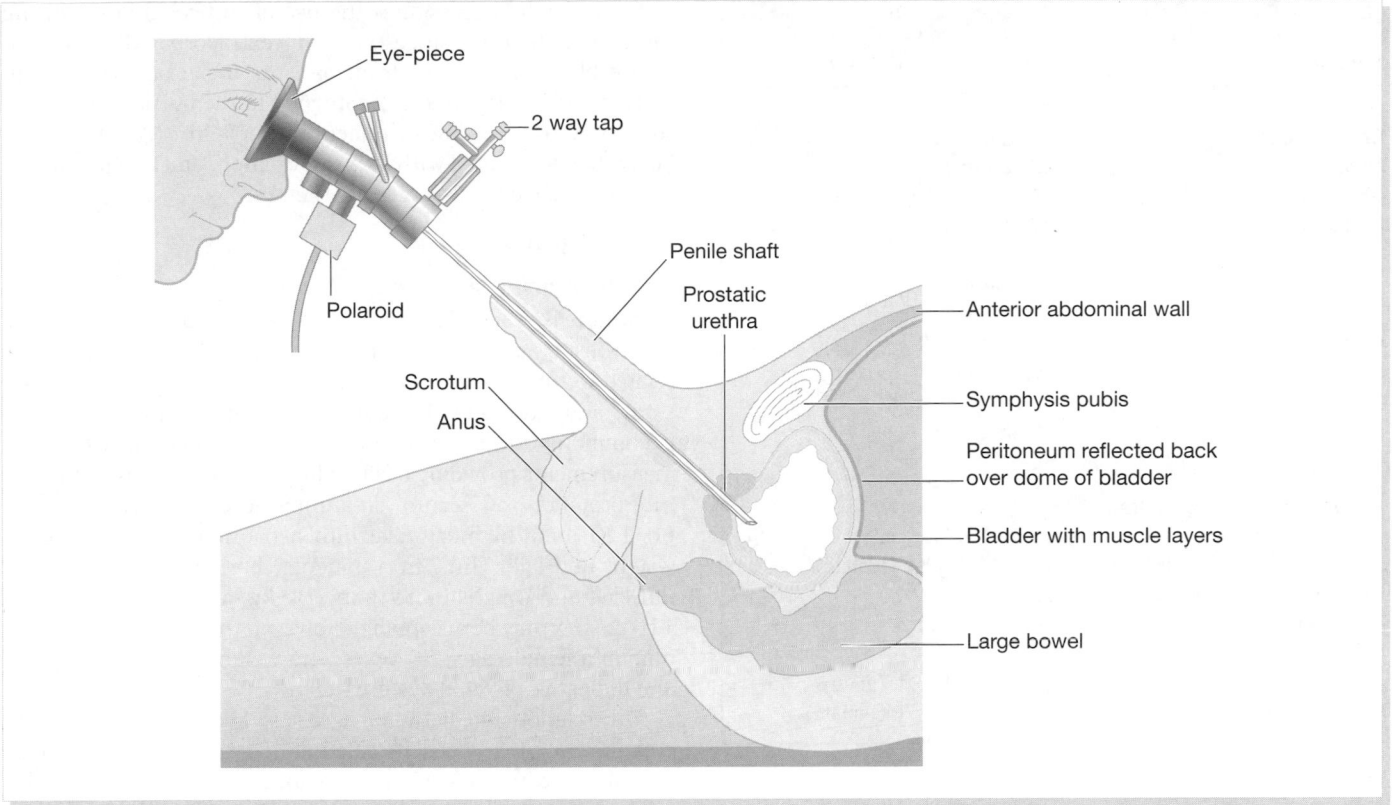

Figure 24.9 Cystoscopy.

now allows cystoscopy to be performed on both an in-patient and outpatient basis. Flexible cystoscopy is performed under local anaesthetic, commonly with gel containing lidocaine (lignocaine) instilled intraurethrally prior to the procedure. Bladder biopsy may be performed as part of the procedure; or where cystoscopy is part of the follow-up of patients with superficial bladder tumours, removal of tumour(s) may be performed. Where a general anaesthetic is required, patient preparation will include a period of fasting and safe recovery from anaesthesia (see Ch. 29).

URODYNAMIC STUDIES

Urodynamic studies are used to assess the function of the urethra, bladder and sphincters. Uroflowmetry measures both peak and mean urine flow rates during micturition with a flow meter. In females, the normal flow rate is 20–40 mL/s and in males it is 15–30 mL/s. Accurate measurement of flow rate is facilitated by a voided volume greater than 150 mL. Thus, patients are encouraged to have a full bladder when attending for this test.

Evaluation of urine flow can be combined with cystometry. The latter will measure residual urine volume, bladder capacity, detrusor muscle pressures and the volume at which a desire to void occurs.

This test requires urethral catheterization (insertion of a catheter into the bladder), and it is important that the urine is sterile prior to this procedure. Catheterization of the vagina (women) or rectum is also required as part of this procedure to measure intra-abdominal pressures, in order to evaluate detrusor muscle activity. Assessment of sphincter muscle activity can also be undertaken as part of this procedure.

Further coverage of urodynamic studies is provided in later sections (see also Ch. 12 and 'Further reading', p. 702).

BLOOD TESTS

Both haematological and biochemical blood tests provide information about renal function. Nurses should know the normal values for standard haematological and biochemical tests (see Table 24.3, p. 670). The reference range of normal values may vary locally, as indeed may the units of measurement expressed. In addition, the results of blood tests are always interpreted within a clinical context. Thus, while a given blood result may be outside the normal reference range, it may be considered 'normal' in certain situations. One example of this is estimation of serum K^+. The normal range for serum K^+ is 3.3–4.7 mmol/L, and a value outside this range would be considered abnormal. However, in the patient having long-term haemodialysis, a pre-dialysis serum K^+ of up to 6.0 mmol/L and a postdialysis serum K^+ less than the bottom of the range, while abnormal, are both common and acceptable.

Haematological tests
Haemoglobin

Red blood cells that carry haemoglobin are produced in the bone marrow. In adults, the rate of production is dependent on the activity of a hormone (growth factor) called erythropoietin

Table 24.3 Normal blood values

Parameters	Value – reference range
Biochemical parameters	
Creatinine	60–120 µmol/L
Urea	2.5–6.4 mmol/L
Sodium	135–143 mmol/L
Potassium	3.3–4.7 mmol/L
Calcium	2.1–2.6 mmol/L
Chloride	97–106 mmol/L
Phosphate	0.8–1.4 mmol/L
Bicarbonate	22–28 mmol/L
Cholesterol	3.5–5.7 mmol/L
Triglycerides	0.45–2.0 mmol/L
Total protein	60–80 g/L
Albumin	35–55 g/L
Haematological parameters	
Haemoglobin	13.5–18 g/dL (male)
	11.5–16.5 g/dL (female)
Platelets	$150–400 \times 10^9$/L
Leucocytes	$4.0–11.0 \times 10^9$/L
(white blood cells)	
Erythrocytes	$4.5–6.5 \times 10^{12}$/L (male)
(red blood cells)	$3.8–5.3 \times 10^{12}$/L (female)

(see Ch. 18). Primarily peritubular cells in the cortex of the kidney produce erythropoietin, and production is controlled by a negative feedback mechanism. These cells are sensitive to the partial pressure of oxygen (Po_2). When Po_2 falls, the cells respond by increasing production of erythropoietin, which in turn acts on the bone marrow to increase red cell synthesis. Increased red blood cell production normally results in an increase in haemoglobin and thus oxygen-carrying capacity. Once Po_2 sensed by the peritubular cells has returned to normal limits, erythropoietin production declines to baseline levels.

Where there is loss of renal functional mass, as happens when the kidneys have been damaged by disease, synthesis of erythropoietin by the kidney decreases, and may cease entirely. In chronic renal disease, the effect of this is chronic underproduction of red blood cells (anaemia, see Ch. 18) and, if uncorrected, a persistent hypoxic state, with its attendant cardiovascular sequelae (see Ch. 19).

Since the late 1980s, a human recombinant form of erythropoietin has been available for clinical use and has had a significant impact on the ability to manage the anaemia associated with chronic renal disease.

Coagulation studies

Coagulation studies include assessment of bleeding and clotting times – prothrombin time (PT), activated partial thromboplastin time (APTT), international normalized ratio (INR) – plasma levels of fibrinogen, and platelet count (see Ch. 18). Abnormality of haemostasis (see Ch. 18) is common in chronic renal dysfunction, for two principal reasons. The first is that renal dysfunction induces mixed abnormalities of haemostasis, such that a propensity both to bleed and to clot may be observed in the patient. Secondly, replacement of renal function with haemodialysis (see

p. 690) usually necessitates the use of anticoagulants during the dialytic therapy, since this is an extracorporeal treatment where blood is removed from patients to be passed through external tubing before being returned to them. Altered haemostasis may also be a feature of acute renal failure (ARF), particularly when associated with liver dysfunction, and in sepsis where there is damage to vascular endothelium.

Biochemical tests
Serum creatinine

Creatinine is produced endogenously as a by-product of muscle metabolism, and the quantity produced in a 24-hour period is related to total muscle mass. The production rate is fairly constant, and normally the kidneys clear creatinine. Creatinine is commonly used as a marker for renal function, with serial measurements providing a clinically useful indication of change. Interpretation of serum creatinine levels (reference range 60–120 µmol/L) must take into account the patient's body weight and age. Thus, in a patient who is young, fit, heavily muscled and weighs more than 100 kg, a serum creatinine of 110 µmol/L may be acceptable. However, the same serum creatinine in a female aged 50 years who weighs 50 kg is abnormal and indicative of renal dysfunction.

The relationship between age, sex, body mass and serum creatinine can be used to calculate the creatinine clearance rate, which can be used to provide an estimate of the GFR. This estimate can be made using a blood sample only. The lower normal limit for creatinine clearance is 77 mL/min per 1.72 m² (body surface area).

Serum urea

Urea is formed as a by-product of protein metabolism in the body. Unlike creatinine, the serum urea fluctuates as a function of protein intake. It is not used as a clinical marker of renal function in the way that creatinine is. However, measurement of the serum urea level is useful in a number of contexts, e.g.:

- to determine a patient's catabolic rate, and as such can form the basis of dietetic recommendations for optimal protein intake
- to determine dialysis adequacy
- to guide the dialysis treatment plan for a patient undergoing a first haemodialysis, particularly in ARF.

Serum electrolytes

Samples are commonly taken to measure the level of electrolytes in the blood of patients with renal problems. You will remember from the earlier discussion about the formation of urine in the nephron just how important is the kidneys' role in electrolyte homeostasis. The four electrolytes, Na^+, K^+, Ca^{2+} and phosphate (PO_4^-), are outlined here and readers are directed to Chapter 8, which provides a fuller description.

Sodium

Sodium is the main positively charged electrolyte in extracellular fluid (ECF). Dietary intake (see Ch. 11) accounts for the daily sodium load, and extracellular concentrations are maintained by the activity of the kidney. Hypernatraemia ($Na^+ >143$ mmol/L) may result from depletion of vascular volume, or disordered renal tubular handling of sodium. Hyponatraemia

$(Na^+ < 135 \text{ mmol/L})$ may be related to vascular volume overload (dilution hyponatraemia) or excessive loss of sodium.

Potassium

Potassium is the main positively charged electrolyte in the intracellular fluid (ICF). Like sodium, potassium is ingested in the diet (see Ch. 11) and its concentrations, both intracellular and extracellular, are adjusted by the activity of renal tubular cells. Alterations in serum potassium levels outside the normal range have serious implications, and both hypokalaemia $(K^+ < 3.3 \text{ mmol/L})$ and hyperkalaemia $(K^+ > 4.7 \text{ mmol/L})$ give rise to cardiac arrhythmias (see Ch. 19). Hyperkalaemia is a feature of both ARF and chronic renal failure (CRF), and it must be treated as an absolute clinical priority. In the absence of renal function, the most efficient means by which to remove excess potassium is with dialysis (see pp. 690–691).

Calcium and phosphate

Abnormal levels of calcium and phosphate are common in patients with CRF, and may also be a feature of some causes of ARF (e.g. rhabdomyolysis where massive damage to muscle occurs, such as with crush injuries). In CRF, serum evaluation of PTH levels may be requested in addition to levels of calcium and phosphate, because it controls calcium and phosphate homeostasis.

Other blood tests

- Serum levels of the enzyme alkaline phosphatase provide an indication of bone turnover (see Ch. 27) and may be requested in patients with CRF.
- Serum levels of the enzyme acid phosphatase may be measured where there is suspicion of bony metastatic spread from prostate cancer.
- Prostate-specific antigen (PSA, see p. 700).

URINE TESTS

Urine may be examined and tested in the laboratory for a variety of abnormalities. In order to ensure accurate results, nurses must make sure that the correct specimen is obtained using the appropriate container and that patients and all staff are aware if urine is being collected over a 24-hour period and whether an early morning specimen of urine (EMSU) is required. Readers are directed to the suggestions for further reading.

- Urine microscopy will identify the presence of blood cells (red and white), casts, crystals and bacteria. If bacteria are present, urine culture to identify the type of bacteria is indicated, and antibiotic sensitivity. A variety of methods are used to collect urine to test for the presence of infection and ascertain which antibiotics are likely to be effective, e.g. midstream specimen of urine (MSSU), catheter or nephrostomy tube specimen (see Guidelines for Care Priorities box 24.1) or EMSU (see below, renal tuberculosis).
- Urinary electrolytes, urea and albumin.
- Cytological examination, for abnormal cells, is usually undertaken on three EMSUs collected on consecutive days.

(Observation and dipstick tests on urine are discussed on page 663.)

GENERAL DISEASE PREVENTION AND HEALTH EDUCATION

General advice to maintain a healthy urinary system should include the following:

- Maintain a daily fluid intake of about 3 litres consisting primarily of water.

 GUIDELINES FOR CARE PRIORITIES

24.1 Collecting specimens of urine

Midstream specimen of urine (MSSU) and clean-catch specimens of urine

In order to obtain these, you will need a sterile universal container, and gloves if you are going to assist patients. If patients can perform the collection of this independently, you should provide clear instructions. They should be advised to wash their hands prior to obtaining the specimen, and to open the sterile container following this, without touching the inside of either the container or its lid. Female patients should be advised to separate the labia majora using the index and middle fingers of one hand, and men to retract the foreskin if they are not circumcized during specimen collection. In order to obtain the specimen, patients should be advised to commence urination and then to place the container in the stream and collect urine. The container can then be placed to one side while urination is completed. Following handwashing, the lid of the container should be placed securely and without touching the inside of the lid. The identity of the patient and type of specimen should be clearly shown on the universal container. The specimen, with relevant request form, is placed in the appropriate plastic bag and dispatched to the laboratory.

Catheter specimens of urine (CSU)

These are obtained from the specimen port on the catheter drainage bag, using a sterile needle and syringe. Where possible, it is preferable not to open a closed urinary drainage system for specimen collection.

Collecting a urine specimen from a nephrostomy tube(s) attached to a drainage bag where there is no available specimen collection port

In order to do this, you will need to open the closed drainage system and allow urine to drip from the nephrostomy tube into a sterile container. Every care must be taken to ensure that the risk of introducing infection via the nephrostomy tube is minimized. This includes nurse handwashing prior to collecting the specimen and ensuring that you have a clear and clean field in which to work.

- Reduce caffeine intake and only drink alcohol in moderation, and within the recommended weekly limits (see Ch. 23).
- Urinate frequently during the day.
- Urinate following sexual intercourse.
- Personal hygiene is important. Uncircumcised males should be taught at an early age how to retract the foreskin in order to clean the glans. Daily washing of this area with soap and water is all that is required. Females should be taught from an early age to clean the urinary meatus from front to back.
- Pelvic floor exercises should be taught to both males and females, and encouragement given to perform them (see Ch. 12).

Those individuals who are at increased risk of urinary system problems, such as those who have recurrent UTIs, diabetes, known structural urinary abnormality and after renal transplant, should know when to seek assistance or advice. For example, nurses need to ensure that these individuals are able to recognize signs of UTI or other infections that can result in additional physiological stress. Staying healthy may also mean taking medications, e.g. antihypertensives or antibiotics, or keeping to a prescribed diet.

URINARY SYSTEM DISORDERS

URINARY TRACT INFECTIONS: CYSTITIS AND PYELONEPHRITIS

Urinary tract infections (UTIs) are usually isolated or rarely repeated events and are commoner in women than in men (see below). There is significant morbidity associated with recurrent UTI and in infections occurring in patients who already have abnormal urinary tract structure or function. UTIs may be either uncomplicated, when they occur in patients with a normal lower urinary tract, or complicated, when there is structural and/or functional problems affecting the lower urinary tract.

Aetiology and pathophysiology

The microorganisms most commonly associated with UTIs are bowel flora, with *Escherichia coli* and other coliforms accounting for some 68% of cases. In young women, *Staphylococcus epidermidis* and *S. saprophyticus* are causative organisms in some 20–30% of cases. Transfer of these normally occurring commensal bacteria to a site where they become pathogenic (disease-forming) is usually by the ascending transurethral route, although they may also be blood-borne, or transferred via a vesicocolic fistula (abnormal communication between the bladder and bowel) (Hooton 2000).

The development of a UTI can be summarized as follows:

Entry of bacteria. The perineum and periurethral area are heavily colonized with bacteria. There is thus an ample reservoir of potentially pathogenic organisms surrounding the area where the urethra opens externally. Females have short urethras and the transfer of bacteria transurethrally may be spontaneous or facilitated by sexual intercourse (so-called 'honeymoon cystitis') or catheterization. The relatively long urethra in males provides some degree of protection against transurethral bacterial

transfer, although, as in females, catheterization is a potential source of transfer (see p. 674).

Multiplication of bacteria in the bladder. Normally urine in the bladder is sterile. This state has been attributed to mucosal defence mechanisms and the 'flushing' effect that normal bladder voiding has. Urinary stasis and incomplete bladder emptying are contributory factors in the development of UTIs.

Clinical presentation

Some patients will have bacteria in their urine without symptoms – asymptomatic bacteriuria (see below). The symptoms associated with UTIs arise as a sequel to the body's inflammatory response to bacterial entry. Commonly, individuals with cystitis (lower UTI) report frequency and dysuria (painful micturition). The urine may have an odour often described as 'fishy', with haematuria and suprapubic pain also reported. Changes in behaviour, such as confusion in older people, may be indicative of UTI. Symptoms such as fever, loin pain and nausea/vomiting are suggestive of infection that has ascended via the ureters into the renal pelvis and the kidneys to cause pyelonephritis.

Asymptomatic bacteriuria

This is the presence of greater than or equal to 100 000/mL of the same bacterial species in two or more consecutive MSSUs, without symptoms. A number of studies have shown that non-pregnant women with uncomplicated asymptomatic bacteriuria either spontaneously rid themselves of bacteriuria or change the bacterial species. While the significance of, and need to treat, asymptomatic bacteriuria are still debatable, there is agreement on a number of points. The first is that it is important to distinguish between asymptomatic bacteriuria in pregnant and non-pregnant women. Asymptomatic bacteriuria in pregnant women is treated with antibiotics (e.g. nitrofurantoin), because having the condition in the first trimester is associated with the development of upper urinary tract infection in the second and third trimesters. Secondly, asymptomatic bacteriuria that is complicated by an abnormal urinary tract or by co-morbidity (e.g. diabetes mellitus), or which occurs in immuno-suppressed patients (e.g. following kidney transplantation) is also treated with antibiotics, again because of the risk of ascending infection.

Investigations

A urine specimen (MSSU) is obtained for microscopy, culture and sensitivity (see p. 671). Generally, a bacterial count of >100 000 per mL of the same microorganism is indicative of bladder infection. However, this should not be taken as an absolute figure since recent studies have shown that up to a third of patients with active infection may have bacterial colony counts lower than this (Hooton 2000). There may also be a positive result for nitrite on dipstick urinalysis.

In the setting of recurrent UTI, or where post-treatment urinalysis remains abnormal, urodynamic studies may be indicated to exclude the presence of abnormality of the lower urinary tract. In children, this is mandatory following a proven first episode of bacteriuria. A micturating cystogram is indicated in adults to investigate abnormal bladder voiding.

Medical management: cystitis and pyelonephritis

Treatment of uncomplicated cystitis (lower UTI) is with antibiotic therapy (e.g. nitrofurantoin, cefalexin, trimethoprin or amoxicillin). This may be either a 3-day regimen or a single-dose treatment.

Pyelonephritis is also treated with antibiotics on an outpatient basis, unless the clinical condition of the individual warrants hospitalization. In the latter case, inability to maintain oral hydration, take oral medications, severe pain and high fever (> 38°C) are suggestive of a requirement to hospitalize. Management will include:

- pain relief
- i.v. fluids and antibiotics
- antiemetics as necessary.

Urine culture both preceding and following drug therapy is mandatory. If there are clinical signs indicative of septicaemia (see Ch. 9) then blood cultures will be drawn.

Treatment of complicated UTI centres on antimicrobial treatment with subsequent evaluation of urologic function and correction of risk factors if possible.

▶ Nursing management: cystitis and pyelonephritis

Recurrent episodes of uncomplicated UTI should prompt review of patient hygiene, fluid intake and micturition patterns (see Health Promotion box 24.1). Cranberry juice has been promoted as prophylaxis against the development of UTIs, although empirical data to support this are scant (Hooton 2000).

Nursing care of patients with pyelonephritis is essentially supportive and focuses on:

- Assisting patients to maintain adequate hydration. It may be difficult for them to meet their fluid intake needs, particularly in the setting of nausea, emesis, fever or pain. Intravenous hydration may be required. Patients'. i.v. fluid requirements are assessed according to level of hydration/fluid deficit, urinary output and patient size. Minimum standards of care associated with the administration of i.v. fluids include ensuring that the type, volume and rate of fluid are administered as prescribed, observation of the i.v. cannula site for signs of inflammation (redness, heat) or extravasation, observation of urinary output, and accurate documentation of fluid intake and output. All NHS Trusts will have an i.v. policy, and nurses should be familiar with its contents. If patients are able to tolerate it, oral intake should be encouraged, with sips of water, for example, or ice chips offered regularly.
- Making patients comfortable and relieving pain. Loin pain and dysuria with or without frequency are distressing symptoms for patients. Analgesia may be required, e.g. paracetamol (may also be prescribed for its antipyretic effect), and patients' response to this should be monitored, with alterations to the type and/or frequency of administration made if required. Ensure that patients can easily access toileting facilities. This may involve placing a commode beside their bed. Cool drinks (if tolerated) help with personal hygiene and a fan should be made available to patients. Antiemetic administration (e.g. prochlorperazine) may also be required.

HEALTH PROMOTION

24.1 Avoiding UTI

Key preventative strategies include:

- Attention to personal hygiene
- Use of two different towels to dry the genital and anal regions
- Passing urine following sexual intercourse
- Maintaining hydration (> 3 L/day, with water accounting for the majority of this)
- Passing urine frequently during the day
- Passing urine just before going to bed
- Avoiding the use of potentially irritant toiletries
- Reducing intake of caffeine and alcohol since both are bladder irritants
- Increasing intake of cranberry juice, which may acidify the urine and thus inhibit bacterial growth. However, care should be taken when providing this advice, as increased urinary acidity can diminish the effectiveness of concurrent antibiotic therapy
- Seeking advice from a health professional if symptoms (e.g. dysuria) of UTI occur.

Further reading

Cantagallo A, Castelli M. Cost-free prevention to asymptomatic bacteriuria in diabetic women: two hands two towels. Diabetes Care 2001; 24(2): 412–413.

Kerr KG. Cranberry juice and prevention of recurrent urinary tract infection. The Lancet 1999; 353(9153): 673.

- Monitoring of patients' cardiovascular system, temperature, pulse, respirations, overall fluid balance and pain experience. The frequency of these observations should reflect the severity of the illness.
- Administration of i.v. antibiotics. This may be necessary and, as noted above, readers are advised to familiarize themselves with the local i.v. policy. Usually i.v. antibiotic administration will only be required for 24–48 hours, after which time response to antibiotic therapy should be evident and oral administration of antibiotics can begin. Nurses should ensure that patients are aware of the importance of completing the course of antibiotics after discharge.

REFLUX NEPHROPATHY (CHRONIC PYELONEPHRITIS)

The principal predisposing cause of reflux nephropathy is incompetence of the one-way valve system where the ureters enter the bladder. This defect may be unilateral or bilateral. Readers will recall that the ureters enter the bladder obliquely, forming the vesicoureteric junction. Normally, during voiding of the bladder, contraction compresses the vesicoureteric junction, sealing it off and preventing reflux of urine back up the ureters – vesicoureteric reflux (VUR). Incompetence of this valve system allows reflux of urine up the ureters (ureteral jet). In addition, it leads to incomplete bladder emptying, since once the person has voided, the urine that refluxed into the ureters flows back to the bladder. Stasis of urine in the bladder predisposes to infection, and persistent reflux of infected urine up the ureters results in damage to the renal parenchyma (renal tissue). The defect is present in infants and young children, and confirmed bacteriuria in the young should be thoroughly investigated. Early detection and treatment can minimize or prevent renal damage in later life. Prompt treatment of UTI and low-dose prophylactic antibiotic therapy (e.g. low-dose trimethoprim at night) are the mainstays of management of this condition. Treatment of the structural abnormality may also include surgical re-implantation of one or both ureters to form a competent valve.

INFECTION ASSOCIATED WITH INDWELLING URINARY CATHETERS

The incidence of bacteriuria associated with indwelling urinary catheters increases with the length of catheter placement. In the context of catheterization of longer than 30 days, bacteriuria is almost universal. Gram-negative septicaemia in the hospitalized patient is closely associated with the presence of an indwelling catheter (Stamm & Hooton 1993).

In view of this, preventative measures to reduce catheter-associated infection are warranted. From a nursing perspective, the latter includes:

- sterile catheter insertion
- strict attention to personal hygiene in the catheterized patient
- strict adherence to maintenance of the closed collecting system.

Catheterization should only be undertaken when necessitated by patient needs (see Reflective Practice box 24.2).

Urinary catheterization of both women and men is an established nursing role. While the procedure is relatively simple, it is not without risks, and the well-informed nurse should be aware of these and be able to justify the rationale for catheterization, type of catheter (see Guidelines for Care Priorities box 24.2) and drainage system selected, and also be able to plan both short- and long-term care of patients with indwelling catheters.

Urinary catheters may be inserted via the urethra (urethral catheterization) or via an abdominal approach above the level of the symphysis pubis (suprapubic catheterization). The choice of route is influenced by both the reason for catheterization, and particularly in the case of long-term catheterization, patient needs and physical abilities.

RENAL ABSCESS

Cortical abscess

The causative microorganism of cortical abscesses is commonly *Staphylococcus aureus* and the transmission route is blood-borne (haematogenous). There is good response to antibiotics and abscess drainage is not usually required.

Corticomedullary abscess

Corticomedullary abscess formation usually results from ascending infection from the lower urinary tract and is associated with abnormal function. The abscess may penetrate deep through the renal parenchyma and perforate the renal capsule, ultimately forming a perinephric abscess (abscess around the kidney).

24.2 Is catheterization always necessary?

Urinary catheterization is highly associated with the development of bacteriuria, and thus careful consideration must be given to its use.

Student activities
- Consider the following statements and make a note of your response to them:
  — Urinary catheterization is the only way to accurately measure urinary output
  — Incontinence in older people is best treated by urinary catheterization
  — The risk to patients associated with urinary catheterization is negligible.
- Outline your evidence for agreeing or disagreeing with the above, and discuss this with another student on your course. Explore any differences or similarities between you. Identify any areas where you think you need further information.

Further reading
Godfrey H, Evans A. Catheterization and urinary tract infection: microbiology. Br J Nurs 2000; 9(11): 688–690.
Penfold P. UTI in patients with urethral catheters; an audit tool. Br J Nurs 1999; 8(6): 362–364, 366, 368.

Investigation will include a CT scan to locate the site of the abscess. Causative organisms include those usually associated with infection of the lower urinary tract (e.g. *E. coli*). Aspiration and drainage of pus with concomitant antibiotics are the principal treatments. The potential for Gram-negative septicaemia is very real, and close attention to monitoring of cardiovascular status, respiratory function and overall fluid balance is a necessary nursing function.

RENAL TUBERCULOSIS

Tuberculosis (TB) is a multisystem bacterial disease caused by several types of mycobacteria, e.g. *Mycobacterium tuberculosis* (see Ch. 20). In the developed world it is more common in older people and specific groups (e.g. those of Indo-Asian origin), although a rise in incidence in the younger population associated with human immunodeficiency virus (HIV) infection has occurred over the last two decades, and also in those who are socially disadvantaged, such as rough sleepers. Renal TB is usually blood-borne and occurs secondary to infection elsewhere in the body (usually the lungs).

Clinical presentation

Frequency, dysuria, haematuria and nocturia (waking to pass urine at night) account for some 80% of the clinical features seen. Sterile pyuria (pus in the urine) and microscopic haematuria are also notable features. There may also be general features of TB such as weight loss and pyrexia. However, patients can be asymptomatic, and diagnosis serendipitous, rather than actively sought.

24.2 Catheter selection

The factors that influence choice of catheter (size, balloon infill size and material) include the indication for catheterization, patient needs and the likely duration of catheterization.

Catheter length and Charriere (Ch) size

Urinary catheters come in two adult lengths: female (23–26 cm) and male or standard (40–44 cm). The longer length must be used on male patients for urethral catheterization, because of the length of the male urethra.

It may also be used for female patients. The shorter 'female' length can only be used for female patients.

Charriere size refers to the external diameter of the catheter. This may also be referred to as French gauge or French units. A Charriere unit is 0.33 mm, thus a 12Ch catheter is approximately 4 mm, a 16Ch is 5.3 mm, etc. As a general rule, you should choose the smallest diameter that will provide adequate urine drainage. Smaller Charriere size allows the mucus produced by paraurethral glands to drain away easily and exerts less pressure on the internal wall of the urethra. A larger diameter catheter is usually required after surgery when haematuria with clots is anticipated.

Balloon infill size

Balloon infill sizes for indwelling catheters vary from 2.5 to 5 mL in paediatric catheters, 10 to 30 mL in adult size catheters, and greater than 50 mL in some specialist urological catheters. Again, the rule is that the smaller the balloon infill, the better. For general use, a 10 mL infill is preferable. In the catheterized patient, the filled infill balloon rests on the bladder neck. If it is overfilled, or where there is a high balloon infill, the weight exerted on the bladder neck and pelvic floor will be increased.

Catheter materials

Catheters that are being utilized for short- or medium-term use (up to 4 weeks) are commonly made of Teflon-coated latex. For longer-term catheterization, more specialized (and more expensive) catheters are used; they may be made of silicone, latex coated with silicone, latex coated with a hydrogel or a hydrated polymer. The latter usually have a life span of 12 weeks. Catheters used for intermittent self-catheterization may be composed as either polyvinyl chloride (PVC) or plastic.

Further reading

Getliffe K. Care of urinary catheters. Nurs Stand 1995; 10(1): 25–31.

Robinson J. Urethral catheter selection. Nurs Stand 2001; 15(25): 39–42.

Winn C, Thompson J. Catheterisation: the scope of professional practice. Nurs Stand 1997; 12(13–15): 57–64

Investigations

Diagnosis can be confirmed in a number of ways:

- Positive culture of mycobacteria from a series of EMSUs. Usually between three and five early morning specimens are obtained. This method is relatively slow, since it takes up to six weeks or more for microcolony growth to be visible.
- Polymerase chain reaction (PCR) and soluble antigen fluorescent antibody (SAFA) tests on patient serum are now available as rapid methods of confirming diagnosis.

Medical management

In the past, nephrectomy was the only treatment available for renal tuberculosis. Currently, treatment is with a combination of bactericidal drugs, each of which is active against a specific group of *M. tuberculosis* (Maher et al 1997). Antituberculous drugs include:

- isoniazid – pyridoxine is always prescribed with this as prophylaxis against the development of peripheral neuropathy, a known side-effect of isoniazid
- rifampicin – patients should be informed that red/orange discoloration of the urine is associated with this drug
- pyrazinamide
- streptomycin
- ethambutol.

All of these drugs have unpleasant side-effects, including gastrointestinal upset, rashes and flu-like symptoms. However, it is imperative that each is taken as prescribed for the duration of the prescription.

The pharmacological treatment of TB is biphasic (initial and a continuation phase). In the initial phase, drug treatment aims to decrease the bacterial population quickly. For this phase a combination of three or more drugs is used (e.g. rifampicin, isoniazid, pyrazinamide and ethambutol) and is usually continued for 2 months. Combined preparations are available for use (e.g. rifampicin, isoniazid and pyrazinamide). In the continuation phase, a reduced schedule of medications (e.g. two drugs in combination) is continued for 4 months, or longer if there is drug resistance.

Failure to complete the prescribed course may result in incomplete eradication of *M. tuberculosis* and increases the potential for the development of drug resistance.

▶ Nursing management

One of the key features of care for people with renal TB is enabling patients to comply with the drug therapy regimen, especially following discharge. The ability and willingness of the patient to take medications should not be taken for granted. The discharge planning process involves:

- an assessment of the patient's understanding and acceptance of the requirement for the prescribed drug regimen
- identification of potential barriers to compliance with the drug regimen – this includes the individual's home and

social circumstances, ability to read and follow the dose regimen, and the identification of support requirements. A number of these drugs can be provided as fixed-dose combinations of two or more drugs. Combining drugs is simpler for the patient and may increase compliance and reduce the potential for dosing errors.

Multidisciplinary support involving the family, district or practice nurse, social worker and language interpreter, if required, must be planned and in place prior to discharge. All patients require follow-up outpatient care, and care should be taken to ensure patients are aware of plans for this.

NEPHROLITHIASIS

Nephrolithiasis (renal calculi) is the formation of stones within the kidney. Stones may be found within the renal tubules or renal pelvis, ureters and bladder. There are a number of different types of renal stones, classified according to composition, e.g. calcium, urate, cystine. Renal calculi range in size from small to large staghorn calculi that can obstruct the collecting system.

Aetiology and pathophysiology

Renal calculi are more common in men than in women, and are predominantly found in Caucasian individuals. A number of predisposing factors to stone formation have been described:

- supersaturation of the urine with the constituents of a specific stone (e.g. calcium)
- persistent production of concentrated urine consequent to dehydration, e.g. those who work or live in hot climates, or older people unable to access adequate fluids
- failure of factors present in the urine to inhibit crystallization (e.g. urinary pH can influence propensity to form stones) (Mandel 1996).

Certain drugs are known to potentiate stone formation (e.g. salicylates, glucocorticoids and loop diuretics such as furosemide [frusemide]).

Clinical presentation

The clinical presentation depends on the site of the calculus, the presence of infection and/or urinary tract obstruction. Ureteric colic is classically associated with renal calculi. The severe flank (loin) pain generated frequently has a sudden onset and then gradually intensifies. Pain may radiate to the groin, testes or labia majora in women. Renal calculi of less than 5 mm diameter can be passed spontaneously with adequate patient hydration. Larger stones usually require urologic intervention for removal. Calculi that are sufficiently large to obstruct the urinary tract may present with the signs and symptoms of ARF (see p. 685), particularly if there is bilateral obstruction or underlying chronic renal dysfunction.

Specific investigations

- Ultrasound, CT scans and plain X-ray film of the kidneys, ureters and bladder can be used to determine the presence of the calculus, its size, position and any obstructive dilatation in the urinary tract
- Blood samples to assess renal function

- Biochemical screening for metabolic causes of calculus formation, including serum calcium, phosphate, oxalate, uric acid and PTH levels
- Urine samples are taken to determine the presence of infection
- A 24-hour urine collection to determine urinary calcium, phosphate, oxalate and uric acid
- In renal colic or following urologic intervention, the urine should be strained in order to catch any small stones/gravel passed. Stones passed in the urine or physically removed should be sent for analysis of their constituents
- Review of patient medications should also be undertaken, since there are drugs known to potentiate stone formation (see above).

Medical/surgical management

The treatment of calculi obstructing the ureter involves elimination of obstruction, pain relief (usually with strong opioid analgesics since renal colic is excruciatingly painful), and treatment of infection with antibiotics. Elimination of obstruction is dependent on the site of obstruction. Upper urinary tract obstruction can be treated with percutaneous nephrostomy tubes. These are inserted with ultrasonic guidance under local anaesthetic through the flank to lie with their tips within the collecting system of the kidney. One of the particular benefits of nephrostomy tube insertion is that it facilitates subsequent radiologic evaluation of the urinary tract (nephrostogram).

Urologic interventions to remove renal stones are also dependent on the site and size of stone. Stones in the lower ureter can be pulverized (broken into small particles) using a number of techniques, including shock-wave lithotripsy, lasers, and electrohydraulic or pneumatic lithotripsy. Insertion of a nephrostomy tube for 1–5 days is usual where any of the latter three techniques have been used. Stones in the upper ureter can be pushed upwards into the renal pelvis, and again pulverized using one of the techniques mentioned.

A stone within the kidney which is too large to pass down the ureter and which is not treatable using one of the described techniques may require open surgical removal (nephrolithotomy).

Shock-wave lithotripsy

This involves the use of high-energy shock waves, applied externally and aimed at a stone in the kidney or ureter. These waves cause the stone to break into small pieces that may then be passed in the urine or retrieved endoscopically. Cardiac monitoring is required during shock-wave lithotripsy for two reasons – firstly to synchronize the shock-wave pulse with the R wave of the PQRST complex, and secondly to monitor for cardiac arrhythmias (see Ch. 19). A double J stent may be inserted into the collecting system as part of this procedure to allow for the passage of stone fragments greater than 5 mm.

> ▶ **Nursing management: patients with a nephrostomy tube**

Nursing interventions specifically associated with caring for the patient following nephrostomy tube insertion include the following:

- Checking the insertion site for bleeding or urine leakage. The nephrostomy tube(s) will be secured to the skin with a suture, and an occlusive dressing applied following insertion. If the nephrostomy tube is patent, the area around the insertion site will be dry. If there is urine leakage, this may be related to external obstruction of the tube (e.g. the patient sitting on the tube) or internal blockage (e.g. by a clot). While it is possible to check patency of the tube by instilling no more than 5–10 mL of normal saline through it using a 10 mL syringe, this procedure should never be undertaken in the absence of specific medical instruction, since it carries the risk of trauma to the renal pelvis and the potential to introduce infection, particularly if the urine is not sterile. Ensure that the nephrostomy tube is secure and that it cannot be pulled out of position.
- Ensuring adherence to a closed collecting system, to minimize the risk of infection. A collecting bag for urine will be attached to the nephrostomy tube on insertion. If hourly monitoring of urine output is required, this may be exchanged for a urinometer (collection system with integral measuring). In either case it is important to ensure that all connections are secure and that unnecessary manipulation of the closed system is avoided.
- Measuring and recording all urinary output via the nephrostomy tube(s). Haematuria can be expected following nephrostomy tube insertion usually for the first 24–48 hours. Gross haematuria with or without clots is abnormal. Sudden cessation of urine output, particularly where there has been urine flow in excess of 0.5 mL/kg per hour, may be related to tube blockage or dislodgement.

RENAL TRAUMA

Traumatic damage to the kidneys and urinary tract is associated with blunt trauma (e.g. road traffic accident or assault), deceleration trauma (e.g. road traffic accident or fall from a height) or penetrating injury (e.g. stab or gunshot wound). Blunt trauma to the kidneys is the commonest of these, and is classified as grade I to grade IV, where grade I signifies bruising of and around the kidney, and grade IV signifies fracture of the kidney and loss of integrity of the renal artery and/or vein. Grades I and II renal injury are further classified as minor and are usually treated conservatively, if the patient is haemodynamically stable. Grades III and IV are major injuries that will warrant surgical exploration, repair if possible, and nephrectomy if repair is impossible. Investigations performed will include CT scan, and in some centres intraoperative 'single-shot' intravenous urography (pyelography – IVU/P) is performed to assist evaluation of the renal injury.

MALIGNANT TUMOURS OF THE KIDNEY

Tumours may affect renal cells and the transitional epithelium (urothelium) that lines the urinary tract from the renal pelvis to the urethra. The commonest renal malignancy in adults is renal cell carcinoma that arises from the proximal tubular epithelium. Malignant renal tumours are commoner in males and are rarely seen before the fourth decade.

Pathophysiology

Renal cell carcinoma is usually unilateral, and the tumour may be solitary or multiple. These are highly vascular tumours. Metastatic spread may be local to the renal veins, or to lymph nodes, bone, liver and lung. As with all malignancies, prognosis is dependent on tumour differentiation and the presence or absence of metastatic spread (see Ch. 33).

Clinical presentation

Early signs include pyrexia of unknown origin, disordered coagulation and a raised erythrocyte sedimentation rate (ESR). Haematuria, loin pain and a palpable mass in the flank are typical features on late presentation.

Investigations

The investigations used to confirm diagnosis include renal ultrasound and CT scan. Renal angiography can be used to identify abnormal circulation associated with the tumour.

Medical/surgical management

In the presence of unilateral disease and an acceptable level of function in the other kidney, removal of the affected kidney (nephrectomy) is the treatment of choice. Partial nephrectomy may be undertaken if there is abnormal renal function in the other kidney. Chemotherapy is primarily used to control metastatic spread (see Ch. 33).

It is important to note that nephrectomy may be undertaken for a number of reasons other than as a primary treatment for renal cell carcinoma. Other indications include:

- uncontrollable renal haemorrhage, e.g. as a complication of renal biopsy or severe blunt renal trauma (see above)
- to remove a healthy kidney for transplantation (live-related renal transplantation)
- to remove a transplanted kidney which has been severely damaged by immunological responses.

The surgical approach for nephrectomy of a native kidney is usually lateral, with an incision made over the 11th or 12th rib, or abdominal. Nephrectomy of a transplanted kidney is undertaken through an incision made over the kidney in the right or left iliac fossa where it has been placed (see p. 694).

> ▶ **Nursing management: the patient undergoing nephrectomy**

If the situation/condition allows, preoperative preparation of patients should include, as a minimum, an explanation of the procedure and what they should expect postoperatively. All patients who undergo nephrectomy will require i.v. access, urinary catheterization and monitoring of cardiovascular function and peripheral oxygen saturation in the postoperative period (see Ch. 29).

Patients undergoing nephrectomy in order to donate a kidney for transplantation may well have a number of concerns surrounding the loss of a vital organ and the future impact that this may have on health. In this particular case, the evidence suggests that there is a slightly higher incidence of asymptomatic low-level proteinuria in later life. In those who undergo nephrectomy for other reasons (e.g. staghorn calculus, renal cell carcinoma), and who may not have normal function in the remaining kidney, there is an increased risk of subsequent renal failure.

Management of postoperative pain is an essential part of nursing care for these patients. Nephrectomy is a painful procedure, and postoperative pain management (e.g. patient-controlled analgesia, PCA) is ideally discussed and planned with each patient (see Chs 7 and 29). Nephrectomy is subdiaphragmatic and patients will naturally attempt to minimize pain by avoiding turning, coughing, deep breathing or mobilization. All these activities are required postoperatively and the patient's ability to contribute to these is enhanced by effective pain relief.

Preoperative assessment by the physiotherapist is ideal in order that patients are prepared to undertake the required postoperative exercises. With the assistance of the physiotherapist, they will be encouraged to perform deep breathing exercises and, in some centres, use an incentive spirometer postoperatively. Unless there is a clinical contraindication, patients should be assisted, with effective pain management, to commence ambulation from the first postoperative day. This is in order to reduce the risks of chest infection or thromboembolic complications (deep vein thrombosis and pulmonary embolus). A number of centres prescribe prophylactic heparin and use anti-embolism stockings postoperatively to minimize the risk of thromboembolic episodes (see Ch. 29).

A potential complication associated with nephrectomy is puncture of the pleura surrounding the lungs, resulting in pneumothorax. If this occurs, patients will require insertion of a chest drain to facilitate lung re-expansion (see Ch. 20). The potential for pneumothorax should be borne in mind, and alterations in respiratory effort or peripheral oxygen saturation warrant investigation.

Postoperative monitoring of cardiovascular status, vascular volume and urinary output is essential. In the early postoperative period, maintenance of hydration will require i.v. fluid administration. Adjustments to the rate and volume of i.v. fluids are made in accordance with urinary output, blood pressure and CVP if a central line has been inserted. Fluid loss through drainage tubes should also be included in the overall assessment of volume loss. Close adherence to fluid inputs balanced with fluid outputs is especially important where there is underlying renal dysfunction. Oral hydration should not commence until there is evidence of normal bowel sounds. In the early postoperative period, it is unlikely that oral intake will be sufficient to replace all losses.

Both the incision site and drainage tube(s) are monitored for blood loss. Some loss of blood through drainage tubes is to be expected during the first 24–48 hours, but the volume and the rate of drainage should decline gradually. Any increase in blood in drainage or increased volume or rate must be reported. In the absence of any complicating factor, wound drains are generally removed within 72 hours postoperatively, following surgical review. Wound closures (sutures or staples) can usually be removed by the tenth postoperative day.

As with any surgical procedure, discharge planning following nephrectomy is essential in achieving good patient outcomes (see Health Promotion box 24.2, Ch. 29).

UROTHELIAL (TRANSITIONAL CELL) TUMOURS

The commonest malignancy of the lower urinary tract is transitional cell carcinoma arising in the urothelial tissue. It can arise in the renal calyces, renal pelvis, ureters, bladder and urethra, since all are lined with transitional epithelium (or urothelium). Transitional cell carcinoma occurs more commonly in men, and like malignant renal tumours is rarely seen before the fourth decade. Transitional cell carcinoma of the bladder is commoner than malignancy at other sites within the lower urinary tract.

 HEALTH PROMOTION

24.2 Discharge planning after nephrectomy

Patients should be advised to avoid strenuous exercise such as going to the gym or running. However, they should start gentle exercise, such as walking, as they feel able. A gradual return to the preoperative activity level should be discussed. Lifting of weights in excess of 3 kg should be avoided for 6–8 weeks following nephrectomy. Advice regarding driving will depend upon patients' general health and age, the reason for surgery and the wishes of the surgeon.

For both men and women, it is important to ensure that there is support available in the home to provide assistance with childcare, shopping, cooking and cleaning, for at least the early post-discharge period. Adequate rest periods during the day, and sleep are essential components of postoperative rehabilitation.

Patients are advised to have a balanced diet that includes the nutrients needed for wound healing and to prevent constipation (see Ch. 11). Advice regarding fluid intake will depend on the reason for nephrectomy.

All patients will require follow-up surgical review as an outpatient. Other considerations will depend on the nature of the necessity for nephrectomy. Thus referral to a cancer support group will be appropriate for patients who had a nephrectomy for cancer. For those who undergo nephrectomy of a transplanted kidney, renal replacement therapy will be inevitable (see p. 689). Referral to the dialysis nursing team should have taken place preoperatively, but referral to renal dieticians and counselling services are also requirements. The loss of a transplanted kidney may be difficult for patients to accept and deal with. However, it is also possible that some patients will greet transplant nephrectomy with resignation, and perhaps a measure of relief. The needs and requirements of patients have to be both assessed and addressed on an individual basis.

Aetiology

A number of predisposing factors have been described, including:

- cigarette smoking – toxic metabolites are excreted in the urine
- exposure to industrial carcinogens such as aniline used in dyeing
- exposure to certain drugs (e.g. cyclophosphamide)
- chronic inflammation.

Clinical presentation

Clinical presentation depends on the site of the tumour and the presence of metastatic spread. Both bladder tumours and transitional cell tumour of the kidney and ureter can present with painless haematuria. Cystitis may be a feature in women, and prostatism (dysuria, perineal or groin pain and painful prostate) in men.

Investigations

- Urine samples will be sent for cytological examination to detect the presence of abnormal cells.
- Urodynamic studies may provide evidence of obstruction.
- Cystoscopy and examination under anaesthesia are standard investigations for suspected bladder tumours, since these allow for direct visualization and manual assessment of the bladder wall depth. Biopsy and histological examination are essential for a number of reasons – confirmation of diagnosis, degree of cell differentiation, and to ascertain the depth of tumour penetration.

Tumour classification is important, since the degree of local, invasive and metastatic spread will influence the treatment given and determine the likely prognostic outcome for the patient.

Medical/surgical management

Nephroureterectomy (removal of the kidney and ureter) is undertaken for renal pelvis and ureteric tumours. The nursing management following nephroureterectomy is similar to that for nephrectomy (see p. 677).

Bladder tumours may be classified as either superficial or invasive. Treatment of superficial bladder tumours includes diathermy and transurethral resection of the tumour. Chemotherapy given intravesically (into the bladder) and regular check cystoscopies are adjunctive therapies. Intravesical bacillus Calmette-Guérin (BCG) and mitomycin (cytotoxic antibiotic) are both used in treating patients who are diagnosed with carcinoma-in-situ. Mitomycin is usually administered at 6-weekly intervals because one of its side-effects is delayed bone marrow toxicity.

Treatment of invasive bladder tumours includes:

- transurethral resection of tumour
- partial cystectomy – may entail the removal of up to half the bladder. In the initial postoperative period, bladder volume capacity is small (< 70 mL), but increases over the months following surgery
- total (radical) cystectomy with the creation of urinary diversion – a radical procedure associated with significant morbidity and mortality that increases with age (see below)
- palliative therapy without surgical intervention – regardless of the patient's age, tumour with extensive invasion of surrounding organs may be inoperable, and in this case, palliative care is the treatment option (see Ch. 34).

Any decision to proceed to total cystectomy must weigh the benefit to the patient against the associated risks. In older people, radiotherapy may be a preferred option. Total cystectomy always requires the creation of a urinary diversion. This may be achieved with the insertion of bilateral nephrostomy tubes or by the surgical creation of a urinary diversion, e.g. by the formation of an ileal conduit or a continent internal urinary pouch. The formation of an ileal conduit (also termed a urostomy) involves the implantation of the ureters into a short segment of ileum, and the ileum is then brought out to open onto the anterior abdominal wall as an ileostomy (see Fig. 24.10, p. 680).

A number of factors influence the type of urinary diversion chosen, including age, physical and mental condition of the patient, likely prognostic outcome and presence of chronic bowel disorders.

▶ Nursing management

Intravesical BCG or mitomycin

This involves passing a urethral catheter through which the prescribed agent is instilled. Following this, the urinary catheter is either clamped or removed, and patients asked not to pass urine for 2 hours. During that time, patients should be asked to change position every 15–30 minutes, lying on either side, supine and prone. After 2 hours, they may void. Oral intake of fluid should be increased (3 L) following this procedure to promote flushing of the bladder. Dysuria is a frequent complaint following this procedure, but should resolve within 48 hours (Swibold 1999). Urine that contains BCG or other chemotherapy agents should be discarded in accordance with local hospital policy for cytotoxic agents (see Special Issues box 24.1, p. 680).

Radical cystectomy with urinary diversion

Radical cystectomy with ileal conduit is a major surgical procedure.

Preoperative care

Usually, this is a planned procedure and, as such, allows time for patient preparation. Physical preparation should include advice on smoking cessation and ensuring that dietary intake meets the current nutritional recommendations. Dietary supplementation may be required if the usual daily intake is insufficient. Patients should be encouraged to remain active and undertake their normal daily activities. Psychological preparation should anticipate patients' need to understand the nature of the procedure and the likely outcomes. When faced with such a potentially life-altering procedure, individuals can find it difficult to retain and process information provided. For this reason, it is important to assess the level of understanding of patients and family members, up to and including the immediate preoperative stage, and to provide remedial information and support if these are required.

Urinary diversion with formation of an ileal conduit means that patients will need to accept and care for a stoma (urostomy) that opens onto the anterior abdomen. Preoperative assessment must include the ability to self-care. Preoperative referral to a stoma therapy nurse specialist (if this is an anticipated outcome) and patient support group should be offered to all patients. It is

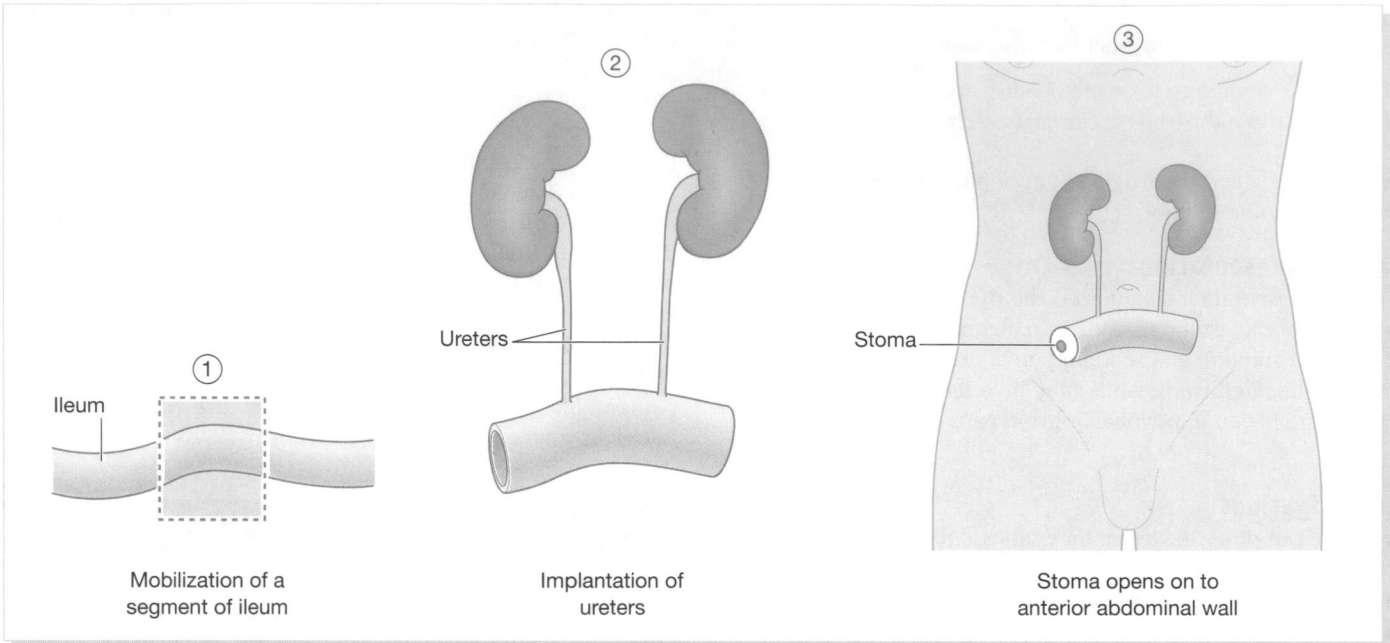

Figure 24.10 Ileal conduit.

 SPECIAL ISSUES

24.1 Safe use of intravesical BCG and mitomycin

The BCG now available for bladder instillation is a live attenuated strain derived from *Mycobacterium bovis*. The administration of BCG stimulates a local inflammatory immune response within the bladder that acts to destroy the abnormal cancer cells. The use of BCG for bladder instillation is contraindicated in patients with active tuberculosis.

Cytotoxic means poisonous to cells, and these drugs are given as chemotherapy agents precisely for that effect on cancer cells. However, they can also cause damage to normal tissue, and the way in which these drugs are handled must reflect that risk. Both BCG and mitomycin should be handled in accordance with recommendations for handling cytotoxic drugs. These include the following:

- Staff trained in the preparation and use of cytotoxic drugs should reconstitute these.
- Protective clothing, including gloves, aprons and eye protection, should be worn.
- Required first aid in the event of accidental exposure, e.g. inhalation, should be specified.
- Pregnant women should not handle cytotoxics.
- All materials used in the preparation and administration of cytotoxic drugs must be disposed of carefully and in accordance with hospital guidelines for disposal.

Further reading

Bohle A, Rusch-Gerdes S, Ulmer AJ, Braasch H, Jocham D. The effects of lubricants on viability of bacillus Calmette-Guérin for intravesical immunotherapy against bladder carcinoma. J Urol 1996; 155(6): 1892–1896.

normal for patients and their families to be anxious about this procedure. Patients should be involved in decisions regarding placement of the stoma, which needs to be sited so that they can both see and reach it, and so that it can be securely fastened and free from constraint by the patient's usual clothes. The stoma therapy nurse specialist and others who have had this procedure performed provide an important resource for patients who are seeking an open and honest discussion about, for example, changes in body image, ability to be sexually expressive, and coping following discharge home (see Reflective Practice box 24.3).

Expected hospital stay is approximately 10–14 days and patients should be made aware of this so that they can attend to personal arrangements. Assessment of each patient's home circumstances is also helpful at this early stage so that anything that may impinge on the discharge process is identified, and the need for post-discharge support is anticipated.

Following admission, all patients will have blood drawn for full blood count, full biochemical profile, and blood group and cross-match. A chest X-ray and ECG are also usually performed. Thigh-length anti-embolus stockings may be ordered and, if this is the case, patients should be measured accurately to ensure that the appropriate size is provided. Physiotherapy referral should take place preoperatively and patients instructed in the performance of deep breathing exercises and the use of an incentive spirometer, if appropriate.

Where urinary diversion using a segment of bowel is anticipated, patients will usually undertake some preoperative bowel preparation prior to admission (see Ch. 29). Preoperatively, they should have clear fluids only.

Pain control and how this will be achieved are discussed preoperatively with patients. Epidural analgesia is commonly used in this setting to control pain (see Chs 7 and 29). Nurses should inform patients that a nasogastric tube (because of paralytic

24.3 Altered body image

The ways in which individuals perceive themselves and the extent of their perception of individual 'control' over their bodies have important behavioural consequences within health care provision. The presence of chronic illness or sequelae to disfiguring surgery can present significant challenges to the person's body image.

Student activities
Read the following articles: Borwell (1997)and Price (1998). Use the information provided in these articles to perform an assessment of your own body image.

- Would you be comfortable answering all these questions if someone else was asking them?
- Is your body image fixed, or does it alter? What factors influence this?
- What other observations, apart from answers to verbal questions, do you think are necessary for a holistic assessment of a patient's body image?
- How will you integrate this information into your future practice?

Further reading
Borwell B. Psychological considerations of stoma care nursing. Nurs Stand 1997; 11(48): 49–55.
Price B. Cancer: altered body image. Nurs Stand 1998; 12(21): 49–55.

ileus associated with handling the bowel), i.v. access, i.v. fluids and drugs, and wound drains (1–2 usually) are normal features of the postoperative period.

Postoperative care
Postoperative observations include blood pressure, pulse, respiration, temperature and usually oxygen saturation. The condition of the stoma should also be noted (see below). Assessment of pain control is ongoing and adjustments to analgesia made as patients require.

The nasogastric tube is allowed to drain freely and should be checked to ensure that it is securely attached to the patient. Urinary output will be monitored and adherence to a closed drainage system is maintained. Patients remain nil-by-mouth and hydration with i.v. fluids will be required until bowel sounds have returned (usually after 3–4 days). Local procedures with regard to maintaining and monitoring i.v. access, and changing i.v. cannulae and giving sets should be followed.

Anticoagulation therapy with subcutaneous heparin is usually prescribed. In common with other operative procedures, it is important that patients are encouraged to move around in bed, and to get out of bed from the first postoperative day. Good pain control facilitates the latter. Observation of abdominal wound and drainage tubes is also undertaken. Wound closures can usually be removed 7–10 days postoperatively.

Following formation of an ileal conduit, the stoma should be observed for size, shape, colour and the presence/absence of oedema. Ureteric stents may have been inserted during the operation to maintain patency of the ureters while the ureteric anastomoses are healing. Stents may be seen protruding through the opening of the stoma. The presence of these should be noted in both the nursing documentation and the record of the surgical procedure in the hospital notes.

The newly formed stoma should be moist and red. Stomal oedema is expected in the early postoperative period. Changes in the colour of the stoma, e.g. if it becomes dusky red, cyanotic or pale, are indicative of vascular insufficiency. If you note these, check that the flange/baseplate around the stoma is not constricting it. Document (in the nursing or multidisciplinary notes) the change in appearance, and verbally report this to the senior ward nurse and surgical team.

Initially, nurses will perform stoma care, but the responsibility for this is gradually transferred to patients, such that they are competent to self-care prior to discharge. Patients should be encouraged to contribute to the care of the stoma early in the postoperative period. This can begin with encouraging them to acknowledge its presence and explaining what you are doing when attending to the stoma, such as cleaning it or changing or emptying the collecting bag. Patients should be encouraged to provide feedback on the comfort and ease of use of the stoma flange and bag so that this can be used to inform decisions as to which product is best for the individual. There is a range of urostomy products available.

On discharge, the nurse must ensure that patients have a supply of equipment required for stoma care. Depending on local arrangements, additional supplies may be delivered to the home or obtained through prescription. Stoma therapy nurse specialists will usually visit patients frequently in the postoperative period to assess progress and identify individual care or support requirements on discharge home. Follow-up home visits by the stoma therapy nurse specialist and assessment of patients in the home environment are important aspects of transferring, and supporting the transfer of, responsibility for stoma care to patients.

Care of patients having a continent internal urinary pouch
During this procedure, bowel (e.g. ileum or ascending colon) is mobilized and used to create a sac-like reservoir for urine. The ureters are joined to this reservoir. The pouch is externalized for access with a surgically created one-way valve that opens onto the skin. The capacity of this reservoir is usually at least equal to that of the bladder. The reservoir is drained of urine by catheterization through the one-way valve. As with the formation of an ileal conduit, preoperative bowel preparation is required.

The urinary pouch is catheterized once its formation in theatre is complete. This ensures free flow of urine from the ureters through the urinary pouch postoperatively. Free flow of urine out of the pouch minimizes the potential for distension while ureteric anastomoses and other suture lines are healing. Maintaining catheter patency postoperatively is extremely important. Catheter irrigation with normal saline can be used to either prevent or treat blockage. In either case, it is important that the irrigation volume is prescribed.

DIABETIC NEPHROPATHY

Diabetic nephropathy is the renal disease associated with diabetes mellitus (see Ch. 17). Diabetic nephropathy is now the commonest cause of end-stage renal failure (ESRF) worldwide (Friedman 1997).

Epidemiology

The prevalence of ESRF in type 1 diabetes is well defined. Prevalence increases with duration of diabetes. The peak is reached 20–25 years following diagnosis of type 1 diabetes. Thereafter, it declines to around 10% in those who have had type 1 diabetes for more than 40 years. The prevalence of ESRF in type 2 diabetes is less well defined. This has been attributed to the significant cardiovascular comorbidity and mortality associated with this patient group. In essence, while renal dysfunction may be a feature, these patients are more likely to die from cardiovascular complications before they reach ESRF.

Aetiology, pathophysiology and clinical presentation

Risk factors for the development of ESRF in the diabetic population may be summarized as:

- racial group – in the UK, for example, the prevalence of diabetes is higher in the Asian population than in Caucasians
- duration of diabetes
- hypertension
- hyperglycaemia
- cigarette smoking.

Diabetic nephropathy is characterized by disruption to the normal structure of small blood vessels (microvasculature). These structural changes in the glomeruli result in functional abnormalities. In type 1 diabetes, the stages in the evolution of diabetic nephropathy have been well described (Mogensen 1976), and the description of pathologic change that follows makes specific reference to diabetic nephropathy in this group of patients. However, recent evidence suggests that there is comparable pathologic evolution in type 2 diabetes.

While not all diabetics will develop ESRF, the progressive renal damage associated with diabetes can be ameliorated by good glycaemic control and maintaining normal blood pressure.

Stages

- Changes in renal function may be seen at the time of diagnosis of diabetes. There is an increase in kidney size (nephromegaly), glomerular size increases and the GFR increases accordingly.
- Within the next 2–5 years after diagnosis of diabetes, structural changes within the kidney occur, with changes in the glomerulus and PCT cell hypertrophy. The latter has been associated with elevated blood glucose levels and other metabolic changes associated with diabetes. In addition, there is a reduction in the negatively charged glycosialoproteins, leading to a diminution of the electrostatic barrier within the glomerulus (see p. 656).
- Microalbuminuria (albumin excretion in the range of 20–200 µg/min) appears between 5 and 15 years after the diagnosis of diabetes because the electrostatic glomerular barrier is less effective. This level of albumin excretion is not detectable on standard dipsticks used in practice. There are commercially available dipsticks that can measure albumin excretion in the 20–200 µg/min range. In the absence of these, a 24-hour urine collection for albumin excretion may be performed. Changes in blood pressure levels may also occur at this stage.
- The fourth stage in the evolution of diabetic nephropathy occurs between 10 and 20 years after the diagnosis of diabetes. At this stage, the blood pressure is usually elevated and urinary albumin loss may be large enough to result in the development of nephrotic syndrome (see p. 684). A gradual decline in the GFR accompanies this stage.
- The fifth and final stage, the development of ESRF secondary to diabetic nephropathy, occurs with duration of diabetes in excess of 20 years. The mortality rate for diabetic patients who receive dialysis therapy for ESRF is higher than for non-diabetics.

▶ Nursing and medical management

In terms of renal function, treatment of diabetic patients principally involves managing risk factors, monitoring renal function, and timely preparation of patients if dialysis, or indeed transplantation, is required. Ideally, the management of these patients is collaborative and equally shared between medical and nursing staff (from both diabetes and nephrology specialties) and patients themselves. In common with other chronic diseases (see Ch. 35), patient compliance with the treatment prescribed is a major determinant of treatment success or failure.

Management of risk factors includes:

- *Control of hypertension.* Angiotensin-converting enzyme (ACE) inhibitors (e.g. captopril) and, more recently, ACE-II receptor antagonists (e.g. irbesartan) have become the treatment of choice in the control of hypertension. ACE inhibitors confer two principal benefits. Firstly they can reduce the quantity of microalbuminuria; and secondly, they lower systemic blood pressure. There is good evidence that treatment with ACE inhibitors or receptor antagonists should be instigated even in the absence of hypertension, in those who have microalbuminuria (EUCLID Study Group 1997).
- *Blood glucose control.* The importance of this cannot be overemphasized. There is a clear relationship between poor glycaemic control (see Ch. 17) and the development of multisystem complications of diabetes, including renal disease. Recent guidance from NICE (2002) recommends a glycosylated haemoglobin of 6.5–7.5% (see Ch. 17). Poor glycaemic control may also cause problems during dialysis (see below).
- *Monitoring renal function.* This includes serial measurements of serum creatinine, urea and electrolytes, and haemoglobin. Patients should be encouraged to maintain a record of body weight and to stop smoking, as the vasoconstrictive effect of cigarette smoking compounds small vessel disease (microangiopathy).

In ESRF requiring long-term renal replacement therapy, the available treatments include haemodialysis, peritoneal dialysis and renal transplantation (see p. 689). However, there are some specific points worth highlighting with respect to diabetic patients requiring dialysis. Poor glycaemic control in this patient group reduces ability to maintain restriction in daily fluid allowances. This is because hyperglycaemia increases serum osmolality and thus stimulates thirst. Peripheral neuropathy and abnormal physiological responses to circulatory volume reduction may additionally complicate fluid removal during dialysis.

GLOMERULONEPHRITIS

Glomerulonephritis is an autoimmune disease and is associated with immunologically mediated injury to the glomerulus and surrounding structures. The clinical manifestations of glomerulonephritis may be restricted to renal involvement, or renal involvement may arise as part of a multisystem disease process (e.g. systemic lupus erythematosus, SLE – see Ch. 27) and vasculitis. Glomerulonephritis is classified into several types, e.g. focal, diffuse, membranous, according to the histologic appearance of renal tissue obtained by biopsy (see 'Renal biopsy', p. 667). Each of these classifications is associated with clinical signs on presentation, although correlation is not absolute, and different prognostic outcomes.

Pathophysiology

Glomerular damage associated with glomerulonephritis arises from deposition of circulating antigen–antibody complexes within the glomerulus, the formation of these immune complexes within the glomerulus itself, or the deposition of anti-glomerular basement membrane (GBM) antibody within the glomerulus. Once in situ, these immune complexes elicit a complex inflammatory reaction that includes complement activation, fibrin deposition and neutrophil infiltration. It is the severity of the damage related to this inflammatory reaction that is the principal determinant of glomerular injury.

Clinical presentation

A number of factors will influence presentation, including renal involvement in multisystem disease and the extent of the glomerular injury. Some types of glomerulonephritis are associated with rapid deterioration in renal function to ESRF. Commonly, patients with glomerulonephritis present acutely, with no previous history of renal dysfunction, but manifesting signs and symptoms of ARF (see p. 685). Presentation may be associated with a history of pulmonary haemorrhage, as in anti-GBM disease (Goodpasture's disease) with the presence of anti-GBM antibody, a history of epistaxis (associated with Wegener's granulomatosis; see Ch. 21), or a history of recent throat infection with beta-haemolytic *Streptococcus*. Hypertension may be a feature of presentation.

Investigations

- Renal ultrasound usually reveals normal-sized kidneys, and a normal collecting system.
- Urinalysis (if there is output) will be positive for protein and may also be positive for blood. Proteinuria is the most significant indicator of glomerular disease.
- Renal biopsy will be undertaken to determine the cause of acute renal function deterioration (see above).

Box 24.3 Serologic markers of autoimmune disease

- Anti-glomerular basement membrane antibody (anti-GBM)
- Antineutrophil cytoplasmic antibodies/cytoplasmic (cANCA)
- Antineutrophil cytoplasmic antibodies/perinuclear (pANCA)
- Antinuclear antibody (ANA)
- Anti-doublestrand DNA antibody
- Complement 3 and complement 4 (C3 and C4)

- Blood tests will be carried out to determine renal function and for a number of serological markers of autoimmune disease (see Box 24.3).

Medical management

Medical management priorities are dictated by the clinical presentation.

- Loss of renal function is supported by dialysis, primarily to manage fluid, electrolyte and acid–base imbalances. Haemodialysis may be undertaken as acute renal replacement therapy.
- Anaemia secondary to blood loss and coagulation abnormalities are corrected with transfusion of the appropriate blood cells.
- Immunosuppressive drugs (e.g. corticosteroids, cyclophosphamide), with or without plasma exchange (see Special Issues box 24.2) or immunoadsorption to reduce circulating antibody titres, are prescribed to depress the immunologically mediated inflammatory reaction.
- Hypertension, if present, is controlled with anti-hypertensive therapy (e.g. nifedipine).

▶ Nursing management

Nursing care priorities are similarly determined by the patient's condition. In the early post-admission period, these will

 SPECIAL ISSUES

24.2 Plasma exchange

Like the dialytic therapies, this is an extracorporeal treatment. Plasma exchange may be used as an adjunctive therapy for a range of disease states, e.g. glomerulonephritis. However, the common denominating factor between all of these will be a requirement to reduce or remove abnormal immunoglobulin that has been generated as a result of an autoimmune process (autoantibody). Essentially, this therapy removes plasma from the patient and replaces it with fresh frozen plasma (FFP) or human albumin solution, or a combination of both. The principle behind this is that plasma containing autoantibody is removed and replaced with plasma that does not contain autoantibody. A number of plasma exchanges are required to reduce circulating antibody titres and concomitant immunosuppressive drug therapy is prescribed.

necessarily focus on close observation of vital signs (temperature, pulse, respiration, blood pressure and oxygen saturation), strict attention to fluid balance, with maintenance of euvolaemia, and provision and monitoring of prescribed therapies. The latter may include haemodialysis, plasma exchange, oxygen therapy or blood transfusion.

There are a number of factors that should be borne in mind when caring for patients having immunosuppressant therapy. Immunosuppressive drugs modify normal immune responses and thus patients are at increased risk of infection. Opportunistic infection, e.g. with cytomegalovirus (CMV), may be a sequel to immunosuppression and carries significant morbidity. Where the drug cyclophosphamide is to be used as part of the immunosuppressive regimen, patients must be informed of the known side-effects – specifically, that it may cause infertility. It is important to give patients the opportunity to have oocytes or spermatozoa collected and preserved for future use prior to drug administration.

Patients will always require nephrological surveillance following discharge. Slow progressive deterioration in renal function is a feature of many forms of glomerulonephritis (Feehally & Johnson 2000). Patients may experience long-term remission of their disease with immunosuppressive therapy, or alternatively present with acute exacerbations.

NEPHROTIC SYNDROME

Nephrotic syndrome is a manifestation of glomerular damage and is characterized by proteinuria, hypoalbuminaemia (low level of albumin in the blood) and gross oedema. It is a sequel to glomerulonephritis. Disruption of the glomerular structure by inflammatory damage results in loss of protein in the urine. This, and the consequent hypoalbuminaemia, leads to oedema through two mechanisms. A fall in plasma oncotic pressure (normally albumin contributes to oncotic pressure) means that when fluid in the capillaries moves out of the vascular compartment and into the interstitium it is unable to return and stays in the interstitial spaces. Loss of vascular volume stimulates the renin–angiotensin–aldosterone system, resulting in increased renal retention of sodium and water, thus compounding the problem.

Medical management

The medical management centres on reducing proteinuria and controlling oedema, blood pressure and other associated physiological disruptions. Treatment for oedema will include diuretics (furosemide [frusemide], a loop diuretic, is commonly used) and, in the absence of an adequate response to this, furosemide with concurrent administration of human albumin solution. The level of furosemide dosage (maximum 500 mg/day) is considerably greater than that usually seen in practice. The principle behind the combination of these two is the following. Albumin will raise the plasma oncotic pressure, facilitating the movement of interstitial fluid back into the vascular compartment; forced diuresis by the diuretic will then facilitate the removal of fluid from the vascular compartment. Disordered lipid metabolism is also a feature of nephrotic syndrome, and patients may be prescribed a lipid-lowering agent, e.g. simvastatin.

▶ Nursing management

Oedema is commonly the most obvious patient problem on admission. Patients may be grossly oedematous. Assessment of their physical activity level is important, and risk assessment for pressure ulcer formation should be performed (see Ch. 10). Any identified requirements for pressure-relieving aids should be met. Patients are encouraged to take regular and gentle exercise around the ward/corridors whilst in hospital, because gross oedema and coagulation abnormalities predispose them to venous thrombosis. Anticoagulant prophylaxis may be required both during hospitalization (heparin) and as a long-term therapy (warfarin) (see Ch. 19). If patients are unable to exercise, a referral should be made to physiotherapy services, with subsequent planning and performance of assisted exercises.

During treatment with high doses of furosemide (frusemide) and albumin, it is essential that overall fluid balance be closely monitored, since there is an associated risk of profound intravascular depletion. Maintenance of accurate fluid balance charts, monitoring of vital signs, with central venous pressures if these are required, and daily weighing are nursing responsibilities.

Formal nutritional assessment is undertaken for these patients (see Ch. 11). Protein loss can be up to 30 g/day in the urine and this needs to be replaced. Oral supplementation of the diet with protein-rich drinks or fortified food may be prescribed, and it is important that nurses monitor the intake of these.

As with other chronic illness, assisting patients to cope with the demands of both their disease and its treatment is an important aspect of nursing care. This will encompass information on drug therapy and the importance of adequate nutrition and regular attendance for outpatient follow-up.

TUBULOINTERSTITIAL DISEASE – INTERSTITIAL NEPHRITIS

Tubulointerstitial disease may be acute or chronic. Acute tubulointerstitial nephritis may arise as a result of an infecting microorganism directly invading renal tissue (e.g. *Streptococcus*, adenovirus) or as a result of local (renal tissue) response to a systemic infection (hypersensitivity reaction). It may also be associated with systemic diseases such as SLE. Chronic tubulointerstitial disease has more commonly been associated with misuse of analgesics, so-called 'analgesic nephropathy', and prolonged exposure to non-steroidal anti-inflammatory drugs (NSAIDs), gold salts and herbal medicines.

Medical management

Management is determined by the clinical presentation. If patients present in ARF, treatment priorities are dictated by a requirement to support remaining renal function, minimize further renal damage, and/or replace renal function with dialysis, until the renal lesion heals. Treatment with corticosteroids may be instigated. If patients present with CRF, interventions are dictated by the magnitude of renal functional loss.

POLYCYSTIC KIDNEY DISEASE

Adult polycystic kidney disease (APKD) is an inherited multisystem disease characterized by multiple cyst formation in the kidneys and other body sites, including the liver and meninges. Inherited as an autosomal dominant trait, it affects both sexes equally. There is usually a history of familial renal disease, and familial death from subarachnoid haemorrhage (see Ch. 14) may also be reported.

Pathophysiology

As the individual ages, there is increased formation of cystic lesions within the kidney. These undergo progressive enlargement and are distributed in both kidneys. Normal renal tissue is compressed, and progressive deterioration in renal function occurs.

Investigations

Investigation for the presence of APKD may be instigated following confirmation of this diagnosis in a sibling or parent, or following investigation for recurrent UTI, or the diagnosis of extrarenal manifestations of APKD (see below). The diagnostic criteria for individuals with a known family history of APKD have been described as (Ravine et al 1994):

- < 30 years old – two cysts either unilaterally or bilaterally
- > 30 and < 60 years old – two cysts in each kidney
- > 60 years old – more than four cysts in each kidney.

A diagnosis of APKD should be accompanied by ultrasound evaluation of siblings and offspring.

Clinical presentation

Symptoms may be secondary to renal or extrarenal manifestations of APKD. Renal manifestations include:

- abdominal or flank pain due to compression, cystic haemorrhage, infection or renal stones
- cyst haemorrhage – a common complication and may occur with or without haematuria
- UTI – commonly caused by coliforms (see p. 672)
- renal stones.

Extrarenal manifestations include:

- polycystic liver disease – enlargement of the liver and compression of surrounding intra-abdominal structures (see Ch. 23)
- vascular abnormalities – aneurysms affecting intracranial (see Ch. 14) and coronary arteries, and dissecting aneurysms of the thoracic aorta (see Ch. 19)
- valvular heart disease (VHD) – commonly mitral valve regurgitation (see Ch. 19).

Medical management

There is no curative treatment available for APKD and management involves surveillance of renal function with:

- control of hypertension
- control of acidosis (see Ch. 8)
- prevention of hyperphosphataemia (excess phosphate in the blood)
- treatment of hyperlipidaemia
- adequate nutritional intake
- non-opioid analgesia – sclerosis of cysts or surgical decompression can be undertaken for chronic debilitating pain associated with cysts

- prompt treatment of UTIs
- urological intervention for renal stones
- treatment of haemorrhagic episodes
- timely preparation of the individual for dialysis or renal transplantation, if ESRF develops.

RENAL FAILURE

Renal failure is classically differentiated into acute and chronic. In either case, loss of normal renal function results in an inability to maintain fluid, electrolyte and acid–base homeostasis. Where there is CRF, additional sequelae to functional derangements of the kidney develop over time. Symptoms that arise from loss of renal function are collectively referred to as the uraemic syndrome.

ACUTE RENAL FAILURE

Acute renal failure (ARF) is defined as a sudden loss of renal function that is potentially reversible.

Aetiology

Causation of ARF may be classified as pre-renal, renal and post-renal.

Pre-renal

Pre-renal causes are principally those that reduce kidney perfusion with blood, resulting in hypoxic damage. Thus any situation in which there is loss of circulatory volume or alteration to cardiac output can result in functional disruption of the kidneys (see Chs 9 and 19).

Renal

Renal causes include damage to the renal parenchyma by nephrotoxins (e.g. opaque contrast medium), diseases such as glomerulonephritis, or hypoxia resulting from prolonged and uncorrected underperfusion of the kidney. Acute tubular necrosis (ATN) is a term commonly associated with ARF. It signifies damage to renal tissue as a result of oxygen deprivation.

Post-renal

Post-renal causation is essentially obstructive. Obstruction to urine outflow can occur at any level, from the tubules to the urethral meatus. Obstruction may be secondary to stricture, renal calculi, prostatic hyperplasia, tumours or retroperitoneal fibrosis (e.g. following radiotherapy).

Pathophysiology

Acute renal failure typically occurs in patients hospitalized for other conditions, and the incidence of ARF as a primary cause of patient presentation is low (Liano & Pascual 1996). For both pre-renal causes of ARF and the majority of cases of renal ARF, the primary precipitating cause of renal damage is hypoxia that arises as a consequence of renal ischaemia. When circulatory volume is ineffective, systemic and local renal mechanisms act to preserve the GFR and renal blood flow (see 'Further reading', p. 702). If compensatory mechanisms fail to restore circulatory volume and renal perfusion then hypoxic damage to renal cells becomes inevitable.

The pathology associated with post-renal obstructive causation of ARF also results in alterations to the GFR, although through a different mechanism. Obstruction to outflow results in an increase in intratubular hydrostatic pressure, as urine literally backs up behind the obstruction. This increase in pressure is transmitted to the level of the glomerulus and eventually leads to cessation of glomerular filtration.

Investigations and medical assessment

Medical assessment of patients who present with ARF centres on acquiring a detailed patient history, including review of medical hospitalization notes, evaluating renal function with serological (creatinine, full blood count and haematocrit) and ultrasonic investigations, urine volume and analysis, and physical examination. Underlying each of these is the search for answers to the points noted below (Iglesias & Liebertal 2000):

- whether this is ARF or an acute exacerbation of chronic renal dysfunction
- the presence or absence of renal obstruction
- assessment of vascular volume – this includes 'effective' vascular volume (volume in vascular compartment) and 'non effective' volume (fluid lost from the capillary bed but not from the body). For example, in septicaemia, damage to vessel walls allows fluid to leak from the capillary bed into the interstitium (oedema), causing a reduction in effective vascular volume (see Ch. 9)
- presence or absence of a major vessel occlusion (e.g. thromboembolism in renal artery)
- evaluating evidence of parenchymal disease other than that caused by hypoxic injury
- review of medications, specifically those associated with nephrotoxicity or those known to alter glomerular functions (e.g. NSAIDs).

Once the cause has been determined, appropriate medical interventions are prescribed.

Clinical presentation – course of ARF

The course of ARF can be divided into three stages, as described below.

Initial stage

This stage includes alteration to urine volume, or, in the case of non-oliguric ARF, alteration in the chemical characteristics of urine, fluid, electrolyte and acid–base imbalance. Patients' level of mentation may be depressed, as a result of metabolic toxins, poor oxygenation or acid–base disturbance. Respiratory changes caused by acid–base imbalance or pulmonary oedema may be noted (see Chs 8, 9 and 20).

Maintenance stage

The maintenance stage is characterized by oliguria (very little urine output) or anuria (no urine output). GFR will be at its lowest and is generally assumed to be < 10 mL/min during this phase, which can last for more than 2 weeks. However, as a general rule, the longer the oligo-anuric phase, the poorer the prognosis in terms of restoration of renal function.

Recovery (diuretic) stage

During this stage, there is a gradual increase in urine output to diuresis and a fall in the serum creatinine. Volumes of urine in excess of 2 L can be passed. Patients lose both salt and volume during this stage, and strict attention to replacement of volume excreted, and preservation of circulatory volume is mandatory. Patients frequently require i.v. hydration early in the diuretic phase in order to keep pace with the volume of replacement intake required. Oral hydration is always encouraged where possible, and care should be taken to ensure that patients do not replace urine excretion solely with water, since this will compound urinary salt loss and render them hyponatraemic (low serum sodium level, see Ch. 8).

Medical management

Treatment of ARF involves restoration of kidney perfusion pressures through restoration of effective vascular volume, minimizing further renal injury by elimination of iatrogenic (prescribed drugs) toxins, specific treatment for the cause of renal failure, and instigation of dialytic support (see p. 693) if this is required, to assist management of fluid, electrolyte and acid–base disturbances.

▶ Nursing management

Nursing care of the patient in ARF encompasses monitoring of cardiovascular function, fluid status and respiratory function. Nutritional status and the need for supplementary feeding must be assessed. Commonly, these patients are highly catabolic and require adequate protein-calorie intake (see Ch. 11). All patients should have baseline and then continuous assessment of skin integrity performed. Pressure-relieving beds or aids should be provided if the assessment dictates (see Ch. 10). There is an increased risk of infection for these patients as a consequence of ARF and the interventions (central venous lines, drugs) required as part of their treatment. Central and peripheral venous access lines should be changed in accordance with local policies and removed as soon as they are no longer required. Urinary catheters are rarely, if ever, necessary during the oligo-anuric phase and should be avoided altogether, if possible, to minimize the risk of infection.

ARF and its treatment, particularly where this involves the use of extracorporeal treatments (see p. 693), is a frightening and anxiety-inducing experience for both patients and families. Care must always be taken to ensure that every effort is made to inform and include patients and family members in the treatment process.

CHRONIC RENAL FAILURE

Chronic renal failure (CRF) is chronic irreversible loss of renal function. A patient with CRF may or may not need renal replacement with dialytic therapy, but in ESRF, failure to replace renal function will result in death. Renal function can be considered as a linear scale with normal renal function at one end and ESRF at the other. Individual levels of renal function or chronic dysfunction may lie anywhere along this scale (see Fig. 24.11).

Symptoms associated with progressive decline in renal function become worse the closer to ESRF the individual is on the scale. CRF affects every body system and much of the medical

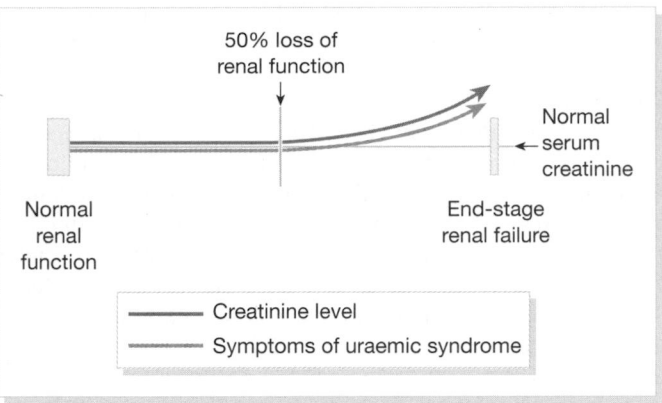

Figure 24.11 Renal function as a linear scale. Up to a 50% loss of renal function, the changes in the serum creatinine may be relatively small. With continuing deterioration of renal function, the serum creatinine begins to rise, and the symptoms of uraemia become increasingly evident.

and nursing intervention associated with caring for these individuals is focused on symptom management and assisting patients to live with the disease.

Aetiology

Any condition that disrupts the normal structure and function of the kidney may eventually lead to CRF. Important causes include reflux nephropathy, glomerulonephritis, tubulointerstitial disease, APKD, diabetes and SLE, some of which are discussed above.

Clinical effects of declining renal function

Electrolyte, acid–base and fluid imbalance

The ability to maintain electrolyte homeostasis is progressively diminished by chronic decline in renal function. In the early stages of CRF, control of sodium and potassium are unproblematic. Many patients retain normal levels of sodium, although as renal failure progresses, a decrease in salt intake is usually advised. This is principally because ingesting large quantities of salt will generate thirst and thus make adherence to any fluid restriction more difficult.

Inability to maintain potassium balance is a feature of the later stages of CRF. Generally, the GFR will be < 10 mL/min before hyperkalaemia develops. Disordered calcium and phosphate homeostasis occur relatively early in CRF and is universal where the GFR is < 25 mL/min. The development of renal bone disease (renal osteodystrophy) is a sequel to this. There is increased bone turnover with skeletal disruption, hyperphosphataemia and raised plasma levels of PTH. The effects of disordered calcium and phosphate metabolism are minimized through control of serum phosphate levels and maximization of calcium absorption from the gut. Phosphate binders are prescribed to bind dietary phosphate, and a vitamin D analogue is used to maximize dietary calcium absorption. Management of metabolic acidosis with oral sodium bicarbonate or, where the patient is on dialysis, dialysate bicarbonate also contributes to management of renal osteodystrophy.

Acid–base disturbances worsen as renal function declines. Patients who progress to ESRF requiring dialysis will have chronic metabolic acidosis, with respiratory compensation (see Chs 8 and 20).

The ability to maintain fluid homeostasis also diminishes as renal function declines. In the absence of renal function, the only way to control fluid balance is with dialysis and fluid restriction. As a general rule, the recommended fluid intake restriction for those on dialysis is the volume of any residual urine output plus 500 mL to replace insensible fluid loss (see Ch. 8).

Cardiovascular effects

Cardiovascular comorbidity is one of the most important determinants of survival on dialysis. The majority of deaths in this patient group occur as a result of cardiovascular complications related to both the systemic effects of CRF and treatment with dialysis. Chronic fluid overload of the vascular compartment is associated with hypertension, left ventricular hypertrophy and left ventricular dilation (see Ch. 19). Uncorrected anaemia both contributes to and compounds the latter (see Ch. 18). Disordered carbohydrate and lipid metabolism contribute to the development of atherosclerosis in this patient group. Complications associated with excessive blood flow through arteriovenous fistulae (see p. 691) for dialysis can result in high output cardiac failure. Decreased myocardial blood flow in coronary artery disease may be worsened by haemodialysis, particularly where the patient is also anaemic. If the primary cause of CRF was an autoimmune process, certain antibodies may directly damage the myocardium.

Respiratory effects

Respiratory effects may include pulmonary oedema (see Ch. 20) associated with volume overload (high pressure pulmonary oedema), or sepsis where fluid leaks out of the pulmonary capillaries (so-called low pressure pulmonary oedema). Respiratory compensation for metabolic acidosis, evidenced by an increase in alveolar ventilation, is frequently observed.

Renal anaemia

Renal anaemia associated with CRF is secondary to failure of erythropoiesis (see pp. 669, 670 and Ch. 18) as less erythropoietin is produced. Replacement of endogenous erythropoietin with human recombinant erythropoietin (rhuEPO) is now a standard treatment. Prior to commencement of treatment with rhuEPO, evaluation of iron stores in the body is undertaken; if these are depleted, iron replacement is prescribed.

Alterations in immune system

Alterations in immune system function are seen in patients with CRF. Delayed hypersensitivity and functional abnormality in white blood cells have been described. Immunosuppressive drug therapy will also affect the immune system.

Nutritional effects

Protein calorie (energy) malnutrition occurs in a significant number of patients with CRF. The relationship between malnutrition and increased morbidity and mortality in this patient group is now well described. There are a number of factors that influence nutritional status: those related to renal dysfunction and those caused by treatment with dialysis. Uraemia (excessive amounts of urea and other nitrogenous waste material in the blood) is associated with nausea and anorexia and these two alone will decrease food intake. Patients often complain that they have a metallic taste in their mouth, and stomatitis and gingivitis are particularly problematic (see Ch. 22). Alterations in gastric motility, gastric irritation and gastric bleeding are seen. Immune system function will be further compromised by malnutrition. Haemodialysis removes intact amino acids and also induces catabolism. Peritoneal dialysis leads to albumin loss at each bag exchange. This loss is further exacerbated by the presence of peritonitis (inflammation of the peritoneum). Adequate nutrition and calorie intake of 35 kcal/kg is important in this patient group. While protein restriction has been a feature of medical management of CRF, the benefit of this strategy has to be weighed against the strong evidence for

GUIDELINES FOR CARE PRIORITIES

24.3 Protein intake in chronic renal failure

Restriction of protein intake has been a feature of the medical management of chronic renal failure (CRF) in the past and remains controversial in the CRF patient population who are not on dialysis. The personal opinion of individual nephrologists will determine whether or not protein is restricted. However, continuous nutritional assessment should be a particular feature of care in this setting, to monitor for signs of patient malnutrition. The evidence currently available underlines the fact that protein restriction in the dialysis patient population carries significant risk in terms of increased patient morbidity and mortality.

Patients having dialysis have increased protein intake requirements. Both the dialytic therapies (haemodialysis and peritoneal dialysis) predispose patients to protein loss. For example, loss of the protein albumin across the peritoneal membrane is a 'normal' feature of continuous ambulatory peritoneal dialysis (CAPD), with some 5–15 g lost per day. This loss can increase up to 30 g if peritonitis is present. During haemodialysis, losses of intact amino acids of 8–12 g per treatment have been described.

The current guidelines for protein intake in the dialysis patient population are:

- for the patient having haemodialysis: 1.2 g/kg per day
- for the patient having CAPD: 1.2–1.5 g/kg per day.

It should be noted that these recommendations are greater than the 0.6–0.75 g/kg per day recommended for the normal healthy individual.

Further reading

Blake PG et al. Clinical practice guidelines for adequacy and nutrition in peritoneal dialysis. J Am Soc Nephrol 1999; 10 (suppl 13): S311–S321.
Chertow GM. Assessing the nutritional status of patients with end-stage renal disease. Semin Dialysis 1997; 10(2).
Daugirdas JT, Ing TS. Handbook of dialysis, 2nd edn. Boston: Little Brown; 1994.
Kim Park Y. Comparison of nutritional status between peritoneal dialysis and haemodialysis patients. Peritoneal Dialysis Int 1999; 19(suppl 2).

increased mortality and morbidity where there is protein calorie malnutrition (see Guidelines for Care Priorities box 24.3).

Reproductive effects

Altered menses, menorrhagia and amenorrhoea are all reported symptoms in females (see Ch. 25). Men experience alterations in sperm production and motility. Loss of libido is experienced by both sexes, and men may experience erectile dysfunction. These alterations to sexuality and fertility can profoundly alter patients' self-perception. Women of child-bearing age experience difficulty in both conception and the ability to carry a pregnancy to term. A successful pregnancy while on long-term dialysis treatment is rare.

Drugs and renal disease

Since the majority of drugs are excreted via the kidneys, renal impairment has a significant impact on drug clearance. In addition to altered clearances, other aspects of pharmacokinetics are affected by renal dysfunction (see Box 24.4). Dialysis and haemofiltration (see below) will remove drugs and their metabolites. The extent to which this occurs is dependent on molecular size, water solubility, volume of distribution, and the degree to which an administered drug is protein-bound. Alteration to drug dosage may be required to achieve therapeutic levels, and timing of administration may need to coincide with a specific intradialytic period.

The decision to commence dialysis as long-term renal replacement therapy is influenced by a number of factors (see Ethical Issues box 24.1). Failure of medical and dietetic interventions to manage fluid, electrolyte and acid–base balance, to control hypertension and maintain adequate nutritional status are all

---

Box 24.4 Pharmacokinetics affected by renal dysfunction

Absorption from the gastrointestinal tract
Gastrointestinal absorption of drugs can alter in uraemia, as a consequence of changes to the normal acidity of gastric juice. Drugs whose absorption is pH-dependent (e.g. folic acid or ferrous sulphate) will be affected by this.

Volume of drug distribution and protein binding
The volume of distribution for a given drug is affected by changes in vascular volume, alterations in the proportion of fat as a percentage of total body weight, and alterations in plasma protein levels. Where drugs are normally protein-bound in the body, a decrease in plasma albumin, for example, decreases the number of available binding sites, and thus the proportion of free to bound drug changes. Phenytoin and digoxin are examples of two drugs whose volume of distribution is significantly altered by changes in plasma albumin levels.

Drug clearance
The extent to which any drug or its metabolites are excreted by the kidneys is determined by the GFR. Thus, decline in GFR will give rise to accumulation of a given drug, with the potential for toxic plasma levels.

ETHICAL ISSUES

24.1 Dialysis provision

Provision and government funding of dialysis as renal replacement therapy is lower in the United Kingdom than in many other European countries and the United States.

Student activities

Consider the following:

- Do you think long-term dialysis should be available to all who require it? On what ethical principles do you base your argument?
- Under what circumstances, if any, would it be ethical not to commence dialysis in a patient in end-stage renal failure?
- Do you think patients who fail to comply with the prescribed therapeutic regimen for dialysis (this includes taking medications, attending for/performing dialysis, adhering to fluid and diet restrictions) should be withdrawn from a dialysis programme?

Further reading

Chandna SM, Schulz J, Lawrence C et al. Is there a rationale for rationing chronic dialysis? A hospital based cohort study of factors affecting survival and morbidity. Br Med J 1999; 318: 217–223.

considerations. The patient's subjective experience of uraemia is also taken into account. Ideally, commencement of dialysis should be a planned event. A planned multidisciplinary approach to preparation of patients for dialysis is preferable. Educative and supportive nursing roles are vital in pre-dialysis nursing care provision and will continue when dialysis commences.

RENAL REPLACEMENT THERAPIES

The term renal replacement therapy is used to describe the dialytic therapies (haemodialysis, haemofiltration, peritoneal dialysis) and renal transplantation. In relation to the dialytic therapies, the term is something of a misnomer, particularly in the context of long-term dialysis. Dialysis cannot fully replace normal renal function and offers at best a means to palliate some of the symptoms associated with loss of renal function. In addition, to be effective, dialysis therapy must not only be accompanied by a range of dietary and pharmacological interventions, but also requires considerable patient compliance (see Reflective Practice box 24.4).

Any decision to instigate long-term dialysis therapy must take into consideration the significant morbidity and mortality associated with this treatment, and balance this with patients' own perceptions of quality of life (Chandna et al 1999). As a treatment for ARF, the use of dialysis therapy may be less problematic, since it is used primarily as a short-term, supportive therapy. Once renal function is restored, the requirement for dialysis ceases.

R|Я REFLECTIVE PRACTICE

24.4 Personal views and beliefs about patient compliance

Patient compliance with treatment regimens is a major issue in chronic renal failure. The literature suggests that patient non-compliance is an issue that nurses have difficulty with on many levels, including ethically and in terms of its impact on service provision. In order to plan care and support patients' attempts to live with chronic illness and its many demands, it is important that nurses consider their own beliefs and attitudes toward patient compliance and non-compliance.

Student activities

- Make a note of what compliance and non-compliance mean to you.
- Take time out to reflect on your experiences in caring for a patient who was deemed to be compliant, and one deemed to be non-compliant:
  - How did these two patients make you feel in terms of your ability to provide nursing care?
  - Did you approach these patients differently?
  - How did you know that one was compliant and the other non-compliant?
  - Did this influence you in any way?

- Consider the following statements, and make a note of your reaction to them:
  - Patients with CRF should always follow the treatment regimen prescribed because the possibility of death is very real if they do not.
  - Compliance with a treatment regimen does not guarantee freedom from complications of a given disease process, so why should patients follow them?
  - Nurses only ever act in the best interests of their patients so patients should comply with their advice.
- Now read the following articles, and with reference to their contents, reflect on the notes that you have previously made: Cameron (1996), Wainright & Gould (1997) and Wichowski & Kubsch (1997).

Further reading

Cameron C. Patient compliance: recognition of factors involved and suggestions for promoting compliance with therapeutic regimens. J Adv Nurs 1996; 24(2): 244–250.

Wainright S, Gould D. Non-adherence with medications in organ transplant patients: a literature review. J Adv Nurs 1997; 26(5): 968–977.

Wichowski H, Kubsch S. The relationship of self perception of illness and compliance with health care regimens. J Adv Nurs 1997; 25(3): 548–553.

A successful kidney transplant offers the best opportunity to restore normal renal function for those with ESRF. However, life following transplantation may be no less difficult for the individual than it is for the person having long-term dialysis. Renal transplantation brings with it an absolute requirement to adhere to immunosuppressive drug therapy regimens, with their attendant side-effects, and the constant awareness that survival of the transplanted organ is limited. The latter is perhaps best explained when one considers that the 1-year survival for a transplanted kidney is approximately 90%, the 5-year survival is approximately 70%, and the 10-year survival only approximately 50%. Despite the huge advances that have been made in immunosuppressive therapy over the last 20 years, its impact on long-term renal transplant survival has been relatively small. However, managing rejection of a transplanted kidney is not the primary barrier to transplantation today – it is the lack of donor organs. While the number of those awaiting renal transplantation has risen year on year, the number of cadaveric donor organs available for transplantation has remained fairly static. Essentially, demand has outstripped supply. More recently, there have been attempts to encourage live-related kidney donation (see p. 694) and inter-spouse (where compatible) donation in the adult population affected by ESRF.

Haemodialysis

Haemodialysis is an extracorporeal treatment that enables removal of fluid and solute from the body. The two processes involved are diffusion (for solutes) and ultrafiltration (which removes water). Access to the circulation is required to establish the extracorporeal circuit, and this may be provided by a central venous catheter or an arteriovenous fistula (see section below on venous access). Blood is drawn from the body and pumped around a closed circuit through an 'artificial kidney' (dialyser), and thence returned to the body (see Fig. 24.12). The dialyser has two compartments, one for the blood and one for dialysis fluid (dialysate). A semipermeable membrane separates these two compartments, either formed of bundles of hollow fibres or a bundle of flat sheets. Normally, there is no direct contact between the blood being pumped along one side of the membrane and the dialysis fluid being pumped in the opposite direction (countercurrent flow) along the other side.

Removal of water and solute from the blood occurs across the semi-permeable membrane of the dialyser. The factors that determine solute removal via the dialyser can be summarized as:

- the size and shape of solute molecules
- solute concentration differences between the blood on one side of the semi-permeable membrane, and the dialysis fluid on the other – for example, creatinine is a small solute molecule that will be in high concentration in the patient's blood. Creatinine is not a component of the dialysis fluid. The concentration gradient thus favours the movement of creatinine from the blood across the dialyser membrane and into the dialysis fluid compartment
- hydrostatic pressure derived from the force exerted by the blood pump pushing blood through the extracorporeal circuit
- the frequency of presentation of a given solute to the dialyser membrane – essentially what this means is that the faster the blood pump speed (mL/min), the greater the total volume of blood, and therefore the amount of solute that is

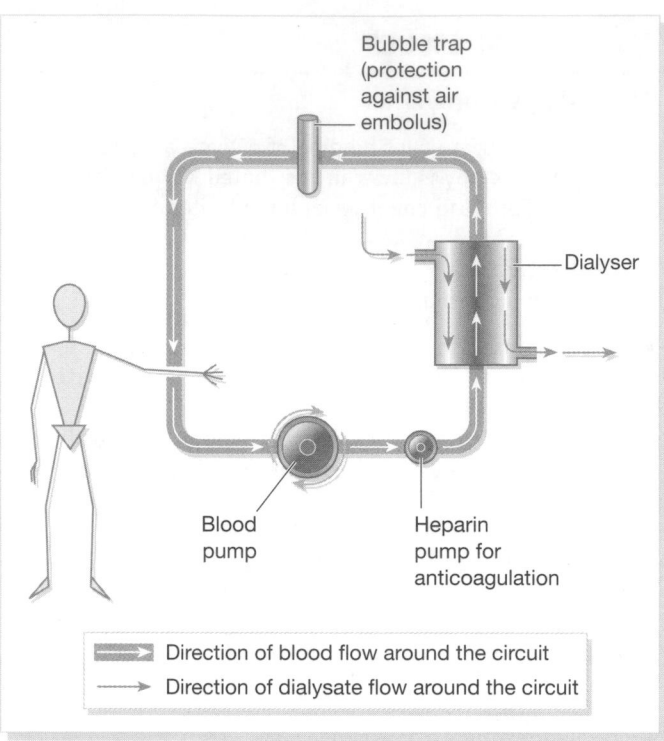

Figure 24.12 Extracorporeal circuit for haemodialysis (artificial kidney).

presented to the dialyser membrane. This in turn increases the likelihood of that solute moving from the blood and into the dialysate compartment.

Dialysate is a physiological solution and, in general, solute movement across the dialyser tends to be from the blood compartment into the dialysate compartment, with one notable exception. Bicarbonate is now a standard component of dialysis fluid, and the dialysate concentration of this is approximately 35 mmol/L. Metabolic acidosis, and thus bicarbonate depletion, is a feature of ESRF, and pre-haemodialysis serum levels of bicarbonate are usually abnormally low. Thus, the concentration gradient across the dialyser membrane, between the blood and dialysate, favours the movement of bicarbonate into the blood compartment. This is the principal means by which bicarbonate deficit in the ECF is replenished in these patients.

Removal of water is achieved by programming the dialysis machine to generate a negative 'suction' pressure within the dialysate compartment of the dialyser. This acts to pull water across the dialyser membrane from the blood compartment (ultrafiltration). Volumetric scales within the dialysis machine monitor the volume of water removed in this way constantly over the duration of a defined dialysis session.

The volume of water to be removed during each dialysis session is determined primarily by the patient's 'dry weight', interdialytic fluid gain and blood pressure. 'Dry weight' is the term used to signify the body weight at which a patient on haemodialysis is normotensive, euvolaemic and has no dependent (ankle) or pulmonary oedema. At the beginning of each haemodialysis session, the patient is weighed. The difference between this predialysis weight and the patient's weight at the end of the previous dialysis session is the interdialytic weight gain. For example, assume dry weight = 70 kg, postdialysis weight for previous session = 70 kg, and predialysis weight = 73 kg; the interdialytic weight gain is 3 kg (equivalent to inter-dialytic fluid intake), and this volume will be removed during the subsequent dialysis session to return the patient to the 'dry weight', unless clinical observations dictate otherwise.

The majority of patients having haemodialysis will dialyse for 3.5–5 hours, three times a week. Some will attend an in-hospital dialysis unit for treatment, while others dialyse themselves at home (home haemodialysis).

The dietary, and in particular fluid, restrictions associated with haemodialysis are especially problematic for patients. All renal units have dedicated renal dieticians who play a significant part in the care of people with renal dysfunction. Dietary restriction aims to reduce the ingested load of potassium, sodium and phosphate primarily. Fluid restriction is a necessity since, in the absence of normal renal function, fluid balance can only be achieved by dialysis. As a general rule, the amount of fluid allowed in a 24-hour period is 500 mL (to cover insensible loss) plus the volume of any residual urine output. For many patients, this equates to a fluid restriction of around 1–1.5 L/day and is very difficult to maintain. Accurate measuring of fluid intake is complex and all fluid, e.g. milk used on cereals, must be included.

Venous access for haemodialysis

Venous access is an important component of haemodialysis as a treatment. Patients having haemodialysis recognize this and can be, naturally, very protective of their venous access. Such access may be secured by means of a venous catheter or the formation of an arteriovenous fistula (see Fig. 24.13), the latter being the access of choice in long-term haemodialysis. Formation of an arteriovenous fistula involves a minor surgical procedure during which an artery and a vein are anastomosed. The commonest sites are radial artery to cephalic vein in the forearm, or brachial artery to one of the superficial veins in the upper arm. Anastomosis diverts blood flow from the artery and into the vein. As a result of increased blood flow through a vessel that has less elastic tissue than an artery, the vein dilates. The combination of increased internal diameter, increased blood flow and superficial-ization of the vein renders it suitable for repeated puncture with large-bore fistula needles and able to sustain the blood pump speeds required for dialysis (300–450 mL/min).

A functioning arteriovenous fistula is usually easily visible on either the forearm or upper arm. Some have very prominent vessels and some patients may find the change in body image upsetting. Blood flow through the fistula can be felt (slight buzz/thrill) by placing a hand lightly on the fistula. Similarly, blood flow through the fistula can be heard with a stethoscope.

Formation of an arteriovenous fistula presupposes that the patient has blood vessels that are suitable for anastomosis. If this is not the case, or where there are other contraindications, venous access will be secured with a central venous catheter. In long-term haemodialysis, the central venous catheters used for this purpose are usually dual-lumen with low thrombogenicity (ability to induce clot formation, e.g. silicone-based materials are used in their manufacture). The site of insertion is commonly the right or left subclavian vein, and the catheters are tunnelled under the skin. Nurses should be familiar with local protocols for caring for this type of central venous catheter.

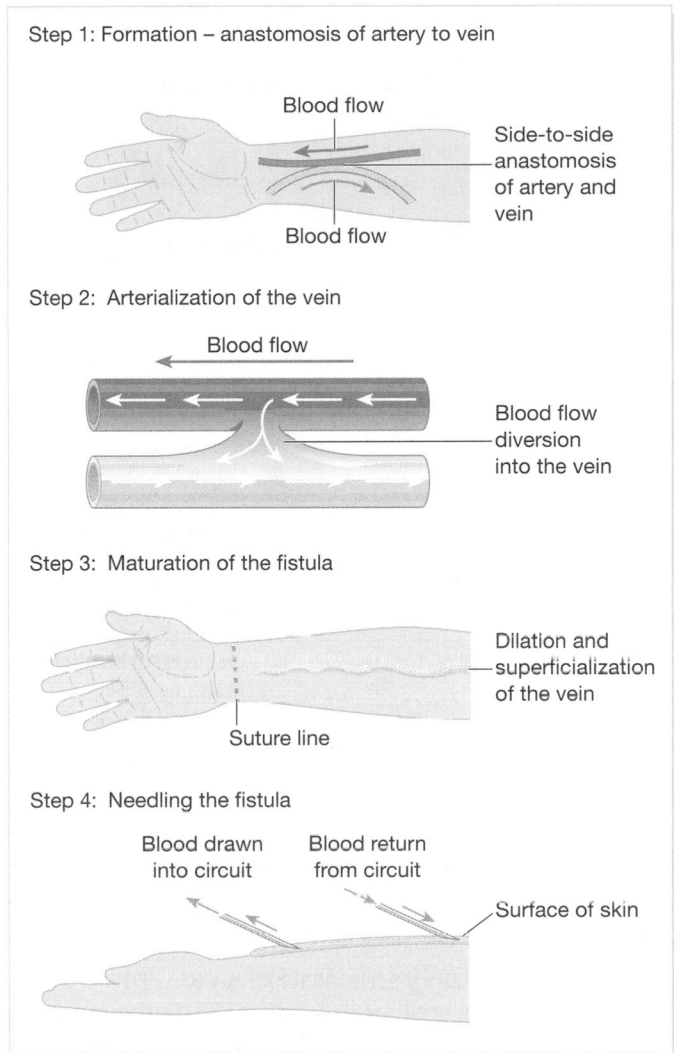

Step 1: Formation – anastomosis of artery to vein

Blood flow

Side-to-side anastomosis of artery and vein

Blood flow

Step 2: Arterialization of the vein

Blood flow

Blood flow diversion into the vein

Step 3: Maturation of the fistula

Dilation and superficialization of the vein

Suture line

Step 4: Needling the fistula

Blood drawn into circuit

Blood return from circuit

Surface of skin

Figure 24.13 Arteriovenous fistula.

Venous access failure is a significant contributor to morbidity and mortality in patients having long-term haemodialysis. Thus, preservation and protection of venous access are vital facets of patient care. Venous access for haemodialysis is precisely that, and neither arteriovenous fistulae nor central venous dialysis catheters should be used for other purposes (e.g. blood sampling).

Peritoneal dialysis

Like haemodialysis, peritoneal dialysis (PD) utilizes the process of diffusion to achieve movement of solute from blood to dialysate across a semi-permeable membrane. In the case of peritoneal dialysis, the semi-permeable membrane used is the peritoneum. The peritoneal capillary bed provides the blood flow, and thus presents solutes for diffusion, and the peritoneal cavity provides the compartment for dialysate fluid (see Fig. 24.14, p. 692). A permanent indwelling catheter, a Tenchkoff catheter, provides access to the peritoneal cavity. The Tenchkoff catheter is inserted through the anterior abdominal wall to lie with its tip above the peritoneum in the abdominal cavity.

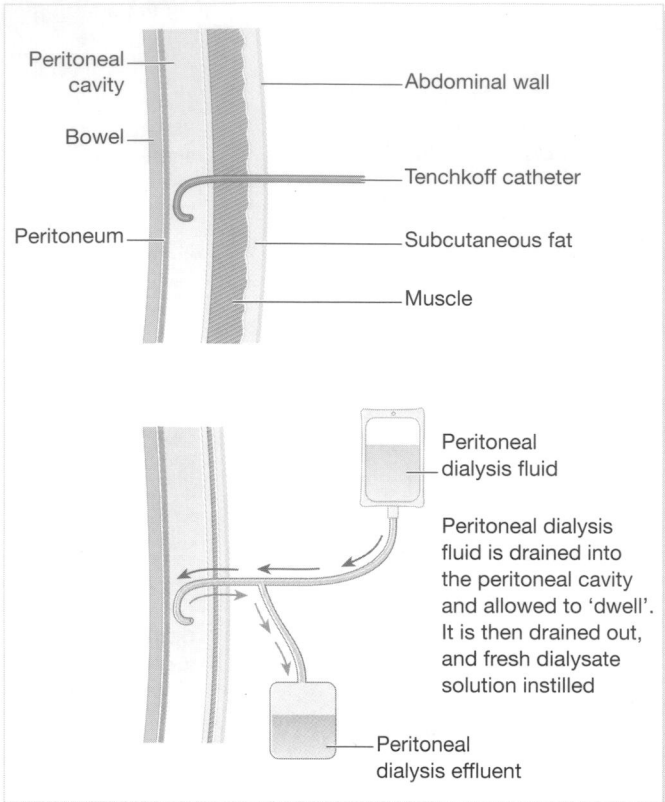

Peritoneal cavity
Bowel
Peritoneum

Abdominal wall
Tenchkoff catheter
Subcutaneous fat
Muscle

Peritoneal dialysis fluid

Peritoneal dialysis fluid is drained into the peritoneal cavity and allowed to 'dwell'. It is then drained out, and fresh dialysate solution instilled

Peritoneal dialysis effluent

Figure 24.14 Peritoneal dialysis.

A number of terms are used to describe PD, including:

- continuous ambulatory peritoneal dialysis (CAPD)
- continuous cycling peritoneal dialysis (CCPD) – this requires the use of a machine to cycle fluid into and out of the peritoneal cavity
- automated peritoneal dialysis (APD).

Dialysate fluid used for PD comprises sterile water and solutes in physiological solution. Two-litre bags of this are commonly used, although this volume depends on individual patient requirements, and thus more or less volume may be used. The PD procedure is called an 'exchange' and involves the following:

1. Dialysate fluid is instilled into the peritoneal cavity.
2. It is allowed to dwell there ('dwell time') for a period of time sufficient to allow solute movement between blood and dialysate fluid to occur.
3. The dialysate effluent is then drained out of the peritoneal cavity.

Removal of water by PD is achieved by the use of peritoneal dialysate containing different concentrations of dextrose. The three concentrations of dextrose commonly used are 1.36, 2.27 and 3.86%. Dextrose in the peritoneal dialysate provides an osmotic force that draws water from the patient across the peritoneal membrane. The greater the concentration of dextrose used, the greater the osmotic force generated, and thereby the more water that will be removed. If an exact estimation of fluid removal by peritoneal dialysis is required, this is achieved by weighing the bag of dialysate both prior to and following the

exchange procedure. The difference in weight between these two readings is the volume of water removed or, in some circumstances (e.g. hypovolaemia, hyperglycaemia), retained. Box 24.5 provides a sample regimen for PD.

Patients and/or their carers perform PD exchanges at home. The benefits associated with this treatment include patient control over treatment and the portability of PD, so that patients can work or travel and bring their dialysis with them. The length of time that a patient can be away from home is limited by the ability to carry all the equipment required for the duration of time away. Patients receiving CAPD wishing to go on holiday need to arrange for the transfer of sufficient quantities of equipment to the holiday destination, even if this is overseas. The renal care provider (hospital renal department) arranges this through the company that normally delivers supplies to the patient at home.

While CAPD is perceived as beneficial by many patients, and less restrictive than haemodialysis, it also places a burden of responsibility on patients and their families. Part of the ongoing care for these patients must therefore include continuous assessment of their ability (and that of their family) to manage their own treatment. Strict attention to personal hygiene, hand-washing and a non-touch technique when performing a bag exchange or caring for the exit site of the Tenchkoff catheter are essential. Exit site infection is an important problem of long-term PD (see Fig. 24.15).

In common with haemodialysis, PD is associated with significant morbidity. One of the commonest complications of PD is peritonitis. In this patient group, peritonitis is characterized by abdominal pain, fever and thick cloudy dialysis effluent (normally clear). If peritonitis is suspected, it is usual to send a 10 mL sample of dialysis fluid effluent for microscopy, culture and antibiotic sensitivity tests. The causative microorganisms include *Staphylococcus aureus* and *S. epidermidis*, which are normal skin commensals. Repeated episodes of peritonitis may damage the peritoneum such that it is no longer suitable as a dialysing membrane. If this occurs, then the individual is faced with a number of choices, including conversion to haemodialysis and withdrawal from dialysis as a treatment.

Treatment of peritonitis is with antibiotics. These may be given orally (e.g. ciprofloxacin), intravenously (e.g. vancomycin),

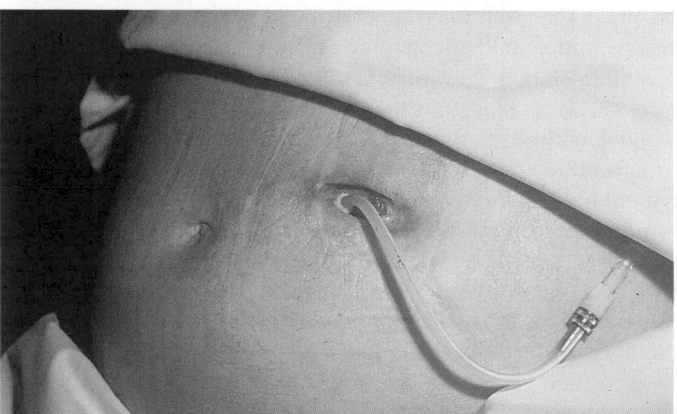

Figure 24.15 Exit site infection. (Reproduced with kind permission from Johnson & Feehally 2000.)

Box 24.5 Sample regimen for peritoneal dialysis

Peritoneal dialysis procedure

- Number of daily exchanges – 4 × 2 litre exchanges: morning (on rising), midday, late afternoon and bedtime
- Patient to weigh daily in the morning
- Dialysate bags to be used – 2 × 1.36% and 2 × 2.27% dextrose
- Dwell time for daytime bags 3–4 hours: patient may perform an exchange on going to bed and dialysate fluid remains in peritoneal cavity overnight or may perform an exchange, then drain out and cap off (seal) Tenchkoff catheter so that the peritoneal cavity is empty of fluid overnight
- Tenchkoff catheter exit site/dressing cleaned and changed daily

Dietary and fluid allowances

- Caloric energy requirements are equivalent to those of a healthy person of equivalent age, sex and physical activity
- Protein intake – 1.2 g/kg ideal body weight with 70% of intake from high biological value proteins (ones containing the essential amino acids)
- Protein supplementation if unable to ingest sufficient or following episode of peritonitis

- Restricted intake of foods containing potassium, e.g. dried fruit, bananas, crisps
- No salt added to food
- Restricted intake of foods containing phosphate balanced against need to maintain adequate intake of protein (protein contains phosphate)
- Fluid restricted to volume of residual urine output over 24 hours plus 500 mL to cover the insensible loss. Usually restriction is in the region of 1–1.5 L.

Medications

- Phosphate binders – to inhibit phosphate absorption from the gut
- Antihypertensive drugs if hypertension is not volume-dependent
- Vitamin D analogue – to replace lack of active vitamin D
- Vitamin supplementation – to enhance dietary intake and replenish those lost across the dialysis membrane
- Antibiotics may be injected into the peritoneal dialysate bag for subsequent instillation into the peritoneal cavity (e.g. gentamicin) if peritonitis is present
- Human recombinant erythropoietin (rhuEPO) given subcutaneously to replace loss of endogenous erythropoietin production

---

or injected into the peritoneal dialysate bag for subsequent instillation into the peritoneal cavity (e.g. gentamicin). All episodes of peritonitis should prompt a review of the patient's bag exchange technique, with remedial action taken if required.

Regular reassessment of patients' ability to cope with the treatment and of their home circumstances should also be undertaken.

Haemofiltration and haemodialysis in ARF

In ARF, haemofiltration and haemodialysis may be used to replace renal function. Both are extracorporeal therapies, and access to the central circulation is usually achieved with a dual-lumen central venous catheter. The care of the catheter and exit site is outlined in Guidelines for Care Priorities box 24.4. Sites of catheter include the internal and external jugular vein (right and left sides), and the femoral vein. In practice, the subclavian vein tends to be the least favoured site primarily because of the relatively high risk of lung puncture with pneumothorax on insertion.

The extracorporeal circuit used for haemofiltration is similar to that used in haemodialysis (see p. 690) and consists of blood lines through which blood flows, a pump to drive blood round the circuit and a dialyser (or filter) that has two compartments. However, the semi-permeable membrane used for haemofiltration is thinner and has slightly larger pore sizes. As for haemodialysers, the semi-permeable membrane is either arranged as bundles of hollow fibres or flat sheets. Blood in the extracorporeal circuit flows either through or along these, respectively. At commencement of a haemofiltration treatment, the compartment outside the hollow fibres contains normal saline, which is used to prepare the extracorporeal circuit for use. However, once

 GUIDELINES FOR CARE PRIORITIES

24.4 Vascular catheters used for haemodialysis or haemofiltration

It is worth keeping in mind that the combination of a catheter with direct access to the patient's central circulation and the diminished ability to fight infection associated with renal failure (or other organ failure) increases the risk of infection. Most centres will have a clinical guideline for the care of central venous catheters for dialysis or filtration and nurses should be familiar with local protocols. However, the following general guidance is likely to be included.

General guidance

- As a general rule, vascular catheters that are inserted for the purpose of dialysis or filtration should not be used for any other purpose.
- The exit site of the catheter, and the limbs of the catheter, should be cleaned with, for example, an alcohol-based scrub solution as part of the commencement of haemodialysis or filtration procedure.
- A semi-occlusive dressing (e.g. OpSite) may be used to dress the catheter exit site.
- When not in use, the vascular catheter is usually 'heparin-locked' (i.e. a quantity of heparin equal to the volume of the internal diameter of both limbs of the venous catheter is injected into the limbs and left in place to prevent clotting in the catheter) and protected by wrapping gauze swabs around the limbs and securing with tape.

the haemofiltration treatment has started, this compartment will contain an ultrafiltrate of the patient's blood.

Haemofiltration is a convective therapy, whereby the combination of a membrane of relatively high porosity and the hydrostatic pressure generated by blood being pumped along the blood circuit pushes water and solute across the membrane from the blood, forming an ultrafiltrate of the blood. This is essentially the same process occurring normally within the glomerulus of the kidney. Ultrafiltrate thus obtained drains into a collecting bag and is discarded. Fluid and solute removed from the patient in this way are replaced, via the extracorporeal circuit, with a sterile physiological solution, so-called haemofiltration replacement fluid. The patient's circulating vascular volume can be adjusted or left unchanged, simply by giving more than, less than, or a volume of replacement equal to that removed through the haemofilter.

The decision to instigate renal replacement in ARF is based on the presence of:

- hyperkalaemia
- vascular volume overload and/or pulmonary oedema
- metabolic acidosis.

Both haemofiltration and haemodialysis will remove solute and water, and rectify bicarbonate deficits. However, a number of additional factors dictate the use of one rather than the other. Haemodialysis is an intermittent therapy that can achieve rapid removal of solute and water, whereas haemofiltration is a continuous therapy, but the rate of solute removal is slower than with haemodialysis. In practice, the choice between haemodialysis or haemofiltration in ARF is made on an individual basis.

Renal transplantation

The surgical procedure for renal transplantation involves placement of a kidney from a donor into a recipient. The transplanted kidney is placed extraperitoneally, in either the right or the left iliac fossa. The renal artery of the donor kidney is anastomosed to the recipient's internal or external iliac artery, and the renal vein of the donor kidney to the recipient's iliac vein. The donor ureter is tunnelled into the recipient's bladder (see Fig. 24.16).

A number of factors are taken into consideration when determining whether or not transplantation should be undertaken. Thus, the ideal transplant recipient is medically fit, well nourished, adequately dialysed, normotensive, has no active disease (e.g. HIV or HBV infection, TB, UTI) and is competent to take immunosuppressive drugs.

As part of the preparation for renal transplantation, blood samples are drawn to determine the patient's ABO blood group and individual tissue type, based on genetically determined human leucocyte antigens (HLAs) present on the surface of most cell types. HLAs are important in transplantation, since they are involved in the recognition of a transplanted organ as 'non-self' (see Westwood 1999).

Renal transplantation always takes place between an ABO-compatible donor and recipient. Tissue type compatibility between donor and recipient is assessed prior to transplantation and, where possible, recipients receive a kidney from a donor whose tissue type most closely matches their own.

The donor must also be free from infection or other disease that could be transmitted to the recipient (e.g. CMV, HIV, HBV,

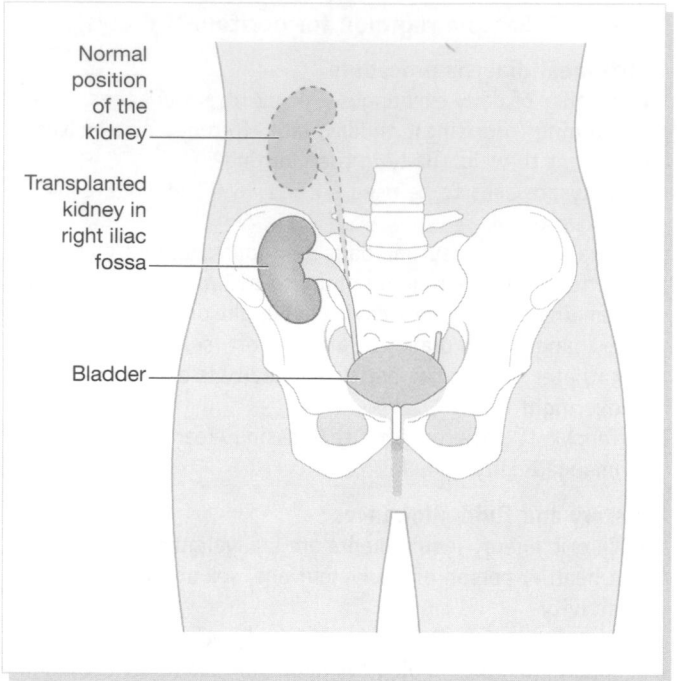

Figure 24.16   Position of transplanted kidney (right iliac fossa)

etc.). Once transplantation has been performed, patients are required to take immunosuppressive drugs to prevent rejection.

Currently, the majority of adult renal transplants undertaken in the UK involve transplantation of a kidney donated by an individual who has been declared brain stem dead (cadaveric transplants). The criteria for testing and confirming brain stem death are extremely stringent.

In recent years there has been an impetus to increase live-donor transplantation. All transplantation in the UK is governed by the Human Organ Transplant Act 1989 and associated Regulations (1989 and 1998). There is, in addition, a specific medicolegal framework in place to protect live donors of kidneys where the donor and recipient are not genetically related. The Unrelated Live Transplant Regulatory Authority (ULTRA) oversees the latter. Permission to perform renal transplantation between a living unrelated donor and recipient can only be granted by ULTRA. ULTRA acts to prevent coercion to donate a kidney, and the buying and selling of organs for transplantation, which are reported to occur in some countries (see Ethical Issues box 24.2).

In the case of live donation, donors undergo medical assessment to ensure fitness to donate. The assessment includes examination of their renal function. Abnormal renal function, active disease, such as diabetes, and infectious diseases (see before) will preclude kidney donation. Donors must also undergo psychological assessment to establish competence to make a decision to donate and that they are acting without coercion. Again, if these basic requirements are not met, kidney donation is precluded. It is also important to note that throughout assessment, the health care professionals involved must act in the best interests of the donor.

A live-donor kidney transplant has a number of benefits. Nephrectomy (donor) and transplantation (recipient) take place

ETHICAL ISSUES

24.2 Kidneys for sale

The sale of kidneys for transplantation is a highly contentious issue. In many countries, sales of kidneys for transplantation, from both adults and children, take place. Radcliffe-Richards et al (1998) make a case for re-opening the debate surrounding the sale of kidneys for transplantation, and present this from an ethical perspective. Drukker (1998), Soper (1998) and Velasco (1998) are a sample of some of the many comments that followed publication of the Radcliffe-Richard et al article.

Before you read any of these (and they are well worth reading), ask yourself the following questions:

- If you lived in abject poverty, with little of no resources to provide care for yourself or your family, what would you be willing to do to improve your lot in life?
- Is selling a kidney allowing someone else to take advantage of you?
- Can a parent consent to the sale of a kidney on a child's behalf?
- How would you feel about caring for a patient whom you suspected had donated a kidney for money?
- How would you feel about caring for the recipient of that kidney?

References

Drukker A. Organ donation and sales, The Lancet 1998; 352 (9126): 483–484.

Radcliffe-Richards J, Daar AS, Guttman RD et al. The case for allowing kidney sales. The Lancet 1998; 351(9120): 1950–1952.

Soper C. Organ donation and sales. The Lancet 1998; 352(9126): 484–485.

Velasco N. Organ donation and sales. The Lancet 1998; 352 (9126): 483.

almost in tandem, and usually in adjoining operating theatres. Once the kidney is removed, it is taken into the transplant theatre, flushed through with special kidney perfusion fluid and then immediately placed into the recipient and anastomosed to the recipient's blood supply. The duration of hypoxia is short, and thus hypoxic damage is minimal. Usually these kidneys begin to produce urine as soon as the blood vessel anastomoses are complete and the kidney reperfused, and continue to do so in the postoperative period. Long-term graft survival is good in live donation.

Specialist renal centres offering renal transplantation maintain a list of those awaiting transplantation. There is also a national waiting list that is administered by the UK Transplant Support Services Authority (UKTSSA) based in Bristol. When the kidneys of a cadaveric donor are offered for transplantation, the local renal centre undertakes tissue typing of the donor organs. The results are matched against the information held in UKTSSA databases, and potential recipients for transplantation are identified. These individuals may be anywhere within the UK. Commonly, the local centre retains one of the donated

kidneys for transplant if there is a suitable recipient. If not, both kidneys are dispatched for transplant elsewhere in the UK.

▶ Nursing management

Patients who are called for transplantation experience a complex mix of emotions, from joy and relief that the wait is over, to fear and anxiety about the procedure and what it will mean for their future life (Franklin 1997). Care should be taken during the admission procedure to present clear and factual information to patients. In addition to obtaining the standard information required during an admission procedure, the following are specific aspects of pre-transplantation patient assessment.

The majority of patients who present for renal transplantation are having long-term dialysis therapy. It is important that a requirement for dialysis or fluid removal by ultrafiltration is identified early in the admission procedure. If either is required, transplantation cannot proceed until these treatments are performed. The two parameters that are most important in the pre-transplantation period are fluid status and serum potassium, and assessment of both is mandatory. All patients should be weighed. Differences between weight on admission and the prescribed 'dry weight' in patients having long-term dialysis must be identified, and medical assessment of the significance made. Dialysis is indicated if the serum potassium is > 5.5 mmol/L.

Prior to transplantation, evaluation of biochemical and haematological parameters is undertaken. In addition to these, blood samples are drawn for repeat tissue typing and a cytotoxic cross-match. The purpose of the latter is to check whether or not the potential recipient has pre-formed antibodies specific to donor antigens. Previous transplantation, pregnancy or blood transfusion will have exposed the recipient to foreign antigens, with subsequent specific antibody formation. For a cytotoxic cross-match, serum from the recipient is mixed with donor cells (from the spleen or lymph nodes). If the donor cells die then they have been attacked by recipient antibody; this is a positive cytotoxic cross-match and means that the kidney is not suitable for the potential recipient. A negative cytotoxic cross-match is thus mandatory.

Patients' dialysis history should be obtained prior to transplantation, and the relevant dialysis nursing team informed of the admission for transplantation. It is good practice also to inform the nursing team responsible for acute dialysis on the ward area of the admission, so that they can prepare for a potential change in clinical workload should a patient require dialysis postoperatively.

All patients and their families require an explanation of what should be expected in the post-transplant period. This includes requirements for monitoring vital signs and fluid status, how the function of the renal transplant will be monitored, and commencement of immunosuppressive therapy.

Post-transplantation, patients are cared for on the ward area, usually in a high-dependency area for 2–4 days. Maintaining adequate perfusion of the transplanted kidney (graft) and provision of immunosuppressive therapy are care priorities in the post-transplantation period. Close assessment of haemodynamic status, with continuous monitoring of vital signs and assessment of fluid status, are specific nursing responsibilities. CVP measurements are usually performed at least for the first

24–48 hours. Fluid intake and output are measured hourly. All intake volumes are adjusted hourly to maintain euvolaemia with reference to the observed blood pressure, CVP, urine and wound drain output. Any changes in these parameters must be reported (e.g. haematuria, increased blood loss through the wound drain, changes in urine volumes). Intravenous 'renal dose' dopamine is a standard therapy in some centres. At this dosage, dopamine, which is inotropic at higher doses, enhances renal perfusion through dilation of the renal arterial network. Colour Doppler renal ultrasound may be performed within the first 24 hours to assess graft perfusion.

Serological assessment of graft function, using the serum creatinine as a marker, begins immediately after transplantation (see below). Postoperatively, monitoring of electrolytes, particularly potassium, and haematological tests are performed. Postoperative dialysis will be required if there is fluid overload, hyperkalaemia or delayed function of the graft.

Adequate pain relief is essential. However, care must always be taken with dosage, since the absence of normal renal function may lead to the accumulation of drug metabolites to toxic levels. As with nephrectomy (see p. 677), deep breathing exercises, the use of an incentive spirometer and first postoperative day ambulation are components of care. Physiotherapy review and support are essential both pre- and postoperatively, and good pain control increases the effectiveness of physiotherapy. Assessment of the nature, site and extent of pain relief should accompany the medication administered. New onset of pain over the graft site may be a symptom of arterial or venous occlusion of the graft.

Immunosuppression predisposes patients to infection. Opportunistic infection, e.g. with CMV, is relatively common, and the incidence increases where immunosuppressive therapy is increased to prevent rejection. Because of immunosuppression, usual signs of infection, e.g. pyrexia, may not be present. Immunosuppression also has an impact on wound healing, and skin closures are usually left in place for approximately 10 days.

Following renal transplantation, patients have to take what may appear to them as a bewildering array of medication (see Box 24.6). The importance of compliance with immunosuppressive drug therapy cannot be overemphasized. Graft rejection associated with non-compliance is a known postoperative complication (Rovelli et al 1989). Nurses play a major educative role in familiarizing patients with drug regimens, ensuring that they know when and when not to take each drug, dose requirements and the drug action. Education of patients toward competent self-medication begins on admission. Assessment of competence must always be performed prior to discharge.

Monitoring graft function is an essential component of post-transplant care. This begins postoperatively and continues for the life span of the graft. The serum creatinine is the principal marker used for this purpose. Rejection of the graft is possible at any time following transplantation. Rejection episodes may be classified as hyperacute, accelerated acute, acute and chronic (see Box 24.7).

Renal transplantation does not offer a 'cure' for renal disease. While it conveys potential for improvements in quality of life, and the possibility of physiological and psychosocial rehabilitation, it can also present patients with additional stressors. One of the commonest stressors identified in this group of patients is

---

> **Box 24.6 Drug groups commonly prescribed in the early post-transplant period**
>
> - Immunosuppressants (e.g. ciclosporin, tacrolimus, prednisolone, mycophenolate mofetil, azathioprine) – suppress rejection of transplanted kidney. Usually used in combinations
> - Antibacterial (e.g. co-trimoxazole) – prevention or treatment of bacterial urinary tract infection
> - Antifungals (e.g. fluconazole, amphotericin or nystatin) – prevention or treatment of fungal infection
> - Antituberculous drugs (e.g. isoniazid) – prophylaxis against tuberculosis needed in some immunosuppressed patients to prevent reactivation of latent tuberculosis. (**NB.** Pyridoxine [vitamin B_6] is also prescribed to prevent peripheral neuropathy [side-effect of isoniazid])
> - Antivirals (e.g. aciclovir or ganciclovir) – prevention or treatment of viral infection
> - Broad-spectrum antibiotics – perioperative prophylaxis or treatment of infection

---

fear of rejection with subsequent loss of a functioning graft (Frey 1990). When one considers the statistics describing long-term graft survival (see p. 690), this fear is entirely reasonable and representative of a fear of loss of control over one's health and life. Other well described stressors, including side-effects associated with immunosuppression, changes in body image and medical complications of transplantation, have significant impacts on patients' perceptions of quality of life (Welch 1994). It is important that nurses caring for these individuals plan interventions that aim to support their attempts to develop positive coping strategies and perception of control.

DISORDERS OF THE PROSTATE GLAND

BENIGN ENLARGEMENT OF THE PROSTATE

Benign enlargement is due to hyperplasia (growth of new cells) of the prostate and is known as benign prostatic hyperplasia (BPH). It occurs most often in males over 60 years of age.

Aetiology and pathophysiology

The aetiology of this condition is unclear. BPH distorts the prostatic urethra and obstructs bladder outflow. Bladder compensation for outflow obstruction results in hypertrophy of the bladder muscle (detrusor), so that increasingly higher intravesical pressures are generated to force urine past the obstruction. Ultimately, bladder dilation ensues and the muscle becomes hypotonic (force of contraction diminishes).

Clinical presentation

Frequency of micturition and nocturia are common early symptoms. Alterations in urine outflow with reduced force of stream, delay or difficulty in initiating urination, and post-urination dribbling are often present. Overflow incontinence secondary to acute urinary retention is also described (see Ch. 12).

Box 24.7 Types of rejection following renal transplantation

Hyperacute rejection

This catastrophic rejection occurs intraoperatively, on revascularization of the transplanted kidney. It is caused by the presence of pre-formed cytotoxic antibodies specific to donor antigen, or the presence of anti-ABO blood group antibodies. The transplanted kidney becomes cyanotic, flaccid or hard, and rupture is a possibility. There is no treatment for this type of rejection, and if it occurs, the graft is removed immediately. Cytotoxic cross-match (see p. 695) is performed pre-transplantation to prevent hyperacute rejection.

Accelerated acute rejection

Usually develops within the first 5 days following transplantation and is also associated with pre-sensitization to donor antigen. The onset of this may be heralded by a decrease in urine output and a sharp rise in the serum creatinine, where previously there had been a urine output and a falling serum creatinine. Biopsy of the transplanted kidney (see p. 667) may be undertaken to confirm the diagnosis. Treatment of this involves adjustment to the immunosuppressive drug regimen. However, like hyperacute rejection, prevention is preferable. Those who are most at risk include patients who have been previously transplanted, women who have had several pregnancies, even if these

have not been carried to term, and patients who have had multiple blood transfusions. Pre-sensitization secondary to blood transfusion is much less problematic, as since the advent of erythropoietin, the need for transfusion has greatly reduced. Pre-transplantation induction with immunosuppressive therapy and increased postoperative immunosuppressive dosage are strategies employed for at-risk patients.

Acute rejection

Episodes can occur at any point following transplantation. This is a systemic inflammatory disorder. A rise in the serum creatinine may be the only indication that this is occurring. Diagnosis is confirmed by biopsy of the transplanted kidney. Treatment involves adjustments to the immunosuppressive drug regimen.

Chronic rejection

This is associated with delayed graft function in the postoperative period secondary to hypoxic injury (acute tubular necrosis, ATN), early or multiple acute rejection episodes, and inadequate immunosuppression (either because insufficient has been prescribed or because of non-compliance). Chronic rejection leads to persistent deterioration in renal function, with return to life on dialysis as the end-point.

Investigations

These include urine culture, serological evaluation of renal function, renal and prostatic ultrasound, and cystoscopy. Urodynamic flow studies may also be performed to determine alterations in urine outflow. Physical examination will include abdominal palpation and rectal examination. Blood sampling for evaluation of PSA levels may also be undertaken if malignancy is suspected (see p. 700).

Medical/surgical management

Treatment is dependent on the clinical presentation of the patient. In acute retention, relief of pain and outflow obstruction are priorities. Suprapubic catheterization through the abdominal wall will be required if urethral catheterization is not possible (see Guidelines for Care Priorities box 24.5).

Episodes of acute retention indicate the need for resection of the prostate. Transurethral resection of the prostate (TURP) using an electric cautery is associated with lower morbidity and shorter hospital stay than open prostatectomy. In BPH, a third pathological prostatic capsule grows outwards from the midline, compressing the normal part of the gland. TURP involves chipping out the abnormal capsule. Open prostatectomy may be required where the prostate is too large to be resected transurethrally. Types of open prostatectomy include:

- retropubic prostatectomy – the prostate is accessed through a suprapubic incision; the bladder is retracted upwards to expose the prostate behind the pubis
- transvesical prostatectomy – the prostate is approached through the bladder using a suprapubic incision

- perineal approach to prostatectomy may be used in some countries.

Anti-androgen (against testosterone) drugs such as finasteride may be used in some cases to reduce the size of the prostate to improve urine flow rate.

▶ Nursing management: TURP

Patients need a full explanation of the operative procedure and the requirement for bladder irrigation via a urethral catheter in the postoperative period. They should be forewarned that initial urine drainage would be bloodstained. The urologist will have explained the potential risks associated with TURP, and as part of preoperative preparation nurses must ensure that patients understand the risk (albeit very small) of incontinence, erectile dysfunction and disordered ejaculation associated with this procedure (see Ch. 25). The consequences could have significant implications for quality of life and psychosexual relationships postoperatively. Patients should also be encouraged to perform pelvic floor exercises (see Ch. 12), both pre- and postoperatively. These exercises will help them to overcome postoperative urine dribbling.

In the immediate postoperative period, nursing care is focused on observation of vital signs for haemorrhage, providing effective pain relief, maintaining an accurate record of fluid intake and output, and ensuring patency of the three-way indwelling urinary catheter inserted following TURP. Catheter patency is maintained with a closed bladder irrigation system (see Fig. 24.17, p. 698).

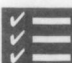

GUIDELINES FOR CARE PRIORITIES

24.5 Suprapubic catheterization

- Patients need a full explanation of the procedure and the opportunity to ask questions.
- A thorough assessment of patient needs and physical and cognitive abilities is essential, especially in situations where the catheter is for long-term use and patients/carers will be required to care for it at home.
- The catheter will be inserted after the use of a suitable anaesthetic (see Ch. 29); usually a local anaesthetic is used. The catheter is initially secured to the skin by a suture.
- The insertion site is treated like any other surgical wound – it is dressed according to local protocols, usually a semi-occlusive, transparent dressing. The site is observed for signs of inflammation and infection (e.g. redness, swelling, discharge) and complaints of pain are noted.
- The catheter/drainage system is secured to the patient's clothing so as to prevent any tension on the insertion site, and in a way that maintains free drainage.
- Catheter patency is checked as with a urethral catheter and patients are asked to report pain or leakage from around the catheter. A blockage is reported and managed according to local protocols such as by bladder washout.

- The suprapubic catheter drains into a collecting bag and is maintained as a closed system to minimize the risk of infection.
- Any signs or symptoms of UTI (e.g. cloudy urine, haematuria, suprapubic pain, pyrexia) are reported and urine is sent for microbiological examination if infection is suspected.
- Discharge planning for patients going home with the catheter will include education about handwashing, emptying the bag, maintaining system integrity, looking for signs/symptoms of infection or blockage, obtaining supplies and caring for the insertion site. Nurses must check that patients are competent to self-care, and in situations where this is not possible, arrangements are made for the community nursing service to undertake this care.

Further reading

Gujral S, Kirkwood L, Hinchliffe A. Suprapubic catheterization: a suitable procedure for clinical nurse specialists in selected patients. BJU Int 1999; 83(9): 954–956.

Peate I. Patient management following suprapubic catheterization. Br J Nurs 1997; 6(10): 555–562

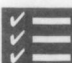

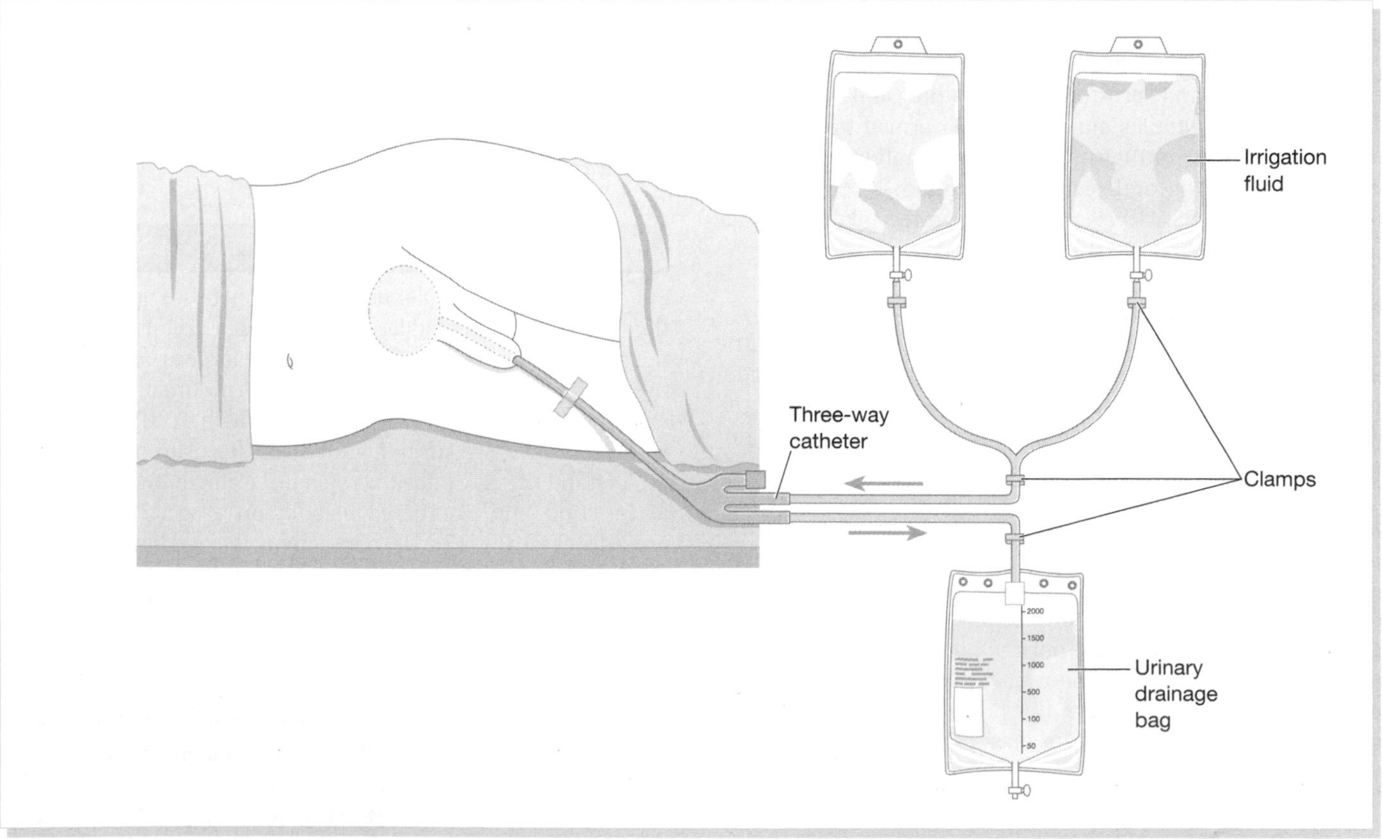

Figure 24.17 Continuous bladder irrigation.

Irrigation fluid (glycine irrigation solution 1.5% is the solution of choice) is allowed to flow into and out of the bladder constantly in the early postoperative period to prevent outflow obstruction associated with blood clots or prostatic debris. The rate of irrigation fluid inflow should be sufficient to give clear or rosé (slightly pink) drainage.

Nurses should be alert to the risk of TUR syndrome (hypervolaemia and hyponatraemia) caused by the absorption of glycine irrigation fluid into the bloodstream. This may lead to a variety of serious circulatory, e.g. cardiac arrhythmias, and cerebral disturbances. Symptoms are variable but may include headache, nausea and vomiting, dyspnoea, chest pain, blurred vision, disorientation and changes in consciousness, pulse (bradycardia) and blood pressure (hypotension or hypertension). For further information, readers are directed to suggestions for 'Further reading', see Steggall (1999) (p. 702).

Monitoring of urine output is complicated by bladder irrigation, since both urine and irrigation fluid pass out of the catheter. Thus strict attention must be paid to the volume instilled and the volume drained on an hourly basis, with urine output calculated accordingly. For example, if 2 L were instilled over a 1-hour period, and 2.2 L is the total volume drained, the urine output for that hour was 200 mL. A drainage volume less than that instilled should prompt assessment of catheter patency. The medical staff should be informed if catheter obstruction is suspected. A manual bladder washout, using sterile irrigation fluid (e.g. sodium chloride 0.9% solution) and a 60 mL syringe attached to the urinary catheter, may be initiated according to local protocols. While some resistance to instillation of fluid by this method can be expected in the presence of debris or a clot, it is important that irrigation fluid is not forced into the catheter. If it is not possible to clear the obstruction, the urologist should be informed, who will usually insert a replacement catheter.

Infection is a potential complication and signs such as cloudy urine or pyrexia should be reported. Urine will be cultured and, if infection is detected, the appropriate antibiotics prescribed.

The length of time that the urinary catheter remains in situ following TURP will depend on the urologist's preferences, the procedure performed and the speed of patient recovery. Following removal of a urinary catheter after TURP, it is necessary to observe patients for signs of acute urinary retention (bladder pain and distension, difficulty in passing urine). Incontinence, usually temporary, but in some cases persistent, can be expected following TURP. Patients having problems maintaining continence should be referred to the appropriate nurse specialist or other health professional. They should be advised of this, and every effort made to ensure that they are assisted in dealing with that incontinence (e.g. advised to urinate frequently, use pads to absorb urine leak) in a manner that preserves their personal dignity. Bladder spasm and/or rectal pain may also be experienced postoperatively. Antimuscarinic drugs may be prescribed to alleviate bladder spasm, e.g. hyoscine butylbromide or propantheline bromide.

Constipation should be prevented to avoid excessive straining during defaecation; early mobilization, adequate oral fluids and a diet containing sufficient fibre will usually achieve this.

Patients will usually have an outpatient follow-up appointment. Discharge planning will include advice about avoiding heavy lifting, straining and vigorous physical activity for about a month (see Ch. 29 for a general discussion). Patients should understand the importance of seeking medical advice if they experience difficulty or pain on passing urine, or have cloudy or bloodstained urine, as these may indicate an infection. Information about resuming sexual activity should be offered sensitively as some patients and their partners will be particularly anxious. Nurses should ensure that patients understand the urologist's advice. Generally sexual activity may be resumed after 6 weeks but some urologists recommend that patients wait until after the follow-up consultation. Patients are advised to abstain from sexual activity if their urine is cloudy or bloodstained.

PROSTATE CANCER

Prostatic carcinoma is one of the commonest malignancies in males in the UK. With over 21 700 new cases each year, it is the second most common male cancer in the UK (Cancer Research UK 2002).

Aetiology

Presentation is rare before the sixth decade and most prostatic cancers occur in men aged over 60 years. Men of African descent have a higher risk of developing prostate cancer. Both viral and hormonal factors have been implicated in the aetiology of this disease (see Ch. 33). High fat consumption and vitamin D deficiency have also been suggested as contributory factors. There may be a genetic predisposition, and men with a first-degree relative with prostate cancer diagnosed at a young age are at higher risk. Men exposed to radiation, such as at work, may have an increased risk.

Clinical presentation

The presentation has many features in common with BPH and includes:

- frequency and nocturia
- urgency
- hesitancy starting, poor stream and dribbling
- dysuria
- haematuria or bloody semen.

Some patients will present with cystitis and prostatitis. Acute retention may also be a feature. Symptoms associated with metastatic spread to the bones include weight loss, anorexia, anaemia and bone pain, such as backache. Some patients with advanced disease may present with signs of uraemia (see p. 687) caused by the cancer obstructing the ureters.

Investigations

These will include:

- rectal examination to assess size, shape and tenderness of prostate
- transrectal or transperineal biopsy of the prostate for histological examination
- serologic assessment of renal function, acid phosphatase and PSA (see Evidence-based Practice box 24.1)
- urodynamic studies
- prostate and renal ultrasound
- X-ray of the pelvis or lumbar spine to detect bony metastases
- radioisotope scans for further investigation of bone involvement.

EVIDENCE-BASED PRACTICE

24.1 Prostate-specific antigen screening

Prostate-specific antigen (PSA) is a protein substance produced almost exclusively by epithelial cells in the prostate gland. High serum levels of PSA are associated with diseases of the prostate, including adenocarcinoma, BPH and prostatic inflammation. Advocates of PSA screening in the male population hold that PSA screening can lead to early detection of prostate cancer, and thus early intervention. Barry (2001) suggests that PSA screening is controversial because there is a lack of evidence that early detection and intervention result in reduced mortality. General recommendations regarding PSA screening made in this article include:

- Men aged between 50 and 75 years should be made aware of the availability of PSA screening and be provided with sufficient information regarding this test, and possible outcomes, such that they can make an informed choice as to whether or not they wish to be screened.
- Early PSA screening should be offered to men in high-risk groups from the age of 45 years onwards. This includes those who have a family history of prostate cancer and those of African descent.

Student activities
- Find out what facilities exist in your area for men to obtain PSA testing.
- What counselling is available for men who decide to have PSA screening?

References
Barry MJ. Prostate-specific-antigen testing for early diagnosis of prostate cancer. New Engl J Med 2001; 344(18): 1373–1377.

Further reading
O'Connor A, Rostom A, Fiset V et al. Decision aids for patients facing health treatment or screening decisions: a Cochrane systematic review. Br Med J 1999; 319(7212): 731–734.

Medical/surgical management

Management will depend on the type, stage and extent of the cancer (see Box 24.8 and Ch. 33 for further discussion of the classification and grading system of tumours), and the health and general wishes of the patient. Management options (with some nursing considerations) are described below.

Watchful waiting

Prostate cancer can be slow-growing and for some patients (especially very old men, where anaesthetic/operation risk is high or where the likely risks/side-effects of treatment outweigh the anticipated benefits), a 'wait and see' approach may be appropriate. If this approach is taken, then regular medical follow-up and serial estimation of PSA levels are required. Nurses need to be aware that patients and their families may require considerable psychological support in order to assist their attempts to live life with cancer.

Box 24.8 Stages of prostate cancer growth. (Adapted from www.cancerbacup.org.uk/info/pros/pros-7a.htm)

Spread of prostate cancer growth is usually divided into four stages (T = tumour):

- Stage 1 (T1) – the tumour is within the prostatic capsule and cannot be felt on rectal digital examination, but the PSA level may be raised
- Stage 2 (T2) – the tumour is within the prostatic capsule but can be felt on rectal digital examination. PSA levels are raised and prostate ultrasound may allow visualization
- Stages 3 and 4 (T3/T4) – the tumour has extended beyond the prostatic capsule to surrounding tissue.

Stages 1 and 2 are further defined as 'early' prostatic cancer. Stages 3 and 4 are further defined as 'locally advanced' prostatic cancer. The term metastatic cancer refers to tumour invasion of lymph nodes, bone or other body tissues.

Surgery

Radical prostatectomy is performed in those patients whose cancer remains confined to the prostatic capsule, and is thus essentially a treatment for early prostate cancer (see Box 24.8). This procedure involves removal of the entire prostatic capsule and surrounding structures (e.g. lymph nodes and seminal vesicles). Radical prostatectomy is not usually undertaken where there is local invasive spread or advanced metastatic spread. Hormonal therapy and radiotherapy are commonly used in the latter cases. In cases of advanced prostatic cancer where urinary outflow obstruction develops, TURP (see p. 697) to relieve obstruction may be undertaken.

Radiotherapy

This may be used when an operation is contraindicated, or to reduce the size of the prostate to minimize urinary problems. Radiotherapy procedures used in the setting of early prostatic cancer include external beam radiotherapy and brachytherapy. The latter procedure involves implanting radioactive 'seeds' in the prostate. In late stage prostatic cancer, radiotherapy can be used to palliate pain associated with bony metastases.

Hormonal therapy

Androgens (male sex hormones) stimulate the growth of prostatic cancer cells. It therefore follows that decreasing androgen levels will depress prostatic cancer growth. This is the basic premise on which the use of hormonal therapy for prostatic cancer is based. Androgen suppression can be achieved surgically by bilateral orchidectomy (removal of the testes and hence the major source of testosterone) or by the use of drugs that, in effect, medically 'castrate' the patient, such as gonadorelin analogues (e.g. goserelin, buserelin) and anti-androgen drugs (e.g. flutamide). Gonadorelin analogues can cause an initial increase in cancer progression with the risk of obstructing the ureters, spinal cord compression (see Chs 14, 27, 33 and 34) and bone pain. Where this is thought likely, an anti-androgen drug can be given concurrently, or a bilateral orchidectomy may be performed. A decision to undergo bilateral orchidectomy is not an easy one to make, irrespective of any benefits it may confer. The procedure is irreversible and carries the additional disadvantages of loss of libido and erectile dysfunction. The psychological impact that this procedure may have on the man's body image and perception of self, particularly in the context of coming to terms with a life-threatening condition, can be traumatic. Patients may choose not to undergo this surgical procedure and opt instead for medical therapy. All of these drugs used as hormonal therapy are associated with side-effects (e.g. nausea, hot flushes, gynaecomastia [male breast enlargement], hepatic dysfunction and glucose intolerance) in addition to loss of libido and erectile dysfunction. It is important that patients and their families are given clear, factual information on the risks, benefits, and likely side-effects associated with hormonal therapies, in order that their choices are informed.

Chemotherapy (e.g. fluorouracil)

Chemotherapy may be used if the cancer is hormone-resistant or if hormone therapy has stopped working.

▶ Nursing management: radical prostatectomy

Radical prostatectomy is a planned surgical procedure. Like other situations in which there is the benefit of time to help prepare the patient and family for a potentially life-altering procedure, every effort should be made to ensure that the patient receives information not just about the procedure, but also about the likely aftermath. Again, it is worth bearing in mind that patients and their families may not retain information, and patient knowledge and understanding of this procedure and its potential sequelae should be continuously assessed and amended as appropriate. Moore & Estey's (1999) study found that lack of information about the post-surgical period following radical prostatectomy had a detrimental impact on quality of life perception. Incontinence (albeit usually temporary), erectile dysfunction and bladder spasm (see p. 699) are reported as significant concerns for men in the postoperative period. The occurrence of these and management strategies should be discussed preoperatively, with the patient's ability to manage these postoperatively assessed and supported.

The surgical approach for radical prostatectomy may be either retropubic or perineal. Preoperative preparation should include assessment by the physiotherapist, practice of deep breathing exercises and the use of an incentive spirometer if this is to be used. Patients should also be taught how to perform pelvic floor exercises and encouraged to do these. Anti-embolic prophylaxis with low-molecular-weight heparin is commonly used. Observation of vital signs and overall fluid balance is as for other major surgical procedures. All patients who undergo radical prostatectomy will require intravenous hydration in the early postoperative period.

Following removal of the prostate at operation, the urethra is re-sutured to the bladder around an indwelling urinary catheter. In this instance, the urinary catheter acts not only as a conduit for urine from the bladder, but also as a 'stent' around which healing of the urethra and bladder neck occurs. For the latter reason, it is important that the urinary catheter does not become dislodged postoperatively, and it is therefore usually sutured in place. The urinary catheter is left in place for up to

3 weeks postoperatively. Wound drains are usually removed by the third postoperative day. Early (first day) postoperative ambulation is important and is facilitated by adequate pain control.

Removal of the urinary catheter following radical prostatectomy is usually accompanied by incontinence. In the majority of men, this is temporary and improves over time. However, patients should be prepared to expect this, and encouraged to continue the performance of pelvic floor exercises. The use of incontinence pads should be discussed with patients. Referral to a specialist continence nurse may be required. Erectile dysfunction is also common following radical prostatectomy. Men should be encouraged to discuss the treatment options open to them (e.g. sildenafil may be prescribed, see Ch. 25).

The care of patients who have undergone radical prostatectomy does not end with discharge home. Surgical follow-up is required on an outpatient basis, and surveillance of the efficacy of the surgical procedure is required. PSA levels, in particular, are monitored and these should become non-detectable if all prostate cells have been removed. Elevated PSA levels in the postoperative period indicate disease recurrence and the need for additional therapy (e.g. hormonal therapy).

SUMMARY: MAIN POINTS

- Nursing patients with disorders of the urinary system requires an understanding of the structural and functional characteristics of this system.

- The nursing roles that can be undertaken and developed in this area of practice are diverse and professionally and personally rewarding.

- The requirement for a multidisciplinary approach to care is well defined in this area of practice.

- Nurses can make a significant impact on the quality of a patient's life through education, counselling, support and specialist practitioner roles.

- A number of disorders of the urinary system are persistent and have a profound effect not just on the patient's quality of life (e.g. incontinence, requirement for dialysis, cancer), but also on life expectancy.

- Disorders of urinary system function can be life-threatening, e.g. ARF, and it is important that patients receive prompt and effective treatment.

- Caring for patients with acute dysfunction of the urinary system requires close attention to overall fluid balance, cardiovascular and respiratory function, in addition to supporting any loss of ability to maintain fluid, electrolyte and acid–base balance, with haemodialysis or haemofiltration.

- The treatments associated with disorders of the urinary system can be life-altering and require considerable adaptation and compliance on the part of patients.

- The issue of patient compliance (with dietary restrictions, fluid restrictions and medication) is significant, particularly since non-compliance can have severe adverse consequences.

SELF-TEST: CRITICAL THINKING ACTIVITIES

1 Think of any one observation or test that you perform as part of the patient admission procedure that will give quantitative data about renal function. Are you able to interpret this?

2 You are caring for a 75-year-old gentleman who is awaiting radical cystectomy with urinary diversion. He says that he feels very unsure about having this procedure and thinks that he might be better off without it. He asks for your opinion. What would you say?

3 You are caring for a 55-year-old man who had a cadaveric renal transplant 6 hours previously. He has been passing < 30 mL of urine/hour postoperatively. Intravenous fluids have been administered at a rate of 300 mL/hour for the last 6 hours. You note that the patient's CVP and blood pressure are rising.
— What do you think might be happening?
— What will you do about it?

FURTHER READING

Cattell WR (ed). Infections of the kidney and urinary tract infection. Oxford clinical nephrology series. Oxford: Oxford University Press; 1996.

Dowsett DA. Psychological needs of adult patients following renal transplantation and implications for care. EDTNA-ERCA J 1996; 22(2): 2–7.

Fillingham S, Douglas J (eds). Urological nursing, 2nd edn. London: Baillière Tindall; 1997.

Jakobsson L, Loven L, Hallberg I. Sexual problems in men with prostate cancer in comparison with men with benign prostatic hyperplasia and men from the general population. J Clin Nurs 2000; 10(4): 573–582.

Johnson RJ, Feehally J (eds). Comprehensive clinical nephrology. London: Mosby; 2000.

Nicholson M, Bradley JA. Renal transplantation from living donors. Br Med J 1998; 318(7181): 409–410.

Nicol M, Bavin C, Bedford-Turner S, Cronin P, Rawlings-Anderson K. Essential nursing skills. London: Mosby; 2000.

Patemman B, Johnson M. Men's lived experiences following transurethral prostatectomy for benign prostatic hypertrophy. J Adv Nurs 2000; 31(1): 51–58.

Shaw C, Williams K, Assassa PR, Jackson C. Patient satisfaction with urodynamics: a qualitative study. J Adv Nurs 2000; 32(6): 1356–1363.

Smith T (ed). Renal nursing. London: Baillière Tindall; 1997.

Steggall M. TUR syndrome – a risk after prostatic surgery. Prof Nurse 1999; 4(5): 323–326.

Westwood O (ed). The scientific basis for health care. London: Mosby; 1999.

USEFUL WEBSITES

www.cancerbacup.org.uk – British Association for Cancer United Patients (BACUP)

www.prostate-cancer.org.uk – Prostate Cancer Charity

www.nephronline.co.uk – Renal Education

www.suna.org – Society of Urologic Nurses and Associates – *some excellent information on this site concerning urinary diversion procedures and their care*

www.argonet.co.uk/body/ – The British Organ Donor Society

www.edtna-erca.org – The European Dialysis and Transplant Nurses Association

www.renal.org – The Renal Association

REFERENCES

Cancer Research UK. Specific cancers. Prostate cancer. Online. Available: http://www.cancerresearchuk.org. 2002.

Chandna SM, Schulz J, Lawrence C et al. Is there a rationale for rationing chronic dialysis? A hospital based cohort study of factors affecting survival and morbidity. Br Med J 1999; 318: 217–223.

Cook R. Urinalysis. Nurs Stand 1995; 9(28): 32–37.

Daffern K, Hillman KM, Bauman A, Lum M, Crispin C, Ince L. Fluid balance charts: do they measure up? Br J Nurs 1994; 3(16): 816–820.

EUCLID study group. Randomised placebo-controlled trial of lisinopril in normotensive patients with insulin dependent diabetes and normoalbuminuria or microalbuminuria. Lancet 1997; 349: 1787–1792.

Feehally J, Johnson RJ. Introduction to glomerular disease: pathogenesis and classification In: Johnson RJ, Feehally J, eds. Comprehensive clinical nephrology. London: Mosby; 2000.

Franklin P. Renal transplantation. In: Smith T, ed. Renal nursing. London: Baillière Tindall; 1997.

Frey GM. Stressors in renal transplant recipients at 6 weeks after transplantation. ANNA 1990; 17: 443–446, 450.

Friedman EA. Dialytic therapy for the diabetic ESRD patient; comprehensive care essentials. Semin Dialysis 1997; 10: 193–202.

Hooton T. Urinary tract infections in adults. In: Johnson RJ, Feehally J, eds. Comprehensive clinical nephrology. London: Mosby; 2000.

Human Organ Transplants Act. London: HMSO; 1989.

Human Organ Transplants (Unrelated Persons) Regulations. London: HMSO; 1989.

Human Organ Transplants (Establishment of Relationship) Regulations. London: HMSO; 1998.

Iglesias J, Liebertal W. Clinical evaluation of acute renal failure. In: Johnson RJ, Feehally J, eds. Comprehensive clinical nephrology. London: Mosby; 2000.

Johnson RJ, Feehally J (eds). Comprehensive clinical nephrology. London: Mosby; 2000.

Liano F, Pascual J. Epidemiology of acute renal failure: a prospective multicenter community based study. Kidney Int 1996; 50: 811–818.

Maher D, Chaulet P, Spinaci S, Harries A. Standardised treatment regimens. Treatment of tuberculosis: guidelines for national programmes, 2nd edn. Geneva: WHO; 1997.

Mandel N. Mechanism of stone formation. Semin Nephrol 1996; 16: 364–374.

Mogensen CW. Renal function changes in diabetes. Diabetes 1976; 25: 872–879.

Moore KN, Estey A. The early post-operative concerns of men after radical prostatectomy. J Adv Nurs 1999; 29(5): 1121–1129.

National Institute for Clinical Excellence (NICE) Guidelines. Diabetes (type 2) and renal disease. Online. Available: http://www.nice.org.uk or http://www.nelh.nhs.uk. 2002.

Parsons R. Imaging. In: Johnson RJ, Feehally J, eds. Comprehensive clinical nephrology. London: Mosby; 2000.

Ravine D, Gibson RN, Walker RG. Evaluation of ultrasonographic diagnostic criteria for autosomal dominant polycystic kidney disease 1. Lancet 1994; 343: 824–827.

Rose BD. Clinical physiology of acid–base and electrolyte disorders, 4th edn. New York: McGraw-Hill; 1994.

Rovelli M, Palmeri D, Vossler E, Bartus S, Hull D, Schwiezer R. Non-compliance in renal transplant recipients. Transplant Proc 1989; 21: 833–834.

Stamm WE, Hooton T. Management of urinary tract infection in adults. New Engl J Med 1993; 329: 1328–1334.

Swibold L. Maintenance therapy with bacillus Calmette-Guérin in clients with superficial bladder cancer. Urol Nurs 1999; 19(1): 38–41.

Valtin H, Schaefer J. Renal function, 3rd edn. Boston: Little, Brown; 1995.

Welch G. Assessment of quality of life following renal failure. In: McGee H, Bradley C, eds. Quality of life following renal failure: psychosocial challenges accompanying high technology medicine. Reading: Harwood Academic Publishers; 1994.

Westwood O (ed). The scientific basis for health care. London: Mosby; 1999.

25 Nursing patients with sexual health and reproductive problems

Jacky Cotton, Mark Jones, Martin Steggall

> 'I thought the examination would be awful and so embarrassing. But the nurse was really gentle and explained everything that she was doing. She also made sure that no one would come in during it. I won't be so worried next time.'
>
> *(Patient)*

THIS CHAPTER WILL HELP YOU

- Understand the structure and function of the normal female and male reproductive structures

- Describe the nursing assessment of women and men with disorders of the reproductive structures or sexual health problems

- Describe the variety of gynaecological and male health disorders including sexually transmitted infections – aetiology, pathophysiology, clinical presentation and medical management

- Describe the nursing management for common disorders

- Describe the care required for women undergoing gynaecological surgery

- Describe the care of men undergoing surgery of the reproductive structures

- Demonstrate an insight into the psychological, emotional and social effects of reproductive and sexual health disorders

- Show an appreciation of the legal and moral implications of caring for patients with reproductive and sexual health disorders

- Understand the role of specialist nurses in reproductive system disorders and sexual health problems.

KEYWORDS

Endometriosis	Non-judgemental attitude
Erectile dysfunction	Oophorectomy
Hysterectomy	Penile cancer
Hysteroscopy	Preoperative assessment
Infertility	Rapid/premature ejaculation
Laparoscopy	
Men's health	Salpingectomy
Menorrhagia	Sexual health
Menstrual cycle	Testicular cancer
Menstruation	Women's health

INTRODUCTION

This chapter covers the common sexual and reproductive disorders. The gender-related topics are discussed separately in the two main sections – women's health and men's health. A third section provides an outline of issues such as contraception, infertility (subfertility) and sexually transmitted infections that affect both women and men. An introduction to human immunodeficiency virus (HIV) infection is included here, although its transmission is not exclusively through sexual contact.

Women have particular health needs linked to their complex reproductive system and problems can develop over a wide age range, from puberty to after the menopause. Many of these problems may not be life-threatening but can adversely affect the quality of the woman's life, having physical and psychological effects. When women are referred to a gynaecologist, the consultation may have to be undertaken in a relatively short time and nurses have a vital contribution to make in reassuring the women and reducing embarrassment. With advances in both medical techniques and technology, many treatments previously carried out on an in-patient basis are now undertaken as day cases or even in outpatient departments. Those procedures that do still require in-patient admission are performed with much shorter convalescent periods and women are discharged earlier back to their home and family.

The majority of women requiring hospital treatment are admitted as planned elective admissions. However, there are occasions, particularly with problems associated with early pregnancy, when patients may be admitted as an emergency. In both circumstances, nurses must be able to establish a rapport quickly to provide support in what can often be an embarrassing and distressing situation.

The women's health section aims to provide information about the commonest gynaecological disorders, diagnostic investigations, medical management and the role of the nurse in providing nursing care.

The emphasis on men's health is a relatively recent phenomenon and has changed its focus from treatment to that of prevention, returning the responsibility of health to the individual, with the expectation of empowering men. Several components can be considered to define men's health:

- biological – concerned with diseases that affect men only, e.g. testicular and prostatic (see Ch. 24) cancers
- behaviour – identifying the concept of risk and risk-taking
- social context of sexuality – what it means to be a man.

The above elements impact on men's perception of health and ill health. Despite the promotion of men's health, there remains an anomaly between the perceptions of health/illness between the genders.

Evidence suggests that there are more boys than girls born every year, yet the male life span is shorter. Men visit the doctor less often than women, even though men have a higher rate of admission to hospital; these data indicate that men's health is a serious but overlooked issue, both by the individual and by Government health policy, evidenced by the national breast and cervical screening programme for women, but no national strategy for testicular cancer screening.

WOMEN'S HEALTH

ANATOMY AND PHYSIOLOGY OF THE FEMALE REPRODUCTIVE SYSTEM – AN OVERVIEW

The female reproductive system can be divided into two parts: the internal genitalia (see Fig. 25.1), which comprises the ovaries, uterine (fallopian) tubes, uterus and vagina, and the structures of the external genitalia (pudendum).

The female reproductive system has a complex role:

- producing ova or oocytes (female gametes or germ cells) in a process known as oogenesis
- providing the site for insemination and fertilization by a sperm
- providing an environment suitable for the nurture and development of the fetus.

OVARIES

The female gonads or ovaries produce the cells destined to become ova (more properly called oocytes until penetration by a sperm) and secrete the female sex hormones, oestrogens and progesterone, and small amounts of male androgens. The almond-shaped ovaries lie on the lateral pelvic walls, one on either side of the uterus, to which they are attached by ovarian ligaments. The ovary has a thin covering layer under which is the fibrous tunica albuginea enclosing an outer cortex and the

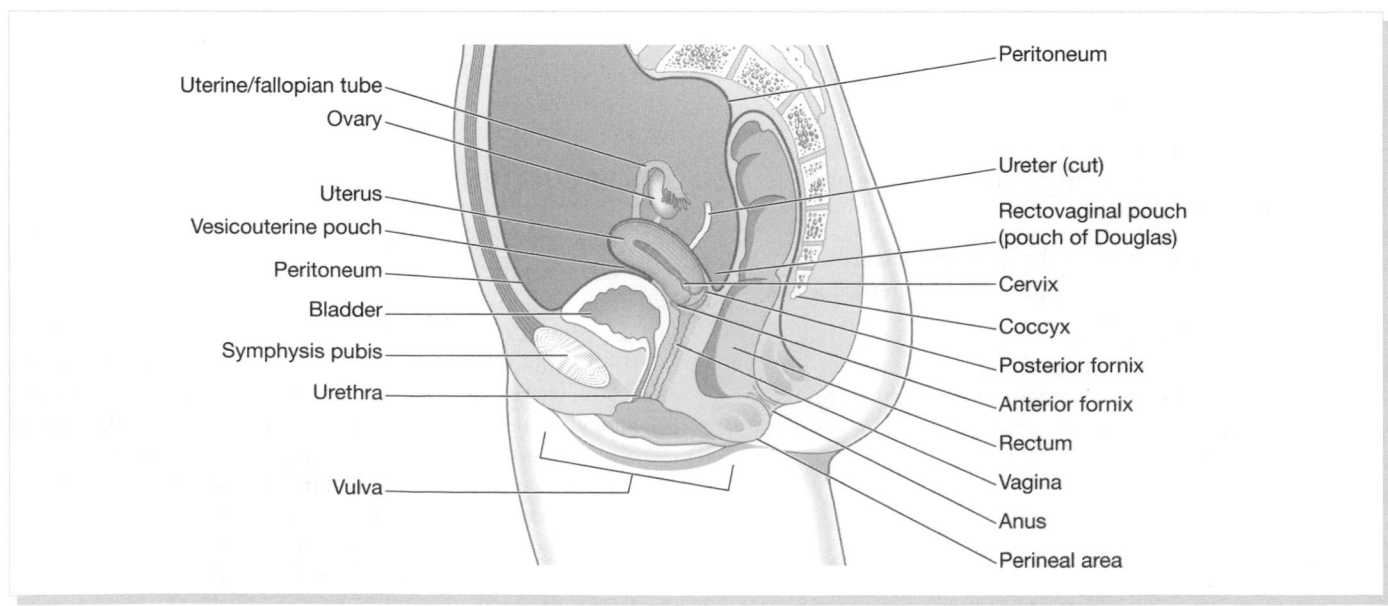

Figure 25.1 *Female reproductive structures (midsagittal section).*

inner medulla. The follicles containing oocytes are in the cortex. The ovary varies in size during the ovarian cycle and contains follicles at different stages of maturation – primary, maturing, mature Graafian follicles and a structure known as the corpus luteum (yellow body) that forms after the ovum is released at ovulation.

Female sex hormones

Oestrogens (oestradiol, oestrone and oestriol)

These are steroid hormones produced from cholesterol. They are secreted by the ovaries, the placenta and, in small amounts, the adrenal glands. Oestrogens control reproductive function – oogenesis and follicle maturation – development of female secondary sexual characteristics and pubertal growth spurt, and growth and maintenance of reproductive organs. Oestrogens also have wider metabolic influences, such as that on blood lipids (see Ch. 19) and calcium homeostasis, demonstrated by the increase in osteoporosis (see Ch. 27) after the menopause.

Progesterone

This is another steroid hormone secreted by the ovary and placenta. It is the 'gestation hormone' that prepares for and maintains pregnancy.

Ovarian cycle and oogenesis

The entire stock of oocytes are present at birth, albeit in an immature state. Oogenesis is a complex process involving mitosis, a first meiotic division that is interrupted by a long resting stage, and a second meiotic division that is only completed if the secondary oocyte is fertilized by a spermatozoon (see Fig. 25.2).

The maturation of oocytes occurs on a cyclical basis, commencing at puberty and continuing until the climacteric. The cycle of events occurring in the ovaries is controlled by two gonadotrophins (hormones influencing the gonads), follicle-stimulating hormone (FSH) and luteinizing hormone (LH), and by other hormones such as inhibin (see Fig. 25.3, p. 708). FSH and LH are released cyclically from the pituitary gland in response to gonadotrophin-releasing hormone (GnRH) from the hypothalamus.

Normally the ovarian cycle lasts for around 28 days but may vary between 21 and 35 days. The changes occurring in the ovary can be divided into two phases: follicular (days 1–14), which includes ovulation, and luteal (days 14–28). Changes in cycle length are reflected in the follicular phase, as the luteal phase remains unchanged.

Follicular phase

Follicle development produces a mature Graafian follicle ready to release a secondary oocyte at ovulation. FSH and LH stimulate initial follicular maturation. At this stage, the follicle produces a small amount of oestrogen that inhibits further secretion of FSH and LH by negative feedback. The hormone inhibin further reduces FSH. Oestrogen, however, increases the local effects of FSH and LH on the follicle where development continues and oestrogen levels rise. As oestrogen plasma levels reach a critical point, they no longer inhibit the hypothalamus/anterior pituitary and now cause the release of more LH and FSH. Around midcycle, there is a sudden surge of LH that causes ovulation and the formation of the corpus luteum. The increase

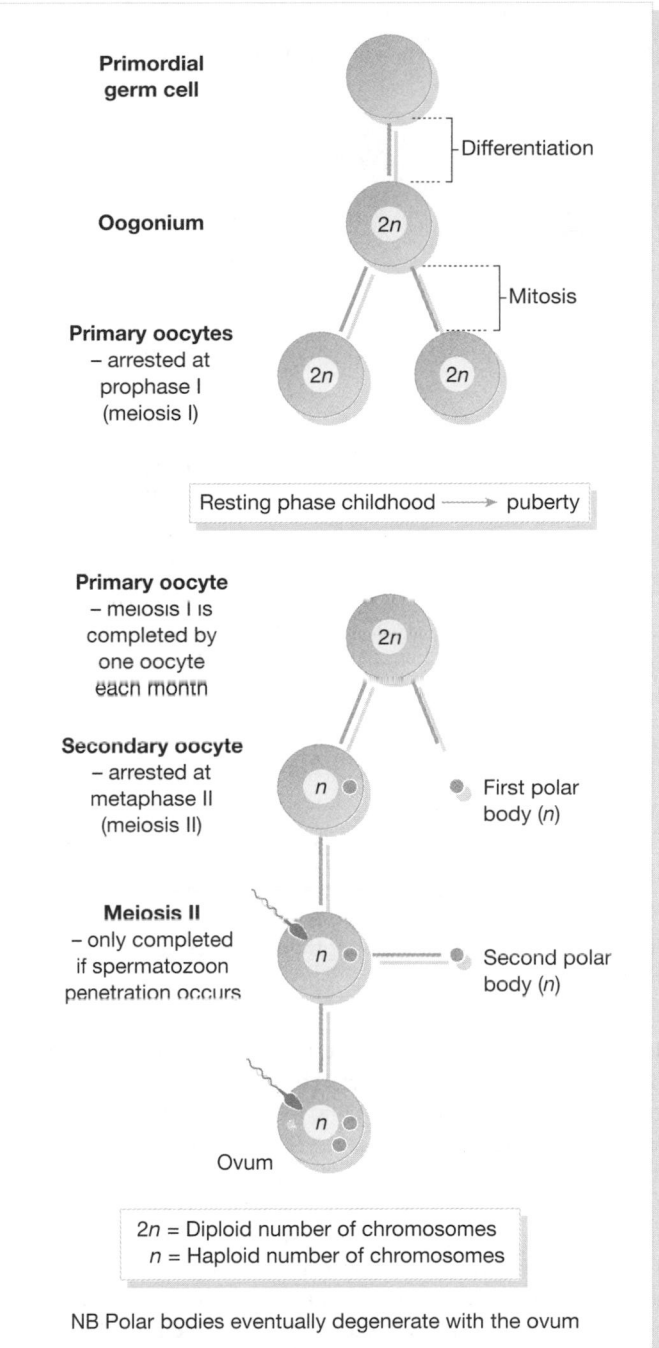

Figure 25.2   Oogenesis.

in LH causes the Graafian follicle to discharge its secondary oocyte into the abdominal cavity from where it enters the fimbriated end of a uterine tube. Ovulation marks the end of the follicular phase.

Luteal phase

The ruptured follicle collapses and fills with blood clot. Various cells form a hormone-secreting structure known as the corpus luteum. The corpus luteum secretes progesterone and oestrogen, which prepare the body for possible pregnancy and prevent the release of further LH and FSH. The life of the corpus luteum

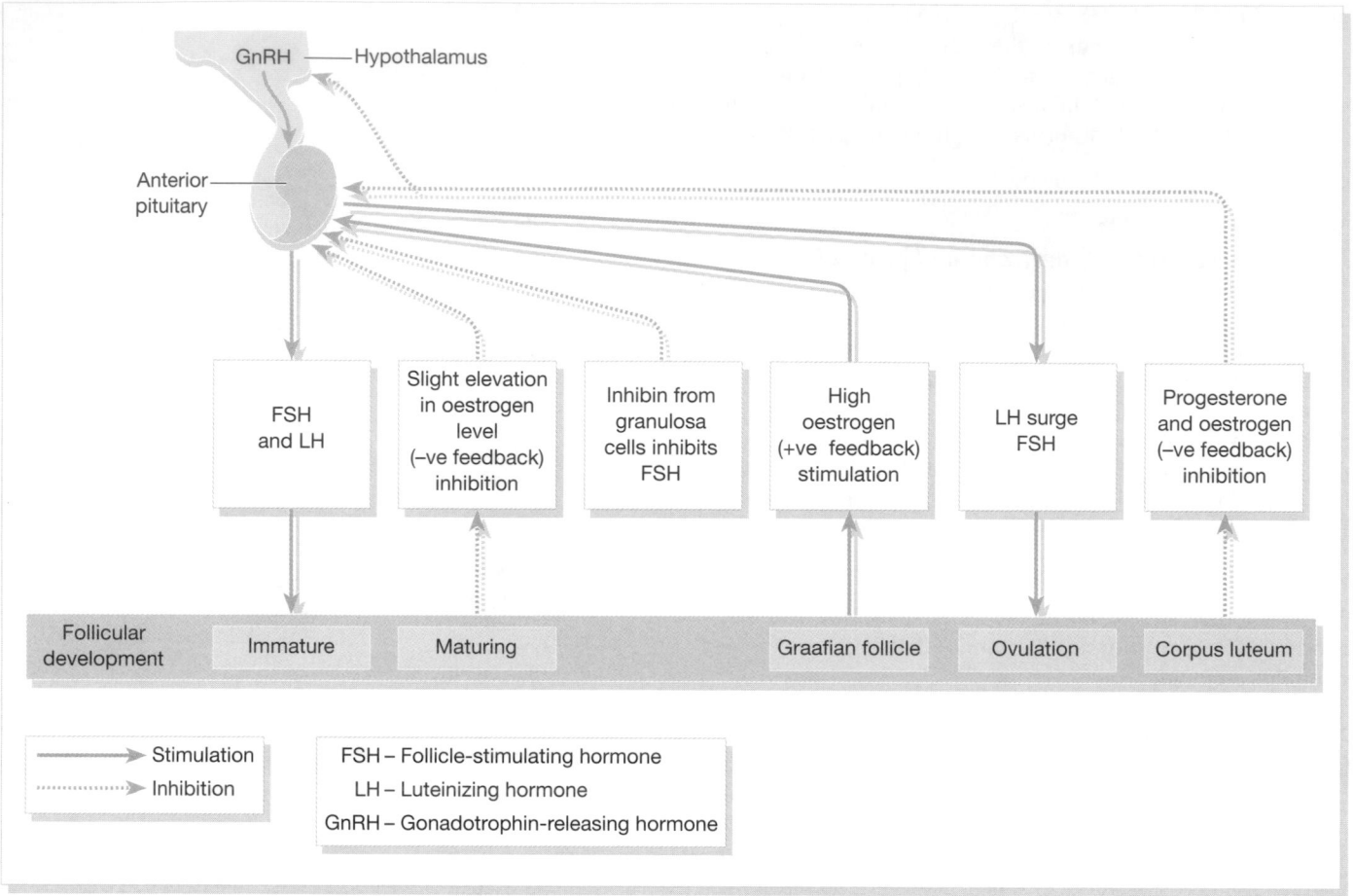

Figure 25.3 Hormonal control of the ovarian cycle.

depends on whether the oocyte released at ovulation is fertilized. Where no fertilization occurs, the corpus luteum only lasts for about 12–14 days due to a fall in LH levels resulting in reduced oestrogen and progesterone production. This means that the ovarian hormone inhibition is removed and the pituitary secretes FSH and LH and a new ovarian cycle commences. The area left is filled with scar tissue and becomes the corpus albicans (white body). However, if the oocyte is fertilized, the corpus luteum functions to maintain the pregnancy until hormones from the placenta and fetus take over.

UTERINE/FALLOPIAN TUBES

The two uterine tubes (fallopian tubes) extend laterally either side of the uterus. They open into the peritoneal cavity, which means infection from other parts of the reproductive tract can spread to the pelvic cavity and cause pelvic inflammatory disease (PID; see p. 732). Each tube has a funnel-like infundibulum ending in the fimbriae (finger-like projections) which help to move the oocyte into the tube, a dilated ampulla where fertilization usually occurs, an isthmus and an interstitial part within the uterine wall which is very narrow (1 mm) (see Fig. 25.4). The uterine tubes have a middle layer of smooth muscle that contracts to help convey the oocyte towards the uterus. The lining is highly specialized with ciliated cells and secreting cells.

The beating cilia move the oocyte towards the uterus and the secretions keep the oocyte and sperm in good condition ready for fertilization. The uterine tubes have an abundant arterial blood supply from the ovarian and uterine arteries. This good blood supply (vascularity) can lead to considerable haemorrhage if an ectopic pregnancy ruptures the tube (see p. 729).

UTERUS

A healthy uterus is pear-shaped and approximately 7.5 cm long, 5 cm wide and 2.5 cm thick, but may be slightly larger following pregnancy. The uterus is a pelvic organ located between the bladder and rectum. Normally it is anteverted (inclined forward) and anteflexed (bent forward) over the bladder (see Fig. 25.1, p. 706). The uterus is maintained in this position by various ligaments (round, cardinal, uterosacral and pubocervical ligaments), the muscles of the pelvic floor (see Ch. 12) and the pelvic peritoneum. The ligaments also support the uterus and cervix, and the bladder and urethra. The supporting structures also maintain continence, assist with micturition and defaecation, and stretch during childbirth.

The thick-walled uterus is a hollow muscular organ which has a fundus (top), corpus (body) and cervix (neck) (see Fig. 25.4). The two uterine tubes insert laterally into the uterus at the cornua below the fundus, and the cervix projects into the vagina.

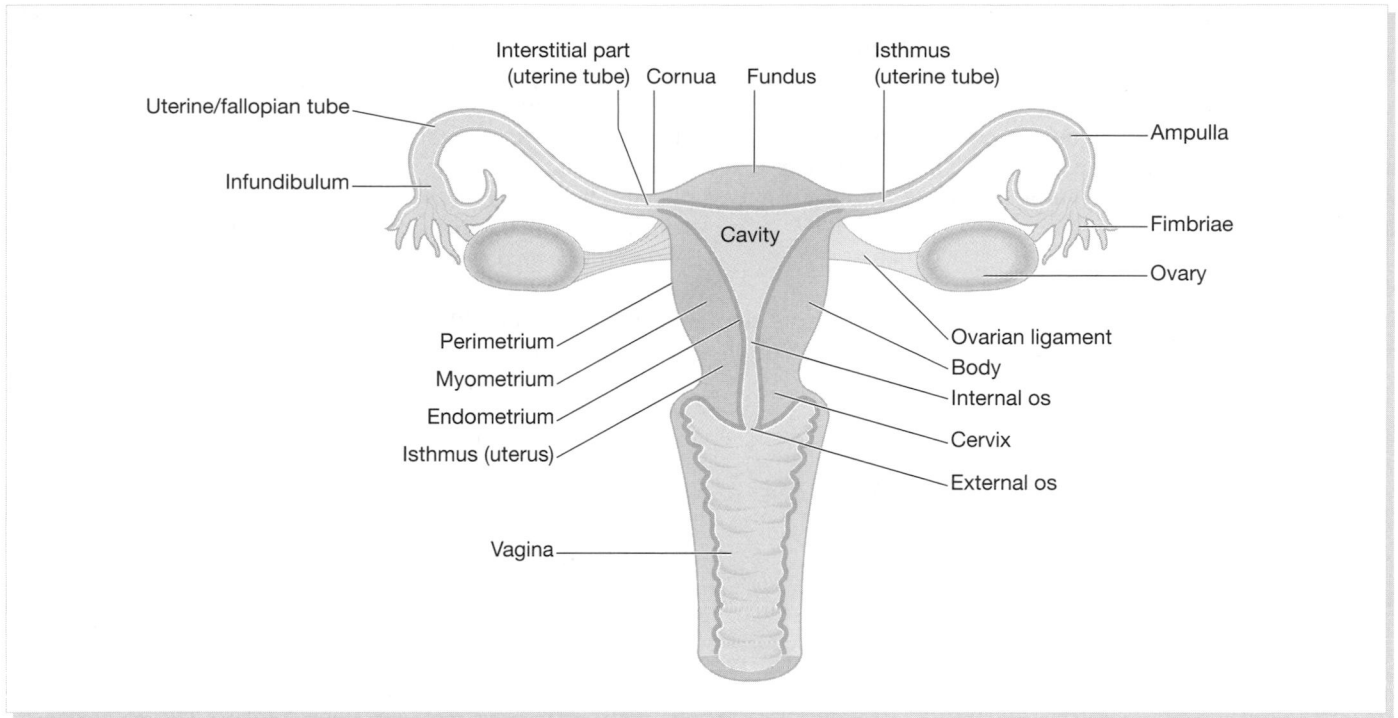

Figure 25.4 Female reproductive structures (anterior view).

The uterus gets an abundant blood supply from two uterine arteries. The branches running up to the fundus are convoluted so as to allow for uterine enlargement during pregnancy.

The uterus has three layers:

■ *perimetrium* (a fold of peritoneum) – drapes the uterus to form an outer covering; this also forms the broad ligament which covers and supports the uterine tubes. The pelvic peritoneum forms the vesicouterine pouch between the uterus and bladder and the rectovaginal pouch (also called the rectouterine pouch or pouch of Douglas) between the vagina/uterus and rectum (see Fig. 25.1, p. 706)
■ *myometrium* – a middle, smooth muscle layer
■ *endometrium* – the mucosal lining of the cavity of the uterus, this has many blood vessels and glands (see Fig. 25.5). During the reproductive years, from the start of menstruation (the menarche) to the end of menstruation (the menopause), the endometrium undergoes cyclical changes in response to ovarian hormones, and if fertilization occurs, the embryo implants into a specially prepared endometrium.

The endometrium has two layers – the stratum basalis, which is fixed, and the stratum functionalis which regrows after being shed every 28 days or so during menstruation (see p. 710).

Arcuate arteries (branches of the uterine arteries) send radial branches to the endometrium. These radial arteries form straight arteries, which supply the stratum basalis, and coiled (spiral) arteries, which supply the stratum functionalis and degenerate with each menstrual flow.

The cervix is mostly fibrous tissue. The lining of the endocervical canal is columnar epithelium but changes to stratified

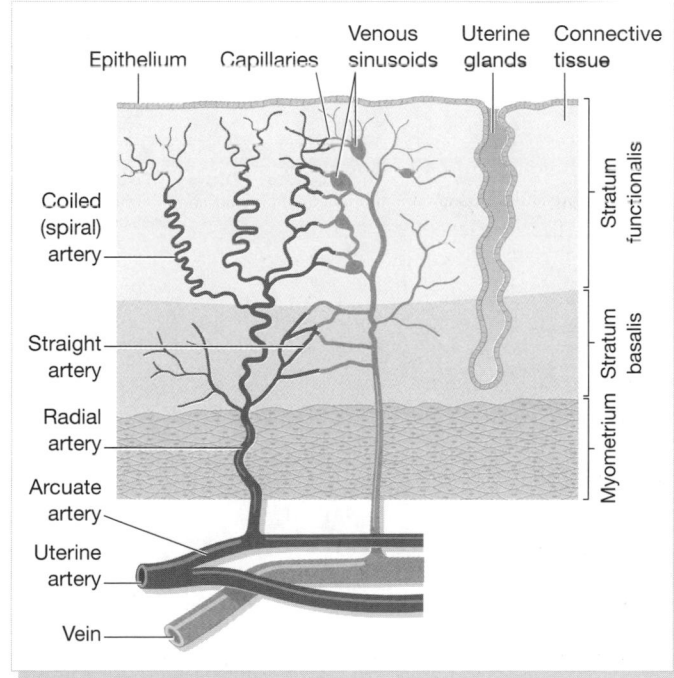

Figure 25.5 Endometrium.

squamous epithelium in the part of the cervix (ectocervix) that protrudes into the vagina, which offers some protection from trauma, e.g. during intercourse. During the reproductive years, oestrogen stimulates basal cell proliferation in the epithelium of the ectocervix. The change from one type of epithelium to another occurs in an area known as the squamocolumnar junction (SCJ). The cervix has two openings: the internal os into the uterine cavity, and an external os which opens into the vagina (see Fig. 25.4, p. 709).

The type and quantity of mucus produced by the cervical glands change during the menstrual cycle. Examination of this mucus forms the basis of a 'natural' method of family planning (see p. 757).

Menstrual (uterine) cycle

The menstrual cycle describes the events occurring as the endometrium responds to ovarian hormones (see Fig. 25.6). It

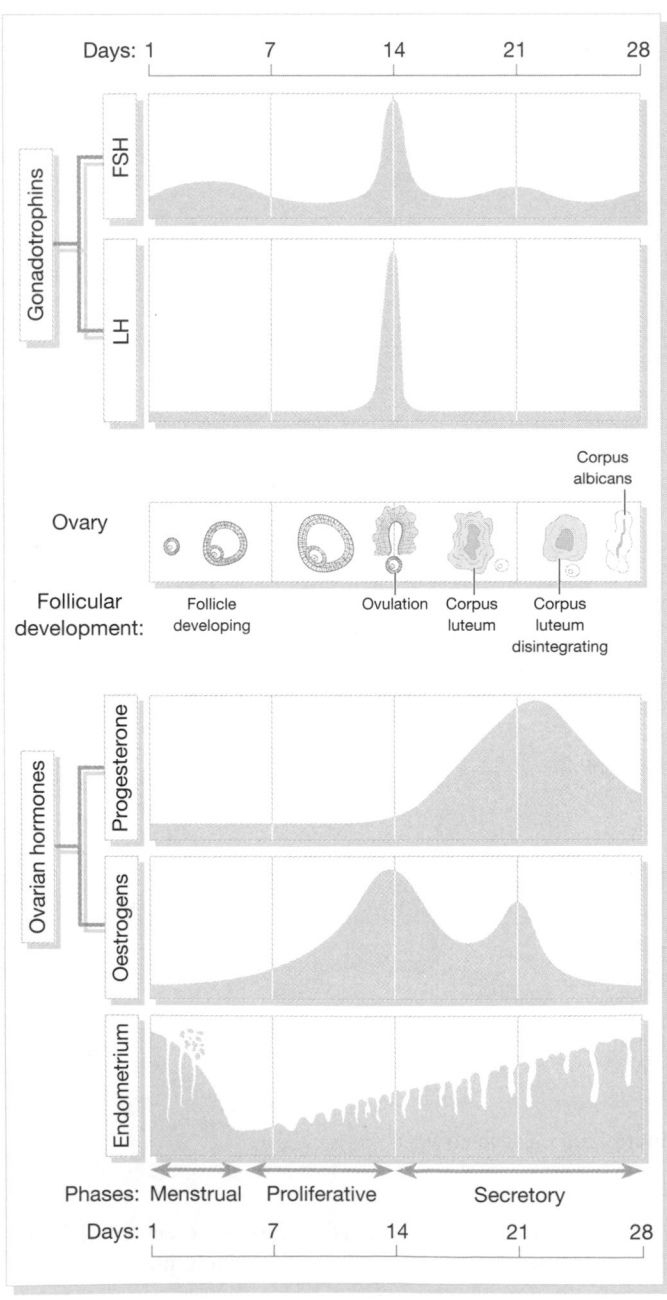

Figure 25.6 Menstrual/uterine cycle (with hormonal and ovarian events).

corresponds to the ovarian cycle (see p. 707) and is normally repeated every 28 days (range 21–35 days) or so during the reproductive years (except during pregnancy). The menstrual cycle is all about preparing the endometrium in case an oocyte is fertilized. The menstrual cycle is usually described in three distinct phases: proliferative, secretory and menstrual. By convention the first day of menstrual bleeding is counted as day 1 of the cycle, although the menstrual phase is at the end of the cycle, so as to provide an obvious landmark.

Proliferative phase

This corresponds to the follicular phase of the ovarian cycle and commences when menstrual bleeding has stopped. Only the endometrial stratum basalis remains after menstruation. Oestrogen causes the regeneration of the stratum functionalis. This phase ends with the maturation of a Graafian follicle and ovulation around day 14. By now the endometrium is approximately 2 mm thick. Cervical mucus changes from a thick plug blocking the cervix to copious amounts of thin slippery mucus through which the sperm can move more easily.

Secretory phase

This phase starts after ovulation, corresponds to the luteal phase of the ovarian cycle and lasts about 14 days. The endometrium is now influenced by progesterone. The glands enlarge and secrete glycogen, which is intended to sustain an embryo during implantation. The endometrium is now 5 mm thick. The spiral arteries grow larger and become more coiled. Cervical mucus gets thicker and blocks off the cervical canal in order to protect an embryo if implantation occurs.

Without fertilization, the reduction in hormones from the corpus luteum leads to spasm in the spiral arteries, caused by prostaglandins that are normally inhibited by progesterone and oestrogen. Arterial spasm causes the endometrium to degenerate as it is deprived of nutrients and, later, autodigestion by enzymes. This leads (about 24 hours later) to menstrual bleeding. The spiral arteries dilate and bleed into the necrotic stratum functionalis, which breaks away.

Menstrual phase

This is the last phase of the cycle (but remember it is taken as day 1 of the cycle). Menstrual flow contains blood, other fluids and endometrial debris, and usually lasts for 3–6 days. Vaginal loss during menstruation, which is usually around 75 mL (only half is blood), varies considerably and is extremely difficult to assess objectively. In order to replace this blood loss, women need more dietary iron than men during the reproductive years (see Ch. 11). Excessive menstrual loss (menorrhagia) is a common cause of iron deficiency anaemia (see Ch. 18). Fibrinolysins stop menstrual blood clotting within the uterus, which ensures that the redundant stratum functionalis is completely discharged through the cervix. As menstruation starts, prostaglandins cause the uterus to contract and expel the blood. These contractions result in the discomfort/pain (dysmenorrhoea) experienced by some women.

Body temperature

Body temperature may vary during the menstrual cycle, with a small fall coinciding with the LH surge occurring just before ovulation. Progesterone from the corpus luteum then increases the metabolic rate and body temperature rises about 0.5°C. This lasts until menstruation. Temperature changes are a rough guide to the timing of ovulation in some women.

VAGINA

The vagina is the passage extending from the cervix to the vulva (see Fig. 25.1, p. 706). The front wall is about 7.5 cm long and is close to the urethra and bladder, and the posterior wall, which is longer at 9 cm, has contact with the rectum and the rectovaginal pouch. The vaginal wall is arranged in folds (rugae) which allows for considerable stretching during intercourse and childbirth. The protrusion of the cervix into the vagina forms four fornices (deep gutters); the deep posterior fornix receives the semen during coitus. The vagina runs up and backwards at an angle of 45°, a point to remember when inserting instruments or teaching patients about vaginal medication or contraceptive diaphragms. The hymen (perforated membrane) partially covers the distal vaginal orifice; the hymen is usually ruptured during the first intercourse, or by tampon use.

The vagina has an outer layer of fibrous tissue, a layer of involuntary muscle, a loose areolar layer and a tough stratified squamous epithelial lining. The vaginal mucosa has no secretory glands; some fluid may leak through the walls, but most vaginal moisture is provided by cervical mucus and that produced during sexual arousal.

The lower part of the vagina is sensitive and is supplied by the voluntary pudendal nerve, and the upper part is supplied by autonomic sympathetic fibres.

During the reproductive years, the vagina is acidic (pH 4–4.5) due to lactic acid produced by bacteria (*Lactobacillus* species) of the normal body flora. The lactic acid helps to protect the vagina from many pathogenic microorganisms.

VULVA

The vulva comprises the structures of the external genitalia (or pudendum) (see Fig. 25.7). There is a fatty pad, the mons pubis, over the symphysis pubis. This is covered with terminal pubic hair from puberty. The vulva is bounded by two fatty outer folds, the labia majora, which merge posteriorly with the perineal skin. These are skin-covered and have many sebaceous glands (see Ch. 28); pubic hair grows on the outer part, but not on the inner surface. Within the protective outer labia are two smaller folds called the labia minora. They are formed from smooth skin and enclose the vestibule. Anteriorly the labia minora fuse to form the prepuce which covers the clitoris, and posteriorly they form the fourchette. The clitoris contains erectile tissue and has an abundant nerve supply. It is extremely sensitive and is involved in the female sexual response.

The vestibule contains the openings of the urethra and vagina and the vestibular glands; two tiny Skene's glands (lesser vestibular glands) open into the urethral meatus and two larger Bartholin's glands (greater vestibular glands) open into the vaginal orifice. Bartholin's glands produce mucus, secretion of which increases during sexual stimulation to facilitate coitus.

The area extending from the fourchette to the anal canal is called the perineum. It consists of muscle, fat and connective tissue and is important in providing attachment to the muscles of the pelvic floor (see Ch. 12).

NURSING ASSESSMENT

Most women present with benign gynaecological disorders. Many women may be anxious that they have cancer or are infertile and need compassion and understanding at all stages of diagnosis and treatment. Most women have consulted their

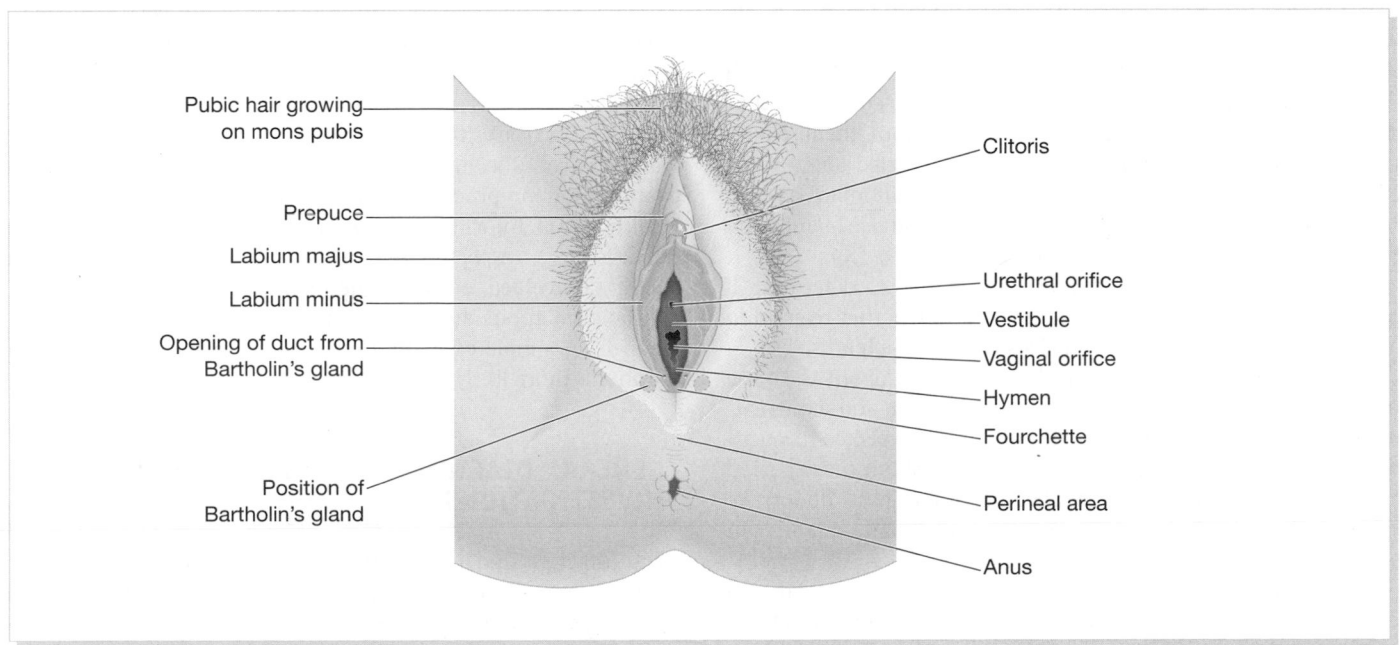

Figure 25.7 External genitalia (female).

GP on at least two occasions prior to being seen by a gynaecologist or specialist gynaecology nurse. A nurse must take an accurate nursing history and assessment, using the opportunity to build a rapport with the woman and understand her personal, social and cultural circumstances. These can all have a bearing on the woman's current and future sexual and gynaecological health.

PHYSICAL ASSESSMENT

Many who attend a gynaecology unit will be relatively healthy women with busy lives. An assessment of menstrual cycle must be carried out and the start and possible end of menstruation ascertained in order to build a full picture of each woman's problem and to assess nursing needs. The obstetric history and history of any relevant surgery will help in assessing any current problems. Many patients with infections will have a high temperature and feel tired. Patients with malignant tumours often complain of tiredness and lethargy, as do women with anaemia due to abnormal bleeding linked to their periods. Women with postmenopausal symptoms will complain of hot flushes, irritability, night sweats and loss of libido. Concurrent conditions can play an important part in gynaecological disease and should be recorded along with any medications used by women. Physical examination will be undertaken by either the medical staff or a specialist gynaecology nurse (see p. 713). Other tests ordered by the health professional may include ultrasound scanning and blood tests (see pp. 713 and 715).

SOCIAL ASSESSMENT

It is always important for nurses to ask patients about their social circumstances. The rapport built at this time enables nurses to discover any factors in a woman's family, friends and work background that may affect her condition. Patients also have the opportunity to discuss any fears about how their family will function if they require hospital treatment. Often, it is the women in the family who organize other members and ensure their lives operate smoothly. They may have performed all the household duties for many years and may be concerned that the family will not be able to function without them. Many women will also be mothers and may be worried about child care and the mutual separation. This can be a major factor when considering treatment options, and practical advice about such treatment options may help to allay some of these fears.

By careful questioning, nurses will be able to determine if patients require any additional support and whether referral to other agencies such as social services would be helpful.

Women in employment may be concerned about the time needed away from work caused by the disorder and any treatment. If surgery is required, advice about the expected recovery period will enable them to inform employers about the expected length of absence. However, in all cases, nurses must undertake this questioning in a sensitive and non-judgemental manner in order to put patients at their ease.

Treatment choices may depend on a woman's social and financial circumstances, particularly in the case of subfertility, where certain treatments in the UK are largely only available in the private sector.

It is often necessary to take a sexual history and to ascertain partnerships for support reasons or, in the case of some infections, for contact tracing (see 'Sexually transmitted infections', p. 760). This should be done with great sensitivity and nurses must be aware of the potential emotional consequences for the people concerned.

PSYCHOLOGICAL ASSESSMENT

Until a firm diagnosis is established, a woman may fear she has cancer. Cancer is a very common disease and many people will have some experience of it, either directly or indirectly (see Ch. 33). Gynaecological cancers are uncommon but this will not stop women being concerned that they may have a malignant disease. The role of the nurse is to ensure that patients are fully informed of the plans for investigations and treatment, explaining the rationale behind them. Talking with the patient and her family and friends can help nurses to build a picture of the woman and how she has coped with health problems in the past. Knowledge of any experiences she has had, perhaps of the illness or death of someone close to her with a related problem, can help in developing a plan to get her through this experience.

Listening and communication skills are extremely important in combating nervousness and helping patients to deal with alterations in body image and fears they may have about treatment. Open questions provide an opportunity for them to express fears and talk about experiences that cause anxiety. Embarrassment and severe stress at being examined may have deep-seated roots, which patients may or may not disclose. Patience and understanding are of far more importance in retaining a sense of worth and value than simply telling patients to relax. Such phrases should be avoided, as it is a reflex to tense muscles when afraid or anxious. Explanation of the value of an examination in finding the cause of the problem, keeping patients informed at all stages of the procedure and reassurance will help them through intrusive tests.

The giving and receiving of information are personal needs, which should be respected by nurses. Not all patients wish to know the details of treatment or its consequences. Although this is not ideal, it is the way in which these people wish to cope with their current situation. However, it is important that these women have sufficient information in order to give consent to an examination or procedure being carried out (Department of Health 2001). Information should be given to and received from patients in a respectful way that is understandable. Jargon should be avoided, even if patients are health care workers. It can be ambiguous and a nervous person is unlikely to understand it. A simple explanation delivered in a non-patronising manner is more likely to be understood.

GENERAL DIAGNOSTIC TESTS AND MEDICAL INVESTIGATIONS

Diagnostic tests and medical investigations are used together with a complete medical history and general examination in order to make a diagnosis and to monitor diseases and the efficacy of treatment. Nurses need to have a basic knowledge of common investigations and any special preparation. This is important as it allows them to provide explanation and support for patients and families and to ensure that patients are adequately prepared, and that the investigation is safe and successful.

GYNAECOLOGICAL EXAMINATION

Gynaecological examination is a fundamental investigation in determining causes for gynaecological disorders. It is one of the most intimate and potentially embarrassing investigations a woman will ever undergo (see Guidelines for Care Priorities box 25.1). There are two types of examination that can be undertaken: bimanual vaginal examination and speculum examination.

Bimanual vaginal examination

This examination is used to ascertain the origins and degree of pelvic pathology and pain. Two forefingers are gently placed in the woman's vagina while she is in a prone position, and the examiner's other hand is placed on the abdomen. Both hands are then used together to feel for abnormalities of the internal genitalia, such as ovarian cysts or fibroids.

An assessment of the cervix and all four 'corners' (fornices) of the vagina is made. The uterus is palpated for size, position, shape and any pain. The ovaries are palpated gently for their position, size and associated pain (see Fig. 25.1, p. 706). The presence of pelvic masses can also be determined from this examination.

Speculum examination of the vagina and cervix

The woman is placed flat on her back with her knees bent and ankles together. Then she is asked to separate her knees so that a Cuscoe (bivalve) speculum can be gently inserted into the vagina (see Fig. 25.8A, p. 714). The blades of the speculum are separated to stretch the vaginal walls and visualize the cervix. The examination is used to assess the cervix for disease or bleeding and for obtaining a cervical smear. Various examinations can be undertaken by the insertion of a speculum and visualization of the cervix (e.g. in sexually transmitted diseases, cases of infertility and assessing for contraception). A Sims' speculum (see Fig. 25.8B, p. 714) is used for assessment of vaginal or uterine displacements and for removal of foreign objects from the vagina and is inserted into the vagina with the woman lying on her left side. All investigations of the vagina and cervix will involve the use of a speculum.

IMAGING TECHNIQUES

Ultrasonography

An ultrasound scan (USS), which uses sound waves, can be helpful in identifying abnormalities of the internal genital tract. It can be performed by a radiographer, doctor or nurse who has undergone appropriate training in order to interpret the findings. The investigation can be done using a probe either on the woman's abdomen or placed vaginally. For transabdominal scanning, the woman must have a full bladder and this can

GUIDELINES FOR CARE PRIORITIES

25.1 Gynaecological examination

Good practice has been based in the past on common sense and courtesy. This involved explaining to the woman why a vaginal examination was necessary, undertaking the examination in a private room in a professional and gentle manner. However, the Royal College of Obstetricians and Gynaecologists (2002) have developed guidelines to ensure that medical staff provide a service that offers respect and dignity to the woman. These guidelines should also apply to nurses and midwives who have been trained to undertake this procedure to ensure the woman is given the best possible care. Recommendations include:

- Full explanation of the reason the clinician considers vaginal examination is necessary.
- Verbal consent gained from the woman prior to the examination. If this is not done, the examination could constitute an assault.
- Women should be offered warm and private changing facilities to undress.
- There should not be an undue delay between undressing and the examination.
- A chaperone should be present for all pelvic examinations irrespective of the gender of the clinician. Traditionally chaperones have been present with male clinicians, but now should be present at all examinations. This provides the woman with additional support during this

embarrassing procedure and a witness for the clinician. Increasingly, allegations have been made against clinicians and their conduct during intimate examinations and the presence of a chaperone will prevent this occurring. This poses a challenge for practice where practice nurses or midwives have traditionally undertaken such an examination on their own.

- Interruptions should not be allowed during the examination. Other staff should not be able to enter the room and bleeps, phone calls or messages should be discouraged during this time.

It is important to remember that the woman must be treated with the same dignity and respect if she is under anaesthetic as she would if she were awake. Vaginal examination at this time, particularly by nursing or medical students, must be discussed with the woman before surgery and her permission sought. This should be recorded in the notes.

Gynaecological examinations are uncomfortable and embarrassing but often necessary, so the woman must be treated with dignity, respect and privacy during such a procedure.

Reference
Royal College of Obstetricians and Gynaecologists. Gynaecological examinations: guidelines for specialist practice. London: RCOG Press; 2002.

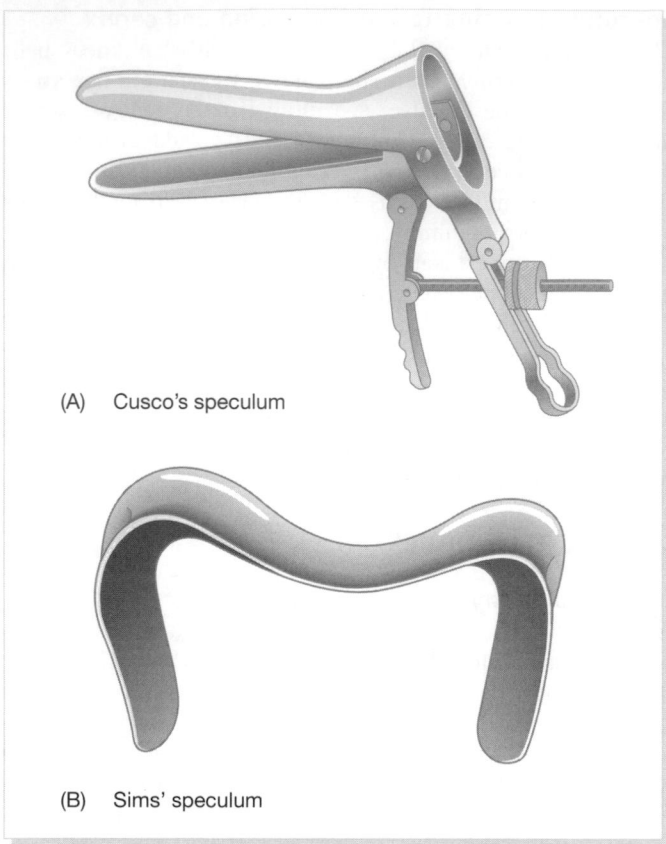

(A) Cusco's speculum

(B) Sims' speculum

Figure 25.8 Vaginal specula. (A) Cuscoe's speculum; (B) Sims' speculum.

cause discomfort. Ultrasound scanning is particularly useful in diagnosing problems in early pregnancy, disorders of the uterus including the endometrium and myometrium, and disorders of the ovary such as cysts or other masses.

X-rays

An X-ray, such as hysterosalpingography (uterosalpingography), is a radiological examination of the uterus and uterine tubes and, as such, is undertaken in the X-ray department. Contrast medium is introduced through the cervix and a series of X-rays are taken to follow the passage of the medium through the tubes. This is used to check the patency of the uterine tubes as part of fuller investigations for infertile couples (see p. 758). A hysterosalpingogram will only show the presence of any blockage in the tube and not any pelvic pathology.

CT/MRI

Computed tomography (CT) and magnetic resonance imaging (MRI) are both used in the investigation of gynaecological diseases.

MICROBIOLOGY

High vaginal swabs

High vaginal swabs (HVS) are taken to investigate the presence of any pathogenic bacteria that may affect the woman's health.

For most bacteria, a dry cotton bud is inserted high into the vagina, using a speculum, and a gentle sweep of the tissues is made. The swab is then removed and placed in transport medium and sent for microbiological examination. For investigation of *Chlamydia*, another swab is inserted into the cervical os and gently turned to capture some endocervical cells. This swab must be placed in special solution before sending it to the microbiology laboratory. These cells are then investigated for the presence of the *Chlamydia* organism, which lives within cells.

CYTOLOGY – CERVICAL SMEAR

This is also known as the Pap smear. It involves removing a sample of cells from the cervix and fixing them on a glass slide that can then be examined in the laboratory for abnormalities. This procedure is often carried out by nurses, both in hospitals and in general practice, who have been trained and are competent to do so. The smear is obtained by using a Cuscoe speculum to visualize the cervix, and then rotating a spatula (usually wooden) against the cervix to scrape off a thin layer of cells. These cells are smeared onto a glass slide and alcohol fixative added to prevent them from drying. The labelled slide and specimen request form with all the patient's details completed are then sent to a cytology laboratory. This procedure can be uncomfortable and embarrassing, so nurses must explain thoroughly what is involved and try to put patients at ease. At the end of the procedure, patients must be informed when the results are expected to be available, in order to minimize the anxiety experienced whilst waiting.

A national cervical screening programme has been developed in order to reduce the incidence and effects of cervical cancer. Premalignant disease of the cervix can be treated relatively easily and effectively if detected before it develops into an invasive malignancy. It is important that women comply with this and so it is the responsibility of the nurse involved with taking the smear to make the experience as comfortable and reassuring as possible. If women are subjected to an unpleasant experience, they will be less likely to participate in the programme and return for further smears when required.

COLPOSCOPY

An abnormal cervical smear result may require patients to be referred for a colposcopic examination, depending on the grade of the abnormality. Patients are referred to a specialist colposcopy clinic where their cervix can be examined closely using a low-powered microscope known as a colposcope which magnifies the cells of the cervix. This is a particularly worrying time for them, as often they will associate having an abnormal smear with having cancer and so nurses must be empathetic. A national programme has been developed to train nurses as colposcopists and the number of accredited nurse colposcopists is now greatly increasing.

During the consultation a specially coated metal speculum is used which is compatible with electrical diathermy treatment if required. The cervix is then viewed through the colposcope for abnormalities. Cervical mucus is removed using a cotton wool ball soaked in saline attached to sponge-holding forceps, exposing the cervical epithelium. Acetic acid is applied and the cervix is then observed for any colour change. Normal epithelial cells remain pink due to their structure, which contains very little protein within the small, central nucleus. Changes in the cells of an abnormal smear are known as dyskaryosis. This is a condition in which the cell structure becomes altered with an enlarged nucleus which stains very dark with cytological and histological stains. It is also known as cervical intraepithelial neoplasia (CIN). Dyskaryotic cells have much larger, protein-based nuclei which change to white under the influence of mild acids (like putting dilute vinegar onto egg white). The density of the aceto-white corresponds to the level of epithelium affected and the relative size of the nuclei. The grade of abnormality found determines what further treatment, if any, is required.

Iodine is also applied to assess the amount of cytoplasm within the cells. Normally, the colour change is a dark even brown due to the presence of starch in the cell cytoplasm. However, if the cells are dyskaryotic, because the enlarged nuclei contains increased amounts of protein, there is little cytoplasm in the cell. The resulting colour change is a much lighter beige colour. This confirms the presence of dyskaryosis in the cells.

LAPAROSCOPY

Laparoscopy involves inserting a laparoscope via the umbilicus into the pelvis (see Fig. 25.9). A laparoscope is an instrument that allows the operator to visualize the pelvis and internal female reproductive system either by direct vision or, more commonly, via a television screen as a camera is attached to the eyepiece of the laparoscope. The abdominal wall is inflated by introducing carbon dioxide into the pelvic cavity to enhance the view of the pelvis. Further incisions will be made in the lower quadrants close to the pubic hair line to enable other instruments to be inserted to grasp or move pelvic organs to enable a close examination of all areas of the pelvis.

If the laparoscopy is part of investigations for infertility, the patency of the uterine tubes can be assessed by injecting methylene blue dye through the cervix; the operator notes how quickly the tubes fill with the dye and whether the dye comes out of the end of the tubes, indicating they are patent.

BLOOD TESTS

Full blood count

A full blood count is commonly undertaken, particularly for women suffering with excessive menstrual bleeding in order to exclude anaemia. The test will identify haemoglobin level, white cell and platelet counts. If a woman is anaemic, iron therapy is usually advised, although not all women can tolerate this. It should be noted, however, that unless the cause of the anaemia, such as heavy periods, is also treated, the condition could become chronic (see Ch. 18).

Hormone levels

Various hormones can be measured through blood tests. A clotted venous blood sample can be used to determine levels of hormones such as progesterone and oestrogen in confirming a diagnosis. For example, oestrogen levels in the form of oestradiol can give an indication of ovarian function and whether a woman is menopausal. Thyroid function tests may also be undertaken, as abnormalities in thyroid hormone levels can affect other hormone levels within the negative feedback mechanisms controlled by the pituitary gland (see Ch. 17).

Tumour markers

Blood samples can be tested for the presence/level of various tumour marker substances, including CA-125 for ovarian cancer and β-hCG (human chorionic gonadotrophin) for choriocarcinoma. (Please note that β-hCG is also a tumour marker for some types of testicular cancer – see p. 745.)

GENERAL DISEASE PREVENTION AND HEALTH EDUCATION

Although many gynaecological disorders are not directly preventable, a healthy lifestyle can influence and improve many of the symptoms. Nurses should take any opportunity to explain the benefits of following a healthy lifestyle in order to take some responsibility for health.

Obesity is becoming an increasing problem in the UK and other developed countries and advice about an appropriate diet and increase in exercise should be given if the woman is overweight. This is particularly important if the woman requires surgery and a general anaesthetic as there is an increase in surgical morbidity in obese patients. Often surgery is more difficult due to the additional layers of subcutaneous fat and the woman may be anaesthetized for longer with the associated risks of chest infection. Fat has a reduced blood supply and so there may be delayed postoperative healing with an increased risk of abdominal wound infections developing, particularly if the wound is sited under a large skin fold. Adipose tissue is also known to secrete oestrogen and so additional fat layers can cause an increase in oestrogen secretion. A slow and sustained weight loss with an appropriate exercise programme should be

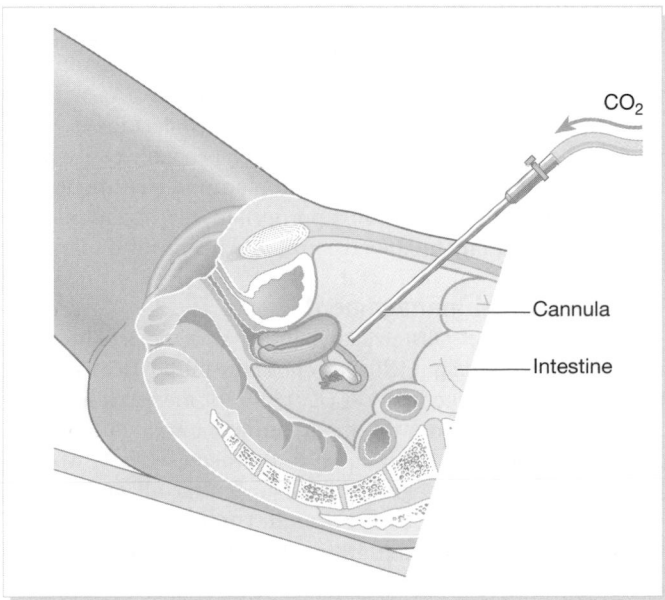

CO_2

Cannula

Intestine

Figure 25.9 Laparoscopy.

recommended and will have additional benefits for the woman's general health.

Whilst advising about exercise regimens, special attention should be given to explaining the need and technique of pelvic floor exercises. This is particularly important after childbirth, but with a new baby to look after, a new mother may not see it as such. Lax pelvic floor muscles result in lack of support to other pelvic structures, particularly later in life, and can cause continence problems (see p. 724 and Ch. 12).

Smoking is known to have several adverse effects on a woman's health. It has been associated with changes in cell structure, resulting in abnormal cervical smears, and is a risk factor for women who require a general anaesthetic for any gynaecological surgery. Women should be encouraged and supported in smoking cessation and advised about diet, as they are often concerned that if they give up smoking, they will put on weight.

Unprotected sex, particularly with several different partners, can cause gynaecological problems. In addition to an unwanted pregnancy, there is an increased incidence of abnormal cervical cytological changes and women are at risk of contracting a sexually transmitted disease. This can cause pelvic inflammatory disease, which may be associated with pelvic pain and vaginal discharge or may be a silent infection such as *Chlamydia* with few symptoms but resulting in internal tubal damage. The incidence of HIV and AIDS continues to increase and HIV can be contracted during heterosexual sex. Women, particularly young women, should be advised to consider only having intercourse in stable relationships or, if having casual sex, always to use a barrier method such as condoms to reduce the risk of infections.

As mentioned previously, there are several aspects of lifestyle that can affect the cytology of the cervix. For this reason, it is important that women participate in the national screening programmes, so that any changes can be detected and treated early in the disease progression. Nurses should explain fully the reasons for, and benefits to, women participating in this programme, as usually they will not experience any symptoms and so may not see the need for it.

COMMON DISEASES/DISORDERS AFFECTING THE FEMALE REPRODUCTIVE SYSTEM

MENSTRUAL DISORDERS

Following the onset of menstruation at puberty (the menarche), until cessation of periods at the menopause, most women will experience some dysfunction of their normal menstrual cycle. These disorders are usually caused by hormonal imbalances that affect the normal feedback mechanisms. The commonest disorders are outlined in Table 25.1.

Aetiology, pathophysiology and clinical presentation

Disorders of menstruation which result in no, or infrequent, periods are usually investigated and treated as part of other endocrine disorders or for infertility. However, it is the disorders that cause excessive bleeding (menorrhagia) that are more common and can seriously affect quality of life. One in 20 women

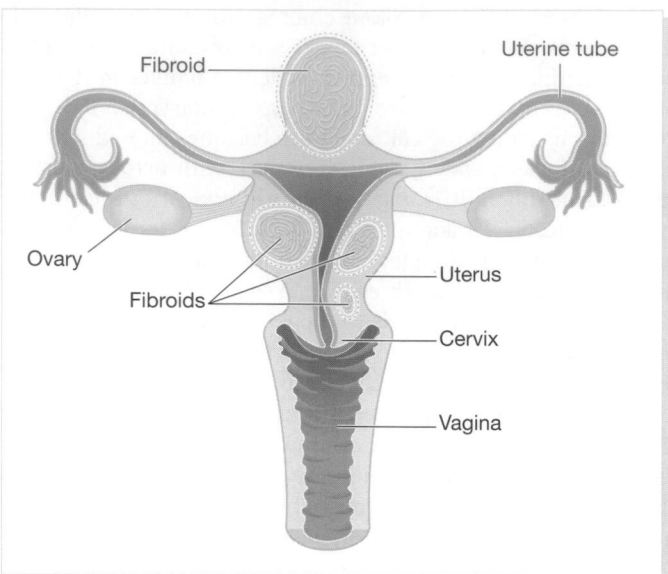

Figure 25.10 Common position of fibroids.

aged 30–49 years will consult her GP with menorrhagia (RCOG 1999). Organic causes include endometrial polyps which can develop in the lining of the uterus, or leiomyomata, also known as fibroids, which are benign oestrogen-dependent tumours that develop in the myometrium (uterine muscle layer) (see Fig. 25.10). Fibroids can cause menorrhagia, due to the increase in surface area of the endometrial cavity, and increased period pain due to uterine contractions squeezing against them. Fibroids are thought to occur in up to 20% of women aged over 35 and, because they are oestrogen-dependent, will decrease in size after the menopause. Fibroids may be asymptomatic and women unaware of having them. However, they can be detected on ultrasound scan and on examination – the uterus may feel enlarged. They are more common in African Caribbean women.

Specific investigations (see Table 25.1)

When a woman is referred to a gynaecologist, a full history will be taken that enables her to articulate the symptoms that are actually causing her the most problems. As with all gynaecological disorders, it is important to undertake a pelvic and abdominal examination to ascertain a probable cause prior to ordering further investigations and planning treatment. The gynaecologist will ensure all appropriate investigations are carried out, including full blood count and ultrasound scan.

Medical/surgical management

The Royal College of Obstetricians and Gynaecologists has produced evidence-based guidelines for both the initial (RCOG 1998) and secondary management (RCOG 1999) of menorrhagia. The guidelines for initial management outline investigations and medical treatment that should be undertaken when a woman presents with menorrhagia. This ensures that all appropriate medical treatment, e.g. with hormones (see Table 25.1), has been undertaken in the community before referral for specialist opinion. Referrals to a gynaecologist that may result in surgical intervention should only be undertaken when other medical options have been tried. It can take several months of monitoring

Table 25.1 Menstrual disorders

Disorder and definition	Possible causes	Specific investigations (as appropriate)	Treatment (as appropriate)
Amenorrhoea Absence of menstruation – may be primary (never had a period) or secondary (menstruation ceases after periods commenced)	Primary • Genetic and chromosomal defects, e.g. Turner's syndrome • Pituitary failure (see Ch. 17) • Cryptomenorrhoea – bleeding is hidden within uterine cavity	Blood tests to check for genetic or endocrine defect Examination under anaesthetic to exclude physical defect	Referral to endocrinologist Surgery to allow menstrual blood flow
	Secondary • Pregnancy • Metabolic/dietary, e.g. anorexia nervosa • Ovarian cysts/tumours • Pituitary disorder • Stress	Pregnancy test USS, skull X-ray Blood tests for hormone levels, e.g. FSH, LH, oestradiol, prolactin	Dependent on results but could include monitor diet, etc; surgery to remove tumour; treatment of endocrine disorder
Oligomenorrhoea Irregular infrequent menstruation	• Endocrine disorder • Lack of ovulation • Polycystic ovary syndrome (PCOS)	USS Blood tests for hormone levels, e.g. FSH, LH, oestradiol	Treatment of cause
Dysmenorrhoea Pain experienced during menstruation – commonly affects girls and young women aged 16–26 years	Increased uterine contractions during menstruation due to excess of prostaglandins	Laparoscopy to exclude organic disease	Oral contraceptive pill (OCP); pain-killers which inhibit prostaglandin formation, e.g. mefenamic acid
Premenstrual syndrome (PMS) A group of symptoms experienced prior to onset of menstruation, including water retention, weight gain, breast tenderness, pain, mood changes (irritable, angry), loss of concentration, etc.	Cause unknown. It is thought to be linked to endocrine imbalance and/or fluid retention	Identification of symptoms through discussion	No one treatment effective for all; depends on severity Suppression of female hormones is helpful but cannot be prescribed long-term Diuretics Various self-help measures, e.g. evening primrose oil, stress management, complementary therapies, etc.
Menorrhagia Heavy bleeding during regular cycle, usually every 28 days	• Dysfunctional uterine bleeding • Endometriosis • Uterine fibroids, polyps • Thyroid disorder	USS Blood tests for haemoglobin, thyroid function and hormone status Hysteroscopy; endometrial biopsy, dilatation and curettage	Depends on cause. Medical treatment includes hormonal (e.g. OCP, HRT) and non-hormonal (e.g. prostaglandins) Progesterone can be used locally on intrauterine devices (e.g. levonorgestrol) Surgical treatment includes removal of organic cause (e.g. polypectomy, endometrial ablation, hysterectomy)
Metrorrhagia Heavy bleeding, usually irregular and frequent	• Dysfunctional uterine bleeding • Uterine fibroids, polyps	USS Blood tests for haemoglobin, thyroid function and hormone status Hysteroscopy; endometrial biopsy, dilatation and curettage	As for menorrhagia
Dysfunctional uterine bleeding Excessive uterine bleeding where no organic cause is found	Abnormal function of control mechanisms of menstrual cycle	As for menorrhagia and metrorrhagia to exclude organic lesion	As for menorrhagia excluding polypectomy

to assess whether medical options have been effective and women can sometimes feel that symptom relief is taking a long time to achieve. Hormonal imbalances can often be treated medically, but if an organic cause is found, this will usually require surgical removal.

The gynaecologist checks that medical treatments, if appropriate, have been undertaken, as surgery (with its inherent risks) should be a final treatment option. If an organic cause is detected, then the appropriate surgical treatment will be discussed fully with the patient. Alternative treatments, the risks of surgery and the risks of not undertaking surgery must be discussed fully so that patients can be involved in the decision and give fully informed consent.

Hysteroscopy, dilatation and curettage

An instrument known as a hysteroscope is introduced into the uterine cavity via the cervix in order to view the endometrial cavity (see Fig. 25.11). This can be either under direct view or by connecting a camera to the hysteroscope and viewing the image on a television screen. This procedure has traditionally been performed under general anaesthetic but is increasingly being undertaken as an outpatient procedure. Once a good view of the endometrium has been obtained, any cervical or endometrial polyps identified can be removed under direct vision, a procedure known as polypectomy. Following hysteroscopy, an endometrial sample may be taken during a procedure known as dilatation and curettage (D&C). The cervix is dilated using metal dilators, a curette is then introduced into the endometrial cavity and the endometrium is shaved off. Hysteroscopy often cannot be performed when a woman is menstruating as it is difficult to get a good view of the endometrial cavity. Uterine perforation is a potential complication (see p. 740).

Endometrial ablation

Ablation or destruction of the endometrium, usually using a form of heat, is now commonly used as an alternative to hysterectomy. This technique using surgical endoscopy developed

rapidly in gynaecology during the late 1980s and 1990s (Sutton 1993). It can be carried out as a day case with much less inconvenience to the patient than undergoing major surgery. Sutton (1993) estimated that nearly 80% of procedures requiring laparotomy could be achieved by minimally invasive surgery. However, these procedures often take longer in the operating theatre, require expensive new technology and both nursing and medical staff gaining new skills in the procedures and care. Consequently, minimally invasive techniques have not completely replaced more traditional forms of surgery.

Heat can be generated to destroy the endometrial cells by laser, rollerball, loop electrode or by water. In the latter case, a catheter is inserted into the uterine cavity and an outer balloon is filled with water that is then heated to 87°C for 7 minutes. This relatively simple and cheap treatment can now be done as an outpatient procedure. The endometrial cavity should be smooth to perform this procedure safely, without the presence of submucous fibroids (see p. 716). The woman should have a hysteroscopy performed to assess this before undertaking ablation. In some instances, medication is prescribed to make the endometrium atrophic prior to this procedure. The lining to be removed becomes compact and easier to destroy, making the procedure easier to perform.

Endometrial ablation is a relatively new procedure and published information on long-term effects of treatment has only recently started to become widely available. A study by Macdonald (1993) involving 187 patients who underwent endometrial ablation showed that, following the procedure, 54% had amenorrhoea, 25% had light loss and 9% had moderate loss. Thirty-two (17%) patients required repeat ablation and 18 (10%) required hysterectomy.

Hysterectomy

This operation is usually performed for menstrual disorders that have failed to respond, to the patients' satisfaction, to other forms of treatment. An organic cause, such as fibroids, may also have been diagnosed which can only be treated effectively by surgical removal. It is important that women are not persuaded to undergo this surgery unless they feel mentally prepared to accept it. This is a significant life event as it ends a woman's ability to reproduce and, although she may not want any more children, the finality can have a profound effect on some women's feelings of sexuality.

The operation is performed through an abdominal incision and involves removing the uterus. This is known as a total abdominal hysterectomy (TAH). The ovaries and tubes may also be removed (bilateral salpingo-oophorectomy, BSO) or the cervix left in situ (subtotal hysterectomy, STAH). Removal of healthy ovaries often depends on the age of the woman. Once removed, the woman will undergo a surgically induced menopause and may require hormone replacement therapy (HRT) for several years. Healthy ovaries in a woman aged in her 30s or 40s are usually left in situ. However, this decision should be reached by mutual agreement between the woman and her surgeon, as many women have very strong views about maintaining their ovaries.

Hysterectomy is also performed by the vaginal route. This may be used for benign conditions such as fibroids with laparoscopic assistance (laparoscopic assisted vaginal hysterectomy, LAVH) or to treat uterine prolapse (see p. 724).

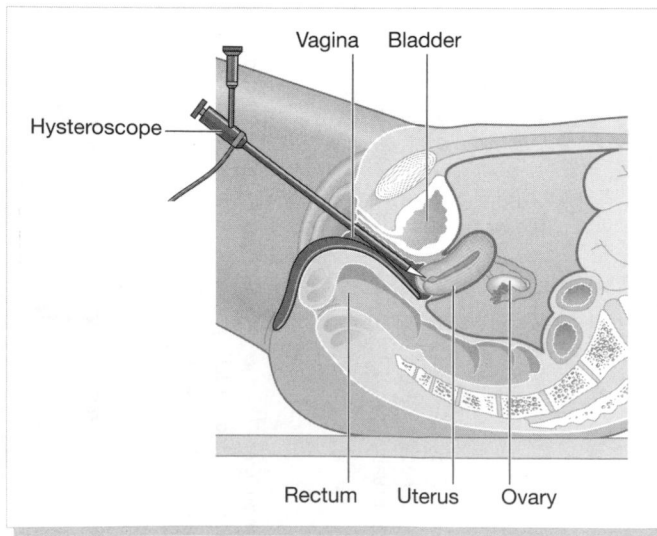

Figure 25.11 Hysteroscopy.

Myomectomy

Where a woman requires surgical removal of fibroids but wishes to remain fertile, a myomectomy may be performed instead of a hysterectomy. The presence of fibroids can have an adverse effect on the woman's fertility by affecting implantation of the embryo or causing miscarriage or preterm labour.

Myomectomy involves cutting into the myometrium and shelling out the fibroid. Because the myometrium is very vascular, there is a risk of significant haemorrhage during surgery. The woman must be counselled fully that she will have blood cross-matched and may require a blood transfusion (see Ch. 18), but if haemorrhage cannot be controlled, then there is a high risk that the uterus may have to be removed at the time of surgery. The fibroids may recur after surgery.

▶ Nursing management – an overview

Nursing care for women admitted for elective gynaecological surgery is explained in detail in a later section (p. 736). However, during preoperative assessment, if the woman is suffering from menorrhagia, particular attention should be paid to a haemoglobin level reduced due to heavy menstrual loss. Treatment of low haemoglobin will depend on the clinical need of the woman. Surgery may be deferred and the woman treated with iron supplements such as ferrous sulphate. This is not always appropriate as the woman's haemoglobin level may continue to fall as she will still be having heavy periods. In individuals in whom the haemoglobin levels are extremely low, a blood transfusion may be necessary. This may be done 2–3 weeks before surgery. It is not advisable to transfuse routinely immediately prior to or during surgery as this increases the risk of the development of venous thrombosis (see Ch. 19).

On arrival, a nurse should be assigned to the woman to introduce her to the unit, enabling a close relationship to develop that will help to reduce any fears and anxieties the woman may have. Discharge planning, if not initiated at the preoperative assessment clinic, should be started now to ensure support arrangements for the woman on discharge are in place. Other preoperative care may include shave, bowel preparation, fasting, attending to hygiene needs, preoperative checks and administration of drugs to prevent infection or venous thrombosis (see Ch. 29).

On return to the ward following surgery, the nurse must regularly monitor vital signs to detect any early changes in the woman's condition. Close attention must also be paid to any additional treatment, such as intravenous infusions, indwelling catheter or abdominal vacuum drain. This care is detailed in the later section on gynaecological surgery. The woman will experience pain and so this must be monitored closely, along with the effectiveness of prescribed analgesia.

On the days following hysterectomy, the woman is encouraged to mobilize early and commence self-caring as soon as possible to reduce the risk of developing complications. Depending on the support available to her at home, she is likely to be discharged 4–5 days after her surgery. Some units operate an early discharge policy, with support at home from visiting hospital nurses. The nursing care for myomectomy is similar to that required by a woman who has undergone a hysterectomy.

BENIGN TUMOURS OF THE FEMALE REPRODUCTIVE STRUCTURES

Benign tumours of the female reproductive tract are relatively common.

Aetiology and pathophysiology

The commonest growths in the uterus are either endometrial polyps or fibroids in the myometrium (see p. 716).

Benign growths on the ovary are usually cysts. Benign ovarian cysts are often asymptomatic and may be found during a pelvic examination or ultrasound for another purpose. Consequently the true incidence is unknown, but Girling & Soutter (1997) describe ovarian cysts as being the fourth most common cause of gynaecological hospital admissions.

The cysts commonly form after some slight dysfunction during maturation of follicles and ovulation (see p. 707). Cysts may develop either in a follicle or in the corpus luteum and are usually fluid-filled. A dermoid cyst often causes great interest as it is lined by stratified epithelium and contains structures made up of similar tissue – cartilage, hair, sebaceous tissue or even teeth!

Clinical presentation

As mentioned previously, many cysts are asymptomatic but women can present with abdominal pain, particularly if the cyst has twisted. This is known as torsion and is usually treated as an emergency as there is a risk of rupture of the cysts, causing internal haemorrhage.

Specific investigations

These include:

- pelvic examination
- ultrasound scan
- blood test for CA-125 (tumour marker for ovarian cancer) – this is done to exclude the risk of malignancy. If the CA-125 level is raised, it is indicative that the cyst could be malignant and so management should be for suspected cancer until it is proved otherwise.

Medical/surgical management

Follicular and corpus luteal cysts rarely require treatment, as they tend to resolve spontaneously over 2–3 months. However, if it is thought that a cyst has twisted or ruptured, emergency surgery may be necessary to remove the cyst and control any bleeding, usually by laparotomy. Occasionally, if the cyst has become integral to the ovary, the latter may need to be removed (oophorectomy). A woman presenting with unexplained abdominal pain must have a urinary pregnancy test performed to exclude an ectopic pregnancy (see p. 729).

▶ Nursing management

Nursing care of a woman having surgery involves physical preparation for theatre and postoperative care as described for a woman undergoing major gynaecological surgery later in the chapter. However, the woman and her relatives may be extremely anxious due to pain, being admitted as an emergency, concerns about surgery and the effect on her future fertility. The nurse must maintain a calm and supportive manner and explain fully all procedures to the woman so she is reassured about what to expect during her admission. The woman may be fit for discharge 2–3 days after surgery.

MALIGNANT TUMOURS OF THE FEMALE REPRODUCTIVE STRUCTURES

Detection and treatment of gynaecological cancers have developed in recent years, resulting in improved survival rates. The way cancer services are delivered, particularly in England, has been modernized through the publication of national guidelines (Department of Health 2000) that ensure that women receive treatment in cancer centres by medical and nursing staff who specialize in that condition and undertake appropriate care on a regular basis. In gynaecology, guidelines recommend that all ovarian cancer patients should be treated in cancer centres (Haward 1999).

However, to receive such a diagnosis has a devastating effect on a woman and her family. Cancer can occur in any part of the genital tract but is extremely rare in the vagina or uterine tube. Consequently, only cancers of the vulva, cervix, endometrium and ovary are described here.

VULVAL CANCER

Aetiology and epidemiology

This is a relatively uncommon disease occurring in approximately 1.8 per 100 000, although it increases to 20 in 100 000 over the age of 75 (Luesley 2001). It is thought to develop from either the effect of human papilloma virus (HPV) or from other inflammatory disorders of vulval tissue such as hyperplasia. Smoking is known to be a risk factor, particularly with HPV.

Pathophysiology

The pathology of vulval cancer depends on how advanced the tumour is and the extent of involvement with other structures. The most common form is squamous cancer which accounts for up to 90% of all vulval cancers. These cancers usually involve the labia and sometimes the clitoris and spread is locally to adjoining tissue and lymph nodes. Luesley (2001) describes how up to 30% of cases have lymphatic metastases at the time of diagnosis.

Specific investigations and clinical presentation

Women often delay seeking a medical opinion due to embarrassment. Clinical presentation includes pruritus (itching of the vulva), ulcers or, in more advanced cases, a mass.

A diagnosis is obviously essential in order to determine the appropriate treatment for any vulval lesion. Direct inspection by a specialist gynaecology oncologist is essential, followed by a biopsy for histological examination. The cancer may be quite advanced and a biopsy not required, so definitive surgery may be undertaken straight away.

Medical/surgical management

Surgical treatment is the commonest form of management, as it is necessary to remove the tumour in order to alleviate symptoms. However, radiotherapy may be indicated either before surgery or following surgery but is not usually indicated as sole treatment. Traditionally, surgery was nearly always radical in nature, particularly if there was node involvement. However, surgery has been modified to reduce morbidity but still achieve beneficial outcomes. Wide local excision of the cancer with bilateral inguinal node dissection, if necessary, is now undertaken, although if the cancer and tissue affected cover a large area, radical vulvectomy may be indicated. This involves dissecting away the invasive lesion, skin, subcutaneous fat, the vulva and inguinal and femoral nodes.

▶ Nursing management

Once a diagnosis is suspected, even before it is confirmed, patients will require the support of a specialist nurse who has developed the appropriate knowledge and skills in oncology. The specialist nurse will be able to provide information and advice about treatment in terms patients will be able to understand at a time of acute anxiety in the outpatient setting. This support will then continue during treatment. Patients may still be sexually active and may be worried about the effect surgery will have on their relationship with their partner. In some cases, specialist counselling is required and couples may require referral to a psychosexual counsellor, although this resource is not readily available in some areas.

On admission for surgery, both ward and specialist nurses should be involved with patient care to provide the appropriate support. Routine preoperative care, as described later in the chapter, will be undertaken although it should be noted that the majority of patients admitted with this condition will be older women and may have additional needs because of this.

Postoperatively, routine observations must be undertaken to monitor the patient's condition. A urethral catheter will be in situ and if there has been surgery to remove lymph nodes, there may be drains left in situ until drainage is minimal.

Wound care can vary between units and there appears to be little published research to recommend the optimum approach. Modifications in radical surgery seem to have had a positive effect in reducing the amount of wound breakdown which was synonymous with vulvectomy. This is an area in which nurses often take the lead in determining the most appropriate wound care. Commonly, following bathing or showering, the wound area is dried with a hairdryer (taking care not to burn patients) to avoid the wound damage/discomfort that can occur as a result of direct drying of the area. However, if infection is present, this practice is contraindicated, as the hairdryer can inadvertently blow microorganisms into the air, with an attendant risk of cross-infection.

Surgery involving the lymph nodes increases the risk of lymphoedema developing in the leg; unable to drain satisfactorily, lymph accumulates in the interstitial tissue. Most cancer centres have a nurse who specializes in treatment of lymphoedema, who is able to offer advice and help with fitting specialist stockings. Patients should be advised to take special care of the legs, avoiding accidental damage or injections to the tissue.

The ongoing support of patients following surgery, particularly in dealing with the emotional impact of having been treated for cancer and undergoing a major change in body image, is a crucial part of the role of gynaecology oncology nurse specialists.

CERVICAL CANCER

Epidemiology

Cancer of the cervix affects approximately 4200 women in the UK annually (Hughes 2001). The incidence is falling due to the introduction of the screening programme mentioned earlier, as abnormalities are being detected whilst in a pre-invasive state. The screening programme recommends women between the ages of 20 and 60 years old have a cervical smear routinely every 3–5 years. The frequency may be increased in high-risk women or where early abnormalities have been found.

Aetiology

The exact aetiology is unknown although there are several risk factors that have been identified, as follows:

- early onset of sexual activity
- multiple sexual partners
- cigarette smoking
- immunosuppression
- sexually transmitted (acquired) disease, particularly human papilloma virus (HPV).

The outer part of the cervix is lined with stratified squamous epithelium and the inner part is composed of columnar epithelium which lines the uterine cavity. The point at which these two meet is known as the squamocolumnar junction. The area where the skin lining the outside of the cervix changes to the glandular epithelium of the endocervical canal is known as the transformation zone, and this is the commonest site of cervical cancers.

Pathophysiology

Approximately 80–90% of cervical cancers involve squamous cells. Others include adenocarcinomas, with sarcomas and melanomas being less common. Abnormalities are graded histologically and cytologically to give an indication of the extent of the disease. Pre-invasive disease is graded as CIN I, II or III, describing the amount and type of abnormality. Pre-invasive disease is usually treated in the colposcopy clinic and often does not require hospital admission.

FIGO (International Federation of Gynaecology and Obstetrics) provides a classification staging cancer of the cervix from 0 (pre-invasive disease) to IVb (distant metastasis), as follows:

0   Pre-invasive disease
I   The cancer is confined to the cervix
II   Involvement of the vagina except the lower third, or infiltration of the parametrium. No involvement of the side wall
III Involvement of the lower third of the vagina with extension to the pelvic side wall
IV   Extension of the cancer beyond the reproductive tract.

Within the classification there are further descriptions involving the size of a lesion and extent of spread that may have occurred.

Clinical presentation

Cervical screening will often identify abnormalities that have yet to cause symptoms, allowing early treatment to be instigated.

However, even following a recent normal smear, symptoms can develop that indicate cervical cancer. These include postcoital bleeding (bleeding after intercourse), postmenopausal bleeding and an offensive persistent bloodstained vaginal discharge. Advanced tumours may be easily identifiable on inspection of the cervix.

Specific investigations

These are usually undertaken in the colposcopy clinic. Women with an abnormal smear will be referred for a colposcopy appointment. This involves examination of the cervix under a low-powered microscope to identify abnormalities in the cervix.

In order to confirm the diagnosis histologically, a biopsy may be taken from the cervix. This may be either a small punch biopsy or a large loop excision of transformation zone (LLETZ). Because of the size of area excised during LLETZ, this can be a treatment as well as a diagnostic procedure. The histologist can examine the biopsy to ensure that the lesion is completely removed and assess the severity of the CIN more accurately by looking at individual cells under a microscope at high magnification. If invasive disease is confirmed then staging of the disease will be required in order to decide on the appropriate treatment. Staging involves undertaking an examination under anaesthetic, cervical biopsy, cystoscopy (see Ch. 24), sigmoidoscopy (see Ch. 22) and chest X-ray. These investigations will give a clear indication of the extent of disease and location of spread.

Medical/surgical management

The management options include surgery, radiotherapy and chemotherapy, and these may be used alone or in combination depending on the grade and stage of the cancer (see Ch. 33). Patients are discussed at a multidisciplinary tumour board meeting where specialist doctors, nurses, pathologists and radiologists evaluate the results of these investigations and then agree appropriate treatment.

The decision as to whether treatment is curative or palliative will depend on how far advanced the disease is. Unless the disease is advanced to stage 1B2 or above, radical surgery is usually recommended. This includes a Wertheim's hysterectomy whereby the uterus, tubes, ovaries and upper third of the vagina are removed. This may be followed by radiotherapy depending on the histology results. For more advanced disease, where a cure is unlikely, palliative radiotherapy will be offered, with additional chemotherapy being considered, as it has been shown to increase survival rates (see Ch. 33). If cervical cancer should recur, further radical surgery may be considered, including exenteration and the removal of further vaginal and pelvic tissue.

▶ Nursing management

Women with cervical cancer will need to be referred to a gynaecology oncology nurse specialist who can provide in-depth explanations of procedures, disease and planned management. This should be commenced in the outpatient clinic when a suspected diagnosis is made and continued through their in-patient stay. General nursing care both pre- and postoperatively is explained later, but because of the extensive nature of this surgery, patients will require a higher dependency of care immediately postoperatively. They may need particular observation for the development of paralytic ileus and will have a nasogastric tube which requires careful monitoring. A large component of nursing care will include sensitive psychological support of patients and their partners. Remember that patients have to deal not only with undergoing major surgery that may have an effect on their sexuality but also with a diagnosis of cancer and an uncertain prognosis. The clinical nurse specialist can offer practical advice and coping mechanisms in these circumstances. Women who undergo radiotherapy following surgery must be offered advice about potential sexual dysfunction subsequently (Jefferies 2002a). Nurses will also be able to support them through palliative care should treatment not be successful (see Ch. 34).

ENDOMETRIAL CANCER

Aetiology and epidemiology

This is the second most common gynaecological cancer and treatment, if begun in the early stages, has a high success rate. Postmenopausal women are most at risk and the majority of cases present in women aged 65–75 years.

Other risk factors include:

- obesity
- late menopause
- smoking
- oestrogen-only HRT
- parity – less than a third of cases are childless.

Pathophysiology

The endometrium becomes thickened due to cell hyperplasia. In a postmenopausal woman, the endometrium should be smooth and very thin. Hyperplasia can be simple or complex, and although this is a forerunner to cancer, surgical treatment is advised to prevent cancer developing. Endometrial cancer is usually an adenocarcinoma.

Clinical presentation

The woman usually presents with vaginal bleeding, which may be sporadic or show only as light spotting, and so may be ignored in the first instance. However, vaginal bleeding is not normal for postmenopausal women and they should be encouraged to seek medical advice. Other causes of postmenopausal bleeding (PMB) include cervical or endometrial polyps and atrophic vaginitis due to lack of oestrogen, which causes the vaginal tissue to be friable and fragile. Because of the risk of endometrial cancer, any woman presenting with postmenopausal bleeding must be investigated urgently to exclude cancer. Only approximately 7–10% of women investigated for postmenopausal bleeding will have endometrial cancer.

Specific investigations

Following consultation and pelvic examination, an ultrasound scan is required to check the thickness of the endometrium and other abnormalities. An endometrial biopsy will be obtained; this can be done either as an outpatient, where a small sample is obtained, or under general anaesthetic following a hysteroscopy.

This has the advantage of direct view of the endometrium but has the added risk of a general anaesthetic. In many units now, hysteroscopy is being undertaken as an outpatient procedure.

Medical/surgical management

Surgical treatment is usually recommended for both hyperplasia and cancer. The planned management will be total abdominal hysterectomy and bilateral salpingo-oophorectomy, whereby the uterus, tubes and ovaries are removed in case of local spread. A high proportion of these cancers are grade 1 due to early diagnosis and no further treatment is required. For more advanced cancers, a course of radiotherapy may be prescribed postoperatively.

▶ Nursing management

Nurses provide vital support to women who may be distressed having received a diagnosis of either cancer or pre-cancer. Reassurance can be given about the success of treatment, particularly if the disease is in the early stages. Patients may already have been admitted for hysteroscopy and D&C and so may already know the unit and staff. However, they will be undergoing a major operation this time and may be worried about the effect on their general health, particularly the anaesthetic. Older women may also have other medical conditions which will need careful monitoring by the nurse, and particular attention should be paid to discharge arrangements as they may live alone and not have good family support. Pre- and postoperative care for a woman undergoing TAH and BSO is described on pages 719 and 736–739.

OVARIAN CANCER

Aetiology and epidemiology

Ovarian cancer is the most common gynaecological cancer and results in the death of 4000 women every year in the UK (Acheson & Chan 2001). Owing to the fact that almost 75% of women present with advanced disease, survival rates are extremely low and have not shown any improvement despite advances in medical knowledge and technology. The incidence is highest in industrialized countries, particularly North America and northern and western Europe. Ovarian cancer predominantly occurs in older women who have undergone the menopause. Risk factors for developing the disease include:

- nulliparity – never having had children
- genetic factors – particularly where first-degree relatives have had breast or ovarian cancer
- late menopause.

Pregnancy, breast-feeding and oral contraceptive are thought to offer some protection against ovarian cancer.

Pathophysiology

There are three main types of ovarian cancer which can be diagnosed by histological examination: epithelial, sex cord (gonadal stroma) and germ cell tumours. Epithelial tumours are the most common and account for nearly 90% of all ovarian cancers. These are further graded into three groups according to the level of cell differentiation (see Ch. 33):

- grade 1 – well differentiated
- grade 2 – moderately differentiated
- grade 3 – poorly differentiated.

FIGO has also provided classification of the stages of ovarian cancer linked to the locality and extent of the disease in a similar manner to cervical cancer.

Clinical presentation

As mentioned previously, many women present with advanced disease. There is an insidious onset of the disease with lack of obvious symptoms. There has been much interest in developing a screening programme, but to date a definitive pre-invasive screening test has yet to be identified. If a woman does experience symptoms, they are often vague and can include:

- abnormal vaginal bleeding
- abdominal distension
- pressure symptoms on other pelvic organs, such as urinary frequency
- gastrointestinal symptoms
- abdominal ascites in advanced disease.

Due to the vagueness of symptoms, the disease can be confused with other causes, such as 'middle-aged spread', irritable bowel or stress.

Specific investigations

A thorough history must be taken, followed by abdominal and pelvic examination. In advanced disease, the mass can be palpated and ascites (fluid in the abdomen) may be present. Other tests include:

- ultrasound scan of the pelvis and abdomen – helpful in identifying abnormalities of the ovary
- blood tests – a full blood count and biochemical profile to check renal and liver function and presence/level of CA-125, a tumour marker which is often elevated in ovarian cancer
- chest X-ray to check for pleural effusion (fluid in the pleural space), or secondary deposits of cancer to the lungs
- CT or MRI may be undertaken to examine for lymph node involvement and further metastases.

Medical/surgical management

The management of ovarian cancer is complex and should only be carried out in a recognized gynaecological centre with specialist medical, nursing, laboratory and radiological staff who are experienced in providing care for women with this disease (Haward 1999). This ensures patients have a competent, experienced multidisciplinary team to deliver their care.

Once a provisional diagnosis has been made using results from the above tests, surgery is usually indicated in the form of a laparotomy. This can be particularly useful for obtaining a definitive histological diagnosis, providing a surgical cure in early stages and removing part of the tumour or debulking prior to chemotherapy. In some cases, such surgical debulking is undertaken followed by chemotherapy to shrink the cancer and then further surgery to remove as much tissue as possible. During laparotomy it is usual to remove the uterus, tubes, ovaries and greater omentum (part of the peritoneum). Samples

of lymph nodes close to the uterus are also taken to check for local spread. Histological examination is the only method of obtaining a definite diagnosis of ovarian cancer.

Chemotherapy is also an important treatment, particularly in advanced disease where surgery alone will not provide a cure. Many different chemotherapy drugs have been used since the 1980s, but the drugs of choice currently are platinum-based, such as cisplatin or carboplatin with paclitaxel – a plant alkaloid derived from the bark of the western yew. As with many cytotoxic drugs, these can have many side-effects and toxic effects on the kidneys and nervous system.

Due to the relatively high morbidity of this cancer, units must either provide or have access to palliative care services. This does not mean cessation of treatment, as often palliative treatments are required to improve the quality of life. In particular, patients may develop ascites or pleural effusions which require draining to alleviate acute abdominal distension or breathlessness.

▶ Nursing management

As with other gynaecological cancers, the role of the oncology nurse specialist is paramount in ensuring patients and family members are provided with emotional support, through information and advice, during this difficult time. A recent study demonstrated the positive impact nurses can have at this time (Jefferies 2002b). Referral to other agencies for additional support and information about resources such as the Macmillan nursing service or Cancer BACUP (see 'Useful websites', p. 767) can be arranged by the nurse specialist.

When patients are admitted for surgery, it is imperative that all the investigations described previously have been performed and results are available. They will require routine preoperative care prior to undergoing major surgery (described below). However, in addition, they will require bowel preparation, usually with a stimulant laxative such as sodium picosulfate (see Ch. 29), in case a colostomy is required if local spread includes the bowel (see Ch. 22). Postoperatively they will require close monitoring of their general condition and, due to the complex nature of the surgery, may require care in a high-dependency unit (see Ch. 31). The physical care delivered by nurses will take priority in the first few days after surgery, but it is important to appreciate that the emotional needs of both patients and family members must be addressed throughout care. They will be fearful about recovery having undergone such extensive surgery and will be anxious about receiving histology results. Bad news, particularly relating to these results, should be delivered in a quiet location, if possible away from a busy ward, with both the consultant and nurse specialist present. The need for further chemotherapy will reinforce that surgery has not been curative and nurses must be able to support patients during this stressful time.

If chemotherapy is required, this should be provided in a specialist centre by nursing staff who are experienced in both administering the drugs and monitoring side-effects. These can be short-term (e.g. nausea or vomiting) or long-term (e.g. renal toxicity). In many centres, the chemotherapy unit is an integral part of the oncology department.

Palliative care is an area where specialist nurses are able to take a lead (see Ch. 34). They are able to support patients when they experience distressing symptoms and offer relief for these symptoms. Pain relief may be necessary, as may drainage of fluid in the abdomen or lungs. Bowel obstruction can also develop in terminal stages and nurses can offer advice about fluid and dietary intake.

Oncology nurse specialists will have an in-depth knowledge of this disease and its progression. They will also have excellent communication skills and will be able to provide appropriate information and advice to meet the emotional needs of both patients and close family members. It must also be recognized that working in this area can be extremely stressful for nurses; they must therefore be able to develop their own coping mechanisms to avoid becoming burnt out (see Ch. 6). Many units have systems in place to support staff and clinical supervision can be helpful for nurses to exchange concerns and discuss possible solutions.

UTERINE DISPLACEMENT AND PROLAPSE

Uterine displacement, whereby there is prolapse of the uterus or vaginal walls, is an extremely common disorder. The true incidence is not known as many women cope with the symptoms and do not seek medical help, often because of embarrassment. Women who do seek medical help often find the examination acutely embarrassing and will need the support of the nurse. A GP may be able to treat the symptoms but often, if surgical management is indicated, the woman will be referred to a gynaecologist.

Aetiology

This disorder, which is also known as uterovaginal prolapse, occurs when the muscles become lax and are unable to support the pelvic organs in their anatomically correct position. This often happens after the menopause and with the loss of oestrogenic effects on pelvic muscles and other tissues. It can be caused by:

- stretching of muscle and fibrous tissue during pregnancy and childbirth
- increased intra-abdominal pressure, e.g. chronic cough, obesity, heavy work/lifting
- predisposition to stretching of ligament tissue thought to be due to erect position.

Improvements in obstetric care and reduction in length of labours have contributed to a reduction in the incidence of this disorder.

The types of uterovaginal prolapse are described in Table 25.2 (see also Fig. 25.12).

Clinical presentation

Women commonly describe a feeling of 'something coming down' when they have a prolapse. Because of the close proximity to the bladder and bowel (see Fig. 25.1, p. 706) there may be associated dysfunction such as stress incontinence, frequency of micturition or difficulty in passing urine or stool. In stress incontinence, a woman leaks urine when the intra-abdominal pressure is raised, e.g. during coughing, sneezing or laughing.

Specific investigations

On examination the doctor will be able to see or feel either the uterus in its abnormal position or a bulge in the vaginal wall, depending on which structure is involved. A detailed history of previous obstetric experience and symptoms will inform the doctor which pelvic structures may be involved, but a vaginal examination is required to confirm this. Stress incontinence can often be demonstrated by asking the patient to cough and, although this is a useful test, it can be acutely embarrassing and the nurse must be sensitive to this.

Medical/surgical management

Treatment will depend on the severity of symptoms, the health status of the patient and her fertility. Surgical treatment will not be considered for women who have not completed their family,

Table 25.2 Commonest types of uterovaginal prolapse		
Type	**Area affected**	**Description**
First degree	Uterus	Uterus descends from normal position into the vagina
Second degree	Uterus	Uterus descends from normal position outside vulva. Cervix becomes ulcerated
Third degree	Uterus	Complete prolapse of uterus outside body – also known as complete procidentia
Cystocele	Uterus, anterior vaginal wall and bladder	Uterus prolapses but stays in pelvis. Bladder prolapses (herniates) into the vagina through anterior vaginal wall (see Fig. 25.12A)
Urethrocele	Uterus, anterior vaginal wall and urethra	Uterus prolapses but stays in pelvis. Urethra herniates through anterior vaginal wall
Rectocele	Uterus, posterior vaginal wall and rectum	Uterus prolapses but stays in pelvis. Rectum prolapses (herniates) into vagina through posterior vaginal wall (see Fig. 25.12B)
Enterocele	Uterus, posterior vaginal wall and pouch of Douglas	Uterus prolapses but stays in pelvis. Pouch of Douglas (peritoneal pouch behind uterus) herniates through posterior vaginal wall. Small bowel may also descend

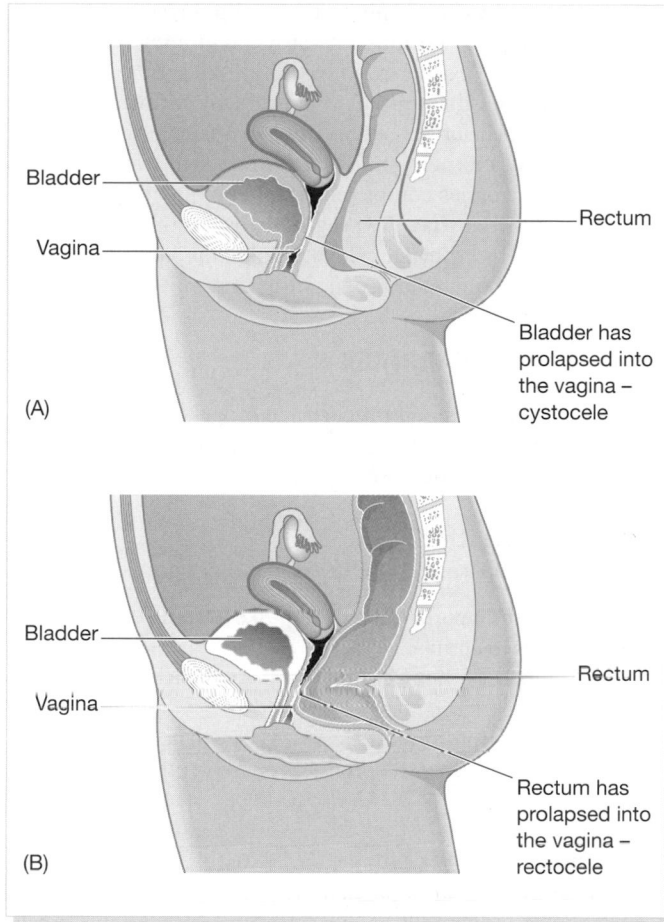

Figure 25.12 Uterovaginal prolapse. (A) Cystocele; (B) rectocele.

as further pregnancies will undo any benefits gained by surgery. In these instances, and for older women who may not be fit for a general anaesthetic, insertion of a ring pessary made of smooth plastic may be the most appropriate treatment. The pessary is inserted into the vagina and sits at the top, supporting the uterus. If tolerated, it can be an excellent solution and will need replacing at 6-monthly intervals. Surgical treatment includes making an incision into the vaginal wall and inserting sutures into the fascia to provide additional support to the pelvic structures. Support of the bladder involves repair of the anterior vaginal wall, known as anterior colporrhaphy or repair. Support of the rectum involves repair of the posterior vaginal wall, known as colpoperineorrhaphy or posterior repair. Hysterectomy via the vaginal route is usually undertaken for a uterine prolapse.

▶ Nursing management

As mentioned previously, women presenting with uterovaginal prolapse are often acutely embarrassed. In addition, older women may find discussion about their condition distressing. For these reasons, nurses must be extremely sensitive to their emotional needs and offer support and reassurance. Often women think they are alone in suffering from this condition and reassurance about how common the disorder is can often be

helpful. Nurses have an important role in the outpatient clinic during initial examination and if a pessary is to be inserted. If surgery is indicated, patients are admitted for a major operation and will require a hospital stay of 4–5 days depending on their physical condition and support at home. Following surgery, they are likely to have a gauze pack in the vagina and a urinary catheter due to the close proximity of surgery to the bladder. Nurses must, in addition to monitoring the general condition of the patient following surgery, closely observe the vaginal pack for any bleeding through it. The amount and type of urine produced and draining via the catheter must be closely monitored to ensure there are no problems following surgery. The vaginal pack will be removed the following day and the catheter removed after 48 hours. Close attention must then be paid to urinary output to ensure patients do not develop urinary retention. Other aspects of postoperative care are described on pages 737–739.

Although the nurse's role in treatment of uterovaginal prolapse is important, the nurse also has a vital role to play in health promotion. Educating women about doing pelvic floor exercises, particularly after childbirth, is vital as this can reduce the risk of the woman developing a prolapse and its distressing symptoms in the future (see Ch. 12).

PROBLEMS OF EARLY PREGNANCY

SPONTANEOUS MISCARRIAGE

In the UK, a miscarriage is defined as the spontaneous expulsion of the fetus or products of conception before 24 weeks of pregnancy. It is defined by the World Health Organization (WHO) as the expulsion of an embryo or fetus weighing 500 g or less, which equates to a pregnancy of about 22 weeks' gestation. The term abortion is also used for miscarriage, although in practice it is more common to refer to this disorder as a miscarriage. Women can become distressed if the term abortion is used, as this is synonymous with a deliberate termination of pregnancy. It is known that at least a fifth of all pregnancies end in miscarriage, although this figure is likely in reality to be much higher as many early miscarriages occur before pregnancy has been confirmed and it may be considered as a delayed period. The majority of miscarriages occur during the first 12 weeks of pregnancy (the first trimester), when the embryo is undergoing major development into the fetal state. Medical and surgical care has changed rapidly during recent years and the nurse has a vital role to play in the psychological support of the woman and her partner during this extremely stressful time, as it is now recognized how important this aspect of care is in helping a couple come to terms with the loss of their baby. Most gynaecology units now have specialist 'early pregnancy assessment units', where specialist nurses can provide both assessment and supportive skills in the diagnosis and treatment of women suffering from a miscarriage.

THREATENED MISCARRIAGE

This is when the pregnancy is 'threatening' to miscarry and is extremely common.

Aetiology and epidemiology

Approximately 700 000 threatened miscarriages occur every year, but for 50–75% the pregnancy will continue to full term with no adverse effects (Allan 1995). The actual causes are unclear, particularly when the pregnancy continues with no further problems. Problems with the development of the embryo or fetus may result in the threatened miscarriage progressing to a full miscarriage.

Clinical presentation

- Slight, irregular bleeding – the loss will often be dark, stale blood; the bleeding is usually from the placental site, which can be extremely alarming.
- Mild or no pain.

Specific investigations

After consulting her GP in the first instance, the woman will be referred urgently, usually to an early pregnancy assessment unit, for further investigations to confirm the state of the pregnancy. A urinary pregnancy test will be undertaken. Recent developments in these tests have produced urine dipsticks that are extremely sensitive to levels of human chorionic gonadotrophin (hCG) in the urine. This is a hormone produced by trophoblastic tissue (eventually forms the placenta) and can be detected in the blood and urine. The sensitivity of these tests means that early pregnancies can now be confirmed at only 4–5 weeks of gestation. The woman will be gently examined vaginally. During this examination, the examiner would expect the cervical os to be closed and the uterus to be enlarged to the size equivalent to dates of the expected pregnancy. An ultrasound scan would be arranged to confirm the presence of a fetal heart. The probability of a threatened miscarriage developing into a miscarriage is much lessened if a fetal heart is identified. However, there are often occasions when women present with vaginal bleeding very early in pregnancy and even the most sophisticated ultrasound equipment cannot detect the fetal heart.

Medical/surgical management

There is no specific treatment for a threatened miscarriage and there is no evidence to indicate that bed rest or refraining from intercourse will influence the outcome. However, from a psychological perspective, reducing strenuous physical activity can be suggested if the woman wants to contribute to the outcome. It is likely that if the pregnancy is going to abort, this can happen at any time, whether the woman is resting or not, but if she was indulging in strenuous physical activity at the time of her miscarriage, she is likely to blame herself. The woman does not need to be admitted to hospital but may return in 2 weeks' time for further assessment and ultrasound to confirm development of the fetus.

▶ Nursing management

This is a particularly anxious time for patients and their partners, particularly if the pregnancy has been planned. Nurses are obviously unable to guarantee the outcome of the threatened miscarriage but must ensure that patients are provided with appropriate information and are fully informed. It is important to include partners in this, as their needs can be overlooked whilst all the physical examinations and investigations are undertaken. Nurses working in early pregnancy assessment units will require excellent counselling skills but all nurses caring for patients throughout their clinical pathway must be aware of the need for sensitivity and to keep the couple fully informed to reduce their anxieties. Nurses will not be able to eliminate their worries completely – this can only happen when patients are assured that the pregnancy is continuing without adverse effects – but they can play a significant part in providing the psychological support needed at this time.

INEVITABLE MISCARRIAGE

This is when a threatened miscarriage progresses to a full miscarriage. As the term suggests, it is inevitable and there is no treatment to prevent the miscarriage.

Clinical presentation

Symptoms develop from a threatened miscarriage, as follows:

- lower abdominal pain, often cramp-like in nature, as the uterus starts to contract
- vaginal bleeding – heavier and the loss will be bright red and fresh
- on vaginal examination, the cervical os will be opening or already open to allow the products of conception to be expelled.

Management

An ultrasound scan is not particularly useful, as once the os has opened, the products will be expelled. The miscarriage can be either complete or incomplete and these are described below. There is a risk that whilst having a miscarriage, the woman can bleed heavily from the placental site and so medical intervention is often required in order to stabilize her overall condition to prevent hypovolaemic shock (see Ch. 9).

COMPLETE MISCARRIAGE

In this instance, the woman has passed all products of conception, including the fetus, fetal sac and placental tissue and the uterus is now empty.

Clinical presentation

Patients may present with a history of heavy, fresh vaginal bleeding with strong abdominal pains, both of which have now subsided. They may also report that they have passed something vaginally, often whilst on the lavatory, and if the products have been collected, a fetus or fetal tissue may be seen. On vaginal examination, the cervical os is now closed again and the uterus is smaller than the gestational dates as it has contracted following the miscarriage. An ultrasound scan may be undertaken to confirm that the uterine cavity is now empty.

Medical/surgical management

Often no further medical treatment is required and patients should be informed that any bleeding will settle within the next few days. If the bleeding becomes heavier, they suffer further abdominal pain or show any signs of vaginal infection, patients should contact the hospital again, as there may be retained products of conception within the uterus. Retained products of conception will prevent the uterus contracting and bleeding may continue. There is also a risk that the retained tissue can become infected causing endometritis (inflammation of the endometrium), which can develop into pelvic sepsis.

Again the nurse's role here is to reassure patients and ensure that they understand what has happened and what may happen during recovery. It is important that the loss of this pregnancy is acknowledged by the nurse and appropriate support offered.

INCOMPLETE MISCARRIAGE

In this case, there has been a miscarriage but not all the products of conception have been expelled from inside the uterus. The presence of these retained products (fetal tissues, membranes or blood clots) prevents the myometrium from contracting around the blood vessels at the placental site. Consequently, there is a danger of heavy bleeding unless the products are removed.

Clinical presentation
- Moderate to intense lower abdominal pain as the uterus contracts.
- Uterine contractions will cause the cervical os to open as in an inevitable miscarriage.
- Vaginal bleeding – the loss may be heavy, fresh and bright red. It is likely the patient will require emergency hospital admission for treatment to stop the bleeding.

Specific investigations
On admission, a vaginal examination may confirm that the cervical os is open and the pregnancy cannot be saved. An accurate history of symptoms should be recorded and so it is unlikely that an ultrasound will be required, although in some instances, where it is unclear whether the os is opening, one may be ordered. A blood test must be taken for a full blood count and to determine the blood group. The full blood count will indicate if the woman is becoming anaemic through the vaginal bleeding. The blood group must be known for two reasons. Firstly if the woman is Rhesus-negative she will require an injection of anti-D immunoglobulin. The blood group of the fetus is unknown and if it should be Rhesus-positive, there may be mixing of fetal and maternal blood, resulting in the formation of antibodies to Rhesus-positive antigens that would endanger future pregnancies. An injection of anti-D immunoglobulin will act prophylactically and prevent this potential reaction in the maternal blood. Secondly, if the bleeding continues, the woman may require an urgent blood transfusion so the sample is used to ascertain her blood group and the serum saved within the haematology laboratory. This serum is then immediately available for cross-matching should an emergency blood transfusion be required.

Medical/surgical management
The usual management for an incomplete miscarriage is the surgical removal of the products of conception, although there are medical and conservative treatments (see below). A surgical approach is usually the treatment of choice due to the potential for rapid and acute haemorrhage. There is also a potential for

retained products of conception to become infected and cause endometritis. Evacuation of retained products of conception (ERPC) is usually carried out as an emergency or urgent procedure, under a general anaesthetic. Using a curette, the remaining products of conception are removed from the uterine cavity. Patients must be counselled before this operation about potential complications. The uterus, being in a pregnant state, is much softer and more vascular than a non-pregnant uterus, thus increasing the risk of perforation during ERCP. Conversely, because gynaecologists are aware of this potential risk, the surgeon may be too gentle and may miss some of the products. If this should occur, it will be confirmed by an ultrasound. Patients might then require a second operation and this should be performed by a more senior, more experienced gynaecologist.

▶ Nursing management

When admitted with an incomplete miscarriage, patients and their partners will be extremely upset as they would not have expected this outcome for the pregnancy. The nurse's role is vital in ensuring they receive full explanations of all procedures and are able to understand and participate in all decisions about treatment. The nurse must provide a sensitive and empathetic support to both parties. Once a decision has been made that surgery is required, the nurse must ensure that patients are prepared in a safe and effective way for operation (see below). Whilst preparing patients for theatre physically, the nurse must continue to provide the psychological support required, as these emergency preparations can be alarming.

Before discharge home, patients must be given the opportunity to discuss their fears and anxieties about the miscarriage. Although it is unlikely that in a future pregnancy they will miscarry again, it is not helpful at this stage to talk of future pregnancies, as they will require time to grieve for the loss of this baby, however early in gestational age. The nurse requires counselling skills to provide appropriate support at this time. It is often difficult to gauge what language to use when discussing the pregnancy loss and what is appropriate for individual women. Some women find talk of fetus or products of conception helpful as they come to terms with the loss by accepting that this pregnancy had not actually developed into a baby. However, others find it distasteful and are caused further distress by professionals not referring to the pregnancy as their baby. This requires skill in assessing appropriate language so any further distress is minimized.

Often women are able to go home on the same day as the surgery. This will enable them to get back to their families as soon as possible, but written information should be provided for them to take home for later perusal. This should include contact telephone numbers for further support should they require it, such as the Miscarriage Association (see 'Useful websites', p. 767). Some units have nurses who provide further counselling and support for women who miscarry after they have gone home and this should be offered before discharge.

BLIGHTED OVUM

This occurs when a gestation sac develops without an actual fetus. It is thought to be caused by an imperfect sperm fertilizing the oocyte. The resulting conceptus is unable to develop properly or implant and a miscarriage occurs. The first a woman may be aware there is a problem is when the blighted ovum is detected on ultrasound scan when no yolk sac or embryo can be seen. There is no urgency for treatment, unlike inevitable miscarriage, as the sac will eventually be aborted spontaneously. However, patients may require considerable psychological support as they would have had no idea there was anything wrong with the pregnancy until it was detected on the scan. They should be reassured that this is unlikely to happen in a future pregnancy.

MISSED MISCARRIAGE

This is also known as early fetal demise and occurs when the fetus dies but is retained rather than being expelled as in inevitable miscarriage.

Clinical presentation

There may not be any obvious symptoms, although women often express anxieties that they no longer feel pregnant. Vaginal bleeding, if it occurs, is usually a dark brown stale discharge. After the fetus dies, the hormones produced during the early stages of the pregnancy decrease, particularly hCG, which is responsible for symptoms of pregnancy such as nausea and vomiting, tender breasts and change in appreciation of certain foodstuffs. However, whilst placental tissue survives, there will still be secretion of this hormone and so the urinary pregnancy test remains positive. An ultrasound scan may indicate the absence of a fetal heart. In order to exclude a very early pregnancy, the crown–rump length (CRL) must be greater than 6 mm. The CRL (crown of the fetal head to the rump or bottom of the spine) is used as a landmark for measuring fetal development. If the CRL is less than 6 mm, then the woman should be rescanned at least 1 week later and local guidelines often recommend 2 weeks later to see if there has been any further development from the baseline measurement. If there is no development and still no fetal heart is seen, a diagnosis of missed miscarriage is made even if urinary pregnancy test remains positive.

Medical/surgical management

Once a diagnosis has been made, there is no medical urgency for intervention and patients should be counselled fully and offered conservative, medical or surgical treatment, as described below.

Conservative treatment

Patients allow nature to take its course and wait for a spontaneous miscarriage to occur. A full explanation must be given of what to expect in terms of bleeding, pain and the appearance of the products of conception. Women must be given details and contact phone numbers of the hospital in case the pain or bleeding becomes excessive. An ultrasound scan is arranged for 1 week later to assess for retained products of conception. Although this is a natural option and offers women the opportunity of being in control of their bodies with an alternative to medical or surgical treatment, many women cannot cope with the psychological effects of carrying a dead baby for what could be several weeks. For these women, another treatment option may be more appropriate.

Medical treatment

These treatments have developed over recent years and have been shown to be extremely effective. It involves giving patients a combination of the antiprogesterone drug mifepristone and prostaglandin E either orally (e.g. misoprostol) or vaginally (e.g. gemeprost) (RCOG 2001). The first dose of mifepristone is usually given whilst patients are in the early pregnancy assessment unit; they then return to the ward for completion using misoprostol 36–48 hours later. They must be counselled fully about the effects of the treatment, explaining that there will be some bleeding and that they may even miscarry at home. Any products passed must be examined closely for fetus, membranes and placental tissue to ensure there are no retained products. Patients must feel comfortable about being able to return to the hospital at any time should they start to miscarry before the second dose. An advantage of this treatment is that general anaesthetic is not required, but women will have to experience a process during the expulsion of the products similar to labour.

Surgical treatment

This involves admitting patients for a surgical evacuation of the uterus as described earlier. In some cases, because the cervix has not dilated spontaneously as in an inevitable miscarriage, patients may be given prostaglandin E in order to soften the cervix prior to surgery. They should be prepared for theatre as described earlier.

Any tissue removed in hospital through any of these procedures will be examined histologically in the laboratory to confirm pregnancy and detect any gestational trophoblastic disease such as hydatidiform mole (see below). It will not be possible for these tests to detect the cause of the miscarriage.

▶ Nursing management

The nurse's role is primarily one of supporting patients and ensuring they are fully informed of the risks and benefits of each option. This will enable them to make an informed choice as to which is the most appropriate. The nurse must ensure that women understand what may happen to them and what action to take to reduce alarm and distress, particularly if they are at home. The nurse should also explain that it is unlikely that a reason for the miscarriage will be determined, particularly as it happens in such a high proportion of pregnancies and is equally likely whether it is the first or any subsequent pregnancy.

RECURRENT MISCARRIAGE

This is defined as three or more consecutive spontaneous miscarriages. Primary recurrent miscarriage occurs in a woman's first and subsequent pregnancies and secondary recurrent miscarriage is when a woman has had at least one successful pregnancy but then miscarries all subsequent pregnancies.

There are thought to be several causes of recurrent miscarriage (Whitton 2001), including:

- anatomical – including congenital abnormalities
- hormonal
- immunological
- hereditary thrombophilias

- genetic
- infection
- psychological.

Specialist gynaecological units may have pre-pregnancy nurse counsellors who can support patients and also take a detailed history and order specific investigations. Due to the possible causes of recurrent miscarriage, these tests are usually of a specialist nature, such as genetic and blood screening for lupus and clotting disorders. This can obviously be an extremely worrying time for women, who will be concerned not only that they will not be able to carry a pregnancy to full term but also about their own health. This is why specialist nurses are often required to provide the advice and support to women who have suffered with recurrent miscarriage.

HYDATIDIFORM MOLE

This is also known as a molar pregnancy or gestational trophoblastic disease. As suggested by the last term, it occurs when the trophoblastic tissue develops abnormally.

Aetiology and epidemiology

Hydatidiform mole is a relatively uncommon abnormality of pregnancy and the incidence varies in different countries. It is relatively common in some equatorial regions and much rarer in the northern hemisphere. It is thought to occur in between approximately 1 in 1200 to 1 in 2000 pregnancies in the UK, although the incidence is much higher among women of Asian origin (Govan et al 1993). In a complete mole there is no fetus, just an abnormal proliferation of trophoblastic tissue, and in a partial mole, there is a fetus present but it has an abnormal chromosome makeup.

Clinical presentation and investigations

Patients will have a positive pregnancy test and may be suffering excessive vomiting in pregnancy (hyperemesis gravidarum) due to the excessive amounts of hCG being secreted by the abnormal trophoblastic tissue. There may be slight vaginal bleeding. On examination the uterus may feel larger than would be expected for the dates, due to the proliferation of tissue inside. On ultrasound scan, no fetal heart will be seen, but instead there will be an enlarged placental site which is often described as looking like a bunch of grapes. A blood test to assess the β-hCG will reveal levels much higher than would be expected for the dates of the pregnancy.

Medical/surgical management

Once the diagnosis has been made, the molar pregnancy must be removed as, in a small proportion of cases, the mole can progress to a cancer known as choriocarcinoma. This is done surgically and the tissue removed is sent for histological examination. Once a definite diagnosis has been made on histology, patients will need to be followed up regularly to ensure choriocarcinoma does not develop. Due to the relatively small incidence of molar pregnancies, there are only three specialist centres in the UK (London, Sheffield and Dundee). Women are referred to the centre closest to their home and the levels of hCG in their blood and urine are monitored regularly. They will be given advice about contraception and the need to refrain from a further pregnancy until their levels of hCG have been monitored for long enough for doctors to be sure they have not suffered any lasting effects from their molar pregnancy (see www.hmole-chorio.org.uk). It is expected that hCG levels will have returned to normal after 4–6 months.

▶ Nursing management

Initially, nurses need to reassure patients about the pregnancy loss and inform them about the need for follow-up. Patients will obviously be extremely concerned about the possibility of developing cancer and will need reassurance that the likelihood of this happening is very small. Once referred to a specialist centre, a specialist nurse will be able to provide in-depth information, advice and support throughout the follow-up period. Once the levels of hCG have returned to normal, patients are advised that they can resume trying for a further pregnancy.

ECTOPIC PREGNANCY

In an ectopic pregnancy, the fetus develops outside the uterine cavity. The commonest site for an ectopic pregnancy to implant is in the uterine tube, but it can occasionally occur in the abdominal cavity or the uterine cervix.

Aetiology and epidemiology

The incidence of ectopic pregnancy is difficult to quantify but was estimated by Irvine et al (1994) as approximately 1 in 60 pregnancies, although this figure is much higher than other reported incidences. Ruptured ectopic pregnancy can still be a cause of maternal mortality and because of this, all suspected cases are treated extremely seriously until a differential diagnosis has been made.

Identified risk factors for developing an ectopic pregnancy include:

- previous sterilization
- previous ectopic pregnancy
- history of pelvic inflammatory disease
- previous tubal surgery
- smoker
- infertility.

Pathophysiology

During the early stages of pregnancy, the fertilized ovum rapidly divides and develops while it passes through the uterine tube prior to implanting in the uterine cavity approximately 6 days after fertilization. In ectopic pregnancy, there is a delay in transferring the fertilized ovum along the uterine tube and consequently, when it implants after 6 days, it is still in the tube and not in the uterine cavity. This delay can be caused by decreased motility of the tube smooth muscle, by a blockage in the tube or by damage to the cilia (microscopic hairs that line the tube and waft the fertilized ovum along its length). A blockage may be caused by scar tissue following a previous pelvic infection, such as gonorrhoea or chlamydia. Sperm are often able to pass a partial blockage in order to reach the oocyte, but the larger fertilized ovum cannot pass it on the return journey. Previous pelvic infection can also damage the cilia and smoking can have a detrimental effect as well. Compared with non-smokers, women who smoke are twice as likely to have an ectopic pregnancy and it is thought that nicotine paralyses the cilia in the same way that it does in the respiratory passages.

Clinical presentation

Because the pregnancy implants in the lining of the tube and continues to develop as if it were in the uterus, a woman with an ectopic pregnancy will exhibit early signs of pregnancy due to production of hCG and will have a positive urinary pregnancy test. Although she may have missed a regular period, she may give a history of dark brown loss around the time of an expected period and this can cause confusion when trying to assess gestational age. The embryo will continue to develop, but when it fills the lumen of the tube, the tube will be stretched and the woman will experience lower abdominal pain. A more worrying sign is if the woman complains of shoulder tip pain, usually an indication that the tube is rupturing or has already ruptured. The bleeding from this site irritates the diaphragm, causing referred pain across the shoulders via the phrenic nerve. It is usually abdominal pain that will make a woman consult her GP, who will refer her for further investigation urgently at a hospital.

Specific investigations

Differential diagnosis can be a problem in these cases, particularly if patients present at A&E with lower abdominal pain, as a diagnosis of ectopic pregnancy is sometimes not considered (Confidential Enquiries into Maternal Deaths in the UK 2001). However, an ectopic pregnancy should always be suspected until proved otherwise. A urinary pregnancy test should always be undertaken to determine whether a woman is pregnant and an ultrasound scan will also be extremely useful. It is unlikely a tubal pregnancy can be positively identified on scan, but a positive pregnancy test and lack of uterine pregnancy seen on scan is highly indicative of ectopic pregnancy. Levels of hCG in the blood can also be estimated and this is a helpful additional test. The level of β-hCG in a viable intrauterine pregnancy doubles approximately every 2 days. In ectopic pregnancy and spontaneous miscarriage, the rise is much smaller. On pelvic examination, women may experience moderate to severe pain when the cervix is palpated, known as cervical excitation. None of these tests should be used solely to diagnose an ectopic pregnancy, but must be used in combination with an accurate history of the symptoms.

Medical/surgical management

Once an ectopic pregnancy has been diagnosed, it must be removed due to the devastating effect it will have on the mother's health – the pregnancy cannot be saved. Recently there have been developments in medical management of ectopic pregnancy by the introduction of drugs directly into the gestation sac, which is left inside the uterine tube for absorption. The drug commonly used is methotrexate (an antimetabolite cytotoxic drug) although other drugs, such as potassium chloride, can be used. For a woman to receive medical treatment, she must be haemodynamically stable and must have an unruptured ectopic pregnancy. Treatment consists of several injections of methotrexate on alternate days and patients must be made aware of the potential side-effects of the drug and have easy access to the unit in case further problems develop.

Surgical treatment is most frequently the management of choice due to the urgent need for treatment. A laparoscopy is undertaken under general anaesthetic to confirm diagnosis and also remove the pregnancy. If an ectopic pregnancy is detected, an incision will be made in the tube and the pregnancy removed. The cut in the tube is left open and will heal spontaneously. If tubal damage is considerable or bleeding is difficult to control, the tube may have to be removed (salpingectomy). In most instances, this can be done laparoscopically, but in some cases an open laparotomy may be required to ensure haemostasis.

▶ Nursing management

Surgery for ectopic pregnancy is always undertaken as an urgent operation and depending on the condition of the woman; if the tube ruptures then it is a surgical emergency that requires immediate intervention. This can be alarming for both patients and their relatives, as the condition can deteriorate rapidly, causing a life-threatening situation that must be responded to calmly but effectively by nursing and medical staff. Once a diagnosis has been confirmed, the nurse's role is vital in monitoring patients. Regular observations must be made of pulse and blood pressure to assess any changes in condition that may be caused by internal bleeding. The frequency will depend on the patient's condition but may be every 15 minutes initially. Vaginal loss and level of pain must also be closely assessed and any changes reported immediately to medical staff so patients can be reviewed. In addition to monitoring the physical condition, nurses must also be sensitive to patients' psychological needs. Along with their partner, they will be extremely anxious about their physical condition, which may become life-threatening at any time, but they will also have lost their baby. It is important that patients are not treated as just another surgical case; they must be given the support required by someone who has suffered a pregnancy loss. Postoperatively the nurse will monitor the blood pressure and pulse regularly and ensure the pain is assessed appropriately so that adequate analgesia can be given.

Patients who have undergone laparoscopic surgery are often fit enough to go home the following day. Nurses must ensure not only that are they physically fit enough for discharge but also that they are given information about further support available once they are at home. As for someone who has suffered a miscarriage, it is important that, if a woman is Rhesus-negative, she has an injection of anti-D immunoglobulin to prevent sensitization to any fetal blood cells (see p. 727 and Ch. 18). Nurses should also be able to offer advice about future pregnancies. Although the effects of this ectopic pregnancy may not directly affect future pregnancies, there will be a continued risk of a further ectopic pregnancy if the tube remains, because the factors that caused this ectopic pregnancy will still be present. As with all other causes of pregnancy loss, nurses must provide a sensitive but professional approach to ensure patients and their partners feel supported through this distressing time.

TERMINATION OF PREGNANCY

In Great Britain, termination of pregnancy (TOP) is regulated by the 1967 Abortion Act, which was further amended in 1990. The number of terminations recorded in 1996 in Great Britain was almost 200 000 and the majority of these were in the first trimester of pregnancy. The Abortion Act states that a pregnancy can be terminated up to 24 weeks of gestation and that two doctors must agree that certain criteria are fulfilled, unless in an emergency situation where a termination is required to save the life of the mother. These criteria include:

- The continuation of the pregnancy would involve risk to the life of the pregnant woman greater than if the pregnancy were terminated.
- The termination is deemed necessary to prevent any permanent injury to mental or physical health of the pregnant woman.
- The pregnancy has not exceeded its 24th week and its continuation would involve risk greater than if the pregnancy were terminated to the physical and mental health of the woman.
- The pregnancy has not exceeded its 24th week and its continuation would involve risk greater than if the pregnancy were terminated to the physical or mental health of any existing children of the pregnant woman.
- There is a substantial risk that if the child were born it would suffer such physical or mental abnormalities as to be seriously disabled.

A woman discovering that she has an unplanned pregnancy is faced with decisions that are intensely personal and individual to her own circumstances. The pregnancy should be confirmed by undertaking a urinary pregnancy test and, although distressing, if there is any doubt about gestational age, an ultrasound scan should be undertaken. This will confirm dates and is important in determining what form of termination would be undertaken if this is the decision the woman reaches.

Medical/surgical management

Prior to undergoing termination, women should be extensively counselled about the options for their pregnancy. These include continuing with the pregnancy with support, continuing with the pregnancy and then allowing the baby to be adopted or terminating the pregnancy. There are many specialist clinics that can provide counselling and also arrange referral to appropriately licensed centres should a decision be taken to undergo termination.

Following an in-depth consultation and examination with a specialist, once a decision has been made to terminate the pregnancy, there are two alternative management options: surgical or medical.

Surgical TOP

The majority of terminations are carried out surgically before the 12th gestational week by suction dilatation and curettage. This can be carried out as a day-case procedure, which is often convenient for women who may wish to conceal their pregnancy and termination. The procedure is usually carried out under a general anaesthetic and so women must be assessed as fit. Prior to surgery, a gemeprost pessary may be inserted to soften the cervix. The operation involves dilating the cervix and removing the products of conception using suction. After this procedure, women are allowed to recover from the anaesthetic and then discharged home when satisfactory. If a woman's

blood group is Rhesus-negative, she must be given an injection of anti-D immunoglobulin to prevent any sensitization that may affect future pregnancies.

Medical TOP

Mifepristone can be administered in licensed premises for pregnancies up to 63 days of amenorrhea and also in the second trimester, i.e. 13–20 weeks' gestation. This drug causes detachment of the embryo, contractions in the uterine muscle and opening of the cervix by blocking the effect of progesterone. It can be administered as an outpatient and women are then admitted 2 days later for administration of prostaglandin. The care is similar for women who receive gemeprost for a missed miscarriage.

Late TOPs

There are still women who require a termination much later in their pregnancy, e.g. where fetal abnormality has been diagnosed, and in those women and girls who had their pregnancy diagnosed earlier but who may have wished to conceal it, or who have been scared and not known where to get help. In these instances, surgical suction termination is not an option and any surgical procedure will involve destruction of the fetus and removing the products in parts. This is often unacceptable to many health professionals and not offered in many units. Medical termination involves administration of mifepristone followed by vaginal prostaglandins, which induces labour. A woman will require pain relief for this procedure and it can often be extremely distressing.

▶ Nursing management

Women undergoing TOP will need support and a non-judgemental attitude to be demonstrated by nurses. Nurses and other staff who do find it difficult, through personal or religious beliefs, to reconcile this treatment are able to raise their conscientious objection and should not be made to participate in the actual process of termination. However, they could be required to participate in the general care of such women and, if this is a personal problem, they should think extremely carefully before choosing to work in a gynaecology unit where women undergoing TOP are likely to be treated. As mentioned earlier, this is an extremely distressing decision and not one that is made lightly by the woman in question, so she will require a supportive and professional approach from the nursing staff (see Reflective Practice box 25.1, p. 732).

Regardless of the type of termination, patients will require effective pain relief and careful monitoring to ensure there is no excessive bleeding during and following the procedure. It is the nurse who will be caring for these patients and observing them closely for signs of haemorrhage. Any products passed must be closely examined by the nurse to ensure that there are no retained products in the uterus. Individual units will have developed their own guidelines for the length of time women are required to stay after their termination. Nurses must be aware that, although women may be desperate to leave the unit, they must be physically fit and receive appropriate information prior to discharge. There will be a vaginal discharge for several days afterwards and women should use sanitary towels, not tampons,

25.1 Caring for a woman undergoing termination of pregnancy

Caring for a woman who has decided to terminate her pregnancy can be extremely emotive and can often cause health professionals to question the reasons behind the woman's decision.

Imagine a young woman has been admitted to your ward for a termination of her 9-week gestation pregnancy. She is not married, nor does she have a steady relationship. She has a history of depression that has previously been treated with medication but her social circumstances cause her great anxiety and she feels she needs to commence medication again. You are not sure she has thought this action through fully. You have been asked to admit her.

- How do you think the woman will be feeling on admission?
- What is the nurse's role during her admission and lead up to surgery?

- What methods of communication must nurses be aware of when caring for this woman, particularly if they do not agree with the woman's decision?
- How do you think the attitude of the nurse can affect the patient?
- What information do you think is particularly important to be discussed with the woman before she is discharged home?

Student activities

- Obtain and read a copy of the form that, under the Abortion Act 1967, must be completed by two doctors who have examined the woman and agreed to the termination. This details the criteria under which a termination may be legally undertaken.
- Consider which criteria might be applicable to support her decision.
- Discuss with colleagues how you would feel personally if you were caring for this woman.
- Discuss with colleagues how you would deal with a request for information about her surgery from her relatives.

---

to reduce the risk of infection. For this reason, they should also refrain from intercourse whilst bleeding. Their next period should occur 4–6 weeks after the termination. Although the time available to nurses is short, they should, where appropriate, discuss future contraception, especially in cases where the pregnancy was unplanned.

INFECTIONS OF THE FEMALE REPRODUCTIVE TRACT

Sexually transmitted (acquired) infections (STIs) are described below but there are other infections that affect the female genital tract. It is important these are diagnosed and treated appropriately to prevent further complications developing, such as pelvic infection or infertility. These are generally described by the area of the tract they affect.

VAGINITIS

During the reproductive years, the vagina normally produces acid secretions that help to prevent infection. Infections tend to be more common when the pH is modified, such as at puberty or after the menopause, during pregnancy, or with antibiotic therapy, etc. The following are common infections of the vagina:

- Trichomoniasis – caused by the protozoon *Trichomonas vaginalis* (see p. 762 for further detail).
- Candidiasis (thrush) – a fungal infection usually caused by the yeast *Candida albicans* (see p. 762 for further detail).
- Bacterial vaginosis – infection caused by overgrowth of the vaginal commensal microorganisms, such as *Gardnerella vaginalis*. Women complain of a grey-white vaginal discharge that has a 'fishy' odour. The nature of the

discharge can be very distressing and women are embarrassed and acutely aware of the associated odour. This type of infection might be associated with an increased risk of late miscarriage or preterm delivery. Treatment is with oral metronidazole or clindamycin cream vaginally.
- Atrophic vaginitis – occurs in postmenopausal women, causing thin bloodstained discharge. It is essential that cancer of the endometrium is excluded as the cause of postmenopausal bleeding.

CERVICITIS AND ENDOMETRITIS

Sexually transmitted (acquired) infections can cause cervicitis, e.g. gonorrhoea can infect the cervix then ascend to infect the uterus and tubes. Chlamydia can cause the same problems but is often asymptomatic, so women are often not diagnosed. There are now plans to introduce routine screening for chlamydia (see p. 763), particularly in patients undergoing TOP. There are not usually any bacteria occurring naturally in the endometrium. Acute endometritis can develop due to ascending infection from the external genitalia or the presence of retained products of conception, resulting in a smelly vaginal discharge and some abdominal pain. Pus can collect in the uterine cavity (pyometria) and will often require draining surgically. In all cases, antibiotics will be required.

SALPINGITIS AND PELVIC INFLAMMATORY DISEASE

Salpingitis (inflammation/infection affecting the uterine tubes) develops from ascending infection as described above and can cause acute abdominal pain. Early diagnosis is essential, otherwise patients can develop acute inflammation of the tubes or pelvis, a condition known as pelvic inflammatory disease (PID).

In the acute phase, this can result in severe abdominal pain and fever which may require patients to be admitted as an emergency and treated with intravenous antibiotics. Long-term damage to pelvic organs can result, which can cause infertility, among other things.

TOXIC SHOCK SYNDROME

Toxic shock syndrome (TSS) can occur when an infection develops in the genital tract and the bacterial toxins produced cause septicaemia and toxic shock. It has been associated with tampons that have been left in the vagina for extreme lengths of time. The absorption of toxins into the bloodstream can result in multiple organ dysfunction, e.g. renal or liver, and so must be treated promptly (see Special Issues box 25.1 and Ch. 9).

> ▶ **Nursing management: genital infections in women**

Women must be informed about the long-term sequelae of suffering from infections and the need for early diagnosis and treatment. Nurses have a duty to ensure that women understand the importance of sexual health and the impact it can have on general health. Nurses must be able to discuss sexual issues in a frank but professional manner, encouraging patients to respond to open questions.

A non-judgemental attitude is essential, particularly when discussing a woman's sexuality, as not all women will be in steady heterosexual relationships. Support and advice must be given at a time when women may feel particularly embarrassed and worried about the effects on their general health.

OTHER GYNAECOLOGICAL CONDITIONS

ENDOMETRIOSIS

Endometriosis is the deposition of endometrium outside the uterine cavity. This tissue responds to hormonal influences during the menstrual cycle as does normally sited endometrium, resulting in bleeding from the deposits which can cause adhesions.

Aetiology and epidemiology

The true incidence is unknown as symptoms are not always indicative of the severity of the disorder, but it has been estimated at 3–7% of women. There appears to be a higher incidence in higher socioeconomic groups but this may be linked to that social group delaying pregnancy and being more health-conscious. Incidence appears to peak between 30 and 45 years of age and is only ever seen during reproductive years. The actual cause of endometriosis is unknown although there are two theories. The first is that it is caused by the deposition of endometrium in the pelvis that has travelled along the tubes during menstruation instead of being expelled via the cervix, a process known as retrograde menstruation. The second theory is that peritoneal mesothelium undergoes some changes and transforms into tissue similar to endometrium.

 SPECIAL ISSUES

25.1 Toxic shock syndrome

Toxic shock syndrome (TSS) is a rare illness caused by bacterial infection which, although seen in immunocompromised patients, is associated with menstruating women who use high-absorbency tampons. It is not contagious, but if left untreated can cause major complications and even result in death.

The most common bacterium to cause this infection is *Staphylococcus aureus*. Although the use of tampons is not necessarily a cause itself, it is thought to facilitate the condition. This is particularly true for high-absorbency tampons that may be left in the vagina for prolonged periods.

Symptoms can occur suddenly and health professionals should be aware that, although rare, toxic shock might be a cause of the following symptoms:

- pyrexia – 38.8°C or higher
- rash that resembles sunburn
- dizziness and light-headedness
- muscle aches
- watery diarrhoea.

Within 48 hours, if the patient is not admitted to hospital for emergency treatment, the infection will become progressively more severe with hypotension, shock and multiple organ dysfunction which may be fatal (see Ch. 9). Desquamation (peeling of the skin) typically occurs on the palms and soles 1–2 weeks after the onset of the illness.

The woman will require emergency treatment so needs to be admitted urgently. Hypotension must be treated with intravenous fluids, and i.v. antibiotic therapy must be started immediately.

Advice to women

This condition can be prevented by good hygiene whilst menstruating.

- Hands must be washed before inserting a tampon into the vagina particularly if the type used does not have a disposable applicator.
- Tampons should be changed regularly and not just when there is leakage. For this reason, the use of tampons with minimum absorbency should be advocated. Many manufacturers of tampons now include an information leaflet with their product.
- If a woman has ever suffered from TSS, she should not use tampons but instead should use external protection such as pads. The new generation of sanitary pads are extremely absorbent, less bulky and more acceptable to women and should be encouraged.

Pathophysiology

The amount and spread of endometrial deposits in the pelvis vary considerably, from a few restricted to one local area to many seedlings spread throughout the pelvis. The commonest sites are on the ovary, peritoneum of the pouch of Douglas, sigmoid colon, broad ligament and uterosacral ligament, although it can be found on other pelvic structures as well. The deposits can appear as raised cystic structures, commonly brownish-black in colour due to the stale blood contained in them.

Clinical presentation

Clinical presentation varies considerably and, as mentioned previously, severity of symptoms does not always reflect the severity of the disorder. In some women, a diagnosis is made incidentally when they undergo surgery for another reason. One of the commonest symptoms experienced is pelvic pain, which can be linked to periods due to pelvic irritation caused by internal bleeding or can occur at other times due to pelvic adhesions. It can also cause disturbance to the normal menstrual cycle and infertility and it is often diagnosed during infertility investigations for tubal patency.

Specific investigations

The only definitive investigation to diagnose endometriosis is by laparoscopy, where all the pelvic structures can be examined closely to assess the number and location of endometriotic deposits.

Medical/surgical management

Management includes treating the symptoms and, as the condition is oestrogen-dependent, medical treatment is aimed at reducing the secretion of oestrogen or opposing its action. The following therapies can be used to halt the effects but will not completely cure it:

- progestogens – side-effects can include irregular bleeding and weight gain
- combined oral contraceptive pill – taken continuously for 3 months
- danazol – a steroid related to testosterone that has anti-oestrogen and androgenic effects. Side-effects include amenorrhoea, weight gain, hirsutism and deepening of voice. It cannot be given over the long term, owing to the irreversible nature of some of the side-effects.

Surgical treatment is usually now undertaken laparoscopically and the aim is to destroy the lesions. Due to the delicate nature of some of the structures where endometriosis is found, e.g. the colon, bladder or rectum, it is not possible to remove them surgically. New techniques are now used to vaporize the deposits with heat and this can be delivered extremely accurately in the form of diathermy or laser. There are currently studies in progress to assess the efficacy of uterosacral nerve ablation, where the uterosacral nerve is divided to relieve severe pelvic pain.

▶ Nursing management

Initial referral and discussions are carried out on an outpatient basis, so nurses only have a short time available to reassure patients and ensure they have appropriate information if endometriosis is suspected. This can be alarming for patients, particularly because of the possibility that fertility may be affected. A diagnostic laparoscopy can be undertaken as a day-case procedure, but if actual laser treatment is planned to destroy deposits during this operation, patients may require an overnight stay. They may also, in this instance, require bowel preparation, e.g. with sodium picosulfate, a stimulant laxative, on the day before surgery. This will ensure the bowel is empty and reduce the risk of damage during the surgery, particularly if there are deposits on the bowel. The effects can be acutely embarrassing and nurses must be sensitive to patients' feelings. Nurses must ensure that pre- and postoperative care is carried out so that patients are prepared safely for theatre and monitored closely following the operation. Nurses are in an excellent position to provide both physical and psychological care to patients and to support them during treatment.

POLYCYSTIC OVARY SYNDROME

Polycystic ovary syndrome (PCOS) is a complex syndrome characterized by oligomenorrhoea, infertility, hirsutism and sometimes obesity.

Aetiology and epidemiology

Polycystic ovary syndrome is thought to be caused by an abnormal function of the hypothalamo-pituitary-ovarian axis. The normal feedback mechanism does not function properly, resulting in relatively high levels of luteinizing hormone (LH) and low levels of follicle-stimulating hormone (FSH). Oestrogen levels are similar to those in the early follicular phase of the menstrual cycle and as a result women do not ovulate (anovulation). There are abnormalities associated with androgen hormone (testosterone) production, levels in the blood and clearance. There is also reduced sensitivity to insulin and consequently the insulin levels in the blood are raised (hyperinsulinaemia). The actual incidence is unknown, although studies have shown figures of up to 20% of a normal population. Stein and Leventhal first described the syndrome in 1935 and their names are still synonymous with features of the disorder.

Pathophysiology and clinical presentation

The actual pathophysiology of the disorder is unknown although it is thought that there may be some genetic influence that can account for the condition in a proportion of women. The syndrome causes certain symptoms that on their own may not be indicative of the disorder but a combination of them indicates this may be the problem.

Clinical features include one or more of the following:

- menstrual disorders – can range from amenorrhoea/oligomenorrhoea to menorrhagia
- hirsutism
- acne
- obesity
- infertility.

Women find this a particularly embarrassing condition, especially as the androgenizing effects can have a considerable impact on their physical appearance.

Specific investigations

There is no definitive investigation, but diagnosis is usually made on clinical features. In addition, multiple follicular cysts are seen on the ovaries on ultrasound scan. Hormonal blood tests may indicate a raised LH:FSH ratio and abnormal testosterone levels.

Medical/surgical management

Treatment is usually aimed at relieving the symptoms and preventing long-term side-effects such as type 2 diabetes mellitus (see Ch. 17). A woman being investigated for infertility who is not ovulating may be given clomiphene to induce ovulation. If amenorrhoea is a problem, the oral contraceptive pill can be given. Weight loss has been shown to improve symptoms and reduce hirsutism. Cosmetic therapies such as depilatory treatments (e.g. creams or electrolysis) may be effective and are important in increasing a woman's self-esteem. Recently, metformin has been used to manage the hyperinsulinaemia with some success.

Surgical treatment to induce ovulation by removing a wedge of ovarian tissue during an open laparotomy was first described by Stein and Leventhal in 1935. This has since been revived and developed as a laparoscopic procedure whereby laser or diathermy is used to drill holes in the ovary. This procedure, known as ovarian drilling, is thought to reduce androgen levels by releasing androgens from the punctured follicles, which in turn affects the delicate hormonal feedback mechanisms.

▶ Nursing management

The majority of the management of a woman with PCOS will be an outpatient setting and so the nurse must provide support for the woman whilst she undergoes various investigations and treatments. She may need to attend hospital on a regular basis to assess effectiveness of treatment and the nurse must be aware of how distressed the woman may become as she receives the results of investigations and the implications for her future fertility and lifestyle become a reality. Women may need information about and want to discuss ways of dealing with unwanted body hair, particularly that on the face. The woman may require admission for laparoscopy and the nurse's role includes her care before and after surgery (see below). The woman may be suffering from infertility and so sensitivity must be used as for any woman who is experiencing problems with conceiving naturally (see p. 758).

PROBLEMS ASSOCIATED WITH THE CLIMACTERIC AND POSTMENOPAUSAL PROBLEMS

All women approaching the menopause (last period) or 'change', as it is commonly referred to, will be affected by the climacteric, a time when ovarian failure results in a decline in production of female hormones. It is worth remembering, however, that the climacteric is a normal event, even if some women will experience problems. The average age of the menopause is thought to be 50–51 years and this has remained constant over many centuries and across different parts of the world. Premenopausal women who have their ovaries removed

surgically, destroyed with radiotherapy or 'switched off' with drugs (see Ch. 26) will experience the menopause.

Physiological events

Ovarian decline results in a failure to ovulate and consequently the ovary no longer produces progesterone. This affects production of other hormones and for a short time gonadotrophin levels rise but then eventually all ovarian activity ceases. The lack of oestrogen causes the internal genitalia, ovaries, uterus and vagina to shrink. Tissue lining these structures becomes very thin, the vaginal acidity decreases, labia shrink and pubic hair disappears.

Clinical presentation

During the climacteric, women may experience a combination of symptoms, some of which will cause them to seek help from a health professional, including:

- vasomotor symptoms – including hot flushes, night sweats, palpitations, insomnia
- psychological symptoms – including irritability, lack of concentration, reduced libido, depression
- irregular bleeding – including an increase in interval between periods, diminishing periods or missed periods.

The sustained lack of oestrogen can have long-term effects, including:

- atrophy of vaginal and urethral mucosa leading to a decrease in vaginal acidity which increases risk of infection, vaginal dryness and soreness on intercourse (dyspareunia), and urinary symptoms such as urgency, frequency and cystitis (see Ch. 24)
- uterovaginal prolapse (see p. 724) caused by atrophy and changes in pelvic floor muscles and supporting ligaments
- osteoporosis – a reduction in bone mass which makes women more susceptible to fractures (see Ch. 27). The absence of oestrogen causes faster turnover of tissue, which reduces bone mass
- cardiovascular disease – oestrogen is thought to protect women from arterial disease as there is a marked increase in the incidence of coronary heart disease and strokes in postmenopausal women
- changes to hair and skin, and breast atrophy.

Specific investigations

A careful history recording the patient's symptoms will give a good indication that these are due to the menopause. Hormone levels can be checked in a blood test and these will indicate a reduction in oestrogen and progesterone. An increase in FSH may also be seen, although these levels can fluctuate considerably during the climacteric and a single result may not be relied upon.

Physical examination may also provide information about the progress of the symptoms. If osteoporosis is suspected, a bone densiometry scan can be undertaken to detect bone mass.

Medical management

Medical intervention, if required, usually involves hormone replacement therapy (HRT). However, many women feel that the climacteric is a natural progression in their life and may just require advice and information about current signs and symptoms. For others, it is a significant event and they will want help with distressing symptoms such as hot flushes, and to delay the onset of long-term effects. For this group, HRT can be prescribed in various forms, including tablets, skin patches, implants and gels. Topical vaginal creams to counter atrophic changes in the vaginal mucosa are appropriate for some women. As mentioned above, unopposed oestrogen with no progesterone therapy can cause hyperplasia of the endometrium. Consequently, women with an intact uterus must be prescribed combined oestrogen/progesterone HRT, but this may result in a regular bleed which is not acceptable to all. Women who have had a hysterectomy will only require oestrogen.

The only absolute contraindication for HRT is a history of an oestrogen-dependent malignancy such as breast or endometrial cancer. It can also be contraindicated in uncontrolled hypertension and past venous embolism, but each woman's circumstances must be considered individually.

Side-effects are caused by either the oestrogen or progesterone components of the HRT and can include breast tenderness, bloating, fluid retention and headaches. Many women are concerned about developing breast cancer and many studies have been undertaken examining the effect that HRT has on this disease. There does appear to be a slight increase in the risk of developing breast cancer for those on HRT, but it is thought that the prognosis for these cases is better than if the women had not had HRT.

Although the benefits of long-term HRT have been shown particularly in the prevention of osteoporosis and cardiovascular disease, women often start HRT to deal with menopausal symptoms then gradually reduce and discontinue them.

Other drugs used during the climacteric include:

- selective oestrogen receptor modulator (SERM), e.g. raloxifene – used for the prevention and treatment of osteoporosis; it has no effect on vasomotor symptoms
- clonidine (antihypertensive drug) – may reduce hot flushes
- bisphosphonates such as etridonate – used in the management of osteoporosis (see Ch. 27).

Readers should consult the *British National Formulary* (http://www.bnf.org.uk) for more details about individual drugs.

▶ Nursing management

Specialist nurses in both outpatient departments and primary care now run menopause clinics, where they provide advice on how women can deal with their symptoms. Women often find it extremely helpful to talk through their symptoms with a nurse, particularly if that nurse is female. The menopause often occurs at the same time in a woman's life as other significant events, such as children leaving home or elderly parents becoming more reliant on her. There are many different HRT preparations and a woman may have to try several types before she finds one that suits her. She will require considerable support during this time, as she may feel disillusioned if her symptoms persist. Nurses can also monitor any side-effects.

Some women decide to use complementary therapies to alleviate distressing symptoms and nurses should support this decision whilst being mindful that some herbal medicines may interact with prescription medicines. Self-help groups can also be helpful in increasing a woman's control over symptoms and in increasing her self-esteem. Women are often receptive to health education at this time and nurses can take the opportunity to stress the importance of exercise, healthy diet (with sufficient calcium), maintaining correct weight, smoking cessation, maintaining hobbies and interests, and attending for cervical and breast screening (see above and Chs 26 and 33). Women will also need advice about contraception during the perimenopause. Ovulation, and hence conception, may occur after the last period, so women wishing to avoid pregnancy should use contraception for up to 2 years if their last period occurred before the age of 50, or for 1 year if it occurred after the age of 50.

NURSING MANAGEMENT OF PATIENTS UNDERGOING GYNAECOLOGICAL SURGERY

The majority of gynaecological operations are undertaken as planned elective admissions and nurses are able to prepare women both physically and psychologically prior to their admission. Following surgery, women are being discharged back to their family earlier, which speeds recovery and reduces postoperative complications (Taylor et al 1993). Operations are generally classified as major (those that require in-patient admissions, e.g. hysterectomy) or minor (including day-case procedures such as laparoscopy). Further detailed information about perioperative care is provided in Chapter 29.

PREOPERATIVE ASSESSMENT

Preoperative assessment is undertaken prior to admission. This ensures that patients are fit to undergo a general anaesthetic and surgery and gives nurses time to discuss with patients the planned surgery and the relevant risks and benefits. Nurses can reinforce the need to stop smoking or at least to cut down prior to surgery. Thorough psychological preparation of patients will reduce anxiety and aid recovery (Wilson-Barnett 1979). It reduces the need for women to be admitted the day before the planned major surgery.

Nurse-led preoperative assessment clinics have been introduced in many units. Nurses assess women's health status, working within clinical guidelines that recommend when referral to medical staff should be made. Nurses are able to undertake a holistic assessment, looking at women's physical, psychological, social and spiritual needs. However, it is important that nurses are aware of their accountability and responsibility in this area, and they must ensure that they are supported legally by their trust through vicarious liability.

Physical assessment
This ensures women are physically fit to undergo a general anaesthetic and surgery. A health questionnaire can be used for patients to record relevant details, including:

- previous surgical history, noting any problems encountered with anaesthetics

- medical conditions, especially heart or lung problems such as angina or asthma, or hormonal conditions such as diabetes or thyroid disorders. Nurses must check for undiagnosed conditions such as cardiac failure or hypertension
- current medication, particularly any recent corticosteroids. Any hormone preparations must also be noted
- allergies/sensitivities to drugs, additives, latex, and dressings and tapes
- last menstrual period – this must be recorded to prevent surgery being performed on a woman in the early stages of a pregnancy.

Based on these observations, nurses may order further diagnostic investigations such as full blood count, group and save serum, electrocardiogram (ECG) and chest X-ray. Patients may also require auscultation of the heart and lungs, which should only be performed by a doctor or a nurse who has undergone appropriate training (UKCC 1992). Written informed consent must be obtained prior to surgery and in some areas this is now being obtained by nurses who have undergone further education to work at specialist level (UKCC 1992).

Psychological assessment

Admission to hospital for surgery, combined with the perceived effect on a woman's femininity, can be an anxious experience. Nurses must use their experience and skills to support patients by providing them with appropriate information. They must assess how much information each patient requires, as some women may want to know only the minimum about their impending surgery.

Giving details about planned procedures during hospital stay can do much to reduce anxiety, particularly about general anaesthesia. An informed explanation by the nurse, combined with a visit from a member of the theatre staff, can do much to allay these fears (Martin 1996).

Patients are often concerned about postoperative pain. An explanation should be given by the nurse about analgesia options and their administration. Many units now use patient-controlled analgesia (PCA) for gynaecological patients (see Ch. 7).

Social assessment

This should be started at preoperative assessment to enable nurses to give appropriate information to women about planning for their family and work commitments during both the hospitalization and recovery periods. The commencement of discharge planning will allow patients to plan with their partner and family their needs on discharge (Raleigh et al 1990) and they should be given an estimated discharge date. Written information should also be given to reinforce the information discussed.

Spiritual assessment

Gynaecological surgery, especially removal of the reproductive structures, can be very upsetting for many women. It should be remembered that for women of certain beliefs and cultures, having their uterus removed will be a bereavement and they will need time to grieve. Support and time should be given to

enable such women to express any fears, and visits of spiritual advisors from their home environment, if appropriate, should be encouraged.

PREOPERATIVE CARE

On the day of surgery, routine preoperative checks should be made in preparation for theatre. Results of any diagnostic tests must be available for medical staff to review to ensure that patients are still medically fit for surgery. Nurses will have the opportunity to build a rapport with patients by undertaking the unit's normal admission procedure when they arrive. Physical preparation includes:

- Removal of pubic hair – this may be necessary if the incision is going to be along the suprapubic hairline. The risk of infection is reduced by using a depilatory cream, but if a shave is to be performed it should be done on the day of surgery to reduce the colonization of the skin by commensal organisms. Women should be encouraged to perform this themselves if they so wish, but a nurse may need to supervise the procedure.
- Bowel preparation – this is now considered to be unnecessary by many surgeons but depends on the extent of planned surgery. Normal bowel function may be affected postoperatively for a while and so women should not be grossly constipated. Patients often complain of painful wind and constipation following major surgery and this can be difficult to treat if already constipated. In this case, glycerin suppositories the evening before surgery may be helpful. For complex surgery in close proximity to the bowel, preparation with stimulant laxatives may be given to empty the bowel.
- Fasting times – these will depend on local policy (see Ch. 29 for a very full discussion).
- A bath or shower (in hospital, a shower is preferable) – this should be taken prior to surgery to reduce the number of commensal organisms on the skin.

Prior to patients leaving the ward area for the operating theatre, routine checks must be undertaken, including the following:

- The wrist band, which has each patient's name and unique hospital registration number, should be checked against the medical notes and the request slip from the theatre assistant who collects the patient.
- The patient should have a good understanding of what the operation entails and the consent form should have been signed. This must not be done after a premedication has been given, as the patient will suffer from a reduction in mental acuity.
- Loose or crowned teeth noted and dentures would be removed. Any prostheses should also be removed. Spectacles and hearing aids may be removed after the patient is anaesthetized and stored safely until her recovery.
- Premedication should be prescribed if the woman is undergoing major surgery, which may include prophylactic antibiotic therapy and thromboembolic prophylaxis. A mild hypnotic may be given to relax the patient.

POSTOPERATIVE CARE

On return to the ward following surgery, routine observations of vital signs form a baseline, enabling nurses to monitor patient progress closely. The frequency of these recordings will depend on the extent of surgery and include:

- pulse and blood pressure to detect primary haemorrhage
- wound site observed for visible bleeding and the sanitary pad should also be checked for abnormal amounts of bleeding.

Patients who have undergone minor day-case surgery should be encouraged to mobilize when they feel able and should be offered water and then light food such as toast. They should not be discharged until it is clear that there are no ill effects from the surgery and anaesthetic, they are able to tolerate fluids and diet, and have passed urine.

Patients who have undergone major surgery such as hysterectomy will require a more intensive level of postoperative care as they will be more incapacitated by the surgery. They will be unable to tolerate fluids immediately postoperatively and so an intravenous infusion will be in situ to prevent dehydration and to provide vascular access should haemorrhage occur. The nurse must routinely check the rate and type of infusion fluid with the prescribed regimen, inspecting the cannula site for signs of inflammation. An indwelling catheter may be in situ to prevent retention of urine and pressure on the surgical site by an over-full bladder. The catheter and drainage bag should be checked for free drainage and the urine should be checked for volume and colour. Small amounts of concentrated, dark urine may indicate dehydration and haematuria, while obviously bloodstained urine may indicate damage to the bladder or ureters during surgery. If patients are not catheterized, any urine voided must be recorded to observe for urinary retention. A record of all fluid intake and output is maintained.

There may be a vacuum drain in the pelvis postoperatively to prevent a haematoma forming, and the amount and type of exudate drained should be noted (see Ch. 29).

Strong analgesia such as morphine will be administered intravenously either by a continuous syringe driver, the rate of which can be altered by nursing staff, or by a pump that can be controlled by patients themselves. PCA systems enable patients to be in control of their medication. A safety lockout device prevents the system from being operated continuously and delivering an overdose. Morphine can cause nausea and respiratory depression and so both of these side-effects must be monitored closely (see Ch. 7).

On subsequent days, patients should be assisted to return to full self-caring as soon as possible, but will need assistance in mobilizing and meeting their hygiene needs particularly on the first postoperative day. Non-opioid analgesics are usually sufficient. Nurses should reinforce and encourage the deep breathing, abdominal and pelvic floor exercises taught by the physiotherapist. As patients recover, plans can be finalized for discharge.

Women are likely to require a minimum of 6 weeks off work and many require longer. Advice should be given about increasing their activity at home. It is important they do not adopt the role of 'invalid' once home, as further complications might occur.

 HEALTH PROMOTION

25.1 Discharge following day-case gynaecological surgery

Information to be given to patients will be mainly linked to recovery from the anaesthetic. The following are recommended guidelines used in most day-case units:

- The woman should have tolerated fluids and light diet before discharge.
- She must have passed urine prior to leaving the ward.
- Explanation must be given that the anaesthetic may take 24–48 hours to be cleared from the body.
- A responsible adult must accompany the patient home in case she collapses on way home.
- A responsible adult must accompany the patient the night after surgery in case she is taken ill during the night. She should not be alone with young children for this reason.
- The woman must have ready access to a phone overnight and contact numbers, should help or advice be needed.
- Extra care should be taken for 24–48 hours after the operation in circumstances such as driving a car, drinking alcohol or operating machinery as the anaesthetic can affect coordination and reflexes.

- The woman should arrange to have some pain-killers in the house such as paracetamol or ibuprofen.
- Women who have undergone laparoscopy must be warned of potential referred shoulder pain as well as abdominal pain. This is due to carbon dioxide used during the operation collecting under and irritating the diaphragm.
- Advice should be given about care of a wound, what type of sutures have been used and, if they need removing, when she should visit her practice nurse for this.
- The woman will be likely to have vaginal loss and should be advised not to use tampons initially because of the risk of infection. This is particularly relevant if she has had any surgery to the cervix. In this instance, she should be advised to refrain from sexual intercourse and using tampons for 6 weeks.
- She may be able to return to work after 2–3 days depending on the type of surgery she has had. Often women who have undergone laparoscopy require up to a week to recuperate fully and she should be warned that she might feel tired for a few days due to the anaesthetic.

Postoperative discharge advice

Patients will require information about how they should expect to feel and about their recovery prior to discharge. Nurses will be able to reassure them and give them guidance in language they and their family members can understand. This will differ according to the type of surgery. For advice after day-care surgery, see Health Promotion box 25.1. Discussion should be backed up with appropriate written material.

Women who have had major surgery are likely to be discharged several days after the operation depending on the surgery involved. The discharge information and advice are discussed with patients to ensure that they are adequately prepared for discharge and, again, written material is provided (see Health Promotion box 25.2).

Postoperative complications

Complications can occur following gynaecological surgery and, although not common, nurses must be aware of the relevant signs and symptoms to ensure early intervention and treatment (Table 25.3, p. 740). They can occur in hospital or at home and patients may have to return to the ward after discharge for reassurance and monitoring.

 HEALTH PROMOTION

25.2 Discharge advice after major gynaecological surgery

The advice and information given to women going home after major surgery will depend on the type and extent of surgery, but will include:

- That she will be reviewed either in the outpatient clinic or, increasingly, at her own GP's surgery 6 weeks after her operation to ensure healing is complete. This appointment should be arranged before she leaves.
- Any drugs she needs to continue at home, such as a course of antibiotics, should be prescribed and given to the woman with a full explanation about how she should take them. Any of her own drugs she has brought in with her should be returned to her.
- Advice about the care of her wound is important, and in clean, healing wounds there is usually no need to wear a dressing. However, the area should be carefully dried after bathing. She should be warned that the wound may itch for several months and if she is worried to contact the practice nurse.
- Arrangements should be made for removing sutures if there are any still in situ.
- Alteration to diet, reduction in normal pattern of exercise and analgesia containing codeine increase the risks of the woman becoming constipated. It may be painful if she has to strain at stool and can cause damage to surgery such as posterior vaginal repairs. Advice should be given about drinking sufficient water, taking a high-fibre diet and being alert for the development of constipation.
- It is important that the woman does not return home and become an invalid. She should continue abdominal/pelvic floor exercises as advised by the physiotherapist. Exercise should be encouraged in small amounts, increasing on a regular basis, as she feels stronger. Walking is an excellent mode of exercise but the woman should be advised not to walk too far at first, as she will have to walk back home when she may feel extremely tired. If she participates in regular exercise such as aerobics or tennis, she will be able to return to these by 6 weeks. Swimming should be avoided until the wound has healed completely because of the risk of infection.
- Driving a motor vehicle should not be attempted until the woman is able to sit comfortably in the driver's seat and practise an emergency stop, at least 2–3 weeks after she has gone home. This procedure may cause abdominal discomfort and the natural response may be to lift the leg from the brake pedal to protect the abdomen. This is not recommended during this procedure! It may be useful for the woman to check with her insurance company whether there are any restrictions on her policy whilst she is convalescing.
- After 6 weeks, most major surgical sites have healed completely. However, after a hysterectomy some women will still feel tired and, if they have a physically demanding job, may require up to 10–12 weeks away from work to convalesce fully.
- Sexual intercourse should be avoided for 6 weeks if there has been vaginal surgery, particularly to the vaginal vault as in TAH. When the woman does resume sexual relations, she should be encouraged to take the lead and feel in control, as she may be apprehensive about discomfort.
- It is important that she returns to normal family life as soon as possible. This is an excellent opportunity for her family to repay all the hard work she has done over the years for them, by pampering her and doing the housework and cooking. She should be advised against any heavy lifting or vacuuming for at least a month, but can then start to increase the activities as she is able. Ironing can be done sitting down but is much better if she can get the family to do it for her!

Table 25.3 Postoperative complications – gynaecological surgery

Complication	Cause	Observations, signs and symptoms, and management
Primary haemorrhage	This can occur after any surgery due to incomplete haemostasis	Regular observations of pulse, blood pressure, vaginal loss and wound site must be carried out postoperatively to detect any signs of surgical shock. Any such changes in the woman's condition must be reported to medical staff. Fluid intake must be increased and an intravenous infusion should be initiated if not already in place
Uterine perforation	This may occur when an instrument is introduced into the endometrial cavity. The instrument may be pushed through the fundus of the uterus, causing a perforation. If this is noted at the time it occurs, a laparoscopy may be performed to assess the extent of the perforation	Frequent observations of pulse, blood pressure and abdominal discomfort must be carried out postoperatively. Uterine perforations usually resolve spontaneously. Prophylactic antibiotics may be prescribed
Bowel and bladder perforation	These can occur either during open abdominal surgery or laparoscopy due to the close proximity of the pelvic organs	The nurse must closely observe the woman's general condition, urinary output, pulse and blood pressure. Peritonitis may develop after bowel perforation and, as this is a potentially life-threatening complication, urgent treatment may be required. A urinary catheter will be required in the case of bladder perforation. Antibiotics will be prescribed to resolve any infection
Urinary retention	Can develop postoperatively as oedema; sutures and handling of the organs can all contribute to bladder dysfunction	Urinary output postoperatively must be recorded and if the woman is unable to void urine, it may be necessary to pass a urinary catheter. Nursing staff in many units are now trained to use a bladder scanner in order to assess the amount of urine in a woman's bladder without having to insert a catheter
Urinary tract infection	Can develop after bladder catheterization or if the woman is unable to empty her bladder fully following surgery	Signs include dysuria, frequency, burning and stinging on micturition, difficulty initiating micturition and incomplete emptying of the bladder. A midstream specimen of urine should be sent for microscopic examination and culture to confirm the presence of infection. Antibiotics specific to the bacteria cultured should be prescribed
Chest infection	Risk factors include prolonged anaesthetic, underlying chest conditions such as chronic bronchitis or asthma, smoking, reduced mobility and shallow breathing due to abdominal pain	Prevention or risk minimization is essential, such as smoking cessation, effective pain management, early mobilization and physiotherapy. Nurses need to be alert to changes in breathing patterns, cough (with or without sputum) and pyrexia. Antibiotics and physiotherapy will be prescribed and nurses can ensure that women support an abdominal wound during coughing in order to reduce discomfort. The increase in abdominal pressure caused by coughing postoperatively can be detrimental to any vaginal repair surgery
Wound infection – may occur at any surgical site		Signs to observe for include inflammation – redness, swelling, pain and there may be exudate apparent at the site. A swab for microbiological examination should be taken of any exudate present and the area kept clean and dry. Specific antibiotics should be prescribed and the wound checked daily
Deep vein thrombosis (DVT) and pulmonary embolism (PE)	Can develop following abdominal and pelvic surgery. Guidelines produced by the Royal College of Obstetricians and Gynaecologists for thromboembolic prophylaxis assist in identifying risk factors and appropriate treatment (RCOG 1995) (see Chs 19 and 29)	Preoperative precautions such as anti-thromboembolic stockings and/or subcutaneous heparin can minimize risks. Signs of DVT include pain, inflammation, swelling and redness in the calf, but signs may be minimal or absent, particularly when the pelvic veins are involved. Treatment includes i.v. heparin and then oral warfarin. PE may present as chest pain or the woman may collapse, suffering a cardiac arrest. Complaints of chest pain especially postoperatively must be investigated thoroughly

(Cont'd)

Table 25.3 *(cont'd)*

Complication	Cause	Observations, signs and symptoms, and management
Anaemia	Caused by blood loss during or immediately after surgery	A full blood count should be checked and iron therapy is recommended, especially if the woman has undergone a hysterectomy. She will no longer be losing menstrual blood and her body will be able to restore haemoglobin levels during convalescence. A blood transfusion is only indicated if the haemoglobin level is excessively low due to the associated risks of blood-borne infections
Secondary haemorrhage	Can occur at surgical sites 10–14 days postoperatively due to infection	Readmission and haemostasis may be required if haemorrhage is excessive, but usually treatment of the infection with broad-spectrum antibiotics is sufficient

MEN'S HEALTH

ANATOMY AND PHYSIOLOGY OF THE MALE REPRODUCTIVE TRACT – AN OVERVIEW

The male reproductive tract consists of the testes, scrotum, vas deferens (ductus deferens), ejaculatory ducts, prostate, urethra, penis, their accessory ducts and glands, and an extensive venous and nerve plexus (see Fig. 25.13).

The two testes (testicles) are the primary sex organs (gonads) of the male. During embryological development, the testes are located near the kidneys. By 35–40 weeks' gestation they have moved from the abdomen to the scrotal sac. The migration appears to occur independently of hormones, i.e. as the fetus grows or enlarges, the attachment of the testes in the body draws them down into the scrotum. However, a specific hormone, müllerian-inhibiting hormone (MIH), may play a role, since absence of MIH is related to failure to descend.

The function of the testes is to produce sperm (spermatozoa), i.e. spermatogenesis (see pp. 742–743) and hormone production. The scrotum, ducts, glands and the penis are termed the accessory reproductive organs, since they assist the passage and delivery of sperm to the female reproductive tract.

TESTES

The testes (singular: testis) are each suspended by a spermatic cord within the scrotum (a bag of pigmented skin and fibrous tissue) on the exterior of the male body. The spermatic cord, which passes through the inguinal canal, encloses blood vessels, lymphatics, nerves supplying the testes, and the vas deferens.

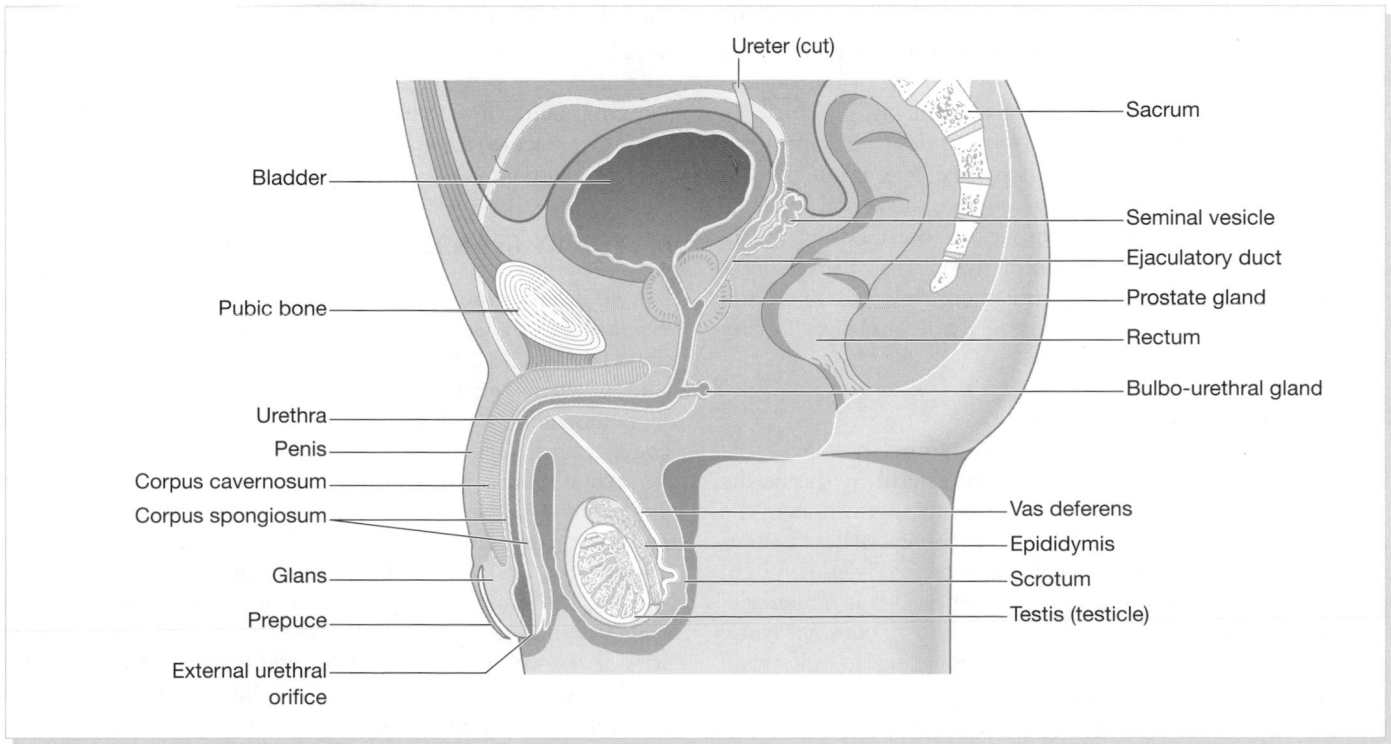

Figure 25.13 The male reproductive tract.

Sperm production and survival are dependent on a constant temperature around 4–7°C less than 'core' body temperature – hence the position of the testes in the scrotum. The testes are not affected by increased core temperature since there is a system of heat exchange. As the warmer arterial blood enters the testis, the proximity of the veins is such that heat moves from the artery to the cooler venous blood from the scrotum. Cooling of the testes is further augmented by extensive sweat glands in the scrotum. Although this anatomical location has physiological benefits in keeping the testes cool, there is an increased risk of a testis rotating, causing obstruction of the blood supply; this is known as torsion (see p. 750).

The oval-shaped testes are approximately 4 cm long and 2 cm in diameter and should normally feel smooth. The testes is covered by the tunica vaginalis (a double membrane) and the fibrous tunica albuginea (see Fig. 25.14).

The testes produce spermatozoa (spermatogenesis, see Fig. 25.15A) and hormones. Spermatozoa pass on the male's genetic material, while the hormones maintain reproductive function. Androgens are the most important of these hormones, e.g. testosterone; however, oestrogens, inhibin and activin are also produced. The testes are complex organs allowing distinct production of two separate activities. This is achieved through anatomical compartmentation of the testes.

Sperm develop in the tubules in association with Sertoli cells that support and nourish the sperm-producing germ cells, whereas androgens are made between the tubules in the Leydig cells (interstitial cells). A barrier that develops at puberty, called the blood–testis barrier, separates these two compartments. This barrier is permeable to some fluids and electrolytes, but is functionally significant in that it prevents sperm from leaking out into the systemic and lymphatic circulation that would elicit an immune response (Johnson & Everitt 1995).

This barrier also allows the sperm to mature in a carefully controlled environment. The maturation of sperm is called spermiogenesis and involves the change in shape of the spermatocytes (sperm cell) into the characteristic form (see Fig. 25.15B). Spermatocytes drain into seminiferous tubules that converge to form a tubulus rectus that allows passage of sperm into the rete testis. Sperm exit the testis through efferent ducts and enter the epididymis (coiled tubule on the back of the testis). The epididymis assists in the maturation of the sperm so that after a stay of approximately 20 days, the sperm have matured and become motile. At ejaculation, the epididymis contracts, forcing the sperm into the vas deferens.

Testicular hormone production

The main testicular androgen is testosterone. It is a steroid hormone formed from acetate and cholesterol in the Leydig cells. Testosterone is responsible for initiating maturation of the reproductive organs, secondary sexual characteristics, such as hair distribution and deepening of the voice, and is also thought to be involved in libido (sex drive), although this is a matter of conjecture, since low serum testosterone *per se* does not cause erectile dysfunction. In addition, testosterone exerts widespread anabolic (growth-promoting) effects.

Approximately 10 mg of testosterone is secreted every day into the bloodstream, although some also enters the lymphatic system. This lymphatic drainage allows testosterone to enter the

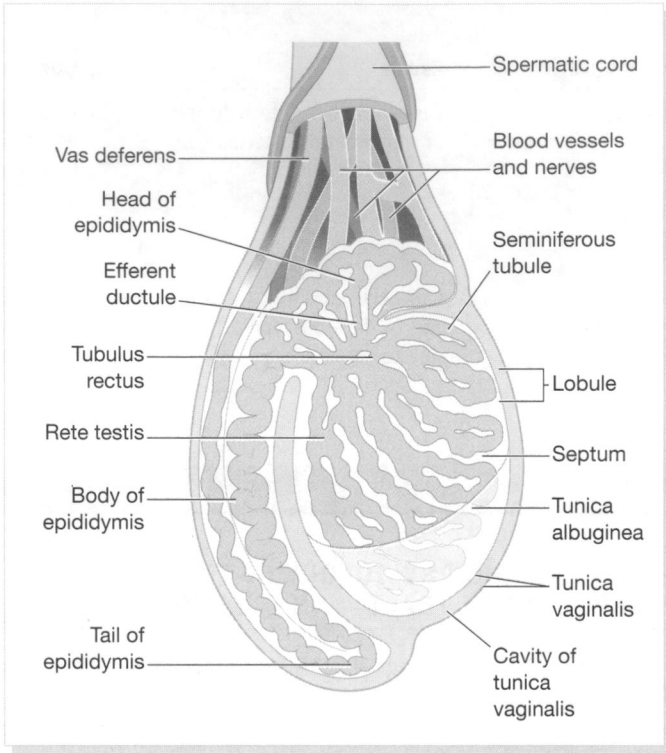

Figure 25.14 Testis (sagittal section of testis and associated epididymis).

male accessory glands. In addition, testosterone is lipid-soluble, which means that it easily crosses the cellular barriers and enters the seminiferous tubules.

A large proportion of testosterone is converted to dihydrotestosterone by the enzyme 5-alpha-reductase in Sertoli cells. Note that one of the theories for prostatic enlargement is hormone dependency: a common treatment modality is by 5-alpha-reductase inhibitors.

ACCESSORY GLANDS AND DUCT SYSTEM

The vas deferens (also called the vas or ductus deferens) delivers the sperm to the seminal vesicles that lie behind the prostate gland (see Fig. 25.13). Secretion from the seminal vesicles contains nutrients, enzymes and prostaglandins, and contributes approximately 60% of the volume of semen (fluid plus sperm). The sperm then enters the ejaculatory duct that passes through the prostate gland, emptying into the urethra.

The prostate (see also Ch. 24) is a firm body that is part glandular, part muscular and is situated immediately below the urinary bladder, at the commencement of the urethra. The prostate gland secretes enzymes, including fibrinolysin, an acid phosphatase that 'activates' the sperm, and forms around 30% of the volume of semen. In addition, the bulbourethral gland (Cowper's gland) secretes a fluid that 'neutralizes' the acid left over in the urethra from urine. The pH of the semen is slightly alkali to combat the remaining acid in the urethra and vagina.

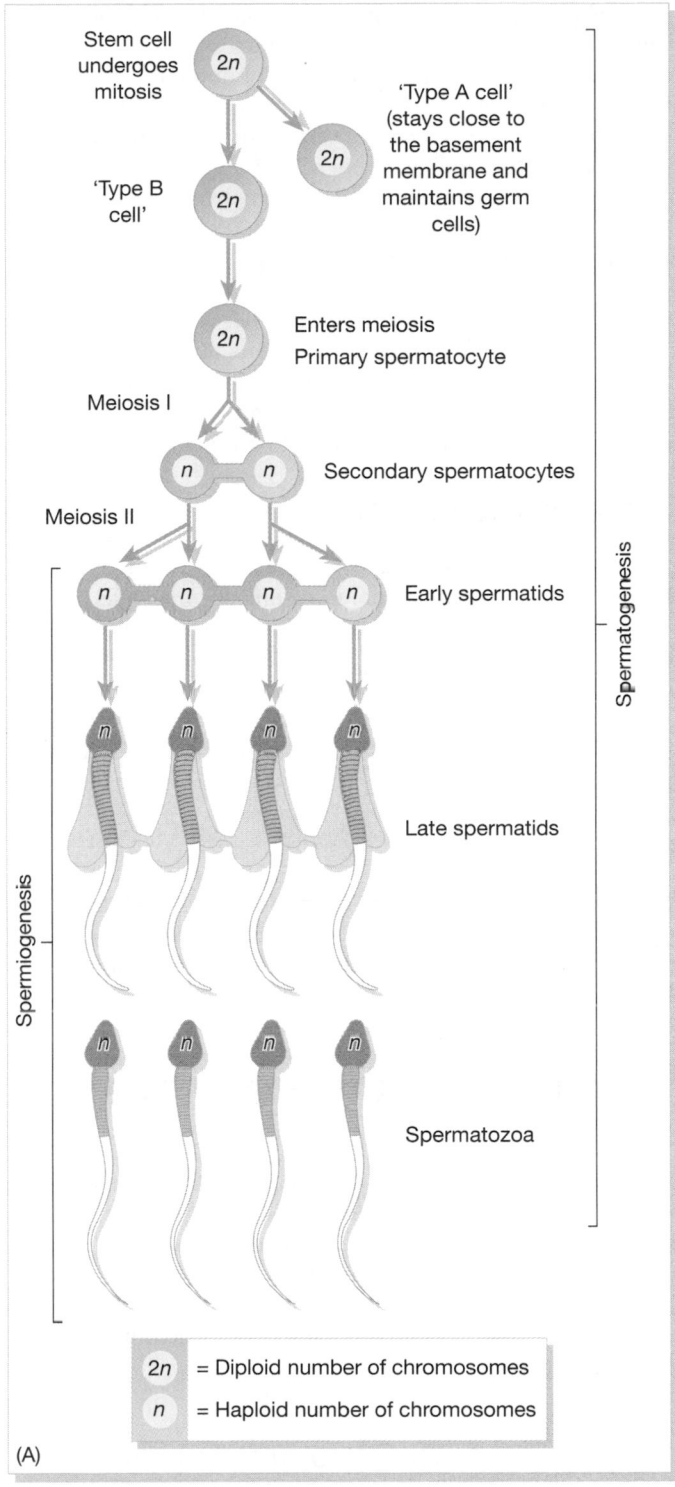

(A)

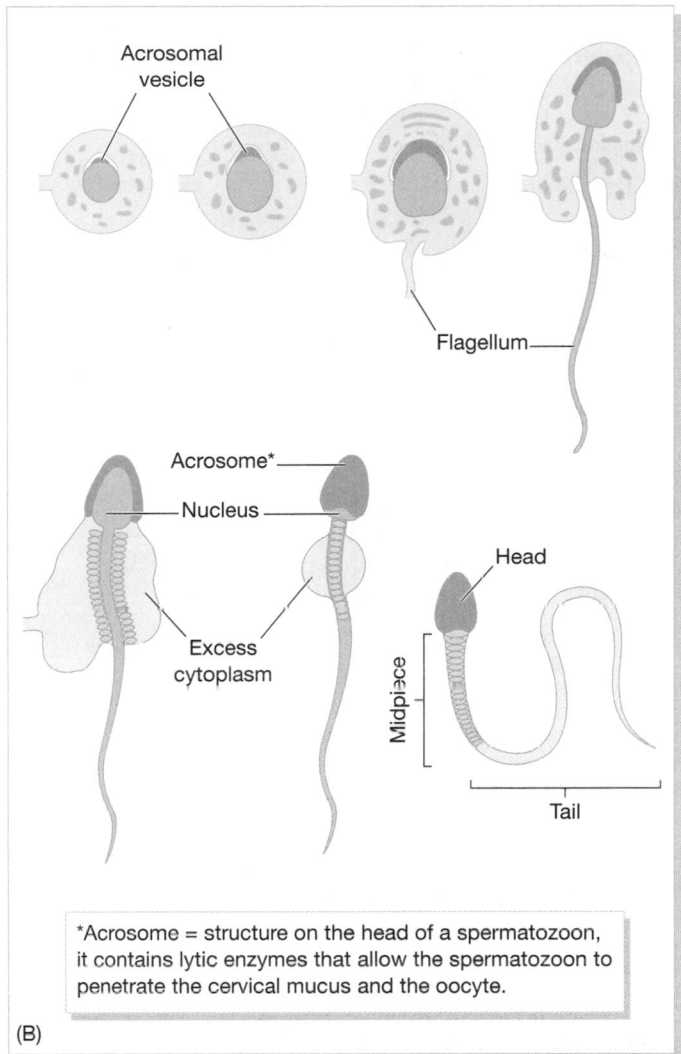

*Acrosome = structure on the head of a spermatozoon, it contains lytic enzymes that allow the spermatozoon to penetrate the cervical mucus and the oocyte.

(B)

Figure 25.15 Sperm production. (A) Spermatogenesis; (B) spermiogenesis – from cell to functional sperm.

The normal volume of ejaculate is approximately 5 mL, containing 50–150 million sperm/mL and secretions from the seminal vesicles and prostate. Sperm production continues throughout the lifetime and hence there is a continued ability to remain fertile despite increased age. Although the volume of semen and the number of sperm decrease as the frequency of ejaculation increases, the quality of the semen may improve in that semen that has remained in the vas for long periods of time loses motility.

PENIS

The penis, through which the spongy (penile) urethra runs, has a root embedded in the perineum and a body/shaft that terminates at the glans penis. The glans is normally converted with a loose double fold of skin known as the prepuce (foreskin). Note that, in some cultures, removal of the prepuce, known as circumcision, is routinely performed, and that in these cultures penile cancer is extremely rare; however, such surgery is not without complications (see p. 752).

The penis consists of three columns of erectile tissue – a single corpus spongiosum and paired corpus cavernosum – that contain vascular spaces, connective tissue and involuntary muscle (see Fig. 25.16, p. 744). It is the corpora cavernosa that fill with blood from the pudendal artery during erection.

Physiology of penile erection

The physiology of erections is poorly understood. However, a blood supply, nerve supply and desire are 'core' components of the erectile response. Erection is not essential for ejaculation.

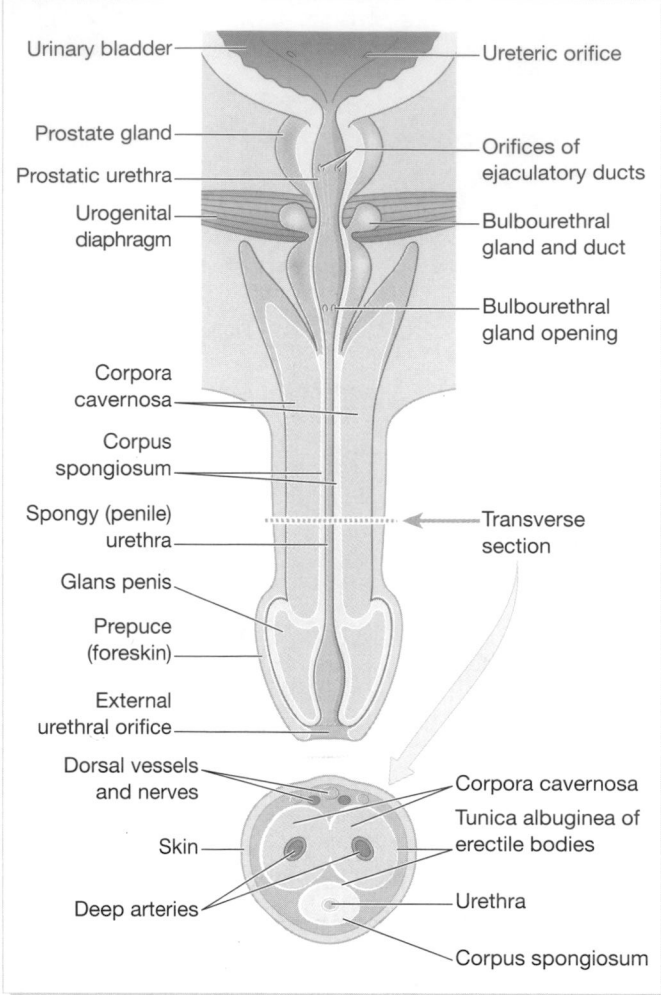

Urinary bladder
Prostate gland
Prostatic urethra
Urogenital diaphragm
Corpora cavernosa
Corpus spongiosum
Spongy (penile) urethra
Glans penis
Prepuce (foreskin)
External urethral orifice
Dorsal vessels and nerves
Skin
Deep arteries

Ureteric orifice
Orifices of ejaculatory ducts
Bulbourethral gland and duct
Bulbourethral gland opening
Transverse section
Corpora cavernosa
Tunica albuginea of erectile bodies
Urethra
Corpus spongiosum

Figure 25.16 Structure of the penis (longitudinal–coronal).

Erection depends on adequate filling of blood at or near systolic blood pressure as well as various muscles that increase the strength of the erection above that attainable by blood pressure. Erections occur when the arteries dilate, allowing increased blood flow in to the corpora cavernosa, resulting in engorgement of the penis. Chemical modulators, such as nitric oxide, mediate part of this response and currently treatment options are focused on the action of these chemicals.

NURSING ASSESSMENT

Nursing assessment in men's health is often related to the specific condition that the man presents with. Often, a general history of the presenting complaint will reveal the nature of the problem, e.g. pain in the testis may indicate torsion, treatment for hypertension may cause erectile dysfunction, etc. However, many of the conditions discussed in this section may be in addition to the presenting complaint. Focused questioning may elicit a previously undiagnosed issue, and therefore knowledge of the common side-effects of treatments or medication will provide valuable tools for assessment.

The ability to carry out a holistic nursing history and assessment is an important tool, allowing nurses to take account of individual physical, psychological, social and cultural circumstances. All of these can influence a patient's reproductive and sexual health. Nurses need the skills to question sensitively, thus ensuring that embarrassment and emotional distress are minimized and the data obtained are complete.

PHYSICAL ASSESSMENT

Nurses should note the general appearance of the patient, such as signs of weight loss, pallor or obvious discomfort. Routine measurements of weight and baseline vital signs and urinalysis are undertaken. Physical examination, e.g. of the testes, will be undertaken by either the medical staff or a specialist nurse.

PSYCHOLOGICAL ASSESSMENT

Psychological state should form part of the assessment. However, nurses can anticipate some anxieties, such as the fear of cancer, change in body image or loss of sexual function, and offer support by giving clear explanations about investigations and treatment and providing opportunities for patients and their families to ask questions. Some patients derive benefit from contact with an appropriate self-help group and nurses can give them contact details.

SOCIAL ASSESSMENT

Nurses should ascertain who patients live with and the extent of their support networks. In some situations (e.g. a STI or infertility), a sexual history will be taken, and again this requires skill and sensitivity.

GENERAL DIAGNOSTIC TESTS AND MEDICAL INVESTIGATIONS

Each condition warrants specific tests and investigations in addition to history and examination. Table 25.4 shows some general investigations that may assist in diagnosis; however, specific tests are detailed in the accompanying text. Nurses should be familiar with the preparation and procedure for general diagnostic tests so that they can give patients sufficient information about what to expect.

DISEASE PREVENTION AND HEALTH PROMOTION

Men's health is generally undervalued, by men themselves and by the providers of health care. Yet it is clear that men die, on average, 6 years earlier than women, are three and a half times more likely to die from coronary heart disease under the age of 65 (see Ch. 19), have a suicide rate at least double that of women, are more likely to smoke, drink alcohol and be overweight and are more likely to contract HIV/AIDS. These statistics reflect that men are greater risk-takers than women. This is also reflected in health care services, as men are less likely to turn up for health checks than women and are more likely to

Table 25.4 General diagnostic tests – men's health

Investigation	Indication	Significance
Urine test, e.g. midstream specimen of urine	Detect presence of infection	May detect presence of infection, blood or indicate the nutritional/hydration status of the patient
Blood tests		
Full blood count	Detect elevation in white cell count	Elevated white cells in the presence of infections
Urea/electrolytes	Assess renal function	Should be normal provided the kidneys are not compromised
Hormone profile	Specific hormone assays are available to assist in diagnosis, e.g. testosterone for erectile dysfunction	Depends on the condition, but may assist in diagnosis
Alpha-fetoprotein (AFP), lactate dehydrogenase (LDH) and β-hCG	AFP, LDH and β-hCG are tumour markers for some testicular cancers	The amounts in the serum can be used to monitor disease progression and response to treatment
Ultrasound scans (USS), computed tomography (CT)	Assessment of genitourinary system	May indicate the presence of a tumour in the testes, for example
Biopsy	Assess histology	Allows staging and grading of tumours

be seriously ill before accessing health care. Men also generally take fewer steps to improve their health. These differences are also affected by social status, which demonstrates inequalities in health between men and women and between health and wealth.

If men's health is to improve, it is important for health and social policy to be targeted specifically at men. Any health initiative, however, must be based on men's own expectations, beliefs and experiences of health and must not be from the perspective of the health professionals.

Public policy initiatives should be considered in order to reach more of the population, and strategies should be developed for health promotion delivery in appropriate settings such as places of employment, sport and fitness venues and social environments. Local drop-in centres should be developed with the involvement of men, who should be consulted on their perceived needs. Informal approaches, e.g. using humour, to allay fears and reduce the risk of embarrassing situations can be a useful strategy. It is also critical that liaison between men and health care professionals be central to all decision-making strategies.

Many opportunities exist for carrying out health-related work with men, but barriers do exist amongst men and health care workers, and within policies and society. However, it is clear that men are now more motivated to improve their health and that many health professionals are breaking down the barriers. It is clear that social and health policies are improving men's health and that health professionals have a better chance than before to ensure that men are given the health care they need and that inclusive strategies of health promotion and education are slowly evolving.

TESTICULAR PROBLEMS

TESTICULAR CANCER

Testicular cancer is relatively rare but represents the most common malignancy in males under 35 years of age (Brewster 2001). It is one of the most curable solid tumours and its current treatment serves as a useful framework for the combination therapy advocated in the treatment of other malignancies (see Ch. 33).

Improvements in survival in testicular cancer have been attributed to effective diagnostic techniques, improved tumour markers, effective medication and modifications in surgical technique. There has been a decrease in patient mortality from more than 50% before 1970 to less than 10% in 1996 (Ritchie 1998).

The testes contain several types of cells, each of which may develop into one or more types of cancer. It is important to distinguish these types of cancer from one another because they differ in their prognosis (the outlook for chances of survival) and in the ways they are treated.

Epidemiology and aetiology

The incidence of testicular cancer has been found by Power et al (2001) to be increasing in England and Wales, which is consistent with the increases seen in other developed countries. However, the average annual rate (age-adjusted) of testicular cancer is highest in Scandinavia (Denmark, Norway), Switzerland, Germany and New Zealand; intermediate in the USA and the UK; and low in Africa and Asia (Muir & Nectoux 1979). It is rare before puberty and commonly occurs in the mid-20s; 1 in 10 tumours occurs in association with cryptorchism (undescended testis) (Blandy 1998). Approximately 2–3% of testicular tumours are bilateral, occurring either simultaneously or successively.

Factors implicated in the development of testicular cancer are described below.

Age
Overall, the highest incidence is noted in 20- to 40-year-old men, making these cancers the most common solid tumour in men between 20 and 34 years of age and the second most common in the age group 35–40 years in the USA and UK (Ritchie 1998). Germ cell tumours commonly occur in the 20–45 year age group, whereas seminomas occur in the 35–45 year age group. Yolk sac tumours have been found in males less than 10 years, and lymphomas can occur in men over 60 years of age.

Racial
White males are four times more likely to develop testicular cancer than black males. The incidence in African-Americans is approximately one-third that of whites, but 10 times that in black Africans. In Israel, Jewish men have around an eight-fold higher incidence of testicular tumours in comparison with non-Jews (Ritchie 1998).

Genetics
Nicholson & Harland (1995) reported that one-third of all testis cancer patients are genetically predisposed to the disease.

Hormones
James (2000) has suggested that testicular cancer may be related to a suboptimal androgen level.

Pathophysiology
Cancer may arise from any of the cell types in the testis but the most common cancers arise from germ cells. Over 90% of testicular cancers develop in germ cells ('germ' = seed; the term refers to the role of male germ cells in producing sperm cells). There are two main types of germ cell tumours (GCTs) in men: seminomas and non-seminomas. Many testicular cancers contain features of both types. Because of the way these mixed tumours grow, spread and respond to treatment, they are classified as being non-seminomas.

Most invasive testicular germ cell cancers begin as a non-invasive form of the disease called carcinoma in situ (CIS) or intratubular germ cell neoplasia. It is estimated that it takes about 5 years for CIS to progress to the invasive form of germ cell cancer. When a cancer becomes invasive, its cells have penetrated the surrounding tissues and may have spread through either the blood or the lymphatics to other parts of the body.

The involvement of the epididymis or spermatic cord may lead to pelvic and inguinal lymph node metastasis, whereas tumours confined to the testis usually spread to retroperitoneal (behind the peritoneum) nodes. The progression of the disease has been summarized as follows (Ritchie 1998):

- Spontaneous progressions are rare.
- Germinal testis tumours should be considered malignant.

- Local spread to the epididymis or spermatic cord occurs in around 10–15% of patients, and increases the risks of lymphatic or blood-borne metastasis.
- Lymphatic metastasis is common to all forms of testis tumours.
- Distant metastasis results from either direct vascular invasion or tumour emboli from lymphatic metastasis.

Seminoma
About half of all testicular germ cell cancers are seminomas. They develop from the sperm-producing germ cells of the testis. There are two main subtypes of these tumours, distinguished by their appearance under the microscope: typical (or classic) seminomas and spermatocytic seminomas. Over 90% of seminomas are of the typical subgroup. Most spermatocytic tumours grow very slowly and usually do not metastasize (spread to other parts of the body). The average age of men who are diagnosed with spermatocytic seminoma is 65 years, about 15 years older than the average age of men with typical seminomas.

Non-seminoma germ cell cancer
These cancers tend to develop earlier in life than seminomas, usually occurring in men in their 20s. The main types of non-seminoma germ cell cancers are embryonal carcinoma, yolk sac carcinoma, choriocarcinoma and teratoma. Most tumours are mixed and have at least two different cell types. This does not change treatment. All non-seminoma germ cell cancers are treated in the same way. This means that the exact type of non-seminomatous testicular cancer a person has is not that important.

Stromal tumours
Tumours can also arise in the supportive and hormone-producing tissues, or stroma, of the testes. Such tumours are known as gonadal stromal tumours. They account for 4% of adult testicular tumours. The two main types are Leydig cell tumours and Sertoli cell tumours.

Leydig cell tumours
These develop from normal hormone-producing Leydig cells. They often produce androgens, but in some cases produce oestrogens (female sex hormones). Although most Leydig cell tumours do not spread beyond the testis and are cured by surgical removal, a small number do metastasize. Metastatic Leydig cell tumours have a poor prognosis, since they do not respond well to chemotherapy or radiotherapy.

Sertoli cell tumours
These develop from normal Sertoli cells. As is the case with Leydig cell tumours, they are usually benign, but if they spread they tend to be resistant to chemotherapy and radiotherapy.

Secondary testicular tumours
Secondary testicular tumours are those that start in another organ and then spread to the testis. Lymphoma is the most common secondary testicular cancer. The prognosis depends on the type and stage of lymphoma. The usual treatment is surgical removal, followed by radiation and/or chemotherapy. Cancers

of the prostate, lung, skin (melanoma), kidney and other organs can spread to the testes. The prognosis for these cancers is usually poor because they generally spread widely to other organs as well. Treatment depends on the specific type of cancer.

Clinical presentation

Presentation is usually with a lump or painless swelling in one testis, which may have been found incidentally by the patient himself or his sexual partner. The 'classic' description is that of a lump, swelling or hardness of the testis. Approximately 30–40% of patients complain of a dull ache or heavy sensation in the lower abdomen, anal or scrotal area. In addition, patients may present with gynaecomastia (breast development), back pain or inflammation (Blandy 1998). Only in around 10% of patients is pain the presenting feature, and on rare occasions infertility is the presenting feature (Ritchie 1998).

Specific investigations

Diagnosis is by examination, blood tests, ultrasound, computed tomography (CT) scan and exploration. Examination of the testis is by palpation between thumb and forefingers. The 'normal' testis is homogenous (smooth) in consistency, freely movable, and separate from the epididymis. Any firm, hard or fixed area within the testis should be considered suspicious.

Ultrasound is a rapid, non-invasive and reliable technique that excludes hydrocele or epididymitis (see p. 750) and should be used in patients suspected of having a testicular tumour. In addition, a CT scan would be used to identify lymph node and pulmonary metastases. Most patients will undergo chest X-ray to identify metastases.

Tumour markers alpha-fetoprotein (AFP), lactate dehydrogenase (LDH) and beta-human chorionic gonadotrophin (β-hCG), which are secreted by yolk-sac cells and trophoblastic cells, should be assessed. In patients with non-seminomatous testis tumour, approximately 60% will have increased AFP and approximately 50% increased β-hCG. Sensitivity of any test or marker varies with the amount of tumour burden. Determinations of AFP and β-hCG, together with other staging modalities, have helped to reduce the understaging error in testis tumours markedly.

Staging of testicular cancers is by the TNM (tumour, nodes, metastasis) classification (see Ch. 33).

- T stage – determined after histological examination of the entire testis
- N stage – lymphatic spread occurs via the testicular vessels that drain to the para-aortic (near to the aorta) lymph nodes at the level of the origin of the renal arteries; CT scan can assess such involvement
- M stage – venous spread can occur early in the disease, typically to the lungs, liver and bone if trophoblastic elements are present.

The tumour size and the amount of disease found in the lymph nodes and/or other body systems assist the medical staff in determining the disease stage. TNM staging may be supported with histopathological grading.

Testicular cancer spreads by local invasion to the epididymis, spermatic cord and, rarely, the scrotal wall.

Medical/surgical management

Treatment modalities include:

- surgery – orchidectomy (removal of a testis), either partial or total
- chemotherapy
- radiotherapy.

Surgery is curative in up to 80% of cases (Brewster 2001). Further treatment will be dependent on histology; therefore these treatment modalities can be used alone or in combination, although benign tumours need no treatment other than orchidectomy.

Generally survival of patients with germ cell tumours is related to the stage at presentation and therefore the amount of tumour burden as well as the effectiveness of subsequent treatment.

One feature of testicular cancers that influences the efficacy of treatment is that they originate from germ cells, which are generally sensitive to radiotherapy and a variety of chemotherapeutic agents. Furthermore, the germ cells retain the ability to differentiate into benign growth phases.

Although the disease progresses swiftly, there is often a predictable pattern of spread that makes diagnosis easier, but perhaps the most significant feature is that the disease occurs in young men without co-existing pathologies who can tolerate multi-modal treatment (Ritchie 1998).

Selection of treatment options depends on the relative advantages and disadvantages of different regimens. Combination therapy has been credited with treatment successes, but the current accuracy of clinical staging (see Table 25.5) and the ability to recognize treatment failure by relatively 'simple' tests such as ultrasound and AFP/β-hCG, mean that the patient's progress can be accurately measured and new treatment started swiftly if necessary.

Because more than 50% of the patients with testicular cancers present with metastatic disease, further treatment following orchidectomy is usual. For residual para-aortic node enlargement after chemotherapy, retroperitoneal lymph node dissection may be curative (Brewster 2001).

Following orchidectomy, treatment depends on the tumour type, pathological risk factors for stage I disease and clinical prognostic factors for advanced disease. The cure rate is excellent for stages I and II, irrespective of treatment adopted; however, the pattern of relapse (rate, timing and site) can be influenced by the therapeutic policy. For metastatic disease, survival depends on clinical factors and treatment (Laguna et al 2001).

▶ Nursing management

All patients will undergo orchidectomy, but some will require additional chemotherapy or radiotherapy depending on the staging of the disease. Staging can only be made once the testis has been removed, which presents a challenge to nurses caring for these patients, since the latter will have significant anxieties concerning their recovery that cannot be answered until the histology report has been received.

The nursing care can be considered to span several phases, which include preparation for surgery, postoperative complications such as wound infection, and long-term factors such as

Table 25.5 Staging – testicular cancers

Stage of disease	Extent	Management
Stage I	Confinement of the tumour is within the testis. This is determined by lymph node dissection, which will identify microscopic metastasis	If metastases have been found, the lymph nodes can be removed, which may cure those with small volume disease (Blandy 1998). Where larger amounts of tumour are present in the lymph nodes, chemotherapy is given afterwards and this is normally based on CT scan staging. If the tumour is a seminoma, prophylactic radiation to the retroperitoneal lymph nodes can give 100% cure with stage I seminomas (Blandy 1998)
Stage II	There is lymph node involvement below the diaphragm level	All patients are given chemotherapy to start with then followed carefully
Stage III	There is supradiaphragmatic lymph node involvement	All patients are given as much chemotherapy as they can tolerate; if a mass remains after two or three cycles of treatment, it is removed surgically (Blandy 1998)
Advanced disease	Widespread metastases	Additional surgery, chemo/radiotherapy may be required (as palliation). The use of 'aggressive' treatments at this stage depend on the wishes of the patient, and the preferences of the consultant, particularly if further surgery is contemplated

coping with a diagnosis of cancer, loss of sexual function and changes in body image.

Preparation for surgery

Moynihan (1987) suggests that, at the time of diagnosis, fear of death is the most frequently expressed anxiety by patients; therefore supportive measures by way of information-giving and allowing time for them to express their fears may need to be a nursing priority in caring for these patients.

Orchidectomy is surgical removal of the testis by scrotal incision; patients will need to be prepared for surgery in the normal way (see Ch. 29). Specific care issues relating to these patients include storage of sperm (cryopreservation using extremely low temperatures), potential for infection and loss of body image. Cryopreservation would normally be offered and must be arranged prior to surgery, even if the surgery is expected to be unilateral, since chemotherapy or radiotherapy may subsequently be used that can affect fertility. Prosthesis use must also be discussed prior to surgery.

Postoperative care

Patients are normally in hospital for up to 5 days following surgery. Wound care and assessment for infection are in accordance with established nursing practice (see Ch. 29), but normally patients will be advised to wear a scrotal support for the immediate postoperative period.

During this recovery period, patients will require nursing time to express their feelings and thoughts regarding the diagnosis and treatment, especially any perceived change in body image.

Various definitions of altered body image exist but all have as a core theme the impact of change on the body taken in context within the society in which we live. It is generally accepted that the three elements of the 'self' that may change are:

- loss of psychological self
- loss of physical self
- loss of sociocultural self.

Testicular cancer and its treatment can be said to involve all of these 'losses' (Blackmore 1989).

Any diagnosis of cancer will engender a fear of death and disability, and therefore there is loss attached to the psychological self. Cancer itself remains a stigmatized disease; the expectation of society is also death, but coupled with this is a fear of embarrassment when the cancer is in the genital region.

Individuals will require time off from their paid employment, which may have financial consequences for the family. In addition, the fear of infertility/change in sexuality may have a profound impact on this group of patients.

Physical loss includes the change in body image from scarring, loss of the testis, hormonal changes and side-effects from the treatment, including sore skin, hair loss, etc. Patients with testicular cancer may be anxious about sexual function post-surgery. Van Basten et al (1999) found that sexual dysfunction is common initially after treatment, but a comparison between orchidectomy alone and orchidectomy plus chemotherapeutic agents found that erectile function improves after 1 year.

Orchidectomy will not necessarily result in reduced fertility or sexual performance but there is some evidence to suggest altered fertility. Fosså & Kravdal (2000) found that men with testicular cancer were subfertile both before and after diagnosis. Furthermore, Møller (1998) reported that men with testicular cancer sired more daughters before and after diagnosis; therefore hormone levels may be reduced although this may not affect fertility *per se* (James 2000).

Chemotherapy

If the histology result shows that the tumour has not spread then patients will not require any further treatment; however, evidence of spread (metastasis) would necessitate chemotherapy.

The chemotherapy commonly used in testicular cancer is a combination of bleomycin, etoposide and cisplatin (platinum-based), which is abbreviated to BEP. Such chemotherapy is not without risks despite its high cure rate. There is evidence showing dose-related toxicity from the bleomycin, and secondary leukaemia associated with etoposide, although this is rare (Bozcuk et al 2000). The common side-effects of BEP include rash and increased pigmentation, hypersensitivity (fevers, chills), pulmonary fibrosis, mucositis, leucopenia, alopecia, nausea and vomiting, diarrhoea, renal toxicity, electrolyte disturbance (hypomagnesaemia), visual disturbances, etc. Clearly any side-effects will need specific nursing intervention and evaluation in the care plan (see Ch. 33). Readers are advised to consult an up-to-date drug reference (e.g. eBNF 2003 – http://www.bnf.org.uk) for more detailed information.

The chemotherapy regimen normally lasts up to 5 days depending on the type of chemotherapeutic agent used. The following additional care is required:

- anti-emetics and analgesia will need to be evaluated for efficacy
- mouth care must be provided, given the potential for mouth ulcers
- advice from the dietician should be sought if weight loss/altered eating pattern is reported
- regular cardiovascular and respiratory assessment (temperature, pulse, blood pressure and respiratory rate) for identification of arrhythmias and respiratory difficulty
- regular blood testing to assess electrolytes and full blood count.

Other treatment

Some patients with metastatic seminoma will require radiotherapy to para-aortic lymph nodes. Residual retroperitoneal lymph node enlargement may need surgical dissection. This form of treatment may leave a patient with erectile dysfunction and ejaculatory disorders (see pp. 752–756).

Summary

Patients must be prepared for the body image changes, be familiar with the risks, side-effects and likely postoperative course of an orchidectomy, the side-effects of chemo/radiotherapy and any further management that may be required. Many patients will require some form of long-term support to rationalize their experiences. Patient support groups can be beneficial to these patients either as a self-help group or facilitated formally by a counsellor.

The role of the nurse can be considered in several contexts: hospital-based, clinical nurse specialist and community-based. The hospital-based and clinical nurse specialist roles have been identified above but the community role has yet to be elucidated.

The increasing incidence of testicular cancer in England and Wales poses a health education/promotion issue. Recent evidence from Webb & Holmes (2000) found that there is role confusion amongst health care professionals as to who performs patient education for testicular self-examination (TSE). The need clearly exists for patient education through programmes such as increasing awareness and TSE (see Health Promotion box 25.3 and Fig. 25.17). This is a role that could be undertaken by community nurses/practice nurses.

 HEALTH PROMOTION

25.3 Testicular self-examination (TSE)

Procedure

It's easiest to examine your testes after a warm bath or shower has relaxed the scrotal tissues.

- Support your scrotum in the palm of one hand. Note the size and weight of your testes. This will help you to detect any changes in the future. It's normal for one testicle to hang slightly lower than the other.
- Examine each testicle in more detail by rolling it between your fingers and thumb. Press firmly but gently to feel for any lumps, swellings or changes in firmness.
- Don't worry if you find the epididymis, a tube that carries sperm to the penis. This can be felt at the top and back of each testicle.

It is best to examine yourself about once every month or two. It's also important not to become obsessed with self-examination – remember testicular cancer is uncommon. But if you do find anything unusual, don't wait for it to disappear or start throbbing – see your doctor as soon as possible.

Student activities

- Consider construction of a poster for your ward or department promoting TSE.
- Find some existing posters/leaflets that promote TSE.
- Modify the design to suit your particular clinical area – think about the client group. Do you need to think about communication methods for non-English speakers, or the needs of marginalized groups such as men with learning difficulties, asylum seekers or serving prisoners?

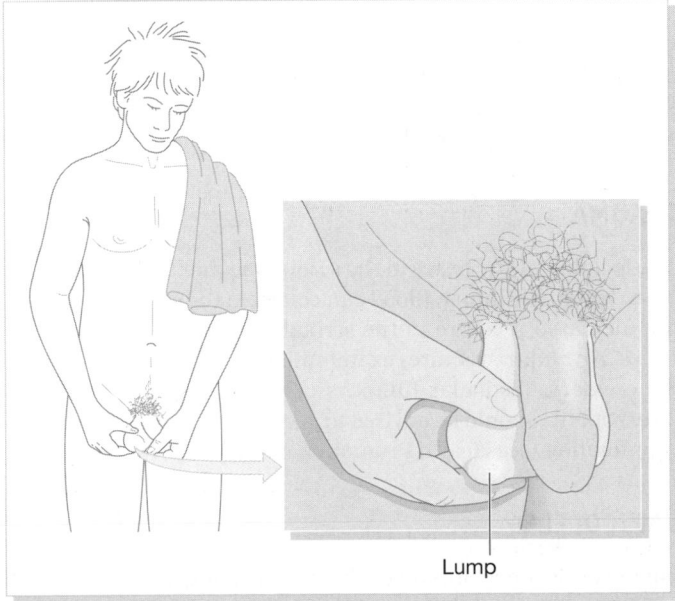

Figure 25.17 Testicular self-examination.

UNDESCENDED TESTES

An undescended testis is one that has failed to migrate to the correct position in the scrotum. The types of undescended testis are ectopic, where the testis may be found in the abdominal wall or near the base of the penis, and incomplete, where the testis is mobile (i.e. it can move up and down).

The complications of undescended testes are:

■ torsion
■ infertility
■ cancer.

Ectopic and incomplete descent of the testes require surgical mobilization by orchiopexy, i.e. mobilization of the testes into the scrotum. Most male infants' testes will descend within 12 months of birth. If the testes have not descended after 12 months, an orchiopexy is normally required. This is usually performed before the child reaches 3 years (Blandy 1998). Failure to correct undescended testicles can lead to infertility and cancer. If an undescended testis were found in an adult male, an orchidectomy would be required, given the risk of developing cancer.

TORSION

Torsion is the rotation of the testis on its spermatic cord that results in occlusion of the veins and arterial blood supply. If left untreated, infarction of the testis follows, resulting in infertility.

The clinical features of torsion include pain and swelling; the scrotum becomes tender, red and swollen. It is essential to untwist the testis before it dies from ischaemia, and therefore urgent surgery is required. A scrotal incision is made under general anaesthetic, and the testes are untwisted and 'fixed' to the scrotal wall. If ischaemia has occurred, an orchidectomy will be required.

▶ Nursing management

Specific nursing care includes bed rest, effective analgesia and advice concerning infertility and orchidectomy.

TRAUMA

The location of the testes in the scrotal sac makes them vulnerable to traumatic injury. Blood can collect in the scrotum, producing increased pressure in the scrotal sac that may damage the testes. Any injury requires examination and evacuation of blood if necessary. Testicular tumours can occur post-injury; therefore, patients should be advised to perform regular testicular self-examination (see Health Promotion box 25.3, p. 749).

VARICOCELE

Varicocele is the dilatation of the veins leading from the testis. It has been suggested that this dilatation depresses sperm production and leads to reduction in testis size, but there is no evidence for this (Blandy 1998).

HYDROCELE

This is accumulation of fluid in the testis because of obstructed lymphatic drainage. The testis may be explored under general anaesthetic to exclude more sinister conditions, but hydroceles *per se* rarely require treatment.

INFECTION AND INFLAMMATION

EPIDIDYMITIS

Epididymitis is inflammation of the epididymis. There is acute inflammation and pain. It is a bacterial infection and the micro-organisms responsible are usually *Escherichia coli* or *Chlamydia trachomatis*, although in rare circumstances tuberculosis and recent urological surgery have also been implicated.

It is important to differentiate between epididymitis and torsion, given the urgent surgical management of the latter. This can be assessed by Doppler ultrasound since epididymitis (an inflammation) would increase blood flow, whereas torsion (occlusion) would decrease it. The complications of epididymitis include:

■ abscess formation
■ testicular infarction
■ altered fertility.

Medical management
This includes:

■ bed rest
■ scrotal support/elevation
■ analgesia
■ antibiotics.

ORCHITIS

Viral infection, particularly mumps, can cause swollen, painful testes as well as pyrexia. It occurs in 20% of men who contract mumps after puberty; it is normally unilateral and subsides after approximately 10 days (Brewster 2001).

Although orchitis resolves on its own, patients will require similar supportive intervention to those listed for epididymitis. Specific complications include testicular atrophy, and fertility may be affected if both testes are involved.

PROSTATITIS

Acute or chronic bacterial infection can cause prostatitis (inflammation of the prostate). Patients report general malaise, fever and acute cystitis. It can occur at any age and typically causes pain in the suprapubic and perineal region, in addition to urinary frequency and urgency.

Full investigation is important as some patients with prostate cancer will present with cystitis and prostatitis (see Ch. 24). Investigations include an ultrasound of the urinary tract and rectum, prostate-specific antigen (PSA), cystoscopy and biopsy (if necessary). Treatment and complications are similar to those listed for epididymitis.

PENILE PROBLEMS

PENILE CANCER

Cancer affecting the penis is usually squamous cell carcinoma.

Epidemiology and aetiology

It is an uncommon cancer, representing 1% of male cancers in Europe and the USA, but up to 10% of malignancies in some African and South American countries (Gloeckler-Ries et al 1990). It is a disease more common in men aged over 60 years, but it can occur in young men. This development of the disease may be related to religious practices, since circumcision at birth is thought to confer complete immunity from this malignancy. Adult circumcision is not thought to confer any protection.

The development of the disease has been attributed to chronic irritation by smegma, a by-product of bacterial action on desquamated cells, and phimosis (tight foreskin that is not easily retracted), which makes cleaning of the glans penis difficult (see Fig. 25.16, p. 744).

Pathophysiology

There are various types of premalignant lesions that appear on the glans penis. These may be chronic red or pale patches and are considered premalignant changes. They include:

- leukoplakia – solitary or multiple whitish plaques that often involve the meatus
- balanitis xerotica obliterans – a whitish alteration seen on the prepuce that is common and usually benign. If the balanitis affects the glans, it can cause meatal stenosis
- erythroplasia of Queyrat – a form of carcinoma in situ of the glans and skin that resembles balanitis. It is diagnosed by biopsy and can be cured by laser therapy or 5-fluorouracil cream (5-FU). If this premalignant lesion is neglected, it may progress into cancer
- Buschke–Löwenstein tumour – a giant form of condyloma acuminatum, from papilloma viruses, that always progresses into invasive cancer.

These premalignant lesions found on the glans or prepuce grow locally beneath the prepuce prior to invading the urethra and corpora cavernosa (see Fig. 25.16). Eventually the cancer will spread into the perineum and pelvic cavity. Metastasis to the inguinal lymph nodes is slow. Blood-borne metastasis is rare but may involve the lungs or liver.

Investigations

Normally the diagnosis is not in doubt since the lesions are visible; however, biopsies can be performed if necessary to establish the depth of invasion and grade of the tumour. A chest X-ray, bone scan and CT scan will detect the presence of metastases. Staging of the tumour is by the TNM classification system; most penile cancers are low grade (see Ch. 33).

Medical/surgical management

The options for treatment are radiotherapy, chemotherapy and surgery. Combined approaches are often employed with some success, although the low incidence of this malignancy makes evaluation of treatment regimens difficult.

Circumcision (excision of the prepuce, see p. 752) would normally be performed to avoid further irritation and to establish the extent of the premalignant or malignant lesions. Partial or total penectomy (amputation of the penis) is then required. With partial penectomy, approximately 2 cm of the penis is left. Total penectomy requires excision of the scrotum and formation of some type of urostomy (see Ch. 24). If lymph nodes are involved, removal may be required and this is often done in combination with radiotherapy or chemotherapy.

 Nursing management

Partial or total penectomy will result in a profound change in body image in the patient. The patient and his partner will need time to accept the diagnosis of cancer, its implications in terms of treatment and the long-term changes that will occur in his relationship. Close liaison and involvement from the psychosexual counsellor and erectile dysfunction team will assist the patient and partner in coping with the change in body image and sexual function that will result from partial or total penectomy (see Reflective Practice box 25.2).

Reconstructive surgery of the penis is possible following partial penectomy, once patients are confirmed as being cancer-free. Formation of a neopenis (new penis) is with a radial forearm flap and prosthetic implant. This site is used because the skin is relatively sensitive, hairless and has a good blood supply.

REFLECTIVE PRACTICE

25.2 Penile cancer: profound change in body image

Penile cancer is uncommon, but the treatment can be disfiguring, resulting in a profound change of body image. A common treatment for advanced penile cancer is partial or total penectomy (amputation of the penis) depending on the extent of the tumour.

- How do you think the changes in body image will affect the patient?
- How can the nurse support the patient in coming to terms with this change in body image/function?
- What services does your clinical area have to assist these patients, i.e. counselling, specialist nurses, etc.
- Do you think the patient will ever have a sexual relationship again?
- How do you think this change will affect the patient's relationships?

Student activities

- Read the article by Blackmore (1989), which discusses the key issues in change of body image.
- Discuss treatment options with the psychosexual counsellors and specialist nurses in erectile dysfunction – what criteria are there for reconstructive surgery, i.e. prostheses?

Reference

Blackmore C. Altered images. Nurs Times 1989; 85(2): 36–39.

A good cosmetic and functional result can be gained and should be offered to patients (Lynch & Schellhammer 1998). Formation of a phallus in patients following a total penectomy is more difficult, although there are some encouraging results using the techniques mentioned above.

Nurses need to be aware of the specific postoperative complications of partial/complete penectomy and plan appropriate nursing interventions, including:

■ haemorrhage – nurses should observe wound dressing for blood loss and perform regular cardiovascular observations, including pulse, blood pressure, respirations and colour, until stable
■ potential for infection – the wound is observed for signs of infection (e.g. redness), and temperature is measured regularly to detect pyrexia; ensure that the patient's catheter is cleaned daily according to local protocols
■ potential for oedema – keep a supportive dressing in situ for at least 24 hours; assess wound daily.

(See Box 25.1 for complications following circumcision.)

PHIMOSIS AND PARAPHIMOSIS

The term phimosis refers to non-retractility of the prepuce of the penis, and narrowing of the preputial ring, resulting in difficulty in passing urine. Phimosis may be a congenital anomaly, but is more commonly associated with repeated episodes of infection, which, because of scarring, give rise to the preputial narrowing.

Paraphimosis occurs where there is a narrow preputial ring that can be pulled back behind the glans penis, but cannot be pulled forward easily. If the prepuce cannot be returned to its normal position, circulation in the glans becomes constricted, with swelling and considerable pain and discomfort. Unresolved compression of the glans penis can result in gangrene of the glans penis.

Paraphimosis can occur following catheterization and patient hygiene (see Special Issues box 25.2).

Medical/surgical management

Manual reduction with local anaesthetic, or in some cases light general anaesthesia, can be performed, but if unsuccessful an emergency circumcision will be required.

Box 25.1 Complications of circumcision and required intervention

- *Pain* – requires local anaesthetic, such as lidocaine (lignocaine)-based gel, or systemic analgesia
- *Erection* – may require benzodiazepines to limit the likelihood of erection, e.g. diazepam
- *Oedema* – close-fitting underwear with non-absorbent dressing should be applied; in addition, the penis should remain upright
- *Bleeding* – check wound for blood loss; excessive blood loss may require further surgical intervention
- *Wound infection* – observation of wound site; nature and colour of any discharge and raised temperature should be considered suspicious and reported immediately

---

 SPECIAL ISSUES

25.2 Preventing paraphimosis

The prepuce (foreskin) is routinely retracted to allow cleansing of the glans penis, limiting the chance of irritation and infection, but if it is not returned to its normal position following catheterization or during bed bathing, paraphimosis easily occurs. Nurses must ensure that self-caring patients, health care assistants and other carers are aware of the importance of repositioning the prepuce after retracting it to facilitate washing and drying of the glans penis.

Nurses need to observe for signs of inflammation such as redness or swelling and report any difficulty in repositioning the prepuce.

Circumcision may be required for phimosis, paraphimosis and balanitis (inflammation of the glans penis and the prepuce), although in some cultures this is performed as a matter of routine. As discussed in the section dealing with penile cancer, circumcision at an early age can provide 'immunity' from this type of cancer. However, it is not without its complications (see Box 25.1).

PROBLEMS WITH SEXUAL FUNCTION

ERECTILE DYSFUNCTION

Erectile dysfunction (ED) is a common condition that is thought to have an annual incidence in men of between 15 and 20%. It can be defined as the inability of a man to gain an erection of sufficient quality for intercourse. This definition supersedes the older term, impotence, although such a definition is still used by the lay public.

The causes of ED have historically been divided into organic and psychogenic factors, i.e. conditions known to affect nerve or blood supply and those where 'stress' can cause failure.

Assessment of erectile function or concerns about ED can be elicited during the nursing assessment by focused questioning, and referral made to the specialist ED clinic for advice and treatment.

Aetiology

The causes of ED and the associated risk factors are often multiple, with psychological, neurological, endocrinological, vascular, traumatic and iatrogenic components (see Boxes 25.2 and 25.3). The exact role played by lifestyle/medical events has yet to be fully elucidated, although smoking, hypertension, hyperlipidaemia, diabetes mellitus and the presence of vascular disease have been proposed as potential risk factors.

Problems with potency are frequently multifactorial in origin. Psychogenic ED is self-perpetuating: each failure increases the associated anxiety levels and can lead to the continual failure to have erections. This is the commonest cause of intermittent ED in young men, although it is usually secondary to organic dysfunction from middle age onwards.

Box 25.2 Risk factors for erectile dysfunction

Organic
- Diabetes mellitus (see Ch. 17)
- Smoking (see Ch. 20)
- Post-urological treatment (see Ch. 24)
- Post-myocardial infarction (see Ch. 19)
- Renal transplant/dialysis (see Ch. 24)
- Hypertension (see Ch. 19)
- Anti-hypertensive drug therapy
- Spinal injury (see Ch. 14)
- Pelvic injury
- Neurological diseases, e.g. Parkinson's disease (see Ch. 14)

Psychogenic
- Stress (see Ch. 6)
- Bereavement
- Relationship difficulties
- Pressure to perform
- Iatrogenic
- Personality

Box 25.3 Drugs implicated in the development of erection failure (Jackson et al 1999)

Cardiovascular
- Thiazide diuretics
- Beta-blockers
- Calcium antagonists
- Centrally acting agents, e.g. methyldopa and ganglion blockers
- Digoxin
- Lipid-lowering drugs
- ACE inhibitors

Psychogenic
- Tranquillizers
- Anxiolytics and hypnotics
- Tricyclic antidepressants
- Selective serotonin reuptake inhibitors

Endocrine
- Anti-androgens
- Oestrogens
- Luteinizing hormone-releasing hormone (LHRH)
- Testosterone

Miscellaneous
- H_2-receptor antagonists, e.g. cimetidine and ranitidine
- Metoclopramide
- Carbamazepine

Recreational drugs
- All recreational drugs

Up until the 1980s, psychogenic causes were attributed as the aetiology in up to 90% of cases of ED. Opinion now favours changes in blood flow as the key factor in ED, with alterations in blood flow to and from the penis the single most important cause.

Recent evidence suggests that there is a marked delay (up to 5 years) between onset of symptoms and seeking treatment. A common finding was that those patients with an organic cause to their dysfunction also had significant psychogenic factors that influenced the condition and its treatment.

Publicity about solutions to sexual problems such as sildenafil (Viagra) has also enabled men to seek help. However, there is still a gap between onset of problems and receiving treatment, which demonstrates that, despite the myth that our society is open about sexuality, there are enormous barriers of embarrassment and fear of humiliation that delay men seeking help.

Erectile dysfunction as communication

For a certain group of men, ED is a form of communication, a way of signalling to themselves, if not to others, that something needs attention in their personal or emotional lives. It is commonly an expression of negative feelings – sadness, anger, guilt, worries, etc. – particularly for those men who do not express their feelings verbally. All these states are known to have an inhibiting effect on the erectile mechanism. Unless these issues are also addressed during the consultation, the medication may provide an erection, but does not always help the man to achieve his goals in terms of having a mutually satisfying sexual relationship with a partner.

Erection failure is not always precipitated by a crisis in the presenting patient's life. Where there is a partner, it is also important to explore that person's situation and feelings about the sexual relationship. For many men, loss of erections is a response to anger or to negative feelings perceived in the partner.

Nursing assessment

Hospitalization for any reason can raise significant fears and anxieties in patients. Some surgery will have an impact on body image, whereas the treatment for certain diseases can cause unwanted side-effects. Both present a challenge to the nurse caring for such patients.

In the light of the conditions and medications listed in Boxes 25.2 and 25.3, many patients are at risk of developing ED. Specific questioning may be of benefit for patients with or potentially suffering from ED (see Reflective Practice box 25.3). Questions may include: 'I notice that you are taking the drug _____. Some men can have difficulty with erections after taking this medicine. Have you had any trouble?'. Alternatively, patients may be undergoing a specific operation that may affect this activity of living. Questions such as the following are helpful: 'Are you aware that some men have difficulty gaining or sustaining an erection or ejaculating after this operation?'. A detailed assessment would not be required; patients could be asked if they would like to be referred to the nurse specialist in ED, and further advice and information sought.

Currently there are specialist practice nurses running ED clinics either independently or in combination with medical or psychology colleagues. Patients referred to these services would be specifically assessed using a focused history sheet (see Table 25.6), enabling the nurse to accurately assess the history of the erection problems and discuss the various treatment options in detail.

REFLECTIVE PRACTICE

25.3 Assessment of erectile dysfunction

You admit a patient on to your ward who is taking enalapril maleate for hypertension. When assessing him using a framework/model of nursing, he seems evasive and embarrassed. What questions could you ask to elicit whether he has erectile dysfunction related to his medication?

Think about situations where you have had to ask questions about sensitive issues – what approach worked well and what would you change next time?

Student activities

- Do you have a urology clinical nurse specialist who deals with ED?
- How would you access them and what details would be required for the referral?
- What treatments are available for ED? Are there any restrictions on who can receive these medicines by NHS prescription?

Medical/surgical management

Irrespective of the cause of ED, there are only a limited number of treatments available. These include drugs, vacuum devices, surgery and psychosexual therapy.

Drug treatment

Apomorphine hydrochloride

This drug acts on dopaminergic receptors to increase the blood flow to the penis. It may take up to six doses before a benefit is seen. It is contraindicated in unstable angina, and renal or hepatic failure.

Sildenafil citrate

Sildenafil citrate may also need up to six doses before benefits are seen. It is a phosphodiesterase type V inhibitor and increases blood flow to the penis. Contraindications include concurrent use of nitrates, a myocardial infarction (within 3 months) and stroke.

Alprostadil (prostaglandin E_1)

Alprostadil increases blood flow to the penis. Intraurethral alprostadil such as 'Medicated urethral system for erections' (MUSE) may be used. It is essential to massage the urethra for up

Table 25.6 Erectile dysfunction (ED) assessment (Steggall & Gann 2002)		
Assessment	**Rationale**	**Implications for treatment**
General history		
Surgical and medical history, and current medication	Clues to organic causes of ED	Assess blood or nerve damage
Allergies	Interaction with treatment	Interaction with treatment
Tobacco use	Assess vascular damage	Give lifestyle advice
Alcohol use	Desensitizes the individual to stimulation	Potential to affect success of treatment
Specific history		
Description of the problem	Erection failure, loss of desire, or rapid ejaculation	Guides management
Duration of problem	Clues to performance anxiety	Guides management
Gradual or sudden onset	Organic or psychogenic	Gradual onset suggests an organic cause, whereas sudden onset suggests a psychogenic cause
Early morning tumescence (swelling/turgidity)	Is the blood supply intact?	May need locally acting medication if blood flow is poor
Libido	Assess desire	Often absent in long-term ED; possible compensatory mechanism
Is penetration possible?	Assess strength of erection	Assesses blood flow; may indicate 'strength' of medication required
Current sexual relationship	Need to know if there is some sexual activity	Absence of intimacy is important – for the treatment to work, some type of sexual stimulation is required
Psychological factors	Anxieties inhibit function	Feelings of 'impotence' in other areas will be reflected in sexuality – need to resolve underlying problem
Social problems (particularly prior to onset of problem)		
Does the partner know of the person's visit?	Status of relationship	Address unresolved issues with both partners

to 10 minutes after administration. Contraindications include sickle cell disease and bleeding disorders. A barrier method of contraception should be used if the sexual partner is pregnant. Intracavernosal injection of alprostadil, e.g. Caverject, Caverject dual chamber or Viridal Duo, is also used. It is essential to provide full teaching of injection technique and support/discuss patient anxieties. It is contraindicated in patients taking warfarin or with bleeding disorders.

Vacuum devices

It is important to teach correct technique and reinforce that the vacuum needs to be inflated slowly. There are no contraindications, but patients must be competent to remember to remove the constriction ring within 30 minutes. It works non-pharmacologically by drawing blood into the corpus cavernosum under pressure. Blood is held in place by a constriction band.

Surgery (prostheses)

Various prostheses are available. The prosthesis is an artificial implant that replaces the corpus cavernosum. Erection is then possible 'on demand'. Any contraindications depend on the patient's fitness for surgery.

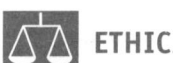 **ETHICAL ISSUES**

25.1 Inequalities in the management of erectile dysfunction

Men with diabetes, prostatic conditions and certain neurological problems are treated by NHS prescription for erectile dysfunction (ED), but it has been identified that ED is more frequently associated with cardiovascular disease yet this group are excluded from NHS prescription treatment.

These patients are referred to a hospital consultant for prescription under the 'severe distress' banner, which is not dealt with by the family GP. This burdens the hospital with the cost of treatment. However, no specific budget has been provided to hospitals allowing them to prescribe medication for ED; indeed, 'severe distress' has yet to be defined. Some hospitals have made unilateral decisions not to see patients under the 'severe distress' umbrella, because the hospital has to meet the cost of the medication, creating a postcode inequality.

Student activities
- Should the NHS treat men with ED?
- Do you think the GP should manage this condition?
- Do you think the GP surgery should fund treatment for ED for all patients?
- How do you think being referred to a hospital will affect the patient, i.e. fear and embarrassment, travel costs, etc.
- What cultural differences can you think of that may affect treatment?

Further reading
Hackett G. Sexual health: the cost effective management of erectile dysfunction. Men's Health J 2002; 1(3): 84–86.

Psychosexual therapy

A behavioural programme with counselling of underlying issues is another form of management. It involves weekly or regular attendance, with 'homework' that breaks the pattern of failure, removes anxiety and restores confidence. This type of treatment will not be appropriate or acceptable to some men, as it may be culturally unacceptable.

The efficacy of these treatments is variable and dependent on patient motivation. There is also evidence indicating that time taken to teach injection technique or application of these options can improve patient acceptability and efficacy.

Not all patients can be treated by NHS prescription (see Ethical Issues box 25.1). The UK government has restricted NHS prescriptions to certain conditions and circumstances (see Box 25.4). Those men who do not 'fulfil' these criteria must seek a private prescription from their GP. Treatment options for this group of patients is often influenced by cost. Prior to April 2002, vacuum pumps were not included in the approved medications/treatment for NHS prescriptions, but this anomaly has now been corrected.

The Department of Health guidelines for the prescription of these medications includes research from Johnson et al (1994), who report that the average number of times that the 40- to 60-year-old age group have intercourse is once a week, and therefore suggest that GPs prescribe to reflect this.

Unfortunately, such guidelines fail to recognize the effect that delayed treatment and performance anxiety has on this group of patients. Considering that the average time to seek treatment is 5 years, any medication will be unlikely to be successful on the

---

Box 25.4 Included conditions in the Department of Health guidelines for the treatment of erectile dysfunction where NHS prescriptions can be issued
(Adapted from Department of Health 1999)

Condition
- Diabetes mellitus
- Multiple sclerosis
- Parkinson's disease
- Poliomyelitis
- Prostate cancer
- Radical pelvic surgery
- Renal failure treated by dialysis or transplant
- Severe pelvic injury
- Single gene neurological disease
- Spinal cord injury
- Spina bifida

Additional circumstances
- Men who were receiving a course of NHS treatment for erectile dysfunction on 14 September 1998

Treatment included
- Apomorphine hydrochloride
- Sildenafil citrate
- Intraurethral pellets (MUSE)
- Intracavernosal injections (Caverject or Viridal)
- Vacuum devices

first few occasions, since the individual will be under extreme pressure to 'perform' (Steggall & Gann 2002).

Recent evidence from Heaton et al (2002) indicates that it is the sixth dose of apomorphine hydrochloride that is most likely to be efficacious; therefore, rigid adherence to the prescribing guidelines will have implications on successful and rapid outcome, possibly exacerbating fear of failure and performance anxiety.

Some clinics recommend that patients take medication more than once a week, using the rationale that this will reduce the anxiety related to the expected efficacy of the medication and pressure to perform. This rationale is thought to influence treatment, i.e. improve the success of the treatment, because when the patient and his partner are relaxed there is less performance anxiety.

▶ **Nursing management**

The majority of erectile dysfunction treatment will be carried out on an outpatient basis using oral, intraurethral or intracavernosal preparations or vacuum devices. If these treatments are unsuccessful, patients may opt for a penile prosthesis or implant. The advantages of this approach include erection available 'on demand', no external devices or medication required for erections and ease of use. However, there are disadvantages that must be considered, namely the risks associated with surgery, mechanical failure, infection, pain, erosion or tissue breakdown, and migration and extrusion.

The prosthesis is implanted completely into the body, replacing the corpus cavernosum. The incision is subcoronal (behind the head of the penis) although this depends on the choice of prosthesis and the urologist's preference.

The specific postoperative nursing care required for the insertion of a penile prosthesis includes:

- pain relief with the provision of adequate analgesia and antiemetic drugs for nausea and vomiting
- regular temperature assessment and wound observation for signs of infection
- anticipation of effects associated with altered body image and coordinated review by a clinical nurse specialist and psychosexual counsellors.

Consistent ED is more likely than not to be the consequence of primary organic pathophysiology in conjunction with secondary psychological factors (Goldstein 1991). Performance anxiety plays a large part in maintaining erection problems, whatever the cause. The erectile function is impaired at the moment the man becomes anxious. This means that notwithstanding the reason for the ED, once a man has a failure and is aware of the possibility of future failures, even when he presents with medical factors that may contribute to his ED, there will also be a psychological component maintaining the difficulties.

To approach assessment and treatment from the purely medical point of view is to deny an important aspect of ED and limit its successful outcome. Effective communication between nurses and patients is an important aspect of managing this condition.

RAPID EJACULATION

Premature or rapid ejaculation is a common male sexual problem affecting an estimated 29% of the sexually active population aged 18–55 (Laumann et al 1994). This complaint is often ascribed to anxiety, in which ejaculation and orgasm occur before desired due to lack of control during sexual activity. Studies indicate that there is hypersensitivity of the penile skin in individuals with rapid ejaculation.

The most widely used definition of rapid ejaculation is the Diagnostic and Statistical Manual – IV (DSM-IV) which is based on a physiological model originating from Masters & Johnson (1970) (see Box 25.5).

Differential features in diagnosing rapid ejaculation are:

- onset or duration – whether lifelong or acquired
- context or range – whether generalized (in all situations) or situational (only some situations).

Assessment of rapid or premature ejaculation would normally be undertaken by the specialist ED nurse.

Management
Treatment for rapid ejaculation includes:

- the start–stop and squeeze technique in a cognitive-behavioural model
- selective serotonin reuptake inhibitors (SSRIs)
- local anaesthetics
- constriction devices.

The major confounding factor in the treatment of rapid ejaculation is accurate assessment.

The normal male reproductive physiology is to lose an erection after ejaculation; most men present to the erectile dysfunction clinic with ED and are found, on closer questioning, to have rapid

---

Box 25.5 Definition of premature ejaculation (DSM-IV criteria for premature ejaculation)
(American Psychiatric Association 1994)

Criterion A
Persistent or recurrent ejaculation with minimal sexual stimulation before, on or shortly after penetration and before the person wishes it. Factors such as age, novelty of the sexual partner or situation and recent frequency of sexual activity must be taken into account.

Criterion B
The disturbance causes a marked distress or interpersonal difficulty.

Criterion C
Premature ejaculation is not exclusively the result of the direct effects of a substance (e.g. withdrawal of opiates).

ejaculation. Treatment using therapies that improve erection quality have little or no effect on rapid ejaculation; therefore, patients do not find any benefit from these treatments.

There is no quick 'cure' for these patients. Some therapies, such as behavioural therapy which involves masturbation, are unacceptable to certain cultures. These patients may be helped by SSRIs, but this is only a short-term measure since SSRIs are used for their side-effects alone. Once the constriction band has been used, there is little chance of patients regaining ejaculatory control; they often lose the ability to recognize the point of inevitability.

This group of patients require specialist assistance from the urology clinic using a combined medical and psychosexual modality approach. Of key importance, however, is the identification of ED, so that appropriate referral and assessment can be made.

SEXUAL AND REPRODUCTIVE ISSUES AND DISORDERS AFFECTING WOMEN AND MEN

SEXUAL HEALTH ISSUES

With sexual activity commencing in teenagers at younger and younger ages, it is important that people engaging in sexual intercourse have a basic understanding of sexual function. This will help them to remain healthy, prevent transmission of diseases outlined below and prevent unplanned, unwanted pregnancies. This should commence in school with related sex education, and school or community nurses now frequently visit local schools and colleges to deliver this. Casual sex has major implications for contracting disease and is known to be a risk factor in cervical cancer, so advice should be given about the risks of multiple partners.

Sexual dysfunction can cause major problems between couples and what starts as a small incident can develop into something much bigger, causing considerable discord and distress. The commonest problems include:

- anorgasmia – failure to achieve orgasm, more often experienced by females than males
- dyspareunia – painful intercourse which may be superficial at the introduction of the penis, or deep due to the penis causing pressure at the vaginal vault
- vaginismus – contraction of vaginal muscles when the penis is introduced which makes intercourse impossible. This can also be seen when a doctor or nurse attempts to examine a woman vaginally
- erectile dysfunction and rapid ejaculation (see p. 752).

Several of these disorders can be helped by talking through the problem with a sympathetic health professional, who can also offer advice about various techniques that may assist. However, often specialist help is required and the couple may benefit from referral to a psychosexual counsellor specializing in the area of sexual health. Unfortunately there are often insufficient counsellors available for the number of couples who require help, particularly as people are becoming less embarrassed about seeking help for these intensely personal problems.

CONTRACEPTION

It is thought that over 5 million women in the UK seek contraception or family planning advice each year (Clayton & Newton 1988). This is an important aspect of sexual health as it reduces the number of unplanned pregnancies when used effectively. This is especially important in the teenage population, as the age at which girls become sexually active is decreasing. It is a high priority of the World Health Organization due to the worldwide effect that current population growth will have in the future.

Types of contraception

These can be classified by the way they act. The objective is to prevent implantation of a fertilized egg, which can be achieved by the following methods:

- *Barrier methods* – prevent fertilization by keeping the sperm and oocyte apart. They include condom, female condom, diaphragm and cervical cap
- *Hormonal methods* – prevent ovulation or implantation if an oocyte is fertilized. They include oral contraceptives, either combined oestrogen/progesterone or progesterone only (mini-pill); local progestogens by injection or subdermal implants; and vaginal rings releasing oestrogen and progesterone. Levonorgestrel (two oral doses 12 hours apart) is used for emergency hormonal contraception within 3 days (72 hours) of unprotected intercourse (see Special Issues box 25.3)
- *Intrauterine contraceptive devices* (IUCDs or IUDs) – prevent implantation. Various devices are available. They may be inert or release progestogen. A copper-containing IUCD can be used as an emergency contraception if inserted within 5 days of unprotected intercourse. Women should be checked for STIs
- *Natural methods* – include the rhythm method, whereby intercourse is avoided at the time of ovulation, or the withdrawal method, where the man withdraws the penis from the vagina before ejaculation
- *Spermicides*, such as nonoxynol, in the form of foams, pessaries and sponges – may be used with barrier methods
- *Permanent method* – e.g. female sterilization or male vasectomy.

With so many methods available, a careful assessment of the couple's needs and medical conditions is required to ensure that the most appropriate method for them is chosen. The commonest reason for contraception failure is non-compliance by one or other partner so it is essential to use a form they are both comfortable with. Individuals who have multiple sexual partners should be advised to use a barrier method to provide additional protection against contracting STIs and cervical changes. Women who choose sterilization must be carefully counselled about failure rate and risk of ectopic pregnancy if it does fail. Importantly, they, along with men undergoing vasectomy, must accept the permanency of this form. Female sterilization is carried out under a general anaesthetic via a laparoscopy and care is similar to that for any woman undergoing laparoscopy. Vasectomy is usually carried out under local anaesthetic and so is preferable to female sterilization because there are fewer risks.

25.3 Emergency hormonal contraception

Nurses in many settings from schools and colleges and accident and emergency departments to GP surgeries will be involved with girls or women who require emergency hormonal contraception, commonly known as the 'morning after pill'. It is important that nurses have sufficient information to answer women's questions, particularly now that this drug is increasingly available, e.g. from pharmacies. In addition, nurses should discuss the use of more reliable contraception in the future.

- Levonorgestrel is used. This is taken as two oral doses 12 hours apart, but it must be started within 3 days (72 hours) of unprotected intercourse.
- No more than 16 hours should elapse between the two doses.
- Levonorgestrel can make the woman feel very nauseated. If the woman vomits within 3 hours of taking levonorgestrel, she can have a replacement tablet.
- Women need to know that their next period may not come on time (early or late) and that she should use a barrier method of contraception until her next period starts.

When to seek medical advice
- If the woman has pain in the lower abdomen, she should seek medical help at once
- If the next period is unusual, e.g. very heavy or light, lasts fewer days than normal or doesn't come
- If she has any other worries.

▶ Nursing management

Apart from the surgical methods, all other forms can be prescribed in the community. Nurses trained in family planning can provide both assessment of women and counselling about the different types of contraception available. Information about side-effects, efficacy and failure rates must be explained in detail and in language the women can understand. Instruction in the correct use of the contraception can have a significant impact on its success. Nurses are now developing skills and knowledge in prescribing which can enable them to provide holistic care in family planning. They are able to monitor the woman's use and provide advice about any side-effects, offering alternatives if required.

INFERTILITY

This is also known as subfertility and can be defined as the inability of a couple to conceive spontaneously.

Aetiology and epidemiology
The length of time a couple have been trying for a pregnancy is important and it is usually considered to be a problem if they have not conceived after 1 year of unprotected intercourse. It is further defined as:

- primary infertility – the couple have never had a pregnancy previously
- secondary infertility – the couple, either together or with other partners, have previously conceived although this pregnancy may not have continued to produce a live baby.

It is estimated that up to 1 in 4 couples may experience problems achieving a pregnancy at some time, and up to 1 in 6 couples will seek specialist advice. In some instances, no actual cause can be found. This demonstrates the large scale of this problem and in recent years major advances in health care technology have provided many more treatment options for both sexes. Many of these advances have major moral and ethical implications and these must be considered with the couple when treatment options are being discussed.

In normal conception, a sperm is required to pass through the cervix, uterine cavity and uterine tubes to meet and fertilize a 'ripe' oocyte that has been released from the ovary. The fertilized ovum then needs to pass through the uterine tube and implant in the hormone-prepared endometrium lining the uterus. Although this sounds relatively straightforward, all factors in this pathway must be present to achieve a successful pregnancy. If one or more of these is absent or not functioning correctly, the couple will be unable to conceive.

Specific investigations
Investigations into possible causes of infertility are based around discovering which part of the pathway may be preventing conception. These can be divided into two areas:

- hormonal – this involves checking that gametes (sperm and oocytes) are being produced
- mechanical – this will involve checking there are no obstructions to the gametes meeting.

When a couple is referred by their GP to a specialist, both partners must be seen together, as this is a problem affecting the couple, not just the woman or man, and both must be fully included and investigated. An accurate history is taken from both partners and will include their medical history, previous surgery, sexual activity (both current and past), previous STIs, family history, alcohol, smoking and use of recreational drugs, and lifestyle/exercise. In addition, details will be recorded of the woman's menstrual, obstetric and contraceptive history and of any previous pregnancies by the man. Each partner will undergo a full physical examination that will include inspection of the external genitalia and a pelvic examination of the woman. The information sought from the couple can be extremely embarrassing for them and so questions must be handled in a sensitive manner. However, individuals may not have disclosed details of previous pregnancies, terminations, STIs and past sexual activities to each other and sometimes this sort of information will only be divulged when the couple are apart, e.g. during a specific test or examination. In many units, specialist nurses undertake this history-taking. Once this initial assessment has been undertaken further, more specific investigations will be planned. Investigations are designed to look at:

- ovulation
- tubal patency
- spermatozoa production.

Ovulation

The following investigations will confirm whether the woman is ovulating:

Basal body temperature (BBT). Secretion of progesterone by the corpus luteum causes a rise in BBT by 0.5°C. The woman records her BBT (on waking) throughout her menstrual cycle. The BBT falls slightly just before ovulation with the LH hormone surge and then rises after ovulation as progesterone is secreted by the corpus luteum.

Blood tests for hormone levels. As mentioned previously, the corpus luteum formed after ovulation secretes progesterone. The serum progesterone peaks in the midluteal phase and so a blood sample is taken on day 21 of the cycle. It is important to record the date of the onset of the next period in order to interpret these results accurately.

Endometrial biopsy. Histological examination of an endometrial biopsy taken in the luteal phase should reveal secretory changes if the woman has ovulated.

Serial ultrasounds. These can be used to assess the development of ovarian follicles and subsequent ovulation. This method is also used to assess development of follicles during treatment for ovulation induction.

Tubal patency

These investigations are aimed at detecting any tubal blockages or adhesions distorting the tubes, so they are not in alignment with the ovaries.

Hysterosalpingogram. This will only show the presence of any blockage in the tube and not any pelvic pathology.

Laparoscopy and tubal dye. A laparoscope is used to visualize the pelvis and female reproductive system. Methylene blue dye is injected through the cervix and the operator assesses how quickly the tubes fill with the dye and whether the dye comes out of the end of the tubes indicating they are patent.

Spermatozoa production

Semen analysis is undertaken to check the number, motility and morphology (form) of spermatozoa. The man produces a sample either at home, in which case he must keep it warm until delivery to the hospital for analysis, or more usually in the specialist unit. The volume of semen, the number of spermatozoa present, their motility and the percentage of abnormal spermatozoa are all measured. It is often recommended to repeat the semen analysis again as spermatozoa production can be affected by physical changes such as an acute infection several weeks previously.

Medical/surgical management

Management of the disorder depends on the cause, if one is discovered. There are many treatment options and all are termed assisted conception. These are outlined in Table 25.7, page 760. However, funding for assisted conception treatments is not universally available throughout the NHS (see Ethical Issues box 25.2).

▶ Nursing management

Specialist nurses have developed skills in both counselling and undertaking procedures in infertility clinics that enable couples to receive continuity of care throughout their treatment. A nurse working in an infertility unit must have the capacity to be both advocate and counsellor to the couple and discuss fully with them all available options during the initial pre-treatment assessment. There is considerable scope for nurses to develop their role and additional skills in infertility care. The discussions will include much embarrassing and personal information and so the nurse will need to be very sensitive to the couple's feelings and anxieties. Many people who experience difficulties in conceiving find this acutely distressing as they may never have considered that once they decided to start a family, there would be a problem.

 ETHICAL ISSUES

25.2 Infertility treatment

Couples who have not been able to conceive but who have had over a year of unprotected intercourse are often referred to a specialist unit for further investigations. Investigations such as ultrasound, hysterosalpingogram, laparoscopy to check tubal patency and semen analysis to check the content and morphology of the sperm are often carried out on the NHS.

The results of these investigations may reveal that the best and possibly only chance of achieving a pregnancy is through assisted conception techniques. However, funding for these procedures are not universally available on the NHS and there are many different options as to how treatment is funded, including:

- All treatment, including medication, has to be paid by the couple.
- Treatment costs are paid by the couple but the health authority funds the drugs.

- The health authority may fund a limited number of treatments each year. Because the number of these funded treatments is far below the actual demand, criteria are applied to determine who on the waiting list will have their treatment paid for.
- Some units operate egg donation schemes whereby women who agree to donate some of their eggs produced during ovulation induction will pay a reduced cost for treatment.

Student activities
- Should the NHS fund all infertility treatment?
- Should there be specific criteria for treating couples, such as whether they already have any children?
- Do you think there should be an age limit for treatment and, if you do, what would you consider it should be?
- Do you agree that incentives should be offered for donating gametes, such as reduced costs for treatment?
- What do you think should happen to surplus embryos produced during assisted conception procedures?

Table 25.7 Common assisted conception treatments

Disorder	Treatment	Description of treatment
Ovulatory disorder	Clomifene	Non-steroidal, anti-oestrogen oral tablet. Acts on hypothalamus and increases pituitary gonadotrophin production. Effective in inducing ovulation in approximately 80% of women, and up to 50% of these will conceive
Ovulatory disorder	Follicle-stimulating hormone (FSH)	Daily injections to induce ovulation. Follicles mature, hCG injection to release eggs, followed by intercourse
Tubal blockage	Tubal surgery salpingostomy	Can be done laparoscopically or by laparotomy to remove blockages, particularly at fimbrial end. Salpingostomy involves stitching back fimbrial ends to form opening at end of tube
Pelvic adhesions	Division of adhesions	Can often be done laparoscopically but may need to undergo open surgery via laparotomy. Adhesions are divided to free up tubes and ovaries so both are aligned
Unexplained infertility	Artificial insemination by partner	Woman is given treatment to induce ovulation and produce up to three oocytes. Semen is introduced through the cervix
Low/absent sperm count	Donor insemination (DI)	Semen from screened donor introduced through the cervix
Unexplained infertility	Gamete intrafallopian transfer (GIFT) – one tube must be functional	Woman has ovulation induction using gonadotrophins to produce several follicles. Oocytes collected before ovulation either transvaginally or laparoscopically under general anaesthetic. A maximum of three oocytes plus a medium containing motile sperm are transferred to the functional uterine tube. Thus fertilization occurs in the normal site
Unexplained infertility	Zygote intrafallopian transfer (ZIFT) – one tube must be functional	As for GIFT but this time fertilization occurs in the laboratory (*in vitro*). The fertilized oocyte is transferred to the functional tube about 18–24 hours following insemination. A further variation is tubal embryo transfer (TET) where the transfer takes place 48 hours following insemination
Unexplained infertility Tubal blockage	*In vitro* fertilization (IVF)	Known as 'test tube baby'. Woman has ovulation induction using gonadotrophins to produce several follicles. Oocytes are collected before ovulation, either transvaginally or laparoscopically under general anaesthetic. Best sperm is selected from fresh sample and introduced to oocytes in the laboratory. Resultant embryos (maximum three) are introduced to uterus at 4–8 cell stage for implantation. Donor eggs can also be used if there are problems with ovulation. Additional embryos can be frozen for use at later date
Sperm disorder	Intracytoplasmic sperm injection (ICSI)	Sperm is obtained via ejaculate or directly from testis. In the laboratory a single sperm is injected into the centre of an oocyte obtained as in IVF procedure

Once the initial assessment has been undertaken and a plan of management agreed with the couple and medical staff, the nurse can also undertake many of the investigations. Serial scanning is required during all stages of ovulation induction to assess the development of follicles and ensure the ovaries are not becoming over- or hyperstimulated. Nurses who have received appropriate training and are competent in the procedure (NMC 2002) can undertake this test, which will offer a more flexible service for the woman, often being able to be fitted in around the woman's work commitments. This is particularly important, as many couples do not want work colleagues, family or friends to know they are receiving infertility investigations or treatments. Confidentiality is a key aspect of assisted conception and all NHS and private infertility units must be licensed by the Human Fertilization and Embryology Authority (HFEA) and must comply with their standards in order to practise.

Couples undergoing treatment for infertility embark on a roller-coaster of emotion, ranging from hope and joy to extreme disappointment and distress when treatments are unsuccessful. This is an extremely emotive clinical area to work in and the nurse plays a pivotal part in providing advice and support to ensure couples' expectations are fully informed and realistic. Women and men undergoing surgical procedures for both investigation and treatment will require the nurse's skill in both pre- and postoperative care. Once individuals are fit for discharge, the nurse must be able to give appropriate advice as to what to expect during recovery and when normal social and work functions can be resumed.

Although there can sometimes be much heartache working with infertile couples, it can be extremely rewarding when treatment is successful and the couple achieve a pregnancy which continues to term and a live baby.

SEXUALLY TRANSMITTED INFECTIONS

Sexually transmitted infections (STIs), now more commonly known as sexually acquired infections (SAIs), are an ancient and common problem. There are various theories for the advent of these infections. One prominent one is that with the advent of travel, discovery and war, people from different cultures with different immune systems came into close contact and ill-prepared immune systems were suddenly confronted with new bacteria to recognize, fight and kill. Without effective medicines, such infections flourished. When these discoverers and soldiers returned to their native lands, they brought with them 'new' bacterial infections that easily swept through society.

SAIs have carried a significant social stigma throughout the ages; various acts of legislation, such as the Contagious Diseases Act – 1864, confirmed the ignorance and abhorrence of these infections and sought to 'blame' individuals (usually women) for their spread. Acknowledging the tendency of fighting men to fraternize, in 1916 Public Health (Venereal Diseases) Regulations heralded free and confidential SAI clinics for all. The result of this legislation was that gonorrhoea and syphilis became less common in the UK, compared with industrialized countries that still stigmatized these infections. With the advent of penicillin came a major breakthrough in treating SAIs that may have contributed to the sexual freedom of the 1960s. Since this time, the human immunodeficiency virus (HIV) has become the feared SAI. Again society has looked for scapegoats for this infection, often incorrectly blaming those on the periphery of society.

The current trends in SAIs show that cases are still rising despite public health programmes (see Health Promotion box 25.4) and the availability of contraceptives and barrier methods such as condoms. Risk factors for SAIs include young, single individuals, those who have multiple sexual partners, who do not use barrier contraceptives and live in metropolitan areas. The numbers of all episodes of SAIs continues to increase in the UK.

The role of the nurse in a sexual health setting involves several key concepts, irrespective of the infection that patients present with. A diagnosis of any SAI can raise significant anxieties, not only from the diagnosis but also from the need to know the type of sexual act involved. It is essential to provide open, non-judgemental care, responding to the needs of the patients. Counselling services are important for patient support, particularly when patients are deciding whether to have a test for HIV. Effective counselling both before and after tests should be offered to patients. Sexual health centres maintain a policy of confidentiality that often allows previously hidden sexual expression from the patient or client.

Often contact tracing is required to limit the spread of the disease, managed by anonymous cards that are sent requesting attendance at the nearest sexual health clinic. These cards record a 'code number' that will indicate which treatment is required. Health advisors attached to sexual health clinics organize contact tracing.

The common sexually acquired/transmitted infections are discussed below, with some generalized treatment strategies; however, since this field of health care is evolving (particularly so with HIV), the drugs indicated are a rough guide rather than fixed treatment regimens, since in this dynamic area therapies

 HEALTH PROMOTION

25.4 Safe sex

Promoting sexual health or a safe sex campaign can be a difficult process. Peer pressure, empowerment, legal aspects and information-giving are just a few problems that are commonly encountered by health professionals, but the biggest barrier to health promotion is embarrassment. Practitioners are embarrassed to ask patients about their sexual activity, and patients are too embarrassed to ask for advice; no information is given and the spread of sexually acquired infections, unwanted pregnancies and HIV infection continues.

The only safe way of 'having sex' is masturbation. Any sexual act that involves exposure to, or transfer of, bodily fluids carries a risk. Using a condom, whether for vaginal, anal or oral sex, dramatically reduces the chances of problems, although it does not remove the chances altogether. The condom should be worn throughout the sexual encounter, i.e. before penetration, and using alternative methods of contraception, such as the diaphragm, may not be as effective.

Intercourse is often a spontaneous event, and therefore both partners should be responsible for their sexual health; this may be achieved by both having condoms in their possession and acknowledging the effects of alcohol on inhibition.

A general guide to safe sex includes:

- Avoid casual sex
- If you don't want a child, use a condom
- If you're not having intercourse with your regular partner, use a condom
- If in doubt, don't have sex.

often change. Of fundamental importance is an accurate sexual history (see Guidelines for Care Priorities box 25.2).

GENITAL WARTS

External genital warts are caused by various types of human papillomavirus (HPV) and are very common. HPV is passed by close physical contact (skin to skin) and is almost always through genital contact, although warts in the oral cavity are not uncommon. The HPV attacks squamous epithelia and mucous membranes of the cervix, vagina, vulva, penis, anal cavity and oral cavity. The warts appear as pink or whitish lumps, either singly or in groups. These groups have been divided into three categories: pointed (acuminata), rounded (papula) and flat (macula).

Clinical presentation

The signs and symptoms of genital warts include genital lumps, bleeding, itchiness and sometimes hyperpigmentation; therefore diagnosis can be made visually. In some cases, however, the incubation period can be up to 18 months, and therefore DNA testing will be required.

25.2 Taking a sexual history

Gaining an accurate sexual history is vital for the effective treatment of patients and their sexual partner(s). Nurses should emphasize that information is confidential and ask questions in a sensitive and non-judgemental way. Patients may ask why certain information is required and the nurse should be able to give a full explanation.

Information required
- Presenting complaint
- History of presenting complaint
- Symptoms:
  — discharge: amount and colour
  — associated symptoms
  — bowel or bladder symptoms
  — duration of symptoms
- Partners:
  — are they sexually active?
  — condom use
  — type of sex (e.g. oral, vaginal or anal)
  — regular or casual partners
  — other partners in the last 3 months
  — sex with same or opposite sex partners
  — sex work (have you been paid for sex)
  — partners from overseas
- Contraception – method and correct usage
- Previous SAI diagnoses:
  — what was diagnosed and when?
  — how was it treated?
  — compliance
  — treatment of partner (possibility of re-infection)
- Menstrual history – date of last menstrual period and duration
- Past medical history – serious medical conditions and operations
- Smear history – last cervical cytology and result
- Drug and social history – allergies/all medication (prescribed and over-the-counter), tobacco, alcohol and illicit drugs.

Management

Patients should always be tested for other SAIs. Treatment is aimed at removing visible warts since it is impossible to eradicate the virus. The treatment options include solutions and creams containing podophyllin, or its major active constituent podophyllotoxin, or cryotherapy. Podophyllin is a cytotoxic topical solution that is applied two to three times per week to the wart. The solution is left in situ for 4–6 hours and then washed off. Care should be taken not to allow the solution to affect the surrounding skin (protected by using a covering of soft paraffin), to reduce the chance of damaging the skin. Podophyllin should not be used in pregnancy or during breast-feeding.

Cervical warts may require colposcopy and/or cryotherapy (see p. 714) and oral warts are treated by cryotherapy. This technique freezes the wart with liquid nitrogen, resulting in cell necrosis.

Normally, contact tracing would form a routine part of the patient assessment, but since incubation may be delayed, this is often futile in these individuals.

CANDIDIASIS (VAGINAL THRUSH)

The causative organism is usually *Candida albicans* and most women will have an episode in their lifetime. The yeast *Candida albicans* normally lives in the gut, mouth and genital tract, thriving in warm, moist and dark environments. The vagina can be considered an ideal environment for growth of this infection, since semen, menstrual blood, pregnancy and feminine hygiene products can all change the pH of the vagina. These changes in pH create an imbalance that predisposes to the development of thrush. Additional risk factors include diabetes mellitus, thyroid disease, iron deficiency, oral contraceptive, antibiotic therapy and immunodeficiency.

Transmission can be by sexual intercourse, during foreplay and by oral/genital contact. Men are more likely to acquire the infection during sexual activity, whereas women acquire it as a result of their predisposing factors. The incubation period is between 2 and 5 days.

Clinical presentation

Signs and symptoms include intense pruritus (often worse at night), vaginal soreness, white patches on the vulva/vagina, sometimes dysuria, creamy white vaginal discharge and balanitis in men, although these signs are non-specific. Diagnosis is by examination and microbiological investigation.

Management

Antifungal drugs such as clotrimazole, miconazole and nystatin are commonly used as creams and pessaries in the management of this condition. Systemic treatment may be necessary if symptoms persist. Sexual partners with symptoms should also be treated as they may cause re-infection.

Some patients prefer to use many traditional and alternative therapies, e.g. oral garlic supplements and dietary changes.

TRICHOMONIASIS

Trichomonas vaginalis (a protozoon) causes trichomoniasis, and is exclusively a sexually acquired disease in adults. This is a very common sexually acquired infection, living as a parasite that causes disease in the genital tract, affecting the vagina and urethra. Transmission is by contact with vaginal or seminal fluid; although there is no evidence that transmission occurs via infected materials, this protozoa can last for several hours outside the body.

Clinical presentation

The signs and symptoms include profuse vaginal discharge (offensive, yellow, thin, frothy and irritating), dysuria, vulval soreness and lower abdominal pain, although men can remain asymptomatic. The incubation period can be up to 4 weeks, although this can be dependent on the menstrual cycle. It can be difficult to diagnose in men due to the lack of distinct symptoms, and although there are difficulties, it is vital to contact trace.

Management

Diagnosis is by examination (the vaginal walls and cervix may be inflamed), high vaginal swab and assessment of pH. Treatment options include the antibiotic metronidazole, given to both partners over 5 days. This should be taken with food; alcohol and sexual activity should be avoided during the treatment programme.

CHLAMYDIA

Chlamydia is caused by the bacterium *Chlamydia trachomatis*. It is the most common sexually acquired infection in the UK (Public Health Laboratory Service 2002). It is particulary common in young, sexually active women (16–24 years). Chlamydia is a serious disease and has a number of complications, therefore early detection and treatment are important. Treatment is relatively simple, once the infection has been detected.

Clinical presentation

Many patients with chlamydia are asymptomatic – 80% of women and 50% of men. However, women may present with:

- postcoital or intermenstrual bleeding
- purulent vaginal discharge
- lower abdominal pain
- proctitis.

The presentation in men includes:

- urethral discharge
- dysuria
- testicular/epididymal pain
- proctitis.

Testing for chlamydia now involves the use of molecular biological tests to detect chlamydial DNA in urine, vaginal, cervical and vulval swabs. A national screening service for chlamydial infection is proposed for the UK and various sites offering urine tests will be phased in during 2002–2003.

The most common complication in men is epididymitis. In women the infection spreads up the reproductive tract and leads to pelvic inflammatory disease (PID), endometritis, salpingitis, tubal damage and chronic pelvic pain. PID increases the risk of ectopic pregnancy and infertility (see pp. 729–730).

Management

Sexual intercourse should be abstained from during the treatment programme. Antibiotics such as doxycycline can be used provided the patient is not at risk of pregnancy or is breast-feeding. Alternative treatment can be with erythromycin.

Partner notification must be discussed with patients. It is essential that all recent (last 3 months or previous partner if longer) and current sexual partners should be informed and advised to attend for assessment. Without treatment the reproductive system of both sexes can be severely damaged, in addition to the continued transmission of the infection.

GENITAL HERPES

This is a highly contagious viral disease transmitted through close physical or sexual contact and is caused by the herpes simplex virus (HSV). There are two types of HSV, both of which infect the skin and mucous membranes: HSV-1, which commonly causes cold sores, and HSV-2, which infects the genital areas.

Clinical presentation

The virus attacks the outer layer of the skin, forming characteristic blisters with clear fluid inside. Prior to the formation of these blisters, however, the skin often becomes 'tingly' or more sensitive. The period between infection and signs of the disease is approximately 7 days. In addition to the signs described above, patients may complain of fever, joint/muscle pain and cystitis.

Management

There is no cure for HSV – once infected the individual is always a carrier of the virus. It lies dormant around nerve roots, but in the presence of a weakened immune system, the virus reactivates. Patients should be given advice about mild painkillers, e.g. paracetamol, resting and taking extra fluids during the systemic disturbance associated with the primary infection. Treatment with aciclovir (topical or oral route) may help to prevent the formation of blisters. The blisters should be kept dry and clean.

Since transmission of HSV is through close contact, a barrier (condom) method of contraception should be used. Even though there are no blisters or ulcers visible, the virus can be passed on during sexual intercourse, oral sex (from a cold sore to the genitals), and via the vulva when giving birth (this does not include caesarean section).

GONORRHOEA

Gonorrhoea is caused by the bacterium *Neisseria gonorrhoeae*, which infects the mucosal surfaces of the genital tract, rectum and oropharynx. The infection is always transmitted by sexual contact (however, eye infections can occur in infants during birth, and gonococcal vulvovaginitis in young girls can result from sexual abuse). The incubation period is around 24 hours, but can take up to 5 days, and is highly infectious. Currently gonorrhoea is most commonly seen in minority ethnic groups, homosexuals and younger women (Nicholas & Weston 1999). Uncomplicated gonorrhoea is the second commonest bacterial SAI (Public Health Laboratory Service 2002).

Clinical presentation

The signs and symptoms of gonorrhoea depend on the site of infection but include urethritis (causing dysuria and purulent discharge), cervicitis (causing vaginal discharge), proctitis with discharge and pharyngitis. However, many patients, especially women with uncomplicated infection, are asymptomatic. It is important to note that:

- 85% of men with urethral infection develop symptoms within 2 weeks
- rectal infection may be asymptomatic
- pharyngeal infection may be asymptomatic
- cervical infection in women is often asymptomatic.

Complications of gonorrhoea include formation of abscess, epididymitis, prostatitis and urethral strictures in men. Women may develop endometritis, ovarian abscesses, salpingitis and infertility, and bartholinitis. Gonorrhoea is diagnosed by microbiological examination of a swab of the discharge to identify the microorganism. In addition, patients need to be screened for chlamydia and trichomoniasis.

Management

Treatment options vary, but single-dose antibiotics such as intramuscular procaine penicillin with probenecid (delays renal clearance of the drug) or oral amoxicillin with probenecid are given when the microorganism is sensitive to penicillin. Oral ciprofloxacin is used for penicillin-resistant microorganisms.

Single-dose treatment is useful in appropriate circumstances, as it overcomes problems of non-compliance.

Patients are asked to abstain from sexual activity until a second test confirms that treatment has been effective. The opportunity should be taken to advise patients about the use of condoms in preventing the spread of SAIs.

Contact tracing with partner notification must be discussed with patients but it is essential that all recent (last 3 months or previous partner if longer) and current sexual partners should be informed and advised to attend for assessment.

SYPHILIS

Syphilis is caused by the bacterium *Treponema pallidum*. In adults it is spread through close sexual contact. Congenital syphilis occurs by vertical transmission from mother to fetus.

The number of cases of primary and secondary syphilis (particularly in men who have sex with men) has risen in the UK over recent years (Public Health Laboratory Service 2002).

Clinical presentation

Syphilis has four stages: primary, secondary, latent and tertiary (see Box 25.6). However, some authorities use the terms early or late syphilis. It is worth noting that in many individuals there may be no clinical signs of syphilis (latent syphilis).

Infectious syphilis includes primary, secondary and latent stages, but patients are highly infectious during the first two stages. Diagnosis is by close medical history, since the disease is often acquired abroad. Primary syphilis is diagnosed by microbiological confirmation of the presence of the microorganism in exudate obtained from the ulcer (chancre). Serological tests are used to detect the presence of antibodies, e.g. fluorescent treponemal antibody absorbed test (specific test), rapid plasma reagin test (non-specific test).

Management

The antibiotic chosen and duration of treatment depend on the disease stage; intramuscular procaine penicillin or oral erythromycin if allergic to penicillin, or oral doxycycline and oxytetracycline are used. Patients having penicillin should be warned about the possibility of having a Jarisch–Herxheimer reaction. This is characterized by fever, chills, nausea, muscle pain, dizziness and headache. It is possibly caused by toxins released when the microorganisms are destroyed. The reaction occurs within a few hours of having the penicillin and is usually short-lived.

Box 25.6 The stages of syphilis – clinical presentation

Primary
Two to four weeks after exposure, a papule develops (at the site of infection), which ulcerates, becoming a hard, painless ulcer known as a chancre. There is swelling of local lymph nodes. The ulcer is highly infectious. The ulcer usually heals within a few weeks.

Secondary
A few months after the ulcer has healed, there may be a generalized 'flu-like illness, with fever, sore throat, and non-specific pain. Clinical signs of secondary syphilis may be present and include generalized lymph node enlargement, skin rashes, warty areas (condylomata lata) in the perianal and other moist body sites, and mucosal ulcers in the mouth/external genitalia (also called 'snail-track' ulcers)

Latent
The person is well but serological tests for syphilis are positive. This stage may last for years.

Tertiary
Tertiary syphilis is characterized by deep ulcers (gumma) affecting the skin, bones and organs, and further cardiovascular and neurological effects:

- Cardiovascular problems include aneurysm formation in the ascending aorta
- Cerebral vascular changes increase the risk of strokes and dementia
- Neurosyphilis may lead to tabes dorsalis (ataxia with loss of coordination and abnormal sensation in the legs) and general paralysis of the insane (GPI).

Patients should also abstain from sexual activity during antibiotic treatment and continue to use a barrier method (i.e. condoms) at least until blood tests show that the infection has passed. However, the benefits of condom use in preventing further infection should be stressed.

HUMAN IMMUNODEFICIENCY VIRUS

An introduction to human immunodeficiency virus (HIV) and acquired immune deficiency syndrome (AIDS) is provided here, but readers should also consult specialist books (see 'Further reading', p. 767) and Chapter 13 for details of universal precautions, the transmission of blood-borne viruses and guidelines to follow in the event of exposure to HIV, such as through needlestick injuries. The management of HIV infection and AIDS is evolving all the time and readers are encouraged to consult authoritative journals and websites for the latest information.

The immune system provides specific resistance or defence from harmful substances that have 'invaded' the body. This is a complex system that involves recruitment of white blood cells or lymphocytes that respond to substances that actively harm the body, either by surrounding them so that no further damage can occur or by killing them. The activation of lymphocytes requires antigens.

There are two basic types of lymphocytes: T cells and B cells. B cells produce antibodies. Each antibody recognizes a particular antigen and binds to it. When this occurs, it signals to the immune system to attack the invading organism. T cells make proteins called receptors that recognize specific antigens, but these receptors remain on the surface of the cells.

There are two types of T cells: killer or cytotoxic cells (T_{killer}) and helper (T_{helper}) cells. Killer cells bind directly to cells carrying an invading organism, attacking and (hopefully) killing them. Helper cells interact with B cells, helping them to respond to antigens. These T cells have specific markers on their surface. CD-8 is found on T_{killer} cells whereas CD-4 is found on T_{helper} cells. These markers are functionally useful in that they can be easily counted, thus indicating the presence of an infection. Both B cells and T cells freely circulate through the bloodstream and lymphatic system.

HIV is a retrovirus, meaning that it contains RNA which, by reverse transcriptase enzymes, makes a viral DNA copy of the RNA. This is able to integrate into the host cell DNA where it changes the chromosomes, and replication of further viral RNA occurs. This means that there is a constant supply of new virus. These exit the cell, by a process termed budding, and move on to infect more cells.

A particular feature of retroviruses is that they do not kill the cells they infect. HIV depletes T cells (specifically, T_{helper} cells) of the immune system that normally stimulate the immune response. Without the means to mount an immune response, the host is open to a wide variety of opportunistic infections that do not normally produce disease. It is these infections that are so detrimental to patients. However, not all HIV patients will develop AIDS, implying that there is some resistance to HIV-associated immune system suppression.

HIV is transmitted through sexual contact, in blood or blood products and other body fluids, and by vertical transmission perinatally.

Clinical presentation

Infection with HIV can cause non-specific illnesses such as fever, malaise, lymphadenopathy and rashes. Within 6 weeks, antibodies to core and surface proteins can be observed, although there is some evidence to indicate that these antibodies can take longer to be developed. Antibodies can be detected (once expressed) by blood tests, e.g. enzyme-linked immunosorbent assay (ELISA). This is not highly specific for HIV infection, and a positive test is usually repeated and followed by the more specific Western blot test to confirm the diagnosis.

Patients may remain asymptomatic in the early stages of the disease process, but may have generalized lymph node swelling. Opportunistic infections can follow which commonly affect mucous membranes, e.g. candidiasis, affecting the mouth, oesophagus and lungs. Other opportunistic infections include pneumonia, caused by *Pneumocystis carinii*, tuberculosis (see Ch. 20), cytomegalovirus infection and *Cryptococcus neoformans*, causing meningitis and lung disease. As the disease develops, weight loss, fevers and night sweats are commonly found.

Patients with HIV are also prone to develop malignancies such as Kaposi's sarcoma (characterized by new blood vessel growth producing red, brown or purple lesions, often on the skin but with metastatic potential) and non-Hodgkin's lymphoma (see Ch. 18).

Management

The management of HIV is drug-based. Treatment is with antiviral drugs such as zidovudine (azidothymidine, AZT), which can prevent the spread of the disease to other cells. Additional aims of treatment include prevention or treatment of opportunistic infections (such as fluconazole for candidiasis), augmentation of the immune system, and support to patients. Antiviral drugs are usually given in different combinations depending on the stage of the disease, and include:

- Nucleoside reverse transcriptase inhibitor (anti-retroviral), e.g. zidovudine (azidothymidine, AZT), didanosine (DDI), zalcitabine (DDC). These drugs replace components needed for DNA replication and so halt the further replication of viral DNA. The benefits include the slowing of the infection in the T cells, allowing partial restoration of the immune system (note that our immune cells are replenished every 3 months).
- Protease inhibitors, e.g. amprenavir, ritonavir, saquinavir.
- Non-nucleoside reverse transcriptase inhibitors, e.g. efavirenz and nevirapine.

SUMMARY: MAIN POINTS

- Women suffering with gynaecological disorders often experience embarrassing symptoms.

- Initial investigations will involve obtaining a detailed history of symptoms and previous history followed by a pelvic examination. The nurse must provide empathy and support to ease the woman's anxieties during examination and provide relevant information.

- Many disorders are linked to problems with early pregnancy so the nurse requires a sound knowledge of pregnancy and its development.

- Surgical options are often the management of choice for many conditions. The nurse must ensure preoperative assessment has been undertaken and that the woman is fit for surgery and general anaesthetic.

- The nurse has a vital role in preparing women safely for theatre and in monitoring their condition postoperatively to ensure early detection of any complications.

- Nurses provide women with relevant information about their care in hospital, planned operation and procedures, and advice on discharge.

SUMMARY *(cont'd)*

■ It is clear that men and the health care professions generally undervalue men's health, evidenced by an increased mortality and morbidity in men compared with women. It has also been identified that men take greater risks with their health.

■ There are many reasons for these statistical differences, which have been discussed in this chapter, and nurses must take into consideration not only medical and nursing history, but also the social context, e.g. the man's social status, employment background and education.

■ Nurses need to understand that men generally perceive health in relation to fitness and masculinity and not disease and its prevention, whereas women perceive the opposite. This has implications in the delivery of care in all care settings, and the design of health promotion and education packages. There is clearly a demand for innovative action in men's health, i.e. if men will not go to the clinic, the clinic must go to them.

■ Many conditions that have been identified in this chapter need not affect the health of men, since some of them are preventable or treatable in the early stages of the disease. This has personal, economic and social consequences that affect society, which are continually ignored.

■ The unique role of the nurse is an excellent opportunity to promote men's health by direct questioning, information notices and provision of literature, irrespective of the environment in which care is delivered, e.g. hospital, community, leisure and employment.

■ Some of the treatment options discussed should be considered as a guide only, as each man should have an individualized care package that meets his needs. Despite the perceived promotion of men's health, there remains a discrepancy between the literature, clinical practice and the male population.

■ It is hoped that the conditions discussed in this chapter will provide an insight into the nursing care and management of men in the various care environments.

■ The number of women and men affected by SAIs continues to rise and with it serious health problems, such as infertility, which affect individuals and communities. SAIs remain a major public health issue.

■ Nurses have an important role in the prevention, detection and management of SAIs. This role includes health promotion, providing explanation and information, supporting patients through diagnosis and treatment, and providing open, non-judgemental care that meets individual needs.

■ Many specialist nurses practise in the areas of women's, men's and sexual health, e.g. oncology, infertility and erectile dysfunction.

SELF-TEST: CRITICAL THINKING ACTIVITIES

1 Farida (not her real name), who is 40 years of age and has 3 children aged between 6 and 17 years, has been admitted with a diagnosis of menorrhagia, causing her to be anaemic. She is to undergo a major operation tomorrow. You are allocated to admit her and also provide her care the following day.
   — What operation do you think she is likely to be having?
   — Why is Farida anaemic?
   — What information would you give her about the ward?
   — What types of assessment and what investigations would have been done in the preoperative assessment clinic?
   — What information would you give her about her impending surgery?
   — How would you deal with a question from Farida about whether she should have her ovaries removed?
   — What preoperative care would you need to ensure has been undertaken in order for her to have a general anaesthetic safely?
   — On return from theatre, what care will Farida receive and what postoperative observations will be undertaken? Give reasons for undertaking these observations.
   — What information will you give to Farida before she is discharged?

   — What complications can occur after a major gynaecological operation?

2 What are the common causes of erectile dysfunction?
   — What are the treatment options available for erectile dysfunction?
   What are the common investigations for testicular cancer, i.e. blood tests, and what is their significance?
   — How would you plan a teaching programme for testicular self-examination?
   What are the priorities of managing paraphimosis?
   What are key features of a sexual history?

3 Critical thinking analysis:
   — Why do you think there is a higher mortality and morbidity rate in the male population?
   — Do you think men's health promotion strategies have been successful? Give reasons for your answer.
   — Why do you think treatment for erectile dysfunction has been restricted by the UK government to a few selected medical conditions? Why have these been selected and not others?

FURTHER READING

Adler MW. ABC of sexually transmitted diseases, 4th edn. London: BMJ Publishing Group; 1998.

Adler MW. ABC of AIDS, 5th edn. London: BMJ Publishing Group; 2001.

Andrews G (ed). Women's sexual health. Edinburgh: Baillière Tindall; 2001.

Davidson N, Lloyd T. Promoting men's health; a guide for practitioners. Edinburgh: Baillière Tindall; 2001.

Department of Health. The national strategy for sexual health and HIV. London: Department of Health; 2001.

Ewles L, Simnett I. Promoting health; a practical guide, 5th edn. Edinburgh: Baillière Tindall; 2003.

Fillingham S, Douglas J. Urological nursing, 2nd edn. London: Baillière Tindall; 1997.

Gangar E (ed). Gynaecological nursing: a practical guide. Edinburgh: Churchill Livingstone; 2001.

Garden OJ, Bradbury AW, Forsythe JLR. Principles and practice of surgery, 4th edn. Edinburgh: Churchill Livingstone; 2002.

Harrison T, Dignan K. Men's health: an introduction for nurses and health professionals. Edinburgh: Churchill Livingstone; 1999.

Luesley D (ed). Common conditions in gynaecology. London: Chapman Hall; 1997.

Mallett J, Dougherty L (eds). The Royal Marsden Hospital Manual of Clinical Nursing Procedures, 5th edn. Oxford: Blackwell Science; 2000

Moulder C. Miscarriage: women's experiences and needs. London: Pandora; 1990.

Nicol M, Bavin C, Bedford-Turner S, Cronin P, Rawlings-Anderson K. Essential nursing skills. London: Mosby; 2000.

O'Mahony P. A question of life: its beginning and transmission. London: Sheed and Ward; 1990.

Smith JR, Barron BA. Gynaecological oncology. Oxford: Health Press; 1999.

Wells D, Clifford D, Rutter M, Selby J. Caring for sexuality in health and illness. Edinburgh: Churchill Livingstone; 2000.

Wilson H, McAndrew S (eds). Sexual health: foundations for practice. Edinburgh: Baillière Tindall; 2000.

USEFUL ADDRESSES

The Amarant Trust

11–13 Charterhouse Buildings
London EC1M 7AM
Tel: 020 7401 3855
Helpline: 01293 413000
Provides information, self-help for women undergoing menopause

Women's Health

52 Featherstone Street
London EC1Y 8RT
Enquiries: 020 7251 6580
Produces wide range of leaflets giving advice on women's health issues. Will provide further contacts for women requiring support following hysterectomy

USEFUL WEBSITES

www.agum.org.uk/filingcab – Association for Genito Urinary Medicine

www.bbc.co.uk/health/mens/ – BBC men's health website

www.cancerbackup.org.uk/ – Cancer BACUP

www.hmole-chorio.org.uk – Charing Cross Hospital – *information about hydatidiform mole for patients and health professionals*

www.endo.org.uk – Endometriosis Society – provides self help and information for patients and health professionals, with local groups (helpline: 0808 808 2227)

www.caritasdata.co.uk/Charity4/ch007274.htm – ISSUE (The National Fertility Association) – *provides information and support for couples with fertility problems*

www.malehealth.co.uk – Men's Health Forum – *information and advice for men*

www.miscarriageassociation.org.uk/ – Miscarriage Association

www.nat.org.uk – National AIDS Trust

www.nos.org.uk – National Osteoporosis Society – *patient information about issues relating to osteoporosis and menopause*

www.orchid-cancer.org.uk – Orchid Cancer Appeal – *information about testicular cancer*

www.rcog.org.uk – Royal College of Obstetricians and Gynaecologists – *details of all professional standards, guidelines and current issues in gynaecology*

www.roysocmed.ac.uk/pub/std.htm – Royal Society of Medicine

www.tht.org.uk – Terrence Higgins Trust

REFERENCES

Acheson N, Chan KK. Epithelial ovarian cancer. In: Shafi M, Luesley D, Jordan J, eds. Handbook of gynaecological oncology. Edinburgh: Churchill Livingstone; 2001.

Allan A. Types and causes of miscarriage. Modern Midwife 1995; 5(3): 27–30.

American Psychiatric Association. Diagnostic criteria from DSM-IV. Washington, DC: American Psychiatric Association; 1994.

Blackmore C. Altered images. Nurs Times 1989; 85(2): 36–39.

Blandy J. Lecture notes on urology, 5th edn. Oxford: Blackwell Science; 1998.

Bozcuk HS, Ravi R, Turner B et al. Computed tomography 21 days after chemotherapy, three-dimensional estimates of metastatic volume and the need for surgery in patients with germ cell cancer. Br J Urol Int 2000; 86: 707–713.

Brewster S. Urological oncology. In: Brewster C, Cranston D, Noble J, Reynard J, eds. Urology: a handbook for medical students. Oxford: Bios Scientific Publishers Ltd; 2001, ch 9.

Clayton SG, Newton JR. A Pocket Obstetrics and Gynaecology, 11th edn. Edinburgh: Churchill Livingstone; 1988.

Confidential Enquiries into Maternal Deaths in the United Kingdom. Why mothers die 1997–1999. London: RCOG Press; 2001.

Department of Health. Treatment for impotence. HSC 1999/148. London: Department of Health; 1999.

Department of Health. The NHS cancer plan. London: Department of Health; 2000.

Department of Health. Good practice in consent implementation guide: consent to examination or treatment. London: Department of Health; 2001.

Fosså SD, Kravdal Ø. Fertility in Norwegian testicular cancer patients. Br J Cancer 2000; 82: 737–741.

Girling JC, Soutter WP. Benign tumours of the ovary. In: Shaw RW, Soutter WP, Stanton SL, eds. Gynaecology, 2nd edn. London: Churchill Livingstone; 1997.

Gloeckler-Ries LA, Hankey BF, Edwards BK (eds). Cancer statistics review 1973–1987. National Cancer Institute, National Institutes of Health Publications No. 90-2789. Bethesda: National Institutes of Health; 1990.

Goldstein I. Foreword. In: Kirby R, Culley CC, Webster GD, eds. Impotence diagnosis and management of male erectile dysfunction. Oxford: Butterworth-Heinemann; 1991.

Govan ADT, McKay Hart D, Callander R. Gynaecology illustrated, 4th edn. Edinburgh: Churchill Livingstone; 1993.

Haward R. Improving outcomes in gynaecological cancer. London: NHS Executive; 1999.

Heaton JPW, Dean J, Sleep DJ. Rapid communication: sequential administration enhances the effect of apomorphine SL in men with erectile dysfunction. Int J Impotence Res 2002; 14: 61–64.

Hughes C. Cancer of the uterine cervix. In: Gangar EA, ed. Gynaecological nursing: a practical guide. Edinburgh: Churchill Livingstone; 2001.

Irvine LM, Hicks JL, Blair-Bell, Setchell ME. The incidence of ectopic pregnancy in the City and Hackney health district of London 1990–1991. J Obs Gyn 1994; 14(1): 29–34.

Jackson G, Betteridge J, Dean J et al. Systemic approach to erectile dysfunction in the cardiovascular patient: a consensus statement. Int J Clin Pract 1999; 53(6): 445–451.

James WH. A possible cause of testicular cancer. Br J Cancer 2000; 82(12): 2022–2023.

Jefferies H. The psychosocial care of the patient with cervical cancer. Cancer Nurs Pract 2002a; 1(6): 19–25.

Jefferies H. Ovarian cancer patients: are their informational and emotional needs being met. J Clin Nurs 2002b; 11(1): 41–47

Johnson A, Wadsworth J, et al. (1994) Sexual attitudes and lifestyles survey. UK 1990–1991. In: Department of Health. Treatment for impotence. HSC 1999/148. London: Department of Health; 1999.

Johnson MH, Everitt BJ. Essential Reproduction. 4th edn. Oxford: Blackwell Science; 1995.

Laumann EO, Gagnon JH, Michael RT, Michaels S. The social organisation of sexuality. Chicago, IL: University of Chicago Press; 1994.

Luesley DM. Vulval cancer. In: Shafi M, Luesley D, Jordan J, eds. Handbook of gynaecological oncology. Edinburgh: Churchill Livingstone; 2001.

Lynch DF, Schellhammer PF. Tumors of the penis. In: Walsh PC, Reyik AB, Vaughan ED, Wein AJ, eds. Campbell's urology, 7th edn. Philadelphia: WB Saunders; 1998, ch 79.

Macdonald R. Audit applied to endometrial ablation. In: Sutton CJG, ed. New surgical techniques in gynaecology. Carnforth: Parthenon; 1993.

Martin D. Pre-operative visits to reduce patient anxiety: a study. Nurs Stand 1996; 10(23): 33–38.

Masters WH, Johnson VE. Human sexual inadequacy. Boston: Little, Brown; 1970.

Møller H. Trends in sex ratio, testicular cancer and male reproductive hazards: are they connected? Acta Pathol Microbiol Scand 1998; 106: 232–239.

Moynihan C. Testicular cancer: the psychosocial problems of patients and their relatives. Cancer Survey 1987; 6(3): 477–510.

Muir CS, Nectoux J. Epidemiology of cancer of the testis and penis. National Cancer Institute Monographs 1979; Nov: 157–164.

Nicholas H, Weston A. Gonorrhoea: symptoms and treatment. In: Weston A, ed. Sexually transmitted infections: a guide to care. London: Nursing Times Books; 1999.

Nicholson PW, Harland SJ. Inheritance and testicular cancer. Br J Cancer 1995; 71(2): 421–426.

Nursing and Midwifery Council (NMC). Code of professional conduct. London: Nursing and Midwifery Council; 2002.

Pilar-Lagunam M, Pizzocaro G, Klepp O, Algaba F, Kisbenedek L, Leiva O. EAU Guidelines on testicular cancer. Eur Urol 2001;40(2):102–110.

Power DA, Brown RS, Brock CS, Payne HA, Majeed A, Babb P. Trends in testicular carcinoma in England and Wales 1971–99. Br J Urol Int 2001; 87(4): 361–365.

Public Health Laboratory Service. HIV and STIs: epidemiology. Online. Available: www.phls.org.uk. 2002.

Raleigh EH, Lepczyc M, Rowley C. Significant others benefit from pre-operative information. J Adv Nurs 1990; 15: 941–945.

Ritchie JP. Neoplasms of the testis. In: Walsh PC, Retik AB, Vaughan ED, Wein AJ, eds. Campbell's urology, 7th edn. Philadelphia: WB Saunders; 1998, Vol 3, pp 2411–2452.

Royal College of Obstetricians and Gynaecologists (RCOG). Report of RCOG working party on prophylaxis against thromboembolism in gynaecology and obstetrics. London: Chameleon; 1995.

Royal College of Obstetricians and Gynaecologists (RCOG). The initial management of menorrhagia – national evidence based guidelines. London: RCOG; 1998.

Royal College of Obstetricians and Gynaecologists (RCOG). The management of menorrhagia in secondary care – national evidence based guidelines. London: RCOG; 1999.

Royal College of Obstetricians and Gynaecologists (RCOG). Management of early pregnancy loss. London: Chameleon; 2001.

Steggall MJ, Gann SY. Assessing patients with actual or potential erectile dysfunction. Professional Nurse 2002; 18(3): 155–159.

Sutton CJG (ed). New surgical techniques in gynaecology. Carnforth: Parthenon; 1993.

Taylor J, Goodman M, Luesley D. Is home best? Nurs Times 1993; 89(37): 31–33.

United Kingdom Central Council. The scope of professional practice. London: UKCC; 1992.

Van Basten JPA, ven Driel MF, Hoekstra HJ et al. Objective and subjective effects of treatment for testicular cancer on sexual function. Br J Urol Int 1999; 84(6): 671–678.

Webb V, Holmes A. Urological cancers: do early detection strategies exist? Br J Urol Int 2000; 86(9): 996–1000.

Whitton A. Early pregnancy disorders. In: Ganger EA, ed. Gynaecological nursing – a practical guide. Edinburgh: Churchill Livingstone; 2001.

Wilson-Barnett J. Stress in hospital. Edinburgh: Churchill Livingstone; 1979.

26 Breast disorders

Helen Barlow

'She's having a mastectomy tomorrow and I really want to support her but I'm not sure how I will react when I see it. The Breast Care Nurse says it's quite common for partners to feel like this and has promised to be there when we see it for the first time'.

(Patient's partner)

THIS CHAPTER WILL HELP YOU

- Understand the structure and function of the normal breast and how it is altered by breast disease

- Describe the nursing assessment of patients with breast disorders

- Describe the variety of breast disorders with respect to aetiology, pathophysiology, clinical presentation and medical management

- Describe the nursing management of each disorder

- Demonstrate an insight into the psychological, emotional and social effects of breast disorders

- Understand the role of the specialist breast care nurse.

KEYWORDS

Breast reconstruction	Mammogram
Body image	Mastalgia
Chemotherapy	Metastases
Gynaecomastia	Palliation
Hormone therapy	Radiotherapy
Lymph nodes	Tamoxifen
Lymphoedema	Triple assessment

INTRODUCTION

Powerful sexual stereotyping has meant that breasts are symbolic of feelings of warmth, motherhood, affection and femininity (Ch. 25). It is therefore not surprising that deviations from 'normal' can cause changes in self-image, low self-esteem, embarrassment, feelings of unattractiveness and reduced libido (Fallowfield & Clark 1991).

Breast disease is extremely common, and because of this, the majority of health care professionals will come into contact with it. Nurses have an important role at all stages of breast disease, from health promotion and screening to terminal care (Ch. 34). They can support both patients and carers (Ch. 6) and also act as a resource to other health care professionals (Ch. 3). Approximately 90% of women referred to a breast clinic have benign disease, but all fear cancer. Breast cancer remains the most common malignancy in women (Ch. 33). One in 12 women will develop the disease during their lifetime and there are over 30 000 new cases per year in the UK (CRC 1996). It is essential that women have an accurate diagnosis in specialist breast clinics. Historically, inequity of care has been highlighted in breast cancer. For example, a woman's treatment, and therefore survival, could depend on where she lived. The Calman-Hine Report (Calman & Hine 1995) has sought to address this through research-based evidence to guide care. This advocates the use of protocols, so that all women have the same high standard of care across the country. This work is ongoing and change is slow, but developments include the start of specialization and recognized breast clinics.

OVERVIEW OF ANATOMY AND PHYSIOLOGY

THE NORMAL BREAST

The structure of the female breast (mammary gland) is related to function, which is the production of nourishment for a baby, initially colostrum and then milk. It is considered to be a modified sweat gland, which rests on the anterior rib cage.

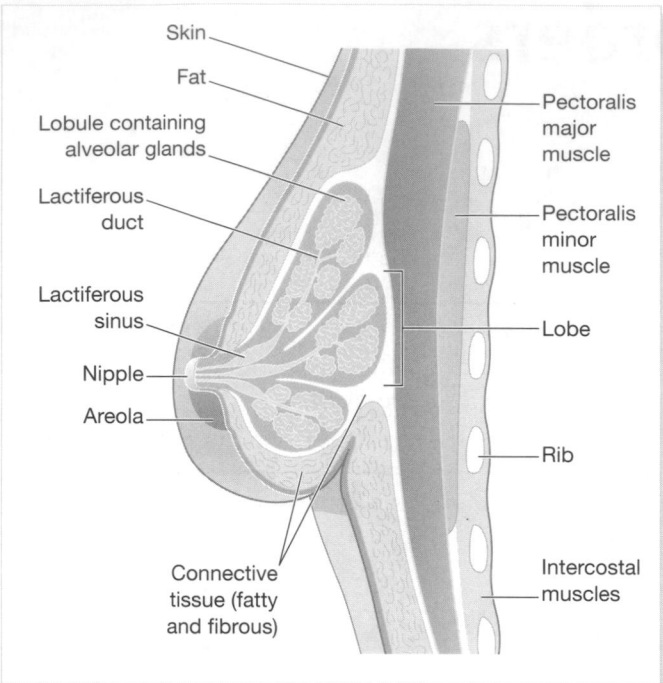

Figure 26.1 Lateral view of the breast.

Breast tissue consists of about 15–20 lobes arranged around the nipple. These consist of lobules of alveolar glands where milk is produced (Fig. 26.1). The lobules drain into lactiferous ducts which form dilated lactiferous sinuses at the nipple. The nipple, surrounded by the pigmented areola, contains small muscle fibres that react to stimulation and temperature. There is an extensive lymphatic system within the breast, which drains to regional lymph nodes in the axilla and to other nodes. The lymphatic drainage is significant to the way that breast cancer spreads so effectively around the body. The breast is a highly vascular organ, served by the axillary artery and the internal mammary artery.

Several pituitary and ovarian hormones influence the breast. During each menstrual cycle, the breasts undergo changes associated with the hormones oestrogen and progesterone. Milk secretion is stimulated by prolactin, and oxytocin is concerned with milk ejection or 'let down'.

NURSING ASSESSMENT

The vast majority of women presenting with breast disorders will have benign disease. Most, however, fear it will be cancer and need to be treated with care and compassion at all stages of the diagnostic and treatment phase. Most patients will have presented to their GP with a specific breast problem. Where GPs feel it is indicated, patients are referred (routine or urgent) to a specialist breast clinic for further assessment. As soon as such a referral takes place, patients will begin to fear that there is an underlying tumour in their breast. In reality, 90% of referrals are for benign disorders, but until a woman receives her diagnosis, it is difficult to dispel this fear.

In the UK, the breast-screening programme targets all eligible women (between the ages of 50 and 70 years) for 3-yearly mammography (breast X-ray) checks. This can be a source of anxiety since it may pick up small cancers in women who have no physical signs. The nurse in a screening clinic should bear in mind that the routine screening programme could suddenly give a 'well woman' a diagnosis of cancer. In the event of unsatisfactory mammograms, a woman may be recalled to the clinic for repeat films. The recall system may cause unnecessary anxiety in women and information about when they are likely to receive their results should be given.

Male breast disorders are relatively uncommon in comparison to female disorders, but they do occur and nurses need to consider the effect this can have on a man. Breast disease is associated with females and men may feel that their sexuality is threatened and may feel stigmatized.

The nursing assessment of patients with breast disorders may occur in the clinic setting or in hospital and will include several aspects, as described below.

PHYSICAL ASSESSMENT

Most patients will be otherwise well, especially if they have come through the screening programme. Patients later diagnosed as having a malignancy may recall feeling more tired than usual, but for others the diagnosis may be a complete surprise since they had been feeling so well. Patients who have breast infections may feel systemically unwell, with a raised temperature and general lethargy. Concurrent conditions should always be assessed and any current medication recorded. Patients will always undergo a breast examination, either by medical staff or by nurses trained in breast examination.

SOCIAL ASSESSMENT

It is always important to establish who patients live with and what support networks they are able to access through family and friends. For some women, child care may be a huge consideration, especially when considering treatment options. Likewise, travel issues may influence choice – not all patients have access to a car. It has not been uncommon for women to opt for a mastectomy rather than a lumpectomy with radiotherapy, because attending the radiotherapy centre involved a 2-hour journey. Financial issues should be explored, especially if the patient is the main wage earner. Referral to social workers should be made where appropriate to ensure access to available benefits. Self-help groups may also be of benefit to some patients (see 'Useful addresses').

PSYCHOLOGICAL ASSESSMENT AND COPING SKILLS

Most people know of someone who has died of breast cancer, either directly or perhaps through the media, and until they have received a firm diagnosis of a benign disorder, there will be an underlying fear of the unknown. The nurse can help to allay these fears by always making sure that patients are fully informed about what is happening to them. Nurses should try and spend time talking to patients, and accompanying friends or relatives, to establish how they have coped with previous

> **Box 26.1 Promoting disclosure by patients** (adapted from Maguire 1995)
>
> There are effective ways of getting patients to talk about how they are really feeling:
>
> - Ask open direct questions, not closed questions
> - Ask questions with a direct psychological focus; do not use leading questions
> - Ask single questions, not multiple ones
> - Summarize as you are talking
> - Be empathetic
> - Make educated guesses
> - Do not offer advice or concentrate on physical issues

medical interventions. This may highlight any patient fears, such as coping with a potential change in body image or even a dislike of needles. Basic communication skills are paramount and nurses should make time to talk and, much more importantly, listen to patients (Ch. 3). Most patients will be nervous in a health care setting and some may feel self-conscious or embarrassed.

Giving adequate and relevant information is one way of allaying fear, but asking open questions and dealing with this group of patients with compassion are also essential. Ward nurses are well placed to pick up signs of psychological distress. Likewise, clinic nurses may build up relationships with patients that allow them to probe gently or to notice any behavioural changes. It can sometimes be difficult to tell if a patient is abnormally anxious. The breast care nurse (BCN) specialist is useful in situations like this and can often provide the extra time and support in the clinic setting. There are some basic points to observe when talking to patients to promote disclosure, and these are outlined in Box 26.1.

The amount and content of the information required by patients will vary and it is important to assess individual information requirements. Some patients are happy to follow the paternalistic biomedical health care approach, while others will come armed with the latest research and information from the internet. You need to check that patients understand what is happening to them and why. Check their understanding throughout the visit and back it up with written information when appropriate (Ch. 3). Many patients do not absorb what they are being told, but written information should not be a substitute for verbal communication. Always make sure they have a contact number in case they need to ask more questions. Often this will be the BCN's number. Check their understanding especially if they are signing a consent form for a procedure. Informed consent should be exactly that. Consider also that not all patients can read the written information. Poor literacy skills are not uncommon and some patients will not understand English. Use of an interpreter or close family member can aid communication, but sensitivity to cultural considerations is important. For example, it may be inappropriate for a male family member to see a female patient undressed, and some female patients prefer not to see a male doctor. Patients with learning disabilities need particularly careful explanation and may find it helpful to have a carer with them. The way in which you impart information will vary according to who is receiving it. Never

 EVIDENCE-BASED PRACTICE

26.1 The benefits of having access to a breast care nurse specialist

Studies conducted in the early 1980s (Maguire et al 1980, 1983) support the view that access to counselling from a specialist BCN can reduce psychiatric morbidity and improve social recovery after mastectomy.

A group of 152 patients newly diagnosed with breast cancer and about to undergo mastectomy were randomized to be followed up by specialist nurses or to have routine care alone. The studies report that in the control group, non-specialist nurses could only identify 15% of these patients who had developed psychiatric morbidity, whereas the specialist nurses identified 90% of patients with psychiatric or social problems and referred 75% on for further expert help. This resulted in a fourfold reduction in psychiatric and social morbidity in the experimental group 12–18 months after surgery.

The two studies are summarized in Faulkner & Maguire (1994).

References

Faulkner A, Maguire P. Talking to cancer patients and their relatives. Oxford: Oxford University Press; 1994.

Maguire P, Tait A, Brooke M, Thomas C, Sellwood R. The effect of counselling on the psychiatric morbidity associated with mastectomy. Br Med J 1980; 281: 1454–1456.

Maguire P, Tait A, Brooke M, Thomas C, Sellwood R. The effect of counselling on physical disability and social recovery after mastectomy. Clin Oncol 1983; 9: 319–324.

assume anything – the nurse with a breast lump may be as petrified as the next patient and know nothing about the tests and procedures she may undergo.

ROLE OF THE BREAST CARE NURSE

Breast cancer is now a high profile cancer and the complexity of the disease calls for a specialist multidisciplinary approach to its management. The BCN is an important part of that team. The profound psychological effects of breast cancer and the fact that this was seldom identified were highlighted in Maguire et al (1978). Further studies showed that a specialist nurse could reduce psychiatric morbidity (Maguire et al 1980) (see Evidence-based Practice box 26.1). The 1980s also saw women's expectations of health care changing, with scope for choice in treatment options and involvement in their care. This led to the development of the clinical nursing speciality of breast care nursing in the UK (Thomson 1989). From the early 'mastectomy nurses', there are now clinical nurse specialists (CNS) in breast care nursing (BCN).

In the early 1980s there was an increasing emphasis on the importance of quality of life issues and psychological health, in promoting a quick recovery and patient satisfaction. Patient participation in treatment options needed the input of BCNs to ensure that informed choice was an option.

The role of any clinical nurse encompasses the four aspects outlined by Tiffany (1990), namely clinical, research, teaching and consultant. Patient care is central to the role. General nurses should utilize the BCN to enhance the care they give and to access the experience and knowledge of their specialist colleague. Conversely, BCNs need to share knowledge and keep staff updated with patient progress and new research in breast care issues. The two roles should be mutually supportive. BCNs may be involved in direct patient care, e.g. dressing wounds and examining patients.

All aspects of breast cancer care should be research-based and nurses need to take an active role in initiating research projects to improve patient care. Designated breast units will undertake clinical trials and BCNs may need to act as neutral but supportive information-givers (Barlow 1995).

The specific execution of the specialist role will vary between BCNs to meet the needs of the population; however, some common principles apply:

- needs to make contact with the patient as early as possible
- should be easily accessible
- should be experienced and knowledgeable in all aspects of breast disease
- should be the patient's advocate and refer to clinicians when appropriate
- should be able to offer formal counselling and support and refer appropriately for further psychological support.

The BCN is now an established member of the specialist breast care team working with multiprofessional colleagues.

DIAGNOSTIC TESTS AND INVESTIGATIONS

The majority of patients presenting with breast disorders will undergo the tests and investigations described in Figure 26.2. In order to reassure patients and prepare them for the diagnostic process, it is important for nurses to have a basic understanding and knowledge of what happens in each test.

HISTORY

As well as a general history of current medication and illnesses, the doctor needs to establish details of any risk factors for breast cancer. These will include:

- family history of breast cancer and, if so, the age at presentation
- the age of the menarche (first menstruation) and, if relevant, age at the menopause (last menstruation)
- age at first pregnancy (if relevant)
- use of contraceptive pill and for how long
- if any children were breast-fed and for how long
- use of hormone replacement therapy (HRT) and for how long.

The duration of any breast sign or symptom is important, since cysts may appear very rapidly, whereas a breast cancer tends to grow slowly.

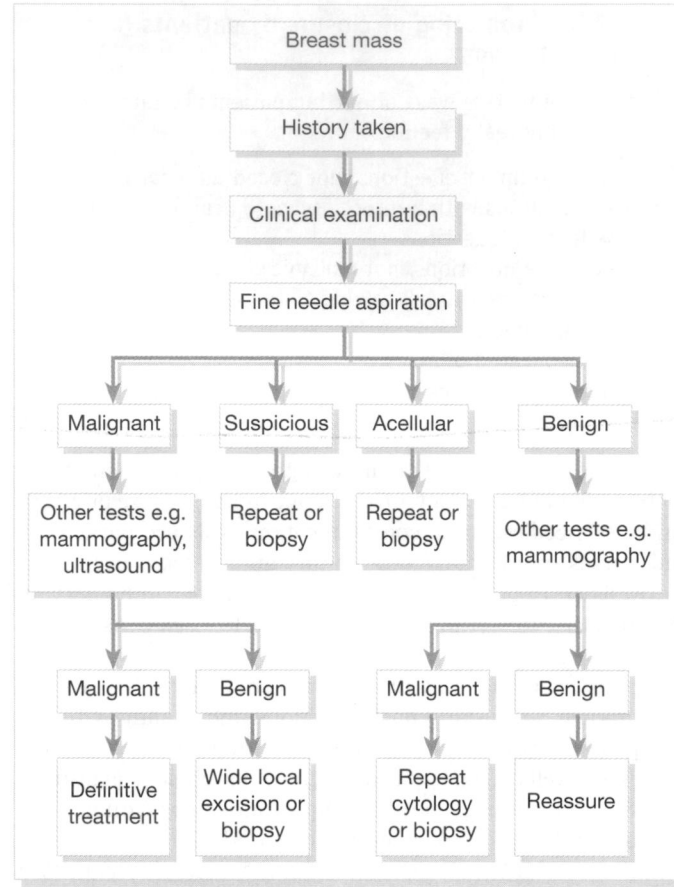

Figure 26.2 Diagnosis of a breast mass. Investigations and referral mechanisms for a palpable breast lump.

CLINICAL EXAMINATION

The patient will have a full clinical examination, with breast palpation and palpation of the axillary and cervical lymph nodes. This will be done by either a doctor or a specialist nurse trained in breast examination. Any signs of a lump, dimpling or puckering will be noted. Any palpable lesion will be measured with a tape measure. The nodal areas are checked also by palpating under the arms and in the neck, although this is not an accurate way to assess for node disease.

FINE-NEEDLE ASPIRATE

A fine-needle aspirate (FNA) can differentiate between solid and cystic lesions. A fine needle, attached to a syringe, is inserted into the lump and the plunger pulled upwards. A local anaesthetic may be used. The material obtained is then mounted on a slide ready to be reported by pathology.

IMAGING – MAMMOGRAPHY AND ULTRASOUND

Mammography is a special X-ray technique which can aid diagnosis and is also used in the national screening programme to detect impalpable lesions in the breast. The breast is compressed between two plates and so can be rather uncomfortable. Mammography is of little value in women under 40 years of age because their breasts are generally too dense. In older women, cancers show up as dense areas on film.

Ultrasound is the preferred option for younger women, where high-frequency sound waves are beamed through the breast and turned into images. Cancers usually show up as indistinct outlines while benign lesions have well demarcated edges.

TRIPLE ASSESSMENT

Triple assessment is the name given to the combination of clinical assessment, imaging and FNA. The Clinical Outcomes Group (COG 1996) state that triple assessment should be available for women with suspected breast cancer at a single visit.

OTHER TESTS

The remaining tests are used according to the need to establish a diagnosis.

Core biopsy

A small core of tissue is obtained from a mass using a cutting needle technique. This is done under local anaesthetic.

Open biopsy

Open biopsy should only be performed in patients who have undergone imaging, FNA and, if appropriate, core biopsy and in whom no definitive diagnosis has been reached. The lump will be removed under general anaesthetic and sent for examination to the histology department.

Frozen sections, where the surgeon waited for a histology report on the lump in theatres with the patient anaesthetized, are no longer in routine use. Fortunately the days are gone where it was usual for a woman not to know if she would return from theatres with her breast or not. Improved diagnostic tests have removed any need for frozen sections and the associated damaging negative psychological impact.

ONE-STOP CLINICS

Some breast units operate one-stop clinics. A woman will have all these diagnostic tests and a diagnosis at one visit. This is extremely useful for the woman with benign breast disease. There may, however, be disadvantages for women with a malignant breast lump. These women may find that a one-stop clinic does not allow them time to prepare for the shock of a breast cancer diagnosis. Research into the psychological effects of receiving a quick malignant diagnosis is ongoing.

GENERAL DISEASE PREVENTION AND HEALTH EDUCATION

Health promotion has an important role to play in the planning, coordination and implementation of a breast screening service. An enormous amount of work is required to ensure that eligible women attend.

OLDER ADULTS–NURSING PRIORITIES

26.1 Breast cancer and older women

A woman's age should not mean that she is offered different treatments from those offered to a younger woman with similar clinical requirements. The vast majority of breast cancers occur in older women, yet women have to request mammography after the age of 70:

- 80% of breast cancers occur after the menopause (Carrol 1998)
- 40% of all breast cancers occur in women aged over 70 years
- They should receive similar medical treatment as younger women, since very few are absolutely unfit for surgery or radiotherapy
- Many older women are unhappy about losing a breast, yet there can be an ageist approach to offering this group surgery or breast reconstruction
- Sexuality issues still need to be addressed and considered
- Also consider concurrent illnesses that could mask metastases, e.g. bone pain could be dismissed as arthritis.

Reference
Carrol S. Breast cancer. Part 1: aetiology. Prof Nurse 1998; 13(10): 721–723.

The screening programme does not routinely check women over the age of 70 years, even though this group of women has specific health needs (see Older Adults–Nursing Priorities box 26.1).

BREAST SCREENING PROGRAMME IN THE UK

Primary prevention for breast cancer is currently a distant prospect, but screening (secondary prevention) is the alternative approach to reduce mortality from breast cancer.

In 1987, the UK government accepted the recommendations of the Forrest report (Forrest 1986) and set up a national screening programme. This followed extensive research in several European countries (Tabar & Gad 1981) which suggested that mammography screening could reduce breast cancer mortality.

Current data indicate that the reduction in mortality is greatest in women aged 50–70 years. There are currently no data to suggest that screening in the under-50 age group is of any benefit. Women within the 50- to 70-year-old age group are identified from GP lists and are sent specific screening appointments. Women who are over the age of 70 can arrange an appointment through their GP. The current UK screening programme is organized as illustrated in Box 26.2.

Woman should be informed of a normal mammogram within 2 weeks of the test. Where there is an abnormality, the radiologist will consult with the surgeon and further diagnostic tests will be carried out. At this stage a proportion of patients will be found to have a benign condition, e.g. a cyst. Those who require pathology results will be given an appointment to receive them. When women are recalled for assessment, they are understandably frightened. They often have no symptoms and are otherwise well. The primary role of the nurse in the assessment clinics is to provide information and support and to provide a contact number for the BCN.

Screening uptake

Over 70% of the target population need to accept their screening invitation if a screening programme is to reduce mortality significantly. The reduction in mortality is estimated to be around 25% (Vessey 1991). The current recall for screening is 3 years, but the most appropriate interval has yet to be determined. The rate of interval cancers climbs rapidly between the second and third year. Some areas have notoriously low uptake for the breast-screening programme (see Reflective Practice box 26.1). In some cases this can be as low as 47%, notably in areas with lower socioeconomic groups.

The success of any screening programme must involve the compilation of accurate lists of patients' names and current addresses, how enthusiastic the GP is about screening, and education in the community about the local screening programme. Practice nurses and those in the primary health care setting are in a good position to provide information about the programme. It remains difficult to target certain groups, e.g. travellers, since they do not appear on any GP lists (see Special Issues box 26.1).

Benefits of breast screening

Compared with symptomatic cancers, cancers detected by screening are smaller and more likely to be non-invasive. Early diagnosis from screening identifies breast cancers at the stage when the chances of developing metastases are smaller.

Breast awareness

Breast awareness is the term used to describe the process of a woman getting to know her breasts better, so that any changes in them will be spotted sooner. Breasts may naturally have a lumpy feel and it is important that women are aware of what is normal for them in terms of how their breasts look and feel. They should look at and check their breasts regularly (after a period if still menstruating) to achieve this. They should be reassured that changes detected are not always signs of breast cancer – many women will have a breast problem at some stage, due to hormonal changes (see Health Promotion box 26.1).

HIGH-RISK PATIENTS – GENETIC ISSUES IN BREAST CANCER

For a small percentage of women, a family history is recognized as an important risk factor for breast cancer. Up to 5% of breast cancers in Western countries are due to genetic predisposition. About a third of these familial cases are thought to be due to mutations in the BRCA1 gene. The younger the patient who presents with breast cancer, the greater the likelihood that it will be due to an inherited predisposition. This risk also increases where a high number of first-degree relatives (mother or sister) have breast or related cancers, such as cancer of the ovary or colon, or sarcomas (Evans et al 1994).

Where three first-degree relatives have early-onset or bilateral breast cancer, the risk of inheriting the gene is close to 50%. About 80% of gene carriers develop breast cancer in their lifetime. These genes can also be inherited through the father.

Family history clinics have now been set up in most health regions. These clinics offer risk assessment, screening and counselling. High-risk families are offered screening from the age of 35 years or 5 years earlier than the first family breast cancer. Screening will usually take the form of an annual clinical breast examination and mammography. For those at very high risk of developing breast cancer, prophylactic mastectomy may be considered; however, this is not widely used in the UK at present. The implications of prophylactic surgery for a woman are enormous. Immediate reconstruction will be offered as well as preoperative counselling. For a woman who may have watched several young close relatives die from breast cancer, surgery can be a real option, however extreme. Trials of preventative tamoxifen (an anti-oestrogen that competes with oestrogen at receptor sites) are also underway in an attempt to reduce breast cancer in high-risk groups.

There is a need for more uniform protocols for screening in this group and further research in gene therapy to treat or even prevent breast cancer (see Ethical Issues box 26.1).

SPECIAL ISSUES

26.1 Breast screening and marginalized groups

The targets outlined in the NHS Breast Screening Report (Vessey 1991) state that the screening programme will prevent about 25% of deaths from breast cancer in the population of women invited for screening. If this is to be achieved, the numbers attending must be increased and it will be necessary to ensure that all women in the age group for screening are actually invited to attend. Efforts to include women who may be marginalized or difficult to reach should start with the identification of these groups before looking at strategies to reach them.

Groups that may need targeting are as follows:

- minority ethnic groups
- women with learning disabilities
- homeless women
- women living in residential or nursing homes
- women with mental health problems
- women in prison
- low income groups
- older women
- travellers
- refugees.

These groups may be reached as follows:

- through accurate population lists; however, these may not be very useful as many of these women are not registered with a GP, nor do they appear on the electoral roll

- good GP liaison
- taking information out to the women
- providing accessible information for women who cannot read
- providing information in different languages and large print
- using interpreters
- making contact with community or religious leaders where appropriate
- working with nurses working in prisons, practice nurses, primary care nurses and A&E nurses
- working with midwives and health visitors
- working with the social services: social workers and care workers
- working with voluntary groups, charities and community groups.

Student activities
- Can you think of other ways to reach these groups?
- How can programmes be maintained once these groups have been reached ?
- What difficulties might there be?

Reference
Vessey M. Breast cancer screening: evidence and experience since the Forrest Report. Sheffield: NHS BSP Publication; 1991.

 HEALTH PROMOTION

26.1 Breast awareness

Women should be encouraged to look and feel (with a flat hand) for the following changes and remember that breast tissue extends into the axilla. They also need to consider the hormonal changes that occur through the life span, e.g. menstrual cycle, pregnancy and after the menopause when they feel softer:

- any dimpling or puckering on the breasts
- skin changes, e.g. 'orange peel' skin, redness or more prominent veins
- any change in the shape (the contour) or size in either breast
- any lump or thickening in either breast or axilla
- any change in either nipple, including any discharge, eczema around the nipple or change in shape or prominence
- any changes in sensation, such as an odd or different feeling in the breast or nipple.

 ETHICAL ISSUES

26.1 Screening for breast cancer in high-risk groups

There are several issues surrounding the screening for breast cancer in high-risk women which need to be considered, as described below.

Ethical considerations
- Consider the effects on individuals
- Consider the effects on the immediate family
- Consider the effects on first-degree female relatives who may also be at increased risk

Cost implications
- Consider the increase in demand and the fact that high-risk groups are responsible for a small percentage of breast cancers

Legal and social implications
- Who should have access to the test results?
- Consider the implications of this for obtaining life insurance and mortgages
- Consider the implications for decisions about relationships and having children

COMMON DISEASES/DISORDERS AFFECTING THE BREAST

The incidence of benign breast disorders is common and 90% of all women referred to a breast clinic will have a benign disorder. Many breast changes are physiological and are related to normal cyclical development, e.g. changes that happen during the reproductive and perimenopausal years. In all cases, cancer needs to be excluded and women should therefore be seen in specialist breast clinics. Until they can be reassured, women will always fear the worst and will need information and support from health care professionals.

BREAST PAIN

Up to 50% of all women who present at breast clinics do so with breast pain (mastalgia) and/or lumpiness. Breast pain is rarely a symptom of breast cancer and only 7% of women with breast cancer have breast pain as their only symptom (Mansel 1995).

Aetiology, epidemiology and clinical presentation

Although there is a relationship with the menstrual cycle, hormonal studies have not revealed any clear differences in patients with mastalgia. They have been found to have abnormal blood fatty acid profiles, but the role of diet in mastalgia remains unclear.

Breast pain may be cyclical or non-cyclical. Two-thirds of women have cyclical pain; the remainder have non-cyclical pain. Patients with cyclical pain are premenopausal (mean age 34 years), whereas non-cyclical mastalgia affects older women (mean age 43 years). In cyclical mastalgia, women often report the following in the days before menstruation:

■ discomfort
■ increased breast size and heaviness
■ tender lumpiness
■ increasing pain from mid-cycle that only improves at menstruation.

Physical activity can increase the pain. The menopause relieves cyclical mastalgia.

The pain of non-cyclical mastalgia has a more random pattern and can occur in the chest wall or the breast. The pain is more localized and is described as 'drawing' or 'burning'.

A patient history is needed and a clinical examination must be performed to exclude breast lumps. If no lump is present, further investigations are not indicated.

Medical/surgical management

The impact of the breast pain on quality of life should be taken into account. If treatment is being considered, patients should keep a pain chart for 2 months to assess the pattern and duration of their pain.

In cyclical mastalgia, reassurance that symptoms are not indicative of breast cancer and an explanation are all that is needed in 85% of patients. Stopping the oral contraceptive pill can sometimes relieve symptoms. For the remainder there are currently three drugs that can be prescribed: gamolenic acid, bromocriptine and danzol (Fig. 26.3).

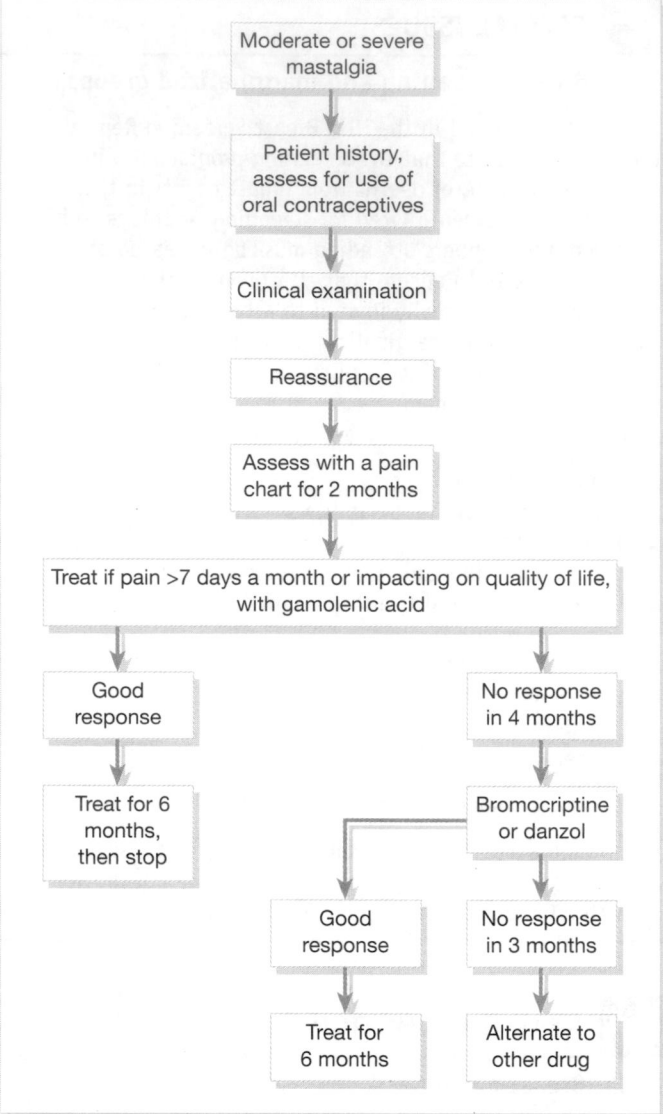

Figure 26.3 The treatment of breast pain. A protocol for treating mastalgia.

The location of non-cyclical breast pain must be established. Patients with a persistent localized pain can be treated successfully by injections of local anaesthetic into the area and a corticosteroid injection. Some women report that wearing a good support bra 24 hours a day helps.

Local surgery to trigger spots in the breast should be avoided since it generally exacerbates the pain.

▶ Nursing management

The results of treatment for breast pain are often slow and nurses need to support women and ensure that they are adequately informed about treatment options. During initial investigation, patients need psychological support, as they often fear their pain is due to malignancy. Advice on bras is an important aspect of the nurse's role. Many women notice an improvement when they are actually measured into a correctly fitting bra and others may require different bra sizes throughout their menstrual cycle.

INFECTION

Breast infections are now less common due to improved hygiene. It is most common in women aged between 18 and 50 years and can be divided into lactation- and non-lactation-associated infections.

Aetiology, epidemiology and clinical presentation

Lactation infection most frequently occurs within the first 6 weeks of breast-feeding. The most commonly isolated micro-organism is *Staphylococcus aureus*, a skin-associated infection. There is pain, swelling and tenderness and there may be a history of cracked nipples.

There are several different non-lactating infections:

- Periareolar infection is most common in young women (mean age 32 years). Smoking appears to be a factor in the aetiology of periareolar infection – 90% of women presenting with periareolar infection smoke cigarettes. There is inflammation or an established abscess. Patients may have pain and nipple discharge.
- Mammary duct fistulae can develop after abscess drainage or biopsy. Breast abscesses are often associated with underlying conditions such as trauma, diabetes (Ch. 17) and corticosteroid treatment. There is inflammation and an external opening on the breast with pain and discharge.
- Primary infections present as a cellulitis of the skin on the breast. This often affects the lower half of the breast and is commonly seen in women with large breasts and where personal hygiene is poor. It is commonly seen after radiotherapy to the breast and *Staph. aureus* is the usual causative microorganism.

Specific investigations

Breast cancer should be excluded in any patient with an inflammatory lesion that is solid on aspiration or that does not settle despite adequate antibiotic treatment.

Medical/surgical management

The principles for treating breast infections are as follows:

- appropriate antibiotics
- hospital referral if the infection does not settle
- aspiration of any abscess prior to surgical drainage.

▶ Nursing management

The patient who presents with a breast infection will be in varying degrees of discomfort and alarmed at the redness and soreness on her breast. Pain assessment (Ch. 7) and treatment are priorities, as well as checking adherence to the treatment prescribed. The woman who is trying to breast-feed may fear that she will have to stop breast-feeding because of the pain and infection and will need the nurse's support. She may need reassurance that the prescribed antibiotics are safe for her to use whilst feeding and should consult her midwife or health visitor.

Some women may be embarrassed because they feel unclean and may be upset that they have an infection in an area they consider of sexual significance. This may lead to isolation from their partners and keeping their breast hidden. Reassurance should be given that a full course of an appropriate antibiotic will resolve the problem.

CONGENITAL BREAST DISORDERS AND VARIATIONS IN NORMAL BREAST DEVELOPMENT

Until puberty, the breast is identical in girls and boys. Growth normally starts in girls around the age of 10 years. Common disorders include:

- supernumerary nipples and breasts
- hypoplasia of the breast (under proliferation of the breast tissue)
- juvenile hypertrophy (over proliferation of the breast tissue)
- gynaecomastia (male breast development).

Aetiology and epidemiology

Between 1 and 5% of men and women have supernumerary nipples and (less frequently) breasts. The extra nipples develop along the milk line, which runs from the axilla to the inguinal region just under the normal breast. Extra breasts usually occur in the lower axilla.

With breast hypoplasia one breast may be considerably smaller or totally absent. This creates breast asymmetry and is usually due to a defect in the pectoral muscle. The vast majority of patients who have breast hypoplasia have a pectoral muscle defect.

Uncontrolled overgrowth of breast tissue can occur in adolescent girls. Their breasts may start to develop normally and then continue to grow. It is relatively common and usually there is no sign of any endocrine abnormality. It only requires investigation if there are other signs of sexual maturation. There may, however, be psychological effects because the girl is different from her contemporaries.

Gynaecomastia is benign and reversible and commonly occurs in puberty; 30–60% of boys aged 10–16 years will have gynaecomastia, but it normally reverses spontaneously in 80% of cases. It causes this age group considerable distress due to embarrassment at having a noticeable breast. In adult men it commonly occurs between the ages of 50 and 80 years and should always be fully investigated. Anabolic steroids can cause gynaecomastia and 8% of cases are caused by liver cirrhosis, since the liver is unable to deal with naturally occurring oestrogens.

Specific investigations

Breast enlargement in older men requires a careful history and examination. Recent progressive breast enlargement without pain or any cause requires further investigation, such as mammography and FNA, to exclude malignancy.

Medical/surgical management

- Supernumerary nipples and breasts – no surgical treatment is required unless requested by the patient for cosmetic reasons
- Hypoplasia of the breast – breast augmentation may be offered (see p. 790)

- Juvenile hypertrophy – reduction mammoplasty is the preferred treatment option
- Gynaecomastia – breast dissection may be offered where the condition does not resolve spontaneously.

▶ Nursing management

Patients with this group of disorders usually suffer social embarrassment, pain in some cases and the inability to perform normal activities.

Surgery improves their quality of life and should be more widely available. The nurse can help by referring patients with breast hypoplasia to the BCN, who may be able to provide a prosthesis to enhance the smaller breast. Good bra support is essential.

The embarrassment for young male patients presenting with what is seen as a 'woman's problem' is a major issue. They should be reassured that surgery will resolve it. Referral for psychological support may be indicated if there is evidence of depression or sexual difficulties.

BENIGN TUMOURS

Benign breast disease accounts for the majority of women passing through a breast clinic. The most common disorders are fibroadenomas, cysts and papillomas. Figure 26.4 depicts the final diagnosis of palpable breast lumps.

Aetiology, epidemiology and clinical presentation

Fibroadenomas occur from the menarche and are most common below the age of 30 years. They consist of fibrous and epithelial cells and present as small mobile lumps. In very young women under 20 years of age, they account for 60% of all palpable symptomatic breast masses.

Cysts rarely occur below the age of 35. The majority of women in their 40s will have microscopic breast cysts, but a few

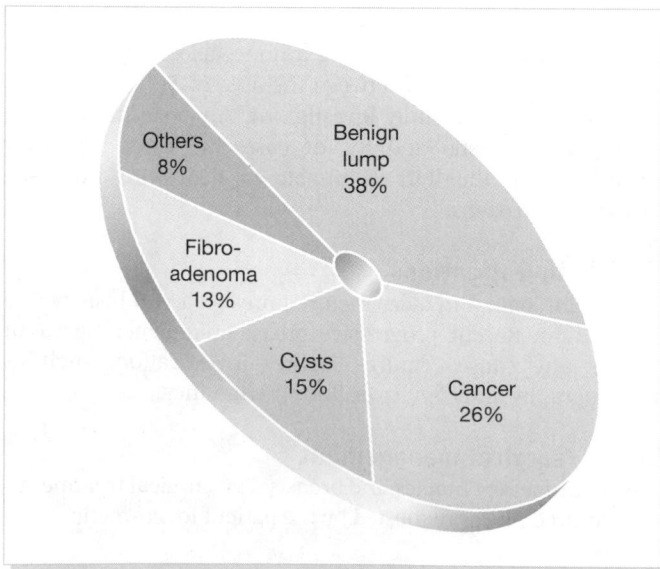

Figure 26.4 Final diagnosis of palpable breast lumps. (Adapted from Dixon & Mansel 1995.)

will become clinical lumps which are smooth and discrete and often painful. Cysts are distended, convoluted lobules, occurring most frequently in perimenopausal women and are often detected during routine screening. Cysts have no malignant or premalignant characteristics on histology.

Duct papillomas are composed of papillary connective tissue and can be single or multiple and are very common. They have minimal potential for malignant changes. They most often present with bloodstained nipple discharge. An underlying nodule will be palpable behind the areola or a thickened duct may be felt.

Specific investigations

A definitive diagnosis of fibroadenoma can be made by a combination of FNA, clinical examination and ultrasound. Cysts have characteristic halos on mammography and are easily diagnosed with ultrasound. Diagnosis is established by FNA. Non-bloodstained aspirate does not need to be sent for cytology and the cyst should disappear after aspiration.

Medical/surgical management

Fibroadenomas greater than 4 cm in diameter tend to be excised. Excision of fibroadenomas is not needed in women under 40 years of age, unless requested by the patient, since they tend to decrease in size or disappear spontaneously.

Cysts are both diagnosed and treated by aspiration and if the cyst disappears completely on aspiration no further treatment is required. Any remaining lump must be investigated.

Duct papillomas are treated surgically by microductectomy (duct removal).

▶ Nursing management

Whilst the diagnosis and treatment of benign disorders can be relatively straightforward, the time between presentation and diagnosis can be interminable for women and this group of patients benefit from the one-stop clinic. As always, clear information and support are paramount. Patients may require information regarding scars and whether they can be treated as day cases.

NIPPLE DISORDERS

Nipple disorders are common and include:

- inversion
- discharge
- eczema
- Paget's disease.

Aetiology, epidemiology and clinical presentation

Nipple inversion is reported in up to 40% of women and is often noticed in the teenage years (Mansel & Bundred 1995). Young women may lack the tissue supporting the nipple. During the reproductive years, inversion may be due to duct distension (ectasia) and is often bilateral. An underlying carcinoma can also cause nipple inversion.

Nipple discharge accounts for 5–10% of all referrals to a breast clinic. It is significant only when it occurs spontaneously and especially if it involves a single duct, which should be investigated. Bilateral and milky discharge from several ducts of the nipple should be disregarded and women reassured. Bloodstained discharge is indicative of an underlying papilloma, but may indicate a ductal carcinoma. A coloured single duct discharge is often due to a duct ectasia.

Nipple eczema usually begins on the areola and skin and causes intense itching.

Paget's disease is characterized by an inflammatory eczematoid change of the nipple associated with breast cancer. It affects women in a similar age range to that at which other breast cancers present and is often associated with delayed diagnosis. It develops on the nipple and spreads outwards and is usually moist, non-scaly and unilateral. It is not as itchy as eczema. Microscopically there are large malignant cells in the epidermis and usually an underlying breast cancer.

Specific investigations

Mammography is indicated in nipple retraction and discharge, with duct exploration only if there are abnormalities. A biopsy should be taken in addition to mammography where Paget's disease is suspected.

Medical/surgical management

Ductectomy is indicated for nipple retraction or discharge where abnormalities are detected. If an underlying malignancy is causing the problem, further surgery and treatment are indicated.

Topical corticosteroids are used for straightforward nipple eczema (Ch. 28).

Mastectomy with radiotherapy is indicated for Paget's disease with an underlying cancer. Where there is no underlying mass, a wide local excision with radiotherapy is the treatment option.

▶ Nursing management

Education regarding what constitutes a normal nipple is important, particularly for older women. There may be body image problems, leading to embarrassment, and women may need practical advice with dressings and pads if the discharge is profuse. Where cancer is the underlying cause, women will need support in dealing with this (see below).

MALIGNANT TUMOURS

Breast cancer remains the commonest malignancy for women and is the commonest single cause of death for women aged 35–54 years (CRC 1996). Mortality from breast cancer was greater than that for lung and colorectal cancers in England (Department of Health 1998) (Fig. 26.5).

Breast cancer has a high prevalence and health care professionals will have frequent contact with those affected. Breast cancer receives high media exposure and there are now many support groups. Although certain groups appear to be at higher risk, the disease is indiscriminate, affecting all ages and both men and women.

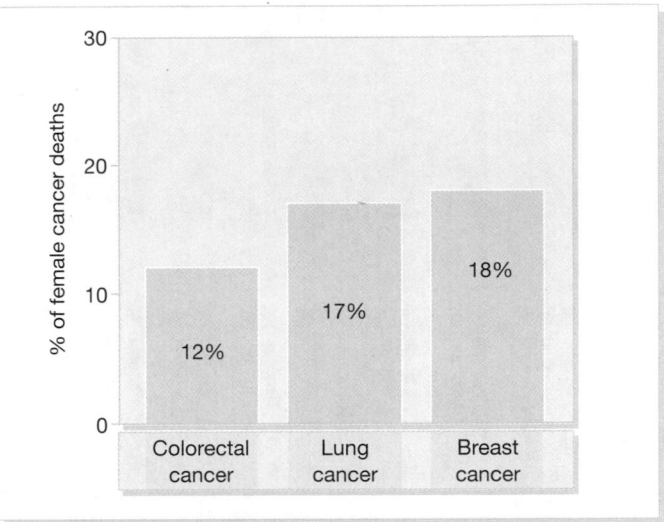

Figure 26.5 Major causes of cancer deaths in women (during 1996 in England). Source: Department of Health 1998.

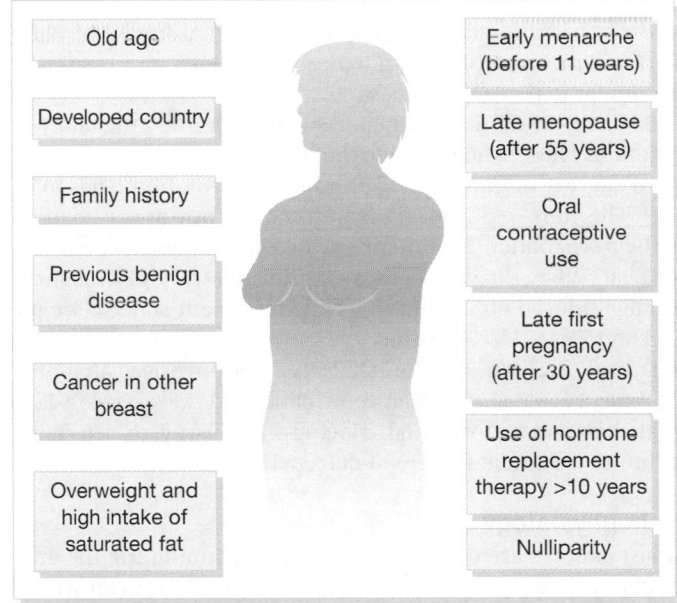

Figure 26.6 Risk factors for breast cancer.

Aetiology and epidemiology

There are over three-quarters of a million new cases of breast cancer worldwide each year. In the UK, 1 in 12 women will develop the disease. The aetiology is unknown, but certain risk factors have been identified (Fig. 26.6). Many of the factors are associated with a moderately increased risk. Nurses should bear this in mind, since patients may feel guilty and anxious when, in fact, their individual risk is very small.

In the UK, breast cancer mortality is one of the highest in the world, but recent research findings have shown a decrease (Peto et al 2000). There is a marked variation in the incidence of breast cancer around the world (Fig. 26.7). About 1% of all

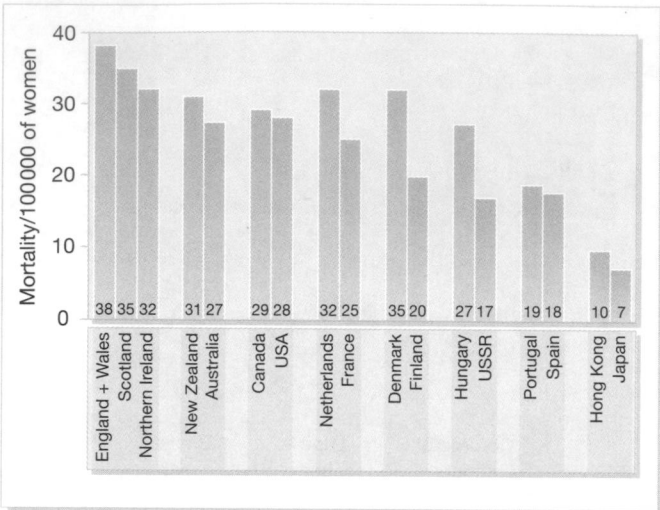

Figure 26.7 The mortality for breast cancer by country. (Adapted from McPherson & Heel 1995.)

breast cancers occur in men. It is generally a disease of older men and the presentation, diagnosis, prognosis and treatment are similar to those for women.

About 1–2% of all breast cancers occur during pregnancy or lactation. There is no evidence that these breast cancers are any more aggressive than others, although presentation tends to be later. This may be due to women attributing any breast changes to their pregnancy. Treatment during the first two trimesters is surgical. When diagnosis occurs in the final trimester, labour is usually induced at 32–34 weeks and treatment started (see pp. 783 and 784).

Ductal carcinoma in situ (DCIS) is a non-invasive carcinoma that may become invasive in some patients. Widespread DCIS is treated by mastectomy and trials are underway to determine optimum treatment for screen-detected DCIS.

Pathophysiology

Breast cancers are derived from the epithelium lining the duct lobular unit, e.g. adenocarcinoma. Cancers that remain within the duct unit are classified as in situ or non-invasive, whereas those that extend outside the basement membrane of the ducts and lobules are invasive. Malignancy of connective tissue origin, e.g. sarcomas, are rare. Metastatic spread from other cancers to the breast is also rare (Ch. 33). Other less common types of breast cancer include lymphomas and phyllodes tumours.

Clinical presentation

The majority of breast cancers present as a lump. All lumps should be investigated, although the majority will not be malignant. Most breast cancers are painless at presentation, but around 20% of women will feel some discomfort or altered sensation.

A locally invasive breast cancer may cause puckering or dimpling. This is why breast awareness incorporates looking for changes. Some breast cancers may present with an indrawn nipple or discharge. A small number of breast cancers present with an enlarged axillary lymph node. Lymphatic system involvement may be indicative of metastatic spread. It may represent other disorders and should always be investigated.

The screening programme will pick up very small, non-palpable tumours. This group of women may have little idea that they have breast cancer.

Inflammatory carcinomas of the breast (locally advanced tumours) present with redness, swelling and breast pain. The skin resembles that of an orange with fine indentations and is referred to as peau d'orange. It may be mistaken for infection; hence the importance of referring women to a breast unit if the condition does not respond quickly to antibiotics.

Specific investigations

The general investigations – history, examination, mammography, ultrasound, FNA and biopsy – are those already outlined above (pp. 774, 775). Once malignancy is confirmed the following investigations are performed to exclude the presence of metastases:

- blood tests – full blood count, liver function tests, calcium levels and urea and electrolytes
- chest X-ray
- bone scan and liver ultrasound – where there is clinical evidence of metastases, these may be performed to assess metastatic spread to bone and/or liver.

Disease staging is important in determining the best treatment option and assessing treatment efficacy. The TNM staging method assesses tumour size, presence of nodes and any metastases (Ch. 33). Other staging tools are available, but one of the most important prognostic indicators in breast cancer is the status of the lymph nodes. Women with no lymph node involvement have 70% survival at 5 years, compared with 30% survival for those with node involvement. Other prognostic factors are the tumour size, oestrogen receptor status and grade. The higher the grade and size, the poorer the prognosis, since risk of metastases is increased.

Hormone receptor assays are now performed on excised breast cancer specimens to establish if the tumour is oestrogen receptor (ER)-positive. Those women with ER-positive tumours are more likely to respond to hormone treatment. Over 65% of postmenopausal women and 30% of premenopausal women will be ER-positive.

Medical/surgical management

Once breast cancer has been diagnosed, the following may influence the choice of treatment:

- Overall health status – good health enables women to withstand intense treatments
- Patient choice
- Age – some may be too frail to undergo treatment
- Extent of local disease – surgery may not be viable in extensive local disease due to poor healing potential
- Tumour size – large tumours may mean that local surgery, e.g. wide local excision, is not possible
- Premenopausal women tend not to respond as well to hormone therapies unless they are ER-positive
- Lymph node involvement – the more lymph nodes that are involved, the more likely a woman is to receive chemotherapy

- Metastatic disease – may exclude a patient from some clinical trials. Where cure is not possible, palliative treatment should concentrate on quality of life and reducing side-effects becomes a priority (Ch. 34).

For many years there were only modest improvements in survival despite advances in treatment modalities; however, there has been a marked reduction in mortality recently, which is attributed to several improvements in early detection and treatment (Peto et al 2000).

There are four main treatment modalities that may be used alone or (more usually) in combination:

- surgery
- radiotherapy
- chemotherapy
- hormone therapy.

Surgery

Most women will undergo some type of surgery regardless of other treatment modalities they may have. Over the years, surgery has become less radical since it is no longer believed that breast cancer is a local disease. Data have suggested for some time that survival is not improved by extensive surgery (Hardy 1988) and that it is much more of a systemic disease. Surgery may be used for a variety of reasons (see Box 26.3).

Surgery aims to eradicate the primary lesion with a good cosmetic result and minimize the risk of local recurrence. Where possible, women will have a choice regarding the type of surgery they undergo. Women who opt for breast conservation (lumpectomy or wide local excision) will require postoperative radiotherapy. There is no difference in local recurrence between lumpectomy with radiotherapy and mastectomy (Fisher et al 1989). However, some women may not be suitable for conservation due to tumour size or position (Fig. 26.8).

Other women may feel unable to make the decision. Fallowfield et al (1986) found that there was no significant difference in the anxiety and depression rates of women opting for either mastectomy or breast conservation. What was important was that the women were offered a choice. Those offered a choice were less prone to depression than those who were not.

There are several types of breast surgery available:

- *Radical mastectomy* (rarely performed) – removal of the entire breast, pectoral muscles and axillary lymph nodes. Breast reconstruction should be offered to all women after mastectomy
- *Modified radical mastectomy* – removal of the breast, removal or division of the pectoralis minor muscle and axillary node clearance
- *Simple mastectomy* – removal of the entire breast
- *Axillary dissection* – varies from the removal of a node to a full clearance, but a sample usually contains four nodes. It enables treatment planning and aids prognostic information. The greater the number of lymph nodes involved, the poorer the prognosis and the more likely it is that chemotherapy will be required. The removal of the axillary lymph nodes is a contributory factor in the development of lymphoedema. The sentinel node may be used for diagnostic purposes. This involves the injection of radioactive colloid or dye into the skin above the tumour; images are taken as the colloid passes

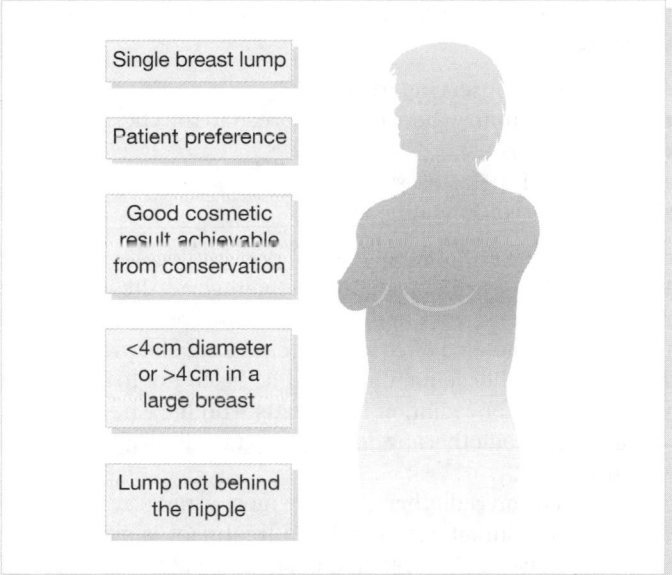

Figure 26.8 Suitability for breast conservation (some reasons that allow women a choice between mastectomy and wide local excision).

into the lymph channels. A small probe locates the most active lymph node: the sentinel node. If the sentinel node is clear of cancer, then no tumour cells should have reached the axilla and axillary surgery is not needed. Clearly the benefits of avoiding axillary surgery are great, but the technique is still undergoing validation in the trial setting.

- *Palliative surgery* – may be used to control local fungating lesions (see p. 787).
- *Conservative surgery* – wide local excision or lumpectomy. The tumour and a margin of normal tissue are removed.

Chemotherapy

Chemotherapy (Ch. 33) can be used to treat all stages of breast cancer. Surgery will treat the localized tumour, but undetectable micrometastases may be present. These may be eradicated with systemic chemotherapy.

Chemotherapy can be used preoperatively (neo-adjuvant) to reduce tumour size. This may facilitate breast preservation when previously the tumour was too large. Adjuvant chemotherapy is commonly used after primary surgery for premenopausal patients and for postmenopausal patients with lymph node involvement.

Palliative chemotherapy can be used in advanced breast cancer, but benefits must outweigh potential side-effects. The response to treatment is assessed by measuring the tumour on scan, X-ray or by palpation.

Combination chemotherapy is most often used, e.g. cyclophosphamide, methotrexate and fluorouracil (CMF). It is given intravenously in an outpatient setting. Newer drugs are increasingly available, e.g. paclitaxel and trastuzumab (monoclonal antibody), which are used to treat advanced breast cancer. The side-effects of each drug differs and should be regularly monitored. Nausea and vomiting should be anticipated and adequate antiemetics prescribed (Chs 33 and 34).

Radiotherapy

Radiotherapy (Ch. 33) may be used in a variety of situations, including:

- after breast-conserving treatment
- after mastectomy where there is spread to the chest wall
- large tumours
- palliation of metastases
- local control of fungating lesions.

The aim of radiotherapy is to prevent local recurrence. Although the specific techniques may vary, the aim is to irradiate the chest wall and any remaining breast tissue. The axilla is not irradiated after axillary clearance since it increases the risk of lymphoedema. Care must be taken not to exceed the maximum dose of radiation in patients who have had previous radiotherapy. Radiotherapy does not start until surgical wounds have healed.

External beam radiotherapy is the most usual way and treatment is as an outpatient. Individual treatment is planned and patients receive daily irradiation for a prescribed number of doses. Local treatment usually means that side-effects are limited to the area being treated. There may be some redness, itching and desquamation (skin peeling) in women with very sensitive skin, but 'radiation burns' are rarely seen with improved techniques and dosing. Women do, however, often complain of tiredness during therapy.

Hormone therapy

The growth of many breast tumours is stimulated by oestrogen. If the source of oestrogen production is removed or inhibited, 50% of breast tumours will shrink or die. The ovaries are the major source of oestrogen in premenopausal women, and therefore they are either removed surgically or 'switched off'. This can be done chemically with goserelin, an analogue of gonadotrophin-releasing hormone (in which case the effects are reversible), or by irradiation. In postmenopausal women the sources of oestrogen are adipose tissue and the adrenal glands. Tamoxifen can be given to block the effects of oestrogen by binding to tumour oestrogen receptors. Drugs called aromatase inhibitors, such as formestane, can be used to block adrenal oestrogen production in postmenopausal women. Hormone therapy is used curatively and for palliation in advanced disease.

Follow-up

Women are followed up with annual mammography after the completion of treatment for primary breast cancer. They will be encouraged to contact the breast team should they have any worries.

▶ Nursing management

The nursing management of women with breast cancer is enormously challenging. There are many aspects to consider and a wealth of information to impart and support to give. There is, however, very little in the literature regarding the impact of male breast cancer. Men have to cope with the fact that the disease is associated with women and this may lead to problems with body image and sexuality. It is a rare disease and men can feel very isolated.

The specific nursing management will vary according to which treatment modalities are used.

Breast surgery

Patients having surgery will need information preoperatively (Ch. 29). Women face a huge threat to their body image and femininity, as well as coping with a life-threatening disease. A specialist nurse may support ward- and clinic-based nurses in assessing a patient's needs and fears.

Women having breast surgery require routine postoperative care (Ch. 29), pain relief and observations, e.g. for bleeding. In addition, their care will involve:

- wound and drain management
- observation for wound healing and signs of infection, e.g. pyrexia, wound inflammation
- referral for physiotherapy
- care for the affected arm (see 'Lymphoedema' p. 785).

Women may need support when viewing the wound for the first time. Partners and children will also need explanation and support. Where appropriate, a temporary prosthesis is fitted prior to discharge. This is especially so for those patients not having breast reconstruction who will have a permanent prosthesis when their wound has healed. This is usually done by the BCN. Women and their families are made aware of self-help groups if appropriate.

Chemotherapy

The nurse must prepare patients, and monitor them, for drug side-effects (see Reflective Practice box 26.2). These will vary according to regimen. Chemotherapy can have a profound effect on self-image. Hair loss is a common side-effect and women will need practical help and support in dealing with this. Early referral for a wig is important. Chemotherapy can also cause fatigue and a loss of concentration, impairing ability to work. Libido may decrease due to menopausal symptoms, e.g. hot flushes and vaginal dryness. All of this comes on top of previous surgery with its physical and emotional effects.

Women will often need advice on contraception or the use of hormone replacement therapy. Chemotherapy can cause

REFLECTIVE PRACTICE

26.2 Nicola

Nicola (not her real name) is a 40-year-old woman who is married with two young children. She works full time as a teacher. She was recently diagnosed with breast cancer and underwent a lumpectomy and axillary node clearance 8 weeks ago. She is now on her second course of CMF chemotherapy and is also taking tamoxifen. Nicola feels very tired and tells you that she is having hot flushes during the day and wakes most nights drenched in sweat.

Student activities
- What factors could be contributing to her fatigue?
- What could be the cause of her menopausal symptoms?

---

amenorrhoea, but women should continue to use non-hormonal contraception. Periods return after treatment but the timing can vary. In perimenopausal women, chemotherapy can precipitate the menopause and periods may not return. Women wishing to have children are generally advised to wait as long as possible after treatment, since 80% of relapses occur within 2 years. Pregnancy will not alter the course of the disease.

Radiotherapy

Women and their families may have misconceptions regarding radiotherapy and will need explanation about what a course of radiotherapy entails. They will need information about skin care during and after treatment. This usually involves washing the area with water only and not using soaps or creams during treatment. Women should be warned about the fatigue associated with radiotherapy, both during treatment and well after it has finished. Patients should also be informed that there might be daily travel involved if they are outpatients; transport may be an issue. Support must be ongoing and involve other health care professionals as appropriate.

Hormone therapy

Many hormone therapies cause menopausal symptoms. Nurses should provide accurate information and education with regard to symptom management. Symptoms vary and include hot flushes, vaginal dryness, depression, weight gain, menstrual disturbances and libido changes. As well as preparing patients for these potential side-effects, the nurse should assist in accurate symptom monitoring so that treatments can be changed where appropriate. This may involve asking patients to complete questionnaires regarding symptoms and monitoring their weight. Some of the newer drugs, e.g. anastrozole, have a lower side-effect profile than the older therapies.

Up to 30% of women with breast cancer develop anxiety or depressive illness within a year of diagnosis. Psychological morbidity further increases when radiotherapy or chemotherapy is used (Maguire 1995). Patients are often reluctant to mention their feelings and nurses should promote disclosure of such problems (see Box 26.1). The introduction of the BCN at diagnosis can reduce psychological morbidity (see Evidence-based

Practice box 26.1). Referral should be made to a psychiatrist/psychologist if women exhibit signs of depression. Patients who are anxious respond to support and understanding, but in severe cases they may need medication.

METASTATIC SPREAD AND OTHER PROBLEMS

RECURRENT BREAST CANCER

When breast cancer returns, it can be more traumatic than the initial diagnosis. Health care professionals should remain realistic and be honest with patients, remembering that many women live for years with metastatic disease (spread to distant sites). The most common sites for metastatic spread are brain, lung and liver, and there may be local recurrence. There is a risk of hypercalcaemia (Chs 8, 17, 33 and 34) or spinal cord compression (Chs 33 and 34) with bone metastases, both of which are oncological emergencies.

Secondary cancer can develop shortly after initial diagnosis or after many years. The nature of breast cancer is such that it is frequently present over many years with episodes of recurrent disease.

At routine follow-up, patients are examined and a thorough history taken. Patients highlight many recurrences themselves, since they are aware of any changes. Specific investigations will be tailored to the clinical presentation. Routine blood tests are done, but scans are only performed where clinically indicated.

Management may involve the treatment options previously mentioned. Other treatment options, such as surgery for pathological fractures or pleural taps for pleural effusion, may be indicated for symptom control. It is important to continually assess patient response to treatment and for them to be fully involved in decision making.

Nurses need all their communication skills to help women come to terms with recurrence (Chs 3 and 34). Women may feel cheated that the disease has returned or angry at going through the primary treatment for apparently little gain. Metastatic disease progresses very rapidly in some women, but many women continue to lead full lives with chronic breast cancer, having treatment when their condition dictates. Fears should not be dismissed and support for the patient and her family is paramount. Specific nursing care is tailored to individual needs and proposed treatment.

LYMPHOEDEMA

Lymphoedema is swelling of the arm on the affected side. It occurs, to some degree, in around a third of women who have treatment for breast cancer. The swelling can be unsightly, uncomfortable and cause problems with clothes and mobility, and for many is a constant, distressing reminder of the cancer.

Lymphoedema may be primary (congenital problems with the lymphatic system) or secondary. Secondary lymphoedema is most often due to the interruption of lymphatic flow. Breast cancer treatments, such as surgery and radiotherapy, cause trauma to the lymphatic system, resulting in a low output or failure of the system (Földi et al 1985).

Lymphoedema is a chronic and incurable condition. There appears to be a lack of data concerning the incidence and current reliable figures are not available (Woods 1993). In the first year after treatment, Kissin et al (1986) found that 25–38% of patients developed lymphoedema, whereas Hoe et al (1992) found an incidence of 7.6%. In a literature review, Logan (1995) suggests that the prevalence is 25–28% in women treated for breast cancer.

Pathophysiology

Hodkinson (1992) described the physiological changes that occur in lymphoedema. The lymphatic system regulates the environment of tissues by removing many substances, including protein and water, and returning them to the general circulation. There are changes in these processes in lymphoedema. When lymphatic flow is compromised, proteins cannot be effectively removed from the tissues distal to the blockage, causing them to stagnate in the interstitial fluid. In turn, this high protein content causes fluid to accumulate by osmosis (Földi et al 1985). A protein-rich oedema arises and fluid circulation in the limb is reduced. Congestion of the tissues with excess proteins may lead to cellulitis. Untreated, the inflamed tissue becomes fibrosed and the skin becomes hard with loss of elasticity. Stasis of a protein-rich oedema increases the risk of infection. The mechanical removal of fluid is compromised by the loss of tissue elasticity and may lead to loss of limb function.

Clinical presentation

Clinical presentation may vary from a slight swelling of the fingers to a heavily swollen and congested limb. There may be infection present, pain and loss of function. Even in mild cases of lymphoedema, patients may complain of loss of fine movements such as doing up buttons (see Fig. 26.9).

Medical/surgical management

A firm medical diagnosis of lymphoedema must be made prior to treatment. There are other causes of swelling that must be excluded prior to commencing any treatment. This will include

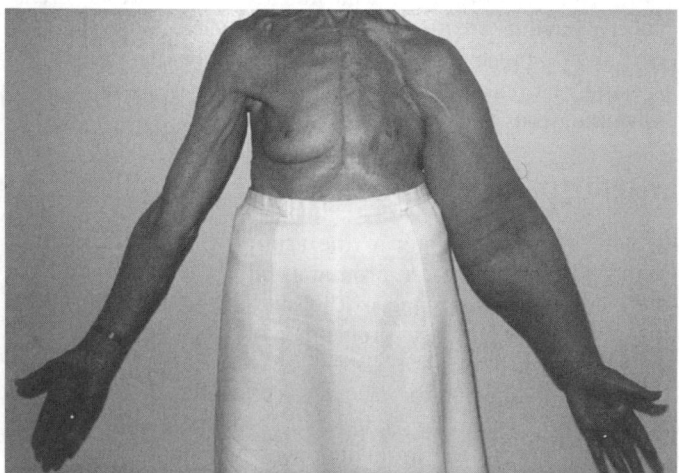

Figure 26.9 Gross lymphoedema of the arm. This patient has gross lymphoedema following a radical mastectomy and radiotherapy years before. (Reprinted from *A Slide Atlas of Breast Diseases*: Mansel R, Bundred N, 1999, by permission of Mosby Ltd.)

assessing the patient for signs of cellulitis, thrombosis or a low serum albumin, all of which may cause a swollen arm. Pain should be investigated since this can indicate active disease or a deep vein thrombosis in the axillary vein.

It is not possible to replace damaged lymphatic vessels and cure the condition. There are a variety of treatments available. Most surgical procedures for lymphoedema are intended to debulk the volume of skin and subcutaneous tissues of the affected limb, or to form lymphaticovenous anastomosis in order for the vein to transport lymph. Early results may look favourable, but do not contribute to the long-term restoration of normal physiology. The drawbacks are impaired healing and the risk of infection (Földi et al 1985).

The use of diuretics should be discouraged since, although initial fluid loss may suggest an improvement, the condition may be exacerbated as the protein part of the lymphoedema is left behind in much higher concentrations, worsening inflammation and fibrosis (Badger 1987).

Infection should be managed with antibiotics prior to starting any massage and containment treatments. Recurrent infections are common and patients can feel very unwell with cellulitis. If the lymphoedema is due to active disease, medical management may include chemotherapy, radiotherapy or hormone manipulation to contain any tumour compressing the lymphatic system.

Some patients may experience pain with lymphoedema due to the compression and stretching. Adequate assessment of this should be made and analgesia prescribed.

▶ Nursing management

Lymphoedema responds much better when detected early and when patients are compliant with their treatment. Any management must include continuous assessment which involves regular limb measurement and assessment of hosiery for a correct fit, patient education, treatment and evaluation.

There are four main areas of treatment, which should be used simultaneously:

- Skin care – aims to prevent infection and inflammation, which can lead to lymphatic damage and a worsening of the lymphoedema. Patients should be advised about minimizing risks. This includes avoiding minor skin injuries, treating cuts immediately and consulting a doctor if the arm becomes infected, and keeping hands and nails clean. It can also mean avoiding having blood taken from the affected arm.
- Exercise – normal use of the limb should be encouraged to improve lymph drainage. Passive (if patients are unable to move their arm) or specific exercise can be used to increase joint mobility; however, excessive use may cause vasodilatation and increased lymph flow.
- Massage – radioisotope studies have shown that massage is effective in increasing the uptake of fluid in the lymphatics (Földi et al 1985). The technique used is not vigorous, as this would increase blood flow to the area, but a gentle technique known as manual lymphatic drainage (MLD). This technique assumes that fluid can only be removed effectively if it can be taken up by unaffected lymphatics beyond the area of lymphoedema. Fluid will re-accumulate if containment hosiery is not used.

■ Containment hosiery or bandaging – this increases the interstitial pressure and aids absorption by the pumping action of the muscles. It is not intended to force fluid out of the limb by compression and is therefore used in conjunction with massage and exercise. Hosiery and bandaging are the two methods of containment. Hosiery is used long-term for mild uncomplicated lymphoedema. It is an elastic arm sleeve, which exerts a pressure of about 25 mmHg. Any improvement gained will be lost if a patient does not comply with treatment or if the sleeve does not fit properly. It should be worn all day and taken off at night. Bandaging is used for more complicated lymphoedema and gross swelling. The aim of treatment is to restore the limb to a more reasonable shape, size and condition so that compression hosiery can be used (Badger 1987). Bandaging involves daily high compression treatment, where most of the fluid reduction occurs in the first 4 days. Indications for bandaging are lymphorrhoea (leakage of lymph through the skin), oedematous fingers and broken skin.

Lymphoedema is a distressing and disabling condition, with no predictability regarding its onset. It may occur soon after breast cancer treatment or several years later. It can have both physical and psychological effects. A woman may experience pain or discomfort that may cause her to use the limb less, which compromises her ability to perform normal activities of living or maintain independence. There may be a cost and time impact as she is forced to visit the hospital for treatment. Feelings of embarrassment at such a visible reminder of the disease are not uncommon (Salter 1989). Physical problems often lead to psychological problems, as a result of altered body image.

FUNGATING LESIONS

Breast cancer is the most common cancer to fungate, i.e. to ulcerate through the skin (Ch. 10). This acts as a constant reminder to patients of their disease (Fig. 26.10).

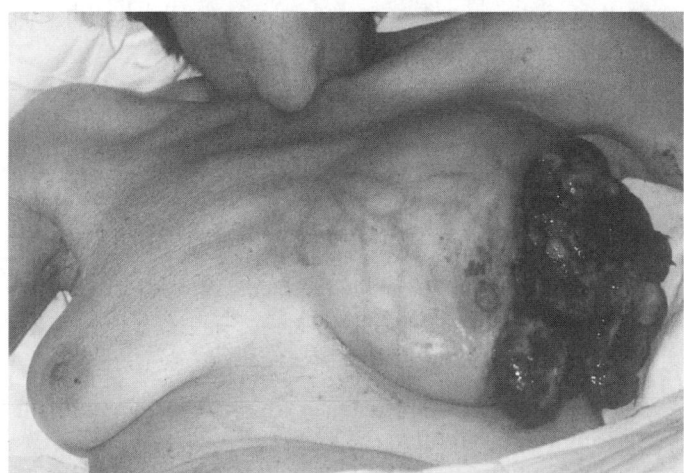

Figure 26.10 Fungating breast lesion. Locally advanced breast cancer. (Reproduced with kind permission from the Department of Medical Illustration, Christie NHS Hospital Trust, Manchester.)

Pathophysiology

Fungating wounds are the result of the cancerous infiltration of epithelium and the surrounding blood and lymphatic vessels. As the tumour develops and grows, necrosis may occur.

Clinical presentation

Presentation of a fungating breast normally falls into one of three categories:

■ a rapidly progressing breast cancer (usually inflammatory breast cancer);
■ a local recurrence;
■ a late presentation where a woman ignored a lump for many years. The fungating lesion may first present as a nodule, as a fungus-like lesion or an ulcerating crater. A woman may have noticed that her skin becomes dry, red, shiny or itchy. Areas of unhealing broken skin may develop and begin to discharge. Untreated, the area will ulcerate and discharge, with the risk of infection and bleeding.

Medical/surgical management

There are few specific investigations aside from confirming the histology of a breast cancer and suitability for any subsequent treatments. Initial management will include establishing the clinical history to identify how the disease has progressed and any concurrent diseases. The management of fungating lesions should be realistic and acceptable to patients. It is rarely intended to be curative. The primary aim, therefore, is always comfort and the promotion of quality of life. A multidisciplinary approach is essential and may include:

■ Radiotherapy – often the treatment of choice and is very effective in symptomatic control. It will be a very short course, or even a single fraction, so side-effects will be minimal.
■ Chemotherapy – may reduce the size of the tumour and will reduce pain and irritation. Combination agents may be used but consideration is given to balance the efficacy against side-effects, such as nausea and vomiting.
■ Hormone manipulation – may reduce symptoms of patients with hormone-responsive tumours.
■ Laser treatment – can be useful for reducing pain and necrotic tissue and aiding granulation. This can sometimes enable the ulcer bed to be excised and grafted (Ch. 10).
■ Surgery – may be possible after one or more of the above treatments. The side-effects and risks of surgery should be carefully considered.

▶ Nursing management

The aim of nursing management is often palliative and a nursing assessment must take into consideration issues such as physical limitations that may influence wound management, available support and patients' knowledge of their disease. The management of a fungating lesion must be realistic and agreed by both patient and carers. The family may require more practical help if patients wish to be managed at home, with access to specialist help as required. The progression and management of the disease should be fully discussed so that patients can always be in control of treatment options.

GUIDELINES FOR CARE PRIORITIES

26.1 Fungating lesions

The following issues need to be addressed:

- *Wound assessment* – both initial and ongoing.
- *Control of odour* – swabs for microbiology should be taken to exclude infection. Treatment with systemic or topical antibiotics, e.g. metronidazole, may be indicated. Debridement (removal of necrotic tissue) using specific dressings or surgery may control offensive odours. Choosing an appropriate dressing, e.g. activated charcoal dressings, is necessary. Very basic nursing interventions, such as providing clean bedding and fresh air, can help to reduce odours.
- *Haemostasis* – haemorrhage is always a risk and dressings should be wet with warm 0.9% saline prior to being removed. Obviously great care must be taken to avoid traumatizing the lesion, and the use of alginate dressings (Ch. 10) can reduce bleeding.
- *Exudate* – choosing the appropriate dressing for the amount of exudate and helping the patient with extra pads and suitable clothing.
- *Debridement* – this may be undertaken with specific occlusion dressings, such as hydrocolloids (Ch. 10), but surgery may be necessary.
- *Pain control* – this is a priority and can be achieved by a moist wound environment, analgesia (Ch. 7), soaking the dressing prior to removal and reducing the number of dressing changes.
- *Dressings* – choosing the correct type of dressing is vital and depends upon thorough and ongoing assessment of the lesion.
- *Comfort* – any dressing or nursing intervention must provide comfort and be acceptable to the patient.

A nursing assessment should explore emotional aspects, such as patients' fears. There may be feelings of guilt, because the initial breast lump was ignored, and social stigma or shame because of the change in body image, discharge and offensive smell. Over 20 years ago, Doyle (1980) wrote about how patients might feel with part of their body rotting – the smell, the reaction of others and knowing that it signifies a lingering death. There may be problems with relationships because of a perceived loss of attractiveness and inhibitions.

The choice of dressings will be governed by the characteristics of the lesion and what is comfortable and acceptable to the patient; a detailed account of dressings and their uses can be found in Chapter 10. The management of fungating lesions is described in detail in Guidelines for Care Priorities box 26.1.

BREAST RECONSTRUCTION

Breast reconstruction is an operation to create a breast form that replaces breast tissue removed by surgery for breast cancer. Reconstruction will not produce an identical breast shape with the same sensitivity, but dressed, women will look the same as

REFLECTIVE PRACTICE

26.3 The availability of immediate breast reconstruction

In some parts of the UK, immediate breast reconstruction is not available for women undergoing mastectomy. This may be due to a variety of reasons: resource implications where a health authority has selected other priorities, lack of skilled staff or the views of surgeons who do not offer it.

Student activities
- How do you feel about this inequity of service provision?
- What is the policy in your local area regarding the availability of immediate breast reconstruction to women having a mastectomy for breast cancer?

before. Women may have immediate breast reconstruction at the time of their mastectomy or delayed reconstruction. For many women, living without a breast can be difficult, and psychologically a breast reconstruction can improve their body image. Some women find an external prosthesis unacceptable and they may benefit from a breast reconstruction. Most women, regardless of age, are eligible candidates for a breast reconstruction and the choice should be left to them as to whether to undergo this surgery (Dean et al 1983). However, immediate breast reconstruction is not always available (see Reflective Practice box 26.3).

TYPES OF BREAST RECONSTRUCTION

Reconstruction can be performed using a variety of methods:

- using a woman's own body tissue
- using implants
- a combination of the two methods.

The reconstruction method used will depend upon the type of mastectomy, how recently radiotherapy was given (it may impair tissue healing if very recent), the stage of the cancer when it was discovered and a woman's general health and previous operations.

Flap reconstruction

This method uses a flap from the woman's back, abdomen or buttocks to create a breast mound. Depending on the site, the flap is either tunnelled to the breast area under the skin, remaining attached to its blood supply, or it is surgically removed and transferred to the breast area (a free flap). A free flap involves microsurgery to rejoin the blood vessels to the blood supply at the new site.

TRAM flap

A flap of muscle and skin is taken from the abdominal wall, rotated and tunnelled up to the breast area (Fig. 26.11). There is usually enough tissue to match a larger breast without needing an additional implant. Scarring on the abdomen will be horizontal and oval on the breast. This operation is available to women after radical mastectomy or radiotherapy (or both).

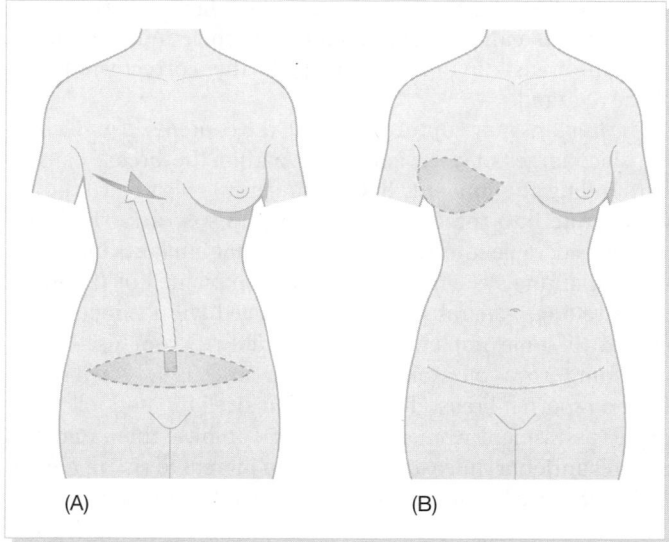

Figure 26.11 A trans-rectus abdominis flap reconstruction (TRAM flap). The rectus abdominis muscle is tunnelled from the abdomen to the chest wall.

Latissimus dorsi flap

A flap of latissimus dorsi muscle and skin from the back, directly behind the operated breast, is rotated and tunnelled just below the axilla and placed on the chest wall (Fig. 26.12). The skin from the back supplements that already on the chest, creating an envelope for the muscle, which can then be bulked out with an implant if necessary. There is a scar on the back, which can sometimes be hidden by a bra strap, and an oval scar around the breast.

Implant surgery

Implants are used for subcutaneous breast reconstruction. All the breast tissue is removed, but the skin and nipple are usually retained. An implant is then placed beneath the skin. This feels and moves like a real breast. The scar will run either horizontally across the breast or under the breast. This operation can also be used to increase breast size or where breast tissue is removed prophylactically in women who are at high risk of developing breast cancer. An implant can also be used to lift a healthy breast to match the reconstructed breast.

A submuscular breast reconstruction may be appropriate in a small breast. An implant is placed beneath the muscles covering the chest. It is unsuitable if a woman has had radiotherapy or if all the muscle has been removed in a radical mastectomy. In these instances, a breast reconstruction using tissue expansion to stretch the skin is indicated. It may require two operations and will take about 6 months to complete. An inflatable silicone bag is inserted beneath the skin and muscle of the chest and is partially filled with sterile saline via a valve. Fluid is added at intervals in outpatients until the size is slightly larger than the normal breast and then left for about 3 months. The saline-filled bag is removed and replaced by an implant at a second operation. Tissue expansion can also be achieved using an implant with an inflatable inner chamber. This does not need to be removed, but the valve is removed, usually under local anaesthetic as a day case.

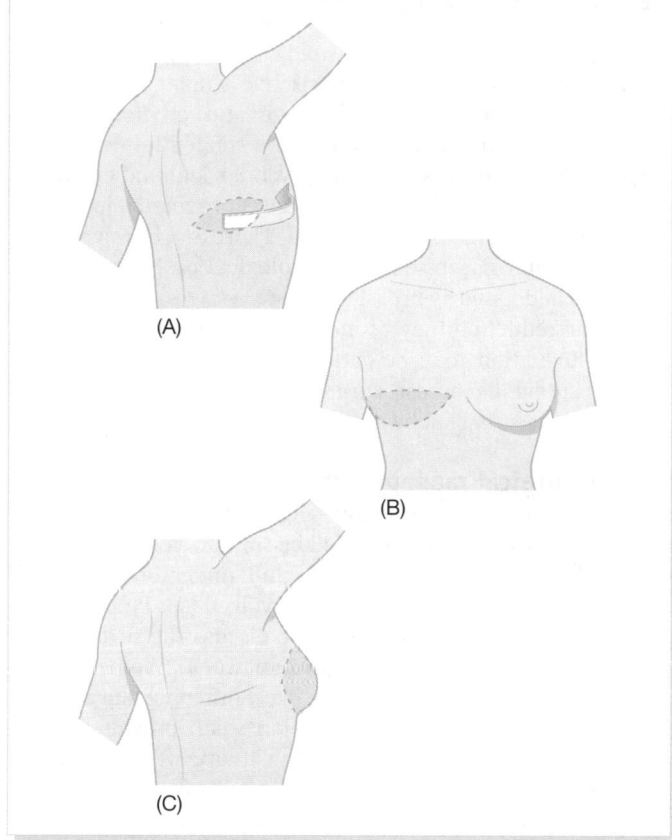

Figure 26.12 Latissimus dorsi flap. The latissimus dorsi muscle is transferred with its own blood supply to the front of the chest. It is tunnelled under the axilla.

Types of implants

Breast implants come in many shapes and sizes, with different inner and outer materials. All implants have an outer pliable silicone envelope, which encloses either a liquid (saline) or soft silicone gel. In addition to these fillers, hydrogel and soya oil have also been used (see p. 790). The outer casings may be rough or smooth. A capsule forms around the implant (non-body tissue) as part of a normal body reaction.

Nipple reconstruction

A nipple can be reconstructed, but this is usually done at a later date so that it matches the position of the nipple on the natural breast. A nipple can be reconstructed using the skin on the reconstructed breast, skin from behind the ear or from the other nipple, or it may be tattooed on. Good artificial nipples are available which can be stuck onto the reconstructed breast.

Surgery to the other breast

Surgery on the natural breast may sometimes be recommended to achieve better symmetry. This may mean reducing the natural breast or lifting it to avoid the natural droop. Often nipples will have to be repositioned and this can lead to a reduction or loss of sensation. Some women decide to avoid surgery with the consequent scarring on the natural breast, whilst others want as close a match as possible.

BREAST AUGMENTATION AND REDUCTION

Breast augmentation can be used to enlarge, reshape or rebalance breasts that differ in size or shape. Implants are inserted as described previously. Age and pregnancy often change breast shape and size and some congenital defects can also be addressed in this way. The psychological and emotional benefits can be considerable in this subset of women, leading to enhanced body image and self-esteem. There are, however, some women who have deep-seated psychological problems that are not always addressed by breast surgery.

A breast reduction may be indicated for medical or cosmetic reasons. Reduction may be performed to even up the breasts following previous breast surgery, or it may be performed bilaterally to ease backache in the larger breasted woman.

Medical/surgical management

For any type of breast reduction, augmentation or reconstruction, the medical management will be similar. The medical staff should ensure that women have a full understanding of all aspects of this surgery and the risks involved (see below). There should be opportunities for women to discuss the surgery with the surgeon and have their questions answered. Women should have realistic expectations as to the likely outcome. Surgery can never replace a natural breast. Implants can provide a better shape, but there may be loss of sensitivity. Where possible, women should be able to see photographs of other patients, talk to them and also have an opportunity to talk to a BCN. The overall health of the woman should be discussed, including any factors that may affect healing, e.g. drug therapy, smoking and alcohol use. This is especially important where a TRAM flap is planned, since flap necrosis may occur. Previous breast surgery and complications from surgery should be assessed.

Potential problems and complications
Wound infection

Infection may complicate any surgery and would be treated with antibiotics. Occasionally it is necessary to remove an implant and replace it later. In extreme cases the flap can be lost.

Scarring

Flap reconstructions may cause additional scarring.

Implant problems

Implants may deflate, requiring further surgery for removal and replacement. Contraction of the capsule or scar tissue may tighten and squeeze the implant, resulting in changes to breast shape, pain and hardness. The implant may need to be removed or corrected. Implants need to be replaced when, or if, they wear out. Implants can sometimes shift from their initial position, giving the breasts an unnatural look. Further corrective surgery will be required.

The implant may rupture releasing the contents, e.g. silicone. The silicone gel may be contained within the breast capsule surrounding the implant, but if the capsule also tears the gel will migrate into the body. Fortunately this is rare. There has been considerable interest in the effects that implants may have on the immune system. Women have complained of tiredness, joint swelling, general aches and enlarged lymph nodes. This has led to some implants being withdrawn from use. Those containing soya oil were withdrawn in 1999, when some women reported breast discomfort and swelling, and following further assessment women were advised to have them removed as a precautionary measure because an increased risk of cancer could not be excluded (Department of Health 2000).

Screening

Some implants make mammography difficult to perform. Clinical examination should still be performed and this may be useful in flap reconstructions to detect any local recurrences.

Breast-feeding

There is no reason why a woman cannot breast-feed successfully from the unaffected side following breast reconstruction. She may need extra support from her midwife to establish breast-feeding.

Loss of sensation

Loss of sensation to both the breast and the nipple may occur after any breast surgery and can have implications for body image and expression of sexuality.

▶ Nursing management

All women should have the choice about whether to undergo some form of elective breast surgery. It is the nurse's role to ensure that each woman has been fully informed about the options available to her, the expected outcomes and the potential risks. Practical issues such as returning to work, bra styles and exercises must be discussed. Assessment of body image and the involvement of partners is important.

Postoperatively there is no specific nursing care, except checking of the wound for warmth and colour to ensure that it is well perfused, checking for signs of infection, such as pyrexia, and monitoring drainage.

SUMMARY: MAIN POINTS

- The majority of women who present to a breast clinic have benign disease, but all will need adequate investigation and explanation.

- Breast patients need the support of a specialist breast care team who have undergone specialist training and who can access triple assessment and specialist opinion.

- Early diagnosis enables malignancies to be treated more effectively and patients with benign disease to be reassured quickly.

- Women are aware that inequities in service provision exist and that there is still a lack of consensus as to treatment. The quest for optimum standards is the concern of all health care professionals. The development of protocols and service monitoring will aid this, as will the collection of data to monitor outcomes.

- Patients are entitled to a choice and need the support of a specialist nurse to facilitate this. Psychological support and quality of life issues are vital components of nursing care.

- We cannot prevent breast cancer, so screening remains one of the main ways to detect early disease. Uptake needs to be improved to ensure that all eligible women attend.

- Breast cancer can affect all ages, races and both sexes. The effect on individuals, families and friends is enormous and can create a state of uncertainty.

- The media is full of miracle treatments, deaths from breast cancer and survival rates. Effective information and support are essential.

- The search for more effective breast cancer treatments continues. Clinical trials involving high-dose chemotherapy and other drug therapies are currently in progress in the UK.

- As outcome monitoring becomes more prevalent and equity of access to high-quality services improves, we will be moving towards effective breast cancer treatment.

SELF-TEST: CRITICAL THINKING ACTIVITIES

1 Find a care pathway (for example Northwest Nursing and PAMs Pathways in Cancer Care) for a woman who finds a breast lump (later diagnosed as malignant). Follow her journey from her visit to the GP through to discharge.

2 What investigations/interventions will she undergo in the preliminary stages until she has surgery, and which health care professionals should she meet?

 ## FURTHER READING

Denton S. Breast Cancer Nursing. London: Chapman and Hall; 1996.

Early Breast Cancer Trials Collaborative Group. Treatment of early breast cancer 1985–90. Oxford: Oxford University Press; 1990.

Kirshbaum M. The development, implementation and evaluation of guidelines for the management of breast cancer related lymphoedema. Eur J Cancer Care 1996; 5(4): 246–251.

Luker KA, Beaver K, Leinster SJ, Owens RG, Degner LF, Sloan JA. The information needs of women newly diagnosed with breast cancer. J Adv Nurs 1995; 22: 134–141.

Luker KA, Beaver K, Leinster SJ, Glynn Owens R. Information needs and sources of information for women with breast cancer: a follow up study. J Adv Nurs 1996; 23: 487–495.

Maslin A. A survey of the opinions on 'informed consent' of women currently involved in clinical trials within a breast unit. Eur J Cancer Care 1994; 3: 153–162.

 ## USEFUL WEBSITES

www.breastcancercare.org.uk – Breast cancer care
www.breastcare.co.uk – Breast care campaign

www.churchillmed.com/journals/breast/jhome.html
www.healthgate.com

✉ USEFUL ADDRESSES

BACUP
3 Bath Place
Rivington Street
London EC2A 3JR
Tel: 0800 181 199

Cancerlink
70 Brittania Street
London WC1X 9JN
Tel: 020 7833 2451
Asian language line: 020 7713 7867

REFERENCES

Badger C. Lymphoedema: management of patients with advanced cancer. Prof Nurse 1987; 2(4): 100–102.

Barlow H. What is good practice in breast cancer care? IHSM Network 1995; 2(24): 5.

Calman K, Hine D. A policy framework for commissioning cancer services. London: Department of Health; 1995.

Cancer Research Campaign (CRC). Factsheet 6.1–6.6. London: CRC; 1996.

Clinical Outcomes Group (COG). Cancer Guidance Sub-group: the NHS COG breast guidelines. Guidance on commissioning cancer services. Improving outcomes in breast cancer. London: Department of Health; 1996.

Dean C, Chetty U, Forrest AP. Effects of immediate breast reconstruction on psychological morbidity after mastectomy. Lancet 1983; 1(8322): 459–462.

Department of Health. Our healthier nation (green paper). London: The Stationery Office; 1998.

Department of Health. Warning issued to remove trilucent breast implants (press release 2000/0326). Online. Available: http://www.open.gov.uk/doh/dhhome.htm 26 Mar 2000.

Dixon J, Mansel R. Congenital problems and aberrations of normal breast development and involution. In: Dixon J, ed. ABC of breast diseases. London: BMJ Publishing Group; 1995.

Doyle D. Domiciliary terminal care. The Practitioner 1980; 224: 577–582.

Evans DGR, Fentiman IS, McPherson K et al. Familial breast cancer. Br Med J 1994; 308: 183–187.

Fallowfield L, Clark A. Breast cancer. London: Tavistock and Routledge; 1991.

Fallowfield L, Baum M, Maguire GP. Effects of breast conservation on psychological morbidity associated with diagnosis and treatment of early breast cancer. Br Med J 1986; 293: 1331–1334.

Fisher B, Redmond C, Poisson R et al. Eight year results for a randomised clinical trial comparing total mastectomy and lumpectomy with or without irradiation in the treatment of breast cancer. N Engl J Med 1989; 320(13): 822–828.

Földi E, Földi M, Weissleder H. Conservative treatment of lymphoedema of the limbs. Angiol J Vasc Surg 1985; 36(3): 171–180.

Forrest AP. Breast cancer screening report to the Health Ministers of England, Scotland and Northern Ireland. London: DHSS; 1986.

Hardy JD. Hardy's text book of surgery, 2nd edn. London: JB Lippincott; 1988.

Hodkinson M. Lymphoedema: applying physiology to treatment. Eur J Cancer Care 1992; 1: 2.

Hoe AL, Iven D, Royle GT, Taylor I. Incidence of arm swelling following axillary clearance for breast cancer. Br J Surg 1992; 79(3): 261–262.

Kissin M, Querci della Rovere G, Easton D, Westbury G. Risk of lymphoedema following the treatment of breast cancer. Br J Surg 1986; 73(7): 580–584.

Logan V. Incidence and prevalence of lymphoedema: a literature review. J Clin Nurs 1995; 4(4): 213–219.

Maguire G. Psychological aspects. In: Dixon J, ed. ABC of breast diseases. London: BMJ Publishing Group; 1995.

Maguire G, Lee E, Bevington D, Küchemann C, Crabtree R, Cornell C. Psychiatric problems in the first year after mastectomy. Br Med J 1978; 1(6118): 963–965.

Maguire G, Tait A, Brooke M, Thomas C, Sellwood R. The effect of counselling on the psychiatric morbidity associated with mastectomy. Br Med J 1980; 281: 1454–1456.

Mansel R. Breast pain. In: Dixon J, ed. ABC of breast diseases. London: BMJ Publishing Group; 1995.

Mansel R, Bundred N. Colour atlas of breast diseases. London: Mosby-Wolfe; 1995.

Mansel R, Bundred N. A slide atlas of breast diseases. London: Mosby-Wolfe; 1999.

McPherson K, Heel C. Breast cancer – epidemiology risk factors and genetics. In: Dixon J, ed. ABC of breast diseases. London: BMJ Publishing Group; 1995.

North West Nursing and PAMs Pathway in Cancer Care. www.nwrocancer.org.uk/NWRefDoc.htm#Pathways

Peto R, Boreham J, Clarke M, Davies C, Beral V. Correspondence – UK and USA breast cancer deaths down 25% in year 2000 at ages 20–69 years. Lancet 2000; 355: 1822.

Salter M. Altered body image. London: John Wiley; 1989.

Tabar L, Gad A. Screening for breast cancer – the Swedish Trial. Am J Radiol 1981; 138: 219–222.

Thomson L. Breast Cancer. In: Tschudin V, ed. Nursing the patient with cancer. London: Prentice Hall; 1989.

Tiffany R. Specialisation in nursing. Nurs Stand 1990; 5(2): 26–27.

Vessey M. Breast cancer screening: evidence and experience since the Forrest Report. Sheffield: NHS BSP Publication; 1991.

Woods M. Patients' perceptions of breast cancer related lymphoedema. Eur J Cancer Care 1993; 2: 125–128.

27 Nursing patients with musculoskeletal disorders

Mike Smith

> 'When she broke her hip I thought she'd be in bed for weeks. But she was sitting out of bed when I went in yesterday and has just rung to ask me to bring her shoes because she's going to start walking tomorrow! Apparently slippers can be dangerous to walk in.'
>
> (Patient's carer)

THIS CHAPTER WILL HELP YOU

- Describe the normal and altered physiology relating to the patient with a musculoskeletal disorder

- Identify the origins of musculoskeletal conditions

- Identify common modalities of management of musculoskeletal conditions

- Assess the patient with a musculoskeletal condition in relation to the development of appropriate nursing diagnosis

- Identify appropriate nursing actions related to a specified diagnosis

- Recognize the need for programmes of health promotion in the prevention of musculoskeletal conditions and related secondary health complications.

KEYWORDS

Arthroscopy	Joint
Avascular necrosis	Kyphosis
Bone mineral density	Myopathy
Cast	Orthosis
Dislocation	Osteoporosis
Extension	Prosthesis
External fixator	'RICE'
Flexion	Scoliosis
Fracture	Subluxation
Intra-articular	Traction

INTRODUCTION

The term orthopaedics gained in popularity towards the end of the 19th century and, deriving from the Greek words *orthos* (straight) and *paedios* (child), was used to describe the management of a child with a physical deformity. It is somewhat ironic, therefore, that of those requiring musculoskeletal intervention at the beginning of the 21st century, perhaps the most significant proportion is the older adult population, a group that continues to grow as a proportion of the whole. Generally speaking, these days musculoskeletal conditions comprise a wide range of patient situations and relate to impairments of the neuromusculoskeletal system.

The use of traction, casts, orthotic devices (e.g. splints), prostheses, bandaging, external fixators and mobility aids is common across a wide range of musculoskeletal disorders and nurses will encounter them in many areas of practice in the community and in hospital. The specific nursing management associated with these interventions is discussed early in the chapter and appears before specific disorders are covered.

ANATOMY AND PHYSIOLOGY OF THE MUSCULOSKELETAL SYSTEM – AN OVERVIEW

An overview of the skeleton, bone, long bones, joints and skeletal muscle is provided, and readers requiring further information are directed to 'Further reading' section where some suggestions are provided.

THE SKELETON

The skeleton may be divided into two distinct parts, namely the bones of the axial skeleton and those of the appendicular skeleton. The axial skeleton comprises the skull, vertebral column, sternum and ribs. The appendicular skeleton comprises the pectoral girdle (clavicles and scapulae), upper and lower limbs and the pelvic girdle.

Bone

Bone is a highly vascular, specialized type of mineralized connective tissue, and together with cartilage comprises the skeletal system. Healthy adult bone is composed of compact (cortical) bone, a hard, dense bone, and cancellous (trabecular) bone, which is light and spongy in structure. Bone has the following functions:

- provides mechanical support and is the site of muscle attachment, so allowing movement to occur
- protects body organs, e.g. heart, lungs, brain and spinal cord
- contains red bone marrow (cancellous bone in adults), which is the site for the formation of some blood cells (see Ch. 18)
- storage of minerals, notably calcium and phosphorus.

Four types of bones can be described:

- long, e.g. femur
- short, e.g. carpal bones
- flat, e.g. scapula
- irregular, e.g. vertebrae

Gross structure of a bone

Using a long bone as an example (see Fig. 27.1), there are several key components present:

- Diaphysis – the shaft of the bone
- Epiphysis – the proximal end of the long bone
- Metaphysis – lies between the proximal epiphysis and the diaphysis
- Growth or epiphyseal plate – this is where the bone grows until around the early 20s
- Articular hyaline cartilage – this covers the proximal ends of the epiphysis that articulates within a synovial joint
- Periosteum – dense irregular connective tissue forming the outer covering of bone containing blood vessels and bone-building cells
- Endosteum – dense irregular connective tissue which lines the medullary cavity
- Medullary cavity or marrow cavity – this contains yellow bone marrow; yellow marrow is composed mainly of adipose tissue
- Sharpey's fibres – these secure the periosteum to the underlying bone (not shown in Fig. 27.1).

It is noteworthy that flat, short and irregular bones lack medullary cavities.

There are bone markings visible on the periosteum that provide a surface for muscle attachment, facilitate fit between bones, and create an opening for passage of blood vessels or nerves.

For further classification of bones, bone formation (osteogenesis), bone remodelling and homeostasis, readers are directed to the suggestions in the 'Further reading' section.

Ageing and bone

There are two main effects of ageing on bone tissue:

- Loss of calcium – demineralization of bones (osteoporosis) in females commences after the age of 30 years, but accelerates after the menopause. Decreases in oestrogen levels may

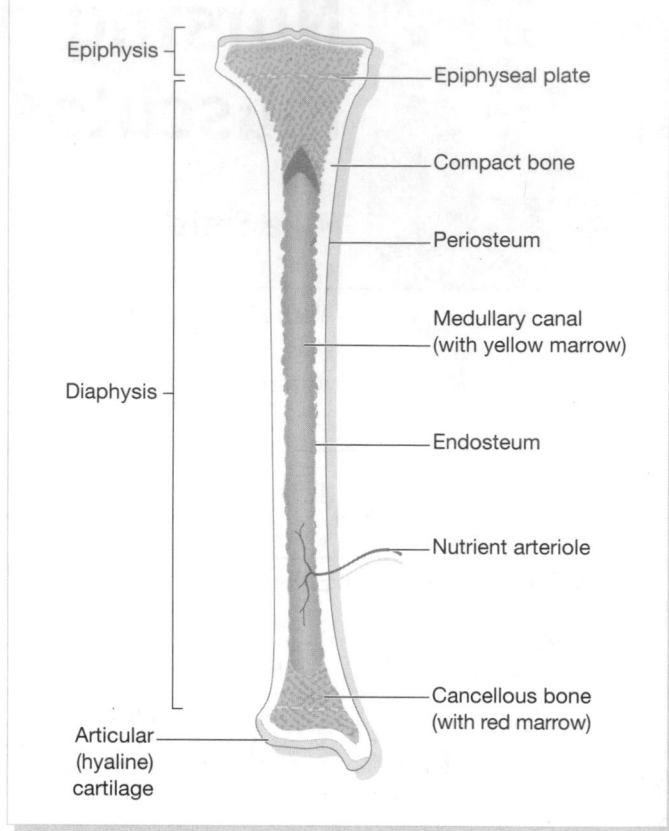

Figure 27.1 Structure of a typical long bone.

cause as much as 30% loss of calcium by the age of 70 years. In males the onset of osteoporosis occurs later, more commonly after the age of 60 years
- Decreased protein synthesis (collagen) – collagen provides bone tensile strength, and therefore loss of collagen during the ageing process results in bones becoming brittle.

JOINTS

Joints (the articulation of two or more bones) can be classified according to a combination of structural and functional characteristics:

- fibrous joints – immovable joints, e.g. sacrum
- cartilaginous joints – partially movable joints, e.g. vertebrae, pelvis
- synovial joints – freely movable joints, e.g. hip and knee.

It is noteworthy that no joint is truly freely movable, but rather has a specific broad range of motion or movement (ROM). The fibrous joint capsule, associated ligaments, and the design of the particular bones that comprise the joint restrict the particular movement of any joint

Ligaments are strong, tough collagenous fibres that serve to reinforce the joint capsule through binding the articular ends of bone together. They may be inside (intra-articular) and/or outside (extra-articular) the joint capsule. By nature, ligaments are relatively inelastic and prevent excessive movement of the joint. If ligaments are stretched they will not rebound.

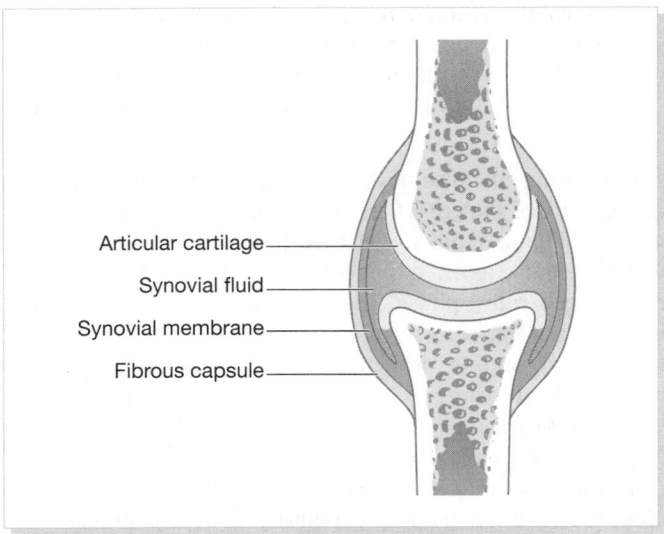

Figure 27.2 A typical synovial joint.

- Articular cartilage
- Synovial fluid
- Synovial membrane
- Fibrous capsule

In synovial joints there is an interfacing layer of articular hyaline cartilage, and a synovial capsule surrounds the joints. A synovial membrane lines the capsule and covers all the non-articular surfaces inside the joint; therefore, in health, the bones in such a joint do not have direct contact (see Fig. 27.2). This thin membrane secretes a clear, oily, lubricating fluid into the synovial cavity.

Thus, during movement of the joint, cartilage and synovial fluid protect bone tissue. The effect of this is to:

- dampen vibration
- reduce shock
- reduce friction
- create smooth movement.

Fibrous sacs filled with synovial fluid, known as bursa, also help to reduce friction and facilitate movement. They are located near joints in muscle, between tendons and bone, and between bone and skin.

The different types of synovial joint with examples and the movement possible are summarized in Table 27.1.

The stability of joints is determined by the nature of the articular surface, sockets and grooves, the number of stabilizing ligaments (i.e. the more ligaments, the stronger the joint), and the amount of muscle tone; the presence of looser, stretchable joint ligaments is often termed 'double-jointed'.

There are various types of movement that joints can perform: gliding, angular, circular and special (see Box 27.1).

SKELETAL MUSCLES

There are close to 700 skeletal muscles in the body. These are formed from striated, voluntary muscle tissue and are usually responsible for moving bones. Additionally they have the ability to react quickly, but, equally, they will tire quickly. The characteristics of muscle tissue are outlined in Box 27.2.

Table 27.1 Types of synovial joints

Type of synovial joint	Movement	Example
Gliding	Short, gliding movement; back-and-forth or side-to-side movements	Wrist, ankle, vertebral
Hinge	Angular movement allowed in only one direction	Elbow, interphalangeal, knee
Pivot	Limited to rotation around an axis of one bone on another bone	Ring of the atlas around the peg of the axis (cervical vertebrae) Proximal radioulnar joint allows for rotation of the forearm (supination and pronation)
Condyloid	No rotation allowed, but back-and-forth or side-to-side movement	Metacarpophalangeal joint
Ball and socket	Allows the greatest range of motion	Hip, shoulder
Saddle	Permits a wide variety of movements	Carpometacarpal joint of the thumb

---

Box 27.3 Muscle groups

- *Agonists* – muscles contracting and causing movement, e.g. flexor muscles of the thigh (hamstrings) bring lower leg towards thigh
- *Antagonists* – muscles that perform opposing actions, e.g. quadriceps and hamstrings. Therefore, the movement produced by one can always be reversed by another. Antagonism also limits and controls motions
- *Synergists* – groups of muscles that contract together to accomplish the same body movement, e.g. quadriceps group, contraction of which causes extension of the leg

---

The functions of skeletal muscle are as follows: movement, posture and heat production. The range of contraction of a muscle is dependent on its length, and the power of a muscle depends on the number of muscle fibres present.

Skeletal muscle often works in groups and these groups are named according how they work (see Box 27.3). Additionally muscular movement is always opposed or aided by gravity, it requiring more effort to move against rather than with gravity.

Tendons attach muscle to bone and are made of collagen fibres which, by their nature, resist stretch and are flexible. They are avascular (without a blood supply) and so appear white and, as a consequence, heal very slowly following injury.

MUSCULOSKELETAL CONDITIONS, MOBILITY AND NURSING ASSESSMENT

The major objective when nursing a patient with a musculoskeletal condition is usually the restoration of mobility (Davis 1994). People need to be able to move to perform all the activities of daily living. In this particular patient population, and in the absence of other pathology, it is reduced mobility that is likely to be the cause of problems relating to toileting, eating, social interaction and the ability to maintain personal hygiene, and problems in these areas will increase the likelihood of secondary complications. Psychological consequences of reduced mobility, such as fear of falling (Resnick 1999), may occur directly as a result of the current condition or as a consequence of a previous fracture (e.g. fractured neck of femur) and is clearly an issue for older people.

Additionally, other impairments, particularly of a neurological nature, such as cerebrovascular accident (CVA) (see Ch. 14) or spinal cord injury, may be further complicated by the presence of a musculoskeletal condition.

Musculoskeletal problems may also occur secondary to other pathology, e.g. shoulder pain in the paralysed limb of a patient with hemiplegia (paralysis affecting one side of the body) or quadriplegia (paralysis affecting all four limbs).

Assessment of the person with a musculoskeletal condition must take into account all of these issues:

- What are the causes of reduced movement and how may these be reduced or removed?
- What activities (functional and social) do the reduction of mobility impact upon and how may these be resolved?
- What potential secondary complications may develop as a result of the reduced mobility and how may the risk of these be limited?

The nature of musculoskeletal disease determines that, for the majority of patients, there will be a variable period of time between diagnosis and surgery. In elective cases, diagnosis will usually be made as an outpatient and, in most cases of trauma, in the preoperative phase. There is much that can be done to promote desirable postoperative patient outcomes in this period. Based on this premise, it seems logical that nursing assessment and indeed interventions to improve outcomes, e.g. education regarding the care of casts, should occur during this period, not simply preparation for surgery.

In the case of elective admissions, the concept of pre-admission clinics is gaining popularity; however, nurses could have a greater role in this. As well as determining fitness for anaesthesia, the following could be part of that process:

- Assessment, improvement and maintenance of good general health to ensure optimum fitness for surgery and the postoperative period
- Assessment and education relating to secondary complications and how to prevent them occurring
- Appropriate and considered drug therapy that may impact on the patient's current situation, i.e. explanation of the likely drug therapy needs postoperatively. It is arguable that this might improve compliance following discharge
- Assessment of postoperative rehabilitation needs. Education with regard to likely requirements, e.g. brace wearing, care of plaster, postoperative exercise, showing the patient an external fixator, should be commenced. The ability of patients to accept such measures will surely be improved in many cases, rather than waiting until the postoperative period when they are recovering from surgery and possibly experiencing discomfort and inconvenience
- Assessment of the need for devices that enable activities of living to be undertaken. In some cases, use of these could be practised prior to surgery, e.g. crutches, raised toilet seats.

In the case of the trauma patient, the duration of time to surgery may be more limited, depending on the particular condition and the availability of operating theatre time. However, there is still much of the above that could be undertaken.

There is a compelling case for the involvement of nurses in the assessment, care and preparation of patients with musculoskeletal disorders at the earliest stage following diagnosis.

THE ORIGINS OF MUSCULOSKELETAL CONDITIONS

As stated above, the origins of musculoskeletal conditions may be primary or secondary to other conditions. Table 27.2 summarizes the originating causes of the majority of musculoskeletal conditions, which form the framework for this chapter.

Table 27.2 Origins of musculoskeletal conditions

Origin	Example
Inflammatory disorders	Rheumatoid arthritis (RA)
Metabolic disorders	Gout
Muscle disorders	Muscular dystrophy
Joint disorders	Osteoarthritis (OA)
Back problems	Prolapsed intervertebral disc (PID)
Connective tissue disorders	Systemic lupus erythematosus
Bone disorders	Osteoporosis
Bone tumours	Sarcoma
Infections	Osteomyelitis
Spinal curvature	Scoliosis
Trauma	Fractures and soft tissue injuries

GENERAL DIAGNOSTIC TESTS AND MEDICAL INVESTIGATION

PHYSICAL EXAMINATION

The physical examination of the affected part(s) is a fundamental element of musculoskeletal assessment. Nurses should be aware of a particular joint's range of movement, the signs and symptoms of specific musculoskeletal injuries or conditions, and the symptoms of common associated complications, e.g. compartment syndrome. This is essential not only in helping to ascertain a diagnosis, but also in being able to assess a situation that is changing, e.g. in multiple trauma. Additionally, there is the need to avoid making a condition worse through inappropriate management; for example, attempting to take an injured joint through the normal range of movement too soon may affect healing, increase patient pain or cause further damage to the affected part.

There are many 'named' tests for particular musculoskeletal conditions. Table 27.3 provides some examples, but it is worth pointing out that these comprise only a few of the more commonly used tests. Some of the tests will be referred to in the relevant sections concerning specific musculoskeletal conditions later in the chapter.

X-RAY

The plain X-ray or radiograph is a vital part of the diagnostic armoury. Prior to any surgical intervention, after any actual or suspected injury and at regular intervals during a patient's health care episode, the X-ray remains a key tool. Densities, relationships between different bones, continuity of bone and bone contour are all key features that may indicate the presence of a musculoskeletal condition. Although it may not be necessary for a nurse to have an in-depth knowledge regarding the interpretation of X-rays, one could argue that in the role of educating patients about their particular condition, a basic knowledge is advantageous at the very least. Clearly those in nurse practitioner or clinical nurse specialist posts will require a deeper understanding in order to fulfil their roles (see Reflective Practice box 27.1).

Bone mineral density (BMD) can be measured using dual-energy X-ray absorptiometry (DXA). This can be used to identify individuals with osteoporosis.

COMPUTED TOMOGRAPHY (CT SCAN)

In CT scanning, an X-ray beam passes through the body part at the different angles of rotation. This information is transformed into a cross-sectional image. Significantly more information can be gained via CT scan than with traditional X-rays, although not to the same degree as MRI (see below).

Intravenous (i.v.) contrast may be given to outline vascular structures and assess the enhancement characteristics of pathological processes.

No special physical preparation is normally required for CT scanning other than for abdominopelvic scans where contrast may be used. It is beneficial to explain to patients what will happen to them to facilitate compliance during the procedure, and most imaging departments produce patient information materials that the nurse can use.

MAGNETIC RESONANCE IMAGING (MRI)

Magnetic resonance imaging is based on the interaction between nuclei of hydrogen atoms occurring abundantly in all biological tissues and the magnetic fields generated and controlled by the MRI equipment. The images produced provide detailed information regarding the majority of body tissues.

MRI examination is useful in musculoskeletal and neurological conditions because observation of soft tissues as well as bone is advantageous in diagnosis and planning medical intervention.

The main contraindications to MRI examinations are cardiac pacemakers, cochlear implants, epidural electrodes, ferromagnetic aneurysm clips and some other metal implants. Relative contraindications include first trimester pregnancy and claustrophobia. Once again, therefore, psychological preparation as well as ascertaining the presence of any of the physical contraindications are vital prior to the procedure.

ULTRASOUND

Quantitative ultrasound (QUS) can be used to identify individuals at risk of hip fracture caused by osteoporosis.

BLOOD TESTS

A variety of blood tests, e.g. full blood count (FBC), erythrocyte sedimentation rate (ESR), C-reactive protein, rheumatoid factors and muscle enzymes, may be indicated in specific musculoskeletal conditions, e.g. rheumatoid arthritis and myopathy. Where appropriate, these will be discussed in the relevant sections of this chapter.

Table 27.3 Common physical examination diagnostic tests

Test	Procedure and possible diagnosis
Adam's sign	In scoliosis the patient bends over. No straightening of the curve would indicate a positive result. A straightening of the curve would indicate a negative result
Anterior drawer	The knee is flexed to approximately 90° and the proximal tibia is pulled forward. If excessive movement is found, it is indicative of a tear of the anterior cruciate ligament
Apley test	Whilst in a prone position, the knee is flexed 90°. While compressing the knee, the lower leg is rotated in both directions. If this manoeuvre elicits pain, it is likely that a meniscal tear is present
Apprehension test	The shoulder is forcefully abducted and externally rotated. Patients who have experienced either dislocation or subluxation of the shoulder will become extremely apprehensive
Chest expansion test	Chest expansion is measured from maximal exhalation to maximal inspiration. An expansion of less than 2.5 cm is indicative of forms of arthritis, which can affect the spine and rib cage, most commonly ankylosing spondylitis
Clonus	The foot is dorsiflexed, resulting in repetitive, uncontrolled up-and-down motion of the ankle. A positive test indicates pressure upon the spinal cord
Impingement test	The shoulder is forcefully abducted or abducted and internally rotated, causing the greater tuberosity to press against the undersurface of the acromion. A positive test indicates impingement syndrome
Lachman test	The knee is flexed to approximately 20° and the proximal tibia is pulled forward. Excessive motion of the tibia anteriorly is indicative of a tear of the anterior cruciate ligament
Lasegue's test	If flexion of the hip of the affected limb is not painful, but extension of the knee while the hip is flexed is painful, this would indicate sciatica and spinal cord nerve root compression
McMurray's test	The patient lies supine with knee fully flexed and the foot is rotated fully outward and the knee is slowly extended. A painful 'click' indicates a tear of the medial meniscus of the knee joint. Inward rotation of the foot with pain indicates a tear in the lateral meniscus
Patellar apprehension test	The knee is slightly flexed, the examiner attempts to push the patella in a lateral direction. Patients who have experienced a subluxation or dislocation of the patella will become very apprehensive at this point and attempt to stop the examiner from completing the test
Posterior drawer	The knee is flexed to 90° and the proximal tibia is pushed posteriorly. Excessive movement is indicative of a tear in the posterior cruciate ligament
Quadriceps inhibition	Pressure is placed over the superior aspect of the patella and the patient is asked to perform a straight leg raising manoeuvre. Pain and grinding with this manoeuvre are indicative of chondromalacia of the patella
Straight leg raising	With the knee extended and the patient supine or seated, the hip is flexed (with the leg straight). A positive test results in pain in the sciatic nerve distribution and suggests a disc herniation
Supraspinatus isolation	Abducting and forward flexing the arm with the forearm in internal rotation tests strength of abduction of the shoulder. This isolates the supraspinatus muscle. If weakness is demonstrated, this test is very suggestive of a rotator cuff tear
Trendelenburg test	The patient stands erect with back to the examiner and is instructed to lift one leg and then the other. When weight is supported by the affected limb, the pelvis on the healthy side falls instead of rising. A positive test indicates gluteus medius weakness or a dislocated hip

R|Я REFLECTIVE PRACTICE

27.1 Role of the specialist orthopaedic nurse

Does your orthopaedic area have nurse specialists? What specialist orthopaedic skills and knowledge do they possess which enables them to fulfil their role. Are there any roles which could be added that you think would improve the experience for patients, improve outcomes and be of benefit to non-specialist nurses, e.g. in educating staff or patients in hospital or in the community?

ELECTROMYOGRAPHY

An electromyogram (EMG) is usually performed to measure the electrical activity of the muscle. It involves placing a small needle into the muscle and recording the muscular activity on an oscilloscope.

SURGICAL DIAGNOSTIC TECHNIQUES

The major surgical diagnostic technique employed in musculoskeletal conditions is diagnostic arthroscopy. Additionally, many surgical procedures can be performed through an arthroscope, making them popular with both surgeons and patients due to the reduced invasiveness in comparison to 'open' surgery. Reduced postoperative complications and reduced length of hospitalization are two obvious advantages.

Biopsy of muscle tissue may be used in the diagnosis of some myopathies (see p. 811).

GENERAL DISEASE PREVENTION AND HEALTH EDUCATION

It is worth making brief reference to health promotion and education related to orthopaedic conditions, as such programmes are often run by, or in collaboration with, nurses. Essentially these fall into two categories, namely interventions in trauma prevention and interventions in non-traumatic musculoskeletal problems. The former, often combined with legislation, has certainly reduced the severity of some injuries as well as incidence. For example, seatbelt legislation has reduced the severity of cervical spinal cord injury sustained in motor vehicle accidents, and alteration in sports equipment, training techniques and formal rehabilitation programmes has reduced the occurrence, and just as importantly recurrence, of certain sports-related injuries.

In non-traumatic conditions, public education programmes have gone some way to try to reduce the incidence and severity of certain conditions. Osteoporosis is an example of this, where initiatives to reduce falls, hormone replacement therapy and screening programmes may have had a positive impact on the health of older women who are at particular risk of this condition. The obvious threat of osteoporosis is the possibility of pathological fracture (fracture associated with existing bone disease), commonly of the hip, in elderly women (Lappe 1998). Unfortunately, evidence of the efficacy of such programmes in the literature is sparse, and the fact that the population is ageing makes acquiring such evidence more complicated.

GENERAL NURSING CONSIDERATIONS – PATIENTS WITH MUSCULOSKELETAL DISORDERS

There are numerous interventions and treatment modalities that cross specific boundaries and are commonplace throughout many musculoskeletal conditions (see Fig. 27.3). It is worth exploring the general principles of nursing management for some of these (traction, casts, orthotic devices, mobility aids and external fixators) as it could be argued that it is these that form the basis of knowledge deemed specialist orthopaedic practice.

NURSING PATIENTS IN TRACTION

Traction is generally used to counteract the potential or actual problems caused by the pull of muscles on a damaged bone or joint. The purpose of traction may comprise any one or more of the following:

- to maintain or achieve correct alignment of injured bone
- to prevent development or deformity, or reduce existing deformity
- to immobilize a damaged joint

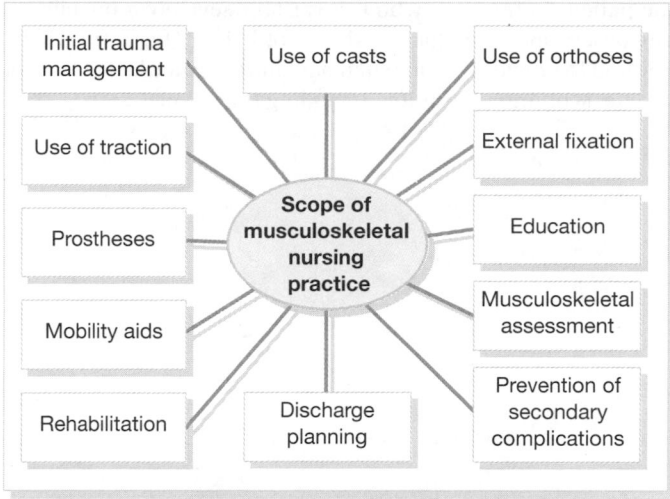

Figure 27.3 Scope of musculoskeletal nursing practice.

- to relieve pain through attaining normal anatomical alignment and reduce muscle spasm around the injury site
- (occasionally) to protect underlying tissues and structures. An obvious example would be the patient with cervical traction in which the aim is protection of the spinal cord.

Clearly the type of traction utilized will be dependent on the particular condition. Although it is not within the remit of this chapter to give details of the alternative forms of skin or skeletal traction (see Fig. 27.4), reference will be made as appropriate within specific sections. However, it is worth outlining the basic principles that the nurse should consider when caring for patients with skeletal traction in situ:

- Care of the pin site (see Special Issues box 27.1).
- Observe skin condition, particularly areas in contact with splints (e.g. Thomas' splint) or frames. For example, the skin under the ring of a Thomas' splint can be damaged if swelling is severe.
- Observe the traction cord for fraying.
- The knots at the weight end of the cord should be reinforced with Elastoplast or similar non-stretch tape. It should be ensured that the knots applied to the traction are not touching any pulley, as this will reduce or completely remove the pull of any traction.
- Pulleys should run freely and be lubricated as necessary.
- Weights/water bag should be hanging freely and not touching the floor. Again weights touching the floor will remove any traction effect.
- Traction systems should be preferably set up, or at a minimum supervised, by the relevant senior medical personnel.
- The nurse should be present during setup to offer assistance as required and support to the patient. For example, to most patients, the insertion of metal pins into bone will be a new and potentially frightening experience. It may be of benefit if pictures of other patients in traction are shown to the patient prior to application.
- The rationale and timescale for use should be clearly explained, and the nurse should check that the patient has understood and answer any questions.

The patient in traction, who is invariably severely immobilized, may be less able to perform activities of living. The nurse will be required to provide care for such patients and should be aware of the effects of immobilization, including the following:

- breathing difficulties in the patient with ankylosing spondylitis
- eating and drinking problems in the patient who has forced immobilization on flat bed rest (see Ch. 11)
- sleeping problems caused by pain (see Chs 4, 7) and inability to change position
- circulatory complications, e.g. deep vein thrombosis (DVT) in those with reduced lower limb mobility (see Ch. 19)
- potential for development of pressure ulcers (see Ch. 10)
- potential for constipation (see Ch. 22).

NURSING PATIENTS IN A CAST

The three varieties of cast – plaster of Paris, resin reinforced plaster bandages and water-activated polymerizable casts – serve the same purpose, i.e. to immobilize the affected part until healing has occurred, so protecting against further damage.

General principles of care

Plaster of Paris will take a minimum of 24 hours to attain its full strength. The cast should be supported by a soft surface throughout this period, e.g. pillows. A hard surface may result in pressure problems underneath the cast. Artificial heating to facilitate drying should be avoided, as the cast is likely to become brittle.

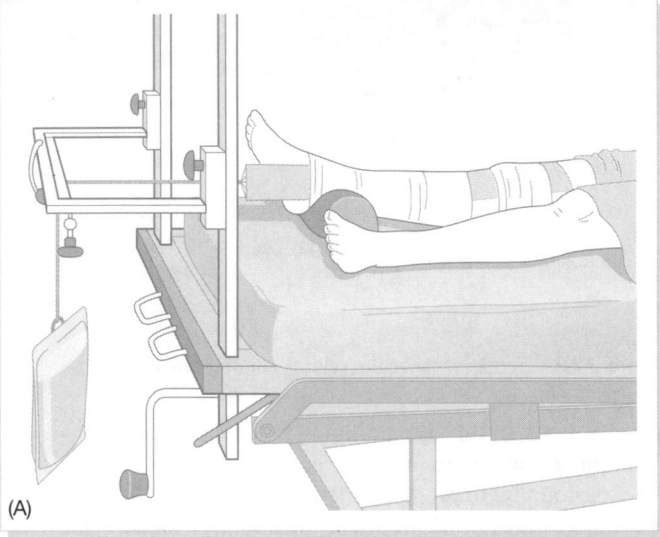

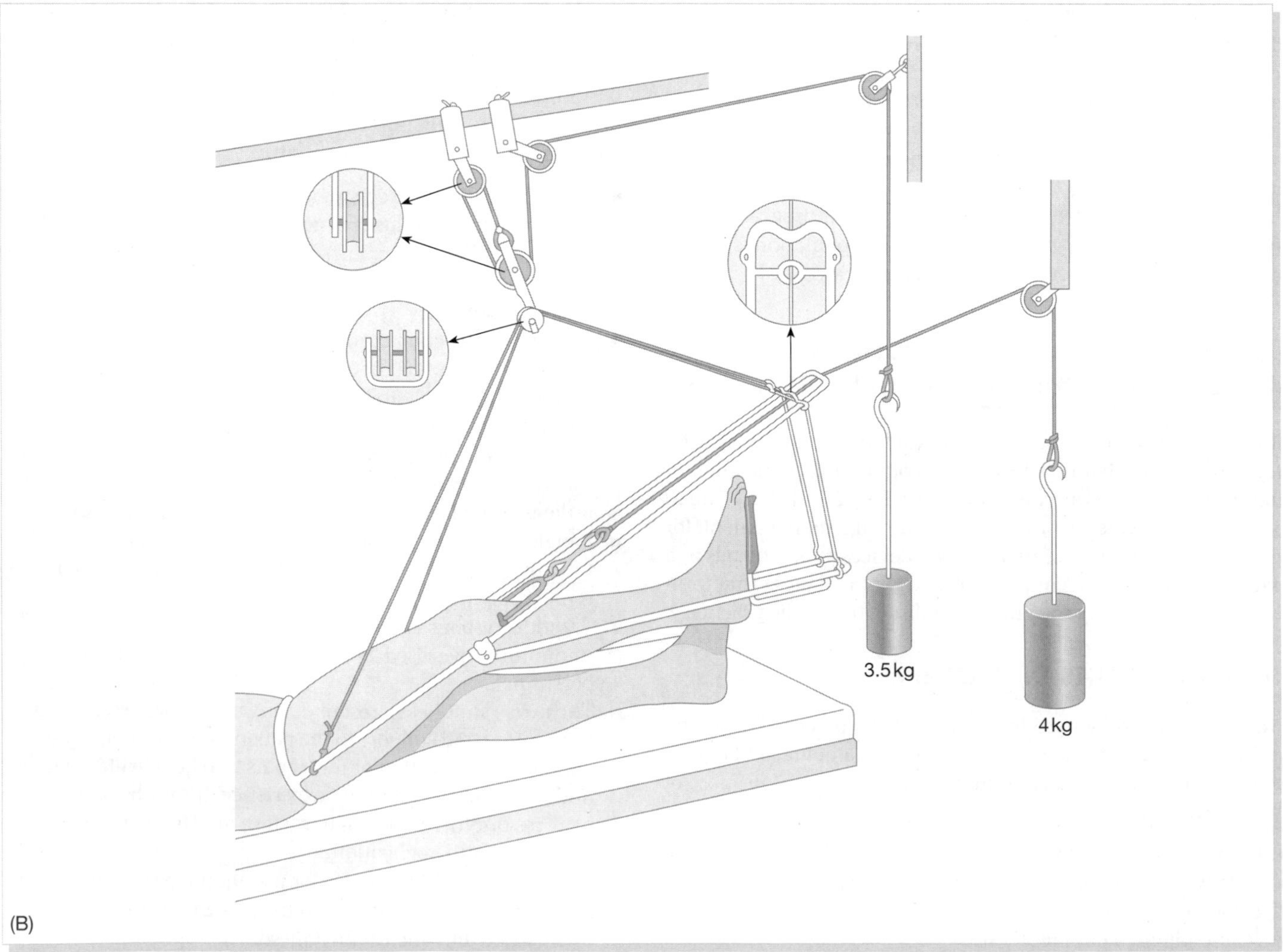

(A)

Figure 27.4 (A) Straight leg skin traction. (B) Skeletal traction.

(B)

SPECIAL ISSUES

27.1 Care of pin sites

Pin sites and the surrounding skin should be frequently observed. The pin sites should be symmetrical. Any disruption or bulging may indicate that the pins are slipping and should immediately be reported to medical staff. The tightness of skeletal traction pins should be checked by the medical staff daily, as a minimum, in the initial period following application. Following the initial period, local protocols will determine the frequency of the checks; often these relate to the specific site of pin insertion.

Observations for signs of pin site infection (e.g. redness, swelling) are undertaken, which is an obvious concern (Sims & Saleh 2000). The amount and type of any drainage are noted and a small dry dressing may be applied if this is substantial. The cleaning of pin sites should be carried out according to the local protocol. There have been many debates in the area of orthopaedic nursing relating to pin site care and research has been inconclusive (McKenzie 1999). Even studies into the type of cleaning fluid have been inconclusive. Most clinical areas utilize normal saline or chlorhexidine solution for cleaning. The dressing used, if at all, and whether scabs are left on or removed will be dictated by local policy.

References

McKenzie LL. In search of a standard for pin site care. Orthop Nurs 1999; 18(2): 73–78.

Sims M, Saleh M. External fixation – the incidence of pin site infection: a prospective audit. J Orthop Nurs 2000; 4(2): 59–63.

During this drying period, the extremities of the relevant limb should be inspected on a 2-hourly basis, testing each digit for temperature, colour, sensation and mobility. Acute compartment syndrome (see p. 829) may be caused through the application of a cast that is too tight, and so it must be ensured that the cast is impairing neither circulation nor nerve transmission. Any adverse observation should be reported immediately to the appropriate medical staff, plaster technician or nurse within the hospital. Those patients who have been discharged should be instructed to return to their accident and emergency (A&E) department if there is any evidence of neurovascular (relating to nerves and blood vessels) impairment. Once the cast has dried, the frequency of such observations may be reduced to a twice-daily basis.

Complaints of pain beneath a cast by the patient should always be acted upon. The nurse must ascertain the potential cause of the pain. It may be from the initial injury or site of surgical intervention, in which case the appropriate prescribed analgesia should be administered. However, pain may also be the result of a developing sore underneath the plaster, as a consequence of swelling of the affected limb or application of a cast that is too tight (potentially highlighting the need for increased frequency of neurovascular observations in the limb). In any case, such a situation merits immediate consultation with the plaster team or medical staff.

It is worth noting that casts on limbs that are paralysed, e.g. in clients with CVA or spinal cord injury, should always be bi-valved (split) and kept in place with a crepe bandage wrapped around them. This should be removed on a daily basis to inspect the skin, as the major symptom, pain, of a developing sore or a tight cast will be absent.

The cast should be kept dry even during meeting hygiene needs. A cast that gets wet may become soft so potentially reducing effectiveness. During bathing or any activity where the cast may get wet it may be temporarily covered with a plastic bag.

Patients should be strongly discouraged from putting items down the side of the cast to relieve itching. The potential resulting trauma to the skin may initiate development of a sore or crease the lining of the plaster, resulting in increased pressure over that area. It is worth noting that severe irritation may be as an adverse reaction to the material in the cast or lining and, if suspected, should be reported. A rise in body temperature or offensive smell may also be an indicator of sore development and should be investigated (McCann & Gruen 1997).

A window may be cut in the plaster to facilitate changing of dressings or to check for potential sore development. This is quite commonplace and well within the scope of most able plaster technicians and some experienced orthopaedic nurses.

Exercising the affected limb should be commenced only after the cast is completely dry. These exercises are commonly prescribed by the physiotherapist, and will be supervised by the nurse over the 24-hour period.

A cast that has become loose will be ineffective and should be renewed.

Clients who are discharged from hospital with a cast should be issued with a set of appropriate and comprehensive instructions that cover all of the above points. These should always be fully explained and comprehension checked by the nurse, rather than assuming patients will understand the written instructions. Ideally these should be available in different languages, depending on the make up of the local community.

NURSING PATIENTS FITTED WITH ORTHOTIC DEVICES

In general terms, an orthosis is an external device used to correct, control or counteract the effect of an actual or developing deformity. Common types of orthosis the nurse may encounter in patients with musculoskeletal conditions include braces, callipers and splints. Such orthoses may be used as follows:

- to provide postoperative restriction of movement following spinal surgery
- to provide stability during mobilization of the paralysed or weakened limb
- to compensate for dissimilarity of leg length, e.g. alterations to footwear
- to rest an affected body part until healed, e.g. use of a cock-up splint to rest tenosynovitis in the wrist.

Ideally a qualified orthotist should be involved in the design and fitting of the appropriate device to meet the specific needs of individual patients. Formal follow-up by an orthotist to solve actual or potential problems should be organized and contact details be available should the nurse or client suspect that the device is not functioning properly.

General nursing care of clients wearing an orthosis comprises a few key points. Patients should be educated regarding the donning, removal and care of the orthosis as appropriate. Although this may be provided initially by the orthotist, constant reinforcement is essential. This should also include relevant exercise both in and out of the orthosis. Additionally the nurse should be able to offer practical advice regarding the effects on and potential restrictions to the activities of clients that may result through wearing the orthosis, e.g. maintaining personal hygiene, elimination and dressing. Clearly this demonstrates the need for education not only of patients, family members and others, but also of nurses directly involved in the care of such patients.

After initial prescription and wearing of a new orthosis, the skin condition should be checked on removal of the orthosis. The nature of most orthotic devices is that they must fit the patient properly if they are to achieve their purpose. Any orthotic device that is too tight may cause undue pressure and ultimately may result in the development of sores. In the long term, any weight gain in the client may result in the same outcome. This is a particularly vital observation in those patients who have a degree of sensory impairment of the affected limb or body part.

Patients may need constant psychological support, again particularly in the early stages of wearing the orthotic device. Although significant improvements have been made in achieving a more acceptable appearance, many clients may find that the altered body image that may result from the wearing of a new orthosis requires some period of adjustment. An approach that has been successfully used in such situations is constant reference to the benefits of wearing the device, particularly so with an orthosis which is designed to enable increased function. Additionally, preparing the patient for wearing the device through the provision of pictures or contact with similar patients may aid in the reduction of anxiety.

As with the wearing of a cast, patients should be instructed to report immediately any numbness or pins and needles that may indicate the onset of neurological impairment.

NURSING PATIENTS WITH A PROSTHESIS

While orthotics refers to the wearing of a device that enhances limb function, prosthetics refers to replacement of a particular body part with an artificial device in order to perform an articular function. Probably the most obvious example is the use of a prosthetic limb following amputation (see Chs 17 and 19). As with orthoses, there is a debate regarding the importance of function versus cosmetic appearance. Such decisions may be based on what the person wants to do socially, as this will determine which aspects are important in prosthetic design. For many, both function and appearance will be important, and it seems essential that any decision made by the prosthetist should be in full consultation with the client and the rest of the health care team.

Ongoing skin care issues tend to be related to the contact of the stump with the prosthesis and problems can result from friction, increases in pressure due to swelling, or the potential moist environment caused by poor hygiene or temperature changes. Such problems should be avoided as they may have a negative impact on the health, function and social activity of the person.

As well as the health issues associated with wearing of a prosthesis, in order to enable optimum function patients must be taught to care for the 'mechanics' of the prosthesis. Generally the prosthesis should be kept clean, all joints should be fully operational and lubricated, and there should be access to a prosthetist should any problems occur.

BANDAGING AND STRAPPING

There are many techniques for bandaging and strapping that are used according to the location and type of injury sustained or condition. As a general rule, many of the principles relating to casts are also applicable to bandaging and strapping. The aim must be to support or partially immobilize the affected part to allow healing, whilst preventing the potential pressure and neurovascular problems. In many cases, strapping is used in sporting activities. Although these may offer little in the way of actual physiological protection from further injury, they may prevent further injury through acting as a reminder to the person to restrict movement when playing a sport.

Stump bandaging

Following amputation, the earlier the prosthesis is fitted, the better it is for the amputee. One of the challenges facing the amputee and the health care team is oedema of the stump. The use of a rigid dressing is an intervention that aims to control oedema (Smith 1999).

Patients are taught the proper technique for bandaging during their time in hospital and are generally expected to be self-caring in this area following discharge home if functional ability permits. Clearly the knowledge of stump bandaging and the ability to pass these on to patients are fundamental roles in the nursing management of the amputee (Donohue 1997).

In recent years, elastic shrinker socks have commonly been used instead of bandages. Although some may consider that they are not as effective as a properly applied bandage, they are easier for the patient to apply and may therefore produce a better outcome than a poorly applied bandage.

Whether a bandage or a shrinker sock is used, it should be removed at least three times daily and the stump should be massaged vigorously for 10–15 minutes. The bandage or sock must be reapplied immediately after the massage. Applying the correct technique for a stump bandage is extremely important in using a prosthesis successfully (see Fig. 27.5). Clearly the technique will differ slightly for below-knee amputations, but the principles remain the same.

USE OF MOBILITY AIDS

Crutches

It is important to know how to adjust crutches and to instruct patients correctly in order to avoid problems caused by improper usage (see Reflective Practice box 27.2). Potential problems include reduced mobility, pain, excessive fatigue, compromised safety, and damage to the axillary nerves.

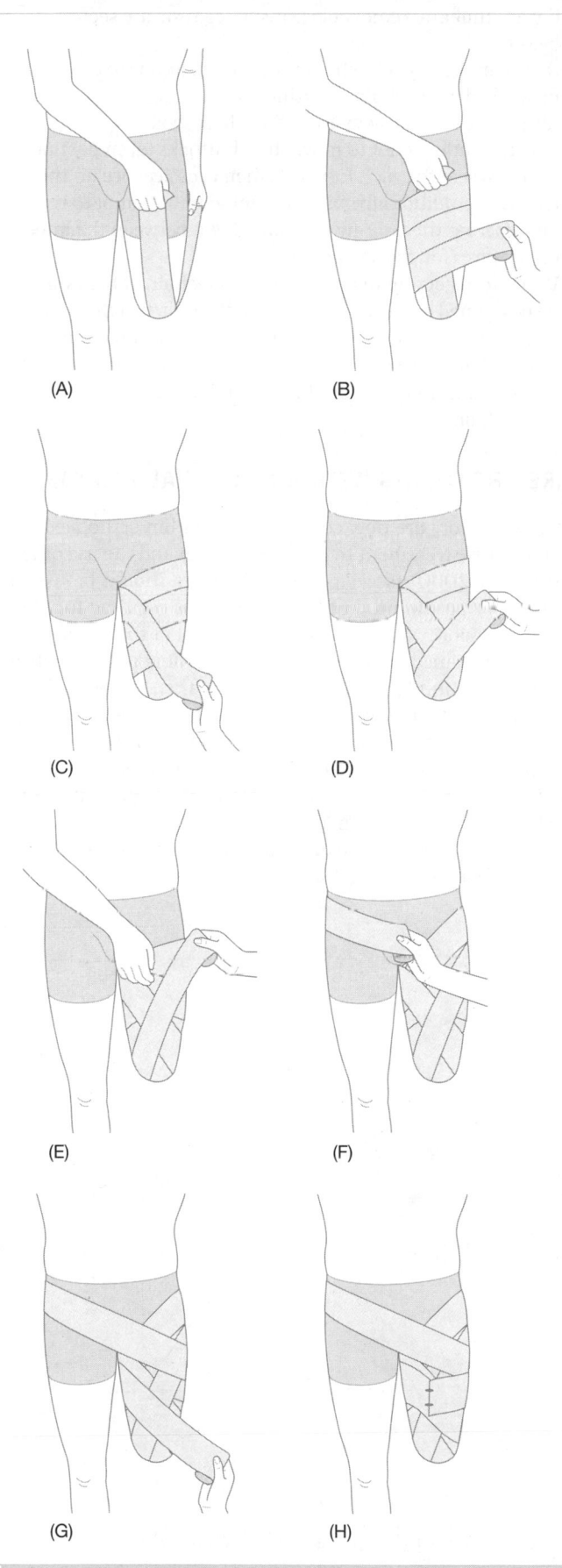

(A)

(B)

(C)

(D)

(E)

(F)

(G)

(H)

Figure 27.5 Technique for stump bandaging – above-knee amputation. (A) Begin at the front of the stump. Cover the bottom of the stump and continue upwards towards the top of the back of the stump. (B) Wrap two to four diagonal turns around the stump. This keeps the bandage over the end of the stump in place. (C) Take the bandage down towards the bottom of the stump and begin a figure-of-8 pattern, from the underside of the stump upwards to cover the sides of the stump. (D) Pressure should be directed evenly upwards and outwards from the end of the stump as you wrap. (E) Take the bandage from the front, inside of the thigh and wrap upwards and outwards across the front of the hips. (F) Carry the wrap around behind the hips at the level of the iliac crests. (G) Return the bandage wrap to the stump and finish wrapping with more figure-of-8 turns. (H) Anchor the end of the bandage at the upper front part of the thigh, with safety pins, clips or adhesive tape.

R|Я REFLECTIVE PRACTICE

27.2 Mobility aids

Use of mobility aids is a fundamental part of musculoskeletal rehabilitation. Nurses have a central role to play in the use of mobility aids over the 24-hour period, but it often appears to be taken for granted that nurses will be able to perform this role.

Student activities
Look at the recommendations for safe use of crutches and wheelchairs as outlined in this chapter.

- What do you think is the nurse's actual level of knowledge relating to these?
- Think about a client or patient who used either crutches or a wheelchair – were the safety recommendations always followed?

The adjustment of crutches is important and the tops of the crutches should be adjusted to two finger-widths below the patient's axillae. The patient should have the wrists straight and elbows bent 25–30°; the weight should be on the palms on the handgrips.

When using crutches, patients should be instructed as follows:

- Wear well-fitting, low-heeled shoes with non-slip soles.
- The weight should be supported on the handgrips, with the elbows slightly bent. The axillary pad should be 'squeezed' between the upper arms and ribcage.
- The first stage is to move the crutches and injured/weaker leg 30–40 cm ahead of the 'good' leg.
- The good leg should be swung to about 30–40 cm ahead of the crutches.
- With the weight on the 'good' leg, patients should move the crutches to the first position.
- When going up stairs the weight should be on the handgrips while the good leg is moved up one step. The body weight should be on the stronger leg while the crutches and the weaker leg are moved up to the same step. If the stairway has a handrail, this should be used for safer support instead of one of the crutches.

- If patients tire and need to rest, they should sit down or lean against a wall rather than shifting the weight onto the axillae.
- To go through a door on crutches, patients should face the door and turn their body slightly at an angle to it so the door will be clear of the feet as it opens. The doorknob should be turned with one hand while patients support themselves on the crutch with the other. As the door opens, the crutch tip should be placed against the door to keep it open.

Wheelchairs

The nurse has a key role in enabling patients a degree of mobility through the use of wheelchairs, while at the same time ensuring that patient safety is maintained. The following are general principles relating to safe wheelchair use – as manual wheelchairs are the type the nurse will most commonly encounter in hospital when caring for patients with musculoskeletal conditions, the focus is on these, but the principles apply equally to powered chairs:

- Wheelchairs should only be used if in a good condition.
- Putting heavy loads on the back of a manual wheelchair may alter the balance of the chair and increase the likelihood of tipping.
- Beware of caster flutter, which is the rapid side-to-side motion of the caster. This usually happens at high speed, such as when going downhill. It can throw the patient forward out of the chair.
- Always lock the brakes before the patient gets in or out of the chair.
- Avoid injury by lifting the footplates up before getting the patient in or out of the chair.
- Always point the casters in the forward position before the patient's position in the chair is changed, i.e. leaning forward or to the side. To do this, move the wheelchair forward and then reverse it in a straight line.

- Ensure that any removable arms or leg rests are secure before use.
- Do not make any adjustments or modifications to a prescribed wheelchair or cushion.
- Keep loose objects away from the wheel spokes.
- Instruct patients not to move their buttocks (even partially) from the seat to reach forward when their feet are on the footrests. Additionally patients should not attempt to retrieve objects from the floor by reaching down between the knees.
- Check tyres for proper pressure.
- When transferring to and from a wheelchair, patients should be positioned as close as possible to the seat/bed they are transferring to. Point the casters in the same direction as the seat/bed. Remove or flip back the wheelchair armrests on the transfer side and position the legs in the direction of the wheelchair.

CARE OF PATIENTS WITH AN EXTERNAL FIXATOR

External fixators are now commonplace within orthopaedics as an alternative treatment to internal fixation and the use of traction (Santy 2000) (see Fig. 27.6). Patients should be assisted with proper positioning, utilizing pillows as required for elevation and support. Neurovascular assessment of the affected limb must be performed on a regular basis according to local policy – as a rule of thumb, hourly for 2 hours, then 2-hourly for 12 hours, then reducing to 6-hourly should be sufficient. Details of pin site care are provided in Special Issues box 27.1 (see p. 801).

It is often advisable to administer analgesia prior to adjustment of pin torque and wound care to facilitate patient comfort in what can be very painful procedures.

The patient should be educated regarding all of the above to enable self-care following discharge.

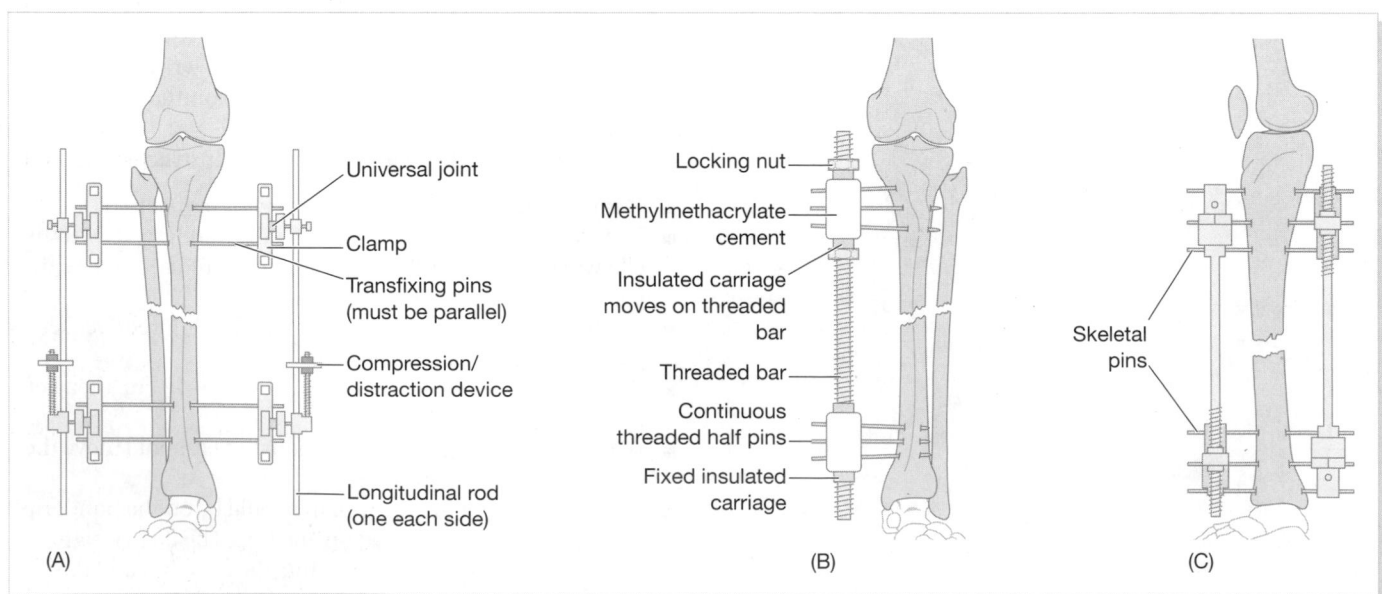

Figure 27.6 External fixators. (A) Universal day frame. (B) Portsmouth external fixation bar (Denham external fixation compression). (C) The Belfast fixator.

COMMON DISEASES/DISORDERS AFFECTING THE MUSCULOSKELETAL SYSTEM

This section aims to take the reader through the scope of common musculoskeletal conditions. This is not an entirely comprehensive list and each topic could merit a chapter on its own in a specialist musculoskeletal text.

Surgical techniques, as well as medical interventions, are utilized in musculoskeletal conditions. In some cases, these will be a 'last resort', when all other health care techniques have failed to produce a positive outcome, e.g. chronic back pain, and in others they will be the primary intervention, e.g. joint replacement. Many different surgical terms are used and nurses will need to have a basic understanding of common musculoskeletal operations so they can reinforce the information given to the patient by the surgeon (see Box 27.4). Patients will also require specific information about the operation, e.g. the site, dressings, packs and drains. The various surgical techniques will be referred to in the chapter as they apply to specific conditions.

INFLAMMATORY DISORDERS

BURSITIS

Bursitis is inflammation of a bursa.

Pathophysiology and aetiology

There is inflammation presenting as an effusion of clear fluid within the sac, which may be caused by mechanical irritation or infection (Butcher et al 1996). The former is the more common and is associated with repetitive trauma or friction. Particularly frequent locations include the common 'bunion' over a metatarsal head, in the subacromium, patella ('housemaid's knee') or olecranon ('tennis elbow').

> **Box 27.4 Common surgical techniques used in musculoskeletal conditions**
>
> - *Arthrodesis* – surgical fusion of a joint
> - *Arthroplasty* – remodelling of a joint often including a prosthesis (i.e. an artificial part that is fitted to or implanted into the body to replace a damaged part)
> - *Arthrotomy* – surgical opening of a joint
> - *Fasciotomy* – division of the fascia (connective tissue under the skin, and surrounding and separating muscles)
> - *Meniscectomy* – removal of the meniscus
> - *Osteotomy* – surgical division of a bone
> - *Sequestrectomy* – excision of dead bone (sequestrum)
> - *Synovectomy* – excision of synovial membrane, or its destruction by medical means using radiocolloids such as yttrium-90
> - *Tenosynovectomy* – removal of a tendon sheath
> - *Tenotomy* – surgical division of a tendon

Clinical presentation

The patient presents with an area of redness and tenderness around the joint and limited movement of the joint with varied degrees of reduced function depending on severity. There is often a history of repetitive movement and increasing pain and loss of function.

Medical/surgical management

In the majority of cases, management of bursitis is to rest the affected part until the inflammation has subsided and to control pain with non-steroidal anti-inflammatory drugs (NSAIDs). Occasionally the sac may be aspirated. In recurrent bursitis, a hydrocortisone injection (Pronchik & Heller 1997) may be indicated; patients may experience an increase in pain for 8–12 hours following injection. Severe cases may require surgical intervention through excision of the bursa to obtain relief.

The less common infective bursitis is treated through surgical drainage and antibiotics.

▶ Nursing management

Nursing management focuses on three key issues: pain control, regaining previous mobility of the affected part and patient education, e.g. strategies for avoiding repetitive movement. In infective bursitis, similar nursing management issues exist with the addition of wound management and monitoring of temperature.

TENOSYNOVITIS

Tenosynovitis is inflammation of the synovial lining of a tendon sheath. The most common location of tenosynovitis is in the wrist, although it may occur in other tendons, e.g. patellar, Achilles. Again the most common aetiology is repetitive movements of the affected area. There is tenderness along the affected tendon sheath that is exacerbated by movement, associated reduction in function, and mild inflammation around the area.

▶ Nursing management

Nursing management includes education regarding pain medication (usually NSAIDs), avoiding repetitive movement and the need for rest, often using a splint.

RHEUMATOID ARTHRITIS

Rheumatoid arthritis (RA) is inflammation of many joints (polyarthritis). It usually affects the smaller peripheral joints, before involving larger joints accompanied by general ill health. Many authorities prefer the term rheumatoid disease to describe the complexities of a joint disease that can involve most body systems, e.g. the lungs.

Pathophysiology and aetiology

The exact aetiology of RA is unknown but it is thought to have an autoimmune component. Additional contributory factors may include heredity, emotion and viral infection. Eventually it leads to varying degrees of joint destruction and deformity, with

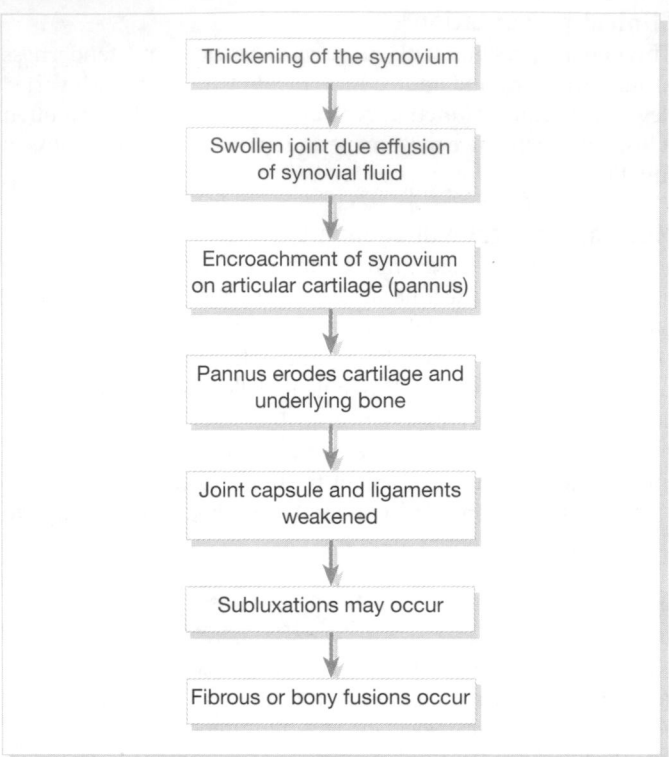

Figure 27.7   Progression of rheumatoid arthritis.

associated muscle wasting, as well as systemic effects. The progression of the joint disease is outlined in Figure 27.7. It has been reported that the incidence of RA increases with age, and although clinical symptoms do not appear to be age-related, they are often less severe in older people (Ramsburg 2000). However, the combination of RA, at whatever severity, with other impairments can obviously cause additional problems in nursing older people.

Clinical presentation

Common presenting features of RA include pain and stiffness of affected joints resulting in mobility problems and reduced function in the sufferer. Usually the pain and stiffness are more severe early in the day. There may be low-grade pyrexia, often with general malaise and anorexia, all of which further compromises the patient's ability and desire to function at full capacity and contribute to secondary complications, e.g. pressure ulcer development. Additionally, involvement of the non-articular connective tissues may be present, resulting in degenerative lesions, e.g. in muscles, tendons and blood vessels. These again may have an impact on the functional abilities of the client.

Specific investigations

- Analysis of synovial fluid
- Blood tests such as ESR as an indicator of inflammation
- Serological tests, e.g. presence of rheumatoid factors, antinuclear antibodies (ANAs)
- X-rays, CT and MRI.

Additionally patients will have blood, urine and other tests to monitor for possible drug side-effects, e.g. FBC and liver function tests during therapy with sulfasalazine.

Medical/surgical management

Medical management of RA usually involves drug therapy, often utilizing a combination of NSAIDs, simple painkillers, and early use of disease-modifying anti-rheumatic drugs (DMARDs) such as sulfasalazine, methotrexate, hydroxychloroquine, penicillamine and parenteral gold salts. Other drugs that modify the immune system may be used, e.g. azathioprine and ciclosporin. More recently, selective immunosuppressants, e.g. etanercept and infliximab, have been introduced on a limited basis. They act by inhibiting the activity of tissue necrosis factor. Etanercept appears to have good efficacy without the major side-effects associated with the anti-rheumatoid drugs (Luong at el 2000). Corticosteroids are used, but long-term administration is associated with serious side-effects, e.g. osteoporosis (see p. 819).

Specialist physiotherapy (exercise, heat, the use of splints) and traction may be used to prevent or treat deformity, and facilitate pain relief and rest. Occupational therapy, environment modification and the provision of mobility aids will be required in some cases.

Surgical options for the patient with rheumatoid arthritis include the following:

- tenosynovectomy – can often prevent a tendon from rupturing if inflamed
- surgical repair of a ruptured tendon – to restore joint function
- synovectomy – less often used and may only be of benefit if performed before cartilage destruction occurs
- joint arthroplasty – performed when there is significant destruction of the bones resulting in loss of function, or there is significant pain in the joint, limiting function. Used when RA has grossly affected the hip or knee joints. Shoulder arthroplasty has some success when medication fails to produce a good outcome
- arthrotomy – may also be performed in patients aged less than 50 years
- arthrodesis – sometimes performed in patients with significant joint pain or loss of function. It is especially useful in patients with significant wrist pain (Anderson 1996). It may also be used where the ankle or vertebral joints are affected.

▶ Nursing management

A thorough nursing assessment is required for the patient with RA and would include:

- degree of reduced mobility related to the condition and level to which this affects other tasks
- assessment of pain (see Ch. 7), including severity, location and activities that exacerbate it
- impact on activities of living related to reduced function
- level of knowledge relating to the condition, potential for secondary complications and measures to prevent these, and medications
- issues relating to body image
- disturbance of sleep pattern (see Ch. 4)
- optimum functional goals
- the social implications of the above.

Nursing intervention would therefore include assisting with diagnostic and progress investigations, referral to dietician, occupational therapist and physiotherapist for review, and reporting progress (in the ward, clinic and primary care settings) of prescribed regimens and treatment modalities to other team members.

Assistance with meeting hygiene and nutritional needs will need to be provided according to the disease progression and the individual disability. The nurse will assist the patient with mobility according to the prescribed rehabilitation regimen, and education and setup will be provided regarding use of aids to functional independence.

Additionally any knowledge deficit relating to any aspect of condition will be met through formal patient education (Brus et al 1997). Nurses should ensure that patients are aware of the side-effects associated with certain drugs, e.g. weight gain with corticosteroids, and the importance of reporting side-effects and attending for specific monitoring. For example, patients having gold therapy will require regular monitoring for blood disorders, or proteinuria indicating renal damage.

Monitoring and evaluation of strategies to relieve pain and disturbance in sleep pattern and pain should be performed.

Discharge planning and follow-up are vital, including referral to the appropriate community professionals. Obviously the patient undergoing surgical intervention will require the appropriate pre- and postoperative care as covered in the section on joint replacement.

ANKYLOSING SPONDYLITIS

Ankylosing spondylitis is a progressive inflammatory disease of unknown aetiology. There is gradual stiffening of the axial skeleton, sacroiliac joints and pubic symphysis with loss of joint space and fusion. It primarily involves the spine but may involve other joints. It is seen more commonly in men than in women (2:1 ratio).

Clinical presentation

The onset is usually gradual, with the eventual presenting picture being a marked difference in the individual's physical appearance:

- The thoracic spine becomes stiff and 'rounded' and the cervical spine grows rigid
- Spinal changes lead to reduced chest expansion and vital capacity, which will affect breathing
- Debilitating pain
- Decreased mobility with related problems.

Medical management

Management of any acute phases is usually through administration of NSAIDs. Hospitalization related primarily to the condition is usually for a review of the condition or chest infection.

Any respiratory infection must be managed through the administration of i.v. antibiotics. Analgesia will be prescribed for those in pain. Provision of a firm mattress should be seen as essential, and patients may also be advised to wear a spinal orthosis to maintain the best possible alignment of the affected areas.

▶ Nursing management

A variety of potential problems may occur in being able to perform activities of daily living, due to the reduced mobility, and nurses should plan to assist as necessary. Assistance in meeting hygiene, nutritional and eliminatory needs, to varying degrees, may be required during a period of illness.

Altered body image will be an important issue for many patients and their families. Nurses can offer support by providing opportunities for discussion, helping individuals to develop coping strategies and, where necessary, referring patients for specialist help, e.g. psychosexual counselling.

Key to nursing management of a patient with ankylosing spondylitis is to limit bed rest, as this may encourage further fusion of the vertebrae. Where the person with ankylosing spondylitis is admitted for another reason, the requirement to limit bed rest must be borne in mind, as problems in nursing following any illness will be compounded if long-term mobility is reduced by prolonged immobilization. Good posture is generally also indicated. An exercise programme designed to increase muscle strength will also be of benefit, the nurse's role being to reinforce any physiotherapy-prescribed regimens and report progress to the relevant therapist.

Prior to discharge from hospital, the patient should be educated in the use of any spinal orthosis, prescribed medication and strategies to maintain mobility and optimum respiratory function.

METABOLIC DISORDERS

GOUT

Gout is a metabolic disorder in which the amount of uric acid in the blood is raised. Acute arthritis can result from inflammation caused by urate crystals in the joint.

This debilitating and painful condition more commonly presents in men over the age of 40 years, although it can affect adults of any age. Gout generally affects older women, usually after the menopause.

Pathophysiology and aetiology

Uric acid is a metabolite formed when purines (derived from the digestion of nucleoproteins) are broken down in the body. Normally, uric acid enters the blood and is excreted into the urine by the kidneys. In gout, the high level of uric acid in the blood (hyperuricaemia) may be due either to excess uric acid production or to an inability to excrete uric acid in the urine.

In either case, excess uric acid can stay in the body and form needle-like crystals. When these crystals are deposited in a joint, they cause inflammation and the painful joint swelling associated with gout. A similar condition, termed pseudogout, may occur if crystals of calcium pyrophosphate dihydrate enter a joint.

Certain other conditions, especially affecting the blood, and treatment with some cancer drugs can cause higher levels of uric acid and are termed secondary gout. Certain food products are high in uric acid (e.g. offal, meat extracts and fish roe) and alcohol causes increased levels, by producing lactic acid that competes with uric acid for excretion. Also renal failure can lead to high uric acid levels, as can the use of diuretics (see Ch. 24).

Episodes of gout may be either exacerbated or brought on by:

- drinking too much alcohol
- overeating
- surgery
- sudden, severe illness
- crash diets
- joint injury
- chemotherapy.

However, gout is a complex disorder and often the exact aetiology remains unclear.

Clinical presentation

Gout causes sudden, severe attacks of pain and tenderness, redness, warmth and swelling in some joints. It will usually affect one joint at a time, the most common site being the big toe. However, gout may also occur in the feet, knees, ankles, hands, elbows and wrists.

The initial attack of gout usually comes on suddenly, often at night. Typically the pain lasts 5–10 days and then stops. Following an attack of gout, the person may go for weeks or months with joints that are pain-free and seem normal. Some people never have another attack, but for others the pain and swelling can come back as suddenly as before, occurring more often and in more joints (Pittman & Bross 1999). Some people with chronic gout develop lumps beneath the skin called tophi. A small number of people with gout will additionally develop renal calculi.

Specific investigations

- Physical examination and medical history – affected joints will be painful on palpation and inflamed. Tophi may be present in the pinnae of the ears and metacarpal joints.
- Blood test to measure serum uric acid level.
- Joint fluid analysis to check for presence of urate crystals.

Medical management

Medication used in an acute attack may include colchicine, NSAIDs and corticosteroids. Long-term control and prophylaxis are with allopurinol (prevents build-up of uric acid) and the uricosuric agents (increase kidney excretion of uric acid) probenecid and sulfinpyrazone. Regular prophylactic treatment may be of some benefit in those with recurring attacks of gout.

▶ Nursing management

Nursing assessment will explore:

- the degree of acute pain
- any knowledge deficit relating to the condition
- the extent of reduced mobility.

Nursing management therefore has the objectives of monitoring and controlling the symptoms with a review of diet to reduce the purine intake and administration of prescribed medication. The patient will need education related to medication and potential side-effects, e.g. gastrointestinal disturbance with high-dose NSAIDs, and the inclusion of a dietician within the team is essential.

MUSCLE DISORDERS

This section will provide an overview of the myopathies and myasthenia gravis.

MYOPATHIES

The myopathies (diseases of muscle) are a diverse group with many causes and different presentations and effects.

Pathophysiology and aetiology – an overview

Myopathies are diseases that affect skeletal muscle and can be caused by several different factors (see below). At an advanced stage of some myopathies, however, there are often effects on smooth and cardiac muscle tissue.

It is known that certain myopathies are caused by genetic or endocrine defects; however, the sequelae of events leading to the condition are less well understood. For the inheritable myopathies, researchers are studying the DNA to try to locate the exact place where the defect occurs. Gene therapy involving the insertion of normal DNA to correct the defect that is causing the condition may be a potential treatment for the future. Various biochemical processes that occur regularly in muscle cells are also being studied, in an effort to understand better how defects in these processes lead to disease. The sequelae in the development of a myopathy and the response to treatment depend on the particular specific condition. For example, the muscular dystrophies develop at a very early age, whereas others usually develop later in life.

Inherited genetic defects

These are either autosomal or X-linked, and dominant or recessive, e.g. the muscular dystrophies and other inheritable myopathies (see Tables 27.4 and 27.5). Although many of these develop in childhood, the majority of patients will survive into adult years; hence their inclusion within this chapter. When a defective autosomal gene causes a disease, females and males are affected equally. Most of the inherited myopathies are caused by a defect of an autosomal dominant gene. However, defective recessive X-linked genes cause most of the muscular dystrophies, such as Duchenne muscular dystrophy (DMD), which predominately affects males. Most individuals with DMD die from respiratory and cardiac complications during early adult life.

Familial periodic paralyses are inherited disorders associated with hypo- and hyperkalaemia (low and high levels of potassium in the blood). All involve periodic attacks of muscle weakening and none are lethal. The muscles function normally in between attacks. Several genetic defects have been linked to hyperkalaemic periodic paralysis, some of which are also linked to myotonia and paramyotonia congenita (see Table 27.5). Attacks vary in severity and tend to decrease as a person grows older. Hypokalaemic paralysis usually appears in adolescence

Table 27.4 The muscular dystrophies

Type	Defect	Patient groups	Effects
Duchenne muscular dystrophy (DMD)	Recessive gene on the X chromosome	1:3000 male births	Muscle weakening often when boy is 4–5 years of age. By 12 years can no longer walk. Weakened cardiac muscle. Often death by early adulthood
Becker muscular dystrophy (BMD)	Recessive, X-linked gene that codes for dystrophin	Develops during adolescence or adulthood	Can be as for DMD but progression much slower
Emery–Dreifuss muscular dystrophy (EDMD)	Recessive gene on the X chromosome	Affects children and young teenagers	Affects the shoulder, upper arm and shin muscles and can cause heart complications. Progresses slowly
Limb-girdle muscular dystrophy (LGMD)	Recessive gene on either an autosomal or X chromosome	Onset anywhere from childhood to middle age	Slow progressive weakening of the shoulder and pelvic muscles. Usually eventually causes cardiac and pulmonary complications
Fascioscapulohumeral muscular dystrophy (FSH or FSHD), also known as Landouzy–Dejerine muscular dystrophy	Defect of an autosomal dominant gene	Onset anytime from childhood to early adulthood	It is a slow progressive weakening of the facial, shoulder and upper arm muscles. Often experience bouts of rapid deterioration
Myotonic dystrophy (DM) or 'Steinart's disease'	Defect of an autosomal dominant gene	Anytime from childhood through middle age	Involves both the proximal and distal muscles, so can affect the feet, hands, as well as the face and neck. Slowly progressing condition. May have difficulties swallowing and suffer from sleeping disorders. Most suffer from cardiac arrhythmias
Oculopharyngeal muscular dystrophy (OPMD)	Defect of an autosomal dominant gene	Adults through middle age	Slowly progressive disease that first affects the eyelid and throat muscles and causes swallowing difficulties
Distal muscular dystrophy (DD)	Defect of an autosomal dominant gene	Adults 40–60 years of age	Progressive weakening of the hands, forearms and lower legs. Not life-threatening
Congenital muscular dystrophy (CMD)	Defect of an autosomal dominant gene	Starts at birth	Causes general weakening of the muscles and joint deformities. Very slow to progress. In severe form (Fukuyama), affects mental function

Table 27.5 Other inheritable myopathies

Type	Patient population	Effects
Central core disease	Early infancy	Slowly progressive skeletal muscle disorder that is not life-threatening. The muscle fibres associated with the disease have a light inner core surrounded by a dark circle. Symptoms include hip displacement, an inability to jump and run smoothly, and general weakening of the muscles
Myotonia congenita or Thomsen's disease	Develops in people from infancy to childhood	Non-progressive muscular disorder. Characterized by stiff muscles that take a long time to relax after contraction. It is generally not painful. The muscles that are affected (arms, legs and face) do not weaken, rather they enlarge
Paramyotonia congenita or Eulenberg's disease	Evident at birth	Characterized by stiff muscles that take a long time to relax after contraction. Non-progressive and it does not cause muscle weakening. Often triggered by cold temperatures. The hands become clumsy, the face rigid, and the muscles in the forearm stiff
Myotubular myopathy, or centronuclear myopathy	Evident at birth to infancy	Slowly progressive disease that causes drooping of the eyelids, foot drop, facial weakness, and assorted other muscle weakness. The weakened muscles usually do not have any reflexes at all. It is rarely fatal
Nemaline myopathy or Rod body disease	Develops from birth to adulthood	Non-progressive, usually non-fatal. Symptoms include weakening of the leg, arm and trunk muscles and some weakening of various facial and throat muscles. Affected muscles usually do not have good reflexes. There is a particularly severe type of nemaline myopathy that, if present at birth, causes death due to breathing complications

through young adulthood and seems to be triggered by strenuous exercise and high carbohydrate intake, as well as various medications. Strenuous exercise, as well as cold temperatures, also triggers hyperkalaemic periodic paralysis.

Exercise and certain drugs also trigger periodic paralysis in the presence of a normal potassium level (normokalaemic).

Endocrine myopathies

Undersecretion (hypothyroidism) or oversecretion (hyperthyroidism) of thyroid hormones may lead to the development of myopathy (see Ch. 17). Neither type is fatal. They differ with respect to the muscles affected and whether the muscle wastes away or is simply weakened. Hyperthyroid myopathy leads to weakening and wasting of the muscles, especially in the shoulders and hips, and possibly also the eyes, whereas hypothyroid myopathy results in muscle weakening in the legs and arms. The muscles may become enlarged. Often treating the underlying endocrine abnormality helps to relieve the muscle symptoms.

Inflammatory myopathies

These include polymyositis (PM) and dermatomyositis (DM). Both PM and DM are characterized by weakening of the neck and limb muscles, muscle pain and swelling. Inflammatory myopathies are autoimmune disorders where healthy muscle fibres are attacked, causing inflammation, which in turn damages the muscle. It is not known what triggers this autoimmune response. Some people with PM and DM may develop other disorders, such as cardiac arrhythmias, pulmonary disease, gastrointestinal problems, osteoarthritis and cancer.

PM causes muscle ache, cramp and tenderness. The severity and progression of these types of myopathy vary considerably. PM can occur at any age in either sex, but it is more common in children and in women between the ages of 40 and 60 years. Muscle weakening is often quite marked and may fluctuate over weeks to months. It is often worse in the neck, arms and upper portion of the legs, making it difficult to stand up from a sitting position. Many patients also experience fever, malaise and anorexia.

DM is characterized by a skin rash, as well as all of the common muscular symptoms of PM. The rash is a purple discoloration around the eyes and on the cheeks but may also be found on other parts of the body. Eventually the skin becomes thin and fragile. DM most commonly develops in children and will progress through to adulthood. People who have DM are at an increased risk of developing cancer.

Biochemical (metabolic) myopathies

Biochemical abnormalities in muscle tissue can cause weakness and fatigue. The biochemical (metabolic) myopathies are a group of diseases characterized by the absence of a particular substance, such as an enzyme that is essential for normal muscle functioning. In many of these disorders, the symptoms increase after exercise, and people may experience severe muscle pain during exercise. This is usually due to a lack of oxygen and the absence of the chemicals necessary for maintaining the energy level of the muscle. There are numerous metabolic muscular disorders. Two examples are McArdle's disease and phosphofructokinase deficiency.

McArdle's disease (also known as phosphorylase deficiency) is caused by an enzyme deficiency due to a genetic defect. It usually develops in adolescence and is characterized by cramps after exercise, and sometimes by muscle weakening. Most people can avoid progression of the disease by avoiding strenuous exercise, although about one-third of all people with McArdle's disease eventually experience permanent muscle weakening.

Phosphofructokinase deficiency A deficiency of the enzyme phosphofructokinase (Tarui's disease) is also genetic in origin. Symptoms include cramping after exercise and sometimes muscle weakness. The primary goal in treating metabolic myopathies is simply to avoid situations, like exercise, that promote muscular pain and weakness.

General clinical presentation – an overview

- The common outcome in almost all myopathies is a weakening and atrophy of the skeletal muscles, particularly in the proximal muscles closest to the centre of the body, such as those in the thigh and shoulder. Distal muscles are as a general rule less affected by myopathies unless the condition is at an advanced stage. Although the specific clinical features of the muscular diseases depend on the particular myopathy, some generalizations can be made. A weakening of the skeletal muscle is the primary symptom of most myopathies, with some noticeable exceptions such as myotonia and paramyotonia congenita – two inheritable conditions in which weakening does not occur; rather the muscles enlarge and do not relax after contracting.
- Individuals may initially feel fatigued doing only very light physical activity. Walking and climbing stairs may be difficult for many patients because of the involvement of the muscles in the pelvis and legs which are needed to stabilize the trunk. Patients often find it difficult to get up out of a chair and have trouble walking. Some patients may fall.
- Muscles might be tight and stiff and there may be muscle pain, cramping, tenderness or aching feelings.
- Muscles atrophy as the disease progresses.
- Various other signs indicative of a potential myopathy include skin rash, endocrine abnormalities, cardiac problems and mental dysfunction.

In the later stages of the disease, if the cardiac muscle is affected there may be arrhythmias, or cardiomyopathy and subsequent congestive heart failure (see Ch. 19). When the respiratory muscles start to weaken, a person can develop significant breathing difficulties (see Ch. 20).

Specific investigations

Generally, diagnosis involves several outpatient tests to determine which type of myopathy is present. Sometimes it is necessary to wait until the disease progresses to a point at which the exact syndrome can be identified. In such cases, the term 'non-specific myopathy' is often utilized.

- A complete family history will help to reveal the chances that the disease is an inheritable myopathy.
- A full neurological examination is undertaken and involves testing coordination, deep tendon reflexes (e.g. knee jerk reaction), ability to walk, and ability to get up from a sitting

position. In some cases, patients will be tested for the existence of a myotonia (see above) by having them squeeze their hand muscles and observing for any signs of failure to relax.

- A serum enzyme test might be done to measure how much muscle protein is circulating in the blood. For many myopathies, there is increased muscle protein in the blood when the muscles are weakened. These proteins include creatine kinase (CK) – an especially important diagnostic protein for Duchenne muscular dystrophy – lactic dehydrogenase (LDH) and pyruvate kinase (PK). Usually, a serum enzyme test is helpful only at the early stages of the disease, when the sudden increase of protein in the blood is conspicuous. Later, as muscle tissue wastes away, there is less and less protein to circulate and so the amount in the blood falls to an apparently normal level.
- The level of potassium in the blood may be determined for those patients in whom periodic paralysis is suspected.
- DNA may be collected from the blood as well, in order to evaluate whether one of the known genetic defects is present.
- An electromyogram (EMG) is usually done to measure the electrical activity of the muscle. This provides information about which particular muscles are weakened. It is especially helpful for diagnosing myotonia and paramyotonia congenita.
- A muscle biopsy and consequent biochemical analysis may be undertaken to look for cellular and protein abnormalities. This is especially helpful for diagnosing certain types of myopathy.

Medical/surgical management – an overview
Inherited myopathies

Treatment for myopathy is limited to slowing progression of the disease once it has occurred. Unfortunately, there is no cure available and current management focuses on the symptoms. Drugs and physiotherapy are both used to alleviate muscular discomfort. Researchers are seeking gene therapy treatments for inherited disorders, such as DMD, for which no cure exists.

For people with breathing problems, whether caused by muscular dystrophy or another myopathy, an incentive spirometer might improve breathing function (see Ch. 20), and appropriate antibiotics are prescribed for chest infections.

Treatment for contractures includes physiotherapy, good limb positioning and different kinds of bracing, all used as preventative measures. The patient and/or the family should be taught relevant exercises to reduce the risk of contracture development as part of a formal education programme. Baclofen and other skeletal muscle relaxants may be given to reduce the spasticity that contributes to their development. Sometimes surgery is necessary in very severe cases.

There is currently no known association between diet and muscle disease, but it may be recommended that people with myopathies try to keep body weight within an acceptable range to avoid overexerting their muscles.

Inflammatory myopathies

The inflammatory myopathies such as PM and DM are usually treated with drugs, particularly corticosteroids, e.g. prednisolone,

that suppress the action of the immune system. Daily prednisolone is used initially in high doses, and then slowly tapered to the lowest dose that relieves the symptoms.

▶ Nursing management of inheritable myopathies

Nursing management involves education regarding nutrition, exercise and medication (Janus 1996), assistance with affected activities of daily living and education to allow carers to take on this role following discharge. In the case of the progressive conditions, this must be made clear to both the patient and health and social services so that provision can be made for increasing support at home and in other community settings.

People with myopathies should visit their doctor at least annually, depending on how the disease progresses, and this should be organized as part of discharge planning. Physiotherapy to limit the effects of muscle weakening will often be ongoing and is often performed by patients or family. Nurses will therefore assist in the education of patients and family members/partners to enable this to occur. Assessment of the home environment and provision of aids to daily functioning will be undertaken by the occupational therapist. In those with respiratory involvement, any equipment to facilitate pulmonary function should be prescribed and the patient educated in the use of equipment related to these.

Genetic counsellors can provide information on the risk of passing on the disease to children. Again the nurse is in an ideal position to provide referral for this and other specialist services, including local education services.

Patients and family members should be advised on support groups related to their condition, which will be in a position to provide appropriate advice and support (see 'Useful addresses and websites').

MYASTHENIA GRAVIS

Myasthenia gravis is a neuromuscular autoimmune disease that causes a weakening of the voluntary muscles.

In myasthenia gravis, abnormal antibodies bind to receptors at the neuromuscular junction and initiate a series of events that prevent the neurotransmitter acetylcholine (ACh) from binding and transmission of the impulse to the muscle fibres, and as a result the muscle fibres cannot contract.

The distinctive features of myasthenia gravis include a fluctuating weakness in the muscles that move the eyeball and keep the eyelids open, some of the muscles involved with facial expression, chewing, swallowing and breathing, and muscles in the neck, arms and legs. Sometimes the symptoms may be so severe that a person is unable to breathe without mechanical ventilation (Putman & Wise 1996) (see Ch. 31).

Management is with anticholinesterase drugs such as pyridostigmine to delay the breakdown of ACh, and immunological treatment. This includes thymectomy (removal of the thymus gland which is usually abnormal), plasma exchange to remove antibodies, corticosteroids and immunosuppressants such as azathioprine. Patients are advised to plan for rest periods and avoid fatigue.

JOINT DISORDERS

SEPTIC ARTHRITIS

Septic arthritis (pyogenic) or suppurative arthritis is an infection of the joint by pus-forming bacteria.

Pathophysiology

The bacteria enter the joint from the bloodstream, and this can occur in early adulthood although more commonly it tends to be a condition affecting infants and young children. If untreated, the bacteria cause destruction of the cartilage covering the bones forming the joint, with eventual destruction of the joint.

Early complications in adults range from systemic effects of potential septicaemia, possibly even death, to localized problems with destruction of the cartilage or avascular necrosis.

Clinical presentation

- Severe acute pain
- Pyrexia
- Joint movement is usually restricted by the pain
- Spasm of the muscles surrounding the joint is often present.

Specific investigations

An FBC reveals an increase in white blood cells, with elevated ESR and C-reactive protein. The latter two tests indicate the level of acute inflammation in the body. Blood cultures will often be taken to identify the responsible organism.

X-rays are taken in the early phase, which may indicate the presence of fluid in the joint. An MRI can also confirm the presence of fluid in the joint, as well as inflammation of the joint lining.

Aspiration of fluid from the joint is often helpful in identifying the organism involved and antibiotic sensitivities.

Medical management

Treatment consists of immediate drainage of the joint. The knee can be drained adequately with arthroscopic lavage, but a hip joint often needs to be drained and irrigated in open surgery (arthrotomy). Intravenous antibiotics are a necessity.

▶ Nursing management

This involves:

- assisting in the investigations required for diagnosis
- assessment and control of pain
- administration of prescribed i.v. antibiotics
- monitoring temperature, pulse and respiration to assess response to treatment and to detect systemic problems
- assisting patients in meeting hygiene needs whilst symptoms persist.

OSTEOARTHRITIS

Osteoarthritis (OA) is a degenerative disorder that affects the articular surfaces of a joint.

Pathophysiology and aetiology

There is a widely suggested correlation between the development of OA and increasing age. Consequently OA is commonly present in older patients to some degree (Simon 1999). It may be classified as primary (or idiopathic), often affecting more than one joint and seen in older people, or secondary, which is usually associated with a previous history of joint injury or disease, e.g. RA, childhood disorders such as scoliosis and avascular necrosis, and often restricted to one joint.

Clinical presentation

Symptoms are predominantly pain and stiffness, but these tend to occur at any stage during the day, particularly after periods of immobility or rest. Clearly the severity of symptoms will be dependent on the specific progression of the disease and location according to the individual patient.

Medical/surgical management

Non-operative management relies on symptom control through the use of analgesic and anti-inflammatory drugs, the use of aids for walking or activities of living affected by the relevant joint, and physiotherapy and exercise to strengthen muscles that may be weakened. Individuals are advised to maintain body weight within an acceptable range to reduce the impact of obesity on joint condition. As with RA, a small degree of OA that would not normally have an impact on an individual's ability to undertake tasks in daily life may contribute to a disability following the development of other impairments. In severe cases, surgical procedures, commonly arthroplasty or hemiarthroplasty, are used in OA of both the hip and knee.

Joint replacement surgery

The replacement of knee and hip joints is commonplace and represents a significant proportion of orthopaedic management in older people. There are a variety of prostheses available for implantation. Cemented prostheses utilize an agent called polymethylmethacrylate to keep the prosthesis in place, whereas uncemented prostheses have a porous surface that allows bone ingrowth to occur, thus securing the new hip joint.

Such replacements are utilized in patients with severe arthritis, resulting in major disability as regards reduced mobility. Total hip replacement (THR) may also be used to treat avascular necrosis of the femoral head, failure of previous surgery and congenital hip deformity. Total knee replacement (TKR) may also be used in congenital knee deformity and severe intra-articular injury (Martin et al 1998).

▶ Nursing management of the patient with OA

Nursing assessment of the patient with osteoarthritis would include (Kee et al 1998):

- assessment of the degree of reduced mobility related to the condition and the level to which this affects other tasks, e.g. functional incontinence
- assessment of pain, including severity, location and activities which exacerbate it
- impact on activities of living related to reduced function

- level of knowledge relating to the condition, potential for secondary complications and the means by which to prevent these, and medications
- effects on body image
- disturbance of sleep pattern
- optimum functional goals
- the social implications of the above.

Nursing intervention is again multifaceted (Nolan & Nolan 1998) and depends on whether the patient undergoes surgical intervention. Assistance will be required with meeting hygiene and nutritional needs until patients are able to regain their optimum independence in these. Education will need to be provided regarding the condition itself, use of aids to functional independence, e.g. walking aids, medication or orthoses. Formal programmes should be in place in the clinical area for this patient population to ensure a consistently good standard and comprehensive coverage of all of the above aspects.

Assistance will be required with mobility according to the prescribed rehabilitation regimen, including strategies to reduce the likelihood of prosthetic dislocation if a knee or hip arthroplasty has been performed (see below). Progress in the ward and other settings of prescribed regimens and treatment modalities should be reported to other team members.

The nurse will be required to monitor and evaluate strategies to relieve pain and disturbance in sleep pattern.

Finally formal discharge planning and follow-up should be undertaken, including involvement and referral to appropriate community professionals.

Specific nursing management – joint replacement surgery

Preoperative nursing management of patients having replacement arthroplasty incorporates physical preparation for anaesthesia, including preoperative health checks, and patient education relating to the surgery and what to expect in the postoperative phase. This should include an explanation of mobility and strengthening exercises that are used following surgery.

Immediate postoperative management (see Ch. 29) will involve recovery from anaesthesia, including administration of oxygen therapy, monitoring vital signs such as pulse for signs of haemorrhage, effective pain control and observation of local wound and drain management protocols in the first instance. Later care involves monitoring for pressure ulcer development (based on preoperative assessment of risk), administration of prophylactic antibiotics and measures to prevent deep vein thrombosis, e.g. anticoagulants (see Ch. 19).

Preventing dislocation of the prosthesis is paramount in the early stages following surgery. Following TKR, patients should avoid hyperextension, rotation and acute flexion of the knee joint. Partial weight-bearing is normally allowed initially, progressing to full weight-bearing as tolerated by the individual patient and providing there are no signs of potential dislocation. When mobilization commences, a knee brace should be worn to limit these movements. Patients, and nurses when assisting, should adhere strictly to the prescribed gait training during this rehabilitation phase. Leg strengthening exercises, including quadriceps (large four-part extensor muscle of the anterior

thigh) tightening and the use of a continuous passive movement, are standard interventions both to enable early mobility and to reduce the swelling around the knee joint.

Similarly, following THR, measures must be implemented to decrease the likelihood of prosthesis dislocation. Some surgeons will insist on at least 24 hours' strict bed rest following surgery. In reality, it will often take at least this long for some older patients to recover from the anaesthetic sufficiently to commence mobilization. Patients must avoid situations that may result in adduction (movement toward the midline of the body) of the affected limb. An abduction (movement away from the midline) wedge/pillow or the placing of two to three pillows between the legs would be standard means to achieve this. Patients will be turned, maintaining the legs in this position, often with the pillows still in place. Patients must not cross their legs or move the operated limb past the midline. They should avoid rotation and reduce hip flexion. Some surgeons may prescribe initial restrictions on bed head elevation for the first days postoperatively. The standard would be to ensure that patients do not flex the leg past 90°. They should therefore be instructed not to reach down to put on shoes/socks, the bed should be raised to at least mid-thigh level prior to patients getting up, and elevated toilet seats and high chairs should be used.

Partial weight-bearing will be permitted initially and will increase to full weight-bearing according to what patients can tolerate, the prosthesis type and surgeon preference. When transferring, e.g. from a bed to a chair, patients will be instructed to pivot on the non-affected leg.

In either case, should dislocation be suspected due to severe pain, abnormal leg position and an inability to move with a potential deterioration in neurovascular status, the management is the same whether for knee or hip replacement. Patients should be returned to bed and bed rest maintained; X-rays should be ordered of the affected leg. Prosthesis dislocation is most commonly treated by further surgery, or occasionally closed reduction (e.g. using traction) will be used.

HALLUX VALGUS

Hallux valgus (bunion) is a common deformity, where the great toe is deviated laterally to overlap the second toe, and the first metatarsal bone is deviated medially, causing a prominence to form on the medial aspect of the metatarsophalangeal joint.

Pathophysiology, aetiology and management

A bursa forms over the area as a result of the constant irritation and inflammation, forming a painful bunion. There may be some degree of foot pronation ('flat feet') associated with the condition. Many factors may come into play to cause the problem, including foot structure – hereditary or acquired from wearing narrow stylized shoes that crimp the toes. Most cases are mild and asymptomatic, and do not need treatment. These patients should be educated in the wearing of shoes with lots of toe room and no heels. If there is a flat foot, a shoe insert to correct the foot pronation may help to prevent progression of the disease. In more severe cases, surgical correction may be needed.

▶ Nursing management

Nursing management consists of education relating to symptom management, choice of footwear, the use of orthoses and prevention of potential skin problems. In those who progress to surgical intervention there is additionally nursing care of the wound following surgery, effective pain control and generally a longer period of hospitalization as the patient is assisted in regaining optimum mobility.

ENTRAPMENT NEUROPATHY

There are various situations in which a nerve becomes trapped with effects that include sensory abnormalities, muscle weakness and wasting, and pain. It is beyond the scope of this book to cover all such events and only carpal tunnel syndrome is discussed.

CARPAL TUNNEL SYNDROME

The carpal tunnel runs under the ligaments connecting the bones on either side of the wrist. The median nerve that controls hand muscles and tendons, which enables the fingers to be bent, passes through this tunnel. Carpal tunnel syndrome results when the tunnel becomes narrow and the nerve is squeezed against bone and ligament.

Pathophysiology and aetiology

The primary cause is most often wear and tear and swelling of the tendons from overuse. Carpal tunnel syndrome is common in people who have jobs or hobbies requiring repeated hand motions, e.g. assembly workers, computer operators, and those who play racquet sports. It may be associated with hypothyroidism and diabetes mellitus (see Ch. 17).

Clinical presentation

Transient alterations in sensation in the hand are usually the first sign: tingling, burning and numbness are the common complaints. They occur most often early in the morning or during the night and may disturb the patient's sleep pattern if severe. Eventually, the hand becomes weaker and the pain is constant and extends up the arm.

Medical management

Management depends on severity, but in any case the patient should be advised to discontinue the activity that led to the condition developing. A splint may be of benefit, and NSAIDs are commonly used. Oral corticosteroids may be prescribed and occasionally a corticosteroid injection is effective. As a last resort surgery to relieve pressure on the nerves may be necessary.

▶ Nursing management

Nursing management involves control of pain, education regarding the wearing of the appropriate splint and postoperative care of the wound if the patient progresses to surgery.

BACK PAIN AND PROBLEMS

Back problems are a major cause of days lost from work, inability to undertake activities of living, inconvenience and pain.

MUSCULOSKELETAL BACK PAIN

The most common type of back pain is musculoskeletal in origin, resulting from some mechanical problem with the back muscles, bones, joints or ligaments.

It is usually a result of abuse, overuse or underuse of the back. Individuals with occupations requiring excessive lifting, bending and heavy work on a routine basis may be more prone to develop this condition. Nurses have been prime candidates for back problems in the past, due to poor handling techniques and lack of specialist equipment.

In addition, the ageing process commonly contributes to the development of back pain. As the person ages, bony spurs (osteophytes) develop on the vertebrae that project outward. The vertebral joints become inflamed and the ligaments may thicken. The intervertebral discs begin to wear away or dehydrate and the annulus of the disc starts to deteriorate. All of these various changes can cause pain, and as with any pain there is decreased mobility in the affected part.

Back pain will often also occur as a result of other pathologies, e.g. RA, secondary tumour, osteoporosis and infection.

INTERVERTEBRAL DISC DEGENERATION AND HERNIATION

A 'slipped disc', or more correctly a herniated or prolapsed intervertebral disc, most commonly occurs in the lumbar and cervical areas. These are the areas of the spine that have the greatest mobility and consequently where the discs are more prone to damage. When abnormalities occur in the thoracic spine, they usually reflect some sort of disease affecting the spinal nerves or cord rather than a disc exerting pressure.

The pressure that the disc puts on the nerve roots usually causes neurological symptoms in addition to the pain. A person may feel numbness, tingling, burning, aching or a shooting pain down a limb. Some patients may develop motor weakness. These various neurological symptoms are known as 'radicular' symptoms (i.e. relating to the nerve root).

Damage in the lumbar region is often termed sciatica because these processes can irritate the sciatic nerve, the largest nerve in the body extending down through the buttock and the leg to the foot.

If the herniated disc material compresses the spinal cord itself and not the nerve roots, other symptoms can include weakness along one entire side of the body, numbness, and bowel or bladder complications. The particular symptoms depend on which neurological pathways are affected.

SPINAL STENOSIS

Spinal stenosis is a bony narrowing of the spinal canal. It may occasionally be congenital but more commonly is acquired secondary to disc degeneration, subluxation (partial dislocation) of the posterior facet joints or even following previous spinal fusion. Spinal stenosis usually develops in adults over the age of 50 years.

Symptoms are similar to those for other types of back problems and range from a dull backache to the more severe pain that shoots down the lower limb. The pain is usually felt when standing or walking and disappears when a person sits down or bends forward at the waist and is more commonly diffuse if central, or sciatic if a lateral stenosis is present.

OTHER CAUSES OF BACK PAIN AND PROBLEMS

Rheumatoid arthritis

When RA affects the back, it usually involves the cervical and lumbar spine. This causes severe neck and back pain as well as the inability to move these normally very mobile parts of the back. Vertebral osteophytes may lead to spinal stenosis, which results in pressure on the spinal cord and nerves.

Primary tumours

Primary tumours affecting the spine can develop in the bone marrow, bone, nerve roots, spinal cord or the meninges. Metastatic tumours commonly originate from tumours in the lung, breast, prostate and kidney, but may arise from other sites. Both primary and metastatic tumours can compress the spine or nerve roots and cause significant pain. The spinal cord has limited space inside the spinal column, so even a very small tumour can exert enough pressure to cause problems, such as spinal cord compression (SCC), which results in serious neurological damage if diagnosis and treatment are delayed (see Chs 33 and 34). The general management of bone tumours is covered below.

Infection

Infection can arise in the vertebrae, the discs, the meninges or the spinal fluid. In addition to back pain, people with infections usually have a fever as well as abnormalities in their blood. Some infections can cause SCC.

Osteoporosis

This is the most common cause of vertebral fractures in older people, especially older women (see below). Patients may develop chronic back pain, as well as multiple bony fractures. Osteoporosis is covered in more detail on page 819.

Disorders elsewhere in the body that may be mistaken for musculoskeletal syndromes

These include aortic dissection (see Ch. 19), pancreatic disease (see Ch. 23), pneumonia (see Ch. 20), kidney and bladder diseases (see Ch. 24) and uterine disorders (see Ch. 25). However, these only account for about 1 in 200 people who visit their doctor for low back pain.

THE PATIENT WITH BACK PAIN

Specific investigations – back pain and problems

A medical history and complete physical and neurological examination are usually the most helpful tools for making a correct diagnosis. Patients should be questioned regarding onset of the back pain, how it affects activities of daily living, whether it results in any other symptoms apart from the direct pain itself, and what exacerbates or lessens the pain.

A neurological examination involving testing of all muscle groups, sensory testing for pain and light touch and reflex testing will be performed to ascertain neurological involvement and to ensure that no other underlying neurological condition is present. Patients will be asked to move through a full range to test spinal mobility.

A set of spinal X-rays should be able to detect any fractures, inflammation from RA, and any significant degeneration of the intervertebral discs.

An MRI scan will provide additional information regarding potential disc disease, spinal cord pathology, infectious processes, spinal stenosis and spinal tumours.

Although less common these days, a myelogram or CT scan may also be performed, particularly if a patient is unable to have MRI.

In some patients, neurophysiological testing may be helpful for diagnosing the cause of back pain. These tests include EMG and nerve conduction velocity (NCV) evaluation, which help to determine whether a particular nerve root and the muscle that it supplies are abnormal.

Management

The main treatment for back pain caused by muscle or ligament strain or stiffness is restricted bed rest combined with appropriate back-strengthening exercise and pain control. It is worth stressing that too much bed rest can make the situation worse. Gentle exercise is important for increasing circulation to the area and for strengthening the muscles to minimize likelihood of recurrence.

Medication used to relieve acute back pain includes mild pain relievers such as paracetamol, aspirin and ibuprofen, or stronger prescription drugs for more severe pain. NSAIDs, including ibuprofen, help to relieve pain and decrease inflammation in the soft tissues and other structures. They can be used to treat arthritis flare-ups, disc disease, muscular pain and traumatic injuries. Usually they are taken orally, although some can be given by injection. The major side-effect of NSAIDs is significant gastrointestinal problems, particularly ulcers. Patients with previous gastrointestinal problems may be better advised to use alternative methods of pain relief.

Other anti-inflammatory drugs that work much like the NSAIDs but without the unpleasant gastrointestinal side-effects include celecoxib (a selective inhibitor of the enzyme cyclo-oxygenase 2). Tramadol, which has opioid effects, is usually reserved for short-term back pain but can be used to treat chronic pain if other drugs are ineffective, e.g. for neuropathic pain (see Ch. 7) caused by a tumour exerting pressure. Side-effects include dizziness and light-headedness. Narcotics can be used for short-term pain relief and are appropriate for patients who experience the severe pain of disc herniation or trauma. However, if no other drug works, narcotics are sometimes necessary to relieve chronic back pain. They can be administered orally or transdermally. The potential complications from narcotic usage include dependence, withdrawal reactions, an altered mental status and constipation.

Muscle relaxants (e.g. orphenadrine and diazepam) are often used to treat muscular spasm or related neurological problems and are often combined with NSAIDs for pain relief. The major side-effect of extreme sleepiness may be helpful if a person is having difficulty sleeping due to back discomfort. Tizanadine is used to treat muscular spasticity as well as chronic back pain, especially musculoskeletal back pain.

In patients with chronic back pain, the tricyclic antidepressants, e.g. amitriptyline, are often administered in low doses. They may be indicated in patients who experience numbness, burning, aching, and throbbing or stabbing pains that shoot down the limbs. Side-effects include drowsiness, dry mouth and constipation.

Gabapentin has proven extremely helpful in the management of many forms of chronic pain. Like the tricyclic antidepressants, it is especially helpful if there are any signs of irritated nerve roots and it is often taken in combination with a tricyclic antidepressant. It has minimal side-effects, including mild drowsiness.

Physiotherapy and occupational therapy

Physiotherapy is often a part of the rehabilitation and treatment of back pain. The goals of physiotherapy are to minimize discomfort, restore normal movements and help return patients to their previous level of functioning or the highest level possible. The particular technique that is used depends on personal choice, as well as the severity of the pain and extent of immobility. For some of these techniques, e.g. spinal manipulation, there is little clear evidence of efficacy but it may be beneficial in some patients. A range of techniques may be used:

- Exercises include bending and stretching the muscles and spine, as well as endurance strengthening.
- Massage increases circulation to the area and includes traditional techniques, as well as neuromuscular massage therapy and the use of hand-held devices.
- Ultrasound may also increase blood flow.
- A cold application, e.g. an ice pack, to the painful area is a good way to relieve pain within the first 48 hours. After this, using a hot water bag or heating pad on the painful area, or soaking in a hot bath, will probably provide some relief.
- Spinal manipulation – use of one's hands to apply force to the back so that the spine can be moved and adjusted.
- Occupational retraining programmes led by an occupational therapist may help individuals gradually resume their previous work roles.

Surgical intervention

Surgery is not always effective in the treatment of most types of back pain. Most back pain, especially lower back pain, is self-limiting and goes away with proper care. Clearly, though, some people have more serious conditions and/or still experience pain or other problems despite other forms of therapy. When surgery is performed, its purpose is usually to relieve pressure on neurological structures or to eliminate particular movements that are causing pain or leading to some other dysfunction. Surgery should be considered only after a complete physical and neurological examination and should be based on the clinical symptoms, as well as the results of the various imaging (X-ray, MRI and CT) and other tests to determine fitness for anaesthesia.

Surgery is indicated in about 10% of patients, e.g. those having recurrent episodes of sciatica.

Nowadays, most discectomies (termed a microdiscectomy) are performed through a small laminectomy (surgical procedure, which includes removal of a portion of the lamina, to provide more room in the vertebral canal) and an operating microscope. This has reduced postoperative recovery time and hospital stay considerably.

Surgery is often necessary in patients who have certain spinal infections or tumours, as well as in trauma patients whose spine is clearly unstable and requires major intervention (see Ch. 14). Infections, tumours, trauma and spinal instability are usually treated with spinal fusion.

Some surgical procedures involve implanting specialized systems that deliver a constant rate of medication or stimulation to the spinal area. These implantable 'pumps' can deliver narcotics or other substances directly to the spinal area to relieve pain. Direct drug delivery, as compared with oral administration, has the advantage of fewer side-effects. Surgically implanted spinal cord stimulators modulate the pain response, so that patients feel less pain than they would otherwise.

▶ Nursing management

Nursing management is dependent on the particular treatment modality utilized. It will involve administration of drug therapy, psychological support, identification of functional and social goals with patients and other health care team members, education regarding use of orthosis and self-care, and pre- and postoperative care in those who undergo surgery.

Even with all of the above, it may not be possible to completely remove a patient's pain. In such circumstances, patients often enter a chronic pain cycle in which the focus of their attention in life becomes almost exclusively the pain itself, resulting not only in physical symptoms but also in major life changes. Employment and relationships both at home and outside may all suffer. Many dedicated chronic pain clinics have now been set up which attempt to enable sufferers to live with the pain, commonly based on the principles of good rehabilitation goal-setting techniques. Through removing the focus on the pain and empowering patients to get on with their lives, the pain experience, although often still an issue, becomes less disabling and the individuals become more participative and constructive members of society.

The nurse's role in managing chronic back pain is clearly dependent on the particular treatment modality employed. Education will be required regarding techniques to perform activities of daily living despite the pain, administration of analgesia or other pain management techniques and dealing with the psychosocial aspects that may be associated with chronic back pain. Indeed, there are nurse counsellors who may receive a referral within some specialist rehabilitation units.

For those requiring surgery, preoperative care ensuring fitness for operation and postoperative assistance with activities until patients are able to resume these are key areas of nursing intervention. Additionally patients will often be prescribed a brace to be worn for a specified period of time. Principles of care for patients wearing an orthosis as previously outlined in this chapter (p. 801) form the basis of nursing care.

CONNECTIVE TISSUE DISORDERS

Connective tissue disorders form a large, diverse group of complaints. Systemic lupus erythematosus is an important example and is discussed in some detail.

SYSTEMIC LUPUS ERYTHEMATOSUS

Systemic lupus erythematosus (SLE) is a chronic inflammatory autoimmune disorder that may affect many systems, including the skin, joints and internal organs.

Pathophysiology and epidemiology

The primary role of the immune system is to control body defences in the actual or potential presence of some threat, e.g. pathogenic microorganisms. In SLE, as with other autoimmune diseases, these defences are turned against the body when antibodies that are produced attack body cells. These antibodies damage the body's blood cells, tissues and organs, causing chronic diseases. The mechanism or cause of SLE is not fully understood.

The disease affects eight times as many women as men. It may occur at any age, but appears mostly in people between the ages of 10 and 50 years. The incidence is four out of 10 000 people. African-Americans and Asians are affected more often than other races. Certain drugs may also cause SLE. When this occurs, it is known as drug-induced lupus erythematosus and is usually reversible when the medication is stopped.

Clinical presentation

The course of SLE may vary from a mild episodic illness to a severe fatal disease. Symptoms also vary widely with the individual and are characterized by remissions and exacerbation. At the onset, only one organ system may be involved. Additional organs may become involved later. SLE affects different organs in different ways.

It would be rare for a person with SLE not to have joint pain and swelling, and most will develop rheumatoid arthritis. The joints primarily affected are the fingers, hands, wrists and knees. Death of bone tissue can occur in the hips and shoulders and subsequently results in further pain in those areas.

Around 50% of persons with SLE develop a malar 'butterfly' rash, commonly located over the cheeks and bridge of the nose. A more diffuse rash may appear on other body parts that are exposed to excessive sunlight. Other skin lesions, such as patchy colour, or nodules can occur.

SLE commonly affects the kidneys and in about half of patients this will result in chronic inflammation (nephritis) where the eventual outcome may be chronic renal failure necessitating renal replacement therapy (see Ch. 24).

Around a quarter of patients with SLE will have some degree of neurological involvement. Mild mental dysfunction is the most common symptom, but any area of the brain, spinal cord or nervous system can be affected. Fits, psychosis, organic brain syndrome, numbness and tingling, and headaches are some of the varied nervous system disorders that can occur.

Blood disorders are common and affect around 85% of those with SLE. Thromboembolic conditions such as CVA and pulmonary embolism (see Chs 19 and 20) may occur. Often

platelets are decreased, or antibodies are formed against blood clotting factors, which may cause significant bleeding, e.g. haematuria, haemoptysis and epistaxis. Anaemia is also common.

SLE can cause pericarditis, endocarditis or myocarditis (see Ch. 19). Pleural effusions and pleuritic pain may also occur in some patients. Patients may present with chest infection and/or shortness of breath as a result.

Other signs and symptoms include (Leach 1998):

- pyrexia, fatigue, malaise, weight loss
- enlarged lymph nodes
- muscle pain
- mouth ulcers
- dysphagia, nausea and vomiting, abdominal pain
- visual disturbances
- hair loss
- fingers that change colour upon pressure.

Specific investigations

Diagnostic tests to determine the presence of SLE and ascertain the level of involvement on various body organs will include some or all of the following, depending on the presentation:

- blood tests – ANA
- chest X-ray – for pleuritis or pericarditis
- chest auscultation – pericardial or pleural friction rub
- urinalysis for blood or protein
- FBC, ascertaining possible decreases in some cell types
- kidney biopsy
- neurological examination.

Medical management

There is no cure for SLE. The presence and severity of symptoms related to the effects of the disease on specific organs will ultimately guide treatment modalities in each individual patient.

Prognosis for people with SLE has improved over recent years. Many respond well to drug therapy and the disease is managed to ensure that only a mild illness is present. Women with SLE who become pregnant are often able to continue the pregnancy safely to term and deliver normal infants, provided severe renal or cardiac disease is not present and the SLE is under treatment.

Although the 10-year survival rate exceeds 85%, patients with severe brain, lung, heart and kidney involvement have the worst prognosis in terms of survival or, as a minimum, the presence of major disability.

Mild disease resulting in a rash, headaches, fever, arthritis, pleurisy and pericarditis will require drugs, other therapies and interventions. Some of the following may be used:

- NSAIDs – for arthritis and pleurisy
- topical corticosteroids – for skin rashes
- hydroxychloroquine – for skin and arthritis
- other pain control strategies, e.g. TENS
- light sensitivity is managed with protective clothing, sunglasses and sunscreen.

Severe or life-threatening manifestations (haemolytic anaemia, extensive heart, lung, kidney and central nervous system involvement) often require treatment by specialists in the specific area.

Systemic corticosteroid therapy or medications to suppress the immune system may be prescribed to control the various manifestations of severe disease. As a last resort, where corticosteroid therapy fails, cytotoxic drugs may be considered.

▶ Nursing management

Nursing the patient with SLE may be complex due to the variety of systemic effects of this condition. Nursing intervention includes assisting in investigations, initial assessment and ongoing monitoring for the aforementioned potential involvement of body systems and prescribing plans of care accordingly. Patients must be educated not only in the prescribed treatment but also to have an input into self-detection of potential secondary health problems relating to the condition.

Additionally the nurse should be aware of the support for patients and families available following discharge (see 'Useful addresses and websites'). Joining a support group where members share common experiences and problems can help to reduce the stress of the condition.

BONE DISORDERS AND INFECTION

PAGET'S DISEASE (OSTEITIS DEFORMANS)

Paget's disease of bone is associated with increased bone reabsorption and production.

Pathophysiology

This condition of unknown origin tends to affect men more than women and occurs primarily in young adults to middle age. The sequelae of events resulting in the disease commences with an increase in osteoclast (bone reabsorption cells) activity, which results in increased bone reabsorption. Osteoblasts (bone-producing cells) repair the loss, which results in a relatively rapid turnover with bone anatomy that may be deformed, enlarged and/or highly vascular. Hypercalcaemia may develop as a result of the increased calcium load in the blood (see Chs 8 and 17). This 'pagetoid' bone is brittle and susceptible to pathological fracture. It commonly affects the lumbosacral vertebrae, pelvis, femur, tibia and skull.

Clinical presentation

Presentation of Paget's disease can be divided into three broad categories. Approximately one-third of patients will be unaware until the disease is discovered on X-ray. Another third will have bone deformity but will be asymptomatic and therefore require no intervention. The final third will be symptomatic and, depending on the sites affected, may present with bowed legs, kyphosis (exaggerated curvature of the spine, in the flexion/ extension axis) and an enlarged cranium (but not face). Hearing may be impaired and pain on pressure is common.

Skin temperature may be elevated due to the increased vascularity of the affected bone.

In severe cases, a high cardiac output may result in a degree of cardiac failure (see Ch. 19), particularly in older people who have had the disease for some time.

Pressure on the brain or cranial nerves due to cranial enlargement, or SCC in those with vertebral involvement, may lead to neurological symptoms such as alteration in motor function or sensation.

Specific investigations

- Blood tests – serum alkaline phosphatase level (high levels are associated with increased severity of Paget's disease), calcium level
- X-ray and bone scans – help to confirm diagnosis.

Medical/surgical management

Goals of treatment include controlling pain and reducing inflammation with NSAIDs. Replacement of the pagetoid bone with normal bone may be assisted with the use of drugs such as calcitonin and disodium etidronate (a bisphosphonate). With such treatments, remission for several months at least is a frequent outcome. Some surgical management may be useful in symptom control in severe cases, e.g. spinal decompression, as well as management of pathological fractures.

▶ Nursing management

Nursing interventions will involve assisting with investigations, education of the patient about prescribed treatment modalities, and pre- and postoperative care in those who undergo surgery (Lewis et al 1999). Patients must be educated about all aspects of the disease to minimize the effects of symptoms on their daily lives and to facilitate compliance with drug regimens. Additional assistance may be required in the activities of daily living in those patients who have progressed to develop neurological symptoms.

OSTEOGENESIS IMPERFECTA

Osteogenesis imperfecta refers to a group of hereditary disorders characterized by fragile bones that result in multiple fractures at birth or during childhood.

Pathophysiology and aetiology

The incidence is one per 10 000 live births. A genetic defect causes abnormal formation of type I collagen, found in bones, teeth, sclera and ligaments. In the bones, this causes severe osteoporosis. The severe forms (types II and III) are usually inherited as an autosomal recessive gene, whereas the milder forms (types I and IV) are autosomal dominant. Babies with type II disease usually die during the first few weeks of life.

Clinical presentation

The symptoms vary in severity and are classified using genetic type, and clinical and radiographic characteristics.

Signs and symptoms include:

- fractures following only moderate trauma
- blue sclera
- early hearing loss
- multiple deformities – severe bowing of long bones, triangular faces, short stature (severe in some types) and scoliosis (lateral curvature of the spinal column).

Specific investigations

In most cases, the diagnosis is not in doubt, given the genetic, clinical and X-ray manifestations. However, in some cases of type I disease, where the diagnosis is not clear, a skin biopsy with tissue culture of the fibroblast may be necessary.

Management (team approach)

There is no cure for this condition, so treatment is directed to preventing and treating fractures and deformities through adolescence and into early adulthood. Treatment consists of physiotherapy, splinting and bracing, castings and orthopaedic surgical correction when indicated. Non-musculoskeletal conditions, e.g. hearing loss and dental problems, are obviously referred to the appropriate specialists.

Nursing management therefore incorporates education regarding lifestyle, prevention of complications, medication prescribed and the use of any orthosis prescribed.

OSTEOMALACIA

Osteomalacia is failure of the normal mineralization process of bones (in children this condition is known as rickets).

Pathophysiology and aetiology

A soft weak skeleton develops due to a loss of calcium, with associated pain and bowing of the legs and the potential for pathological fracture. People at risk include those with dietary deficiencies, particularly in relation to intake of vitamin D, malabsorption (e.g. coeliac disease, chronic pancreatitis), following gastrectomy and those having reduced exposure to sunlight.

Medical management

Treatment is with large doses of vitamin D orally and monitoring of serum calcium level. Ultraviolet radiation may be of benefit in severe cases. Corrective surgery and/or bracing may be prescribed in those with deformity and education is required to ensure compliance in those wearing a brace on a long-term basis. The patient may be referred to a dietician to ensure that nutritional deficiencies are addressed.

▶ Nursing management

Nursing intervention is primarily in the role of educator. Education regarding wearing a prescribed brace (see p. 801), diet and medications is vital.

OSTEOPOROSIS

Osteoporosis is a condition causing a reduction in bone mass.

Pathophysiology and aetiology

This reduction in bone mass is a direct result of bone resorption exceeding bone formation and results in bones that are porous, brittle and fragile. Consequently there is an increased risk of fracture, notably:

- Colles' fracture
- compression fractures of the lower thoracic and lumbar vertebrae
- neck of femur fractures.

It is more prevalent in women than in men, associated particularly with the hormonal changes occurring following the menopause (Goss 1998). Osteoporosis does affect men but usually at an older age than women.

Other aetiological factors include:

- long-term corticosteroid use
- hyperthyroidism
- hyperparathyroidism
- long-term immobility associated with the reduction of weight-bearing, e.g. paraplegia, long-term casting
- nutritional deficits related to vitamin D and calcium deficiencies
- liver cirrhosis
- osteogenesis imperfecta (see p. 818)
- rheumatoid arthritis (see p. 805)
- diabetes mellitus
- malignancy.

Osteoporosis is essentially asymptomatic until a fracture occurs, although it will result in a decrease in height associated with ageing.

Medical/surgical management

The prevention of osteoporosis is a major public health issue with an ageing population. Health promotion, and detection (using dual-energy X-ray absorptiometry, DXA) and treatment of osteoporosis are vitally important (see below). Management of osteoporosis is directly related to the injury sustained and specific injuries are covered elsewhere in this chapter.

It is essential that a full assessment of the condition be undertaken to ascertain whether it has developed as a result of hormonal changes or from some other pathology.

▶ Nursing management

The main aspects of nursing management include:

- review of the diet, involving an increased intake of calcium, protein and vitamin D; this is often worthwhile
- administration and education relating to medication, e.g. oestrogen hormone replacement therapy for women and bisphosphonates
- advice and encouragement to take weight-bearing exercise and increase general activity
- advice about reducing alcohol intake and smoking cessation, as both excess alcohol intake and smoking are associated with osteoporosis
- advice aimed at preventing accidents and falls.

Arguably more than any other specific musculoskeletal condition, osteoporosis has benefited from prevention as a result of health promotion programmes. National campaigns have resulted in a greater public awareness, hormone replacement therapy as standard for women in their middle years and mobile monitoring services in many areas. Many of these nursing interventions, including advice about accident prevention, are performed by those working in community settings or outpatient departments (see Health Promotion box 27.1).

HEALTH PROMOTION

27.1 Preventing falls and accidents

Consider the traumatic injuries sustained by older people in your current area of practice. Many of these relate to existing musculoskeletal or neurological conditions, e.g. osteoporosis and stroke.

Student activities
- What suggestions can you make regarding accident prevention that may reduce either severity or incidence?

Further reading and resources
Gillespie LD, Gillespie WJ, Robertson MC et al. Interventions for preventing falls in elderly people (Cochrane Review). In: The Cochrane Library, 4. Oxford: Update Software; 2001.
Royal Society for the Prevention of Accidents – www.rospa.co.uk

OSTEOMYELITIS

Osteomyelitis is inflammation of bone tissue (commencing in the marrow), usually caused by acute or chronic bacterial infection.

Pathophysiology and aetiology

The pathogenic organisms, usually bacteria, gains access to bone tissue by one of three main routes:

- haematogenous – blood-borne from infection elsewhere in the body, e.g. respiratory infection
- from erosion of adjacent soft tissue infection, e.g. extensive pressure ulcer (see Ch. 10)
- direct bone contamination, e.g. surgery, open (compound) fracture.

The most common pathogen responsible for osteomyelitis is the bacterium *Staphylococcus aureus*, probably accounting for 70–80% of cases. Other bacteria commonly associated with osteomyelitis are *Proteus* and *Pseudomonas* spp.

The infection results initially in inflammation, increased vascularity and oedema. Blood vessels supplying bone tissue become thrombosed within 3 days, and consequently bone ischaemia and necrosis result. These pathological changes extend into the medullary cavity and under the periosteum where a bone abscess forms. Even if an acute episode is successfully treated, the resulting cavity may be subject to recurrent infections in the long term. This is termed chronic osteomyelitis.

Clinical presentation

Acute osteomyelitis results in:

- pain – this may become excruciating on movement, particularly as the infection spreads to adjacent soft tissues
- redness
- swelling
- pyrexia.

Specific investigations
- Blood tests – an FBC will show an increase in white cells and a raised ESR
- Blood cultures – to identify the causative organism and ascertain antibiotic sensitivities
- X-rays – to show cavities and sequestra (areas of dead bone).

Medical/surgical management

Goals of care in the patient with osteomyelitis include management of the bone infection, reduction of pain and facilitating adherence to prescribed regimens of treatment.

Management therefore comprises administration of i.v. antibiotics, aspiration of pus from the infected area, if possible, and possibly surgical debridement (removal of damaged tissue and foreign material) and irrigation of cavities.

Chronic osteomyelitis will present as recurrent episodes of pain, inflammation and swelling and reduction in functional ability. X-rays will demonstrate large irregular areas of bone with cavities and sequestra. Management comprises antibiotics to treat the infection for 6 weeks and then potentially sequestrectomy under general anaesthesia.

▶ Nursing management

Nursing management of the patient with osteomyelitis comprises wound management post-surgical intervention and administration of prescribed antibiotics (often i.v.). Nurses should monitor the patient's condition and vital signs, e.g. temperature, closely to assess response to treatment and detect systemic complications.

Pain should be monitored, prescribed analgesia administered and its efficacy assessed on a regular basis. Patients will require assistance with hydration, nutrition and hygiene needs during a period of acute illness until they are well enough to perform these without help. Management will also include the restoration of optimum mobility, education regarding prescribed medication and finally ensuring discharge planning and follow-up arrangements are made.

BONE TUMOURS

Bone tumours may be benign, malignant sarcomas or metastatic carcinomas. In bone there are two potential responses to the tumour: either increased osteoclast activity with associated bone loss and weakening or, more commonly, increased bone formation around the tumour as a consequence of increased osteoblast activity.

It is not uncommon for benign tumours to become malignant if left untreated.

A variety of symptoms may be present and depend on the particular tumour type and extent; however, pain and deformity with potential reduction in functional ability are common symptoms across all the tumour types.

Investigations
- History of symptom development and physical examination for deformity and pain

- X-rays, bone scans and CT scans
- Biopsy (often under general anaesthesia) to ascertain the tumour type once the presence of a tumour has been confirmed.

BENIGN TUMOURS

The common types of benign tumour include:

- *Osteochondroma* – the most common of the benign tumours, it usually forms at the end of long bones, e.g. in the knee and shoulder. Results in mild and medium pain with potential functional deficit in the affected joint if it is extensive
- *Enchondroma* – a benign tumour of the hyaline cartilage that causes mild pain. There may be the potential for pathological fracture
- *Osteoidosteoma* – generally restricted to young adults and is commonly associated with severe pain
- *Giant cell tumours* – initially relatively pain-free, they commonly invade local tissues. They are soft tumours but tend to be very haemorrhagic.

Medical/surgical management

Surgical intervention is usual and focuses on restoration of bone continuity of the affected area, comprising excision and, in some cases, bone grafting. As osteomyelitis (see p. 820) is a particular concern, prophylactic antibiotics are commonly prescribed.

▶ **Nursing management**

Postoperative management adheres to general principles of orthopaedic surgery of the affected part. This will comprise appropriate pain management, immobilization and elevation of the affected part until healing has occurred. Observations of vital signs and fluid balance are continued as appropriate. Neurovascular assessment of the affected limb should be performed on a regular basis according to local policy. Prophylactic antibiotics are administered as prescribed and the nurse should ensure that patients understand the importance of taking the full course if early discharge is likely.

MALIGNANT BONE TUMOURS

Malignant bone tumours may be primary or result from metastatic spread from the primary site.

Types, pathophysiology and management
Osteosarcoma

This is the most common of the malignant bone tumours and is most frequently found in the lower end of the femur, upper tibia and upper humerus. It affects males more than females and occurs predominantly in the 10–25 year age group. It may also occur subsequent to Paget's disease in older patients. Unfortunately, mortality rates are high, with the tumour often metastasizing to the lungs. Signs and symptoms include severe pain, swelling around the affected area, immobility and, as the tumour progresses, weight loss and general malaise. Clearly in tumours that have metastasized there will be symptoms related to the secondary site. Management is often a combination of radical surgery, such as amputation, with additional chemotherapy.

Chondrosarcoma

This is a malignant tumour of hyaline cartilage. It is generally slow-growing compared with other tumours and large. It affects men more often than women, and the common sites include the pelvis, ribs, femur, humerus and spine. If left untreated for a long time, it may metastasize to the lungs, but this is uncommon, as patients tend to seek help before this happens as they develop pain and the tumour affects functional ability. Survival rates are comparatively high with surgical excision or amputation of the affected part.

Multiple myeloma

Multiple myeloma is a malignancy of plasma cells. The bone marrow is the principal location, although the kidneys, spleen, lymph nodes and liver will also be involved as the condition progresses. As there is erosion of the marrow cavity and bone cortex, the most common symptom is that of severe bone pain. There will be swelling, tenderness and pain, with the potential for pathological fractures around the bone lesion. In cases involving the spine, mild pain may result as compression fractures of the lumbar vertebrae occur. (Myeloma is covered in depth in Chapter 18.)

Metastatic bone tumours

These commonly arise from carcinoma affecting the kidney, breast, prostate, ovary and thyroid, and are often diagnosed following investigation of pathological fracture. Bone scans will generally confirm diagnosis. In such cases, surgery may be used to correct the fracture, but otherwise management is usually palliative as the primary site is often well developed at this stage.

▶ **Nursing management**

The nursing management of patients with malignant tumours is covered extensively within other chapters (see Chs 33 and 34). Any radical surgery involving the need for a prosthesis or orthosis will require education and psychological preparation for both patients and their families (see pp. 801, 802). Pain relief is obviously a major concern and the psychological aspects of nursing patients with a bone tumour are immense.

Patients managing changes in mobility and body image, and a diagnosis of cancer will require considerable support from the multiprofessional team. Nurses can assist patients with rehabilitation and coping strategies by working closely with physiotherapists, occupational therapists, specialist oncology nurses and, if necessary, specialist palliative care nurses.

TRAUMA – AN OVERVIEW

In the UK, trauma is the leading cause of death in people under the age of 35 years. It is vital that expert management at the scene and in the A&E department is undertaken to enhance the possibility of survival and, in the medium term, the potential for recovery from any traumatic injuries sustained.

Interventions implemented to improve outcomes for the trauma patient include:

- formal hospital-based trauma response protocols for those with major injuries, e.g. pelvic injury
- mobile trauma teams who attend at the scene and stabilize the patient's condition before transfer to the A&E department
- concentrating specialist trauma expertise in larger units
- increasing the knowledge and skills of those initially attending trauma, e.g. paramedical training for ambulance personnel
- advanced trauma life support training for other professionals.

More detailed information relating to primary surveys, immediate resuscitation of the patient with multiple injuries and nurse-led management of minor injuries can be found in Chapter 30.

SPORTS INJURIES

The cost to health services of sports-related injuries both nationally and internationally is substantial due to their frequency. Much has been spent on health promotion relating to playing sport in order to reduce both the incidence and severity of injury (Watson 1997). Some common-sense ways of preventing or reducing the risk of sports injuries are outlined in Health Promotion box 27.2.

Some of the sports injuries discussed below also occur in nonsporting situations. Readers are advised to consult the fracture section, where some injuries are discussed in a different context, and note the differences in aetiology and management needs and priorities.

Sprains and strains form the major group of sports injuries. Therefore prior to exploring specific regional sports injuries,

 HEALTH PROMOTION

27.2 Prevention of sports injuries

Many common-sense measures can reduce the incidence of sports-related injuries and include the following:

- Maintain a healthy weight
- Play within the rules
- Practise safety measures to help prevent falls
- Wear the correct shoes that fit properly
- Replace sports shoes as soon as the tread wears out or the heel wears down on one side
- Do stretching exercises daily
- Be in proper physical condition to play a sport
- Warm up and stretch before participating in any exercise or sporting activity
- Wear appropriate protective equipment when playing
- Avoid exercising or playing sports when tired, unwell or in pain
- Run on even surfaces

it is worth discussing some general principles related to these conditions.

SPRAINS AND STRAINS

Sprains

A sprain is an injury relating to the stretching or tearing of ligaments. It is not uncommon for a sprain to involve more than one ligament. The severity of the injury is dependent on both the extent of injury to each single ligament (i.e. whether the tear is partial or complete) and the number of ligaments involved.

Pathophysiology and aetiology

A sprain can result from a fall, a sudden twist, or a blow to the body that forces a joint out of its normal position. This results in overstretching or tearing of the ligament(s) supporting that joint. Typically, sprains occur when people fall and land on an outstretched arm, slide, land on the side of their foot, or twist a knee with the foot planted firmly on the ground.

Although sprains can occur in both the upper and lower parts of the body, the most common site is the ankle. Ankle sprains often occur during sports or recreational activities and are thought to account for around 85% of the ankle injuries occurring in the UK.

Clinical presentation

A sprain may be classified according to mechanism and symptoms as follows:

- *Grade I* (mild). There is over-stretching or slight tearing of the ligaments with no joint instability. A person with a mild sprain usually experiences minimal pain, swelling and little or no loss of functional ability. Bruising is absent or slight, and the person is usually able to put weight on the affected joint
- *Grade II* (moderate). This results in partial tearing of the ligament and is characterized by bruising, moderate pain, and swelling. A person with a moderate sprain usually has some difficulty putting weight on the affected joint and experiences some loss of function
- *Grade III* (severe sprain). This results in a complete tear or rupture of a ligament. Pain, swelling and bruising are usually severe, and invariably the patient is unable to put weight on the joint.

Specific investigations

Taking a thorough history of the injury is vital in the diagnosis of a sprain, including specific details of forces and direction of the affected joint at the time of injury. Joint stability, movement and the ability to weight-bear will also be examined. An X-ray may be needed to rule out fracture. MRI may very occasionally be used to differentiate between a significant partial injury and a complete tear in a ligament. X-ray and MRI are used in grade II and III sprains.

Strains

A strain is an injury caused by twisting or pulling a muscle or tendon. Severity of a strain ranges from a simple overstretching of the muscle or tendon, to a partial or complete tear.

Pathophysiology and aetiology

Strains can be acute or chronic. An acute strain is caused by trauma or an injury such as a blow to the body. Additionally, and a particular issue in some types of employment, it can be caused by improper lifting or overstressing of the muscles. Chronic strains are usually the result of overuse, i.e. prolonged, repetitive movement of the muscles and tendons.

Contact sports such as football, hockey, boxing and wrestling put people at risk of strains. Gymnastics, tennis, rowing, golf and other sports that require extensive gripping can increase the risk of hand and forearm strains. Elbow strains sometimes occur in people who participate in racquet sports, throwing and contact sports.

Clinical presentation

Symptoms of a strain typically include pain, muscle spasm and muscle weakness. There can also be localized swelling, cramping or inflammation and, with minor or moderate strains, usually some loss of muscle function. Severe strains that partially or completely tear the muscle or tendon are often very painful and disabling.

Medical/surgical management of sprains and strains

The majority of patients with sprains and strains will not require hospitalization and will be managed through the A&E services initially and outpatients on an ongoing basis. X-rays will almost always be taken to exclude an associated fracture. MRI and CT scan may also be utilized, particularly if surgical intervention is potentially indicated.

Essentially, treatment for sprains and strains is similar and can be thought of as having two stages. The goal during the first stage is to reduce swelling and pain. At this stage, patients are usually advised to follow a 'RICE' regimen (rest, ice, compression and elevation) for the first 24–48 hours after the injury. NSAIDs, such as ibuprofen, are often prescribed to help decrease pain and inflammation.

The second stage of treating a sprain or strain is rehabilitation. Clearly the goal of rehabilitation is to improve the condition of the injured part in order to restore functional ability. The health care provider, usually a physiotherapist, will prescribe an exercise programme designed to prevent stiffness, improve and maintain normal range of motion, and restore the joint's normal flexibility and strength. Range of motion or movement refers to the arc of movement of a joint from one extreme position to the other. Therefore, range-of-motion exercises help to increase or maintain flexibility and movement in muscles, tendons, ligaments and joints.

If the patient remains in a hospital environment during this stage, the nurse will be expected to assist in the continuation of the prescribed programmes. It is essential therefore that clear written guidelines be made available in the patient notes to assist all in this role.

The duration of the programme will often be weeks and therefore will usually continue past the patient's discharge date from hospital. It is therefore vital that patients are familiar with all the prescribed exercises and, by discharge date, can perform these without supervision.

The final goal is the return to full daily activities, including sports when appropriate. Patients must work closely with their health care provider or physiotherapist to determine their readiness to return to full activity. Sometimes people are tempted to resume full activity or play sports despite pain or muscle soreness. Returning to full activity before regaining normal range of motion, flexibility and strength increases the risk of re-injury and commonly results in a chronic problem.

The amount of rehabilitation and the time needed for full recovery after a sprain or strain depend on the severity of the injury and individual rates of healing (Webborn et al 1997). For example, a moderate ankle sprain may require 3–6 weeks of rehabilitation before a person can return to full activity. With a severe sprain, it can take 8–12 months before the ligament is fully healed.

INJURIES TO JOINTS

Injuries to joints may be caused by sporting activities, falls, accidents at home and work, road accidents, etc. and may be associated with other injuries such as ligament tears. There are three types of joint injury, namely:

- subluxation (partial dislocation) – active treatment is often not required
- dislocation – the joint must be reduced and immobilized until the soft tissues have healed, and in severe cases may require open repair
- fracture dislocation – often requires fixation of bony fragment.

Individual joint injuries are discussed in the relevant parts of the chapter as appropriate.

REGIONAL SPORTS INJURIES – UPPER LIMB

Rotator cuff tendinitis and tears

Rotator cuff tendinitis and tears are common disorders affecting some of the muscles controlling movement of the arm and shoulder. Rotator cuff tendinitis and tears are often collectively known as 'impingement syndrome'.

Pathophysiology and aetiology

The rotator cuff is a group of four muscles (teres minor, infraspinatus, supraspinatus and subscapularis) that function to stabilize the shoulder and allow the arm to move through a full range of motion. The subacromial bursa lubricates the muscle tendons. Impingement occurs when inflammation or bony spurs narrow the space available for the rotator cuff tendons. The syndrome is divided into three stages:

- stage I – swelling and mild pain
- stage II – inflammation and scarring
- stage III – partial or complete tears of the rotator cuff.

Rotator cuff tendinitis and tears occur from either a sudden violent movement of the shoulder or chronic overuse. Sports commonly associated with this diagnosis include tennis, swimming, softball and football.

Clinical presentation and investigations

A diagnosis of impingement syndrome is considered when patients complain of pain with overhead arm activities such as a tennis serve. A physical examination of the patient will reveal weakness of the rotator cuff muscles and commonly show a decreased range of motion of the shoulder (a painful arc). X-rays are taken to evaluate the bones of the shoulder. Occasionally, an MRI or shoulder arthroscopy is used to confirm the diagnosis (Cohen & Williams 1998).

Medical/surgical management

Most cases of impingement syndrome will respond to rest, anti-inflammatory medication and a directed course of physiotherapy. Resolution of symptoms typically takes several weeks. Return to full activity may, however, take several months depending on the severity of the problem. Occasionally, a local corticosteroid injection may also be used to help alleviate pain in older patients.

If non-operative measures fail to control the pain and restore full function, surgery may be indicated either to remove the scarred and inflamed tissue (bursitis) and/or to enlarge the space available for the rotator cuff by shaving down spurs (subacromial decompression). Repair or reattachment of torn rotator cuff tendons may also be necessary. This may be performed using arthroscopic surgery, which is indicated in patients with severe inflammation and partial rotator cuff tears. Open surgery is more often required for patients with complete rotator cuff tears.

Shoulder dislocation

A shoulder dislocation occurs when the humeral head slips out of its socket (glenoid cavity – see also 'Fractures', p. 828).

Pathophysiology and aetiology

Anterior dislocations are most common. When this occurs, the anterior inferior labrum (cartilage that stabilizes the shoulder) is frequently torn (a Bankart lesion). A dent in the humerus bone (Hill–Sachs lesion) may accompany the Bankart lesion in severe dislocations. Shoulder dislocations can also occur posteriorly and inferiorly. Repeated dislocations and multidirectional shoulder instability are also possible.

Falling is the most common cause of a new shoulder dislocation, but can also occur if the arm is forcibly moved into an awkward position during a violent action such as tackling in rugby. If a dislocation or subluxation occurs with only minor force, recurrent or multidirectional instability must be considered.

Clinical presentation and investigations

Shoulder dislocation is diagnosed when a patient presents with a history of a fall with subsequent pain around the shoulder. Typically there will be bruising, a visible deformity (flattened lateral shoulder outline), patients will support the arm and will be unwilling to move it because of the pain. X-rays are used to confirm the dislocation and rule out any fracture around the shoulder.

Medical/surgical management

For first-time dislocations, reduction under local anaesthesia, a sling and activity restriction for 3–4 weeks comprise the standard form of treatment. A supervised physiotherapy programme is also beneficial to regain full range of movement and activity and to prevent further dislocations by aiming to strengthen the

muscles around the shoulder and upper back that help stabilize the shoulder joint.

For young patients, there is a high risk of recurrent dislocation. For these patients with repeated dislocations, surgery may be indicated. The surgery involves repairing and tightening the structures within the shoulder that were damaged during dislocation. Although an open reconstruction is still the most common procedure, arthroscopic reconstruction techniques are evolving and may be utilized more commonly in the near future.

Frozen shoulder (adhesive capsulitis)

A frozen shoulder is defined as loss of both active (movement without assistance) and passive (movement with assistance) motion, and the correct medical term is adhesive capsulitis.

Pathophysiology and aetiology

The motion loss in frozen shoulder is due to tightening and thickening (fibrosis) of the ligaments and other supporting structures of the shoulder. These changes result in restriction of movement that can severely limit function.

A frozen shoulder may arise after a fracture or other arm injury. It may also be related to a rotator cuff tear, degenerative arthritis or previous shoulder surgery. Many cases of frozen shoulder, however, do not have a known cause. These cases are called idiopathic or primary adhesive capsulitis. Despite not having a known cause, primary adhesive capsulitis can be associated with systemic disorders such as diabetes and cardiovascular disease.

Clinical presentation and investigations

Most cases of frozen shoulder follow a specific pattern. Initially, there is an acute phase that is characterized by significant pain, difficulty sleeping and significant functional impairment. A progressive stiffening phase, when the shoulder motion worsens, follows this. The final phase is the resolution or 'thawing' phase identified by the gradual return of both motion and function. The overall course is variable but can last 12–24 months.

If there is loss of both active and passive movement on physical examination, the diagnosis of a frozen shoulder can be made. The patient will also describe a pattern of pain that is at times severe and at other times mild. The overall function of the shoulder in the acute phase of a frozen shoulder is poor. X-rays are taken to rule out other shoulder disorders such as degenerative arthritis. MRI may also occasionally be used to further evaluate the shoulder.

Medical/surgical management

Anti-inflammatory medications, stretching and physiotherapy are the primary non-operative treatments. Local corticosteroid injections may also form part of non-operative treatment. Manipulation under anaesthesia may be required if non-operative measures fail.

Fractured clavicle

The clavicle (collar bone) is one of the most commonly fractured bones in sports. The common causes are a fall or a direct blow to the bone. Almost any sport can be associated with clavicular fractures, but football, rugby and hockey are the most common (see also 'Fractures', p. 828).

A fracture of the clavicle is diagnosed from a history of a fall associated with pain and deformity around the shoulder, and there will be some swelling. X-rays are used to confirm the fracture. Rarely, further investigation by CT scan may be needed.

Medical/surgical management

Most clavicular fractures can be treated with an arm sling, or a figure-of-eight splint. The typical time for healing is approximately 6–8 weeks. Restriction of sporting activity during this time period is important for healing.

The indications for surgery include open (compound) fractures, severely displaced fractures and some fractures of the lateral part of the clavicle, which may involve some form of a pin or a plate and screws.

Proximal humerus fracture

These are discussed within the section on fractures (p. 828). Generally sports injuries that cause proximal fractures of the humerus occur in contact sports following a fall or a direct blow from a collision. Occasionally, there may be an associated shoulder dislocation.

Some forms of protective sports bracing or padding may prevent some proximal humerus fractures, but the restrictions such protection imposes on most activities considered to have a higher degree of risk may make their use impractical.

Epicondylitis

Epicondylitis is inflammation of the muscles and tendons around the elbow that control the wrist and hand, and even partial tearing of the forearm muscles (see also bursitis). It can occur if the structures are subjected to excessive or repetitive stress. It would usually arise from overuse of the tendons and muscles. Occasionally, it may begin after a sudden, traumatic movement of the elbow or wrist. It may affect the structures at the lateral (outer) or medial (inner) aspect of the elbow.

Lateral epicondylitis ('tennis elbow') is associated with tennis, other racquet sports and weight training. Incorrect technique or handle size in racquet sports may also lead to this disorder.

Medial epicondylitis ('golfer's elbow'), which is primarily an overuse injury, may occur after a sudden, traumatic movement of the elbow or wrist. Golf and improper lifting techniques are commonly associated with this disorder.

Clinical presentation

In lateral epicondylitis there is pain and tenderness on the lateral aspect of the elbow. The onset of pain from the inflammatory process may arise and progress suddenly or gradually. The pain will worsen with any attempt either to play racquet sports or lift heavy objects.

Medial epicondylitis is characterized by pain and tenderness on the medial aspect of the elbow and also may arise and progress suddenly or gradually. Direct pressure over the beginning portion of the muscles that control the wrist and hand reproduces the pain.

Ruling out nerve injuries or other disorders around the elbow is essential. X-ray may be used to check the state of the bones in the affected area.

Medical/surgical management

Most cases of epicondylitis will respond to rest, anti-inflammatory medication and activity restriction. A compressive forearm band that reduces the tension at the elbow is also frequently used. Physiotherapy designed to stretch and strengthen the forearm muscles after controlling the inflammatory phase may be of added benefit. A local corticosteroid injection may be tried if the plan outlined above fails to alleviate the symptoms.

Surgical intervention may be considered following failure of non-operative measures. A number of procedures have been designed to excise the inflammatory and scar tissue. Repair or reattachment of the remaining tendon to its origin on bone at the elbow may also be required.

Acromioclavicular (shoulder) separation

An acromioclavicular (AC) separation is an injury to the ligaments that connect the clavicle to the acromion (part of the scapula).

A fall on the point of the shoulder is the typical mechanism. A direct blow to the shoulder or a fall on an outstretched hand may also produce one. Football and hockey are common sports associated with AC separations.

Clinical presentation

An AC separation is diagnosed by a history of pain, tenderness and swelling at the AC joint. If the injury is severe, significant deformity may occur. X-rays are taken to confirm the injury and rule out fractures around the shoulder.

Medical/surgical management

Most patients can be treated with a sling and activity restriction followed by a physiotherapy programme. Recovery may take 6–8 weeks or perhaps longer. Surgery and internal fixation (using a screw) may be indicated in injuries involving a complete tear.

Maintaining good strength and stability of the shoulder and upper back muscles may help prevent some AC separations, and information regarding this should be part of any rehabilitation programme to minimize the risk of recurrence.

Biceps tendon tear

A biceps tendon tear is a rupture at its insertion into the elbow at the radius. Ruptures at the elbow are usually due to a sudden violent straightening force applied to an arm that is trying to bend. This can happen when a heavy object falls on the arm, an attempt is made to catch an object with an open hand, or during contact sports or martial arts.

Clinical presentation

Biceps tendon tears are diagnosed by a history of an injury associated with immediate pain in the front of the elbow. A 'snap' or 'pop' may also occur. Typically, there is bruising and swelling in the elbow. Other common presenting problems include a difficulty in fully straightening the elbow or weakness in bending the elbow. Usually, a biceps tendon tear can be diagnosed through the history and physical examination. Occasionally, however, MRI is needed to differentiate between a partial and a complete tear.

Medical/surgical management

Non-operative treatment consists of gentle range-of-motion exercises and anti-inflammatory medication. This type of treatment typically results in the return of at least 60% of the normal strength of the biceps tendon. Operative treatment is indicated for patients who wish to try to restore original strength to the biceps tendon. The surgical reconstruction is complicated, involving an associated risk of potential damage to the nerves and blood vessels of the elbow and hand, and should only be performed by an experienced surgeon. After the repair, the patient is splinted for a period of time and then begins a structured rehabilitation programme under the direction of a physiotherapist.

Fractures of the distal radius and/or ulna

Again, these are discussed in the section on 'Fractures'. Falls and direct contact are common aetiologies in sporting activities.

REGIONAL SPORTS INJURIES – LOWER LIMB

Hip flexor injury (iliopsoas injury)

The iliopsoas (comprising the iliacus and psoas muscles) is a large muscle that begins deep within the pelvis and inserts into the top of the femur, enabling flexion at the hip.

Typically hip flexor injury occurs as a result of hyperextension of the leg at the hip. It can occur with almost any sport, but is particularly common in tackling in rugby and collisions in football when a player is attempting to kick a ball.

Clinical presentation

Patients will present with a sudden sharp pain in the groin area. Bending or flexing the hip against resistance on examination increases the pain. Often, in severe injuries, patients cannot put weight on the affected leg.

Medical/surgical management

Almost all hip flexor injuries can be treated with rest and a progressive rehabilitation programme. This consists of 3–4 days of RICE and then gentle stretching followed by strengthening exercises. Depending upon the severity of the injury, patients may be able to resume light training within 4 weeks.

Hamstring strain

The hamstring muscles (semimembranosus, semitendinosus, and biceps femoris) span the back of the thigh and insert into bone around the knee. These muscles function together to help flex and control the knee. Hamstring strains ('pulled hamstring') are very common and typically occur while running or jumping, among other activities. Sprinting and football are sports commonly associated with hamstring strains. A lack of warm-up and stretching prior to activity is a common cause amongst amateur athletes.

Clinical presentation

Commonly there is a history of a sudden onset of pain in the back of the leg above the knee, and there is pain while walking and tenderness around the area of the muscle strain. Additionally if the injury is severe, a balled-up portion of the muscle may be felt or even seen along the back part of the thigh under the skin.

Medical/surgical management

Almost all hamstring strains can be treated without surgery. Immediate management is with RICE for the first 2 days with control of pain, and gradual and gentle restoration of range of movement occurs over the first week. Flexibility will be increased over the following week through quadriceps and hamstring stretches and thereafter return to various activities will be dependent of the individual patient.

Knee injuries – an overview

The knee joint is stabilized by four ligaments: the anterior cruciate ligament (ACL), posterior cruciate ligament (PCL), medial collateral ligament (MCL) and lateral collateral ligament (LCL). These ligaments function in collaboration with the muscles and menisci (semilunar cartilages of the knee) to help control motion in the knee.

Damage to these structures, resulting in knee injuries, is the most common of all joint injuries in sporting activity. Falls from heights or a blow to the knee during almost any contact sport can result in a fracture. As well as the conditions discussed below, which are predominantly acute sporting injuries, there are other overuse injuries, e.g. iliotibial band friction syndrome, articular cartilage injury (osteochondritis dissecans) and patella tendinitis ('jumper's knee'). These are beyond the scope of this chapter but may be seen in an orthopaedic or sports clinic environment.

Anterior cruciate ligament tear

Located in the centre of the knee, the ACL is a strong band of tissue that limits the chance of hyperextending the tibia beyond the femur. An ACL injury may result from a violent rotation often combined with sudden deceleration, which can occur when the person undertaking the sporting activity plants a foot and suddenly changes direction. The ACL can also tear if the knee is hyperextended. Therefore, almost any sport that involves jumping, cutting or twisting movements involves a risk of an ACL rupture. Basketball, skiing, football and rugby are among the most common sports associated with this injury.

Patients may describe feeling a 'popping' in the knee at the time of injury. There will be immediate swelling with significant effusion and reduced ability to fully straighten the knee immediately after the injury. ACL injuries often occur in association with fractures or a meniscus tear. The Lachman test is the best way to assess a knee for an acute ACL tear (see Table 27.3).

Medial collateral ligament tear

The MCL helps to prevent outward movement of the leg at the knee. Common causes of MCL injury include a hard blow to the outer aspect of the lower thigh, buckling the knee inward, and during any motion that forcefully moves the leg outward at the knee, e.g. in football, rugby or skiing. There is pain accompanied by mild-to-moderate swelling along the inner aspect of the knee. MCL injuries are sometimes associated with injuries involving the ACL, PCL or meniscus, and this should be borne in mind during examination.

Posterior cruciate ligament tear

The PCL is located in the back of the knee and is responsible for limiting backward movement of the tibia. PCL tears are relatively rare as an isolated injury and occur most often in rugby players, hockey players and skiers. A tear of the PCL may occur via two classic mechanisms. The first is falling on a bent knee, pushing the tibia backwards and tearing the PCL. The second mechanism is when the knee is hyperextended. Finally, the PCL may be torn in conjunction with the ACL via a violent twisting of the knee.

PCL injuries are diagnosed by eliciting a history of one of the above mechanisms. The physical examination will show moderate knee swelling and pain with motion.

Meniscus tear

The menisci deepen the joint surfaces, help to stabilize the knee and act as shock-absorbers. Tears can result from a sudden traumatic injury such as a violent twisting of the knee. Tears may also occur without significant trauma due to repeated small injuries to the cartilage or degeneration in older patients. These injuries can occur during almost any sport or activity. Injuries to the menisci may also be associated with ligament injuries such as a MCL sprain or ACL tear.

Meniscus tears are typically associated with pain along the inner or outer aspect of the knee, with mild-to-moderate swelling. Patients will often describe clicking or locking of the knee. X-rays are taken to rule out fractures and an MRI scan may be used to confirm the tear.

Overview of medical/surgical management of knee injuries

Many knee injuries will respond to *conservative non-operative* treatment regimens, which may include:

- RICE
- anti-inflammatory drugs to control pain and reduce swelling
- aspiration of the effusion, which may accelerate recovery
- physiotherapy after pain and swelling subsides – a programme is prescribed to increase range of motion of the knee and to strengthen specific muscle groups, e.g. quadriceps and hamstrings. Sport-specific drills in the later treatment stages help to restore balance and coordination
- a brace may be used prior to commencing physiotherapy and is advised when resuming sports-related activities.

Components from this regimen are indicated for patients with limited activity goals or with partial tears.

Operative treatment is indicated for:

- individuals whose knee 'gives way' during daily living activities
- those wishing to return to sports involving cutting and twisting
- sporting professionals
- those with severe injuries, e.g. complete tears or injuries involving damage to more than one structure, ligament or meniscus
- injuries that fail to respond to conservative treatment.

The combination of minimally invasive surgical techniques and more aggressive rehabilitation has improved the outcomes for knee surgery such as ACL reconstruction. The three most common ways to reconstruct the ACL are with a bone-patellar tendon-bone autograft (a graft using tissue transplanted from one site to another in the same individual), a hamstring

autograft, or with some form of allograft (a graft using tissue transplanted from a donor of the same species) such as patellar tendon and Achilles tendon. Screws or other devices are then used to secure the graft in position inside the knee.

Rehabilitation begins within a few days of surgery. Restoring full range of motion of the knee is the initial goal, often with the use of a brace. Strength, endurance and coordination drills are added as the patient improves. Typically, patients may return to activities of daily living with 1–3 weeks and progress to full sporting activity in 6 months depending upon the surgeon's preference and the patient's recovery (Clasby & Young 1997).

MCL and PCL tears associated with damage to other ligaments may require surgical reconstruction. Meniscus tears that do not respond to conservative regimens and those associated with ACL injuries are treated surgically. Arthroscopic surgical techniques are used to remove or repair the torn cartilage. Several surgical techniques are available, the most common being partial removal of the meniscus (meniscectomy) or repair.

Problems affecting the Achilles tendon – an overview

The Achilles tendon is the common distal tendon of the gastrocnemius and soleus muscles of the calf and inserts into the calcaneus. It may become inflamed (tendinitis) or may tear.

Achilles tendinitis

Excessive running and jumping, especially without proper stretching and strengthening, are the most common causes of Achilles tendinitis. Uphill running, in particular, can precipitate this condition.

Achilles tendinitis is diagnosed by a history of pain behind the ankle when engaging in running or jumping. It is confirmed by tenderness over the Achilles tendon and weakness when testing the calf muscles.

Most cases of Achilles tendinitis can be treated without surgery. Rest, anti-inflammatory medication and stretching are the initial non-operative measures. Physiotherapy in combination with orthotics (shoe inserts) may also be needed. If surgery is indicated, this consists of removing the degenerated portions of the tendon followed by an aggressive postoperative rehabilitation programme. Warming up before exercising and proper stretching are essential to the prevention of Achilles tendinitis.

Achilles tendon tear

Achilles tendon tears typically occur during sports that involve cutting and jumping, such as basketball, tennis or rugby. These tears are the result of a violent contraction of the large calf muscles and usually do not involve any contact with another player. In some cases, Achilles tendon ruptures occur after a long history of Achilles tendinitis.

Achilles tendon tears are diagnosed by a history of a sudden injury followed by a 'pop' felt behind the ankle. The tear is confirmed by squeezing the calf muscles. If the foot does not move, the tendon is probably torn. Occasionally, an MRI or ultrasound is needed to establish that the tendon is indeed ruptured.

For inactive patients, patients who are unsuitable for surgery or those who do not wish to accept surgery, non-operative care is given. This care involves a cast for 4–6 weeks followed by rehabilitation. The risks of non-operative care include a higher risk of re-rupture and possible loss of strength with 'pushing off' activities.

For active patients, surgical reattachment of the torn tendon is recommended. It involves a 75–100 cm incision behind the ankle, suturing the torn tendon ends together and then splinting for 4–6 weeks. The risks inherent in the postoperative period include infection, poor wound healing and scarring. The benefits are a lower risk of re-rupture and a better chance of restoring full power to the leg.

Ankle sprain

The talus bone and the ends of the lower leg bones (tibia and fibula) form the ankle joint. Lateral and medial ligaments support this joint.

Pathophysiology and aetiology

Most ankle sprains happen when the foot turns inward as a person runs, turns, falls or lands on the ankle after a jump, often on an uneven surface. Equipment and surface conditions may therefore also play a role. This type of sprain is termed an inversion injury. One or more of the lateral ligaments are injured, usually the anterior talofibular ligament. The calcaneofibular ligament is the second most frequently torn ligament. Most sprains stretch or tear the lateral ligaments of the ankle. Occasionally, the ligaments in between the bones of the ankle rupture, and rarely only the medial ligament will tear. Sports most commonly associated with ankle sprains include basketball, rugby and football.

Clinical presentation

Ankle sprain should be considered when patients give a history of 'turning' their ankle accompanied by sudden pain and swelling. A physical examination will reveal point tenderness over the injured ligaments with bruising.

Medical/surgical management

Most ankle sprains can be treated conservatively with RICE. A short course of muscle strengthening and balance exercises is essential in order to prevent repeat sprains. Occasionally, surgery is needed to re-establish the stability of the ankle to either repair or reconstruct the ligaments.

Ankle fracture

Ankle fractures result when the ankle is forced inward or outward past its normal range of motion. Modes and mechanisms of injury are as for sprains but with more severe forces at the time of injury (see 'Fractures' below).

▶ Nursing management of the sports injury

Many of the less severe sports injuries will be managed within the A&E department and as an outpatient. Initial assessment would be as for any patient. In addition to RICE, as previously described, patients will require education regarding cast or splint prior to discharge home as well as follow-up instructions.

In the main, those attending orthopaedic wards tend to be those requiring surgical intervention or more extensive investigation or rehabilitation. Preoperative nursing management will therefore comprise a continuation of the principles of RICE, preparation for surgery (see Ch. 29) and assistance with any further investigations.

Postoperative management will obviously be injury-specific as regards the exact treatment modalities and prescribed mobility regimens. The nurse's role will be to assist in the rehabilitation of the patient over the 24-hour period, ensuring treatment modalities are adhered to. Patients will need to be educated about their particular orthosis, if required, or about care of a cast, use of mobility aids and medications required to minimize pain and facilitate return to pre-injury function in all aspects of self-care. A key part of the rehabilitation of sports injury is that of prevention of recurrence; education on reducing risk in the future is therefore also a pivotal nursing role. A useful tactic may be to explore the sequence of events leading up to the current injury, examining what went wrong and assisting patients to devise strategies accordingly.

FRACTURES

A fracture is a break in the continuity of a bone.

CLASSIFICATION

Broadly speaking, fractures may be classified into two types:

- open (compound) – a fracture in which a laceration in the skin or mucous membranes communicates with the fracture haematoma, thus providing a route for the entry of bacteria to the fracture site
- closed (simple).

There are essentially three causes of fracture:

- trauma – direct or indirect
- stress or fatigue fractures – caused by repeated stresses with excessive frequency
- pathological fractures – occur in an abnormal or diseased bone resulting in a fracture caused by limited force, e.g. osteoporosis, tumour (see p. 819, 820).

There are various ways in which to describe a fracture in terms of the mechanical forces involved. The commonly used descriptions are provided in Box 27.5.

Another means by which fractures may be classified is according to the pattern of the fracture as it presents on an X-ray (see Box 27.6).

Box 27.5 Descriptions of fractures

- *Shift* – loss of alignment in the cortices of the shaft
- *Angulation* – loss of normal longitudinal axis of the shaft; this may be anterior, posterior, medial or lateral
- *Shortening* – this may be due to overlap of the fracture fragments or to impaction at the fracture site
- *Rotation* – this refers to the rotation of the distal fragment along the long axis of the bone, which may be external or internal
- *Distraction* – rarely arises from the injury but may be due to excessive manipulation during the treatment

Box 27.6 Fracture patterns

- *Comminuted* – at least three fragments present
- *Greenstick* – these occur in children, a common site being the forearm. The bone is only fractured half through on the convex side of the bend
- *Transverse* – runs at right angles to the long axis of bone, often as a result of direct trauma
- *Oblique* – fracture line is less than 90° to the long axis of bone, often as a result of indirect trauma
- *Spiral* – fracture curves in spiral fashion, again usually through indirect trauma
- *Complicated* – surrounding organs or structures are damaged
- *Avulsion* – may be produced by a sudden muscle contraction or ligamentous attachment pulling off the portion of bone to which it is attached
- *Depressed* (commonly to the skull) – as a result of a sharp localized blow
- *Compression* (crush) – commonly applied to vertebral bodies or ankle; usually indirect trauma, e.g. falls from a height
- *Segmental* (double fracture) – fractured at two distinct levels
- *Impacted* – one fragment is driven into another; may occur in high-impact long bone fractures, e.g. femur or humerus

CLINICAL PRESENTATION

The signs and symptoms of a fracture include:

- local pain and tenderness
- swelling
- bruising
- crepitus (grating noise heard when the broken bone moves)
- deformity, including shortening
- abnormal mobility of the affected part
- loss of functional ability to perform daily living tasks
- soft tissue damage.

FRACTURE HEALING

The process of fracture healing is summarized in Figure 27.8 (see also Ch. 10, wound healing). As a general rule of thumb, a fracture should heal in 8 weeks. This can be doubled in lower limb fractures, and take half the time in children. The healing process may be slower or perhaps even incomplete in older people (Gillies 1999). The risk of poor healing is a major indication for surgery despite the increased anaesthetic risks, because of the potentially life-threatening effects of prolonged immobilization through bed rest.

Two primary factors that may promote fracture healing and that the nurse may directly influence are:

- promotion of adequate nutrition – particularly protein, vitamins A, C and D, and calcium
- promotion of patient compliance with immobility and interventions designed to restrict movement of the affected

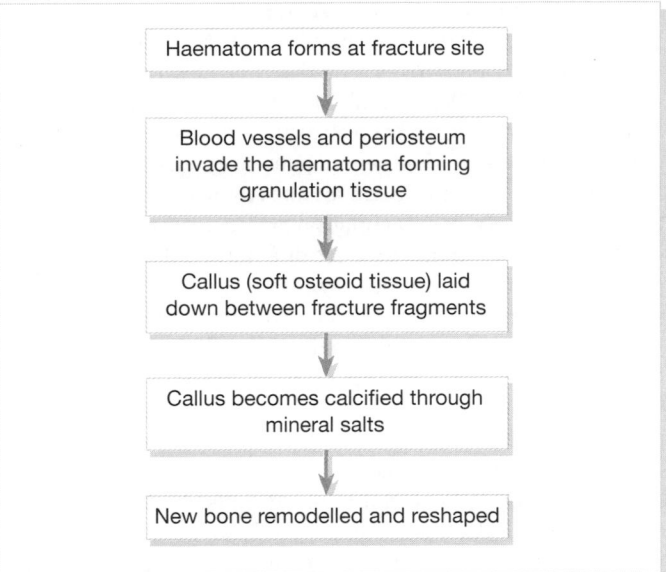

Figure 27.8 Fracture healing.

area – excessive mobility of a fracture site may delay the healing process and may result in non-union of a fracture.

COMPLICATIONS OF FRACTURES

The complications of fractures may be classified as immediate (at the time of injury), early (within hours or days) and late (within weeks or months).

Immediate complications of fractures

- Haemorrhage – blood loss from bone itself combined with loss from damage to surrounding tissues, e.g. tibia (0.5–1.5 L), femur (1–2.5 L), pelvis (1.5–3 L)
- Damage to arteries and nerves, e.g. brachial artery and median nerve in supracondylar fracture of the humerus (see p. 825), aorta in fractures of thoracic (T) vertebrae (T4–5), or in fractures of the sternum
- Damage to surrounding tissues, e.g. pneumothorax in rib fractures, spinal cord damage in vertebral fractures, brain injury in skull fractures (see Ch. 14).

Early complications of fractures

- Wound infection
- Fat embolism – this may occur, particularly with multiple fractures of long bones. Patients will present with petechial haemorrhages affecting the skin and mucosa within 72 hours of injury, hypoxia, restlessness, tachycardia and mental confusion
- Generalized problems of immobilization, e.g. pressure ulcer, DVT, chest infection
- Compartment syndrome – acute compartment syndrome may occur in any muscle compartment but in the context of musculoskeletal conditions is more commonly associated with limb fractures. This condition is caused by an increase in the tissue pressure due either to bleeding into the soft tissues or to oedema and inflammation within the

compartment. The increase in compartment content results in a rise in tissue pressure above that of the capillary pressure. This leads to decreased perfusion with subsequent ischaemia. The affected limb may be pale, painful, pulseless or have altered neurological sensation, and in all cases patients complain of increased pain on extension of the affected limb. Diagnosis can also be confirmed through measuring intra-compartmental pressures; if this is greater than 40 mmHg in the presence of a normal diastolic pressure then compartment syndrome is present. Treatment involves urgent decompression through fasciotomy (division of the fascia [connective tissue] surrounding and separating muscles). Hence the nursing intervention in compartment syndrome involves:

— monitoring neurovascular status of the affected limb (see Reflective Practice box 27.3)
— informing medical staff of any deficits obtained in the neurovascular assessment
— post-surgical wound management following fasciotomy.

Late complications of fractures

- Delayed union – when the fracture does not unite within the expected time
- Malunion – when the bone has united soundly but in the wrong position. Surgery may be required depending on potential disability and outcome
- Non-union – may not be a serious problem in non-weight-bearing bones. A painless, false joint may occur. Internal fixation or bone grafting may be required
- Deformity
- Secondary osteoarthritis of adjacent and distant joints
- Aseptic/avascular necrosis – this may occur particularly following fractures to the femoral head, scaphoid and talus; it results from disruption to the blood supply to the bone following the fracture. The joint is destroyed following collapse of the bone. It will result in pain and stiffness in the affected joint.

OVERVIEW OF THE MANAGEMENT OF FRACTURES

There are six common treatment modalities in fracture patients:

- non-rigid methods of support, e.g. slings, bandages, strapping

R|Я REFLECTIVE PRACTICE

27.3 Neurovascular assessment

Assessment of 'colour, warmth, sensation and movement' is often recorded in patient care plans and commonly involves placing a tick in a box on an observation chart.

Student activities

- Do you and your colleagues know why this is done?
- How easy is it to assess a quality such as warmth or colour?
- What level of change should be reported to the medical staff?

- continuous traction – skin or skeletal types
- plaster fixation
- internal surgical fixation
- external surgical fixation
- casts/bracing.

The specific implications for nursing of individual treatments are discussed earlier in this chapter.

Indications for surgical management of fractures

There is much debate in the medical literature about whether to manage fractures through surgical or non-surgical (conservative) techniques. As a general rule, the following seven criteria are used to determine whether patients would benefit from surgical intervention:

- the presence of open (compound) fractures
- where closed manipulation is unlikely to be successful in reducing the fracture
- if the fracture is unstable, i.e. the ligaments and surrounding structures are unable to support the affected part in its natural alignment
- time factor, e.g. if non-operative management involves prolonged immobilization, or in patients with metastatic disease
- soft tissue management
- management of complications, e.g. vascular or head injuries
- surgical skill available.

Further indications are provided, where appropriate, in specific descriptions of fracture management.

FRACTURES OF THE LOWER LIMB

Fractures to the femur and severe fractures of other lower limb bones affect people of all ages. In older adults, they often occur as a result of falls and may be associated with osteoporosis. High-impact road accidents are a common cause in younger adults. The general principles of nursing management following these fractures are similar, although the degree to which life is threatened will depend often on the presence or otherwise of associated injury.

Intracapsular fractures of the femoral neck

Intracapsular fractures of the femoral neck are one of the most common fractures in the older population. The usual cause is a fall on the area of the greater trochanter and is particularly seen in women aged between 60 and 80 years.

Femoral neck fractures may be classified as follows:

- grade 1 – incomplete impacted fracture of the femoral neck
- grade 2 – complete undisplaced fracture
- grade 3 – complete fracture with moderate displacement
- grade 4 – complete fracture with severe displacement.

Patients will present with moderate to severe pain in the hip, the limb may be shortened and externally rotated, and they will be unable to walk.

Surgical management

Generally the principles of optimum treatment are a successful reduction and fixation, and early mobilization. Older people with grade 1 and 2 fractures are commonly treated with AO screws, and those with grades 3 or 4 are treated with a hemi-arthroplasty. In younger patients, all grades are usually managed with AO cannulated screws.

Intertrochanteric fractures of the femur

These fractures are, by definition, extracapsular. As with fractures of the femoral neck, they are invariably caused by falls onto the greater trochanter. The fracture runs between the lesser and greater trochanter and the proximal fragment tends to be displaced.

These fractures are treated by surgical reduction using a dynamic hip screw.

▶ Nursing/surgical management – hip fractures

Following an extensive systematic review of available evidence, the Scottish Intercollegiate Guidelines Network (1997) produced a national clinical guideline for use in Scotland for the management of older people with a fractured hip. The recommendations from the review are outlined in Guidelines for Care Priorities box 27.1.

The use of hip protectors to reduce the incidence of hip fractures in older people who are likely to fall and/or have established osteoporosis is currently being evaluated (see Evidence-based Practice box 27.1).

Femoral shaft fractures

This is usually a fracture of young adults, often following road traffic accidents, and the fracture pattern may vary considerably depending on the cause (see Box 27.6). A spiral fracture is usually produced by a fall in which the foot has been anchored whilst a twisting force is transmitted to the femur. Transverse and oblique fractures are often due to direct trauma. In addition, the fractures may be comminuted or segmental. Femoral shaft fractures tend to result in significant haemorrhage and up to 1.5 litres may be lost from the fracture alone. Clearly, if other injuries are present, which is common, further haemorrhage from other injuries will usually result in hypovolaemic shock (see Ch. 9).

Surgical management

Urgent fluid replacement, pain relief and immobilization of the fracture, often in a Thomas' splint, should be the initial objectives of emergency management.

There are various methods of treatment, which include traction, traction followed by bracing, intramedullary nailing or external fixators.

Supracondylar fractures of the femur

These are the result of either direct trauma or, in older people, a fall. On examination of the patient, the knee will be swollen and very painful. The fracture is seen just above the femoral condyles on X-ray, and the pattern is commonly transverse or comminuted, with the distal fragment often tilted backwards. The risk of acute compartment syndrome is significant and therefore neurovascular assessment is paramount.

Distal femoral fractures

Fractures that are only slightly displaced or which reduce easily with the knee in flexion may be treated satisfactorily by skeletal traction through the proximal tibia. If closed reduction fails, open reduction and fixation with a dynamic condylar screw may be needed.

Postoperatively there must be radiological evidence that the fracture has united prior to unprotected weight-bearing.

 GUIDELINES FOR CARE PRIORITIES

27.1 Management of older people with a hip fracture

(Adapted from National clinical guideline: Management of elderly people with a fractured hip – Scottish Intercollegiate Guidelines Network 1997.)

Summary of recommendations
Prevention
- Calcium and vitamin D supplements in older people/ house-bound
- Prescribe bisphosphonates for older people with evidence of osteoporosis
- Hormone replacement therapy (HRT) for postmenopausal woman
- Weight-bearing exercise
- Discourage smoking and excess alcohol

Prevention of falls
- Interventions, e.g. certain types of balance exercise for those identified at risk
- Polypharmacy should be avoided

Preoperative management
- Rapid transfer through A&E departments, e.g. 'fast-tracking' (see Ch. 30)
- Pressure-relieving mattresses available
- Surgery performed within 24 hours
- Prophylactic antibiotic cover
- DVT prophylaxis

Postoperative management
- Monitor and relieve pain
- Supplemental oxygen
- Maintain adequate hydration
- Early mobilization
- Multidisciplinary collaboration in management

Student activities
Look at the Scottish recommendations relating to hip fracture following a systematic review. In the context of ensuring that management of patients is based on best evidence, compare one aspect of current practice in your clinical area against the recommendations, e.g. calcium and vitamin D supplements for the house-bound, surgery within 24 hours, the use of pressure-relieving mattresses or adequate hydration.

EVIDENCE-BASED PRACTICE

27.1 Hip protectors as protection against hip fractures in older people

Parker et al (2001) report seven randomized or quasi-randomized controlled trials comparing the use of hip protectors with a control group to determine whether they reduce the incidence of hip fractures in older people after a fall.

Main points

- Over 3500 participants, living at home or in a variety of care settings.
- The studies involved older people in Scandinavia, UK, Australia and Japan.
- A summation of the results from six trials produced an incidence of hip fractures as follows: 2.2% in those wearing hip protectors, and 6.2% in the control groups. It was not possible, however, to show whether the difference between the treatment and control groups was statistically significant, because many participants were allocated according to the care setting (cluster randomization).
- The authors report that no important adverse effects of wearing the protectors were reported.
- Long-term compliance was poor.

Conclusions

- Hip protectors appear to lessen the risk of hip fracture in high-risk groups.
- It is not known if the results can be generalized to other populations.
- The reviewers state that cost-effectiveness is unclear, but results from trials in progress may resolve this issue.
- User acceptability is a problem in terms of practicality and comfort.

Student activities

- Find out if hip protectors are used in your area of practice.
- What practical aspects of wearing the protectors might be a problem for the older age group, often with mobility and other problems, who are most likely to benefit?
- Search the nursing literature for articles describing the use of hip protectors and pay special attention to accounts of minimizing practical problems.

Reference

Parker MJ, Gillespie LD, Gillespie WJ. Hip protectors for preventing hip fractures in the elderly (Cochrane Review). In: The Cochrane Library, 4. Oxford: Update Software; 2001.

Tibial plateau fractures

These generally occur in road traffic accidents or may be due to a fall from a height in which the knee is forced in either direction. Six types of fracture pattern are described.

Medical/surgical management

Management will be dependent on the fracture type and will involve traction, bracing or surgical intervention, with open reduction, plating and bone grafting (often taken from the iliac crest) if significant depression is present.

Fractures of the patella

Fractures of the patella are more commonly associated with direct trauma following a fall on the knee. Management will depend on whether or not the fracture is displaced. Undisplaced fractures may be managed in a cast for 4 weeks. Displaced fractures will usually require surgery, which often involves the use of circalage wire and screws, or K-wire with tension banding if there is disruption of the extensor mechanism.

Fractures of the tibia and fibula

Open fractures of the tibia are more common than in any other long bone due to the tibia's subcutaneous location. Blunt trauma is the major mode of injury, the fracture pattern being variable depending upon the exact nature of the injury. Fractures of the shaft of the tibia are often of a spiral pattern, as they are usually caused by rotational forces. Fractures resulting from direct trauma, often in road traffic accidents, frequently involve associated fractures of the fibula. If the fibula is intact then there is usually little displacement of the tibial fracture. In this case, the fracture may often be managed conservatively with an above-knee cast. Fractures of the fibula alone may be due to direct violence or may occur in association with external rotation and abduction injuries of the ankle. It is therefore important to exclude ankle injuries in the presence of fibular fractures.

Medical/surgical management

As with other fractures, different fracture patterns will necessitate different methods of treatment. The objectives of management are to:

- limit soft tissue damage and preserve skin cover
- monitor for compartment syndrome
- obtain fracture alignment
- preserve the function of the adjacent joints.

Treatment modalities for these injuries are:

- plaster application following reduction
- skeletal traction by insertion of a pin in the calcaneus (os calcis) with subsequent immobilization in plaster
- internal fixation by means of plates or intramedullary devices
- external fixation, e.g. using Ilizarov frame (see p. 804).

The indications for operative management of tibial shaft fractures include:

- associated intra-articular and shaft fractures
- open fractures
- major bone loss
- neurovascular injury
- compartment syndrome
- floating knee.

Box 27.7 Classification of ankle fractures

- *First degree* – a fracture of one malleolus, no talar shift with a stable ankle mortise
- *Second degree* – bimalleolar fracture or a fracture of one malleolus with ligament tear leading to instability of the ankle
- *Third degree* – trimalleolar fracture with instability in the mediolateral and anteroposterior direction
- *Fourth degree* – suprasyndesmotic fracture of the fibula, possible tearing of the inferior tibio-fibular ligament and diastasis
- *Fifth degree* – vertical impaction fracture of the distal articular surface of the tibia

Fractures of the ankle

The ankle is usually injured by indirect forces applied with the foot externally rotated, inverted or everted. The important factor in ankle fractures is the stability of the ankle mortise. The classification of ankle fractures is outlined in Box 27.7.

Medical/surgical management

If the mortise is stable, i.e. no abnormal movement of the talus is possible, the injury is usually easily managed. The aim of treatment in such cases is to protect the ankle until healing has occurred. However, if the mortise is disrupted then it must be reconstructed and held until bone and soft tissue healing is complete.

The aims of treatment are to restore the position of the talus within the ankle mortise, to ensure the joint line is parallel to the ground, the articular surface is in normal congruity and to stabilize the fracture until healing has occurred. Open reduction and internal fixation will achieve this aim in the majority of injuries where there is at least a second-degree fracture.

When there is a fracture dislocation of the ankle, nerves and blood vessels are likely to be compromised by the displaced bone. It is vital that the dislocation is reduced immediately using opioid analgesia and inhaled Entonox. This should be done within the A&E department if possible – time should not be wasted obtaining X-rays (Dellacorte et al 1994). It is not important that exact anatomical reduction is achieved as long as the skin tension is reduced and the circulation is restored. Following reduction, the foot is stabilized in a below-knee back-slab.

▶ Nursing management – lower limb fractures

A full primary and secondary survey is necessary in all cases following trauma (see Ch. 30). Nurses will be involved in the coordination or administration of standard preoperative interventions that comprise the following:

- ensuring venous access
- i.m. or i.v. analgesia, e.g. morphine with an antiemetic
- a pillow placed under the affected limb or splint may make the patient more comfortable
- monitoring of neurovascular status
- monitoring of vital signs
- X-rays of the limb – in addition, a chest X-ray and ECG may be needed

- FBC, urea and electrolyte levels, and also group and cross-matching will be required for all injuries likely to proceed to surgical intervention
- consent for surgery, starve for trauma list and inform theatre
- provision of information and support for patient and family.

Postoperative nursing management includes monitoring of neurovascular status and for other secondary complications, e.g. fat embolus, DVT, pressure ulcer (Hefti 1995). Pain control and evaluation of the effectiveness of prescribed regimens are vital. Often a patient-controlled analgesia system will be utilized in the early postoperative period (see Ch. 7). The nurse may be required to assist in undertaking further tests or tests on the patient's progress, e.g. follow-up radiological or blood investigations.

Assistance with activities of daily living is required until patients are able to resume these independently. If they are unable to do this at discharge, the nurse will be responsible for educating them to be verbally independent, i.e. to be able to dictate their needs to others, as well as for training of relatives and/or carers. This includes providing assistance with regaining optimum mobility according to the prescribed regimen. This may include particular movements conducive to prevention of dislocation of a prosthesis, e.g. a hip prosthesis (Santy 1998).

Education of the patient, e.g. regarding the wearing of specific orthoses, care of casts, medication and prevention of secondary conditions, is a fundamental role which will vary according to the specific condition and treatment modality. Collaborative working with other health care professionals is vital, particularly with regard to reporting patient progress with prescribed treatment, with particular reference to mobility goals.

Patients will often require psychological support in adapting to alterations in body image. Sometimes these alterations will only be temporary, e.g. in the case of an external fixator, but at other times, e.g. in the case of amputees or those with altered neurological function, they will be permanent.

Finally, referral to community services and discharge/ follow-up planning are essential, particularly in older orthopaedic patients who may require additional home support. There are some examples of early discharge and 'hospital at home' schemes, e.g. for hip fractures, whereby patients are discharged early with additional community nursing and carer support whilst still undertaking some of the rehabilitation exercises and mobility regimens. Older patients should be specifically followed up to address the issues of the prevention and treatment of osteoporosis and to aim to reduce the incidence of falls.

UPPER LIMB INJURIES – FRACTURES AND DISLOCATIONS

Upper limb fractures affect all age groups. In older people, they often result from falls onto the outstretched hand and may be associated with osteoporosis, e.g. wrist fractures. In younger adults, they may be caused while playing sport, or in road traffic accidents or accidents at home or at work.

Nursing management of upper limb injuries requiring surgery is consolidated and covered after the discussion of individual injuries. Readers should consult the section on 'Nursing patients in a cast' for the principles of care for patients requiring a cast (p. 800).

Fractures of the clavicle

Fractures of the clavicle most commonly occur as a result of a fall onto the shoulder or onto the outstretched hand (see also 'Sports injuries', p. 822). The midshaft of the clavicle is the most frequent location of fracture, and the resulting clinical picture is that of the distal fragment of the clavicle pulled down by the weight of the arm, whilst the proximal fragment is displaced superiorly by the action of the sternocleidomastoid muscle (large muscle of the neck).

Medical management

Patients will require immobilization in a sling/collar and cuff and will require analgesia until the pain subsides over the next couple of weeks. Active shoulder movement should be commenced after this time within each patient's comfort levels. Reassurance needs to be given that swelling around the fracture site over the subsequent weeks is normal and due to callus formation.

Shoulder dislocation

Although the shoulder joint can be dislocated either anteriorly or posteriorly, anterior dislocations account for 96–98% of the total. Posterior dislocations are more often missed. Anterior dislocations may occur as a result of a fall onto the hand (see also 'Sports injuries', p. 822). The humerus is driven forwards, resulting in tearing of the joint capsule or avulsion (forcible wrenching away) of the glenoid labrum. Diagnosis will be confirmed by X-ray and neurovascular status of the arm must be tested.

Medical/surgical management

Reduction of the dislocation is performed in most cases within the A&E department using sedation, or general anaesthetic where the shoulder has been dislocated for some time or reduction under sedation has failed. Following reduction and recovery from the sedating drug or anaesthetic, patients are discharged wearing a collar and cuff for up to 3 weeks. Analgesia is prescribed for pain control.

Active movement may then be commenced. However, patients must not laterally rotate and abduct the arm for another 3 weeks, as that particular movement may result in further dislocation.

Fractures of the proximal humerus

These occur primarily in older women with osteoporosis who fall on the outstretched hand. In the majority of cases, the displacement is not marked and treatment causes few problems.

Management for most cases comprises analgesia and rest in a broad-arm sling, until the pain has subsided to a level whereby mobilization can occur.

If there is major displacement of three or more fragments, patients will usually require admission and surgical intervention, commonly for an open reduction and internal fixation. Compartment syndrome is a risk and neurovascular assessment should be performed both pre- and postoperatively. In rare cases,

hemiarthroplasty may be required, and in those who are very elderly there may be a decision to treat conservatively in hospital, should it be deemed that there is a considerable risk associated with anaesthesia.

Fractures of the shaft of the humerus

Fractures of the shaft of humerus are commonly caused by a fall onto the hand (leading to a spiral fracture), falling onto the elbow (resulting in oblique or transverse fractures), or direct trauma (leading to a transverse or comminuted fracture). There is a risk of associated damage to the radial nerve, so neurological status must be regularly evaluated through testing the patient's ability to extend the wrist and move the metacarpophalangeal joints.

Medical/surgical management

Fractures of the humerus are commonly managed with a back-slab type cast from shoulder to wrist with the elbow flexed to 90°. The arm is then supported in a collar and cuff sling. The cast can be reduced to just above the elbow after 2–3 weeks.

If the fracture is simple, a collar and cuff may be used to support the arm while the fracture heals and the patient can be reviewed in the fracture clinic. Patients are admitted to hospital if the fracture pattern is more complicated, the arm is grossly swollen or the pain cannot be controlled by simple analgesia at home.

If conservative treatment is not indicated, surgery may be needed to stabilize the fracture. This may involve intramedullary nailing or plating depending on the fracture pattern and the surgeon's preference.

Supracondylar fractures of the humerus

Supracondylar fractures involve an area between the condyles at the lower end of the humerus. They are most often seen in children. The distal fragment may be displaced posteriorly (more common) or anteriorly. Posterior displacement suggests an extension injury usually due to a fall on the outstretched hand. The jagged end of the proximal fragment may poke into the soft tissue anteriorly and thereby compromise the brachial artery or the median nerve. Neurovascular assessment is important, e.g. the radial pulse should be checked in the affected arm, plus observations as outlined above. The fracture can be clearly shown on a lateral view X-ray.

Medical/surgical management

Fractures with no displacement are treated in a sling for 2–3 weeks with the elbow flexed to more then 90°.

Displaced fractures must be reduced as soon as possible under general anaesthesia, and stabilization with K-wires may be needed. Post-manipulation X-rays are done to assess the reduction, position and degree of any deformity present.

Fractures of the head of radius

Radial head fractures are usually caused by a fall onto the outstretched hand which forces the elbow into valgus (angulation away from the midline) and pushes the radial head against the capitulum (condyle of the humerus). There is pain on rotation of the forearm and tenderness on the lateral aspect of the elbow.

Medical/surgical management

Treatment of undisplaced fractures involves placing the arm in a collar and cuff for 3 weeks. Flexion and extension of the elbow are encouraged but rotation is allowed to come back on its own. Single large fragments may be reduced using an AO screw. Severe comminuted fractures may be treated with excision of the radial head or prosthetic replacement.

Fractures of the olecranon process of the ulna

Two types of injury are commonly seen: a comminuted fracture due to a direct blow or fall onto the elbow; and a clean transverse fracture due to a fall onto the elbow whilst the triceps muscle is contracting. The fracture enters the articular surface and also damages the articular cartilage.

Medical/surgical management

A lateral X-ray is essential to show details of the fracture pattern. Comminuted fractures in older people are treated with an arm sling, with further X-rays at 1 week to exclude displacement. With transverse fractures, the extensor mechanism should be repaired, which can be carried out by tension banding of the fracture.

Fractures of the shaft of radius and ulna

These fractures are common in road traffic accidents. A twisting force caused by a fall onto the hand produces a spiral fracture, with fractures at different levels in the two forearm bones. Direct trauma usually produces a transverse fracture at the same level.

Medical/surgical management

In adults, reduction is difficult and position is usually lost even in a cast. Therefore, they are most often treated by plating of the fracture. Postoperatively a cast is applied with the elbow flexed to 90° for 6 weeks. Although acute compartment syndrome can occur in the majority of fractures, those of the forearm are particularly susceptible (see 'Nursing management' below).

Single forearm bone fractures

Fractures of the shaft of the radius or the ulna alone are relatively uncommon and are usually caused by a direct blow. Ulna shaft fractures are rarely displaced, whereas radial fractures may have a degree of rotary displacement. Radial shaft fractures are treated conservatively with a cast (usually above the elbow). The position of the forearm for cast application varies, being:

- supinated (palm upwards) for fractures of the upper third of the radius
- neutral for middle third fractures
- pronated (palm downwards) for lower third fractures.

Ulnar fractures may be treated conservatively or surgically depending on the fracture pattern.

There are several types of fractures to the forearm; two of the more common wrist injuries are the Colles' fracture and the Smith fracture.

Colles' fracture

This is a transverse fracture of the distal radius with dorsal displacement ('dinner-fork' deformity) of the distal fragment, occurring within 2.5 cm of the wrist joint. It is one of the commonest fractures in older people (see Reflective Practice box 27.4). The fracture occurs due to a fall onto the outstretched hand in extension. X-rays show dorsal displacement, radial displacement and impaction of the distal fragment. Undisplaced fractures are treated with a dorsal back-slab, which is converted to a complete cast when the swelling has subsided, often following attendance and review at a fracture clinic.

Displaced fractures are reduced under anaesthesia. The hand is grasped and traction is applied in the length of the bone; sometimes extension of the wrist to disimpact the fracture may be needed. The distal fragment is then restored to its normal position by applying pressure over the dorsum of the wrist whilst applying flexion, ulnar deviation and pronation to the wrist. If a reduction is not maintained then an external fixator may be applied, although this is relatively rare.

Smith fracture ('reverse Colles' fracture')

In this fracture, the distal fragment is displaced towards the volar (palm) aspect of the wrist. It is generally caused by a fall on the back of the hand. Reduction of the fracture is the opposite of that for the Colles' fracture and subsequently the forearm is placed in a cast with the wrist in extension.

Injuries to the carpus and metacarpus

Carpal injuries

Scaphoid bone injuries account for almost 70% of injuries to the carpus (eight bones of the wrist). The common mechanism of injury is a fall onto the dorsiflexed hand. There is tenderness in the anatomical snuffbox (natural depression on the back of the hand by the wrist). Various X-ray views will be taken of the carpus. It may not be possible to confirm diagnosis using X-rays at this stage; however, if there is any degree of suspicion based on injury history and physical examination, the forearm should be placed in a scaphoid plaster. Check X-rays will be performed at 2 weeks post-injury, when diagnosis may be confirmed if a sclerotic margin around the fracture is present. It is important to look for angulation of the distal fragment since this may cause non-union of the fracture.

Undisplaced fractures are treated with a scaphoid plaster, which extends from the upper forearm to the distal metacarpal with the wrist in dorsiflexion; the thumb is incorporated into the cast up to the distal phalanx whilst in a 'glass-holding' position. Open reduction and compression screws are used to treat displaced fractures.

Fractures of the metacarpus (five bones of the hand)

The fifth metacarpal is commonly damaged due to a punch. Treatment is most often conservative with a wool and crepe dressing, analgesia and review in the fracture clinic. If the fracture is angulated more than 40°, manipulation will be needed.

R|Я REFLECTIVE PRACTICE

27.4 Colles' fracture: the practical difficulties

'I realized that my wrist was broken immediately I had fallen – it looked very strange (the classic "dinner fork" deformity of a Colles' fracture they said in A&E). At the A&E I was given a sling and two paracetamol tablets and after an X-ray the fracture was reduced and supported with a back-slab plaster. The following day, as an X-ray revealed a satisfactory alignment, the full plaster was completed. My wrist and lower arm were uncomfortable and ached but were not very painful. I was given an information sheet comprising many "do nots" – i.e. do not get the plaster wet, do not place in direct heat, do not probe or cut the plaster – and advice to contact A&E immediately if the hand was unduly painful, swollen or discoloured. I was told to exercise my hand and arm and attend for checks.'

'I left the hospital contemplating 5–6 weeks' minimal restriction due to the plaster being on my dominant right arm. Within hours my idea of mild inconvenience was overtaken by an inability to cope with everyday living activities. I found it difficult to wash, shower and bathe using only my left hand. It was difficult to clean myself after using the lavatory, and putting on a bra, socks or tights was impossible. Eating and cutting up food was a nuisance. I could not drive, sign for cards or cheques and even the mouse on the PC was a problem. All this reduced my independence, especially as my arm ached and was sore and the plaster was very heavy.'

'I considered the "do not" list and advice given. What should I do if I was not to get the plaster wet? How was I to get washed and dressed? Would I ever wear anything but the oldest bra, put on like a contortionist? How was I to prepare meals? What did "exercise my arm and hand" actually mean? What was "discoloured"? Should I eat any special diet to help healing? Could the fracture indicate the start of osteoporosis?'

Student activities

Reflect on the practical problems experienced by this patient after a relatively simple fracture.

- How well do you think you would have coped in similar circumstances?
- What suggestions and information might the nurse have given her to help overcome some of the problems with activities of daily living?

Think about the usefulness of the advice given to this patient, i.e. exercise the hand, and contact the A&E if it becomes discoloured.

- What further points would you have discussed with her to support the written instructions and ensure a better understanding of the advice and its importance?

▶ Nursing management – upper limb injuries requiring surgical intervention

The general principles are the same as for lower limb injuries, although obviously the types of treatment modality, prescribed rehabilitation regimen and the ability of the patient to perform activities of daily living independently will differ. Preoperative management will focus on a complete assessment, including the presence or otherwise of associated injury, pain control and preparation for surgery as appropriate.

Postoperative nursing management will include monitoring of neurovascular status. This is particularly pertinent for injuries to the forearm or for patients in an arm cast who are at major risk of compartment syndrome. Other secondary complications mentioned for lower limb fractures as less likely to occur following upper limb injury. The patient's pain should be controlled within tolerable limits and evaluation of the treatment utilized should be performed.

Assistance may be required in undertaking further or progress tests, e.g. follow-up X-rays or blood investigations.

Until patients are able to resume activities of daily living independently, assistance with these will be required. Again, if they are unable to do this at discharge, the nurse will be responsible for educating them to be verbally independent, i.e. to be able to dictate their needs to others, as well as for training of

relatives and/or carers. Usually carers would only be employed in the most chronic of upper limb conditions. Some activities of living are likely to be affected until healing has occurred, even in injuries that are not severe. Clearly this will be more of an issue in those with both arms affected. Patients will require assistance in regaining optimum mobility of the upper limb according to the prescribed regimen and reports of patient progress with prescribed treatment and mobility regimens will need to be given to other health care professionals.

The nurse must provide psychological support to patients and their families as they adapt to alterations in body image. These alterations may be either temporary (e.g. in the case of an external fixator) or permanent (e.g. in the case of amputees or those with altered neurological function).

Discharge planning includes ensuring that community support is available and that any follow-up arrangements are made. A fundamental part of preparation for discharge is education about the specific condition and treatment modality (see Health Promotion box 27.3). This includes advice regarding specific orthoses, care of casts, medication and prevention of secondary conditions. In older patients, whose fracture may have been due to a fall, investigation of causes should be undertaken in an attempt to minimize the likelihood of recurrent falls and fractures. Again the issues surrounding osteoporosis should be addressed as necessary.

HEALTH PROMOTION

27.3 Preventing secondary complications or recurrence

Education of patients about the prevention of secondary complications or recurrence of injury is a vital part of the discharge planning process for those with musculoskeletal conditions. There is an obvious difference between giving someone an information leaflet and actually educating that person.

Student activities

Reviewing current practice in your area, choose two or three issues on which you 'educate' patients and look at the process.

- Do you simply give information, or are patients educated?
- What are your thoughts about the quality of any written information given?
- Make recommendations for improvement.
- Think about how other ways of giving information, such as the internet, could be used effectively.

(See also Reflective Practice box 27.4.)

SUMMARY: MAIN POINTS

- The role of the nurse in managing the patient with a musculoskeletal condition requires both specific technical skills and underpinning knowledge of conditions.

- Many of the practical skills are based on general principles and are adapted according to the particular condition with which the patient presents. Such skills include managing the patient with restrictions in mobility, e.g. in traction, wearing a cast, orthosis.

- Additionally, skills are required in facilitating a return to optimum mobility, e.g. the use of walking aids or safe wheelchair use.

- The underpinning knowledge of pathophysiology and treatment modalities is useful in the education of patients and other nurses, and allows an increasing rationalization of care regimens, which may have been lacking in previous years.

- Nurses need to acquire skills and knowledge relating to the acute physiological events following trauma and in the immediate postoperative stage, as well as those required for rehabilitation. These include education, psychological support, coordination in discharge planning and evaluation not only of care prescribed by nurses, but also of regimens prescribed by other health care professionals.

- This combination of skills and vast breadth of knowledge required is a challenge to orthopaedic nurses internationally if optimum patient outcomes are to be achieved.

SELF-TEST: CRITICAL THINKING ACTIVITIES

1 Sanjay complains of pain under his cast (fractured tibia treated by skeletal traction):
   — What are the likely causes of his pain?
   — What questions will you ask him regarding the pain and any other symptoms?
   — What observations will the registered nurse ask you to commence?

2 Patients having joint replacement are at risk of prosthesis dislocation. What measures would you take during the postoperative period to reduce this risk in a patient having a total hip replacement?

FURTHER READING

Brooker CG. Human structure and function, 2nd edn. London: Mosby; 1998.

Dandy DJ, Edwards DJ. Essential orthopaedics and trauma, 3rd edn. Edinburgh: Churchill Livingstone; 1998.

Davis P. Nursing the orthopaedic patient. Edinburgh: Churchill Livingstone; 1994.

Hill J. Rheumatology nursing – a creative approach. Edinburgh: Churchill Livingstone; 1998.

Kakulas BA. Problems and solutions in the rehabilitation of patients with progressive muscular dystrophy. Scand J Rehab Med 1999; 39(suppl.): 23–37

McQuillan KA, Flynn MB, Hartsock RL, Von Rueden KT, Whalen E. Trauma nursing from resuscitation through rehabilitation, 3rd edn. Philadelphia: WB Saunders; 2001.

Maher AB, Warner Salmond S, Pellino TA. Orthopaedic nursing, 2nd edn. Philadelphia: WB Saunders; 1998.

Smith MJ. Rehabilitation in adult nursing practice. Edinburgh: Churchill Livingstone; 1999.

Wiesel SW, Delahay JN, Cyrus P, Rizzo RD. Principles of orthopaedic medicine and surgery. Philadelphia: WB Saunders; 2001.

  USEFUL ADDRESSES AND WEBSITES

Arthritis Care
18 Stephenson Way
London NW1 2HD
www.arthritiscare.org.uk

Chartered Society of Physiotherapy
14 Bedford Row
London WC1R 4ED
www.csp.org.uk

College of Occupational Therapists
106–114 Borough High Street
London SE1 1LB
www.cot.co.uk

Disabled Living Foundation
380–384 Harrow Road
London W9 2HU
www.dlf.org.uk

Lupus UK
St James House
Eastern Road
Romford
Essex RM1 3NH

Muscular Dystrophy Campaign (MDC)
www.muscular-dystrophy.org

National Osteoporosis Society
PO Box 10
Radstock
Bath BA3 3YB
www.nos.org.uk

Royal Association for Disability and Rehabilitation (RADAR)
Unit 12, City Forum
250 City Road
London EC1V 8AF

Royal Society for the Prevention of Accidents (RoSPA)
Cannon House
Priory Queensway
Birmingham B4 6BS
www.rospa.co.uk

Scoliosis Association (UK)
2 Ivebury Court
325 Latimer Road
London W10 6RA
www.sauk.org.uk

REFERENCES

Anderson RJ. The orthopedic management of rheumatoid arthritis. Arthritis Care Res 1996; 9(3): 223–228.

Brus H, van de Laar M, Taal E, Rasker J, Wiegman O. Compliance in rheumatoid arthritis and the role of formal patient education. Sem Arthritis Rheum 1997; 26(4): 702–710.

Butcher JD, Salzman KL, Lillegard WA. Lower extremity bursitis. Am Family Phys 1996; 53(7): 2317–2324.

Clasby L, Young MA. Management of sports-related anterior cruciate ligament injuries. AORN J 1997; 66(4): 607, 609–610, 612.

Cohen RB, Williams GR Jr. Impingement syndrome and rotator cuff disease as repetitive motion disorders. Clin Orthop Rel Res 1998; 351: 95–101.

Davis P. Nursing the orthopaedic patient. Edinburgh: Churchill Livingstone; 1994

Dellacorte MP, Birrer RB, Grisafi PJ. The acutely painful foot and ankle (part 1): traumatic injuries. Emerg Med 1994; 26(11): 46–48, 51–52, 55–58.

Donohue SJ. Lower limb amputation 3: the role of the nurse. Br J Nurs 1997; 6(20): 1171–1172, 1174, 1187–1191.

Gillies D. Elderly trauma: they are different. Aus Crit Care 1999; 12(1): 24–30.

Goss GL. Osteoporosis in women. Nurs Clin North Am 1998; 33(4): 573–582.

Hefti D. Complications of trauma: the nurse's role in prevention. Orthop Nurs 1995; 14(6): 9–16.

Janas J. Muscular dystrophy. Nurs Pract Forum 1996; 7(4): 167–173.

Kee CC, Harris S, Booth LA, Rouser G, McCoy S. Perspectives on the nursing management of osteoarthritis. Geriatr Nurs: Am J Care Aging 1998; 19(1): 19–28.

Lappe JM. Prevention of hip fractures: a nursing imperative. Orthop Nurs 1998; 17(3): 15–26.

Leach M. Signs and symptoms of systemic lupus erythematosus. Nurs Times 1998; 94(13): 50–52.

Lewis T, Tesh AS, Lyles KW. Caring for the patient with Paget's disease of the bone. Nurs Pract 1999; 24(7): 50, 53, 57.

Luong BT, Chong BS, Lowder DM. Treatment options for rheumatoid arthritis: celecoxib, leflunomide, etanercept, and infliximab. Ann Pharmacother 2000; 34(6): 743–760.

McCann S, Gruen G. Fracture blisters: a review of the literature. Orthop Nurs 1997; 16(2): 17–24.

Martin SD, Scott RD, Thornhill TS. Current concepts of total knee arthroplasty. J Orthop Sports Phys Ther 1998; 28(4): 252–261.

Nolan M, Nolan J. Arthritis and rehabilitation: developments in the nurse's role. Br J Nurs 1998; 7(1): 22–24, 37–39.

Pittman JR, Bross MH. Diagnosis and management of gout. Am Fam Phys 1999; 59(7): 1799–1806.

Pronchik D, Heller MB. Local injection therapy: rapid, effective treatment of tendinitis/bursitis syndromes. Consultant 1997; 37(5): 1377–1380, 1386–1389.

Putman MT, Wise RA. Myasthenia gravis and upper airway obstruction. Chest 1996; 109(2): 400–404.

Ramsburg KL. Rheumatoid arthritis. Am J Nurs 2000; 100(11): 40–43.

Resnick B. Falls in a community of older adults: putting research into practice. Clin Nurs Res 1999; 8(3): 251–266.

Santy J. Rehabilitation of the patient with a hip fracture: facing the challenge. J Orthop Nurs 1998; 2(1): 11–15.

Santy J. Nursing the patient with an external fixator. Nurs Stand 2000; 14(31): 47–52, 54–55.

Scottish Intercollegiate Guidelines Network. National clinical guideline. Management of elderly people with a fractured hip. Edinburgh: SIGN; 1997.

Simon LS. Osteoarthritis: a review. Clin Cornerstone 1999; 2(2): 26–37, 55–60.

Smith MJ. Amputation: the transition from hospital to home. Nurs Times 1999; 95(47): 52–53.

Watson AWS. Sports injuries: incidence, causes, prevention. Phys Ther Rev 1997; 2(3): 135–151.

Webborn ADJ, Carbon RJ, Miller BP. Injury rehabilitation programs: "What are we talking about?". J Sport Rehab 1997; 6(1): 54–61.

28 Nursing patients with skin problems

Jill Peters, Shirley McKeon, Fiona Pringle, Jane Watts, Amy Winsor

> 'When he went into the care home I was worried they wouldn't look after his skin properly. He mustn't use soap and has to have lots of moisturiser. I was relieved when they asked me to bring in what he usually has so that they can order the right stuff.'
>
> (Patient's relative)

THIS CHAPTER WILL HELP YOU

- Carry out an assessment of the skin
- Describe and document a presenting skin condition
- Describe and carry out common investigations
- Identify common signs and symptoms
- Assess, plan and undertake the nursing care of patients with skin conditions
- Describe the psychological impact of skin disease and plan care accordingly
- Undertake patient education about specific chronic skin conditions.

KEYWORDS

Blister	Macule
Bulla	Nodule
Cutaneous	Papule
Dermis	Petechia
Emollient	Plaque
Epidermis	Pruritus
Erythema	Purpura
Excoriation	Pustule
Exfoliation	Vesicle
Fissure	

INTRODUCTION

Nurses will meet patients with skin disorders in every area of practice. This chapter aims to provide the knowledge and understanding to be able to assess any patient's skin whether or not it is the primary problem and thus assist the person in maintaining skin integrity. The skin as an organ provides information about many aspects of the general health of patients, e.g. nutritional status (Ch. 11), hydration status (Ch. 8), how they have aged (Ch. 32) and assessment of risk to skin integrity (Ch. 10). General principles of skin care and common conditions are covered here, but with over 2000 different skin conditions, readers may need to consult specialist texts for information about some of them.

The majority of patients with skin conditions are cared for in the community or on an outpatient basis. You may find that you have been caring for patients in relation to another condition (not of the skin) when you make a nursing diagnosis which requires that you implement care to improve the integrity of the skin or relieve symptoms. The concept of self-care lends itself very much to these patients, and can range from patients taking part in decisions about treatment to them actually carrying out the treatment in full themselves.

Self-care offers patients with a skin condition the opportunity to stay in control and nurses can help by supporting and encouraging them to be as independent as possible.

ANATOMY AND PHYSIOLOGY – AN OVERVIEW

The basic anatomy and physiology of the skin are discussed in Chapter 10 along with wound healing and age changes. However, as we are dealing here with conditions affecting the skin and its appendages, we need to look in more detail at certain aspects, e.g. the epidermis, pilosebaceous units, sweat glands, nails and the protective role of the skin as part of the body's innate defences.

The skin has two layers, the superficial epidermis and the dermis (true skin), which are attached to the subcutaneous (below the skin) layer or hypodermis and fatty tissue. It has several functions:

- protection – physical/chemical/biological barrier
- sensation (see Ch. 14)
- thermoregulation (see Ch. 5)
- metabolism – synthesis of vitamin D (see Ch. 11)
- excretion (small role)
- absorption of substances, e.g. some drugs
- storage of water and energy.

A healthy intact skin is therefore vital to physiological homeostasis. In Chapter 10 you will find a discussion of the role of the skin in non-verbal communication in terms of the emotions, e.g. blushing, and clues to age and health status.

EPIDERMIS

The epidermis has several layers of stratified epithelium through which cells progress, losing water and protein as they go. What you see on the surface of the skin are dead cells continually being shed and forming most of the dust at home.

The epidermis comprises several special cell types:

- keratinocytes – produce keratin, a tough fibrous protein found in epidermis, nails and hair; they contain lipids
- corneocytes – contain water-retaining substances and natural moisturizing factor
- immune cells called Langerhans' cells (dendritic cells)
- melanocytes that produce melanin.

The epidermis has five layers:

- stratum corneum (horny layer)
- stratum lucidum (clear layer) – not present in all areas
- stratum granulosum (granular layer) – overlays the germinative zone
- the stratum spinosum (prickle layer) – one part of the germinative zone
- stratum basale (basal layer) – the other part of the germinative zone, which contains the melanocytes.

If you imagine the stratum corneum as a wall, then the corneocytes are the bricks, and these are held together by the lamellar lipids as the mortar (see Fig. 28.1). The lipid barrier

helps the corneocytes to retain water. The swollen corneocytes prevent cracks forming between them. However, any disruption to the epidermal lipids leads to water loss and cracking that permits penetration by irritants and allergens which can initiate an immune response.

Epidermal renewal and keratinization

Renewal occurs as the stratum corneum, which is continually shed (desquamation or exfoliation), is replaced by new cells formed in the stratum basale. The new cells migrate through the layers over a period of around 35 days. During renewal, epidermal cohesion is maintained by the desmosomes (special junction between cells able to withstand mechanical stresses) that bind keratinocytes together and help to prevent structural damage. The cells of the stratum granulosum contain keratohyalin, the precursor of keratin. The cells undergo several changes as they migrate upwards: the nucleus disintegrates, keratinization occurs (addition of keratin) and there is flattening. As a result, the stratum corneum comprises dead cells containing keratin. Renewal is most rapid during childhood; it stabilizes in adult life and then declines with advancing age. This is a relevant point when you consider the time needed for the skin to heal in older people. Next time you make your bed, observe the dust; this comprises exfoliated epidermal cells. It is merely a nuisance at home, but in a surgical area it is a potential infection risk, as microorganisms present in the exfoliated epidermal cells can be transferred to wounds when the dust is disturbed.

Normal pigmentation

A mixture of substances – haemoglobin, melanin and carotene – gives skin its normal colour. Untanned Caucasian skin is pink due to haemoglobin in the blood. The presence of varying amounts of the brown-black pigment melanin accounts for different shades of skin, hair and iris colour. This includes racial differences, pigmented areas such as the scrotum, areola/nipples, moles, freckles and the changes that occur when Caucasian skin tans. Melanin production, by specialized epidermal cells called melanocytes, is stimulated by hormones and ultraviolet (UV) radiation. Carotene found in the stratum corneum and the dermis contributes to normal skin colour in people of Asiatic origin. Rarely, however, yellow-orange discoloration can be associated with a high intake of carotene-rich foods.

PROTECTIVE ROLE OF THE SKIN

Many skin functions are protective, e.g. prevention of water loss, thermoregulation, detection of harmful stimuli. Intact skin also provides physical, chemical and biological barriers against harmful agents.

Physical

The skin keeps out microorganisms and is able to withstand the harmful effects of some chemicals, e.g. weak acids, and alpha ionizing radiation does not penetrate it. The stored fat layer also offers some protection against trauma.

Chemical

The normally acid secretions form a chemical barrier (acid mantle) that protects against some microorganisms. Both sebum and sweat may have bactericidal properties.

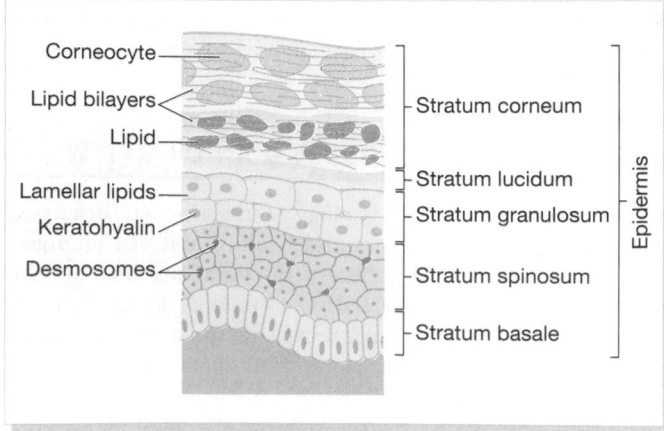

Figure 28.1 Detail of the epidermis.

Biological

The normal bacterial flora (surface and in the deeper layers) of the skin protects against infection (see Ch. 13). These commensal microorganisms, which are well adapted to their environment, tend to prevent other, more harmful microorganisms becoming established. It is worth remembering that the skin flora changes after admission to hospital, resulting in diminished protection. Langerhans' cells and other immune cells are also part of the biological barrier, and hopefully deal with pathogenic microorganisms that do get past the frontline defences.

SKIN APPENDAGES

Pilosebaceous unit

A pilosebaceous unit comprises a hair, its follicle and the associated sebaceous gland.

Hair and follicles

Hair protects the skin, has a minimal role in thermoregulation and is used in the expression of sexuality.

The hair follicles are formed from epidermal tissue that grows down into the dermis or subcutaneous layer. Hair, which is formed from keratinized cells, comprises a growing region (bulb) at the base of the follicle, a root and the shaft visible above the surface of the epidermis. Each hair follicle is associated with an involuntary muscle, the arrector pili, controlled by sympathetic nerve fibres, which causes the hair to stand more erect, giving gooseflesh when cold or frightened.

There are three types of hair:

- lanugo – the soft, downy hair sometimes present on newborn infants, especially when they are preterm; it is usually replaced before birth by vellus hair
- vellus – short downy hair found on most hair-bearing parts of the body except the scalp, axillae and external genitalia
- terminal hair – coarse pigmented hair of the scalp and eyebrows. During puberty, terminal hair replaces the vellus hair of the axillae and external genitalia in both sexes and forms body and facial hair in males. The amount of terminal body hair varies between individuals.

Hair growth is cyclical: there is a period of growth, then a resting phase before the old hair is shed and a new hair develops. Individual hair follicles remain active for varying times and those on the scalp may function for years.

Sebaceous glands

These are particularly abundant on the face, neck and back. Sebaceous glands secrete sebum, a fatty substance containing cholesterol and other lipids. The glands usually disintegrate to discharge sebum into hair follicles but some discharge directly onto the skin surface. Sebum waterproofs the skin and helps to keep hair and skin supple and resistant to cracking. It may have some bactericidal/fungicidal properties. The activity of sebaceous glands increases during puberty and is especially stimulated by the action of androgen hormones. Bacterial action on sebum, with associated blockage of the follicles, inflammation and bacterial infection, leads to the development of acne (see p. 851). The activity declines in older people, which renders the skin more prone to dryness and damage and reinforces the

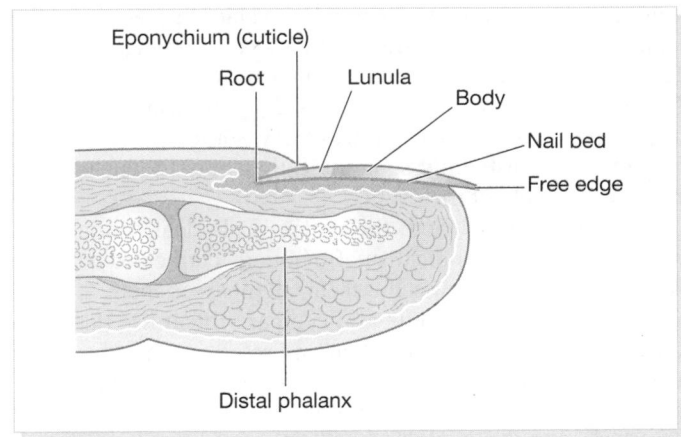

Figure 28.2 Section through the distal phalanx and nail.

view that older people need particular care to maintain skin integrity (see pp. 848–849).

Sweat glands

Sweat glands are of two types: eccrine and apocrine. Eccrine sweat glands are the most abundant, especially so on the forehead, palms and soles of the feet. They produce watery sweat that exits via a sweat duct to empty on the skin surface through pores. The principal function of eccrine sweat glands is thermoregulation. Sweat contains electrolytes (sodium and chloride), metabolic waste, and food and drug residues, and has a small role in excretion. Water is also lost by diffusion (insensible loss), and this, with sweat, may amount to between 800 and 1000 mL/day under normal conditions in a temperate climate. In situations where sweating is excessive, or skin integrity is breached, as in burns, there is great risk of fluid and/or electrolyte imbalance and hypovolaemic shock (see Chs 8 and 9).

Apocrine sweat glands are located in the external genitalia, groin, axillae and areola. These glands do not become active until puberty when they start to produce thicker sweat which, when subjected to bacterial action, has a distinctive musky odour.

Ceruminous glands are modified sweat glands present in the external auditory canal. They produce cerumen (wax) that traps particles and prevents them entering the ear (see Ch. 16).

Nails

The nails are keratinized sheets that protect the distal ends of the digits and are used in some fiddly tasks (see Fig. 28.2). They are derived from epidermal cells and each nail grows on a vascular nail bed. A nail has a root, a body and a free edge. At the proximal edge, the nail is thickened to form the white lunula that is covered by the cuticle (eponychium). An abundant capillary network in the dermis means that in health the nail appears pink.

NURSING ASSESSMENT

The environment is important in the assessment of any patient, but this is particularly true when assessing patients with a skin condition. The examination should take place in private and the room should be warm. Natural light is ideal, but where artificial lighting is necessary it should not alter the natural skin colour. Sometimes a magnifying lamp is used. In the ward/outpatient setting the nurse should be aware of how sound travels and that others may be listening, something that may inhibit patients from speaking about their skin.

The nurse should note the patient's physical bearing and posture – it may be indicative of emotions connected with the skin disease, such as low self-esteem or embarrassment.

It is essential to examine and compare the entire skin – no lesion/rash should be looked at in isolation The chance of detecting a melanoma is 6.4 times greater with a complete skin examination than with a partial examination of just exposed skin (Peters 2001). Patients should be asked to undress to their underclothes after a suitable explanation. Nurses must be sensitive to cultural and religious needs. Some patients may experience embarrassment, especially if they see the problem as being local, e.g. a rash on the legs.

It is important to document that the skin examination has been completed and the findings regarding its condition, not just because the patient has a skin disease but as a baseline observation. Recording your findings in the nursing notes is essential for the next nurse, so that the previous status of the patient will be known and the nurse can adjust care accordingly.

COLLECTING INFORMATION

A great deal of information can be obtained by asking patients about the skin complaint and how it affects their life. This should be recorded in their own words.

- What is their existing knowledge base?
- What do they understand about their treatment and its outcomes?
- Explore symptoms to provide you with insight into the patient's perceptions and expectations of the consultation/admission.
- Identify the 'patient experience' and ascertain their agenda.

Although patients may have presented with a skin problem, you need to consider a holistic review of all systems. A skin condition may be indicative of systemic disease (e.g. intense itching or pruritus could be due to jaundice – yellow discoloration of the skin, sclerae and mucosae; see Ch. 23). Alternatively, a patient may be too embarrassed to mention the real problem unless specific questions are asked, e.g. vulval soreness could be a symptom of skin disease, rather than the sexually transmitted infection that the patient fears (see Ch. 25).

A holistic review also needs to consider the psychological impact of skin diseases, and questionnaires such as the Dermatology Life Quality Index are useful tools (Finlay & Khan 1994).

The use of scales can provide information about the intensity of symptoms and can indicate their remission or exacerbation. A scale of 0–10 (where 0 represents the best a patient's skin has been, and 10 the worst) can be used to assess the intensity of itch, dryness or erythema (redness of the skin due to vascular congestion) etc., as well as exploring what aspects are difficult for the patient.

THE PHYSICAL EXAMINATION

The physical examination should be systematic, and gentle but sure movements should be used to avoid causing discomfort or pain.

It is important to use the senses when examining the skin, e.g. look, touch and smell. Nurses need to be thorough and not just accept what they are told; for example, a patient may not associate a rash under the breasts with plaques (elevated flat-topped lesions) on the elbows. Or patients may deny scratching but excoriation (loss of skin substance due to scratching) is present. The nurse may elicit further information by asking questions that include:

- Is there a particular time of day or night when the itch is worse?
- Does scratching disturb sleep?
- Have you taken anything to help the itching?

Figure 28.3 provides some common examples of skin lesions.

Skin assessment should be carried out as part of the admission process in which you can also gain information about patients' nutritional and hydration status, as well as assessing the potential risk of pressure ulcer development (see Guidelines for Care Priorities box 28.1; also see Ch. 10).

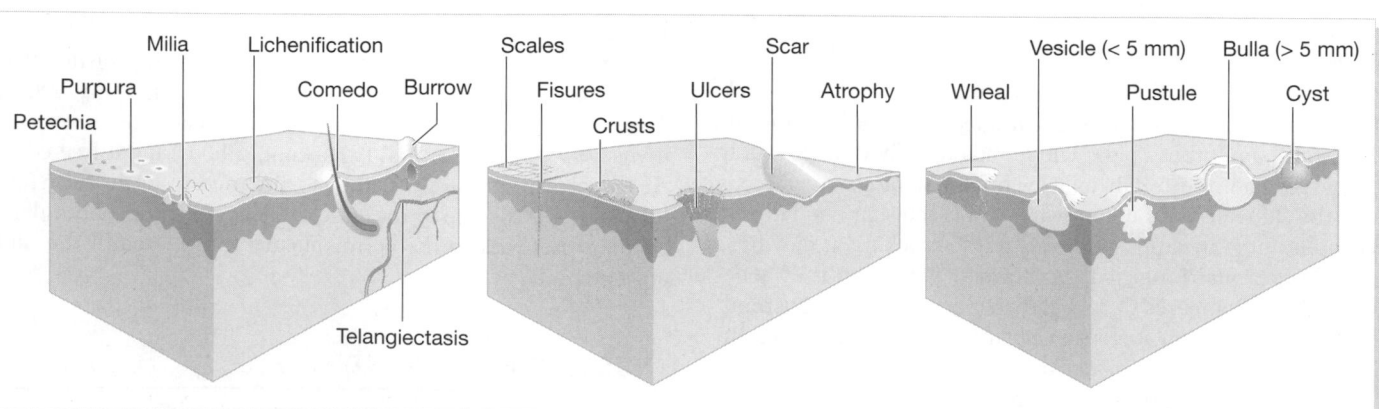

Figure 28.3 Common skin lesions.

GUIDELINES FOR CARE PRIORITIES

28.1 Physical examination and skin assessment

1. Wash hands.
2. Ensure that the patient is involved and is aware of reasons for assessment.
3. Ensure privacy for patient.
4. Organize good lighting.
5. Gloves only need to be worn if contact with bodily fluids is involved.
6. Examine all of the skin, including mucosae, nails and hair. Palpate with fingertips gently but confidently. Light surface palpation allows you to assess the texture and extent of any lesions.
   — Start with the fingernails, moving to finger webs, palms and dorsum of the hands, moving up both arms to the axilla – note the state of the cuticles; check the nails for pitting, lifting (onycholysis) or extra lines; check both flexural and extensor sides of the arms, and the axilla for lesions or damage
   — Now examine the scalp. Part the hair to examine the hair shaft and assess hair texture – note any bald patches behind the ears and signs of hair thinning at the hairline
   — Examine all areas of the face – note any obvious lesions. Check all areas including the eyelashes and brows, the nasolabial folds, the oral mucosa and tongue
   — Now examine the trunk using a systematic approach to ensure that no area is missed. Commence under the chin, into both axillae, and down the chest wall across the abdomen to the pelvic area
   — Examine the feet and front of the legs. Check the toenails as before. Examine in between the toes, and the dorsum and sole of the feet for moles and other lesions before working up the front of the legs
   — Examine the back and the back of the legs by asking the patient to turn over or stand so you can examine the skin from the nape of the neck to the feet. Again a systematic approach ensures that no areas of skin are missed
   — Examination of the genitalia should be respectful and gentle (see Ch. 25). Ask the patient to manoeuvre and to point to the areas of concern. Gloves should be worn where contact is anticipated (see Ch. 13).
7. Document findings using body charts.
8. Deal with specimens (correct container, labelled correctly and dispatched to laboratory)
9. Plan of care.
10. Time-frame for implementation of care.
11. Review and evaluate progress.
12. Wash hands.

Further reading
UKCC. Guidelines for records and record keeping. London: UKCC; 1998.
RCN. Standards of care for dermatology patients. London: RCN; 1995.

Distribution and configuration of skin lesions

The distribution and configuration of the skin lesions will provide clues to the diagnosis. The primary lesion, such as a rash, is identified and its position noted, and also whether it is localized to one area or more generalized (see Box 28.1). Endogenous (from within the body) rashes are usually symmetrical, whereas exogenous rashes (from outside the body) may affect only one side of the body. Where the cause is sun exposure, there will be unaffected areas that were shaded, e.g. under the chin. In some conditions, e.g. pemphigus, the lesions typically affect both the skin and oral mucosa. There may be a demarcation to indicate the extent of the condition, such as at the wrists with allergy to latex gloves.

Any findings should be related to the age of your patient and the expected physiological changes that occur with normal ageing (Ch. 32). Learning to recognize what is normal across the age spectrum and what is unusual comes with experience.

Box 28.1 Describing lesions by configuration and distribution (configuration is the arrangement or pattern of lesions in relation to other lesions, whereas the distribution is the arrangement of lesions over an area of skin)

Annular	Shaped like a ring	Nummular or discoid	Shaped like a coin
Asymmetrical	Unilateral distribution of lesions	Polymorphous	Lesions display variable forms
Confluent	Lesions merge	Punctate	Marked by the points or dots
Diffuse	The lesions are widely spread over different parts of the body	Serpiginous	Snake-like
Discrete	Lesions are separate from others	Solitary	Single lesion
Generalized	Widespread distribution	Satellite	Single lesion situated close to a larger group
Grouped	Lesions in clusters	Symmetrical	Bilateral distribution of lesions
Gyrate	Ring spiral shape	Zosteriform	Distribution of lesions is band-like along a dermatome (area of skin innervated by sensory nerve [afferent] fibres from the cutaneous branches of a particular spinal nerve)
Iris lesion	Concentric rings		
Linear	Lesions in a line		
Localized	Lesions in limited, well-defined areas		

Changes in skin colour and pigmentation

It is important to be aware of the range of colours (differences in pigmentation) of human skin. Skin types can be based on a person's own estimate of sunburning and tanning (phototypes) (Fitzpatrick et al 2001):

- skin type I – always burns
- skin type II – sometimes burns, always tans
- skin type III – always tans, never burns
- skin type IV – Mediterranean skin
- skin type V – brown skin
- skin type VI – black skin

During assessment of the skin, the nurse should observe for changes and abnormalities, remembering that natural pigmentation will affect the appearance of the change (see Box 28.2).

Loss of pigmentation can occur following inflammatory changes and is often seen after eczema and herpes zoster in individuals with darker skin colour (skin type IV–VI). An understanding of the normal pigmentation allows detection of change; palpation is often useful in darker pigmented skins (Baxter 1993). Inflammation in black skin may also lead to other physical changes, e.g. the skin may become more papular (raised and spotty) with an increase in the risk of scarring.

DOCUMENTATION

Clear documentation is essential; the nurse needs to record findings even if the skin is intact and well hydrated, thus establishing a baseline from which to measure (see p. 844).

A body map is used to record the distribution, location and size of any mark, lesion or wound, along with any landmarks such as tattoos or scars (see Fig. 28.4). The body map provides a visual record of the patient's skin and the extent of any skin disease. A closer examination and documentation of the lesions should be done following the initial general assessment.

Questions can be asked during this time, e.g. 'Has there been any change (improvement or worsening) on your current treatment?' Patients often volunteer information that they had not thought important.

GENERAL DIAGNOSTIC TESTS AND MEDICAL INVESTIGATIONS

Nurses undertake many general investigations after appropriate training and assessment, and some are able both to initiate and to carry out certain investigations. It is the responsibility of the practitioner carrying out the procedure to ensure that the patient understands the implication of the procedure and makes an informed choice to give verbal consent. The framework illustrating how the patient was counselled should be written in the nursing notes. An important role for all nurses is always to talk patients through the procedure first. This would include a discussion of how uncomfortable/painful it may be, what their skin will look like afterwards and how healing may occur.

Investigations assist with the process of elimination or act as supporting evidence for a working diagnosis.

MICROBIOLOGICAL INVESTIGATIONS

Bacteriological investigations

A skin swab for microscopy, culture and antibiotic sensitivity is taken to determine the presence of either primary or secondary bacterial infection (Ch. 13). (Note that in some skin conditions the pus is sterile, e.g. pustular psoriasis.) Distinguishing between colonization and infection is essential, as wounds colonized by bacteria will heal without antibiotics (see Ch. 10), whereas infected skin will require antibiotics. Using the correct method to take and transport the skin swab is vital if the laboratory is to detect infection and identify the bacteria responsible (see Guidelines for Care Priorities box 28.2).

Virology tests

Tests are used to detect primary infection, e.g. herpes zoster (shingles), or secondary infection, such as herpes simplex virus (HSV) complicating eczema and resulting in eczema herpeticum (see p. 864). A special virology transport medium is used for samples undergoing serology tests for HSV. If a vesicle (small fluid-filled blister < 5 mm in diameter) is present, the roof is pierced and a swab taken. When an immediate result is required

---

Box 28.2 Skin changes in pigmented skin (adapted from Hughes & Van Onselen 2001)

- **Cyanosis** (blue discoloration of the skin and mucosa caused by poor oxygenation) – in individuals with dark skin this may only be detected by ash-grey lips or by checking the nail beds. Skin changes may only be obvious in severe cyanosis
- **Erythema** – in darker skin this may present as a purplish tinge (difficult to see in dark area), macular change, local or more diffuse changes. Increased warmth associated with inflammation, or the tight skin and hardening (induration) of deep tissues can be felt
- **Inflammation** – hyperpigmentation may occur in black or brown skin, but lighter areas may be seen on the tip of the nose and in front and behind the ears. Again increased warmth can be felt

- **Jaundice** – in patients with darker skin this may be detected by yellowing of the sclerae, junction between hard and soft palate and on the palms of the hands
- **Oedema** – lightens the skin, weals appear pale. Palpation will detect the tight skin and increased warmth of oedema
- **Pallor** – this may be manifest in black skin as ash-grey, and in brown skin as yellow-brown
- **Purpura** (discoloration caused by the extravasation of blood into the skin or mucosae), either petechia (small, purple or red haemorrhagic spot) or ecchymosis (large bruise) – appears as jet-black in brown skin

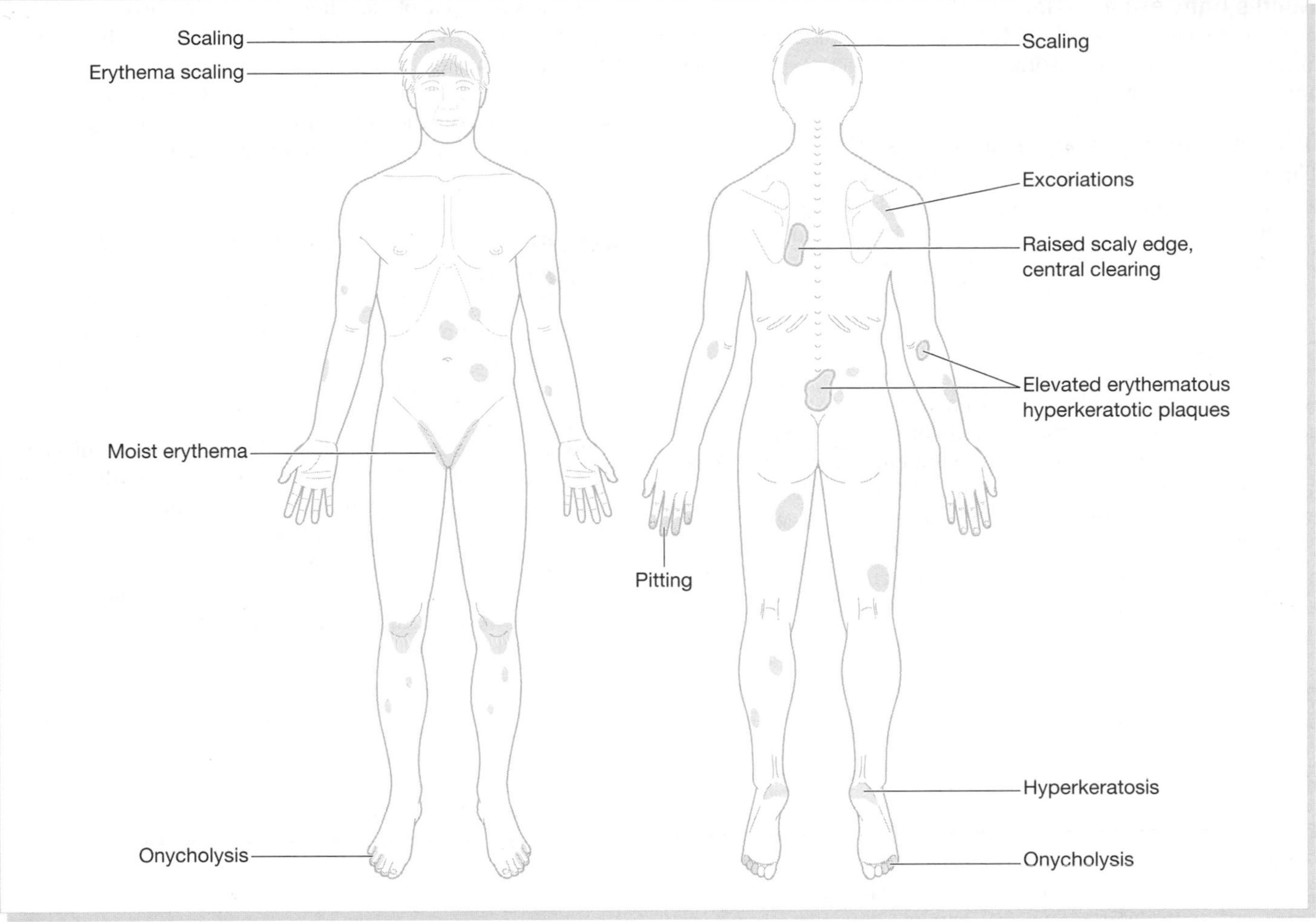

Scaling

Erythema scaling

Scaling

Excoriations

Raised scaly edge,
central clearing

Moist erythema

Elevated erythematous
hyperkeratotic plaques

Pitting

Hyperkeratosis

Onycholysis

Onycholysis

Figure 28.4   Body map showing documentation of skin lesions.

 GUIDELINES FOR CARE PRIORITIES

28.2 Obtaining a skin swab

1. Ensure that the swab tip is moistened with either sterile normal saline or transport medium so that you pick up microbial cells.
2. Rotate the swab between the fingers in a zigzag motion across the wound/skin; this collects cells from an adequate depth and ensures maximum coverage of the swab tip. If pus is present then swab that.
3. Put the swab into the transport medium, add the patient's details to the container and indicate the body location from where the swab was taken. Check that the request form is complete.
4. Arrange prompt transportation to the laboratory.
5. Results are usually available within 24 hours. However, testing for methicillin-resistant *Staphylococcus aureus* takes longer (see Ch. 13).

Further reading

Committee Members of the Wound Care Society. Wound care procedures. J Wound Care 1993; 2(2): 77.

and the laboratory has facilities for direct cytology, a Tzanck smear may be taken. This involves smearing the contents of a blister on a glass slide, which should be placed in alcohol to preserve the quality of the material and then transported to the laboratory.

Mycology

Mycology investigations assist in the diagnosis of fungal infections, supporting clinical findings or providing a definite diagnosis to ensure the correct systemic or topical therapy. The most common reason for treatment failure is misdiagnosis (Goodfield 1998), and therefore skin scrapings, nail clippings or hair debris should be sent to the laboratory:

- Skin scrapings are obtained by using a blunt blade at 45° to scrape skin cells (without cutting the patient's skin) onto black filter paper. To prevent the loss of specimens during opening in the laboratory, it is not sealed with adhesive tape.
- Nail clippings are obtained with nail clippers on to black filter paper.
- Hair debris – a stiff toothbrush is used to collect skin, exudate and hair.

Wood's light examination

A UV light with a nickel oxide filter is often used to identify fungal infections such as ringworm, some bacterial infections and to assess skin pigmentation.

Ovasites and parasites Sellotape test

This involves placing a strip of Sellotape across the anal orifice at night in an effort to trap any worms as they emerge. It is an awkward test to undertake and can be very embarrassing for the patient. Educating patients so they can apply the tape themselves can minimize this.

SKIN BIOPSY

A punch biopsy provides a full-thickness excision of the skin down to the fat. A biopsy may be used for suspected skin cancers to ascertain diagnosis and inform treatment. Biopsy is very useful for inflammatory rashes or skin infiltrates, when multiple biopsy can be taken with ease. It is common practice to biopsy both affected and unaffected skin for comparison. Skin samples are sent for histological interpretation, culture for bacterial infections and immunofluorescence testing for autoimmune conditions.

The nurse's role in this minor surgical procedure, which can be done in the community, may involve patient preparation and assisting the doctor, or by performing the biopsy.

PATCH TESTING

This investigation is usually carried out in most dermatology departments. Allergy patch testing is one of the investigations to detect contact allergy of type IV – delayed cell-mediated hypersensitivity. The patch consists of hypoallergenic tape containing aluminium discs, each containing a different allergen. The investigation is quite time-consuming for the patient, with several appointments in 1 week to read the tests.

BLOOD TESTS

Routine blood tests, such as a full blood count, may be used to check general health. Specific tests may be done if a systemic disease is suspected of causing skin symptoms, e.g. thyroid function tests if hypothyroidism is implicated as the cause of pruritus (see Ch. 17).

A radioallergosorbent test (RAST) may be used in allergy testing; it measures the amount of specific immunoglobulin E (IgE) produced against a suspect allergen, e.g. peanuts.

GENERAL DISEASE PREVENTION AND HEALTH EDUCATION

Preventing moisture loss from the skin, and therefore consequent drying, is key to maintaining healthy skin. It is also important to protect the skin from adverse weather and sun damage, as well as trauma, e.g. burns.

The skin has a natural moisturizing factor. This substance, which attracts water to it (humectant), is present in the skin and is protected by lipid material that balances the transepidermal water loss, keeping the skin flexible and smooth. If the natural moisturizing factor is removed from the stratum corneum through excessive washing with soap, it loses its capacity to bind water. When the moisture content of the stratum corneum falls below 8–10%, it becomes dry, rough and cracked.

Various factors influence the hydration of the stratum corneum, e.g.:

- environmental conditions
- dehydration (see Ch. 8)
- nutritional deficiency (see Ch. 11)
- chronic venous insufficiency (see Chs 10 and 19)
- ageing (Ch. 32) (see Older Adults: Nursing Priorities box 28.1).

Various synthetic detergents and soaps can remove the lipids from the epidermis.

The level of cleanliness is high in today's society but over-washing of the skin can lead to dryness because the alkaline soaps remove the natural oils that keep the skin hydrated. One study clearly demonstrated that using a soap substitute instead of soap in an older population reduced skin dryness, redness and flaking (Hardy 1990).

OLDER ADULTS: NURSING PRIORITIES

28.1 Dry skin

Normal age-related changes that affect the skin's ability to remain an effective barrier, e.g. development of dry skin, occur in 80% of people over 60 years of age.

Factors likely to affect skin function in older people
- Lifestyle
- Anaemia (see Ch. 18)
- Diabetes (see Ch. 17)
- Thyroid dysfunction (see Ch. 17)
- Alcohol intake
- Environmental factors

Specific nursing priorities in emollient therapy for older adults includes:
- Choice of appropriate emollient
- Check for allergies
- Consider patient preferences
- Take account of patient's dexterity and mobility – can he/she open the container and reach relevant body areas to apply the emollient?
- Safety issues, e.g. falls caused by a slippery bath or poor balance – consider need for assistance, e.g. community nursing service

NB. Blood screening would be required if there was no improvement after emollient therapy.

MAINTAINING HEALTHY SKIN
(see Reflective Practice box 28.1)

Ways in which skin can be kept healthy are as follows:

- Use of medicated bath oils and soap substitutes – however, it is important to choose one that is suitable for the patient's skin. Safety issues must be considered, as some products can make the bath/shower slippery
- Bathing/showering daily – this is recommended but the length of time in the water should be restricted to 10–15 minutes. Longer immersion times lead to skin dehydration and white, wrinkly skin that is easily damaged
- Regulating bath water temperature – the temperature of the water should be tepid or equal to body temperature. Immersion in hotter water causes capillary dilatation and increases water loss through evaporation
- Careful drying – the skin should be gently patted dry with no heavy rubbing. This is especially important in the case of newly healed skin (wounds, skin grafts) or in older people with very fragile thin skin (Ch. 32)
- Use of a topical emollient (moisturizer that stays in the skin) – this should be lightly applied to the skin using smooth strokes (following the direction of hair) so that the skin glistens. Keeping water in the skin reduces the formation of fissures (cleft or split). Emollients imitate the action of the lipid barrier by permeating the corneocytes and enhancing water-carrying capacity (Cork 1997). Gentle application avoids friction and protective skin changes. Making evidence-based decisions about which emollients to use and the frequency of application in a variety of situations is difficult, as very little research has been undertaken. Personal preference can guide the choice of emollient but nurses should always ask patients about any allergies. Frequency of application depends on the level of dryness, e.g. 2-hourly applications over a short period may be

appropriate if the skin is very dry. This regimen should quickly rehydrate the stratum corneum and reduce itchiness. As the skin improves, the frequency of application can be reduced, e.g. to twice daily. On exposed areas like the face, neck and hands, the application may need to be more frequent, especially for those who do 'wet work', such as catering, hairdressing or nursing. Drying the hands thoroughly after washing is vital.

INFLAMMATORY SKIN DISORDERS

Nursing diagnosis can be used in the management of patients with inflammatory skin disorders to enhance their quality of life. Providing health education about the condition is a key role for the nurse. Dermatological care is labour-intensive and this gives the nurse the opportunity for prolonged patient contact and a chance to talk.

ATOPIC ECZEMA

Atopic eczema is an inflammatory skin condition affecting both the epidermis and dermis. It is acute, subacute or more usually chronic inflammation with pruritus (Fitzpatrick et al 2001).

Aetiology and epidemiology
The precise aetiology is unclear but there is an immunological factor in many cases. Atopic individuals who have a genetic predisposition to asthma (see Ch. 20) and hay fever (see Ch. 21) also develop eczema. They produce a specific abnormal immunoglobulin (IgE) in response to common environmental allergens. Eczema affects anywhere between 1 and 10% of the general population (Williams 1994).

Some of the triggers for atopic eczema are clearly identified in the environment or lifestyle of patients:

- house dust mite
- animal dander can also trigger eczema in some individuals
- stress and tiredness caused by increased scratching (thought by many to be a trigger)
- illness or other event that overloads their coping mechanisms
- increase in body temperature can cause itching
- change in environmental temperature, such as going from a hot room to the cold outdoors, or vice versa
- weather conditions – the skin dries in winter, sun and wind exposure also causes skin dehydration
- alcohol intake has a diuretic effect and can cause skin dehydration 12–24 hours after consumption. Alcohol also causes skin capillaries to dilate, causing flushing and increased itch
- bacterial infections.

Pathophysiology and clinical presentation
Acute atopic eczema presents with erythema, itching, oedema, papules (raised lesions or scaly, crusted, keratinized or macerated surface < 1 cm), vesicles, excoriation, exudating lesions, crusting or scaling but with no defined borders. Adults with chronic atopic eczema have more scaly (hyperkeratotic) skin, which can be hyperpigmented from previous inflammation; the epidermis

28.1 Skin care

After reading the section about maintaining a healthy skin, reflect on the skin care given to patients you have nursed in non-acute settings, e.g. nursing homes.

Student activities
- What type of soap or soap substitute was used?
- Did patients have individualized skin care?
- How many patients used emollients (moisturizers)?
- What advice was given to patients about the length of time they should spend in the bath?
- What was the temperature of the bath water? Did it exceed body temperature?
- Did the care differ from that outlined in the chapter? If the answer is yes:
  — Can you identify any reasons for these differences?
  — Suggest some small changes that would encourage the maintenance of healthy skin.

thickens (lichenification) as protection against friction and damage caused from repeated scratching but there is less erythema and fewer vesicular eruptions.

Medical management

This includes:

- Topical therapies – topical corticosteroid preparation, new topical immunosuppressants, soap substitute, bath oil (may include an antiseptic agent), emollients
- Systemic therapies – antibiotics for clinical infection, antihistamines to aid sleep, immunosuppressants.

▶ Nursing management

Adults diagnosed with eczema can be very angry, looking for a cure and finding it very difficult to come to terms with the condition. Those who had eczema as children are presumed to know about the condition and how to care for their skin but need as much input to support and educate them so they can gain control and be able to initiate their own treatment when required.

Adjusting the environment and avoiding allergens and triggers

The identification of triggers or known allergens is important for patients in order to adjust their environment and avoid triggers where possible.

House dust mite. It thrives in the warm, comfortable environment created by double-glazing, central heating and wall-to-wall carpeting. Mite faeces left in mattresses and soft furnishings causes the allergy. The use of mite-impermeable covers (microporous) over mattresses and pillows is recommended. Frequent washing of bedding, damp dusting and vacuuming (non-bag machines or those with filters) are also helpful. If possible, someone without eczema should do the washing up and housework.

Animal dander. Simple actions, such as avoiding animals or not allowing companion animals on the bed or in the bedroom, can help. Prick testing can confirm these allergies but a clear history is sufficient.

Stress and tiredness. Find ways of reducing stress, such as exercise (see Ch. 6). Worsening eczema is frustrating, disturbs sleep and often leads to anger and further anxiety. It is important for patients to recognize the need for rest and adequate sleep. Nurses can encourage the use of prescribed sedating antihistamines to reduce scratching at night.

Diet. Considerable research has failed to find a causal link between diet and most cases of eczema (Carman 1999). Food intolerance is often mistaken for allergy in patients' searches for an answer to their eczema. However, if there is true IgE sensitization with anaphylaxis then a Medic-Alert bracelet is recommended.

Changes in temperature. This can be dealt with by wearing layers of clothing that can be removed or added to, as conditions change, and more frequent application of emollients if skin is becoming drier. The texture of emollient can be changed as the seasons change.

Irritants. Avoidance can be difficult as patients come into contact with irritants in everyday life. At work there may be chemicals that are airborne, air conditioning can cause dryness, and having a window with the sun shining through can cause overheating. In the home, household cleaning products can irritate either because of the chemical make-up of the product or because of detergent effects. Wearing protective gloves may be helpful or, alternatively, domestic chores should be delegated.

Alcohol. Avoidance can be difficult but beneficial.

Infections. A skin swab should be taken for sensitivity, although 90% of infections are staphylococcal and 10% are streptococcal. Advise on use of antiseptic emollients. Avoidance of people with cold sores thus reducing the exposure to herpes viruses (see p. 855).

Scratching. It has to be recognized that there is a difference between the sensation of itch and the behaviour of scratching. Often the patient with chronic eczema talks of scratching all the time as a habit and behaviour modification may be required.

Skin care and treatments

A whole care package is essential if patients are to be empowered towards self-care. Nurses need to be sure that patients can initiate the level of intervention required to ensure remission of the flare.

An explanation about the use of topical therapies improves patient outcomes and quality of life. The following are used in combination when the skin has flared. However long-term topical emollient therapy should be continued even when the skin is controlled (Holden et al 2002):

- Soap substitute that both cleanses and hydrates (available at all sinks)
- Bath oil – recommend daily bath or wash to cleanse and hydrate the skin, using tepid water
- Emollient (moisturizer) – patient preference; apply hourly if skin is very dry, reducing the frequency as the skin improves. Use oil-based emollient if skin is very dry, but creams if the skin is sore or moist. Moisturizing removes the scale on the surface that would otherwise block the penetration of topical medication. For patients with arthritis, emollients are available in a pump dispenser
- Topical corticosteroids – potency depends on severity of the condition and location and is reviewed after 5 days with a view to reducing it if potent or very potent used. Mild-to-moderate potency corticosteroids can be used for longer but must be regularly reviewed (Greaves & Gatti 1999)
- Impregnated bandages – if free from infection, these are effective for hydration and cooling the skin, and can act as a physical barrier to reduce damage to fragile skin from scratching. Hydrocolloid dressings can be useful for localized protection of the skin from picking or scratching, but it is advisable not to use topical corticosteroids underneath in case occlusion increases the potency and leads to atrophy
- Antiseptic/oxidizer (potassium permanganate) – can be used in soaks/bath (as a light pink solution) for moist weeping skin. It is used for 10 minutes twice daily for 3–5 days, stopping once the skin is dry
- Wet wrap dressing – should only be used under direct supervision that allows a review of skin condition every 24–48 hours. They should not be used for more than 2 weeks without consulting the patient's dermatologist. There are two different types of wet wrap in use and neither has been

fully evaluated. The concept behind them is to intensely rehydrate and cool the skin, calming the itch while the wet wraps are in situ; the skin should not become dry.

STASIS (GRAVITATIONAL OR VARICOSE) ECZEMA

Gravitational stasis eczema is a chronic eczematous condition affecting the lower leg and associated with chronic venous insufficiency (see Chs 10, 19). It mainly affects older people.

Epidemiology and aetiology
Williams (1994) cites a study from the USA that suggested that around 1% of the population had a clinically significant eczema that was not atopic eczema or contact dermatitis.

This type of eczema is often accompanied by chronic venous insufficiency. It can, on occasions, become acute due to infection.

Pathophysiology and clinical presentation
- Inflammation – redness, warmth, etc.
- Dryness
- Skin fissuring
- Severe oedema may be present with bullae (large watery blisters). Thus the combination of eczema and ulceration can be complicated by itch, infection and superimposed contact dermatitis.

Medical management
The underlying aetiology is identified by Doppler examination and, if indicated, compression bandaging will be considered (see Ch. 10). Oral antibiotics are prescribed for infection. Consideration is given to other conditions such as diabetes (see Ch. 17) that can affect healing.

▶ Nursing management

It is important to advise patients of the need for regular leg exercises to improve the calf pump mechanism to improve venous return, and elevation to reduce oedema. Walking regularly and wearing support stocking are to be encouraged so long as patients are able to remove them daily to wash and moisturize their legs to prevent the build-up of dry hyperkeratotic skin. For topical therapy see 'Atopic eczema' (p. 850).

CONTACT DERMATITIS

Contact dermatitis is a generic term applied to acute or chronic inflammatory reactions to substances that come into contact with the skin (Fitzpatrick et al 2001). It can be classified as:

- contact irritant dermatitis caused by chemical irritants, e.g. detergents, etc.
- contact allergic dermatitis as a result of an allergen (antigen) that causes a type IV delayed cell-mediated hypersensitivity following a previous exposure to the allergen, e.g. rubber, nickel, etc.

Clinical presentation and specific investigations
The presentation can vary from severe pruritus to erythema, papules and vesicles which initially occur at the site of contact,

which may give clues to possible causes, e.g. around the neck where a necklace has been worn. Contact dermatitis is often wet and prone to secondary infection. In chronic irritant dermatitis, fissuring, scaling and maceration can occur. It is more common in people who do wet work, e.g. hairdressers, engineers, nurses and cleaners. Substances that frequently cause irritant reactions include detergents, solvents, water and even body fluids, e.g. exudate from a leg ulcer can cause maceration of the surrounding skin.

Referral for allergy patch testing is a useful investigation, especially supportive for a patient who may have an occupational contact dermatitis.

Medical management
Management combines use of topical therapies (see 'Atopic eczema', p. 850). In very severe cases, systemic corticosteroids would be used.

▶ Nursing management

Management involves supporting patients through allergy patch testing. If an allergen is identified then it is important that patients understand now to avoid that substance. This might mean checking the content list of every product they use in the house, e.g. for perfume that is present in foods and shampoos. If they are allergic to rubber, it is important for all other health care professionals to know this, e.g. dentists. Sometimes patients develop a type 1 antibody-mediated (anaphylaxis) allergy. This will necessitate the provision of a Medic-Alert bracelet and patients or a relative should be taught how to administer adrenaline (epinephrine).

ACNE

Acne is inflammation of the pilosebaceous units, particularly those on the face and trunk. The peak onset in males is 17–19 years and in females is 16–17 years. It is generally more severe in males. Late onset occurs more frequently in women and can be related to polycystic ovary syndrome (Ch. 25). The aetiology is multifactorial and includes hormone effects, especially androgens, increased keratinization blocking the hair follicle and increased sebum production.

Acne is a condition that can be treated, but in adolescence it is often trivialized as growing up spots or related to diet; 85% of all teenagers experience some degree of acne. Some patients suffer devastating social and psychological effects. Cuncliffe (1994) describes a useful assessment tool – Assessment of psychological and social effects of acne (APSEA).

Clinical presentation
Acne manifests itself in several different forms:

- comedones (open blackheads and closed whiteheads)
- papules
- pustules (pus-filled lesion < 1 cm)
- nodules (rounded, elevated solid lesion > 1 cm)
- cysts
- pitting
- hypertrophic scars.

Box 28.3 Treatment for acne

Benzoyl peroxide (topical)
Antimicrobial and anticomedonal properties. Effective on both inflamed and non-inflamed skin. Can initially cause redness and peeling

Retinoids (topical), e.g. tretinoin
Decreases the retention of cornified material in the follicular canal, can cause mild skin irritation and care needs to be taken when exposed to ultraviolet radiation such as sunlight

Topical antibiotics, e.g. clindamycin
Mild-to-moderate acne, can be used in combination with the two treatments above. Can cause mild irritation and requires twice-a-day application

Azelaic acid
Antibacterial and anticomedonal, is applied twice a day, causing redness and scaling (reduce applications if this occurs)

Systemic antibiotics, e.g. minocycline
Act against *Proprionobacterium acnes* (a normal skin commensal) and reduce the free fatty acid content of the surface lipids. Choice of antibiotic may depend on resistance and tolerance of the antibiotic. Advise girls taking the oral

contraceptive pill that the contraceptive effect may be reduced during the first month of antibiotic treatment. Patients should be advised that it takes 6 weeks before an improvement is seen and reassessment should occur after 3 months

Anti-androgen hormone therapy
Used with young women who do not respond to systemic antibiotics and give a history of exacerbation related to menstrual cycle

Isotretinoin (retinoid) (topical and oral)
This inhibits sebum production, comedonal formation, reduces the number of *P. acnes* and the inflammatory response. It can only be prescribed by a hospital dermatologist and requires close monitoring because of potential side-effects. Isotretinoin is teratogenic (causes fetal abnormalities) and sexually active women must have access to effective contraception both during treatment and for 6 months afterwards; pregnancy should be excluded prior to starting treatment. Can cause severe dryness, nose bleeds and joint pain; liver function and lipid levels should be monitored as they can be affected by this drug and bloods tests are carried out before commencing and at intervals during treatment

Exacerbation can be caused by topical or oral corticosteroids, oral contraceptives, lithium, greasy cosmetics, etc. It may be classified as mild, moderate and severe. Factors influencing severity include persistent disease, poor response to therapy, scarring and patient anxiety.

Medical treatment
The treatment of acne is summarized in Box 28.3.

▶ Nursing management

The nursing diagnosis may be based on supporting patients and educating them so that they optimize therapy and reduce the disease processes. These patients often have low self-esteem and do not necessarily seek medical attention because others trivialize it. It is important that regular review of therapy is undertaken, so that dosage can be increased or therapy changed if effectiveness is limited.

At every opportunity nurses should reinforce the importance of effective treatment to manage the condition. They should increase the patients' understanding of the inflammatory process, so that they do not pick or squeeze spots as this lengthens the healing time and can lead to permanent scarring.

Nurses have a vital role in ensuring patients understand that the drugs used may have local or systemic side-effects. For example, they should check the patients' knowledge about the need to avoid UV radiation (or use a suitable sunscreen or cover up) with topical retinoic acid, and the need for effective contraception with systemic isotretinoin (and for 6 months after treatment).

ROSACEA

Rosacea is a chronic acneform disorder of the facial pilosebaceous units plus an increased reactivity of capillaries to heat, leading to flushing and finally telangiectasia (dilation of small blood vessels) that may progress to the appearance of continuous flushing. It occurs in the over-30s and is more common in women.

The flushing can be stimulated not only by heat but also by the intake of spicy food and alcohol, which can restrict dietary intake. As rosacea progresses, lymphatic failure can result from sustained inflammation in the tissues. Men may develop rhinophyma (enlargement of the nose). This can be cosmetically disfiguring and is the main reason people seek medical help.

Medical management
Medical management comprises both topical and systemic drugs, and surgical treatments (see Box 28.4).

Box 28.4 Treatment for rosacea

- **Topical** – antibiotics, e.g. metronidazole, erythromycin, clindamycin, applied as creams or gels. They often cause peeling and gel form is preferred
- **Systemic** – antibiotics, e.g. minocycline. In severe cases isotretinoin can be used (see Box 28.3 for side-effects)
- **Surgical treatments** – laser therapy may be used to minimize the effects of telangiectasia. Plastic surgery may be needed for rhinophyma

▶ Nursing management

Nurses can support and educate patients to optimize treatment and reduce the effects of rosacea. Avoidance of known heat triggers is advised, e.g. heat when cooking. The use of sunscreens is advised, as 70% of patients find their skin deteriorates after sun exposure. Patients are advised to avoid alcohol and foods that cause flushing. Stress can exacerbate rosacea and nurses can help patients to manage stress (see Ch. 6). Camouflage make-up may be acceptable to some patients. Laser therapy can be of some assistance in correcting the damage caused by flushing and telangiectasia. It is important that patients have realistic expectations for laser therapy.

LICHEN PLANUS

Lichen planus is an acute or chronic inflammatory dermatosis (skin disease) involving skin and/or mucosae.

Clinical presentation

It is characterized by violaceous (violet), shiny, flat-topped papules on the skin, and milky-white papules in the mouth. Both can have a lacy, white surface pattern. Lichen planus can occur on previously traumatized skin (Koebner phenomenon). This condition is very itchy. An acute flare may cause the spread of papules over days, or more insidiously over weeks. The lesions stay for months to years. There are many variations, including those with bullous type eruptions, or they may even be drug-induced eruptions that mimic lichen planus. Diagnosis is important if the treatment is to be effective; however, it is self-limiting and does burn itself out. Management comprises the use of topical emollients and topical corticosteroids (see 'Atopic eczema', p. 850).

▶ Nursing management

Reassurance and support are key to this group of patients, as well as advising effective use of topical therapies to relieve symptoms. Patients with darker skins may be left with post-inflammatory hyperpigmentation, which can cause embarrassment and require camouflage for exposed areas.

PRURITUS

Pruritus (itchy skin) is a symptom with many causes. Persistent itchy skin can be like pain, difficult to control and capable of dominating the patient's day-to-day existence.

Aetiology

A full examination and appropriate investigations are required to consider the possible causes, which include:

- age changes
- underlying dermatosis, e.g. atopic eczema (see p. 849)
- infestation, e.g. scabies (see p. 859)
- adverse drug reaction
- blood diseases (see Ch. 18)
- liver or biliary disease (see Ch. 23)
- endocrine or metabolic condition (see Ch. 17)
- cancer.

Pathophysiology and clinical presentation

The mechanism of itch depends on the underlying cause, e.g. in obstructive jaundice the itch is caused by an increase in bile salts in the blood.

There may be no skin lesions seen on examination and patients may feel concerned that they are wasting the health professional's time and need reassurance. Constant scratching damages the skin and it is important to explore whether there were any lesions present before the patient started scratching. The scratching behaviour can be very distressing; patients may have disturbed nights and the lack of sleep can be detrimental to well-being. It can also affect other family members, who feel helpless. The physical trauma to the skin causes the release of chemicals, e.g. histamine, that stimulate further itchiness.

Pruritus can be localized, e.g. in the anal area (pruritus ani), or may involve the whole skin surface. Although physiological skin changes do occur with age (drier and more itchy), investigations should be undertaken to exclude pathological causes for pruritus. Over time, the skin may have been stripped of natural lipids by excessive use of alkaline soap.

▶ Nursing and medical management

Basic investigations should be undertaken as a routine, e.g. weighing to identify unusual weight loss, and urinalysis to detect abnormalities such as glycosuria (glucose in the urine), indicating the possibility of diabetes. Medical management depends on the underlying aetiology, but will include symptom control where possible, e.g. topical emollient with antipruritic effects, antihistamines and possibly low-dose antidepressants to aid sleep and lift mood. However, itchy skin is a subjective experience for each patient (see Reflective Practice box 28.2).

Simple changes, e.g. using soap substitute and introducing an emollient, may correct the problem, but if this fails further investigations should be considered. A vital nursing role is the

R|Я REFLECTIVE PRACTICE

28.2 Itchy skin

Itchy skin, or pruritus, causes distress and misery to many people. Reflect on the effects of the continuous itch–scratch cycle on quality of life. Consider how it might impact on self-esteem, relationships and everyday activities, such as choosing what to wear, and working, sleeping and leisure activities. What self-help measures are available (ask someone with pruritus or, if you have suffered yourself, think about what measures helped you)?

Student activities

Think about a patient you have nursed who had pruritus and couldn't stop scratching.

- What caused the itching?
- What local measures were taken to relieve the itching, and did they work?
- How did you help the patient to stop scratching?
- Were drugs prescribed, if so, what?

support of patients undergoing investigations, reassurance and advice depending on the diagnosis (see 'Atopic eczema', p. 850, for topical therapies; and 'General disease prevention and health education', pp. 848–849, for factors causing dry skin).

URICARIA

Urticaria (nettle rash) is a transient (< 24 hours), itchy, skin eruption consisting of areas of erythema and weals.

Aetiology

It may be caused by allergies to drugs [e.g. non-steroidal anti-inflammatory drugs (NSAIDs), angiotensin-converting enzyme (ACE) inhibitors] and foodstuffs, infections, physical events such as sun exposure and cold, or thyroid disease, vasculitis, etc. However, for most patients with chronic urticaria there is no identifiable cause (idiopathic).

Medical management

This depends on the underlying aetiology and may be aimed at symptom control or the management of vasculitis, etc. Chronic urticaria is treated with non-sedating antihistamines daily for 6 months, stopping to see if it has burnt out. If it has not improved, the drugs are continued for another month before stopping again.

▶ Nursing management

Reassurance should be given and strategies to reduce the symptoms discussed, e.g. avoidance of hot baths and use of clothing to keep skin at a constant temperature. The possibility of over-the-counter medications triggering urticaria should also be discussed. Patients may be asked to keep a food diary if sensitivity to a particular food is suspected. If a food-related cause is identified, the nurse should emphasize the need to avoid that particular agent.

SEBORRHOEIC DERMATITIS

Seborrhoeic dermatitis is chronic inflammatory dermatosis.

Aetiology and epidemiology

The yeast-like fungus *Pityrosporum ovale* plays a role in the inflammatory process and increase in scaling that occurs. Seborrhoeic dermatitis is more common in males, with an incidence of 2–5% of the population (Fitzpatrick et al 2001). It often occurs as a presenting feature in patients with HIV infection.

Clinical presentation

Seborrhoeic dermatitis is characterized by itchy skin, redness and scaling occurring in areas of high sebaceous gland activity, e.g. the face and scalp and skin folds. There is severe dandruff.

▶ Nursing and medical management

Patients need practical advice about topical applications and information about triggers like stress that can cause an exacerbation. Reassurance can be given that exacerbations are easily controlled by increasing frequency of treatment.

Management comprises topical therapies:

- Shampoo containing an antifungal element, or imidazoles can be used on scalp and trunk (avoiding eyes), daily initially and then less frequently for control.
- Removal of sticky scales – applying olive oil followed by gentle teasing of the scale from the scalp; this may be repeated over a week until the scalp is clear and then used to maintain clearance.
- Topical antifungal cream/ointment – this is effective if the area is very inflamed; in flexural areas a combination antifungal/corticosteroid or antibacterial/corticosteroid cream can be used. Initially, use a twice daily application and then a reduced application to keep clear. The corticosteroid cream is stopped once inflammation has cleared and the antifungal cream is used alone.
- Topical emollient.

INFECTIONS AND INFESTATIONS OF THE SKIN

When the intact skin or mucosae is broken, it becomes vulnerable to a host of invasive microorganisms that include bacteria, viruses and fungi (yeasts). Some organisms limit their activity to the skin, whereas others may cause systemic illness, particularly if treatment is delayed (see Ch. 13).

Normally the body is protected from infection by an elaborate system of defences, including:

- intact skin and mucosae
- a system of cells, e.g. various white blood cells that destroy microorganisms that breach the physical barrier
- the ability to mount an inflammatory response (acute or chronic)
- an immune response that recognizes and destroys microorganisms.

Whenever cells are damaged or destroyed, a series of cellular and vascular events is set in motion, known as the inflammatory response (see Ch. 10). This is a protective mechanism intended to contain or eliminate invading microorganisms and pave the way for healing and a return to normality.

The major signs of inflammation are:

- redness – due to vasodilatation
- heat – due to vasodilatation
- swelling – due to the accumulation of fluid (extravasation)
- pain – caused by chemical mediators released by damaged tissue
- loss of function – in the case of the skin, the inability to maintain the hydrolipid film.

BACTERIAL SKIN INFECTION

Bacterial infections occur when microorganisms gain entry to the dermis via a break in the epidermis. Infections caused by *Staphylococcus* or *Streptococcus* produce a pustular infection characterized by acute inflammation and the formation of pus, e.g. boils (furuncles), impetigo, etc.

Infection of soft tissue is called cellulitis. It is characterized by a well-differentiated area of redness, swelling and heat, and may follow a bite, other trauma or a blood-borne infection. Erysipelas is a severe debilitating form of cellulitis caused by *Streptococcus pyogenes*.

Medical management

Skin swabs for microscopy, culture and sensitivity should be taken if there is clinical evidence of infection. Impetigo and cellulitis are normally treated with systemic antibiotics as a matter of urgency without waiting for the results of microbiological swabs. Pain relief should be prescribed as required.

▶ Nursing management

Nurses often see the clinical signs of infection and hear patients complain of increasing pain. Reassurance and explanation should be provided for any investigations and the results. If there is an area of redness, it should be marked using a marker pen to draw around the edge, so that any spread can be clearly seen and re-marked. Affected limbs should be elevated to reduce swelling. Patients should be observed for any changes in general condition, e.g. increase in temperature. Nurses should ensure that prescribed antibiotics and pain relief are administered and that patients in the community are advised to finish the course of antibiotics and to report any worsening of the infection.

VIRAL SKIN INFECTIONS

A brief outline of viral skin conditions is provided and readers should consult specialist texts if they require more information. Viruses may invade the epidermis directly through a break in the skin, e.g. viral warts, from the bloodstream as in chickenpox (varicella), or through the peripheral sensory nerves, as in the case of shingles (herpes zoster).

Aetiology and clinical presentation
Papilloma viruses

The human papilloma virus (HPV) causes epidermal cells to grow more quickly and produce the typical hyperkeratotic lesions associated with warts. Common viral warts (verrucae) of the hands and feet and other non-mucosal surfaces are, as their name suggests, common, spontaneously resolving with the development of acquired immunity. If the virus invades the mucosae, particularly of the genitalia, it produces numerous moist, soft, vascular warts called condylomata acuminata. These warts are spread by sexual contact and may become malignant. In those people with impaired immune response, the proliferation rate is greatly increased (see Ch. 25).

Herpesviruses

The same virus, varicella zoster virus (VZV), is responsible for both chickenpox (varicella) and shingles (herpes zoster) and those who have shingles have had chickenpox previously. The virus lies dormant in the sensory nerve and is reactivated at a later date either spontaneously or following a failure of the immune defence systems. The virus invades the epidermis by moving along the nerve branches and confines itself to one sensory nerve. This is demonstrated by severe pain followed by a cutaneous, vesicular (blistering) rash in the dermatomes innervated by the cutaneous branches of that particular spinal nerve, or in areas supplied by a cranial nerve (see Ch. 14). The VZV can invade the trigeminal nerve (Vth cranial nerve) leading to a facial rash and corneal ulceration (see Ch. 15).

The herpes simplex virus (HSV-1) produces blisters in the epidermis around the mouth (herpes labialis – cold sores), and a related virus HSV-2 affects the genitalia (see Ch. 25).

The severity of herpes infections depends on the state of the person's immune system; the effects may be much more severe in debilitated individuals, especially those with impaired immunity, and at the extremes of age. People with atopic eczema (see p. 849) are included in the high-risk group, particularly those whose condition is poorly controlled. The invasion of eczematous skin by the herpes viruses may result in a generalized herpetic eruption affecting both skin and mucosae and can be life-threatening unless prompt diagnosis is made and appropriate treatment is given (see also p. 864).

▶ Nursing and medical management

If treatment for common viral warts (of the hands and feet) is initiated, chemicals such as salicylic acid are used, or cryotherapy with liquid nitrogen for plantar warts. If chemicals are used, great care must be taken to protect the surrounding skin.

If shingles is detected within the first 48 hours, patients are treated with an oral antiviral, e.g. aciclovir; however, if the signs are missed then topical therapies to reduce skin discomfort with analgesia are used. Reassurance and explanation of how the virus affects the nerve and the issue of pain control, which can extend to over 18 months, is needed. Any blisters are aspirated with a sterile needle and potassium permanganate soaks are used to dry the area. Smoothing emollient is used to ease the inflamed skin.

HSV-1 can be cultured from fluid taken from the lesions (see before). Topical antiviral drugs, such as aciclovir or penciclovir, are used in cream form to treat HSV-1. However, intravenous systemic treatment with antiviral drugs, e.g. aciclovir, may be indicated for immunocompromised individuals and those with atopic eczema. HSV-1 can also involve the cornea to cause inflammation and ulceration (see Ch. 15). A referral to an ophthalmologist is required whenever a herpesvirus has involved the cornea, to prevent scarring.

Nurses should follow local control of infection protocols but the nursing team will need to provide support for patients and family especially those who need to be isolated (see Ch. 13). They will need reassurance about physical change in their appearance and nurses should stress the importance of not scratching or picking, to reduce the possibility of scarring. The nurses' role includes caring for the intravenous site, administering medication and monitoring effectiveness, e.g. pain relief (see Ch. 7).

FUNGAL INFECTIONS

Fungal infections (mycoses) affecting the skin, hair and nails (dermatomycoses) are caused by several groups of fungi, including dermatophytes and yeasts (candidosis and pityrosporum). The effects they cause may be further subdivided into two groups:

- superficial mycoses that do not generally provoke a significant host response

■ cutaneous mycoses, where, although the fungus is confined to the stratum corneum, there are pathological changes, e.g. erythema and inflammation.

Some of the fungi that cause these infections are present in the environment, and others have an intimate association with humans and are part of the normal flora of the skin and gut, e.g. the yeast *Candida albicans*. In addition there are a few fungi that have evolved to the point where they are almost completely reliant on the human host for survival, e.g. the dermatophyte that causes scalp ringworm (tinea capitis).

The diagnosis of a fungal infection is usually suspected on clinical signs (see below) but can be confirmed by Wood's light examination, or by sending skin scrapings, hair or nail clippings to the laboratory for examination. It therefore follows that the quantity and quality of the material gathered for examination are critical.

Fungal infections and reinfection of the skin, hair and nails can be the cause of considerable distress to patients, and nurses can offer advice about simple measures that may help in prevention (see Health Promotion box 28.1).

Dermatophytosis (tinea)

Dermatophytosis is an infection of the skin caused by dermatophytes. The dermatophytes are three related genera of fungi that cause tinea or ringworm infections of the skin, hair and nails:

■ Epidermophyton (nail and skin)
■ Microsporum (hair and skin)
■ Trichophyton (hair, nail and skin).

 HEALTH PROMOTION

28.1 Dermatomycoses; prevention of infection and reinfection

The prevention of infection and reinfection are based on personal hygiene and clothing rules designed to minimize spread of the pathogen and to avoid direct contact with infectious material.

The following measures will counter the risk factor profile of dermatomycoses:

● Wash and dry susceptible areas of skin thoroughly on a daily basis.
● Change underwear and socks daily, and if possible not wearing the same shoes each day.
● Do not share clothing, towels, brushes and other personal items.
● Minimize contact with pathogens, e.g. by wearing sandals in public areas, such as swimming pools and shower areas.
● Avoid trauma to the skin caused by poorly fitting shoes and clothing.
● Prevent softening and thinning of the skin's horny layer caused by over-washing.

If infection occurs, seek treatment early and notify possible contacts, encourage them to implement treatment. This will help to contain the infection and prevent reinfection.

Dermatophytes may originate from the soil, from animals such as cats and horses, or from humans. An important characteristic of dermatophytes is their restriction to dead, keratinized tissue in the epidermis.

Tinea (ringworm) infections are usually classified according to the body part affected:

■ tinea capitis – ringworm of the scalp
■ tinea barbae – ringworm of the beard
■ tinea faciei – ringworm of the smooth, hairless skin (glabrous) of the face
■ tinea corporis – ringworm of the body
■ tinea cruris – ringworm of the groin
■ tinea pedis – ringworm of the foot, or athlete's foot
■ tinea manuum – ringworm of the hand
■ tinea unguium – ringworm of the nails, or onychomycosis caused by dermatophytes

The term ringworm is a misnomer, as no 'worms' are involved. It is important to convey this to patients, so that they may understand the nature of the infection. Details of some types of tinea are given in Table 28.1.

Another type of tinea is described – dermatophyte infection modified by systemic or topical corticosteroids (tinea incognito) given for pre-existing disease or given mistakenly for the treatment of a misdiagnosed tinea. The clinical diagnosis of dermatophyte infection relies heavily on the presence of a well-defined inflammatory response. Such a response may be almost totally suppressed by corticosteroids – there is no inflammation, scale or accompanying itch. It has been postulated that at the same time the immune response may diminish the host's resistance to infection. This means that the infection is less likely to be diagnosed and the patient is rendered more susceptible to infection. The history should give the first clue to recognition of the condition, and the sites affected offer another clue to the possibility of diagnostic error. In some cases, taking samples is difficult as the corticosteroid application reduces the amount of scaling. The patient should be instructed to stop treatment for a few days and with the next inflammatory response scaling increases, making clinical diagnosis easier and facilitating the taking of samples.

Medical management

Most local dermatophyte infections are treated with a topical antifungal cream such as one of the imidazole group, e.g. clotrimazole and miconazole. Systemic antifungal treatment is required for tinea capitis, tinea unguium and for more generalized skin infection; for example, treatment might involve using one of the triazole group, such as itraconazole, orally for 3 months, or as two or three short courses. Oral antibiotics may be required for secondary bacterial infection.

▶ Nursing management

General management involves reassurance and education about avoiding recurrence by completing treatment courses even when the skin looks clear, by improving personal hygiene (suggested sensitively if appropriate), and by not sharing personal items, e.g. hair brushes, shaving equipment, flannels or towels, sports clothes, etc. Patients should be advised to avoid scratching,

Table 28.1 Tinea infection – described by location

Tinea infection and site	Aetiology and pathophysiology	Clinical presentation	Specific investigations
Tinea capitis – affects the scalp	Population movement is largely responsible for the introduction of new species to a country or region (Hay et al 1996). In urban areas of the UK, the predominant species are spread between people (anthropophilic) If hair infection is to occur then invasion of the stratum corneum of the scalp skin must first develop. Trauma assists inoculation, and is followed, some 3 weeks later, by clinical evidence of hair shaft infection. It is likely that scalp hair acts as a trapping device, as do oily hair preparations The infection spreads to other follicles and for a variable period of time persists but does not spread further. Finally there is a period of regression that may or may not be accompanied by an inflammatory response	The appearance may vary from confluent greyish scale with or without hair loss to annular scaly patches with broken hair or loss of hair, to a severe painful highly inflammatory mass covering a large area of the scalp In all types there is some inflammation, hair loss or patches of broken hairs. The most severe inflammation is usually seen with animal (zoophilic) infections There is kerion formation (painful boggy mass), with loose hairs Commonly there is pus discharge from the follicles and rarely sinus formation Thick crusts may form and adhere to surrounding hairs causing matting of the hair Lymphadenopathy is frequently found, as is secondary bacterial infection	Some species are visible using a Wood's light Hair sample for laboratory examination
Tinea barbae – affects the bearded area of adult males	Usually caused by dermatophytes of animal origin (zoophilic), e.g. T. verrucosum, T. mentagrophytes	Annular shape may be difficult to recognize and the erythema accompanied by papules and pustules and not much scale Loose hairs in infected areas that are easily plucked out for examination Hair stumps broken off close to the skin may also be seen	Hair and skin scrapings sent for laboratory examination
Tinea corporis – affects the limbs and trunk. Typically on exposed areas of skin, unless it has spread from an existing site, e.g. the scalp	Caused by fungal hyphae or spores from active lesions on an animal or another human being deposited on the skin of a susceptible person The incubation period may be 1–3 weeks before the host produces a tissue response	Lesions are often unilateral, asymmetrical and characteristically annular, well defined and with a raised edge. They may be single or as plaques where several lesions coalesce into one Inflammation and the presence of scale are extremely variable In some cases, vesicles or bullae (blisters) may be present	
Tinea cruris – affects the inguinal folds (groin and upper thigh), and less frequently the gluteal folds and natal cleft	It thrives in the warm moist conditions found at the sites listed It predominates in adolescents and young adults; men are more susceptible than women Sweating, maceration and poor personal hygiene all contribute to infection There are several routes of transmission: auto-infection from foot to groin via a towel; sharing of towels and sports clothing; and direct contact with an infected individual	Predominant symptom is itching. In the early stages there is an erythematous plaque with a curved well-demarcated edge that extends down the thigh There may be scaling, and minute pustules. The skin eruption is often unilateral or asymmetrical Excoriation is common in response to the itching	
Tinea manuum – commonly on the palm of the hand. If the dorsal surface of the hand is affected, it should be considered as tinea corporis	Caused by any species of dermatophyte fungus Often those with tinea pedis cross-infect themselves. The prevalence of tinea manuum is directly related to the degree of tinea pedis in the population Special mention should be made of infections that begin under rings, watches or where there is anatomical deformity, or occupational usage that causes maceration between the fingers. In these instances, infection may occur without obvious foot involvement	Lesions are dry and scaling. They are asymmetrical	

(Cont'd)

Table 28.1 *(continued)*

Tinea infection and site	Aetiology and pathophysiology	Clinical presentation	Specific investigations
Tinea pedis – (commonest fungal infection in the UK). Initially a toe web space infection (NB. Athlete's foot is a term used by some to describe any form of toe web intertrigo. For this reason tinea pedis or foot ringworm is preferred)	Maceration of the toe webs from the wearing of shoes predisposes to this condition. There is a higher incidence in males, thought to be due in part to the wearing of heavier and more occlusive footwear. There is a marked absence in those who habitually go barefoot. Frequent hosing down of poolside areas and communal showers, and in some areas the provision of antifungal powder have proved effective in reducing the incidence	Characterized by fissuring, peeling and maceration of the lateral toe web spaces, sometimes involving the undersurface of the toes and joint crease. Itching is a common feature, especially in warm environments	Skin scrapings are taken to make a positive diagnosis and should be repeated if a negative result is incompatible with the clinical picture
Tinea unguium – affects the nail plate. Toenails are more commonly affected than fingernails	Often associated with tinea pedis and tinea manuum. Nail plate invasion occurs either from the lateral nail fold or the free edge. A nail that has been traumatized and nails in older people where linear growth is slow both seem to be susceptible to infection. Poor peripheral circulation is thought to play a part in both susceptibility to infection and resistance to treatment	Gradually the nail becomes opaque, yellow and crumbly. Eventually there is nail thickening and destruction of the nail plate may occur	

as this can spread infection to other areas and lead to secondary bacterial infection.

Specific care in particular types of tinea is as follows:

- Tinea capitis – reassurance that completion of an effective treatment course could prevent further inflammation, scarring and hair loss. Regular hair washing with an antifungal shampoo and combing with an awareness of how it could be spread to others. A wig may be required until hair has regrown.
- Tinea manuum – appropriate handwashing and making sure hands are dried properly, especially under rings.
- Tinea pedis – footwear can be treated in addition to local antifungal treatment. Particular attention to foot hygiene, e.g. changing socks/tights daily. Infected people should avoid walking barefoot in communal areas. Swimming pools and changing rooms are a major source of infection and should be avoided by those with foot infections. This is not always feasible as many infections are asymptomatic.
- Tinea unguium – advice about nail care and regrowth (new clear nail could be visible after 9 months).

Superficial *Candida* infections (candidosis, candidiasis)

Candidosis is caused by a yeast infection and may affect the skin, nails and mucosae. The most common pathogen is *Candida albicans*, although other species may cause infection in humans. It is known colloquially as 'thrush'. Candidosis may also affect the gastrointestinal tract (see also Ch. 22), the genital tract (see Ch. 25) and, more rarely, the respiratory tract.

Superficial *Candida* infections occur worldwide, but there are regional patterns of disease prevalence, e.g. interdigital candidosis of the feet is more common in the tropics, whereas candidosis of the nails is more frequently seen in colder climes.

There are many factors known to predispose to candidosis and an underlying reason for infection can generally be found, for example:

- patients taking broad-spectrum antibiotics
- patients who are immunocompromised, e.g. cancer chemotherapy, HIV infection, etc.
- older people – due to declining immune function.

Details of common types of candidosis are presented in Table 28.2.

Pityriasis versicolor – *Malassezia* yeast infection

Pityriasis versicolor is a mild, chronic yeast infection of the skin.

Aetiology and epidemiology

Pityriasis versicolor in most cases represents a change in the relationship between human host and resident yeast flora. The causative organism, *Malassezia*, does not invade the hair shaft, nails or mucous membranes.

It affects both sexes equally, and all races, but there is a difference in susceptibility at different ages. In tropical areas,

Table 28.2 Candidosis

Site	Clinical presentation	Medical management	Nursing management
Oral candidosis (thrush)	Splitting at the corners of the mouth in angular cheilitis is an important and common sign of candidosis and occurs frequently in those with ill-fitting dentures	Topical anti-yeast preparations, e.g. nystatin suspension or pastilles Oral antiseptics	Assessment of general health (awareness if immunocompromised) Regular mouth hygiene, dental care, well-fitting dentures
Candidal intertrigo	Prominent red rash – groin and the upper thighs, which may be spotted with satellite pustules and papules. May occur in other sites, e.g. under the breasts and umbilicus	Topical anti-yeast preparations, e.g. nystatin cream, or an imidazole, e.g. clotrimazole cream	Discussion about personal hygiene, to complete the course of topical preparations, not to stop too soon
Interdigital candidosis	White soggy-looking skin in the interdigital spaces, which is superficially eroded Secondary infection with bacteria is a common complication	Topical anti-yeast preparations – see above Antibiotics for secondary infection	Ensure skin is dried thoroughly after wetting Complete the course of topical preparation Use of emollients to improve the lipid barrier for occupations with wet work, e.g. nursing
Candidosis of the nails	The condition presents as painful swellings around the nail fold that may sometimes discharge pus The lateral nail border may be undermined with nail destruction and separation in severe cases	Oral anti-yeast preparations, e.g. itraconazole	It commonly affects those patients whose job involves continuous wet work, e.g. washing up Discuss how nails should be cut and filed so cuticles remain intact

it is far more common and as many as 40% of some populations may be affected.

Clinical presentation

It is characterized by scaly hypo- or hyperpigmented macules (stain < 1 cm with a flat surface that does not blanche), mainly on the upper trunk and arms. The term versicolor is apt because, in the untanned white skin, affected areas are darker than normal, but fail to respond to UV radiation exposure, and in tanned or black skin, the abnormal skin is usually paler. This variation in pigmentation may remain for several months after spontaneous resolution or treatment but without the scaling.

▶ Nursing and medical management

If the patient is very concerned and the skin is uncomfortable then anti-yeast creams may help (see above). Intractable infections may need a course of oral itraconazole.

Most patients are seeking reassurance about the variation in pigment and just need to know that it will resolve. To prevent recurrence, the use of anti-yeast shampoos as a body wash prior to going to a hot climate might be useful.

INFESTATIONS

SCABIES

Scabies is caused by infestation with a minute arthropod mite, *Sarcoptes scabiei hominis* (itch mite).

Aetiology and pathophysiology

The mite is passed from person to person during close physical contact, and in severe infestations from contaminated clothing and bedding. The female mite burrows under the stratum corneum to lay eggs, leaving a small visible track on the skin. The larvae emerge from the skin after 3–5 days and become adults in around 17 days. The mites feed and multiply as they move through the skin. The chemicals produced by elimination cause intense irritation in the skin, which in turn provokes scratching, a primary feature of this condition. It should be noted that it might take up to 4 weeks to mount this allergic response so it is possible to be infected in the absence of any symptoms.

The primary sites of entry are in the finger webs, natural skin folds and pressure areas. In time, all areas of the body may be affected, except the head, neck and soles of the feet.

Acquired immunity to scabies is almost non-existent and recurrent attacks are common, and especially in 'at risk' groups, which include immunocompromised individuals, those in institutions such as prisons and nursing homes, and individuals whose personal hygiene and lifestyle put them at risk.

Clinical presentation

- Characteristic burrows
- Intense itching (worse at night and when hot)
- Eczematous changes and secondary infection from chronic itch–scratch cycle
- Papules – may form due to persistent damage to the skin from scratching.

Medical management

The treatment of scabies consists of using chemical pesticides, e.g. aqueous preparations of permethrin or malathion, which need only one application if applied effectively. Treatment with other preparations may need repeat applications. Topical corticosteroid may be applied to ease the irritation caused by treatment.

It is important to identify the index case and treat all contacts and family members at the same time, whether or not they have signs of scabies. Sedating antihistamines may be prescribed to help patients sleep. Antibiotics may be required for secondary bacterial infections.

▶ Nursing management

Topical anti-scabetic treatment should be applied after bathing to a clean dry skin. It should be applied to all skin from the neck downwards. The gluteal cleft, genitalia, umbilicus, flexures, finger and toe webs and nails must not be overlooked and the hands require particular attention. If the hands are washed for any reason then the treatment must be reapplied. The treatment should be allowed to dry and left on the skin for 24 hours. All clothing, bedding (sheets, duvet covers and pillow cases) used during the treatment time should be laundered. The ordinary wash cycle of a machine will suffice. It may be necessary to repeat these procedures 5–7 days later.

PEDICULOSIS

Pediculosis is infestation with lice:

- head louse *(Pediculus humanus capitis)*
- body/clothing louse *(Pediculus humanus humanus)*
- pubic (crab) louse *(Phthirus pubis)*.

The body louse is a major carrier of epidemic typhus, trench fever and relapsing fever.

The body louse and head louse are almost identical in appearance. Infestation with body lice is rare in developed countries, except in rough sleepers and others unable to change and launder their clothing. In contrast, the head louse maintains a high profile amongst schoolchildren everywhere and affects all socioeconomic groups, and adults may also be affected.

Pubic lice are transmitted almost entirely by sexual contact. This louse differs from the others by being shorter and fatter with two huge hind claws that are designed to cling to widely spaced hairs in the pubis region; all short body hair may be infested.

Head lice

Head lice transmission is primarily from head to head contact. The role of shared hats, brushes and combs is debatable; the lice can live for several days off the scalp but may be so damaged that they cannot infest or reproduce on another host.

Clinical presentation

- Pruritus is the main symptom but may only be apparent with large numbers of lice.
- Persistent scratching may result in secondary bacterial infection and lymphadenopathy.

- The presence of eggs (nits) cemented to the hair shaft; initially the main sites are behind the ears and the nape of the neck. The eggs are laid close to the scalp and it is possible to postulate the timescale of infestation from the presence of eggs or egg cases along the hair shaft.
- Live adult insects are often not seen on clinical examination, as they are hard to detect if they have just had a blood meal.
- Presence of bite reactions and excoriations.

▶ Nursing management

Detection is the first step and the best way of finding lice is by using a fine-tooth comb on damp clean hair. This can be made easier by applying conditioner to the hair before checking.

1. Have a sheet of white paper to hand and a good light source.
2. Comb through the hair with an ordinary comb first to disentangle the hair.
3. Part the hair into sections.
4. Using the detector comb with the teeth close to the scalp, carefully draw it through the sections of hair.
5. Any lice present can be seen on the comb or the white paper.
6. Continue to work your way around the head, combing each section.

This physical removal of the lice will not remove the eggs but may damage them. Treatment is only needed if live lice are found.

Chemical treatment with lotions, e.g. malathion, is another treatment option. Individuals with eczema and/or asthma should use aqueous solutions instead of those in alcohol. Chemical shampoos should not be used as they are too dilute and do not kill the eggs. These treatments are considered safe but should only be used in moderation. No one chemical is recommended; rotational policies of various insecticides have not proved effective in preventing resistance. Take advice from the pharmacist as to the current chemical of choice. The instructions for use should be followed exactly and the nurse should be able to explain these to patients and ensure that enough treatment is given to treat all cases. Lotions should be allowed to dry naturally on the hair. A hairdryer must never be used, as alcohol-based solutions may ignite the hair and the heat may degrade the chemical insecticide. All family members should be checked and all those with live lice treated at the same time. Repeat treatment after 7 days will kill any lice that have hatched from untreated eggs.

The scalp and hair should be checked daily after treatment; if very small lice are found, treatment has not been effective. If mature adults are found then re-infection has taken place.

Repeated physical removal – 'bug busting' – is a safe method of treating, as it breaks the life cycle by constantly removing immature lice (nymphs) as they hatch. It is not effective against eggs and needs to be repeated every 3–4 days for a period of 2 weeks. Chemical treatments should not be used to prevent infection.

Body and pubic lice

The treatment of pubic lice is best done with aqueous solutions of the same chemicals used for head lice, as alcoholic solutions may irritate the genitalia. The instructions included with the treatment should be complied with and repeated after 7–10 days.

Eyelash infestation is treated by application of petroleum jelly (e.g. Vaseline) – three times per day for a week should remove and kill the eggs.

Treatment of body lice involves the removal and laundering of clothing in a high-temperature wash and ironing the seams of clothing to kill both lice and eggs. Bathing the host will remove any live lice from the body. The most common cause of treatment failure is inadequate treatment and failure to treat all contacts so that reinfestation occurs.

BENIGN SKIN CHANGES

CYSTS

A true mucocutaneous cyst is a closed sac lined by epidermally or adnexally derived epithelium and filled with a liquid or semi-solid material derived from that epithelium (Fitzpatrick et al 2001).

Pathophysiology
Skin cysts may be:

- epidermoid (epidermal) cyst – commonest cyst, derived from the epidermis
- trichilemmal (sebaceous) cyst – second most common, seen most often on the scalp
- epidermal inclusion (dermoid) cyst – traumatic implantation of epidermis within the dermis.

▶ Nursing and medical management

Skin cysts may be excised, e.g. if they catch on clothing or are unsightly. If they are to be excised, it is important that patients understand the procedure, and that they will have a scar to replace the lesion; also that if it is in the mantle (shoulders, neck, face and ears) region, the likelihood of keloid development is increased. Patients with pigmented skin have an increased risk of keloid development (Fitzpatrick et al 2001).

KELOIDS

Keloids and hypertrophic scars are exuberant fibrous repair tissue following a cutaneous injury. Hypertrophic scars remain confined to the site of original injury whereas a keloid extends beyond this site. The upper mantle of the body is most susceptible to keloid formation, as are those with dark skin.

Medical/surgical management
The management of keloids may include:

- silicone dressings – soften and reduce scar bulk
- intralesional corticosteroids – monthly injection may reduce bulk and flatten, and reduce pruritus or sensitivity
- cryotherapy – use of liquid nitrogen can debulk the keloid
- re-excision – but recurrence rates are higher and resulting scars are often larger than the original scar. Silicone gel could be applied immediately after surgery.

▶ Nursing management

These patients require support, as they will be very self-conscious of their body image. They may already have low self-esteem if the keloids are caused by acne, and it is important that the underlying pathology is treated prior to dealing with the scars. Advising patients of the risk of scarring for cosmetic surgery is important.

Nurses may administer the intralesional injections. Another nursing role is to supervise and teach patients how to apply the silicone gel dressing. This is applied daily for at least 3 months. A piece of dressing is cut to the size of the scar and applied, with the patient wearing it for a minimum of 12 hours a day. Depending on the make of dressing, it can be re-washed and re-applied for up to 14 days.

Camouflage may be the only solution to cover the lesions.

DISORDERS OF KERATIN SYNTHESIS

PSORIASIS

Psoriasis is a chronic, non-infectious, inflammatory disease.

Aetiology
The aetiology is complex, but genetic, immunological and skin factors are involved. The genetic predisposition affects 1.5–2% of the population of the Western world (Fitzpatrick et al 2001).

Various factors can cause exacerbation of psoriasis:

- trauma – psoriasis appears on skin damaged by scratching, surgery or tattoos, etc. (Koebner phenomenon)
- drugs such as beta-blockers and antimalarials can exacerbate the condition. Stopping systemic or potent topical corticosteroids can cause the skin lesions to 'rebound'
- throat infection with beta-haemolytic streptococcal throat often triggers guttate psoriasis
- sunlight – condition worsens in about 10% of patients
- emotion – emotional upset can cause some exacerbations
- disease – HIV infection, for example, can exacerbate the disease.

Pathophysiology
The proliferation rate of epidermal cells is increased and the process of keratinization is abnormal. The keratinocytes progress through the layers of the epidermis much more quickly, and the epidermal turnover time is drastically reduced.

Clinical presentation
Psoriasis has several clinical expressions (erythrodermic, pustular and guttate) but is most commonly characterized by well-defined erythematous plaques bearing large adherent silvery scales. Classical sites include the scalp, knees, elbows and sacral area, but it can be generalized. The nails are commonly affected, with onycholysis and hyperkeratosis under the nail.

Psoriasis may be associated with joint disease (arthropathy) and 5–8% of those with psoriasis are affected, especially those with pustular or erythrodermic psoriasis (Fitzpatrick et al 2001; see Ch. 27).

Medical management

Communication between the health professionals is key to the management of psoriasis. The primary care team manages the majority of patients but some will receive care in specialist units.

Both topical and systemic strategies may be needed to control symptoms.

Topical therapy

- Soap substitute, bath oils (choice includes coal tar additives)
- Emollients – removal of keratin scale enables the absorption of topical medication (see 'Atopic eczema')
- Corticosteroids (see 'Atopic eczema') – used to reduce erythema. Only mild-to-moderate potency corticosteroids should be used, as corticosteroids can make the psoriasis unstable, and cause the skin to thin
- Combination of mild-to-moderate potency corticosteroids and coal tar solution
- Salicylic acid used in combination with emollients to remove hyperkeratotic skin from soles or palms
- Coal tar (shampoos, bath oils, creams and ointments) – can be messy and smelly and is often used under supervision in day care units
- Dithranol (paste, ointment, cream and lotions) – application must be precise to prevent burning of normal skin, and staining whatever it touches. Can be used as short contact at home or under supervision of a day care unit
- Vitamin D – fairly easy to use and does not stain but can cause irritation; initially makes the plaques red and exfoliate more. Vitamin D combined with a potent corticosteroid may be used daily for 4 weeks before reverting to vitamin D alone. The time to become effective varies with different products and patients should know this or they will stop too soon. Patients should be aware of the total dose of preparation used in a week because of the potential to absorb calcium
- Vitamin A – application must be precise to prevent irritation. It is greasy and can smudge if applied just before bed (leave 30 minutes)
- Phototherapy (UV radiation) – there are three types of treatment: UVB, UVB narrow band and PUVA (long-wavelength UV radiation with oral or topical psoralen, a naturally occurring photosensitive substance). Treatments may be whole-body or just to localized areas. If patients fail to respond to topical therapies, the second phototherapy treatment can be used in conjunction with systemic therapy such as retinoids.

Systemic therapies

Systemic therapies may be used where other therapies fail. They include:

- methotrexate (cytotoxic drug) – requires close monitoring of blood count, liver and renal function. Patients should report any cough or breathlessness
- ciclosporin (immunosuppressant drug) – patients need education to recognize signs of infection that may be hidden by the therapy.

▶ Nursing management

An assessment of patients' needs should include education needs, the psychological impact of the disease, as well as whether they live alone or not. Treatments will only be effective if used correctly, and incorrect use may produce unnecessary side-effects. Some patients need systemic therapies that require regular blood test to monitor side-effects and support from the nurses. An understanding of each patient's needs and lifestyle will enable the nurse to plan an effective and workable regimen (Watts 1999). Living with a chronic illness can be draining and providing support for patients and their families is key to maintaining their motivation.

DISORDERS OF PIGMENTATION

An imbalance of normal pigment or the presence of abnormal pigments can cause abnormal pigmentation.

Disorders of pigmentation may present as hypo- (less colour) or hyperpigmentation (more colour), and may be congenital or acquired. Any disorder of pigmentation will alter patients' body image and may have a profound impact on their psychological well-being.

Pigment changes can follow any skin inflammation, e.g. hypopigmentation associated with eczema or psoriasis, etc. It may also occur after a burn or cryosurgery. The more severe the inflammation, the more likely the pigment is to decrease rather than increase. Problems are also more likely to develop in people with dark skins. Repigmentation will usually occur, but this may take many months.

Hyperpigmentation caused by inflammation is common in conditions such as lichen planus and eczema, and following cryosurgery. As with hypopigmentation, it can clear but may take many months.

There are many rare conditions that alter pigmentation, but some of the more common disorders are outlined below.

ALBINISM

Albinism is genetically defined hypopigmentation, secondary to a defect in the melanocyte. It can affect the skin, hair and eyes. The skin in light-skinned people will become very light and the hair white to cream or yellow, or even vibrant red, whereas dark-skinned individuals will have large pigmented freckles over a pale background in light-exposed areas and the hair may become yellow or yellowish brown. The eyes are also affected and lack pigment. Photophobia is a problem and individuals may squint.

Medical management

There is no cure and management focuses on monitoring and preventing complications such as skin cancers, which can arise from the lack of sun protection. Eyes also need to be checked regularly as problems such as cataracts can develop.

▶ Nursing management

Nurses must be aware that this condition can alter body image, and ensure that all health professionals understand that it is not contagious. Patients need advice and information about sun protection, e.g. clothing and sunscreens, as well as eye protection. Patients should be advised to check their skin for changes and to attend regularly for checks for skin cancer or ocular complications.

VITILIGO

Vitiligo is a depigmentation disorder of the skin characterized by patchy loss of colour.

Epidemiology and aetiology

Vitiligo affects 2% of the population worldwide, regardless of race or gender (Halder & Young 2000). It is not contagious and it is most likely that a particular gene is associated with vitiligo. Bhatia et al (1992) found a higher prevalence of vitiligo in relatives of patients than in controls.

Although the exact cause is unclear, it is known that hormonal changes, excessive stress and damage to the skin can act as triggers in predisposed individuals.

Clinical presentation

Patches of vitiligo are always whiter than the rest of the skin and are caused by loss of melanocytes. Patches can appear anywhere on the body, but usually appear in a symmetrical pattern. Vitiligo can also cause white patches in scalp hair, eyebrows, eyelashes, beard and body hair, but apart from the colour difference, affected areas will look and feel the same as normal skin or hair. Some patches of vitiligo will repigment spontaneously, although there is always a risk of relapse, whereas other patches will never repigment.

Medical management

There is no ideal treatment and current treatments can be difficult, lengthy and do not alter the underlying cause.

Areas of vitiligo lack protection from the sun and are therefore at risk of sunburn, which can cause the condition to spread. Patients should be advised to cover up and/or wear high-protection sunscreens (factor 25 or above).

Topical corticosteroids may be used on patches to try and stimulate repigmentation. They are more effective on new and smaller patches, but long-term side-effects mean they cannot be used continuously. Phototherapy has been used on vitiligo for many years with varying degrees of success. PUVA (see p. 862) is a treatment in which the patient's skin is sensitized to light by the use of psoralen, which can be oral or topical, and then irradiated with UVA radiation. Not all patients will respond to this treatment, but those who do may regain some or all of their pigment. Treatment can be for up to a year. Unfortunately, most patients relapse after a few years of stopping treatment.

Bleaching is a drastic treatment and is not considered unless over 70% of the body is affected with vitiligo. In this treatment, the normal areas of skin are bleached to try to obtain a more even skin colour over the body.

▶ Nursing management

Vitiligo does not affect physical health initially, but psychological effects can be devastating. It is neither painful nor itchy, but there can be a tendency for it to be trivialized by health professionals and the general public (Agarwel 1998). However, vitiligo can be a great psychosocial handicap and cause considerable distress to sufferers and their families. Many people with vitiligo feel isolated, have a poor body image and lack self-confidence; some can become depressed and withdrawn. Teenagers are particularly vulnerable, as are some brown-skinned individuals, who may be stigmatized and ostracized.

Nurses who are well informed about vitiligo are able to give support to patients. They need to understand the physical and psychological problems experienced by patients. Problems should never be trivialized and time should be allocated to listen to them.

Some practical considerations for nurses to take into account include the following:

- Inform patients that vitiligo is not contagious.
- Offer advice on sun care to reduce the risk of burning and photo damage.
- Inform and advise patients of the availability of cosmetic camouflage (this information should be available in the local dermatology department). Patients can be taught by specially trained individuals to blend and apply camouflage preparations to give good cosmetic results. This can help some patients to face the world and regain some of their confidence. Although it can be effective, it is time-consuming, may rub off on clothing and needs to be applied daily.
- Support patients using topical corticosteroids or having phototherapy by being aware of side-effects and the likely duration of treatment.
- Inform patients about the Vitiligo Society (see 'Useful addresses', p. 875).

CHLOASMA

Chloasma is a common acquired light or dark brown hyperpigmentation occurring on light-exposed areas, usually the face. It is usually associated with pregnancy or the oral contraceptive. Treatment for this is not always helpful but bleaching agents containing hydroquinone may be helpful. Protecting the lesions from the sun with a high-factor sunscreen will reduce their prominence and may prevent further lesions.

FRECKLES AND LENTIGINES

Freckles are examples of hyperpigmentation. They are well demarcated, brown macules, usually less than 5 mm in diameter. They proliferate and darken with sun exposure. Freckles are extremely common and no treatment is needed.

Lentigines are larger dark brown macules (1–10 mm across). Simple lentigines often appear in adolescence and are common in older people ('liver spots'). They are harmless but should be distinguished from more serious conditions such as skin cancer. Pigment is also disordered in certain malignant conditions such as malignant melanoma (see p. 868).

▶ Nursing management

Benign pigment lesions increase in number as an accumulative effect of sun exposure. The use of clothes, shade and sunscreens may reduce the impact. These are cosmetic but often cause distress. Support and advice are required but unfortunately earlier sun exposure during childhood does the damage and these effects cannot be reversed in adults.

VASCULAR DISORDERS

HAEMANGIOMAS

Haemangiomas of the skin are one form of birthmark, e.g. 'port wine' stain. They are benign proliferations of the vascular endothelium. With early diagnosis and laser management of haemangiomas, there are few residual problems in adulthood.

However, in 20% of capillary haemangiomas ('strawberry' naevus) there are complications, including (Linward 1999):

- bleeding
- ulceration
- visual impairment
- interference with respiration
- deformity and disfigurement.

Intervention is required which may influence these patients psychologically as they become more aware of their own appearance. If treatment of the haemangioma was delayed then the cosmetic effect may be more noticeable and the desire to have corrective surgery may be an issue.

Port wine stains of the face can affect ocular function, and later in life patients can develop glaucoma. This is open to debate so regular ophthalmologist review is necessary (Atherton 1992).

TELANGIECTASIA (CHERRY ANGIOMAS)

There is a hereditary (autosomal dominant) haemorrhagic telangiectasia affecting blood vessels, especially those in the mucosa of the mouth and gastrointestinal tract. This disease is frequently heralded by recurrent epistaxis that appears in childhood. Small, pulsating, macular and papular, discrete but multiple vascular telangiectasias are seen on the lips and tongue.

Management focuses on controlling epistaxis and gastrointestinal bleeding. Laser surgery may be used to destroy the abnormal vessels. Nursing would be tailored to individual patients depending on their prognosis.

BLISTERING SKIN DISORDERS

A blister is a fluid-filled lesion arising in the skin. A lesion of less than 5 mm diameter is termed a vesicle, and one greater than 5 mm diameter a bulla. The accumulation of fluid is either within the epidermis or immediately subepidermal. There are many causes of blisters and the diagnosis of a blistering condition is made from the patient's history as well as the appearance and distribution of the blisters. Where diagnosis is unclear, a skin biopsy will show histologically where the blister lies within the skin and so aid diagnosis.

There are three main types of bullae (see Fig. 28.5):

- subcorneal bullae – located just underneath the stratum corneum, e.g. bullous impetigo

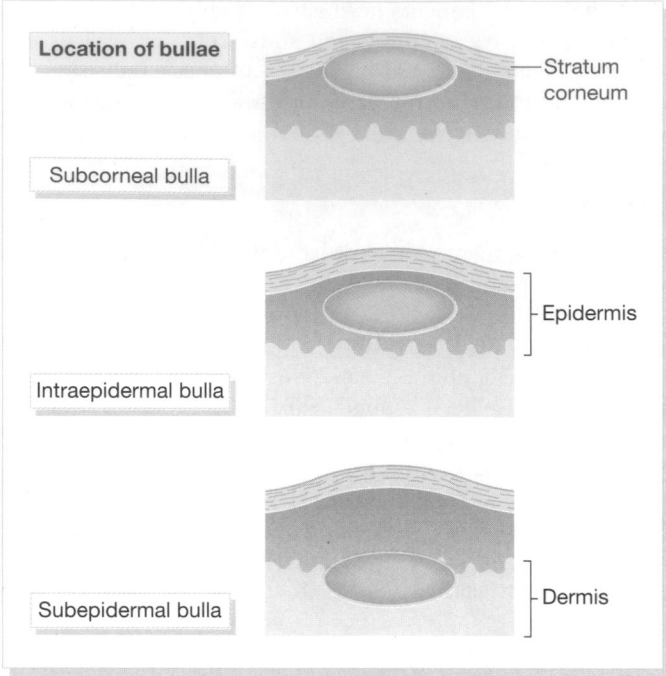

Figure 28.5 Types of bullae – location.

- intraepidermal bullae – located in the centre of the epidermis, e.g. acute eczema, pemphigus and viral blisters
- subepidermal bullae – just under the epidermis within the dermis, e.g. bullous pemphigoid, epidermolysis bullosa.

INFECTIVE BLISTERING DISORDERS

Infective blistering disorders are treated according to their origin or cause.

Bullous impetigo
This is caused by *Staphylococcus aureus*. The blisters are subcorneal, burst easily and may contain pus. Antibiotics are given orally and often topically as well.

Bullous cellulitis
Excessive oedema caused in cellulitis of the lower limb often results in erosion and ulceration. Patients with leg ulcers are prone to recurring infections of the soft tissue and require hospitalization for intravenous antibiotics.

Eczema herpeticum
This is a serious condition that occurs when existing eczema becomes infected with HSV-1. Groups of small vesicles form in clusters on areas of eczema and normal skin. They have a typical punched-out appearance and can spread rapidly over large areas of the body. Patients may feel very unwell. Antiviral agents are administered, and in severe cases these are given intravenously in hospital. Patients remains hospitalized until the blisters start to subside and they feel better. Isolation is essential due to the infectious nature of eczema herpeticum (see Ch. 13).

► Nursing management: infective blistering disorders

If an infective cause is suspected, swabs should be taken for bacterial culture and sensitivity and/or for viral cultures. The aim is to treat the cause and let blisters dry and the skin heal underneath. When a lesion is very weepy, potassium permanganate solution applied as soaks may act as an antiseptic and also as a drying agent. Thick crusts may form from the fluid as the blisters burst in impetigo; these may need to be soaked off with warm water or saline solution to make the patient more comfortable. Nurses need to monitor antibiotic (intravenous, oral and topical) therapy.

Bacterial and viral blistering disorders are usually highly infectious and advice needs to be sought and given on avoiding spread of the infection. The HSV-1 responsible for eczema herpeticum can spread easily through close bodily contact. Patients need to be warned of this and given advice on using separate towels, flannels and clothing. Health professionals and patients with eczema should be aware that a simple cold sore (see p. 855) could cause eczema herpeticum in adults with eczema. When they have active lesions, they should avoid contact with such patients.

AUTOIMMUNE BLISTERING DISORDERS

Autoimmune blistering disorders are rare and the causes remain unknown. They can have a devastating effect on affected individuals. Due to their rarity, they are not always easily diagnosed and in some instances can be life-threatening if severe or left untreated.

Bullous pemphigoid

This is the most common autoimmune blistering disorder. It is generally a disease of older people and occurs in those aged 60–80 years. Blisters appear on normal or slightly urticated (raised and red) skin. The blisters are subepidermal and therefore quite tense and usually seen intact. Commonly the blisters develop on the limbs. Blisters can develop anywhere on the body, although the mucosae, e.g. the mouth, are not usually affected (Watts 2001). Treatment involves high-dose systemic corticosteroids and topical corticosteroids to the lesions. Systemic corticosteroids may be needed for several years to reduce the disease process. Eroded areas should be swabbed and sent for culture and, if needed, appropriate antibiotics should be prescribed.

Pemphigus

Pemphigus affects a younger age group (usually 40–60 years of age). Prior to the use of systemic corticosteroids, the condition had a 75% mortality rate within the first year. The blisters are intraepidermal and very fragile. Often no intact blisters can be seen as they burst, leaving open eroded areas. The lesions particularly affect the scalp, face and axilla, and the mucosae of the mouth and genitalia are often also affected.

Even before the diagnosis is confirmed on skin biopsy the patient commences high doses of systemic corticosteroids and once the blistering has subsided the dose is gradually reduced and systemic immunosuppressive drugs introduced. If blistering recurs the corticosteroid dose would be increased again.

► Nursing management: autoimmune blistering disorders

- Make regular assessments of the skin and check for new blisters; record results.
- Keep skin clean with a daily bath when possible; mild antiseptics, e.g. potassium permanganate solution, can be added.
- Emollients are applied with great care, so as not to enlarge existing lesions and to prevent causing further lesions.
- Large tense blisters, e.g. in pemphigoid, may need aspirating (see Fig. 28.6 and Guidelines for Care Priorities box 28.3).
- Topical treatments, e.g. corticosteroids, should be applied very gently as prescribed.

GUIDELINES FOR CARE PRIORITIES

28.3 Aspirating blisters associated with skin conditions

Tense fluid-filled bullae can be uncomfortable and painful. Blisters should not just be burst with a sterile needle but should be emptied by aspiration. The blister roof should be left intact as this will cover the raw area underneath and will aid re-epithelialization.

Method (see Fig. 28.6)
1. The blister should be aspirated using an appropriately sized needle. A large needle may traumatize the blister more than is necessary and one that is too small may allow the blister to refill soon after aspiration.
2. The syringe with needle should be positioned near the roof of the blister and the fluid gently aspirated from the blister.
3. Some of the fluid is sent to the microbiology laboratory for culture and sensitivity if infection is suspected.

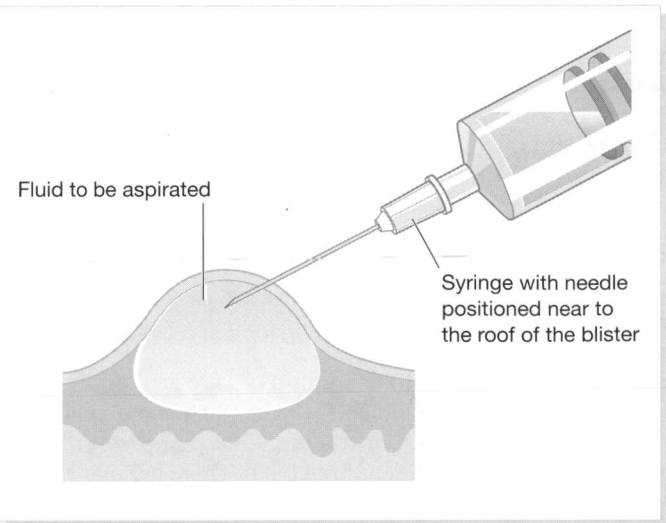

Figure 28.6 Correct technique for aspirating a blister.

- Large eroded areas may need protection, and non-adherent dressings such as paraffin gauze can be applied. Dressings are secured by gently bandaging into position; tape should not be used directly onto the skin.
- Systemic therapy with corticosteroids should be closely monitored and any side-effects noted. For example, daily blood pressure reading and urinalysis for glycosuria should be undertaken.
- Oral fluids should be encouraged when possible, and if intravenous fluids are necessary, this must be monitored, keeping an input and output record.
- Where oral lesions occur, patients need frequent attention to oral hygiene and mouthwashes should be encouraged.
- The diet should be monitored and soft food provided when necessary. A referral to a dietician or specialist nutrition nurse may be necessary.

It should be remembered that both bullous pemphigoid and pemphigus can, in some cases, be life-threatening, as can the secondary effects of the systemic treatment. These patients require the skills of a dermatological trained nurse.

DERMATITIS HERPETIFORMIS

Dermatitis herpetiformis is a rare, chronic, intensely itchy condition. It can affect all age groups but especially the young and middle-aged. Patients also have gluten intolerance.

Clinical presentation

There are groups of red papules, weals and small vesicles. The condition is so intensely itchy that these are very quickly scratched and intact vesicles are rarely seen.

Medical management

Specific management includes:

- systemic dapsone (a drug used in leprosy) – this is effective, but has serious side-effects such as haemolytic anaemia and leucopenia (see Ch. 18), and regular blood checks are necessary
- sedating antihistamines – these may help to relieve itching
- gluten-free diet.

▶ Nursing management

Prescribed emollients and topical corticosteroids should be applied regularly and gently to the skin. Nurses should ensure that patients are referred to a dietician for advice on a gluten-free diet. Continual support and encouragement will be needed especially in helping patients to maintain a gluten-free diet, as they often find this diet particularly hard to follow.

EPIDERMOLYSIS BULLOSA

Epidermolysis bullosa (EB) is a group of rare genetically determined skin disorders in which the skin can separate following minimal everyday friction or trauma. EB encompasses a group of conditions that are present from birth. There are many forms but the most severe are due to abnormalities of the structures anchoring the epidermis to the dermis. This defect allows blisters to develop easily at the site of trauma.

▶ Nursing management

It is especially important to minimize trauma, to prevent contractures and web formation between digits, and to combat secondary infection. It is a severe and chronic condition and specialist medical and nursing advice needs to be sought when caring for adults with this condition. The DEBRA support group produce useful publications for patients and health care professionals (see 'Useful addresses', p. 875). A nurse specialist is employed by the charity to support the patients and the nurses caring for them when admitted to hospital. These patients in middle adulthood require regular surgical procedures for release of contractures and excision of skin cancers.

STEVENS–JOHNSON SYNDROME AND TOXIC EPIDERMAL NECROLYSIS

Stevens–Johnson syndrome (SJS) and toxic epidermal necrolysis (TEN) now appear to be different forms of disease within the same spectrum (Roujeau 1994). Usually these diseases are related to drugs and they tend to be induced by the same drugs, including sulphonamides, anticonvulsants and NSAIDs. In both these conditions, the skin blisters so badly that it can come away in sheets and leave large eroded areas.

Pathophysiology

In SJS there is extensive blistering of the mucosae, including the lips, eyes, mouth and genitalia. Patients are very unwell and up to 10% of the epidermis will detach from the dermis.

TEN is the most severe blistering disorder, with a mortality rate of around 30%. More than 30% of the epidermis detaches from the dermis. The lesions develop very quickly and there is a widespread sheet-like loss of the epidermis, leaving dark red oozing dermis (Watts 2001). Infection is the main cause of death.

▶ Nursing and medical management

A multidisciplinary team approach to the care of these patients is vital. Severe blistering conditions can be viewed as acute skin failure. Patients with these conditions are usually cared for in specialist dermatology units, intensive care units or burns units. Patients follow a clinical course similar to that of extensive second-degree burns.

As with severe burns (see p. 871), fluid, electrolytes and proteins are lost through the skin. Treatment and nursing care are mainly symptomatic with fluid replacement, antibacterial therapy and nutritional management, as described below:

- Fluid replacement is carefully monitored and accurate records of input and output kept (see Chs 8, 9 and 31).
- Electrolyte balance is monitored through regular blood testing and corrected with appropriate intravenous fluid replacement.
- Pain relief – patients with extensive skin loss have severe pain and this may be hard to control. Prescribed analgesia should be given regularly and especially before any procedures are undertaken.
- It is preferable for the patient to be fed either orally or nasogastrically, as parenteral nutrition offers another

portal of entry for infection. The advice of the dietician and specialist nurses should be sought.

- Patients should be observed for signs of infection and swabs taken where necessary. Antibiotic therapy should be instigated if appropriate.
- Patients are unable to maintain normal body temperature due to skin damage, so the environment temperature should remain constant at around 30–32°C.
- Physiotherapy is important, and anticoagulants may be necessary, for patients who are immobile for long periods of time.
- Patients should be nursed on a bed that reduces pressure to the skin.
- The skin needs to be kept well lubricated at all times to prevent sticking and rubbing and to maintain comfort. Bland emollients should be gently applied directly to the skin or to dressings, which are then applied to open lesions and secured by bandaging.
- Patients with severe disease and their relatives will need considerable help and support in coping with the situation. Time must be made for listening and talking to the patients and their relatives.

SKIN TUMOURS

Skin tumours may be benign, or premalignant, or malignant (cancers). Both benign and malignant types are linked to excessive exposure to UV radiation. In the UK there are 46 000 new cases of skin cancer each year and the disease is responsible for about 2000 deaths (Cancer Research UK 2002). Most of these cancers are either preventable (see Health Promotion box 28.2) or curable if they are diagnosed at an early stage. Initial skin screening occurs in primary care settings with a referral to a hospital dermatological department as appropriate. Some hospitals offer pigmented lesion clinics but all skin cancer patients are prioritized.

BENIGN TUMOURS – SEBORRHOEIC KERATOSES

Seborrhoeic keratoses are benign tumours common in Caucasians and are often accepted as a normal change of ageing.

Clinical presentation
Usually these are non-pigmented brown or black nodules, which have the characteristic appearance of being stuck on the skin. They occur in older people and on sun-exposed sites, the most typical sites being the face, bald scalp and back of the hands. The surface of seborrhoeic keratoses is waxy and sometimes scaly.

▶ Nursing and surgical management

The keratoses may be removed by curettage (after local anaesthetic), or cryotherapy may be used if there are several small lesions. A doctor or specialist dermatology nurse may undertake removal.

 HEALTH PROMOTION

28.2 Safe sun behaviour

Whatever type of skin cancer patients have, there is much the nurse can do to support them and provide education about good sun habits. The aim of successful health promotion advice is to reduce sun exposure and prevent sunburn and should be aimed at all groups, not just those diagnosed with skin cancer. The sun produces three types of UV radiation: UVB that causes reddening and burning of the skin; UVA that causes chronic photodamage and ageing; and UVC, which is normally blocked by the ozone layer, but which is produced by some welding processes (Cancer Research UK 2002).

Patients need education about preventing excess sun exposure and sunburn, which helps to reduce the risk of skin cancer:

- Know your skin type – people with skin types I–III and those with moles and freckles are most at risk from sun exposure, but people with dark skin (types IV–VI) can also suffer sun damage.
- When out in the sun, people (especially children) should be encouraged to wear loose T-shirts. The cloth should be tightly woven to provide maximum protection from the UV radiation. Hats with a brim should also be worn to protect the face.

- It is advisable to avoid the sun between 11.00am and 3.00pm when the UV radiation from the sun is most intense.
- Even on cloudy days, a third of the sun's rays can penetrate the cloud cover, so it is important to seek shade under a parasol or tree. However, this is not always easy to achieve – e.g. carers sometimes forget to move older people seated in the shade when the sun shifts, and it is difficult to restrict children sent out to play during the lunch break at school.
- Patients should be encouraged to use a sunscreen. The sun protection factor (SPF) on the container of sunscreen gives some indication as to the time that can be spent in the sun without becoming burnt compared with the time if no sunscreen is used. Sunscreens should block both UVA and UVB radiation. A sunscreen with 15 SPF is generally considered to provide adequate protection (Ley 1997).
- Avoid the use of sun beds (Cancer Research UK 2002).
- Take extra care when visiting areas close to the equator, and at high altitudes where UV radiation is more intense.

References
Cancer Research UK. Sun and UV light. Melanoma skin cancer. Available. Online: http://www.cancerresearchuk.org. 2002.
Ley S. Sunscreen for photo protection. Dermatol Therapy 1997; 4: 59–71.

Nurses should ensure that patients understand and consent to the minor surgical procedure, and that they understand any specific wound care. Wounds should granulate within 7 days with good cosmetic effect.

MALIGNANT TUMOURS – SKIN CANCERS

There are three types of skin cancer: basal cell carcinoma (BCC), squamous cell carcinoma (SCC) and malignant melanoma. BCC and SCC are termed non-melanoma skin cancers (NMSCs). Kaposi's sarcoma is also discussed in this section because it commonly involves the skin.

BASAL CELL CARCINOMA

Basal cell carcinoma, or 'rodent ulcer', is the most common skin cancer. The commonest cause of BCC is prolonged sun exposure over many years. Individuals who work outside, e.g. farmers or builders, or those with light skins living near the equator, are more at risk of developing a BCC in later life.

Pathophysiology and clinical presentation

Basal cell carcinoma occurs mainly on sun-exposed sites, the most common being the nose, inner canthus and temple, but the tips of the ears and backs of the hands may be affected. They are most commonly seen in those over 60 years of age who present with a history of a non-healing facial lesion that has grown slowly over the preceding 2 or 3 years.

Untreated BCC will ulcerate and erode surrounding tissue including cartilage and bone. However, although BCC can cause extensive local damage it almost never metastasizes.

Surgical management

Early detection and excision are vital for BCC given the potential for tissue destruction. The diagnosis of BCC is usually confirmed following a punch biopsy and histopathological examination. A wide surgical excision of the tumour is then performed under local anaesthetic. For recurrent tumours and those with difficult to define edges, Mohs' micrographic surgery is performed (Ratner et al 1994). Treatments using laser light to destroy the previously photosensitized cancer cells are available in some centres. Annual skin screening by the general practitioner is advised.

SQUAMOUS CELL CARCINOMA

Squamous cell carcinoma is an invasive carcinoma which, untreated, may metastasize. The most common cause of SCC is damage caused by prolonged exposure to UV radiation; however, it also occurs after contact with known carcinogens, such as arsenic, used in some industries.

Clinical presentation

Squamous cell carcinoma is more prevalent in older people and particularly those with fair skin and hair. Patients usually present with a history of a fast-growing lesion on an area of skin that shows signs of sun damage, such as the face, neck, hands and forearms.

Medical/surgical management

A biopsy is taken to confirm the diagnosis prior to a wide excision being performed. In the very elderly or frail patient, radiotherapy may be used but this is not a first-line treatment, as it may further damage the skin and thus encourage new tumours to develop. Patients are examined for lymph node involvement at the time of diagnosis and at every follow-up appointment. Regular follow-up with a dermatologist is usual.

> ▶ **Nursing management: non-melanoma skin cancers**

Nurses are well placed to offer patients further reassurance about prognosis, treatments and cosmetic effects. BCC is curable but surgery becomes more extensive if the cancer has ulcerated. Patients with SCC may require further support if they need treatment for lymph node involvement.

Health promotion is a key role of the nurse (see p. 867) and advice about the use of hats and clothes in general, sunscreens and self-screening should be given as patients have the potential to develop another lesion.

MALIGNANT MELANOMA

Malignant melanoma is a serious form of skin cancer that affects the melanocytes. It accounts for 10% of all skin cancers (Cancer Research UK 2002). The numbers of people with melanoma are increasing yearly (Pedlow et al 1997). Unlike other skin cancers, melanomas tend to occur in younger people and are most common in those aged 40–60 years. In people under 35 years, melanoma is the fifth most common malignancy in men and the third most common in women (Cancer Research UK 2002). Exposure to UV radiation, especially in people with type 1 skin, is the most important cause.

Pathophysiology

Melanoma starts in the epidermis and occurs as a new mole or a change to an existing one. More rarely they can develop under a nail or in the eye. Melanoma is the most dangerous skin cancer, as it has the capacity to metastasize rapidly via the lymph and the blood to liver, lung or brain.

Clinical presentation

Malignant melanomas are classified into four main groups. Each differs slightly but all have some of the following features:

- change in size – a mole enlarges or a new mole appears
- change in shape and an irregular border in a previously symmetrical mole (round or oval), or a newly developed, asymmetrical mole with irregular edges
- change in colour – variation of brown or black pigment in old mole, or newly acquired mole may be speckled
- inflammation of mole or surrounding skin; rare in benign moles
- crusting or bleeding not seen in normal moles unless traumatized
- change in sensation – pain, tenderness or itch
- diameter larger than 7 mm; most benign moles are smaller than this.

Medical/surgical management

Treatment, management and prognosis depend on tumour depth. This is measured as the Breslow depth (Breslow 1970) – vertical measurement taken through the thickest part of the tumour, from the granular layer in the epidermis to the deepest melanoma cell. Complete excision of any pigmented lesion causing concern should be performed and the excised lesion sent for histopathological examination. To reduce the risk of recurrence, a 1 cm margin around the lesion should be excised.

At the time of diagnosis, the patient should undergo a complete physical examination. All other moles should be checked and a photographic record kept. Lymph nodes should be palpated and a chest X-ray performed. Usually the patient will be followed up every 3–4 months for the first 2 years, then 6-monthly and eventually yearly. If at any stage lymph node involvement is detected, a fine-needle biopsy should be carried out to check for malignancy. Radiotherapy, chemotherapy and biological therapies (see Ch. 33) may also be used in certain situations.

▶ Nursing management

Every patient reacts differently to the diagnosis of cancer and it is normal to go through several stages of adjustment (see Ch. 33). Once diagnosed with melanoma, psychological support for patients and their families is vital. Patients often find it difficult to come to terms with the lack of physical treatment available for melanoma although research is ongoing. However, contact with a support group known as Marc's line (see p. 875) can be helpful. Depending on staging they may need the support of Macmillan nurses (see Chs 33 and 34).

It is most important for this group of patients to realize that they cannot afford to sunbathe or burn again. Skin screening and follow-up by a dermatologist are essential as there is the potential to have another cutaneous primary lesion.

KAPOSI'S SARCOMA

Kaposi's sarcoma is a multisystem vascular malignancy characterized by mucocutaneous violaceous lesions and oedema as well as involvement in nearly any organ (Fitzpatrick et al 2001). Many individuals who develop Kaposi's sarcoma are immuno-compromised to some degree, especially those with HIV disease (Smith et al 1998).

▶ Nursing and medical management

Management focuses on symptom relief and not cure. Combination systemic antiviral therapy has been effective in arresting the progression of the disease with a decrease of incidence (Nunley 2000). Localized interventions may be useful, especially around the disfigurement of lesions, and nurses may be involved in carrying out cryotherapy or laser therapy.

Support of the patient is primarily the role of the nurse, acting as an advocate for informed choice regarding therapy and motivation to continue with therapy, as adapting to life around regular medication can be very difficult.

ABNORMAL HAIR GROWTH

Hair may fall out, grow excessively, or grow in an abnormal site – all of which can lead to distress. A detailed account is beyond the scope of this chapter and readers needing more detail should consult a specialist text.

ALOPECIA

Literally, alopecia means a fall of hair. Several different types are described:

- Androgenic alopecia (male pattern baldness), the onset and severity of which is genetically determined
- Endocrine and nutritional factors, e.g. hypo/hyperthyroidism, diabetes, malnutrition and anaemia, can cause poor hair growth or thinning of hair leading to alopecia (see Chs 11, 18 and 17)
- Telogen effluvium caused by stress/serious illness/childbirth
- Drug-induced, e.g. cytotoxic drugs, warfarin, heparin, retinoids (see p. 852), etc.
- Alopecia areata – generalized or localized sudden hair loss, more common amongst patients with Down's syndrome, autoimmune disorders, etc.
- Trauma – visible broken hairs, twisting or pulling of hair (underlying psychological distress)
- Fungal infections – tinea capitis with kerion (see p. 857)
- Scarring alopecia – permanent hair loss related to an underlying dermatosis or infection.

Medical management

Treatment will depend on the diagnosis and underlying cause. Investigations may include blood screen for ferritin, thyroxine and male hormone levels. Bacterial or fungal infections (see pp. 854–859) are treated according to type. Inflammatory dermatosis would be treated with topical potent corticosteroids or intralesional corticosteroids.

▶ Nursing management

Hair (including eyebrows, lashes and beard) is very much part of the human identity and self-esteem. Hair loss causes great psychological distress and thus reassurance and support are required not only through the treatment phase but also during the regrowth phase. In the short term, the patient may benefit from having a wig fitted. Any treatment programme should be fully explained as well as the importance of completing the course of therapy. Support via a patient support group may also be of benefit to the patient and family.

HIRSUTISM

This is excessive terminal hair growth in an androgenic (male) pattern, e.g. face, chest, inner thighs, external genitalia, etc., due to increased androgen activity in a female. A full examination and investigation should be carried out to identify the cause.

▶ Nursing management

Treatment depends on the underlying cause, e.g. systemic anti-androgen drugs, or local cosmetic interventions, e.g. hair removal (shaving, depilatory creams, waxing, electrolysis) or bleaching. Practical advice and psychological support are the cornerstones of nursing care. Clear explanations of specific investigations are needed and support if the scope for resolution is limited. Nurses can offer support while monitoring potential side-effects of systemic therapy and managing those symptoms.

HYPERTRICHOSIS

This is excessive terminal hair growth in a non-androgenic pattern. It can occur in either sex. There are several types:

- symptomatic hypertrichosis as a sequel to or manifestation of a variety of pathological states
- acquired universal hypertrichosis, where hair pattern is normal but hairs are larger and coarser than usual
- drug-induced hypertrichosis, with uniform growth of fine hair over extensive areas of the trunk, face and hands, etc.

Depending on the underlying cause (possible malignancy), investigations and treatment chosen would need to be fully explained with realistic outcomes so as not to give false hope.

▶ Nursing management

Nurses should offer support. Access to NHS electrolysis is limited and treatment is prolonged and patients often resort to bleaching the hair or using cosmetic products. Contact with a support group can be helpful.

NAIL AND NAIL FOLD PROBLEMS

Nail problems may be a manifestation of systemic disease, e.g. spoon-shaped nail in anaemia (see Ch. 18) or splinter haemorrhages in the nail with infective endocarditis (see Ch. 19), or may be caused by a local skin condition such as tinea unguium or psoriasis.

PARONYCHIA

This is inflammation of the proximal and lateral nail folds. The cuticles may have disappeared and the folds are swollen and sore. People who regularly immerse their hands into hot water are susceptible to developing this, particularly those with diabetes (Peters 2001). *Candida* infections can also cause very painful paronychia (see pp. 859). Any infection is treated with the appropriate antimicrobial drug.

▶ Nursing management

Nurses should explain to patients how frequent wetting of the skin can cause paronychia and encourage the use of gloves, emollients and nail care to promote regrowth of the cuticle to enable the skin barrier to function again. Patients are advised to avoid causing trauma to the cuticle during nail care. It is worth reminding patients that it can take 9 months to grow a new nail.

SKIN REACTIONS WITH SYSTEMIC DISORDERS

There are many skin reactions associated with systemic diseases but only xanthomas and drug eruptions are outlined.

XANTHOMAS

These are collections of lipid material in the skin and tendons. The clinical presentation varies and includes yellow-brown, pinkish or orange macules, papules, nodules or infiltration of tendons. Xanthoma may appear on the eyelids, buttocks, knees, elbows and in the Achilles tendon and those of the fingers. This is disfiguring and has a significant psychological impact on the patient.

A xanthoma may be a sign of a primary or secondary hyperlipidaemia (see Chs 17 and 19) and blood should be taken to monitor lipids and cholesterol.

There may be some limited surgical removal but recurrence is not uncommon. Nurses can offer support and advice, scarring can occur after surgical intervention and camouflage may be helpful. In addition, patients may need further support if hyperlipidaemia has been diagnosed and diet modification and drugs have been prescribed.

DRUG ERUPTIONS

Obtaining a detailed history of any medication is an essential part of assessment. Adverse drug reactions (ADRs) can be unpredictable but the nurses' role in advising patients on how and when medications are taken and prompt reporting of any ADRs may minimize discomfort and more serious effects. It is also important to discuss any over-the-counter (OTC) products as well as complementary therapies that are perceived to be safe because they are natural. Early reporting of any reaction is particularly important in dermatological patients who may be more prone to adverse reactions, because their skin may be dryer, fragile and fissured.

The list of drugs known to cause drug eruptions is extensive so a review of drugs and guidance on preventing ADRs in the relevant national formulary or pharmacopoeia is advised. Nurses should, however, be familiar with ADRs associated with drugs commonly used in their area of practice.

There are several different types of drug eruption and some are outlined below:

- Fixed drug eruption – an adverse cutaneous reaction to an ingested drug, characterized by a solitary (or sometimes multiple) plaque, bulla or erosion. It is usually asymptomatic but may be pruritic or burning. If the patient is rechallenged with the same drug, the lesion recurs on the same site within hours of ingestion. Lesions persist if the drug is not stopped otherwise they resolve within days to weeks. Drugs most commonly implicated in a fixed drug eruption include tetracyclines, sulphonamides and quinine. Some foods and food colouring in foods or tablets produce similar effects
- Urticaria, e.g. ACE inhibitors
- Acne-like lesions, e.g. systemic corticosteroids
- Purpura, e.g. sulphonamides
- Pigmentation, e.g. oral contraceptive

- Hair loss during cancer chemotherapy
- The serious condition TEN (see p. 866), e.g. anticonvulsants
- Some drugs increase photosensitivity, e.g. phenothiazines, tetracyclines, thiazide diuretics and psoralens, etc. Photosensitizing reactions are more common in dermatological patients but advising patients to take extra care or to keep sun exposure to a minimum reduces this likelihood.

BURN INJURIES

Burn injuries have a variety of aetiologies and potentially cause death or lead to injuries that have a lifelong impact on patients and their families. Therefore it is vital that effective treatment is begun swiftly after injury to minimize damage to the skin and related structures (Richard 1999). It would be better still, of course, to prevent such injury (see Health Promotion box 28.3).

 HEALTH PROMOTION

28.3 Preventing burn injuries

Burn injuries are potentially life-threatening and they cause severe pain and disfigurement. Most accidents can be prevented, but this requires both national campaigns and interventions by government and such bodies as the RoSPA, and specific health education from the nurse.

Nurses in primary care are instrumental in improving accident prevention. They may lead the field in exploring the common causes of burn injury and encouraging the public to inspect their home for dangers, such as faulty electrical wiring and unguarded fires. Commonly it is people's lifestyle that produces accidents, e.g. smoking in bed or hurriedly drinking a cup of tea that then accidentally spills over an older person to cause a potentially serious burn. Barbecues and bonfires must be used with care and petrol must never be used to make lighting easier. Irons should not be left unattended, or hot fat in a chip pan on the cooker.

The workplace is another area where burn injuries occur and health and safety should be paramount. For example, COSHH details the correct usage and storage of chemicals that should be adhered to at all times.

The general public should be made aware of the dangers of burn injury and the means to prevent accidents. The most common place for an accident to occur is in the home, so effective health education is required to keep it a safe haven.

However, it is not possible to prevent all burn injuries and nurses can increase knowledge of effective first aid measures and the need for prompt referral to medical care in order to minimize the extent of the injury and possibly save life.

Resources

Control of Substances Hazardous to Health Regulations 1999 (COSHH) (see HSE)
Health and Safety Executive (HSE) – www.hse.gov.uk
Royal Society for the Prevention of Accidents (RoSPA) – http://www.rospa.co.uk

TYPES OF BURNS

- Wet heat (scalds) caused by hot baths/hot water, e.g. kettles, saucepans or drinks
- Hot fat burns from cooking fat
- Burns from bonfires, barbecues and fires caused by smoking in bed (often linked to alcohol consumption). Petrol poured over a barbecue or bonfire causing flashback onto the person nearest the fire
- Hot objects, e.g. a radiator
- Radiation, e.g. sunburn
- Electrical burns from poorly maintained electrical appliances. There may be no obvious skin damage but usually an entry and exit point are present. Electrical burns may cause cardiac arrhythmias and these patients should have cardiac monitoring for at least 24 hours post-injury (see Ch. 19)
- Chemical burns caused by acids and alkalis often result in extensive skin damage. The antidote for the chemical should be known and used to neutralize its effects
- Inhalation injury occurs from exposure to hot gases, explosions, head and neck burns, or being confined in a smoke-filled room. Inhalation injury should be considered and dealt with swiftly. Oxygen therapy should be administered as quickly as possible and the extent of airways damage assessed. The patient may require assisted ventilation within a burns unit or intensive care unit (Carrougher 1997).

FIRST AID

The person should be removed from the source of the burn to a safe place. Regardless of cause, the injured part should be bathed in copious amounts of cool water. Time should not be wasted in taking off clothes as this may cause further injury and pain. However, they should be removed where there are chemicals on the clothes (Atkins 1999a). Patients should be kept warm and receive medical attention as soon as possible. If patients are on fire, roll them on the ground to put out the flames. Do not put yourself in danger, e.g. do not enter a house on fire – always call the fire brigade.

ASSESSMENT OF BURNS

Burns are assessed using both depth and percentage of body surface area affected.

Depth

The patient's skin should be examined to assess the depth and extent of the burn.

- *Superficial burn* (only involves the epidermis) – red, painful and has capillary refill. Heals spontaneously and leaves no scars
- *Partial thickness/deep dermal burn* (involves epidermis and upper dermis) – red, blistered and has sensation. It blanches under pressure and heals in 14–28 days. Some scarring may occur according to genetic disposition. Sometimes partial-thickness burns require skin grafting. There is an infection risk

■ *Full-thickness burn* – involves all the layers of the skin and may include subcutaneous fat, muscles and bone. It is white, charred and may have a leathery appearance. Thrombosed veins may be visible. There is little sensation as the nerves are damaged and scarring occurs. Skin grafts are required to promote healing. There is an infection risk.

Remember that the injury may deepen over time if the heat of the original cause of the burn remains. Alternatively, this may be due to infection or dehydration (Atkins 1999b).

Body surface area

The rule of nines chart can be used initially to assess the percentage body surface area involved (see Fig. 28.7). A more accurate assessment can be made using one of several more precise charts, e.g. the Lund and Browder chart (see Fig. 28.8). Adults with 15% or more body surface area involvement should receive fluid resuscitation in a specialized burns unit.

An aid for assessment when the injury is not clearly demarcated is that the patient's palm is considered to be 1%.

INITIAL MANAGEMENT

The ABC of resuscitation is given priority as necessary (see Chs 19, 30 and 31). Patients are kept warm to encourage good perfusion. Following assessment of the burn injury, an intravenous cannula is inserted in order to replace fluids, the burn is cleaned and covered with a non-adherent dressing as appropriate, and pain is controlled.

Abnormal fluid loss from the intravascular to the interstitial space may cause hypovolaemia (see Chs 8 and 9). This must be dealt with as soon as possible. Fluid replacement should be given according to the agreed local formula of the burns unit, e.g. the Muir and Barclay formula:

$$\text{Volume} = (\% \text{ burn area} \times \text{body weight}) / 2$$

This figure is the volume required in each of six time periods over the first 36 hours (timed from the injury, Atkins 1999a). In addition, the haematocrit is checked at the end of each time period to further inform decisions about fluid replacement. However, the patient who does not require intravenous fluid resuscitation should be encouraged to drink at least 3 litres/day (Carrougher 1997).

Pain control is vital. Burns are usually of mixed depth, so even when most of the burn is full-thickness, some pain will be experienced due to areas of superficial and partial-thickness burns. Opiates are useful for pain control. Non-opiates may be used in the less extensive burns (see Ch. 7).

Some patients with full-thickness burns may require urgent attention to relieve restriction around a limb or the chest caused by eschar (scab formed by tissue destruction). An escharotomy is performed to save the limb or allow chest expansion. This should only be performed by a plastic surgeon specializing in burns.

▶ Nursing and medical management

The nursing care of a burns patient is complex. It involves working closely with the multidisciplinary team – doctors, physiotherapists, dieticians – and the family to support the patient

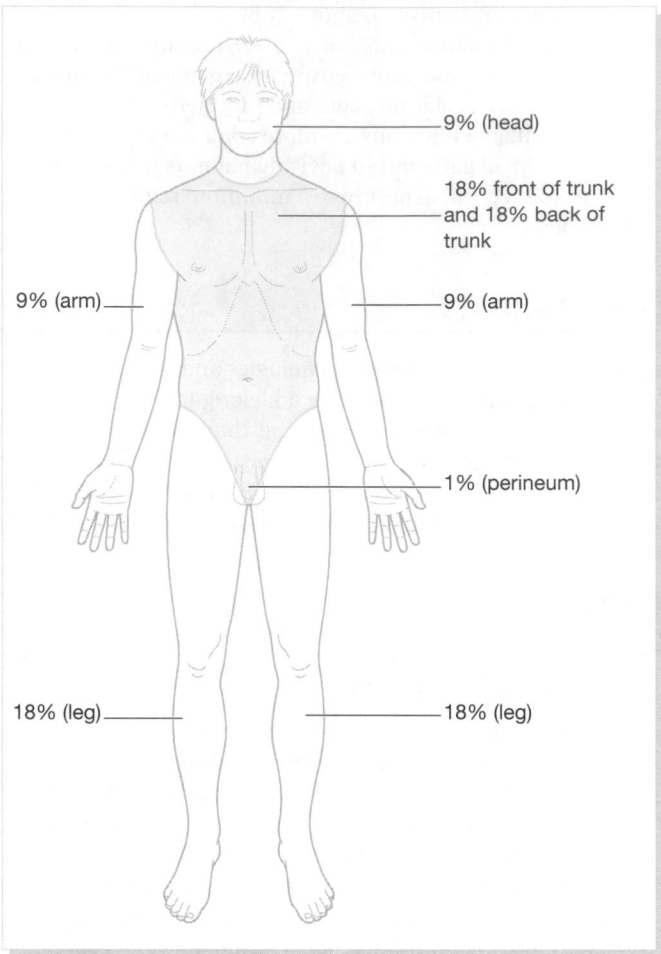

Figure 28.7   Rule of nines.

psychologically and physically. Treatment may take months and nurses are well placed to provide continuity and ongoing support. The nurse is involved in all aspects of patient care, including monitoring, which allows the care team to alter therapy accordingly to need.

Monitoring

The patient requires constant nursing monitoring with accurate records of fluid intake and output. It may be necessary to catheterize the patient and monitor hourly urine output to detect renal failure (see Ch. 24). The fluid replacement regimen will be altered according to the patient's response monitored through blood pressure, pulse, respiratory rate, urinary output and sometimes invasive monitoring such as central venous pressure (see Ch. 9). Temperature is monitored for signs of infection.

Preventing hypothermia

The patient with burns has suffered skin loss and the body's ability to maintain temperature homeostasis will depend on the surface area involved. Room temperature is maintained between 28 and 30°C to prevent heat loss from the damaged area, and also to reduce further evaporation of fluid from a weeping burn. Body temperature is monitored and patients observed for signs of hypothermia (see Ch. 5). Abnormalities are reported and treated as appropriate.

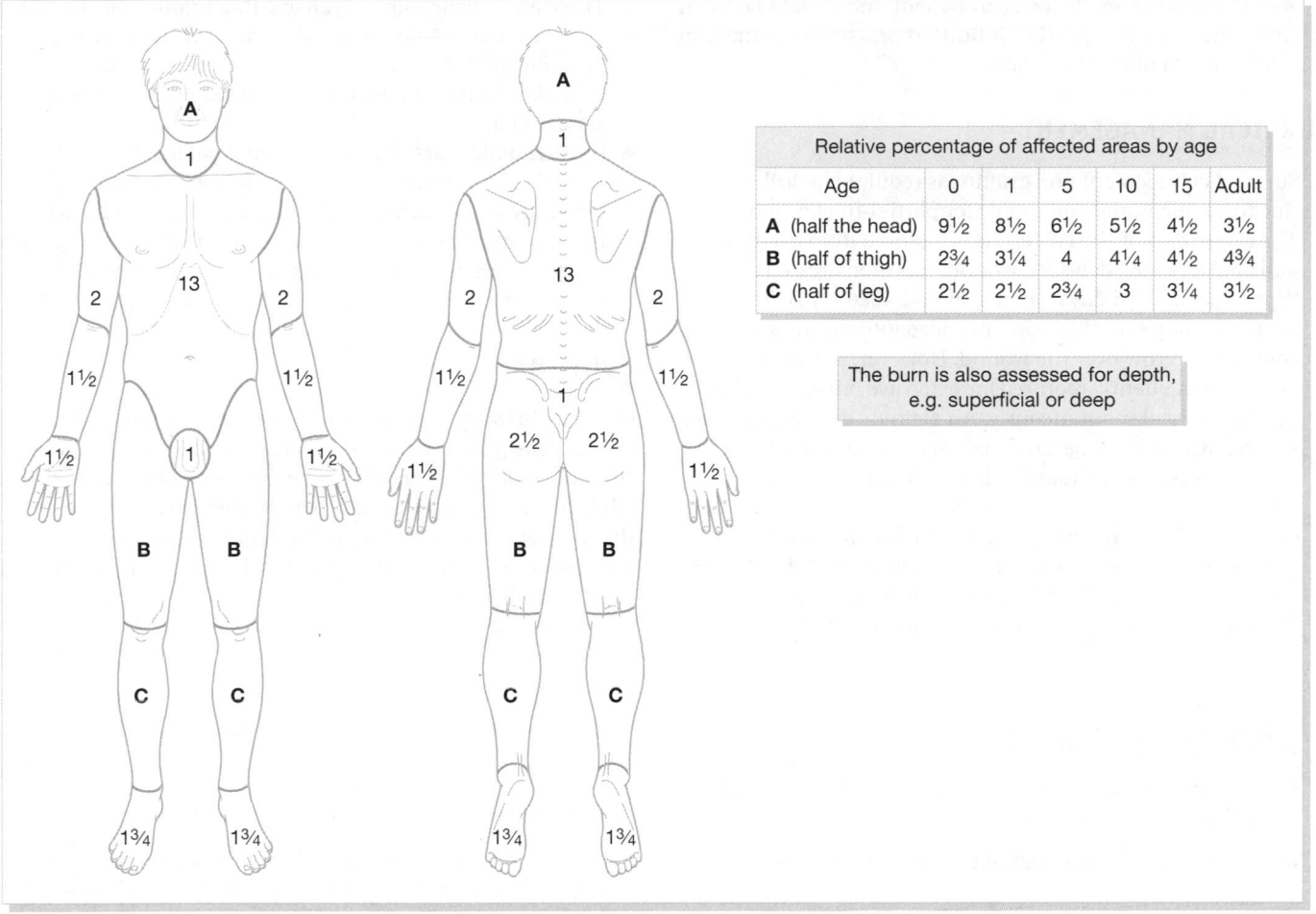

Relative percentage of affected areas by age						
Age	0	1	5	10	15	Adult
A (half the head)	9½	8½	6½	5½	4½	3½
B (half of thigh)	2¾	3¼	4	4¼	4½	4¾
C (half of leg)	2½	2½	2¾	3	3¼	3½

The burn is also assessed for depth, e.g. superficial or deep

Figure 28.8 Lund and Browder burn assessment chart. Note that areas marked A, B and C change during growth.

Nutrition

The burns patient requires a diet high in energy and protein to promote healing and to replace albumin lost from the damaged skin. Patients with extensive burns may need two or three times their normal calorie intake to overcome the catabolic state. The delivery of increased dietary needs may necessitate the use of enteral or parenteral nutrition (see Ch. 11).

Pain control

Ongoing pain control is essential for the burn patient's psychological well-being, and also to encourage movement to prevent contractures and other complications. Nurses should regularly assess pain intensity and the efficacy of prescribed analgesics (see Ch. 7). A patient's fear of pain is often greater than the pain sensation. It is important to ensure that patients receive appropriate pain relief, e.g. during potentially painful procedures.

Wound care

In the patient with burns, the natural barrier to infection is breached and the injury should be kept clean and covered in a non-adherent dressing to prevent further skin damage. However, facial burns are not covered, and hand burns are treated using plastic bags containing silver sulfadiazine or saline. The principles of effective wound care should be adhered to, viz. that the wound should be kept warm, moist and clean (see Chs 10 and 29). Dressings should be non-adherent and absorbent. Patients should be kept comfortable and dressings should be changed if strikethrough occurs.

It is imperative that no creams or ointments are applied to a burn before it is seen by the plastic surgeon, as they will mask the nature of the burn.

- Superficial burns are kept clean and warm – simple non-adherent dressings should be applied and kept intact for 2 or more days to promote spontaneous healing
- Partial-thickness and full-thickness burns may be dressed with absorbent, non-adherent wound dressings. Extra pads should be applied to absorb excess fluid and secured with a cotton or tubular bandage. These should be changed daily and an antimicrobial cream applied directly to the injury to prevent infection with *Pseudomonas aeruginosa*. Wound swabs should be taken at each dressing change and antibiotics prescribed as indicated.

The dressing regimen changes as the body heals and will focus on the protection of fragile granulation tissue, and the issue of support dressings and clothing to reduce the impact of hypertrophic scars. Treatment for hypertrophic scarring commences with emollient application several times a day. Pressure garments are tailor-made for each patient and should be worn for 24 hours to exert a gentle continuous pressure over the skin to reduce, soften and flatten the scar.

SURGICAL MANAGEMENT

- Surgical debridement and grafting is required for full-thickness burns and commonly for partial-thickness burns. The upper part of the epidermis is removed from a donor site and applied to the debrided wound. It is then dressed and kept intact for 3–5 days when it should 'take'. A 100% take is rare but any skin that has embedded into the injury should continue to grow over the wound. However, repeat skin grafts are frequently required for extensive burns. The *donor site* should heal spontaneously. An alginate dressing and pad secured with a bandage could be used and left for 10–14 days. By this time it should be healed and have no need of further dressings.

- Cultured skin – a sample of the patient's skin is taken, grown under laboratory conditions, and then applied to the wound. This is suitable where burns are so extensive that there is insufficient intact skin to use for a split-skin graft.

There are now dressings available that mimic cultured skin and are a useful adjunct to split-skin grafts and cultured skin (Purna 2000). It is now also possible to obtain skin from skin banks and use this to promote granulation in a similar manner.

- Hypertrophic scars often result from healing of partial-thickness or full-thickness burns. They are red, raised, unsightly and often very itchy. Contractures develop when they occur over a joint. Surgical reconstruction is frequently needed, especially to excise contractures. Patients with severe burns often require many such operations.

BODY IMAGE

Changes in body image lead to loss of confidence and self-esteem. The person with a scar often has to endure unpleasant reactions from other people. Some may overcome this with ease while others find it too much to bear. There are self-help groups that help burn patients and their families to cope. The nurse is a key person in enhancing patients' self-esteem by encouraging discussion about their fears and exploring coping strategies or by referring them to a self-help group or counsellor (Jobling 2001).

SUMMARY: MAIN POINTS

- Assessment of the skin is important as an indicator of general health and well-being.

- Nurses will encounter patients with skin conditions in every area of practice.

- There are numerous opportunities for health promotion, e.g. safe sun behaviour, skin screening and maintaining skin integrity.

- Nurses have a key role in educating patients about treatments and promotion of good skin care.

- The support that nurses provide for patients can help to overcome psychosocial effects of chronic skin disease and have a positive effect on well-being.

SELF-TEST: CRITICAL THINKING ACTIVITIES

1 Look at either a discharge plan for a patient being discharged home after intensive treatment for acute atopic eczema, or a care plan for a patient with a chronic skin condition being managed in a community setting:
  — What areas are included in the plan? Consider the rationale for each area covered.

  — What opportunities are taken to promote skin health?
  — Which health professionals or other agencies are involved in the management?
  — What changes would you consider making to the plan and why?

 ### FURTHER READING

Hughes E, Van Onselen J (eds). Dermatology nursing: a practical guide. Edinburgh: Churchill Livingstone; 2001.
Papadopoulos L, Bor R. Psychological approaches to dermatology. London: The British Psychological Society; 1999.
Penzer R. Nursing care of the skin. Oxford: Butterworth-Heinemann; 2002.

White G, Cox N. Diseases of the skin. A colour atlas and text. London: Mosby; 2000.
Williams H. Dermatology health care needs assessment. Oxford: Radcliffe Medical Press; 1997.

✉ USEFUL ADDRESSES

Acne Support Group
First Floor, Howard House
The Runway, South Ruislip
Middlesex HA4 6SE

British Allergy Foundation
Deepdene House
30 Bellegrove Road
Welling
Kent DA16 3BY

British Dermatology Nursing Group
BAD House
19 Fitzroy Square
London W1P 5HQ

Bullous Pemphigoid Support Group
17 Barley Mount
Redhills
Exeter EX4 1RP

DEBRA (International Patient Support Group)
Debra House, Wellington Business Park
Duke's Ride, Crowthorne
Berks RG45 6LS
www.debra.org.uk

National Eczema Society
Hill House
Highgate Hill
London N19 5NA
Tel: 0870241 3604
www.eczema.org

Pemphigus Vulgaris Network
Flat C, 26 St German Road
London SE23 1RJ
(SAE required for information)
www.pemphigus.org – *shared website with*
National Pemphigus Foundation

Psoriasis Association
Milton House
7 Milton Street
Northampton NN2 7JG
Tel: 01604 711129

Vitiligo Society
125 Kennington Road
London SE11 6SF
www.vitiligosociety.org.uk

The Wessex Cancer Trust's Marc's Line
Marc's Line Resource Centre
Salisbury District Hospital
Salisbury SP2 8BJ
www.k-web.co.uk/charity/wct/wct.html

REFERENCES

Agarwal G. Vitiligo: an underestimated problem. Family Practice 1998;15(Suppl 1):s19–23.

Atherton DJ. Naevi and other developmental defects. In: Champion RH, Burton JL, Burton JL, 5th edn. Textbook of dermatology. Oxford: Blackwell Scientific; 1992, pp 305–373.

Atkins S. Dousing the flames. Nurs Times 1999a;95(34):29–31.

Atkins S. Burns assessment and initial management. Nurs Times 1999b;95(35):46–48.

Baxter C. Observing the skin. Commun Outlook 1993;Jan:19–20.

Bhatia PS, Mohan L, Pandy ON, Singh KK, Arona SK, Mukhija RD. Genetic nature of vitiligo. J Dermatol Sci 1992;4:180–184.

Breslow A. Thickness, cross sectional area and depth invasion in the prognosis of cutaneous melanoma. Ann Surg 1970;172:902–908.

Cancer Research UK. Sun and UV light. Melanoma skin cancer. Available. Online: www.cancerresearchuk.org. 2002.

Carman C. Clinical evidence – atopic eczema. Br Med J 1999;318:1600–1603.

Carrougher GJ. Management of fluid and electrolyte balance in thermal injuries: implications for perioperative nursing practice. Semin Perioper Nurs 1997;6(4):201–209.

Cork MJ. The importance of skin barrier function. J Dermatol Treat 1997;8(Suppl 1):S7–13.

Cuncliffe WJ. New approaches to acne treatment. London: Martin Dunitz;1994.

Finlay AY, Khan GK. Dermatology quality of life index. Clin Exp Dermatol 1994;19:310–316.

Fitzpatrick TB, Johnson RA, Wolff K, Polano MK, Suurmond D. Colour atlas and synopsis of clinical dermatology, 4th edn. New York: McGraw-Hill;2001.

Goodfield M. Superficial infections. Prescriber J 1998;38:183–189.

Greaves MW, Gattin S. The use of glucocorticoids in dermatology. J Dermatol Treat 1999;10:83–91.

Halder RM, Young CM. New and emerging therapies for vitiligo. Dermatol Clin 2000;18:79–89.

Hardy MA. A pilot study of the diagnosis and treatment of impaired skin integrity: dry skin in older persons. Nurs Diag 1990;1(2):57–63.

Hay RJ, Clayton YM, De Silva N, Midgley G, Rossor E. Tinea capitis in south-east London: a new pattern of infection with public health implications. Br J Dermatol 1996;135:995–998.

Holden C, English J, Hoare C, Jordan A, Kounacki S, Turnbull R, Staughton RCD. Advised best practice for the use of emollients in eczema and other dry skin conditions. J Dermatol Treat 2002;13:103–106.

Hughes E, Van Onselen J (eds). Dermatology nursing: a practical guide. Edinburgh: Churchill Livingstone; 2001.

Jobling R. Psychological issues in dermatology. In: Hughes E, Van Onselen J, eds. Dermatology nursing: a practical guide. Edinburgh: Churchill Livingstone; 2001.

Linward J. Haemangiomas. British Dermatology Nursing Group Distance Learning Pack. London: British Dermatology Nursing Group; 1999.

Nunley JR. Cutaneous manifestations of HIV and HCV. Dermatol Nurs 2000;12(3):163–169.

Pedlow P, Walsh M, Patterson C, Atkinson R, Lowry W. Cutaneous malignant melanoma in Northern Ireland. Br J Dermatol 1997;76(1):124–126.

Peters J. Assessment of the dermatology patient. In: Hughes E, Van Onselen J, eds. Dermatology nursing: a practical guide. Edinburgh: Churchill Livingstone; 2001.

Purna SK, Babu M. Collagen based dressings – a review. Burns 2000;26(1):54–62.

Ratner D, Grande DJ. Moh's micrographic surgery: an overview. Dermatol Nurs 1994;6(4):269–273.

Richard R. Assessment and diagnosis of burn wounds. Advances in wound care. J Prevention Healing 1999;12(9):468–471.

Roujeau JC. The spectrum of Stevens-Johnson syndrome and toxic epidermal necrolysis: a clinical classification. J Invest Dermatol 1994;102:S28–30.

Smith C, Lilly S, Mann KP et al. AIDS related malignancies. Ann Intern Med 1998;30(4):323–344.

Watts J. Update: psoriasis. Prof Nurse 1999;14(9):623–626.

Watts MJ. Care of the acutely ill patient. In: Hughes E, Van Onselen J, eds. Dermatology nursing: a practical guide. Edinburgh: Churchill Livingstone; 2001.

Williams HC. Is atopic eczema really on the increase. Dermatol Today 1994; 3: 6–7.

SECTION 4

Specific Areas of Adult Nursing

29 Perioperative nursing   879

30 Nursing patients in the accident and emergency department   923

31 Nursing critically ill patients   947

32 Nursing older adults   967

33 Nursing patients with cancer   985

34 Nursing patients who need palliative care   1021

35 Nursing patients with chronic (long-term) illness and disability   1047

Perioperative nursing

David Morris, Karrie Ward

> 'It wasn't until I saw the patient anaesthetised that I really realised just how important the pre-op checklist is. The patient is so vulnerable and totally reliant on us to get it right'
>
> *(Student nurse)*

THIS CHAPTER WILL HELP YOU

- Understand the principles and practice of dynamic patient assessment within the perioperative process

- Have a raised awareness of how nurses may provide patients with a safe, dignified and comfortable passage through the perioperative process

- Recognize the dynamic relationship between the three stages of the perioperative process

- Identify the roles of those involved in providing quality care throughout the surgical process

- Develop and enhance knowledge of surgical procedure and associated nursing interventions

- Appreciate the psychological impact of surgery as a potential stressor.

KEYWORDS

Ambulation	Interdisciplinary care
Anaesthesia	Patient education
Asepsis and infection control	Pain and symptom management
Assessment	Perioperative care
Communication	Post-anaesthetic recovery
Consent	
Day-care surgery	Safety
Deep vein thrombosis	Skin preparation
Dignity	Wound care and drains
Discharge planning	

INTRODUCTION

Surgery may be considered as a specialty of medicine whereby patients require operative or invasive intervention. The perioperative period (entire surgical experience from pre-admission to discharge) is the source of a great deal of the anxiety and distress felt by the hospitalized person. Numerous studies have identified fears of the anaesthetic, loss of dignity, pain and simply losing control of the ability to function as major stressors for patients. It is imperative then that the perioperative nurse has the knowledge, awareness and skills to act as patient advocates and ensure the safest, most dignified and most comfortable passage through this process.

This chapter provides readers with the essential knowledge required for nursing in a perioperative environment. Where appropriate, traditional practices are challenged or at least reassessed in the light of current clinical evidence. The essential interdependency between nurses and staff working in all phases of the perioperative process is emphasized throughout the chapter. Problems experienced by patients in a particular perioperative phase may have their origin or effect in another phase, such is the dynamic nature of surgical nursing. Issues relevant to the preoperative period will be reviewed and the potential for improved pre-surgery preparation will be explored. For many people, not least nursing students, a visit to the operating theatre is a source of fear and anxiety. The use of apparently complex terminology may compound feelings of insecurity. A review of common surgical terminology is provided in Box 29.1. Excellence in the operating theatre can have a major positive influence on patient outcome. Methods of anaesthesia and their implications for postoperative patient management will also be examined. Surgical, and more specifically operating room, care is often described in terms of process, procedure and task. The endless struggles for the perfect core plan (standardized care plan) or care pathway bear testimony to this ethos. Certainly surgery is relatively discrete and transient, having a well-defined beginning and end; it relies on the adherence to many universal principles for practice. Yet for the recipient of these processes, such an experience is always unique.

Box 29.1 Surgical terminology

Surgical terminology can appear a complex and confusing second language. However, it is possible to promote understanding from a review of the commonly used prefixes and suffixes (examples are given in the last column).

Prefixes

Angio-	of a vessel	angiography
Arthro-	of a joint	arthroplasty
Broncho-	of a bronchus	bronchoscopy
Chole-	literally, of gall or bile	cholecystectomy
Colo-	of colon	colostomy
Cysto-	sac or bladder	cystectomy
Gastro-	of stomach	gastrostomy
Hepat(o)-	of the liver	hepatitis
Lipo-	of fat	lipoma
Litho-	of stone	lithotomy
Rhino-	of the nose	rhinoplasty
Thoraco-	of the chest	thoracotomy

Suffixes

-ectomy	excision of	mastectomy
-graphy	picture of	radiography
-itis	inflammation of	appendicitis
-ostomy	opening or passage	ileostomy
-otomy	to cut into	laparotomy
-orraphy	to repair	herniorraphy
-oscopy	to visualize with light	cystoscopy
-paxy	to crush	lithopaxy
-pexy	fixation of	orchidopexy
-plasty	to refashion	mammoplasty
-stasis	state of inertia	haemostasis
-therm	with heat	diathermy

This chapter provides many examples of good practice and evidence-based care, but hopefully never loses sight of the individuality of those we care for. Ultimately, this chapter relies on the practitioner to reflect and perhaps act on its content, which hopefully provides the springboard for discussion and deeper enquiry to the ultimate benefit of the person undergoing surgery.

THE CONTEXT AND CLASSIFICATION OF SURGERY

Surgery is performed for different reasons and with varying degrees of urgency. With the advent and continual refinement of minimally invasive endoscopic techniques, many surgical procedures are diagnostic in nature. The use of a fibreoptic endoscope in the visualization of gastrointestinal, genitourinary and respiratory tracts and bony joints is commonplace. Surgery may also be considered as curative, ablative (amputation or excision of a body part or tissue) or reparative, whereby the identified or diagnosed source of a problem is excised, repaired, refashioned or reconstructed to promote the patient's quality of life.

The timing of intervention may differ according to the identified level of urgency. Surgery may be elective, preferably performed at a time of optimum benefit to the patient, or it may be an urgent or emergency procedure to save life, preserve function or reduce the risk of longer-term complication or disability.

Surgery in all its forms may take place in a variety of settings, from the GP surgery and outpatient clinic to the community hospital and larger specialist surgical centres. However, whenever and wherever surgery is performed, the nursing and medical management in this perioperative process will always be the same: to provide the safest, most effective and efficient service for the patient.

DAY SURGERY

Recently there has been a massive increase in day surgery, both in the UK and globally. Such are the numbers of people undergoing day-care surgery that nursing activity in this area is now considered a nursing specialism, with an increasing number of post-registration educational programmes reflecting this emphasis. The criteria for defining the concept of day surgery is perhaps best provided by the Royal College of Surgeons (1992) guidelines, which describe day surgery as appropriate for the patient who is admitted for an operative procedure, requiring the facility for postoperative recovery, yet not requiring an overnight hospital stay.

Most day surgery units in the UK are typically open from 8.00am to 6.00pm. Clearly the implications for the type of surgery that can be carried out within such time spans will be substantial. It is worth noting, too, that the term ambulatory surgery (patients will walk in and walk out) is often used interchangeably with day surgery.

There are, however, a number of minor operative procedures which are commonly performed as day cases. Hernia repair, dental extraction, minor gynaecological surgery and excision of skin lesions and lipoma are regularly carried out in day units, as are many endoscopic procedures, such as cystoscopy (see Ch. 24), bronchoscopy (see Ch. 20) and gastroscopy (Ch. 22). The breadth and extent of these procedures vary between surgical centres and are constantly reviewed as techniques and technology advance.

The massive increase in day-care surgery may be explained from both a sociopolitical and a professional perspective. Considered by the UK government to provide a cost-effective strategy that would reduce waiting lists, guidelines and targets for the number of day cases to be undertaken are set and devolved to local NHS Trusts. There have been major technological advances in surgery and the development of minimally invasive techniques. Endoscopic equipment and ever-improving anaesthetic and pharmacological protocols have all provided impetus to this strategy. Part of the reason for the increase in the number of day surgery units is that patients generally prefer it. The benefits to patients are outlined in Special Issues box 29.1.

There are also benefits to the NHS, as follows:

- In-patient beds are not required, allowing sicker patients access to care.
- Risk of cancellation due to bed shortages is no longer a direct issue.
- Costs are reduced with no overnight stay.
- The development of specialist-trained staff in day surgery units can only further reduce the potential for readmission.

SPECIAL ISSUES

29.1 Benefits of day surgery

- Reduced waiting list times
- Increased number of patients treated
- Patients benefit from being able to go home
- Reduced disruption to normal lifestyle
- Fixed date for surgery
- Greater patient control and improved psychological effects
- Maintenance of personal privacy through going home

■ Direct referral of patients to the day unit by GPs is becoming increasingly common, so avoiding the need for a consultant outpatient appointment. Similarly, many units now take direct referral from optometrists who have diagnosed cataract problems (see Ch. 15).

Despite the clear advantages, there are implications of day surgery for both patients and nurses. There is a potential for patients to feel inadequately prepared in terms of informational and educational support (Otte 1996). Post-discharge symptom management and continuity of care can be variable and the added pressure on primary care services in the community may be problematic. The surgical process can become 'conveyor belt'-like, a characteristic that both patients and nurses may dislike, and the patient care focus may be lost. Yet nurses are recognizing and rising to these challenges and demands, and ever-increasing targets will require them to continue to do so.

Clearly not all surgical procedures, nor indeed patients by virtue of their health status, are either eligible or suitable for day surgery. Most NHS Trusts will have local policies and protocols that determine patient suitability and access to day surgery. It is worth noting that whilst health problems associated with the older adult often negate their potential for day surgery, age should not in itself be considered a barrier (see Older Adults: Nursing Priorities box 29.1).

OLDER ADULTS: NURSING PRIORITIES

29.1 Perioperative issues for the older adult

Stereotypical assumptions often stigmatize older people as being physically and intellectually incapacitated and a liability to both society and the health care system. However, the reality is that most older people are independent, physically healthy and mentally astute.

General issues

- Old age does not automatically equate with ill health. However, as people age there is a higher incidence of conditions requiring surgery. Ageing will, by definition, be associated with an increasing incidence of degenerative disease such as cancer, coronary heart disease, musculoskeletal and neurosensory disorders.
- Changes in social and family structures mean that many more people are living alone and without the direct support of their family. Trends towards early discharge place added burden on informal carers and professional support services.
- Advances in operative and anaesthetic technique make surgery a safer and more viable choice of treatment leading to an increase in the overall number of older patients undergoing surgery.
- Overall perioperative mortality rates have improved greatly in the past 40 years. However, overall mortality in the older patient remains five to 10 times greater compared with those under 65 (Arron et al 1992). Surgical mortality rates are 55% higher in those aged over 65 (Nolan 1992).
- Slower recovery and longer hospital stays are features of post-surgical care of older patients.
- The older patient is more at risk from postoperative complications.

Specific care issues

Whilst accepting that older patients are individuals with their own specific needs and problems, it would be irresponsible not to recognize that there are normal and expected changes associated with the ageing process that might influence surgical recovery.

Perioperative assessment, then, must facilitate the detection of specific problems that might affect the older person so that appropriate interventions may be initiated. The following aspects might form the focus of assessment and subsequent care management:

Skin and tissue viability
Skin loses elasticity with age and the decrease of the subcutaneous fat layer predisposes to pressure ulcer development and the potential for hypothermia.
Perioperative considerations: assessment of pressure ulcer risk, use of appropriate pressure-relieving aids on the ward and in theatre, monitoring body temperature, nutritional status.

Sensory function
Diminished lens elasticity and transparency affect vision. Hearing acuity decreases and vestibular changes may lead to dizziness and loss of balance.
Perioperative considerations: ensuring the patient can access hearing aids, spectacles, etc. If necessary, provide written information in large text format, physical support and specific safety precautions.

Respiratory function
Lung elasticity and chest muscle strength decrease, leading to reduced chest expansion and decreased vital capacity.
Perioperative considerations: preoperative chest physiotherapy, respiratory function screening, positioning to facilitate chest expansion and oxygen support as required.

(Cont'd)

Cardiovascular function

Cardiac output decreases, arteries are less elastic with sclerosis of vessel walls. Diminished response to physiological stress and changes in blood pressure.

Perioperative considerations: cardiac screening (ECG), careful monitoring of vital signs, deep vein thrombosis (DVT) prevention therapy, caution with fluid balance, avoiding overload, and early ambulation.

Musculoskeletal function

Muscle atrophy, joint stiffness and decrease in bone density, degenerative vertebral change.

Perioperative considerations: careful positioning on theatre table, encouragement of early ambulation, provision of mobility aids and observation for prolonged spinal/epidural effects.

Renal and genitourinary function

Reduced renal blood flow and glomerular filtration rate, prostatic enlargement and reduction in bladder capacity. Loss of pelvic and bladder muscle tone.

Perioperative considerations: observation of urinary output and possible urinary retention, encouragement of oral fluids as appropriate, early ambulation and observation for prolonged drug effects.

Gastrointestinal and hepatic function

Decreased gut motility, loss of teeth, taste sensation decreases, reduction in saliva, decreased gut motility and reduced hepatic function.

Perioperative considerations: nutritional status, appetizing and edible diet, reviewing period of perioperative fasting, monitoring of bowel motility and peristalsis, early ambulation, observation for prolonged drug effects.

Neurological function

Decrease in neurons and cerebral blood flow, cognition learning speed and memory, but no change in intelligence.

Perioperative considerations: allow more time for instruction and teaching purposes, treat with appropriate respect, observe for toxic or prolonged effects of medication.

References

Arron M, Martin G, Webster J. Perioperative care of the elderly. Comprehens Ther 1992; 18: 4–10.

Nolan T. Surgery in the elderly: lowering risks by understanding special needs. Postgrad Med 1992; 91(2): 199–208.

All patients should be assessed for suitability using non-ageist criteria. Both surgeon and anaesthetist must be in agreement on the choice of day care as a safe and appropriate environment for the patient. The American Society of Anesthesiologists (ASA 1963) provides a framework that has been accepted as the most convenient, and consequently most commonly used, classification of physical health status. The anaesthetist assesses the patient's condition and a status rating is identified. The grades range from grade 1, a normal healthy individual, to grade 5, a moribund individual not expected to survive with or without an operation. The classification is used in conjunction with broader considerations below, and a decision about suitability for day-care surgery is made.

Issues likely to influence suitability and acceptance for day surgery

- Relatively fit and healthy (fulfils appropriate ASA criteria)
- Benefits the patient more than in-patient treatment
- No evidence of chronic health problem likely to adversely affect recovery (e.g. chronic obstructive pulmonary disease [COPD], cardiovascular disease, unstable diabetes)
- Length of procedure and amounts of anaesthetic required
- The presence of appropriate social and home support
- Patient acceptance
- Surgical procedure unlikely to cause excessive bleeding, or postoperative pain, nausea and vomiting.

Pre-admission assessment and admission

All patients scheduled for day-care surgery attend a pre-admission clinic for assessment. Ideally this will take place a week or so before surgery is planned so that appropriate blood samples may be taken, consent obtained and any further investigations instigated. A medical selection and investigation tool is used (see Fig. 29.1).

On admission to the day unit, patients will be shown to an appropriate waiting area and orientated to the environment and the proposed surgical process. A preoperative assessment will be undertaken following similar principles as for in-patient admission. Specific preparation will depend on the procedure to be performed. However, general safety aspects, including fasting, informed consent, skin preparation and recording of baseline vital signs, will remain essential.

Anaesthesia in day care has had a major influence on the ability to perform surgery and safely discharge patients home soon afterwards. The days of patients being so disorientated, nauseated and generally unwell after surgery that lengthy recovery was inevitable have gone. Non-barbiturate induction agents such as intravenous (i.v.) propofol and maintenance vapours such as sevoflurane are metabolized rapidly and allow rapid recovery (see Table 29.1). In addition, a better understanding of the mechanisms of postoperative pain and nausea and vomiting have allowed more effective management. Commonly, antiemetics such as ondansetron or cyclizine are

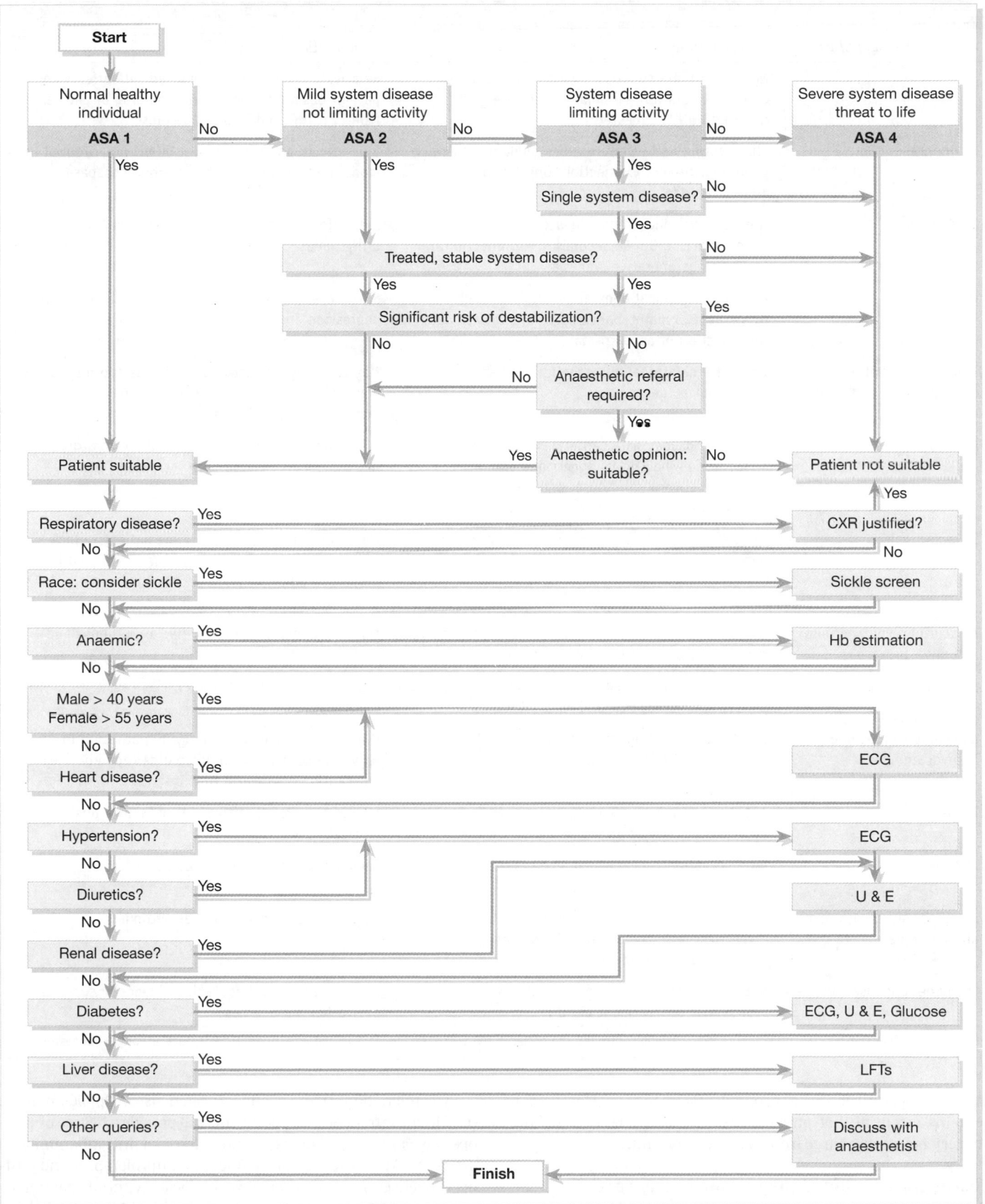

Figure 29.1 Medical selection and investigation algorithm (used in day-care surgery). (Reproduced with kind permission from Whitwam 1994.)

Table 29.1 Commonly used perioperative anaesthetic agents and other drugs

Anaesthetic agent/drug	Action and uses	Comments
Propofol	Non-barbiturate sedative/hypnotic. Rapid onset and short duration. Minimal 'hangover' effect. Reduced PONV suggested	Relatively expensive, but reduced side-effects and patient desirability make this the drug of choice. Painful if injected into small veins
Thiopental sodium	Short-acting barbiturate used as induction agent. Usually given by i.v. injection. Onset of action 10–20 seconds	Side-effects and slow recovery limit its potential in modern anaesthesia. May cause bronchospasm
Midazolam	A benzodiazepine used as induction sedative. Onset of action 30–60 seconds in i.v. injection. Provides postoperative amnesia	Side-effects include bronchospasm and cardiac arrhythmias
Halothane	Potent inhalational general anaesthetic used primarily as a maintenance agent and occasionally for induction of anaesthesia	Slow onset and slow recovery. May cause cardiac depression and arrhythmias. Toxic to liver
Isoflurane, sevoflurane, enflurane and desflurane	Volatile inhalational anaesthetics used as maintenance agents	May cause hypotension, arrhythmias and respiratory depression. Implicated in the onset of malignant hyperthermia (rare) – see Chapter 5
Nitrous oxide	Used with oxygen as a carrier gas for the potent anaesthetic inhalational agents and enhances their effect. Very rapid onset and recovery time. Used for GA and for pain control in local procedures.	Good analgesia with minimal cardiorespiratory depression. Associated with increased PONV
Suxamethonium	Ultra-short acting (3–5 min) depolarizing muscle relaxant. Onset within 30–60 seconds	May cause muscle pain. In some patients a lack of the enzyme pseudocholinesterase will lead to prolonged paralysis and apnoea. May cause malignant hyperthermia (see Ch. 5)
Atracurium, vencuronium and mivacurium	Short-, medium- and long-acting non-depolarizing muscle relaxants. Effects last 15–60 minutes	May cause hypotension, cardiac arrhythmias and bronchospasm
Morphine, fentanyl	Opioids commonly used for intra- and postoperative pain relief via i.v., PCA and regional routes	Causes respiratory depression. May cause bronchospasm
Lidocaine (lignocaine), bupivacaine	Local anaesthetic agents used for local infiltration and for SP/EP anaesthesia	May cause cardiac irregularity. Hypotension in regional use. Used with adrenaline (epinephrine) but caution if injected to extremities
Naloxone	Antagonist used to reverse untoward respiratory depressant effect of opioids	Should be carefully titrated to minimize analgesia reversal
Neostigmine	An anticholinesterase which reverses the effects of non-depolarizing muscle relaxants	Causes bradycardia, increased secretions
Atropine, glycopyrronium and hyoscine	Anticholinergic (muscarinic receptor antagonist) given to reverse the negative effects of anticholinesterase above	May cause tachycardia and arrhythmias
Cyclizine, ondansetron	Antiemetics that may be given orally or i.v. for prophylaxis or treatment of PONV	Expensive agents. Debatable evidence of superiority over other antiemetics

GA, general anaesthesia; i.v., intravenous; PCA, patient-controlled analgesia; PONV, postoperative nausea and vomiting; SP/EP, spinal or epidural anaesthetic.

given preoperatively as a prophylactic measure. However, it remains essential that patients are sufficiently recovered from surgery before discharge from the day-care unit.

Postoperative pain management in day care

Postoperative pain control is especially important following day surgery where patients need to be comfortable on discharge. Analgesia should be commenced early and may be given preoperatively as a pre-emptive control strategy.

A combination of medication is often used. Opioids may be used in the intraoperative period and will provide a degree of postoperative analgesia. The use of non-steroidal anti-inflammatory drugs (NSAIDs) such as diclofenac and ibuprofen pre- and postoperatively is common, providing analgesia without sedation or the side-effects of nausea and vomiting which might delay recovery. Paracetamol may be useful for minor operation pain relief or may be used in combination with codeine for stronger pain relief. It is essential that patients are given appropriate verbal and written information on the effects, dosage, side-effects and contraindications of their prescription prior to discharge. An adequate supply of medication should be prepared for them to take home.

Pain management is a major concern for both staff and patients, and many units will provide a follow-up telephone call service to patients in order to evaluate the effectiveness of pain and symptom relief regimens.

Criteria for discharge

In the event that patients do not recover as rapidly as expected, a protocol that allows overnight admission to hospital must be in place. Patient satisfaction audit tools will regularly be used as an indicator of the success of the day-care process. In many centres, patients will be given the telephone number for the day unit so that any concerns postoperatively may be resolved. Criteria for discharge from day unit include:

- vital signs stable
- tolerating oral fluids without undue nausea or vomiting
- has appropriate and adequate medication to take home
- has been provided with postoperative education/instruction
- has passed urine
- pain control effective
- no signs of bleeding
- has transport and a suitable person present for a minimum of 24 hours following discharge.

GENERAL PREOPERATIVE CARE

Preoperative care is the stage of perioperative care concerned with the physical and psychological preparation of a patient before surgery. The aims of preoperative care are to:

- ensure that patients are in the optimum physical and mental condition to undergo surgery
- establish fitness for anaesthesia and ability to withstand the operation
- identify and minimize the risks of perioperative complications.

PREOPERATIVE ASSESSMENT

Preoperative assessment is undertaken to fulfil the aims stated above. In the case of acute/emergency surgery where the underlying problem may be life-threatening, the time available for preoperative assessment is more limited. However, whilst by necessity assessment and investigation are more selective, rapid and focused on immediate and often life-preserving needs, general principles of assessment are still maintained. For the majority of patients, preoperative assessment is often undertaken before admission to hospital and may take place in a variety of settings. In recent years, many hospitals have introduced preadmission clinics for this purpose, although their exact focus is variable. They provide an opportunity for patients to be assessed for their fitness for anaesthesia, and have any necessary investigations, e.g. blood or electrocardiography (ECG) (see Ch. 19), performed prior to admission for elective surgery. Such preadmission assessments enable patients who are deemed to be fit for surgery to be admitted as planned. For those who are deemed

unfit for surgery and in need of further investigations, their admission can be postponed, which means another patient can take their place, consequently avoiding unnecessary cancellations of operations for patients already admitted.

Patients awaiting elective surgery are usually invited to attend pre-admission clinics approximately 2–4 weeks, and preferably no more than 6 weeks, prior to the planned date of admission. Whilst some clinics are run solely by medical practitioners predominately to assess patients in advance, other departments employ specialist nurses to begin the preparation of patients for operation. The expansion of the nursing role has allowed nurses to take on many of the tasks previously undertaken by doctors, such as the taking of bloods. This has given nurses in the pre-admission clinic an ideal opportunity to provide patients with information and advice about their impending operation. In this respect, nurses can play a crucial role in preparing patients psychologically for surgery.

Assessment is essentially a collaborative and interdisciplinary process. Data from a number of sources may be utilized to formulate plans of care that meet the specific and individual needs of the surgical patient. These will include primary care notes, nursing and medical notes, professionals allied to medicine, relatives and patients themselves.

It is also an opportunity for patients to participate and for their needs and views to be taken into account. It is likely that assessment data will have considered a number of key areas:

- status of pre-existing pathology
- detection of unknown conditions
- patient's psychological state and awareness of surgery
- current medication, allergies/sensitivities and any relevant family history, e.g. malignant hyperthermia (see Ch. 5). The findings are documented according to local protocols
- potential for postoperative complications
- baselines for intra- and postoperative monitoring
- identification of ongoing assessment and monitoring tools
- referral to specialist support
- social status and discharge support
- cultural and spiritual needs (see Special Issues box 29.2).

ESTABLISHING FITNESS FOR SURGERY AND ANAESTHESIA

Preoperative assessment establishes the nature, extent and severity of both known pre-existing disease and previously unknown medical problems. Whilst this is often the responsibility of medical practitioners, nurses also have a vital contribution to make in this respect. Information obtained in the nursing assessment is also relevant to the general risks associated with anaesthesia and surgery. Any abnormalities in observations should be communicated to the medical staff.

The extent of screening and investigations will depend on the condition and age of the patient, the nature of surgery to be performed and local policy. Whilst it is vital not to stereotype all older people as at risk, statistically those over 65 years of age are more susceptible to postoperative complications (see Older Adults: Nursing Priorities box 29.1, pp. 881–882). Medical assessment regardless of age may include a number of physiological investigations:

29.2 Culture and the perioperative experience of patients

Patients arrive from many different social, economic, religious, racial, ethnic and cultural origins and will react to the perioperative process in different ways. As a member of the perioperative team, the nurse needs to have an understanding of the concept of culture and its diversity.

Key points
- Variations are evident in the definition of culture. Allen (2000) suggests that culture is broader than race or ethnicity. Culture also encompasses social, economic and religious facets.
- The following factors influence cultural differences: religion, age, gender, sexuality, ethnicity and social class.
- People's cultural identity influences their health beliefs and practices and their perceptions and reactions to illness.
- By being non-judgemental in their approach and open-minded to cultural differences, nurses can meet the needs of individual patients.

Cultural aspects that might influence patient–nurse interaction in the perioperative period
- Beliefs about health and illness including the meaning that the patient attaches to surgery
- Use of language – verbal and non-verbal communication
- Spiritual and religious beliefs
- Personal space
- Gender and role
- Eating and drinking habits and dietary taboos
- Attitudes about the body and personal clothing, such as keeping the head covered. Attitudes about modesty and which areas of the body can be exposed or should be covered
- Personal cleansing practices
- Attitudes and beliefs about elimination
- Customs regarding the expression of sexuality
- Sleeping habits
- Beliefs and responses to pain
- Beliefs about death and dying

Student activities
- How might you define the term culture?
- What examples of cultural diversity have you seen in practice?
- How may cultural differences influence perceptions and experiences of surgery?
- How can nurses demonstrate respect for other people's cultural beliefs?

Reference
Allen H. Culture: the social context of surgery. In: Manley K, Bellman L, eds. Surgical nursing: advancing practice. Edinburgh: Churchill Livingstone; 2000, ch 10.

- chest X-ray
- ECG
- blood tests, including full blood count, haemoglobin, urea and electrolytes (see Chs 8 and 18).
- group, save and cross-match as appropriate (depending on likelihood of haemorrhage)
- sickle cell test for those at risk of sickle cell disease (see Ch. 18)
- neurological examination
- urinalysis
- baseline measurement of temperature, pulse, respiration (TPR) and blood pressure (BP), weight and body mass index (BMI).

Identified abnormalities that might adversely affect surgical recovery are corrected preoperatively. Anaemia will need to be corrected, possibly with a blood transfusion. If there is any indication of a fluid or electrolyte imbalance, this may need to be corrected with an intravenous infusion.

Abnormalities of TPR and BP should be recorded and reported, as critical variations may mean postponing surgery. These recordings serve as a baseline and are compared with those performed in the immediate and ongoing postoperative recovery period. It is, however, important to allow time for patients to settle into their new environment before doing the observations, as most patients are naturally a little anxious on arrival at the ward. Consequently, their BP might be raised, thus giving inappropriate data for a baseline standard (see Ch. 6).

Routine screening of urine may detect the presence of renal disease or diabetes mellitus. Untreated or poorly managed diabetes can lead to many serious health complications (see Ch. 17).

Perioperative care for diabetic patients will ideally begin before arrival in the operating department. Due to the wide range of potential problems and complications associated with diabetes, a comprehensive medical assessment of patients and their suitability for surgery will have been undertaken. Diabetes may affect virtually all body systems, but damage to nerves and blood vessels, in particular, may predispose to a number of potential problems in the perioperative period. The medication (oral hypoglycaemics or insulin) required by patients with diabetes is discussed in the section dealing with preoperative fasting (p. 893).

The date of the last menstrual period (LMP) will be ascertained in female patients of child-bearing age. The effects of anaesthesia on the embryo/fetus can be significant and, if pregnancy is confirmed, surgery may be postponed. A pregnancy test may be undertaken to investigate this possibility in the potentially pregnant patient. From both aesthetic and possibly sociocultural perspectives, it is useful to be aware of menstrual status to promote and maintain appropriately dignified and sensitive care.

It is important to establish whether patients are taking any medication. For those patients on long-standing medication, such as corticosteroids or essential treatment for epilepsy, cardiac disease and hypertension, arrangements will be made for them to continue taking these. If they are prescribed these medications orally, they will need to be administered with water. Occasionally, the same medications will need to be provided via a different route over the perioperative period whilst patients are fasting.

Most importantly, patients are also asked if they have any known allergies and their patient documentation is checked. Allergies may include those to:

- drugs or additives
- plasters, tapes or dressings
- latex – these allergies are becoming more common and any sensitivity to this should also be established and documented.

ASSESSING THE POTENTIAL FOR AND PREVENTING POSTOPERATIVE COMPLICATIONS

Identifying the potential for and preventing postoperative complications is an important element in preoperative preparation.

Infection and skin preparation

Many surgical techniques involve incisions that breach the skin, one of the innate defences against infection (see Ch. 28). This allows the potential entry of microorganisms through the wound during or after surgery. Prior to the pioneering work of Semmelweiss in 1847, who identified the links between the standard of handwashing and sepsis, and Joseph Lister in 1863, who applied Pasteur's 'germ theories' in his explanation of postoperative wound infection, many patients died of surgical sepsis. Contemporary understanding of microbiology has led to a dramatic reduction in mortality, but awareness and vigilance remain essential in protecting surgical patients from infection. The skin is populated by a number of microorganisms, which can be classified into two categories: commensals (resident microorganisms or normal flora) and transient organisms.

Commensal or resident organisms are naturally occurring and are non-pathogenic when they remain in their normal environment. Commensal organisms are found throughout the body, e.g. *Escherichia coli* (*E. coli*) in the bowel. Skin commensals, e.g. *Staphylococcus epidermidis*, are generally found in the dermal layers of the skin within hair follicles and sweat glands. However, these may become pathogenic when introduced into other tissues.

Transient microorganisms are acquired through touch or direct contact and can generally be removed by thorough washing as they are loosely attached to the skin.

Preoperative skin preparation aims to minimize the risk of wound infection by rendering the operation site as free from microorganisms as possible. This is achieved by thorough skin cleansing and possibly hair removal from the operation site preoperatively as well as topical skin preparation in theatre.

Skin cleansing

Patients are usually advised to shower prior to surgery. For day-care surgery or for admissions on the day of surgery, such advice may have been provided in pre-admission clinics or written instructions. The hair should also be washed if possible, as hair can act as a reservoir for microorganisms, and attention also given to the cleanliness of the nails. In hospital, having a shower may be preferable to taking a bath, as there may be a risk of cross-infection from microorganisms already present in hospital baths. Patients will be provided with a clean theatre gown prior to arrival in the theatre. Sometimes caps, socks and paper knickers are also made available. Whilst there appears to be little valid literature to support their use as infection control mechanisms, they may be useful in preserving comfort and dignity. Much of the debate concerning skin cleansing can be traced back to Joseph Lister, who advocated the use of carbolic soap as an antiseptic. Today the bathing versus showering issue and the use of antiseptics as preoperative cleansing agents continues. Research has focused on the use of specific skin antiseptic agents such as chlorhexidine 4% for preoperative cleansing. Many studies have compared the use of non-medicated soap with chlorhexidine, for example, as well as the use of other agents such as iodine (Byrne et al 1991). The studies suggest that patients who shower using chlorhexidine achieve a greater degree of bacterial decontamination compared with other skin-cleansing agents (Garibaldi 1988). However, there are many inconsistencies in the methodology of these studies, so no firm conclusions can be drawn. Furthermore, other research studies (Leigh et al 1983, Byrne et al 1994) have shown a direct association between a reduction in skin flora and the incidence of postoperative wound infection, but the results of these studies are again inconclusive. Patients who are carriers of, or are colonized or infected with, methicillin-resistant *Staphylococcus aureus* (MRSA) should use an antiseptic detergent for bathing, and the advice of the infection control team should be sought about other precautions required during the perioperative period.

Hair removal

Extensive debate and research have focused on the issue of hair removal and its potential for reducing wound sepsis, although again much is inconclusive. Operation site shaving is an area of practice historically steeped in ritual. As recently as the 1980s, surgeons were instructing nurses in 'nipple to knee' shaving prior to hernia repair and appendicectomy.

The rationale for hair removal is based on the premise that hair harbours microorganisms and its presence may also obscure the operation or incision site. The practicality of placing and securing wound dressings has also been considered as an issue. However, the act of shaving potentially increases the risk of infection to the patient because of the likelihood of sustaining cuts and nicks in the shaving process. Skin abrasions sustained in this way provide an entry site for microorganisms, thus increasing the risk of postoperative wound infection (Jepson & Bruttomesso 1993). Surgical shaving of the operation site is a skilled procedure and it is important to remove the hair without causing skin injury.

There is also some debate about the best method to remove hair. Shaving has historically been the method of choice, yet has consistently been reported as leading to higher rates of wound infection when compared with other methods (Small 1996). If shaving is to occur then a wet shave is preferable to a dry shave, as it is much less traumatic to the skin. If shaving is necessary, it should be performed as close to the surgery as possible. Consequently, patients may well be shaved once they have arrived in the operating theatres rather than on the ward.

The use of clippers has been compared with shaving in a comparison of infection rates (Alexander et al 1983). Patients who had hair removed using clippers on the morning of the operation had a lower infection rate than either those who had been shaved the night before or on the morning of surgery, or those who had had hair removed with clippers on the night before their operation. Jepson & Bruttomesso (1993) suggested that hair be left on the body unless it interfered with surgical access. Where hair removal is necessary, they suggest that methods other than shaving be used.

More recently, the use of depilatory creams has been advocated as an alternative to mechanical hair removal methods. Results suggest it to be a non-traumatic, effective and low-risk method. However, patients need to use these creams with care. A patch test for allergy or sensitivity to such creams must be carried out prior to use.

In summary, the evidence appears to support a non-interventionist approach. If depilation needs to take place, the use of clippers or depilatory creams is preferable to shaving.

The physical, cultural and emotional effects of shaving on the patient must be respected. For some religions and cultures, the removal of body hair may be contrary to spiritual well-being and alternatives must be considered. Hair removal is potentially embarrassing and undignified and causes considerable discomfort when hair regrows.

It has become common practice in some clinical settings to ask patients to shave, clip or apply creams to their own operation site. Yet for many it is a difficult or uncomfortable task. It is essential to ensure that, whatever technique is utilized, appropriate individual assessment of the patient is undertaken. Evidence of pre-existing skin infection or inflammatory disorders, coagulation problems, dexterity or visual problems may influence the choice of technique. Small (1996) cites a case report in which a man died of sepsis resulting from cuts sustained after being asked by a nurse to use clippers to remove abdominal hair. The patient had a pre-existing skin infection, which was considered influential in his demise.

Malnutrition and nutritional assessment

Many patients who are admitted to hospital are already nutritionally compromised and indeed deteriorate during hospitalization (see Ch. 11). Surgical patients are at particular risk of developing malnutrition. Whilst the nature of the surgical procedure and the presence of pre-existing disease are clearly influential, a number of generic risk factors may be identified:

- inadequate nutritional assessment
- prolonged preoperative fasting
- stressful effects of surgery on the body
- prolonged restriction of oral fluid and diet postoperatively
- inadequate and inappropriate reliance on isotonic intravenous fluids, such as normal saline, that do not provide sufficient energy (see Ch. 8)
- low priority afforded to nutritional aspects of care.

The effects of malnourishment have been associated with delayed wound healing, the development of pressure ulcers (see Ch. 10), impaired respiratory function, reduced immune response and prolonged hospitalization.

Nutritional assessment requires a collaborative approach to ensure all patients are screened for malnutrition risk and to identify those requiring additional nutritional support. Referral to dieticians and nutritional nurse specialists may take place prior to admission. For patients with gastrointestinal disorders, cancer or undergoing major surgery, preoperative nutritional support can positively influence surgical outcome. More emphasis is now being placed on the use of a structured nutritional assessment aided by the use of documentary scoring tools to provide an objective predictor of risk.

Patients should always be weighed routinely on admission as part of this nutritional assessment. This baseline measure allows nursing staff to monitor the nutritional state and progress of patients. It also allows for accurate drug dosage calculations to be made on the basis of body weight. Dependent on the surgery to be performed, individual fasting regimens need to be planned for patients, which acknowledge the adverse effects of prolonged fasting (see p. 893).

Deep vein thrombosis

Hospitalization, surgery and prolonged bed rest all have the potential for an enforced reduction in mobility. Previously, an operation meant an enforced period of bed rest for unnecessary long periods of time; however, now the emphasis has changed to early postoperative mobilization. Despite these changes in practice, the development of deep vein thrombosis (DVT) still poses a risk to surgical patients. DVT is probably the greatest single threat to successful postoperative recovery and is the most common cause of pulmonary embolism (PE). A DVT occurs when a thrombus (clot) develops in one of the deep veins of the body and attaches itself to the wall of the vessel (see Ch. 19). This occurs most commonly in the lower limbs, and more specifically the femoral and popliteal veins, but also in the pelvic veins. The thrombus formation may result in diminished blood flow with associated local symptoms. More critically, a thrombus or part of it may break free of the vessel, travelling via the circulation to other parts of the body. Commonly an embolus resulting from a DVT will become lodged in a pulmonary vessel, causing a PE.

Autar (1996) recognizes DVT to be a largely preventable occurrence, and clearly an understanding of the factors that might precipitate this condition will aid prevention. Three key factors (Virchow's triad) have been identified as predisposing to the formation of venous thrombosis:

- venous stasis
- hypercoagulability
- blood vessel damage.

Autar (1996) identifies several high-risk categories, including increasing age, increased BMI, immobility, trauma, existing peripheral vascular disease, oestrogen therapy and surgery.

Particular surgical procedures increase the risk of thrombosis – pelvic operations are more likely to be complicated by thrombosis due to localized trauma to the pelvic veins. Craft & Upton (1992) identify gynaecological surgery in women over 40 years old and orthopaedic surgery as particular risks. Initial assessment of risk and therapeutic strategy is likely to involve medical and nursing collaboration. Specific risk assessment tools for DVT now exist and these may provide predictive indices for those most at risk.

Preventative approaches to DVT focus predominantly on four interventions:

- subcutaneous (SC) heparin therapy
- anti-embolism stockings
- limb physiotherapy exercises
- early postoperative mobilization.

The use of anticoagulants has been shown to reduce the incidence of DVT in surgical patients. For those identified as being at risk, a prophylactic regimen may be achieved by administration of subcutaneous injections of heparin. A commonly used regimen requires a dose of 5000 units 2 hours before surgery, then every 8–12 hours (once or twice daily) for 7 days or until the patient is fully ambulant.

The administration of prophylactic heparin may be used in conjunction with the application of graduated compression stockings. Agu et al (1999) report stockings to reduce the relative risk of DVT by 64% in surgical patients. They confirm the findings of many studies which state that stockings combined with low-dose heparin perform better than stockings or heparin alone. It is important to note that anti-embolism stockings must be correctly measured and applied. There is little evidence available to recommend a particular style of stocking. However, thigh-length stockings are reported to be more expensive, more difficult to fit accurately and apply, and less well tolerated by patients than knee-length stockings. Poorly fitting stockings may be constrictive and diminish blood flow, leading to reports of ischaemia, thrombosis and even gangrene, particularly in patients with existing disease such as diabetes or peripheral vascular disease. Ideally, patients should continue to wear stockings until discharge or until they are fully mobile. Commonly, stockings may fall down or are removed by patients, who are unaware of their benefits. It is essential, then, that patients be fully informed as to the purpose of the stockings to aid compliance.

Chest infection

Whilst the major cause of perioperative death is cardiac-related, the greatest cause of perioperative morbidity is pulmonary complications (McKnight 1994). The potential for postoperative chest infection is diminished through appropriate management. Prior to surgery, a patient's respiratory status is reviewed and an assessment of the potential for developing chest infection is made.

Patients considered to be most at risk are those with a pre-existing chronic respiratory disease, such as asthma or COPD, or long-term smokers (see Ch. 20). Mobility-related problems due to existing systemic disorders or potential problems related to the location and duration of surgery to be performed also pose a risk. Patients undergoing surgery and, more specifically, general anaesthesia are at increased risk of developing pulmonary complications.

Smoking irritates the mucosa and damages the lining of the respiratory tract. Chemicals in cigarettes permanently destroy the cilia that normally clear mucus upwards for expectoration. Inability to maintain this protective mechanism can lead to the potential for secretions to be retained in the lower respiratory tract (see Ch. 20). Smokers need advice on the reduction or, better still, cessation of smoking. Ideally patients should cease smoking at least 2 weeks prior to surgery. For some the impending surgery can provide a positive focus and a reason to consider cessation. In reality, it is unlikely that most smokers will follow such advice and it could be argued that smoking cessation is unlikely to be successful at times of increased stress and anxiety. Hospitalization and surgery can provide an excellent focus for opportunistic health education. However, it would be both unethical and immoral, and ultimately unlikely to achieve long-term success, if scare tactics are used when patients feel vulnerable. Any advice or information requested and any decisions made by patients should be respected without prejudice or value judgement.

Inhaled gases and drugs used in anaesthesia to inhibit secretions, such as atropine, will have a drying effect on the respiratory tract. Muscle-relaxing drugs and the use of mechanical ventilation may limit full lung inflation and reduce the capacity for deep breathing. Surgery and any associated pain often inhibit mobility and patients' ability and desire to fully expand their lungs. This may lead to an accumulation of mucus in the bronchioles which consolidate, therefore making it difficult to expectorate. These retained secretions inhibit gaseous exchange precipitating respiratory distress. Additionally these secretions provide an ideal environment for bacterial infection.

Investigations prior to surgery may include chest X-ray, blood gases and a lung function assessment. The anaesthetist will assess the patient and the choice of anaesthetic may be influenced by the results of this assessment. It is likely that at-risk patients will be referred to the physiotherapist preoperatively. This will involve the instigation of deep breathing and coughing exercises designed to promote maximal lung inflation and the expectoration of secretions. Patients should be given advice regarding how to avoid putting strain on the incision and will be taught how to support the wound when coughing. The nurse has an active role in this interdisciplinary intervention, both providing reinforcement to the educative aspects of therapy and fulfilling the lead role in the absence of the physiotherapist.

PSYCHOLOGICAL PREPARATION FOR SURGERY

Whilst surgery may be routine for nurses, to patients it is often perceived to be a formidable undertaking, associated with particular fears and anxieties (see Reflective Practice box 29.1).

The experience of hospitalization induces concerns for some patients, particularly as they are in an environment that leads to an enforced loss of independence and reduced control. Separation from family and usual support groups, disruption to normal lifestyle and the associated fears of treatment are all major stressors (see Ch. 6 and 'Further reading' section).

For many patients, this will be a new experience and not knowing what to expect can lead to fear of the unknown. Interestingly, previous experience of surgery does not guarantee that anxieties will be lessened. For some, previous knowledge of surgical procedures and knowledge of what to expect may lead to an anticipatory anxiety. This has clear implications for the manner of preparation and is discussed later.

Whilst patients often have a disproportionate perception of risk, it must be recognized that despite advances in surgical technique and anaesthesia, no procedure or surgical intervention is without risk.

29.1 Perioperative fears

The following list includes some of the common fears experienced by patients prior to anaesthesia and surgery:

- Being put to sleep and not waking up
- Waking during surgery
- Feeling pain while under the effects of the anaesthetic yet unable to communicate
- Pain postoperatively
- Inappropriate behaviour whilst under the influence of anaesthetic
- Talking and personal disclosures under anaesthetic
- Postoperative nausea or vomiting
- Diagnosis and outcome of surgery
- Disfigurement and changes to normal body image
- Loss of control and dependency on others
- Fears of dying
- Loss of dignity

Student activities

Reflect on the list.

- If you have had surgery which, if any, of these fears troubled you the most?
- If not, look at the list and think which would cause you most anxiety?
- What interventions by health professionals would best allay these fears?

Physiological effects of stress and anxiety on surgical patients

Stress and anxiety are multifaceted concepts, which can have major implications for patients (see Ch. 6). For the surgical patient, these emotional reactions are associated with physiological responses that increase the likelihood of postoperative complications occurring. Classic nursing studies have demonstrated the association between surgical intervention, stress, anxiety and the quality of recovery (Hayward 1975, Boore 1978).

An increased level of chemicals found in the body postoperatively has been considered a clear indication that surgery has a definitive impact on the body. Cortisol (a corticosteroid), the catecholamines adrenaline (epinephrine) and noradrenaline (norepinephrine), and antidiuretic hormone (ADH) have all been implicated. The presence of these chemicals is widely believed to be detrimental to patient well-being. Increased levels may result in raised BP, pulse rate and further risk of cardiac arrhythmias, consequently placing the patient as a higher surgical risk. The stress response ultimately inhibits the immune system and leads to a decreased white blood cell count, thus counteracting the ability to fight infection. The increase in cortisol may delay healing.

The effects of stress can be summarized as:

- raised levels of adrenaline (epinephrine) and noradrenaline (norepinephrine), cortisol and ADH
- diminished recall and memory

- increased pain perception
- reduced white blood count (WBC)
- immune system inhibition.

Anxiety manifests in different ways – agitation and an overly talkative demeanour are common indications of stress, yet withdrawal and aggression can also be symptomatic. Stress and anxiety have the potential to interfere with the effectiveness of nurse–patient communication (see Ch. 3). Patients' ability to recall and comprehend information may be diminished; consequently they may be unable to process, absorb or retain all the verbal information that they are given.

Patients display a wide range of coping techniques and these have the potential to enhance or interfere with their adaptation to the process of surgery. A refusal to accept or to confront any emotionally threatening aspects of surgery is common. Fears about the diagnosis found at surgery or the effects of surgery on body image, for example, are major concerns.

Anxiety is often assumed to be a passive state that is both an undesirable and unhelpful response to stress. There is an alternative view that insufficient arousal (anxiety) is as detrimental as too great a level of arousal. Effectively, there is an optimal level of arousal or anxiety, which may be beneficial in helping the individual prepare and adapt positively to the forthcoming event.

▶ Nursing management: stress and anxiety

Surgery is a critical life event and an understanding of how individuals respond to crisis is useful. Assessment will require the nurse to identify patients' understanding of their problem, coping behaviours and any support networks. Psychological preparation encompasses assessing levels of anxiety and assisting patients in understanding and ultimately accepting the proposed surgery. This may be achieved by the provision of verbal and written information based on a previous assessment of what patients want to or need to know and their existing level of understanding. The following areas might be discussed:

- specific perioperative tests and investigations
- the sequence of events on the operation day, including time of operation and necessary preparation
- transfer to operating theatre and where the patient will wake up; this information may be supported by a preoperative visit
- nursing interventions required in the immediate and continuing postoperative periods
- likely drains, intravenous infusions, catheters, nasogastric tubes
- the management of pain and nausea/vomiting postoperatively
- patient expectations in terms of mobility
- preparations for discharge and likely postoperative follow-up.

Patient education

Because a fear of the unknown is a major perioperative stressor, provision of information and explanation in the form of patient teaching can help to decrease stress and anxiety, and increase feelings of control. Patient education begins as soon as patients enter the health care system. Information and advice are likely to be provided in primary care where GP and practice nurse collaborate in patient care management prior to referral or admission to hospital. Outpatient and pre-admission clinics provide a further opportunity for patient education, and on admission additional interaction may take place. Ideally, specific patient education relevant to the proposed elective surgery should take place well in advance. This allows patients time to digest and retain information, as well as the opportunity to ask questions.

Some patients are content to allow the health professional to take control and to make decisions on their behalf. However, it must be recognized that in a contemporary and consumer-led society, patients are rarely content to be passive recipients, preferring an active role. This can be seen in the proliferation of health-related internet sites providing information on virtually every health topic. Whilst the quality and monitoring of this information are very variable, most patients with internet access will already have some level of knowledge. It is important that health professionals recognize that the wholly uninformed patient is rare, but they must ensure that patients' understanding is accurate and appropriate. Therefore the goal of patient education is to develop a partnership that provides patients with sufficient knowledge to make informed decisions. The application of these concepts will empower patients and increase feelings of control.

The quality of patient education has traditionally been very variable and often ineffective (see Ch. 2). The UK NHS has produced good practice guidelines for conveying patient information (Department of Health 2001), recommending that all communication must be clear, easily accessible, understandable, honest and respectful to the consumer and cost-effective. For surgical patients, these principles can be applied to provide quality information in all aspects of communication.

Good practice in surgical patient education (see Ch. 3) includes the following:

- Identify existing level of knowledge.
- Ensure a conducive environment (e.g. privacy, quiet).
- Be sensitive to cultural needs.
- Involve family, partners and carers where appropriate.
- Be aware of factors that influence successful education (e.g. stress, pain, confusion).
- Understand that spaced repetition of information is often better than a 'one-off' delivery.
- Avoid the use of jargon or overly technical terminology.
- Written information, supplied in the appropriate language, should be used to support information provided verbally.
- Ensure readability of written information and alternatives for patients who do not read.

CONSENT

Obtaining consent prior to an operative procedure is an essential aspect of pre-surgical management from both an ethico-legal and a humanitarian perspective.

Consent may be defined as the giving of approval to a particular course of action. However, without an understanding of the implication of that action, any consent will remain uninformed.

For consent to be valid, patients must:

- be competent to make a decision
- have received appropriate and sufficient information
- not be acting under duress.

The NHS Plan (Department of Health 2000) identified the need for change in the way patients give consent to treatment, care and research. Consent issues were apparent in several high-profile revelations, including the alleged failure to provide sufficient information regarding morbidity and mortality rates in paediatric cardiac surgery at Bristol Royal Infirmary. These occurrences serve to remind health professionals of the understandable lack of public tolerance for poor quality information or evasive, if well-meaning, reassurances.

As a consequence, the UK government has introduced new consent-to-treatment forms and a model for consent to treatment (Department of Health 2001). This publication provides explicit guidance in issues of consent and, along with its associated documents addressing specific client groups, should be essential reading for all nurses working in surgical care. For a review of some of the key issues, see Health Promotion box 29.1.

In surgical nursing, as in other areas of health care, obtaining consent to treatment or procedure is integral to everyday nursing activity. Indeed, without consent, even touching patients might be considered a trespass against them, i.e. battery or assault.

The exact nature of informed consent has developed substantially over the years, although it remains a contentious issue for both medical staff and lawyers. For patient consent to fulfil the requirements of both the law and the professional bodies, it must be informed. In English law, consent can be obtained through implied, verbal or written means, although there is no legal distinction between these forms (Dimond 2001).

Implied consent, whilst open to misinterpretation, is obtained on the premise that recipients have agreed to treatment by their actions or behaviour. Patients who roll up their sleeves in the presence of a phlebotomist would provide implied consent to the provision of a blood sample. Such an act comprises legally valid evidence of consent, but from a professional perspective is satisfactory only for the more trivial or minimal of interventions. The essence of informed consent is the patient's awareness of the implications of the proposed action. The consent may be a verbal agreement, but for reasons of documentation and the ability to provide evidence of the process, written consent is most desirable.

A consent form signed by both the patient and the operative practitioner is evidence of an interaction between the two. As such, it is likely to provide the only acceptable evidence that informed consent has been obtained. It will provide a permanent record implying that the patient was made aware of the proposed procedure, its consequence, possible risks and any alternatives. It is worth noting that a nurse may well undertake the operation. The increasing number of clinical nurse consultant appointments in colorectal work, for example, has seen them undertaking invasive operative procedures. Within the consultation, the patient has both legal and moral rights. Rights in consent include:

- right to quality information
- right to know alternatives
- right to ask questions
- right to consult others/second opinion
- right to have time to consider options
- right to changing one's mind.

HEALTH PROMOTION

29.1 Good practice in consent

Issues

- Patients have traditionally adopted a passive role in surgical treatment decision-making
- Many patients are not fully informed prior to surgery
- Patients have both legal and moral rights to make informed choices
- Nurses are in an ideal position to promote patient participation and empowerment through patient teaching
- Patients will make different treatment choices in response to similar health scenarios

Background

Recent well-publicized events have highlighted the need for information sharing and transparency in decision-making. *The NHS Plan* (Department of Health 2000) consequently promised action to ensure consent procedures reflected the rights of the patient in decision-making. The *Good Practice in Consent Implementation Guide* (Department of Health 2001) asks NHS trusts to implement a new consent policy incorporating new consent-to-treatment documentation and patient information leaflets. The document provides guidance and a series of questions that may be asked of health professionals. Nurses have a pivotal role in working in partnership with patients to ensure they receive the very best quality information. Patient teaching can ensure patients are aware of, and comfortable with, asking questions of the surgeons and staff involved in their care. The questions below may provide a structured framework for this purpose.

Questions about the treatment

- What are the main treatment options?
- What are the benefits of each of the options?
- What are the risks, if any, of each option?
- What are the success rates for different options – nationally, for this unit or for the surgeon?
- Why do you think an operation (if suggested) is necessary?
- What are the risks if I decide to do nothing for the time being?
- How can I expect to feel after the procedure?
- When am I likely to be able to get back to work?

Questions about how treatment might affect the patient's future state of health or lifestyle

- Will I need long-term care?
- Will my mobility be affected?
- Will I still be able to drive?
- Will it affect the kind of work I do?
- Will it affect my personal/sexual relationships?
- Will I be able to take part in my favourite sport/exercises?
- Will I be able to follow my usual diet?

References

Department of Health. The NHS Plan. London: HMSO; 2000.

Department of Health. Good practice in consent implementation guide: consent to examination or treatment. London: DoH; 2001 (Also online. Available: www.doh.gov.uk/consent).

Many patients, despite the provision of written consent, are not always fully aware of the implications of the surgery being undertaken. This is perhaps not surprising in a highly pressured environment and a combination of low staffing levels, increased throughput and workload have contributed to this scenario. Clearly this is an unsatisfactory situation with the potential for unnecessary distress and inappropriate surgical management.

Traditionally patients were obliged to adopt a passive stance in their health care. Yet contemporary society, and health care in particular, places an increasing emphasis on the consumer taking an active role in decision-making. The surgical nurse has a professional responsibility and is in a prime position to empower the patient by encouraging equal participation and partnership in decision-making.

Age and factors reducing potential for informed consent

Patients can sign the consent form if they are of the legal age of 16 years and above and/or have the mental capacity to understand fully all that is involved (see Dimond 2001). If they are unable to sign the form, the parent or legal guardian may do so. Where an adult lacks mental capacity either temporarily or permanently to give or withhold consent, no one has the right to give approval for a course of action. However, treatment may be given if it is considered to be in the patient's best interests so long

as an explicit refusal to such action has not been made by the person in advance. The consent form must be signed before any premedication is given and, in signing the form, patients give their consent to the administration of an anaesthetic and performance of surgery. This includes a signed declaration by the medical practitioner that the nature and purpose of the proposed operation has been explained.

PREOPERATIVE SAFETY MEASURES

The importance of preoperative preparation cannot be overemphasized. With over 3 million operations being performed every year, the potential for untoward occurrences is ever apparent. Preparation for surgery must be based on best practice and must be respectful of both safety and the effects of pre-surgical protocols on patient comfort. Issues of fasting, bowel preparation and safety, including patient identification, are of particular prominence and importance.

Fasting prior to surgery

The purpose of fasting is to reduce the volume of gastric content at induction of anaesthesia and consequently to reduce the risk of postoperative nausea and vomiting (PONV). When patients are unconscious and anaesthetized using muscle relaxants and sedatives, the muscle tone is reduced. This affects the respiratory muscles, the gastro-oesophageal (cardiac) sphincter between the stomach and oesophagus, and the muscles of swallowing. Essentially the normal reflex functions that allow the conscious patient to respond safely to regurgitation are lost. Food or fluid in the stomach may reflux during the administration of a general anaesthetic and there is a risk of inhalation of stomach contents through the open larynx into the lungs leading to aspiration pneumonia of varying severity (often termed Mendelson's syndrome). With adequate preparation, aspiration is a relatively rare occurrence in healthy patients undergoing elective surgery (Maltby 2001) and the majority of clinically significant cases occur in emergency, trauma, obstetric and abdominal surgery.

The length of time necessary for safe fasting has long been debated. As long ago as 1883, Joseph Lister recommended that there be no solids in the stomach but that clear fluids could be taken up until 2 hours before surgery. Consequently, most medical texts recommended 6-hour fasting for solids and 2–3 hours for liquids. During the 1960s in the USA, the nil by mouth from midnight protocol was applied to both solids and liquids and was widely accepted as *de rigueur* and implemented throughout the world as standard pre-surgical instruction.

Concern about the risk of pulmonary aspiration may have been fuelled by fears of litigation, but for whatever reason there emerged a number of research studies that attempted to provide scientific evidence for this protocol (e.g. Shevde & Triveldi 1991). Two factors considered critical in the occurrence of inhalation were a pH of gastric aspirate less than 2.5 and a volume greater than 25 mL. Yet other researchers found that a light meal of tea and toast only 2–3 hours before surgery had no effect on the volume or pH of gastric content. Chapman (1996) concluded that gastric volume and pH are independent of a fluid fast beyond 2 hours and suggested that patients can safely be offered fluids up to 2 hours preoperatively.

Clearly there is a lack of consistency in the research findings, although a generally consistent protocol for practice appears to be emerging. Although the stomach takes longer to digest some foodstuffs than others, and there is variation in gastric emptying time, it is usually complete for most meals in 4–5 hours. Consequently, the protocol for fasting that has frequently been adopted is 4 hours for fluids and 6 hours for food. In the case of patients requiring emergency surgery, it is not always possible to ensure that they have been fasted for a safe period of time, and in these circumstances alternative strategies need to be considered (see pp. 897 and 899).

Many patients are fasted for unnecessarily lengthy periods. An early study by Hamilton Smith (1972) showed that patients were fasted preoperatively for varying lengths of time, and often for much longer than necessary, sometimes for 13 hours or more. More recently, Chapman (1996) demonstrated that despite advances in knowledge, inconsistencies in fasting procedures still persist.

In practice, many nurses persist in the ritual of starving all patients from midnight in preparation for morning surgery, giving patients on the afternoon list a light breakfast at 6.00 or 7.00am. The result of fasting all patients on the same operating list from the same time and not adopting more individualized fasting regimens is that the last patient on the list is starved for much longer than the first (see Reflective Practice box 29.2 and Ch. 11).

R|Я REFLECTIVE PRACTICE

29.2 Personal observations on preoperative fasting

A critical incident detailed by a qualified nurse revealed that an older woman admitted with a hip fracture was expecting surgery on one day but this was cancelled. The operation was eventually performed the following day, which meant that the lady in question was fasted for a total of 16 hours. The consequences of such prolonged fasting times are not insignificant for such a patient.

Student activities
Find out the following:

- Is there a local policy for preoperative fasting in your clinical area?
- How long are patients fasted for in your hospital?
- Does this vary from ward to ward or between patients?
- Who makes the decision as to how long patients should be fasted for?
- How would you respond to the patient who informs you that he has not complied with the nil by mouth regimen?
- What information is given to patients about preoperative fasting?
- Why do you think that clinical practice is not always congruent with evidence-based practice?

Fasting for the recommended period of 4–6 hours is unlikely to be detrimental to any other than the most frail, those who are critically ill or those at the extremes of the life span. The main complication of prolonged fasting is dehydration and electrolyte imbalance, which can be a particular problem in older people and the very young (see Ch. 8).

The effects of prolonged fasting include:

- confusion – caused by fluid and electrolyte imbalance
- dry mouth, hunger and thirst – patients can have frequent mouthwashes but must be advised not to swallow any of the fluid. Thirst and hunger can affect patients psychologically and potentially cause distress, especially if they do not understand or are not made aware of the reasons for fasting
- headache and nausea – due to the fall in blood glucose; this may be problematic and reported by the patient.

The effects of prolonged fasting may be a particular concern for diabetic patients. Ideally they should be placed first on the operating list to minimize the effects of perioperative fasting on blood glucose levels. The anaesthetist will give specific instructions regarding changes to the usual timing or dose of oral hypoglycaemic drugs or insulin. In some cases, i.v. fluids are commenced preoperatively and patients will have regular blood glucose monitoring.

Patients need to be informed of the reasons for preoperative fasting and this information should be reinforced with relatives, ensuring they understand its significance and thus encouraging compliance. A study by Thomas (1987) found that many of the patients studied had not received any explanation or information as to why they were being fasted, nor how long they should fast for.

A nil-by-mouth sign is placed above the patient's bed so that all staff are aware. All fluids and edibles such as sweets and fruit are removed from the bedside. If for any reason, a patient has failed to comply with the nil-by-mouth regimen, the surgeon and anaesthetist must be notified.

Nurses cannot be unaware of the research and recommendations, yet they continue to set wide parameters in their fasting regimens. A number of explanations can be offered for the persistence of traditional and anecdotal practice. Fear of changes in the order of an operating list and perceived unpredictability of the operation time are major barriers to individualized care. Theatre times are often only approximate and the duration time of operations cannot be predicted. For those patients requiring emergency surgery, the operating time is often even less predictable.

The use of a standard regimen such as nil by mouth from midnight clearly does not subscribe to a philosophy of individualized care management. Patients could be offered light snacks and fluid at any time of the day or night. However, this often does not take place. The fear of litigation in the case of a mistake has resulted in an ultra-cautious and conservative approach to fasting management. Confusion over whose responsibility it is to instigate better practice (nurses or anaesthetists) may also be an issue. It would be inaccurate to assume that individualized fasting regimens have not been adopted at all. Good practice is evident in many areas where nurses and anaesthetists have both attempted to implement changes in practice. However, the issue appears to be a lack of uniformity in fasting practices.

Bowel preparation

Patients undergoing gastrointestinal tract or pelvic surgery may require specific preparation of the bowel. This often involves the administration of an oral laxative, bowel cleansing solutions or the administration of an enema or suppositories. Commonly used oral solutions, e.g. Picolax, are prescribed orally with water the morning and afternoon prior to surgery the following day. The medication acts rapidly to evacuate the bowel. Consequently, surgery may be performed in an environment with a much lower risk of faecal contamination and subsequent infection. Additionally, the use of bowel preparatory agents preoperatively may reduce the risk of PONV and discomfort caused by abdominal distension. It is likely that patients will also be prescribed antibiotic cover, e.g. cefuroxime or metronidazole, to reduce the bowel flora, further lessening the risk of infection caused by faecal contamination during surgery. It is important to recognize that these purgative regimens can cause some distress to the patient, as the drug effect is often rapid and unpredictable. For patients who may already have a pre-existing bowel condition, this can prove an embarrassing and uncomfortable experience. If bowel preparation is used, nurses need to monitor and record the results and effectiveness of this, as well as ensuring access to the lavatory and the opportunity to wash and attend to hygiene needs.

Immediate preoperative measures

Patients in the operating theatre are unable to communicate effectively or to control their environment. Consequently a number of preparatory measures are instigated just prior to transfer to the theatre to ensure patient safety. The attending nurse records these on a standardized checklist. Cosmetics, including facial make-up and nail varnish, are removed as they can mask natural skin colour, which might prevent detection of cyanosis or extreme pallor. The reasons and significance for this should be explained to patients.

The presence of dental caps, crowns or dentures that may become damaged or dislodged during the induction of anaesthesia, or even lost during transfer to and from the operating theatre, must be ascertained and recorded. Jewellery should ideally be removed prior to operative procedures to prevent loss or damage. These are stored safely according to local protocols. Many patients are reluctant to remove their wedding rings or are unable to do so and these can be covered with adhesive tape. Similarly the presence of prostheses such as hairpieces, contact lenses, limbs and breasts should be identified, recorded and removed if appropriate. However, it is essential that the dignity of the patient be preserved. If patients are reluctant to remove any accessory or prostheses and appear distressed, they should be reassured that it will be acceptable for removal to take place in the anaesthetic room or theatre. Head covering (required by some cultures), hearing aids and spectacles might be left in place until patients are anaesthetized. Any items removed must be recorded and stored appropriately according to local policies.

Patients are asked to empty their bladder preoperatively in order to prevent incontinence during the operation (and injury to the bladder during an abdominal or pelvic operation).

Premedication

Prior to anaesthesia, the use of a premedication agent may be prescribed. A commonly used drug for premedication is temazepam given orally with a few sips of water if required. Temazepam is a sedative given to promote relaxation and reduce apprehension, and may induce drowsiness. The use of such drugs has largely superseded intramuscular injections of papaveretum, pethidine and hyoscine for premedication.

Anticholinergic (muscarinic receptor antagonist) drugs such as atropine may be prescribed as premedication to dry up salivary and bronchial secretions. Patients must be warned that a dry mouth is normal and is a positive indicator that secretions have been suppressed. It is essential that the nurse clearly informs patients of the effect of drugs used and instigates appropriate comfort and safety measures.

If a premedication is prescribed, it is usually administered 45 minutes to 1 hour prior to the time of operation. The nurse must always check that written consent for operation has been obtained by the relevant health professional before administering any premedication drug. Patients should be asked to stay in bed and advised to use the call system if they need any assistance. Some patients who are admitted the night before surgery may be prescribed sedation to ensure that they are rested at the time of operation and therefore better prepared to withstand the stress of surgery.

Other commonly prescribed medications given preoperatively are antibiotics. These may be given if there is an infection present or as a prophylactic measure over the perioperative period (see above). In fasting patients, these may be given rectally or intravenously. Similarly, anticoagulant drugs used as prophylaxis in the prevention of DVT and PE may be prescribed at this time.

PATIENT TRANSFER, SAFETY AND IDENTIFICATION ISSUES

Patients are transferred to the operating department with an escort. Ideally this should be a registered nurse known to them who has knowledge of their condition and any individual needs. In practice, and depending upon local policy and protocols, patients are often transferred with a health care assistant or a student nurse as escort. It is essential that the escort is fully aware of the implications of this role and has had the appropriate preparation for this activity. Information regarding the journey to theatre, including the use of lifts or noisy corridors, should be explained. This is especially important where sensory impairment is an issue.

It is essential that the correct patient leaves the ward for the correct operation. Checking the patient wristband and all corresponding biographical details such as name, unit number and date of birth will act as confirmation of correct identity.

The following documentation accompanies the patient to the theatre:

- consent form
- patient's medical notes
- nursing notes and care plans
- X-rays
- completed preoperative checklist
- observation charts
- medication chart
- current blood results.

Traditionally, patients have been transferred to the operating department on a trolley. However, even this most traditional of rituals is being called into question. Influenced perhaps by the transportation changes seen in day-case/ambulatory surgery, where patients often walk to the operating department, Turnbull et al (1998) report how patients given the option of walking to the operating department appeared to demonstrate reduced anxiety and increased relaxation. The researchers suggest the element of control and perceived autonomy to be crucial elements of these results. Interestingly, the managerial/financial benefits of fewer staff required during transfer and the reduced potential for excessive manual handling involvement should prove an added efficiency motivation. By necessity, however, many patients will arrive in the operating department on a trolley, or preferably on their bed as this negates the need for excessive transfer activity. Care should be taken to ensure that patients are suitably covered in order to preserve warmth and dignity.

Identification

On arrival at the operating department, a member of the theatre team will greet the patient. Dependent on local protocols, this may be an operating department nurse or an operating department practitioner (ODP). The practitioner will confirm through the documentation and through interactions with both the patient and the escort, patient identity, the nature and site of operation and any other information deemed relevant. The wearing of identity bracelets on the wrist (or wrist and ankles in accordance with local policy) also serves to reinforce confirmation of the identity of the patient. In some circumstances, the operation site is also marked (e.g. left inguinal hernia repair) by the medical practitioner prior to surgery and preferably at the time consent is obtained. This may also be confirmed at this time.

Depending on patients' wishes and on local protocols, escorts may remain with them until they are anaesthetized or even during surgery carried out under local or regional anaesthesia. Most patients will benefit from having a familiar face with them during this very anxious period. For the sensory impaired patient or for those who cannot speak the national language, this can be a particularly stressful time. The presence of a member of staff or volunteer who can use sign language or a foreign language interpreter will greatly enhance the communication process. The emergence of preoperative visiting by operating department nursing staff as a now commonplace activity is likely to prove particularly beneficial if visiting perioperative nurses can make contact with patients. A member of the perioperative team or the accompanying escort must remain with patients until the commencement of anaesthetic induction, or until transfer into the operating room. At this stage, the aim of the staff is to provide the most conducive environment for patients and place them at ease. This is not a time for idle chat and escorts need to take the lead from patients and respond to any concerns or questions they may have.

INTRAOPERATIVE CARE

Nursing care in the intraoperative period is a skilled and highly responsible activity. Patients are wholly dependent on the surgical team and are unable to control even the most basic function. For the operating department nurse, a knowledge of anaesthesia, physiological responses to surgery, infection control, prevention of complications and surgical hazards is critical in patient management.

Effective, efficient and smooth running of the operating department requires cohesive, coordinated and skilled management. Whilst local practices may differ, it is likely that most operating departments will function utilizing a multidisciplinary, multiskilled and collaborative approach to management. For the best quality care, surgeons, anaesthetists, nurses, ODPs, ancillary and support staff such as radiographers will bring their own unique skills together to provide a mutually complementary framework, with each member of the team being respectful of colleagues' needs and worth. Whilst the medical staff and those professions allied to medicine have relatively well defined roles, it is worth noting that role demarcation is often much less distinct when contrasting the nursing and ODP roles. Previously, nationally certificated operating department assistant (ODA) training programmes were developed in a further attempt to free the nurse to address direct care activity. This 2-year programme equipped the ODA with the skills required to function in an anaesthetic or surgical assistant role. In practice, this apparent role demarcation was rarely seen, and the nursing and ODA contribution was often difficult to clarify. The Bevan (1989) report confirmed that the ODA and the nurse were interchangeable and that common training should be developed. Today the title of ODP describes those who complete a 2-year training programme that provides a comprehensive academic and practical education. Included in this are aspects such as psychological care, moral and ethical studies and the nature of caring that might be considered traditional nursing activity.

There are, however, aspects of operating department practice that could potentially benefit from the developments occurring elsewhere in nursing, e.g. specialist and advanced practitioners.

ANAESTHESIA

Anaesthesia may strictly be defined as an absence of feeling. In practice, anaesthetics are of course somewhat more complex and may usefully be described as general, regional or local in nature. Some of the most common agents used in anaesthesia are outlined in Table 29.1 (p. 884). Choice of anaesthetic method will be determined by numerous factors, including patient condition and suitability, therapeutic advantage, postoperative management and anaesthetist choice.

Local anaesthesia

Local anaesthesia (LA) involves the use of agents designed to block nerve impulse transmission in localized sensory nerve endings. Strictly speaking, LA may be described as a regional technique, as the effect is in a specific anatomical region. Furthermore, the local anaesthetic agents used, such as lidocaine (lignocaine) and bupivacaine, will also be used for regional blocks. However, for practical purposes, surgery under LA is generally considered to involve topical or well-defined localized tissue infiltration, usually in the conscious patient.

The use of LA is often naively considered to be without risk and requiring little anaesthetic nursing management. While it is true that the majority of LAs are administered without adverse effect, the potential for problems must be recognized and managed. Aside from possible allergic or anaphylactic reaction, large doses of local anaesthetic agents have the potential for cardiac toxicity and tachycardia, nausea and dizziness. Such occurrences are not uncommon and appropriate monitoring of vital signs is required following the use of LAs.

Perhaps the most commonly used local anaesthetic agent is lidocaine (lignocaine), either plain or containing adrenaline (epinephrine). Adrenaline prolongs the anaesthetic action and reduces bleeding through its vasoconstrictive properties. Adrenaline-enhanced local anaesthetic agents should be avoided in anaesthetic blocks of peripheral extremities such as toes, fingers and penis. The vasoconstrictive effects can be very potent and may cause tissue ischaemia and subsequent necrosis.

Regional anaesthesia

Most minor topical procedures will utilize a local anaesthetic agent administered directly into those tissues to be incised. On occasions when the amount of the agent required to ensure anaesthesia might be excessive, a regional block may be required. Regional anaesthetics are also designed to provide a pain- and sensation-free environment in a specific region of the body but will provide this over a greater area of tissue than is practicable with local infiltration anaesthesia. They include caudal, Bier's block and spinal and epidural.

Caudal

Caudal anaesthetic may be considered to be a modified epidural injection. For caudal anaesthesia, the local agent is injected into the epidural space through the caudal canal in the sacrum. The anaesthetic is very localized and does not produce the systemic effects of spinal and epidural anaesthesia. Because of their ease of use, caudal anaesthetics are commonly employed for perineal and genital pain relief.

Bier's block

Bier's block involves the intravenous injection of local anaesthetic into an extremity, i.e. a limb that has been exsanguinated using a rubber elasticated (Esmarch) bandage and a double-cuffed pneumatic tourniquet, applied to prevent arterial blood re-entering the vessels. With an upper time limit for the tourniquet of around 90 minutes, the surgeon is able to operate on a limb that is both sensation-free and presents a bloodless field. The primary care consideration involves the potential toxicity from release of LA into the bloodstream that may occur at deflation of the pneumatic cuff. It is essential that the technique is only undertaken by appropriately trained and experienced practitioners and with equipment that has had a thorough safety check. It must be remembered that any LA, by its very mode of action, will affect sensory and possibly motor function. Care must be taken to ensure the patient comes to no harm whilst vulnerable and unable to perceive sensation or maintain muscular control.

Epidural and spinal anaesthesia

Spinal and epidural injections are commonly employed in modern anaesthesia and involve the injection of LA and/or analgesic into either the subarachnoid or epidural space, usually accessed between the lumbar vertebrae. Whilst there are a number of fundamental differences in technique, spinal and epidural anaesthetics share many similarities in purpose and effect (see Table 29.2). The spinal anaesthetic is injected into the subarachnoid space (see Fig. 29.2B) to mix with the cerebrospinal fluid (CSF). The epidural injection is inserted into the epidural space (see Fig. 29.2B) and has no contact with the meninges. The injection has an anaesthetic effect on tissues distal to the site of injection and is commonly used for abdominal, pelvic, lower limb, orthopaedic and perineal surgery.

A spinal or epidural anaesthetic may be considered for a number of reasons, including:

- It is non-irritant to the respiratory tract and therefore useful where respiratory disease exists.
- Patients may be awake if desirable, e.g. during a caesarean section.
- It is useful in an emergency where preoperative preparation is limited.
- It provides some muscle relaxation.
- It promotes early mobilization.
- It is useful in hepatic disease (see Ch. 23) where general anaesthetic agents may be toxic.
- It allows postoperative analgesia – short-term for spinal and longer-term if an epidural catheter is used.
- The hypotensive effect provides a therapeutic reduction in intraoperative bleeding, alleviating the need for blood transfusion.

Local anaesthetic agents, e.g. lidocaine (lignocaine), are commonly used for injection. The sympathetic nerve blockade produced by these agents can promote profound hypotension and

Table 29.2 Comparison of spinal and epidural anaesthesia

Feature	Spinal	Epidural
Most common needle placement for lower torso surgery	Lumbar space 2–5	Lumbar space 2–5
Site of injection	Into cerebrospinal fluid (CSF) in subarachnoid space	Into epidural space
Common injection agent	Bupivacaine, lidocaine (lignocaine)	Bupivacaine, lidocaine (lignocaine)
Volume of agent	2–3 mL	10–30 mL
Needle bore	Very fine	Wider bore
Hypotensive effect	Very marked	Marked
Use as a single dose	Yes	Yes
Potential for divided dose and catheter placement	No	Yes – catheter commonly inserted for postoperative pain relief
Operator difficulty	Relatively easy	More difficult
Significant complications	Post-injection CSF leak, haemorrhage, infection	Haemorrhage, inadvertent dural puncture

patient assessment and preparation for this procedure must take this into account. Prior to injection, i.v. access is established and i.v. therapy commenced. In addition, ECG and BP monitoring equipment will be sited to ensure constant monitoring of cardiovascular status. Cardiopulmonary resuscitation equipment must be immediately available should any catastrophic hypotensive episode or toxic reaction occur. An i.v. dose of a vasoconstrictive agent such as methoxamine must also be available to reverse the vasodilatory effects of the anaesthetic.

Patients may be positioned on their side with their knees drawn up (see Fig. 29.2A), or sitting up and leaning forward. This promotes lumbar spine flexion and vertebral separation and facilitates access for the needle or cannula. The injection area is prepared using an antiseptic solution, and a local infiltration of anaesthetic around the site for needle insertion is commonly used to numb the skin. For both spinal and epidural anaesthesia, the choice of insertion is usually between the second and fifth lumbar vertebrae (L2 and L5) (see Figs 29.2C and D).

To provide the regional anaesthesia, a suitably sized needle is inserted using strict aseptic principles. For the spinal injection, in particular, introduction of microorganisms into the CSF may have life-threatening implications. The anaesthetic agent will bathe the nerves adjacent to the site of injection, producing blockade, and within a few minutes both sensory and motor function will be lost. The level and extent of blockade will depend on a number of factors including the volume, strength and type of anaesthetic agent used. In addition, the position in which patients are placed in the minutes after injection will determine the nerves to be affected. Gravity will take precedence until the solution is 'fixed' in the tissues. The speed of injection and the presence of raised intra-abdominal pressure, which may increase the spread of a spinal anaesthetic, are also influential factors.

It must also be recognized that not all patients are fit or suitable for spinal and epidural anaesthesia. The following, for example, are contraindicated:

- uncooperative patients
- unstable cardiovascular status
- existing hypotension

- existing blood clotting disorder
- raised intracranial pressure (see Ch. 14)
- unstable or uncertain spinal anatomy, e.g. previous spinal fracture
- local skin sepsis, or generalized sepsis
- neurological disease.

Whilst the use of spinal and epidural anaesthetics is commonly very safe and with minimal risk, the potential for complication must never be underestimated.

▶ Nursing management: following spinal and epidural anaesthetic

Management focuses on safety and patient comfort. Whilst the exact nature of care will differ between these two types of anaesthesia, there are common aspects of care. The assessment and monitoring of neurological and cardiovascular status are paramount. Frequent and regular review of BP and pulse will identify the extent of induced hypotension. Assessment of sensory and motor function will provide evidence of the persistence of blockade. Bladder function and tone, for example, may take some time to become fully re-established, requiring periodic assessment of comfort. Similarly, nurses must be alert to patients' inability to feel the presence of pressure or heat and the potentially serious consequences of that. With the use of fine-bore needles, haemorrhage or leakage of CSF is a rare but significant occurrence. The presence of persistent headache may indicate evidence of a leak of CSF.

Patients will be encouraged to assume a recumbent position, resting quietly with subdued lighting. Analgesia may be prescribed and fluid replacement can help reduce headache. If symptoms persist, the injection of a venous blood sample from patients into the epidural space surrounding the leak (blood patch) may be performed. The subsequent rise in intrathecal (within the meninges) pressure will usually provide rapid relief.

Following spinal injection, the needle will be removed; however, epidural injection allows the anaesthetist to insert a cannula into the epidural space for ongoing, longer-term pain management (see Ch. 7).

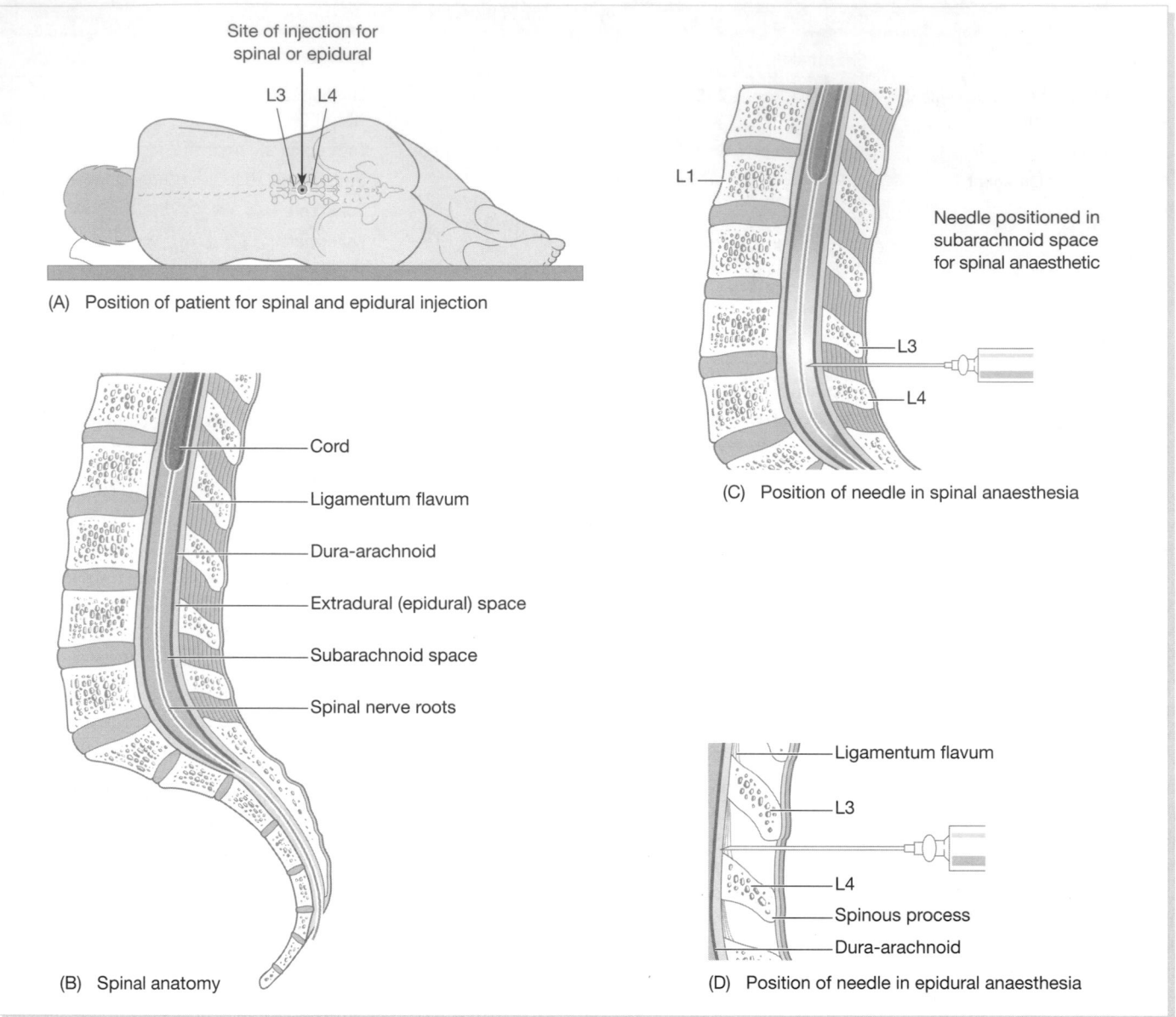

Figure 29.2 Spinal and epidural injection.

General anaesthesia

All patients scheduled for surgery will undergo an anaesthetic assessment prior to their arrival in the operating department. For many, the use of general anaesthesia (GA) will be the method of choice. GA is characterized by a medication-induced, reversible state of unconsciousness. The three key elements ('triad') of anaesthesia are the states of analgesia, sedation and muscular relaxation. The triad may be achieved through a variety of means but a combination of i.v. and inhalational agents are most commonly used. The process of anaesthesia involves three distinct phases: induction, maintenance and reversal (see pp. 899–900).

Airway maintenance

Any procedure altering the level of consciousness has the potential to compromise the airway. Consequently, the process of anaesthesia often requires the use of an airway maintenance

device (AMD). There are a number of different types of AMD, used according to patient airway requirement (see Fig. 29.3).

Oropharyngeal airways

Oropharyngeal airways such as the traditional rubber or plastic Guedel are commonly used for short-term airway maintenance in minor surgical procedures and postoperative airway management (see Fig. 29.3A). Oropharyngeal airways function by preventing the tongue from falling back and occluding the throat. They are often used in conjunction with an anaesthetic face mask that focuses anaesthetic gases and/or oxygen to the nose and mouth for passive inhalation. Nasopharyngeal airways are also available (see Fig. 29.3B).

Laryngeal mask airway

The laryngeal mask airway (LMA) is used in cases where patients can breathe spontaneously or where assisted ventilation is

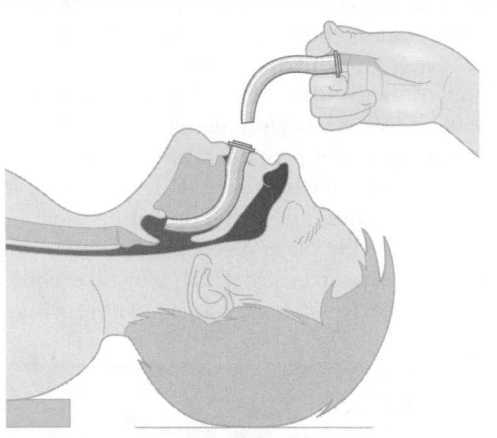

(A)   Insertion of Guedel oropharyngeal airway

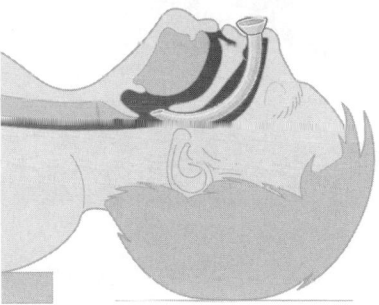

(B)   Position of nasopharyngeal airway

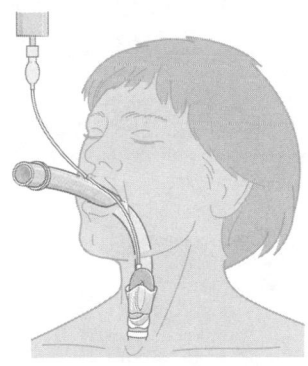

(C)   The laryngeal mask in situ

Laryngoscope

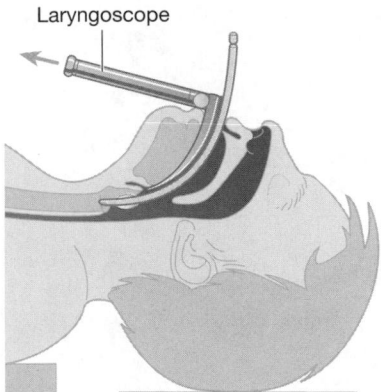

(D)   Endotracheal tube insertion

appropriate and can be maintained. It is relatively easily inserted and because the inflated cuff sits over and masks the larynx, there is no trauma or damage to the vocal cords or throat (see Fig. 29.3C). The LMA is not ideally suitable in procedures requiring patient repositioning during surgery or where manipulation of the neck (e.g. in thyroidectomy, see Ch. 17) is required. Such activity has the potential for dislodging the mask. Furthermore, emergency surgery and procedures in which there is a high risk of regurgitation and aspiration of gastric contents are not ideal scenarios for LMA usage either. The trachea is not occluded using this device and aspiration may be a concern.

Endotracheal tube

An endotracheal tube (ETT) is designed to provide optimal anaesthetic delivery and minimal risk of aspiration. In the anaesthetic room, a short-acting muscle relaxant, such as suxamethonium, may be used to allow the tube to pass through the vocal cords. The ETT, which may be cuffed or non-cuffed, is inserted nasally or orally and passes through the larynx and vocal cords and down the trachea (see Fig. 29.3D). The tube may be attached via various connections to an anaesthetic circuit or ventilator, rebreathing circuit or breathing bag (e.g. Ambu-bag), or simply left open to allow patients to breathe spontaneously. The cuffed tube incorporates a balloon or cuff which, when inflated in the trachea, provides an occlusive seal, thus preventing any fluid draining into the lower airway and lungs. The ETT is ideal where:

- airway maintenance is difficult due to anatomical features
- alternate methods of airway maintenance are inappropriate due to the length of operation
- long-acting muscle relaxants are used
- there is poor airway access due to operating position
- there is face or neck trauma.

In cases where neck manipulation during surgery is required, specially reinforced or armoured ETTs may be used to prevent the airway becoming compromised. The ETT does have the greatest potential of the AMDs for causing sore throats and hoarseness following surgery, due to trauma to the throat and vocal cords.

Anaesthetic induction

Critical to the success of any anaesthetic is the preparation of both the patient and the anaesthetic environment. In the anaesthetic room, appropriate cardiovascular and respiratory devices, such as electrocardiograph electrodes, pulse oximeter (see Chs 8, 9 and 31) and temperature monitors, are attached to the patient. Following induction, specific activity such as the fitting of eye protectors prior to laser surgery will also be instigated.

Induction involves the administration of sleep-inducing drugs to provide sedation during surgery. Whilst inhalational agents may be used, e.g. in needle-shy adults and small children, the i.v. route is most common. Previously the most commonly used induction agent was thiopental sodium, a short-acting barbiturate. Today, it is probably propofol, which produces a short-acting but very rapid loss of consciousness.

Figure 29.3 Airway maintenance devices.

There is a high risk of regurgitation and aspiration in emergency anaesthetic induction situations where there has been no preoperative fast, or where there is raised intra-abdominal pressure, as in pregnancy. In such cases, a technique that applies pressure to the cricoid cartilage may be employed at the time of anaesthetic induction and ETT intubation (see p. 899). Known as Sellick's manoeuvre, patients are placed in a supine position and pressure is applied to the anterior cricoid cartilage of the larynx in order to compress the underlying oesophagus between the trachea and the vertebra. This has the effect of preventing the passage of fluid from the oesophagus into the oropharynx and subsequent inhalation. Once the oesophagus is occluded, the ETT can then be passed with the aid of a laryngoscope and the ETT cuff inflated. This is a critical manoeuvre requiring appropriate training. Incorrect placement of the fingers and undue pressure can actually occlude the trachea and damage the cartilage.

Anaesthetic maintenance and reversal

Significant improvements in anaesthetic and surgical techniques have seen major reductions in perioperative morbidity statistics. In the UK, the surgical unit managers and anaesthetists have a responsibility to ensure that the most appropriate equipment and most contemporary techniques are used. Accordingly, patients will be monitored throughout surgery for any signs of physiological disturbance. Assessment and recording of cardiovascular, neurological and respiratory function, including oxygen saturation and carbon dioxide levels, are maintained throughout the anaesthetic. Throughout surgery, an optimal level of sedation achieved at induction will be maintained and may be complemented with the use of analgesics and muscle relaxants (see Table 29.1, p. 884). These may be either inhalational or i.v. agents, or more commonly a combination of both. These agents, supplemented by oxygen and usually nitrous oxide, complete the triad and allow patients to be sedated and pain-free and for body muscle to be relaxed, so enabling adequate surgical access.

As surgery is completed, the effects of anaesthesia, or more usually of muscle relaxation, may need to be reversed and an anticholinesterase such as neostigmine may be given. Should reversal of narcotic analgesia be required due to respiratory depression, an antagonist such as naloxone may be given, although this will of course reduce postoperative analgesic effect.

PATIENT MOVEMENT AND ISSUES OF IMMOBILITY

Movement of the anaesthetized patient requires an awareness of both the safety aspects for the patient and the health and safety requirements of operating department staff. The HSE Manual Handling Operations Regulations (1992) provides the legislation and guidance to support safe manual handling in all settings. They set out specific responsibilities for both employees and managers, which should promote a safe system of work. Key aspects of the regulations include:

- the implementation of a safe handling policy
- appropriate assessment of handling risk
- provision of suitable equipment
- appropriate training programmes
- appropriate staff supervision.

Whilst an in-depth review of manual handling technique is outside the remit of this chapter, it is worth noting that operating theatres have a high potential for manual handling-related injuries. Much of the equipment used in the department is very heavy and can be awkward to manoeuvre easily. There is often a need to move patients, but patients may only be able to participate or help preoperatively in transfers between bed, trolley or table, and not in positioning on the operating table. The need to move patients quickly often discourages staff in the use of specific equipment to aid transfer which may take a little time to prepare. However, there is ample scope for improving practice

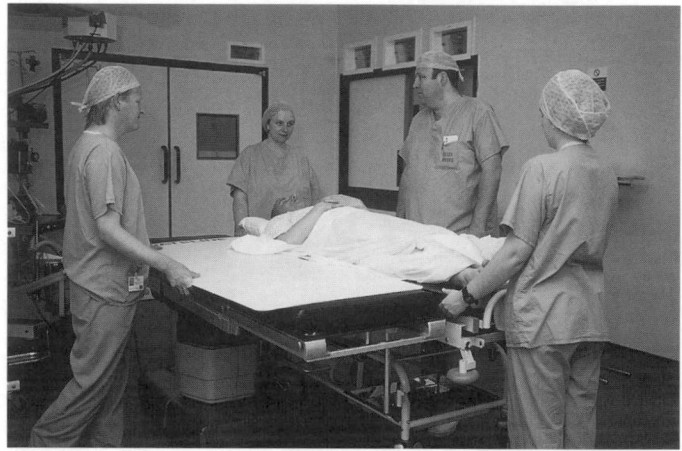

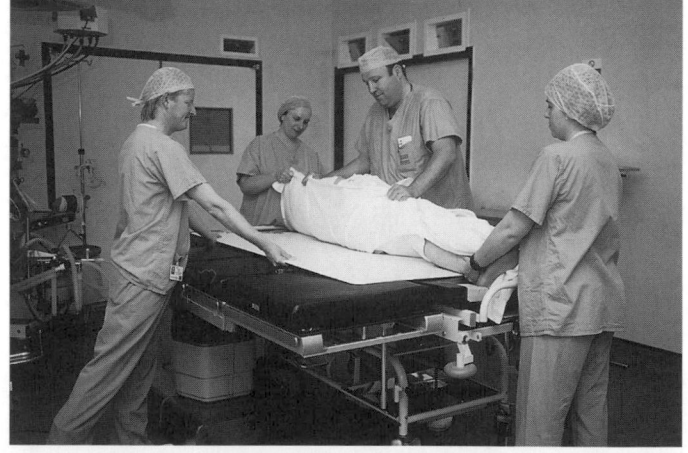

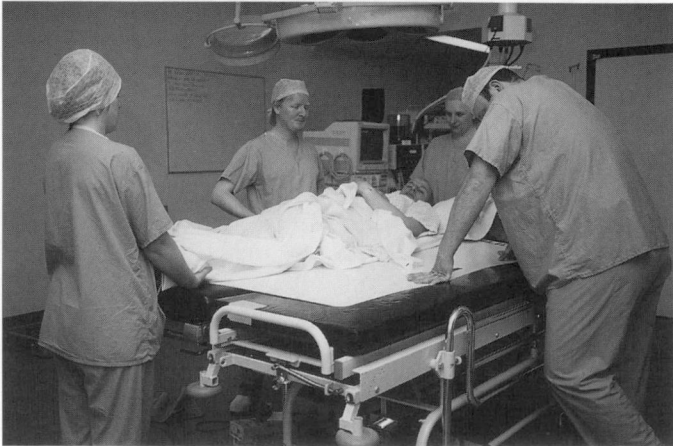

Figure 29.4 Patient-assisted transfer (PAT) slide.

and the modern operating department utilizes a range of equipment, resources and protocols in promoting the safety of staff and patient.

Essentially, the need for minimal handling is paramount and a reduction in the number of patient transfers is deemed to be instrumental in achieving this. In many surgical units, patients are transferred to the operating department on their own bed and are transferred to the operating table and back to the bed following surgery, so reducing the potential for accidents. Where there is a need to transfer patients, equipment is available to minimize risk. The traditional practice of transferring patients using a stretcher canvas and poles is both dangerous and positively discouraged and is highly unlikely to be seen today. The use of sliding aids, e.g. patient-assisted transfer (PAT) slide, in conjunction with a low-friction nylon-sliding sheet is a much safer approach to transfer (see Fig. 29.4).

Patient positioning

On arrival in the operating theatre, patients will be placed in a position appropriate to the need for surgical access and anaesthetic integrity (see Fig. 29.5). The likely access indications for specific positions are:

- supine (most commonly used general position) – abdominal, cardiac, thoracic
- prone – cervical spine, back, rectal area, dorsal aspects of extremities
- Trendelenburg – varicose veins, pelvic surgery
- reverse Trendelenburg – head and neck, shoulder
- lithotomy – perineal, vaginal, endoscopic urological
- lateral – upper chest, kidney and ureter
- jackknife – spinal, pilonidal sinus procedure, haemorrhoidectomy

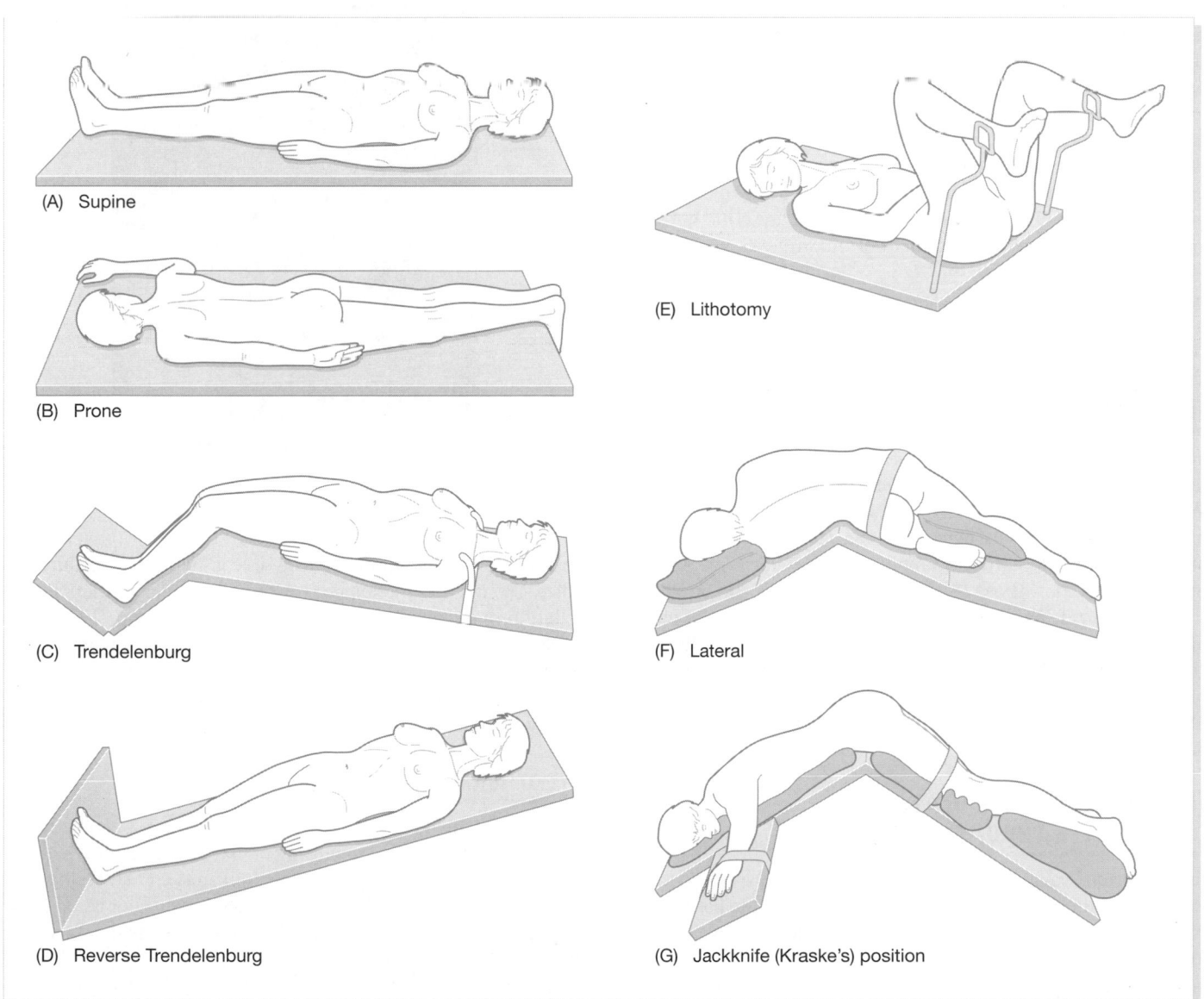

(A) Supine

(B) Prone

(C) Trendelenburg

(D) Reverse Trendelenburg

(E) Lithotomy

(F) Lateral

(G) Jackknife (Kraske's) position

Figure 29.5 Table positions commonly used in surgery.

Whilst the need for optimal surgical access is clearly essential for successful surgery, the dexterity/mobility of each individual patient must be assessed. Anaesthesia will render patients sedated and pain-free. In such a state, it is essential that they are not manipulated into positions likely to lead to postoperative discomfort or even longer-term damage, such as nerve or joint trauma. Similarly the potential for damage or injury caused by the equipment used to maintain that position must be minimized and eradicated. Inappropriate hyperabduction of the arms, for example, may result in severe damage to the brachial nerve plexus. Limbs must be positioned carefully and care taken to ensure that the potential for stretching or for direct pressure on the soft tissues or bony prominences is minimized. A number of resources may be used, e.g. foam or gel pads, to relieve pressure and the risk of injury.

DIGNITY

The need to maintain patient dignity cannot be over-emphasized. Patients should never be exposed for any longer than surgical access requires. Apart from issues of dignity, minimizing exposure will conserve body heat. Equally, the operating room is not the place for physical examination, other than that for which consent has been obtained. Whilst patients are unlikely to have retained auditory sensation, any dialogue concerning them should be both respectful and pertinent to their care. To manage aspects of patient dignity as we would like to be treated ourselves not only promotes a professional care ethic but also encourages the humanistic element of nursing.

PRESSURE ULCER PREVENTION

Historically the development of pressure ulcers has been considered a phenomenon specific to the bed-bound patient (see Ch. 10). More recently, the potential for the development of this problem has been identified as an intraoperative issue. There are a number of specific factors that might contribute to this distressing and costly occurrence in the operating room. Whilst anaesthetized, patients' BP will invariably fall, leading to reduced perfusion of oxygen to the peripheral tissues. The associated lack of body movement and the constant physical pressure placed on those tissues in contact with the operating table will provide an ideal environment for pressure ulcer development. The type of mattress used may have little influence. Defloor & deSchuijmer (2000) carried out a comparative study of operating table mattresses and concluded that none of those tested reduced pressure significantly to prevent pressure ulcer development.

INTRAOPERATIVE PREVENTION OF DEEP VEIN THROMBOSIS

Inappropriate surgical interventions may predispose to DVT. Pressure on the calf muscles caused by inappropriate positioning on the operating table combined with the effects of hypotensive anaesthetic agents and increased coagulability as a result of surgery may exacerbate the potential for thrombosis (Tyrell et al 1995) (see p. 888). It is standard practice to utilize an intermittent external pneumatic compression system during surgery

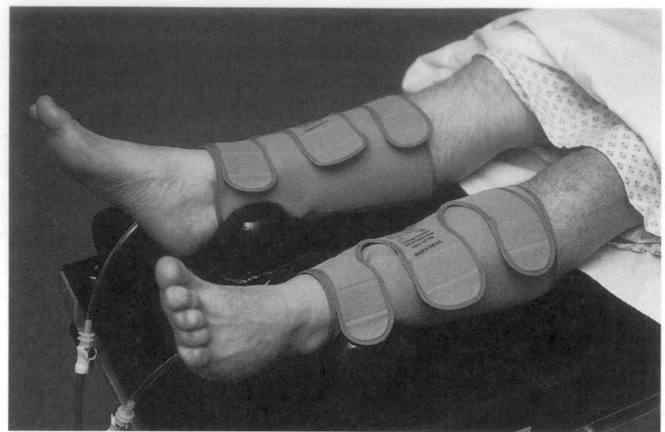

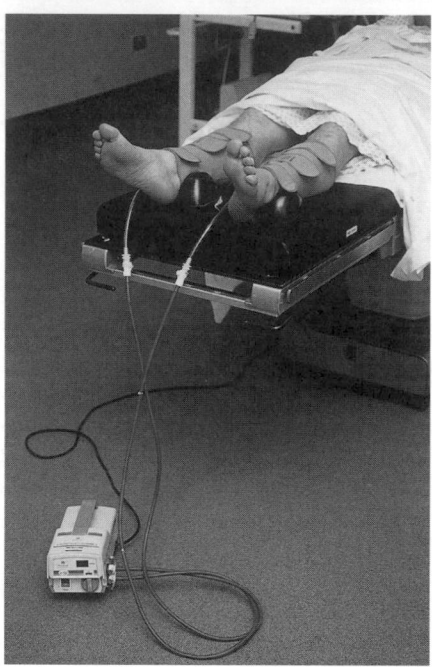

Figure 29.6 Flotron stockings.

unless specifically contraindicated, e.g. where DVT already exists. The device functions by process of a cyclical inflation and deflation of a pair of pneumatic stockings (see Fig. 29.6). The subsequent compression in the calves decreases the potential for venous stasis. In addition, the use of sponge-filled pads placed under the heels can prevent both undue pressure on the calf and reduce the risk of pressure ulcers to the heel.

HYPOTHERMIA

Normal body heat regulation is achieved through a combination of behavioural means, e.g. putting on a woolly hat, and through homeostatic thermoregulatory mechanisms, e.g. shivering (see Ch. 5). Such processes allow us to increase body heat when environmental temperature falls and to increase heat loss when conditions are hot. For the patient undergoing surgery, there is the potential for these mechanisms to be inadequate. In consequence, if not compensated for, an outcome of many surgical procedures is clinical hypothermia.

There are a number of factors with the potential to adversely affect perioperative thermoregulation and contribute to hypothermia (core temperature < 35°C):

- lack of clothing
- body exposure during surgery
- radiated heat loss through open wounds
- lengthy surgery, immobility and muscle inactivity
- inability to shiver due to the effects of muscle relaxants
- reduced metabolism
- use of cold antiseptics, i.v. or irrigational fluids
- blood loss and/or shock (see Ch. 9)
- peripheral vasodilatation following spinal or epidural anaesthesia leading to cooling
- poorly regulated operating room temperature and convectional heat loss.

Whilst a state of surgical hypothermia may be therapeutic in some specialist surgical procedures, e.g. cardiac and neurological surgery, for the majority of patients a reduction in body temperature is usually viewed as an adverse condition.

There are a number of adverse physiological effects of perioperative hypothermia (see Ch. 5). If hypothermia is not compensated for, there is the potential for both myocardial and central nervous system depression. Additionally, a lowered basal metabolic rate and subsequent diminished heat production may lead to a reduction in carbon dioxide production and a depressed respiratory function (see Ch. 20). Dennison (1995) further emphasizes how glucose metabolism and protein catabolism, glomerular filtration rate and calcium balance may all be adversely affected by the reduced metabolic rate.

Drug metabolism may be reduced, adversely influencing the effectiveness of perioperative medication. This may reduce or curtail the effects of analgesia, antiemetics and other therapeutic agents with obvious detriment to the patient. Kurz et al (1995) evaluated the consequences of intraoperative hypothermia concluding that the effects are generally modest in the younger and healthier patient. However, for those at the extremes of the life span, there is a substantially higher risk (Surkitt Parr 1992). Older patients, in particular, may also have a reduced shivering reflex ability, and when combined with other risk factors highlighted (see Older Adults: Nursing Priorities box 29.1 p. 881) this represents a real challenge for the perioperative nurse.

▶ Nursing management

Body temperature may be monitored throughout the perioperative process to identify deviations in thermoregulatory mechanisms. Depending on the nature of surgery, this may be achieved using either invasive technology, such as oesophageal temperature probes, or non-invasively with a tympanic membrane thermometer. The operating room is maintained at an ambient temperature of 20–22°C. The temperature is regulated to accommodate both the staff, who work under hot lights and in extra layers of surgical attire, and the scantily clad patient in an often flimsy surgical gown. Despite the careful regulation of ambient temperature within the operating room, the risk of hypothermia is always present. This can be prevented or at least diminished by a number of nursing interventions. Nursing

activity that ensures that only essential patient exposure (for therapeutic or operating reasons) occurs will help to promote normothermia (normal temperature). The use of warming devices when transfusing or infusing fluids may also reduce hypothermia.

The major cause of hypothermia is the redistribution of blood from body core to the peripheral tissues. Reducing the redistribution is the key to maintaining normothermia. The most common method for achieving this is using the concept of cutaneous warming. Approximately 90% of body heat is lost through the skin surface. To minimize this loss, cutaneous warming may be employed using passive or active methods.

Passive insulation

This utilizes insulation material or equipment such as cotton blankets, drapes and space blankets. A layer of still air between the patient's skin and the insulating material provides the barrier to heat loss. Heat loss can be reduced by up to 30%. Comparisons between the use of plastic bags, cotton and paper sheets, specialized thermal drapes and reflective space blankets reveal few clinically significant differences in effectiveness. The use of warmed blankets shows no clinical advantage over non-warmed blankets although patient preference for the former might justify this practice.

Active cutaneous heating

This involves the application of artificially generated heat to patients using various systems.

Warming mattresses are used but have limitations; relatively small areas of warming mattresses are in contact with the skin, and as patients lie on the mattress, the skin will be compressed and less able to absorb heat via the peripheral capillaries. Extreme caution should be taken when using such devices, which typically operate at temperatures of 37–40°C.

Forced air systems that deliver warm air via a fan or blower unit have been shown to be more effective in reducing hypothermia and outperform warming mattresses by a significant degree. However, fears that forced airflow may increase bacterial circulation in the operating room have limited their use. They are also an expensive option.

Radiant heating units generate heat via heated metal surfaces or by incandescent bulbs. They are advantageous in that no direct contact with the patient's skin is required. They are proven to provide excellent protection against heat loss and hypothermia. Problems in set-up and intraoperative access to the patient limit its use in adult care.

PROCEDURAL SAFETY ISSUES

Patient safety is a crucial aspect of the theatre nurse's role. Because patients have very little, if any, ability to control their environment, nurses must act as patient advocate to ensure they are not exposed to environmental or surgically related hazards.

Within the theatre, a number of clearly defined roles are apparent, although these may be fulfilled by interchangeable professional identities:

- surgeon and surgical first assistant
- anaesthetist and anaesthetic assistant

- scrub practitioner
- circulating practitioner
- supporting personnel, e.g. perfusionist, radiographer.

The surgeon and the anaesthetist may each have an assistant to aid in the surgical procedure or anaesthetic process, respectively. Whilst the anaesthetist will commonly have a nurse or ODP for assistance, the surgical assistant may be another member of the medical staff or a nurse or ODP who has undertaken appropriate training for the role.

Completing the basic team will be the scrub and circulating (or floor) practitioners. The scrub person will, as their name suggests, undertake a surgical scrub and will don gown and gloves prior to surgery. This practitioner, who may be a nurse or an ODP, has responsibility for the preparation of the instrumentation and equipment for a particular case or for a list of cases. The scrub person will be responsible for monitoring and maintaining standards of asepsis, dignity and patient safety, as well as anticipating and providing surgical instruments appropriately during surgery.

The circulating nurse does not undertake a surgical scrub but works in partnership with the scrub person in promoting safety and comfort of the patient and the surgical team. The primary functions of the circulating person will be to provide extra swabs, sutures and instruments to the scrub person as required. The circulating person is also generally involved in keeping records of fluid loss and of maintaining nursing documentation.

On completion of surgery, the scrub and circulating personnel have the responsibility of ensuring that all records are complete, any specimens are accurately labelled and stored, and the patient is transferred for post-surgical recovery in a safe and dignified manner.

Accounting for swabs, needles and instruments

It is clearly essential to ensure that swabs, needles and instruments used during the operation procedure are not inadvertently left inside the patient. It is the responsibility of the scrub nurse to inform the surgeon that such counts have been completed and that all equipment is accounted for. Swabs and surgical packs are manufactured with an X-ray-opaque metallic strip integral to the gauze. This allows visualization of the swab by X-ray should it become misplaced within the patient. It is recommended by the National Association of Theatre Nurses (NATN) that such checks are carried out prior to the commencement of the procedure to establish the baseline. The scrub nurse will continue to monitor the number, and whereabouts, of all equipment during the procedure and will carry out all formal checks with the circulating practitioner upon closure of any body organ or cavity and on final skin suturing.

Haemostasis

Despite the development of minimally invasive techniques and the use of hypotension-inducing anaesthetic agents, the potential for blood loss and its adverse effects on the patient remains. In order to minimize blood loss, the surgeon will utilize a number of techniques. Initially, oozing or bleeding may be surgically clamped or direct pressure applied using swabs or surgical packs. As a permanent measure, the surgeon will use one of two techniques: ligatures or diathermy.

Whilst it is possible, and indeed common practice, to use the diathermy unit as a cutting tool for dividing muscle fibres, it is primarily a tool for haemostasis (arrest of bleeding). Electrodiathermy involves the application of an electrical current via a pair of specially insulated dissecting forceps to provide heat at the bleeding site at a temperature sufficient to cauterize and effectively seal the bleeding vessels. There are two types of diathermy equipment used in the operating theatre (see Fig. 29.7):

- *Unipolar diathermy* is more frequently used for major surgery. This unit uses only one cable and consequently both tips of the forceps are active. Because the discharged current is unable to return to the diathermy unit via the cable, a grounding plate is secured to the patient and the current may then flow via the plate back to the diathermy machine to complete a safe electrical circuit.
- *Bipolar diathermy* is used when the surgeon requires great precision in the coagulation of the bleeding vessels. Frequently used in surface surgery such as cosmetic and minor ENT procedures (see Chs 16 and 21), the forceps used to grasp the bleeding vessels are smaller and finer than those used for general surgical diathermy. The electrical current travels down the active element of a double cable to one tip of the forceps. The current passes across to the other tip and burns tissue held between the forceps. The current returns to the electrosurgical (diathermy) unit via the inactive element of the cable.

It is essential to ensure that theatre staff are fully conversant with the testing and use of electrosurgical equipment. Diathermy is potentially hazardous, and the main risk is one of thermoelectrical burns (see Ch. 28). Whilst the modern design of diathermy units minimizes the potential for accidents, the siting of the patient plate should be reviewed throughout surgery to ensure it remains in full contact with the skin. Should the plate become dislodged, an alarm should sound and the electrical output should stop. However, it is essential to ensure that patients are not in contact with any metallic structure through which electrical current could feasibly travel, leading to the potential for a burn. Diathermy plates must be sited over a well-vascularized and hairless area of skin to promote the flow of current, e.g. the

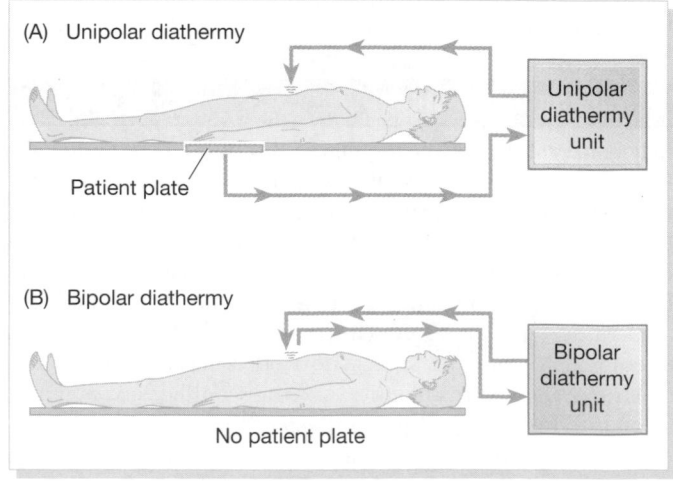

Figure 29.7 Unipolar and bipolar diathermy.

thigh. It is also essential that the plate is kept dry, ensuring that body fluids or the antiseptic solutions used in skin preparation do not compromise the contact between plate and skin.

PREVENTING INFECTION IN THE OPERATING THEATRE

By the nature of clinical activity in the operating department, the potential for infection is high. Universal precautions should be taken throughout the department to minimize risk (see Ch. 13). Gloves and aprons should be worn for all patient contact activity and particular care taken over the handling of instruments, sutures, blades and surgical specimens. To complement the use of universal precautions, a number of protocols are adopted in the promotion of asepsis and the reduction of cross-infection.

Skin preparation

Appropriate preparation of the patient is a significant factor in minimizing the risks of infection and sepsis. As discussed earlier, adherence to evidence-based principles of general hygiene, shaving and skin preparation may all promote asepsis. Final preparation of the incision site will take place in the operating room with the application of an antiseptic solution. For common incision sites and the anatomical regions of the abdomen, see Figure 29.8.

The most commonly used preparations are iodine-based solutions and chlorhexidine gluconate, used in an alcohol base for general purposes and in an aqueous base for more sensitive areas of the body such as face or genitalia. It is essential to ensure that any alcohol-based solution has fully dried on the skin and that no pooling of fluid has occurred. Pooling in the umbilicus is a particularly common occurrence. The use of diathermy in such a situation has the potential to ignite the alcoholic fluid, causing burn injuries. It is also worth noting that some topical antiseptics may contain a staining dye, which identifies the coverage of the solution on the body. With normal washing these dyes may take some days to remove completely. Consequently their use is contraindicated on distal areas of the limbs where observation of skin colour for cyanosis or pallor may be masked by the dye.

Handwashing and surgical scrub

In most general hygiene situations, a simple 10–15-second handwash with soap and water or an aqueous antiseptic solution is adequate (see Ch. 13), However, for a surgical scrub, a more rigorous, extensive and lengthy technique is required. Whilst the technique of handwashing is universal, the process will be supplemented by a forearm wash and a sterile nailbrush will be used for the first scrub of the day. The whole process should take 2–3 minutes.

Surgical gloves

Attempts to provide a physical barrier between the operating department staff and the patient is a major strategy in infection control. Surgical gloves are worn both for the protection of the wearer and to minimize the potential for microorganism transmission to the patient. It is important to note that glove wearing does not negate the need for appropriate handwashing. It has been regularly reported that increase in operating time is directly

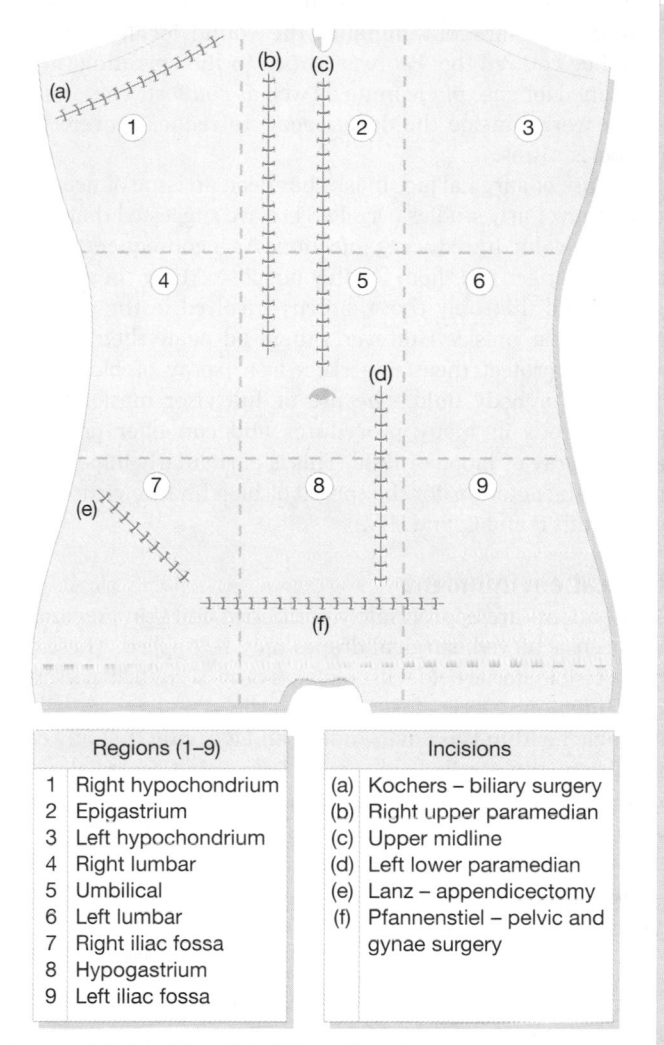

Regions (1–9)		Incisions	
1	Right hypochondrium	(a)	Kochers – biliary surgery
2	Epigastrium	(b)	Right upper paramedian
3	Left hypochondrium	(c)	Upper midline
4	Right lumbar	(d)	Left lower paramedian
5	Umbilical	(e)	Lanz – appendicectomy
6	Left lumbar	(f)	Pfannenstiel – pelvic and
7	Right iliac fossa		gynae surgery
8	Hypogastrium		
9	Left iliac fossa		

Figure 29.8 Abdominal regions and incision sites.

associated with diminishing glove integrity. Some studies show that obvious visible tears or less obvious perforations can occur in over 50% of surgical cases (Naver & Gottrup 2000). The use of gloves has been implicated in skin irritations and allergies due to latex sensitivity. Where possible, latex-free gloves and indeed a latex-free environment should be created to minimize risk. Gloves that are covered in a fine powder or film to aid application should be avoided, or the powder removed before operative use, as it has been implicated in the formation of adhesions and granuloma in patients.

Surgical clothing

The use of surgical gowns may also reduce the potential for cross-infection. However, a plastic apron should be worn beneath the gown if manufactured from a permeable non-repellent cotton material with the potential for saturation. The technique for donning gown and gloves should ideally follow a closed method that reduces the potential for self-contamination following surgical scrub. This is a technical skill almost unique to this environment and requires appropriate training and supervision initially.

The wearing of a theatre cap or hood may be useful in preventing loose hairs contaminating the wound. Ideally, facial hair should be covered too. Footwear worn in the operating theatre is designed for ease of cleaning as well as comfort. These should not be worn outside the department, to reduce movement of microorganisms.

The use of surgical face masks has been an issue of debate for some years. Early studies (Orr 1981) have suggested that masks are of no value in reducing infection. As a consequence, many units no longer use them for this purpose. Many theatre units recommend that only those directly involved in the operation need to wear masks. However, others advocate their use as a barrier to protect theatre workers from spray of blood, bone chippings or body fluid. The use of full visor masks may be advantageous in many procedures and can offer protection against spray of blood or fluid. This is particularly important in limiting the potential for the spread of blood-borne viruses such as hepatitis B and C, and HIV.

Surgical environment

Once patients are appropriately positioned and skin preparation has been achieved, surgical drapes may be applied. These provide a visible sterile field within which only 'scrubbed' personnel may function. Sterile instrument trolleys and tables will be assembled within this environment and it is vital that any compromise of this sterile field is reported so that remedial action may be taken. It is similarly essential that all surgical instrumentation, sutures and dressings be confirmed as sterile using visual and written criteria.

Airborne contamination will increase with the movement of the surgical team. As a consequence, the number and movement of staff within the theatre should be kept to a minimum during surgery.

The correct environment is essential to minimize airborne infection as well as enhancing staff and patient comfort. The temperature within the theatre should be frequently monitored and ideally remain constant at 20–22°C with a relative humidity of 45–55%. An airflow system that provides frequent air exchanges (at least 15/hour) is recommended. This is achieved in a unidirectional airflow system environment that depends on the air pressure in the operating room being greater than that elsewhere in the department. Clean air enters the theatre through central vents and is expelled through calibrated vents to the exterior. This prevents microorganisms from gaining entry to the theatre. In some surgical specialties (e.g. joint replacement – see Ch. 27) that require ultimate regard for asepsis, closed tents may be employed to diminish risk further.

Sterile instruments

Fibreoptic endoscopic and laser technology as well as major developments in more traditional instrumentation have resulted in the inventory of instruments and equipment in a modern operating department becoming vast. Much of this equipment is very expensive and the need for cost-efficient protocols for decontamination and sterilization of items deemed suitable for reuse is paramount. It is essential, then, that such methods are safe for both the equipment and those involved in its processing.

In recent years, the potential spectre of cross-infection, the real rise in the incidence of infection and problems of HIV, hepatitis B and MRSA have led to an increase in single-use items of equipment (see Ch. 13). These include dressings, sutures, cannulae, injection needles, gowns, gloves and patient airway equipment. The uncertainty surrounding the transmission of new variant Creutzfeldt–Jakob disease (vCJD) has precipitated the use of disposable instrument sets for some types of high-risk procedures in a bid to reduce to an absolute minimum any risk of spread via the nervous and lymphoid tissues. Tonsillar, appendix, neurological and ophthalmic surgery has been affected in this manner. From the perspective of both infection control and general safety, single-use items have much to commend them, although their use may prove financially very costly. Understandably, the reuse of equipment within the NHS is tightly regulated. Staff need to be aware of whether an item may be reused and, if so, how many times and following what means of decontamination. The consequences of not adhering to these protocols can be catastrophic for both patients and nurses. Recent media reports about the reuse of disposable endotracheal tubes and the potential for subsequent equipment malfunction highlight the importance of conforming to manufacturer, Department of Health and local guidelines.

SUTURES

The term suture relates to any material used to sew or secure body tissues and there are a variety available to the surgeon during surgery. Sutures may be used to bring the wound edges together, secure structures and tissues to ensure strength, and to secure drains. They may be used with a needle to provide access through the tissues or as a ligature to tie off a vessel or body structure. Suture material may be synthetic or produced from the living world – silk and animal tissues are regularly used. Choice of suture will be determined by the operative procedure requirements, the type of tissue to be sutured, the condition of the patient's tissues and the surgeon's preference.

Suture material may be conveniently classified as absorbable or non-absorbable in nature. The advantages and limitations of both types are given in Box 29.2, and some of the most commonly used sutures and their properties are described in Table 29.3. The absorption rate of the suture will be determined by the nature of the material and any chemical coating. This chemical causes an inflammatory response and enzyme action at the suture site. Absorbable and non-absorbable suture materials have specific characteristics that may make one more suitable than others.

Further considerations in suture choice include the thread strength and the type of needle used to introduce it. Strength of thread in the UK is based on British Pharmacopoeia (BP) index. Needles may be traumatic, in which case they must be threaded by the operator, or atraumatic, where the thread is swaged or bonded to the needle. In the case of atraumatic needles, the most commonly used type, only one thread is drawn through the tissue, thereby reducing trauma. The body of the needle may be round, triangular or flat, and the tip or point may be described as having a cutting or non-cutting edge(s). In practice, the surgeon's preference is a major factor in suture choice.

Box 29.2 Advantages and disadvantages of absorbable and non-absorbable sutures

Absorbable sutures

Advantages
- Completely absorbed
- No need to remove
- No foci for irritation
- Neat scar line

Limitations
- May absorb too quickly, so weakening healing
- May cause reaction/allergy
- Limited evidence of current tensile strength

Non-absorbable sutures

Advantages
- Remain in tissues when desirable to do so
- Strengthen tissues

Limitations
- Need to be removed
- Disturb healing process
- Scarring
- Sinus formation
- Potential for abscess

Table 29.3 Characteristics of absorbable and non-absorbable sutures

Absorbable				Non-absorbable			
Material	Tissue reaction	Absorption	Common uses	Material	Tissue reaction	Tensile strength	Common uses
Plain catgut	High	5–10 days	Fat	Nylon	Low	High	Muscle repair, skin
Chromic catgut	Moderate to high	10–21 days	General internal	Silk	High	Good	Drain security
Vicryl	Low	80 days	Skin	Prolene	Low	Fair	Muscle repair, skin
Dexon	Low	90 days	Skin	Linen/cotton	High	Good	Internal ligature
PDS	Low	180 days	General	Ethibond	Moderate	High	Anastomosis of synthetic graft
				Steel clips and staples	Low	High	Skin, anastomoses

POSTOPERATIVE CARE

Postoperative care consists of ensuring that patients are nursed in the greatest possible comfort, kept free from hazards and complications during the postoperative period, and encouraged to take an increasing responsibility for their own care/health until complete recovery is effected.

Following surgery patients will be transferred to a unit providing specialist care in post-anaesthesia management. Depending on the type of surgery and the patient's health status, this may be an intensive care unit (ICU), a high-dependency unit (HDU) or specialized postoperative recovery room. Management of the critically ill patient in the ICU and HDU is discussed in Chapter 31. The annual National Confidential Enquiry into Perioperative Deaths Report (2001) clearly recognize the importance of a well-staffed and equipped specialist postoperative recovery unit in reducing perioperative mortality and morbidity rates. Standards of staffing and resources should conform to national guidelines for safe post-anaesthetic nursing care. A one-to-one nurse–patient ratio is desirable, although changes in patient dependency level may require an increase in this ratio. Alternatively, as a patient's condition improves, the level of intensive support may be reduced. The postoperative recovery unit should be sited close to the theatres. It should provide adequate space for the anticipated throughput of patients and should be equipped with appropriate lighting so that changes in skin colour can be noted.

IMMEDIATE POSTOPERATIVE CARE – RECOVERY UNIT

Patients will be transferred to the specialist postoperative care unit accompanied by the attending theatre nurse or ODP and anaesthetist. Prior to admission the nurse will have prepared the environment to receive the patient and ensured that the following equipment is available:

- resuscitation trolley
- laryngoscope and a range of artificial airways
- range of oxygen masks, catheter mounts and tubing
- suction catheter, tubing, sterile water, gauze and gloves
- pulse oximeter and BP monitoring equipment
- temperature monitoring equipment and warming devices
- vomit bowls and tissues.

The recovery nurse will obtain full patient details, including the surgery performed, anaesthetic history and any specific postoperative instructions. A comprehensive assessment of the patient's condition is performed and documented according to local protocols. However, it is likely that the following will be addressed:

- ability to maintain airway
- cardiovascular and respiratory function
- orientation and consciousness levels
- provision of warmth
- management of pain and PONV (see pp. 910–911)
- prevention of injury, e.g. falls

- management of specific needs resulting from surgery
- emotional state and need for reassurance that the surgery is over.

The structured and systematic assessment of patients will pay particular attention to airway, breathing, circulation and consciousness (ABCs). To monitor general recovery, the vital signs of BP, temperature, pulse rate and volume, and respiratory rate should be recorded at 15-minute intervals, postoperatively unless otherwise instructed, until the patient's condition is stabilized. This enables any deviation in condition to be detected when compared with the baseline observations that were established preoperatively.

Airway and breathing assessment

Airway obstruction is a major postoperative concern in the unconscious patient and is often due to the tongue falling back against the posterior pharynx. Effective management of this problem may be achieved through a number of complementary strategies. Providing the surgery allows, patients are nursed in the lateral (recovery) position, to facilitate airway management and minimize the risks and effects of aspirating vomit. Forward displacement of the jaw and a gentle backward tilting of the head will maintain patency of the airway.

If patients are unable to fully maintain their own airway, an artificial airway may be inserted, if not already in situ, to facilitate the management of this crucial stage of recovery. The most commonly used oral airway is the Guedel type, which may easily be removed by patients as consciousness returns.

It is essential that the nurse in the recovery unit is able to recognize signs of impaired respiratory function, which may be due to either partial or total airway obstruction.

Airway obstruction

Airway obstruction may result directly from the presence of a foreign body that prevents air entering the lungs on inspiration. Alternatively it may be an inflammatory or protective response to airway trauma. Signs of airway obstruction range in severity and may include (from mild to severe):

- restlessness
- mouth breathing
- confusion, agitation and anxiety
- changes in respiratory rate
- noisy or laboured breathing
- exaggerated use of accessory muscles of the neck and abdomen
- absence of breath sounds and chest movement.

If obstruction is suspected, an immediate examination of the mouth and throat must be performed to identify and remove any mechanical obstruction to breathing. Any artificial airway that is present (see Fig. 29.3, p. 899), such as an ETT, LMA or Guedel airway, should be examined for an obstructed lumen. Suction equipment must be used to remove any oral or nasal secretions, vomit or blood to ensure a clear airway.

Laryngospasm is also a relatively common occurrence postoperatively, in which the laryngeal muscles contract causing a reflex closure of the vocal cords. This occurs as a protective reflex action against foreign material (e.g. secretions and artificial airways) or trauma. Often occurring as the patient emerges from the anaesthetic, it may be exacerbated by the irritant effects or incomplete reversal of the anaesthetic agent and the trauma of intubation or extubation. Laryngospasm may be identified by the characteristic stertorous and laboured noise on inspiration known as stridor. Patients require a calm and reassuring approach from the nurse, who must ensure there is no mechanical obstruction of the airway. Oxygen should be administered via an appropriate mask at a high concentration, e.g. 10 L/min, or as prescribed. Persistent stridor or signs of progressive airway distress will require the immediate attention of the attending anaesthetist.

Any airway obstruction has the potential for producing hypoxia. Defined as low oxygen tension in the tissues, this may be assumed to be present when the oxygen saturation falls below 90%. A non-invasive pulse oximeter applied to the patient's digit provides an indication of the oxygen saturation levels in the blood and is now standard postoperative monitoring procedure. Ideally, oxygen saturation rates should be above 95%, although a number of factors may affect patient ability to achieve this level. Where oxygen saturation levels in the blood are lowered, cyanosis of the peripheral extremities, particularly the lips, finger and toenails, may also be present. Severe anoxia will lead to a centralized cyanosis seen in the tongue and surface tissues. It must be remembered, however, that evidence of cyanosis may be absent in hypovolaemic shock when patients will exhibit increasing pallor (see Ch. 9).

Oxygen therapy

Most postoperative patients will receive oxygen for a variable period of time, ranging from a few minutes to several hours depending upon individual circumstances in a bid to improve effective oxygen exchange. Oxygen should be administered in accordance with anaesthetic instruction via a correctly fitted clear, soft mask that fits over the nose and mouth, or via nasal cannulae. Humidification is recommended to reduce the drying effect of oxygen on the upper airways. Oxygen prescription is dependent on an assessment of the patient's existing pathology. Patients with COPD, for example, lose their sensitivity to carbon dioxide as a respiratory trigger, relying instead on hypoxia to trigger ventilation. Whilst there remains some controversy in the treatment of this disorder, caution should be exercised in the postoperative period. Delivery of even moderate amounts of oxygen may cause potentially fatal respiratory depression (see Ch. 20).

Temperature and shivering

The most common method for monitoring temperature in the immediate postoperative period is the electronic aural thermometer, which measures temperature at the tympanic membrane. A phenomenon often associated with hypothermia (see p. 901) is postoperative shivering. Although shivering is an important homeostatic mechanism, it produces other considerations for the surgical nurse. It is a common feature following anaesthesia characterized by involuntary muscular activity, which can result in particularly violent tremors. Shivering has been linked to the use of volatile anaesthetic agents, particularly halothane. To some extent, regional anaesthetic techniques have also been implicated. Similarly the use of cold fluids in urological surgery may be a contributory factor. Shivering raises the metabolic rate and greatly increases oxygen demand. Management usually requires the use of warming techniques to promote normothermia (see p. 903) and oxygen therapy to meet increased metabolic demand.

Circulatory assessment

Cardiovascular homeostasis may be disturbed by both anaesthesia and the operative procedure. Most general anaesthetic agents have cardiac depressant effects and can produce cardiac irritability, hypotension and alteration in cardiac output (see Ch. 19), manifested by changes in the heart rate and arrhythmias. Epidural and spinal anaesthetics also produce hypotension (see p. 896). Any invasive surgical intervention involving an incision may potentially lead to blood loss. Major loss of blood and body fluid is the most likely cause of hypovolaemic shock in the surgical patient.

Shock

Clearly the need for skilled and accurate assessment of cardiovascular status is paramount. Whilst the effect of anaesthetic hypotension is generally self-limiting, prolonged or excessive blood and fluid loss may lead to hypovolaemic shock and will require early detection and prompt treatment.

Hypovolaemic shock is a complex, life-threatening process of haemodynamic dysfunction which may result in diminished tissue perfusion. For the surgical nurse, an understanding of the potential causes and the physiological processes involved (see Ch. 9) is essential in early diagnosis of the shocked patient. Failure to recognize and treat the circulatory failure may lead to metabolic disturbance, multiple organ dysfunction and death. Signs of hypovolaemic shock include the following:

- decreased BP
- tachycardia
- thready, weak pulse
- cool and clammy skin
- reduced urine output
- restlessness and confusion
- air hunger (deep sighing respirations).

Primary haemorrhage occurring during surgery is the most likely precursor to shock. However, reactionary haemorrhage is not an uncommon occurrence. Most anaesthetics have a hypotensive effect. As the patient's BP rises postoperatively, bleeding from vessels and damaged capillary beds, apparently intact during surgery, may occur. This might be a particular concern following anaesthetic procedures designed to reduce BP during surgery. Anaesthesia for prostatic, gynaecological and some ENT surgery commonly utilizes this technique. Similarly, ligatures that appear secure may be prone to slippage if placed under pressure. As BP rises, the potential for a reactionary haemorrhage exists. Some superficial capillary bleeding from the wound edges is to be expected as the BP returns to normal.

In the immediate postoperative period, observation of the wound site is crucial. If significant bleeding is discovered, the original dressing should not be removed. If practicable, manual pressure should be applied to the bleeding site, a pressure pad applied and medical opinion sought. However, evidence of continued and excessive bleeding may require further medical intervention or even a return to the operating theatre.

The primary medical consideration in caring for patients in hypovolaemic shock is to restore oxygen delivery to the tissues and to correct the underlying cause of the bleed. Patients may require intravenous blood volume replacement in the form of crystalloids, whole blood and packed cells or, if these are not immediately available, blood plasma expander solutions. Intravenous infusion enables patients to receive fluids by the quickest route, thus increasing intravascular fluid volume immediately in emergency situations. The nurse's first priority is to implement the medical prescription and to monitor its effect. However, it is imperative in urgent and emergency situations that the nurse does not forget the individual undergoing the crisis. Patients in shock are likely to be anxious, distressed and even confused and disorientated, and the provision of clear and appropriate explanation is crucial in alleviating their fears.

Assessing consciousness

With recent advances in anaesthetic technique, many patients will be conscious or semiconscious on arrival in the recovery unit. However, it is essential that nurses remain with them until they are fully conscious. Specific management of the patient airway and positioning are discussed above, but return to consciousness will include the ability to breathe without the use of an artificial airway. Level of consciousness may be further confirmed by a patient's response to commands, reaction to stimuli and the ability to verbalize responses. Depending on local policy and the nature of surgery, a formalized neurological assessment tool may be used (see Ch. 14). The last sensory input to diminish and the first to return is hearing. Consequently, the environment should be suitably quiet and nurses should avoid any inappropriate discussion of patients or their condition. Unconscious and semiconscious patients are unlikely to be able to maintain a safe personal environment. Trolley or bed rails may be used to prevent falling. Returning spectacles or hearing aids to patients will enhance communication and orientation. Nurses must provide reassurance and support at frequent intervals, orientating patients to their surroundings and reinforcing the fact that the surgery is now over.

Discharge from recovery unit

Whilst it is recognized that many factors, both clinical and organizational, are likely to influence local policy in the decision to transfer patients back to the ward, all guidelines or criteria must reflect the necessity for safe discharge and transfer. It should always be borne in mind that patients are likely to be moving from a high-dependency area with appropriate staff/patient ratio to a less intensive clinical setting. Most units will utilize a scoring system to assist in assessment of discharge criteria (Aldrete & Kroulik 1970).

A suitably qualified member of the recovery team should undertake discharge from the recovery room (see Guidelines for Care Priorities box 29.1). Subsequent handover should involve an appropriately qualified member of the ward nursing staff, who will receive information about the nature of the operation, i.v. fluids, drugs, the presence of tubes/drains, special instructions and anything else that is relevant to the patient's condition. Patients discharged from the recovery room will be accompanied by all completed relevant paperwork, including nursing and anaesthetic records, operation notes and completed

29.1 Discharge criteria from recovery units following general anaesthetic

- Patients must be able to protect their own airway
- There is no evidence of haemorrhage, internal or external
- A minimum of three stable observations have been obtained, consistent with preoperative readings and individual patient assessment
- Body temperature is relatively normal for that individual and shows no evidence of hypothermia or pyrexia
- No patient should be discharged from the recovery unit with a low oxygen saturation level and should remain in the recovery room for a minimum of 15 minutes following the withdrawal of oxygen therapy
- The patient's pain/nausea level has been assessed and controlled with prescribed analgesia/antiemetic drugs and nursing measures

- All patients should be kept in the recovery unit for a minimum of 30 minutes following administration of opioid analgesia administered by any route
- All adult patients will remain in the recovery unit for a minimum of 30 minutes
- All patients who are admitted to the recovery unit still intubated will be kept in the recovery room for a minimum of 30 minutes following extubation of the endotracheal tube
- Observations of respiration, oxygen saturation level, pulse and blood pressure will be recorded at 5-minute intervals for the first 15 minutes following extubation
- Patients having a blood transfusion will be kept in the recovery room for a minimum of 1 hour following the commencement of the transfusion, and respiratory and pulse rates, blood pressure and temperature will be assessed every 15 minutes.

discharge notification where appropriate. Written prescription for oxygen therapy, intravenous fluids and postoperative medication should all be completed prior to transfer in order to facilitate continuity in care.

MANAGING POSTOPERATIVE PAIN

The Royal College of Surgeons and the College of Anaesthetists' (1990) report was pivotal in drawing attention to the fact that postoperative analgesia was not always adequate. Recommendations included the instigation of acute pain service teams and a radical review of current pain management practices (see Ch. 7). Whilst progress is being made, many patients continue to experience moderate to severe pain following surgery (Audit Commission 1997) (see Reflective Practice box 29.3).

There is no shortage of research identifying the association between pain management and a safe, uneventful surgical recovery. Patients in pain will be reluctant to move and mobilize (see below), and for many, the primary strategy in dealing with this is to remain still. However, immobility is implicated in the development of DVT, chest infection, urinary and gastrointestinal disturbance.

Patients in pain are likely to suffer the effects of sleep deprivation (see Ch. 4). Closs (1992) reported that pain was the most common cause of disturbed sleep in patients after abdominal surgery. Many patients felt that tiredness accentuated their postoperative pain and that sleep reduced pain intensity. Almost all patients believed that sleep enhanced their overall postoperative recovery.

Patients have historically been dependent on nurses for information about the effects of surgery, including pain, and for administration of pain relief. Despite the availability of pain assessment tools, a wealth of clinical research and a much greater emphasis on pain management in educational programmes, deficits in pain assessment remain evident (see Reflective Practice box 29.3).

Factors associated with inadequate postoperative pain management (see Ch. 7) include:

- suboptimal medication within a variable dose prescription
- fear of addiction
- inadequate/inappropriate choice of pain relief method
- influence of subjective perceptions of patients' pain, e.g. operative procedure
- reluctance or inability to use pain assessment tools appropriately
- discrepancy between patient and nursing pain assessment
- over-reliance on objective indicators of pain to verify patients' reporting of discomfort.

Essentially, patients' perceptions and subsequent control of this aspect of the surgical process are overridden by the nurse. Yet nursing perceptions of the extent and severity of patient pain may be based on very subjective beliefs, such as cultural background. If objective measures used by the nurse, such as raised BP, sweating or distress, are not consistent with the patient's description, nursing assessment will often prevail. Such indicators can obviously be misleading and often modified by adaptive and coping mechanisms. Pain, then, is often what the nurse considers it to be.

A number of pain assessment tools exist in practice and some variants are described in Chapter 7. All these tools provide multidimensional measurement of intensity, location and type of pain, allowing continuous review and evaluation of the effectiveness of pain intervention.

The use of pain assessment tools provides patients with an opportunity to take an active role in pain management, promoting a feeling of control. This participative and collaborative alliance enhances the nurse–patient relationship as well as providing an evaluative mechanism for the success of individual regimens.

Patient-controlled analgesia (PCA)

Traditional 4- to 6-hourly intramuscular analgesic prescriptions have little justification in modern pain management. The peaks and troughs such regimens provide only reduce the chances of achieving adequate analgesia. In addition, such regimens

R|Я REFLECTIVE PRACTICE

29.3 Pain management

Despite major advances in minimal access surgery, pharmacology and administration technology, patients fear pain above almost any other aspect of surgical management.

Points for reflection

- Do patients ever ask you whether a procedure or operation will be painful? How do you respond?
- Do you anticipate some patients to be more likely than others to complain of pain? If so, why?
- If patients complain of pain but you see no behavioural or non-verbal evidence of this, how easy is it to accept their word?

Student activities

- Identify a patient you have nursed who has complained of pain. Make a note of the sequence of events, beginning with the patient complaining of pain to its resolution. What did you discover and what are the implications?
- Do you ever feel that asking patients if they are in pain is likely to raise their awareness and prompt them to answer yes?

- Read Schafheulte et al (2001) and consider the questions below:
  — Can you identify any organizational barriers to effective pain management?
  — Does your organization employ nursing pain specialists? How might they influence pain management strategies?
  — Are patients using epidural or PCA technology in your setting regularly assessed and monitored for the effectiveness of their pain relief?
  — Reflect on the pain assessment tools you have used or seen in use. How effective are they? Which ones do you feel work best, and why?
  — Do you feel pain management to be generally effective in your ward/setting?
  — Can you think of ways in which pain management could be improved?
  — Record your ideas in your portfolio and refer to these regularly.

Reference

Schafheulte EI, Cantrill JA, Noyce PR. Why is pain management suboptimal on surgical wards? J Adv Nurs 2001; 33(6): 728–737.

---

are often inflexible, poorly prescribed and build in a significant delay between the request for, and the eventual administration of, the drug.

PCA devices have become an essential tool in the management of postoperative pain (see Ch. 7). The intravenously sited PCA is probably the most commonly used for demand dosing. More recently, epidural infusion, delivering analgesia at a constant rate, has become very popular, although so far this is usually controlled by a professional rather than by the patient.

The PCA system will be commenced in the operating theatre or, more commonly, the recovery room. Whilst the potential benefits are discussed in Chapter 7, it is worth noting that not all patients will wish to participate in this regimen. Patient selection is therefore a critical element in achieving success. It is the surgical nurse's responsibility to assist in this selection and subsequently to monitor and evaluate pain control. It is also important that nurses monitor vital signs, in particular respiratory rate, the slowing of which may indicate respiratory depression.

Management of postoperative nausea and vomiting

The management of pain should be considered in conjunction with the control of PONV. Certain surgical interventions predispose patients to PONV and anaesthetic agents also contribute to this discomfort. The management of PONV ideally begins in the preoperative period. It is becoming increasingly common practice to administer prophylactic antiemetics prior to surgery. Ondansetron has proved particularly useful, due to its lack of sedative and hypotensive side-effects. Cyclizine, too, has been used successfully for the same purpose. Despite the success of preventative medication, many patients will still experience PONV and need to be monitored for this. Indeed, the use of opioids

may contribute to the onset of nausea. Antiemetics should therefore be considered as an important adjuvant therapy in achieving optimum postoperative pain relief (see Evidence-based Practice box 29.1, p. 912; see also Ch. 7). Nurse specialists in pain control and symptom management have also played a crucial role in developing and advancing practice in these aspects of care.

PARALYTIC ILEUS – NASOGASTRIC INTUBATION

Any surgical procedure that involves extensive handling of the bowel has the potential to disrupt normal bowel motility (or peristalsis). Whilst reduced motility can be a normal consequence of abdominal surgery, an absence of peristalsis is of greater clinical concern. The bowel continues to secrete intestinal juices whilst motility is diminished or absent, leading to an accumulation of fluid with the potential for causing distress. Additionally, any surgical incision or anastomosis (join) performed on the bowel may leak, particularly if distension occurs. The absence of muscle tone in the bowel is termed paralytic ileus and is a not infrequent complication of abdominal surgery, peritonitis and inflammatory bowel conditions. It can be exacerbated by chemical derangement such as hypokalaemia (see Ch. 8), diabetes and uraemia (see Ch. 24). Paralytic ileus is characterized by the accumulation of gas and gastrointestinal secretions, diminished or absent bowel sounds and decreased passage of flatus and abdominal distension. If the condition persists, patients may also complain of nausea and vomiting.

Whilst the condition is self-limiting, there is often a need to take measures to reduce and limit its development. Prophylactic measures may be planned for surgery where paralytic ileus is anticipated or where there is a potential for bowel leakage.

EVIDENCE-BASED PRACTICE

29.1 Postoperative nausea and vomiting

Bibby (2001) discusses the management of PONV in patients with PCA. The choice of antiemetic drugs is discussed and the possibility of adding these to the PCA solution. Other factors contributing to nausea in patients using PCA are cited. A useful summary for the management of PONV and a framework for practice have been provided.

Key issues
- PCA is (incorrectly) assumed to contribute towards the increase of PONV
- Predictive factors in the incidence of PONV have been identified
- A predictive risk assessment may identify the probability of PONV occurring and informs prescribing of prophylactic antiemetics
- Patients receiving opioids benefit from prophylactic antiemetic therapy

- Variable practice exists in the administration of antiemetics to PCA patients
- The practice of mixing antiemetics in PCA solutions is questionable
- Ondansetron should not be considered superior to other antiemetics. The practice of using different antiemetics concurrently is now an established rule for best practice
- Non-invasive strategies should be considered in the management of PONV

Student activities
Read Bibby (2001) and the key points. Consider how PONV has been managed in your own surgical placement and how these practices compare to the recommendations cited in the paper.

Reference
Bibby P. Post-operative nausea management and patient controlled analgesia. Br J Nurs 2001; 10(12): 775–780.

Alternatively, treatment can be initiated for patients who develop paralytic ileus or bowel leakage unexpectedly in the postoperative period.

The primary management involves bowel decompression by removing the secretions and accumulated gas from the gastrointestinal tract with a nasogastric tube. This will ideally be passed in the operating theatre so as to instigate early treatment as well as to minimize the discomfort of passing the tube in a fully conscious patient.

The gastrointestinal secretions are removed by either intermittent aspiration or continuous drainage. Intermittent aspiration requires that the tube be aspirated manually at frequent intervals using a syringe. If continuous drainage is required, the tube is attached to a drainage bag.

The colour and amount of the aspirate will be measured and recorded on the patient's fluid balance chart. Although aspiration is not a sterile procedure, the nurse must follow infection control procedures when emptying and collecting the drainage. Strict handwashing protocols must be adhered to before and after the procedure and an apron and gloves should be worn throughout. The tube will remain in situ until bowel function resumes, which is confirmed by bowel sounds and patient reports of passing flatus.

It is important to ensure that the tube is held in place comfortably and securely, and the use of hypoallergenic tape to anchor the tube is recommended. Regular checks should be made for signs of pressure or soreness affecting the nose. Allowances need to be made for patient movement and the tube needs to be fixed to the patient's clothing so as to avoid tension on the nose. It is worth noting that the sight of a nasogastric tube may cause psychological distress to both patients and their relatives. In addition, the tube is a further physical discomfort following major surgery. Some patients will find coughing more difficult.

Patients will be nil by mouth or having only restricted fluids or ice to suck. Consequently they will be unable to experience the pleasures of eating and tasting food and will often complain of a very dry mouth. Frequent rinsing of the mouth and oral hygiene will help to keep it clean. The mouth and nose should also be inspected regularly and appropriate oral and nasal hygiene implemented. The use of a non-irritant lubricant gel on the area where the tube exits the nose may reduce any soreness from friction that is sometimes present, particularly in longer-term therapy.

FLUID BALANCE MAINTENANCE AND MONITORING

In the postoperative period, a major goal of care is to restore normal fluid homeostasis as soon as possible. Fasting prior to surgery and the potential for intraoperative fluid loss may disrupt patients' ability to maintain an adequate fluid intake. Anaesthetic agents, airway maintenance devices, oxygen therapy and the prolonged fast are likely to produce a very dry mouth and throat. It is therefore important to reinstate oral fluids as soon as possible. Unless medically contraindicated, patients are able to resume these as soon as full consciousness and swallowing and cough reflexes return. Exceptions to this include some types of oral, dental and endoscopic procedures following the use of a local anaesthetic throat spray that might inhibit these reflexes.

Intravenous infusions

In some situations, patients' oral intake may be restricted. In addition, fluid loss from nasogastric tubes and wound drains may increase the potential for development of fluid and electrolyte imbalance. Intravenous fluids are commonly prescribed until patients are able to maintain adequate fluid intake, for a number of reasons:

- rehydration following bleeding or fluid loss
- inability to tolerate oral fluids
- gastrointestinal surgery
- postoperative sedation and ventilation
- venous access for drug administration
- redress of electrolyte imbalance.

Patients with a large draining wound or fistula (abnormal opening or tract between two organs or structures) may also lose excessive amounts of fluid containing protein and electrolytes. Systemic or wound infection will lead to inflammatory responses and a subsequent rise in metabolic rate. This is likely to cause a rise in body temperature, resulting in sweating and thus increasing the requirements for fluid intake.

The prime responsibility of the surgical nurse in caring for the patient with an i.v. infusion is to ensure that the fluids are administered safely and in accordance with medical instruction. Reliance on volumetric pumps, ensuring accurate fluid delivery, has removed the need to regulate i.v. infusion flow manually. However, nurses should still observe that pumps are infusing the fluid correctly. The fluid output as well as input is monitored and the patient assessed for signs of over- or under-hydration (see Ch. 8). Circulatory overload might be identified by distension of the neck veins or the patient complaining of dizziness, headache or dyspnoea. The i.v. cannula site should be observed for any signs of inflammation, extravasation or infection that might indicate the need to re-site the infusion.

Monitoring patients' reactions to i.v. additives such as antibiotics, if prescribed, is also essential. The nurse who acts as an advocate for the patient should also consider the positioning of an i.v. infusion. Siting the infusion in the non-dominant arm can help patients to feel more in control, thus enhancing their self-esteem, self-care ability and dignity. Intravenous fluids provide little nutritional value, and therefore the need for alternative sources of nutrients must be considered; this is discussed below.

POST-SURGICAL NUTRITION AND FASTING

Adequate nutrition is essential for surgical recovery. Delayed wound healing, pressure ulcer development and reduced immune response have all been associated with postoperative malnutrition (Wells 1994). It is essential, then, to reinstate normal nutritional intake as soon as possible. For the majority of patients having relatively straightforward, uncomplicated surgery, a normal diet may be resumed almost immediately. However, for patients who are restricted in their desire or ability, or by enforced postoperative fasting, further nutritional support must be provided. This may be in the form of enteral and parenteral nutrient administration (see Ch. 11).

The practice of postoperative diet and oral fluid restriction and the timing of its subsequent resumption have been challenged and the perceived benefits of this practice questioned. Even in bowel surgery, the traditional regimen of increasing oral fluid intake by 30 mL over a period of time has been shown to have little benefit in resting the bowel and protecting the anastomosis. Lewis et al (2001) demonstrated that enteral feeding within 24 hours of gastrointestinal surgery is well tolerated and that there is no benefit in keeping patients nil by mouth. Whilst further research is required in this area, consideration needs to be given to current practices.

POSTOPERATIVE RENAL/URINARY ISSUES

An adequate state of hydration is necessary to ensure a good fluid output, thus minimizing the risk of urinary stasis and subsequent urinary tract infection (UTI).

Surgery is associated with urinary output problems for a number of reasons. Physiologically, hypovolaemia, hypothermia and the body's reaction to the surgical stressors may lead to circulatory, perfusional and hormonal disturbance and decreased urine production. Other factors that may influence urinary inhibition or output in the surgical patient include:

- reduced mobility
- bed rest
- effects of spinal, epidural or general anaesthesia on bladder muscle tone
- embarrassment, privacy and dignity issues
- dehydration or reduced oral input
- underlying pathology or disease, e.g. prostatism, pelvic surgery
- physiological effects of surgery
- pre-existing renal problems
- effects of surgery on adjacent structures (e.g. bowel surgery)
- inadequate pain control.

Depending on the nature of the surgery performed, some patients return from surgery with a urinary catheter in situ. Catheterization may be required, for instance, following lower abdominal, pelvic or rectal surgery, in order to empty and maintain decompression of the bladder. Additionally, a urinary catheter will allow accurate measurement of output in patients for whom fluid balance management is critical. A catheter may also be used in patients in whom the anticipated postoperative level of consciousness is expected to cause difficulties with eliminatory self-care. Patients having major cardiac, vascular and neurological surgery, for example, may be sedated for a period of time following surgery.

Urinary retention can commonly occur following surgery and nurses must be alert to any evidence of ensuing discomfort or distension of the bladder so that appropriate action can be taken. Mobilizing patients, where appropriate, and providing privacy can encourage micturition. The sound of running water may also be helpful. Catheterization may be indicated postoperatively for the relief of urinary retention when all other appropriate interventions have been unsuccessful. However, it is worth noting that this is an invasive procedure associated with the risk of urinary tract infection (see Ch. 24). The safe insertion, assurance of patency, and prevention of complications such as UTI are key nursing skills. Nurses need to ensure that an accurate fluid balance record is maintained and that the volume and characteristics of urine output are recorded. The nursing role includes an appreciation of patients' possible embarrassment at being catheterized as well as the more obvious functions of safe and effective catheter management.

CONSTIPATION

Immobility allied to the effects of medication, reduction in fluid and nutritional input may predispose to diminished bowel motility. Constipation with painful retained wind is a common postoperative problem that may be alleviated by increasing fluid intake and by early mobilization programmes. Although a bowel action may not be expected immediately after surgery, especially where the bowel has been emptied preoperatively or following gastrointestinal surgery. However, the nurse must still ascertain from patients whether they have had a bowel action. If constipation occurs, a diet that includes non-starch polysaccharide (fibre) may be required. The use of aperients and suppositories, however, should only be considered as a secondary option.

POSTOPERATIVE DEEP VEIN THROMBOSIS

Preoperative assessment and instigation of relevant prophylactic or therapeutic activity will have reduced the potential for DVT. As a preventative measure, early mobilization is a primary nursing goal and should be preceded by instigation of active leg exercises. These should encourage regular flexion and extension of both the ankles and knees, and rotational exercises for the ankles as soon as possible following surgery. Passive limb exercises are imperative in those unable to comply. The physiotherapist is vital in promoting patient compliance with the limb exercise regimen, as well as providing educative support to the nursing staff.

The use of prescribed anti-embolic compression stockings must be maintained until full mobilization is achieved. They may be used in conjunction with prophylactic heparin therapy (see p. 888). Regular subcutaneous injections of heparin may be associated with localized pain and bruising and patients should be monitored for these effects. Injection sites should be rotated to minimize pain and tissue trauma. It is essential to document this rotation to ensure continuity and communication in care.

There are a number of classic diagnostic features of DVT and, if detected, the thrombosis may be accompanied by localized pain, tenderness or swelling. Tissue overlying the affected site may be reddened and warm or hot to the touch and the patient may be pyrexial. Thrombosis development in deeper vessels, such as a femoral or iliac vein, may predispose to the entire limb becoming swollen, tender and cool, due to arterial spasm and lymphatic obstruction. It is worth noting that the majority of DVT episodes actually present no obvious signs or symptoms (Wallis & Autar 2001). However, the ability to recognize its occurrence postoperatively is essential.

Patient education, stressing the need for reporting symptoms, is likely to promote speedy and potentially life-saving treatment of the disorder. Should the surgical nurse have any suspicion of the presence of DVT, it is imperative to reassure the patient and ensure bed rest is maintained until medical diagnosis and treatment can be instigated. The affected limb should be kept inactive to reduce the risk of a thrombus breaking free and entering the systemic circulation causing a PE. This may be recognized by complaints of pleural pain, haemoptysis, respiratory distress and signs of shock requiring urgent medical treatment (see Ch. 19). Further medical management of DVT and PE is discussed in Ch. 19.

POSTOPERATIVE CHEST INFECTION

As discussed earlier, respiratory morbidity is the most common postoperative complication. Reduced mobility, pain and the effects of anaesthesia may all potentiate its occurrence. The effects of a chest infection may range from a relatively minor discomfort in the otherwise healthy adult, to a life-threatening condition and pneumonia in the susceptible patient. Preventative activity is the primary focus for the management of chest infection. The pathological aspects are discussed in Chapter 20.

Evidence of chest infections is commonly seen within 48–72 hours following surgery. Signs of a chest infection may include the following:

- productive cough with green, infected sputum
- increased respiratory rate and dyspnoea
- pyrexia and tachycardia
- chest pain on inspiration and coughing
- cyanosis in advanced cases.

Medical and nursing activity is aimed at both treatment and symptom management. A sputum specimen will be sent for culture and sensitivity and antibiotic treatment based on microbiology results commenced. The build-up of secretions in the bronchioles will compromise effective gaseous exchange, resulting in reduced oxygen uptake and retention of carbon dioxide. Oxygen may be administered to reduce the effects of hypoxia. Aggressive physiotherapy is commenced that aims to encourage expectoration, deep breathing and subsequent elimination of obstructive secretions. Nursing activity is aimed at reducing the effects of the infection and the side-effects of treatment. Patients should preferably be nursed in an upright position to facilitate maximum chest expansion. Deep breathing exercises will allow air to move beyond the plugs of mucus and so enhance the effects of coughing. Exercises should be practised as regularly as the patient's condition permits, but preferably before meals to prevent the nausea and vomiting associated with excessive coughing and sputum production.

Analgesia may usefully be given to reduce pain associated with coughing and deep breathing. For many patients, i.v. and epidural PCA systems can play a major role in enhancing painless chest physiotherapy. Patients should be advised to support their wound whilst coughing to reduce the stress on the suture line.

However, it is vital to consider the surgical conditions in which coughing and subsequent rise of intracranial pressure may be detrimental, e.g. some types of ophthalmic and neurological surgery. Those undergoing some forms of ear and nose surgery may also require modification to the coughing technique because of changes in eustachian tube pressure and risks of haemorrhage, respectively.

The drying effect of oxygen must be considered and humidification is commonly employed to reduce this. Rigorous and frequent attention to mouth care is strongly indicated to reduce the potential for oral discomfort and disease.

WOUND MANAGEMENT

A key aim of care is to achieve wound healing as soon as possible with minimal complication and scarring. Healing achieved by primary intention is the preferred and most commonly utilized method of choice in uncomplicated surgery (see Ch. 10). Primary intention means that the wound edges are held together with sutures, clips or staples until the wound has healed sufficiently. Depending on site and purpose, skin staples and clips will usually be removed between 5 and 7 days, and non-absorbable sutures 5–10 days, following surgery. When there is evidence of infection or difficulty in closing skin edges, the surgeon may choose not to close the wound and to allow all or part of it to heal by secondary intention. Similarly, should a wound fail to heal, or if dehiscence (see p. 918) occurs, it may be resutured, a process often termed tertiary healing.

Wound assessment

Assessment should reflect the nurse's understanding of the factors that influence wound healing and its management and is likely to involve a documented assessment tool. Regular assessment will identify both the potential for and evidence of wound complications such as infection and dehiscence (see pp. 917–918).

Wound dressings

An understanding of the functions of wound dressings is essential if wound management is to be evidence-based. Key functions of dressings are:

- prevent the entry of microorganisms but allow gaseous exchange
- absorb exudate
- retain warmth and humidity for optimal wound healing
- protection of the wound and closure materials
- aesthetic purposes, e.g. concealment
- wound compression, e.g. to control bleeding
- support and immobilization.

The literature is ambiguous with regard to the length of time a dressing should remain intact. However, it should be retained for as long as the above functions are required. Appropriate healing will occur relatively quickly. The initial inflammatory stage of healing describes the formation of an occlusive epithelial layer or scab, which in primary intention healing is seen along the incision line (see Ch. 10). In uncomplicated wounds, this is likely to occur within 72 hours of surgery. The wound dressings may be removed at this time in the absence of any complication or therapeutic need. Whilst patients may not wish to view the wound in the initial stages of healing, it is useful to advise that some itching along the incision line is a normal aspect of the healing process. Such sensations may last for some months following surgery, until healing is complete.

A wide range of commercial dressings is available and provide for a multitude of wound requirements. Wound dressings utilized postoperatively will meet the general criteria (see above and Ch. 10) but may also fulfil specific patient and nursing requirements.

Factors to consider in wound dressing choice include:

- effectiveness in achieving wound healing
- ability to observe the wound
- patient comfort
- hypoallergenic
- ability to remove without undue distress or wound trauma
- cost-effectiveness and availability.

In the absence of evident complications, the dressing should remain intact and undisturbed until removal. The practice of lifting and replacing dressings is a common and unsatisfactory occurrence and one that predisposes to both wound infection and delayed healing (Wilson 1995).

The choice of dressing, if dressing change is required, should be reviewed regularly in relation to changes occurring as the wound heals. In more complicated surgical wounds, lengthy or repeated dressing changes are inevitable, but exposure and cleansing with cold solutions will reduce the temperature at the wound surface.

Wound drainage

As surgical recovery progresses, the risk of haemorrhage diminishes but the possibility of its occurrence should remain part of observation. The presence, characteristics and volume of other forms of drainage must be observed and reported. Changes in wound appearance associated with fluid leakage and the presence of malodour may be indicative of complications and delayed healing. Excessive fluid drainage following the removal of a wound drain or leakage from a specific part of the wound may be indicative of a fistula or track originating in deeper tissues or a body cavity. Faecal fistulae can occur following bowel surgery and biliary fistulae after biliary tract surgery. These fistulae may or may not be infected, although their continued presence is likely to increase the potential for contamination to occur. The presence of serosanguinous (serum and blood) drainage from a previously dry incision is suggestive of disruption and may indicate the early stages of wound dehiscence (see p. 918).

Wound drains

A surgical drain is inserted to provide a conduit for the elimination of existing exudate that has formed as a consequence of existing pathology, or to prevent potential complications anticipated as a result of surgery. Essentially, then, drains may be used as a primary therapeutic measure, as in the drainage of an abscess or a haemopneumothorax, or as a preventative measure.

There are a number of types of drain available and choice is generally based on the site and purpose of the drain (see Fig. 29.9). Drainage systems may be classified as open or closed.

Open drainage systems

Open drainage systems are passive systems that rely on posture and gravity as the means of eliminating exudate. Whilst less common than closed drainage systems, they include the Penrose, Yates and corrugated drains. Often used to assist in the drainage of pus and haematoma from an abscess, fistula or sinus in the superficial tissues, these drains will usually divert leakage into a dressing pad or, if there is a substantial volume, into a drainage bag. The drain may be secured to the skin with a suture. On occasion, the suture may be removed and the drain may be partially extracted and continually shortened over a period of time. This is done in a bid to encourage healing to begin beyond the depth of the drain and to minimize the potential for abscess formation. In such situations, a large sterile safety pin may be inserted in the drain so that it does not retract back into the wound, in the absence of the restraining suture. Such a system requires vigilance to minimize or eliminate any leakage onto the skin that may cause excoriation and soreness. In addition, scrupulous attention to handwashing and aseptic technique is essential in limiting the potential for cross-infection (see Evidence-based Practice box 29.2).

Closed drainage systems

Closed drainage systems consist of a length of plastic tube sutured to the skin. The proximal end is placed at the site of

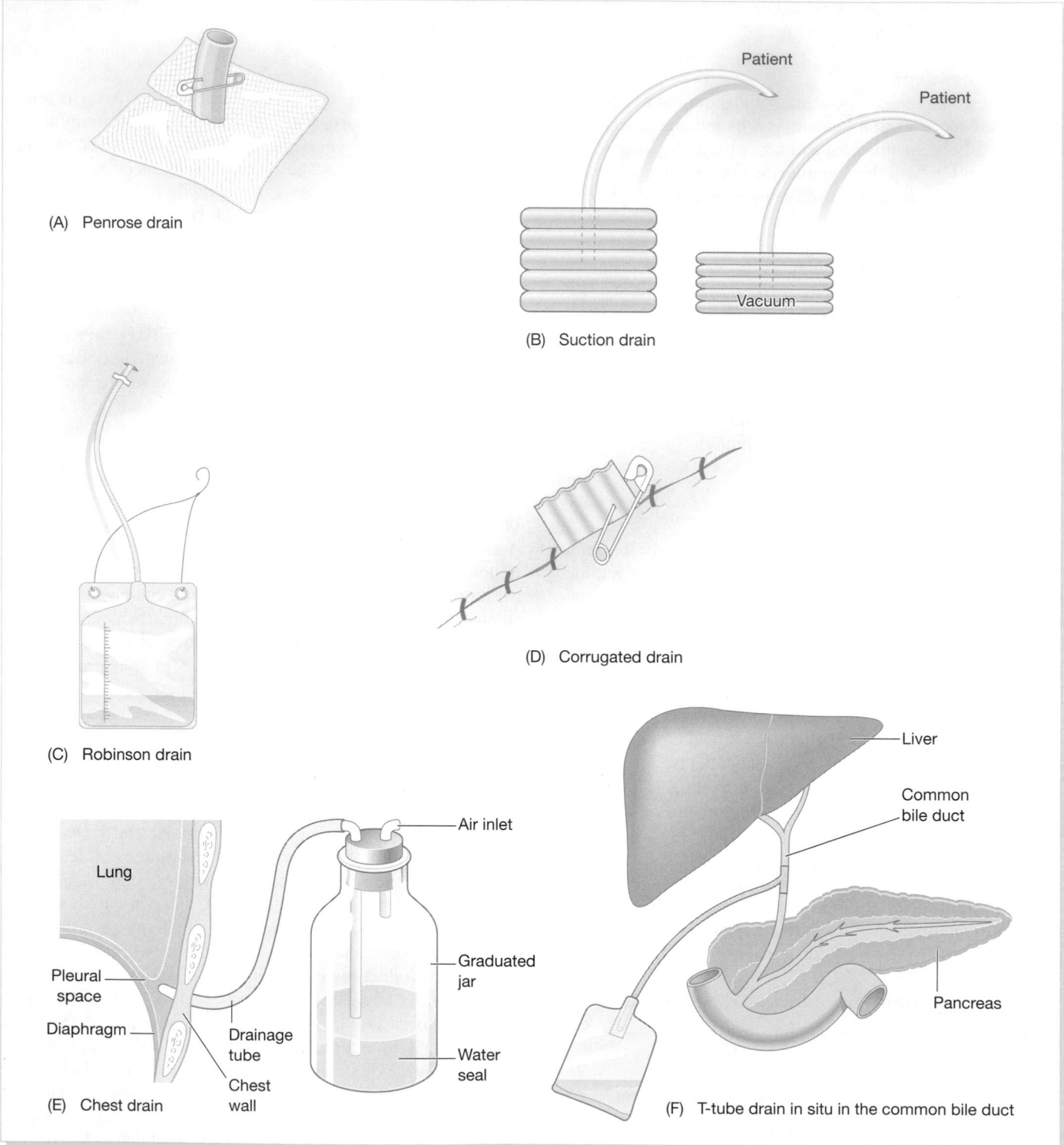

(A) Penrose drain

(B) Suction drain

Patient

Patient

Vacuum

(C) Robinson drain

(D) Corrugated drain

(E) Chest drain

Lung

Pleural space

Diaphragm

Drainage tube

Chest wall

Air inlet

Graduated jar

Water seal

(F) T-tube drain in situ in the common bile duct

Liver

Common bile duct

Pancreas

Figure 29.9 Types of drainage systems.

actual or potential exudate collection. Examples include an anastomosis site, or where a structure has been traumatized or where removal of a structure or tissue has left a potential space within which fluid may gather, e.g. a mastectomy (see Ch. 26). The distal end is attached to a drainage bag. Closed systems have a number of advantages, not least the reduction of the potential for contamination of the drainage tract or site. It is easier for the nurse to monitor the volume and nature of the fluid. Whilst a closed system can be used as a sump drain and provide drainage in a passive manner, it may also be used in conjunction with a vacuum created in the distal part of the closed circuit. Such systems may be self-contained, as in the Microvac and Redivac

EVIDENCE-BASED PRACTICE

29.2 The importance of handwashing in the surgical environment

Parker (1999) reviews the importance of handwashing and the evidence supporting this practice. The correct method of handwashing is detailed and soaps and antiseptic agents are contrasted. Barriers to adequate handwashing are also discussed. The author provides suggestions for enhancing compliance in the clinical area.

Key issues
- Health care workers' hands are strongly implicated in the transmission of nosocomial infection
- Handwashing is acknowledged to be the primary method of controlling infection and the most important single factor in preventing hospital-acquired infection
- Handwashing is often infrequent and inadequate
- An understanding of the rationale underpinning handwashing will increase compliance
- Handwashing technique and length of wash will vary depending on purpose
- The wearing of gloves is wrongly assumed to negate the need for handwashing

Student activities
Read Parker (1999).

- Why is handwashing particularly important in perioperative nursing practice?
- Observe how staff in your current clinical practice area carry out handwashing. Make notes on the frequency and technique of handwashing in relation to specific aspects of care provided.
- Keep a diary of your handwashing activity for one shift.
- Reflect on the result and the effectiveness of your own handwashing technique in relation to the illustration provided on page 718 of Parker (1999).

Reference
Parker LJ. Importance of handwashing in the prevention of cross-infection. Br J Nurs 1999; 8(11): 716–720.

---

systems, or may be attached to an appropriate mechanical suction pump. Unless specific medical contraindications exist, patients should be informed that ambulation should not be affected by the presence of a wound drain.

▶ Nursing management: wound drains

Whilst the type and function of the wound drain may differ, a number of key principles will apply:

- System patency must be monitored regularly – kinking or blockage of the drain may inhibit flow of fluid.
- Ensure that the drain remains anchored and is not liable to retraction or displacement.
- Suction drains only function when perforations in the tube are below the wound surface.
- All exudate is observed, measured and documented. Any concern regarding the volume, consistency, smell or complaints of pain must be reported.
- Aseptic technique is used when handling the wound drainage system.
- All aspects of wound drainage will be explained to the patient and mobility encouraged.
- Wound drains are removed when they have fulfilled their purpose. Generally the level of drainage will be minimal or will have ceased for a suitable period of time.
- Appropriate analgesia and patient preparation will be required prior to drain removal.

Wound infection

Where infection does occur, its extent and the nature of the causative microorganism will influence the colour and consistency of drainage. The presence of purulent exudate or pus will indicate infection and the presence of foul-smelling brown fluid may denote a faecal contamination.

Wound infection is a major cause of discomfort, distress, prolonged recovery and even death. A number of factors have been implicated in the development of postoperative wound infection:

- the nature of surgery and surgical contamination (see Table 29.4, p. 918)
- poor nutritional state
- immunocompromised patient
- excessive obesity
- poor surgical preparation
- length of surgery
- poor nursing and medical practices
- presence of drains.

Careful wound assessment is essential for the recognition of wound infection. There may be systemic evidence of infection, such as pyrexia, tachycardia and malaise, as well as a number of localized signs. Whilst there is some discussion and lack of consensus about the precise criteria for diagnosing the presence of infection, there are a number of clinical signs that may be valid indicators (Cutting & Harding 1994):

- abscess (collection of pus)
- cellulitis (inflammation of skin and soft tissues)
- discharge
- delayed healing
- discoloration
- friable granulation tissue which bleeds easily
- unexpected pain and tenderness
- accumulation of exudate at the base of the wound
- abnormal smell
- wound breakdown.

Table 29.4 Wound classification and potential for wound infection

Wound classification and characteristics	Wound infection and potential for delayed risk	Examples of operations
Clean No inflammation and no evidence of infection. Operative wounds in which respiratory, alimentary and genitourinary tracts are not incised	Low	Breast surgery Hip replacement Inguinal hernia repair
Clean contaminated No sign of existing infection. Respiratory, alimentary and genitourinary tracts are opened but with no breaks in surgical technique or asepsis	Low–raised	Appendicectomy Thoracotomy Hysterectomy
Contaminated Often open or traumatic wounds. Surgical spillage has occurred. May have signs of infection apparent. Major breaks in aseptic protocols	Moderate–high	Perforated appendix removal Bowel resection in perforated bowel Gunshot wounds Gross trauma
Dirty or infected Surgery involves tissues with existing clinical infection. May have retained devascularized or necrotic tissue. Evidence of pus and infective exudate	High–very high	Excision and drainage of abscess Necrotizing fasciitis Gangrenous tissue resection Gross peritonitis

Despite research questioning the accuracy and technique of wound surface swabbing, if infection is suspected a wound swab will be obtained. A recent national surveillance scheme identified the most common bacteria causing almost half of all wound infections to be staphylococci. Of these, 81% were identified to be *Staphylococcus aureus* and 61% of these were methicillin-resistant (NINSS 2000). It is essential that the swabbing technique and subsequent transport of the specimen to the laboratory be appropriately managed according to local protocol and best practice (see Ch. 13).

Wound dehiscence

Dehiscence is a complication that occurs in a primary closed wound, whereby the wound edges separate with possible evisceration of internal organs. It occurs most frequently in abdominal wounds and complete dehiscence may result in evisceration of the intestine, commonly referred to as a 'burst abdomen'.

Patients are frequently frightened that their wounds will tear. Advances in surgical wound management have reduced the incidence of dehiscence but it can still occur. Risk factors include:

- pre-existing disease, e.g. obstructive jaundice, diabetes, cancer
- abdominal distension, e.g. ascites, obstructed bowel
- inadequate nutrition
- obesity
- straining, as in coughing and vomiting
- corticosteroid therapy
- wound infection
- poor surgical technique.

Dehiscence may occur almost immediately after surgery and potentially up to 2 weeks postoperatively. Perkins (1992) distinguishes between early dehiscence, related to suture failure or poor surgical technique, and late dehiscence related to infection.

▶ Nursing management: wound dehiscence

The first indication of wound dehiscence may be a patient complaint of wound leakage and a change in wound tension. Patients often describe a feeling that 'the wound has given way'. An inspection of the wound might reveal that the wound edges are open, and in the case of an abdominal wound, loops of bowel may be protruding from it. The wound is likely to be wet and saturated with serosanguinous drainage. It is likely that patients will require further surgical intervention to repair the wound and appropriate preoperative preparation will be instigated.

Patients should stay in bed and be encouraged to adopt a recumbent semi-Fowler's position (the head of the bed is inclined at a 30° angle). Maintaining this position will help to reduce intra-abdominal pressure and prevent strain on the wound and worsening evisceration. The wound should be covered with sterile wound pads soaked in normal saline warmed to body temperature (37°C). This helps to keep it clean and prevent any exposed bowel from drying out, as well as preserving body heat. An abdominal support or binder may be prescribed to reduce tension and minimize further dehiscence.

Patients will be anxious and probably very frightened. It is important to provide reassurance as to the temporary nature of the condition and the ability to resolve this quickly and effectively. Whilst waiting for a medical assessment to take place, patients' vital signs must be monitored and recorded for signs of shock. Wound swabs may also be taken if there is a clear indication of infection so that appropriate treatment may be started. An i.v. infusion may be prescribed and antibiotics commenced. Relatives should be informed of the change in the patient's condition and advised if further surgery is required. Surgical repair is the usual course of treatment if patients are physically well enough. They will be taken to theatre for irrigation of the wound, possible debridement and closure of the wound. In some instances, where infection is present or difficulties are encountered in achieving closure of the outer layers of the wound, these may be left to heal by secondary intention.

On return to the ward after surgery, patients are monitored for any signs of wound infection (see above), as this is more likely following a second surgical intervention. Nurses should stress the importance of supporting the wound during coughing to avoid strain on the incision.

Although an unusual occurrence, it is important to reiterate that dehiscence may occur after discharge from the relative safety of the hospital, especially with the practice of short hospital stays and earlier discharge. This emphasizes the need for effective liaison with community nurses. Vulnerable patients should be assessed and identified as part of the discharge process and referred appropriately.

MOBILITY AND AMBULATION

One of the most beneficial and yet most underestimated strategies in the prevention of postoperative complications and enhancement of patient well-being is early ambulation. It increases muscle tone and strength, circulatory function and gastrointestinal tone and allows patients to become actively involved in their recovery process. Early mobilization postoperatively has been associated with a reduction in the incidence of DVT, chest infection, constipation, urinary stasis (see p. 913), pressure ulcer development and even depression.

Preparation for mobilization should begin prior to surgery. Patients should be provided with specific information regarding the need for and advantages of early mobilization. Additionally an indication of mobilization expectations may be discussed with them preoperatively. This may enhance compliance and reduce misperception or misinterpretation of what is expected. Ideally mobilization should begin as soon as is practicable after initial recovery from anaesthesia. The nature of surgery may require a delayed or limited level of ambulation in some patients. Those requiring critical care support and also those for whom non-weight-bearing is a requisite of therapy, will be unable to regain independence in mobility immediately. However, the need for active and/or passive exercise activity remains essential if the potential for complications is to be reduced.

DISCHARGE PLANNING

In the past 20 years, there has been a paradigm shift away from institutionalized health care generally and, more specifically, from surgical convalescence units. Allied with the advent of minimal access and ambulatory surgery and the increasing demand on hospital in-patient beds, many patients are discharged into the community almost immediately after surgery. As a consequence, the majority of in-patient surgical admissions are for more major surgery, requiring high-dependency care with even greater implications for early discharge. The aim of successful discharge is to provide a seamless transition of care between the day-care or hospital unit and the community (Department of Health 2000). Preparation for discharge often begins at the time of admission but should ideally start at the first point of contact with the health care system. The NHS Act (Department of Health

1999) provided the framework and legislation for the creation of Primary Care Trusts. Within this structure, GPs are able to work in partnership with the patient and hospital in the booking of surgical care. Patients will be able to decide when they want their operation and consequently discharge planning will become an explicit and integral part of the surgical process. All hospitals will have a discharge policy that is developed by, and agreed with, the appropriate stakeholders, including primary care and social services. In many cases, this may include a telephone follow-up or support service through which patients may seek clarification or advice in aspects of their care or concerns regarding postoperative discomforts.

The aims of quality discharge planning are to:

■ maximize self-care ability
■ prepare patients (and family members/carers) physically and emotionally for discharge to a suitable environment
■ provide appropriate verbal and written information to patients and family members
■ ensure appropriate resources and facilities are in place to meet the individual requirements of patients
■ promote a coordinated and seamless discharge through quality communication between hospital unit and community to ensure continuity of care
■ maintain quality record-keeping and documentation for professional accountability.

One of the primary functions of discharge information is to promote patients' ability to self-care. Throughout the surgical care process the continual provision of clear, appropriate and honest information for patients and, where possible, appropriate family members and carers, will minimize discharge confusion. Inadequate information may contribute to home care needs not being met and poor patient outcomes with the possibility of hospital readmission.

The effectiveness of discharge information is questioned in a literature review (Henderson & Zernike 2001) that identifies a number of factors contributing to its suboptimal quality:

■ lack of time
■ poor understanding of information by patients
■ information not relevant to patient needs
■ information delivered is insufficient or unclear
■ timing of information is often too late or too hurried
■ patient reluctance to ask questions.

Following surgery discharge preparation is likely to require discussion on pain relief and wound care. However, there are many other issues that may need to be addressed (see Health Promotion box 29.2).

Whilst many patient concerns may appear trivial or of little consequence to the health professional, they may be of considerable importance to the patient and should never be underestimated. Concerns may lead patients to seek further help from a health care facility, placing unnecessary pressure on an already stretched service.

The consequences of failure to adhere to the principles and practices of discharge planning may be significant. Discharge is one of the most important aspects of the surgical process. Ultimately, without due regard for its centrality, this part of the surgical process has the potential for undoing much of the care preceding it.

HEALTH PROMOTION

29.2 Preparation for discharge

Successful discharge planning should begin as soon as individuals enter the health care system. An early appreciation of patients' perceptions of their problem, the support systems available to them and their coping abilities is pivotal in identifying resource requirements for discharge. Regardless of whether patients are undergoing a minor procedure in a day-care setting or the most complex of operations, early planning can significantly and positively influence successful recovery.

Inappropriate discharge has been highlighted as a major reason for patient readmission. Poor and non-compliance with health information and medication are strongly linked to the quality of the discharge process. The pressure to meet operating list targets may lead to inappropriately early discharge.

Key educational aspects of a discharge plan

General effects of surgery/anaesthesia
- Driving, lifting and physical activity may be restricted for a period of time
- Need for rest and sleep
- Postoperative depression
- Sleep disturbance, dizziness and drowsiness

Procedure specific advice
- Advice on activity restriction such as not swimming/diving following some ear surgery
- Flying/travel restrictions
- Wearing of anti-embolism stockings

Specific exercise activity
- Explanation of deep breathing exercises
- Pelvic floor strengthening
- Walking and leg exercises

Dietary and nutritional advice
- Foods to be encouraged or restricted
- Alcohol consumption
- Fruit, vegetable and fluid consumption and prevention of elimination problems

Medication
- The nature of drug treatment, dosage, action, side-effects, and special instruction verbally and in written form, e.g. pain relief and anticoagulant therapy

Postoperative complication potential
- Advice on the recognition of bleeding, infection, persistent pain, nausea and vomiting, limb swelling, chest problems and the appropriate action to be taken
- Understanding of when to seek help is confirmed

Nurse- and self-administered treatment
- Information on the frequency, duration and techniques of dressing change
- Care of operation site and expected date of suture/clip/staple removal
- Stoma care
- Catheter management
- Enteral/parenteral nutrition management

Continuing and follow-up care
- Contact details and documentation for community nurses, GP, clinical nurse specialists
- Outpatient and follow-up appointment and possible transport needs
- Contact information for self-help groups

Social support
- Confirmation of arrangements for transport home
- Confirmation of home-based social support

SUMMARY: MAIN POINTS

- Surgery is a critical life event and an understanding of how individuals respond to crisis is crucial.

- The nurse's understanding of psychosocial and emotional aspects of surgery can positively enhance patient recovery.

- The patient undergoing day care and minimally invasive surgical technique has specific needs.

- Accurate and appropriate pain and symptom management will hasten healing, recovery and emotional well-being.

- Adherence to principles of asepsis and infection control is a key tenet of perioperative practice.

- Perioperative nursing activity must always promote empowerment and informed decision-making.

- Patient education is a key feature of surgical care throughout the perioperative process.

- Accurate and appropriate assessment and action throughout the perioperative period can greatly reduce the potential for postoperative complications and patient discomfort.

- Collaboration, partnership and inter-agency working will significantly enhance surgical recovery.

- Surgical consent must be based on the patient making an informed choice.

- Planning for discharge begins at first contact with the health care system.

- Perioperative nursing must be based on best practice rather than on tradition and ritual.

SELF-TEST: CRITICAL THINKING ACTIVITIES

1 Rosa (aged 55) is admitted for pelvic surgery under GA. Identify the risk of this patient developing a DVT and discuss the care required to prevent the occurrence of DVT in the perioperative period.

2 A patient has come to the pre-admission clinic for assessment prior to a hernia repair as a day case in 2 weeks' time. He is very quiet and withdrawn.

— What might be the reasons for this behaviour?
— How might you undertake a preoperative nursing assessment of this man and what information will you need to discuss with him?

 FURTHER READING

Burden N (ed). Ambulatory surgical nursing, 2nd edn. Philadelphia: Saunders; 2000.

Davies R. Psychological, existential and spiritual aspects of surgery. In: Manley K, Bellman L, eds. Surgical nursing: advancing practice. Edinburgh: Churchill Livingstone; 2000, ch 9.

Dimond B. Legal aspects of nursing. Harlow: Pearson Higher Education; 2001

Manley K, Bellman L (eds). Surgical nursing: advancing practice. Edinburgh: Churchill Livingstone; 2000.

Pitts M. The experience of treatment. In: Pitts M, Phillips K, eds. The psychology of health – an introduction. London: Routledge; 1998, ch 5.

REFERENCES

Agu O, Hamilton G, Baker D. Graduated compression stockings in the prevention of venous thromboembolism. Br J Surg 1999; 86: 992–1004.

Aldrete JA, Kroulik D. A post-anaesthetic recovery score. Anesth Analg 1970; 49: 924–934.

Alexander J, Fisher JE, Boyajian M, Palmquist J, Morris MJ. The influence of hair removal methods on wound infections. Arch Surg 1983; 118: 347–352.

American Society of Anesthesiologists (ASA). New classification of physical status. Anesthesiology 1963; 24: 11.

Audit Commission. Anaesthesia under examination: the efficiency and effectiveness of anaesthesia and pain relief services in England and Wales. London: Audit Commission; 1997.

Autar R. Nursing assessment of clients at risk of deep vein thrombosis. The Autar DVT Scale. J Adv Nurs 1996; 23(4): 736–763.

Bevan P. The management and utilisation of operating departments – report of the steering group. Leeds: NHS Management Executive; 1989.

Boore JA. Prescription for recovery. London: Royal College of Nursing; 1978.

Byrne DJ, Phillips G, Napier A, Cuschien A. The effect of whole body disinfection on intraoperative wound contamination. J Hosp Infect 1991; 18: 145–158.

Byrne DJ, Lynch W, Napier A. Wound infection rates: the importance of definition and post discharge wound surveillance. J Hosp Infect 1994; 26: 37–43.

Chapman A. Current theory and practice: a study into preoperative fasting. Nurs Stand 1996; 10(18): 33–36.

Closs S. Post-operative patients' views of sleep, pain and recovery. J Clin Nurs 1992; 1: 83–88.

Craft T, Upton P. Key topics in anaesthesia. Worcester: BIOS Scientific Publishers; 1992.

Cutting KF, Harding KG. Criteria for identifying wound infection. J Wound Care 1994; 3(4): 198–201.

Defloor T, DeSchuijmer JD. Preventing pressure ulcers: an evaluation of four operating mattresses. Appl Nurs Res 2000; 13(3): 134–141.

Dennison D. Thermal regulation of patients during the perioperative experience. AORN J 1995; 61(5): 827–828, 831–832.

Department of Health. The NHS Act. London: HMSO; 1999.

Department of Health. The NHS Plan. London: HMSO; 2000.

Department of Health. Good practice in consent implementation guide: consent to examination or treatment. London: DoH; 2001.

Dimond B. Legal aspects of nursing. Harlow: Pearson Higher Education; 2001.

Garibaldi RA. Prevention of intraoperative wound contamination with chlorhexidine shower and scrub. J Hosp Infect 1988; 11(Suppl B): 5–9.

Hamilton Smith S. Nil by mouth. London: Royal College of Nursing; 1972.

Hayward J. Information: a prescription against pain. London: Royal College of Nursing; 1975.

Health and Safety Executive (HSE). Guidance on manual handling regulations L23. London: HMSO; 1992.

Henderson A, Zernike W. A study of the impact of discharge information for surgical patients. J Adv Nurs 2001; 35(3): 435–441.

Jepson OB, Bruttomesso KA. The effectiveness of preoperative skin preparation. AORN J 1993; 58(3): 477–484.

Kurz A, Sessler D, Narzt E et al. Postoperative thermodynamic and thermoregulatory consequences of intraoperative core hypothermia. J Clin Anaesth 1995; 7(5): 359–366.

Leigh DA, Stonge JL, Mariner J, Sedgwick J. Total body bathing with Hibiscrub (chlorhexidine) in surgical patients: a controlled trial. J Hosp Infect 1983; 4: 229–235.

Lewis SJ, Egger M, Sylvester PA, Thomas S. Early enteral feeding versus "nil by mouth" after gastrointestinal surgery; systematic review and meta analysis of controlled trials. Br Med J 2001; 323: 1–5.

McKnight C. Preoperative assessment of the surgical patient. Care Crit Ill 1994; 10(1): 35–38.

Maltby JR. Preoperative fasting guidelines update in anaesthesia, Issue 12, Article 2. Online. Available: www. nda.ox.ac.uk/wfsa/html/u12/ul1202_01.htm. 2001.

National Confidential Enquiry into Perioperative Deaths. Changing the way we operate. London: NCEPOD; 2001.

Naver L, Gottrup F. Incidence of glove perforation in gastrointestinal surgery and the protective effect of double gloving. A prospective randomized controlled study. Eur J Surg 2000; 166: 293–295.

Nosocomial Infection National Surveillance Scheme (NINSS). Surveillance of surgical site infection in English Hospitals 1997–1999. London: Public Health Laboratory Service; 2000 (Also online. Available: www.phls.co.uk/).

Orr N. Is a mask necessary in the operating theatre? Ann Royal Coll Surg Engl 1981; 63: 390.

Otte DI. Patients perspectives and experiences of day case surgery. J Adv Nurs 1996; 23(12): 1228–1237.

Perkins P. Wound dehiscence: causes and care. Nurs Stand 1992; 6(34): 12–14.

Royal College of Surgeons and the College of Anaesthetists. Pain after surgery. London: Royal College of Surgeons; 1990.

Royal College of Surgeons. Commission on the provision of surgical services. Guidelines for day case surgery. London: Royal College of Surgeons; 1992.

Shevde K, Triveldi N. Effect of clear fluids on gastric volume and pH in healthy volunteers. Anaesth Analg 1991; 72(4): 528–531.

Small SP. Preoperative hair removal: a case report with implications for nursing. J Clin Nurs 1996; 5: 79–84.

Surkitt Parr M. Hypothermia in surgical patients. Br J Nurs 1992; 1(11): 539–545.

Thomas E. Preoperative fasting, a question of routine. Nurs Times 1987; 83(49): 46–47.

Turnbull LA, Wood N, Kester G. Controlled trial of the subjective patient benefits of accompanied walking to the operating theatre. Int J Clin Pract 1998; 52: 81–83.

Tyrell M, Birtel A, Taylor P. Deep vein thrombosis. Br J Clin Pract 1995; 49(5): 252–256.

Wallis M, Autar R. Deep vein thrombosis: clinical nursing management. Nurs Stand 2001; 15(18): 47–54.

Wells L. At the front line of care. Prof Nurse 1994; 9(8): 525–530.

Whitwam JG (ed). Day-case anaesthesia and sedation. London: Blackwell Scientific Publications; 1994.

Wilson J. Infection control in clinical practice. London: Baillière Tindall; 1995.

30 Nursing patients in the accident and emergency department

Lindsay Etherington

'I was with my mentor in resus when he was brought in. His heart stopped as he came through the door and it was incredible to watch. My mentor was the team leader and everyone just knew exactly what to do. There was no panic – the teamwork was amazing. Afterwards we talked it through and I realised why training and updates are so important'

(Student nurse)

THIS CHAPTER WILL HELP YOU

- Explain the role of the accident and emergency (A&E) department and issues of caring

- Understand patient assessment within the role of nurse triage

- Discuss health promotion and the prevention of accidents

- Describe the skills required to manage the A&E department

- Discuss the role of the emergency nurse practitioner

- Discuss the role of the nurse in the resuscitation room and in caring for the patient with major trauma

- Describe the care of the patient with minor trauma

- Discuss social issues in A&E

- Describe the recognition and management of challenging behaviour

- Describe the management of the patient with acute mental health problems

- Reflect upon sudden death and the care of the bereaved in A&E

- Discuss major disaster procedures.

KEYWORDS

Accident	**Emergency**
Aggression	**Resuscitation**
Anxiety	**Trauma**
Assessment	**Triage**
Communication	

INTRODUCTION

This chapter introduces the reader to the care of patients in the accident and emergency (A&E) department. The role of A&E is covered in some depth since debate continues as to whose needs it should serve. Issues raised are closely linked to the care given by A&E nurses and the qualities required to work in A&E.

The process of nursing and the promotion of health, covered in Chapter 1, are related to the A&E setting and patient assessment is considered within the role of triage. Links will be made with Chapter 3 with regard to the use of effective interpersonal skills during the assessment process. Management issues specific to the lead nurse are discussed, as well as the role of the emergency nurse practitioner.

The role of the nurse in resuscitation in A&E is closely considered, as is the environment in the resuscitation room, and the discussion includes the sensitive issue of witnessed cardiopulmonary resuscitation (see Ch. 19). A standard team approach to the patient with major trauma is described alongside some of the special issues within trauma care.

The perceptions of both the patient and the nurse are a regular theme within the chapter and are discussed in relation to the term 'minor' trauma and to the care of this group of patients.

Social problems inform a large part of A&E nursing and some common issues are raised in order to paint an accurate picture of the A&E world. Communication is reiterated in discussions relating to the management of patients with acute mental health problems and confronting challenging behaviour.

Sudden death presents A&E nurses with the immense task of establishing brief relationships with distressed relatives. Bereavement in A&E provides a link to Chapter 34, within the concept of death and dying.

Finally, major disasters are discussed briefly as an issue that extends beyond the A&E department, and includes the role of the A&E nurse in caring for large numbers of injured people.

THE ROLE OF THE A&E DEPARTMENT

The primary function of the A&E department is to receive, assess and treat ill or injured people, quickly, and at any time of the day or night. For many patients, A&E represents the 'shop window' of the organization – the first, and possibly lasting, impression they will have of the hospital.

Some people will be admitted into hospital from A&E. However, the majority will receive treatment for their injury or illness and be discharged back into the community. These would include patients with cuts and bruises, strains and sprains, minor throat and chest infections, rashes and uncomplicated limb fractures. The more serious illnesses the A&E nurse can expect to see include patients with cardiovascular emergencies, such as a myocardial infarction or heart failure, those with gastrointestinal problems, e.g. appendicitis, peptic ulceration, or acute intra-abdominal bleeding, and those with neurovascular emergencies such as cerebrovascular accident (CVA) and meningitis – these are detailed in Chapters 19, 22 and 14 respectively.

Investigations carried out in the A&E department reflect the urgency of the situation, and generally extend only as far as the emergency period demands. Routine investigations are normally carried out once the patient reaches the ward or, if discharged, can be performed by the general practitioner.

Every kind of physical and psychosocial crisis is likely to present itself to A&E, providing links with the entire multi-disciplinary team, inside and outside the hospital environment.

The community surrounding the A&E department varies geographically, and therefore the care delivered should reflect the population who use it. In other words, the socioeconomic and cultural composition of the catchment area, and any dominant industry, should be provided for within the service offered. Specific issues for some A&E departments may include a large homeless population, high prevalence of HIV and AIDS, or drug-related problems. Similarly, an A&E department situated in a seaside location must be able to respond to different types of accidents and emergencies, and may experience dramatic rises in attendance during the summer months.

An emphasis on health care in the community in the UK means that more patients will be treated and discharged, and therefore liaison between A&E, general practitioners (GPs) and community nurses and health services is essential to provide continuity of care and avoid unnecessary readmissions into hospital.

WHO USES A&E?

Each of us has a different interpretation of the word 'emergency'. Should A&E serve only those involved in an accident or emergency, or anyone with a health need?

In fact, there are many reasons why people come to A&E (Rieffe et al 1999). The patient's perception of an emergency is an important issue. Many people are not registered with a doctor, e.g. they may be homeless or part of a transient population, such as visitors to the area. Getting an appointment may be difficult or it may simply be that the hospital is nearer. Most A&E departments are open 24 hours a day, there is no appointment system, and many investigations are immediately available; the attraction is evident. However, no one should have to prove they are an emergency. If patients have a health need and are worried enough to come to A&E, the least they require is reassurance and support.

The name 'casualty' was replaced by 'accident and emergency' following the Platt (1962) report, which suggested that A&E was used by 'inappropriate' groups of patients, who should be treated by their GP. However, attendance figures continue to rise, although there is no single reason for the increase (Audit Commission 1996).

In October, 2001, the UK goverment launched a series of reforms (DOH 2001) as a means of improving access for patients with urgent care needs, and reducing long waits in A&E departments. One of the key recommendations was that acute hospitals should work in partnership with community healthcare providers and local GP surgeries to direct patients to the most appropriate healthcare practitioner. Hospitals were advised to explore the patients' 'journey' through the A&E department to identify blocks in the system responsible for frustating waits. The development of nurse-led Minor Injury Units (MIUs) was encouraged to separate patients into separate treatment flows according to their needs.

These initiatives address the issue of increasing attendance in A&E departments, rather than simply labelling certain groups of patients as inappropriate.

Changing social trends can be monitored in A&E, e.g. the relationship between alcohol consumption and accidents (Walsh 1996), drug misuse, or the pattern of domestic violence.

Part of becoming an A&E nurse involves reading the whole story of the patient, not merely dipping into the chapter of the isolated problem. Holistic assessment is essential in order that the full extent of the patient's problem is identified. Rich experience can be gained as people of every age, culture, class and background, each with their own concepts of health and illness, are represented in the 15 million attendances to A&E departments each year in the UK.

The skilled A&E nurse can comfort the patient with multiple injuries in the resuscitation room, or advise the homeless person with blistered feet, and provide the same level of care for both.

PREHOSPITAL CARE

Prehospital care is described as the care given prior to the patient's arrival in hospital. An unskilled bystander, workplace first-aider or fully qualified paramedic may deliver this. In order to plan appropriate care, the A&E team needs to know what has been done for the patient before he or she arrived.

Challenges such as the weather, time of day, and potential hazards, such as chemical spillage, fire and explosion risks, demonstrate that the prehospital environment is quite different from that of A&E. Demanding situations, such as transporting an obese patient from a high-rise flat with no lift, put both patient and care provider at risk.

Ambulance services have progressed in order to deliver rapid and skilled care to seriously ill or injured patients. Paramedics are trained to carry out advanced skills, such as venepuncture (the puncturing of a vein to take a sample of blood or to inject a drug or fluid) and defibrillation (the application of an electrical current to the heart to restore normal rhythmic contractions).

The types of vehicles used reflect the environment from which the patient is retrieved, and include motorcycles, four-wheel drive vehicles and helicopters, alongside the traditional emergency ambulance.

Information provided by ambulance personnel is an integral part of the assessment process and they should be considered part of the A&E team. An experienced ambulance person will note subtle clues from the patient's home environment, which may influence the management. For example, the older adult who is brought in following a series of falls may be living in squalor because of reduced mobility and independence. Only by having an understanding of the environment from which the patient has been extracted can the A&E team plan care and anticipate psychological and emotional responses.

The prehospital environment is a challenging one. The patient's story does not begin at the doors of the A&E department, but in a world full of obstacles not encountered in the ordered environment of the hospital.

CARING IN THE A&E DEPARTMENT

Almost every person who comes to A&E as a patient or relative will experience some degree of anxiety. Furthermore, one patient with devastating injuries will cope with stoicism and humour, whilst another, perhaps with a cut finger, will be in great distress. It is easy to make assumptions regarding the amount of emotion we feel is appropriate. Yet, there is little relationship between the severity of an injury or illness and the extent of psychological trauma. The essence of A&E nursing is to understand the world from which the patient comes. Their reactions are normal; it is the event that is not.

Cultural background can influence responses to illness, pain and bereavement. Everyday stressors, such as family or work worries, indeed anything that disrupts our daily lives, will affect our ability to cope with the crisis of sudden injury or illness.

All patients in A&E crave communication – acknowledgement of their suffering, information, eye contact, a smile and, for many, the reassurance of touch.

The impression gained by patients in A&E will influence their perception of the hospital and may shape any future experience. A&E nurses must learn, therefore, that their own personal values will not always match those of their patients. To judge people according to the way they look, dress or smell, or even whether they speak English, may result in a serious health problem being overlooked. It will also undoubtedly deepen their existing crisis.

Waiting areas and cubicles in A&E can be sensory wastelands, a reminder that the environment in which we place patients can increase their stress and lead to dissatisfaction. A well-designed waiting room contains comfortable seating, access to toilet and refreshment facilities, reading matter and, above all, written and verbal information regarding waiting times and the function of the A&E department.

A&E is a bewildering place for most people. Their lives have been interrupted, they are anxious, may be in pain, and most will have no previous experience to enable them to cope. A&E nursing requires an open mind, the ability to use intuition, and the skills to provide constant human contact in every situation.

THE PROCESS OF NURSING IN A&E

The nature of the work in A&E means that the process of nursing often occurs as a rapid sequence of events, beginning with the recognition of life-threatening needs. Traditional care planning is inappropriate in the A&E setting, because of the time required to complete extensive paperwork. For most patients, care is promptly planned in the nurse's mind, and implemented according to need.

Many established nursing models do not fit well into an area where speed is of the essence. Nursing assessment and problem identification overlap into the medical model, as specific physiological problems often take priority. However, A&E nursing values the patient as an individual, and part of a family or community, encompassing psychosocial, cultural and spiritual needs.

Many A&E nurses adapt or create their own models of nursing, which are both realistic and reflect their philosophy of care. An experienced A&E nurse knows when a patient is ill, by using intuition or 'gut feeling'. However, an appropriate model enables A&E nurses to clarify what they do and how it is done. Figure 30.1 demonstrates an example of a nursing model, designed specifically for A&E, embracing physiological and psychosocial priorities of care.

NURSING ASSESSMENT IN A&E

TRIAGE

The term 'triage' is derived from the French word *trier*, meaning 'to sort'. In the 17th century, triage referred to quality control of food and was later used to describe the prioritization of injured soldiers in the Napoleonic wars. There is a difference, however, between war and peacetime triage. In battle, the aim was to return soldiers to the front line, so those with serious injuries were left in favour of the 'walking wounded'.

Nurse triage is not merely a means of allocating a category rating to a patient, although pressures on A&E departments to speed up the flow of patients present a difficult task. Decisions have to be made quickly and acted upon. Triage encompasses assessment, prioritization of need, first aid, the initiation of relevant investigations and the provision of health promotion.

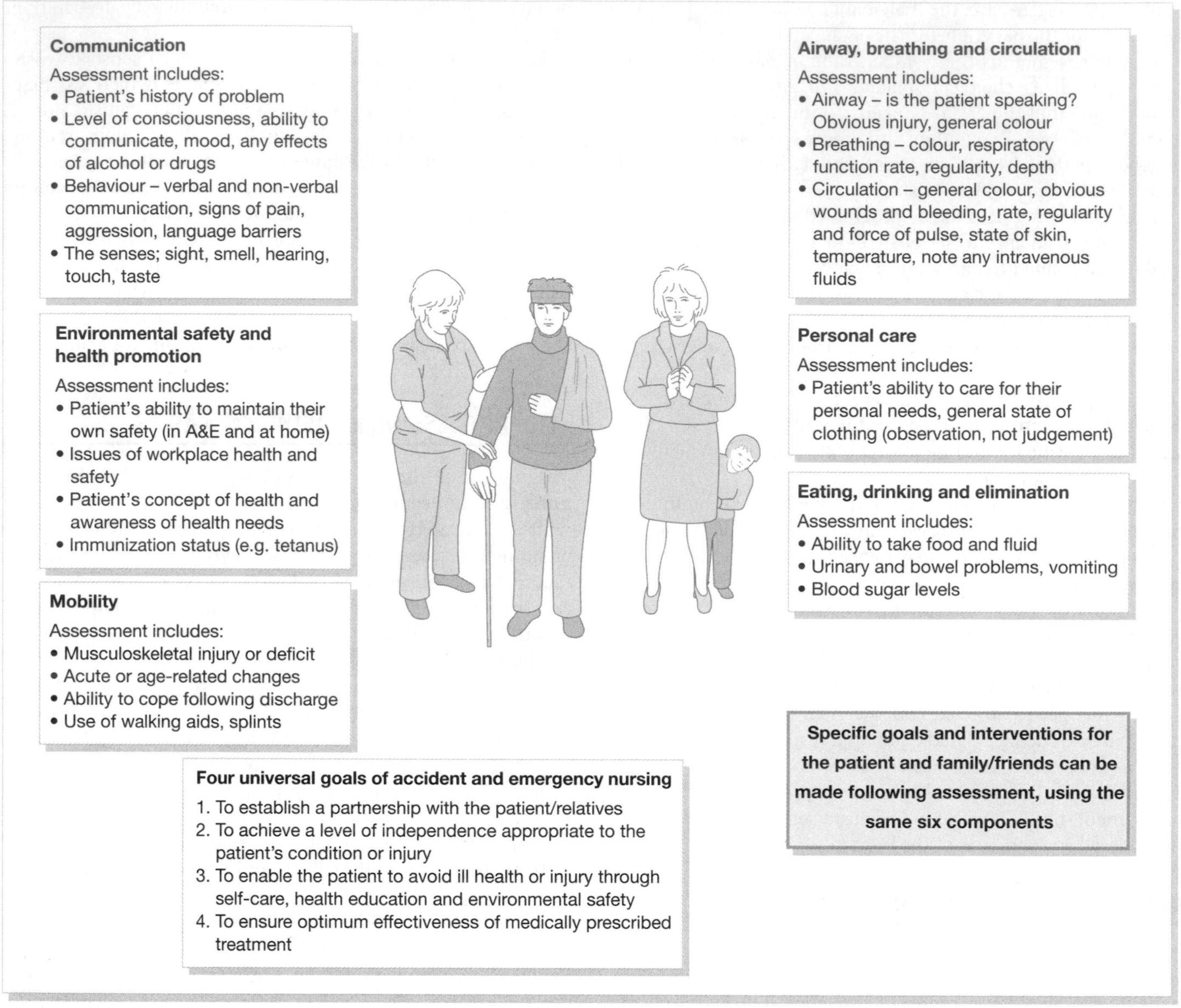

Communication

Assessment includes:
- Patient's history of problem
- Level of consciousness, ability to communicate, mood, any effects of alcohol or drugs
- Behaviour – verbal and non-verbal communication, signs of pain, aggression, language barriers
- The senses; sight, smell, hearing, touch, taste

Environmental safety and health promotion

Assessment includes:
- Patient's ability to maintain their own safety (in A&E and at home)
- Issues of workplace health and safety
- Patient's concept of health and awareness of health needs
- Immunization status (e.g. tetanus)

Mobility

Assessment includes:
- Musculoskeletal injury or deficit
- Acute or age-related changes
- Ability to cope following discharge
- Use of walking aids, splints

Four universal goals of accident and emergency nursing

1. To establish a partnership with the patient/relatives
2. To achieve a level of independence appropriate to the patient's condition or injury
3. To enable the patient to avoid ill health or injury through self-care, health education and environmental safety
4. To ensure optimum effectiveness of medically prescribed treatment

Airway, breathing and circulation

Assessment includes:
- Airway – is the patient speaking? Obvious injury, general colour
- Breathing – colour, respiratory function rate, regularity, depth
- Circulation – general colour, obvious wounds and bleeding, rate, regularity and force of pulse, state of skin, temperature, note any intravenous fluids

Personal care

Assessment includes:
- Patient's ability to care for their personal needs, general state of clothing (observation, not judgement)

Eating, drinking and elimination

Assessment includes:
- Ability to take food and fluid
- Urinary and bowel problems, vomiting
- Blood sugar levels

Specific goals and interventions for the patient and family/friends can be made following assessment, using the same six components

Figure 30.1 The Components of Life model. A model of A&E nursing using six components of life. (Reproduced with permission from Jones 1990.)

Skills include effective communication, objectivity and the ability to make rapid clinical decisions, in order to achieve the best care for every patient. The triage nurse has to avoid being seen as the 'gatekeeper' of A&E, to whom patients must prove that they really are an emergency.

Many A&E departments have a designated triage area, providing some privacy from the rest of the waiting area. However, a difficult balance has to be struck between the preservation of dignity, and visibility and access to and from the triage nurse.

Triage standards

The triage nurse is faced with the difficult task of identifying the sickest patients, whilst providing a service for the large numbers of people whose problem may not be serious, yet who suffer long waits.

A standard triage scale (Crouch & Marrow 1996) was designed to provide five categories of urgency, indicating appropriate waiting times for patients (see Box 30.1).

Triage is a dynamic process. The condition of patients may improve or deteriorate and their need for attention will alter. People in pain require special attention, as their distress can lead to dissatisfaction. Pain relief must therefore be seen as a high priority, which can be altered when the person is more comfortable.

The skills of patient assessment

The purpose of assessment is to know what is normal and what is not. In the A&E setting, this also has to be done with some degree of speed. However, first impressions can be made, not just about the patient, but also by the patient. With

Box 30.1 The standard triage scale. A priority scale developed for national use indicating target waiting times and colour coding for patients between triage assessment and treatment. (Reproduced with permission from Crouch & Marrow 1996.)

- *Immediate resuscitation (red) – patients in need of immediate treatment for the preservation of life.* All patients seen on arrival. These patients would usually be met by a team 'standing by' after prior notification by the ambulance
- *Very urgent (orange) – seriously ill or injured patients whose lives are not in immediate danger.* All these patients should be seen within 10 minutes of arrival
- *Urgent (yellow) – patients with serious problems but apparently in a stable condition.* All these patients should be seen within 60 minutes of arrival
- *Standard (green) – standard A&E cases without immediate danger or distress.* The aim should be for these patients to be seen within 120 minutes. The percentage that can be seen within this time depends on resources available. Few departments in the UK can achieve rates above 80%
- *Non-urgent(blue) – patients whose conditions are not true accidents or emergencies.* If these patients are to be treated in A&E, they should not have to wait more than 240 minutes to be seen. The percentage seen within 240 minutes will depend on the resources available. Patients in this category may be redirected to more appropriate facilities

Department of Health targets state that 90% of all patients attending A&E departments must spend no more than 4 hours from arrival to discharge, admission or transfer (DOH 2001).

this in mind, let us consider some of the skills required to carry out effective triage.

Visual assessment
Significant data can be gathered by observing patients as they approach the triage area. Facial expression, manifestations of pain (see Ch. 7), obvious injury, general colour and state of well-being can be assessed. Establishing eye contact with patients communicates to them that the nurse is interested and cares about their problem.

Listening
Listening is not just lending an ear, but hearing and paying attention. Unfortunately, our ability to concentrate on what is being said to us can be affected by pressures of the workload. There is a danger of appearing impatient and missing vital clues. Further skill is required to assess children and those whose communication is affected, e.g. speech or hearing difficulties, a learning disability or a language barrier (see Ch. 3).

Keeping an open mind avoids false assumptions. For example, the young woman with a head injury may simply have tripped over on her way to work. Alternatively, she may have collapsed because of an eating disorder.

Both what the patient says and does not say are of equal importance, as the real reason for coming to hospital could turn out to be something quite different. The man with shortness of breath may have a respiratory problem, or may be suffering from stress, due to work and family pressures.

Taking an accurate history
Information must be gathered quickly in order to act if the need arises. Obtaining a patient history is more than asking a series of questions. As a triage nurse gains experience, questions are posed which are relevant to the suspected problem.

Making decisions
Decisions are the end result of data gathered during the assessment process. When you choose where to go on holiday, you consider various factors – the climate, journey time, accommodation, etc. Once you have the information, you make your decision. Deciding what is right for the patient in A&E means fitting together the pieces to obtain a full picture, so that priorities of care will emerge.

Being sure
Patients present confusing pictures at times, and the jigsaw pieces may not appear to fit together properly. You must be able to justify what you think you see or hear. A patient who complains of indigestion may in fact have cardiac pain. Symptoms that are at odds with the findings of assessment may be concealing another problem.

The first aim of triage is to identify patients with life-threatening needs. Just as an airline pilot double-checks every piece of information, so should the nurse whose responsibility it is to assess and prioritize the patients in A&E. It is safer to believe the patient is sick until proven otherwise.

The role of triage is a complex one. However, rich insights can be gained into the diversity of people and their behaviour, and triage demands nursing care at its most intricate.

HEALTH PROMOTION AND THE PREVENTION OF ACCIDENTS

The majority of injury and illness seen in the A&E department is not serious, and clearly there is no place for imposing health promotion upon the badly injured victim of a road accident. However, there are many opportunities for health promotion with patients who present with minor problems.

People come to A&E because they have already sustained an injury or are ill, and therefore prevention of disease tends to be secondary in nature, aiming to minimize risk to health by complications of existing injury or illness.

Patients may only perceive advice regarding recovery from their current problem as important, rather than future prevention (Baelz 1979). General health education may not be a high priority for someone whose prime concern is to leave A&E, return home and resume normal life.

Fluctuating workloads in A&E sometimes limit the provision of health education; however, the large number of people who come to A&E every day can benefit from some form of health promotion.

Written health promotion material is useful and should be supplied in other languages, with enlarged print for patients with impaired vision. However, health advice leaflets should augment, rather than substitute, verbal advice. Health promotion videos in waiting areas are popular, although dissatisfaction may grow if the patient is still waiting when the programme repeats itself.

ACCIDENTS

We live in a risk-taking society where people, particularly young adults, drive powerful vehicles, consume alcohol, experiment with drugs and participate in dangerous sport and leisure activities. An accident is an unforeseen or unexpected event, which makes use of the term seem inappropriate. However, the world would be a dull place without some adventure (at least the legal ones), and yet the more we strive for something new, the more we place our health at risk. In 1999, road traffic accidents caused 3423 fatalities and 39 122 serious injuries in Great Britain (RoSPA 2001).

The UK government aims to reduce accidental deaths by 20% by the year 2010 (Department of Health 1999), focusing on the young and older age groups, and specific responsibility for the provision of health promotion was placed on A&E departments.

Health promotion has to be realistic and achievable, and should reflect individual circumstances. There is no point telling the lone parent of three young children to rest a sprained ankle. An assessment of the home situation and any support that may be needed is probably of greater value.

Basic first aid practices need to be reinforced. Many people do not think to place minor scalds and burns under cool running water, or to apply direct pressure to a bleeding wound.

PROTECTING CHILDREN

Whilst this book is directed towards adult nursing, it would be wrong to ignore the importance of protecting vulnerable children, as they represent approximately a quarter of all A&E attendances.

Children should be assessed and treated in designated areas, and cared for by a registered sick children's nurse. Fortunately, the vast majority of accidents and illnesses in children are entirely genuine; however, formal procedures exist should abuse, in any form, be suspected. These include child protection registers and multidisciplinary child protection teams.

There is enormous scope for accident prevention education within the younger age groups. Schemes involving A&E nurses are targeting 10- to 12-year-olds, in the hope of influencing their perception of health and safety before risk-taking behaviour develops (Orzel 1996). Issues include the wearing of cycle helmets and the dangers of drugs and alcohol.

MANAGING THE A&E DEPARTMENT

The nurse in charge or lead nurse in A&E assumes a similar role to that of a traffic policeman – remaining visible, directing the flow, and generally keeping the A&E department as clear and calm as possible. One of the key skills is constant and effective communication.

DIRECTING THE TRAFFIC

A great deal of thought and planning goes into the movement of patients in and out of A&E. The patients who often wait the longest are those with minor injuries, whose need for physical attention is not as high. Nursing and medical team leaders have to maintain a consistent flow for this group, who otherwise run the risk of slipping further back in the queue as each hour passes.

Moving patients around to clear space can be bewildering and impersonal for them. If care is not taken to communicate appropriately, patients may feel they have been forgotten or that they do not matter. Responsibility falls to the lead nurse to ensure patient comfort is attended to, communication is effective, and collaboration takes place within the multidisciplinary team.

DIRECTING THE TEAM

Appropriate rostering and allocation of staff has to reflect fluctuating workloads in A&E. The early morning is often quieter than late evening and shift times may have to alter accordingly. If resources are not used effectively, waiting times will increase, along with patient dissatisfaction.

Responsibility placed upon junior medical staff is enormous, as they encounter illness and injury completely new to them. The lead nurse has a large part to play in providing guidance and support for medical colleagues.

The diversity of problems seen in A&E means that nurses will see patients with variable levels of dependency; for example, someone with acute mental illness or multiple injuries will require considerable nursing and medical input. A nurse with advanced life support training is best placed to care for patients in the resuscitation room, although nurses new to A&E can develop their practice and confidence by working alongside an experienced colleague. This way, skills are passed on, the patient is cared for safely, and the team remains motivated.

Matching the person with the job

Accident and emergency offers enormous scope for the development of nursing skills and the lead nurse is responsible for ensuring that appropriate nursing care is delivered by the right person at the right time.

Many A&E nurses practise wound closure, casting (plaster of Paris), interpretation of electrocardiographs (ECGs) and defibrillation. Some thrive on the excitement of being part of a team in the resuscitation room, feeling this represents what A&E nursing is really about. However, nurses should also consider the risk to pressure areas (see Ch. 10) and other problems caused by waiting for long periods on a hard trolley; this is especially important when older people are in the department (see Older Adults: Nursing Priorities box 30.1). The fundamental aspects of care, such as physical comfort and psychological support, are as much a part of A&E nursing as advanced skills.

Sharing the skills

Learning opportunities in A&E are endless, as just about every speciality is encompassed within the client group.

People with diverse characteristics and interests make up a team; therefore, professional development for A&E nurses

OLDER ADULTS: NURSING PRIORITIES

30.1 Older adults with neck of femur fractures

The majority of neck of femur fractures occur in older adults, usually as a result of a fall. They represent approximately 60 000 A&E cases a year and this figure is likely to increase with an ageing population. Ninety-six per cent of these patients waited on an A&E trolley for longer than the recommended hour (Audit Commission 1996). This increases risks of pressure ulcer development, possibly after lying undiscovered on the floor at home. Immobilization of the injured limb threatens skin integrity. Many patients arrive cold, dehydrated and disorientated. The A&E environment may exacerbate confusion.

A 'fast track' system improves quality of care (Ryan et al 1996, Morley 1998). Priority assessment involves pain relief, fluid replacement and X-rays, before prompt admission to a ward. Early surgery can enhance a favourable outcome.

The nursing assessment and intervention includes:

- effective communication and reassurance
- observations of pulse, respiratory rate and blood pressure
- orientation to environment
- pain assessment and careful positioning of the injured limb to achieve maximum comfort, e.g. in a foam trough
- risk assessment – of pressure ulcer development, safety in A&E, etc.
- use of pressure-relieving mattress
- involvement of relatives and carers
- assessment of previous level of dependency
- general health needs.

References

Audit Commission. By accident or design: improving A&E services in England and Wales. London: HMSO; 1996.

Morley J. The case for 'fast tracking' fractured neck of femur patients. J Orthop Nurs 1998; 2: 91–94.

Ryan J, Ghani M, Staniforth P, Bryant G, Edwards S. 'Fast-tracking' patients with a proximal femoral fracture. J Emerg Med 1996; 13: 108–110.

should be tailored to suit the needs of the individual. Some A&E nurses are skilled in caring for the critically ill, and others demonstrate expertise in caring for older adults or children, or perhaps show a particular interest in wound management.

The A&E environment is an ideal setting in which to study human diversity, and one in which nurses can increase their confidence and skills in relating to people's needs at a time of crisis.

THE ROLE OF THE EMERGENCY NURSE PRACTITIONER IN A&E

The Scope of Professional Practice (UKCC 1992) has enabled experienced A&E nurses to develop their role and enhance the care of patients with less serious injuries, the largest group attending A&E departments.

As waiting times in A&E departments increase, role expansion provides an alternative means of access to health care. Groups of patients are managed by the nurse, from admission to discharge, within locally agreed protocols.

The Royal of College of Nursing (1992) offers a definition of the emergency nurse practitioner (ENP) as 'an accident and emergency nurse who has a sound nursing practice base in all aspects of accident and emergency nursing, with formal, post-basic education in holistic assessment, in physical diagnosis, in prescription of treatment and in the promotion of health'.

Key characteristics of the role are autonomous practice and accountability, providing care independent of direct medical supervision (Dillner 1995). Perhaps the skills which distinguish the role of the nurse practitioner from that of doctor's assistant are those of holistic assessment and the promotion of health and caring, principles which fit within nursing.

Resource management is increasingly important, and cost-effectiveness of role development must be assured, but should not be considered in purely financial terms. A competent A&E nurse, who has received recognized training, has the benefit of expertise and experience to provide continuity of care for patients and their families and to deliver effective health promotion. This is particularly important for those isolated in their need for health care, such as the homeless.

RESUSCITATION IN THE A&E DEPARTMENT

Caring for the critically ill patient, and being part of the resuscitation team, can be one of the most rewarding experiences in A&E nursing.

A resuscitation area is designed for the assessment and treatment of patients whose injury or illness is life-threatening. Equipment is readily available to deal with any eventuality.

Less than 0.5% of patients who attend A&E departments are critically ill or injured (Audit Commission 1996); however, demands upon health care resources to care for them are extremely high. A&E teams must therefore ensure that they are trained, rehearsed and prepared to receive the sickest patients at short notice.

Successful resuscitation depends upon a number of factors, many of which can be influenced by A&E nurses.

THE ENVIRONMENT

Whatever the size of the resuscitation room, A&E nurses can improve patient care by reviewing working practices, equipment, and health and safety issues.

Equipment may be arranged according to the order in which it is required. Think about the ABC of basic resuscitation (see Ch. 19). Items of equipment for management of the airway may be stored next to items for breathing, and so on. Checking and cleaning everything on a regular basis may seem tedious, but is an excellent way to become familiar with the area.

Noise, mess, poor lightening and non-functioning equipment are some of the greatest stressors for the team and the patient, as well as risks to safety. A&E nurses can promote changes that benefit patient care and enhance team performance, simply by examining the way they work.

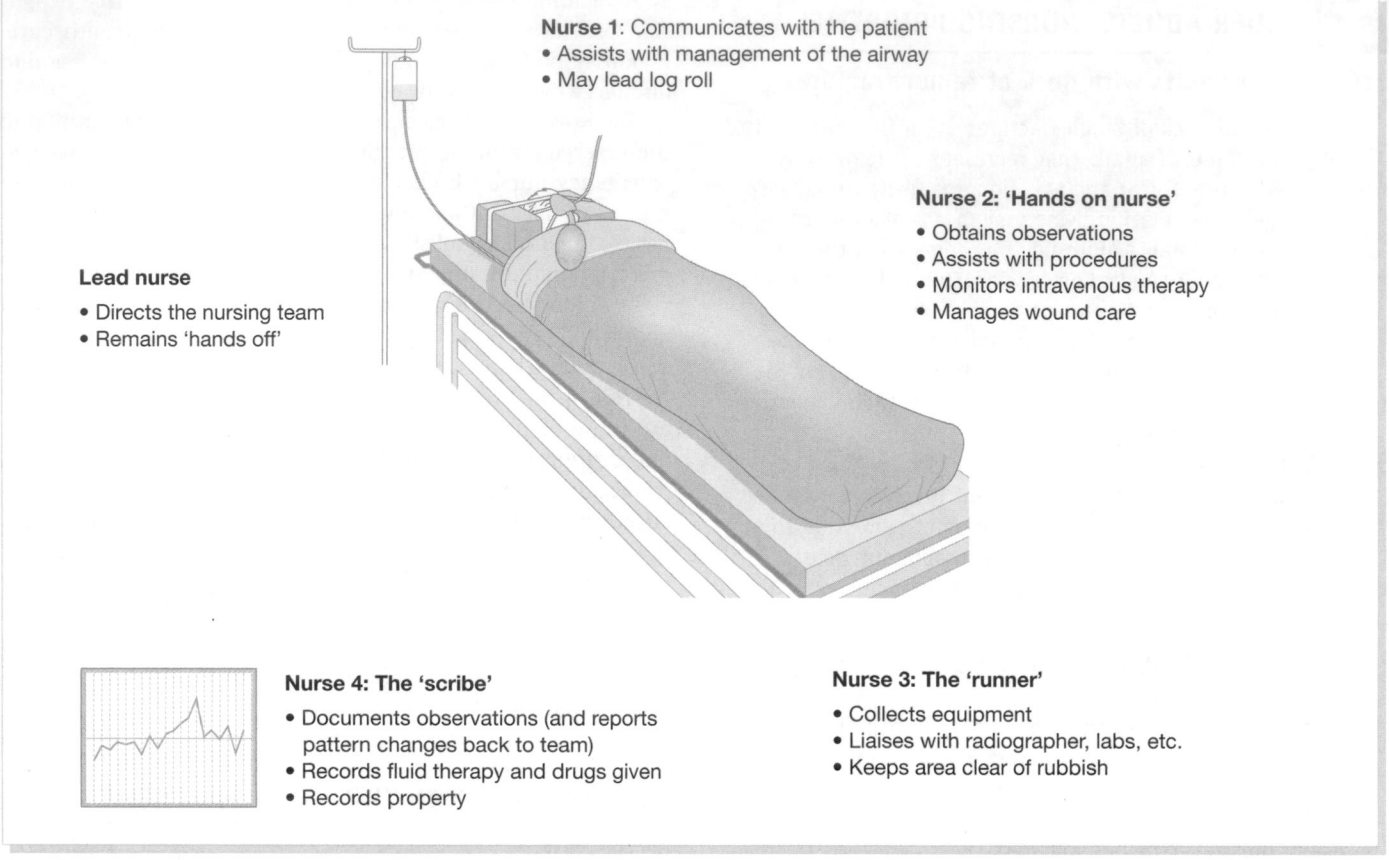

Nurse 1: Communicates with the patient
• Assists with management of the airway
• May lead log roll

Lead nurse
• Directs the nursing team
• Remains 'hands off'

Nurse 2: 'Hands on nurse'
• Obtains observations
• Assists with procedures
• Monitors intravenous therapy
• Manages wound care

Nurse 4: The 'scribe'
• Documents observations (and reports pattern changes back to team)
• Records fluid therapy and drugs given
• Records property

Nurse 3: The 'runner'
• Collects equipment
• Liaises with radiographer, labs, etc.
• Keeps area clear of rubbish

Figure 30.2 The nursing team in resuscitation. An example of roles available to the nurse when caring for the patient in the resuscitation room.

THE TEAM

Resuscitation teams are effective when team members adopt specific, pre-agreed roles, which can be carried out simultaneously (Driscoll & Vincent 1992). A&E nurses can decide the roles most appropriate for them within the team.

The number of staff available varies between A&E departments and is influenced by the time of day. However, effective teamwork is possible with just three people present, if leadership, trust and collaboration are achieved. Figure 30.2 demonstrates some of the roles available to the nurse during resuscitation.

The resuscitation team needs a visible leader, who has the knowledge and communication skills to direct the team members. Many A&E nurses perform this role as well as their medical colleagues. You do not have to observe many teams to realize that the most effective leader is not necessarily the person with the loudest voice.

In order to improve the standard of care and ensure the most efficient use of resources, staff must be given the skills (Mitchell 1999). Supervised practice and formal training in advanced life support methods can achieve this. Simulated patient scenarios are effective, as they actively involve the learner.

Many of the people involved in caring for the critically ill or injured patient have no direct contact with the patient. However, the A&E department would not function without the input of laboratory technicians, porters, cleaners, ambulance crew, the police, clerical staff, chaplains and, of course, the family.

HEALTH AND SAFETY

The speed required to care for critically ill patients may increase the health and safety risks if they are not anticipated. Sharp objects, such as needles, must be disposed of appropriately, as indeed should any rubbish. Staff need to protect themselves from body fluids with a minimum of gloves, water-resistant gowns and eye protection, when caring for the trauma patient.

X-rays are normally obtained in the resuscitation area, and therefore lead aprons or radiation-impermeable screens should be considered standard.

THE PATIENT

The person who has suffered serious injury or illness is in danger, despite best intentions, of being further assaulted by crowds, noise, pain, and threat to their dignity and warmth (see Reflective Practice box 30.1). In the resuscitation room, where speed is of the essence, the execution of nursing tasks can take precedence over vital communication, leaving the patient void of human contact.

REFLECTIVE PRACTICE

30.1 Psychological care of the patient in the resuscitation room

'More urgent voices, speaking with rapid energy, treating me as an object, to be lifted and carried and moved this way and that ... I feel the muscles and movements of people all around me, above me, at my side, behind me. Nobody engages me as a person, speaks with head directed towards me, communicates with me. I exist as a mass, I have physicality, but no personality. I am simply the object of other people's decision. They point their mouths to each other, never towards my head, I am totally present, the centre of all the energetic talking, but I am never included in the discussion, my will, my existence is being violated, I am banished even while in the group.'

Student activities

Consider the emotions and anxieties which may be experienced by the patient in the resuscitation room. How can the A&E team minimize these feelings and prevent further psychological trauma?

Reference

Sachs A. Albie Sachs: The soft vengeance of a freedom fighter. London: Grafton Books; 1990, pp 7–32.

The A&E team has a responsibility to protect the patient, not only from further physical harm, but also from psychological trauma. Talking, listening and touch are some of the most important skills a nurse can use and cannot be underestimated if psychological suffering is to be avoided (Tippett 1994). The patient is likely to feel helpless, out of control, disorientated and isolated, feelings which may be lessened by appropriate use of these basic skills.

Explaining procedures in simple terms and telling patients where they are and what time it is can alleviate much of their anxiety. Importantly, the A&E nurse should remember that unconscious patients might be able to hear what is being said.

Whilst this should be the primary role of a designated nurse, all the team members need to be aware of the psychological impact of being a patient in the resuscitation room.

Pain control should be addressed early, as patients may be unable to ask or may not feel they can ask. Furthermore, their distress may also be heightened by a full bladder, by the cold and by lying on a hard trolley.

Noise levels rise as team adrenaline (epinephrine) levels increase during resuscitation, so keeping the number of people immediately around patients to a minimum reduces the assault upon them and calms the atmosphere.

Removing clothing encroaches on dignity, and loss of body heat is perilous for the seriously ill patient. Pre-warmed intravenous fluids and blankets or carefully controlled overhead heaters are essential pieces of equipment (see Ch. 5).

The resuscitation room is an awe-inspiring place for the nurse new to A&E; however, the small acts of caring are as vital to the patient as the ability to operate the most complicated machinery.

Witnessed resuscitation

Many friends and relatives are present during prehospital resuscitation, only to be prevented from entering the resuscitation room when they arrive in the A&E department.

There are many reasons why relatives are prevented from attending resuscitation, and the issue is a complicated one. In trying to do the best for the patient, health care providers do not want to be seen to fail. In a situation where tension often runs high and difficult decisions have to be made, many staff find it impossible to cope with the presence of relatives. Some fear relatives will become disruptive and therefore hinder the care given to the patient.

Nurses must consider whether the duty of care owed to the patient (UKCC 1996, NMC 2002) extends to the relative. Do we risk harming them as a result of what they might see or hear, things that may remain with them, particularly if the patient dies?

One of the earliest studies proved overwhelmingly that the vast majority of relatives who attended resuscitation gained great comfort from being given that opportunity, regardless of the outcome (Hanson & Strawser 1992). The ability to be there at such a critical time was of enormous importance to them.

Some relatives simply wish to be present in the resuscitation room for a few seconds, to satisfy their need to know that something is being done. Support must be given by a designated nurse, who has received special training, in order to prepare them and to anticipate reactions and unspoken concerns. Wherever possible, the team benefits from time to prepare themselves for relatives coming into the resuscitation room, allowing for bloodstained clothing and distressing wounds to be covered.

The decision to stop resuscitation may be difficult in the presence of family members. However, if guidelines are agreed and followed by the whole team, it is possible to manage the situation sensitively and therefore minimize the distress to the relatives.

Clearly, if witnessed resuscitation is to succeed, all the issues must be addressed by all the team members who will be involved in the patient's care, and who must be able to voice their concerns without fear of reproach (see Ethical Issues box 30.1).

CARING FOR THE PATIENT WITH MAJOR TRAUMA

The arrival of a patient with serious injury presents one of the most challenging aspects of A&E nursing. Trauma transcends all age groups and is the single most common cause of death in people under 40 years of age (Robertson & Redmond 1994).

Primary prevention includes legislation, e.g. compulsory seat belts, crash helmets and the enforcement of motoring legislation. Advanced technology has resulted in safer car design (e.g. driver air bags). However, accidents will happen, violent injury in young adults persists, and the A&E department must be able to deliver the highest standard of care to victims of major trauma.

ETHICAL ISSUES

30.1 Witnessed resuscitation

Mr Roberts (not his real name), a 52-year-old father of two, is brought into the resuscitation room with a cardiac arrest after collapsing at home. The ambulance crew at the scene commenced cardiopulmonary resuscitation. On arrival in A&E, his wife says that she would like to stay with her husband. The physician leading the resuscitation team states that her presence will impede medical efforts and he is not happy for her to be there.

- What are the key issues for Mrs Roberts and the A&E staff?
- How do you feel about the presence of relatives in the resuscitation room?

Student activities

- Outline ways in which witnessed resuscitation could be introduced into the A&E department.
- Explain how a nurse could support relatives when accompanying them in the resuscitation room.

Trauma care in the UK has developed in the last 15 years, since disturbing evidence emerged that 20% of the deaths were avoidable (Royal College of Surgeons 1988). A structured approach was adopted with the principles of (American College of Surgeons 1997):

- rapid assessment
- intervention and resuscitation of life-threatening injury
- appropriate ongoing evaluation and management.

The Advanced Trauma Life Support (ATLS) method (American College of Surgeons 1997) is now practised widely throughout the UK. The airway, breathing and circulation (ABC) approach is used to identify the priorities of care. In other words, a patient with an airway problem is likely to die more quickly than a patient with a breathing problem, and so on.

Where resources allow a team of people to care for the trauma patient, the stages of the process can be carried out simultaneously. The priority is to recognize and deal with injuries from which the patient will die unless quickly treated. If everyone is familiar with a set of protocols and adopts pre-agreed roles, then the patient will receive the highest level of care (Driscoll & Vincent 1992).

NURSING ROLES WITHIN TRAUMA MANAGEMENT

A&E nurses have a large part to play in the assessment and resuscitation of the trauma patient, as they are often the first person to meet the patient. Other roles include (Hadfield 1993):

- communication
- planning
- evaluation
- documentation
- debriefing
- advocacy.

A nurse with minimal experience in A&E can be part of the team, carrying out fundamental aspects of care.

ASSESSMENT AND MANAGEMENT

The A&E department often receives prior warning of a patient's arrival, which allows for the preparation of the resuscitation area and the team.

Initial assessment consists of (American College of Surgeons 1997):

- a primary survey
- a secondary survey
- a definitive care phase.

The primary survey

This is the phase in which the patient is assessed within a straightforward 'ABCDE' system.

A – Airway with cervical spine control

Assessment of the airway includes:

- talking to the patient to assess a response – an unconscious patient is at risk of airway obstruction
- looking in the mouth for signs of obvious injury or vomit
- checking the face for swelling, which may compromise the airway
- noting the patient's general colour.

All trauma patients require a high percentage of oxygen and this must be delivered early. Multiple injuries caused by a fall or speed-related incident, or any significant injury above the shoulders, may also damage the vulnerable neck – the cervical spine. Until this can be excluded, caring for the patient includes immobilization of the whole spine, in particular the head and neck. This is best achieved by application of a semi-rigid neck collar and head restraints, in conjunction with a spinal board (see Evidence-based Practice box 30.1).

B – Breathing and ventilation

There is no point putting air into a punctured tyre and the same applies to a patient's chest. Injuries to the chest may impede oxygenation (see Ch. 20), and some of these are life-threatening. Assessment of the chest includes:

- rate and depth of respiration
- observation of unequal movement of the chest on respiration
- noting the patient's general colour – the trauma patient with impaired ventilation may appear pale or cyanosed (a bluish discoloration, particularly noticeable around the mouth)
- assessing normal entry of air into the lungs – this is done by listening with a stethoscope and comparing both sides (auscultation).

Signs of external injury may indicate underlying damage. For example, visible bruising suggests heavy force was applied to the chest, and therefore the internal organs.

An effective assessment tool for assessment of respiratory function is oxygen saturation measurement, using pulse oximetry recordings (see Chs 9, 20 and 31).

EVIDENCE-BASED PRACTICE

30.1 The use of spinal boards in A&E

- The long spinal board was developed as an extrication device at the scene of an accident. Patients with potential spinal injuries can be slid onto a hard surface and removed from a vehicle. A semi-rigid neck collar and head restraints are applied, and the patient is strapped to the board.
- Many patients remain on spinal boards in A&E for prolonged periods – often due to the anxiety of staff in removing the board before spinal injury can be excluded.
- Advanced Trauma Life Support (ATLS) protocols (American College of Surgeons 1997) state that spinal boards are intended for use before and during transfer only. Removal should be prompt, following exclusion of life-threatening injury.
- Studies show that patients are at risk of developing pressure ulcers over bony areas, e.g. back of head, coccyx and heels (Main & Lovell 1996).
- Lying strapped to a hard spinal board is uncomfortable and frightening. Discomfort may lead to excessive movement and, therefore, further injury.
- A firm trolley mattress is a more comfortable and appropriate support for the spine; or a vacuum mattress, which moulds to the body. A semi-rigid collar and head restraints must still be applied.
- Sexton (1999) suggests trauma-trained A&E nurses can take the decision to remove spinal boards, following agreed criteria. Removal should be carried out using the recognized four-person log roll.

References

American College of Surgeons (Committee on Trauma). Advanced Trauma Life Support Programme. Illinois: American College of Surgeons; 1997.

Main P, Lovell M. A review of seven surfaces with emphasis on their protection of the spinally injured. J Accid Emerg Med 1996; 13: 34–37.

Sexton J. Can nurses remove spinal boards and cervical collars safely? Emerg Nurse 1999; 6(9): 8–12.

C – Circulation with haemorrhage control

The state of the circulation (see Ch. 9) is easily assessed from a few basic observations:

- noting the patient's colour
- level of consciousness
- rate, rhythm and force of the pulse
- noting any obvious external bleeding – like putting air into a punctured tyre, there is little point pouring water into a leaking bath, so any external haemorrhage must be controlled by direct pressure or elevation

Along with oxygen, trauma patients need adequate amounts of warm fluid and debate continues about what is the best fluid for trauma patients. Hartmann's solution, described as a crystalloid solution, is widely accepted, as it has the ability to restore circulation as a temporary measure. Transfusion of compatible blood is the gold standard for many trauma patients.

Blood samples are obtained when the patient arrives, which include full blood count, urea and electrolytes, and blood group and cross-match for transfusion purposes.

D – Disability

Disability is described as the presence of any neurological deficit, which may result from loss of blood (hypovolaemia), oxygen shortfall (hypoxia) or brain injury.

In the initial stages of resuscitation, a brief neurological assessment only is carried out, using the Glasgow Coma Scale. Patients receive a numerical score, which relates to their ability to open their eyes, know who and where they are, and follow simple commands (see Ch. 14). The size and reaction to light of both pupils are also noted.

E – Exposure and environment

At this point, all clothing is removed to allow full assessment of the patient's body, front and back. This has to be done safely and gently. Clothing may have to be cut, which must be explained to the patient beforehand.

The patient is turned over, using a method described as the 'log roll', the purpose of which is to maintain immobility of the entire spine while the patient is turned through a continuous plane. To achieve this immobility, a minimum of four people is required (Advanced Trauma Nursing Course 1999).

This is the ideal time to remove debris from underneath the patient and to straighten sheets, whilst preserving dignity and warmth.

The secondary survey

Once life-threatening injury has been excluded and any resuscitation measures have proved effective, a secondary survey is carried out, during which other injuries are identified, e.g. wounds or fractures.

Anti-tetanus immunization is considered alongside medication such as antibiotic therapy. Pain relief must be addressed early, particularly as many procedures may increase patient distress, and they may injure themselves further by moving around. Intravenous opiates (see Ch. 7), e.g. morphine sulphate, are useful for the trauma patient.

These issues may appear trivial compared with major injuries; however, an overlooked finger fracture could affect a patient's ability to work in the future. A wound infection might be catastrophic for vulnerable patients, such as the older adult and the very young, and patients left in pain throughout their ordeal may endure years of psychological trauma.

The definitive care phase

The definitive care phase is the final stage concerned with the ongoing management of trauma. This may mean transfer to the operating theatre, intensive care unit, ward, or perhaps a specialist unit. During transfer, team members with the relevant skills to continue their care en route should escort patients.

Planning a transfer takes a great deal of thought, even if the patient is moving only a few yards within the hospital. How many times have you left home in a hurry and forgotten something vital? Trauma patients are at their most vulnerable in transit, and should not leave the resuscitation room until all preparations are finalized. This means ensuring that the team taking over their care is informed and ready, equipment is collected and checked, documentation and property are complete, and relatives have been contacted.

Accurate documentation is essential, describing all aspects of care given to a patient. This ensures safe continuity of care and provides an effective communication tool. It is the responsibility of the A&E nurse to ascertain that patients' clothing, personal effects and valuables are documented and safeguarded prior to transfer.

CARING FOR THE PATIENT WITH MINOR TRAUMA

The greatest percentage of A&E attendances are people with injuries that are not very serious.

The development of nurse-led MIUs in the UK offers patients an appropriate alternative access to health care, whilst providing suitably skilled A&E nurses with the opportunity for autonomous and expert practice.

Patients may feel their problem is anything but minor, which explains some inconsistency between the severity of an injury or illness and the extent of their distress. Imagine yourself travelling to a job interview when you fall and cut your leg. Your new clothes are torn and muddy and you arrive in A&E to face a 2-hour wait, knowing you will miss the interview. The intuitive A&E nurse will understand that all patients feel they are an emergency case and need understanding and support, regardless of their problem.

Box 30.2 Acute wounds. The different types of wounds seen in the accident and emergency department

- *Abrasion* – a wound which damages the epidermis as a result of friction
- *Laceration* – a wound which extends through the epidermis, often involving deeper structures. The cut is linear but may have an irregular shape
- *Pretibial* – most commonly seen in the older adult. Laceration caused by tearing of the fragile skin of the shin (pretibial – in front of the tibia bone). Normally closed using adhesive strips
- *Penetrating wound* – may be as small as a puncture. A narrow track is formed, the depth of which is sometimes difficult to assess. Penetrating injuries include stab and gunshot wounds
- *Crush injury* – immensely painful injuries, due to damage to soft tissues, e.g. deckchair injury. Sometimes involve fractures. Require careful management
- *Bites* – produce ragged, sometimes deep wounds that need thorough cleansing. Not normally sutured because of high infection risk, due to high levels of bacteria in human and animal mouths. HIV and hepatitis B transmission must be considered in human bites. Anti-tetanus vaccination status must be ascertained

---

ASSESSING MINOR TRAUMA

Minor trauma injuries include soft tissue injury (sprains, strains and bruising), wounds, scalds and minor burns, uncomplicated fractures, skin rashes, bites and stings.

Assessment should follow a holistic structure, not just that of the injury itself. Table 30.1 outlines the nursing assessment of some common minor trauma problems, using some of the skills covered earlier in the section on triage.

The need for health promotion is evident in the many factors that cause minor injury, and these must be considered when treating and advising the individual, e.g. the welder who does not wear eye protection and incurs an eye injury, and the builder with a head laceration who was not wearing a hard hat on a building site.

Acute wound management

A variety of acute wounds are seen in A&E (Box 30.2). During the day, many of these are work-related, but once night falls, the influence of alcohol increases the number of falls and assaults (e.g. knife and glass injury) (see Ch. 10 for wound healing and care of chronic wounds).

The acute traumatic wounds seen in A&E are considered to be dirty and thorough cleansing is essential. The cleansing agent, e.g. physiological saline 0.9% (normal saline), should be warmed to body temperature and then gently irrigated over and into the wound (see Evidence-based Practice box 30.2).

Abrasions present their own difficulty, as grit can be tattooed into the skin (remember falling off a bicycle as a child). A local anaesthetic gel and soft scrubbing brush are extremely useful for this purpose, and are neither as gruesome nor as painful as they sound. Debris must be removed otherwise infection will occur. Closure of any wound is delayed until it can be assured that contaminants have been removed.

 EVIDENCE-BASED PRACTICE

30.2 Tap water as an irrigation agent for acute wounds in A&E

The most widely used solution for cleansing and irrigating A&E wounds is physiological saline 0.9%. Riyat & Quinton (1997) have shown that tap water can be used as safely for this purpose, as no bacterial colonization was found in tests. The benefits of using tap water include availability, plentiful supply and cost-effectiveness. However, Lawrence (1997) argues that water causes pain in raw tissue and can damage epithelial cells if the procedure is carried out regularly on the same area.

References
Lawrence J. Wound irrigation. Journal of Wound Care 1997; 6(1): 23–26.
Riyatt MS, Quinton DN. Tap water as a wound cleansing agent in accident and emergency. J Accid Emerg Med 1997; 14: 165–166.

Table 30.1 Assessing minor trauma. The assessment of minor trauma using a look, listen and feel approach

	Look for	Listen to	Feel for
Soft tissue injury (is it a fracture?)	Can patients walk, are they clutching a limb? Are they in pain? Deformity, swelling, colour and movement of area	What happened? How much force was involved? Was there a crack? Description of pain	Presence of pulse at site of injury Deformity of bone
Wounds	The type and size of wound, e.g. puncture, laceration, crush. It is old or new, dirty or clean? Is it bleeding? Underlying structures visible, e.g. tendon or bone. How deep is it? Is the patient in pain?	How and when it was caused *Note*: there is a time limit up to when some wounds can be sutured (normally up to 8 h) Was the accident preventable?	Distal pulses when wounds on limbs
Burns and scalds (see also Ch. 28)	The size and depth of burn As a rule, superficial burns are more painful as nerve endings are irritated, whereas they are destroyed in deep or full-thickness burns Visual signs of pain Any skin loss or blistering Colour of burn (red, black, white)	What happened and when? What was the cause? *Note*: electrical burns can be extensive, and not obvious to look at	Sensation in burned and surrounding area – good indication of burn depth – tested using gentle pinprick technique
Rashes	The type of rash (see Ch. 28) How far it extends. Is the patient scratching? Is there lice infestation? *Note*: swelling to the mouth or face, and breathing difficulty, indicate acute allergic reaction and require urgent intervention	When it started. History of new medication, change in diet, soap or washing powder. Any other symptoms, e.g. headache, neck stiffness	Temperature of the skin Is rash raised?
Bites and stings	The site of injury Bite or sting around mouth may endanger the airway Injury over joints and limbs may swell Signs of infection – redness Visual signs of pain	Is there a history of severe reaction to stings in the past? Animal or human bite	Warmth of skin may indicate infection if a bite is old

Most A&E wounds can be managed by what is called primary closure. The skin edges are brought together, using one of the methods outlined in Table 30.2.

Tetanus immunization

Tetanus is caused by the bacterium *Clostridium tetani*, a Gram-positive anaerobic bacterium. High-risk wounds are any wounds that have been contaminated with soil, or human or animal faeces, where the microorganism is found.

Toxins released by the microorganism affect the motor nerves. Ensuing muscle spasm will be fatal if respiratory muscles are involved.

Although immunization programmes in the UK have almost eradicated the disease, the A&E department has a responsibility to identify people at risk. These include the homeless, who may never have completed an immunization course, people whose work places them in contact with the soil (e.g. farmers), and older adults, who were born before vaccination started. This last group also takes part in more gardening activities, and therefore their risk may be higher.

Discharging the patient with minor trauma

Discharge advice requires consideration of a patient's individual social circumstances and concepts of health. Advice is only effective if patients feel it is appropriate and realistic for them. Telling someone to 'go home and rest' assumes they actually have one and, for the thousands of homeless people, is not practical.

When we say 'keep it clean', we need to remember that our idea of clean may not match that of the patient. The self-employed builder with a lacerated arm will probably not be able to keep it immobile or particularly clean. The same applies to the

Table 30.2 Closure of traumatic wounds. Some methods of wound closure in A&E

Method	Indications for use	After-care	Removal times
Sutures (stitches)	A clean wound with minimal tissue loss. Sutures are absorbable and non-absorbable and made from natural or synthetic fibres. Absorbable sutures are normally used internally or inside the mouth	Do not always require a wound dressing, depending on patient comfort and choice. Should be kept dry until removal, although hair can be washed once for most scalp wounds	Scalp: 7 days Face: 3–5 days Limb: 7–10 days Trunk: 7–10 days
Adhesive strips	Superficial lacerations with low tissue damage and wound tension. Better cosmetic result and lower reactions to material than sutures. Easy to apply and less traumatic for patients. Not generally suitable for wounds over joints, hair, or if wound bleeds excessively. Can be used in conjunction with sutures. Applied at intervals to allow wound to breathe	Dressing depends on site and patient comfort and lifestyle. Patient should avoid getting strips wet as they may fall off. Should not be re-applied	Face: 3–5 days Other areas: 5–7 days Pretibial lacerations: at least 10 days May be removed by patient without having to return to A&E
Surgical glue	For single, small wounds with minimal wound tension and bleeding. Edges of the wound are held together, drops of adhesive placed at intervals and held for a further period. Quick and easy to use, once practised. Less traumatic than sutures. Particularly useful for children. Minimal scarring	Normally requires wound to be kept dry for 5 days. Patient should be told to expect a scab to form. Gentle washing after 5 days dissolves scab and residual glue	
Skin staples	As for sutures, but used for linear wounds, i.e. not jagged in shape. Very quick to apply; however, not as accurate in closing wound as sutures. Scarring can be greater	As for sutures. Can be more painful to remove than sutures	7–10 days

chef with a burn, whose job will be offered to somebody else. Neither may disagree with the advice, but their priority is to make a living. Hence, the A&E nurse must offer sound reasons for health guidance and negotiate the minimum level of self-care each patient might achieve.

The choice of dressings and bandages should reflect the patient's lifestyle and ability to cope with having to change or reapply them.

For those patients with a minor injury, inadequate advice may lead to complications and delayed recovery, and we will have failed them if they have to return to the A&E department with the same problem.

SOCIAL ISSUES IN THE A&E DEPARTMENT

It is possible to witness almost every human weakness and suffering in the A&E department, which is often a regular port of call for people who have nowhere else to turn. A fundamental part of being an A&E nurse is to understand the depth of despair that brings some people through the doors.

The following are some of the more common problems encountered by the A&E nurse, a list that is by no means exhaustive.

ALCOHOL-RELATED ATTENDANCE

Alcohol is consumed by at least 90% of the population, and is the most commonly used recreational drug in our society (Taylor & Roberts 1998). Alcohol remains a major factor in road traffic deaths and in the incidence of assaults.

Lack of reasoning makes inebriated patients difficult to assess and treat, as they are more likely to walk out, perhaps with a life-threatening problem, or to become aggressive or violent towards A&E staff.

Patients may face negative attitudes from the people to whom they turn for help. The smell of alcohol on a patient's breath, particularly if he or she is uncooperative, leads us to make assumptions that may not represent a true picture of the situation. Imagine how your breath smells after a couple of drinks at the end of a stressful shift. You trip over on the way home, cut your head and arrive, disorientated, in your local A&E dept. Think of the distress and humiliation you would feel if you were treated as a social outcast.

Rather than assuming that anyone who staggers into A&E smelling of alcohol is merely drunk, we should look for other underlying illness or injury that may be complicated by alcohol. For example, a patient with a head injury is liable to be drowsy and may vomit, both of which could threaten the airway. This is because alcohol depresses the central nervous system. High levels of alcohol can cause patients to stop breathing, and therefore people who are severely intoxicated must be carefully observed, not simply left in the waiting area.

Patients with chronic alcohol dependence sometimes turn to A&E as a route of admission for treatment or 'detox'. Unfortunately, their attendance often occurs after a drinking binge, and most detoxification units will not admit patients when drunk, as their decision-making ability is affected.

Patients who have stopped, or reduced, their alcohol consumption and who are physically dependent on alcohol may attend suffering from alcohol withdrawal. Symptoms include restlessness, nausea, tremor, vomiting, seizures (fits) and hallucinations. These patients can be extremely ill, and many require admission into hospital.

DRUG DEPENDENCE

Walsh (1996) suggests that the use of such terms as 'alcoholic' and 'addict' is judgemental and will influence our treatment of an individual with needs. Few people fit into stereotypes and drug use involves all groups in society. Key issues for the A&E nurse are to be familiar with types of substance misuse and how they affect the patient. Commonly misused substances include:

- opioids, e.g. heroin
- solvents, e.g. glue, lighter fuel
- ecstasy (MDMA)
- amphetamines (speed)
- cocaine and crack
- LSD (acid)
- cannabis (dope, hash).

The greatest priority for patients who have taken any substance is to protect them from further harm. As with the inebriated person, they are a potential danger to themselves and to others, as behaviour can be unpredictable. Therefore, they may have to spend a long time in the A&E department while the effects of whatever they have taken wears off. Particular effects following drug usage are hard to predict as patients may have taken a mixture of substances, tolerance levels vary, and they may be reluctant to give a true history.

Pain relief for patients with a history of drug misuse is covered in Chapter 7.

VICTIMS OF VIOLENCE

Although violent crime has increased over the last 20 years, many cases still go unreported to the police. The A&E department sees the victims (and sometimes the alleged offender) of many violent incidents, and health care professionals often find themselves on the receiving end of verbal or physical aggression.

Shepherd (1998) suggests that the A&E department plays a pivotal role as a source of data on violence in society. For example, A&E nurses are able to provide links with the police and victim support groups in order to empower patients by encouraging the reporting of violence, whilst respecting patient confidentiality and offering care and support.

Domestic violence

We live in a society where violence in the home occurs with alarming regularity, to both women and men. To be attacked by a partner is humiliating and many people will fabricate an accident rather than admit the truth. The courage needed by the patient to tell the real story must be reciprocated with empathy and understanding.

There is little point in telling patients they should leave a violent partner and report the incident. The A&E nurse needs to remain impartial and empower victims of domestic abuse by being aware of support networks available and by offering health promotion information (Lane & Beales 1998). Self-help information can be displayed in waiting areas, and A&E staff should be able to access women's refuges, social services and counselling services.

Assessment of physical injury is the first priority, but a multifocal approach to the care of victims of domestic violence is essential for nurses to be able to offer the support so badly needed.

Rape and sexual assault

Victims of rape and sexual assault, whether male or female, are victims of violence as well as a sexual crime and they require the most sensitive care. In the aftermath of assault, the victim is likely to experience feelings of self-blame, lack of self-esteem and of being unclean. Whatever the circumstances, A&E nurses must be aware of the effect that their own judgements and values can have upon these vulnerable patients.

Dedicated police rape suites in many areas allow victims to be cared for in more appropriate surroundings by specifically trained police officers. Therefore, the A&E department is normally only involved where the victim has sustained physical injury. If rape and sexual assault are reported, the police must be involved immediately, as a police surgeon carries out examination unless serious injury requires medical intervention. Swabs are taken from body orifices, as well as fingernail clippings and blood samples. The victim's clothing will be placed in paper bags to preserve forensic evidence. All of this is carried out with caring and tact, as it adds to the person's distress and humiliation. He or she will, however, be supported by a designated, trained police officer throughout the process, up to the time of any court proceedings.

The decision to report rape and sexual assault to the police must rest firmly with victims. If the police are not involved, a full and accurate history, related only once, is vital. This is followed by gentle examination of injuries, providing time and explanations of all procedures. Blood samples and swabs may be obtained, with patient consent, in case they decide to report the assault at a later date.

Assessment must be carried out in the most comfortable and private area available, with designated nurse support. Advice regarding sexually transmitted infection and emergency contraception should be given. Above all, patients must feel empowered regarding their decision to report the assault or otherwise and must always be given details of a local rape crisis centre.

THE HOMELESS PERSON

The term 'homeless' refers to people living on the streets, in hostels, bed-and-breakfast accommodation and squats. Many of them are large families sharing one room in 'budget hotels', often in appalling conditions. Others may be refugees from one of the increasing number of war-torn areas of the world. The one thing they will all have in common is a need for health care, and for many the only place available to them is the A&E department.

Whilst many GP practices offer excellent community-based care for the homeless, some do not want the problems associated with this group of people and will avoid registering them. Many of the patients themselves will not register with a doctor as they constantly move around, or are present illegally, and therefore attend whichever A&E department is closest at the time.

Many A&E departments employ local GPs to provide primary care, and the role of the primary care nurse in some community areas has been developed to meet these needs.

Homeless people living on the streets are sometimes referred to as 'NFAs' (no fixed abode) or 'dossers', although these terms can add to the negative values placed upon them. Certainly, there are difficulties when caring for the homeless in A&E. Alcohol misuse is a problem and there is the potential for aggression to occur as a result. Homeless people who have been drinking heavily and are injured in any way should never be left in the waiting room simply because they are disruptive or dirty. Their injuries may be serious and they should not be overlooked merely because of assumptions made about them.

The A&E department is open 24 hours a day and the waiting room is warm and relatively comfortable. Turning out a homeless person after treatment, especially during winter, makes the A&E nurse appear heartless, but allowing the person to stay will not solve the underlying social problems. The A&E staff should develop links with the local community, social services and voluntary organizations.

Remember, most people without a permanent home would never choose to be living in the circumstance in which they find themselves.

DEALING WITH CHALLENGING BEHAVIOUR

The A&E department is a minefield of human emotion. There was a time when violence and aggression towards health care professionals was tolerated as being 'part of the job' and little training was offered to deal with challenging incidents. Today, with increasing violence and aggression in health care settings, the UK government and NHS Trusts are adopting a firm stand against those whose behaviour is considered antisocial (Health Service Advisory Committee 1997).

It is unrealistic to believe that all untoward incidents could be eliminated. To understand why, we must first consider some of the reasons why disruptive behaviour occurs (Box 30.3).

Every person who comes to A&E experiences some degree of stress. Some are able to cope with the emotional impact of sudden injury or illness and some are not, whether they be a patient, friend or relative. 'Becoming' a patient or relative results in a loss of control and independence, which leads to a feeling of vulnerability.

A weatherman could not predict a storm without knowledge of prevailing weather conditions. Whereas the storm may be unpreventable, there are many occasions when aggressive and violent behaviour can be avoided. Violence and aggression do not often erupt spontaneously, which means that we usually receive warning signs, should we choose to read them. Sometimes, health care staff get it wrong, and a single incident is distressing for everyone, leaving the staff feeling exposed. However, if environmental and human factors are addressed, dissatisfaction and confrontation might be anticipated and minimized.

HANDLING AGGRESSION

Some patients have expectations that far exceed the capabilities of the service. Challenging behaviour is upsetting at any time, and verbal abuse or threat of physical attack can be just as distressing as actual assault (see Reflective Practice box 30.2). This is particularly distressing when directed at an individual member of staff. Defusing aggression requires effective communication skills (see Ch. 3), including:

- reducing eye contact in this context
- respecting personal space
- lowering voice level
- adopting a non-aggressive body posture.

When defusion skills fail and personal safety is threatened, the emphasis is to remove oneself and others from danger and summon help, from colleagues, security staff or the police.

NHS Trusts are now confronting these problems, by providing staff with the skills to deal with violent incidents and making clear to the public that unacceptable behaviour will not be tolerated. Members of staff need support in the aftermath of an incident, and time to reflect upon the situation constructively, in order to learn from the experience for future practice.

All incidents of challenging behaviour, no matter how trivial, must be fully documented and reported according to individual hospital policy. This provides a record for potential legal proceedings and the basis by which we can examine the cause and effect of aggression in health care, so that it might be minimized in the future.

MENTAL HEALTH PROBLEMS IN A&E

Caring for the patient with mental health problems demands the use of appropriate communication and management skills. A busy A&E department is not an ideal environment for the management of a disturbed person, as nurses often feel anxious and underconfident and may have had little preparation to deal with disturbed and bizarre behaviour, where the use of familiar interventions is ineffective.

Acutely ill patients may be brought in from the streets against their will by the police, or from their homes by desperate friends and relatives. Equally, those with chronic problems often turn to A&E as a means of primary care.

Remember, people with existing mental health problems also have accidents and experience physical ill health, and the reason for their attendance may be physiological. False assumptions

Box 30.3 Causes of challenging behaviour in the accident and emergency department. Some of the internal and external factors predisposing to aggression

What patients bring to A&E
- Any past experiences of a similar situation
- Their own expectations and perceptions
- Cultural values and beliefs
- External influences, e.g. problems at home, child care, work commitments

Physiological causes
- Drug or alcohol misuse
- Drug or alcohol withdrawal
- Head injury, seizure
- Hypoglycaemia or hypoxia
- Mental illness, e.g. schizophrenia
- Infection (particularly in older people)

Pain
- Leaving patients in pain may reduce their coping mechanism further and is distressing for friends and family, who feel helpless. There is no reason why patients should have to wait a long time for pain relief, whether or not they have seen a doctor
- A&E nurses in many departments have been developing their practice in order to meet this need

What happens to patients in A&E
- Their future experience may be shaped depending on the care they receive
- Expectations and perceptions of staff may not match those of the patient, e.g. waiting times or treatment decisions
- Cultural values and beliefs of staff
- External influences, e.g. unpredictable waiting times, noise, distress of other patients

Comfort
- Environmental temperature, hard chairs, access to refreshments, reading material, TV/video, toilets and telephones

Communication
- All A&E patients are worried!
- They need to be told what is happening and why, otherwise expectations can become unrealistic and dissatisfaction grows

Waiting times
- Identified as a prime cause of aggression (Akerstrom 1997)
- The patient's acceptance of the wait is directly related to the issues above
- Initiatives to reduce waiting times include:
  — development of emergency nurse practitioner (ENP) role
  — minor injuries units
  — use of GPs in A&E to treat primary care patients
  — development of nurse roles to benefit patient care, e.g. nurse-requested X-ray service to reduce a secondary wait after seeing the doctor or ENP
- Patients should be informed if the waiting time increases substantially, e.g. the arrival of a seriously ill patient

Note. The two things patients most want addressed are the way they are received by staff and waiting times.

can be made, because of bizarre behaviour and because of difficulty patients may have in expressing symptoms and feelings.

In the countries of the UK, the relevant Mental Health Act allows for the legal detention of individuals against their will, where deemed necessary for their assessment and any ensuing treatment. The decision is made by a doctor, either the patient's GP or a psychiatrist, and an approved social worker. The patient's next of kin may sign the section papers, although this is uncommon nowadays.

Section 4 of the Mental Health Act (1983) is particularly relevant to the A&E department, in which a person may be compulsorily admitted to hospital for 72 hours, during which time an assessment is carried out.

The police may bring a person thought to be suffering from a mental health problem into hospital from a public place. This is referred to as Section 136, where the hospital is considered a place of safety.

CAUSES OF DISTURBED BEHAVIOUR

There are many reasons for acutely disturbed behaviour, some which reflect mental illness and others which are due to physical or metabolic problems, e.g. hypoglycaemia, haemorrhage or head injury. Language barriers or unfamiliar responses to acute

R|Я REFLECTIVE PRACTICE

30.2 Aggression in the A&E department

A young man arrives in A&E late at night. He has sustained a hand injury following a fight in a nightclub. The triage nurse has informed him of a 2-hour wait and the waiting room is full. After an hour, he complains to reception staff that the doctor has already seen people who arrived after him. A while later, he begins to shout at the nurse, stating that the service is unacceptable and that he intends to wait a further 10 minutes before leaving. The nurse informs him that a patient with serious injuries is being treated, the wait may well increase, and that perhaps he should not have been fighting. The patient walks out of the department, saying that he will complain.

Student activities
- What are the key areas for reflection in this incident?
- Discuss some of the factors that may have influenced the patient's aggression.
- How should the triage nurse handle the situation?
- What support will the staff members require following such an incident?

illness, pain or anxiety can cause us to misinterpret behaviour. The physical causes of behavioural disturbance can be considered the same as those that cause aggression and violence (Box 30.3).

An acute psychotic episode is one in which the patient suffers disordered thought processes and an inability to acknowledge what is real and what is not. Symptoms include delusions, illusions, confusion, hallucinations and lack of insight and reasoning. Some conditions precipitate physical and verbal aggression, which compound difficulties in management.

Schizophrenia

People with schizophrenia suffer from disordered thought patterns, dissociation and delusions, and an inability to distinguish reality from imaginings. They are often withdrawn from their surroundings and appear emotionless, although there is a risk of violence as a result of auditory hallucinations (hearing voices).

Depressive illness

Most people suffering from depression do not require hospital treatment, but for some, coming to A&E is a reflection of their despair at a time when they might be contemplating suicide. Patients who suffer from a bipolar affective disorder (manic depressive) experience extremes of mood, swinging from elation to deep depression.

Acute anxiety state

There is a world of difference between normal feelings of anxiety, something we all experience at times, and the extreme acute state for which there may be no obvious cause. People who suffer from panic attacks feel completely out of control and fear they will die. Presentation includes rapid breathing and pulse rate, sweating and carpopedal spasm that increase distress (see Chs 8 and 17). The spasm is caused by a reduction in carbon dioxide (CO_2) levels due to overbreathing (hyperventilation) which leads to a reduction in the amount of available calcium in the blood. Management of hyperventilation involves the patient breathing in and out of a paper bag, so that they re-inhale their own exhaled CO_2. Note that a patient with a life-threatening chest problem (e.g. tension pneumothorax) may be mistaken for someone having a panic attack, and therefore physical causes of breathing distress must be excluded beforehand.

RECOGNIZING THE PATIENT WITH AN ACUTE MENTAL HEALTH PROBLEM

Disruption caused by the behaviour of a disturbed person may be exacerbated if not dealt with calmly and speedily. The patient in the waiting area who is becoming agitated or increasingly inappropriate, threatening or loud may well be psychotic and warrants rapid assessment. The aim of assessment in A&E is to identify those whose need is truly urgent.

An accurate history is vital from all available sources – family and friends, ambulance crew or the police, if involved. Concealment of potential weapons, which may injure the patient or someone else, must be considered, although nurses may risk harm to themselves whilst attempting to remove something from an agitated person.

Society deems what is normal or tolerable behaviour and what is not. Concepts of mental ill health vary and some families deny mental health problems due to shame and stigma. Consequently it may be many years before help is sought.

Deliberate self-harm

Patients who inflict harm on themselves pose a difficult problem for the A&E department. Opinion is divided as to whether there is a link to actual suicide intent, but there is no doubt that nurses often feel inadequate when caring for such patients following an episode of deliberate self-harm (Perego 1999). The patients themselves can be seen as 'undeserving' and face negative attitudes from health care staff.

The reasons why people self-harm vary. Some describe the need to release themselves from intense mood and some use it as a means of communicating to others. For example, people with a severe learning disability have been known to self-harm for this reason. Self-injury is also indicative of religious belief within certain cultures.

Methods of injury include drug overdose, ingestion of harmful substances and objects, and lacerations – usually involving the upper limbs.

Following self-poisoning with any drug, the A&E department will often gain advice regarding treatment from a local or national poisons centre in the UK, as treatment regimens can change. Many drugs turn out to be relatively harmless and the patient may simply require admission into hospital for observation of any untoward symptoms. Other drugs warrant removal from the body, although this depends largely upon the type of drug consumed, the time since ingestion and the condition of the patient.

Methods of removal include emetics (e.g. ipecacuanha), which cause the patient to vomit, gastric lavage (irrigating the stomach with water, introduced via a large oral tube), and antidotes, which are specific to individual drugs.

Blood samples and electrocardiograph recordings (ECG) may be necessary following the ingestion of certain drugs. Regular observations of pulse, blood pressure, respiratory rate and conscious level are vital for many patients, who may become unwell some hours after the event.

Cases of deliberate self-harm represent a large percentage of hospital admissions, many at night, and nurses must be aware of the reasons why people injure themselves in order to be effective in their care. Agreed protocols regarding psychiatric assessment and follow-up, using a multidisciplinary approach, are essential to ensure patients receive the right intervention and support.

Caring for the acutely disturbed patient

Once physiological causes are ruled out, psychiatric support should be enlisted early. If patients have harmed themselves in any way, the initial priority is to attend to serious physical injury.

Patients should be cared for in a quiet area with comfortable seating and access to refreshment and smoking facilities. Wherever possible, a dedicated nurse should remain with or near patients. However, the safety of everyone involved, including that of other patients, must be addressed, so there will be times when the presence of security personnel or police is unavoidable.

Restraint is widely used in some parts of the world. However, restricting patients' freedom by force is not recommended, unless their behaviour is so disturbed that they risk harm to themselves or others. Wherever used, restraint must be kept to an absolute minimum, and only employed as a temporary measure, until appropriate psychiatric assessment is carried out. Sedation is best given with a patient's consent, and again only administered forcibly where deemed in the person's best interest, in order to control the situation. A duty psychiatrist should always make this decision.

Some A&E departments have developed the role of specialist psychiatric liaison nurses, who can assess patients and provide expert guidance, thereby avoiding unnecessary hospital admissions, which may impede a patient's long-term care.

SUDDEN DEATH IN A&E

Caring for the bereaved is a task that leaves nurses feeling emotionally drained. This is particularly so when someone dies following concerted efforts to resuscitate. Breaking bad news in A&E is particularly difficult, as there is little time to form therapeutic relationships and relatives have little time to anticipate their loss (see Ch. 3). The responsibility placed upon A&E nurses in this role is immense and can lead to feelings of inadequacy, particularly when demanding workloads add to the pressure of the situation. But the rapport, however brief, that is established with the bereaved has a far-reaching impact on the grieving process.

Sudden death is a major life crisis. When it occurs, irrespective of age, sometimes with horrific injury, those affected by it can extend beyond family and friends, to A&E staff, the emergency services, survivors and witnesses, many of whom may be work colleagues.

Principles of good practice in bereavement care were recommended by the Royal College of Nursing and British Association for Accident and Emergency Medicine (1995) to guide A&E staff in this difficult area. Examples include the necessity for appropriate facilities for the bereaved, agreed bereavement policies, training and staff support.

People who have already died are sometimes brought into A&E by ambulance, either because they died at home and a local doctor was not available or because death occurred in a public place and resuscitation was considered futile. The A&E doctor certifies (ascertains) death and the body is transferred directly to the hospital or public mortuary. The patient's clothing and belongings are normally removed and documented by mortuary personnel; however, details of the deceased will be recorded in A&E in order to contact relatives.

THE ROLE OF THE NURSE IN CARING FOR THE BEREAVED

The relatives' perceptions of care given will be enhanced by the presence of a dedicated nurse to meet and remain with them until they leave. Early intervention is essential to facilitate anticipatory grief. This means, for example, that if resuscitation looks unlikely to succeed, truthful communication will enable relatives to prepare themselves in some way.

Breaking bad news is discussed in Chapter 3 and the skills required in the A&E setting are no different, except that relatives are likely to be complete strangers to A&E staff. Most A&E departments have a designated room, allowing privacy and comfort, where relatives can obtain refreshment, smoke and use a telephone. The presence of relatives in the resuscitation room has already been raised in this chapter, and A&E nurses need to anticipate individual needs of the bereaved, whose wishes should not be impinged upon by the feelings of staff.

Viewing of the deceased by relatives
Offering bereaved relatives the chance to say goodbye to a loved one is an important part of the grieving process. This need not be in a formal viewing area, as many relatives benefit from seeing the actual place where the patient died (Wright 1999).

If injuries are severe, great comfort can be derived from being able to touch an uninjured hand or foot. To withhold this can lead to disturbing fantasies about the state of the loved one, which remain with the relative forever (Scott 1995).

Few people ever express regret at having seen the body of a loved one, whereas they may not ask, feeling unsure of what is 'allowed'. Empowering relatives to make choices whilst remaining proactive in caring promotes control and aids the grieving process (Wright 1999).

Contacting absent relatives
Sadly, many people who die suddenly do so without the knowledge of their loved ones. Contacting them must be done without delay. The telephone is usually an inappropriate means of breaking bad news; therefore, the police may need to be involved. Police officers are frequently called upon to undertake this role and do so with great sensitivity. Relatives should be advised to contact the A&E department and speak to a named nurse involved in the care of the deceased, so that questions can be answered accurately and relatives can speak with someone who was present at the time their loved one died. The opportunity to visit the department must be offered should they wish it.

Respecting religious and cultural values
When patients arrive alone, being unaware of their background we may unwittingly offend religious and cultural practices when dealing with a body following death. Guidance can be sought from religious leaders in the community, as well as hospital chaplains, who are an invaluable source of support regarding multicultural rites (see 'Further reading', e.g. Neuberger 1994).

Liaising with the coroner
When a death is sudden and unexpected, the law in the UK requires that the appropriate authority be informed, in order for a death certificate to be issued. In England and Wales this authority is the coroner (who is a doctor and/or lawyer) and in Scotland the procurator fiscal. Decisions regarding postmortem examination also rest with the coroner or procurator fiscal, in order to ascertain cause of death. An unnatural event, such as a road traffic accident or suicide, may result in a coroner's inquest (fatal accident enquiry in Scotland), the sole purpose of which is to determine who the person was, and how and when death occurred.

Ensuring accurate documentation

All events, no matter how trivial, need to be recorded. If the death becomes the subject of an inquest/fatal accident enquiry, nursing and medical notes may be produced, and therefore full and accurate documentation is essential.

Relatives will perceive a lack of care if their questions cannot be answered because the people involved have gone home, leaving inadequate documentation.

Details of property should indicate whether clothing was cut or soiled, and whether any jewellery remains on the body. Handing over a bag full of bloodstained clothing is devastating for distraught relatives, and therefore, unless required by the police or coroner, the family may prefer that they are disposed of. Their consent must be obtained sensitively and this documented in the notes.

Ensuring follow-up and support

The Royal College of Nursing (1995) report noted that adequate contact and support for relatives following a death was lacking in many hospitals. We cannot assume that people are able to cope or that support is available. It is not appropriate to blame demanding workloads, since the damage caused is too great.

A&E nurses should not underestimate the importance to relatives of knowing the place where their loved one died, and likewise the people who were present. Contacting relatives the following day, for example, communicates a caring attitude and enables the nurse to anticipate needs and reiterate information given previously.

Normally, the family is required to obtain a death certificate from the relevant authority (see p. 941) and to collect any property from the hospital. This information should be given both verbally and in a written form, with details of a named nurse to contact in A&E.

Bereavement services, hospital chaplaincy, social services and volunteer agencies all provide further support, in particular the GP, who may be well known to the patient and family members.

Caring for the carers

A single death can be as traumatic for the staff involved as any major disaster, and time must be available to reflect before going home. The circumstances may not be unusual, nor the death violent, but everyone responds to loss of life in different ways on different occasions (see Ch. 6).

Caring for a person who dies suddenly, and for the people they leave behind, can be a distressing task, but is also one of the most privileged roles a nurse is called upon to undertake.

MAJOR DISASTERS

A major disaster is an emergency that requires special arrangements and organization by the emergency services, due to the number and/or severity of casualties. Some or all of the emergency services may be involved, and the number of victims may not be vast. However, their accumulated need may be such that the normal workings of the hospital are affected.

Hospitals and emergency services need a formalized and well-rehearsed plan that is familiar to everyone involved.

THE ROLE OF THE HOSPITAL AND A&E DEPARTMENT

Most areas in the hospital are affected in the event of a major disaster, as extra staff, beds and supplies are required. Patients may be discharged home from wards, and theatre lists and outpatient clinics cancelled.

The hospital may be asked to provide a medical and nursing team to assist in the assessment and treatment of victims at the scene of the incident.

The work of the A&E team does not change; there are simply more patients arriving at once. Existing patients are rapidly assessed and are either admitted to a ward or referred to their GP or to another A&E department not involved in the disaster. The same process applies to patients in the waiting area, some of whom could be extremely unwell and must not be turned away.

Seriously injured patients may arrive without identification, and therefore the police become an integral part of the team in order to identify victims and inform relatives.

Documentation normally used in A&E is adapted to save time and each patient will be allocated a specific identification number.

Clothing, debris and body parts may need to be preserved, either for forensic evidence or to assist in accident investigation, as the smallest item could provide clues as to the cause of a disaster.

Communication and the multidisciplinary team

Communication is the key to a successful major disaster plan. The ambulance service normally pre-warns the hospital, providing details of location, number of casualties, types of injuries (e.g. burns) and other hospitals involved.

Visible clothing for the mobile team and lead nurse and doctor in the A&E department is essential for clear identification. A communications centre in A&E led by senior hospital personnel provides liaison between the incident site and the hospital. This allows the A&E team to care for the patients.

No A&E department or hospital is a sponge, and the number of casualties each can absorb is limited. Constant communication between the site and the hospital enables early dispatch of patients to another centre well before saturation point is reached.

Anxious friends and relatives require constant information and support. Privacy must therefore be provided within the hospital and extra telephone lines set up to deal with the deluge of calls.

At some point, all the victims will have been seen in A&E, and their care continued within the hospital or community. The A&E department, having taken a deep breath, must reopen its doors and continue as before. Agreement to 'stand down' and resume normal activity is made between the emergency services and the hospital.

Support and debrief

Some incidents continue for many hours, and the A&E staff rely on normal physiological reactions, e.g. the release of adrenaline (epinephrine), to enable them to endure distressing sights, often for the first time. Once it is over, time must be put aside to reflect and gather thoughts. There may be restrictions due to the need to resume normal running of the service; however, a short debrief is essential for everyone involved to voice feelings and emotions, and thereby make some sense of a highly stressful experience.

Debrief should be managed by someone with the skills necessary to lead it through a constructive process and should be attended by everyone, including ancillary workers and portering staff. A formal review of hospital incident procedure is normally arranged within a few days.

Post-disaster stress is a recognized phenomenon and hospitals have a duty to provide support for any member of staff who needs it (see Ch. 6).

Whilst most patients caught up in a major disaster do not experience any long-term psychological effects, some people will suffer significant distress. Therefore, regardless of the extent of their injury, every patient must be offered some form of review in the ensuing months, to identify those whose need may continue.

SUMMARY: MAIN POINTS

- The A&E department provides emergency care for people with sudden injury or illness. These patients require nursing care which considers the impact of the A&E environment upon their crisis.

- Patient assessment in A&E involves knowing what is normal and what is not, keeping an open mind, and an awareness of the importance of first impressions.

- A&E nurses have a responsibility to undertake health-promoting activities and to offer realistic, individualized education aimed at the prevention of accidents.

- Key skills for the lead nurse in A&E are the ability to remain visible within the team, provide constant communication, and match the right job to the right person at the right time.

- The role of the ENP allows experienced and appropriately trained A&E nurses to undertake autonomous practice in the provision of an alternative service for patients with minor injury and illness.

- People with serious injury or illness require a skilled team, who follow recognized life support protocols within agreed roles. A&E nurses can take the lead in improving practices in the resuscitation room and thereby minimizing psychological trauma suffered by the patient.

- The majority of A&E patients attend with minor illness or injury, although their perception of their problem may differ. Assessment must be holistic and discharge advice relevant to the person's individual environment.

- Many people attend A&E as a result of alcohol or drug problems, homelessness or following violent crime. The A&E nurse requires sensitivity and a non-judgemental attitude when caring for people with a variety of social problems.

- Challenging and aggressive behaviour has many sources, some of which are influenced by the A&E environment. Personal attack is devastating and leaves staff feeling vulnerable, and therefore support is essential.

- A key component in the care of patients with mental health problems is the identification of urgent needs. Justification should always be sought when considering restraint or enforced sedation. Remember, people with mental health problems also experience physical ill health, although their ability to communicate may be affected.

- Bereaved relatives and the staff involved in a sudden death have little time to prepare for its devastating effects. The A&E nurse needs to intervene early to allow for anticipatory grief, and remain receptive to the different needs of those who have lost a loved one.

- A major disaster disrupts the normal function of the hospital; however, the work of the A&E department does not change. Everyone must be aware of their role within a well-rehearsed plan, with an emphasis upon communication and the provision of support after such an event.

SELF-TEST: CRITICAL THINKING ACTIVITIES

1 Imagine you have been asked to design an A&E waiting area:
   — Highlight the issues relevant to the comfort of the patients who are waiting.
   — Provide rationale for each component of your design. How can basic layout of the area affect comfort?
   — Decide upon the order of priority you would choose for each aspect, in case your budget is reduced.
NB. You may be able to arrange a visit to your A&E department (or perhaps a local GP practice), for ideas.

2 The single most common cause of death in young adults (aged 15–24) are road traffic accidents (Department of Health 1999). One of the UK government targets is to reduce the death rate for accidents among this age group by 25% by the year 2005.
   — Outline some of the reasons why accidental deaths are so high in young adults.
   — What contribution can the A&E nurse make to the prevention of accidents in this age group?

FURTHER READING

Bateman R, Wright S. Accident prevention in the A&E department. Accid Emerg Nurs 1999; 7: 164–167.

Blomfield RA. Relatives in the resus room: don't overlook the patient! Accid Emerg Nurs 2000; 8: 52–53.

Dolan B, Holt L. Accident and emergency. Theory into practice. London: Baillière Tindall; 2000.

Morgan J. Introducing witnessed resuscitation in A&E. Emerg Nurse 1997; 5(2): 13–18.

Neuberger J. Caring for dying people of different faiths, 2nd edn. London: Mosby; 1994.

Sbaih LC. Initial assessment in the A&E department. Accid Emerg Nurs 1997; 6: 2–6.

Shepherd JP, Rivara FP. Vulnerability, victims and violence. J Accid Emerg Med 1998; 15(1): 39–45.

Spilsbury K, Meyer J, Bridges J, Holman C. The little things count. Older adults' experience of A&E care. Emerg Nurse 1999; 7(6): 24–31.

Tyrell MP. The nature of aggression and violence in the accident and emergency department. Nurs Rev 1999; 3: 71–75.

Walsh M. Accident and emergency nursing. A new approach, 3rd edn. Oxford: Butterworth Heinemann; 1996.

Walsh M, Dolan B. Emergency nurses and their perceptions of caring. Emerg Nurse 1999; 7(4): 24–31.

Wright B. Caring in crisis, 2nd edn. London: Churchill Livingstone; 1993.

 USEFUL ADDRESSES

Advanced Trauma Nursing Course (ATNC)
Baileys Consulting
Church Street
Charlbury
Oxon OX7 3PR
e-mail: lisahlaw@aol.com

Royal College of Nursing, A&E Association
Royal College of Nursing
20 Cavendish Square
London W1M 0AB

Royal Society for the Prevention of Accidents (RoSPA)
Rospa House
Edgbaston
353 Bristol Road
Birmingham B5 7ST

Trauma Advisory Services (TAS)
PO Box 272
Dorking
Surrey RH4 4FR
e-mail: tas@brake-campaign.demon.co.uk

Victim Support
Cranmer House
39 Brixton Road
London SW9 5DZ

 USEFUL WEBSITES

www.harcourtinternational.com/journals/aaen – Accident and Emergency Nursing

www.doh.gov.uk/capacityplanning/reform.htm – Department of Health

www.emergency-nurse.com/ – Emergency Nurse

www.bmjpg.com/data/aem.htm – Journal of Emergency Medicine

www.trauma.org – Trauma International

REFERENCES

Advanced Trauma Nursing Course (ATNC Committee). Advanced trauma nursing course provider manual. Oxford: ATNC; 1999.

Akerstrom M. Waiting: a source of hostile interaction in an emergency clinic. Qualit Health Res 1997; 7(4): 504–520.

American College of Surgeons (Committee on Trauma). Advanced trauma life support program. Illinois: American College of Surgeons; 1997.

Audit Commission. By accident or design: improving A&E services in England and Wales. London: HMSO; 1996.

Baelz PR. Philosophy of health education. In: Sutherland I, ed. Health education. Perspectives and choice. London: George Allen & Unwin; 1979, 20–38.

Crouch R, Marrow J. Towards a UK triage scale. Emerg Nurse 1996; 4(3): 4–5.

Department of Health. Reforming Emergency Care. London: Department of Health; 2001.

Department of Health. Saving lives: our healthier nation. London Department of Health; 1999.

Dillner L. A matter of chance. Nurs Times 1995; 91: 14 15.

Driscoll PA, Vincent CA. Organising an efficient trauma team. Injury 1992; 23(2): 107–110.

Hadfield L. Preparation for the nurse as part of the trauma team. Accid Emerg Nurs 1993; 1(3): 154–160.

Hanson C, Strawser D. Family presence during CPR. Foote Hospital Emergency Department's nine-year perspective. J Emerg Nurs 1992; 18(2): 104–106.

Health Service Advisory Committee (HSAC). Violence and aggression to staff in health services: guidance on assessment and management. London: HSE Books; 1997.

Jones G. Accident and emergency nursing. A structured approach. London: Faber and Faber; 1990, 21–40.

Lane M, Beales J. Health promotion in relation to domestic violence. Emerg Nurse 1998; 6(1): 26–29.

Mitchell S. Essential skills for life. Prof Nurse 1999; 15(1): 5.

Nursing and Midwifery Council (NMC) Code of professional conduct. London: NMC; 2002.

Orzel, M-N. Injury minimization programme for schools. Accid Emerg Nurs 1996; 4: 139–144.

Perego M. Why A&E nurses feel inadequate in managing patients who deliberately self harm. Emerg Nurse 1999; 6(9): 24–27.

Platt H. National health services accident and emergency services. London: HMSO; 1962.

Rieffe C, Oosterveld P, Wijkel D, Wiefferink C. Reasons why patients bypass their GP to visit a hospital emergency department. Accid Emerg Nurs 1999; 7: 217–225.

Robertson C, Redmond AD. The management of major trauma, 2nd edn. Oxford: Oxford University Press; 1994.

RoSPA. Accident statistics – brief overview. Online. Available: http://www.rospa.co.uk/accstats.htm; April 2001.

Royal College of Nursing. Report of special interest group on accident and emergency nurse practitioners. London: Royal College of Nursing; 1992.

Royal College of Nursing and British Association for Accident and Emergency Medicine. Bereavement care in A&E departments. London: Royal College of Nursing; 1995.

Royal College of Surgeons of England. Report of the working party on the management of patients with major injuries. London: Royal College of Surgeons of England; 1988.

Scott T. Sudden death in A&E. Emerg Nurse 1995; 2(4): 10–13.

Shepherd J. Victims of violent crime. Accid Emerg Nurs 1998; 6(1): 15–17.

Taylor B, Roberts M. Sobering effect. Nurs Times 1998; 94(16): 30–31.

Tippett J. Providing comfort in the resuscitation room. Accid Emerg Nurs 1994; 2: 155–159.

UKCC. The scope of professional practice. London: UKCC; 1992.

UKCC. Guidelines for professional practice. London: UKCC; 1996.

Walsh M. Accident and emergency nursing. A new approach, 3rd edn. Oxford: Butterworth Heinemann; 1996.

Wright B. Responding to autonomy and disempowerment at the time of a sudden death. Accid Emerg Nurs 1999; 7(3): 154–157.

31 Nursing critically ill patients

Mandy Sheppard

> *'I was worried about going to ITU after the operation then this evening a nurse from ITU came to see me and explained what it would be like – what to expect and so on, and said that he would be looking after me. I'm still not looking forward to it but at least I'll know one person when I come round.'*
>
> *(Patient)*

THIS CHAPTER WILL HELP YOU

- Appreciate the continuum of critical care and recognize potential and actual critical illness in the clinical environment

- Understand the physiological compensatory mechanisms of the body, which will assist in the timely detection of critical illness

- Appreciate a range of assessment and monitoring methods which will facilitate diagnosis and patient care and management

- Appreciate the physical and psychological effects of critical illness that inform clinical care and management.

KEYWORDS

Central venous pressure

Continuous positive airways pressure (CPAP)

Critical care continuum

High-dependency unit

Inotrope therapy

Intensive care unit

Mechanical ventilation

Outreach team

Pulmonary artery wedge pressure

Renal replacement therapy

INTRODUCTION

Critical care has been one of the most rapidly developing areas of health care over the past 40 years; it has had to respond to the dramatic changes in our hospitals, staff, patients and the treatments available. The term 'critical care' was once synonymous with 'intensive care' but this is no longer the case. Critical illness is a continuum, of which intensive care forms only a part, at one end. Care of the critically ill patient is relevant to nurses working in all areas including community settings such as nursing homes.

This chapter addresses the development and current context of critical care, underpinning physiological principles, assessment methods and key management strategies of mechanical ventilation, inotrope therapy and renal replacement therapy.

DEVELOPMENT OF CRITICAL CARE

The 1940s saw the development of postoperative recovery rooms, and this resulted in a reduction in the mortality of postoperative patients (Oh 1996). Such patients, particularly in the more immediate postoperative phase, are 'highly dependent' and, as such, recovery areas were, and still are, a form of specialized high-dependency care unit (HDU). Intensive care was not developed until the 1950s, when as a result of a poliomyelitis epidemic (which left many patients in need of respiratory support) mechanical ventilators were developed. This led to the introduction of intensive care, and the intensive care unit (ICU). The term intensive therapy unit (ITU) is also used. The next two decades also saw the development of the coronary care unit (CCU), specialized units offering continuous electrocardiogram (ECG) monitoring for patients after myocardial infarction (see Ch. 19).

In 1967 a report by the British Medical Association (BMA) stated that the care and outcome of seriously ill patients could be improved by the provision of intensive care facilities and during the 1970s and 1980s, many hospitals started to provide

947

such facilities. However, the development of intensive care across the UK was haphazard, often driven by and reliant upon the enthusiasm of local clinicians, and this resulted in a significant variation in terms of size, structure and staffing of units (Association of Anaesthetists 1988). In the 1980s, questions were being asked about intensive care, in particular about the lack of evidence to justify which patients would benefit from it (King's Fund Panel 1989). The same report raised questions about cost versus benefit, and also about the longer-term benefits of intensive care for the patient, both of which would be asked many times again over the next decade. Intensive care, when compared with other hospital services, is an expensive resource in relation to the number of patients treated and was under the spotlight to justify its expenditure (Mohan 1995).

Meanwhile, patients requiring high-dependency care were either 'specialled' by one nurse on a general ward, or nursed in an intensive care unit. This situation highlighted the so-called 'middle band' of patients who were too sick to be cared for in a general ward yet not sick enough to require intensive care. To 'special' such patients in a general ward required extra nurses and resulted in sick patients being scattered throughout a hospital, which was undesirable in both clinical and economic terms. However, if these patients occupied intensive care beds, those that required intensive care would not be able to be admitted.

A study of the provision of intensive care in England during 1993–94 (Metcalfe & McPherson 1995) reported that it differed significantly in hospitals throughout England and that in many hospitals there was no HDU. Consultants who were involved in the study indicated that 65% of the inappropriate admissions to ICU would have been more appropriately admitted to an HDU. The HDU provides a level of care that is higher than it is possible to provide within the general ward environment. The ICU provides a level of care beyond high-dependency care which usually includes mechanical ventilation. The report suggested that more high-dependency care beds were required. In 1996, partly in response to the continuing ambiguity over the difference between high-dependency and intensive care, and the problems of timely access to intensive care, the Department of Health produced the report *Guidelines on Admission to and Discharge from Intensive and High Dependency Units* (Department of Health 1996). The report contained national guidelines regarding the admission and discharge process, what constitutes an ICU and a HDU, and which service is appropriate for which patients. This was followed in 1997 by another report, *Augmented Care Period (ACP) Dataset* (Department of Health 1997), which was designed to provide information about critical care activity in acute hospitals that previously had been unavailable.

Throughout this time, a number of other changes were happening which helped to shape, and in many cases drive, the development of critical care. The progression of medical technology combined with the ageing population and the successful management of many chronic diseases has been significant in producing a patient population with a higher level of chronic diseases. This results in patients being potentially sicker and requiring enhanced levels of care. In addition, a reduced length of hospital stay has produced a greater concentration of these patients. The hospital environment, patient population and activity patterns have changed dramatically. Nurse recruitment, retention and training, and changes in medical working patterns also contributed to these changes. Training for nurses working in critical care also changed, and reflected the ongoing development of this area. In 1972, the Joint Board of Clinical Nursing Studies (JBCNS) was established and provided post-registration courses, including intensive care nursing. In 1979, the English National Board (ENB) replaced the JBCNS and the ENB 100 General Intensive Care Nursing was established. The 1990s saw the introduction of ENB accredited post-registration high-dependency nursing courses.

CLASSIFICATION OF CRITICALLY ILL PATIENTS

The current state and the future development of critical care have been profoundly influenced by a report published in 2000, *Comprehensive Critical Care – A Review of Adult Critical Care Services* (Department of Health 2000). The report contained a number of recommendations that addressed a range of different aspects of critical care and proposed a framework for critical care services. An important concept was highlighted in the report, namely that:

> Comprehensive critical care is the complete process of care for the critically ill which focuses on the level of care that individual patients need rather than on beds and buildings. It is a 'whole systems' approach, which encompasses the needs of those at risk of a critical illness, and of those who have recovered from such illnesses, as well as the needs of patients during the critical illness itself.

A classification of critical care patients was proposed (see Box 31.1).

Box 31.1 Classification of critically ill patients
(Department of Health 2000)

Level 0 Patients whose needs can be met through normal ward care in an acute hospital

Level 1 Patients at risk of their condition deteriorating, or those recently relocated from higher levels of care, whose needs can be met on an acute ward with additional advice and support from the critical care team

Level 2 Patients requiring more detailed observation or intervention, including support for a single failing organ system or postoperative care and those 'stepping down' from higher levels of care

Level 3 Patients requiring advanced respiratory support alone or basic respiratory support together with support of at least two organ systems. This level includes all complex patients requiring support for multi-organ failure

CATEGORIES OF ORGAN MONITORING AND SUPPORT

The classification of critically ill patients (Department of Health 1996) refers to the need for support of organ systems. The categories of organ monitoring and support are described below.

Advanced respiratory support
- Mechanical ventilatory support (excluding mask continuous positive airways pressure [CPAP] or non-invasive, e.g. mask ventilation)
- The possibility of a sudden, precipitous deterioration in respiratory function requiring immediate endotracheal intubation and mechanical ventilation.

Basic respiratory monitoring and support
- The need for more than 40% oxygen via a fixed performance mask
- The possibility of progressive deterioration to the point of needing advanced respiratory support
- The need for physiotherapy to clear secretions at least 2-hourly, whether via a tracheostomy, mini-tracheostomy or in the absence of an artificial airway
- Patients recently extubated after a prolonged period of intubation and mechanical ventilation
- The need for mask CPAP or non-invasive ventilation
- Patients who are intubated to protect the airway, but needing no ventilatory support and who are otherwise stable.

Circulatory support
- The need for vasoactive drugs to support arterial pressure or cardiac output
- Support for circulatory instability due to hypovolaemia from any cause and which is unresponsive to modest volume replacement. This will include, but not be limited to, post-surgical or gastrointestinal haemorrhage or haemorrhage related to a coagulopathy
- Patients resuscitated following cardiac arrest where intensive or high-dependency care is considered clinically appropriate
- Neurological monitoring and support
- Central nervous system depression, from whatever cause, sufficient to prejudice the airway and protective reflexes
- Invasive neurological monitoring.

Renal support
- The need for acute renal replacement therapy (haemodialysis, haemofiltration or haemodiafiltration).

However, within the formal guidelines and definitions, it is important to recognize critical care as a continuum that reflects the fact that patients may become critically ill in a variety of settings and may during the course of their illness move between hospital environments.

Frequently, as the physiological status of the patients becomes increasingly compromised, the input required in terms of interventions, assessment and care rises and the patient becomes more 'dependent'. It is important, though, to differentiate this category of dependency from the person who is dependent through physical disability, i.e. where the physiological status of

the patient is not compromised (Sheppard 2000). Regardless of where the patient is on the continuum, there are implications of critical illness that need to be appreciated and integrated into patient care and management.

CRITICAL CARE OUTREACH TEAMS

The Department of Health (2000) report also emphasized the need to adopt a hospital-wide, coordinated approach and part of this was the provision of outreach services (referred to in the classification of patients as 'critical care team'). These services are designed with three clear objectives:

- to avert admissions to critical care
- to enable discharge from critical care
- to share critical care skills with ward and community-based staff.

To avert admissions to critical care
The early identification of patient deterioration can enable a more timely implementation of treatment and often this can halt any further deterioration. Treatment, with support from the outreach team, may be possible within the ward environment, therefore averting an admission to critical care. If it is not possible or not appropriate to treat the patient in the ward environment, then early identification allows earlier admission to critical care, which can result in an improved outcome. It has been recognized that a failure to do so adversely affects patient mortality and morbidity (McQuillan et al 1998).

To enable discharge from critical care
When patients no longer require critical care, it is essential that there is a timely discharge back to their ward environment, not only for their own well-being but also to ensure appropriate use of resources, i.e. ensuring that critical care beds are available for those who need them. Although patients may no longer require critical care, discharge can still be frightening and can also cause anxiety for ward nurses. The outreach team can provide support for patients, relatives and staff members in this situation (see Ethical Issues box 31.1).

To share critical care skills with ward and community-based staff
To detect patients who are deteriorating requires assessment skills and underpinning knowledge. Another role of the outreach team is to share knowledge and skills and provide training opportunities for ward nurses. This can also prevent the de-skilling of ward staff, which can result if all critically ill patients are nursed in HDU or ICU. For these objectives to be met, a close liaison is required between the outreach and ward teams. Consequently, the development of outreach services also has to consider issues such as the communication and interpersonal skills of the team members.

Some hospitals may call their teams patient-at-risk teams (PARTs). The first implementation of such a team in the UK was at the Royal London Hospital in London and a study revealed that early intervention could decrease the number of cardiopulmonary arrests on the ward and reduce mortality rates (Goldhill et al 1999a; see Evidence-based Practice box 31.1).

ETHICAL ISSUES

31.1 No bed in the ICU

A 75-year-old man, Mr White, is admitted to the hospital via his GP with septicaemia and an acute abdomen. A laparotomy is performed which reveals a ruptured diverticulum with faecal peritonitis. Postoperatively, the anaesthetist contacts the ICU to admit.

At the same time, the ICU is contacted by the accident and emergency department and asked to admit a 22-year-old young man who has been involved in a major road traffic accident.

The ICU has only one empty bed. None of the other patients can be discharged, and it appears that all other ICUs in the locality are full.

It is accepted that the mortality associated with peritonitis and sepsis, particularly in the older patient, is extremely high, but the patient's chances of survival will be greatly reduced if he is not cared for in the ICU. Although the 22-year-old man has severe injuries, his chances of survival are much better than those of the 75-year-old man and he will probably survive without being admitted to ICU, but if he develops any complications he could die if not in the ICU.

In this situation, where two patients require intensive care, one with a good chance of survival, and the other with little chance of survival, which ethical, moral and professional principles should be considered in order to arrive at a decision?

 EVIDENCE-BASED PRACTICE

31.1 The effectiveness of the Patient-At-Risk Team

The first patient-at-risk team (PART) to be set up in the UK was at the Royal London Hospital. Previously, similar teams, known as medical emergency teams (METs), were shown to be effective in The Liverpool Hospital, NSW, Australia. The key objective for such teams is to enable early identification of seriously ill patients on general wards.

A study was undertaken at the Royal London Hospital between 1 June and 30 November 1997, where 69 assessments were made on 63 patients. It was shown that for those patients seen by the PART, the incidence of cardiopulmonary resuscitation before ICU admission was lower, and the incidence of death on the ICU was lower than for those patients not seen by the team.

The early identification and implementation of advice and treatment were shown to improve the outcome and prevent the need for cardiopulmonary resuscitation.

Reference

Goldhill D, Worthington L, Mulcahy A, Tarling M, Sumner A. The patient-at-risk team – identifying and managing seriously ill ward patients. Anaesthesia 1999; 54: 853–860.

EARLY WARNING SYSTEMS

As discussed above, one objective of the outreach team is either to avert or to enable a timely admission to critical care; both require the early identification of patient deterioration. To assist with this, 'early warning systems' have been developed that are designed to identify the patients at risk, by looking at a series of physiological variables (see Box 31.2). It has been shown that 80% of patients admitted to ICU from wards have abnormal heart rates, oxygenation levels and respiratory rates (Goldhill et al 1999b). There are a number of systems in use, but essentially all include assessment of the following physiological variables:

- Respiratory rate: > 25 or < 10 breaths/min
- Systolic blood pressure: < 90 mmHg
- Heart rate: > 110 or < 55 beats/min
- Conscious level: not fully alert and disorientated
- Oxygen saturation: < 90%
- Urine output: < 100 mL over 4 hours.

This objective assessment of the patient, underpinned by physiological values, also provides a baseline of the patient's condition for future reference.

Box 31.2 Patient-at-risk team (PART) protocol
(Goldhill et al 1999a)

(A) The senior ward nurse should contact the responsible doctor and inform them of a patient with:

(i) Any three or more of the following:

- respiratory rate > 25 breaths/min (or < 10)
- arterial systolic pressure < 90 mmHg
- heart rate > 110 beats/min (or < 55)
- not FULLY alert and orientated
- oxygen saturation < 90%
- urine output < 100 mL over last 4 hours

(ii) OR a patient not fully alert and orientated AND a respiratory rate > 35 breaths/min OR a heart rate > 140 beats/min.

(B) A doctor of registrar grade or above may call the team for any seriously ill patient causing acute concern. This will normally be done after discussion with the patient's consultant.

The success of outreach services, and the effectiveness of early warning systems requires acceptance and a hospital-wide approach. The report also recommended that nurses in general wards receive high-dependency care training. This acknowledges the changed patient population and recognizes that to care effectively for these patients, nurses require an enhanced level of skills and knowledge, particularly in patient assessment.

NURSING MANAGEMENT OF THE CRITICALLY ILL PATIENT

Nurses have a pivotal role in the care of critically ill patients. This includes ensuring effective communication and supporting patients emotionally and physically.

COMMUNICATION

The fact that critically ill patients may, during the course of their illness, move to different hospital areas highlights the importance of a 'whole hospital' approach to critical care and the need for effective interdepartmental communication. The relationship between staff and relatives is vital. Relatives will often prefer to remain near the patient for as much of the time as possible. There is understandable anxiety and fear of what could happen. Particularly in the ICU, where the nurse:patient ratio is likely to be 1:1, the dynamics among the nurse, the patient and the relatives becomes key and there is the opportunity for supportive relationships to be established; this can often be extremely important for the relatives.

Relatives and patients require clear communications in order to make informed decisions, but those communications need to be consistent and often repeated (see Ch. 3).

Many critically ill patients require intubation, where an endotracheal tube is passed through the mouth or occasionally through the nose, then through the larynx and into the trachea. Intubation is frequently performed to provide mechanical ventilation. Most, but not all, patients will require sedation in order to tolerate mechanical ventilation and as a result communication can be difficult. Alternative methods such as lip reading, letter boards or, if the patient is able, paper and pen should be explored. A failure to do so can lead to frustration on the part of the patient, staff and relatives and can have an adverse effect on relationships.

THE MULTIDISCIPLINARY TEAM

The size and varied membership of the team means that communication and good working practices are key to the provision of effective patient care. One such communication method is the 'ward round'. Although patients may be assessed on a number of occasions during a 24-hour period, there is usually a more formal assessment made at a specified time of the day where a plan of management and care is also agreed. It is vital that the contributing members of the team have access either to the 'ward round' or at least to the decisions that were made.

There is often a relatively large multidisciplinary team involved in the care of the patient, who may approach or be

R R REFLECTIVE PRACTICE

31.1 Effective communication in critical care

Mrs Brown has been admitted to your ward with a suspected pneumonia. She has been attended by the medical team and has received intense chest physiotherapy. The microbiology department has been closely involved in her microbial treatment.

Mrs Brown's daughter has been in almost constant attendance but has returned home to collect some items for her mother.

Mrs Brown becomes progressively breathless and her S_pO_2 has fallen to 89%. It is decided to transfer her to the HDU. Can you list all of the people that you would need to communicate with regarding this transfer?

approached by relatives, and it can be helpful to maintain a record of communications to the relatives (Wilkinson 1995). Medical staff (e.g. intensivists, surgeons, physicians, anaesthetists, microbiologists, etc.), nursing staff, physiotherapists, pharmacists, technicians and dieticians may be involved (see Reflective Practice box 31.1).

Nurses

Within any critical care area it is usually only the nursing element of the multidisciplinary team that has continuous, 24-hour contact with the patient. Consequently, the nurse often acts as a vital link: facilitating communications between different multidisciplinary team members and between the patient and team members. The critically ill patient requires the specialist skills and knowledge of the various team members; another vital role of the nurse is to coordinate their interventions to avoid overloading the patient and allow adequate periods of rest. Nurses are also responsible for patient comfort and safety through the prevention of complications and the provision of personal care (see p. 952).

Surgeons

Surgical involvement may be required if the patient's original reason for hospital admission was for a surgical procedure and continued surgical management is required, or if the cause for deterioration and critical care is surgical in nature. Some HDUs may be overseen by surgical teams.

Anaesthetists

Most intensive care patients require intubation and mechanical ventilation. Historically, specific intensive care training was unavailable for medical staff and consequently anaesthetists were often the most suitable medical personnel to manage such patients; this remains the case in many ICUs. However, in more recent times, specialized intensive care training has enabled doctors in the UK to become 'intensivists'. Anaesthetists may also play a pivotal role in pain control for postoperative patients or those with more chronic causes of pain.

Physicians

Some ICUs and HDUs may be overseen and managed by physicians. In units that are managed by anaesthetists, intensivists or surgeons, a physician may be asked to provide specific advice on medical problems for individual patients.

Physiotherapists

Physiotherapists may provide specific care for respiratory conditions or for the prevention of respiratory complications, e.g. in the postoperative or immobile patient. Physiotherapists are also required to treat and prevent musculoskeletal conditions, particularly those associated with immobility (see p. 953).

Speech therapists

When patients are intubated, via an endotracheal tube or tracheostomy, speech therapists can assist with alternative methods of communication, such as letter boards or electronic devices. After long periods of intubation, or perhaps after specific disorders (e.g. throat surgery or neurological conditions), some patients may require speech therapy.

Dieticians

Critically ill patients often have specific nutritional requirements which can in some patients be difficult to achieve and problematic; dieticians can provide expert advice on methods, types and problem management.

Radiographers

Particularly where patients are intubated and mechanically ventilated, serial chest X-rays are required to monitor progress and identify problems. Normally, a portable chest X-ray will be performed, to avoid having to move the patient to the X-ray department.

Microbiologists, pathologists and haematologists

Infection may be the reason for the critical illness or it may be a complicating factor. Advice may be sought regarding the suitability of certain antimicrobial or antiviral treatments.

Haematological or biochemical abnormalities may be both a cause and a complication of critical illness and the relevant specialists are often closely involved in the care of critically ill patients.

Technicians

Critical care areas have a relatively high level of equipment, whether for monitoring purposes, such as an ECG monitor, or for treatment purposes, such as a mechanical ventilator. The maintenance and speedy repair of such equipment are vital and dedicated technicians are required. In addition, many critical areas perform a range of blood tests 'in-house' rather than sending them to the hospital laboratories, to enable results to be obtained much more quickly. These include arterial blood gas analysis and electrolyte levels and often these will be the responsibility of a dedicated technician.

DECISION-MAKING AND INFORMED CONSENT

The dependency of patients has implications for their decision-making powers, and this impacts upon the roles of relatives,

friends and professional staff. Patients may be unconscious (in a coma) as a result of their illness, they may have been deliberately sedated or they may have an altered conscious state, perhaps due to metabolic derangement, such as hypoxia, uraemia or extreme electrolyte disturbance. In consequence, they may be unable to make decisions regarding their treatment, and invariably others must take this on. Patient advocacy is concerned with promoting and protecting the interests of patients or clients, many of whom may be vulnerable and incapable of protecting their own interests (UKCC 1996). Although relatives cannot dictate the care or management of their loved ones, or be expected to make difficult decisions on their own, it is in everyone's interest (not least the patient) for there to be a consensus in any decisions which are made.

PERSONAL CARE

The dependency of patients also has an impact upon the degree of nursing care required. At the intensive care end of the continuum, where patients may be heavily sedated, perhaps requiring mechanical ventilation, nursing staff will need to provide total care, in terms of moving the patients' position, washing, bathing, eye care, mouth care and so forth. Encouraging relatives to bring in personal items can be comforting, e.g. a patient's favourite soap or deodorant. It is imperative that all care is provided with dignity, remembering to protect patients' privacy with the use of screens or curtains. Where appropriate, relatives may like to be involved in the care of their loved one. Assessment of patients' needs will inform not only the level but also the frequency of personal care required.

Eye care

The eyes are normally kept moist and infection-free by the production of tears, which are spread over the eyes by blinking and the blink reflex. These can be absent or impaired in the critically ill patient, such as in the following cases:

- where oxygen or CPAP masks are poorly positioned and the patient's eyes suffer from the drying effects of the gas
- where the blink reflex is reduced or absent, such as in sedated or unconscious/semiconscious patients
- patients who are dehydrated, in whom tear production can be reduced
- patients whose eyes remain partially open.

Any potential causes of eye problems, such as dehydration or poorly fitting CPAP masks, should be identified and, if possible, rectified. Where the eyelids do not close completely, the cornea must be protected. The use of hydrogel pads, which move if the eye is opened and so do not touch the cornea, is the preferred method of protection. Artificial tears (hypromellose drops) can be used where tear protection is reduced and sterile water or saline should be used for routine cleansing of the eyes.

Oral hygiene

Critically ill patients require frequent oral hygiene as many of the normal, physiological methods of maintaining this are lost or reduced for the following reasons:

- Sedation or the debilitating effects of the illness itself may render patients unable to perform their own care.

- Eating stimulates saliva production and drinking keeps the mouth moist. In some cases, critically ill patients cannot eat or drink.
- Patients with increased respiratory rates can also have a dry mouth and increased insensible losses associated with respiration, especially if mouth breathing.
- A dry mouth, where the buccal mucosa becomes dehydrated, can also occur in patients with oxygen therapy via a mask and in general dehydration.

Where possible, causative factors should be prevented or treated, e.g. by humidifying oxygen and maintaining a normal fluid balance. The mouth may be moistened using foam sticks and water, but where possible, 'normal' oral hygiene with a toothbrush and toothpaste should be used to clean the mouth.

Effects of immobility

In many situations, the critically ill patient is relatively immobile and is therefore at risk from the many complications of restricted mobility.

Chest infection

This may occur due to reduced secretion clearance, atelectasis (collapse of the alveoli causing a reduction in gas exchange), and ventilation to perfusion (V/Q) mismatches (see p. 955). Measures to prevent chest infections include:

- maintaining fluid balance to prevent drying of pulmonary secretions
- deep breathing and coughing exercises, with adequate pain relief if necessary
- changing patient position regularly to facilitate expansion of the lungs
- suction – oropharyngeal or nasopharyngeal, or via an endotracheal tube or tracheostomy
- mobilizing patients as much as their condition allows
- oxygen and other pharmacological interventions (e.g. antibiotics or bronchodilator drugs) if indicated.

Damage to skeletal structures, muscles and nerves

The absence of weight-bearing exercise on the long bones can lead to reduced bone density and osteoporosis. Muscles can atrophy through lack of use and flexor muscles can shorten, resulting in contractures. Foot drop, where dorsiflexion is decreased, is a common site of damage. Regular physiotherapy, in which the muscles and joints are taken through a full range of movement, should be performed as a preventative measure.

Peripheral nerve damage can result from incorrect positioning, external pressure (e.g. from equipment) or the pressure of another limb (i.e. the uppermost leg when patients are positioned on their side). Care should be taken to ensure careful positioning and avoid undue pressure being placed on peripheral tissues.

Urinary infection and kidney stones

Infection can occur due to urinary stasis, the presence of a urinary catheter and an increase in urinary pH. Nephrolithiasis (kidney stones) can result from increased urinary calcium excretion, related to the skeletal degeneration. Regular changes of patient position, the maintenance of an adequate urine output,

aseptic technique during catheter insertion and regular catheter care are all preventative measures.

Decreased gut motility and constipation

This may be due to many factors, including the severity of illness, drugs or loss of normal eating stimuli. Where possible, enteral or oral feeding should be commenced as soon as possible, and fluid balance maintained (see 'Nutrition' below). Patient mobilization should be commenced as able. Certain drugs, e.g. opiates, can reduce gut motility and lead to constipation. Consideration should be given to alternatives or dose reduction, if appropriate.

Deep vein thrombosis

The risk of deep vein thrombosis and peripheral oedema can result from decreased venous return and stasis. Patient mobilization, limb exercises and low-molecular-weight heparin can minimize the risk (see Ch. 19).

Pressure ulcer formation

Pressure ulcer formation is a particular risk for the critically ill patient. This is in part due to immobility but also due to factors such as vasoconstriction, caused by a reduced cardiac output or the use of constrictor drugs such as noradrenaline (norepinephrine). Chronic conditions such as diabetes may increase the risk of pressure sore formation (see Ch. 17). The patient may be too unstable to turn from side to side because in some this can have a deleterious effect on the heart rate, blood pressure or oxygenation. Preventative measures include:

- early mobilization, provided that cardiovascular and respiratory stability is maintained. Intensive care patients, who may be attached to ventilators and other equipment, can still sit on the edge of their beds, sit out in chairs and perhaps have a short walk
- regular skin assessment and position changes
- early use of pressure-relieving mattresses and specialist beds (see Ch. 10).

NUTRITION

Many critically ill patients require nutritional support because tracheal intubation, sedation and altered conscious levels will prevent them from eating. Where possible, nutritional support should be provided via the enteral route (GI tract) rather than intravenously, as weight gain and nitrogen retention are improved and the incidence of intestinal bleeding is reduced (Dobbs 1992). It has also been shown to maintain gut wall integrity and reduce the risk of sepsis (Raper & Maynard 1992). Enteral feeding can be provided via the following routes:

- nasogastric – a feeding tube is passed into the stomach via the nose
- nasoenteral – a feeding tube is passed into the jejunum via the nose
- percutaneous endoscopic gastrostomy (PEG) – with the aid of a gastroscope, a feeding tube is passed into the stomach and brought out through the abdominal wall. This can also be achieved via the jejunum.

THE EFFECTS OF THE ENVIRONMENT ON THE PATIENT

Any critical illness will be frightening for patients and cause stress, and the critical care environment is likely to cause stress for their family as well (see Fig. 31.1). Stress is a normal physiological response (see Ch. 6). Stimulation of the sympathetic nervous system in the short term is a required response but it can be damaging in the longer term and lead to unwanted side-effects in those who are critically ill. The sympathetic nervous system may be stimulated not only in response to emotional or psychological stress, but also when the physiological systems are stressed, e.g. due to pain or hypovolaemia. This physiological mechanism is key in understanding many of the clinical features exhibited by critically ill patients.

Alteration in sensory perception can occur for a number of reasons, including both a reduction in and an overload of sensory inputs. It is important that patients are given personal space and time, yet not left isolated for long periods. This highlights the needs to plan the care and management for patients over a 24-hour period and not just over the course of one shift. There needs to be a coordination of activities to ensure that patients are allowed to rest without procedures and other interventions for periods of the day, and wherever possible a normal day/night pattern should be created. It is important to rest the GI tract as well and, if possible, enteral feeding should be suspended for at least 4 hours during the night to allow the gastric pH to return to its normal acidic state (Adam & Osborne 1997).

Touch, as opposed to the clinical contact made through nursing or medical interventions, and speech – reminding patients of the date, time and where they are – are extremely important even if they are unable to respond. Critical care environments can be noisy, due to the number of people and amount of equipment, and all efforts should be made to minimize this. Some patients find music (of their personal taste) comforting and relaxing (Chlan 1995). Constant light can also be problematic, and although the care of critically ill patients must continue throughout the 24-hour period, the reduction of activity, noise and light at night to enable sleep is important. Sleep deprivation and alterations in sensory perception can lead to tiredness, confusion, disorientation, hallucinations and delirium (see Ch. 4) (see Reflective Practice box 31.2).

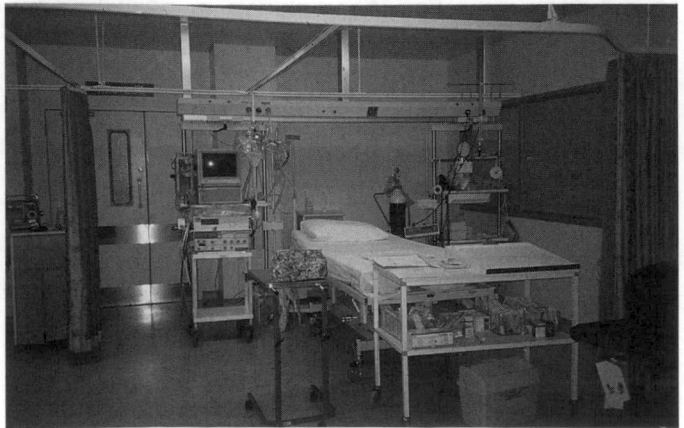

Figure 31.1 The ICU environment.

R|Я REFLECTIVE PRACTICE

31.2 How nurses can influence sensory and sleep alterations in the critically ill patient

Critical care areas are often busy with relatively high numbers of personnel involved in patient care. Critically ill patients also require monitoring and care throughout the 24-hour period, often involving the use of equipment.

Student activities
With the above in mind, and from reading the section regarding sensory and sleep alterations, can you identify:

- What measures could be taken to minimize noise in the area?
- What measures could be taken to ensure that the patient is not constantly interrupted by clinical interventions?
- What measures could be taken to provide sleep for the patient?

PHYSIOLOGICAL OVERVIEW

The respiratory system is responsible for the movement of oxygen into the body and the excretion of carbon dioxide. The pulmonary circulation acts as a conduit between the lungs and the systemic circulation, allowing the movement of oxygen into, and carbon dioxide out of, the systemic circulation. All of these components must be working for cell metabolism to be achieved. In addition, many other body systems facilitate this process, partly by the maintenance of an appropriate physiological environment, e.g. pH balance, electrolyte balance, fluid balance and temperature.

RESPIRATORY SYSTEM

Regardless of whether the patients are self-ventilating, breathing room air or oxygen-enriched air, or are being mechanically ventilated, gases (containing oxygen) enter the trachea and move through the bronchial tree to the alveoli. To transport oxygen and carbon dioxide from the lungs to the systemic circulation, the gases must first be moved into the pulmonary circulation. The movement of gases in and out of the lungs is dependent on the efficient movement of the chest wall and diaphragm. The respiratory centre controls inspiration, while expiration is a passive process that occurs when inspiration has stopped, due to the natural elastic recoil of the lung tissue (see Ch. 20). This passive process of expiration occurs in the same way when patients are mechanically ventilated, i.e. the ventilator inflates the lungs by delivering a volume of gas and when that delivery stops, expiration occurs.

There are two important respiratory mechanisms to be aware of:

- Central chemoreceptors detect an increase in carbon dioxide in the blood supply to the brain and will act on the respiratory centre to increase respiratory effort, in an attempt to excrete the accumulating carbon dioxide

- Peripheral chemoreceptors detect low oxygen levels, and again will act on the respiratory centre to increase respiratory effort.

Consequently, when a patient presents with changes in respiratory rate, depth or pattern, although this may be due to anxiety or physical exertion, causes such as carbon dioxide retention or hypoxia should always be excluded.

The pulmonary capillaries are situated close to the alveoli. Alveoli have a membrane of one cell thickness and this allows the movement of oxygen from the air in the alveoli into the pulmonary circulation, and that of carbon dioxide from the pulmonary circulation into the alveoli. This relationship also highlights a vital physiological requirement for gas exchange: there must be alveolar ventilation, i.e. air entering the alveoli (known as V), and perfusion of the pulmonary capillaries (known as Q). Healthy respiration depends on most alveoli being ventilated and being in close proximity to well-perfused pulmonary capillaries. This is referred to as the V/Q ratio. This should be 1, i.e. a ratio of 1:1 between V and Q. Where there are factors that reduce alveolar ventilation (e.g. pneumonia or pulmonary oedema) or pulmonary perfusion (e.g. pulmonary embolus), a mismatch occurs. Oxygen is then transported around the body bound to haemoglobin, which in turn is carried in red blood cells (erythrocytes) (see Ch. 18). Consequently, assessment and management of respiratory illness in critical care should take the following into account:

- the neurological control of respiration, which may be affected by respiratory depressant drugs, diseases such as Guillain–Barré syndrome or neurological disease or trauma
- the mechanical ability of the chest to respond to neural stimulation, which may be affected by pain or a flail chest
- alveolar efficacy, which can be reduced in long-term respiratory disease (such as chronic obstructive pulmonary disease) or conditions such as a chest infection, where sputum can inhibit the movement of oxygen from the alveoli to the blood
- perfusion of the pulmonary capillaries, which can be adversely affected by profound hypovolaemia or an obstruction to pulmonary blood flow such as a pulmonary embolus (see Chs 19 and 20)
- haemoglobin levels, for the carriage of oxygen.

CARDIOVASCULAR SYSTEM

Once oxygen has passed from the alveoli to the pulmonary capillaries, the blood must be pumped around the body to reach the cells. The left ventricle pumps the blood into the aorta and into the arterial circulation, supplying oxygen to the cells. Carbon dioxide, released by the cells, is carried in the venous circulation back to the right side of the heart. The right ventricle pumps blood into the pulmonary artery and into the lungs to excrete the carbon dioxide and to pick up more oxygen (see Ch. 19).

Cardiac output

Cardiac output is the amount of blood being pumped out of the heart over the course of a minute, which for an adult is in the range of 4–6 L/min. The cardiac output depends upon how many times the heart contracts per minute (heart rate) and how much blood is pumped out of the heart with each contraction (stroke volume). Cardiac output is therefore: heart rate × stroke volume. Three factors influence the stroke volume: preload, contractility and afterload.

Preload

Preload refers to the volume of blood (i.e. circulating volume) that distends the ventricle. The larger the volume of blood in the ventricle, the more the ventricle is distended and the greater the degree of stretch of the muscle fibres. Starling's law states that the length of the muscle fibres determines the force of myocardial contraction. Therefore, an adequate circulating volume is required for cardiac contraction. Where cardiac output is reduced, it is important to ensure that circulating volume is adequate. Fluid challenge, informed by CVP monitoring, is a common method (see Ch. 9).

Contractility

The inherent contractility of the muscle fibres can be decreased by myocardial dysfunction, hypovolaemia, hypoxia, hypocalcaemia and hypomagnesaemia. In the event of a low cardiac output, once an adequate circulating volume (preload) has been established, the next step would be to treat any of these factors. Myocardial dysfunction would commonly be treated with positive inotropic drugs (see p. 962).

Afterload

Afterload refers to the resistance offered to blood leaving the ventricles. Resistance to the right ventricle is from the pulmonary circulation, and to the left ventricle by the systemic circulation. With a poorly functioning left ventricle, even normal resistance can cause the cardiac output to fall. Vasodilating drugs can be administered to relieve systemic resistance.

Blood pressure

Blood pressure (BP) is the product of cardiac output (CO) and peripheral resistance (PR), the resistance supplied by the vessels in the circulation. Therefore BP = CO × PR. The state of the peripheral circulation is influenced by vasomotor tone. An increase in sympathetic activity causes vasoconstriction and an increase in BP. Conversely, a decrease in sympathetic activity causes vasodilatation and a fall in BP. Blood pressure can be maintained as long as resistance is provided to the blood in the circulation. Thus, blood pressure can be maintained in the face of hypovolaemia if the capacity of the circulation (the space that the reduced amount of fluid has to occupy) is correspondingly reduced. The sympathetic nervous system is responsible for reducing the capacity of the circulation through the release of adrenaline (epinephrine), which causes vasoconstriction.

This highlights a situation that may be seen in critically ill patients as a result of sepsis, when they may be hypotensive (which would suggest a reduced cardiac output) and yet have a normal or even elevated cardiac output. Patients may look and feel warm because the peripheral circulation is dilated as a result of sepsis. The hypotension occurs because vasodilatation enlarges the capacity of the circulation and consequently little resistance is provided to the blood, resulting in a fall in blood pressure (see Ch. 9).

Cardiac output (specifically preload) and the maintenance of blood pressure are intimately linked with the volume of fluid in the circulation. The kidneys are responsible for fluid balance by excreting urine and reabsorbing water and electrolytes. The functional unit of the kidneys is the nephron, the first part of which is concerned with filtering arterial blood. Blood that is filtered is known as filtrate and is produced at a rate of approximately 120 mL/min. The kidneys also control electrolyte balance and a significant part of acid–base balance (see Ch. 8). Thus, assessment and management of cardiovascular illness in critical care should take into account:

- *Heart rate and rhythm.* An increase or decrease in heart rate and/or an altered rhythm may reduce cardiac output.
- *Circulating volume,* which must be adequate for the capacity of the circulation. This is important in critical care, as frequently drugs are given that either constrict the circulation (e.g. noradrenaline [norepinepherine]) or dilate the circulation (e.g. sodium nitroprusside). In order to maintain a blood pressure when administering vasodilator drugs, it is important to ensure that as the circulation enlarges, the patient is given sufficient fluid to occupy that space.
- *Blood pressure.* Untreated hypotension can result in the underperfusion of organs, organ ischaemia and finally organ dysfunction (see Ch. 9). Hypertension can result in an increased resistance to the left ventricle (increased afterload) which may reduce cardiac output.
- *Cardiac output, components and derivatives.* The cardiac output and stroke volume can be measured. The degree of vasoconstriction can be assessed by measuring the systemic vascular resistance (SVR; see p. 960).
- *Renal function and fluid balance,* which if not optimized can lead to reduced or increased circulating volumes, both of which can adversely affect cardiac output.

Two compensatory mechanisms are operational when the cardiovascular system is challenged: the sympathetic nervous system and the renin–angiotensin–aldosterone mechanism. The latter is a mechanism that, when activated through hypotension caused by hypovolaemia, will increase the circulating volume. However, if it is activated through hypotension caused by heart failure, the resultant increased circulating volume may serve to exacerbate the existing heart failure (see Ch. 19).

MONITORING AND ASSESSMENT

As discussed above, the body's systems interact with and depend upon each other and this forms the basis for the holistic nature of the care and management of the critically ill patient. For example, a patient may present with a primary respiratory problem that requires immediate attention to prevent further deterioration or to allow the initiation of support therapies such as intubation and ventilation (see below). However, it is also important to optimize the other body systems. For example, it would be illogical to treat only the respiratory system if the cardiovascular system were also failing and unable to transport oxygen to the cells. Critically ill patients are already using many of their homeostatic mechanisms and their physiological reserves are being stretched. One aim of monitoring and assessment is to detect when a patient is compensating and to intervene. Once the patient has exceeded their compensatory reserve, their physiology is more vulnerable and the patient less stable.

PRINCIPLES OF MONITORING AND ASSESSMENT

The term 'monitoring' can be misleading. Monitoring is not just about using equipment, it also includes visual assessment, touch and auditory assessments, and investigations such as blood tests and radiological procedures. Patients will require careful monitoring to:

- assess their condition where there is a general potential for deterioration, e.g. during and after complicated, prolonged surgery in an already compromised patient
- assess their condition where there is a more defined potential for deterioration, e.g. in the presence of arrhythmias post-myocardial infarction (see Ch. 19)
- assess their response to therapy, e.g. changes in central venous pressure (CVP) measurement in response to a fluid challenge (see Ch. 9) or changes in blood pressure in response to inotrope therapy (see p. 962).

Monitoring techniques may be invasive or non-invasive. Invasive techniques, which include urinary catheterization, tracheal intubation or arterial cannulation to facilitate blood gas analysis and arterial blood pressure monitoring, will breach the body's normal defences against infection. Therefore, the risks of infection posed to the critically ill patient must be balanced against the benefits that can be gained. There are also other considerations. For example, a patient who is confused and breathless and requires a central venous catheter to assist with fluid balance estimation will be required to adopt a head-down position during insertion of the catheter. The breathless patient may not be able to tolerate this and the procedure may be more hazardous if the patient is confused. The benefits to be gained from the CVP information have to be balanced against the risks posed to the patient, the most significant of which is a pneumothorax (see p. 960). This can occur during central line insertion due to accidental puncture of the pleura (see Ch. 20). It may be necessary to wait until the patient is less breathless and more lucid and the risks are minimized to such an extent that the procedure is considered beneficial.

When caring for the critically ill, it is crucial that monitoring equipment is used in combination with visual and other means of observation. The body has a wide range of compensatory mechanisms that will be activated when physiological systems are challenged, their purpose being to maintain homeostasis until the challenge is removed. Monitoring equipment may be unable to detect the often subtle changes, which require more fundamental methods such as touch or visual observation. Equally, the body systems interact and react to each system's 'problems'. For instance, in the initial stages of hypoxia, heart rate and blood pressure rise, which is an example of a respiratory problem with cardiovascular effects. This interaction and interdependence must be anticipated in the assessment, care and management of the patient. Trends are also extremely important, and which observations are grouped together in those trends. Rarely does one single physiological value lead to a diagnosis.

Patient history

The patient's history is extremely valuable, and in many cases may have to be gained from relatives or from the medical and nursing notes and verbal handover. The term 'patient history' is important; the medical record is part of this, but we also need to know about patients themselves. The history should not be confined to home, or pre-hospital admission; patients on the critical care continuum may have been in hospital for some time and been transferred between different locations. For example, the assessment of fluid balance in the older patient is frequently informed by the patient history (see Older Adults: Nursing Priorities box 31.1).

Sensory observations

A vital element of patient assessment and ongoing monitoring is to observe and listen to the patient. Observations gained from this activity can be valuable, especially in conjunction with other assessment and monitoring methods. The following are examples of information that can be gained by visual observation and listening, but the list is in no way exhaustive.

Visual observation

- Skin colour – pallor may suggest anaemia or peripheral vasoconstriction; a flushed appearance may be due to vasodilatation
- Skin condition – a rash may be due to the disease process or a drug reaction; bruising in the critically ill may suggest a deficiency in the coagulation system such as disseminated intravascular coagulation (DIC, see Ch. 19). Sweating, particularly on the forehead, is often a sign of respiratory distress

OLDER ADULTS: NURSING PRIORITIES

31.1 Assessing fluid balance in the older patient

There are a number of physiological and physical changes that occur in the older patient which need to underpin fluid balance assessment, including:

- loss of skin turgor
- reduction in saliva production
- decrease in renal function.

The *history* can inform fluid balance assessment:

- the volume of fluids consumed (thirst sensation decreases and the patient may therefore perceive their intake to be adequate)
- mobility – intake could be reduced merely as a result of relative immobility and the associated difficulty of walking to a kitchen
- disability – musculoskeletal disorders (e.g. arthritis) may make it physically difficult to hold a cup or glass
- incontinence – fluid intake may be self-restricted due to the fear of incontinence
- diuretic prescription – long-term use may cause fluid and electrolyte imbalance.

- Mouth breathing, pursed lips and the use of accessory muscles of respiration (i.e. abdominal and sternomastoid muscles) are all signs of respiratory distress
- Mucous membrane colour – a blue tinge (cyanosis) may be indicative of central cyanosis due to hypoxia
- Patient behaviour – confusion, hallucinations or other altered mental states may be observed and can be due to a number of factors, including hypoxia, electrolyte imbalance or sleep deprivation
- Patient movement – use of the accessory muscles of respiration indicates respiratory distress, while a lack of movement may indicate a reluctance to move due to pain.

Auditory assessment

- Respiratory signs – wheezing (on inspiration, indicating an obstructive problem or on expiration, indicating bronchoconstriction), or a 'bubbly' sound due to pulmonary oedema (fluid in the interstitial space)
- The way the patient speaks is also important: is the patient orientated? The breathless patient may only be able to speak two or three words before pausing to take a breath, sentences sound very interrupted.

Touch

- Skin temperature – a cool skin can indicate vasoconstriction, which may be due to hypovolaemia, cardiac failure or an attempt to maintain core body temperature
- Skin condition – a lack of skin turgor (elasticity) may be due to hypovolaemia or, conversely, peripheral oedema may be the result of fluid overload. Caution must be exercised in the older patient where reduced skin turgor may naturally occur as a result of reduced skin elasticity.

RESPIRATORY MONITORING AND ASSESSMENT

As previously discussed, monitoring and assessment should combine information gained by observing and listening to the patient, with clinical parameters. It is often the detection of subtle changes in condition that highlight potential respiratory failure (Field 2000).

Respiratory rate, pattern and depth

- The pattern of breathing is significant and may indicate an underlying condition, e.g. Kussmaul breathing, where both the rate and depth are increased in response to diabetic ketoacidosis (see Ch. 17).
- Increased depth of breathing and use of the accessory muscles of respiration are seen in the early stages of respiratory distress.
- An increased rate of breathing is a normal response to exercise or exertion. However, in the critically ill patient this may be in response to hypoxaemia (low levels of oxygen) or hypercapnia (high levels of carbon dioxide).

Tidal volume

The volume of each breath is known as the tidal volume and the amount that the patient is breathing over the course of a minute is known as the minute volume. Thus the respiratory rate multiplied by the tidal volume is equal to the minute volume. The terms respiratory rate, tidal volume and minute volume are common within the ICU environment where the patient is mechanically ventilated and by manipulating the rate and/or the tidal volume, the minute volume can be changed.

Breath sounds

When listening to a patient's chest, it is important to identify normal breath sounds:

- vesicular – heard all over the lung edges, it is a rustling sound
- bronchial – heard over the trachea, it is loud with a high pitch
- bronchovesicular – heard over major airways, this is a combination of the above two sounds.

This enables the detection of abnormal breath sounds:

- wheezes – when heard on inspiration, these can indicate airway obstruction, and when heard on expiration they can indicate bronchoconstriction
- crackles – usually heard on inspiration, indicating conditions such as pneumonia or pulmonary oedema. Crackles that are heard on both inspiration and expiration can indicate conditions such as bronchiectasis (see Ch. 20).

The absence of breath sounds in one lung or area of the lung may be indicative of pneumothorax, the abnormal presence of air between the visceral and parietal pleura that prevents expansion of the lung.

Pulse oximetry

Pulse oximetry enables a continuous assessment of arterial oxygen saturation, monitored through peripheral arterial capillaries (S_pO_2). Key to its success is the ability to detect peripheral blood flow, and therefore accuracy cannot be guaranteed in any condition that causes a reduction in peripheral perfusion. Vasoconstriction due to extreme cold, drug therapy or in response to a low cardiac output (caused by either cardiac failure or hypovolaemia) is not uncommon in the critically ill patient. The respiratory system is also concerned with the excretion of carbon dioxide, but this is not monitored by pulse oximetry. Hypoventilation will result in less carbon dioxide being excreted during expiration and consequently it accumulates in the circulation. Hypoventilation may be due to a low respiratory rate (e.g. through the depressant effects of systemic opioids on the respiratory centre), or in the end stages of respiratory failure where, although the respiratory rate may remain high, the tidal volume may be severely reduced. The normal S_pO_2 is 95–100%. A S_pO_2 of 90% or less is extremely serious and would suggest ensuing respiratory failure (Woodrow 1999).

Arterial blood gas analysis

Analysis of arterial blood provides information about the oxygenation of the arterial blood and the acid–base status of the patient. Many patients in the ICU or HDU require frequent blood gas analysis and so an indwelling arterial cannula is inserted to avoid repeated arterial punctures. The arterial cannula site must always be visible (i.e. not under the bedclothes) so that accidental disconnection of the tubing can be immediately detected. Because it is arterial blood, the patient could lose a large volume in a short period of time if undetected. For this reason patients with arterial lines must be nursed in an

ICU or HDU where the ratio of nurses to patients allows constant observation of the patient.

The blood sample for blood gas analysis is collected in a special syringe that contains heparin to prevent the sample clotting. The sample is left in the syringe and must be transported to the laboratory for analysis as soon as possible, to avoid changes in the gas tensions (oxygen and carbon dioxide), which would invalidate the results. As discussed earlier, many ICUs and HDUs have their own machines to enable immediate analysis. If the patient does not have an arterial line, an arterial puncture will be necessary. This requires prolonged pressure after puncture (usually about 5 minutes) to stop the bleeding. Arterial blood gases and the normal values are discussed in detail in Chapters 8 and 9.

Interpretation of blood gas analysis

Arterial blood gas monitoring will enable diagnosis of a number of situations, as described below.

Hypoxaemia (Pao$_2$ < 10.0 kPa; normal 10.0–13.3 kPa)

The causes of hypoxaemia are numerous and may be due to an acute event such as pneumonia or pulmonary oedema, or can be a feature of a more chronic respiratory disease such as fibrosing alveolitis. The cause must be diagnosed and treated, while supportive measures are taken. This may include supplemental oxygen via a mask, non-invasive ventilation, or intubation and mechanical ventilation.

Respiratory acidosis (Paco$_2$ > 6.0 kPa; normal 4.6–6.0 kPa)

Respiratory acidosis, where there is an accumulation of carbon dioxide in the circulation (hypercapnia), is invariably due to hypoventilation, the cause of which must be investigated and treated. Where the patient is mechanically ventilated, it suggests that insufficient ventilation is being provided and the minute volume should be increased.

Respiratory alkalosis (Paco$_2$ < 4.6 kPa; normal 4.6–6.0 kPa)

Respiratory alkalosis is where there is a reduced level of carbon dioxide in the circulation (hypocapnia). If the patient is self-ventilating, it can be caused by hyperventilation, as seen in some anxiety states, or in response to conditions such as diabetic ketoacidosis. Where the patient is mechanically ventilated, it suggests that he or she is being overventilated; the minute volume should be reduced.

CARDIOVASCULAR MONITORING AND ASSESSMENT

The heart rate can be assessed either by palpating an arterial pulse or by continuous electrocardiograph (ECG) monitoring. The presence of an ECG monitor should not obviate the need for palpation of the pulse, as this more fundamental method also allows assessment of the pulse volume. The pulse volume refers to whether it feels weak and 'thready' due to low cardiac output, or whether it is strong and 'bounding' due to fluid overload or sepsis. Feeling the pulse also allows assessment of the skin condition to detect whether it is dry with little turgor, indicating hypovolaemia, or the presence of peripheral oedema. Equally, feeling whether the patient is warm or cold to touch, can assess peripheral perfusion. ECG monitoring is common in many hospital areas and is an assessment tool that may be used for patients at all stages of the critical care spectrum (see Ch. 19).

Blood pressure

Blood pressure may be monitored:

- intermittently using a manual sphygmomanometer
- intermittently using an electronic non-invasive blood pressure device (NIBP)
- continuously via an indwelling arterial cannula.

A continuous assessment of blood pressure may be required to monitor the effect of vasoactive drug therapy (e.g. inotropes), or as a reflection of the severity of illness of the patient. NIBP devices are generally reliable within normal blood pressure parameters, but at low pressures they have been shown to over-estimate the BP. Erroneous results can also occur in patients with arrhythmias (Gomersall & Oh 1997).

> ### ▶ Nursing management: the patient with an arterial line

The radial artery is the artery most commonly used for continuous arterial blood pressure monitoring (see Fig. 31.2), although the femoral, brachial and dorsalis pedis artery in the foot can also be used. Key principles for the management of an indwelling arterial cannula are:

- To observe the site for infection. The choice of dressing must allow for visibility of the site and surrounding tissues. Regular inspection should be made of the site and the patient's temperature recorded regularly. Notice should be taken if the patient complains of pain in or around the cannula.
- To maintain stability and safety of the cannula in order to avoid accidental removal with the attendant risk of arterial bleeding. The cannula should be stabilized by an adhesive dressing. The attached tubing should be supported and not allowed to 'drag' on the cannula.
- To be clearly identified as 'arterial' to avoid accidental administration of drugs, which could present a risk of air embolism and damage to the limb distal to the cannula.
- To observe the limb distal to the cannula for perfusion. The arterial line should only be inserted where there is a collateral arterial supply to the distal tissues, i.e. the hand in the case of the radial artery, and the leg and foot in the case of the femoral artery. For example, the presence of a good ulnar pulse should be identified before insertion of an arterial line into the radial artery. Regular inspection of the limb should be carried out, observing colour and, in the case of a femoral arterial cannula, pedal pulse. Any complaint of pain in the distal limb should be investigated.

Urine output and fluid balance

The kidneys normally filter approximately 120 mL/min (see Ch. 24) and after the processes of reabsorption, the final urine output should be a minimum of 0.5 mL/kg/h. When perfusion of the kidneys is reduced, urine output falls. Thus, it is a good indicator of renal function and perfusion, and most critically ill patients are catheterized so that the urine may be measured on an hourly basis.

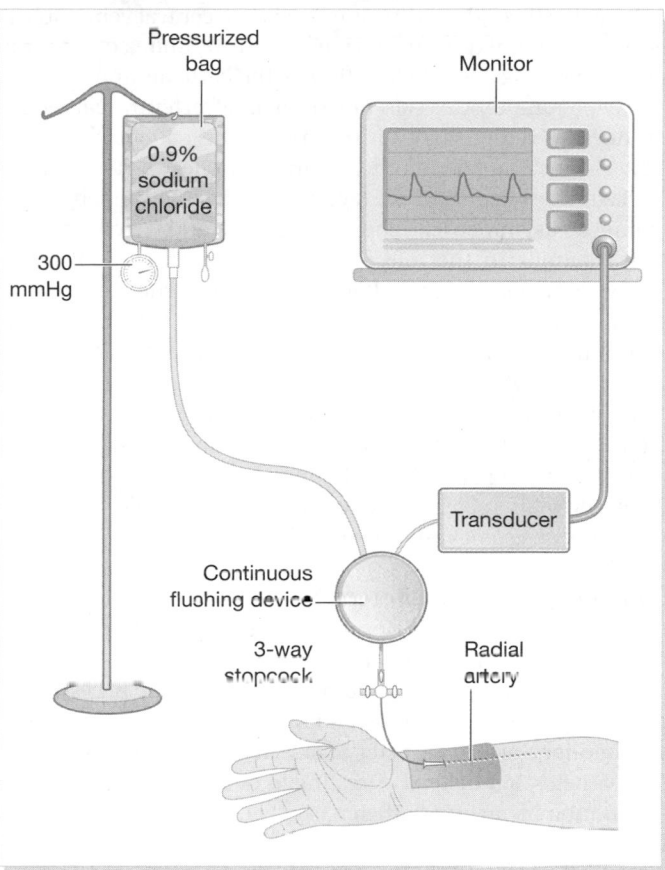

Figure 31.2 Arterial cannula in the radial artery.

Core–skin temperature gradients

The difference between core and skin temperatures can provide a useful indicator of peripheral perfusion. The core temperature can be measured using rectal or tympanic thermometers. The skin temperature can be measured by the application of a monitoring probe to the skin, often the finger or toe. Where cardiac output is reduced, peripheral circulation (via sympathetic nervous system mediated vasoconstriction) is also reduced in order to maintain perfusion to vital organs. The greater the difference between the core and peripheral temperatures, the greater the degree of vasoconstriction (see Ch. 5). However, there are factors unrelated to a reduced cardiac output that can cause cold peripheries (such as cold ambient temperature causing vasoconstriction to conserve heat, or peripheral circulatory problems) and so core–skin temperature gradients must be used in conjunction with other measurements.

Central venous pressure

The central venous pressure (CVP) is commonly used as a guide to the circulating volume, by reflecting the right heart filling pressures. It has significant limitations, partly as it is measuring a pressure (the right atrial pressure) which is then used to reflect a volume. Intracardiac pressures can be affected by a number of factors, including vascular tone, cardiac valve disorders, cardiac failure and pericardial tamponade (see Ch. 19). Consequently the measured pressure may change but may not necessarily indicate fluid imbalance.

Access to the right atrium is gained via a central vein, such as the internal jugular or subclavian. After insertion, a chest X-ray is performed to check the position of the catheter and to check that a pneumothorax has not been inadvertently caused. A key nursing responsibility is to observe the patient closely for clinical signs of a pneumothorax until the chest X-ray has been checked. These signs include tachycardia, hypotension, hypoxia, dyspnoea, asymmetrical chest movement and a reduction in breath sounds to the affected lung. The normal CVP range (in the absence of any influencing factors, such as cardiac failure), when continuously measured using a transducer, is 3–10 mmHg. CVP can also be measured intermittently using a water manometer, the normal values then being 5–12 cmH$_2$O. When measuring the CVP using a manometer, it is important to ensure that the patient is always in the same position. Lying flat is best if the patient's condition will allow, and the point at which the manometer is level with the heart should be marked to ensure consistency (see also Chs 8, 9 and 19).

Pulmonary artery catheters

In the critically ill, the CVP is an inadequate guide to circulating volume and cardiac filling pressures, particularly for the left side of the heart, and in such circumstances it may be necessary to gain a more accurate understanding of the left-sided pressures. A pulmonary artery catheter is inserted in the same way as a CVP catheter, but instead of resting in or near the right atrium, the pulmonary artery catheter (see Fig. 31.3) passes through the right ventricle and into the pulmonary artery. The catheter has an inflatable balloon at its tip which, when inflated with air, allows it to travel onwards into the pulmonary artery until it becomes 'wedged'. This allows the left-sided heart pressure, known as the pulmonary artery wedge pressure (PAWP), to be measured. The normal value is 5–12 mmHg. Low values would suggest reduced left-sided filling pressures (e.g. hypovolaemia), whereas high values might suggest increased left-sided pressures.

There are conditions where the PAWP is not necessarily an accurate reflection of the left-sided heart pressures, and these include raised intrathoracic pressure, mitral stenosis and pulmonary venous obstruction.

Thermodilution cardiac output and derived variables

Pulmonary artery catheters can be modified to allow measurement of the cardiac output. A cold solution is injected into the right atrium and the subsequent decrease in temperature is measured in the pulmonary artery. This allows the calculation of the cardiac output. The modified pulmonary artery catheter can also calculate a number of other variables, including:

- systemic vascular resistance – this provides information relating to the resistance (afterload) being offered to the left ventricle by the systemic circulation. Where the patient is vasoconstricted, the SVR would be high; where the patient is vasodilated (as can be seen in sepsis), it would be low
- oxygen delivery and oxygen consumption – it is important to know if sufficient levels of oxygen are being delivered to the tissues, but, equally importantly, whether the tissues are effectively utilizing that oxygen (oxygen delivery and consumption, respectively).

Doppler ultrasound

Doppler ultrasound can provide an alternative to pulmonary artery catheters to determine the cardiac output. There are a number of approaches that may be used, including suprasternal or transtracheal, or oesophageal. The latter is described here. A probe is placed in the oesophagus parallel to the descending aorta. The ultrasound waves produce a signal consisting of a row of triangles, where each triangle shows the variation in blood flow velocity as a bolus of blood is pumped down the descending aorta. From this, the distance travelled by blood down the descending aorta with each cardiac contraction, and thus cardiac output, can be calculated.

KEY CLINICAL SCENARIOS IN CRITICAL ILLNESS

There are three body systems that commonly require support in critically ill patients, particularly as they approach the intensive care end of the spectrum:

- the lungs with mechanical ventilation
- the heart with inotrope drugs
- the kidneys with renal replacement therapy.

MECHANICAL VENTILATION

When the patient's own respiratory efforts are insufficient to maintain oxygenation and the excretion of carbon dioxide, a mechanical ventilator can be used to provide respiration. Mechanical ventilators (sometimes referred to in lay terms as 'life support machines') can provide varying degrees of respiratory support, ranging from all of the patient's respiratory requirements, i.e. where the patient can make no respiratory effort at all, through to providing support for the patient's efforts, which on their own would not be sufficient to maintain gas exchange.

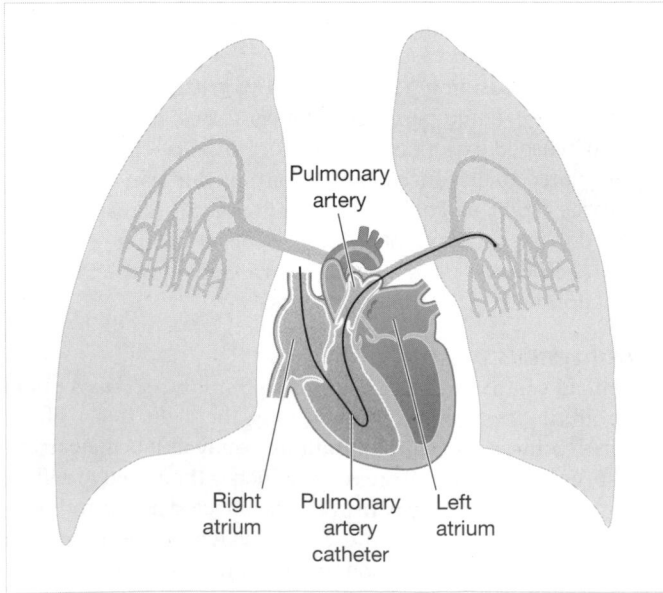

Figure 31.3 Pulmonary artery catheter.

Indications for intubation and mechanical ventilation

- Respiratory failure – where oxygenation and carbon dioxide excretion are inadequate despite maximal therapy (e.g. uninterrupted oxygen therapy via a mask, physiotherapy, antimicrobial drugs to treat infection, good position, etc.)
- After prolonged major surgery, e.g. repair of aortic aneurysm
- After successful resuscitation following cardiopulmonary arrest.

Principles of mechanical ventilation

In order to provide mechanical ventilation, patients must be intubated with an endotracheal or tracheostomy tube. For mechanical ventilation, the endotracheal or tracheostomy tube will have an inflatable cuff which provides an airtight seal to enable ventilation, helps to maintain the position of the tube, and protects the airway from aspiration of gastric contents. The tube is connected to the ventilator via two lengths of ventilator tubing; one arm of the ventilator tubing delivers gas to the patient and the other takes the patient's exhaled gas back to the ventilator. Both will bypass the normal warming, filtering and humidification mechanisms of the nose and nasopharynx and consequently these functions have to be provided artificially. Commonly, either heat–moisture exchangers are inserted into the ventilator tubing, or the inspired gases are warmed and humidified via hot water vapour (see Guidelines for Care Priorities box 31.1).

Mechanical ventilators deliver a set volume of gas (tidal volume) at a set number of times per minute (respiratory rate). The aim is to manipulate the minute volume (tidal volume × respiratory rate) to maintain carbon dioxide levels within normal limits, and the inspired oxygen concentration to maintain

oxygen levels within normal limits. The ventilator uses positive pressure to 'force' the volume of gas into the lungs, causing a pressure within the lungs referred to as the 'airway pressure'. This is monitored closely, as high airway pressures can precipitate a pneumothorax. A range of observations about the ventilator function should be made on at least an hourly basis, and include:

- inspired oxygen concentration
- respiratory rate
- tidal and minute volume
- airway pressure
- humidification
- mode of ventilation.

In addition, it is important to observe the patient's cardiovascular state, oxygen saturation, arterial blood gases, air entry and breath sounds, and general appearance.

Non-invasive ventilation

Non-invasive ventilation does not require patients to be intubated and is indicated when oxygen therapy via an oxygen mask is not sufficient. Non-invasive ventilation can be provided via nasal or facial masks and common examples include CPAP (continuous positive airways pressure) and NIPPV (non-invasive positive pressure ventilation). The latter is usually indicated where hypoxia is accompanied by hypercapnia.

▶ Nursing management

Nurses have a vital role in the prevention of complications and ensuring the safety of the ventilated patient.

Care of the endotracheal tube

The endotracheal tube (see Fig. 31.4) must be secured to maintain its position and to avoid accidental extubation. The commonest method is to use lengths of material tape attached to the tube and secured around the patient's neck (see Nicol et al 2000). The tapes must be tight enough to maintain stability of the tube yet not so tight as to restrict blood flow or cause pressure ulcers.

Compliance with mechanical ventilation

To ensure optimum respiratory therapy, it is vital that patients are compliant with the mechanical ventilator. There are a number of factors that may influence a patient's ability to be compliant, including anxiety, discomfort, inappropriate ventilator settings (e.g. the respiratory rate is too fast or too slow), hypoxaemia or hypercapnia. Although most patients will require some level of sedation whilst being mechanically ventilated, any underlying cause of non-compliance must be dealt with as a priority.

Bronchial hygiene

Bronchial hygiene, by passing a suction catheter down the endotracheal tube, will be required regularly to prevent obstruction of the tube and to remove secretions. Endotracheal suction is an aseptic procedure, to avoid the introduction of pathogens into the respiratory tract. Gloves are worn and a technique used that ensures that the part of the suction catheter that enters the endotracheal tube remains untouched and sterile. The

 GUIDELINES FOR CARE PRIORITIES

31.1 Prevention of nosocomial pneumonia in the critically ill patient

Critically ill patients, particularly those admitted to the ICU, are at a greater risk of nosocomial (hospital-acquired) pneumonia (Santamaria 1998). It is also more common in intubated than in non-intubated patients. Advanced age, immunosuppression and antibiotics can all increase the risk of nosocomial pneumonia.

Preventative measures should include:

- Regular changing of ventilator circuits (every 48 hours)
- The use of anti-bacterial heat/moisture exchangers
- Correct suction procedures
- Strict asepsis during suction and tubing changes
- Handwashing and associated infection control measures
- Removal of endotracheal and nasogastric tubes as soon as possible
- Appropriate antibiotic regimens.

Reference

Santamaria J. Nosocomial infections. In: Gomersall C, Oh T, eds. Intensive care manual. Oxford: Butterworth-Heinemann; 1998, pp. 543–545.

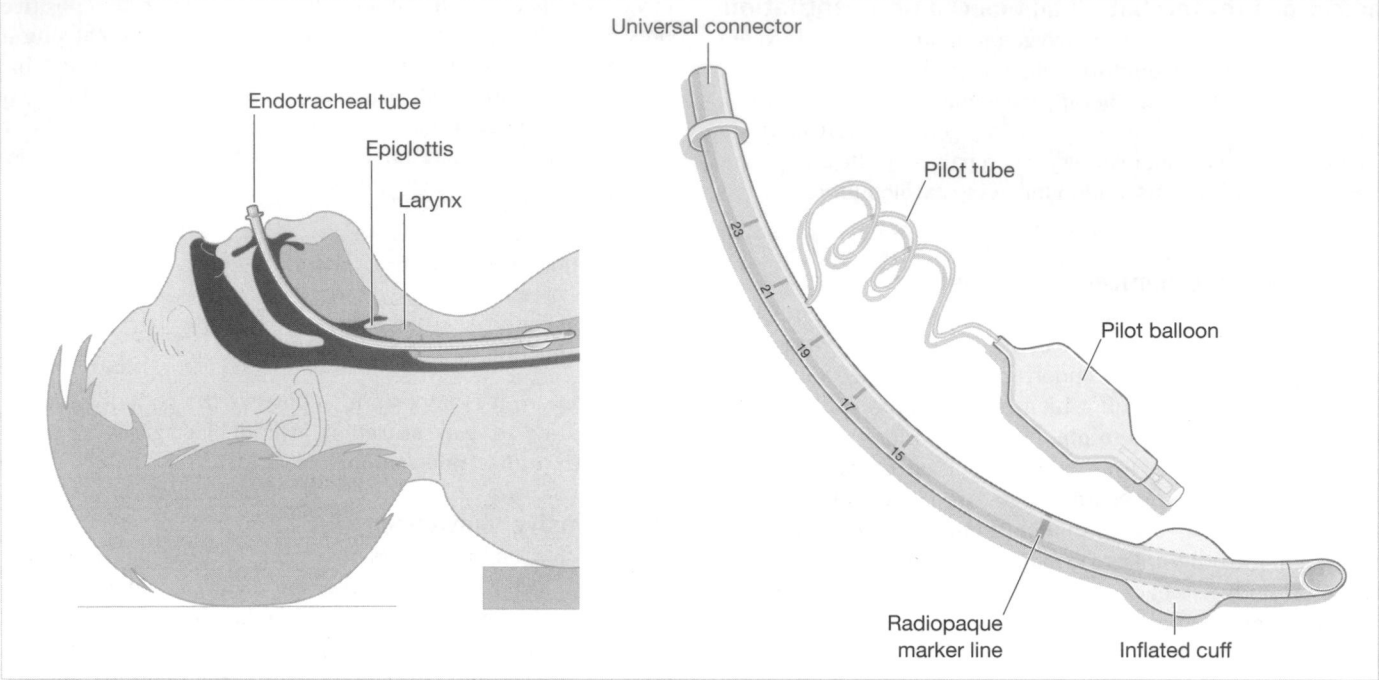

Figure 31.4 Endotracheal tube.

nurse should wear protective clothing (gloves and an apron) and ensure effective handwashing and the correct disposal of equipment. The procedure has potential complications in the critically ill patient, including trauma to the trachea and bronchi, infection, hypoxaemia (due to interruption of ventilation during suctioning) and cardiovascular instability (see Evidence-based Practice box 31.2).

Cardiovascular observations

The application of positive pressure ventilation increases mean intrathoracic pressure, which may cause a fall in venous return (a yet higher CVP reading) and a fall in cardiac output (decreased blood pressure and urine output). Urine output can decrease as a result of a reduced cardiac output but also as a response to increased antidiuretic hormone (ADH) production and activation of the renin–angiotensin–aldosterone mechanism. Therefore haemodynamic monitoring is a significant part of respiratory monitoring.

INOTROPE THERAPY

Inotrope drugs increase the force of contraction of the heart and consequently increase blood pressure. The drugs act upon adrenergic receptors in the body and, in doing so, mimic the effects of natural catecholamines, e.g. adrenaline (epinephrine), as would be seen in a sympathetic nervous system response. Inotropes include drugs such as dobutamine, adrenaline (epinephrine), noradrenaline (norepinephrine) or dopexamine. Dopamine is a drug that has inotropic effects when given at higher doses; it is also commonly used at lower doses (1–3 μg/kg/min) when its effects are limited to the enhancement of renal perfusion. The potential benefits of dopamine against

 EVIDENCE-BASED PRACTICE

31.2 Tracheal suction

Tracheal suctioning is a common procedure undertaken in the critically ill patient. It is necessary to clear secretions and maintain tracheostomy tube patency. There are hazards associated with the procedure and some of the key nursing points are described below.

Prevention of hypoxaemia
● Hyperoxygenation and/or hyperinflation prior to the procedure
● The duration of the procedure should take no longer than 10–15 seconds

Prevention of infection
● Wear aprons, gloves and goggles and wash hands

Prevention of tracheal trauma
● Use a suction catheter where the external diameter is no more than one half of the internal diameter of the tracheal tube.
● Maintain suction pressures of no more than 20 kPa
● The suction pressure should be applied continuously and the suction catheter should not be rotated (i.e. rolled between the fingers)

Reference
Day T. Theory to practice, tracheal suctioning: when, how and why. NT Plus 2000; 96(20): 13–15.

the potential deleterious effects are, however, still debatable (Dobbs & Coad 1999).

Indications for inotrope therapy

Inotrope therapy is used to enhance cardiac contractility in:

- heart failure
- cardiogenic shock – post-myocardial infarction or cardiac surgery
- sepsis – myocardial depressant factor, a mediator thought to be released in sepsis which can reduce the contractility of the ventricles.

▶ Nursing management

- As inotrope drugs are given to improve blood pressure, continuous blood pressure monitoring is required. This is normally via an indwelling arterial cannula.
- Prior to starting inotrope therapy, it must be ensured that patients have an adequate circulating volume. It can be dangerous and cause arrhythmias to attempt to improve contractility in a hypovolaemic patient.
- Inotropes have a short half-life and consequently need to be administered as a continuous infusion. Accuracy is also important and an infusion-regulating device should always be used (see Special Issues box 31.1).

 SPECIAL ISSUES

31.1 Management of syringe drivers

Syringe drivers and infusion pumps have become necessary and commonplace in the management of critically ill patients. Syringe drivers enable the accurate administration of drugs such as sedatives, analgesics, and cardiac and vasoactive drugs. Under- or over-administration of such drugs can lead to under-treatment, adverse effects and even death in the extreme.

Freeflow is one potential problem with syringe drivers and can be caused by leakage of air into the system (syringe or lines), gravity or incorrect placement of the syringe and failure to secure the plunger in the device.

There are a number of precautions for the nurse to take when using syringe pumps, including:

- Being competent to use a particular pump, attending training sessions
- Using the device according to the manufacturer's recommendations
- Using recommended syringes and administration sets, with luer-locks
- Checking that syringes and administration sets are intact, and not cracked or broken
- Checking correct infusion rates and infusion completion times
- Ensuring that the syringe driver is no more than 80 cm above the infusion site
- Ensuring that both the syringe barrel and the plunger are secured and clamped in the pump.

- When commencing inotrope therapy, a low dose should be used initially and gradually increased until the desired effect is achieved. Equally, when aiming to discontinue inotrope therapy, the dose should be reduced gradually and not suddenly stopped.

RENAL REPLACEMENT THERAPY

Renal replacement therapy takes over the functions of the kidneys, primarily in the maintenance of fluid, electrolyte and metabolic balance, and the removal of metabolic waste products. Examples include peritoneal dialysis, haemodialysis and the method used in critical care areas: haemofiltration (see Ch. 24).

Indications for renal replacement therapy

Indications for renal replacement therapy are as follows:

- acute renal failure
- circulatory overload associated with cardiac failure.

In acute renal failure, the key mechanisms of fluid, electrolyte and acid–base balance are lost, and therefore renal replacement therapy aims to support these functions. Continuous haemofiltration is the commonest form of renal replacement therapy, where a double-lumen cannula is inserted into a large vein (e.g. the internal jugular, subclavian or femoral). The patient is attached to an extracorporeal circuit, which takes blood from one limb of the double cannula and passes it through an artificial kidney, removing waste products by the process of ultrafiltration. The blood is then returned to the other limb of the cannula and so to the patient.

While the equipment looks very similar to that used for haemodialysis, the physical processes are very different. Haemofiltration (using ultrafiltration) has to remove an accompanying load of water and electrolytes in order to remove waste products. This water and electrolytes have to be concurrently replaced to avoid hypovolaemia and electrolyte imbalance. Haemodialysis, on the other hand, utilizes diffusion and osmosis, and in doing so is a relatively selective procedure (see Ch. 24).

▶ Nursing management

Safety is paramount as patients are attached to an extracorporeal circuit. The double-lumen cannula must be firmly secured, the circuitry supported, and patients observed at all times. The severity of illness in combination with the movement of large volumes of fluid and electrolytes requires close cardiovascular monitoring of heart rate, blood pressure and CVP (or PAWP). Electrolyte and blood pH values should also be assessed regularly.

To avoid blood clotting in the circuits, and more particularly the artificial kidney, a level of anticoagulation usually has to be achieved. The aim is to anticoagulate the blood in the circuit rather than the patient. Many critically ill patients already have abnormalities of their coagulation and, with the addition of haemofiltration, must be observed for bleeding tendencies such as disseminated intravascular coagulation (DIC) (see Chs 9 and 18).

SUMMARY: MAIN POINTS

- Critical care is a continuum which may begin in the community, or in any of the acute hospital environments; most nurses will care for critically ill patients at some point.

- The HDU provides a level of care that is not possible in the general ward environment. The ICU provides a level of care beyond high-dependency care and usually includes mechanical ventilation.

- Outreach or patient-at-risk (PART) teams and 'early warning systems' can assist in the early identification of critical illness. This enables treatment to be instigated in

the existing environment to avoid further deterioration, or a timely transfer to the HDU or ICU – all of which can reduce mortality and morbidity.

- Particularly at the ICU end of the continuum, there are three body systems that commonly require support in the critically ill patient: the lungs with mechanical ventilation; the heart with inotrope therapy; and the kidneys with renal replacement therapy.

- Monitoring is not only the use of equipment; most importantly, it should also include visual, touch and auditory assessment.

SELF-TEST: CRITICAL THINKING ACTIVITIES

1 Can you identify any of the 'comprehensive care' recommendations in your hospital, e.g. an outreach team, or the use of an early warning system?

2 Think back to a patient that you have nursed who became critically ill:

— What were the physiological changes that signified a deterioration in his or her condition?
— What assessment and monitoring methods were used?

3 There is an increased risk of infection in ventilated patients. Why is this and what can nurses do to minimize the risk?

 FURTHER READING

Darovic GO. Haemodynamic monitoring: invasive and non-invasive clinical application. New York: WB Saunders; 1995.

Hinchliff S, Montagu SE, Watson R. Physiology for nursing practice, 2nd edn. London: Baillière Tindall; 1996.

Hudak CM, Gallo BM. Critical care nursing; a holistic approach, 9th edn. Philadelphia: Lippincott; 1998.

Oh T. Intensive care manual, 4th edn. London: Butterworth; 1997.

Sheppard M, Wright M (eds). Principles and practice of high dependency nursing. Edinburgh: Baillière Tindall; 2000.

REFERENCES

Adam S, Osborne S. Critical care nursing science and practice. Oxford: Oxford Medical Publications; 1997.

Association of Anaesthetists. Intensive care services – provision for the future. London: Association of Anaesthetists of Great Britain and Ireland; 1988.

Chlan L. Psychophysiologic responses of mechanically ventilated patients to music: a pilot study. Am J Crit Care 1995; 4: 233–238.

Department of Health. Guidelines on admission to and discharge from intensive and high dependency care units. London: NHS Executive; 1996.

Department of Health. Intensive and high dependency care data collection – users manual for the augmented care period (ACP) dataset. London: NHS Executive; 1997.

Department of Health. Comprehensive critical care. A review of adult critical care services. London: NHS Executive; 2000.

Dobbs GJ. Enteral nutrition for the critically ill. In: Vincent J-L, ed. Yearbook of intensive care and emergency medicine. Berlin: Springer-Verlag; 1992, pp. 609–619.

Dobbs P, Coad N. The use of dopamine in intensive care. Care Crit Ill 1999; 15(2): 38–41.

Field D. Principles and practice of high dependency nursing. Edinburgh; Baillière Tindall; 2000, pp. 69–109.

Goldhill D, Worthington L, Mulcahy A, Tarling M, Sumner A. The patient-at-risk team – identifying and managing seriously ill ward patients. Anaesthesia 1999a; 54: 853–860.

Goldhill D, White S, Sumner A. Physiological values and procedures in the 24 hours before ICU admission from the ward. Anaesthesia 1999b; 54: 529–534.

Gomersall C. Haemodynamic monitoring. In: Oh TE, ed. Intensive care manual. Oxford: Butterworth-Heinemann; 1997, pp. 831–838.

King's Fund Panel. Intensive care in the United Kingdom: report from the King's Fund Panel. Anaesthesia 1989; 44: 428–431.

McQuillan P, Pilkington S, Allan A et al. Confidential inquiry into the quality of care before admission to intensive care. Br Med J 1998; 316: 1853–1858.

Metcalfe A, McPherson K. Study of provision of intensive care in England. London: School of Hygiene and Tropical Medicine; 1995.

Mohan J. A national health service? The restructuring of health care in Britain since 1979. London: St Martins Press; 1995.

Nicol M, Bavin C, Bedford-Turner S, Cronin P, Rawlings-Anderson K. Essential nursing skills. Edinburgh: Mosby; 2000.

Oh T. Critical care – standards, audit and ethics. London: Edward Arnold; 1996, pp. 11–18.

Raper S, Maynard N. Feeding the critically ill patient. Br J Nurs 1992; 1(6): 273–280.

Sheppard M. The development, role and function. In: Sheppard M, Wright M, eds. Principles and practice of high dependency nursing. Edinburgh : Baillière Tindall; 2000, pp. 4–14 .

UKCC. Guidelines for professional practice. London: United Kingdom Central Council for Nursing, Midwifery and Health Visiting; 1996.

Wilkinson J. A qualitative study to establish the self-perceived needs to family members for patients in a general intensive care unit. Int Crit Care Nurs 1995; 11: 77–86.

Woodrow P. Pulse oximetry. Nurs Stand 1999; 13: 44–46.

32 Nursing older adults

Roger Watson

Cheryl Holman, Sally Roberts (additional boxed material)

'When you're in hospital you expect to have to fit in with their routines so I was really surprised to find that I could have my bath in the afternoon – I thought I'd have to have it in the morning like the others. And I could also get dressed if I felt like it – it makes you feel more human doesn't it.'

(Patient)

THIS CHAPTER WILL HELP YOU

■ Discuss how and why the demographic profile of society is changing

■ Describe what happens to people as they age

■ Discuss the nature of ageism and theories of ageing

■ Describe physiological and psychological changes with ageing

■ Identify the aspects of health related to older people

■ Discuss the consequences of long-term care for older people.

KEYWORDS

Ageing	Long-term care
Ageism	Nutrition
Dementia	Senescence
Demography	Theory
Frailty	

INTRODUCTION

Society is ageing and we are sitting on a 'demographic time bomb', at least according to some sources (Johnston 1999). Accompanying phrases such as the 'greying of the population' and the 'intolerable burden' of the elderly (Warnes 1993) convey a sense of anxiety, on the one hand, and threat on the other, about contemporary demographic trends in the developed world. The fact that people are living longer and healthier lives is one of the successes of modern medicine and sanitation. Nevertheless, there are some challenges for society in having an increasing number of older people. Although increased dependency is not an inevitable consequence of ageing, an ageing society is likely to mean an increase in those requiring nursing care and thus care of the older person is an important area of nursing for most nurses.

National policies not only have a major impact on the availability of resources for the care of older people, but also increasingly set standards and identify performance criteria against which health care provision can be measured (Kopp 2001). National service frameworks are designed to 'set national standards and define service models for a specific service or care group' (Department of Health 1998). In 2001, the government published a *National Service Framework for Older People* which identifies eight key areas (see Special Issues box 32.1). As part of the process of consultation, nurses and other care providers were asked to provide examples of good practice in the care of older people. These examples are incorporated into the national service framework so that others can implement these practices in their own areas.

AGEING

There is no single adequate definition of old age (Tinker 1997). Functionally defined, it may be taken as the age at which a person becomes eligible for a pension from the state and it is this group of people that are commonly referred to as the elderly.

⚡ SPECIAL ISSUES

32.1 The National Service Framework For Older People

The *National Service Framework For Older People* sets minimal standards for the care of older people. It aims to improve quality of care, extend access to services, ensure fairer funding, promote independence and help older people stay healthy. The specific areas of care it addresses are summarized below.

Rooting out age discrimination
NHS services will be provided on the basis of clinical need alone, regardless of age. Social care services will not use age to restrict access to services.

Person-centred care
NHS and social care services will treat older adults as individuals and enable them to make choices about their own care.

Intermediate care
Older adults will have access to a range of services at home to promote their independence and prevent unnecessary admission to hospital. They will also have access to effective rehabilitation services to enable early discharge from hospital.

General hospital care
This is designed to make sure that hospital teams are skilled in recognizing the needs of older adults and collaborate with colleagues who have expertise in the care of older adults.

Stroke
The NHS will work in partnership with other agencies to take action to prevent strokes and provide access to specialist diagnostic services, treatment by specialist stroke services, and secondary prevention and rehabilitation.

Falls
The NHS, in partnership with councils, will take action to prevent falls and other injuries in older adults, and improve the treatment and rehabilitation available for those who have fallen.

Mental health in older people
Older adults who have mental health problems will have access to integrated mental health services to ensure effective diagnosis, treatment and support for them and their carers.

The promotion of health and active life in old age
The health and well-being of older adults will be promoted through a coordinated programme of action led by the NHS with support from councils.

Reference
Department of Health. National service framework for older people. London: DOH; 2001. (Also online. Available: www.doh.gov.uk/nsf/olderpeople.htm).

Pensionable age is currently 65 years for men and 60 for women in the UK, but in line with the rest of Europe, it will become 65 for both men and women by 2020, being gradually phased in from 2010. In the USA, the retirement age is 55 years. Therefore, when looking at tables or graphs of demographic data related to ageing it is essential to know which definition of old age is being used. It should also be understood that, at whatever age old age is considered to begin, it is arbitrary and, largely, socially defined. For example, an athlete would be considered old at 30 in terms of athletic performance but would still have over 30 years of working life left (Posner 1995). There is a further classification amongst those considered to be elderly into the 'old', those aged over 75 years, and the 'very old', those aged over 85 years (Watson 1993). A broader age group that includes those aged 50–74 years is referred to as the 'third age', and this has proved useful for some research purposes (Grimley Evans et al 1993). It should be understood that there is a great variety of experiences and ability amongst all older people (see Reflective Practice box 32.1).

The number of older people is increasing in both absolute and relative terms in the developed and developing countries. This is due to a number of factors, including the increasing life expectancy at birth. This has demonstrably increased throughout the 20th century and is predicted to increase into the 21st century (Disney 1996). However, it is generally the case in

R|R REFLECTIVE PRACTICE

32.1 Contemplating old age

Sometimes contemplating your own old age is difficult. To help you imagine what it might be like, draw a picture of yourself aged 75. When you have completed your drawing, make an analysis of it.

Themes you might notice in your drawing might relate to physical characteristics of old age, relationships, meaningful or fun activities, and connections with people in your past or people who might be significant in your future. You may have surprised yourself by drawing something of a spiritual nature or relating to death. Think about why you represented your old age in the way you did and if possible discuss it with others.

---

developed countries that fertility is decreasing and so the number of older people constitutes an ever-increasing proportion of the population.

The fact that there has been, and is projected to be, a relative and absolute increase in the number of older people has consequences for the individuals who are living longer and for the societies in which they live. There is an increase in dependency among older people and this dependency arises for reasons of physical and mental disability as well as social dependency. While the reasons for this are open to discussion, this increased rate of dependency among older people is a fact. It does not mean that all older people are dependent – in fact the majority are independent – but the dependency does have economic and social consequences. For example, there are increased requirements for health and social care and these must be paid for, depending on the political system, either by individuals or by the state.

Whatever the source of funding for medical and social care, if the relative number of older people is increasing then those who are economically active are becoming inversely proportional to those who require support. The demographic profile of society is changing. Instead of being triangular, with fewer older people at the top of the age range relative to the number of people in the younger age ranges, it is predicted that by the mid-21st century the profile will be almost rectangular (Olshanky et al 1993). The outcome of this changing profile is that those who are economically active have to increase their productivity in order to support older people in their society. In the UK, for example, this is reflected in higher taxes and government spending and in the USA in higher insurance premiums to cover rising costs.

THE PURPOSE OF AGEING

The purpose of old age is unclear. Humans, amongst the animal kingdom, are almost unique in the display of ageing and life beyond their reproductive years (Chritiansen & Grzybowski 1993). The theories of ageing will be covered below but here it is necessary to establish that ageing or senescence (visible signs of ageing) does take place and becomes more evident towards the end of the life span. However, the point at which ageing begins is unclear. Chronological ageing clearly begins at birth and senescence probably begins when development is complete in late teens or early 20s.

Old age is a natural precursor to death and could be taken broadly as an indicator of the end of the active phase and the beginning of another phase of less activity in retirement, leading to completion of life span and death. It is clear that the human life span is finite. Classically this has been set at 'three score years and 10' (70 years) but has been revised upwards as people are beginning to live longer. There is no precise figure for the maximum human life span but it is unusual to find people who live beyond 100 years of age.

Looking at old age in terms of a period of less activity for many and the prelude, however prolonged, to death does not explain its function. There are still parts of the world, principally in the developing countries, where extreme old age is relatively rare and where the experience of older people is different from that in the developed world. Nevertheless, humans have ascribed functions to old age and it is certainly the case for many that it is a time for reflection, for finishing projects and making provision, through wills and covenants, for the next generation. Aristotle saw the process of ageing in terms of a changing balance between the use of the imagination and the application of wisdom (Posner 1995). When viewed in this way, the value of old age to society, in terms of a repository of people who provide stability and who are a source of knowledge, is evident.

HETEROGENEITY OF AGEING

Ageing is not a uniform experience. In fact, there is greater heterogeneity amongst older than amongst younger people in terms of physical, psychological and sociological variables. The physical aspects of ageing may be measured by functional capacity, i.e. measures of independence, mobility, physical vigour and sensory functions. It is possible to demonstrate both a general decline with ageing and considerable heterogeneity amongst older people (Stenhamgen-Thiessen & Borchelt 1993). Some younger old people have very low functional capacity and some very old people have excellent functional capacity. At the extreme end of the age spectrum there are some, described as the 'oldest old', who are extremely healthy and, in many cases, fitter than their much younger counterparts (Peris 1995). In the psychological domain, individual differences in intelligence, personality and social relationships between older people are also observed to be very large (Smith & Baltes 1993). In the socioeconomic realm, considerable heterogeneity amongst older people is observed, with older women being predominant in the lowest income categories (Mayer & Wagner 1993).

One perspective on ageing is that of 'usual' versus 'successful' ageing. In usual ageing, the ageing process is heightened by the experiences and circumstances of life, whereas in successful ageing these so-called extrinsic factors play a minimal or even positive role. There is some evidence that successful ageing can be enhanced, and the factors which contribute towards it include the avoidance of disease, high cognitive and social function and engagement with life (Rowe & Khan 1997). Nevertheless, there would appear to be no elixir of youth, the search for which was really the precursor to the whole field of gerontology (Achenbaum 1995). The only way in which it is possible to slow the effects of biological ageing is to restrict intake of calories (Merry 1999) which is not an acceptable option for the vast majority of people.

THE AGEING EXPERIENCE

Growing old is easy, requires no effort and ends only with death (Sutherland 1999). This somewhat drastic appraisal of ageing, however, masks the many complexities of the process, the variation between the experiences of individuals and the fact that, for an increasing number of people, ageing can be quite a prolonged process due to the scientific and social advances discussed above.

IMAGES OF AGEING

It is easy to present a picture of ageing which is negative. This may be because many people who write about ageing are not themselves old, but look on ageing as a process to be feared and avoided at all costs. Certainly, there are aspects of ageing which are not enjoyable, but our own knowledge of the older people we know, e.g. parents and grandparents, should be enough to demonstrate that it is not altogether a negative experience. For many it is positive and rewarding and when the evidence for usual ageing is sought, it is often not found in terms of mental, physical and social decline. Many older people, despite evidence of the outward signs of ageing, will readily protest that they 'don't feel old' (Thomson 1992).

R|Я REFLECTIVE PRACTICE

32.2 Images of ageing

This box is designed to get you to think about the way that older people are represented in society.

- Think of five words commonly used to describe older people. What do you notice about them – are these words negative or positive?

- Now think of two or three older people from fiction (e.g. characters from novels, paintings, theatre, pantomime or nursery rhymes) from several years ago and next think of two or three older characters from recent novels, radio, television film or theatre. What sort of characteristics do these people display? Are they negative or positive? Have any of the characteristics changed over time?

- Now think of two or three older people currently in the media, e.g. newsreaders, journalists, politicians or actors. Think of some words to describe these people. Are your words negative or positive? How do they compare with the characteristics you found in the fictional characters?

Nevertheless, when you look at advertisements, magazines and the media, it is apparent that we live in a youth-orientated culture, especially in the developed world, where ageing and older people are rarely presented in a positive light. The people used to promote the sale of goods are young and attractive and this applies to the major stars of television, music and cinema. The older few amongst this group are usually youthful-looking either by nature or by design. The nature of what is being advertised on billboards and magazines includes make-up, lingerie and clothes which, if they are not specifically designed for younger people, are designed to hide the effects of ageing such as wrinkled skin and sagging breasts. The majority of such advertising is aimed at women, often by being appealing to men, and it appears that the effects of ageing may be less acceptable in women than in men (see Reflective Box 32.2).

AGEISM

We live in an age where there is considerable discrimination against older people. Some of this discrimination is individual and some is institutional but both demonstrate the phenomenon of ageism. Ageism is simple prejudice on the grounds of age (Blytheway 1995) and it is evident in middle-aged and older people as well as in the young. On an individual level, ageism usually involves the stereotyping of older people as being all the same: infirm, unable to learn and of declining intelligence as they age (Victor 1994). Institutional ageism is represented by, for example, compulsory retirement at a specified age and lack of access to certain medical screening procedures (Sutton 1997). When several aspects of disadvantage in society, such as low income, are taken into account, it has been concluded that ageing is an independent source of inequality between people (Vincent 1995).

Most of us harbour some ageist attitudes, because we are ambivalent towards our own ageing, and such is the extent of ageism in our society that we are unlikely to be immune from this prejudice. Nevertheless, unless we specialize in working with children, as nurses we will work with a great many older people, but sadly the attitudes of nurses towards older people are not always positive (McCabe 1989). Despite our own attitudes, we must do all we can to ensure that our prejudice does not adversely influence the care we deliver. Nurses are often guilty of promoting negative attitudes towards older people by the ways in which they interact with them, e.g. treating older people as if they were infants (Hepworth 1996). It is essential that we try to promote positive attitudes towards older people to our colleagues and to other professionals and, especially, towards the older people in our care.

Promoting positive images of ageing and older people by nurses is not easy. The objectives of working with older people are often misunderstood and frequently undervalued. The emphasis on care, as opposed to cure, does not suit everyone coming into the profession and there is an attendant negative attitude towards working with older people amongst many nurses. Those who work with older people have an important role in tackling such negative attitudes. First they must learn to value their own work – education is a major issue here (Masterton 1997) – and then publicize this area of work through research and publication.

Tackling ageist attitudes is not simply a matter of political correctness with no practical or tangible outcome. There is a world of difference between viewing some of the problems that accompany old age as inevitable and not worth addressing, and learning that it is possible to alleviate many problems and improve quality of life for older people. Related to this is the use of expressions such as 'basic care' in relation to working with older people. This expression should be challenged because there is nothing 'basic' about ensuring that people, who are less able to look after themselves, are well nourished and hydrated, have intact skin and remain continent or, if that is not possible, at least dry and comfortable. Such care is essential and it is always possible to improve delivery of essential care.

CONSEQUENCES OF AGEING

Ageing itself may be effortless but, as many older people will tell you, it does not come alone. There are attendant physical, social and economic changes with consequences for many older people. Some of these changes and the underlying reasons will be covered in the next section, but first, some of the consequences of being old will be considered.

The normal pattern of life events for the vast majority of people is that they grow up and leave their parents to set up their own home, earn their own living and become independent. Accompanied by this independence may be the establishment of a partnership with a member of the opposite sex and the raising of children. In turn, the children seek their own independence and the parents are left at home to complete their working lives before retirement. There is a variety of experience in terms of the relationship between older parents and their children and grandchildren. Generally, considerable contact remains and this is viewed as positive and helpful in a reciprocal way, help with childcare for working mothers being a prime example (Johnson 1995).

Whilst poverty and loneliness are not inevitable outcomes of ageing, retirement and living on a pension often lead to a fall in income for many older people and the loss of family and friends. On the other hand, it also brings about maturity in investments and probably the end of mortgage payments for those who can afford both. However, it has been observed that social and economic differences tend to persist into old age (Thomson 1992).

Loneliness is not an inevitable outcome of old age either (Donaldson & Watson 1996) but is a significant problem for many older people as family members move away from the parental home and friends, family and spouses die. Loneliness is composed of objective elements, such as being alone or isolated, and subjective elements, such as feeling alone. Factors that influence isolation include marital status and lower social class, while feeling lonely is influenced by such things as household composition and health.

While the increasing number of older people is a worldwide phenomenon, it should be appreciated that the experience of retirement is not uniform throughout the world. While it may be discriminating to force people, who may not wish to do so, to retire at a certain age in the developed countries, retirement is a luxury that is not available to many older people in the developing countries. It is common, in developing countries, for a high proportion of older people to remain in work, often through necessity, and to continue to make a valuable contribution to the economy of the country and to their family income. Ironically, with the demographic changes described above, where the developed world may be having difficulty in recruiting younger workers, we may come to depend more on older workers in particular occupations. For example, the myth that older workers are unable to learn and adapt to new working practices has been challenged (International Labour Organization 1992).

INEQUALITY AND AGEING

If there is a 'burden' of ageing, as referred to above, then the responsibility for carrying it falls disproportionately on women. There are more older women than men and they are more likely to live in difficult circumstances such as widowhood and poverty, poorer health and disability (Arber & Ginn 1994). Moreover, while women are more involved in providing care for older relatives at home (Dooghe 1992), it is also the case that much of this care is carried out by older women for their spouses. It is not uncommon for many women to provide care for three generations: their own children, their children's children and their older relatives.

While the range of experience of ageing has been referred to, there is another aspect to this, particularly in the UK, and that is the experience of older people from minority ethnic backgrounds. This is sometimes less than positive, especially when there is a need to seek medical or social help (RCN 1998). The health needs of older people from minority ethnic backgrounds are greater than those of other older people, due to low incomes, poor housing, unemployment and discrimination. Moreover, there are a greater number of older women in minority ethnic groups than in the rest of the population and this may compound the discrimination. They are certainly the major

providers of care to this community. Language differences are often a problem as the women from ethnic minority groups are often discouraged from learning English. However, as stated by the Royal College of Nursing (1998a), this should be perceived as a communication issue to be taken into account and dealt with professionally and sensitively by nurses, not as the patient's problem.

FAMILIES AND OLDER PEOPLE

Nursing is usually concerned with those older people who, for a variety of reasons, lose their independence and require nursing care. Clearly, as the number of older people increases, so the number requiring care will increase. However, in addition to the expected levels of dependency, there are other aspects of modern society that may be exacerbating the need for care among older people. Families used to be less separated geographically and close family members, principally women, carried out a considerable amount of the care for older people who had lost their independence. However, the working population has become more mobile and families tend to become separated geographically. In addition, the number of children relative to the number of older people is declining and women form an increasingly important part of the workforce. Furthermore, divorce is more common providing a greater impetus for the break-up and geographical distribution of families (Dooghe 1992). All these factors mean that older people who lose their independence are now less likely to be looked after by a family member, with the result that an increasing number of older people require care in an institutional setting, or in the community with the support of health care professionals.

SOCIAL, PSYCHOLOGICAL AND BIOLOGICAL ASPECTS OF AGEING

To some extent the social aspects of ageing have been dealt with above in terms of the changes that take place as a person becomes older. While older people are often seen as a repository of wisdom and stability, they are also the focus of discrimination in the form of ageism. Particular attitudes towards older people are often based on misunderstandings of the psychological and biological aspects of ageing. In particular, it is a commonly held that older people are intellectually slower and less adaptable than their younger counterparts due to declining intelligence and because it is felt that they become 'fixed in their ways'. In terms of biological ageing, it is commonly understood that old age is a time of decline in all bodily functions leading to physical weakness and, of course, loss of the ability and desire for sex. Combining such misconceptions about the psychological and biological aspects of ageing conjures up a picture of decay, confusion and ugliness that is a remarkably common stereotype of older people. In this section some of the theories that underpin our understanding of the social, psychological and biological aspects of ageing will be considered. Such evidence as exists to support or refute these theories will then be examined and the reader may be surprised by how different, on the whole, the stereotypical attitudes towards ageing and older people are from the reality.

PSYCHOSOCIAL THEORIES OF AGEING

It is hard to disentangle the social from the psychological aspects of theories of ageing and they are usually considered together under the term 'psychosocial'. Moreover, it should be appreciated that, while there are a number of theories of psychosocial ageing, there is little evidence to support any systematic change in the psychology of people as they become older. This is indicated by the contradictory nature of two well-known theories of psychosocial ageing: disengagement theory and activity theory (Robbins 1986).

Disengagement, activity and continuity theories

Disengagement theory describes a process whereby people gradually disengage from life as they become older. For example, a person may retire from employment and thereby have less involvement with the lives of the people who were also employed in the same company. On the other hand, activity theory describes a process whereby, while people do disengage from certain activities as they become older, they replace these with others as they are able physically and economically to do. For example, there are those who retire from work who take up new hobbies and interests and, indeed, become more active in old age than they were in their younger years. Of course, there is evidence to support both of these theories of ageing and it is certain that, while there are elements of truth in both theories, neither of these could be described as comprehensive.

Lying somewhere between the above theories is continuity theory which describes a process whereby people, as they age, struggle to retain as many of the activities of their younger life as possible. Clearly, there is a wide range of experience amongst older people in terms of activity, which will be dictated by many factors such as ability, motivation and financial status.

Erikson's theory of life span

One theory that attempts to describe the process of ageing, from cradle to grave, is Erikson's theory of the life span in which eight stages (see Box 32.1) to the life process are described. This is in contrast to the above theories which really only consider old age and are not developmental. Erikson's theory incorporates adjustment to the process of ageing and further psychological development as people age.

Each stage represents a choice or conflict, and the way in which that conflict is resolved will affect all subsequent stages. It also affects the development of personality and success in adapting to the world. The internal conflicts in old age are integrity versus despair. Integrity is concerned with a sense of wholeness, uniqueness and worthwhileness, a feeling that one's life has been of value (Schofield 1999). The ultimate stage of Erikson's theory sees the older person reflecting on life and evaluating whether or not it has been a worthwhile and positive experience. If the answer is affirmative then they can die peacefully, but if it is negative then they experience despair before death. Erikson's theory is borne out to some extent by the process of life review whereby older people tend to reminisce more than younger people do in an effort to evaluate the past and their part in it.

The psychosocial theories of ageing presented above are by no means complete but some conclusions can be drawn. None of the theories is comprehensive and none is testable scientifically

Box 32.1 Erikson's theory: the eight stages of life span development

- Basic trust vs. mistrust in infancy
- Autonomy vs. shame and doubt in early childhood
- Initiative vs. guilt in play age
- Industry vs. inferiority in school age
- Identity vs. confusion in adolescence
- Intimacy vs. isolation in young adulthood
- Generativity vs. self-absorption in adulthood
- Integrity vs. despair in old age

because it is not possible to measure some of the concepts upon which the theories are based. It is important, however, to be aware of these theories and their influence on practice. As one observer put it, for example, we often pay lip service to activity theory in the care of older people but our practice promotes disengagement (Robbins 1991).

Intelligence and personality

It is a common misconception that, as people become older, they become less intelligent and that their personality changes such that they become very stubborn and inflexible. Setting aside the profound cognitive decline, or dementia, which occurs in conditions such as Alzheimer's disease, it is simply not true that older people lose their intelligence, nor do they undergo personality changes as a result of ageing. Intelligence and personality are largely a matter of genetics: what you are born with, you take through life (Atkinson et al 1990). What we may perceive as stubbornness in older people may have something to do with their innate personality and will be the result of individual observation. People with a particularly strong personality trait are unlikely to change it or modify it simply because they are getting older. They will have learned that they cannot change their personality and old age may have brought them to the position of accepting the way they are, despite what others may think.

Intelligence has been described as having two components: a fluid component and a crystallized component (Poon & Siegler 1991). Fluid intelligence is the ability to think on one's feet, to approach situations flexibly and to solve problems rapidly. Crystallized intelligence, on the other hand, depends on the application of knowledge and the ability to solve problems by tried and tested methods. It can be seen, therefore, that crystallized intelligence is analogous to wisdom. As people age, they suffer a slight decline in fluid intelligence but no decline in crystallized intelligence (Poon & Siegler 1991). In fact, the overall effect on intelligence is negligible – as people age they depend less on fluid intelligence and more on crystallized intelligence; therefore, the expression 'older and wiser' contains more than a grain of truth (see Reflective Practice box 32.3).

Memory

A classic stereotype of old age is loss of memory and it is true that, as we age, we suffer a decline in memory. Memory is crudely divided into short-term and long-term memory and these allow us to remember recent events and distant events, respectively (Atkinson et al 1990). Clearly there is some interplay between short- and long-term memory, as recent events

REFLECTIVE PRACTICE

32.3 Memory

A person's life history is unique and an important part of their personality. Including life history in an assessment process can lead to more individualized care. In order to try and appreciate the value of this approach, think back to a pleasant memory that you have. It might be helpful to think of public events or personal milestones such as birthdays.

Sharing early memories can be an emotional experience. It can help you to understand more about your patient as a person with a history. Next time you are with an older person, take notice of any memories he or she shares and encourage conversation.

ETHICAL ISSUES

32.1 Disguising medication

If older people become confused or forgetful, they sometimes refuse to take their tablets. If the medication is important to their well-being, do you think it is alright to disguise it in their food?

The UKCC (2001) have stated that 'disguising medication in food and drink can be justified in the best interests of patients who actively refuse medication but who lack the capacity to refuse treatment'. However, the UKCC stresses that every adult must be presumed to have the mental capacity to consent to or refuse treatments unless the patient is unable to understand or retain the information. In exceptional situations, 'covert administration may be considered to prevent a patient from missing out on essential treatment and where the patient is incapable of informed consent' (UKCC 2001). The considerations that should apply in such situations are summarized below:

- The medication must be considered essential for the patient's health and well-being – it must never be simply a convenience for the health care team.
- The decision should be considered as a contingency measure rather than regular practice.
- There should be open discussion beforehand with all involved.
- The involvement of a pharmacist is important.
- The action taken should be fully documented in the care plan and regularly reviewed.
- Regular attempts should be made to encourage the patient to take the medicine voluntarily.
- There should be a clear policy that incorporates the UKCC guidelines.

Reference

United Kingdom Central Council. Register, Number 37, Autumn 2001. London: UKCC; 2001.

---

may become stored, eventually, in the long-term memory while others are forgotten. It is short-term memory that declines with age but, while this can be a significant inconvenience for older people, it does not usually have an adverse effect on their lives. Older people learn to compensate for any decline in short-term memory and it is often the case that this feature of ageing is barely noticeable, especially in familiar surroundings. However, for some older people, age-associated memory impairment is a problem (Deary 1995) and memory loss is a cardinal feature of dementia. It is unclear, however, whether normal memory decline with age, age-associated memory impairment and dementia lie on a continuum. If they do, the conclusion must be that longevity ultimately leads to memory failure. If they do not, then age-associated memory impairment and dementia are distinct conditions.

Dementia

Dementia, which means madness or insanity, is a label which has been applied to a number of diseases that lead, not to madness, but to progressive loss of cognitive function (Watson 1993). Such diseases include Alzheimer's disease, Lewy body disease and cerebrovascular dementia. While dementia is certainly not an inevitable consequence of ageing, there is an association between ageing and dementia such that it is more common in older age groups.

Being progressive, dementia is mild in its early stages with small lapses of memory being ascribed by the individual sufferer and significant others (friends and family) to the effects of ageing. However, the memory loss eventually begins to have a significant negative impact on sufferers and those close to them. Subtle personality changes may take place and noticeable changes in behaviour. For example, the expert cook may begin to forget crucial ingredients from recipes and eventually lose interest in cooking. The keen golfer may give up this activity to sit at home watching television with no apparent explanation.

A most distressing aspect for family members is that dementia sufferers may forget who they are and may become hostile or aggressive towards people who were once familiar. Other aspects of this middle stage of dementia may include loss of social (including sexual) inhibition, leading to embarrassing situations for those around sufferers. Wandering may be a feature of

dementia while sufferers are still active and this may lead to them getting into dangerous situations, getting lost, 'turning night into day' by being up all night wandering around the house and engaging in repetitive behaviour. Clearly this is exhausting and anxiety-provoking for those living with them, and other aspects such as excessive eating and incontinence may have significant adverse economic and social implications.

While it is difficult to describe dementia specifically in terms of stages, it is nevertheless useful to view it in this way. Following on from the early and middle stages of dementia described above, there is a late stage dementia which leads to a very high level of physical dependency and may require the individual to be taken into institutional care. One of the problems sometimes associated with dementia is a refusal to take prescribed medication which leads to difficult ethical decisions about how to persuade confused patients and whether to disguise their medicines within their food or drink. The UKCC provides guidance on this (see Ethical Issues box 32.1).

Depression in old age

Depression is not an inevitable accompaniment to old age. The prevalence of depression in older people is quite hard to determine because definitions of depression differ, but it is thought to be present in older people at a rate comparable with that of the general population (Bond et al 1993). This does not mean that it is a problem that can be ignored in older people. The aetiology of depression in older people may differ from that in younger people and may result from specific incidences of loss such as bereavement, which is more common in older people. The possibility of depression in older people who appear to be suffering from cognitive decline must always be considered, as the symptoms of depression and dementia are remarkably similar in older people and the differential diagnosis between the two can be difficult.

BIOLOGICAL THEORIES OF AGEING

Biological ageing, or senescence, is an indisputable fact with plenty of supporting evidence. There are many classic signs of ageing, some of which become evident even in relatively young people. For example, the loss of hair colour and thinning of hair, the loss of elasticity of the skin leading to wrinkling and reduced joint flexibility are all signs of ageing which are universally displayed, albeit to different extents in people as they age. However, these signs are outcomes of the ageing process which, together with other effects of ageing on the systems of the body, will be considered below. There are many theories of biological ageing and they can be grouped under three headings (Dye 1985): the hereditary theories of ageing, the physiological theories of ageing and the cellular theories of ageing.

Hereditary theories

The hereditary theories are genetic in nature and propose that we are programmed at birth to age and die. Clearly this is true for all humans and may be true for individuals also in terms of rate of ageing and life span. Environmental aspects may play their part by acting on the genetics of individuals; for example, some people may be more prone to certain diseases but may or may not be exposed to them depending on how and where they live. The hereditary theories, in addition to explaining how we age, also offer some explanation in evolutionary terms of why we age and eventually die. The body is designed such that a major effort is expended in the earlier years of life maintaining reproductive potential but it is not designed to withstand the passage of time beyond its reproductive years.

Physiological theories

There are a number of physiological theories of ageing:

- The notion of 'wear and tear' which leads, at different rates between systems and between individuals, to the organs of the body gradually deteriorating as we age and losing capacity to undertake their physiological functions.
- Another physiological theory is based on a decreased ability to maintain homeostasis as the body ages and this leads to a decreased ability to withstand physiological stresses such as dehydration, changes in temperature and other disturbances to the homeostatic balance of the body caused by disease.

- The cross-linkage theory is based on accumulation of metabolic waste products with age that leads to a chemical change in the collagen (the main protein constituent of fibrous tissue) in the body. This change is a chemical reaction leading to cross-linking between amino acids in the collagen and therefore loss of flexibility. This is observable in the skin and in the joints, as mentioned above.
- The immune system has been implicated in ageing because as we age it becomes less capable of fighting infection and may even begin to attack cells of the body – a condition known as autoimmunity. There is evidence for reduced numbers of immune system cells, and autoimmunity has been implicated in diseases associated with ageing, such as type 2 diabetes (see Ch. 17) and rheumatoid arthritis (see Ch. 27).

Although there is considerable evidence, in terms of effects, for the physiological theories outlined above, with the possible exception of autoimmunity, they do not offer explanations of why we age.

Cellular theories

The remaining theories of physiological ageing may be grouped under the heading of cellular theories.

- Cell doubling theory is based on the notion that the somatic (body) cells are only capable of doubling a specified number of times. In other words, the cells of the body age and undergo changes in size, shape and content which are responsible for the ageing process as tissues gradually lose cells. There is evidence to support this in terms of changes that may be observed in cells; moreover, the nervous tissue contains cells that are not capable, under normal circumstances, of undergoing reproduction and this tissue loses cells as the body ages.
- There are theories which focus on the genetic material of the cell, the DNA. These speculate that, with age, the cell is decreasingly able to repair the inevitable errors that take place as DNA is replicated. These errors lead to malfunctions in cell activity. It is observed that parts of the chromosome, the telomeres, which contain DNA that does not code for proteins, shorten with age, but the extent to which this influences ageing is not known.
- Related to the DNA theories there is speculation that ageing takes place by error catastrophe whereby errors accumulating in DNA accumulate in RNA through transcription and in protein through translation. The number of errors in the protein of the cells rises to a critical level beyond which cell function is no longer possible, leading to death of cells and ageing of the body. Puberty and menopause are part of the ageing process and are triggered by some event in the body. This has led to speculation about a pacemaker in the central nervous system which triggers these events and which may also control ageing of cells.
- Free radical theory encapsulates the notion that, with age, the body becomes less able to withstand the effects of oxygen on its DNA and phospholipids (organic molecules important in the formation of the plasma membrane of cells), leading to genetic and cellular damage. Oxygen, despite its crucial role in cell metabolism and the survival of the body, is in fact

a very toxic molecule and during the process of metabolism, and also due to certain pollutants such as cigarette smoke, it is potentially very damaging, as described above. The body certainly has several biochemical mechanisms for handling the toxic products of metabolism involving oxygen, and fewer antioxidants (substances that delay the process of oxidation) are produced as we age.

PHYSIOLOGICAL CHANGES WITH AGEING

As indicated above, the theories of ageing do not explain why it takes place but, while there may be some doubt about the veracity of physiological ageing, its effects are very evident. The most obvious changes are those taking place on the outside of the body where the loss of elasticity in the skin leads to loss of elasticity and wrinkling. Changes in the protein from which the hair is made leads to loss of colour and greying. Other changes take place which are less visible, but any reported changes should be interpreted cautiously because they are, inevitably, the result of comparisons between groups and not usually the result of the study of individuals as they age. Related to the changes that lead to wrinkling of the skin are changes in the tendons and ligaments of the body, which become less flexible. There is also atrophy of the muscles of the body with ageing and the combined effect is reduced strength and flexibility in the musculoskeletal system. In both men and women, particularly older women, bones become demineralized leading to osteoporosis which can be so severe that spontaneous fractures arise (see Ch. 27).

Ageing of organs

The organ that is most adversely affected by ageing is the kidney (see Ch. 24) which, even at a relatively young age, loses its filtration capacity through a reduction in glomerular filtration rate (GFR); there is a much more rapid decline in advanced age. This reduction in GFR leads to a reduction in the ability of the kidney to clear drugs from the body and to cope with changes in water balance. Some subtle changes take place in the liver in terms of its ability to metabolize drugs and it reduces in size with age. However, these changes have no adverse effect.

The capacity of the lungs and the heart both decline with age, but as these two organs are so intimately associated it is hard to determine the effect of ageing on each. Moreover, the functional capacity of the lungs depends on the ability of the thorax to expand and contract and this is influenced by the condition of the musculoskeletal system. Contrary to popular belief, there are no significant changes to the functioning of the gastrointestinal tract; it does not slow down and remains capable of absorption. However, changes in the colon do take place in some older people leading to the formation of diverticula or pockets in the large bowel, which are harmless unless the contents become infected leading to diverticulitis (see Ch. 22).

The nervous and endocrine systems (see Ch. 17) undergo changes with ageing but few of these have any significant effect. Perhaps the most noticeable change takes place in women at the menopause when reproductive capacity ceases. There is some decline in reproductive capacity in men in terms of decreased sperm production but, essentially, sperm production continues throughout life. Impotence, while more common in older men, is not considered to be a normal aspect of ageing. A number of small changes in the nervous and endocrine system occur, such as changes in pain perception and changes in taste. However, although much is often made of these changes, they are small and do mean that older people either do not feel pain or have no capacity to taste food. The eyes and the ears, on the other hand, both decline with age. The lenses of the eyes become more opaque leading to cataracts in some older people (see Ch. 15), and the range of sounds which can be heard becomes restricted due to decreased movement of the bones of the inner ear (see Ch. 16). Again, caution should be exercised in interpreting this last observation: it does not mean that all older people are deaf. However, many older people do use a hearing aid and it is important that it is working and correctly fitted.

FRAILTY

Despite the physical effects of ageing on the body, the majority of older people lead full and independent lives. However, a significant proportion, which increases with age, does become dependent on a higher than normal level of care either at home, in the community, or in institutions such as hospitals or residential homes. Apart from obvious illnesses which can afflict people of all ages, it is not entirely clear what leads to increasing dependence in older people. Older people who require care are often described as 'frail', and indeed 'frailty' is a concept that has received some attention (Campbell & Buchner 1997). Frailty defies accurate definition but implies a lower than normal ability to withstand the physiological stresses that life imposes.

What leads to frailty is unclear but it has been proposed that repeated bouts of illness or disuse of physical functions lead to lowered 'vitality' (Campbell & Buchner 1997). Certainly, there is evidence that some people age better than others and also that specific interventions, such as exercise, maintain and improve physical and mental function. One of the longest standing debates in gerontology is where the normal process of ageing ends and pathology, leading to frailty and dependence, begins.

Immobility, instability, incontinence and mental impairment

However it is defined and whatever its cause, frailty has a number of manifestations (immobility, instability, incontinence and mental impairment) that lead to dependency and these have been described as the four giants of geriatric medicine (Isaacs 1981). The description of the four giants arose because physicians working with older people (geriatricians) are often unable to pin a precise diagnosis on an older person presenting with increased dependency. It is frequently the case that an older person requiring care has a number of underlying pathological conditions; each one is not sufficiently serious to require help with care, but together they contribute towards loss of independence. This concept is described as multipathology and it is mediated via the four giants which are often responsible for the presentation. Of course, they are intimately interrelated and have further adverse consequences if left to develop. Older people may become immobile for a number of reasons, such as a fall (instability) or depression (mental impairment). If the immobility is not alleviated, they will lose muscle tone and bone minerals, which will compound the immobility. The muscle

EVIDENCE-BASED PRACTICE

32.1 Use of bed rails

It is common practice with older people in hospital to use bed rails (cot sides), purportedly to prevent them from falling out of bed. The use of bed rails has been questioned in the past on the grounds of unnecessary restraint, an inability to reduce falls and the potential to cause greater injury than would otherwise occur in their absence (Watson & Brunton 1990). It has been demonstrated in one trial (Hangar et al 1999) that bed rails do increase injury while having no effect on the number of falls and this provides strong support for those who believe that bed rails have little or no place in the care of older people in hospital.

References

Hangar HC, Ball MC, Wood LA. An analysis of falls in the hospital: can we do without bedrails? J Am Geriatr Soc 1999; 47: 529–531.

Watson R, Brunton M. Restrain yourself. Nurs Elderly 1990; 2(5): 21–22.

weakness and bone fragility may then lead to falls, while the immobility may lead to incontinence, isolation, loneliness and depression (see Evidence-based Practice box 32.1).

IMPLICATIONS OF BIOLOGICAL AGEING FOR INDIVIDUALS AND CARERS

Strictly speaking, there are no implications of biological ageing for individuals or carers because ageing is a normal process and, even with some of the normal features mentioned above, it does not necessarily lead to loss of independence and dependence on others. Nevertheless, a proportion of older people are unable, either through illness directly or through frailty, to live independently and do require assistance from either relatives or professional carers such as nurses. The key consequence for such individuals and their carers is the decline in the ability to maintain homeostasis that occurs with old age. This means, as outlined above, that older people are less able to withstand illness and frail older people will be more susceptible to disturbances of homeostasis. A frail older person may miss the normal physiological cues such as change in temperature and water balance. For example, an older person may not sense a fall in ambient temperature and become hypothermic as a result (see Ch. 5). This may be further compounded by immobility if the person cannot use the large muscles of the body to generate heat or even to move to a warmer room. The sensation of thirst declines with age, which is a particular problem in frail older people that can lead to dehydration (see Ch. 8). This is often compounded when frail older people with reduced mobility mistakenly restrict their fluid intake in order to avoid having to visit the lavatory or risk being incontinent (see Ch. 12).

The ageing skin

A particular problem in older people, which is associated with immobility and poor nutrition, is skin breakdown. This results from the normal thinning of the dermis and concomitant loss of elasticity that is part of the ageing process. Dehydration also contributes to skin breakdown. This particular problem is manifested in pressure sores, which range from the superficial, due to damage to and removal of the epidermis, to very deep wounds that may extend down to the bone. Consequently attention must be paid to the condition of the skin, to skin hygiene and to the prevention of pressure ulcers (see Ch. 10). Good diet and hydration play an important role in this, but the key aspect of pressure ulcer prevention is to overcome immobility and loss of skin sensation by encouraging positional change in older people who are at risk. This can be achieved by alternating time spent in a chair with periods of bed rest and short walks – anything that will take the pressure off the skin and restore blood circulation to it.

MEDICINES AND THE OLDER ADULT

Older people often take a disproportionate amount of medicines and this increases with age (Corlett 1996). This is partly due to the increasing incidence of disease and multiple pathology, but older people also tend to undergo fewer investigations for underlying conditions. This may be either because they are reluctant to undergo the investigation or because physicians make a judgement that the conditions are not worth investigating and treating in older people and so they are treated conservatively (by means of drug therapy) instead.

There are some special considerations to be taken into account when drugs are being administered to older people, not least of which is the potential for adverse interactions between drugs. This is compounded by the tendency of many older people to self-medicate with drugs which they are able to buy themselves over the counter at a pharmacy. This can also lead to overdosing with common drugs such as paracetamol, which they may take regularly for pain but which is also present in many common cold and 'flu' remedies and other analgesics.

Pharmacokinetics

The largest influence on drug therapy in older people is physiological and it is mostly a result of the decreasing ability, with increasing age, of the kidneys to filter the blood and excrete drugs from the body via the urine. This means that many drugs that are administered to older people will be present in the blood in larger amounts than in younger people because they are not being excreted as rapidly. Furthermore, the effects of these drugs are prolonged and older people are more prone to adverse side-effects. In order to take this into account, it is usual to reduce the dose of the drug when prescribing for older people and to lengthen the time interval between doses. There are other physiological effects that are relevant to drug therapy in older people but these are minimal compared with the decreased filtration at the kidney (see Special Issues box 32.2).

Compliance with drug regimens

Another aspect of drug therapy in older people is lack of adherence to prescribed drug regimens and there are a number of reasons for this (see Special Issues box 32.3). It has been demonstrated that older people are less likely to understand their drug regimens and often leave a consultation with a physician, where

SPECIAL ISSUES

32.2 Medications and older adults

Taking medicines can be a problem for older people due to some of the physiological changes that take place with ageing. These include:

- Reduced glomerular filtration rate
- Muscle atrophy
- Arthritis
- Failing eyesight
- Confusion and failing memory.

These changes lead to:

- Decreased ability of the kidneys to excrete drugs into the urine
- Higher blood levels of drugs
- Longer-lasting effects of drugs
- Increased side-effects
- Inability to open medicine containers
- Inability to read labels
- Inability to remember or understand drug prescriptions.

The above problem can be alleviated by:

- Prescribing lower dosages of drugs and increasing interval between doses
- Providing drugs in non-childproof containers
- Ensuring that older people understand their drug prescriptions
- Helping older people to understand their drug prescriptions or providing supervision at times when drugs should be taken.

 SPECIAL ISSUES

32.3 Compliance and concordance

Until a few years ago, patients who failed to take their medicines as directed were described as being 'non-compliant'. Health professionals thought non-compliance was a problem caused by the behaviour of irrational patients, who didn't keep to (or perhaps wilfully ignored) the instructions given by their doctors.

Concordance is a new approach to the prescribing and taking of medicines. It is an agreement reached after negotiation between a patient and a health care professional that respects the beliefs and wishes of the patient in determining whether, when and how medicines are to be taken. Although reciprocal, this is an alliance in which the health care professionals recognize the primacy of the patient's decisions about taking the recommended medications.

Concordance has also been called *partnership in medicine taking*. It includes:

- *Sharing beliefs* between patient and professional
- *An explicit agreement* on whether medicines are the best way forward
- *Making the best use of medicines* and their potential benefits – while accepting the limits to those benefits and respecting those beliefs that the patient doesn't want to change.

Website address
www.concordance.org.uk/

---

their drug therapy was explained, with little knowledge of what they were told. This may be due to the often large number of drugs that older people are prescribed, combined with some decline in cognitive ability. Whatever the cause, nurses have an important role to play in helping older people to understand their drug therapy by checking their knowledge of the drugs they are prescribed and ensuring that they know how and when to take them and in what dose. Nurses should also ensure, especially if an older person is being discharged home from hospital with drugs, that these are in appropriate containers. Some older people are unable to open the childproof containers in which many drug prescriptions are packed. This problem can be overcome by packing medicines in non-childproof packages with advice to keep the medications well out of reach of children. Increasingly, medicines are being dispensed in blister packs, which can also be difficult for older people to manage, especially if they suffer from arthritis in the hands.

The use of pre-filled boxes (e.g. 'Dossett' box) provide a safe alternative. These are filled with the correct medication, by a pharmacist or a registered nurse, for the various times during the day, usually for a whole week. This makes it easy for older people to remember to take their medicines at the appropriate times without the need to open a number of difficult containers. It also makes it easier for others to monitor the taking of medicines.

HEALTH AND HEALTH PROMOTION

Health is not an easy concept to define although we are acutely aware when we are deprived of it. Nevertheless, there are a number of definitions of health (see Ch. 1) and most are concerned with a subjective feeling of well-being, an ability to achieve one's own potential and autonomy in so doing (Cartwright 1998). While the area of health promotion in older people is often overlooked, there is no requirement for a separate definition of health for older people as all of the elements of health expressed above apply equally to both old and young. One of the first steps in promoting the health of older people, therefore, is the ability to see them as individuals who still have goals, aspirations and preferences, despite their advanced years.

In terms of physical health, it is unrealistic to expect the majority of older people to be as fit as younger people, but this should not lead to an attitude which says, for example, that there is no point in promoting exercise among older people. Moderate exercise is an excellent example of a health promotion strategy for older people as it maximizes cardiovascular and respiratory capacity, helps to prevent osteoporosis and maintains muscle tone. If this can be achieved, mobility can be sustained for longer in older people, which will have positive physical as well as psychological consequences. Moderate exercise programmes have also been shown to have a positive benefit for older people who are cognitively impaired in terms of promoting cognitive function and reducing urinary incontinence (Watson 1993).

FALLS

Older people are at greater risk of falling than their younger counterparts (see Special Issues box 32.4) and they suffer more serious consequences (Watson 1993). There are many reasons for falls in older people, which can be divided into the intrinsic and the extrinsic. There may be little that can be done to prevent the intrinsic reasons, which include neurological conditions and medications. However, extrinsic factors, such as poor lighting, torn carpets and trailing flexes from electrical appliances, can and should be dealt with wherever possible. There may be financial reasons why some older people maintain their home in an unsafe state, and if money is required to solve such problems, the social services should be contacted.

SEXUAL HEALTH

Health should not be seen solely in terms of fitness; other aspects of normal life such as sexuality are also important to older people. Sexuality does not mean simply engagement in sexual activity, but it is a common misconception that older people do not. The truth is that many couples engage in sexual activity into advanced old age (Watson 1993). Old age may lead to some sexual dysfunction in both sexes, but nevertheless, with appropriate advice and care, sexual activity can be maintained.

NUTRITION AND HEALTH

Any consideration of health in older people would be incomplete without considering diet and nutrition. While obesity is a problem for many older people, and has consequences for the cardiovascular, respiratory and musculoskeletal systems, there is greater concern about under-nutrition, which is quite common, especially in those who are 'at risk' from a social or economic point of view (Department of Health 1992). As mentioned above, some older people will simply take the bad habits of a lifetime, including poor diet and nutrition, into their old age. However, other factors increase the tendency to under-nutrition in older people, including reduced income, bereavement, depression, confusion and immobility. Most commonly, one or a combination of these factors leads to reduced food intake and subsequently protein calorie (energy) malnutrition, the commonest outcome of which is weight loss (see Ch. 11). This is indicative of loss of fat reserves from the body and protein from muscle wastage. The condition leads to fatigue and proneness to skin breakdown and infection. Of course, there are other aspects of under-nutrition, such as vitamin and mineral deficiency, but these are mostly consequent to protein calorie malnutrition.

There is no easy answer to the problem of under-nutrition in older people. Clearly, it needs to be assessed properly and the underlying causes identified. It is pointless telling someone to eat a better diet if he or she lacks the motivation to do so. There is really no specific dietary advice for older people as, contrary to

SPECIAL ISSUES

32.4 Predisposing factors to falls in older adults

Falls are a major cause of injury and disability among older people in the UK and a leading cause of mortality (Department of Health 2001). The following are known to be predisposing factors:

- History of previous falls
- History of chronic illness
- Being female
- Living alone
- Osteoporosis
- Reduced mobility or an unsteady gait
- Unfamiliar surroundings
- Hazards such as loose slippers, rugs, trailing wires
- Alcohol
- Medication, especially if several are prescribed together (polypharmacy)
- Postural hypotension or episodes of dizziness
- Impaired cognition or depression
- Reduced light
- Impaired eyesight
- Lack of safety equipment such as hand rails.

Older people who should be referred to a specialist falls service are those who:

- Have had previous fractures
- Attend an A&E department after falling
- Call an ambulance having fallen
- Have frequent, unexplained falls
- Fall in hospital or a nursing home
- Live in unsafe housing conditions
- Are afraid of falling.

Reference

Department of Health. National service framework for older people. London: DOH; 2001. (Also online. Available: www.doh.gov.uk/nsf/olderpeople.htm).

the commonly held view, their dietary requirements do not differ significantly from that of their younger counterparts. Calorie intake should be regulated according to individual requirements and, if an older person is less active, fewer calories will be required in order to sustain nutrition. It is a common misconception that older people all suffer from constipation, and indeed many older people also believe this. It is not true and if constipation arises in individuals the first line of approach should be to ensure adequate and appropriate diet and adequate fluid intake. Laxatives should be avoided if possible because they become habit-forming and, paradoxically, may lead to constipation as the bowel begins to depend upon them. There are specific problems related to the nutrition of older people in hospital and these are considered below.

There is some controversy about the wisdom of regular health screening of older people in the community (Illife et al

1998). Although screening may lead to early detection and therefore early management of some conditions, it may also turn up problems that cannot be dealt with, and that the older person was previously unaware of, thus raising anxiety needlessly (Cartwright 1998).

▶ Nursing management of older adults

It has been emphasized throughout this chapter that the vast majority of older people do not require any kind of care. Nevertheless, the need for care is greater in older people than in younger people and with the changing demographic profile of the population, an increasing number of older people now require care than in previous years, a trend which is set to continue. Many of the conditions and combinations of conditions that lead to dependency in older people are irreversible and require the help and support of others in order to alleviate or minimize adverse effects. It is often the case, therefore, that when older people become dependent, they require long-term care.

LONG-TERM CARE

Long-term care of older people takes place in four environments: the individual's own home, nursing homes, residential homes and hospitals. Apart from long-term care in hospital, the responsibility for long-term care in the community, which covers home, nursing and residential homes, rests with the local departments of social services. However, apart from residential homes, where the level of dependency is not supposed to be as high as in nursing homes, care is largely delivered by nursing staff and, of course, relatives and friends in the patient's own home. In the last decade of the 20th century, the distribution of responsibility for long-term care of older people has shifted in line with government policy to encourage care in the community (Henwood 1992). The idea behind this was to keep older people out of long-stay hospitals and in their own homes for as long as possible. This was designed to reduce costs in the age of predicted demographic changes and to promote a better quality of life for older people. The reality is that, while long-stay hospital places have duly been reduced, care in the community has mainly taken place in privately run nursing homes and the number of these has increased dramatically in the past decade.

Institutionalization, autonomy and paternalism

Wherever long-term care of older people takes place, including in the home, there are common elements and common problems that need to be overcome. Older people requiring long-term care are less independent than they were previously but this does not mean that they are always totally dependent. Steps must be taken by carers to ensure that dependency is not reinforced. This requires skilled practitioners, as a realistic approach to maximizing and promoting independence is required in order that older people do not become frustrated and even depressed by their lack of ability. Promoting independence does not mean standing back and doing nothing; it means providing the physical and emotional support necessary to enable people to achieve their potential.

Other aspects of long-term care include loss of autonomy and dignity through paternalism and institutionalization (Watson 1993). It is very hard in an institution such as a nursing home, where some element of routine and collective activity is necessary, to avoid institutionalization, but steps must be taken to minimize it. Promoting individual choice, creating a pleasant physical and interpersonal environment with personal possessions, and promoting activities outside of the institution are important factors. Paternalism, which is often the result of the best of intentions, is likewise very hard to avoid. If individuals are dependent and unable to maintain a safe environment for themselves then it is natural to limit their activities and to take decisions for them. Nurses should question the necessity of limiting someone's activity each time it is a possibility and should consider the alternative of allowing some element of risk. In fact, nurses have no right to limit movement or to restrain people unless they are held under the appropriate section of the Mental Health Act. However, maintaining safety is obviously important and it takes sensitive nursing skills to achieve the right balance (see Ethical Issues box 32.2).

Nutrition in long-term care

Removing people from their homes into unfamiliar environments, imposing an institutional regime upon them and taking away their independence often results in adverse psychological consequences. In addition, there are physical considerations in long-term care, primary among these being nutrition. The nutrition of older people in any kind of care is problematic (see Ch. 11) and particularly so in long-term care. Some of the reasons are intrinsic; for example, dementia and stroke, both of which are common among older people admitted to long-term care, are known to have adverse nutritional consequences. Other reasons possibly stem from adverse psychological consequences. In addition, adequate hydration is also a problem for older people in long-term care (see Ch. 8). Encouraging older

 ETHICAL ISSUES

32.2 Paternalism versus risk

Some older people are unable to take decisions for themselves or are liable to put themselves in danger due to chronic confusion. A common cause of chronic confusion is dementia. It is uncommon for older people with dementia to be held under a section of the Mental Health Act, which allows them to be restrained because they are a danger either to themselves or to others.

- How do you feel about having to care for an older person with dementia who is liable to wander away from the relative safety of the ward and on to a busy road?
- At what point, if any, do you restrain such patients from wandering?
- Do you prevent them from leaving the television room, the ward or do you wait until they are about to step on to the road before pulling them back?
- Which of the above alternatives is legal and/or ethical in your view?

people to eat adequately involves a great deal more than simply presenting them with a nourishing diet. If feeding is involved, this requires special skills (see Guidelines for Care Priorities box 32.1). Attention should be paid to individual preferences, where they can be expressed, and to cultural and religious differences between patients, all of which stems from adequate individualized holistic assessment of older people when they are admitted to long-term care.

In terms of hydration, nurses must be imaginative. Fluid intake should be spaced throughout the day and should be varied to include fruit juices, tea, coffee, soup and water as required in order to ensure that each older person receives as close as possible to 1500 mL of fluid daily. The adverse consequences of dehydration include confusion, pressure ulcers and a sore

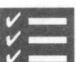

GUIDELINES FOR CARE PRIORITIES

32.1 Feeding older adults

Malnutrition is a problem among older people and can lead to slower wound-healing rates, higher rates of infection and pressure ulcer development. As Weetch (2001) stresses, feeding a patient requires skill and knowledge.

- Offer handwashing and make sure your hands are clean.
- Nurses need to pay attention to the amount being eaten.
- Patients are more likely to eat when with others who are eating.
- The second course should not be put on the table while the first is being eaten.
- Food should be colourful and well-seasoned so that it stimulates the appetite.
- Portion size should be individually adjusted – smaller, more frequent meals are often better.
- Hearing and sight difficulties cause isolation and so spectacles and hearing aids should be checked regularly. If necessary, describe the food.
- Oral hygiene and well-fitting dentures are important.
- Adequate fibre is important to reduce constipation.
- Posture is important when eating – sitting upright with the head inclined forwards is best.
- Occupational therapists should be contacted for advice regarding suitable utensils.
- When feeding, the nurse should be seated in the patient's line of sight and talk calmly, providing verbal and non-verbal encouragement and prompts.
- Appropriately sized mouthfuls should be given – if chewing is a problem, food should be minced or liquidized. Foods should be liquidized separately, not mixed, so that there is a variety of flavours.
- Care must be taken to avoid aspiration of food or drink into the lungs when feeding patients with swallowing problems. Patients at risk need to be taught to cough, without first inhaling, after each mouthful.

Reference
Weetch R. Feeding problems in elderly patients. Nursing Times 2001; 97(16): 60–61.

mouth. At the heart of good nutrition for older people in hospital is assessment and this should involve other professionals, such as the dietician and speech therapist, especially where swallowing is a problem, e.g. after stroke. The occupational therapist also has an important role in adapting utensils and the environment to enable older people to maintain their independence in eating and drinking and preparing meals. The nurse can achieve a great deal by weighing an older person on admission to hospital and continuing this on a weekly basis. Weight and height can be used to work out the body mass index and significant changes in this should be reported (RCN 1998).

An adverse consequence of long-term care is vitamin D deficiency, which results from a lack of exposure to sunlight. This is of particular concern in older people who are immobile or who, due to a tendency to wander, are restricted to indoors. The consequence of vitamin D deficiency is calcium deficiency from bones, already a problem in older people and especially in older women, and this increases the risk of falls and fractures, especially of the hip. All that is required is a few minutes per day in normal daylight to ensure that vitamin D synthesis, which is completed under the influence of ultraviolet light, takes place. It is unnecessary and dangerous for older people to sunbathe or to spend prolonged periods in bright sunlight.

THE OLDEST OLD

The oldest old are those who live to a very advanced age, usually beyond 85 years. As mentioned above, it appears that the maximum life span is around 100 years but the number of people reaching advanced years is increasing. Due to the process of ageing and the adverse effects that it can have, those over the age of 85 include some of the most frail, disabled and vulnerable people in society. On the other hand, the oldest old have survived to very advanced years and they may be unusual in this respect. Indeed, many live extremely active lives displaying physical fitness which would be the envy of those 40 or 50 years their junior (Peris 1995).

CARING FOR THE CARERS

As the requirement for care of older people increases and this burden increasingly falls on the community, an increasing number of older people are cared for by relatives, including spouses, friends, neighbours and significant others. The responsibility for such care often falls upon women and this burden often has adverse physical and psychological consequences. Despite the burden, it is almost universal that those caring for aged relatives or friends will try to keep them out of institutional care for as long as possible. Admitting older people to a nursing home or hospital is often seen as a failure to take care of them properly and as abandoning them to the care of others, which is generally considered inferior to the care they were receiving at home. While an institution can rarely be as good as a home, it has to be acknowledged that the net effect of an admission to institutional care can be positive.

The social aspects of long-stay care are rarely as good but it is often the case that the carer at home could no longer cope with the physical demands of a very frail and dependent older person, which may have had adverse consequences for the person's health. On the way to admission to long-term care, there are such stages as home helps and visits from a district nurse, for specific nursing problems such as leg ulcers or other dressings, and help can be obtained with bathing. In some areas, respite care is available whereby the older person can be admitted to a hospital or nursing home for a week or a fortnight in order that the carer may take a break.

ABUSE

Abuse of older people in care, both at home and in institutions, does occur. In institutions, the abuse, of course, constitutes misconduct or even professional misconduct and may have employment, professional and even criminal implications. Abuse at home, on the other hand, is harder to detect. Abuse takes many forms, e.g. financial, physical, verbal and pharmacological abuse and includes sexual abuse. Abuse at home is often carried out by a family member and is therefore hard to detect. It is also hard to understand but may be the result of frustration and exhaustion through caring for the older person. Abused older people may be reluctant to report that they are being abused, possibly out of fear of the abuse getting worse or possibly because they feel guilty at being a burden to their family.

Nurses are often in the front line for detecting physical abuse when an older person is admitted to a hospital or nursing home. A full physical examination may reveal injuries which are perfectly explicable through falls or other accidents, but there are cardinal signs of abuse such as bilateral injuries and 'pepperpot' bruising (Watson 1993). The nursing response to abuse should be sensitive; the first reaction should not be to call the police – the older person may not want that and the alleged abuser may be suffering from stress with little to be achieved by causing more. The best solution is to approach the local social services in order to ensure that the problem is investigated thoroughly and that an appropriate outcome is reached whereby the older person is no longer abused.

BEREAVEMENT AND DYING IN OLD AGE

It is almost inevitable that older people will become bereaved and certain that they will eventually die, and the way that they cope with this, as they evidently do, is worth considering. Sudden death shocks older people as much as anyone else and is usually accompanied by an initial numbness and a realization that the person, often a spouse, is gone forever. Later, the person left behind may be able to rebuild a life without the deceased (Bond et al 1993). An older person losing a spouse may be left truly alone, due to the geographical separation from family or due to disability, and the subsequent loneliness can be difficult to bear. A great many deaths in old age take place after prolonged illness and the fact that it is expected may serve to alleviate the reaction to it. It should be noted that many older people prefer to be present at the death of a spouse.

There is no 'cure' for these aspects of old age and bereavement but it should not be assumed that older people always cope admirably with bereavement. As nurses, we should be concerned with the dying, and dying older people require as much comfort, pain relief and care as anyone else in the same situation (see Ch. 34).

SPIRITUAL ASPECTS OF OLD AGE

The neglect of spirituality in nursing has often been lamented but this area has been receiving a great deal more attention in recent years. Spirituality is hard to define, particularly when it is devoid of any religious meaning. Nevertheless, many people who are not religious recognize a spiritual side to their lives and this is something that nurses should be aware of in the care of older people. It is certainly the case that old age and the approach of death turns some people towards spiritual matters in the religious sense and this may be more pressing with older than with younger people. However people respond to or recognize that they have a spiritual life, this is something to which nurses should be sensitive and responsive.

SUMMARY: MAIN POINTS

- The care of older people is important for all nurses, not just those working in elderly care settings.

- Old age is arbitrarily defined. The retirement age is usually taken as the age at which people are considered to be elderly but this varies across the world and, in some societies, retirement is rare.

- The purpose of ageing is not clear and humans are almost unique amongst the animal kingdom in surviving beyond fertility. A number of theories have been advanced but there is still little empirical research evidence to support them.

- The process of ageing has been shown to have physical, psychological and sociocultural effects. However, these

are not inevitable and will affect each individual in different ways.

- Attitudes towards older people are often based on negative stereotypes. Nurses are in an excellent position to challenge these stereotypes and promote health in older people.

- Short-term memory declines but not long-term memory, and fluid intelligence also declines but not crystallized intelligence.

- Older adults in long-term care may suffer from institutionalization, confusion, under-nutrition, dehydration and pressure ulcers. High-quality nursing care can positively influence the risk of all of these.

SELF-TEST: CRITICAL THINKING ACTIVITIES

1 Think back to your experience. How many patients over the age of 65 have you cared for? What are the common physiological features of ageing and how may these affect the patient recovering from surgery?

2 Health promotion can be very effective with older people. Think of ways in which you might encourage older adults to maintain their level of mobility.

3 Older people are likely to experience bereavement more often as they get older. Do you think that this means that they accept death and loss more readily than younger people?

 ## FURTHER READING

Biggs S. Understanding ageing. Buckingham: Open University Press; 1993.

Denham M. Continuing care for older people. Cheltenham: Stanley Thornes; 1997.

Hall MRP, MacLennan WJ, Lye MDW. Medical care of the elderly, 3rd edn. London: Wiley; 1993.

Hunter S. Dementia: challenges and new directions. London: Jessica Kingsley; 1997.

O'Mahoney D, Martin U. Practical therapeutics for the older patient. London: Wiley; 1999.

Offerhaus L. Drugs for the elderly, 2nd edn. Copenhagen: World Health Organization; 1997.

Pickering S, Thomson JS. Promoting positive practice in nursing older people. London: Baillière Tindall; 1998.

REFERENCES

Achenbaum WA. Crossing frontiers: gerontology emerges as a science. Cambridge: Cambridge University Press; 1995.

Arber S, Ginn J. Women and ageing. Rev Clin Gerontol 1994; 4: 349–358.

Atkinson RL, Atkinson RC, Smith EE, Bem DJ. Introduction to psychology, 10th edn. San Diego: Harcourt Brace Jovanovitch; 1990.

Blytheway B. Ageism. Buckingham: Open University Press; 1995.

Bond J, Coleman P, Peace S. Ageing in society: an introduction to social gerontology, 2nd edn. London: Sage; 1993.

Campbell AJ, Buchner DM. Unstable disability and the fluctuations of frailty. Age Ageing 1997; 26: 215–318.

Cartwright M. Community perspectives. In: Marr J, Kershaw B, eds. Caring for older people: developing specialist practice. London: Arnold; 1998, pp 213–235.

Christiansen JL, Grzybowski JM. Biology of aging. St Louis: Mosby; 1993.

Corlett AJ. Aids to compliance with medication. Br Med J 1996; 313: 926–929.

Deary IJ. Age-associated memory impairment: a suitable case for treatment? Ageing Soc 1995; 15: 393–406.

Department of Health. The nutrition of elderly people. London: DoH; 1992.

Department of Health. National service frameworks (Health Service circular HSC 1998/074). London: The Stationery Office; 1998.

Department of Health. National service framework for older people. London: The Stationery Office; 2001.

Disney R. Can we afford to grow older? Cambridge: MIT Press; 1996.

Donaldson JM, Watson R. Loneliness in elderly people: an important area for nursing research. J Adv Nurs 1996; 24: 952–959.

Dooghe G. Informal caregivers of elderly people: a European review. Ageing Soc 1992; 12: 369–380.

Dye CA. Assessment and intervention in geropsychiatric nursing. Orlando: Grune & Stratton; 1985.

Grimley Evans J, Goldacre MJ, Hodkinson HM, Lamb S, Savory M. Health and function in the third age. London: Nuffield Provincial Hospitals Trust; 1993.

Henwood M. Through a glass darkly. London: King's Fund; 1992.

Hepworth M. 'William' and the old folks: notes on infantilisation. Ageing Soc: 1991; 16: 423–441.

Iliffe S, Patterson L, Gould MM. Health care for older people. London: BMJ Books; 1998.

International Labour Organisation. An active future for older workers. ILO Information 1992; 28: 14.

Isaacs B. Ageing and the doctor. In: Hobman D, ed. The impact of ageing. London: Croom Helm; 1981, pp 143–157.

Johnson ML. Interdependency and the generational compact. Ageing Soc 1995; 15: 243–265.

Johnston P. Children 'will be outnumbered by elderly in 2008'. Daily Telegraph 1999, 29 May, p 8.

Kopp P. Development of national and local policy in the care of older people. Prof Nurse 2001; 17(2): 111–114.

McCabe BM. Ego defensiveness and its relationship to attitudes of registered nurses towards older people. Res Nurs Health 1989; 12: 85–91.

Masterton A. The continuing care of older people. London: UKCC; 1997.

Mayer KU, Wagner M. Socio-economic resources and differential ageing. Ageing Soc 1993; 13: 517–550.

Merry BJ. A radical way to age. Biologist 1999; 46: 114–116.

Olshanky SJ, Carnes BA, Cassel K. The aging of the human species. Scientific Am 1993; 268(4): 18–24.

Peris TT. The oldest old. Scientific Am 1995; 272(1): 51–55.

Poon LW, Siegler IC. Psychological aspects of normal ageing. In: Sadavoy, J, Lazarus LW, Jarvik LF, eds. Comprehensive review of geriatric psychiatry. Washington: American Psychiatric Press; 1991, pp 117–145.

Posner RA. Aging and old age. Chicago: University of Chicago Press; 1995.

Royal College of Nursing. The nursing care of older patients from black and minority ethnic groups. London: Royal College of Nursing; 1998.

Robbins SE. The psychology of human ageing. In: Redfern S, ed. Nursing elderly people. Edinburgh: Churchill Livingstone; 1991, pp 19–38.

Rowe JW, Khan RL. Successful aging. The Gerontologist 1997; 37: 433–440.

Royal College of Nursing Institute. The use of nutritional standards to improve nutritional care for older adults: a case study. London: RCN; 1998.

Schofield I. Theories of ageing. In: Heath H, Schofield I, eds. Healthy ageing: nursing older people. London: Mosby; 1999.

Smith J, Baltes PB. Differential psychological ageing: profiles of the old and very old. Ageing Soc 1993; 13; 551–587.

Steinhagen-Thiessen E, Borchelt M. Health differences in advanced old age. Ageing Soc 1993; 13: 619–655.

Sutherland S. With respect to old age: a report by the Royal Commission on long term care. London: The Stationery Office; 1999.

Sutton GC. Will you still need me, will you still screen me, when I'm past 64? Br Med J 1997; 315: 1032–1033.

Thomson P. 'I don't feel old': subjective ageing and the search for meaning in later life. Ageing Soc 1992; 12: 23–27.

Tinker A. Older people in modern society. London: Longman; 1997.

United Kingdom Central Council. Register, Number 37, Autumn. London: UKCC; 2001.

Victor CR. Old age in modern society. London: Chapman & Hall; 1994.

Vincent JA. Inequality and old age. London: UCL Press; 1995.

Warnes AM. Being old, old people and the burdens of burden. Ageing Soc 1993; 13: 297–338.

Watson R. Caring for elderly people. London: Baillière Tindall; 1993.

Weetch R. Feeding problems in elderly patients. Nurs Times 2001; 97(16); 60–61.

33 Nursing patients with cancer

Tanya Andrewes

> 'I thought cancer nursing was all about people dying. I was relieved to find this wasn't the case and it was a surprisingly cheerful and positive place. I didn't realise that so many people actually survive cancer and that they can do so much to control pain and sickness nowadays.'
>
> *(Student nurse)*

THIS CHAPTER WILL HELP YOU

- Describe the biological basis of cancer cells
- Describe how cancer develops and spreads
- Discuss the biological basis of cancer treatment and its effects upon patients
- Describe the factors that influence decisions to undergo cancer screening or to make healthy lifestyle changes
- Understand the diagnostic tests used and their potential side-effects
- Critically analyse the nursing role in the care of people with cancer, from diagnosis through treatment to rehabilitation
- Identify strategies for providing supportive nursing care of people with cancer based on the latest available evidence
- Apply ethical principles to situations that may compromise the care/position of people with cancer and their partners
- Understand the specialist nurse roles in cancer care
- Use reflection in order to learn from practice

KEYWORDS

Aetiology	Malignant
Benign	Metastasis
Biopsy	Mutagen
Body image	Neoplasm
Cancer	Oncogenes
Carcinogen	Oncology
Chemotherapy	Proto-oncogenes
Cytology	Radiotherapy
Epidemiology	Rehabilitation
Histology	Screening

INTRODUCTION

Cancer is a significant health problem in the UK, recently overtaking coronary heart disease as the leading cause of mortality (Tattersall & Thomas 1999). 'Cancer' is a recognized medical diagnosis that encapsulates over 200 separate and distinctive diseases. The consequences of each disease are different, as is the prognosis, but for many people the word cancer conjures up the image of a single condition that will cause inevitable pain, sickness and hair loss and ultimately death. Although cancer remains a serious, potentially life-threatening problem, the significant advances in treatment over the last decade have resulted in more effective management, with cure in some cases. Side-effects are no longer deemed to be inevitable and those that present are effectively managed, in most cases, by a range of interventions.

One in three people in the UK will get cancer and one in four people will die from it. A government audit (Calman & Hine 1995) uncovered significant differences in mortality rates between the UK and the rest of the world, and even between different regions within the UK. The report recommended a series of wide-ranging changes related to the delivery of cancer services and the provision of care, recognizing a need for health professionals with specific knowledge and skills in oncology. Cancer services in the UK are now led from regional cancer centres with the facilities to support the site-specific treatment of common and rare cancers. Cancer units within district general hospitals support the cancer centres by treating people with common cancers. The Calman–Hine report (1995) focuses on the need for cancer care to be led by the primary sector, with a particular emphasis on the prevention of cancer and screening since these represent key prognostic factors in cancer diagnosis and treatment.

The British government is committed to improving the services for people with cancer and recently published *The NHS Cancer Plan* (Department of Health 2000), which has been developed by a team of cancer experts in conjunction with patients and cancer care professionals from across the country. This document sets out a strategy for developing existing services, supported by additional funding, with the intention of:

- saving more lives, through proactive health promotion and education, early diagnosis aided by extended access to appropriate screening programmes, prompt referral and treatment by appropriately qualified professional support
- improving outcomes by ensuring access to the best available treatments and ensuring the provision of support by appropriately qualified professionals in the primary care setting
- tackling the inequalities in health that increase the risk of cancer in unskilled workers
- investing in the cancer workforce, through strong research and preparation for the genetics revolution, so that the NHS achieves its full potential in cancer care.

The NHS Cancer Plan reinforces that cancer is largely preventable through the modification of unhealthy behaviours. Nurses are identified as having a fundamental role in reducing the number of people in the population who smoke, at both national and local levels. Furthermore, they are charged with promoting a healthy diet, based on a standard of five portions of fruit or vegetables per day. Since these behaviours are largely associated with social policy and poverty, nurses are expected to be involved in wider policy-making debate at local and national levels.

The measurement of treatment outcomes is considered to be essential and will be ongoing through the work of the National Institute of Clinical Excellence (NICE), who will offer guidance on the use of new cancer drugs. Furthermore, NICE will commission a comprehensive package of guidance between 2001 and 2004 on the organization of cancer services. All parts of the NHS will be expected to implement this. In the future, cancer services will be regularly audited, both independently by the Commission for Health Improvement (CHI) and by the use of peer review teams. The audits will serve to monitor the implementation of national guidelines and ensure quality in cancer service provision. In order to strengthen the coordination and prioritization of cancer research, the National Cancer Research Institute (NCRI) has been created.

The NHS Cancer Plan (Department of Health 2000) supports the idea that implementation of the strategy is dependent upon the specialist education of all professionals engaged in the care of people with cancer.

Nurses will have contact with people who have cancer within a variety of clinical settings – at home or in a health care setting, general or specialized. The provision of sensitive and understanding nursing care develops out of a sound knowledge base about the nature of cancer, and the impact of the diagnosis and therapeutic treatment on patients and their families. 'Cancer' represents much more than a disease to those people directly affected by it. Rather, it is a powerful experience that has profound implications, often leading to a reappraisal of personal values, goals and even life itself. Effective management of the cancer experience, in terms of the symptoms of the disease and the side-effects associated with treatment, serves to improve quality and length of life.

Nurses caring for people affected by cancer require a sound knowledge and understanding of screening, health promotion and health education, therapeutic treatment and the management of its effects, and the physiological, psychological, social, spiritual and economic impact of cancer. This chapter will take the reader through the cancer journey from screening and diagnosis through treatment to rehabilitation. It complements Chapter 34, nursing people with palliative care needs. Background biological information will enable the reader to understand how cancer develops and how it is treated. The latter part of the chapter will focus on the nursing issues associated with the care of the cancer patient, with the emphasis upon nursing interventions. The chapter offers basic knowledge to pre-registration nurses caring for people with cancer and their significant others in a range of clinical settings. It will serve as a revision tool for post-registration nurses, provoking reflection on practice and encouraging wider reading around a range of issues.

AETIOLOGY

Aetiology is the study of factors involved in the development of a specific disease. These may include internal elements or external agents. Aetiology is also concerned with the nature of disease progression and the effects of specific diseases as they invade the human body. Over the past two decades, research into the nature of cancer has resulted in a substantial increase in knowledge about causative factors, the development and the progression of the disease. This knowledge is being used to encourage health-promoting, health improvement and health-maintaining behaviours. Furthermore, it is informing new developments in cancer treatment.

WHAT IS CANCER AND HOW DOES IT OCCUR?

Cancer is a disease of the cells that is characterized by genetic alteration and inappropriate reproduction (Weinberg 1998). The disease is classified according to the originating cell type. Cancer can arise from almost any of the body tissues, whilst maintaining distinct/unique features.

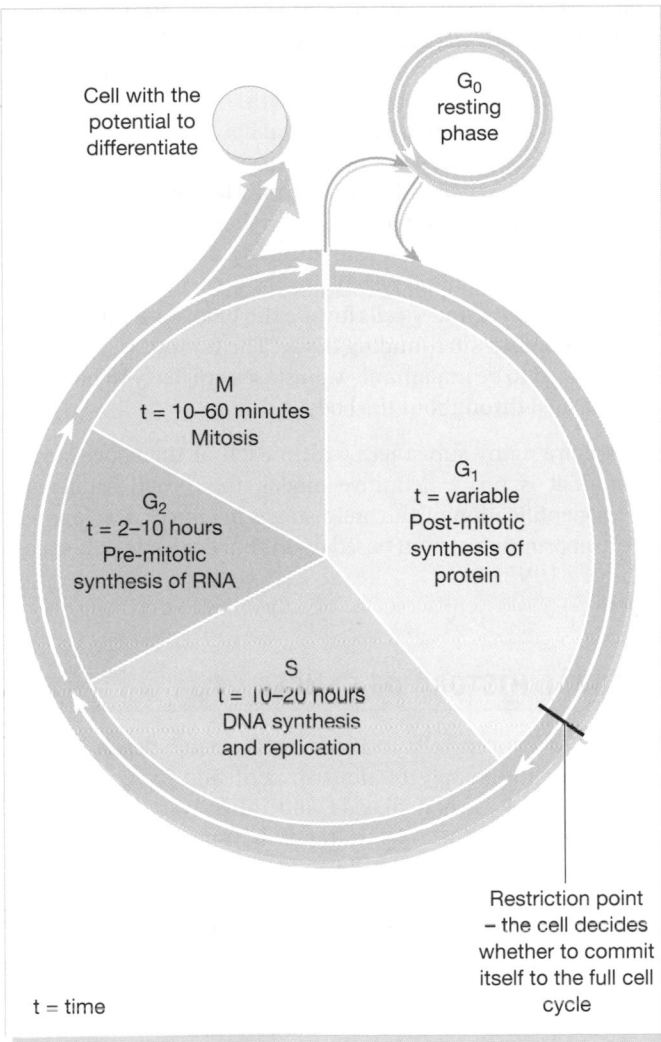

Figure 33.1 The cell cycle.

Differences between normal and cancer cells

Normal cells are created either by mitosis (somatic cells divide to form two identical daughter cells) or by meiosis (a two-stage division resulting in gametes with only one set of chromosomes). The essential difference between normal and cancer cells is that normal cells are closely regulated and divide in a controlled fashion, whilst cancer cells are characterized by uncontrolled growth.

Growth in humans occurs in two phases. The first phase is from birth to maturity when the total number of cells increases as the person grows to full size. The second phase of cell growth occurs between maturity and death, where the number of cells produced is equal to the number of cells that die and thus body size remains relatively constant. Cell growth occurs within a regulated process known as the cell cycle (Fig. 33.1).

Genes directly control the behaviour of individual cells, enabling the creation of body form and function (Weinberg 1998). The body is a community of cells, each one occupying a specific place where it is enabled to perform its tasks for the body. Within the healthy body, cells live in a complex state of interdependence, their division instructed or regulated by hormones and growth factors. Apart from leucocytes which circulate throughout the body undertaking a surveillance role, normal cells maintain their position within the tissue from where they were derived and now function.

Like healthy cells, the cells that form a tumour descend from one common ancestor. They differ from normal cells because they are able to travel around the body and take root in tissues where they would not normally be expected to survive. Normal cells undergo around 50–60 divisions (cell mortality) before they are subject to programmed cell death (apoptosis). The ageing process in the cell is known as senescence and cells that have undergone multiple division are referred to as 'senescent' or old. Once apoptosis is triggered, the cell will die and disintegrate within 1 hour. Weinberg (1998) explains that cell mortality is associated with the degeneration of the telomeres at each end of the chromosomes. Telomeres, which act like the shields at the end of shoelaces to protect the chromosomes from fusion with each other and from fragmentation, shorten progressively with each cycle of growth and division, increasing the potential for cellular damage. Telomeres do not regenerate. After 50–60 cellular divisions they are worn down, causing chromosomes to fuse with one another. This leads to genetic disarray and ultimately cell death.

Cancer cells are often described as immortal. This is because the loss of cell-to-cell contact inhibition enables them to grow and reproduce out of all proportion (Groenwald 1993). Normal cells stop growing once there is a single layer of cells completely covering the space or cavity they are contained within. They are dependent upon the density of the cells surrounding them for growth or inhibition of cellular division. Inhibition occurs because crowding of cells forces competition for vital nutrients that enable cellular division. Cancer cells require lower concentrations of vital nutrients and are more mobile than normal cells so their growth is less density-dependent (Groenwald 1993). Furthermore, cancer cells only require low levels of growth factors in order to divide. This, in addition to the loss of the restriction point in the cell cycle where the cell either decides to rest in G_0 until required, or continue into G_1 and commit to the whole reproductive cycle (Fig. 33.1), means that cancer cells undergo extensive proliferation.

Weinberg (1998) proposes that within the human genome exist a large set of sleeping cancer genes (proto-oncogenes) that play an important part in the day-to-day life of human cells but do not directly cause cancer. If mutagenic carcinogens (chemicals with the potential to cause genetic change within the cells) activate the proto-oncogenes they transform into oncogenes which cause unrestricted growth of the cell and its descendants. Within the normal processes of replication and division of healthy cells, there is a potential for miscopying of the deoxyribonucleic acid (DNA). Consequently one of the daughter cells will receive a mutated gene. Agents that promote cell growth indirectly influence the development of mutations by forcing cells to replicate their DNA. Increased replication incurs an increased potential for the inadvertent development of mutations as a result of miscopying. Consequently the potential to develop cancer is increased.

Cell growth is also regulated by the action of tumour suppressor genes that work like brakes in healthy cells, slowing down replication and division processes. As healthy cells become cancerous they appear to shed or inactivate the tumour suppressor genes, resulting in a defective braking system. Loss of tumour suppressor gene function is a two-step process; both copies of the tumour suppressor gene have to undergo alteration before function is compromised. People can inherit defective versions of a tumour suppressor gene from their parents in the germ cell line, which incurs an inborn susceptibility to the development of cancer. A large number of tumour suppressor genes have now been identified, e.g. the $p53$ gene. $p53$ is present in a mutant form in around 60% of all human cancers. Mutant versions of the $p53$ gene may be transmitted via the germ cell line and it is also susceptible to somatic mutation by exposure to carcinogenic agents.

The development of cancer can therefore be seen as the result of a close relationship between the oncogene, the tumour suppressor gene and carcinogens.

Cancer spread is generally the result of cell immortality rather than increased proliferation. Only 50–60% of cancer cells die during the course of the disease, whereas normally there is 100% turnover. Cancer cells move despite contact inhibition, which allows them to migrate from the site of origin to invade regional and distant tissues via the circulation. It is the secondary cancer (metastases) forming in vital organs, rather than the primary tumour, that has the potential to cause fatal organ dysfunction.

CARCINOGENESIS

Carcinogenesis is the development and spread of cancer. It is characterized by progressive disorganization of architectural structures, which occurs over a variable period of time within each biologic stage (Lynch 1998). Carcinogenesis begins at the molecular level where inherited or acquired errors cause alterations in cellular anatomical and physiological characteristics at subcellular, cellular levels and then ultimately architectural structure and function. Genetic changes are characterized by structural alterations of DNA.

Carcinogenesis was previously thought to be a simple, staged process of tumour progression (Lynch 1998); however, the genetic changes are variable at each level. Progression towards invasive neoplasia is not inevitable. Rather, it is opposed by restorative factors that normally operate in healthy and damaged tissues. Limited cellular damage is repaired, whilst those cells that are beyond repair are culled and replaced as a function of the immune response. Repair is most likely to be effective early in the process, where there is still relatively normal cell structure and function.

Stages in tumour development

Tumour development occurs within an organized multi-step process:

- *Genetically altered cell.* A previously healthy cell sustains a genetic mutation that increases its propensity to proliferate instead of rest.
- *Hyperplasia* (an increase in the number of cells). The altered cell and its descendants proliferate. The appearance remains normal. After 2–10 years of proliferation, 1 in 1 million of these cells sustains further genetic mutation, increasing the propensity for proliferation still further.

- *Dysplasia* (abnormal development of tissues). Proliferation continues. The cells begin to alter in appearance and look abnormal. Occasional further genetic changes occur.
- *Cancer-in-situ* (a premalignant growth). Affected cells look increasingly abnormal. Proliferation continues and abnormal growth becomes apparent. Surrounding tissue is not compromised and the tumour may be contained locally for an indefinite period of time. If further genetic mutations occur, the tumour invades surrounding tissue and infiltrates the blood or lymphatic systems.
- *Invasive cancer.* Cancer cells invade the blood or lymphatic systems and/or surrounding tissue. The tumour is considered to be malignant. Metastases are likely to be established throughout the body.

There are many sub-stages within each of the above stages. Although it is not a definitive model, this broad framework enables identification of the main stages in cancer development and the appropriate action based upon that evidence to be taken (Weinberg 1998).

NATURAL HISTORY OF CANCER

A clump of cancer cells < 1 mm in diameter depends upon diffusion for the supply of nourishment and oxygen and for the excretion of carbon dioxide and other waste products of metabolism. Once the mass extends beyond 1 mm, the cells begin to starve or suffer from the build-up of waste products and the apoptotic (cellular suicide) response is triggered in the presence of $p53$. In order to survive and continue the process of proliferation, the cancer cells need to develop a means to access nutrients and to dispose of waste products. Weinberg (1998) notes how some of the cancer cells in the mass imitate their surrounding cells and acquire the ability to secrete angiogenic growth factors (chemicals that enable capillary growth). Oxygen and nutrients accessed via the capillaries enable the mass to grow rapidly. Tumour development and spread are closely associated with the ability of the cells to secrete these angiogenic growth factors. Those tumours that develop extensive capillary networks are usually destined to grow aggressively and to spread widely. Subsequently, the associated prognosis for the person with an aggressive cancer is poor. In contrast, those tumours with a poor ability to develop capillaries and which are slow-growing pose less risk of metastatic spread, and therefore the associated prognosis is better.

Cancer cells in the middle of a tumour mass often have poor access to the blood supply, and therefore to oxygen, so they become anoxic. Cells cease to grow without oxygen and eventually die if anoxia is prolonged. The apoptotic (cell suicide) response is mediated by $p53$, but where the $p53$ gene has mutated, the cells are able to survive and recommence growth cycles when blood and oxygen supply is restored (Weinberg 1998). This phenomenon is observed when cancer treatment initially serves to shrink a large tumour mass. The blood supply is restored at the centre of the tumour, enabling rapid and unimpeded cellular proliferation so that the tumour begins to grow quickly. Ongoing treatment aims to continue tumour mass reduction in this situation.

MODES OF SPREAD AND PATHOPHYSIOLOGICAL EFFECTS

A tumour mass of 1 cm diameter may contain as many as 1 billion cells, a very small proportion of the total number of cells in the body. A tumour of this size is unlikely to compromise the function of a vital organ and as such is rarely life-threatening. Fewer than 10% of deaths result from the growth of the primary tumour (Weinberg 1998). In order to mobilize and form metastatic deposits in other tissues, the cancer cells must breach the physical barriers of the primary tumour. This is most clearly demonstrated in the case of carcinomas, which constitute the majority of human tumours (Weinberg 1998). Carcinomas arise from epithelial cells, which line many cavities within internal organs and form the outer layer of the skin. Epithelial cells lie upon a basement membrane that separates the epithelium from the connective tissue and the blood circulation. Any invasion through the basement membrane requires it to be broken down and this is achieved by the release of proteases (enzymes that break down protein) from tumour cells. This initial invasion of tumour cells into surrounding tissues results in minimal expansion of the tumour mass (carcinoma-in-situ).

Once the tumour cells populate the tissues underlying the basement membrane, they continue their path of invasion and destruction by dissolving cells that represent a physical barrier. The close proximity to the blood vessels means that they can move to distant sites throughout the body. Whilst some cancer cells use the blood vessels as a means of migration, others prefer to use lymphatic vessels. The ability of tumour cells to invade surrounding tissues is dependent upon the continued production and release of proteases.

The process of metastatic spread is generally fragmented and poorly understood. We do know that metastasizing colon cancer cells often settle in the liver; breast and prostate cancer cells commonly metastasize in the bones; melanoma cancer cells often spread to the lungs; and lung cancer cells commonly settle in the brain tissue. Each time that cancer cells migrate and settle in a new site they are challenged by the presence of growth factors and physical structures to which they are not accustomed. Late in tumour development the mutant genes that programme for invasion and metastatic spread are few and far between. The primary tumour mass may be quite large and can afford to reproduce large numbers of cells with the intent of facilitating tumour spread (Weinberg 1998). Eventually metastatic tumours begin to thrive and compromise function in the organ. It is at this stage that the cancer may become fatal. It is clear that tumour development and spread comprise a complex multi-step process. Spread can be identified locally with the involvement of tissue surrounding the primary tumour, regionally where tumours spread across cavities, or at distant sites when tumour cells travel in the blood or lymphatic systems.

FACTORS THAT PREDISPOSE TO CANCER

The individual risk of developing cancer is influenced by genetic factors and exposure to environmental carcinogens. The investigation of how internal factors, behaviours or environmental factors influence the frequency of cancers in various human populations is the domain of cancer epidemiology. Percival Potts first identified scrotal cancer in men who had previously worked as chimney sweeps in 1775. The cancer was attributed to the coal dust in the chimneys. The link between nasal cancer and the use of snuff was made soon afterwards.

STRESS, EMOTION AND CANCER

The development and progression of cancer are associated with biological and psychological factors. That stress and emotion play a part in the development of cancer is not a new idea. The physician Galen, who practised in Rome in the 2nd century AD, associated 'melancholy' with cancer.

Stress is universally understood to signify the inability of individuals to meet the demands of their environment (Sarafino 1994). A degree of stress is considered to be beneficial since most people function and feel best at an optimal level of arousal. When an individual faces perceived danger, the fight-or-flight response is initiated, activating a range of hormonal (catecholamines and corticosteroids) and neural physiological coping mechanisms (Ch. 6).

Intense stress causes the body to enter a state of resistance. As the individual attempts to adapt to the stress, the level of physiological arousal declines, although it remains high. There may be few outward signs of stress but the ability to resist new stressors may be impaired for some time. Ongoing exposure to intense stress will result in exhaustion. The prolonged physiological arousal weakens the immune system and depletes energy reserves so that resistance is very low. Physiological damage and/or disease are likely to present. Cancer, arising from impaired immune function, is implicated as part of the stress response process (Sarafino 1994).

Personality has also been linked to the development of cancer. The stereotypical cancer-prone personality is seen in easygoing and acquiescent people who repress emotions that might interfere with smooth social and emotional functions (Taylor 1999). These people tend to be inhibited, oversocialized, confirming, compulsive and depressive and have particular difficulty expressing tension, anger or anxiety. Notably, they display denial and repressive behaviours when faced with stressful life events. It is proposed that the cancer-prone personality interacts with stress to produce feelings of helplessness, hopelessness and depression. Stress hormones are produced that suppress immunological function, which increases cancer risk through an increased potential for proliferation of mutant oncogenes.

Personality and stress are not only implicated in cancer development; they also act as indicators of potential disease progression following a diagnosis of cancer. A rapid course of disease, terminating in early death, has been observed amongst polite, non-aggressive, acquiescent individuals. Conversely, a longer course of illness was seen in people who were combative towards the disease and their medical practitioners (Taylor 1999).

CARCINOGENS

Agents that predispose to cancer have the potential to cause genetic mutations (Weinberg 1998). Mutagens cause mutations whilst carcinogens induce cancer. The two processes must be inextricably linked since both are ultimately concerned with the mutation of genetic material. There are two classes of mutagenic agents: those that cause change in germ line cells (spermatozoon or oocyte) and those that alter somatic (body) cells. Mutagenic changes in the germ cell line can be passed on to offspring, but somatic mutations are not. Somatic mutations therefore represent the critical changes that, in the majority of cases, trigger cancer.

Tobacco

Tobacco and diet together account for almost two-thirds of all cancer deaths. Most significantly, they are usually avoidable or correctable. Tobacco is a significant risk factor in the development of a wide range of cardiac and respiratory diseases and cancer. As early as the 1950s, people who smoked were seen to have a risk of developing lung cancer that was 20–30 times that of a non-smoker. Tobacco is implicated in the development of cancers affecting the mouth, throat, oesophagus, bladder, cervix, pancreas, stomach and kidney. It is also associated with the development of leukaemia. After approximately 10 years of non-smoking, an individual has around the same degree of cancer risk as someone who has never smoked.

Tobacco smoke comprises over 3000 chemicals, including nicotine, tar and carbon monoxide. Inhaled tobacco smoke causes paralysis of bronchial cilia, resulting in the loss of protection from infection. It is harmful not only to the smoker, but also to people in the close vicinity (passive smoking).

Socioeconomic status is implicated in the development of cancer. Incidence is highest in social classes IV and V. This trend is reversed in breast cancer, which is more common in social class I. The association between increased cancer risk and social class is based on lifestyle and takes into account dietary factors and behaviours such as smoking and alcohol intake. With the advent of health information in the 1970s, smoking has decreased significantly in the higher social classes compared with the lower social classes. The result is a disproportionately high incidence of lung cancer in people in social classes IV and V (Cancer Research Campaign 1999a). People struggling with problems such as unemployment and poverty may find it hard to stop smoking, because it may aid coping. Programmes of health education and health promotion need to incorporate strategic plans to address the source problems and prevent the creation of a blame culture, which may reinforce negative smoking behaviour.

Diet

There is strong evidence that diet is implicated in the development and progression of many cancers, colorectal cancer in particular. Dietary factors account for 80% of cancers of the large bowel, breast and prostate (Cummings & Bingham 1998). Fruit and vegetable products and high-fibre cereals confer protective benefits against colorectal cancer whilst high consumption of saturated fats significantly increases the risk of colorectal and prostate cancer.

Body weight, body mass index and physical activity

Body weight, body mass index (BMI) and level of physical activity are implicated in the development of cancer, especially colorectal cancer. People who exercise regularly have a reduced risk for developing colorectal cancer. This association is constant even when confounding variables such as diet and BMI are considered. The risk of developing colorectal cancer is significantly increased when BMI is >29 kg/m^2 (Boyle 1998).

Alcohol

Although consuming one or two units of alcohol per day has been shown to reduce the risk of coronary heart disease in certain groups (Ch. 19), heavy alcohol consumption is linked to the development of many cancers. Men who consistently drink more than four units of alcohol a day, and women who drink more than three, increase their risk of developing a range of health problems, including cancer (Ch. 23).

Alcohol is associated with cancers of the mouth, throat, trachea, oesophagus and liver. The potential risk of developing cancer is increased when an individual drinks alcohol and smokes tobacco. The association between alcohol and cancer is thought to be related not to the chemical components of alcohol, but to the calorific content of alcohol or the unhealthy diet of heavy drinkers.

Occupational exposure

Around 4–9% of cancer deaths are attributable to exposure to chemicals at work. The lung is the most common site for occupational cancers (Cartmel & Reid 1993), e.g. long-term exposure to asbestos and coal dust is linked to the development of mesothelioma, a rare lung cancer. Pesticides, vinyl chloride, aromatic amines and arsenic are similarly implicated in the development of cancer.

Pollution

It is difficult to calculate the exact impact of pollution on the development of cancer because there is no absolute certainty regarding the length and level of exposure to pollutants. It is proposed that pollutants in the air, water and food are implicated in the development of 1–5% of all cancers. Links between air pollution and lung cancer are being investigated (Cartmel & Reid 1993).

Radiation

Ultraviolet (UV) radiation is a major cause of non-melanoma skin cancer and is implicated in the development of malignant melanoma. Short-wave UVB rays in the sun and tanning beds are particularly damaging to the structure of DNA (Weinberg 1998). The cumulative exposure to UV radiation is predictive of risk for skin cancer (Cartmel & Reid 1993). Exposure to UV radiation is largely dependent upon geographical location (latitude, altitude and humidity). Protection from UV exposure requires the adoption of personal protective behaviours, particularly avoidance of the sun. If and when people are unavoidably exposed to the sun, they should be encouraged to apply appropriate strength sunscreens and to wear protective clothing.

Exposure to high-dose ionizing radiation, associated with fallout from nuclear installations and also with therapeutic radiation treatment, has been implicated in the development of leukaemia and thyroid cancer (Cartmel & Reid 1993). Occupational exposure to ionizing radiation is highest amongst nuclear power plant workers, physicians, radiographers and air flight crews.

Drugs

Many drugs, including chemotherapy drugs, have been associated with the development of cancer. The action of chemotherapy on DNA is not exclusive to malignant cells and there is a potential for the development of genetic change within healthy cells, which will render them more susceptible to somatic carcinogens. A late effect of chemotherapy treatment (10 or 20 years after initial therapy) is the development of secondary tumours in the blood or lymphatic systems.

The hormone oestrogen has been linked to the development of breast and ovarian cancer. The association focuses on the number of oestrogen-driven proliferative cycles in the uterus and breast. In previous decades the incidence of breast and ovarian cancer was lower. This is attributable to the age at which menstruation commences (menarche) and reproductive practices. The mean age of the menarche is 4–5 years earlier than in the early part of the 20th century because of the improvements in nutrition. There is a decrease in child-bearing and breast-feeding practices, which normally suppress menstrual cycling. The time that a woman spends on reproduction and lactation has drastically reduced during the 20th century and the average woman now will probably have many more oestrogen-driven proliferative cycles than her great-grandmother. The resulting increase in exposure to oestrogen during the reproductive years and the long-term use of oestrogen replacement therapy has been linked to a higher incidence of breast cancer. By comparison, the combined oral contraceptive has been associated with a decreased incidence of endometrial and ovarian cancer.

Infection

There is strong evidence that exposure to some viruses increases the risk of developing cancer. For example, the hepatitis B virus is linked to the development of liver cancer (Markman 1997). Furthermore, there are studies supporting an association between the human papilloma virus and the development of cervical cancer (Cartmel & Reid 1993). A woman can reduce this, the biggest risk factor in cervical cancer, by limiting the number of sexual partners and by insisting that a condom is used when participating in penetrative sex.

HOST CHARACTERISTICS AND CANCER

Age

Cancer is predominantly a disease of older adults. There is a cumulative effect from prolonged exposure to environmental carcinogens and a decline in the ability of immune processes to destroy abnormal cells. Carcinogenesis generally takes place over many years and abnormalities may not manifest until late in life.

Gender

The incidence of non-gender-specific cancer tends to be lower in the female population (Cartmel & Reid 1993). However, the incidence of lung cancer in women is rising as a result of increased tobacco smoking in women, compared with a reduction in men.

Ethnicity and race

Ethnicity and race may have an influence on the risk of developing cancer (Cartmel & Reid 1993). The association is complex and may have more to do with the socioeconomic status of individuals within specific ethnic groups and their degree of choice with regard to health-promoting behaviours. Individuals within every ethnic or racial group are influenced by cultural norms and values that determine attitudes to illness, care seeking and illness prevention behaviours.

PREVENTING CANCER

Preventing cancer requires health protection and health promotion activities. Health protection is concerned with the development of policies to address unhealthy behaviour. Prevention is concerned with screening and active measures such as immunization against transmissible disease. Prevention can take place on three levels: primary, secondary and tertiary. Primary prevention is concerned with preventing the onset of disease and involves raising awareness of risky behaviours. Secondary prevention is concerned with halting the progression of existing and perhaps previously undiagnosed disease, involving activities such as screening. Tertiary prevention is concerned with minimizing the effects of disease or treatment and enabling rehabilitation.

The key factor in preventing cancer is probably 'body awareness'. Individuals should be aware of what their body normally looks like and monitor for suspicious change. Body awareness is also about believing we can help ourselves to adopt a healthy lifestyle. The key activities for health professionals concerned with preventing cancer are the promotion of healthy behaviours and the promotion of body awareness within the population.

As children grow and mature, they are influenced by overt and covert messages about what is acceptable or unacceptable in terms of appearance and behaviour. These messages, influenced by a range of factors, including cultural and peer group norms, role models and the media, reinforce beliefs about health, the body and associated behaviours. Peer group and media influences are strongest when young adults are developing an individual identity and at this time they may imitate unhealthy behaviours such as smoking tobacco, drinking alcohol or sunbathing. Despite widespread limitations on alcohol and tobacco advertising, young people continue to be influenced by their peer group. Where their parents have been, or are, smokers they are more likely to identify with the behaviour and want to try it themselves.

PROMOTING HEALTHY BEHAVIOUR

Most people have an internal perception, influenced by their view of themselves and their activities, about how healthy they are. Younger people feel less concern about their health, linking health almost exclusively with their level of physical fitness. They tend to believe that they will not be affected by cancer and are often unconcerned about participating in unhealthy behaviours. Health promotion seeks to build upon people's existing knowledge, develop their autonomy and enable them to take responsibility for their own health. Although individuals are, to a large extent, responsible for their health, the health-related actions that are adopted within their daily lives are inexplicably linked to the social processes in their lives. Promoting healthy behaviour therefore requires a multiple strategy approach. For example, information is a central factor in encouraging people to change their lifestyle but it is not sufficient to promote change alone. People are often not enabled to change, despite motivation, because of their social circumstances. National policy changes may be required to address these issues, for instance the national imposition of restrictions on smoking in public areas in order to reduce exposure of the wider population to carcinogens (Department of Health 1999).

People assume unhealthy behaviours for a variety of reasons, some of which may be under their control and others which may not. The adoption of specific behaviours is often related to personal perceptions and beliefs about the level of control over their health situation. This is referred to as the health locus of control (Wallston & Wallston 1982). People may believe that they are responsible for their own health/health-promoting behaviours (internal locus of control), or that these factors are controlled by powerful others such as employers, the government or health professionals (external locus of control). Alternatively, they may consider that their health status at any time is the result of chance factors that are out of their control (chance locus of control). Promoting healthy behaviour often requires a change of perception or attitude that allows people to realize they can take positive action themselves and adopt an internal locus of control.

In order to make health-promoting changes that will either prevent the onset of a disease or enable individuals to maintain their health status once disease is present, people need the power to take control of their situation. It is proposed that five specific levels of control are necessary (Sarafino 1994). Nurses are ideally placed to offer appropriate information and support to enable their patients to take control of their situation:

■ *Behavioural control* – the ability to take concrete behavioural actions to reduce the temporal/intensity impact of a stressor. Behavioural control is often employed to enable coping in a relatively short-term situation. For example, patients might ensure that they take prophylactic antiemetic medication before chemotherapy to minimize the experience of nausea and vomiting.

■ *Cognitive control* – the use of thought processes or strategies to modify the impact of the stressor. For example, the patient receiving chemotherapy might employ visualization or relaxation techniques to ward off or to minimize the experience of nausea and vomiting. Cognitive control consistently appears to have the most beneficial effect in the mediation of a stressful life event (Sarafino 1994).

■ *Decisional control* – the opportunity to choose between alternative courses of action. For the cancer patient, this may refer to the choice an individual makes about accepting either conventional or experimental therapy.

■ *Informational control* – the opportunity to seek out information and develop knowledge about a stressful event. Informational control can help to reduce stress by enabling the individual to predict what may happen. Fear of the unknown is lessened and the patient is prepared for what might happen. For the cancer patient this could be related to making an informed choice about taking protective actions such as scalp cooling to minimize hair loss.

■ *Retrospective control* – a search for meaning based on beliefs about who or what caused a stressful event, after it has happened. Retrospective control doesn't give control over the event itself but it helps individuals to modify the stress that they experience by enabling them to perceive the world as an orderly and meaningful place.

IDENTIFYING WARNING SIGNS

Perhaps the most important role in the prevention of and screening for cancer is monitoring and surveillance for changes in body structure and function by individuals. Nurses are central in educating the public about body changes that should be reported to a health professional. Boothroyd (1995) advocates that changes persisting for 2 weeks or longer should be reported, but people who are at high risk of developing cancer and those with acute and/or serious symptoms should be encouraged to report them immediately. Specific changes to look out for include (Sarafino 1994):

• **C**hange in bowel or bladder habit
• **A** sore that doesn't heal
• **U**nusual bleeding or discharge
• **T**hickening of tissue in the breast or the testes, or anywhere else in the body
• **I**ndigestion or difficulty in swallowing
• **O**bvious change in a wart or mole
• **N**agging cough or a hoarse voice.

TYPES AND CLASSIFICATION OF NEW GROWTHS

Any abnormal growth of tissue is referred to as either a neoplasm or a tumour. The tumour may be either benign or malignant, classified after consideration of the following criteria (Richardson 1995):

• anatomical site of the primary tumour and metastases
• tissue type and histology
• grade of malignancy
• extent of tumour progression based on tumour size, degree of invasion and metastatic spread.

BENIGN AND MALIGNANT TUMOURS

Benign tumours are space-occupying lesions. Depending on the space occupied they do have the potential to be damaging or even life-threatening. For instance, they can cause local damage by exerting pressure on surrounding tissue, nerves or the blood supply. Benign tumours in the brain can be life-threatening if they cause this type of damage. Benign tumours tend to grow slowly. The use of the simple suffix 'oma' usually indicates a benign tumour, e.g. a fibroma is a benign tumour of fibrous connective tissue. The term fibrosarcoma is used to describe a malignant tumour of the fibrous connective tissue. There are some exceptions to the rules in the nomenclature system where malignant tumours have the suffix 'oma'. In these cases, the prefix 'malignant' is used to avoid confusion, e.g. malignant melanoma.

Malignant tumours invade and destroy adjacent tissue and form metastases at distant body sites. Tissue infiltration by tumour cells can lead to haemorrhage and life-threatening organ failure. Malignant tumours make additional demands on the body in terms of energy requirements and infection control. People with malignant tumours are susceptible to cachexia resulting from the increased energy required to sustain cellular proliferation. A malignant tumour is normally represented by the use of the word sarcoma or carcinoma.

HAEMATOLOGICAL MALIGNANCY

Haematological malignancy (Ch. 18) is the global term for cancers affecting the bone marrow, which is responsible for the production of blood and lymphoid cells. This group of diseases, which is known collectively as leukaemia, is characterized by disorders of proliferation and maturation in the lymphoid and myeloid cell lines. Acute leukaemias are characterized by abnormal proliferation of immature blood cells with a short natural history of between 1 and 5 months, whereas chronic leukaemias are characterized by an excessive accumulation of ineffective blood cells with a mature appearance. Progression is much slower in the chronic leukaemias and may take between 2 and 5 years (Hoffbrand & Pettit 1993). The consequential overcrowding of immature blood cells in the bone marrow restricts the production and function of normal blood cells and people die because the blood cells cannot sustain the body.

Leukaemia accounts for around 2% of total cancer incidence in the UK (Cancer Research Campaign 1999b). The incidence of acute and chronic leukaemia is roughly equal; however, 90% of new cases are in adults, compared with only 10% in children. Adults commonly develop acute myeloid leukaemia (AML) or chronic lymphocytic leukaemia (CLL). Acute lymphocytic leukaemia accounts for around 80% of childhood leukaemia (Hoffbrand & Pettit 1993). The development of leukaemia is associated with genetic predisposition, particularly with Down's syndrome where there is a 20- to 30-fold risk of developing leukaemia. Environmental exposure to ionizing radiation, chemicals and viruses have been linked to the development of leukaemia and there is a risk of 'secondary leukaemia' following treatment for lymphoma, multiple myeloma, ovarian and breast cancer with chemotherapy drugs.

Acute leukaemia

The most common features of acute leukaemia are an elevated leucocyte count, fatigue, fever and sweating (Markman 1997). Spontaneous bruising and bleeding may also occur. Assessing the disease stage enables appropriate treatment to be planned. Patients are often very sick on presentation and require supportive care in the form of blood and platelet transfusions, prophylactic treatment to prevent potentially life-threatening infection, and cytotoxic therapy to treat the underlying malignancy.

Patients who present with acute leukaemia usually have a central venous catheter inserted to reduce the potential for infection and to facilitate the administration of chemotherapy drugs, antibiotics and blood products. Blood is commonly transfused during the acute phase in order to correct the symptoms of anaemia, such as dyspnoea and fatigue. Patients are also likely to receive platelet transfusions to correct their thrombocytopenia (reduced platelets) and reduce the risk of life-threatening bleeding. The neutrophil (a leucocyte) count is normally reduced as a result of bone marrow infiltration by immature blast cells (Hoffbrand & Pettit 1993) and intravenous antibiotics are administered if signs of infection are present. If the neutrophil count is less than $0.2 \times 10^9/L$ (normal is 2.5–$7.5 \times 10^9/L$) the patient is nursed in a single room. This provides 'protective isolation' from exposure to potentially pathogenic organisms in the environment (Ch. 13). Acquired infections are predominantly bacterial and commonly arise from patients' own bacterial flora (commensals) that normally inhabit their skin, so education and assistance with hygiene is absolutely essential. This aspect of care is particularly significant since an opportunistic infection can quickly progress to life-threatening septicaemia (bacterial multiplication in the blood) in the absence of neutrophils.

Rapid-induction treatment with cytotoxic chemotherapy is required once a diagnosis has been established. The intention is to induce a remission (absence of clinical or laboratory evidence of leukaemic cells). Once remission is confirmed, consolidation therapy is given to eliminate the hidden leukaemic cell population (Hoffbrand & Pettit 1993). Patients with AML will commonly be offered bone marrow transplantation, although this is dependent upon clinical condition, age at presentation and response to induction chemotherapy.

Chronic leukaemia

Chronic myeloid leukaemia (CML) affects equal numbers of men and women between 40 and 60 years of age. Generally there are no predisposing factors, but an increased incidence of CML was apparent following exposure to the atomic bombs detonated in Japan in 1945 (Hoffbrand & Pettit 1993). Presentation of CML includes weight loss, lassitude, anorexia and night sweats. There is usually gross splenomegaly (spleen enlargement). There may be symptomatic evidence of anaemia and thrombocytopenia and gout is common, arising from the metabolism of uric acid.

Patients with CML are commonly treated with the chemotherapy agent busulfan. The dose can be titrated according to the results of regular blood counts, with low-dose administration on a daily basis or high-dose administration once every 4–6 weeks. The chemotherapy reduces the total leucocyte mass and keeps patients symptom-free for long periods. Unfortunately treatment does not delay the transformation into acute leukaemia (Hoffbrand & Pettit 1993). A bone marrow transplant may offer a 50–70% chance of cure from CML in patients who are aged 55 or younger. Chemotherapy treatment in the chronic phase of CML results in a median survival of 3–5 years. Death usually results from transformation into acute leukaemia or infection. Twenty per cent survive for 10 years or more.

SOLID TUMOURS

Lung cancer (Ch. 20)

Lung malignancies may be classified as non-small cell lung cancer (NSCLC), which accounts for around 75% of lung cancer incidence, and oat cell or small cell lung cancer (SCLC). Symptoms include a productive cough associated with haemoptysis (blood in the sputum) and chest pain in the early stages, with wheezing, hoarseness and arm oedema in advanced disease. NSCLC has the potential for cure following surgical resection, but responds poorly to chemotherapy. The key factor in the development of NSCLC is tobacco smoking. The overall 5-year survival rate in NSCLC is around 55% (Markman 1997).

SCLC is characterized by rapid disease progression and early onset of metastatic disease (see p. 988). Maximum anticipated survival is around 4–5 months (Markman 1997). Surgical intervention is rarely appropriate in SCLC because of early metastatic disease. Combination chemotherapy is currently the treatment of choice and may arrest the disease progress to provide limited extension to life. SCLC is the focus of trials with new clinical agents such as gemcitabine, which may increase survival.

Breast cancer (Ch. 26)

The incidence of breast cancer has been increasing in recent years and this may be due to improved screening techniques and the implementation of national screening programmes. That less than two-thirds of women have lymph node involvement at the time of diagnosis (Markman 1997) is a testimonial to advances in cancer research and the effectiveness of screening. The goals of primary treatment are removal of the macroscopic tumour tissue and treatment of microscopic cells around the tumour margins. Surgical intervention remains the mainstay of treatment with an emphasis on the avoidance of radical disfiguring surgery. Hormonal therapy is offered to women who have reached the menopause. There are ongoing studies with tamoxifen (oestrogen antagonist) which has shown benefits in reducing disease occurrence and mortality in women free from metastatic lymph involvement on presentation. Women who do have metastatic lymph involvement on presentation benefit from a 24–30% reduction in recurrence and a 15–20% reduction in mortality with chemotherapy.

Cancer of the cervix (Ch. 25)

Cervical cancer causes significant mortality, second only to ovarian cancer in terms of gynaecological malignancy. It is highly curable if detected in the early stages by treatment with either surgery or radiotherapy, but prognosis is poor once metastases develop. Carcinoma-in-situ (premalignant condition) is commonly treated by either a hysterectomy or radiation. This offers a potential 100% cure rate. Localized invasive disease is treated with radiation or a radical hysterectomy and patients with locally advanced cancer are treated with radiation. Surgery may be offered at this stage, but will depend upon the patient's physical condition at presentation. Radiotherapy is commonly used to treat metastatic disease. Cisplatin remains the mainstay of chemotherapy for metastatic cervical cancer. This controls the disease but does not provide a cure. It is rarely given today since cervical cancer is generally detected at a much earlier stage.

Colorectal cancer (Ch. 22)

Colorectal cancer (CRC) is the fourth most common cancer worldwide. CRC encompasses cancers occurring anywhere within the colon or the rectum. The incidence of CRC is highest in the developed economies of western Europe, North America, Australia, New Zealand and parts of Europe where dietary fat intake is high (Boyle 1998). The incidence is lowest in developing countries such as Africa where the diet is based almost exclusively on vegetables and grain.

Most cases (67–90%) of CRC arise from benign adenomatous polyps, which line the wall of the colon. Approximately 20% of people with CRC have a family history of colon cancer. Some of these are linked to a hereditary disorder, such as familial adenomatous polyposis (FAP) or hereditary non-polyposis colorectal cancer (HNPCC). The risk of people with FAP developing CRC at some time is around 70%, and 10% of people with CRC have a first-degree relative with HNPCC. These observations, combined with the evidence of successful treatment of early CRC, support the case for genetic screening and identification of families at high risk of developing CRC.

CRC affects approximately 50% more men than women (Boyle 1998). It rarely affects people aged under 40 years, but is common in those aged over 70. The incidence is higher in women below the age of 60 and higher in men thereafter. Overall survival from CRC can be as much as 70% following curative surgery for local disease; however, this rate decreases as the extent of disease at the time of surgery increases.

Testicular cancer (Ch. 25)

Testicular cancer is eminently curable, with 99% survival in local disease and around 80% survival in advanced disease. Undescended testes in young boys increases the risk for testicular cancer in later life. This is attributed to the constant exposure of seminal tissue to higher temperatures when situated inside the body, particularly after puberty. Surgical correction of undescended testes is usually recommended to reduce the risk of malignancy.

Testicular cancer presents as a firm but painless mass in the scrotum. Diagnosis may be confirmed by ultrasonography. The treatment of choice is surgical removal of the testis and spermatic cord (radical orchidectomy) via the inguinal canal. This route is taken in order to prevent scrotal contamination by tumour cells at the time of surgery. Surgery is followed up by radiation or cisplatin-based chemotherapy.

Prostate cancer (Ch. 24)

Prostate cancer is the second most common cancer in men in the UK, predominantly affecting those aged over 60 years. Presentation includes dysuria, cystitis or prostatitis, frequency, poor stream, retention of urine. Prostate cancer is generally slow-growing and a no treatment option may be appropriate in older men, since the benefits of treatment may be minimal. Men who present with advanced prostate cancer commonly experience bone pain and weight loss. There may be evidence of uraemia arising from obstruction of the ureters, and disseminated intravascular coagulation (Ch. 9) secondary to metastatic disease in the bones. Locally contained prostate cancer can be treated surgically (radical prostatectomy), with local radiotherapy or with hormone therapy.

Bladder cancer (Ch. 24)

Bladder cancer occurs most commonly between the ages of 60 and 70 years; men are affected more often than women (M:F = 3:1). Bladder cancer is more common in Caucasian individuals. Early-stage superficial tumours have an excellent

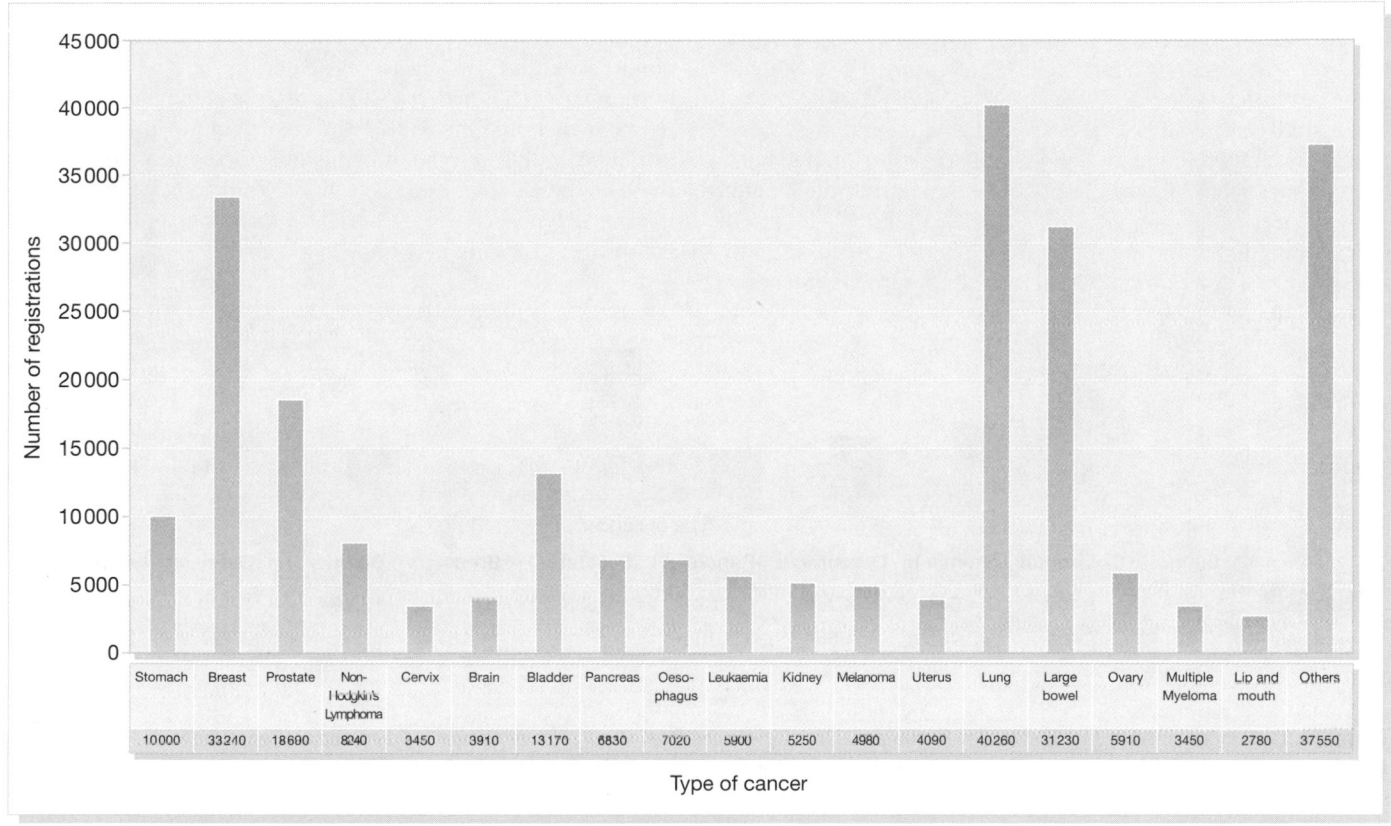

	Stomach	Breast	Prostate	Non-Hodgkin's Lymphoma	Cervix	Brain	Bladder	Pancreas	Oeso-phagus	Leukaemia	Kidney	Melanoma	Uterus	Lung	Large bowel	Ovary	Multiple Myeloma	Lip and mouth	Others
	10000	33240	18690	8240	3450	3910	13170	6830	7020	5900	5250	4980	4090	40260	31230	5910	3450	2780	37550

Figure 33.2   Total UK cancer registrations, 1995 (excluding non-melanotic skin cancer). (Adapted with permission from CRC 1999c.)

prognosis. Presenting features include intermittent and painless haematuria (blood in the urine), dysuria, urinary frequency and urgency. Flank pain may be a feature of advanced disease or may indicate ureteral obstruction. The major risk factor for bladder cancer is tobacco smoking. Chronic bladder irritation from calculi (stones formed from mineral salts) and/or cystitis is also implicated.

Bladder cancer may be treated conservatively by cystoscopy and removal/destruction of a localized tumour, or by radical cystectomy (removal of the bladder) and removal of regional lymph nodes in the case of invasive disease. Aggressive radiation for locally advanced disease confers a long-term disease-free survival of 20–30% (Markman 1997). Intravesicular or systemic chemotherapy increases the length of disease-free survival; however, the 5-year survival for advanced disease is only 10–15%.

EPIDEMIOLOGY

Epidemiological data (Fig. 33.2) provides information about cancer incidence (number of new cases in a population over a given period of time) and cancer prevalence (total number of cases present in an area at a single point in time). The accuracy of data is dependent upon accurate and timely registration of new cancers. The data take approximately 5 years to collate, analyse and publish, therefore statistics are never completely 'up to date'.

COMMON CANCERS

Around 246 000 people were registered with cancer in the UK in 1995 (Cancer Research Campaign 1999b); 70% of cases occur in people aged over 60 years. Lung cancer was the most common male cancer, representing a fifth of all male cancers, and breast cancer was the most common female cancer. The second most common cancer in both men and women was CRC. Prostate cancer is the third most common cancer in men whilst lung cancer ranks third in women. Breast, lung and bowel cancers together account for nearly 50% of all deaths in females with cancer. In men it is lung, prostate and bowel cancers that account for over 50% of all deaths due to cancer. Cancer mortality by gender is depicted in Figure 33.3.

INCIDENCE AND SURVIVAL

Each year, 1 in every 250 men and 1 in every 300 women will be diagnosed with cancer (Souhami & Tobias 1998). The incidence rises steeply with age and 1 in every 100 men over the age of 60 years will be diagnosed with cancer annually. When clinicians evaluate response to cancer treatment they talk in terms of 5- and 10-year survival, i.e. the proportion of patients, with a specific cancer, still alive at 5 or 10 years. Cure is assumed when the expected survival for the treated patient is similar to people of a similar age who have not had cancer (Souhami & Tobias 1998). An older age at diagnosis is associated with a poorer prognosis and survival at 1 and 3 years, from most cancers, is worse in older people (Special Issues box 33.1).

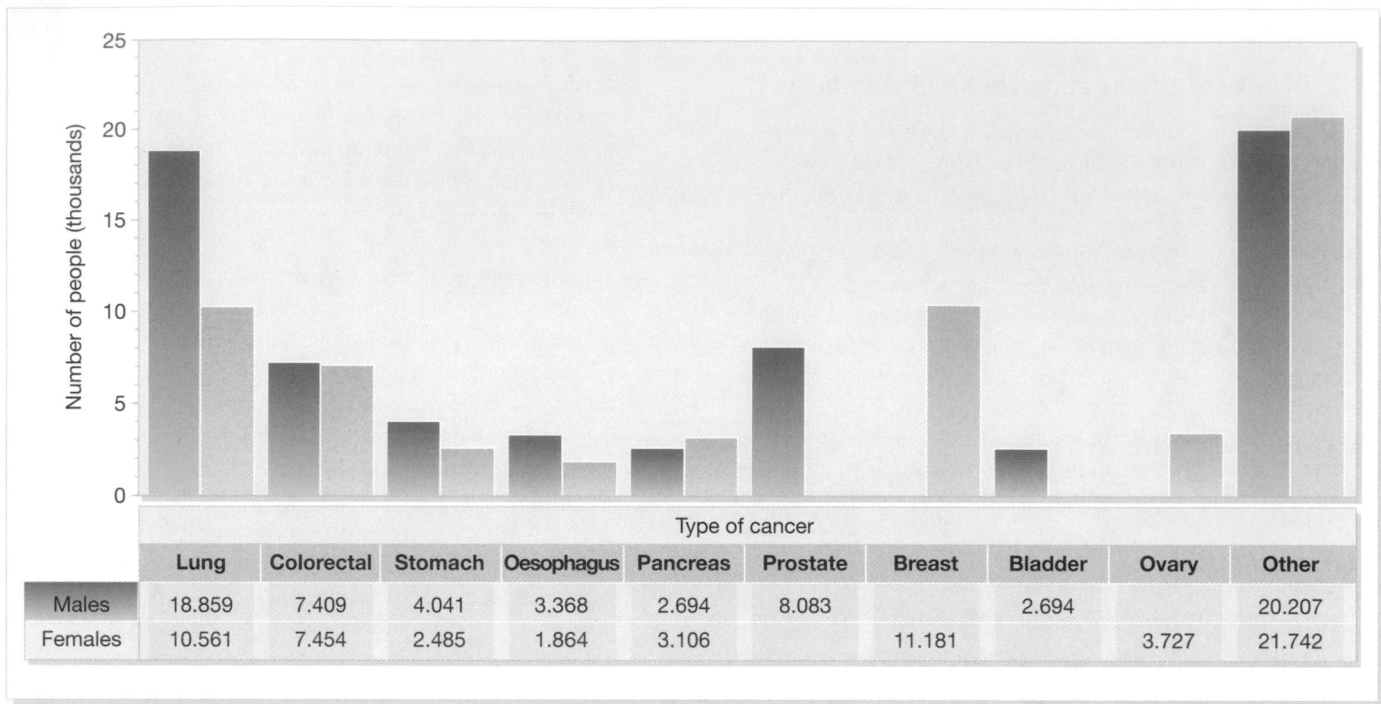

	Type of cancer									
	Lung	**Colorectal**	**Stomach**	**Oesophagus**	**Pancreas**	**Prostate**	**Breast**	**Bladder**	**Ovary**	**Other**
Males	18.859	7.409	4.041	3.368	2.694	8.083		2.694		20.207
Females	10.561	7.454	2.485	1.864	3.106		11.181		3.727	21.742

Figure 33.3 Cancer mortality by gender for England, 1996. (Developed from *Our Healthier Nation – Green Paper* [Department of Health 1998]. Crown copyright material is reproduced with the permission of the Controller of Her Majesty's Stationery Office.)

SCREENING AND EARLY DETECTION

The prevention and early detection of cancer was a key area for action in the *Saving Lives – Our Healthier Nation* strategy (Department of Health 1999). The role of nurses in encouraging screening with either self-test techniques or professional intervention is acknowledged as a central component in reducing cancer deaths.

Screening is concerned with monitoring apparently healthy people with the aim of discovering previously undisclosed disease. Monitoring those people who are at high risk because of genetic predisposition or familial history of cancer is crucial. The aim is to detect actual or potential disease at an early enough stage that the prognosis can be improved through preventative interventions or timely treatment.

Observation is the most widely available technique for cancer screening and is particularly useful for surveillance of the skin, mouth, external genitalia and cervix. Palpation is particularly useful in identifying the presence of lumps, nodules or tumours in breast tissue, mouth, thyroid and subcutaneous tissues. Palpation is also useful for detecting rectal cancer, prostate cancer and ovarian cancer. Enlarged lymph nodes in the neck, groin and axilla are identified by palpation. Internal cancers rely on the use of endoscopic procedures, ultrasound or laboratory tests such as faecal occult blood testing.

Screening is not useful for diseases where there is no early detection test, such as pancreatic cancer, or where there is no recognizable localized stage, such as leukaemia. Although

screening tests able to detect lung cancer are being tested, there is no justification for a national screening programme until the results of larger trials are available since there is no effective treatment for established lung cancer that will prevent the disease or significantly enhance length of life.

Encouraging apparently healthy people to undergo screening is notoriously difficult, since people don't seek medical advice unless they believe they are at risk, or are ill. Nurses have a key role to play in health promotion, alerting people to their risk of developing a disease and explaining the benefits of screening. People choose to undergo or to avoid screening because of perceived benefits or disadvantages: physical; psychological; economic; and political, scientific and organizational (Austoker 1990).

Women have been encouraged to undergo screening with the advent of national cancer screening programmes for breast and cervical cancer. These programmes have been adopted on the basis that early detection of breast and cervical disease leads to prompt treatment, which significantly improves the prognosis and in many cases can achieve complete cure. Prompt treatment is less costly than radical surgical intervention, intensive drug and radiation therapy. Furthermore, preservative treatments reduce the morbidity associated with some cancers and their treatment. This is beneficial since the person with cancer is less likely to have to contend with great changes in body image. However, people who undergo preservative treatments may experience increased anxiety that the disease has not been completely removed and will return.

SPECIAL ISSUES

33.1 Quality of life as an outcome of treatment

As we develop our clinical experience, it becomes easy to assume that 'we know' about quality of life, for we have nursed patients who appear to have, or who state that they have, either 'good' or 'poor' quality of life. We can relate this to their thoughts, their feelings and the actions that they take concerning their illness or their life in general.

Sometimes health professionals make a statement about the quality of another person's life, based either on direct information from the client or on a personal judgement, following an appraisal of the client's situation. Whatever the process, the resultant attitudes and beliefs can directly affect the way that health care professionals interact with the client and their carers.

Student activities

- How do we know what someone's quality of life is?
- Why do we make assumptions about people's lives?
- Make a note of what quality of life means to you – what elements give your life quality?
- Think about a patient who you have nursed recently. Was any reference made to their quality of life?
- Who do you consider was in the best position to measure their quality of life? The patient, his/her family, the doctor, the nurse or somebody else?
- Read the paper by Montazeri et al (1996). This paper examines the key issues in measuring the quality of life of cancer patients. Quality of life is defined and discussed. A historical perspective of measuring quality of life is presented. Measures used to judge quality of life are discussed in terms of validity and reliability.
  Key points:
  — Quality of life may be conceptual (well-being, quality of survival, human values and satisfaction of needs) or operational (ability to fulfil activities of daily living independently)
  — Outcome measures are multidimensional

— Most outcome measures in terms of quality of life are qualitative and subjective but most scales are quantitative. For example, patients may be asked to rate their ability to walk 'a short distance' from a scale of 1 to 4 (where 1 is very difficult and 4 is no problem)
— The outcome of an assessment of the patient's quality of life is dependent upon the time that it is measured and is affected by life circumstances that may or may not be related to the cancer and its treatment
— Quality of life outcomes may not be attributable to a certain treatment, so it is very difficult to make valid generalizations about one specific treatment being better than another
— Qualitative interpretations of quality of life, obtained in an interview with patients, their carers or the clinician, provide stronger data than the use of quantitative measures
— Assessment of quality of life by clinicians correlates poorly with the assessments made by patients themselves; therefore patients are best able to assess their quality of life

(a) Find out what quality of life measures are used in your clinical area. Look through them and consider whether they capture the data that they intend to. If they do not, why not?
(b) Make a note concerning your role in assessing quality of life. How will you ensure that you get accurate data that truly reflect the feelings of the patient?
(c) Find out what happens to quality of life forms after they have been completed. Are they being used effectively?

Reference
Montazeri A, Gillis CR, McEwen J. Measuring quality of life in oncology: is it worthwhile? Eur J Cancer Care 1996; 5: 159–167.

PRINCIPLES OF SCREENING FOR CANCER

Wilson & Jungner (1968) set out some clear principles for cancer screening:

- The condition screened for should pose an important health problem.
- The natural history of the condition should be well understood.
- There should be a recognizable latent or early stage.
- Disease treatment at an early stage should be of more benefit than treatment started at a later stage.
- There should be a suitable test or examination that should be:
  — simple
  — easy to apply
  — reproducible
  — cost-effective

and that should have:
  — high sensitivity (ability to detect abnormality)
  — high specificity (high level of accuracy – results are confirmed as positive or negative)
  — low risk:benefit ratio.
- The test or examination should be acceptable to the population.
- For diseases of insidious onset, screening should be repeated at intervals determined by the natural history of the disease.
- There should be adequate facilities available for the diagnosis and treatment of any abnormalities detected.
- The chance of physical or psychological harm should be less than the chance of benefit.
- The cost of case finding (including diagnosis and subsequent treatment) should be economically balanced against the benefit it provides.

These principles reinforce the importance of screening being acceptable to the general population in terms of convenience and reliability, and to the nation in terms of economic benefits. Screening techniques and programmes are subject to constant evaluation and re-evaluation. An example of this is the national breast-screening programme, which was started in the UK in 1988. The interval at which breast screening is carried out has been determined from ongoing research that has sought to identify the number of interval cancers diagnosed in between each screening, based on intervals of between 1 and 5 years. The screening interval at which the least detectable but presymptomatic disease manifested was found to be 3 years. Those people who are at a higher risk of developing cancer (genetic predisposition or familial history) may undergo screening more frequently (see also Older Adults–Nursing Priorities box 33.1).

65 83 50 71 OLDER ADULTS: NURSING PRIORITIES

33.1 Health surveillance, screening and older adults

Reasons for screening older people
- Cancer is a disease that predominantly affects older people
- Older people are deserving of the same level of cancer screening that the rest of the population receives
- Older people may be cured of cancer as a result of cancer treatment
- Cancer treatment provides effective symptom relief and thus enhances quality of life in the older person

Issues
- Access to older people in the community, for the purposes of screening, may be difficult
- Older people, especially those who are institutionalized or dependent, may not have the opportunity to undergo screening
- Screening for cancer in the dependent older person receives little attention; therefore the older person is placed in a disadvantaged position
- Older people may believe that they do not need to undergo cancer screening
- Early signs of developing cancer may be overlooked

Specific nursing actions required to facilitate screening in the older person
- Target the older person in the community and incorporate health education and cancer screening activities into home visits where possible
- Discuss issues around screening of the older person with colleagues working on the wards and in nursing homes in order to highlight the problems
- Utilize opportunities to reinforce the importance of cancer screening
- Encourage the older person to undertake self-examination techniques, i.e. of the breast, so that problems are identified early

Genetic screening
There is an opportunity, as genetic knowledge increases, to screen most people to identify their risk of developing cancer. The activity of genetic screening must be linked to decreased incidence of cancer and reductions in mortality and morbidity rates. At present, although it is increasingly possible to identify those people who have a 'higher than normal' risk of developing cancer, there is insufficient justification for widespread screening. Based on the principles of screening for cancer, any test should enable interventions that will resolve the potential for disease, will have a beneficial impact on longevity and will enhance quality of life. The use of genetic screening may alert some people to their risk or to the presence of cancer for which there is no effective treatment. Cost implications would be high since there would be an expectation of treatment. The potential for psychological trauma may be increased although the risk is presented as a 'lifetime' risk. The discovery of the BRCA-1 gene and an 85% risk of breast cancer in a young woman means that she will live with that knowledge, although the disease may not develop for a further 40–50 years, if at all (Markman 1997). Furthermore, positive test results may have wider discriminatory implications in terms of employment and securing life insurance.

It is essential that those people who desire, or who require, genetic screening are provided with honest and open information that will enable them to give informed consent. It is important that the potential benefits and harmful consequences of undergoing screening are made clear (Table 33.1).

SCREENING FOR SPECIFIC CANCERS

Lung cancer
There have been many attempts to develop a screening test for lung cancer. Chest X-ray and sputum cytology have been found to be useful in establishing a diagnosis of asymptomatic lung cancer. Screening, however, is not associated with a reduction in mortality (Craddock 1995) because treatment is not yet sophisticated enough to induce a cure. Although treatment may provide symptomatic relief in patients who are relatively well on presentation, the benefit is minimal in terms of survival (Markman 1997). A national screening programme is therefore considered to be unjustified at this time (see p. 996).

Breast cancer
Breast cancer commonly develops in women aged over 50 years of age. The principal test for breast cancer is mammography (radiography of the breast), which allows identification of benign and malignant growths. Mammography has high sensitivity and specificity and has enabled significant reductions in mortality (Austoker 1990). In the UK, the national breast cancer screening programme was set up in 1988 and offers routine screening at 3-year intervals between the ages of 50 and 70 years. Women aged 70 and over may be screened on request.

The single biggest factor inhibiting the uptake of breast cancer screening is considered to be inaccuracy of the data used to identify eligible women. This is especially true in highly populated city areas where people move more often. Another key factor is the approach used to target women from different ethnic

Table 33.1 Benefits and drawbacks of genetic screening (Developed from Markman 1997)

Test result	Implications	Impact
Positive	Leads to increased screening/surveillance appropriate to the individual's needs (e.g. increased frequency of mammography or colonoscopy)	Positive
	Triggers preventative strategies appropriate to the individual's current lifestyle and health beliefs (e.g. alteration in diet)	Positive
	Enables prophylactic surgery to take place (e.g. mastectomy, oophorectomy or colostomy in the presence of familial adenomatous polyposis or hereditary non-polyposis colorectal cancer)	Positive
	Enables individuals to make informed decisions about family planning	Positive
	Enables testing of other family members deemed to be at high/increased risk	Positive
	Causes the individual to be identified and labelled as 'cancer prone', leading to potential employment and insurance discrimination	Negative
Negative	Provides reassurance	Positive
	Reveals that an individual is not at increased risk (although the normal population risk remains)	Positive
	Provides false reassurance that a person is not at risk with the result that that person decides not to undergo regular standard surveillance screening tests (mammography)	Negative
	Leads to false reassurance that there is no genetic element that increases the risk of cancer, when the specific genetic abnormality may be yet to be defined	Negative
	Leads to guilt that a member of the family has escaped the disease whilst other members of the family have not	Negative

groups. The use of appropriate language is considered to be a key factor in encouraging uptake of screening (Craddock 1995).

Screening by mammography is supported by manual breast examination techniques that may be performed by health professionals or by women themselves. Women are taught how to perform breast self-examination themselves which enables self-monitoring on a regular monthly basis. Self-examination is done on the first day after menstruation is finished. Attention is drawn to changes in the breast tissue at the earliest opportunity and prompt investigation and diagnosis can be organized (Ch. 26).

Cancer of the cervix

The natural history of cervical cancer is well understood. Furthermore, the disease is eminently treatable at an early stage and screening has been shown to reduce mortality (see Evidence-based Practice box 33.1). The national screening programme in the UK recommends that women aged between 20 and 64 are monitored by routine cervical smear testing once every 3 years; however, in many areas the interval is being increased. Cervical cancer screening began in the UK in 1964, but was largely ineffective because of sporadic uptake and inefficient follow-up procedures (Craddock 1995). There has been a significant increase in uptake since the introduction of financial initiatives that encourage cervical screening by GP practices. Cervical screening may be a particular issue for some women with certain cultural beliefs and values. In many instances, discussion about sexual health is inhibited and nurses need to identify and tackle the underlying factors that may influence attendance patterns using an individual approach, based on strategies appropriate to each specific community. Female practice nurses now commonly undertake screening and this has been found to be a significant factor in predicting uptake.

 EVIDENCE-BASED PRACTICE

33.1 Exploiting adjuvant therapy to improve survival in cervical cancer

Josefson (1999) analyses the results of three trials where the treatment of cervical cancer incorporated chemotherapy alongside standard radiotherapy treatment. The author proposes that survival could increase by as much as 50% by using adjuvant chemotherapy. It is stated that the report is so significant in terms of service provision that the research papers were posted on the world wide web (www.nejm.org) to facilitate rapid dissemination.

Student activities

- Use the world wide web to access and critically appraise research literature related to your clinical area
- Consider the role of the world wide web in the dissemination of evidence-based practice.
- Meet with your tutor or supervisor and discuss how you can ensure that patients are able to access the best, up-to-date, accurate information that is relevant to their condition, treatment and care.

Reference

Josefson D. Adding chemotherapy improves survival in cervical cancer. Br Med J 1999; 318(7184): 623.

Cervical smear testing (exfoliative cytology) involves visualization of the cervix via a speculum and sampling of superficial cells using a spatula or brush. The sample is examined using a microscope and is also tested for human papilloma virus (HPV) which is implicated in the development of cervical cancer. Changes are noted and a programme of monitoring and observation set up. Those women identified as having changes may undergo further screening using colposcopy (Ch. 25). The screening interval for cervical cancer may be reduced from 3 years and rearranged on an individual basis, determined by the degree of abnormality. The test has high sensitivity and specificity.

Colorectal cancer

Colorectal cancer is eminently detectable and treatable at an early stage. However, poor knowledge, confounded by embarrassment about the nature of the symptoms, often causes late presentation. Screening is extremely effective in those populations at high risk of developing CRC. Children from families affected by FAP may be offered genetic testing from 13–14 years of age. Endoscopy (visual examination of body cavities or orifices) may be used to monitor those people identified as carriers of FAP. Intensive colonoscopic screening in high-risk populations has been demonstrated to reduce CRC mortality from HNPCC; however, the procedure carries significant risk of morbidity through bowel trauma. The tumour marker carcinoembryonic antigen (CEA) is indicative of colorectal cancer when present in the blood at a level above 5 mg/L, and blood testing provides a useful screening tool for CRC. In 1999 the UK government initiated two national pilot schemes to assess the feasibility of CRC screening using faecal occult blood testing and colonoscopy (see Evidence-based Practice box 33.2).

Testicular cancer

The most important test for a testicular tumour is manual testicular self-examination (TSE), performed on a regular monthly basis and/or if there is heaviness and discomfort in the testes. Men's health issues have tended to take a back seat, and lack of knowledge about TSE, confounded by embarrassment associated with procedure, has reduced uptake. It is proposed that as few as 10% of men practised TSE in the past, although this figure may be rising as a result of increased media attention on men's health, particularly through magazines aimed at men. The key roles of the nurse in testicular screening are teaching TSE, encouraging regular screening and prompt reporting of changes.

Prostate cancer

Rectal palpation of the prostate is effective in diagnosing early cancers and is recommended on an annual basis from the age of 40 years. Prostate specific antigen (PSA) is a tumour marker that may be isolated from the blood. Elevated PSA counts may provide evidence of prostatic cancer up to 5 years before a man becomes symptomatic. Confirmation of diagnosis with digital rectal examination or transrectal ultrasound scan is crucial since the specificity of the PSA test is low. Biopsies confirm the presence of prostate cancer in one-third of men with elevated PSA levels. In view of the natural history of the disease, the

---

 EVIDENCE-BASED PRACTICE

33.2 Screening for colorectal cancer using faecal occult blood testing

Towler et al (1998) offers a systematic review of four randomized controlled trials and two non-randomized controlled trials that have examined the effectiveness of faecal occult blood testing (FOBT) as a routine screening tool for colorectal cancer. The potential benefits and drawbacks of using the FOBT are also analysed.

FOBT, which involves obtaining a specimen of faeces and testing for the presence of blood, is the mainstay of colorectal cancer screening in the UK. Aimed at detection of early, asymptomatic CRC it can be carried out in the privacy of a patient's own home, requires minimal disruption to lifestyle, yet provides valuable information. The quality of trial design reviewed was high and screening was seen to result in a favourable shift in the stage distribution of colorectal cancers within the screening group. Those people allocated to screening had an overall reduction in the risk of CRC of around 23%.

The sensitivity and specificity of the test are highly dependent upon the patient's adherence to dietary restrictions prior to undertaking it. In particular, the avoidance of foods containing haemoglobin and myoglobin, such as red and white meat and fish, is a crucial factor for accuracy. It is proposed that the benefits of FOBT screening outweigh the potential harm, i.e. from false-positive tests, for those populations at high risk of developing CRC. More research into the community response to widespread screening and the associated costs is required before a widespread screening programme can be recommended.

Student activities
- Read Towler et al (1998) and identify the factors that make screening with FOBT more accurate.
- How can you use your knowledge to encourage screening and improve the accuracy of the test?
- Consider what skills you would use to encourage a friend to take part in FOBT screening.
- How could you raise the awareness of this screening test in the area where you are working?
- How have the pilot schemes for colorectal cancer screening that started in 1999 begun to inform practice?

Reference
Towler B, Irwig L, Glasziou P, Kewenter J, Weller D, Silagy C. A systematic review of the effects of screening for colorectal cancer using the faecal occult blood test, Hemoccult. Br Med J 1998; 317: 559–565.

incidence of false-positive test results and the potential side-effects of treatment, such as erectile dysfunction, men need to be well informed about their options before undertaking treatment.

Bladder cancer

People deemed to be at risk of bladder cancer as a result of their work receive regular occupational screening. For example, nurses exposed to chemotherapy should have a routine annual urinalysis, which enables observation for mutagenic changes indicative of over-exposure to chemotherapy drugs and/or an increased risk of developing bladder cancer.

The general population should be advised to observe for obvious blood in the urine, which may indicate the presence of either an infection or a bladder tumour. People who have either microscopic or gross haematuria should be screened in order to exclude infection in the first instance. Those people who have evidence of bladder lesions or who are deemed to be at high risk of developing bladder cancer may be routinely monitored by transurethral cystoscopy which enables visualization of the bladder with the opportunity to resect suspicious tissue for biopsy.

DIAGNOSTIC PROCEDURES

A diagnosis of primary or secondary cancer and monitoring of the progress of cancer may be achieved through a variety of tests. In the main these are surgical or imaging interventions. The initial aim is to obtain an accurate diagnosis and confirmation that the patient has cancer and to enable administration of the correct treatment. An accurate histological diagnosis is crucial since different types of cancer are amenable to a range of therapeutic treatment options. Even when people present for health care with metastatic disease, diagnostic tests performed on metastatic lesions offer clinicians information about the primary source of undiagnosed disease. A brief description of some common diagnostic procedures is provided with the rationale for their use.

DIAGNOSTIC TESTS

Aspiration cytology

Aspiration cytology is the removal of fluid via a fine needle and is used to sample abnormal collections of fluid, e.g. in the breast. The emphasis upon non-invasive techniques is one driving force for the use of aspiration cytology, but the technique is also favoured because it is quick and safe. The procedure can easily be performed in the outpatient setting, minimizing the inconvenience to the patient and facilitating rapid investigation. If required, the procedure is carried out in the clinical measurement suite under ultrasound guidance, enabling the clinician to localize the lesion accurately.

Lymph node biopsy

Lymph nodes are likely to be enlarged when the lymphatic system is the site of metastatic disease or primary disease, such as lymphoma (cancer of the lymphoid tissue). In many cases, lymphadenopathy may be the presenting sign of disease. Where

the lymphadenopathy is suspected to be due to metastatic disease, a fine-needle aspiration may be sufficient to provide a histological diagnosis.

Breast biopsy

Breast cancer diagnosis is increasingly based upon the findings of fine-needle aspiration cytology drawn from a palpable lesion in the breast. The procedure enables a quick evaluation of whether a breast lump is fluid (cyst) or solid. If fluid cannot be aspirated from a suspicious breast lump then biopsy and traditional histological examination of the tissue are required.

Skin biopsy

A skin biopsy is performed when primary or metastatic skin cancer lesions are suspected. Those lesions that are suspected to be metastatic or non-melanoma skin cancers, e.g. rodent ulcers, are usually diagnosed using a punch biopsy. Lesions that are suspected to be malignant melanomas are normally diagnosed using a total excision biopsy.

Endoscopy

Endoscopy is the direct visual examination of the gastrointestinal (GI), respiratory, reproductive and urinary tracts. Endoscopy is an invasive procedure, but the development of flexible fibreoptic endoscopic instruments means that the procedure is more acceptable to patients, minimal trauma is caused and the morbidity associated with the procedure is very low. There is, however, a risk of more serious trauma during the procedure, e.g. to the bowel. Furthermore, it is possible to take a biopsy of any suspicious tissue at the same time. The use of endoscopy has cost benefits for the organization, but these have to be balanced against the potential increase in treatment costs as a result of increased diagnosis.

Approximately 95% of malignant tumours of the upper GI tract can be diagnosed by endoscopy; however, the procedure is not infallible and submucosal tumours, in particular, may not be visualized. Endoscopic examination of the duodenum, pancreas or biliary tract is known as endoscopic retrograde cholangio-pancreatography (ERCP). There is a 3–5% risk of developing pancreatitis following an ERCP investigation.

Signs and symptoms of minor rectal bleeding, discomfort or diarrhoea that may indicate an abnormality in the distal colon can be investigated by flexible sigmoidoscopy. When colon cancer is suspected, the procedure of choice is a flexible colonoscopy that enables surveillance of the entire colon. A colonoscopy is potentially more traumatic than a sigmoidoscopy since bowel preparation prior to the procedure is required and the patient needs light sedation during the procedure.

Bronchoscopy using a flexible endoscope is most commonly used to diagnose lung cancer. The procedure can be performed under light sedation in a day care setting, minimizing disruption for patients. At bronchoscopy, the clinician is able to visualize the respiratory tract and biopsy suspicious tissue using small forceps and brushes inserted into the bronchoscope. Alternatively, bronchoalveolar lavage, the process of irrigating the bronchi during endoscopy, enables cytological examination of the aspirated fluid which may contain cancer cells.

A hysteroscopy may be used to examine the cervical canal and uterine cavity in order to identify abnormality. The procedure may be performed without anaesthesia in an outpatient setting, but local or general anaesthesia may be used if biopsy or resection of uterine polyps is required. The uterus is a potential cavity that is normally collapsed and hysteroscopy requires fluid instillation into the uterus to aid visualization. This can cause mild pain and abdominal cramp for up to 8 hours following the procedure, which can be resolved with simple analgesia such as paracetamol. The potential complications of hysteroscopy are infection and uterine perforation.

Bone marrow aspiration and biopsy

Examination of the bone marrow enables diagnosis of primary haematological malignancy or metastatic involvement of the bone marrow. The procedure can be performed under local anaesthetic in an outpatient setting, with samples taken from either the sternum or the iliac crest. The most significant morbidity associated with bone marrow aspiration and biopsy is the risk of bleeding. People who are suffering from thrombocytopenia are at especially high risk and those whose platelet count is $< 20 \times 10^9/L$ (normal $150 \times 10^9/L$) should receive a platelet transfusion whilst undergoing the procedure. It is important to observe for bleeding at the site following the procedure. Simple analgesia such as paracetamol can be given for any pain.

Lumbar puncture

A lumbar puncture enables the diagnosis of secondary disease within the central nervous system. Acute lymphocytic leukaemia is known to metastasize to the central nervous system and lumbar punctures are used to monitor the disease status in these patients. The main problem associated with a lumbar puncture is headache that results from a change in cerebrospinal fluid pressure (Ch. 14). The risk is minimized where the patient remains prone for at least 6 hours after the procedure. Headaches can normally be controlled with simple analgesia and bed rest. There is a potential risk of infection so vital signs should be monitored and pyrexia reported.

Liver biopsy

A liver biopsy enables diagnosis of primary or metastatic disease of the liver. The liver is one of the most common sites for the development of metastatic disease and biopsy is not uncommon. A liver biopsy is performed by inserting a needle, under ultrasound or computed tomography (CT) guidance, to obtain samples able to give an accurate diagnosis. The main side-effect of the procedure is pain at the biopsy site for which analgesia may be required. There is a potential risk of bleeding following the procedure and it is essential for nurses to monitor for and report bleeding, swelling or increased pain in the abdomen or biopsy site.

Imaging

The scope of diagnostic imaging has increased significantly in recent years as a result of technological advances. Clinicians are able to accurately stage the extent of primary tumours and identify metastatic disease without using invasive techniques. This can be particularly useful in planning for either surgical intervention or for radiotherapy.

The imaging techniques that provide the most accurate information are computed tomography (CT), magnetic resonance imaging (MRI) and positron emission tomography (PET), all of which produce highly detailed images. No technique is infallible and false-positive or false-negative results may occur. For example, in the abdomen, false-positive results may be associated with confusion of a mass with non-specified loops of bowel. False-negative results may be due to the inability of the scanner to detect malignant infiltration of normal-sized lymph nodes (Souhami & Tobias 1998). MRI has proved to be more conclusive than CT scanning, particularly for the investigation of the central nervous system. Ultimately, interpretation is largely dependent upon the quality of the scan and the skill of the clinician in image analysis.

Isotope scanning

Scanning with radioactive isotopes is the most effective diagnostic tool for assessing metastatic disease within the bones (Souhami & Tobias 1998). The radioactive isotopes, given by intravenous injection, are taken up by metastatic deposits in bone tissue and show up on a radiograph. The procedure requires patients to lie still for up to 1 hour whilst a series of X-rays are taken and this can be uncomfortable if they have bone pain. The role of the nurse is to prepare patients by providing information and offering appropriate analgesia prior to the procedure. The low-dose isotopes are metabolized by the kidneys and excreted in the urine. They pose a minimal radiation risk.

Laparoscopy

Laparoscopy is visualization of the abdominal cavity using a laparoscope inserted through the abdominal wall. It is used for the diagnosis of suspected ovarian cancer and cancers that involve the peritoneal cavity. Carbon dioxide is instilled into the abdominal cavity to expand it and improve the view of the organs. The procedure is associated with a risk of gas embolus. Furthermore, the gas can get trapped and commonly causes characteristic pain beneath the shoulder blades after the procedure. Preoperative explanation about this phenomenon reduces patient anxiety and pain can be relieved with analgesia and appropriate positioning.

GRADING

Grading is a method of classifying a tumour based on the histopathological characteristics of the tissue. The aggressiveness or degree of malignancy of the tissue is calculated by comparing the level of cellular abnormality and the rate of cellular division with normal cells in the same tissue. High-grade cancer is aggressive and spreads rapidly, whereas low-grade cancer tends to be latent with slow tumour growth and spread. For selected tumours the grade of the disease is more significant than the stage (1–4) as an indicator of prognosis and treatment. In prostate cancer, for example (Ch. 24), a locally confined and well-differentiated tumour requires close observation only. A poorly differentiated tumour requires radical prostatectomy in the absence of lymphatic spread, or radiotherapy if lymphatic spread is confirmed. The grading system for malignant tumours is represented in Table 33.2.

Table 33.2 TNM (tumour, node, metastasis) classification and grading system for tumours (Adapted from Sobin and Wittekind 1997)

Evaluation method	T, N, M	Grade	Classification
Clinical	T (primary tumour)	TX	Primary tumour cannot be assessed
		T0	No evidence of primary tumour
		Tis	Carcinoma-in-situ
		T1, T2, T3, T4	Increasing size and/or local extent of the primary tumour
	N (regional lymph nodes)	NX	Regional lymph nodes cannot be assessed
		N0	No regional lymph node metastasis
		N1, N2, N3	Increasing involvement of regional lymph nodes *Direct extension of the primary tumour into lymph nodes is classified as lymph node metastasis. Metastasis in any lymph node than regional is classified as distant metastasis*
	M (distant metastasis)	MX	Distant metastasis cannot be assessed
		M0	No distant metastasis
		M1	Distant metastasis *M1 may be further categorized, according to the site(s) of metastatic disease, using site coding*
Pathological	$_pT$	$_pTX$	Primary tumour cannot be assessed histologically
		$_pT0$	No histological evidence of primary tumour
		$_pTis$	Carcinoma-in-situ
		$_pT1-_pT4$	Increasing size and/or local extent of the primary tumour histologically
	$_pN$	$_pNX$	Regional lymph nodes cannot be assessed histologically
		$_pN0$	No regional lymph node metastasis histologically
		$_pN1-3$	Increasing involvement of regional lymph nodes histologically *Direct extension of the primary tumour into lymph nodes is classified as lymph node metastasis. A tumour nodule greater than 3 mm in the connective tissue of a lymph drainage area without histological evidence of residual lymph node is classified as a regional lymph node metastasis. Where size is the criterion for classification of $_pN$ (as in breast cancer), the metastasis is measured, not the whole lymph node*
	$_pM$	$_pMX$	Distant metastasis cannot be assessed microscopically
		$_pM0$	No distant metastasis microscopically
		$_pM1$	Distant metastasis microscopically *$_pM1$ may be further categorized, according to the site(s) of metastatic disease, using site coding*
Histopathological	G	GX	Grade of differentiation cannot be assessed
		G1	Well differentiated
		G2	Moderately differentiated
		G3	Poorly differentiated
		G4	Undifferentiated

STAGING

The relationship between the stage of the cancer at the time of diagnosis and the associated mortality and survival underpins the prescription of therapeutic treatment. Tumours are staged according to the TNM (**T**umour, **N**ode, **M**etastasis) system (Table 33.2), which was developed by Pierre Denoix in the early 1950s from the earlier generalized system for the classification of localized, regional and distant (LRD) disease (Sobin & Wittekind 1997). Information about the stage of disease enables the clinician to judge probable mortality and survival. Localized disease is a better prognostic indicator than widespread disease.

Each disease has its own specific classification criteria. Broadly speaking, the classification system enables clinicians to assess, either by clinical (TMN) or pathological investigation (pTMN), the size of the tumour (T), the absence or presence and extent of regional lymph node metastases (N) and the absence or presence of distant metastasis (M). TNM staging may be supported with histopathological grading.

According to the size of the tumour, and based on the extent of disease noted throughout the lymphatic and/or other systems within the body, the clinician determines the disease stage from 0–4 (where 0 = no disease and 4 = advanced disease). The classification system is widely used as criteria for entry into clinical cancer trials where it is important to determine response to treatment in people with different stages of a specific cancer. Using the classification as a baseline measurement enables clinicians to evaluate the outcome of treatment.

TREATMENT MODALITIES FOR CANCER

Surgery and radiotherapy enable localized treatment of cancer whilst chemotherapy and biological therapies have a systemic effect and thus have the potential to treat local and metastatic disease. Apart from surgical interventions, the other treatment modalities all ultimately affect DNA and prevent cancer cell replication. More specifically, chemotherapy and radiotherapy do not merely kill the cancer cells by inflicting massive damage upon the genes, but also create just enough damage to activate the production of *p53* and in turn the apoptosis response (Weinberg 1998). Cancer cells that have lost their *p53* production are seen to be more resistant to treatment because they are less likely to be encouraged into apoptosis. The assault of therapeutic treatment on cancer and indeed healthy cells can result in considerable toxicity, which is best managed at specialist cancer centres and cancer units by skilled professionals (Souhami & Tobias 1998).

SURGERY

Principles of surgical treatment

Surgery is the oldest form of therapy for cancer. Surgical resections for cancer treatment were recorded as early as 1500 BC. The key aim of surgery is removal of the tumour and adjacent tissue in order to eradicate the cancer from the body. Where complete resection is not possible, as much tumour tissue is removed as can be achieved. Reducing the tumour burden enables further treatment with chemotherapy or radiotherapy. In most cases the aim of surgery is cure, but surgery alone cannot effect a cure unless the cancer is confined to its primary site. There is an increasing focus on maintaining or improving quality of life and this overarching aim influences the choice of surgical techniques used. Laparoscopic surgery is used where possible and radical surgery avoided. Surgery may be used not only to remove a tumour, but also to restore form and function and this may be central in rehabilitation following cancer.

Surgery is frequently done to obtain a pathological diagnosis of cancer, grading and staging of the tumour. Where surgery is undertaken for diagnostic purposes, the least invasive method should be applied. There is increasing diagnostic use of fine-needle aspiration and laparoscopic techniques. The use of minimally invasive techniques has reduced associated surgical morbidity. The Calman–Hine report (1995) recommends that all patients with either suspected or confirmed cancer are treated by site specialist surgeons with specific expertise in their area. This is important not only for effective surgical clearance, but in

ensuring accurate staging at the time of surgery where excision is not possible (Souhami & Tobias 1998). This ensures the use of a planned approach to the management of people with cancer.

Surgery may be carried out as the definitive treatment where the primary tumour is localized and small. In some cases, the surgery is combined with a follow-up course of radiotherapy or chemotherapy. The aim of combined (adjuvant) treatment is to eradicate micrometastases that may have already formed and begun circulating throughout the body. Radiotherapy seeks to destroy cancer cells around the surgical margins, whilst chemotherapy seeks to eradicate systemic micrometastases (see p. 1006).

Surgical techniques are commonly used in the treatment of metastatic disease. The metastatic sites most amenable to surgical intervention include isolated hepatic metastases secondary to colon cancer, a single brain metastasis secondary to lung cancer or pulmonary spread from bone cancer. Surgery may be used to provide palliation of the symptoms of advanced cancer. Surgery may be used to drain malignant fluid, e.g. pleural fluid, pericardial fluid and abdominal (ascitic) fluid. Furthermore, surgery can provide relief from the symptoms of cancer by bypassing an obstruction. For example, a shunt (a tube that redirects body fluid from one cavity or vessel to another) may be inserted to relieve biliary obstruction. A colostomy (Ch. 22) enables colon obstruction to be bypassed. The surgical insertion of a percutaneous endoscopic gastrostomy (PEG) tube for artificial feeding directly into the stomach via the abdominal wall, will bypass oesophageal obstruction, enabling the maintenance of an adequate nutritional and hydration intake. Such procedures should improve the quality of life for the person with cancer since the focus on eating is less central and there is less anxiety associated with trying to maintain body weight. Surgical procedures may also be used to achieve pain control, e.g. nerve blocks.

Surgery may be used to treat oncological emergencies such as spinal cord compression, or to support other therapeutic modalities. Common circumstances where surgery is used to support other treatment include:

- insertion of central venous catheters to enable long-term access for chemotherapy, antibiotics, blood products, analgesia and nutritional support
- the placement of intra-arterial, intraperitoneal or intrathecal catheters to support the administration of chemotherapy
- the placement of radiation implants (iridium wires) for direct radiotherapy into the tissues (interstitial radiotherapy) or rods for intracavity radiotherapy (see p. 1005).

Surgery may be undertaken as a means of preventing cancer in those individuals who are found, by genetic testing, to be at high risk. Indeed, some individuals who have a history of familial cancer may choose to undergo prophylactic surgery. Some examples of conditions where prophylactic surgery may be used are familial adenomatous polyposis (FAP), hereditary non-polyposis colorectal cancer (HNPCC), familial breast cancer and familial ovarian cancer. This type of elective surgery should only be considered after full consultation between the surgeon and the patient, with discussion about the potential impact of loss of the body organ and possible alternatives.

RADIOTHERAPY

The discovery of X-rays by Roentgen in 1895 and the discovery of radium by Pierre and Marie Curie in 1898 paved the way for the use of radiation in the treatment of cancer. Prior to this time surgery was the only treatment for cancer (Souhami & Tobias 1998). It is estimated that around 50% of people with cancer receive radiotherapy at some point in the disease process, whether with curative or palliative intent. Radiotherapy may act as the definitive form of treatment or it may be offered to support surgery or chemotherapy, or both (Holmes 1996). The principal advantage of definitive (radical) radiotherapy over surgery is that it preserves form and function, so it is particularly useful for the treatment of head and neck cancers. Radiotherapy is effective for the primary treatment of squamous cell and basal cell skin cancers (Ch. 28), head and neck cancer, cervical cancer, prostate cancer, invasive bladder cancer and lymphomas. In palliation, radiotherapy is effective for the treatment of symptoms associated with lung cancer, brain metastases and spinal cord compression, including nausea and vomiting, dyspnoea and pain.

Pathophysiology

Radiation damages the DNA and leads to cell death, particularly at the M stage of the cell cycle when the cell attempts mitosis (Fig. 33.1). Damage to the DNA is the result of direct radiation damage or from the action of free radicals (unstable compounds that react with DNA molecules) formed when water molecules in the cells absorb radiation. Radiotherapy is usually given in the form of X-rays, gamma rays or electrons and the dose is calculated in grays (Gy), which is a measure of the amount of energy deposited in the target tissue. Radiotherapy is cell cycle-specific with most damage occurring at the G_2 phase when ribonucleic acid (RNA) is synthesized in preparation for cell division and during mitosis where the cell divides to form two identical cells.

Treatment modalities

Radiotherapy may be offered as a definitive treatment with the intention of cure, or as a palliative treatment to alleviate the distressing symptoms of advanced cancer. Since the efficacy and toxicity of radiotherapy are dose-dependent, it is essential to specify the treatment aims. Where there is a realistic potential for cure using radiotherapy, the treatment doses will be higher with a significant risk of short-term morbidity and a small risk of long-term damage to the tissues being treated, such as bowel tissue (Robinson 1995). Palliative radiotherapy seeks to minimize the symptoms of advanced disease without incurring side-effects of the treatment. Approximately 50% of radiotherapy is palliative, for instance, to relieve pain associated with skeletal metastases.

Multiple radiation fields are used to deliver a prescribed dose of radiation, directed at a defined tissue volume that encloses the tumour and surrounding tissue, where there is potential for micrometastatic spread. Healthy tissues respond to the effects of radiation in a similar way to tumour cells, although their recovery is more rapid so that there is an overall differential effect causing tumour cells to sustain more damage and eventually die. The response of healthy tissue to radiation causes

side-effects (see below). In a therapeutic treatment context, the administration of a single radiotherapy dose sufficient to kill the tumour could result in acute radiation exposure, with the manifestation of toxicities that are detrimental to health or even incompatible with life (Holmes 1996). Fractionation, the division of the total radiation dose into smaller doses, given on a regular (e.g. daily) basis seeks to deliver the optimum dose of radiotherapy whilst minimizing direct treatment-related toxicity and late complications.

Teletherapy, where high-energy external beams of radiation are directed at the treatment area, is the most common treatment modality. The treatment, which is similar to having an X-ray, commonly takes a few minutes each day, during which time patients are required to lie still on a treatment table. No discomfort should be felt by patients as a direct result of therapy, but the underlying pathology and symptoms might render the treatment experience uncomfortable. This clearly needs to be a consideration when caring for patients receiving radiotherapy, particularly in the case of palliative radiotherapy for metastatic disease.

Brachytherapy is the delivery of radiation via a radioactive source placed in or on the body. Examples of brachytherapy include caesium-137 intracavity treatment for gynaecological malignancy and interstitial therapy with iridium wires for cancer of the tongue. These techniques enable high-dose radiation to be delivered close to the tumour source.

Systemic therapy involves the oral administration of radioactive isotopes that are preferentially taken up by the target tissue. Examples of systemic therapy include the use of iodine-131 in thyroid cancer.

Side-effects

The action of radiotherapy within the G_2 and M phases of the cell cycle means that side-effects of treatment commonly present in rapidly dividing tissues such as the mouth, bowel and the skin. Notably, the toxicities associated with radiotherapy are localized to the site of the treatment. Early toxicities that commonly present, dependent upon the target treatment area, whilst treatment is ongoing include mucositis (sore mouth), diarrhoea, proctitis (sore rectal area), cystitis, erythema (localized redness of the skin) and alopecia (hair loss). The degree of toxicity is dose-dependent. The administration of radiation treatment is associated with the development of a range of late effects, which manifest after the treatment. These include radiation pneumonitis, a self-limiting effect which can be resolved to some extent with corticosteroids and antibiotics, and the development of secondary solid tumours up to 20 years after primary treatment (Robinson 1995) (see Health Promotion box 33.1).

Safety issues

Some degree of radiological exposure is almost inevitable for those people who work with radiation. Where the radiation is delivered via a sealed source, such as the selectron machine for intracavity treatment of gynaecological cancer, the risk of exposure is minimal. In contrast, nurses caring for patients who receive interstitial or systemic therapy not delivered via a sealed source have a moderately high risk of radiation exposure. Personal contact with patients receiving interstitial or systemic

HEALTH PROMOTION

33.1 Maintaining health during radiotherapy

Issues
- People with cancer can take positive action to either maintain or improve their health status
- Health promotion in the patient with cancer is concerned with maximizing health potential so that treatment is less traumatic and recovery is more rapid

Background
- Radiotherapy treatment is inherently toxic, the degree of toxicity dependent upon the volume of the target tissue, the site and the dose
- Toxicities are largely specific and predictable so that patients can be prepared for their occurrence
- Patients can be taught to manage the side-effects, which offers them control of their situation

Holmes (1997) discusses the concept of health promotion in the broad sense then applies the definitions to the care of the person with cancer. She uses a model to explore the factors that influence patient responses to health promotion initiatives and offers a 10-point plan for helping patients with health promotion.

Key points
- Health is a relative concept with individual meaning
- Health promotion activity is vital to enable patients with cancer to adapt to their illness and treatment and to maximize their potential for good health within the confines of the disease
- Health promotion should focus not only on the immediate effects of the treatment but also on the patient's total needs in terms of having cancer

- Nursing care is holistic, with interventions seeking to achieve cure of the mind and body. Health promotion provides a means to aid psychological adaptation and offers an opportunity for patients to take some control over their situation
- Distress, fear and anxiety may hamper a patient's ability to process information. These are normal reactions that accompany a diagnosis of cancer
- There is a need to present treatment in an honest, positive but realistic light in order to foster hope
- Health promotion requires nurses to offer information and to evaluate the patient's understanding on an ongoing basis, according to changes in the patient's physical and psychological condition that become manifest throughout the cancer journey

Student activities
- Try to speak with a therapy radiographer and clarify what health promotion information/services are offered
- Read the article and identify how some of the side-effects of treatment mentioned above can be minimized or prevented
- With reference to Table 1 (Holmes 1997, p. 398), make a checklist of the questions that you would need to ask in order to assess the patient's current knowledge level and perception of health status
- Make a note of the key areas for health promotion in radiotherapy. Here are a couple to start you off:
  — skin care
  — mouth care.

Reference
Holmes S. The maintenance of health during radiotherapy: a nursing perspective. J Roy Soc Health 1997; 117: 393–399.

---

therapy is avoided until daily checks confirm that the radiation level is within safe limits. Safety standards are laid down for the protection of radiological workers and occupational exposure is limited. Employers are legally obliged to offer protective equipment such as lead aprons and screens, and employees are legally obliged to use the equipment offered. Staff working in wards where radiation is used are required to wear personalized badges that measure their radiation exposure. Radiation badges are monitored by the physics and occupational health departments on a monthly basis. Over-exposure of a staff member normally requires temporary removal from the area to ensure that radiation exposure is reduced to safe and acceptable levels.

CHEMOTHERAPY

The potential for treating cancer has increased since the discovery, between 1940 and 1955, that drugs such as nitrogen mustard (carmustine) could shrink and kill cancer cells. In its first 50 years, cytotoxic chemotherapy has been successful in curing a small number of cancers and improving survival when used as an adjunct to local control measures such as surgery. It is increasingly given before surgery or radiation to shrink the tumour (neoadjuvant therapy). Furthermore, chemotherapy provides effective palliation against the symptoms of advanced disease (Holmes 1996).

Pathophysiology

Anti-cancer (cytotoxic) chemotherapy drugs exhibit their anti-tumour effects through their action on individual tumour cells. Cytotoxic drugs ultimately cause cell death by altering DNA and preventing mitosis or by initiating the apoptotic response. They are classified, according to their precise action on the cell cycle, into cell cycle phase specific (CCPS) and cell cycle phase non-specific (CCPNS) drugs. The CCPS drugs are only active at a particular point in the cell cycle, whilst CCPNS drugs operate anywhere in the cycle.

Cytotoxic drugs are further classified into five groups according to their biochemical action:

- alkylating agents (CCPNS) act to form cross-linkages between the DNA strands, e.g. cyclophosphamide and busulfan
- antimetabolites (CCPS – S phase) block enzymes necessary for DNA synthesis, e.g. 5-fluorouracil and fludarabine

- anti-tumour antibiotics (CCPNS) primarily interfere with DNA function but may also alter the cell membrane, e.g. bleomycin and epirubicin
- vinca-alkaloids and plant derivatives (CCPNS) interfere with DNA replication, e.g. etoposide and vincristine
- miscellaneous agents (CCPNS) work in a variety of ways to alter DNA structure and inhibit replication, e.g. asparaginase and irenotecan.

Cytotoxic drugs are available for administration orally, by injection (intravenous, intramuscular, intra-arterial) and directly into structures such as the bladder (intravesical). Chemotherapy is blood-borne and thus has the potential to treat both primary disease and metastases, which explains its use in a variety of clinical settings from acute to palliative care (Ch. 34).

Treatment schedules

Although cancer develops from a single cell, the genetic events that occur as the tumour grows and spreads throughout the body means that individual tumours vary in their biological and clinical behaviour. Tumours within one patient can vary in terms of the antigens present on the cell surface, the chromosomal abnormalities that present and the response to cancer chemotherapy. For example, a lung tumour might respond to chemotherapy whilst a tumour in the liver does not (Markman 1997). This phenomenon provides a good rationale for the use of combination chemotherapy regimens. Single chemotherapy agents may be effective for the treatment of certain tumours, but only when they are administered in such high doses that life-threatening toxicity results. Combination regimens are selected to exploit the potential of different drugs that are effective against specific tumours and that act at different points in the cell cycle. The result is greater damage to the tumour, but decreased toxicity because drugs with different side-effects are selected.

Cyclical chemotherapy is administered on a regular basis (weekly or monthly) in order to exploit the natural healing process of healthy cells to reduce potential toxicity. Chemotherapy drugs cannot discriminate between healthy and cancer cells and both cell populations sustain damage. Healthy cells repair themselves more rapidly than tumour cells (Holmes 1996). Cyclical chemotherapy regimens are planned so that drugs are administered as soon as the healthy cells have recovered, but before recovery in the tumour cell population. The timing of treatment cycles is crucial since cycles given too frequently cause increased damage to healthy cells and severe toxicity, whilst cycles given too infrequently enable the tumour tissue to recover and even progress.

The use of continuous infusional therapy developed out of observations about the CCPS action of some chemotherapy drugs. 5-Fluorouracil (5-FU) (see p. 1006) is highly effective in the treatment of colorectal cancer. 5-FU exerts its main action during the S phase of the cell cycle, which is relatively short. Furthermore, it has a short half-life of around 20 minutes, which means that each 20 minutes the amount of drug available for use is halved. Therefore, cancer cell damage is far greater when the drug is administered by continuous infusion to ensure that there is a constant stream of the drug available to exploit the cell cycle processes. 5-FU may be delivered continuously over 12 or 24 weeks, with the dose titrated in the presence of diarrhoea.

There is increasing interest in the timing of chemotherapy administration. Many biological processes show variation of activity throughout the day – generally metabolism is more active during daylight and less so when it is dark. The result is an alteration in the rate of chemotherapy metabolism and excretion. It is proposed that administering chemotherapy at specific times in the 24 hours might increase damage to the tumour, but result in less toxicity (Holmes 1997). An example of this is 'chronotherapy', where double dose chemotherapy is administered overnight because cancer cells remain active whilst healthy cells rest. Ongoing research using 5-FU will enable clinicians to evaluate whether this technique is more effective than the conventional continuous infusional 5-FU therapy.

Side-effects

In a similar way to radiotherapy, chemotherapy causes toxicity as a result of its non-discriminatory action on rapidly dividing tissue. The key difference is that the systemic mode of administration results in widespread toxicity rather than the local effects of radiotherapy. Side-effects may be acute at the time of treatment, subacute (short term) 3–7 days after treatment or at least 1 week after treatment (long term). Not all patients will experience all of the common toxicities (Fig. 33.4) since each drug has different actions and toxicities. The level of toxicity is dependent upon the drug(s) used, the treatment schedule, dose, route of administration and the patient (Holmes 1996) (see Reflective Practice box 33.1). It is crucial that patients and their families receive specific information about anticipated effects of their individual treatment regimen.

R|Я **REFLECTIVE PRACTICE**

33.1 Side-effects of chemotherapy

Bob (not his real name) is 79 years old. He had his first dose of chemotherapy 10 days ago and he now wants to report that he feels lethargic. He has noticed that his stools are black in colour and of tarry consistency and he has also noticed small bruises appearing around his ankles.

Student activities

- Why do you think that Bob feels lethargic?
- Do you think his other signs are related to his lethargy?
- What do you think is the cause of the signs he is experiencing?
- How would you assess Bob's understanding about the cause of the signs?
- What advice might you offer him so that he can begin to take control over at least one of the signs?
- Think about another patient that you have nursed in a similar situation – what other problems did he or she have?
- Why do you think these problems occurred?
- What nursing actions did you take to resolve the situation?

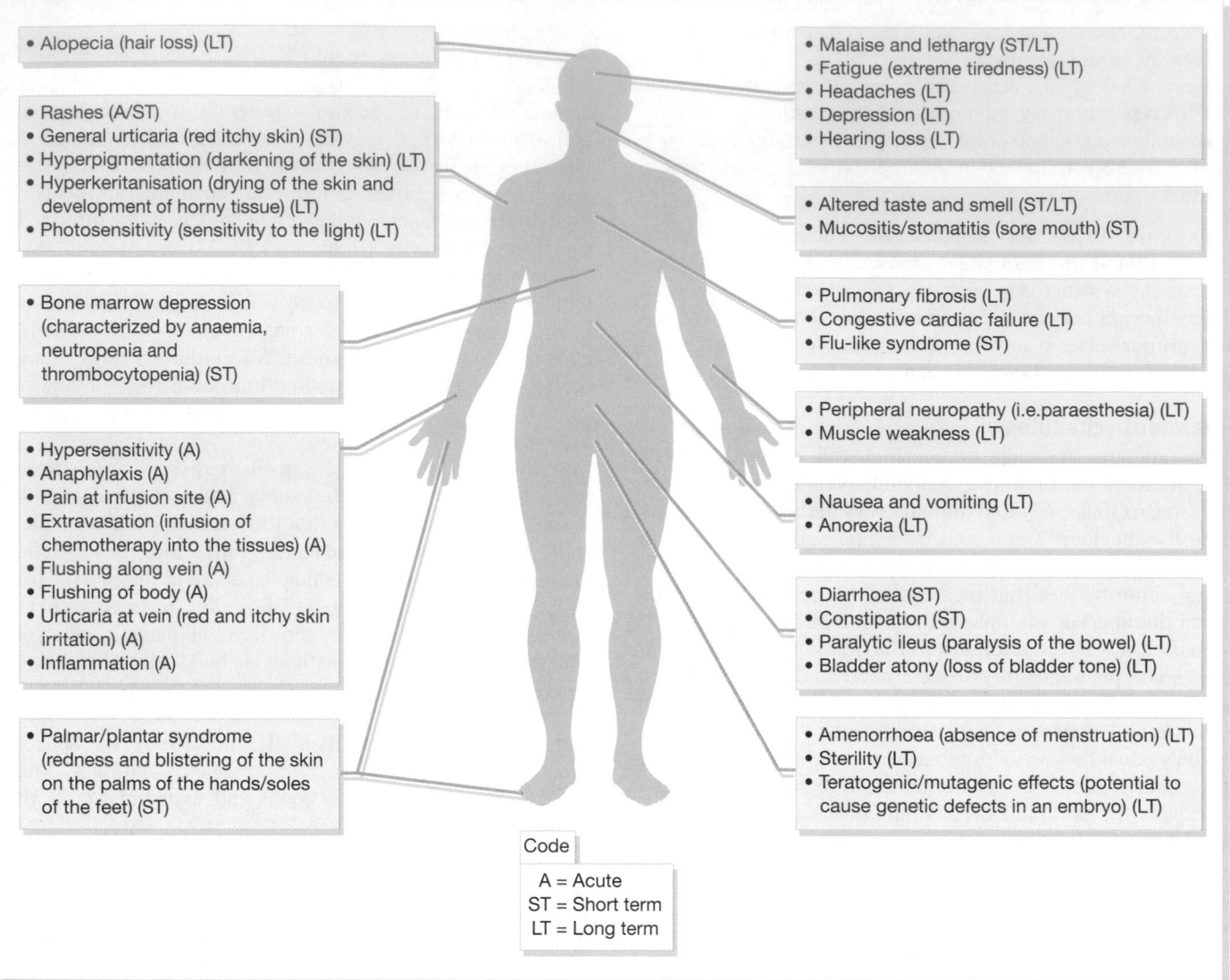

Code
A = Acute
ST = Short term
LT = Long term

Figure 33.4 Effect of chemotherapy-associated toxicity.

Safety issues

Many chemotherapy drugs have the potential to induce mutagenic (genetic changes, i.e. in an embryo or fetus, especially during the first trimester of pregnancy) or carcinogenic changes in healthy tissue. Furthermore, some drugs are extremely irritant. For these reasons, overt exposure to chemotherapy should be avoided. Although nurses handling chemotherapy do not ingest or absorb it directly and therefore only come into contact with minuscule doses compared with patients, it is believed that exposure effects are cumulative (Holmes 1996). Direct contact is avoided by preparing cytotoxic chemotherapy drugs in special preparation facilities that afford maximum protection. Other practical protective measures, such as wearing gloves during administration of chemotherapy, should be routine to minimize the risk of direct contact with the drugs. Chemotherapeutic drugs are usually excreted via the kidney and body fluids should be treated as contaminated. Equipment used for the administration of chemotherapy should be labelled as special waste and incinerated at high temperature in accordance with the control of substances hazardous to health (COSHH) regulations.

Nurses handling chemotherapy drugs on a regular basis should be screened annually for symptoms of exposure to chemotherapy, such as anaemia, neutropenia (reduced neutrophils) and thrombocytopenia. Urine examination for signs of mutagenic change forms part of ongoing monitoring by the occupational health department.

IMMUNOTHERAPY/BIOLOGICAL RESPONSE MODIFIER THERAPY

Immunological and biological response modifier (BRM) therapies are recent additions to the treatment options for cancer. Treatment, which arose after observations that spontaneous regressions of some cancers occurred after bacterial infection, is based on manipulation of the immune system.

Principles of BRM treatment

Biological response modifier therapy recruits the person's immune cells to destroy tumour cells, rather than launching a direct attack.

- Interferons (proteins formed when cells are exposed to viruses) activate macrophages. These immune cells kill invading cells and have antiproliferative properties.
- Interleukins are a group of signalling molecules produced by leucocytes which activate neutrophils and lymphocytes and stimulate antibody production.
- Colony-stimulating factors increase the production of neutrophils and macrophages.

Notably, the association between high dose and degree of response is not seen in BRM, where too high a dose will suppress the desired response (Markman 1997). The effects of BRM therapy may not become evident for several weeks or even months.

Side-effects

Biological response modifier therapy is associated with the development of characteristic toxicities. Chills associated with the first few treatments are common. Patients are advised to dress warmly or to use blankets to enhance their comfort. Fever is also common and may indicate the presence of infection. Paracetamol can provide rapid symptomatic relief. Toxicities affecting the skin include pruritus, erythema at the injection site or dry skin and can be treated with antihistamines and moisturizers. Gastrointestinal toxicities include dry mouth, nausea and vomiting and diarrhoea and commonly result in anorexia. Patients should be encouraged to drink 3 litres of fluid a day and have small frequent meals. Appetite should not be stimulated with corticosteroids since they interfere with BRM therapy.

EMOTIONAL RESPONSES TO A DIAGNOSIS OF CANCER

Psycho-oncology, the study of psychological issues in cancer care, is concerned with facilitating psychological and emotional adaptation to the diagnosis and treatment of cancer. It focuses on assessment of physical, psychological, social, sexual and employment function, measuring deficits against the level of function before the cancer diagnosis.

Until the late 20th century, the association of cancer with death was so powerful that physicians often withheld the diagnosis from the patient and communicated only with the family (Holland 1996). Although there is some residual stigma about cancer and a reluctance amongst the wider population to discuss it, the situation is very different these days (see Reflective Practice box 33.2). Patients and their families have free access to a wide range of information about their disease from health professionals, books, leaflets, helplines and the internet. The stigma of cancer has reduced, but the image of the disease is still quite negative. A diagnosis of cancer commonly evokes feelings of shock and devastation because of its association with death, disfigurement, dependency and inability to protect loved ones (Holland 1996). People diagnosed with cancer may experience a degree of disfigurement or periods of dependence, but this is no different to the losses experienced in other types of enduring illness, such as multiple sclerosis. In fact, advances in cancer treatment have encouraged less radical intervention, the side-effects of cancer treatment can generally be well controlled and

R|Я REFLECTIVE PRACTICE

33.2 Personal views and beliefs about cancer

In order to offer appropriate physical, emotional and spiritual support to people with cancer, nurses need to consider their own views and beliefs.

Student activities
- Make a note of what the word 'cancer' means to you.
- Take a moment to reflect on your experiences of nursing a person with cancer, noting whether they have been positive or negative.
- What kind of language do you use when you think about cancer, i.e. combative?
- What situations do you find the most difficult to handle?
- What do you think you need to do in order to be able to handle these situations better?
- Sit down with your supervisor to discuss your thoughts and plan strategies to enable personal development so that you feel more confident to meet difficult situations.

there is a potential for cure or prolonged remission in many types of cancer. People diagnosed with cancer may well die with it rather than from it.

The psychological impact of a cancer diagnosis is largely dependent on how the disease presents. The process may be very straightforward for those people who have identified early symptoms and sought prompt medical advice. By contrast, the diagnosis may be much more difficult to accept when the case is medically complex, when patients have concealed their symptoms and when patients feel that investigations into their symptoms have not been undertaken properly (Barraclough 1994). The initial response to the cancer diagnosis may be followed by feelings of acute distress, turmoil and depression, which may result in a preoccupation with illness and death, anxiety, anorexia, insomnia and an inability to carry out the activities of daily living. Usually these feelings begin to lessen after several weeks as the person comes to terms with the diagnosis. This process reflects, to some extent, the person's ability to face challenges and life crises. Where distress persists, a psychiatric intervention may be appropriate.

Assessment of emotional state should be holistic in order to identify all factors influencing mood. For example, medication, such as corticosteroids and analgesia, commonly used in oncology may cause mood changes. Although communication has improved tremendously in recent years, the predominant focus of the medical and nursing assessment tends to be on physical symptoms rather than on the psychological and emotional aspects. This may be the result of discomfort and/or embarrassment in dealing with potentially difficult issues (Holland 1996). Open questioning encourages patients to offer far more information and, rather than focusing on how bad nausea has been over the last week or how much hair loss has occurred, the single most important question to ask is 'How are you?'. Situations that prove too difficult to deal with can be referred to an appropriately qualified professional.

In the UK there has been increasing interest in how mind power might affect health. The personal testimonies of many patients attending the Bristol Cancer Help Centre offer evidence that the power of the mind confers protective benefits against cancer progression and may be implicated in cancer cures (Thomson 1989). It is suggested that the therapeutic power of the mind can:

- return the sense of control to the patient, so that harmful biological changes associated with prolonged stress are minimized
- enable the development of positive attitudes and coping mechanisms

- reduce stress levels – promoting optimum hormonal and immunological functioning.

Cognitive techniques for achieving control include meditation, visualization, relaxation, counselling and spiritual healing. Physical intervention is focused on the consumption of a special diet designed to improve immune function, although this idea has proved to be very controversial. The overall intention is to 'fight' the cancer through 'positive thinking'. The language of cancer is highly combative, commonly using terms such as 'courageous fight'. This may be helpful for some people who feel positive that they are fighting, but there is an inference that people with advanced disease who ultimately die from cancer

---

Box 33.1 Roy's Model Assessment – nausea and vomiting (excerpt)

Adaptive mode
1. Physiological – fluid and electrolyte balance

Behaviour
Robert is feeling nauseated following the administration of cyclophosphamide chemotherapy and he has had one episode of vomiting (115 mL of bile-stained fluid).

Direct stimuli
Robert has received cyclophosphamide chemotherapy, which is highly emetogenic.

Indirect stimuli
Robert believes that he will vomit with chemotherapy as a result of his past experience. When he was young, he remembers a family member who received chemotherapy and who had poorly controlled nausea and vomiting.

Nursing diagnosis
- Robert is at risk of dehydration because he is vomiting following the administration of chemotherapy
- Robert expects to vomit as a result of receiving chemotherapy

Nursing intervention
- Administer 5HT$_3$ antagonist antiemetics as per prescription
- Evaluate the efficacy of antiemetics by monitoring the level of nausea and episodes of vomiting
- Administer post-chemotherapy hydration fluids (intravenous) as per prescription
- Maintain accurate fluid balance chart and report deficit in intake of 1 L/24 hours to medical staff in order that the intravenous fluid prescription can be reviewed
- Monitor urea and electrolyte levels in order to identify potential dehydration
- Ensure that Robert has a vomit bowl and tissues to hand and that his call bell is within reach so that he can call the nursing staff for assistance
- Ensure that Robert has privacy when vomiting
- Identify with Robert the factors that make the nausea and vomiting worse and those and that make it better
- Encourage Robert to take small amounts (50–100 mL) of oral fluids on an hourly basis

- Discuss Robert's beliefs about the effects of chemotherapy with him, explain about the action and efficacy of modern antiemetics, and reassure him that nursing interventions will seek to minimize the experience of nausea and vomiting

Adaptive mode
2. Physiological – nutrition

Behaviour
Robert is refusing to eat anything in case he vomits.

Direct stimuli
Robert feels nauseated and he has vomited on one occasion.

Indirect stimuli
Chemotherapy drugs
Robert has been raised to believe that it is better to withhold food if you feel nauseated, and therefore he doesn't want to eat.

Nursing diagnosis
- Robert is at risk of malnutrition since he feels unable to eat as a result of his nausea and vomiting

Nursing intervention
- Administer antiemetics as per prescription (prior to mealtimes) in order to minimize the potential for nausea and vomiting
- Reassure Robert that the nausea and vomiting is temporary
- Monitor nutritional intake and maintain an accurate food chart
- Explain to Robert that it may be helpful to eat small amounts of bland dry food, as this may help to resolve his nausea
- Encourage Robert to supplement his intake by using high-protein drinks as his oral intake in addition to fresh water
- Ensure that there is food available for Robert outside of normal mealtimes in case this is when he prefers to eat or when he fancies some food, i.e. sandwiches can be ordered and delivered on the meal trolley and then stored in the fridge or bread can be toasted
- Encourage Robert's visitors to bring food that he fancies in with them

have not 'fought' against it. Thus, it is essential that nurses treat each patient as an individual and discuss the disease in terms and language that are appropriate to that person.

NURSING MANAGEMENT AND INTERVENTIONS

The key to the nursing management of patients with cancer and their families, friends or carers is effective communication and in-depth holistic assessment. These factors enable the formulation of suitable goals, negotiated between the nurse and the patient, and planning of appropriate nursing interventions to meet the patient's needs.

The nursing assessment of the person with cancer falls into four broad categories – psychological, physical condition and symptoms, knowledge about cancer and its treatment and health surveillance/maintenance behaviours – that can be explored within a formal theoretical nursing framework. The model proposed by Roy (1984) seems particularly appropriate for use in oncology with the adaptation focus. The adaptive modes reflect the areas for assessment described above and go further to explore role function and level of independence. Roy (1984) refers to stimuli that may either hinder or facilitate adaptation to current and future life circumstances. In simple terms, the stimuli may be direct or indirect, as represented in Box 33.1 for the problem of nausea and vomiting. Roy (1984) advocates implementation of the model by first level assessment (identification of maladaptive behaviours), second level assessment (identification of stimuli), nursing diagnosis and establishment of goals in cooperation with the patient, supported by ongoing evaluation of behavioural outcomes and subsequent modification

of nursing approaches. A feature of the model is that underlying stimuli are identified from the start so that intervention is aimed at the source of the problem rather than the symptoms.

COMMUNICATION

Identifying patients' needs (Ch. 3)
Communication is the key factor in identifying the needs of patients, their families and their friends. There has been an increasing focus on meeting patients' communication needs by ensuring a quiet and private environment, frank and honest discussion, and open transfer of information. It is significant that some people with cancer have a desire for openness and information whilst others do not want information, and individual wishes should be respected. Health professionals working with people who have cancer need to be aware of cultural influences on communication, in addition to factors such as learning disability and the requirement to deal sensitively and in collaboration with carers in order to overcome barriers (see Ethical Issues box 33.1).

Addressing spiritual needs
Spirituality pervades every aspect of our being: who we think we are, what we do and how our bodies respond. It influences the way we relate to each other, how we see ourselves and how we interpret our purpose. The experience of illness, and particularly cancer with its image of terminal disease, commonly threatens spiritual beliefs and can cause the phenomenon of spiritual pain. The spiritual challenge may have a negative impact or may be positive in terms of providing an opportunity for reflection, growth and self-development.

 ETHICAL ISSUES

33.1 Communicating with the patient who has a learning disability

Adults with learning disabilities have special needs in terms of communication. Breaking bad news has been identified as a particularly difficult area (see Read 1998).

Issues
- The attitude of many health professionals, carers and/or parents is that people with learning disabilities will not be able to understand what they are being told
- Framing communication so that it can be understood by the person with a learning disability is very challenging and may require assistance from carers and/or parents
- People with a learning disability may have limited vocabulary with which to describe their emotions, so the response to bad news may not be what health professionals expect
- Many health professionals are not familiar with people who have a learning disability

Stephen (not his real name) is 45. He has Down's syndrome. He has just come in with his parents, who care for him at home, to receive the results of tests, which have identified that he has leukaemia. Stephen's parents ask to see the

doctor alone so that they can learn what the diagnosis is. The consultant asks what Stephen's level of understanding is so that he can tell him what is wrong in appropriate language. Stephen's parents reply that he should not be told since he won't understand.

Student activities
- What do you think about the parents' request?
- What level of information do you feel that people with learning disabilities should be entitled to expect?
- Do you think that Stephen should be involved in the discussions? Why?
- How would you deal with the situation so that Stephen became involved?

NB: Remember that each individual patient and each set of circumstances is different. There may be no right answer that can be applied to every situation. Your nursing role ultimately requires you to use professional judgement, based on information from and about patients, their carers and the nursing research, to do what is best for your patients.

Reference
Read S. Breaking bad news to people with a learning disability. Br J Nurs 1998; 7: 86–91.

Spiritual beliefs commonly provide an explanation for the presence of disease and are important in coping with illness. The nurse plays a central coordinating role in the care of the person with cancer and as such is ideally placed to facilitate spiritual support. Sensitive discussion can enable fears and anxiety to be expressed and desired interventions to be planned. Spirituality is often linked with religious beliefs; however, it also reflects a philosophy and belief for living that are independent of religion, and thus has the potential to provide support for non-believers as well as believers from the range of religions. Spiritual resources can include prayer, religious media and people from within the family or the community, appropriate to the person's individual beliefs. The provision of spiritual support is often considered to be difficult and in many cases is not even addressed. The reasons for this include discomfort and embarrassment, fear of intruding on the patient's privacy, fear of being confused – or converted – and fear of getting into a situation to which there are no answers. It is proposed that many nurses who feel unable to provide spiritual care lack an awareness of their own belief system, but this is no justification for not providing appropriate support, which may be facilitated by referral to an experienced professional such as a counsellor or a religious official.

PATIENT TEACHING

Patient teaching is an essential element of cancer care. The provision of succinct information in everyday, understandable language enables people with cancer to understand the disease that they have, its treatment and potential side-effects. Furthermore, education about health maintenance and health promotion behaviours enables people to adapt to and take control of their situation (see Health Promotion box 33.2).

Preparing patient information materials

The information age has led to an exponential growth in the amount of material available for people with cancer to consult, whether in the form of leaflets, journal articles or web-based material. The ease of access to vast amounts of information can be overwhelming and may result in confusion with different statistics and conflicting reports about specific conditions. The situation is likely to get worse with increasing access to the internet and the associated personal freedom to paste any information onto a personal web page. This information can, however, act as a valuable catalyst for discussion about the disease and its treatment. Ultimately, each patient requires honest, up-to-date information that is prepared and presented on an individual basis. This may be in oral or written form, or both, but should ensure that the potential for confusion is minimal. The opportunity to discuss established and new information with the health professionals is critical.

DEALING WITH THE SIDE-EFFECTS OF TREATMENT AND DISEASE

The guidelines below are not intended to offer a definitive guide to symptom control, but they provide an outline of nursing interventions offered for the most common side-effects of

 HEALTH PROMOTION

33.2 Oral hygiene

- Mucositis is a common effect of toxicity associated with chemotherapy and also with radiotherapy to the head and neck region
- It is self-limiting and has a range of adverse consequences since it influences the intake of food and fluids and oral medications
- The maintenance of adequate nutritional levels is vital for healing and recovery of the immunological system following chemotherapy. Mucositis combined with taste changes and anorexia puts the patient at high risk of malnutrition
- Assessment is the key to effective intervention. Oral assessment focuses on elements such as the voice, ability to swallow, colour and moisture of lips and tongue, presence or absence of saliva and presence or absence of ulcers (see Eilers et al 1988)
- A proactive approach to education and care is most effective. Patients are taught how to assess their own oral mucosa so that they can highlight problems promptly
- Prophylactic chlorhexidine mouthwashes are incorporated into a four-times-daily oral care routine. Patients with dentures should remove them whilst attending to their oral hygiene
- The teeth/gums, oral mucosa and tongue are cleansed using a soft toothbrush
- If the oral mucosa becomes very ulcerated and sore, analgesia may be administered in the form of Oramorph or intravenous morphine via the patient-controlled analgesia
- Patients who have severe and prolonged mucositis may require total parenteral nutrition until the oral mucosa recovers (see Goodman et al 1993)

References

Eilers J, Berger AM, Peterson MC. Development, testing and application of the oral assessment guide. Oncol Nurs Forum 1988; 15: 325–330.

Goodman M, Ladd LA, Purl S. Integumentary and mucous membrane alterations. In: Groenwald SL, Hansen Frogge M, Goodman M, Henke Yarbro C, eds. Cancer nursing: principles and practice, 3rd edn. Boston: Jones and Bartlett; 1993, 47–57.

treatment and disease. Further information on management of side-effects is available in Kaye (1994) and in Chapter 34 (see also Special Issues box 33.2).

Nausea and vomiting

Nausea and vomiting is frequently rated as the worst symptom of cancer and its treatment. There are very many factors implicated in the development of nausea and vomiting and multiple causes are commonly identified in the individual patient with cancer. The primary cause is chemotherapy treatment. Chemotherapy drugs are recognized as foreign agents because they attack the body cells so the natural protective mechanism

33.2 Constipation

Constipation is a state in which an individual's pattern of elimination is characterized by hard, dry stool that results from a delay in the passage of food residue. People with cancer are prone to constipation, especially if they are taking opioid medication such as morphine. Even anorexic patients need to have bowel movements to expel faeces formed from the gastrointestinal secretions, cells and bacteria.

Causes of constipation in oncology
- Drugs, especially iron, opioids and tricyclic antidepressants such as lofepramine
- Immobility
- Lack of privacy when using the toilet, commode or bed pan
- Dehydration secondary to poor fluid intake, vomiting, passing large amounts of urine (polyuria) or sweating
- Absence of fibre in the diet
- Hypercalcaemia (serum calcium level above 2.6 mmol/L), which is common in myeloma (bone cancer) and the presence of bone metastases
- Concurrent disease – painful anal conditions, hypothyroidism

Nursing assessment
- What is the cause of the constipation?
- What is the individual's normal pattern of bowel evacuation?
- How does the individual feel about having constipation?

Nursing management
- Plan intervention according to the source of the problem
- Collaborate with the patient to formulate goals and plan appropriate interventions
- Monitor bowel function daily and plan appropriate pharmacological interventions, including the use of stool softeners and stimulants
- Patients taking opioids should be prescribed laxatives as a routine
- A change in the medication may be considered
- The treatment of constipation should be proactive and not reactive

of nausea and vomiting is initiated in an attempt to rid the body of the drugs. The phenomenon of nausea is commonly more distressing than the act of vomiting itself, which often provides some relief from the associated discomfort. Treatment is dependent upon the cause and should take into account that vomiting will inhibit the absorption of oral medications, and therefore alternative routes (intravenous/intramuscular/subcutaneous/rectal) should be used wherever possible.

Traditionally, nausea and vomiting associated with cancer therapy has been treated with dopamine receptor (D_2) antagonists such as metoclopramide, which reduces gastric motility.

Metoclopramide is effective against chemotherapy-induced nausea and vomiting, acting as a D_2 receptor antagonist at low doses and a 5-hydroxytryptamine ($5HT_3$) antagonist at high doses. Its action is enhanced by the addition of the corticosteroid dexamethasone to the drug regimen. High-dose use of metoclopramide is limited because of central nervous system side-effects such as akathisia (the patient feels anxious and cannot sit still – 'dancing feet syndrome') and torticollis (contraction of the neck muscles). Chemotherapy-induced nausea and vomiting is commonly treated with the new $5HT_3$ antagonists such as ondansetron in the first instance; however, this only remains effective for around 48–72 hours after each course of acute treatment. Lorazepam is beneficial for the treatment of anticipatory nausea and vomiting associated with treatment.

Nausea and vomiting can occur as a result of metastatic disease and is associated with raised intracranial pressure secondary to cerebral metastases. This is treated effectively with palliative radiotherapy. Nausea and vomiting secondary to bowel obstruction by tumour may be treated with cyclizine, haloperidol or levomepromazine (methotrimeprazine) (Kaye 1994). In the palliative stage, nausea and vomiting may be treated with a histamine receptor (H_1) antagonist such as chlorpromazine, which acts as a sedative. The cannabinoids (i.e. dronabinol) have similar sedative effects to chlorpromazine but increase the appetite as a side-effect.

Fatigue
Fatigue is a common effect of cancer treatment and of advancing disease. The physiology of fatigue is largely unexplained but the effects are devastating and have a significant impact on the quality of life. Fatigue resulting from anaemia can be resolved with the administration of a blood transfusion. Corticosteroids may be administered in order to increase the sense of well-being but are associated with the side-effects of muscular weakness and wasting. Every person has individual needs and coping styles, but there is evidence that gentle exercise actually helps to relieve feelings of fatigue (Kaye 1994).

Diarrhoea
Diarrhoea is a condition that commonly manifests as a side-effect of treatment (5-FU and irenotecan) or as a sign of gastro-intestinal infection. Infection should be ruled out before commencing treatment with anti-diarrhoeal agents such as loperamide. Loperamide may be underused in the treatment of diarrhoea secondary to abdominal malignancy because of the fear of causing constipation (Kaye 1994). Meticulous hygiene and the use of skin moisturizers may provide relief of burning in the perianal area in the presence of profuse diarrhoea.

Pancytopenia (Chs 13 and 18)
Chemotherapy drugs and radiotherapy treatment cause pancytopenia (a reduction in the total blood cell count), with characteristic production of immature cells from the bone marrow. Pancytopenia manifests as anaemia which causes dyspnoea and fatigue, thrombocytopenia which renders the patient susceptible to spontaneous bruising and potentially life-threatening bleeding, and neutropenia that can lead to infection and potentially fatal septicaemia (see Guidelines for Care Priorities box 33.1).

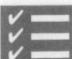

✓
✓ GUIDELINES FOR CARE PRIORITIES
✓

33.1 Nursing care of the patient with neutropenia
(Carter 1994; Campbell & Foody 1995)

- Protection from exposure to pathogens that could cause septicaemia is crucial and therefore the patient with neutropenia (neutrophil count $< 0.5 \times 10^9/L$) is nursed in a protective isolation environment (clean single room or sterile laminar air flow environment where positive pressure is used to filter sterile air through the room)
- Four-hourly observation of body temperature, pulse, blood pressure and respirations
- If the patient is pyrexial on one occasion (temperature $> 38.5°C$), the temperature is recorded 1 hour later.
- If the patient is pyrexial for two consecutive occasions in 1 hour, central and peripheral blood cultures are obtained and broad-spectrum antibiotics commenced (tazocin and gentamicin)
- If the elevated temperature persists for 24 hours or if the patient becomes hyperpyrexial (temperature $> 39°C$), a further antibiotic is added to the regimen (teicoplanin)
- Visitors are restricted to two at any time. They must be well with no signs of infection
- Fresh flowers are discouraged because of the risk of *Pseudomonas* contamination of the flower water. If there are flowers in the room, the water should be changed on a daily basis
- The patient who is neutropenic requires referral to a dietician since there are restrictions on dairy products and some fruit products that harbour microorganisms. Wrapped food, served in single portions, is deemed to be the safest since it hasn't required preparation by another person prior to eating
- The patient is allowed to leave the protective isolation environment when the neutrophil count returns to $0.5 \times 10^9/L$

References
Campbell LR, Foody MC. The administrative issues of an inpatient BMT unit. In: Buchsel PC, Whedon MB, eds. Bone marrow transplantation: administrative strategies and clinical concerns. Boston: Jones and Bartlett; 1995, 39–68.

Carter LW. Bacterial translocation: nursing implications in the care of the patient with neutropenia. Oncol Nurs Forum 1994; 21: 857–867.

Lymphoedema

Lymphoedema is a condition in which lymphatic damage results in the accumulation of lymph in the limbs, which become swollen, heavy and immobile (Badger 1996). The skin can become dry, so moisturizers are applied regularly. Active or passive exercises and manual or electronic lymphatic drainage using massage (Kirshbaum 1996), compression bandaging or a compression pump serve to reduce swelling in the limb and its associated discomfort. Corticosteroids may be administered in the early stages of lymphoedema with some effect, but are largely ineffective once it becomes established (Kaye 1994).

ONCOLOGICAL EMERGENCIES

People with cancer may experience medical emergencies as a result of either the disease process or their treatment. Two of the most common disorders are described below. Other emergency conditions include superior vena cava obstruction (Ch. 34), cardiac tamponade (Ch. 19), disseminated intravascular coagulation (Ch. 9), tumour lysis syndrome and hypercalcaemia (Chs 8, 17 and 34). Refer to Groenwald et al (1995) for further information.

Septic shock (Ch. 9)

Septic shock, characterized by instability of the circulatory system and altered metabolism, arises as a result of systemic invasion of the blood by microorganisms. The incidence has increased with the widespread use of invasive medical devices and the use of corticosteroids and chemotherapy. The potential for septic shock is particularly high in the presence of neutropenia secondary to chemotherapy or radiotherapy. Rapid and aggressive therapy is required since the associated mortality for people with cancer is over 75% (Groenwald et al 1995).

The clinical manifestations of septic shock are tachycardia, fever, rigors, tachypnoea, respiratory alkalosis (Ch. 8) and evidence of poor tissue perfusion in the early stages. Later vasoconstriction causes the skin to cool and become clammy and cyanosis is evident. These symptoms are accompanied by a thready pulse and hypotension. If not treated promptly, acute respiratory distress syndrome (Ch. 20) will ensue, closely followed by coma and death (Groenwald et al 1995).

Septic shock is promptly treated with broad-spectrum antibiotics or, when there has been long-term antibiotic therapy in the presence of neutropenia, with an antifungal agent such as amphotericin. Vigorous fluid replacement is given to expand intravascular volume (Ch. 9). The administration of high-dose corticosteroids within the first 24 hours to reduce the inflammatory response may increase survival rates. Ongoing monitoring of the patient's condition enables evaluation of the efficacy of treatment based on observation of tissue perfusion, oxygenation, renal function and level of consciousness (Ch. 9). The mortality rate associated with septic shock ranges from 50 to 90%, so the importance of prompt diagnosis and treatment is clear.

Spinal cord compression

Spinal cord compression is a malignant process in which a tumour exerts pressure upon the spinal cord or cauda equina causing paralysis below the lesion. With prompt diagnosis and treatment, it is possible to preserve neurologic function and patients who are able to mobilize at presentation and treatment may retain their mobility. People who present having lost their mobility are unlikely to regain it (Groenwald et al 1995). Spinal cord compression develops in around 5% of patients with systemic cancer and 95% of these cases are attributable to metastatic disease of the spine. Lung and breast cancers commonly metastasize to the thoracic spine causing high-level paralysis, whilst gastrointestinal tumours metastasize to the lumbosacral region of the spine.

Over 95% of people with spinal cord compression present with back pain, which may be localized or may radiate (e.g. around the chest or waist). The hallmark feature is that the pain changes in location, intensity and nature (Groenwald et al 1995). Around 75% of people have motor weakness at the time of diagnosis of spinal cord compression, although it is rarely the presenting symptom. Autonomic disturbances, associated with the site of the lesion, include bowel and bladder dysfunction. In the presence of sensory loss, these symptoms indicate progressive disease. The diagnosis of spinal cord compression can be confirmed using myelography (X-ray following injection of a radio-opaque medium into the subarachnoid space) or an MRI scan.

Prompt treatment with radiotherapy, supported with corticosteroids to reduce inflammation, is the key to maintaining function. Notably, the use of corticosteroids may compromise skin integrity and healing ability, so assessment and appropriate intervention to prevent the development of pressure ulcers are crucial (Ch. 10). Ongoing assessment of motor, bowel and bladder function gives some indication of a patient's responsiveness to treatment. Active intervention may be required to assist patients to manage the loss of function. The potential for rehabilitation is dependent upon the level of function that the individual had at presentation and the response to treatment. Nurses have a vital role to play in educating patients about the signs of spinal cord compression so that prompt investigation and treatment can be initiated at an early stage in order that neurological function and therefore quality of life can be preserved (see Evidence-based Practice box 33.3).

DEALING WITH CHANGES IN BODY IMAGE

Body image reflects the view that each one of us presents about how we see ourselves in reality and as an ideal. It is strongly influenced by cultural norms and values, peer and media pressure. It is recognized that illness or treatment that results in an altered body image can invoke temporary or permanent distress associated with that change. This is because body image is related to self-concept, self-esteem and personal identity (Topping 1995).

Promoting adaptive responses

Roy's (1984) model for nursing is concerned with identifying maladaptive responses and proposing nursing interventions designed to reduce the stressful stimulus. Adaptation to alterations in body image is often a long drawn-out process which requires validation, respect and support offered within a non-judgemental relationship. The role of the nurse is to facilitate discussion and the expression of fears and anxieties in a supportive and non-judgemental atmosphere. Information regarding alternative sources of professional and voluntary support that can be used by patients and their partners is critical. Support systems can include the GP, specialist nurses (breast and stoma), a sexual counsellor, patient support groups or formal support networks and helplines.

 EVIDENCE-BASED PRACTICE

33.3 Malignant spinal cord compression

Husband (1998) reports on a controlled prospective study designed to evaluate the degree of delay in referral following the onset of symptoms of spinal cord compression. The report analyses the effects of delay according to the morbidity associated with spinal cord compression in terms of loss of motor and bladder function at the time of treatment.

Key points

- Metastatic malignant spinal cord compression is a common oncology emergency situation which can result in paralysis below the physiological position of the lesion unless treated promptly
- Less than half of the patients admitted to hospital with spinal cord compression retain or regain the ability to walk and around two-fifths require a permanent urinary catheter
- The most important prognostic factor for functional outcome is neurological function before treatment
- The delay from the onset of symptoms (back pain, weakness, pins and needles and bladder dysfunction) to treatment was measured. A longer delay was associated with increased morbidity as a result of the spinal cord compression
- The delay from the onset of symptoms to treatment was found to be significantly longer in patients with an established diagnosis of cancer than those who presented with the spinal cord compression as the symptom of an undiagnosed cancer

- The delay from the onset of symptoms to treatment was reduced when patients presented to the cancer centre rather than to their general practitioner
- The author concludes that, in this study, there was unacceptable delay in the diagnosis, investigation and referral of people with spinal cord compression for treatment, so that there was preventable loss of function before patients underwent treatment
- This remains a common problem. The main causes of delay are failure to diagnose spinal cord compression and failure to investigate and refer for treatment within 24 hours
- Educating patients about the common symptoms of spinal cord compression and encouraging presentation direct to the cancer centre may reduce delay and improve functional status at treatment.

Student activities

- Read the key points above and consider how you could facilitate earlier referral and diagnosis of malignant spinal cord compression, i.e. through education regarding symptoms.
- How does this link in to what you have already read in the chapter?

Reference

Husband DJ. Malignant spinal cord compression: prospective study of delays in referral and treatment. Br Med J 1998; 317: 18–21.

Psychosexual issues

Related to the effects of an altered body image and perhaps compounded by the effects of cancer treatment there is a high risk of people experiencing altered sexual functioning. Particular cancer sites that could predispose sexuality problems include the head and neck, where changes are highly visible, the breast and pelvis where the sexual organs are altered or where there may be vaginal dryness or infertility. Sexual relationships may also suffer as a result of stoma formation. Elements of sexuality that may be affected include role and relationships, functioning and frequency of sexual activity (Topping 1995). The role of the nurse is to provide a forum for discussion appropriate to cultural norms, values and influences and to provide support and reassurance about progress. This serves to assist in the reorientation to the altered body image and to enhance feelings of self-worth and personal autonomy so that patients can take control once again.

REHABILITATION AND SURVIVAL

Rehabilitation is concerned with the restoration of a 'normal' or optimal state of health and the preparation of a disabled or disadvantaged person for employment by vocational counselling or training (Gender 1998). Florence Nightingale (1859) first introduced the notion of rehabilitation in nursing in her proposal that to do as much for oneself as possible reduces feelings of anxiety and aids adaptation and recovery from illness.

The advances in screening and diagnostic techniques that enable and encourage earlier detection of cancer and the advances in therapeutic treatment mean that there is a far greater potential for prolonged remission or even cure from the disease. This has significant implications for people with cancer who are no longer expected to 'turn their face to the wall' and wait for inevitable death. The emphasis instead is on adaptation, rehabilitation and survival. Work remains a very meaningful activity for cancer patients (Berry & Cantanzaro 1992) and nurses are well placed to facilitate treatment schedules that fit in with work patterns wherever possible. Those people who are required to give up work while they undergo cancer treatment find it very difficult to re-establish a position in the workplace. This may be largely due to public attitudes that people with cancer are going to die and cannot work since they are too sick. Although public figures have demonstrated that this is not necessarily the case, attitudinal change is slow. In the meantime nurses can help people with cancer by utilizing the services of rehabilitation specialists who will help patients re-integrate into an adaptation of their previous lifestyle. The major roles of the nurse in rehabilitation are to educate, to listen to patients and their families, and to give and coordinate care, according to the needs identified by patients and their families (Gender 1998).

SUPPORTING FAMILY AND FRIENDS

Family members are most often the main source of support for the person with cancer and the diagnosis of cancer can be as difficult for them as it is for the patient. A stoic attitude towards the disease by the patient may leave carers feeling helpless and frustrated. Depression and anxiety can be as common amongst the significant others of patients as it is in the patients

themselves. The emotional state and mood of people with cancer are commonly reflected in those who are close to them, so that when patients are anxious and depressed, their significant other(s) is also depressed. In most cases, these feelings have not been shared because one person doesn't want to upset the other (Barraclough 1994). Nurses and other health care professionals have a key role to play in encouraging communication and sharing of feelings between patients and their significant others.

Family members and friends often experience feelings of guilt because the person they love has cancer and they do not. The situation often provokes a reappraisal of life and their relationships for them as well as for the person with cancer. Many people experience discord in their life relationships and although the crisis of cancer may act as a catalyst for the resolution of problems, the relationship may also deteriorate and ultimately end. Providing support for the person with cancer can be difficult and carers often feel obliged to put on a brave face and present a cheerful outlook. It is extremely helpful for carers to have personal support from the health professionals and nurses can facilitate private appointments where carers are offered an opportunity to discuss their own feelings. This may be followed up by a meeting with the patient so that mutual grief and distress can be shared openly if this is appropriate for the individuals concerned.

Practical help can be offered to carers in terms of advice, encouragement and even permission to take time for themselves. Nurses can offer advice about, and in many cases referral to, professional and voluntary services such as Macmillan and Marie Curie nursing services, occupational therapists, physiotherapists and social workers. Referral to cancer day centre services may be particularly helpful, offering carers respite and sanctioned time for themselves. Nurses can also advise patients about benefits for which they are eligible, such as attendance allowance (Chs 34 and 35).

MANAGEMENT OF CANCER PAIN

Pain is one of the most feared consequences of cancer. Studies in the USA have indicated that as many as one-third of people receiving cancer therapy and two-thirds of those with advanced cancer suffer from significant discomfort (Foley 1996). Providing relief from pain acts as a goal in its own right, but coincidentally encourages people to continue with cancer treatment that they might otherwise abandon. It is estimated that 95% of cancer pain can be relieved with appropriate pharmacological and non-pharmacological intervention (Chs 7 and 34). Assessment is an essential element of pain control, enabling the collection of objective data about the cause, nature and type of pain, strategies used to resolve it and their effect. It should not be assumed that the pain is due to the cancer and all potential causes should be explored.

The nature of pain experienced by the person with cancer is multi-faceted. The pain stimulus may be defined as having a peripheral, central or psychogenic origin (O'Connor 1998). Cancer pain may arise as a direct result of physiological stimulation or as a result of spiritual distress or anxiety. Cancer pain is significant since it is often all-encompassing and serves to exacerbate other symptoms of the disease, including anorexia and dyspnoea. It is therefore crucial that the underlying cause of the pain, and not just the symptoms, is identified and treated promptly. Pain control may be achieved by the administration of medication; by non-pharmacological strategies such as visualization, relaxation, meditation and massage; or by a combination of pharmacological and non-pharmacological strategies according to the source of the pain and the patient's needs.

PHARMACOLOGICAL STRATEGIES

Pharmacological interventions are offered according to the World Health Organization analgesic ladder (see O'Connor 1998). Patients admitted to hospital with severe pain are given either weak or strong opioids to get the pain under control before a baseline assessment of pain is made. Regular pain assessments enable analgesia to be titrated appropriately (Ch. 34).

Mild pain is initially treated with non-opioid analgesic agents such as paracetamol, with or without the addition of adjuvant drugs such as anxiolytics or antispasmodics, such as lorazepam. If pain persists or increases then mild opioid agents such as co-proxamol are administered, with or without the addition of adjuvant drugs. If pain still persists or increases then strong opioids such as morphine are administered, with or without the addition of adjuvant drugs. The dose of strong opioids is titrated until pain control is achieved.

NON-PHARMACOLOGICAL STRATEGIES

Many people with cancer employ alternative or complementary methods of support in addition to pharmacological intervention. Non-pharmacological strategies for pain control seek to alter the patient's perception of the pain and to reduce stress, exploiting the mind–body relationship. Commonly used interventions include massage, application of heat or cold, transcutaneous electrical nerve stimulation (TENS), imagery, distraction and relaxation techniques (Chs 7 and 34). All of these techniques, which offer patients clear control over their pain, have proved to be effective (O'Connor 1998).

SPECIALIST CANCER NURSE ROLES

Oncology offers many opportunities for the development of specialist nursing roles. The nature of the specialty, which covers all aspects of care from screening through to rehabilitation or death, and the increasing interest in cancer site specialization have led to an abundance of new roles. The clinical nurse specialist roles may be site-specific (breast and stoma care nurses), service-specific (chemotherapy and central venous access service specialist nurses) or research-specific (clinical research nurse).

In general terms, any new role must be developed in the spirit of patient interest and not merely to devolve roles from junior doctors to nursing staff. The specialist nurse role is challenging, with the expectation that the post-holder will integrate clinical, management, research and education functions. The current emphasis on clinical governance enables specialist nurses to maximize their roles in order to develop evidence-based practice with colleagues. A recent development in the UK is the lead cancer and consultant nurse roles, strategic posts focused on developing oncology nursing services for the new millennium. A key role of the lead cancer and consultant nurse is the coordination of specialist nurses within oncology to ensure the provision of a high-quality cohesive service.

ETHICAL DILEMMAS IN CANCER NURSING

ETHICAL PRINCIPLES

The ethical principles of beneficence, non-maleficence, justice and autonomy are applicable in oncology in the same way that they are in all other nursing specialties and all care situations. The main ethical dilemmas in oncology are related to issues of communication and choice. People with cancer are often in a unique position in terms of their treatment requirements. It is common for treatment to follow extremely quickly after diagnosis with little opportunity for communication and this situation can create ethical dilemmas (see Ethical Issues box 33.2).

 ETHICAL ISSUES

33.2 Maintaining confidentiality

Jack (not his real name), aged 46, was told yesterday that he has got lung cancer. You have just been in and put up the chemotherapy for him and he said that he is expecting his wife to come and visit him. He hasn't told her what his diagnosis is. He doesn't intend to tell her and he doesn't want anybody else to tell her.

Student activities
- How do you feel about Jack's request not to communicate his diagnosis to his wife?
- Consider how you might deal with the situation if she approaches you and specifically asks you what is wrong with Jack.
- Would you tell Jack's wife what is wrong with him?
- What would you say if she asked you what the drugs he is having are for?
- What professional guidance do we have to help us deal with this kind of situation?
- What strategies would you use to try to get Jack to start talking to his wife?

Note: Ethical dilemmas are often difficult to handle because there is no black or white, nor any right or wrong answer. You are expected to make a judgement about what is best for everybody involved. Once you have experienced a situation, it becomes a little easier because you have been through something similar, but every patient and every situation is unique and reacting in the same way, in a new or different situation, may produce completely different results. Personal reflection on this type of incident enables you to discuss what was difficult about it and to plan how you would approach it in a similar situation.

Cancer patients and research

Oncology is a rich area for research and the drive for clinical governance is increasing the focus on clinical research. The Calman–Hine report (1995) also highlights the importance of involvement in clinical research. This strong research focus could result in pressure to enrol patients into clinical trials, with the potential for subtle coercion to ensure that targets for recruitment are met. People with cancer already have little enough time to consider their treatment options since it is normally crucial to start treatment promptly. Furthermore, they are renowned for their willingness to enter clinical trials without much opportunity for careful consideration and questioning with regard to other treatment options (Tabak 1995).

The research nurse is ideally placed to ensure that patients are satisfied with the information that they have received and that they have no questions to be answered before trial registration is carried out and treatment started. An essential component of informed consent is that patients sign a form to acknowledge that they can withdraw from the trial at any point. The nurse can facilitate discussion with the physician and ensure that patients' voices are heard and their questions answered.

SUMMARY: MAIN POINTS

- Oncology is an exciting specialty where there is clear evidence of biological research development enabling practice to move forward.

- The key to reducing the incidence of cancer is the adoption of healthier lifestyle practices and relies on nurses taking a lead in health education, health promotion and health policy development.

- Knowledge about the biological basis of cancer treatment enables effective, proactive nursing interventions to be planned.

- The nurse has a key role in educating the person with cancer about their disease, treatment and the associated toxicity.

- The opportunity to reflect upon practice and to consider ethical dilemmas within cancer nursing will have enabled nurses to consider how they can best represent the patient and their interest in the health care setting.

SELF TEST: CRITICAL THINKING ACTIVITIES

Examine the nursing records of a patient who has been admitted to your ward for non-surgical cancer treatment.

1. What framework was used for assessment? Did it cover the areas suggested in the chapter or do you feel that there were data missing?

2. How were the goals and nursing interventions negotiated and planned?

3. What areas are included on the plan? Do you feel there are any gaps?

4. Discuss the care plan with a qualified nurse colleague and highlight the rationale for the areas covered on the plan.

5. What changes would you make to the care plan? Include your rationale for any changes.

 ## FURTHER READING

Costain Schou K, Hewison J. Experiencing cancer. Buckingham: Open University Press; 1999.

Diamond J. C: Because cowards get cancer too. London, Vermilion; 1998

Gates RA, Finks RM. Oncology nursing secrets. Philadelphia: Hanley and Belfus; 1997.

Guerrero D. Neuro-oncology for nurses. London: Whurr Publishers; 1998.

Lind MJ. Cytotoxic chemotherapy. Med Int 1995; 23(10); 422–435.

Rice AM. An introduction to radiotherapy. Nurs Stand 1997; 12(3): 49–56.

Scientific American. What you need to know about cancer. Sci Am 1996; 275(3).

Stuart NSA. Emergencies in cancer. Med Int 1995; 23(10): 445–447.

Wilkes GM, Ingwersen K, Barton Burke M. 1997–1998 Oncology nursing drug handbook. London: Jones and Bartlett; 1997.

REFERENCES

Austoker J. Breast cancer screening: practical guide for primary care teams. Oxford: Cancer Research Campaign; 1990.

Badger C. Treating lymphoedema. Nurs Times 1996; 92: 84–88.

Barraclough J. Cancer and emotion, 2nd edn. Chichester: John Wiley; 1994.

Berry DL, Cantanzaro M. Persons with cancer and their return to the workplace. Cancer Nurs 1992; 15: 40–46.

Boothroyd W. Promoting health and preventing cancer. In: David J, ed. Cancer care: prevention, treatment and palliation. London: Chapman and Hall; 1995, 13–28.

Boyle P. Some recent developments in the epidemiology of colorectal cancer. In: Bleiberg H, Rougier P, Wilke HJ, eds. Management of colorectal cancer. London: Martin Dunitz; 1998, 19–34.

Calman K, Hine D. A policy framework for commissioning cancer services. London: HMSO; 1995.

Cancer Research Campaign. About cancer: reducing risk. London: Cancer Research Campaign; 1999a.

Cancer Research Campaign. About cancer: the facts. London: Cancer Research Campaign; 1999b.

Cancer Research Campaign. The Cancer Research Campaign scientific yearbook 1998/9. London: Cancer Research Campaign; 1999c.

Cartmel B, Reid M. Cancer control and epidemiology. In: Groenwald SL, Hansen Frogge M, Goodman M, Henke Yarbro C, eds. Cancer nursing: principles and practice, 3rd edn. Boston: Jones and Bartlett; 1993, 3–27.

Craddock P. Screening for cancer. In: David J, ed. Cancer care: prevention, treatment and palliation. London: Chapman and Hall; 1995, 48–76.

Cummings JH, Bingham SA. Diet and the prevention of cancer. Br Med J 1998; 317: 1636–1640.

Department of Health. Our healthier nation – green paper. London: Stationery Office; 1998.

Department of Health. Saving lives – our healthier nation. London: Stationery Office; 1999.

Department of Health. The NHS cancer plan. London: Stationery Office; 2000.

Foley KM. Controlling the pain of cancer. Sci Am 1996; 275: 164–165.

Gender AD. Scope of rehabilitation and rehabilitation nursing. In: Chin PA, Finocchiaro D, Rosebrough A, eds. Rehabilitation nursing practice. New York: McGraw-Hill; 1998, 3–20.

Groenwald SL. Differences between normal and cancer cells. In: Groenwald SL, Hansen Frogge M, Goodman M, Henke Yarbro C, eds. Cancer nursing: principles and practice, 3rd edn. Boston: Jones and Bartlett; 1993, 47–57.

Groenwald SL, Hansen Frogge M, Goodman M, Henke Yarbro C. (eds). Comprehensive cancer nursing review, 2nd edn. Boston: Jones and Bartlett Publishers; 1995.

Hoffbrand AV, Pettit JE. Essential haematology, 3rd edn. Oxford: Blackwell Scientific Publications; 1993.

Holland JC. Cancer's psychological challenges. Sci Am 1996; 275(3): 158–161.

Holmes S. Radiotherapy: a guide for practice, 2nd edn. Dorking: Asset Books; 1996.

Holmes S. The maintenance of health during radiotherapy: a nursing perspective. J Roy Soc Health 1997; 117: 393–399.

Kaye P. A-Z pocketbook of symptom control. Northampton: EPL; 1994.

Kirshbaum M. Using massage in the relief of lymphoedema. Prof Nurse 1996; 11: 230–232.

Lynch P. Biology of colorectal cancer: an overview of genetic factors. In: Bleiberg H, Rougier P, Wilke H, eds. Management of colorectal cancer. London: Martin Dunitz; 1998, 1–17.

Markman M. Basic cancer medicine. London: WB Saunders; 1997.

Nightingale F. Notes on nursing. London: Harrison; 1859.

O'Connor L. Cancer pain – providing solutions for current problems. In: Poulton G, ed. Nursing the person with cancer. Melbourne: Ausmed; 1998, 88–106.

Richardson P. What is cancer? In: David J, ed. Cancer care: prevention, treatment and palliation. London: Chapman and Hall; 1995, 1–12.

Robinson MH. Radiotherapy. Med Int 1995; 23: 417–421.

Roy C. Introduction to nursing: an adaptation model. New Jersey: Prentice Hall; 1984.

Sarafino EP. Health psychology: biopsychosocial interactions, 2nd edn. Chichester: John Wiley; 1994.

Sobin LH, Wittekind C (eds). TNM classification of malignant tumours, 5th edn. Chichester: John Wiley; 1997.

Souhami R, Tobias J. Cancer and its management, 3rd edn. Oxford: Blackwell Science; 1998.

Tabak N. Decision making in consenting to experimental cancer therapy. Cancer Nurs 1995; 18: 89–96.

Tattersall MHN, Thomas H. Recent advances: Oncology. Br Med J 1999; 318: 445–448.

Taylor S. Health psychology, 4th edn. New York: Randon House; 1999.

Thomson R. Loving medicine. Bath: Gateway Books; 1989.

Topping A. The scope of cancer surgery. In: David J, ed. Cancer care: prevention, treatment and palliation. London: Chapman and Hall; 1995, 146–173.

Wallston KA, Wallston BS. Who is responsible for your health? The construct of health locus of control. In: Sanders GS, Suls J, eds. Social psychology of health and illness. New Jersey: Erlbaum; 1982.

Weinberg RA. One renegade cell. London: Weidenfeld and Nicolson; 1998.

Wilson J, Jungner G. Public Health Paper no 34. Geneva: World Health Organization; 1968.

34 Nursing patients who need palliative care

Denise Quinton

'I've enjoyed most aspects of nursing but I feel I want to know more about supporting patients and their families when there's no chance of a cure. I've seen the difference that the palliative care team can make – you need a lot of knowledge and specialist skills to do that.'

(Staff nurse)

THIS CHAPTER WILL HELP YOU

- Discuss the development of palliative care, the settings and types of patients
- Recognize common emotional responses to a terminal diagnosis
- Identify support systems for people involved with palliative care
- Discuss associated ethical issues
- Assess a patient needing palliative care and plan care
- Identify the role of specialist nurses
- Discuss common palliative care emergencies
- Identify the variety of cultural and spiritual needs in palliative care
- Identify the care needs of patients close to death
- Identify information and help required by relatives after the death
- Suggest how health care professionals may obtain support.

KEYWORDS

Anticipatory grief
Bereavement
Ethics
Holistic care
Hospice
Multidisciplinary team
Palliative care
Symptom control
Terminal care

INTRODUCTION

Nursing patients with life-threatening illnesses can be very emotional. At some stage in your nursing career, you will meet someone who has been told that he or she is dying. This will be a very difficult time for the patient and the staff. This chapter will look at the holistic care of palliative patients, their families and friends. This will include the physical, psychosocial, spiritual and emotional care of everyone involved. It will be related to other chapters, including those dealing with communication (Ch. 3), pain (Ch. 7) and patients with cancer (Ch. 33), and others dealing with disease processes.

This chapter will help you to think about how to care for palliative patients and their families.

CONCEPTS OF PALLIATIVE CARE

HISTORICAL BACKGROUND

In medieval Europe, death was a familiar concept to most individuals and was accepted as a part of life. The life expectancy in England at the time was around 33 years; of course, nowadays, most people can expect to reach retirement age and well beyond. Perhaps this is why feelings about death and the dying have undergone considerable change in the 20th century, and death has even become a taboo subject in some cultures.

During the 19th century death began to become medicalized; people began going to hospital to die. Consequently, because medicine was about cure, death came to represent failure. Hence curative care was to become the dominant theme of modern health care.

THE DEVELOPMENT OF PALLIATIVE CARE IN THE 20TH CENTURY

Despite the care offered by health professionals in hospitals during the first half of the 20th century, the experience of many users highlighted an overall failure to provide patients with the holistic care required to meet their needs. The social climate gradually changed, however, and led during the 1950s and 1960s to the modern hospice movement and the establishment of specialist nurse practitioners such as Macmillan nurses. These new concepts have changed attitudes towards dying patients, their families and the bereaved.

Palliative medicine and care have became a specialty. In 1990, the World Health Organization (WHO) produced the following definition: 'The active total care of patients whose disease is not responsive to curative treatment. Control of pain, of other symptoms, and of psychological, social and spiritual problems is paramount. The goal of palliative care is achievement of the best quality of life for patients and their families.'

This definition was extended to state that palliative care:

- affirms life and regards dying as a normal process
- neither hastens nor postpones death
- provides relief from pain and other distressing physical symptoms
- integrates the psychological and spiritual aspects of care
- offers a support system to help patients live as actively as possible until death
- offers a support system to help families cope during patients' illnesses and in their bereavement.

It is clear from the above definition that palliative care is not just about cancer. Care is now increasingly being provided for people who have any life-threatening illness, such as acquired immune deficiency syndrome (AIDS), multiple sclerosis and chronic respiratory disease.

THE CARE TEAM

Successful palliative care needs to be delivered within a multidisciplinary framework. It is unrealistic to expect one professional group to provide the holistic care needed by patients and families (Fig. 34.1).

Care is both patient- and family-centred. It should be them, not the professionals, who decide the priorities. This can only be achieved by involving patients and families in decision-making and care. It is therefore important that these parties have the information required for decision-making.

Effective palliative care should be undertaken in every area where people might die, e.g. the residential home, at home, the hospital or the hospice. To achieve this, there has been a gradual development of specialist health care professionals, including hospital and community clinical nurse specialists, doctors specializing in palliative care, and the education of general nurses through specialist courses.

Palliative care is appropriate from the moment it is clear that treatment will be palliative until death. It involves the holistic care of patients and families, and keeps them informed, so that they might decide where to die. The number of people able to be nursed at home with their family and friends is increasing. Specialized care continues after the patient's death until the bereaved family members have started the recovery process.

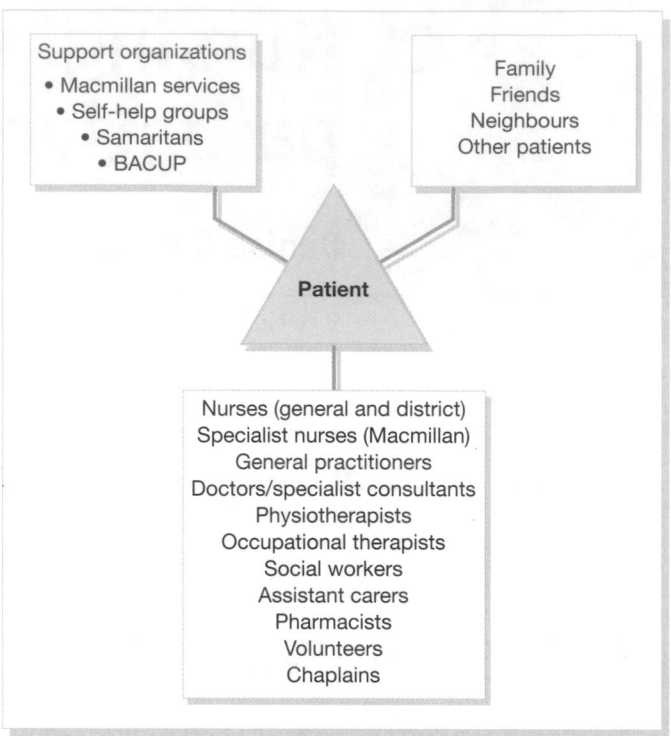

Figure 34.1 The multidisciplinary team involved in caring for the palliative patient.

SETTINGS FOR PALLIATIVE CARE

Palliative care offers a unique combination of support in hospices, hospitals, day centres and at home, each providing for the individual needs of the patient and family.

HOSPICES

In the Middle Ages, a hospice was a place offering hospitality to pilgrims and travellers. They were not associated with the dying until 1876, when the Irish Sisters of Charity opened Our Lady's Hospice to care for such patients, followed 16 years later by St Joseph's in Hackney.

The modern hospice movement really began in the UK during the 1950s and 1960s with two developments: the establishment of the Marie Curie Foundation, and the building of St Christopher's in Sydenham by Dame Cicely Saunders. The central hospice idea combined deeply rooted spirituality with an emphasis on expert medical care, skilled confident nursing and the experienced use of drugs. Dame Cicely Saunders developed the idea of the patient as a family unit and not as an individual.

From this initial movement, the philosophy of hospice care has developed to include control of pain, alleviating symptoms and supporting patients and their families, enabling patients to enjoy an improved quality of life.

The hospice has developed specifically to care for palliative patients and their families. Hospices are not, however, just a place to die, as patients may be admitted for symptom control or to give respite to families before returning home. Some hospices

EVIDENCE-BASED PRACTICE

34.1 Complementary therapies: aromatherapy and massage

The use of touch to relieve discomfort is probably one of the most instinctive therapies in existence. This is perhaps why there has been an increase in the use of complementary therapies such as aromatherapy and massage in palliative care. Practitioners have reported psychological, emotional and physical benefits for patients, relatives and staff.

Vickers (1996) states that complementary medicine appears to be particularly widely used in palliative care. A study conducted in 1992 found that about 70% of UK hospices offer massage and aromatherapy services:

- Massage appears to be of benefit for anxiety, by producing feelings of relaxation, calmness and well-being.
- Practitioners of aromatherapy use aromatic substances extracted from plants. Aromatherapy patients showed a consistent fall in anxiety levels.
- Vickers also discusses the use of acupuncture with pain and nausea.

There are some practitioners who feel that complementary therapies are unorthodox. Trevelyan & Booth (1993) report that complementary therapies have an enormous popularity in the UK. Two schools of thought exist: those of the vitalists and those of the mechanists. The vitalists argue that psychological, physical or spiritual forces are responsible for disease and these forces must be invoked if a patient is to recover. The mechanists, on the other hand, seek a physical cause for illness and will suggest a physical treatment to remedy it. Complementary medicine operates primarily within the vitalist area. The authors investigate the bad press about complementary medicine and how it has failed to satisfy critics. If complementary medicine is to survive in the 21st century, much-needed research evidence that it is effective will be required.

References

Trevelyan J, Booth B. Fringe benefits. Nurs Times 1993; 89(17): 30–33.

Vickers A. Complementary therapies in palliative care. Eur J Pall Care 1996; 3(4): 150–153.

---

have home-support teams which allows continuity of care. In specialist hospices, the ratio of nursing staff to patients is high, and the staff usually have a special interest in palliative care. Hospices can have a varied range of nursing and medical expertise, as well as other members of the multidisciplinary team. Specialties include complementary therapies, bereavement support and specialist nurses (see Evidence-based Practice box 34.1).

Advantages of hospice care

The advantages of hospice care include:

- specialize in palliative care
- provide expertise for difficult problems
- provide a 'seamless' multi-agency service, through partnership with the NHS.

Disadvantages of hospice care

Some disadvantages include:

- may be seen as a place to die
- pressure on places may restrict length of stay
- few diagnostic facilities
- continuity of care can be difficult, without a home-support team
- need to secure funding.

HOSPITALS

Most hospital wards are busy, containing patients who require different philosophies of care. This can make supportive and specialist care difficult to achieve. The facilities can be inadequate, with little or no privacy for the patient or family.

Some hospitals still lack dedicated palliative care services. However, they can provide nursing, medical and surgical expertise, and are able to admit patients 24 hours a day (Evidence-based Practice box 34.2).

Patients who may benefit from hospital admission include those requiring:

- active treatment
- radiotherapy for symptom control
- palliative procedures, e.g. stent insertion for dysphagia
- further investigations.

Around half of the deaths in palliative care occur in hospitals. This has led to the development of consultant-led palliative care teams or specialist nursing teams in some hospitals and sometimes dedicated palliative care beds. The presence of specialist hospital palliative care nurses ensures a better understanding of the specific issues concerning palliative patients. Their role is collaboration with hospital staff in order to enhance the service offered to the patient and families. They also provide advice, support and education for other staff. These developments in hospital-based services improve the palliative care offered to patients and families.

DAY CENTRES

Day care is of particular value for patients not yet ill enough for admission, but who need more than community care support. It offers a complementary service to the hospital, hospice or home. They operate on weekdays and patients visit 1 or 2 days per week, giving their relatives or carers a break.

Day centres provide support by peers, nursing and medical staff. Patients can feel isolated with their disease and these

EVIDENCE-BASED PRACTICE

34.2 Hospice or hospital for palliative care

There are various settings for nursing the palliative care patient and family. All have advantages and disadvantages. Jackman & Millard (1995) state that the goal of palliative care is to achieve the best quality of life for patients and their families. Where people die is clearly not the same as where they are cared for during their last illness. The majority of people with cancer die in hospital – this, despite a widely held professional view that acute hospital wards are poorly equipped for the care of the dying. The authors discuss the advantages and disadvantages of palliative care in the home, hospice and hospital.

In a study of the care of dying patients in general hospitals, Mills et al (1994) concluded that for many, the care observed was poor. There is a need to identify and implement practical steps to facilitate high-quality care of the dying. Much can be learnt from the hospice movement, but such knowledge and skills must be replicated in all settings.

McDonnell (1989), who compared perceptions of patients before and after admission to a hospice, concluded that prior to admission, over half the patients were unaware where they were going. Once admitted the patients' focus seemed to change. They no longer dwelt on their physical distress and fears for the future, but seemed content to discuss short-term plans. Was this because the patients found themselves in a system of care that was person-orientated rather than disease-orientated? An environment must be created in which the dying are heard, because it is only in listening that we can know and learn.

References

Jackman J, Millard P. Care for the dying. Geriatr Med 1995; January: 39–41.

Mills M, Davies HTO, Macrae WA. Care of dying patients in hospital. Br Med J 1994; 309: 583–586.

McDonnell MM. Patients' perceptions of their care at Our Lady's Hospice, Dublin. Pall Med 1989; 3: 47–53.

OLDER ADULTS: NURSING PRIORITIES

34.1 Patient and carer

There are extra problems associated with nursing an older adult at home when the only family carer is old and infirm. Nursing assessment will need to include the carer's ability to manage and the factors likely to influence this ability, which may include the following:

- Weakness and lack of mobility, e.g. due to arthritis, may make it difficult for them to manage stairs, shop and prepare food.
- Cognitive ability, e.g. confusion, may affect ability to cope with medication.
- Sensory defects, e.g. visual impairment, may affect safety.

Specific nursing action may include:

- referrals to other health or social care professionals, e.g. occupational therapist for assessment, provision of aids, moving bed downstairs; and social services for meals on wheels/frozen foods, help with personal care, shopping and cleaning
- district nurse for help with general care, provision of 7-day medicine dispenser, provision of night sitters
- respite care
- support and explanation
- check benefit entitlement.

HOME CARE

As the development of palliative care and hospices has evolved, so has community care. Townsend et al (1990) found that most people, when given the choice, would prefer to die at home. Home is more peaceful and relaxed, and patients have loved ones and their own belongings around them.

The practicalities of nursing palliative patients at home until death will differ according to the availability of resources and the quality of the professionals involved. Nursing patients in their own home requires a very different approach from that needed in hospital or in a hospice, as the patient remains in control of the surroundings. For a patient to be nursed at home, the environment has to be correct and they need support from the multidisciplinary team and family and friends. Communication is essential if the team is to provide quality care for patients and their families at home; everyone must be aware of what is happening and be able to anticipate problems. Remaining at home might not be practical or possible for some patients. The team, including the patient concerned, should discuss the situation and consider the alternatives (see, for example, Older Adults: Nursing Priorities box 34.1).

General practitioners

General practitioners (GPs) ensure continuity of care by coordinating the team. They are aware of the patient's history and know the family. They are available both in the surgery and for home visits. The GP is not always available so it is essential to have good communication to make sure that locum doctors

centres provide opportunities to meet other patients and professionals, who can offer advice and reassurance, promote confidence and provide an opportunity to talk about problems. Day centres run programmes of diversional therapy, with activities as diverse as art, gardening and relaxation techniques.

The nursing needs of the patient can be met, and referrals made to members of the multidisciplinary team, e.g. the physiotherapist. The general condition of the patient can be assessed at each visit and the need for additional services identified. Some day centres have doctors who provide outpatient services where symptoms can be reviewed and treated.

Day care is a rapidly developing service for palliative care patients. It provides support for patients whilst at home and can help to improve their quality of life. However, most importantly, it allows patients to remain at home.

and GP cooperatives are fully aware of the needs of the patient and family.

District nurses

District nurses coordinate nursing care, assessment and provision of equipment, such as pressure-relieving devices and commodes. They assist with general care and support the patient and family.

Macmillan nurses

The Macmillan Fund was founded in 1911 to improve the quality of life for people with cancer and their families. The fund provides nurses, cancer care units, grants, medical support and education programmes, and finances for other charities.

The clinical nurse specialists (Macmillan nurses) are experienced practitioners skilled in palliative care. They offer advice and support to colleagues. By visiting patients and families at home, they can assess them and suggest alternatives to treatment. Support is from referral, by GPs, nurses (community, hospital, hospice) and the family. Normally, support continues throughout a patient's illness and a Macmillan nurse will provide bereavement support for the family after the patient dies.

Marie Curie organization

The Marie Curie organization was established in 1948. They provide centres for patient care and advice, research centres, education departments and a community nursing service. Marie Curie nurses provide a complementary service to the district nurses. They can also provide night sitters, which helps by allowing the family to sleep.

Occupational therapists

Occupational therapists perform home assessments. They can offer practical advice on moving rooms and furniture for safety and easier assess, e.g. moving the bed downstairs or fitting handrails in the lavatory. Such assessment and the provision of aids allow patients to remain independent for as long as possible.

Social workers

Social workers assess the home situation and provide extra help as available and required, e.g. help with personal care. They can ascertain whether patients and their families are receiving their correct benefit entitlement (see p. 1031).

Family

Family members are an important part of the team. They often provide 24-hour care for their loved one and they need support in their caring and emotional role. This can be facilitated by providing information about and contact numbers for specialist nurses and help lines. Time should be allocated for them to discuss their fears and worries.

EMOTIONAL RESPONSES TO TERMINAL ILLNESS

The diagnosis of a terminal illness affects the emotions in many ways and no two patients will have the same emotional response, even where the physical condition is similar.

Many palliative patients, especially those with cancer, will have already come to terms with having a life-threatening illness and all the emotions this provokes. To be told that their illness is now terminal, however, will cause further emotional responses.

Telling patients something unpleasant is never easy, but the way it is told can help the patient and family to cope (Ch. 3). The environment in which the news is delivered, as well as the manner, are important. It should be in private, quiet surroundings, with a gentle approach and manner. The choice of words is crucial, as it is often the first words that are remembered by patients. It is essential to discover what patients know; often they understand the situation and only need confirmation. Those involved should know that the patient is dying, so communication can be honest. In these circumstances, honesty is the best policy with the consequence that hope is not destroyed. Feelings of hope can be re-focused from obtaining a cure to concentrating on the notion that life can be lived to the full in whatever time is left. Where communication is not open and honest, there can be detrimental consequences for family relationships. Everyone needs to be aware of what is happening, since individuals guide their talk and actions according to who knows what and with what certainty.

Glaser & Strauss (1965), in their study of interactions with terminally ill patients, identified four awareness contexts. These refer to the differing levels of awareness about the patient's impending death which may exist between the patient and other individuals:

- *closed awareness* – patients do not recognize that death is impending, although everyone else does
- *suspected awareness* – patients suspect what others know and therefore attempt to confirm or validate their suspicions
- *mutual pretence awareness* – everyone, including the patient, is aware that death is impending, but each pretends to the other that they do not know
- *open awareness* – everyone, including the patient, is aware that death is impending and acts on this knowledge relatively openly.

STAGES OF THE EMOTIONAL RESPONSE

The emotional experience of the patient and family starts from the moment they suspect something is wrong and continues throughout the illness and after the patient's death. Their response to the situation usually covers several stages through which they progress. Responses are very individualized, but Kubler-Ross (1970) proposed the following five stages: denial, anger, bargaining, depression and acceptance. In addition, many people experience fear.

Denial

Denial is a common defence mechanism when patients and families realize the seriousness of their disease. There are various stages of denial, ranging from acknowledging the illness but playing down its seriousness, to a more extreme and sustained form of believing that the illness is not terminal. The extreme form is undesirable as it can lead to communication problems between everyone, and a patient's failure to put practical affairs in order prior to death. Denial may be suspected when patients do not ask questions about their illness despite being given ample opportunity.

Management of denial can involve two approaches:

- collusion – acceptance of the self-deception
- confrontation – challenging feelings and beliefs with the truth.

Fear

Feelings of fear can include anxiety about the unknown, the manner of dying, losing control, pain, being a burden and losing independence. These feelings can hopefully be reduced through communication and explanation, so that patients understand how they will feel and what will happen.

Anger

Anger is a powerful emotion and can be directed at anyone and everyone. It can be a difficult response for the multidisciplinary team to handle. The person who is experiencing anger should be given time and opportunity to vent these feelings. Nurses should listen without responding defensively.

Bargaining

This relates to a feeling that somehow a bargain will prevent the inevitability of death. People feel that if they fulfil their side of the bargain, all will be well; for example, they may say that they will stop smoking if they are spared.

Despair and depression

Despair arises from the loss of hope, leading to sadness. Reassurance and acknowledgement that this is a normal process will hopefully communicate to patients that they are still important. Patients can alter their goals from large ones to small ones, creating aims that it is possible to achieve. Despair and sadness may lead to depression, which is characterized by low mood, fearfulness, the feeling of being a burden, agitation, apathy, social withdrawal, anorexia, weight loss, insomnia, tiredness and pain. Diagnosis of depression can be difficult as many symptoms are also those of advanced cancer. Depressed or unhappy people should be given the opportunity to express their feelings. Depression can be treated with antidepressant drugs, which should be prescribed if depressive illness is suspected (see p. 1039).

Acceptance

Acceptance is the final stage – those who reach it essentially come to terms with what is happening. Along with all these feelings, relatives may experience a phenomenon known as 'anticipatory grief' (Smith 1995). During a terminal illness, the realization that death is imminent dawns on the family as the patient's condition deteriorates. They actually start the grieving process before their loved one has died. This can be something as simple as anticipating what life will be like without the person. It can be considered insensitive, but it is part of the normal adjustment to impending loss.

Prolonged anticipatory grief can be a problem when relatives withdraw, already anticipating the hurt and loss they will feel. This can upset the dying person and result in communication

problems. This period of time is terribly important as it provides opportunities to put right personal and business matters, including making a will, arranging the funeral and expressing feelings.

Hampe (1975) identified the important needs felt by spouses experiencing the stages of anticipatory grief, including:

- to be with and help the dying patient
- to be assured of the comfort of the dying patient
- to be informed of their partner's condition and impending death
- to express emotions
- acceptance, support and comfort from health care professionals and family members.

These needs can be achieved by keeping the relatives informed of what is happening. This preparation for death can be a learning experience for the patient and relatives, as it will hopefully open up communication. Grieving for someone before he or she has died cannot and does not exempt the survivors from all sadness in advance, but it can start the process of relinquishing their loved one.

EMOTIONAL SUPPORT FOR ALL THOSE INVOLVED

Everyone has to die, but with diseases that require palliative care there is usually time for the family members to prepare themselves. Although the dying patient is the centre of palliative care, health care professionals must remember that family and friends will also need emotional support to cope during this stressful time.

Nursing the dying patient and supporting family and friends are stressful occupations for health care professionals. This is especially so in hospices and in the community where the care of these families is continuous. Nurses must therefore be aware of their own emotional responses in order to continue their supportive role.

SUPPORTING THE FAMILY

Support given to the family is support given to the patient. This is important where the family spends long periods of time being with, and caring for, the patient. Many feel that they have to put on a brave face to protect the patient from their distress.

Needs of relatives

Relatives need regular information about the patient's condition and medication changes. There needs to be good liaison among members of the care team and good communication with the patient and family.

Family members may feel the need to be with the patient for as long as, and whenever, they wish. In hospices this is not normally a problem as there is usually open visiting. It can be a problem in hospital with restricted visiting. This is usually relaxed when patients are dying. Unrestricted visiting can, however, create pressure on the family to be with the person for long periods, causing them to become stressed and overtired. Nurses need to be aware of this potential problem.

Relatives may want to care for the dying patient. Nurses need to ascertain how much care they want to give and then support them in this.

The family and friends need encouragement and opportunities to express emotions with one another or with the staff. In hospitals and hospices, health care professionals and counsellors can provide support and help relatives to work through their feelings. Families can be encouraged to support one another, but this may not be possible where relationships are strained. The presence of health care professionals can be helpful. Not everyone wants to talk, but a presence can be comforting.

The feelings experienced by relatives can be exactly the same as those of the dying patient, but not necessarily at the same time. Additionally they may experience anxiety, depression and feelings of guilt because they are well or feel cross with the patient. It is important to help them understand that these feelings are normal.

Caring for the dying person at home can be particularly stressful and the family might feel unable to cope. However devoted and competent, they should not be expected to cope single-handed. The multidisciplinary team can provide practical help and support (see p. 1022). Day centres and in-patient respite care can be beneficial to the carer by providing a break from caring.

SUPPORTING HEALTH CARE PROFESSIONALS

Providing support to the dying patient, family and friends can take its toll on health care professionals. To work effectively they must develop a close and facilitating relationship in which patients and families feel able to express, explore and share their feelings. Inevitably health care professionals are exposed to the distress felt by patients and families. This is part of their everyday life, but continual exposure can be damaging. Unfortunately this can lead to stress and, without adequate coping strategies, health care professionals are at risk of developing health-related problems (Ch. 6).

Health care professionals may exhibit stress in a variety of ways and people have different tolerances to stressful situations. Stress might present as irritability, depression, poor self-esteem, over-involvement in work, sleep disturbance, weight changes, headaches and minor illnesses resulting in time off work. Stress can affect their private life, causing marital or family problems and excessive social activity or misuse of alcohol. Failure to deal with stress can eventually lead to breakdown or burnout. All nurses have a responsibility to notice if the health or safety of colleagues is being adversely affected, which in turn could put patients at risk (see Code of Professional Conduct, clause 8.2, NMC 2002).

Support for the heath care professional is vital and can be achieved by:

- self-monitoring for signs of stress
- talking to colleagues, which is a major source of support for many professionals – this may be on a one-to-one basis or in a group; ideally time is made for reflection
- a relaxed working environment – humour can be part of stress management
- individual counselling, where stress remains a problem – such help should be confidential and health care professionals must not be made to feel guilty if they need help.

There are many organizations offering support to patients, relatives and health care professionals from the time of diagnosis to death. Some organizations are discussed in the section on 'Follow-up support and counselling' (see p. 1043).

ETHICAL ISSUES IN PALLIATIVE CARE

There are many ethical issues in palliative care, including those of informed consent, advance directives, withholding information, feeding, rehydration and euthanasia. Some of these challenging issues are discussed below.

ADVANCE DIRECTIVES

Developments in medical science create dilemmas. New drugs and treatments mean that lives previously lost to disease are now sustainable for indefinite periods of time. Advance directives (living wills), in which people state their wishes in relation to medical treatment and intervention at the end of their lives, will impact on nursing care. They focus on patients being allowed to die rather than being kept alive artificially, but still receiving drugs to relieve pain and distress, even if death is hastened.

An advance directive may be recorded in any form. It can be handwritten and signed by individuals, indicating that this is their choice. There are some advance directives that include a proxy clause, which names a person who will act on the patient's behalf if he or she becomes unconscious or incompetent.

Nurses are increasingly acting as advocates for patients (Ch. 3). They must ensure that patients have all the information required to make decisions. Nurses **must not** be involved in drawing up or witnessing an advance directive, as this can detract from their professional impartiality. Advance directives can help nurses to discuss what individual patients wanted when they are no longer able to do so for themselves (Cowe 1996). The document is legally binding where it takes the form of an advance refusal and the maker is competent at the time of making.

Voluntary groups such as the Voluntary Euthanasia Society provide information and are active in supporting advance directives (see Ethical Issues box 34.1).

ETHICAL ISSUES

34.1 Withdrawing treatment

There are various forms of euthanasia. One type involves withdrawing life-prolonging treatment.

- What are your views on withdrawing treatment in palliative care?
- Do you think advance directives have a role to play in palliative care?

Student activities
Find out what is contained in an advance directive.

ETHICAL ISSUES

34.2 'No more treatment please'

A palliative care patient tells you that she does not want any treatment that prolongs her life. Her condition deteriorates, and the family want intravenous fluids to be commenced as she can no longer drink.

- What ethical issues arise in this situation?
- What do you think the care team should do?

TERMINAL DEHYDRATION AND REHYDRATION

Dehydration is commonly experienced by terminally ill patients. The most frequently observed symptoms are thirst and a dry mouth (Patchett 1998). There is no correct answer as to whether to treat dehydration or not; it must be decided for each individual situation by the patient, relatives and multidisciplinary team.

Reasons for rehydration include increasing alertness and sense of well-being, as fluid and electrolyte imbalance is corrected. Dehydration can be distressing for the patient and for the family fearing that their loved one is thirsty. Where dehydration is due to a reversible condition such as hypercalcaemia (high blood calcium level), hydration should be commenced (see Ethical Issues box 34.2).

Reasons for not rehydrating include the fact that dehydration is a normal part of dying. As patients weaken, they become unable to take fluids. There is no clear evidence that rehydration affects comfort, mental state or survival. Symptoms can be minimized by effective mouth care. Dehydration also reduces gastric and respiratory secretions which may lessen nausea and vomiting, and noisy breathing. Moreover, rehydration may give false hope to the family.

Individual patients should be assessed according to their needs and wishes. Health care professionals should educate the patient and family so they can make informed decisions.

NUTRITIONAL SUPPORT

Nutritional support of dying patients is just as controversial as rehydration. As their condition deteriorates, they become too frail to eat. Many patients exhibit signs of weakness, anorexia and cachexia (extreme emaciation), but this is natural disease progression.

Nutritional support may be administered orally, through a nasogastric tube or gastrostomy tube or via intravenous total parenteral nutrition (Ch. 11). Although palliative patients appear malnourished, there is no evidence to suggest that treatment corrects metabolic abnormalities. Tumour growth may actually be accelerated, thereby increasing the symptoms of cancer (Dunlop et al 1995).

Providing nutritional support may be advisable for some patients who have dysphagia, e.g. patients with oesophageal cancer (Ch. 22), head and neck cancer and motor neurone disease (Ch. 14).

Starting or discontinuing nutritional support must be discussed with all concerned, but where possible it must be the patient's choice. There have been test cases where courts in England and Scotland have ruled on the withdrawal of life-supporting medical treatment, including nutrition and hydration. The first was in 1993 when the House of Lords ruled that doctors could lawfully withhold medical treatment in the case of a patient in a persistent vegetative state.

EUTHANASIA

Euthanasia, when translated literally, means 'good death'. It is only recently that it has come to mean 'the deliberate killing of someone by a fatal intervention'. There are different forms of euthanasia (Ellis 1991); it may be voluntary, involuntary, non-voluntary, active (e.g. by drug administration) or passive (where treatment is withdrawn or not commenced).

The topic of euthanasia is a matter for worldwide debate. Some countries allow euthanasia under strict control. For example, in 1993 the Dutch government approved euthanasia guidelines which, if followed by a doctor, allow immunity from prosecution. In 1995 the Northern Territory of Australia became the first place in the world to legalize euthanasia, but this was subsequently challenged and overturned. Debate continues in the UK where euthanasia remains illegal.

NURSING ASSESSMENT

Assessment is a vital stage of the nursing process. It is the basis for all the other stages and without an accurate assessment, nurses are unable to plan the high-quality, individualized care (Crossfield 1989) to which every patient is entitled.

The purpose of assessment, especially in palliative care, is to establish trust in the nurse–patient relationship and to assess the needs and problems of the patient and family.

During the initial assessment, a great deal of information is obtained from the patient and family. This involves communication skills (Ch. 3), observation and examination. If patients are unwell, it may be necessary to obtain the relevant information from relatives. Assessment is an ongoing process as problems and needs change. Furthermore, what nurses might perceive to be a problem initially might not be considered as such by patients. It is important to remember that some problems are unconnected with their terminal illness, e.g. arthritic joint pains. In palliative care, assessing patients during the first 48 hours can be helpful, after which a care plan is written.

AREAS FOR ASSESSMENT

Breathing

There are many causes of breathlessness, e.g. tumour, pulmonary disease (Ch. 20) and anaemia. An individual assessment is required; some may have a few hours to live and others months. Investigating the cause in a patient with hours to live may detract from alleviating distressing symptoms.

Where appropriate, a detailed history of breathlessness and other problems is obtained. This includes whether it occurs at rest or exertion, and what, if anything, helps, e.g. sitting upright in bed or an armchair.

Examination of the chest may detect problems, such as infection. A chest X-ray can be performed if appropriate and sputum specimens may confirm infection. Blood samples should be obtained for full blood count to check for anaemia. Feelings of fear and anxiety should be investigated as these may exacerbate breathlessness.

The colour of the skin, nail beds and lips should be observed for cyanosis (pale grey-blue colour with blue lips), a sign of hypoxia. If the patient is close to death, there may be some respiratory sounds as secretions fill the trachea (death-rattle).

Oral assessment

An oral assessment should be performed on admission to identify problems and plan care. Where the oral condition is poor, further assessment should be performed daily to detect changes. The following areas should be assessed:

- voice
- swallowing
- lips, mucous membranes, tongue and gingiva
- amount and consistency of saliva
- teeth or dentures (or denture-bearing areas).

Assessment may identify poor hygiene, dehydration, infection, drug side-effects or low platelet counts.

Eating and drinking

Assessment of all aspects of eating and drinking and associated problems (see Ch. 11) is required, and includes:

- changes in appetite or eating pattern
- taste changes, such as a metallic taste
- foods causing indigestion and other upsets
- food preferences
- what help is needed with eating and drinking
- nausea and vomiting
- weight change – loose clothing or tight around the abdomen with ascites. Weighing patients with cachexia may not always be appropriate.

Skin condition and hygiene needs

An assessment of pressure areas and general skin condition is undertaken on admission. The risk of developing a pressure ulcer is assessed using an appropriate risk scale (Ch. 10). The Waterlow (1985) risk scale is well suited to palliative care as it assesses appetite, skin type, weight and special risks such as terminal cachexia, anaemia, paraplegia and medication.

Further assessment should take place at regular intervals and when the patient's condition changes. Identification of patients at risk ensures the appropriate use of resources. Where pressure ulcers are present, their location, stage or grade should be documented and reassessed at each dressing change for signs of change.

Hygiene needs should be assessed, including the level of self-care and the amount of assistance required. Personal preferences are ascertained, e.g. baths or showers. Assisting with hygiene needs provides opportunities to assess the general skin condition. This should include the colour (pallor, redness, jaundice or cyanosis), swelling, dryness, sweating, scratch marks, bruising and weight loss (Chs 10 and 28).

Elimination

Assessment of elimination involves both voiding urine and bowel function (Chs 12, 22 and 24).

Voiding

- Normal voiding pattern and changes
- Presence of frequency, dysuria or hesitancy
- Observation and testing of the urine for abnormal contents, including microbiological examination
- Urinary continence problems
- Whether assistance is needed to get to the lavatory, or whether a commode or urinal is more appropriate.

Bowel function

- Normal bowel function
- Stool bulk and consistency – constipation (see p. 1037) or diarrhoea may be caused by drugs, anxiety, infection and impaction; a stool sample may be required
- Pain, discomfort or bleeding on defaecation
- Faecal incontinence may indicate impaction with spurious diarrhoea
- Presence of a stoma (colostomy, ileostomy) and degree of self-caring and help needed (Ch. 22). Usual routine for stoma hygiene
- Monitor and document bowel function daily.

Mobility, activity and leisure

Assessment includes:

- degree of weakness
- previous occupational therapy and physiotherapy assessments
- difficulty in walking – unaided or use of frame or wheelchair
- ability to climb stairs
- ability to stand and weight-bear
- moving and handling aids in use, such as a hoist
- hobbies, interests and ways of relaxing
- day centre attendance.

Pain

Pain assessment tools (Ch. 7) are useful within the palliative care setting. A pain assessment tool (Fig. 34.2) may include:

- a pain scale, e.g. 0–4 with 0 = no pain and 4 = unbearable pain
- outlines of the body where the patient marks the location of pain
- a key that indicates different types of pain
- what eases pain, or makes it worse.

Additionally the nurse will need to assess:

- non-verbal signs of pain, such as facial expression, posture or rapid breathing
- whether pain disturbs sleep (see Ch. 4).
- previous use and efficacy of analgesia and other pain relief measures (to provide a baseline).

The pain and treatment efficacy must be evaluated regularly with each administration of analgesia and any exacerbation of

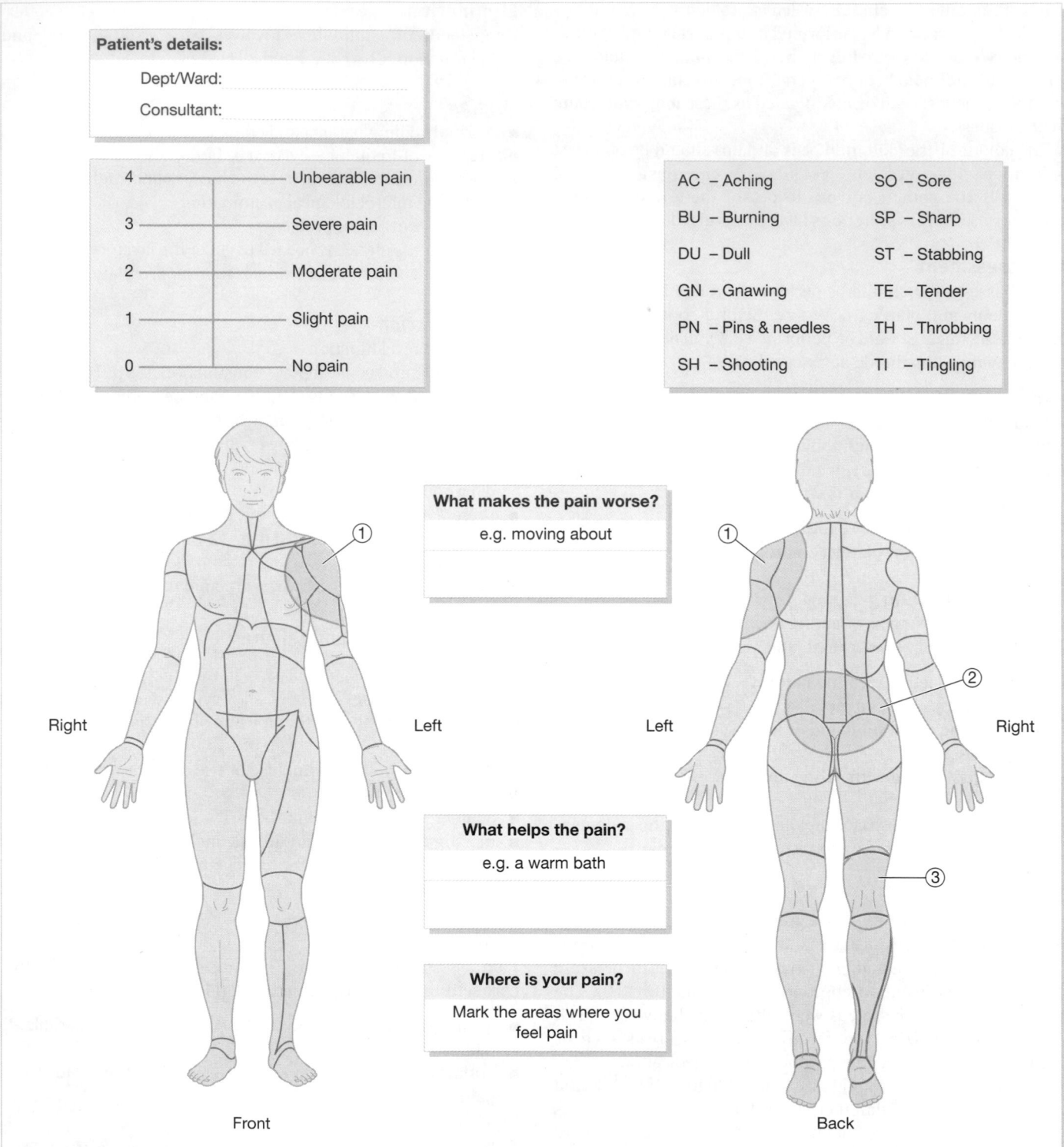

Figure 34.2 Pain assessment tool.

pain. Information including date, time, site and type of pain, pain score and the patient's comments is recorded. Action taken, which may include analgesia or non-pharmacological measures, is also documented. The efficacy of the action should be reviewed 30–60 minutes later.

Sleep

It is important to know the normal sleeping pattern. Patients might sleep for a few hours at night with an afternoon nap, or may sleep all night. Where sleeping tablets have been required at home, it is important that the drug is prescribed during in-patient admissions. Others may settle with a milky or alcoholic drink – health care professionals must weigh the risk of drug interactions with the wishes of a terminally ill patient. The position the patient adopts for sleep is important. Patients with breathing problems usually sleep upright, well supported with pillows. Those too weak to move in bed will require position changes during the night. Some patients sleep in the dark, while others might need a light.

Understanding of illness and self-image

This includes the reaction to admission, e.g. to a hospice. Lack of knowledge about the aims of a hospice can cause anxiety. Where this occurs, the nurse can take the opportunity to allay any fears. It is also important to find out what the patient and family understand about the illness and how they see the future. This provides them with a chance to discuss any problems or anxieties. Knowing what patients know gives health care professionals a baseline from which to work. At first, patients might not talk about their illness, and what they understand is unknown. Later, as relationships develop and patients and their families become more settled, they might start to talk.

Self-image is important. Some patients may not want to undress in front of others or look in a mirror because they dislike their appearance. They may feel that a scar is ugly or be embarrassed by drug-induced hair loss.

Communication, mood and behaviour

It is important to ascertain whether patients and family members understand what is being said to them, e.g. there may a language barrier.

The identification of sensory deficits is vital. Where these exist, the nurse ascertains how patients overcome communication problems. A hearing-impaired person may communicate by sign language (Ch. 16).

Assessing speech is important – people who have had a stroke or who have multiple sclerosis may have slurred speech, making communication difficult. It can take time and good listening skills to understand what patients are trying to say (Ch. 3).

Patients may be confused, which might make it difficult to decipher what they want to say. This may be exacerbated by anxiety and observation of body language may provide clues. Another problem may be poor concentration due to fear, pain or depression (see section on 'Nursing management' below).

Assessing family needs – social and financial

The assessment process gives the health care professional and the family a chance to talk about the situation at home and includes:

- which family members are involved in the care
- input from district nurses and Macmillan nurses
- input from social service carers
- other services – volunteer sitters and respite care
- whether the family are receiving their benefit entitlement.

It is important for health care professionals and social services to cooperate in reducing the number of assessments. This can be achieved by introducing joint multi-agency assessments.

Financial problems can be extremely worrying, especially if the sick person normally supported the household. Relatives may take unpaid leave or even stop working to care for the dying person. There are, however, several benefits to which they may be entitled.

Benefits change from time to time and clarification of entitlement should be sought from the Benefits Agency, Citizens' Advice Bureau or a welfare benefits officer. Claims involving terminally ill people are processed quickly. Benefits include:

- attendance allowance for people aged over 65 years who need help with personal care
- disability living allowance for people aged 16–65 years who need help with personal care and mobility
- invalid care allowance for people aged 16–65 years who spend at least 35 hours a week looking after a person who has claimed or is receiving disability living allowance (certain levels) or attendance allowance.

In addition to state provision, there are grants available from charities, e.g. Marie Curie Welfare Grant Scheme, the Macmillan Fund and charities that assist ex-service people and their families.

Assessing spiritual needs

The provision of holistic care requires that nurses assess and understand the spiritual needs of the patient and family. Stoter (1995) developed a framework for the assessment of spiritual need, which involves:

- patients' self-concept
- their perception of what is happening to them
- their hopes, fears and natural support mechanisms
- the strength and nature of support from family and friends
- the relationships within the family
- patients' views and beliefs in relation to their situation
- their stated religion and/or commitment to religious practice, e.g. special requirements for religious practices
- their cultural background, e.g. special books or food
- their life experience
- assessing their natural defence and coping mechanisms
- their openness and receptivity to help
- assessing their general state of health
- assessing mental and emotional well-being.

▶ Nursing management and interventions

Following assessment, a number of problems may be identified (Table 34.1). This section outlines some of the key nursing interventions required in palliative care.

SYMPTOM CONTROL

The relief of pain and other symptoms is central to the care of patients with life-threatening illness. Symptom control enables many patients to remain active and improves quality of life for them and their families.

Table 34.1 Common symptoms found in advanced cancer. (Reproduced with permission from Kaye P. A-Z Pocket Book of Symptom Control. Northampton: EPL Publications; 1996

Symptom	%
Weakness	95
Pain	80
Anorexia	80
Constipation	65
Dyspnoea	60
Insomnia	60
Sweats	60
Oedema	60
Dry/sore mouth	50
Nausea	50
Vomiting	40
Anxiety	40
Cough	30
Confusion	30
Pressure sore	30
Pleural effusion	20
Ascites	15
Bleeding	15
Depression	10
Drowsiness	10
Itch	5
Diarrhoea	5
Fistula	1

Principles of symptom control

The principles of symptom control include:

- listening to the details as described by patients and families
- asking about all symptoms – there may be many
- where possible, making single treatment changes, otherwise it may be difficult to test effectiveness
- involving the patient and family in decisions and changes
- monitoring symptoms regularly
- remembering that emotions can alter symptoms
- reducing or stopping unnecessary drugs.

PAIN

Cancer is the condition most commonly associated with pain, but there are other life-threatening illnesses that cause pain (Seale 1991). These include AIDS, multiple sclerosis, stroke, and joint disease.

Pain is a very individual experience and is always subjective. It depends on factors ranging from the person's understanding of the illness to previous pain experiences (Ch. 7).

Pain is the symptom that most people associate with cancer, and the fear of dying with uncontrolled pain is foremost in people's minds. Some patients will experience more than one type of pain and it is important to distinguish between the different types of cancer pain. An understanding of the nature of cancer pain is essential for good pain control through selection of appropriate analgesia.

Types of cancer pain

The possibility of several different types of pain makes a thorough assessment vital. It is essential to find out everything about the pain being experienced. A pain assessment tool is very effective (see p. 1029).

Visceral or soft tissue pain

This type of pain is continuous. Causes include infiltration, compression, distension or traction of the viscera. It can result from primary or metastatic tumour growth (Ch. 33). The liver is often a site for metastatic spread and liver pain is a common visceral pain. The pain occurs as the liver capsule is stretched; it is a dull, aching pain in the right upper abdomen, right side and back, which may radiate to the right shoulder. A sudden haemorrhage into liver metastases can cause severe pain.

Bone pain

This is the most common cause of pain in cancer, described as pain on movement. It is caused by metastatic destruction of bone (Ch. 33). Many bone metastases are pain-free and it may be a fracture that first indicates bone involvement (Ch. 27). Pain intensity does not correlate with the number or extent of bone involvement. Pain is usually well-localized, except where nerves are involved or damaged.

Nerve pain

This is described as stabbing or burning that arises from damaged nervous tissue, and from actual or potential tissue damage. The pain may also be produced by a tumour infiltrating or compressing nervous tissue. It can be extremely severe.

Secondary visceral pain

This type of pain includes colicky pain, pleuritic pain, tenesmus and bladder spasms. Colicky pain comes and goes and is followed by a pain-free period. It may result from malignant intestinal obstruction (Ch. 22). Pleuritic pain is sharp chest pain on inspiration, usually due to infection, pulmonary embolus, rib metastases or fracture. Tenesmus is an unpleasant sensation of wanting to defaecate, usually due to rectal cancer or pelvic recurrence. Impacted faeces can cause or worsen tenesmus. Bladder spasms cause severe intermittent suprapubic pain. It can be due to bladder or pelvic tumours, or following radiotherapy for bladder cancer. Urinary infection must be excluded as the cause.

Management of pain

The aim is pain control throughout the 24 hours with an appropriate regimen, an alert patient and minimal side-effects. To achieve this, a knowledge of analgesia and adjuvant analgesics or co-analgesics (drugs and treatments other than analgesics which relieve pain indirectly) is an essential prerequisite.

Knowing the cause of the pain ensures that the correct analgesia is prescribed. Once chosen, the analgesia should be given regularly, with the time interval dependent on the duration of drug action. The dose should be titrated against the pain, so that pain control is achieved with the lowest possible dose.

In 1990, the World Health Organization produced guidelines for the use of drugs that are beneficial to patients with cancer pain. These guidelines (the analgesic ladder) are now widely used by health care professionals (Fig. 34.3).

The non-opioid drugs are the first stage in the treatment of mild pain. If the pain does not respond to these drugs, or is more severe, then patients move onto the next stage – the weak opioid group. Where pain is not controlled with the weak opioids, then patients move onto the strong opioid group. It is important to note that movement can be in both directions. For example, if a patient needed a strong opioid to control the initial pain, it might be possible to reduce the type and strength of analgesia once pain is controlled (possibly with adjuvants).

Only brief details of drugs are offered here. Readers requiring more detail should consult specialist pharmacology books and a national formulary.

Non-opioid drugs

Non-opioid drugs are used for mild pain. They include aspirin which has analgesic, antipyretic and, in higher doses, anti-inflammatory properties. Gastric irritation can occur.

Paracetamol is a synthetic analgesic and antipyretic, but is not anti-inflammatory. It causes little if any gastric irritation. Overdosage may, however, cause potentially fatal liver damage. Patients receiving high doses of opioids can still take paracetamol for a headache or other minor pain.

Weak opioid drugs

Weak opioids are used for moderate pain. These include co-proxamol (dextropropoxyphene and paracetamol) which is generally well tolerated, although it is slightly addictive. Nausea, vomiting and constipation may occur. Dihydrocodeine is an opioid with similar side-effects and is available as a modified-release preparation. A mild laxative might be required with these two drugs to prevent constipation.

Strong opioid drugs

Strong opioids are used for severe pain. These include morphine, which remains the most useful strong analgesic in terminal illness. It is well absorbed by mouth and rapidly distributed through the body. It is effective for continuous pain, but much less so for intermittent pain (see adjuvant analgesics p. 1034). Morphine sulphate can be given rectally. There are three preparations in common use. Morphine sulphate continuous is a controlled-release preparation (tablet or suspension) given 12-hourly. It is not, however, recommended for acute or break-through pain. Controlled-release morphine sulphate capsules are administered once daily, but pain must be controlled prior to converting. Morphine sulphate oral solution or tablets are given 4-hourly. The starting dose depends on the patients' physical condition and whether they have taken other strong opioids for pain control. When morphine is commenced (normally every 4 hours), the effectiveness is continuously reviewed. If the dose is ineffective, a repeat dose may be prescribed and subsequent doses increased.

Giving 4-hourly morphine at night means having to wake patients. They may wake with pain if nurses allow them to sleep. An alternative is to prescribe a double dose of morphine at bed-time, followed 8 hours later by the next routine dose. Once pain is controlled with this regimen, they can be converted to a controlled-release preparation. For example, 4-hourly morphine sulphate solution or tablets converts to morphine sulphate continuous given orally every 12 hours. When patients, converted

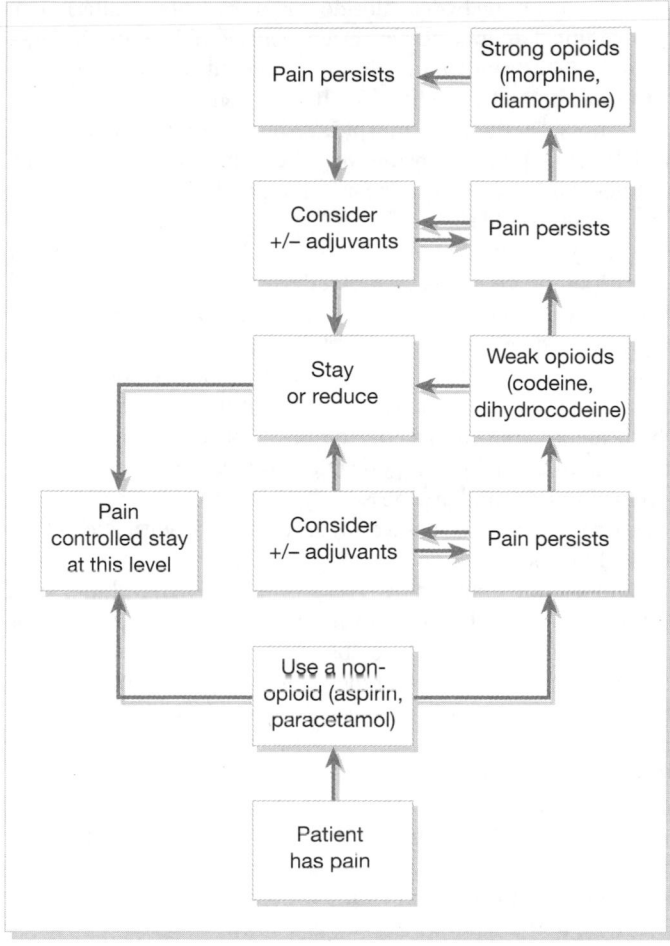

Figure 34.3 Management of pain. (Adapted from WHO 1990.)

to morphine sulphate continuous, get breakthrough pain, a dose of morphine sulphate solution can be given. If the pain becomes uncontrolled again, they should convert to morphine sulphate oral solution and the process of titrating dose against pain is continued until pain control is effective.

Morphine does, however, cause problems, including the following:

- drowsiness
- respiratory depression
- nausea when it is started – an appropriate antiemetic is commenced and then reviewed after 1 week
- constipation is very common and is dose-related – a laxative should always be prescribed
- dry mouth
- confusion and hallucinations
- pupil constriction, especially with high doses
- fear of addiction (will not occur if pain is responding to morphine)
- patients travelling abroad with prescribed morphine may require an export licence (check with the embassy concerned).

Patients may drive whilst taking prescribed morphine, if established on a steady dose that controls their pain without drowsiness (see Health Promotion box 34.1).

Hydromorphone hydrochloride is a fully titratable alternative to morphine. Patients who experience intolerable or unmanageable side-effects with morphine may benefit from a change to hydromorphone hydrochloride. It is a semi-synthetic opioid, with similar actions as morphine, but is more potent. It is available in 4-hourly capsules and 12-hourly slow-release (SR) capsules. The capsules can be swallowed whole or the contents sprinkled onto cold soft food.

Fentanyl patches utilize a transdermal delivery system. Each waterproof patch releases a steady dose over 72 hours and provides equivalent pain control to morphine. It is claimed to have fewer side-effects than morphine, especially constipation.

Buprenorphine tablets can be taken orally or sublingually. The duration of analgesia is 6–9 hours. It has a 'ceiling effect' – which means that increasing the dose above 0.8 mg 8-hourly does not enhance the analgesic effect, but can increase the side-effects of nausea and dizziness.

Dextromoramide is a powerful oral analgesic with effects that last 1–3 hours.

Diamorphine has actions very similar to morphine. It is highly soluble which makes it the drug of choice for injection or subcutaneous infusion. Once absorbed by the body, it is rapidly converted to morphine and reaches a peak level in the blood in about 10 minutes (see 'Parenteral drug administration' below).

Adjuvant analgesics

Adjuvant analgesics are drugs or treatments that may not be analgesics but can help to control pain in some circumstances. They can be used in combination with the opioids. The following are some examples of adjuvant analgesics that can be used according to the type of pain (see p. 1032):

- corticosteroids, e.g. dexamethasone, for liver and nerve pain
- non-steroidal anti-inflammatory drugs (NSAIDs), e.g. ibuprofen, for bone pain
- nerve blocks using local anaesthetic drugs for visceral pain
- antidepressants, e.g. imipramine, for nerve pain
- radiotherapy for bone pain
- anticonvulsants, e.g. carbamazepine, for nerve pain
- antimuscarinics, e.g. hyoscine butylbromide, for colicky pain and bladder spasm
- somatostatin analogues, e.g. octreotide, for colicky pain.

Readers needing more information about adjuvant analgesia are directed to 'Further reading'.

Parenteral drug administration

The subcutaneous route via a syringe driver is preferred for continuous administration of drugs. The intramuscular route can be painful and absorption erratic, whilst the intravenous route is not favoured due to the 'peak' effects of some of the drugs.

A continuous subcutaneous infusion achieves a steady plasma concentration of drugs without the need for regular injections. They may also be used on a temporary basis to control symptoms, e.g. nausea. Drug groups commonly used in syringe drivers include analgesics (opioids), sedatives, antiemetics, corticosteroids and diuretics (see Guidelines box 34.1).

Indications for use

- Persistent nausea and vomiting
- Dysphagia
- Oral route not tolerated

HEALTH PROMOTION

34.1 Going home with morphine sulphate continuous

Information to prevent problems:

- The action of analgesics, when to take them and safe storage
- The drug is prescribed for them and must never be given to another person
- The role of laxatives and when to report any difficulties
- The role of a balanced diet, including fibre-rich foods, if tolerated
- The importance of a gentle exercise and rest
- Safe amounts of alcohol
- The importance of remaining independent, e.g. driving
- The use of breakthrough medication for extra pain and reporting it
- The importance of talking to a health professional about worries

Student activities

Prepare an information leaflet for patients being discharged home on morphine sulphate continuous. The list provided can be used as a starting point.

GUIDELINES FOR CARE PRIORITIES

34.1 Syringe driver

Main points:

- Change syringes every 24 hours
- Syringe drivers 10–50 mm may be used
- Luer lock syringes should be used to prevent disconnection
- Limit the drug combination to two or three and always check compatibility before mixing. Avoid high doses of diamorphine and cyclizine together, as they react
- Use sterile water to mix drugs as it is less irritant. There are, however, some drugs that must be mixed with saline
- Observe the mixed drug solution for any signs of precipitation
- Check the site regularly for signs for redness and swelling. Change site as required
- Check the driver regularly to make sure it is working
- Start oral medication approximately 6 hours before stopping the syringe driver
- Try to avoid boosting the syringe driver as no record is kept, and the total dose of extra drugs needed is not known. If extra medication is needed, use bolus medications
- Remember you can use more than one syringe driver if several drugs are required

- Malabsorption
- Intestinal obstruction
- Altered consciousness
- Severe dehydration.

Advantages

- Avoids regular injections
- Availability of numerous sites, e.g. upper arms and thighs
- Maintains constant symptom control
- Only requires daily loading
- Drug combinations can be administered
- Compact equipment allows mobility.

MOUTH PROBLEMS

Mouth care is important, as oral problems can lead to discomfort and reduced food and fluid intake. Common oral problems include coated tongue, dryness, stomatitis, pain, taste disturbance and halitosis.

Coated tongue

A coated tongue affects taste and feels unpleasant. Loose debris can be removed with mouthwashes, although using a small soft toothbrush with toothpaste is effective. Measures for dealing with heavy coating include dissolving an effervescent vitamin C tablet on the tongue, and using mouthwashes containing sodium bicarbonate, sodium perborate or hydrogen peroxide. Miconazole oral gel can be applied and pineapple slices can clear heavy coating.

Dryness

Dryness (xerostomia) can impede speaking, eating, tasting and swallowing. Reversible causes include mouth breathing, smoking, anxiety, depression, dehydration and drug therapy. Permanent dryness may result from head and neck radiotherapy, surgical desalivation, anaemia and AIDS. Dryness can be relieved by sips of iced water, sucking ice, rehydration, fruit sweets, pineapple, sugar-free chewing gum (stimulates salivation and natural oral cleansing), and the use of artificial saliva.

Stomatitis

Stomatitis is inflammation of the mouth caused by microbial infections. The infection may be caused by opportunistic microorganisms usually associated with systemic illness, lowered host resistance and an alteration in normal flora caused by:

- antibiotics, corticosteroids and chemotherapy
- any immunocompromised state
- altered hormonal and nutritional states.

Infections may be caused by fungi, especially *Candida albicans* (thrush). Candidiasis is treated with antifungal agents, such as nystatin, miconazole (gel, tablets) or amphotericin lozenges. An antiseptic mouth rinse may be valuable in combination with a specific antifungal agent. The mouth should be cleaned prior to taking antifungal medication. Dentures must be cleaned with a brush after each meal, and soaked in antiseptic mouth rinse twice daily. The dentures are left out where oral antifungals are used, to ensure that the entire mouth is exposed to the drug. Oesophageal thrush may occur in the absence of oral thrush.

Viral infections include the herpes simplex virus (HSV). This virus is a particular problem for people with AIDS. HSV, which lies dormant, is reactivated during physiological stress, immunosuppression due to disease or cytotoxic chemotherapy. Treatment is with aciclovir ointment or oral preparation. Ulcers are managed with a soft diet, adequate fluid intake and analgesia as required. Where toothbrushing is painful, an antiseptic mouthwash should be used to control plaque accumulation.

Mouth ulcers may occur in palliative patients and are treated with tetracycline mouthwashes or hydrocortisone lozenges at an early stage. Infected oral malignant ulcers can produce a foul odour. They usually respond to systemic antibiotics, e.g. metronidazole.

Oral pain

Oral pain or soreness may be due to a number of causes: candidiasis (see above), gum disease, ill-fitting dentures, tooth decay, stomatitis, ulcers, trauma and oral tumours.

Topical analgesics have a short duration of action, but they are helpful before mouth care and meals. Severe pain occasionally needs analgesics such as opioids.

Taste disturbances

Taste disturbances can be caused by xerostomia and drugs, especially morphine and chemotherapy. Measures to relieve taste disturbance include effective oral hygiene, fizzy sugar-free drinks with food, avoiding bitter tastes, increasing food flavours (seasoning, herbs, spices, wine or beer in cooking), and fresh fruit and vegetables.

Halitosis

Halitosis may result from poor oral hygiene. It can also be due to infections in the respiratory or gastrointestinal tract, or to vomiting, especially faeculent vomiting. Any infection should be treated and effective oral hygiene implemented, particularly after vomiting.

NAUSEA AND VOMITING

Patients with advanced illness frequently experience nausea and vomiting. These symptoms can be demoralizing and demeaning. Failure to relieve these symptoms results in reduced quality of life for patients and their families.

Physiology of nausea and vomiting

Controlling nausea and vomiting can be difficult and requires an understanding of the physiological mechanisms. The process can be divided into three stages:

1. nausea – an unpleasant sensation felt in the upper abdomen and the throat that may be accompanied by pallor and sweating
2. retching – a rhythmic straining occurring before vomiting and sometimes without vomiting
3. vomiting – where stomach contents are reflexly expelled via the mouth.

Vomiting is initiated and coordinated by two centres in the brain (medulla) – the vomiting (emetic) centre which has overall

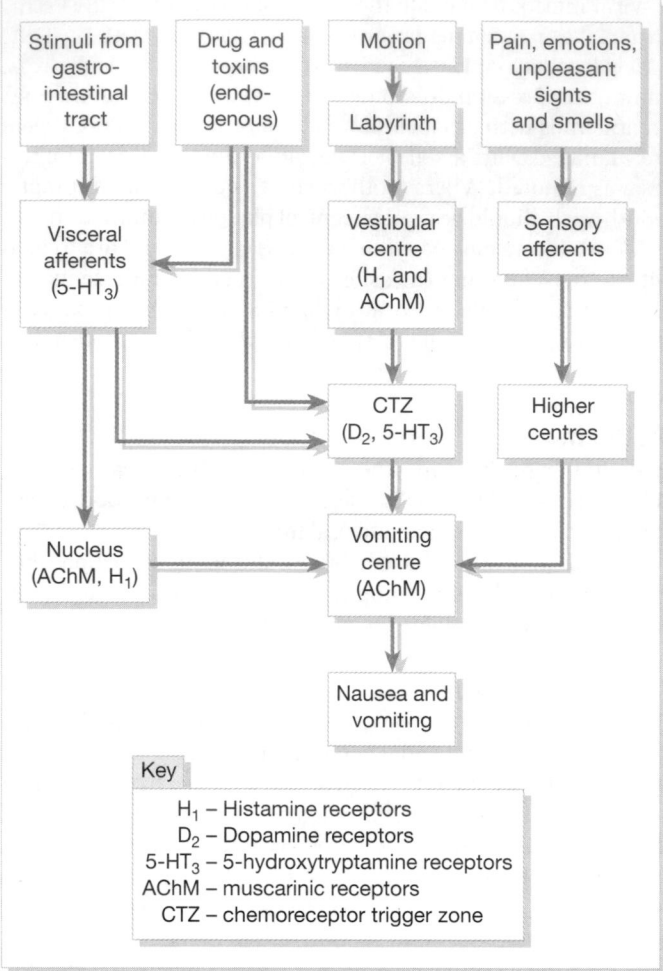

Figure 34.4 Stimulation of the vomiting centre and receptors – simplified.

control, and the chemoreceptor trigger zone (CTZ) which responds to chemical stimuli in the blood and impulses from other areas, such as the visceral afferents. The vomiting centre receives stimulation from various sources (Fig. 34.4):

- cortical pathways (higher centres) via sensory afferents
- vestibular pathways via the labyrinth system
- stimuli from gastrointestinal tract via visceral afferents
- CTZ.

The neurotransmitters involved in vomiting include histamine, dopamine, 5-hydroxytryptamine and acetylcholine. The CTZ and vomiting centre contain receptors able to respond to different stimuli arriving via receptors in other areas, e.g. muscarinic (AChM) and histamine (H_1) receptors in the vestibular nuclei, and 5-hydroxytryptamine (5-HT_3) receptors in the visceral afferents (Fig. 34.4). A knowledge of the receptors is central to controlling nausea and vomiting because each type of antiemetic drug has a different site of action (see below).

Causes of nausea and vomiting

In patients with advanced cancer, the causes of nausea and vomiting (Chs 22 and 33), include:

- drugs, e.g. opioids
- gastrointestinal problems, e.g. gastric stasis
- pharyngeal irritation from coughing and viscous sputum
- radiotherapy and chemotherapy
- hypercalcaemia
- brain metastases
- anxiety and unpleasant sights or odours
- pain
- infection.

Non-pharmacological interventions

Simple non-pharmacological measures can prevent nausea and vomiting, e.g. by positioning the patient away from strong food smells and offering small meals. The nurse should provide effective oral care (see p. 1035).

The use of acupuncture wrist bands may suppress nausea by exerting pressure on a point on the pericardium meridian (Trevelyan & Booth 1994). Diversional therapy such as listening to music or watching television may help. Relaxation, massage, aromatherapy and hypnosis may also reduce symptoms by lowering anxiety levels.

Pharmacological interventions

Antiemetic drugs exert their action in a variety of ways and it is essential to target treatment appropriately. The many types of antiemetics include (Rang et al 1995):

- histamine receptor (H_1) antagonists, e.g. cyclizine, which is used for motion sickness and following radiotherapy to the head or neck
- central dopamine (D_2) receptor antagonists, e.g. metoclopramide, domperidone and thiethylperazine (a phenothiazine), are used for gastrointestinal problems and nausea and vomiting associated with radiotherapy, toxins and opioids
- 5-hydroxytryptamine receptor (5-HT_3) antagonists, e.g. ondansetron, are useful in the management of nausea and vomiting induced by chemotherapy and radiotherapy
- muscarinic receptor antagonists (AChM), e.g. hyoscine, are the drug of choice for motion sickness. They also dry secretions, so may reduce nausea and retching where bronchial secretions are excessive
- synthetic cannabinoids, e.g. nabilone, which are used where other antiemetics fail to control cytotoxic drug-induced vomiting.

Other drugs used in the control of nausea and vomiting include corticosteroids, such as dexamethasone. The mode of action is not fully understood, but may enhance the effects of many antiemetics. They are of value in the management of nausea and vomiting related to organ enlargement through their anti-inflammatory action, especially in cerebral oedema, and possibly by reducing oedema around an obstructive gastrointestinal lesion.

The route of administration of antiemetics is important, as oral drugs are only effective for preventing or treating mild nausea. Persistent nausea or vomiting causes gastric stasis and impedes the absorption of oral drugs. Where this occurs, antiemetics should be given by suppository, injection or subcutaneous infusion.

CACHEXIA AND ANOREXIA

Cachexia is characterized by weight loss, muscle wastage, fat breakdown, anorexia, chronic nausea and generalized weakness. More than 80% of cancer patients develop cachexia before dying (Bruera 1997), and it is most common with solid tumours and dysphagia. In most patients, cachexia is caused by metabolic abnormalities due to tumour products, reduced energy intake and malabsorption.

Anorexia is associated with cachexia. Causes can include nausea and vomiting, mouth infections, constipation (see below), anxiety or depression and drugs.

Management

The management of cachexia and anorexia includes:

- treating the cause, e.g. constipation
- advice from a nutrition nurse specialist and dietician
- small portions of favourite foods and high-energy supplements
- nutritional support (enteral or parenteral) where appropriate and according to the wishes of the people involved (Ch. 11)
- corticosteroids may improve appetite in the short term
- sherry or wine before meals, where appropriate.

CONSTIPATION

Constipation is the passage of small hard faeces infrequently and with difficulty, and is common in cases of cancer and advanced illness. About half of the patients admitted to specialist palliative care units report constipation (Sykes 1993). Patients eating very little still continue to produce bowel waste products and can still become constipated. Assessment is important and is achieved by obtaining a history and examination. A plain abdominal X-ray may also be useful. The following, if present, may indicate constipation:

- general abdominal discomfort, colicky pain or fullness
- anorexia
- nausea and vomiting
- halitosis
- malaise
- impaction/tenesmus/overflow diarrhoea
- intestinal obstruction
- confusion
- urinary retention.

Causes

The causes are varied and include effects of the disease and treatment, and very simple factors such as the use of bedpans. Wright (1974) found that 44% of people using bedpans/commodes became constipated, compared with 26% of those using the lavatory. Other causes are:

- dehydration and lack of fibre
- weakness
- pain
- immobility
- confusion

- lack of privacy, facilities and time
- intestinal obstruction (tumour compresses the bowel)
- hypercalcaemia
- spinal cord compression
- drug side-effects, e.g. opioids and iron.

Management

The management of constipation is not just by the use of laxatives; maintaining good general symptom control contributes to an effective outcome. Being pain-free will increase mobility. Nurses should anticipate problems; for example, opioids cause constipation and therefore patients having opioid analgesia should be given a laxative.

Offering advice on diet and encouraging fluids will also help. Proprietary fibre drinks can be used if patients are unable to tolerate high-fibre diets.

The aim of laxative treatment is comfortable defaecation, rather than any particular frequency of bowel function. The choice of laxative depends on the nature of the stool, the cause of constipation and the condition of the patient. Simple measures like a commode nearby or wheeling to the lavatory may help.

Types of laxatives

There are several types of laxatives (Kaye 1996):

- Bulking agents, e.g. methylcellulose, retain water to produce a soft bulky stool.
- Softeners, e.g. docusate, act by lubricating or softening the faeces; they also act as a weak stimulant laxative.
- Stimulants, e.g. senna, produce peristalsis through local nerve stimulation.
- Osmotic laxatives, e.g. lactulose, increase fluid in the gut lumen through osmosis.
- Combined softeners and stimulants, e.g. co-danthramer, soften the stool and stimulate the colon; they are useful in opioid-induced constipation.
- Rectal preparations are needed when oral laxatives fail or are not tolerated. They should be used if there is no bowel movement for 3 days, but are also useful in treating faecal impaction and preventing constipation in people with spinal cord compression and late stage multiple sclerosis. Rectal preparations are available as suppositories or enemas:
  — Glycerine suppositories soften stools in the rectum, and bisacodyl suppositories, a stimulant laxative, are used when the rectum is full of soft faeces but fails to empty
  — Phosphate enemas act as osmotic laxatives to empty the lower bowel
  — Arachis oil retention enema can be used to soften impacted faeces; however, it may be difficult for the palliative patient to retain the oil.

Alternative methods

Digital disimpaction may be necessary for a loaded rectum, but can be painful so sedatives may be necessary. Disimpaction should be followed by enemas. Great caution is needed to avoid bowel trauma. Abdominal massage can also help to stimulate peristalsis.

INTESTINAL OBSTRUCTION

Intestinal obstruction occurs when the lumen is occluded by tumour or there is a lack of normal propulsion (e.g. paralytic ileus) of intestinal contents (Ch. 22). The signs and symptoms include:

- colic
- abdominal distension (more marked with large bowel)
- continuous abdominal pain
- vomiting (more marked with small bowel)
- no faeces or flatus passed (variable).

Management

There are a number of treatment options available, including surgery (Ch. 22), nasogastric aspiration and intravenous fluids, and symptom control.

Nasogastric aspiration and intravenous fluids are considered in advanced cancer for the severe, distressing vomiting of small bowel obstruction. Symptom control is important for palliative patients. They can be managed well with analgesics, corticosteroids and antiemetics given by continuous subcutaneous infusion.

Palliative patients with obstruction may still be able to drink fluids, which will at least moisten their mouth. Food may be recommended once symptoms have resolved.

BREATHING PROBLEMS

Breathing problems (Ch. 20) are common in patients with advanced incurable disease.

Cough

Patients with a terminal illness can be troubled by a cough – this may be dry or productive with mucus or sputum. The many conditions associated with a cough include heart disease, chronic pulmonary disease, bronchial tumours, pneumonia, neurological disorders and following chest radiotherapy.

Where possible, the cause of the cough should be treated or its effects minimized. Persistent coughing can cause vomiting, syncope, muscle strain, chest pain, rib fractures, insomnia and exhaustion.

Palliative management of cough

Treatment options depend upon the nature of the cough. A productive cough may be managed with drugs – antibiotics for infection, diuretics for heart failure, and hyoscine or scopolamine (transdermally) to dry secretions. Measures to reduce sputum viscosity and aid expectoration include physiotherapy, steam inhalation or nebulized saline, suction, an adequate fluid intake and hot drinks. Expectorants are of little value.

Palliative measures for a dry cough include radiotherapy to reduce irritation from a large bronchial tumour. Corticosteroids may help if the cough is caused by bronchial mass or reversible airways obstruction, and bronchospasm may be relieved with nebulized bronchodilators, for example salbutamol. Drugs that suppress a dry cough include codeine and morphine. Nebulized bupivacaine may help a cough due to bronchial distortion by tumour. Bupivacaine is a local anaesthetic and patients are advised to take nothing orally for 30–60 minutes after administration. Simple measures such as sleeping in a warm room may also help.

Hiccups

Hiccups are a respiratory reflex caused by persistent spasm of the diaphragm. In palliative care this can be upsetting for the patient and family.

Causes include:

- gastric distension
- liver enlargement
- phrenic nerve irritation
- chest infection
- brain tumour
- uraemia.

Management includes rebreathing into a bag or breath-holding to increase carbon dioxide; reducing gastric distension with peppermint water; and increasing gastric emptying with metoclopramide and offering small frequent meals. Other drugs used to treat hiccups may include chlorpromazine, haloperidol, baclofen and nifedipine. Corticosteroids or an anticonvulsant, e.g. carbamazepine, may be used if the cause is cerebral irritation. Radiotherapy may be used to reduce mediastinal nodes. Relief may be gained from inserting a nasogastric tube. Occasionally a folk remedy, such as drinking from the wrong side of a cup, may help.

Dyspnoea

Dyspnoea is a common feature of advanced cancer, heart failure and chronic pulmonary disease. It is a particularly frightening symptom for patients and families (see Reflective Practice box 34.1).

There are many non-pharmacological measures that nurses may use to ease breathlessness, such as helping patients to sit upright in bed or on a chair with cool air blowing onto the face, ensuring a quiet and relaxed environment and enlisting the help of the physiotherapist in teaching patients to make effective use of their respiratory efforts. Relaxation techniques and other complementary therapies can be beneficial.

RR REFLECTIVE PRACTICE

34.1 Dyspnoea and advanced cancer

Mary has advanced cancer of the lung. On admission to a hospice she is extremely short of breath at rest. She is commenced on oxygen therapy and low-dose morphine sulphate solution.

Student activities

- Mary is extremely frightened and feels that she is suffocating. What non-pharmacological measures might be used to help with this situation?
- How would you assess the effectiveness of the morphine sulphate solution, and how does it work?

Treatments options include:

- antibiotics to treat infection
- palliative radiotherapy to reduce tumour mass
- opioids, such as low-dose morphine (oral or via nebulizer), to decrease the respiratory rate and reduce anxiety
- corticosteroids to reduce oedema around the tumour
- anxiolytics, such as a benzodiazepine
- oxygen therapy to reduce dyspnoea at rest. Nasal cannulae are more effective than a mask and allow patients to eat and talk without the oxygen flow being disturbed. Patients who are already breathless may find that a face mask exacerbates the problem.

FUNGATING WOUNDS

Fungating lesions occur when the cancer infiltrates the epithelium resulting in ulceration through the skin to the body surface (Chs 10 and 26). It is usually associated with cancer of the breast, skin, vulva and bladder. Abdominal tumours may occasionally spread through the abdominal wall. Ulceration occurs if lymph nodes at the groin or axilla are affected by spread.

Malignant fungating wounds are very difficult to manage and can cause much distress to all involved. The wound can affect all daily activities, including opportunities to socialize.

Patients may deny there is a problem and may not be seen until the fungating wound is large. They may feel unclean, and are reluctant to let health care professionals attend to the wound. A fungating wound is a visible sign of the cancer.

On a practical level, large fungating wounds require bulky dressings, making it difficult to wear some types of clothing. There may be copious exudate that constantly soaks clothes and bedding.

Management

Patients may experience stress for reasons that include family responses, dressing changes, odour, leakage, bleeding and altered body image (Ch. 6). Stress can be reduced by:

- reassurance and honest explanations for patient and family
- speaking to other patients about the odour
- pain relief, especially at dressing change
- use of the appropriate dressing, to prevent bleeding or to manage exudate without extra bulk
- measures to reduce odour, e.g. charcoal dressings, systemic metronidazole, topical antibiotic and scented candles
- attention to personal care and appearance
- complementary therapies.

Large wounds can sometimes be reduced by surgery, cryotherapy, laser therapy or radiotherapy.

PSYCHOLOGICAL PROBLEMS

Psychological problems can manifest themselves in a variety of ways and at different times (see above). It is important that nurses remember that psychological problems may have a physical cause, such as confusion caused by hypoxia.

Agitation

Agitation at the end of life is very distressing for all concerned and must be dealt with quickly by careful assessment with identification and treatment of the cause, e.g. oxygen for hypoxia. Providing a calm environment, explanation and reassurance for the patient and family are important. Drug therapy may be required, e.g. midazolam or diazepam, and haloperidol for paranoia or hallucinations.

Anxiety

Anxiety occurs when coping mechanisms are inadequate or stress is overwhelming, which can occur when the threat of death is real. Anxiety states may be acute or chronic. The former is usually short-lived and related to a specific situation (Ch. 6). Anxiety is managed by:

- alleviating the underlying cause, e.g. pain, lack of information
- drugs, e.g. tranquillizers, sedatives, antidepressants, neuroleptics and beta-adrenoceptor antagonists
- counselling
- complementary therapies, e.g. relaxation and aromatherapy.

Confusion

Confusion is characterized by decreased attention, disorientation in person, time and place, and inability to act decisively. It can also lead to paranoid delusion, hallucinations, restlessness, drowsiness and aggressive behaviour.

The causes are diverse and include:

- drugs – sedatives, opioids and corticosteroids
- brain tumours
- infection
- metabolic disorders, e.g. hypercalcaemia
- organ failure, e.g. liver
- hypoxia
- extreme anxiety or depression
- retention of urine or constipation
- withdrawal of alcohol, benzodiazepines or barbiturates.

Patients with confusion should be assessed and, where possible, the cause treated. A quiet environment with familiar carers and health professionals is important, as is reassurance and explanation. Sedatives, which may worsen confusion, are only used where symptoms are distressing.

Depression

Depression is estimated to occur in 10% of terminally ill patients (Kaye 1996). Depressive illness can easily be mistaken for natural sadness in response to the circumstances. People with depression may exhibit some of the following:

- changes in sleep pattern – early waking or excessive sleeping
- low self-esteem and feelings of worthlessness
- loss of interest
- weight change
- withdrawal, agitation and delusions
- suicidal thoughts.

Management can include simple support and reassurance or counselling, but antidepressants drugs can be beneficial, e.g. dothiepin, fluoxetine. A specialist psychiatric referral should always be considered where mood improvement fails to occur and suicidal thoughts are present.

EMERGENCIES IN PALLIATIVE CARE

Emergencies in palliative care require prompt treatment to achieve good outcomes. Treatment may not always prolong life, but it should improve quality of life. Before treating an emergency in patients with advanced disease, the following points should be considered:

- the nature of the emergency and whether it is reversible
- the patient's condition
- whether treatment will improve quality of life
- the wishes of the patient and carers.

Emergencies seen in palliative care include fractures, haemorrhage, hypercalcaemia, superior vena cava obstruction, spinal cord compression and seizures.

Fractures

Fractures can occur in patients with advanced disease as a result of minimal trauma, bone metastases and osteoporosis (Chs 27 and 33). The management will include pain control, radiotherapy, immobilization and internal fixation as appropriate.

Haemorrhage

Major bleeding results from erosion of an artery, such as the aorta, carotid artery, or the axillary or femoral arteries from malignant lymph nodes, and can be a terminal event. Management should involve staying with the patient, administering prescribed sedation (diamorphine or midazolam) and supporting the relatives, staff and patients who witness the event. It is important to keep the immediate environment clean and clear of blood or reduce the visual impact by using red or green bedding or surgical towels.

Minor bleeds are dealt with according to site and severity. Supporting the patient and relatives, and ensuring comfort remain the principal nursing aims.

Hypercalcaemia

Hypercalcaemia, which is a serum calcium level > 2.6 mmol/L, occurs in 10–20% of patients with cancer (Chs 8 and 17). It can occur in cancers of the bronchus, breast and some haematological malignancies (Ch. 18). Bone metastases may also cause hypercalcaemia.

The presentation may be insidious with anorexia, nausea, abdominal pain and constipation. There is fatigue, proximal muscle weakness, confusion, drowsiness and coma. Polyuria and polydipsia may be features. High levels require urgent treatment with fluid replacement, bisphosphonates (e.g. pamidronate), diuretics (e.g. furosemide [frusemide]), corticosteroids, and oral sodium cellulose phosphate, which binds calcium and prevents absorption.

Superior vena cava obstruction

Superior vena cava obstruction (SVCO) is usually due to compression by mediastinal nodes or a bronchial tumour (Chs 20 and 33). SVCO is characterized by:

- swelling – neck, face and arms
- headaches (worse on bending over), dizziness or fainting
- venous engorgement – shoulders, scapulae and upper chest
- hoarse voice (laryngeal nerve pressure) and later stridor
- pink eyes
- periorbital oedema
- dyspnoea (tracheal oedema and hypoxia).

SVCO is managed with radiotherapy, corticosteroids and chemotherapy, and where it is a terminal event, diamorphine and midazolam should be administered to control dyspnoea and agitation.

Spinal cord compression

Spinal cord compression (SCC) requires urgent treatment, to prevent neurological damage (Ch. 33).

Seizures

Seizures can occur in patients who have primary or secondary brain tumours (Ch. 14).

ROLE OF SPECIALIST PALLIATIVE CARE NURSES

The role of clinical nurse specialists (CNSs) in palliative care is a fairly recent development, the first Macmillan nurses being employed in 1977. The aim was to improve care for people with cancer and their families and enhance their quality of life.

The CNS influences care outcomes in various ways and specialist practice encompasses:

- clinical – support during illness and bereavement
- consultative – acting as a resource
- education – of patients, carers, colleagues and students
- leadership – for health care professionals
- research – updating of knowledge and evidence-based practice.

CNSs are not primary carers. Rather they seek to equip the primary carers with the skills and knowledge required to provide high-quality care for all patients.

They become involved with patients and families in response to referrals and requests, usually from other professionals. Ideally CNSs should be involved from diagnosis, but large caseloads may make this difficult. CNS contact at diagnosis is particularly desirable to provide information and to help people coping with initial problems. Short-term interventions with patients and families can also be useful when specific problems need several visits, after which they withdraw and leave care management to the primary health care team, until specialist intervention is required again.

Patients and families needing long-term contacts usually have multiple problems or are referred late in their illness. They are usually a highly dependent group, who require considerable intervention from all team members. Accurate assessment, negotiation skills and problem-solving are necessary to ensure that all needs are met.

Palliative care services continue to develop and Macmillan nurses are employed to work in both community and acute hospital settings (wards, clinics, day hospitals).

REFERRALS

Referrals to CNSs need to be timely and appropriate to ensure best use of resources and good outcomes. The appropriateness of referrals is enhanced by ensuring that all staff have an understanding of the role and scope of practice of CNSs. Referrals to the service usually come from professionals, but may come direct from patients or relatives. These, however, are usually only accepted if the GP considers them to be appropriate.

Reasons for referrals

Reasons for referral include:

- advice on symptom control and general management
- concern about the relationship within the family and with professionals
- accessing other services
- financial problems
- to commence pre-bereavement or bereavement counselling
- the patient or family have unrealistic expectations regarding outcomes
- the patient lives alone.

CARE AROUND THE TIME OF DEATH

Terminal care is an important part of palliative care and usually refers to the nursing management of patients during their last few days, weeks, or even months of life, from the point when their condition deteriorated. The focus of care is now the comfort of the patient, and the care of relatives and friends who might already be grieving.

During the final stages of life, there will be increasing weakness and immobility, loss of interest in food and drink, dysphagia and drowsiness. The common signs and symptoms experienced in the final 48 hours are shown in Table 34.2.

Dying can be a lonely experience, as staff or family may avoid the patient because they do not know what to say or do. In hospital this may be further exacerbated because staff are busy and are not able to spend time with the patient and family. With experience, nurses can usually recognize when patients are entering the final stages and are likely to die in the near future, but death can be sudden. Identifying changes in a patient's condition relies on information from everyone involved, including the patient. A peaceful death is important for the relatives as well as the patient, because the memory of the death will remain forever.

As a patient's condition deteriorates, it is important to ascertain whether the family members wish to be present at the time of death. Health professionals must accept and support their decision. Families wishing to be present at the end should be warned that even if they stay, the only sure way is not to leave the patient for a moment. This is difficult as death may occur in

Table 34.2 Terminal symptoms during last 48 hours. (Reproduced with permission from Lichter & Hunte. The last 48 hours of life. *J Pall Care* 1990; 6(4): 7–15.)	
Symptom	**% noted**
Moist breathing – 'death rattle'	56
Pain	51
Agitation	42
Incontinence of urine	32
Dyspnoea	22
Retention	21
Nausea and vomiting	14
Sweating	14
Jerking, twitching	12
Plucking	9
Confusion	9

the short time it takes for a relative to visit the lavatory or have a break. When the final stages last for days, it can leave family members exhausted and emotionally drained. It is important that they are well supported, but being present can make the bereavement process easier. It must also be determined what they want to do after death has occurred.

▶ Nursing management

Although skilled care is required, it is important to recognize that some relatives will wish to participate in caring. Health professionals should facilitate this and offer support.

Explanation to the patient and family is vital and should help to reduce anxiety.

As the patient's condition deteriorates, the need for food and drink lessens. This can cause the family great distress, so explanation is essential. Food is central to life and providing food and feeding can be a loving action. Relatives may still want to feed patients as they lose consciousness, often because they think that food is still beneficial.

The family should also be warned that there might be other manifestations as death draws near, such as changes in the breathing pattern and involuntary movements. A prior awareness of these potential events can reduce feelings of anxiety, if they do occur.

Environment

The environment is important and the atmosphere should be calm and unhurried. Chairs should be placed so as to allow relatives to touch and hold their loved ones. The need for privacy should be anticipated, as should the need for company on occasions. The room does not have to be silent; if desired, the patient's favourite music can be played quietly. Patients unable to speak can still hear and feel, which is why speech and touch are so important. Health care professionals, relatives and friends should be encouraged to talk to the patient, especially as they approach to give care, so as not to startle them.

Skin care and hygiene

Pressure area assessment and care are vital, and the patient should be repositioned every 2–4 hours depending on the type of pressure-relieving equipment in use (Ch. 10). Changing the position of patients relieves stiffness and discomfort as they weaken and cannot move by themselves.

Hygiene is maintained by bed bathing and regular gentle sponging if patients are perspiring. Use of personal toiletries and fresh clothes is important for maintaining comfort and dignity. Relatives can be encouraged to help with hygiene, as it provides a bond by touching and gives them something to focus on. As death approaches, relatives and friends should be told that the patient's skin may feel cold as the peripheral circulation fails and that it may become discoloured and mottled.

Mouth care is essential for the dying patient – a dry and dirty mouth can cause discomfort (see p. 1035). Relatives can also provide the patient with small amounts of water dribbled into the mouth using a syringe and apply lip salve.

Eye care with sodium chloride solution (0.9%) may be required if the eyes are sticky. A patient's eyes may stay open when asleep, resulting in dry eyes, but artificial tears may help.

Coping with restlessness

Restlessness may have several causes that should be investigated before any medication is given. These include tight bedclothes, a blocked catheter or needing to be moved. Pain should always be controlled. Patients may be restless if they have something on their minds, and opportunities to talk through distress may be helpful. Medication may be needed, e.g. midazolam.

Noisy respiration

Respiration may become noisy (death rattle) as the collection of secretions in the throat oscillates with each respiration. The noise does not appear to distress the patient, but may be very upsetting for the family. It occurs when patients are too weak to expectorate these secretions and can be alleviated by changing the patient's position, gentle suctioning or administering anti-muscarinic drugs, such as hyoscine hydrobromide, to decrease secretions.

Medication

Medication should be reviewed as the patient's condition deteriorates and all unnecessary medication stopped. Drugs that should continue include analgesia, antiemetics and other drugs for specific palliation. It may be helpful to use a 24-hour syringe driver to administer medication. Analgesia should never be discontinued even when consciousness is finally lost.

SPIRITUAL, RELIGIOUS AND CULTURAL NEEDS

Spiritual, religious and cultural needs vary from patient to patient. It is vitally important that health professionals are sensitive to the spiritual and any religious needs, and that these are discussed with the patient and family in an appropriate way. Nurses may be asked to arrange visits from religious leaders, provide privacy and opportunity for religious observance and create an environment conducive to the individual patient's spiritual needs.

The importance of health professionals having an understanding, albeit superficial, of the religious beliefs and cultural traditions of their patients cannot be overstated. A patient can derive great comfort from a nurse who has remembered that a

R|R REFLECTIVE PRACTICE

34.2 Pain relief and spiritual needs

Mohammed has been admitted to your ward with severe pain. He hardly speaks any English and is a follower of Islam. Ramadan is due to start in 2 days.

Student activities
- What difficulties might arise with starting oral morphine sulphate solution?
- How would you communicate with Mohammed?
- Think about how you would ensure that Mohammed's spiritual needs are met during Ramadan.

particular day has great religious significance for people of that faith. Nurses must also have a basic knowledge of customs and taboos surrounding death. The last thing nurses normally do for patients is to prepare the body for removal, but for some faiths, having a nurse of a different faith or gender perform last offices would cause great offence and distress to the family. It is essential to ascertain from the patient, family or wider religious community what they require during the last stages and beyond death (see Reflective Practice box 34.2).

It is beyond the scope of this book to cover sufficient detail about all the religious and cultural groups that nurses may encounter in their practice. Readers are encouraged to find out about groups in their locality and are directed to Neuberger (1994) in the 'Further reading' section.

AFTER DEATH

When death has occurred and been verified by medical staff or a senior nurse, the family should be left with their loved one to say their goodbyes. Last offices, performed after death, is the nursing care a deceased patient requires before removal to the mortuary. The family may wish to help with washing the patient and any religious or cultural practices should be followed.

The family should be asked whether they have any favourite clothes they want the deceased to be dressed in. Tubes and catheters should be removed, unless a postmortem is expected to take place, and wounds should be covered with an adhesive plaster to protect staff from body fluid leakage. Pacemakers should be removed unless there is to be a postmortem, and then the mortuary staff should be informed. Identification labels for the deceased and notification of death forms are dealt with according to local policy. The body is usually wrapped in a clean sheet in hospital or hospice prior to transfer to the mortuary. After a death at home, the funeral directors remove the deceased, but occasionally the body is kept at home. A body bag is required where there is leakage of body fluids or if the deceased had certain infectious diseases, e.g. hepatitis or AIDS.

THE OFFICIAL ASPECTS OF DEATH

There are often differences in the way hospitals and hospices deal with a patient's death. Where death occurs in hospital, the relatives return next day to collect the person's property and the medical death certificate. The ward staff may take the relatives to the welfare officer, or they may go directly, and the necessary documents are issued and they are informed about registering the death. If cremation is requested, a special form is completed by a second doctor. In some cases, a postmortem may be necessary.

In hospices, the emphasis changes to the care of the family. Again the family members return the following day to receive the medical death certificate and property. They are normally met by one of the nurses, who spends time with them to assess how they are dealing with the death. A nurse or doctor usually supplies the necessary documents.

If the patient dies at home, the general practitioner confirms death, issues the medical death certificate if possible, and arranges a cremation form if required. A funeral director should be contacted at an appropriate moment either to remove the deceased or to discuss arrangements with the relatives.

REGISTERING A DEATH

Deaths must be registered by the registrar of births and deaths for the sub-district in which it occurred. Normally this occurs within 5 days, unless an extension has been granted. Registration is by appointment, and occasionally the hospital or hospice staff will make an appointment. Where a death is referred to the coroner, the registrar cannot register it until authority from the coroner has been received. A relative of the deceased should register the death, but where this is not possible, another person may do so. The registrar will require information about the deceased, e.g. name, date and place of birth, date and place of death, usual address and occupation.

After registering the death, the registrar will issue the relative with a certificate giving permission for burial or for an application for cremation to be made. Where appropriate, a certificate of registration of death form is issued for social security purposes. Additional copies of the entry in the death register (death certificate) may be needed for the will and other claims.

REPORTING A DEATH TO THE CORONER

Coroners (in England and Wales) investigate any sudden or unexplained death. In Scotland such deaths are reported to the Procurator Fiscal. The following circumstances in palliative care require the death to be reported to the coroner:

- death occurred during surgery or within 24 hours
- a war pension was held
- the deceased had not been seen or treated by a doctor within the last 14 days
- death may be due to an industrial disease
- any suspicious circumstances.

Coroners may authorize registration of the death if they are satisfied that it was due to natural causes or order a postmortem (no requirement for consent). An inquest/fatal accident enquiry may be ordered to investigate the cause of death prior to releasing the body and allowing its registration.

FUNERAL DIRECTORS

Funeral directors are available 24 hours a day, and where a person dies at home they can arrange for the deceased to be removed at any time. Final funeral arrangements should not be made until it is certain that the death will not be reported to the coroner.

Funerals can be expensive and in certain circumstances the Benefits Agency may offer assistance. Banks, building societies or national savings can release funds for funeral expenses, but only with documentary evidence.

Where the deceased had not arranged their own funeral, the funeral directors can make the necessary arrangements. Funeral directors will also arrange for the deceased to be transported within the country or abroad, as required.

ORGAN DONATION

Organ donation can sometimes offer comfort to relatives, as they feel something good has come out of the death. Patients who die from some cancers may still be able to donate selected organs, including corneas, heart valves, trachea and kidneys (in selected patients), but acceptance also depends on meeting the general criteria for organ donation, e.g. age limits and the absence of certain conditions.

FOLLOW-UP SUPPORT AND COUNSELLING

The nurse can help and support family and friends during bereavement by answering questions, listening and helping them to come to terms with their loss, which may require specialist help and counselling.

GRIEF AND BEREAVEMENT

Grief is intensely personal and is a normal and necessary reaction to loss. Although everyone has different experiences, there will be common elements.

A common first response to bad news or loss is shock. This can still occur with an expected death. Shock may last for a week or two, often allowing relatives to cope with the practical funeral arrangements. It can, however, involve denial that is finally confronted by the reality of the funeral. As the shock recedes, the bereaved person begins to feel the physical intensity of the death, and only now can he or she begin to come to terms with the loss.

Both physical and mental manifestations are common and may include shortness of breath, palpitations, dry mouth, anorexia, lack of energy, poor concentration and insomnia (see above). Some might be caused or exacerbated by drugs (prescribed or otherwise) or an increased intake of alcohol. Isolation and loneliness may be experienced as family and friends disperse following the funeral.

According to Worden (1991) there are four basic tasks involved in progressing through the grief process:

- to accept the reality of loss
- to experience the pain of grief

- to adjust to an environment in which the dead person is missing
- to relocate the deceased person emotionally and move on with life.

Experiencing grief can be painful, with feelings of fear, guilt, anger and possibly resentment. Fear can be felt as insecurity and a longing to escape from reality. Most bereaved people feel guilt, e.g. through not having expressed their feelings, or because they wished their loved one would die to prevent further suffering. Anger may be directed at family, health professionals and even the deceased for leaving them.

Adjusting to a new environment can be difficult as well as learning to cope on one's own, perhaps after 50 years of marriage. Combined with an uncertain future, the whole process can be both daunting and frightening.

The final task, of moving on, can take over a year, or much longer in some instances. Although the person left behind may have fully accepted the loss and said goodbye to the deceased, the memories linger.

Abnormal grief

The grieving process may go wrong for a variety of reasons, creating abnormal reactions (Worden 1991) of chronic, delayed or exaggerated grief. Grief may become chronic when there is an inability to relinquish the dead person and mourning is excessive, e.g. a room is preserved as a shrine, which prevents the person returning to normal living.

Delayed (inhibited) grief occurs when normal grieving is postponed by avoiding the painful emotions. This might be achieved by keeping busy, moving house or forming new relationships very quickly. Occasionally there is denial and a complete inability to accept the loss of a loved one. The feelings of grief may return on the occasion of a future loss with greater intensity, as if all the 'bottled-up feelings are let loose'.

A person experiencing exaggerated grief becomes totally overwhelmed by the feelings of loss, often resulting in severe anxiety, depression or dependence on alcohol or drugs.

Presentation of unresolved grief

Unresolved grief may present as:

- persistent depression or false euphoria
- intense emotions when talking about the deceased
- intense grief reactions following a minor event
- continually talking about the loss
- an inability to remove or part with possessions long after the death
- self-destructive impulses and actions.

HELP DURING BEREAVEMENT

Bereavement counselling

Most bereaved people complete the grieving processes with the support of family and friends. Talking about the death and the person can help. There will be some people who need extra help.

Bereavement counselling aims to help them accept the loss by allowing them to acknowledge and express both negative and positive feelings about the deceased. They are supported as they grieve and reassured that their feelings are normal, thus allowing them to understand the need to move on. Counselling may also identify problems such as alcohol misuse or depression.

Support organizations

There are a number of organizations (professional and voluntary) that help during bereavement. Hospices and specialist units sometimes offer bereavement follow-up meetings. Other services include telephone follow-up, support groups or one-to-one counselling. Specialist Macmillan and Marie Curie nurses undertake bereavement visits to ensure that the bereaved person is coping. Some useful information sources are included at the end of the chapter.

SUMMARY: MAIN POINTS

- Palliative care offers a combination of care in a variety of settings, provided by the NHS, social services, charities and volunteers.

- The diagnosis of a terminal illness produces complex emotions in patients and families.

- Providing palliative care can affect health and social care staff emotionally.

- Many ethical issues exist in palliative care.

- Nursing assessment in palliative care aims to establish trust in the nurse–patient relationship and identify any problems experienced by the patient and family.

- CNSs assist the primary carers to acquire the skills and knowledge needed to deliver high-quality care.

- Symptom relief is central to palliative care and the quality of life of patients and families.

- Grief is an intensely personal and normal reaction to loss.

- Understanding the spiritual and cultural beliefs and needs of patients is especially important in palliative care.

SELF-TEST: CRITICAL THINKING ACTIVITIES

1 Select a terminally ill patient who is going home and look at the discharge plan:
   — What areas are included in the plan?
   — Think about the effectiveness of the plan.
   — What changes would you make? Give reasons for and support any changes.

FURTHER READING

Baines M. Drug control of common symptoms. Sydenham: St Christopher's Hospice; 1990.

Barraclough J. Cancer and emotion. Chichester: Wiley; 1994.

Dickenson D, Johnson M (eds). Death, dying and Bereavement. London: Sage; 1993.

Doyle D, Hanks GW, MacDonald N (eds). Oxford textbook of palliative medicine. Oxford: Oxford University Press; 1993.

Kubler-Ross E. On death and dying. London: Tavistock; 1970.

Neuberger J. Caring for dying people of different faiths, 2nd edn. London: Mosby; 1994.

Rang HP, Dale MM, Ritter JM. Pharmacology, 4th edn. Edinburgh: Churchill Livingstone; 1999.

Reynard CFB, Tempest S. A guide to symptom relief in advanced cancer. Manchester: Haigh & Hochland; 1992.

Robbins J (ed). Caring for the dying patient. London: Chapman & Hall; 1992.

Vickers A. Massage and aromatherapy: a guide for health professionals. London: Chapman & Hall; 1996.

USEFUL ADDRESSES

BACUP (British Association of Cancer United Patients)
3 Bath Place
Rivington St
London EC2A 3JR
Tel: 0207 613 2121 (0800 181199 outside London)
Information available from specialist cancer nurses, practical advice, emotional support and various publications

CRUSE – Bereavement Care
Cruse House
126 Sheen Rd
Richmond
Surrey TW9 1UR
Tel: 0208 940 4818
Charity with a network of local branches, offers practical advice and bereavement counselling

Help The Aged
St James Walk
London EC1R 0BE
Tel. 0207 253 0253
Publishes bereavement-related material

The National Association of Bereavement Services
20 Norton Folgate
London E1 6DB
Tel: 0207 247 1080
Provides information of local support agencies

The Samaritans
National number: Tel 0345 90 90 90 (Lo-call); local branch numbers in Phone Book
Charity offering a 24-hour service listening to people who need to talk

The War Widows Association of Great Britain
17 The Earls Croft
Coventry CV3 5ES
Tel: 02476 503 298
Provides advice, help and support to all widows and dependants

USEFUL WEBSITES

www.MarkAllenGroup.com/mag.htm – International Journal of Palliative Care

REFERENCES

Bruera E. Anorexia, cachexia and nutrition. Br Med J 1997; 315: 1219–1222.

Cowe F. Living wills: making patients' wishes known. Prof Nurse 1996; 11(6): 362–363.

Crossfield T. How to formulate patient assessment. Nurs Stand 1989; 3(44): 45.

Dunlop RJ, Elershaw JE, Baines MJ, Sykes N, Saunders CM. On with-holding nutrition and hydration in the terminally ill: has palliative medicine gone too far? A reply. J Med Ethics 1995; 21(3): 141–143.

Ellis P. Euthanasia: the way to a peaceful end? Prof Nurse 1991; 7(3): 157–160.

Glaser BG, Strauss AL. Awareness of dying. Weidenfeld & Nicholson. London; 1965.

Hampe S. Needs of the grieving spouse in a hospital setting. Nurs Res 1975; 24(2): 113–120.

Kaye P. A–Z pocketbook of symptom control. Northampton: EPL Publications; 1996.

Kubler-Ross E. On death and dying. London: Tavistock; 1970.

Lichter I, Hunt E. The last 48 hours of life. J Pall Care 1990; 6(4): 7–15.

Neuberger J. Caring for dying people of different faiths, 2nd edn. London: Mosby; 1994.

Nursing and Midwifery Council. Code of Professional Conduct. London: NMC; 2002.

Patchett M. Providing hydration for the terminally ill patient. Int J Pall Nurs 1998; 4(3): 143–146.

Rang HP, Dale MM, Ritter JM. Pharmacology, 3rd edn. Edinburgh: Churchill Livingstone; 1995.

Seale C. Death from cancer and death from other cause: the relevance of the hospice approach. Pall Med 1991; 5: 12–19.

Smith V. Support for the family in bereavement. In: David J, ed. Cancer care – prevention, treatment and palliation. London: Chapman & Hall; 1995.

Stoter DJ. Spiritual aspects of healthcare. London: Mosby; 1995.

Sykes NP. Constipation and diarrhoea. In: Doyle D, Hanks GW, MacDonald N, eds. Oxford textbook of palliative medicine. Oxford: Oxford University Press; 1993.

Townsend J, Frank AO, Fermont D, Dyer S, Karron O, Walgrave A, Piper M. Terminal cancer care and patients' preference for place of death: a prospective study. Br Med J 1990; 301: 415–417.

Trevelyan J, Booth B. Complementary medicine for nurses, midwives and health visitors. London: Macmillan; 1994.

Waterlow J. A risk assessment card. Nurs Times 1985; 81(48): 49–55.

World Health Organization. Cancer pain relief and palliative care. Technical Report, Series 804. Geneva: WHO; 1990.

Worden WJ. Grief counselling and grief therapy. London: Tavistock; 1991.

Wright L. Bowel function in hospital patients. London: Royal College of Nursing; 1974.

35 Nursing patients with chronic (long-term) illness and disability

Peter Griffiths

'When I saw the words "chronic condition" on my records I thought that was it – the end! But twenty years later I'm still here! It meant I had to change my job and make a few changes around the house but other than that no-one would know.'

(Patient)

THIS CHAPTER WILL HELP YOU

- Define impairment and disability
- Identify the prevalence of chronic disease and disability
- Understand the key challenges facing a person coming to terms with long-term impairment
- Understand how approaches to care for those with chronic illness may differ from those with acute illness.

KEYWORDS

Chronic illness	Handicap
Disability	Impairment

INTRODUCTION

Nursing patients' with chronic illness and disability is a topic that is nearly as big as nursing itself. The older person with multiple pathologies and the young person with paraplegia are obvious extremes. In between fall a range of conditions and approaches to nursing care delivered in a variety of settings. It may well be that the majority of medical conditions and a fair proportion of the surgical ones described in this book are to some degree chronic conditions with the potential to cause significant disability. The 'acute' event of a heart attack (see Ch. 19) can be the first or last step on a career of chronic illness which may ultimately result in disability or death.

Many diseases that were once universally and rapidly fatal are now prevalent as chronic diseases. One of the most striking examples is type 1 diabetes, which, until the availability of insulin, always resulted in a quick death. Those diagnosed with diabetes today can look forward to a long life, albeit one that may be punctuated by acute illness and the disabling consequences of the disease. Even diseases such as HIV infection and AIDS are now often regarded as chronic diseases, since life expectancy has increased dramatically with the advent of new therapies. For many patients seen on hospital wards, the presenting illness is an acute exacerbation of an underlying chronic disorder with which they must live. Studies by the World Health Organization (WHO) suggest that in developed countries like Britain as many years of potentially healthy life are 'lost' to disability as to premature death (Murray & Lopez 1996).

Nurses have always been active in the care of patients with long-term illness and disability but in the future, many of the most advanced nursing roles are likely to be with this client group. Nurses are taking more and more responsibility in both managing and delivering care for clients with chronic illness in a range of settings, including hospital wards, outpatient clinics and GP surgeries. People with severe disability are increasingly receiving almost all their care outside traditional hospitals. Even in long-term care settings such as nursing homes, care can be far more dynamic and challenging than simply 'care-taking', which has often been seen as the main nursing role in the past.

WHAT IS ILLNESS, SICKNESS AND DISABILITY?

DEFINITIONS OF CHRONIC ILLNESS

Chronic illness is not a single entity. The term is used to refer to health problems which persist over an extended period and which are usually (but not always) associated with some degree of disability. The effect on the individual varies despite similar underlying pathology. For example, heart failure may be totally disabling in one person while necessitating only minor adjustments in lifestyle for another. In many respects this is because chronic illnesses are not simply static entities. The disease, the associated disability and the person's response will all change over time.

Nonetheless there are common features. Firstly, chronic illness must be contrasted with acute illness. An acute illness generally has a rapid onset with distinct signs and symptoms which are directly associated with the pathology. For example, a febrile response is elicited by a range of acute infections and is part of the body's attempts to combat invasion of pathogens (see Chs 5 and 13). The signs and symptoms disappear as the disease itself resolves. If the disease does not resolve, the disease is either fatal or it becomes chronic.

A range of definitions has been offered for chronic disease (Curtin & Lubkin 1997). Clearly a chronic disease lasts for an extended period but few definitions specify how long. Many definitions identify the chronic disease as 'incurable' or one from which recovery can only be partial. Since many chronic illnesses are also ultimately life-threatening, the distinction between acute and chronic illness rests in part in the potential for cure but also in the extent to which the person experiences the chronic illness for sufficient time for it to be incorporated into their lifestyle and identity. The defining aspects of chronic illnesses are listed in Table 35.1, along with examples of some disorders that might display those characteristics.

DEFINITION OF DISABILITY AND HANDICAP

Disability is frequently associated with chronic illness. Disability is an emotive and controversial term. For many years WHO's International Classification of Disease Impairment and Handicap (ICDIH) system has provided a standard definition of disability as an inability to function at the level an individual might reasonably expect (Wood 1980). Disability is contrasted with impairment, which is a pathophysiological condition, and handicap, the social disadvantages which occur consequent to the impairment or disability.

However, the ICDIH classification has been widely criticized as focusing too much on impairment as the sole cause of disability and handicap at the neglect of the role society plays in causing disability and handicap (Oliver 1998). An alternative classification is offered by disabled people themselves, who have formulated the 'social model' of disability. According to this approach, there is a simple dichotomy between impairment – 'the functional limitation within the individual caused by physical, mental or

Table 35.1 A definition of chronic illness
(defined by one or more of the following – Strauss 1976)

Definition	Example of chronic illnesses
Permanence	Diabetes Peripheral vascular disease
Residual disability	CVA (stroke) Multiple sclerosis
Non-reversible pathology	Arthritis Osteoporosis
Requires extended rehabilitation	Serious head injury CVA (stroke)
Requires major adaptation in lifestyle	Heart failure Epilepsy
Requires long periods of supervision, observation or care	Breast cancer Asthma

CVA, cerebrovascular accident.

sensory impairment' – and disability – 'the loss or limitation of opportunities to take part in the normal life of the community on an equal level with others because of physical and social barriers' (Oliver 1998). According to this approach, impairment neither directly causes nor justifies disability. Disability is regarded as a form of discrimination against the impaired. Figure 35.1 shows the contrast between these two definitions.

An example of the social causation of disability and handicap is the failure of many organizations to provide adequate access to places of work for those with sight or mobility problems. Even where impairment presents the individual with minimal obstacles, the stigma attached to many chronic diseases and disabilities can cause significant handicap. An obvious example is HIV infection where the individual can suffer significant handicap because of discrimination despite being physically unaffected by the virus. Stigma is attached to many other chronic diseases including cancer and, in many cultures, tuberculosis.

A new classification, the international classification of functioning disability and health (ICF), has recently been devised (WHO 2001), which takes into account some of the criticisms levelled by the social model. The separate classification of handicap is dispensed with. Disability is defined as a loss of function at the level of the individual which is caused by an interaction between personal factors (including impairment) and environmental factors (including discrimination) (WHO 1999).

The value of this view of disability is that it draws attention away from the 'cure' of impairment as the only remedy for disability. This is as relevant to those whose disability is caused by chronic illness as for those whose disability has been caused by accident or congenital conditions and syndromes. For example, chronic illnesses leading to mobility impairment would be far less disabling if wheelchair access to public transport and buildings were universal. The nurse caring for those with disability must be mindful that disability is not simply caused by the person's impairment. Cure of the impairment is frequently impossible and not necessarily the most desirable strategy. However, this does not mean that disability is inevitable or not subject to improvement through nursing care.

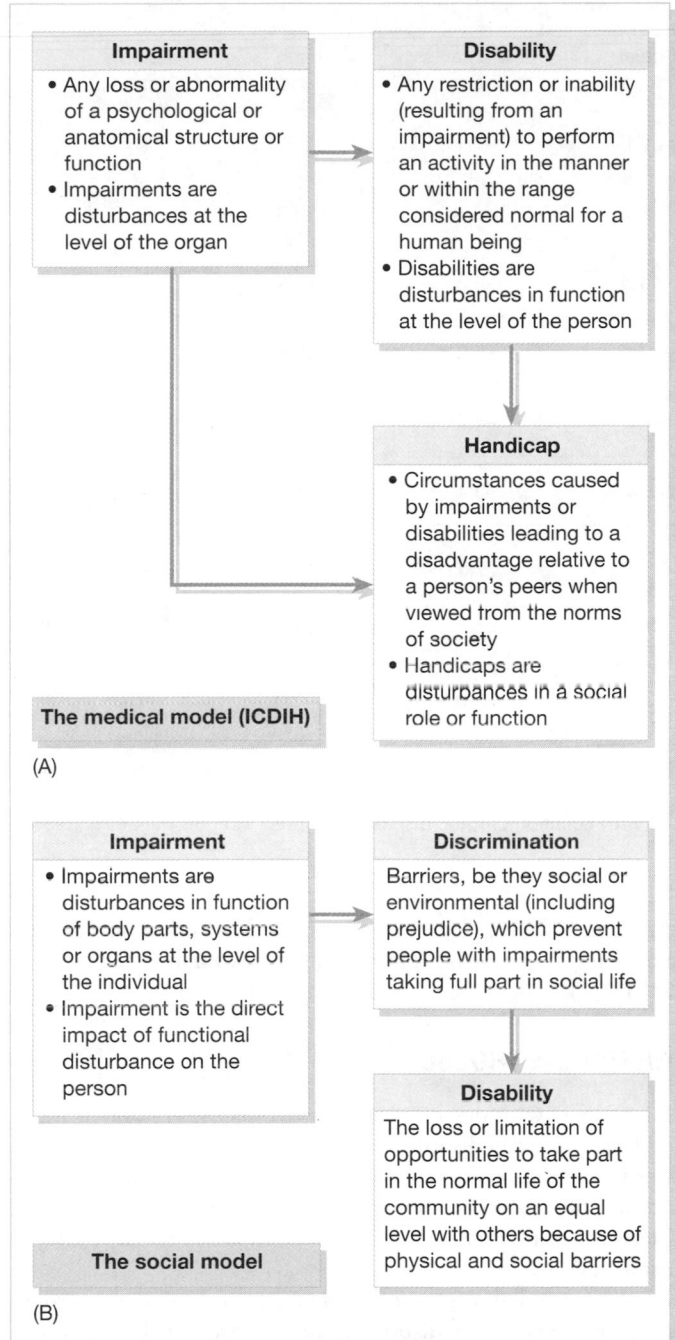

Figure 35.1   Contrasting definitions of disability.

Table 35.2 The leading causes of life-years lost to death and disability in the developed world (Murray & Lopez 1996)

Disease/disorder group	DALYs
Neuropsychiatric disorders	22.0%
Cardiovascular disorders	20.4%
Malignant diseases	13.7%
Unintentional injuries	10.3%
Respiratory disorders	4.8%
Digestive disorders	4.4%
Musculoskeletal disorders	4.3%
Intentional injuries	4.2%
Infectious and parasitic diseases	2.7%
Congenital abnormalities	2.2%

DALY, disability-adjusted life year.

(adjusted for severity). The impact of a particular disease can be measured in DALYs lost.

COMMON CAUSES OF DISABILITY

In developing countries, the leading contributors to the burden of disease are communicable diseases (see Ch. 32), maternal and perinatal disorders, and nutritional disorders (see Ch. 11). Together these account for 49% of all DALYs. The majority of the burden of disease is premature death. In the developed world these conditions account for just 7.8% of the burden of disease (Murray & Lopez 1996). Table 35.2 shows the leading causes of DALYs in the developed world, all of which have considerable potential to cause chronic illness or disability.

THE IMPACT OF CHRONIC ILLNESS

Chronic illness is caused by a range of impairments that affect bodily systems in a variety of ways and does not necessarily lead to disability. The effect of impairment will vary considerably depending on the individual's ability to cope and the severity of the impairment itself. In Britain, 35% of the population report suffering from a long-standing illness and 22% report a long-standing illness that limits their activity; in adults aged 75 and over, this figure rises to 52% (Thomas et al 1998).

Health care professionals may fail to recognize the extent to which many chronic illnesses impact on all areas of a person's functioning. The ability to manage day-to-day activities like shopping and cleaning, the ability to work, care for a family and to enjoy hobbies or the company of others are all frequently affected. The following sections are based on a survey that studied the effects of a range of chronic illnesses on a sample of 9385 adults in the USA (Stewart et al 1989). Their ability to participate in physical activities and contribute to work, home and social life (called functional status) were measured and compared with the functional status of people who attended their doctors but had no chronic illness. In addition their mental health, perception of their own health and pain were also assessed. Figure 35.2 shows the extent to which different illnesses affected people in these areas.

PREVALENCE AND IMPACT OF CHRONIC ILLNESS AND DISABILITY

The relative significance of chronic disease and associated disability has increased in developed countries in response to increases in life expectancy and improved treatment and prevention of communicable diseases. The WHO has used disability-adjusted life years (DALYs) to measure the burden of disease (Murray & Lopez 1996). The DALY is an indicator of the number of years of life lost to premature death or lived with a disability

	Physical function	Role function	Social function	Mental health	Health perception	Bodily pain
Hypertension	0	+1.2	+1.1	−1.1	−3.5	+3.1
Diabetes	−7.6	−9.4	−5.3	+0.1	−12.8	−0.6
Congestive heart failure	−22.5	−28.2	−11.4	−4.3	−13.4	−1.1
Myocardial infarction	−26.2	−33.0	− 11.6	−2.8	−9.9	−2.5
Lung problems	−13.4	−12.9	−7.1	−4.4	−13.0	−4.2
Angina	−15.7	−15.6	−5.4	−3.4	−13.2	−7.3
Back problems	−9.5	−8.2	−2.1	−1.0	−4.3	−10.4
Gastrointestinal problems	−6.7	−14.2	−7.8	−7.3	−13.8	−12.1
Arthritis	−9.3	−10.3	−3.9	−3.0	−7.3	−16.6

Figure 35.2 Change in function (%) relative to general population associated with common chronic disease. (Adapted from Stewart et al 1989.)

One of the most common chronic illnesses is hypertension. Approximately 9% of the UK population receive treatment for raised blood pressure, while a greater number are hypertensive but untreated (Bennet et al 1995). Hypertension seems to have little effect on people's ability to lead a normal life and functional status is hardly affected. However, the person's perception of being healthy is reduced (Stewart et al 1989).

Of the disorders studied by Stewart et al (1989), cardiac disorders (see Ch. 19) seem to have the greatest effect of all on functional status, but diabetes (see Ch. 17), arthritis (see Ch. 27), chronic lung disease (see Ch. 20) and gastrointestinal disorders (see Ch. 22) also significantly reduce all aspects of functional status. Back problems significantly affect physical and role functioning (such as the ability to work) but do not seem to affect social functioning. All the chronic disorders listed in Table 35.1 reduce people's perception of themselves as healthy and, most significantly, also reduce psychological well-being (mental health). Although Stewart et al (1989) did not include people who had suffered a stroke (see Ch. 14) in their sample, there can be little doubt that the impairment and disability can have a massive effect on all aspects of a person's function far beyond the obvious functional limitation caused by hemiparesis.

Negative beliefs about, and the prospect of controlling, impairment can have negative consequences. People who have suffered a myocardial infarction (see Ch. 19) are less likely to attend rehabilitation programmes if they have a negative view of the possibility that their illness can be controlled. A negative view of the consequences of the illness is related to delays in returning to work. Negative attitudes to health are also related to disability in physical, role, social and sexual functions (Petrie et al 1996).

MULTIPLE PATHOLOGY

Many people with one chronic disorder also suffer one or more additional chronic disorders and in many cases the secondary disorders are related to the primary one. Just as multiple acute pathology can significantly complicate treatment in acute conditions so function is additionally impaired with multiple chronic disease.

Those with diabetes have a higher risk of developing cardiac problems, circulatory disorders, stroke (see Ch. 14) or renal disease (see Ch. 24). As discussed earlier, hypertension on its own causes relatively little disability but, if poorly controlled, carries a risk of many other chronic circulatory disorders. Those with impaired mobility are at risk of a range of conditions, including osteoporosis (see Ch. 27) due to reduced loading in weight-bearing bones. People whose mobility is extremely restricted, such as those with paraplegia, are at risk of a range of conditions, including pressure ulcers (see Ch. 10), lung problems, bladder infections and other disorders of the urinary tract.

COMMON FEATURES OF CHRONIC ILLNESS

Perhaps the most striking common feature of chronic illnesses is the tendency for them to become incorporated into a person's identity. People with hypertension identify themselves as less healthy despite suffering few other effects. In other cases, the impact on a person's identity is more fundamental, with challenges to many of the person's most significant social roles, such as breadwinner and parent. These challenges are both internal, as sufferers questions their own ability to cope, and external, as others question and challenge the ability of such people to fulfil normal social roles.

Friends and relatives are often actively involved in care but even when they are not, their lives are likely to be affected, in some cases just as much as those with the impairment. The care of friends and relatives is an important part of the nursing care of those with chronic illness and disability. Their role in the life of the person is of far more significance than that of health care professionals, whose contact is often fleeting.

In an acute illness, the main emphasis is on cure and the majority of effort from the client and therapists is directed toward that end. Chronic illness requires different strategies from both the person with the disorder and the health care professionals. In a chronic illness, disability cannot be relieved or avoided by 'curing' the impairment. Although management of the underlying disorder is of great significance, it is important that effort is invested in developing strategies to minimize disability which may follow from the impairment.

While clients should always be encouraged to become active participants in their health, this is of paramount importance with chronic illness and disability. This requires a significant shift in emphasis by all concerned, including nurses. A passive response to chronic illness may be associated with increased disability. The perception that little can be done to alleviate impairment can impede the person's ability to undertake activities that avoid or reduce disability.

PREVENTION AND REHABILITATION IN CHRONIC ILLNESS AND DISABILITY

During the 1990s, the UK set targets for the reduction of major threats to health (Department of Health 1999), all of which are leading causes of chronic illness and disability. Targets were set for the reduction in rates of accidents, heart disease, stroke, mental illness and cancer. The strategies employed recognized that provision of understandable and credible information to people was a necessary but insufficient way of achieving changes in health at the individual level. In order to reduce the incidence of disease, the social and economic causes such as poverty and social isolation must be tackled. Similarly, the prevention of disability when impairment has occurred is not simply an individual act.

The nursing care of those with a long-term impairment must begin with the identification of the individual and social resources that are available to prevent disability. It is all too easy to focus on what patients cannot do at the expense of what they can do. There is some evidence that traditional approaches to nursing care, particularly in hospital settings, may actually cause disability (Miller 1985). For those who are recovering from a self-limiting illness, dependence on nursing care is unlikely to have long-term consequences. However, if the impairment is long term, e.g. after a stroke, nursing care which focuses on doing for patients what they cannot do for themselves is likely to reinforce dependence and hence disability. Relatives

and friends may also believe this is in the best interest of the patient when in fact such an approach can actively encourage disability.

By contrast, nursing care can be positively therapeutic (Griffiths 1995, Griffiths & Wilson-Barnett 1998). Care that focuses on guiding and encouraging patients in order to adapt and find new ways of achieving their goals independently can actively contribute to prevention of disability for those with chronic impairments. The nurse's role in rehabilitation should be to prevent disability in those with an impairment.

Although the nursing goal may be active participation in care, this is not achieved by simply forcing independence on the person. A study of interactions between staff and older patients in a rehabilitation ward (Waters 1994) clearly demonstrated that nurses wishing to promote self-care must be active facilitators. This is not to be confused with simply leaving people to 'get on with it'. A nurse who simply washes patients who have difficulty washing themselves may be promoting disability. A nurse who simply leaves the same patients to wash themselves is doing nothing but providing the equipment. The nurse who stays with patients and offers guidance, suggestions and some assistance is able to set goals with them, monitor progress and actively promote independence. The care required is supervision and assistance that allows patients to move toward their own goals.

DEVELOPMENTAL, PSYCHOLOGICAL, SOCIAL AND CULTURAL FACTORS IN DISABILITY AND CHRONIC ILLNESS

A range of social and cultural factors affect the way that those with chronic illness or disability are regarded by others and the way they view themselves. These factors can, in turn, strongly influence the extent to which a person is able to adapt in order to prevent impairments leading to disability. As noted above, some regard disability as entirely the product of social forces. The sociologist Erving Goffman's work provides valuable insights. Goffman (1963) described 'stigma' as something that disqualifies a person from being fully socially accepted.

People have expectations of others that allow them to easily accommodate and categorize the social identity of others. Essentially, people have an expectation of what is 'normal' for a person in a particular social situation. Some aspects of chronic illness or disability are stigmatized because they are seen as undesirable but also because they are simply seen as 'abnormal'. They 'spoil' a person's social identity in a society that values being fit and healthy and has an expectation that most people will live long healthy lives (Goffman 1963). The stigma can overwhelm all other appraisals of a person's abilities so that the impairment leads to that person being seen as disabled in ways far beyond the areas of function affected by the illness.

The situation is encapsulated by the question 'Does he take sugar?' asked of the person accompanying the young, fit and cognitively intact person with cerebral palsy who happens to have impairments that affect mobility. The stigma of disability is such that some people simply presume that the person with disability is unable to function normally in any way and therefore cannot usefully fulfil any social role, except that of 'invalid'.

TYPES OF STIGMA

Physical deformity

In many cases it is easy to see the characteristics of chronic illness or disability which can lead to a person being stigmatized. It is obvious to others when a person is using a wheelchair or has a speech impediment. In these cases the stigma is that of physical deformity. A condition such as stroke does not carry a great stigma in itself, although the outward effects may do. Some conditions do not necessarily manifest themselves outwardly, but the knowledge that a person has a particular illness can be enough to stigmatize that person. Both AIDS and cancer (Ch. 33) are associated with a degree of stigma. Both are clearly associated with premature death and for some people this is enough to 'spoil' the social identity of the person with the disease.

Self-inflicted conditions

In the case of AIDS or HIV infection, there is an added stigma which is associated with the perceived responsibility the person has for the condition. The stigma of such 'character blemishes' (Goffman 1963) is also associated with conditions related to alcohol dependence and, increasingly, some smoking-related illnesses.

Prejudice

A third type of stigma is more commonly known as prejudice, where one social group identifies another as in some way deficient on the basis of characteristics such as race, sexuality or religious affiliation. While such stigma does not result directly from chronic illness, some illnesses are (rightly or wrongly) associated with particular social groups who suffer prejudice. An example is the association between male homosexuality and AIDS.

RESPONSES TO STIGMA

People suffering from chronic illness, their family and friends and health care professionals may all be subject to the influence of social stigma. Those who develop a chronic illness or disability will share many of the same norms, values and prejudices concerning stigmatizing illnesses as the society they live in. Just as others may have difficulty accepting them as full members of society, they too may struggle to fully value themselves. While it is important for nurses to be aware of stigma associated with particular conditions, it is clear that the individual nurse working with the individual patient cannot change the wider social values that lead to stigma. However, awareness of the potential effects of stigma can assist nurses to help clients avoid the worst consequences (see Reflective Practice box 35.1).

Disregard

The person subject to stigma may simply attempt to disregard its effect (Saylor & Yoder 1998). As a coping strategy this has positive and negative aspects. On the positive side, choosing to invest little effort in contemplation of the negative responses of others may reflect a confident individual who is well adjusted to the condition. This may be the case with those who have dealt with a stigmatizing condition for a long time. An example of

35.1 The unpopular patient

In 1973, Felicity Stockwell's classic study coined the term 'the unpopular patient' (Stockwell 1984). She identified factors which lead to some patients being 'unpopular' among nurses caring for them. Many of the factors that she identified often apply to those with long-term sickness and disability:

- Many have repeated contact with health care professionals and long hospital stays.
- Their problems are not solved by a simple cure and can be very complex.
- People with long-term impairment are not readily accommodated within the accepted boundaries of the sick role.
- They may be more expert in their own condition or disability than the nurses caring for them.
- In the face of necessary dependence, they may well choose to exert control over their care which can make professionals feel uncomfortable.
- They are often labelled 'demanding'.

Student activities

- Identify a patient you have recently encountered who had a long-term disability.
- Consider how the patient's experience of encounters with professionals differs from that of those with short-term illness.
- How was caring for the patient different from caring for someone whose illness was short term?
- What strategies might you use to recognize the knowledge and expertise of the client and/or carers in planning care?
- What did you find most difficult about caring for this person?
- Did you find the patient 'demanding'?

such disregard may be the determination of a former soldier, who had lost an arm and leg in a mine clearance operation, to undertake an arduous journey through the Himalayas to raise funds for a mine clearance charity. His determination to succeed in an endeavour that others might regard as impossible for him can be seen as an example of disregarding stigma.

However, for those newly diagnosed with a stigmatizing condition, such disregard may be a negative coping strategy, which denies them the opportunity to address the obstacles facing them constructively. A failure to acknowledge the reality of stigma can lead to an increased vulnerability to its effects. The phenomenon of disregard can be paralleled with the 'denial' stage of the grief response.

It is important for nurses to strike a balance between encouraging patients to be self-confident in the face of their own impairment and encouraging the adoption of normal social roles while being realistic about the obstacles.

Resistance

A response related to disregard is resistance. Rather than ignoring the restrictions and stigmas imposed on them, patients actively challenge them. An example of a positive aspect of this response is organized campaigns which have led to improved access to public buildings, particularly for those with impaired mobility. Resistance can be an important step towards autonomy for many people who have become dependent upon others. A negative aspect of this response is the expenditure of energy on angry responses to circumstances that individuals cannot change by themselves. Anger can distance potential sources of social and emotional support.

Isolation

One response to stigma may be to isolate oneself from the source. Again this response can have both positive and negative aspects. Close identification with an 'in' group of friends, family or other people with similar conditions can have a positive effect by reinforcing self-esteem and providing protection from the negative attitudes of others. However, such separation can serve to emphasize the difference between the stigmatized person and others and complete dependence on immediate family or close friends may put undue strain on relationships. In extreme cases, people may withdraw from society completely if they are unable to identify a safe group.

Secondary gains

Individuals may seek to gain maximum benefit from the stigma. For example, they may emphasize their dependence in order to gain maximum help and support. Health professionals generally regard such behaviour as undesirable but it is important that nurses do not simply dismiss it. Rather they should attempt to assess the reasons for behaviour designed to secure secondary gains and be open to the fact that genuine need may exist. If care needs are to be negotiated with clients, nurses cannot simply dismiss their behaviour or perspective of their dependency.

Passing

Some stigmatizing conditions which are not externally apparent provide the opportunity for the response of 'passing' (Goffman 1963). Conditions such as cancer, HIV or diabetes allow sufferers to 'pass' as unaffected by a stigmatizing condition in many aspects of life and thus avoid stigma. This may be advantageous and prevent them from suffering disability as a result of the reactions of others. For example, people with chronic illnesses often fear that their employment will be affected if their employer becomes aware of the condition. However, in some circumstances, such passing may result in behaviour that is detrimental to the individual. For example, a person with diabetes may ignore dietary restrictions or medication regimens in an attempt to hide the disorder from others. Passing can also impede the ability of patients to come to terms with their condition and develop a positive self-image.

Covering

Goffman (1963) describes a further response known as 'covering' in which the impairment is acknowledged but difference from the norm is de-emphasized by downplaying its significance. A person with a diagnosis of cancer may overestimate their prognosis for the benefit of others in order to allow them to be treated as normal since the anxiety provoked in others is reduced.

CULTURAL VARIATIONS

Stigma is a valuable framework for understanding many aspects of how those with chronic illness and disability are treated in our society and in many others. However, the view of those with a particular impairment varies between cultures and between cultural subgroups. Different conditions are associated with stigma to varying extents and the perceptions of particular impairments change over time.

In the developed world, cancer seems to be stigmatized because of its close association with death. Although perceptions may gradually be changing, many cancer patients still experience the situation where friends and acquaintances feel such discomfort that they avoid the person with the disease. In industrialized societies, epilepsy carries great stigma which leads to discrimination in many aspects of life, including employment. In contrast, some sectors of Brazilian society and African tribes revere those with epilepsy, as they qualify for prestigious social roles as witchdoctors or mediums.

The advent of HIV-related disease introduced a new stigma. Within certain groups, notably the gay community in the 1980s, the stigma was similar to that associated with cancer. Within other groups, it carried far more stigma because of prejudice and judgements about behaviours that could label sufferers as responsible for their predicament. In Africa, HIV is associated with heterosexuals and does not carry the same degree of stigma.

It is important that nurses recognize that even familiar cultures contain subgroups, which may lead to a particular impairment being viewed in different ways. Nurses should not simply assume that they know and share the same perspective as their clients.

COMING TO TERMS WITH CHRONIC ILLNESS

Patterson et al (1998), who reviewed a series of studies on patients' adaptation to diabetes, describe the process as one of achieving balance between the management of the disease and the need to have a normal life. This is done by assuming control for the management of the illness and learning about the bodily experience; understanding the cues provided by fluctuating blood sugar facilitates this. In addition, the diabetic person gains a knowledge of strategies which are successful in resolving problems.

Knowledge of the pathophysiology and the rationale for interventions may underpin this and can be shared by professionals. However, the individual expertise of patients is greater than this because of their personal experience and unique insight into their own condition. Developing collaborative, supportive relationships with 'allies' who have a basic understanding of the condition is important and it is clear that nurses might fulfil this role. However, professionals do not fill these roles exclusively. To be successful, the health care professional must have a knowledge of the individual and value his or her experience. The importance of continuity of care for those with chronic illness and disability cannot be over-emphasized. The long-term relationship between nurse and client may be vital in developing a meaningful and constructive therapeutic relationship.

Stages of adaptation

Norris et al (1998) described the process by which those with an alteration in body image or function come to terms with their impairment. Although the process is highly individual, they described three stages that the people tend to move through.

Disruption phase

During the body image disruption phase, they experienced grief and a sense of loss, often accompanied by depression, anger or self-pity. During this stage, denial, avoidance of the truth and attempts to conceal the situation from others are common.

Wishing for restoration

During this second phase, people experience hopefulness, which sometimes drives extreme efforts to alleviate or reduce the impairment. Accompanying this is an intense emotional pain as restorative efforts fail to yield the hoped-for result of cure or removal of the impairment. It is important to recognize that nurses must be careful to strike a balance between encouraging individuals in those things which provide hope while attempting to help them to channel their efforts into activities which are more likely to yield benefit. People who believe that impairments can be cured or controlled are more likely to participate in rehabilitation programmes. Hope is an important motivator and it is important not to simply undermine it even when the client is unrealistic.

Re-imaging the self

The final phase, re-imaging the self, occurs as the person finds a balance between efforts at restoration and the personal costs of those efforts. As this balance is achieved, energy can be expended on developing a positive self-image based on current capabilities rather than on an idealized version of self.

Psychological, social and cultural factors

Various factors influence a person's adaptation to impairment. A person to whom external body image is very important will find it harder to develop a positive self-image. Someone whose self-esteem was already high is more likely to be able to restore it. Those who feel others value them and do not feel stigmatized will be more able to value themselves. It is important that the services offered by health care professionals are acceptable. For example, someone with dark skin is less likely to come to a positive self-image after an amputation if the prosthesis offered is not of a matching skin colour. People whose lives are active and full or who are striving to develop a career may be particularly affected by the long waits that are often endured in hospital outpatient clinics. Services need to be organized in such a way as to value the strengths and respect the needs of the individual, not reinforce powerlessness and the feeling of loss.

It should be noted that there is a marked cultural variation in illness response, which applies as much to chronic as to acute illness. Such cultural variation can influence the extent to which an individual successfully adapts to a particular impairment. For example, it is widely noted that some cultural groups

have a stoical approach to pain until it becomes unbearable, at which point they withdraw from social contact. This may help or hinder adaptation, depending on the severity of the pain.

DEVELOPMENTAL FACTORS

The effect that chronic illness has on an individual's social identity is to some degree affected by the stage of life the person is at. Overcoming impairment and avoiding disability demand considerable effort by people of any age, but particular age groups are recognized as having particular problems associated with impairments. Factors affecting adolescents and young, middle-aged and older adults are addressed below. The problems discussed in each section may be 'typical' of those encountered at a particular stage in life, but many may be encountered at any stage of life. For example, while issues of sexuality may pose particular problems for the adolescent, it is clear that changes in body image or sexual function can have a profound impact on people of any age.

Adolescents

Adolescents may be faced with a new impairment or one that they have lived with for some time. In either case, the challenges of an impairment are complicated by the significant changes in role which occur for all making the transition to adulthood. Growing up involves an increasing independence from parents. A chronic impairment can increase dependence, resulting in an exacerbation in the conflict that often occurs between parents and adolescents. It is certainly vital for health care professionals to recognize that the adolescent's developmental task is independence. There is a danger that channelling all interventions through the parent(s) will delay development and the ability of individuals to assume control of aspects of their lives directly related to the impairment.

Normal adolescent concerns about relationships, appearance and sexuality may be exacerbated by their impairment. Those who have previously successfully managed a condition throughout their teenage life may now find that they need to come to a different balance between normality and the management of a chronic disease as new activities and priorities in life emerge. The young person with diabetes, confronted with friends who discover the joys of late nights, irregular hours and alcohol, may find it hard to balance such temptation with the management of blood sugar. It is unlikely that simple censure and advice to abstain will succeed in this situation. The long-term consequences of poor disease control are likely to carry little weight with the adolescent. Those involved in care need to take a realistic attitude to what might be achieved and seek to assist the person with finding the best balance that can be reached.

Young and middle-aged adults

The period between leaving full-time education and retirement constitutes the largest portion of most people's lives. This period is generally regarded as one in which people become increasingly socially and economically independent and assume a full part in 'normal' society. Individuals assume many changing roles. Individual choices and preferences differ enormously, but work, close sexual relationships and parenting are significant for most people. The ability to fulfil all these roles can be significantly reduced by chronic illness or impairment. In many cases, disability in these areas results from barriers imposed by society.

Disabled people often struggle to secure employment even when their ability to perform a particular job is not affected. The effect of an impairment is generalized in the eyes of others to create disability in spheres where none would otherwise exist. In the UK, legislation was passed in 1995 which was intended to reduce discrimination against disabled people in the job market. The legislation will be fully implemented by 2004; however, attitudes are harder to change. Furthermore, some people with chronic impairment may share the stigmatized view of themselves as unable to fulfil active roles in life. An important aspect of therapy for those experiencing impairments that threaten to cause disability may focus on ensuring that the individual's self-esteem is not undermined.

The ability to form close social and sexual relationships can be impeded by any barrier to situations that allow social interaction. The work environment is a key social meeting place. People may find themselves excluded from other forums of social interaction by their own limitations or those imposed by others. Those whose impairment is readily visible are limited in their ability to 'pass' as normal in many social situations.

The ability to fulfil parenting roles may be impeded by an impairment directly affecting fertility, by barriers to forming relationships with the opposite sex or by difficulties in providing physical, emotional or economic support to a child. Many chronic impairments can reduce the individual's desire or ability to enjoy an active sex life. Spinal trauma is widely recognized as potentially impeding sexual function but many diseases affecting the neurological or vascular systems can also impair sexual function (see Ch. 25), leading to erectile problems in men and reductions in lubrication and sensation in women. Many disorders such as diabetes and heart disease result in specific sexual impairments in addition to general loss of libido associated with reduced energy levels and depression.

It is important that professionals recognize the potential desire of a person of any age and with any impairment to engage in active social relationships, including physical ones. Professionals can be in danger of accepting the limited social roles undertaken by people as their norm when the people themselves may aspire to much more.

Older adults

As the life span increases in a population, the proportion of life spent disabled decreases (Murray & Lopez 1996). In the developed world, a 60-year-old might expect to spend approximately 20% of remaining life disabled. Certainly the proportion of people reporting limiting long-standing illness increases with age. Sixteen per cent of all older people (65 or over) in the UK report some difficulty in mobilizing without assistance and 10% are unable to manage self-care on their own (Thomas et al 1998).

Older people face many additional challenges in dealing with chronic illness. Despite the figures presented above, the majority of older people are well enough to be independent and lead active lives, but irrespective of chronic illness there is a stigma attached to ageing (Ch. 32). Upon retirement, older adults

OLDER ADULTS: NURSING PRIORITIES

35.1 Facilitating self-care

The nursing care of older adults with chronic illness or disability in general differs little from that of the general population with similar problems. Although we have noted particular difficulties encountered by older people in terms of stigma and reduced physiological reserve, this is generally a matter of degree. However, the elderly may be particularly vulnerable to dependence due to a general decline in functional or physiological reserve. Promoting self-care is an important priority.

The settings in which care is delivered often appear to hinder the promotion of self-care. At the same time, the attitudes of some older people to self-care and rehabilitation may present particular challenges for nurses.

- The organization of care for older people can often foster dependence.
- Doing things for patients that they can do for themselves may often appear to be a quicker alternative for nurses in institutional settings such as nursing homes or hospital wards.
- Meeting basic mobility and hygiene needs is often delegated to untrained staff who may fail to recognize the importance of rehabilitation.
- The more active role a patient is expected to take in chronic disease management and rehabilitation can be perceived as a neglect of professional duty.
- Nurses should not assume that anyone wishes to take an active part in their own care. Patient participation should be the subject of careful negotiation.
- Many older people have grown up expecting to take a passive role in health care.
- In part, this is based on historical deference to professionals, in part, the changing profile of diseases and professional attitudes to care
- In addition, many people regard disability as an inevitable part of ageing and may thus be more accepting of it.

Ultimately the amount of personal effort and energy that will be expended on overcoming disability is a matter of choice.

abandon a key aspect of their social identity. Thus they face additional challenges in adapting successfully to chronic illness.

In addition to these external factors, the older person is more likely to suffer disability in the face of impairment. Older people are more likely to have impairment simply through the additional years of exposure to risk factors. Furthermore, lower physiological reserve (the ability to regain homeostasis in the face of physiological stress) as a result of normal ageing renders the older person more vulnerable to disability. Decline in reserves in neurological, musculoskeletal and energy metabolism systems may limit the physical and mental resources that a person can bring to bear (see Older Adults box 35.1).

HEALTH POLICY

Health policy is a rapidly changing area. The last decades of the 20th century saw a significant change in emphasis in UK health policy for the care of people with chronic illness and disability.

Prior to the implementation of the National Health Service and Community Care Act in the 1990s, much of the care of the severely disabled was provided in long-stay wards in hospitals. This was particularly the case for older people. Subsequent to this act, much of the responsibility for organization, funding and provision of care has been passed from health to social services departments. The stated aim of the policy was to move to the provision of care in community settings where possible.

Individual care needs are assessed by a care manager, based on information provided by a range of health and social services professionals, including nurses, and wherever possible individuals are supported and cared for in their own homes. Care assistants employed by social services departments now provide much personal care in the home that was often delivered by district nursing services in the past. Care for those who are unable to manage in their own home is provided in private nursing homes (where professional nursing care is included) or residential homes (where professional nursing, if required, is provided by district nurses just as if the person were in his or her own home). For all but those with specialized health care needs, residential care is the responsibility of social services departments. Test cases in the late 1990s established the NHS's responsibility to fund health care delivered by nurses in private nursing homes.

This policy has tended to focus resources on those who are already dependent rather than providing support to maintain independence. Assessment of need is often not reviewed so dependence is compounded. Services are provided to compensate for disability but not to provide rehabilitation that might help the client become more independent.

A series of new policy initiatives announced in 1998–1999 were designed to change services for those with a disability. In particular, the White Paper *Modernizing Social Services* (Department of Health 1998) proposed a statutory duty of partnership on the NHS and social services. Under these proposals, the two agencies are required to draw up health improvement programmes and invest jointly in services. It is hoped that people with disabilities will no longer be subjected to arbitrary boundaries between the responsibilities of different agencies.

Care is increasingly delivered in people's own homes and rehabilitation, to facilitate hospital discharge or avoid hospital admission, and increasingly takes place outside acute hospital settings, especially in so-called intermediate care settings (Steiner 1997). Nurses could play an active role in these new initiatives through a range of nurse-led services (Griffiths 1997) where nurses take a far more autonomous role in managing patient care.

CARE SETTINGS FOR THOSE WITH CHRONIC ILLNESS AND DISABILITY

Since disability contributes approximately 50% of the burden of disease in developed countries, nurses encounter patients with chronic impairments in a range of settings. As more life-threatening diseases become amenable to treatment, it is quite possible that many more diseases will become perceived as chronic conditions and the significance of chronic illness will rise even further. Many of the most innovative nursing roles in the future will be in the management of chronic disease.

HOSPITAL WARDS

Nurses encounter patients with chronic disorders on a day-to-day basis in hospital wards. Many of the most common causes of hospital admission are related to chronic disease. Nurses in acute hospitals may encounter people at many different stages of their illness.

Those newly diagnosed with a chronic disorder will have significant needs for information about their illness. They may have to come to terms with taking complex medication regimens for the rest of their lives. They may feel that their ability to carry out their normal lives will be significantly altered. Such perceptions may or may not be realistic, but exaggerated assessments of potential disability can become self-fulfilling. For example, individuals who believe that their activities will be severely limited following a heart attack may be reluctant to exercise and are less likely to resume normal roles. Ironically, such behaviour increases the risk of disability and further cardiac problems.

The ability to absorb large amounts of information at a time of acute stress is limited by the very nature of acute ward environments. Nursing priorities are often the needs of the acutely ill and provision of patient information and teaching may not seem a priority. It is also limited by the patient's ability to absorb and retain large amounts of new information. However, it is vital that patients are discharged from hospital with sufficient information to manage their own condition. It is also essential that people with new diagnoses of chronic disease are provided with details of how they can find out more information about their condition.

District nurses, nurse specialists, general practitioners and outpatient clinics are all important potential sources of further information and support, as are voluntary organizations, charities and support groups for patients and carers. The internet is becoming increasingly important as a source of information and as a means of making contact with others who can provide support.

Many patients require practical support after discharge. Nurses need to plan with clients how activities of living, which are supported while in hospital, will be managed at home. Given that hospitals provide food for patients, even patients who appear independent are in fact being supported in their activities of living. Discharge planning is an ongoing activity, which must begin early in a patient's hospital stay. Appropriate referral is important but just as significant is providing the patient with the information required to contact services should additional support be required after discharge.

People who have lived with a chronic illness or disability for some time are likely to have considerable knowledge and experience of their condition. If they have been dependent on a carer, the latter will also have considerable knowledge and experience. Nursing care should be based upon the client's own approach to care where possible and practical. Changes in approaches to care should be undertaken only in negotiation with the client. However, it is important to assess knowledge and understanding

EVIDENCE-BASED PRACTICE

35.1 Managing medication

Many patients with long-term illnesses are discharged from hospital with a range of medications. Stewart et al (1998) studied a group of patients with chronic illness in the 6 months after hospital discharge. The patients they studied were discharged with an average of nearly five different medications. They found that nearly half of the patients failed to adhere to their prescribed regimens and nearly all the patients lacked important knowledge about their treatments.

In a randomized controlled trial of 762 people, they found that a follow-up visit from a nurse or pharmacist 2 weeks after discharge followed by further input for people with poor compliance reduced deaths and readmissions compared with people who simply visited their GP.

Community nurses are in an excellent position to assess medication compliance. This study shows that working with patients to improve compliance can strongly influence their health. It also strongly suggests what has often been suspected, that poor compliance with medications is a significant cause of hospital admission (Stewart et al 1998).

Reference

Stewart S, Pearson S, Luke C & Horowitz J (1998) Effects of home-based intervention on unplanned readmissions and out-of-hospital deaths. Journal of the American Geriatic Society, 46: 174–180.

even when clients appear to have considerable experience. Coping strategies can be based on misunderstanding or outdated clinical knowledge. Contact with acute health services can provide a valuable opportunity for a reassessment of coping strategies. Knowledge of medication is an important area and an acute admission presents an opportunity to assess client knowledge and provide education (see Evidence-based Practice box 35.1).

REHABILITATION SETTINGS AND INTERMEDIATE CARE

Over the past few years there has been an interest in developing alternatives to acute hospital care for patients after the acute phases of illness. In general, patients remain within the acute care system until they are recovered enough to be discharged into their own home. For many people this is quite sufficient and they return home successfully. However, for those with chronic illness or residual disability, immediate treatment of an acute illness is only the beginning of their recovery. After the acute phase has passed, an extended period of rehabilitation and adaptation is required before a person is able to achieve maximum independence.

Increasingly, attention has focused on developing primary care and community-oriented services as alternatives to the provision of health care in hospital. Not only is the acute hospital environment unnecessary for some patients but it may actually be detrimental to recovery for some patient groups. These include the growing number of frail older people and those undergoing a period of rehabilitation following surgery, trauma or an acute episode such as a stroke among others (Griffiths 1995). Health care does not refer only to technical medical care; a range of other professionals contribute to the recovery and maintenance of health. Once medical stability is achieved, therapies other than medicine are increasingly important in determining recovery.

Stroke units have developed to provide people recovering from cerebrovascular accidents with assessment and therapy from a full range of health care professionals, including nurses, physiotherapists and occupational therapists. In these units, medical consultants generally manage care but all members of the multidisciplinary team take an active role. An alternative approach has been the development of 'nurse-led' in-patient units where responsibility for care is fully taken over by nursing staff, though still working closely with the multidisciplinary team. These units have been established to care for people who are recovering from stroke, cardiac problems and even patients whose breathing must be supported by a ventilator, the so-called 'chronically critically ill' (Griffiths & Wilson-Barnet 1998).

In all these settings, nurses take a much more active, therapeutic, role in promoting recovery for their clients than is possible on acute wards (see Evidence-based Practice box 35.2). Such units allow nursing staff to concentrate on rehabilitation, patient education and psychological care, which may be secondary in acute units where the goal of medical cure is emphasized. Since a cure is impossible or unlikely for those with a chronic impairment, this change of emphasis may bring benefits (Griffiths & Wilson-Barnett 1998).

Other new services are being developed in which nurses take a lead in managing or delivering care, including 'hospital at home' schemes where complex and often high-tech care is delivered to patients in their own home.

COMMUNITY NURSING AND PRACTICE NURSING

Community nurses have long played an active part in the care of people with chronic disease and disability. Community nurses may encounter people throughout their chronic illness and are in a unique position to assess their ability to manage in their own environment over an extended period of time. The role of community nurses in the management of chronic illness and disability in their clients has far more significance than professionals whose contact with a person is relatively brief. This is particularly the case with frail older people and others who require ongoing nursing support in their own homes. Assessment of coping and planning, and coordination of the care assistants are vital functions, in addition to the specific nursing treatments such as wound dressings that often initiate contact.

Many practice nurses run clinics for people with conditions such as diabetes or hypertension and take an active role in providing health and lifestyle advice in addition to advice about particular treatments.

EVIDENCE-BASED PRACTICE

35.2 Therapeutic nursing

Since the earliest days of professional nursing, there has been a belief that good nursing care could benefit patients above and beyond the contribution of the medical or surgical treatments which nurses may participate in delivering. The therapeutic contribution of nursing is most significant in areas such as rehabilitation where the nurse's contribution to patient education, promoting psychological well-being and independence in activities of daily living, might be far more important than the effect of any medical treatment. Several experimental studies have attempted to demonstrate this by comparing nursing-led in-patient units (wards where nurses take the lead role in managing and delivering care) with traditional care, for patients with a range of chronic illnesses or disability. Several studies suggest that patients may indeed benefit from this approach to care, although the evidence is by no means conclusive (Griffiths & Wilson-Barnet 1998).

Possible benefits of nursing-led units include:

- patients are less dependent on discharge from hospital
- fewer patients are admitted to nursing homes.

Specialist stroke units have certain similarities in that the focus of care is rehabilitation, although the precise contribution of nursing in these settings is not known. The advantages of specialist stroke units in promoting recovery after stroke has been more clearly demonstrated (Stroke Unit Trialists' Collaboration 1999).

Benefits of stroke units include:

- lower mortality
- less dependence
- fewer patients are admitted to nursing homes.

References

Griffiths P, Wilson-Barnet J. The effectiveness of 'nursing beds': a review of the literature. J Adv Nurs 1998; 27: 1184–1192.

Stroke Unit Trialists' Collaboration. Organised inpatient (stroke unit) care for stroke (Cochrane review). In: The Cochrane Library, Issue 4. Oxford: Update Software; 1999.

NEW NURSING ROLES IN CHRONIC DISEASE MANAGEMENT

A number of relatively new nursing roles are emerging in the care of people with chronic diseases. Nurse practitioners are taking on fuller responsibility for the care of patients with a wide range of conditions, including asthma, bronchiectasis, diabetes, epilepsy, Parkinson's disease and rheumatoid arthritis. They often take full responsibility for managing medication within defined protocols, referring to doctors only when problems emerge. It is believed that a nursing perspective towards care moves the focus from simple disease management to one which enables clients to discuss their wider concerns and issues, which in turn allows for the development of more successful coping strategies. Nurses in these roles are generally able to spend more time with their clients than are doctors.

There is an increasing amount of evidence to support the effectiveness of these roles and it seems certain that they will become increasingly common (Garbett 1996). An example of a nurse practitioner-led programme, developed to prevent disability in frail older people with chronic illnesses, was reported by Leville et al (1998). The nurse meets with clients and develops an individual plan, which identifies risk factors for disability and strategies for self-management of their disease. Clients participate in group educational programmes and are encouraged to be as physically active as possible, thus preventing disability. This simple format of active client involvement and identification of individual strategies for avoiding disability provides a good model for nursing interventions in chronic disease management.

LONG-TERM CARE

Nurses working in long-term care settings have an additional responsibility in patient care over and above all that has been discussed so far. The long-term care establishment is the prime residence of the client. The usual paraphernalia of the clinical environment is detrimental to homeliness and the challenge for nurses is to make it a home. Although most people with long-term illness and disability are able to live independently, some will require long-term care, primarily in nursing homes. Although disability is the reason a person requires such care, it is important to emphasize that a person has abilities. Identification of such abilities is the key to maximizing quality of life in the face of the significant loss of independence that occurs when a person gives up their own home.

Nurses must identify and utilize opportunities to provide social interaction and activities that are preferred by the client. In many cases, relationships with nursing staff are of particular significance and the importance of establishing long-term therapeutic relationships with clients must be considered when arranging work schedules and allocating workload. In all settings where people with long-term impairment are cared for, continuity of care is extremely important.

ASSESSMENT OF CHRONIC ILLNESS AND DISABILITY AND ITS IMPACT ON THE INDIVIDUAL AND FAMILY

MODELS OF NURSING

Concepts and assessment frameworks from a number of models of nursing can provide a valuable structure for nursing assessment and intervention in chronic disease and disability (see Ch. 1). The Activities of Living model provides a framework that can be used to structure an assessment of physical, social and psychological function (Roper et al 1980). The aim of nursing is to promote independence or to assist the individual in coping with dependence on others if this proves necessary. The model does tend to emphasize disability. The Roy 'adaptation' model provides a complex assessment framework (Roy 1976) which emphasizes the ability of the individual to adapt to impairments and disabilities (stressors) resulting from both the individual and the external world. The role of nursing is to promote adaptive responses – physiological, psychological or social – when the person's ability to do so is exceeded. Although the individual's capacity to adapt is intrinsic to this model, the focus of assessment frameworks derived from it has tended to be in the physical domains.

Perhaps the single most valuable model for nursing this client group is Orem's 'self-care' model (Orem 1990). The model describes universal self-care needs, including activities of living and social roles. Ability to meet self-care requirements is balanced against demands for self-care. In terms of this model, chronic impairment may reduce the individual's ability to meet demands but also, as we have seen, can increase the demands themselves as the individual must also cope with externally imposed negative perceptions that lead to stigma and discrimination. The aims of nursing care are described as both reducing self-care demands to a level the person can meet and increasing the person's self-care abilities (see Ethical Issues box 35.1). If this cannot be achieved, nurses should enable others (such as friends or relatives) to meet those needs. Failing this, nurses aim to meet self-care needs directly.

 ## ETHICAL ISSUES

35.1 Promoting self-care

Health policy and professional practice increasingly emphasize independence and self-care. Self-care as a philosophy is closely associated with attempts by governments to control health care expenditure. Enabling independence for those who desire it is rarely questioned as a valid goal, but is it appropriate for everyone? Patients with disabilities may view a nurse's attempt to promote independence as a refusal to provide necessary help. What are your views?

- Is there a conflict between a policy that promotes self-care and the needs of the individual?
- Do patients have a duty to care for themselves if they are able to do so?
- In what circumstances might it be acceptable for a nurse to insist that a patient be independent in activities of daily living?
- Is maximum independence and self-care always desirable?
- Do you think nurses should be concerned about the relationship between philosophies of care and government policy?

Student activities
Debate the proposition: 'It is the nurse's duty to promote maximum patient independence.'

ASSESSMENT OF IMPAIRMENT

Assessment must include a precise description of the nature and history of the impairment(s). Although the medical diagnosis is important and informative, the priority in assessment should be identifying the problems that are manifested in the person. For example, stroke is a medical condition which can cause several different impairments, or indeed none at all. Stroke may lead to one or more problems such as paralysis, difficulty speaking and difficulty understanding language or balance problems.

Concrete descriptions of the difficulties caused are more valuable than simply labelling the person's deficits. The length of time a person has had to cope with a particular impairment is vital in establishing the context in which assessment of adjustment and coping mechanisms will be set. It is vital to identify the understanding of the mechanisms and prognosis of their impairment. Open questions may be helpful to begin such assessments, e.g. 'Can you tell me your understanding of how diabetes affects your body?'.

SECONDARY PREVENTION

For some people, the most significant effect of impairment may be that they are at risk of other impairment or disability. Most people with hypertension are barely affected by the disorder (which is why so many people are undiagnosed). However, they are at considerable risk of cardiovascular disease and stroke. In a controlled trial, between 10 and 14% of untreated hypertensive patients over the age of 70 suffered a stroke or heart attack in a 2-year period (Dahlof et al 1991). The aim of nursing is assessment, monitoring and intervention, to prevent these conditions. Assessment must identify individual risk factors and, in particular, behaviours that contribute to or alleviate risk. The client's knowledge and appraisal of these risks must be assessed in order to guide interventions.

FUNCTIONAL ASSESSMENT

Many scales exist which measure functional abilities in activities of daily living. Although they are often insensitive to problems experienced while a person is relatively independent, they can nevertheless provide a useful structure for assessment and an objective way of measuring progress.

Barthel index
Probably the most commonly used is the Barthel index (Mahoney & Barthel 1965). This index assesses clients' abilities in terms of bathing, personal grooming (cleaning teeth, brushing hair), dressing, feeding themselves, getting to and from the toilet, continence, managing stairs, walking outside and transferring from bed to chair. In all cases where people experience difficulties, the nature of the difficulty should be identified as well as its cause. Where the person is unable to function independently, the sources and extent of help needed should be identified. Assessment of activities of daily living should also include identification of difficulties and sources of support with domestic activities such as washing up, cooking and shopping.

Since disability can be caused by external factors, these should also be assessed. For example, someone may be unable to walk outdoors because they live on the third floor of a block of flats with no lift. The person's immediate home environment forms an important part of assessment of functional ability.

Ten-item abbreviated mental test

Brief structured assessment of cognitive problems using a scale such as the 10-item abbreviated mental test, which includes a structured assessment of memory and orientation, may be added to assessment if difficulties are suspected (Bowling 1995). Problems with communication should also be assessed, along with coping strategies and disabilities that result. It is important, but difficult, to distinguish communication problems which result from specific impairments of speech and language from those which result from global cognitive impairment. For example, people with cerebral palsy may have great difficulty in articulating words but no cognitive problems whatsoever. On the other hand, people with dementia have difficulties in communicating which results from confusion and disorientation in tandem with a gradual decline in the ability to comprehend the world around them.

ASSESSMENT OF COPING AND WELL-BEING

A person's understanding of his or her illness, and beliefs about it, form the basis of an assessment of coping and adjustment to impairment. Clients' views about how others perceive them is an important part of this set of beliefs. In many cases, a very general question such as 'How do you feel about your illness?' can serve to begin an assessment of coping and well-being. Self-esteem is a powerful determinant of adaptation to chronic illness or disability. An assessment of self-esteem forms a significant part of many standard assessments of psychological well-being, and nursing assessment should attempt to identify whether clients' ability to value themselves has been impeded by the impairment. Anxiety and depression often accompany chronic impairment and assessment should include any possible signs of these. Assessment of coping strategies includes identification of how people generally cope with problems, both currently and in the past.

The assessment of coping and well-being should include an assessment of the well-being of carers, who are likely to experience considerable stress which can impact upon their relationship with those they are caring for. Like the person with impairment, they may also move through stages of adaptation akin to the grieving process.

NURSING PRIORITIES FOR OLDER ADULTS: ASSESSMENT OF SOCIAL AND ROLE FUNCTIONS

While it is important to assess disability, the emphasis of assessment should be on the abilities of clients. Their work and leisure activities should be identified in addition to any difficulties associated with the impairment. Strategies used to overcome any difficulties should also be identified. Detailed assessment of financial circumstances may be unnecessary but it is important to identify whether there are any difficulties. It is also important to bear in mind that for many people financial dependency on

the state carries with it great stigma. Others are reluctant to share details of their financial status with professionals and are reluctant to admit to financial difficulties. If problems are identified, further assessment and/or referral (to a social worker or Citizens' Advice Bureau) may be appropriate. Clients with long-term impairment and carers are entitled to many benefits (see Special Issues box 35.1).

Detailed assessment of social role function and issues of sexuality may seem intrusive and may be perceived by clients as an invasion of privacy. However, chronic illness frequently creates difficulties in personal relationships, including sexual ones. In planning care it is necessary to know the people considered to be significant others, including family members, close friends, sexual partners, parents and children. Enquiries about these matters may help to identify key roles the person occupies (such as parent, spouse) and may open up particular lines of enquiry concerning problems experienced. Many of these people may provide crucial sources of physical, social or psychological support and will play an important part in the assessment of resources available.

It should not simply be assumed that close family members are able or willing to provide care. It is vital, where possible, to involve potential carers in the assessment from the earliest opportunity (with the client's permission). Where particular individuals are identified as sources of care, it is essential to include them.

Providing opportunities for the client to discuss general concerns, perhaps at the end of the assessment interview, may help to initiate discussion and identification of particular problems. Questions such as 'Is there anything else you think I should know?' or 'Are there any other concerns you want to discuss?' can provide an opening for a client to raise personal issues. A positive therapeutic relationship established with clients is necessary in order to allow them to raise sensitive issues.

In some cases, direct questioning about topics such as sexuality can give clients permission to raise issues they may otherwise be embarrassed to discuss. A direct question such as 'Has your illness caused any problems in your sex life?' may be appropriate. Many clients need permission to discuss topics such as sexuality and may expect health care professionals to raise the topic if it is appropriate (Larsen et al 1997). Another way of broaching difficult topics is to introduce them in a general manner, such as 'Many people with diabetes experience difficulty achieving erection', or 'Many people with heart disease find that it puts a great strain on their personal relationships'. Written material may save embarrassment for the client but it is important that it is not simply used by nurses to avoid raising topics that they personally find difficult.

NURSING CARE FOR THOSE WITH CHRONIC ILLNESS AND DISABILITY

The nursing care of those with chronic illness and impairment is a topic as broad as nursing itself. The detail of interventions to deal with specific impairments can be found in relevant sections of this book and in specialist texts. However, a number of common principles for nursing care of this group of clients can be identified. The chapter concludes with a discussion of a number

SPECIAL ISSUES

35.1 Benefits and other sources of support

Local social services departments or hospital-based social workers are able to give advice on benefits. However, since routine referral to a social worker may well be unwelcome, it is important that nurses working with patients have some idea of the circumstances in which they may be able to receive benefits and the types of help that may be available. It is generally recognized that many people do not claim benefits to which they are entitled. For some this may be a matter of choice, but frequently people are simply unaware of their entitlements. Organizations such as the Citizens' Advice Bureau (CAB) can also provide considerable help and support. The number for local CABs can be found in the telephone book. The Benefits Agency also provides a confidential enquiry line.

The particular benefits available are complex and changeable. Expert advice should always be sought and nurses should not, and would not be expected to, give anything more that the most general advice. Presented below is a summary of benefits available for the sick or disabled in mid-2002. In general, claimants must have paid National Insurance (NI) contributions. This is for general guidance only.

- **Statutory Sick Pay (SSP)** can be claimed from an employer for up to 28 weeks of illness after the first 4 days.
- **Incapacity Benefit** is available to those under retirement age who are not entitled to SSP, either because they were not working or because their SSP has ended. This benefit is paid at varying rates depending on the particular circumstances.
- **Severe Disablement Allowance** is available to those who have been unable to work for at least 28 weeks irrespective of National Insurance contributions. Those who become disabled after their 20th birthday must be assessed by a doctor.
- **Disability Living Allowance (DLA)** is available to those with long-term mobility difficulties or who require other

help to look after themselves. It is not dependent on someone actually giving the required care. It is also available to parents of children with disabilities. This benefit is not affected by savings or other income the disabled person may have. This benefit is available only to those who became ill or disabled before the age of 65 and is not available to those in residential care.

- **Attendance Allowance (AA)** is similar to DLA but is available to those who become ill or disabled over the age of 65.
- **Invalid Care Allowance (ICA)** is available to those who spend at least 35 hours per week caring for some people receiving AA or DLA. The benefit is means tested and is not available to those in full-time education.
- **Home Responsibilities Protection** is a scheme designed to protect the state pension entitlements of those unable to pay NI contributions because of caring responsibilities.

Special benefits are available to people in particular circumstances such as those who were injured or became ill because of their work or those disabled by vaccinations, and a tax credit (disabled person's tax credit) is available to some disabled people in work.

Other benefits such as income support and housing/ council tax benefit are also of significance to many people with disabilities (or their carers) who are on low incomes. Entitlement to all these benefits depends on a person's income and savings. In general, those in receipt of benefits available to people on low income are entitled to free NHS prescriptions, sight tests and dental care. People with some chronic conditions may get an exemption certificate, which means they are exempt from prescription charges. Those requiring regular prescriptions who are not exempt can purchase a 'season ticket' which will cover an unlimited number of prescriptions over a period of time.

Benefits Enquiry Line: 0800 88 222 00 (textphone: 0800 24 33 55).

---

of approaches to care and interventions that are of particular significance to the care of the chronically ill.

THE CARE TEAM

The most significant members of the care 'team' are those with the impairment and their main carers. People with an established chronic disease or disability have great experience of the disorder and may often know more about the pathophysiology of a particular condition than many professionals with whom they come into contact. In all cases, they will have particular knowledge and experience of managing the impairment as it is manifested in them rather than in general. This may also apply to carers. If patients are to achieve maximum independence, they must also provide the main therapeutic effort.

The role of most professionals is to increase patients' resources to care for themselves or to remove barriers which

impede their ability. If such independence is impossible, it is likely that the main care-giver will be a non-professional relative or friend. In this case the effort of professionals should also include enabling the carer.

The involvement of clients, and where relevant family and friends, is important for the provision of nursing care in all settings but is central to providing care in the face of chronic conditions. Education and information-giving are of particular importance when a person faces a lifetime with a particular impairment (see Health Promotion box 35.1). The goals for care may differ from those identified in acute care and negotiation with the client is of added importance (see Guidelines box 35.1). Client advocacy (see Ch. 3) is of far greater significance when the encounter with health care systems is long term rather than for an illness from which recovery will be complete. Within these broad principles are a number of interventions which apply to large groups of clients with chronic impairments.

HEALTH PROMOTION

35.1 Guidelines for effective teaching

Much nursing intervention in chronic illness and disability is dependent on successful client education. Where a desired behaviour, such as taking medication correctly, is not being performed, the teaching required depends upon a careful assessment of why it is not performed. It may be that the client simply lacks knowledge of correct procedure. Alternatively the correct procedure may be impeded by other factors such as problems of dexterity or it may be perceived as clashing with work or social life. It is only when the client's knowledge and behaviour are carefully assessed that the correct information and intervention can be designed.

When providing information, written or verbal, attention must be paid to the complexity of the language used. Jargon should generally be avoided. Communicating information to clients with communication problems, or whose first language is different from one's own, poses special challenges (see Ch. 3). Providing information is never sufficient in itself. At the very least, the results of any teaching intervention must be carefully assessed and appropriate reinforcement and additional teaching given.

- Teaching should be based on an individualized assessment of information needs which is tailored to the individual's ability to receive information.

- The goal of teaching must be agreed with the client.
- The type of information required is partly determined by the length of time a person has lived with the impairment.
- Knowledge of disease processes and medication should not be assumed even where clients have had a long experience of their disorder (see Evidence-based Practice box 35.1).
- Large volumes of information presented at the point of an acute exacerbation is likely to be an ineffective strategy, but nurses working in acute settings still need to identify when and how vital information will be given.
- In general, all information given should be supported with written materials. Nurses should consider a range of teaching strategies, including group teaching for clients with common concerns.
- Teaching materials including audiovisual packages and computer-assisted learning are available from a variety of sources, including the Health Education Authority in the UK.
- Many charities concerned with particular impairments also have information leaflets and teaching materials available and information is increasingly available over the internet.

 GUIDELINES FOR CARE PRIORITIES

35.1 Goal-setting

With a chronic illness or impairment, the goal of 'cure' is not a realistic one. The goals of care are individual and must be arrived at in negotiation with the client. This is particularly important in chronic conditions since clients' sense of control and mastery is an important determinant of their ability to cope with the condition. Many difficulties can occur when goals are not explicitly agreed between clients and professionals.

- Goals should be set collaboratively between client and professional.
- Goal-setting should begin with a clarification of the role of client and professional in setting and achieving goals.

- The professional's role is to advise the client and help arrive at goals which are neither unrealistically high nor low.
- Long-term goals should have achievable sub-goals so that both client and professional can identify the extent of progress.
- Professionals and clients should identify strategies through which goals will be achieved.
- 'Non-compliance' is often a result of the client and professional working towards different goals.
- Goals must accommodate clients' hopes, expectations and aspirations beyond the management of impairment – their need for 'normality'.
- Clients may be more likely to accept goals identified by professionals if professionals show a willingness to work towards the clients' goals.

PSYCHOLOGICAL SUPPORT – FACILITATING ADAPTATION

Psychological adaptation to impairment is promoted through maximizing independence and control. Where some dependence on others is inevitable, nurses can still facilitate adaptation by promoting control. Several types of personal control have been identified (Taylor et al 1997):

- process control – the ability to participate in the process of health care
- contingency control – people's belief that their actions influence outcomes

- cognitive control – the ability to manage perception of events in order to reduce perceived threat
- behavioural control – a person's ability to directly act and change a situation
- existential control – people's ability to create and perceive meaning in their life in general, and in relation to negative life events in particular.

Miller (1992) identifies the following five interventions that may decrease patients' sense of powerlessness and give them more control over their situation.

Modifying the environment to provide patients with more control

Examples of this can range from the seemingly trivial, such as ensuring that those with impaired mobility have access to call buttons while in hospital, to significant technological adaptations which allow impaired people to control many of the functions of their home independently (e.g. lights, heat and access through doors).

Helping clients to set realistic goals and expectations

Although a disregard of the stigma attached to an impairment may on occasion lead people to achieve remarkable feats, it is also important that nurses use their knowledge and experience to guide patients in setting goals for themselves. A person who has lost limbs might reasonably aim to walk. Someone whose paraplegia was caused by a complete transection of the spinal cord who invests all hopes and aspirations into the goal of walking is at risk of an increasing sense of powerlessness in the face of failure to make progress toward this unrealistic goal.

Increasing patients' knowledge about their illness and its management

The more patients know about and understand their illness, the more they can control events either through self-management or through taking an active part in interactions with others such as encounters with health care professionals. The person with diabetes who is knowledgeable about the condition is able to make more informed choices in managing it and is more likely to achieve good disease control.

Ensuring that significant others (including health professionals) are aware of the potential sense of powerlessness and its negative effects

Well-meaning relatives and health care professionals can often reinforce disability by intervening to help too readily and thus emphasizing powerlessness. On the other hand, pushing a person to be independent in areas that may be too demanding can also reinforce a sense of powerlessness. All involved in care must remember that ultimately the person with the impairment must make decisions about care.

Encouraging the person to talk about their feelings

Giving it verbal expression may reduce the frustration resulting from a sense of powerlessness. In addition to the intrinsic benefit of expressing feelings, it may well be that those around the client are simply not aware of particular things which contribute to a sense of powerlessness.

PROMOTING PHYSICAL ACTIVITY

In addition to promoting psychological adaptation, there may be a considerable demand for physical adaptation. The particular challenges may result from paralysis (e.g. following a stroke) or from fatigue associated with systemic disease (e.g. in the case of renal failure). In all cases, a specific programme of exercise can be of considerable benefit (Kohler et al 1997). Any exercise programme must balance activity with energy conservation. Encouraging general activity within limits can help to strengthen muscles and build stamina. Where possible, gentle exercise such as walking is of benefit. An individual exercise programme should be developed and reinforced. Often a physiotherapist will design this. Where general fatigue is a problem, over-activity when feeling better should be avoided. Modifications to the environment can increase activity, e.g. by allowing access outside the house, or reduce disability associated with restricted mobility. Clients should be encouraged to be aware of their abilities and limits and realistic goals should be set in negotiation with them. There is some evidence that cognitive behavioural therapy may be of benefit in conditions associated with fatigue, including cancer and chronic fatigue syndrome (Kohler et al 1997).

SEXUAL DYSFUNCTION

Difficulties in sexual activity or identity are common in people with chronic illness but are frequently not addressed by health care professionals. Counselling and therapy for sexual dysfunction is a complex and specialized activity but Larsen et al (1997) describe a model that can guide interventions at a number of levels determined by both the needs of the client and the expertise of the professional. The PLISSIT model identifies a series of levels for intervention:

- *Permission for sexual behaviour*. It may be that the only required intervention is to allow the client to express feelings or concerns and to make it clear that sexual activity is possible and permissible. For example, patients with long-term urinary catheters may feel that sexual activity is neither possible nor desirable. Expression of this concern can alleviate anxiety and allows the nurse to make it clear that sexual activity is possible.
- *Limited information-giving* is the provision of concrete general information, such as telling patients with cardiac problems that sudden death during intercourse is rare or that a man with a catheter will suffer no damage as a consequence of erection.
- *Specific suggestion*. This consists of the professional making suggestions that may facilitate sexual activity, e.g. advice on using artificial lubrication for women with conditions leading to reduced vaginal lubrication or planning sexual activity to coincide with the maximum effect of analgesia for those with arthritis.
- *Intensive therapy* from specialists such as a psychologist or sex therapist. This is beyond the scope of general nurses, but nurses can be involved in identifying the need for more specialist input and can facilitate referral.

SUMMARY: MAIN POINTS

- Chronic illness and disability are common and form a large proportion of the 'burden of disease' in the developed world.

- Many of the commonest causes of disease have the potential to become chronic and are often associated with disability.

- Disability is the difficulty a person experiences in taking a full part in the life of the community. Impairment is the direct effect of the disease on the functioning of the body.

- Disability results from factors external to the person (e.g. barriers to mobility) as much as from the impairment itself.

- Many forms of chronic illness or disability have considerable stigma attached to them.

- Chronic illness and disability can affect sufferers deeply in many aspects of their physical, psychological and social function.

- Innovative nursing roles are increasingly being developed to meet the needs of the chronically ill.

- Care must be planned in collaboration with clients and their families.

- Clients' feelings of control are a key determinant of successful adaptation to impairment.

- The nursing role consists of increasing clients' ability to self-care while reducing the external demands upon them.

SELF-TEST: CRITICAL THINKING ACTIVITIES

1 Why does disability form a larger proportion of the burden of disease in developed countries than in the rest of the world?

2 How can the attitudes of others cause increased disability in a person with an impairment?

3 How might your approach to the nursing care of someone with a long-standing disability differ from that of someone with an acute illness?

4 How can nurses prevent disability?

 FURTHER READING

Anderson N. Rehabilitative nursing practice. Nurs Clin North Am 1971; 6(2): 303–309.

Braden CJ. A test of the self-help model: learned response to chronic illness experience. Nurs Res 1990; 39(1): 42–47.

Daly B, Rudy E, Thompson K. Development of a special care unit for chronically critically ill patients. Heart Lung 1991; 20(1): 45–51.

Griffiths P, Wilson-Barnet J. The effectiveness of 'nursing beds': a review of the literature. J Adv Nurs 1998; 27: 1184–1192.

Lubkin I (ed). Chronic illness: impact and interventions, 4th edn. Boston: Jones and Bartlett; 1997.

Miller J. Coping with chronic illness: overcoming powerlessness. Philadelphia: FA Davies; 1992.

Oliver M. Theories of disability in health practice and research. Br Med J 1998; 317: 1446–1449.

Shekleton ME. Coping with chronic respiratory difficulty. Nurs Clin North Am 1987; 22(3): 569–579.

Stewart AL, Hays RD, Wells K et al. Functional status and well being of patients with chronic conditions. J Am Med Assoc 1989; 262(7): 907–913.

Strauss A. Chronic illness and the quality of life. St Louis: Mosby; 1976.

Swanson B, Cronin-Stubbs D, Sheldon JA. The impact of psychosocial factors on adapting to physical disability: a review of the research literature. Rehab Nurs 1989; 14(2): 64–68.

 USEFUL ADDRESSES

Carers National Association
20–25 Glasshouse Yard
London EC1A 4JS
Tel: 020 7490 8818

Provides advice and support to carers of disabled people through a network of local groups (carers' line: 0345 573 369, Mon–Fri, 10–12am and 2–4pm)

USEFUL WEBSITES

www.ace.org.uk/aboutus/default.htm – Age Concern – an organization which provides information and care designed to help older people, including those with impairment to overcome problems

www.dwp.gov.uk/lifeevent/benefits/index.htm – Benefits Agency

www.disabilitynet.co.uk/ – Disability Net – claims to be one of the world's leading internet-based disability information and news services. The site contains a wide variety of information and offers many additional services which are potentially of use to professionals and clients alike

healthpromis.hea.org.uk/ – Healthpromis – the national health promotion database for England. The database contains references and links to a range of sources. These include official publications, surveys, reports, books, research, websites, journal articles and resources (videos, teaching material, software, cassettes and games)

In addition to these, there is a wide variety of support groups and organizations for people suffering from particular impairments. These are often invaluable sources of information.

REFERENCES

Bennet N, Dodd T, Flatley J, Freeth S, Bolling K. Health survey for England 1993. London: HMSO; 1995.

Bowling A. Measuring disease. A review of disease specific quality of life measurement scales. Milton Keynes: Open University Press; 1995.

Curtin M, Lubkin I. What is chronicity? In: Lubkin I, ed. Chronic illness: impact and interventions, 4th edn. Boston: Jones and Bartlett; 1997.

Dahlof B, Lindhom L, Hansson L. Morbidity and mortality in the Swedish Trial in Old Patients with Hypertension (STOP Hypertension). Lancet 1991; 338: 1281–1285.

Department of Health. Modernising social services: promoting independence. Improving protection. Raising standards. London: The Stationery Office; 1998.

Department of Health. Saving lives: our healthier nation. London: The Stationary Office; 1999.

Garbett R. The growth of nurse-led care. Nurs Times 1996; 92(1): 29.

Goffman E. Stigma: notes on management of spoiled identity. Engelwood Cliffs: Prentice Hall; 1963.

Griffiths P. Evaluation of nurse-led in-patient care. Nurs Times 1995; 91(43): 34–37.

Griffiths P. Leading roles. Health Service J 1997; 107: 32.

Griffiths P, Wilson-Barnet J. The effectiveness of 'nursing beds': a review of the literature. J Adv Nurs 1988; 27: 1184–1192.

Kohler K, Schweitert-Stary M, Lubkin I. Altered mobility. In: Lubkin I, ed. Chronic illness: impact and interventions, 4th edn. Boston: Jones and Bartlett; 1997.

Larsen P, Kahn A, Flodberg S. Sexuality. In: Lubkin I, ed. Chronic illness: impact and interventions, 4th edn. Boston: Jones and Bartlett; 1997.

Leville S, Wagner E, Davis C et al. Preventing disability and managing chronic illness in frail older adults: a randomized controlled trial of community-based partnerships with primary care. J Am Geriatr Soc 1998; 46: 1191–1198.

Mahoney FI, Barthel DW. Functional evaluation: the Barthel Index. Maryland State Med J 1965; 14: 61–65.

Miller A. Nurse-patient dependency – is it iatrogenic? J Adv Nurs 1985; 10: 63–69.

Miller J. Coping with chronic illness: overcoming powerlessness. Philadelphia: FA Davies; 1992.

Murray CJL, Lopez AD. The global burden of disease: a comprehensive assessment of mortality and disability from diseases injuries and risk factors in 1990 and projected to 2020. Cambridge: Harvard University Press; 1996.

Norris J, Kunes-Connel M, Spelic S. A grounded theory of re-imaging. Adv Nurs Sci 1998; 20(1): 1–12.

Oliver M. Theories of disability in health practice and research. Br Med J 1998; 317: 1446–1449.

Orem D. Nursing: concepts of practice, 4th edn. New York: McGraw-Hill; 1990.

Patterson B, Thorne S, Dewis M. Adapting to and managing diabetes. Image; J Nurs Schol 1998; 30(1): 57–62.

Petrie K, Weinman J, Sharpe N, Buckley J. Role of patients' view of their illness in predicting work and functioning after myocardial infarction: longitudinal study. Br Med J 1996; 312: 1191–1194.

Roper N, Logan W, Tierny A. The elements of nursing. Edinburgh: Churchill Livingstone; 1980.

Roy C. Introduction to nursing: an adaptation model. New Jersey: Prentice Hall; 1976.

Saylor C, Yoder M. Stigma. In: Lubkin I, Larsen P, eds. Chronic illness: impact and interventions, 4th edn. Sudbury: Jones and Bartlett; 1998.

Steiner A. Intermediate care: a conceptual framework and review of the literature. London: King's Fund; 1997.

Stewart AL, Hays RD, Wells K et al. Functional status and well being of patients with chronic conditions. J Am Med Assoc 1989; 262(7): 907–913.

Stockwell F. The unpopular patient. London: Croom Helm; 1984.

Strauss A. Chronic illness and the quality of life. Saint Louis: Mosby; 1976.

Taylor E, Jones P, Burns M. Quality of life. In: Lubkin I, ed. Chronic illness: impact and interventions, 4th edn. Boston: Jones and Bartlett; 1997, 207–226.

Thomas M, Walker A, Wilmot A, Bennet N. Living in Britain. Results from the 1996 General Household Survey. London: The Stationery Office; 1998.

Waters KR. Getting dressed in the early morning: styles of staff/patient interaction on rehabilitation hospital wards for elderly people. J Adv Nurs 1994; 19: 239–248.

WHO. International classification of functioning disability and health. Online. Available: http://www3.who.int/icf/icftemplate.cfm. Geneva: World Health Organization; 2001.

Wood P. International classification of impairments, disabilities and handicaps. Geneva: World Health Organization; 1980.

Appendix: Normal values

The values below represent an 'average' reference range, in adults, for blood, cerebrospinal fluid, faeces and urine, and should only be used as a guide. Reference ranges vary between laboratories and readers should consult their own laboratory for those used locally.

Blood–biochemistry (venous serum unless otherwise stated)

Test	Reference range	Test	Reference range
Acid phosphatase	0.1–0.6 U/L	Glucose (venous blood, fasting)	3.6–5.8 mmol/L
Alanine aminotransferase (ALT)	10–40 U/L	Glycosylated haemoglobin (HbA$_1$)	4–6%
Albumin	36–47 g/L	Hydrogen ion concentration	35–44 nmol/L
Alkali phosphatase	40–125 U/L	(arterial blood analysis)	
Amylase	90–300 U/L	Iron	
Aspartate aminotransferase (AST)	10–35 U/L	Female	10–28 µmol/L
Base excess	−2 to +2	Male	14–32 µmol/L
Bicarbonate	22–28 mmol/L	Iron-binding capacity total (TIBC)	45–70 µmol/L
(arterial blood analysis)		Lactate (arterial blood)	0.3–1.4 mmol/L
Bilirubin (total)	2–17 µmol/L	Lactate dehydrogenase (total)	230–460 U/L
Caeruloplasmin	150–600 mg/L	Lead (whole blood)	
Calcium	2.1–2.6 mmol/L	Adults	Less than 1.7 µmol/L
Chloride	97–106 mmol/L	Children	Less than 1.2 µmol/L
Cholesterol (total)	Less than 5.2 mmol/L ideal	Magnesium	0.75–1.0 mmol/L
	5.2–6.5 mmol/L mild	Osmolality	275–295 mosmol/kg
	6.5–7.8 mmol/L moderate	Oxygen saturation	More than 97%
	greater than 7.8 mmol/L	PaO_2 (arterial blood analysis)	10.0–13.3 kPa
	severe	pH (arterial blood analysis)	7.35–7.45
HDL cholesterol		Phosphate (fasting)	0.8–1.4 mmol/L
Female	0.6–1.9 mmol/L	Potassium (plasma)	3.3–4.7 mmol/L
Male	0.5–1.6 mmol/L	Potassium (serum)	3.6–5.0 mmol/L
$PaCO_2$ (arterial blood analysis)	4.6–6.0 kPa	Protein (total)	60–80 g/L
Copper	13–24 µmol/L	Sodium	135–143 mmol/L
Cortisol (at 8.00 a.m.)	160–560 nmol/L	Thyroxine (free)	10–27 pmol/L
Creatine kinase (total)		Triiodothyronine	1.0–2.6 nmol/L
Female	30–150 U/L	Transferrin	2.0–4.0 g/L
Male	30–200 U/L	Triglycerides	0.45–2.0 mmol/L
Creatinine	60–120 µmol/L	Urea	2.5–6.4 mmol/L
Ferritin		Uric acid	
Female	14–150 µg/L	Female	0.09–0.36 mmol/L
Male	17–300 µg/L	Male	0.1–0.45 mmol/L
Gamma-glutamyl transferase (GGT)		Vitamin A	0.7–3.5 µmol/L
Female	30–150 U/L	Vitamin C	23–57 µmol/L
Male	30–200 U/L	Zinc	11–22 µmol/L
Globulins	24–37 g/L		

Blood–haematology

Activated partial thromboplastin time (APTT)	30–40s	Mean cell haemoglobin concentration (MCHC)	30–35 g/dL
Bleeding time (Ivy)	2–8 min		
Erythrocyte sedimentation rate (ESR) (adult)		Mean cell volume (MCV)	78–94 fL
		Packed cell volume (PCV)	
Female	0–7 mm/h	Female	0.35–0.47 (35–47%)
Male	0–5 mm/h	Male	0.40–0.54 (40–54%)
	NB. Older people may have higher values	Platelets	150–400x10⁹/L
		Prothrombin time	11–14s
		Red cell count	
Fibrinogen	1.5–4.0 g/L	Female	3.8–5.3x10¹²/L
Folate (serum)	2.0–9 µg/L	Male	4.5–6.5x10¹²/L
Haematocrit *see* PCV		Reticulocytes (adults)	25–85x10⁹/L
Haemoglobin		White cells	
Female	115–165 g/L (11.5–16.5 g/dL)	Differential Total	4.0–11.0x10⁹/L
		Neutrophils	2.0–7.5x10⁹/L
Male	130–180 g/L (13–18 g/dL)	Eosinophils	0.04–0.4x10⁹/L
		Basophils	0.02–0.10x10⁹/L
Haptoglobins	0.3–2.0 g/L	Lymphocytes	1.5–4.0x10⁹/L
Mean cell haemoglobin (MCH)	27–32 pg	Monocytes	0.2–0.8x10⁹/L

Cerebrospinal fluid

Pressure (adult)	50–200 mm water
Cells	0–5 mm³
Glucose	2.5–4.0 mmol/L
Protein	100–400 mg/L
Chloride	120–170 mmol/L

Faeces

Fat content (daily output on normal diet)	less than 7 g/24 h
Fat (as stearic acid)	11–18 mmol/24 h

Urine

Albumin/creatinine ratio (ACR) (used to detect microalbuminuria)	less than 3.5 mg albumin/mmol creatinine
Albumin excretion rate (AER) (used to detect microalbuminuria)	less than 20 µg albumin/min
Calcium (depends on diet)	up to 12 mmol/24 h (normal diet)
Copper	0.2–0.6 µmol/24 h
Cortisol	9–50 µmol/24 h
Creatinine	10–20 mmol/24 h
5-Hydroxyindole-3-acetic acid (5HIAA)	15–60 µmol/24 h
Metadrenaline	0.3–1.7 µmol/24 h
Magnesium	3.3–5.0 mmol/24 h
Normetadrenaline	0.4–3.4 µmol/24 h
Oxalate	
Female	40–320 mmol/24 h
Male	80–490 mmol/24 h
Phosphate	15–50 mmol/24 h
pH	4–8
Potassium (depends on intake)	25–100 mmol/24 h
Protein (total)	no more than 0.3 g/L
Sodium (depends on intake)	100–200 mmol/24 h
Urate	1.2–3.0 mmol/24 h
Urea	170–500 mmol/24 h

Glossary

Abdominal ascites (Ch. 23). Collection of fluid in the peritoneal cavity.

Abduction (Ch. 27). Movement away from the midline of the body.

Access (Ch. 2). A dimension of quality in Maxwell's model which is about accessibility to services for patients, and can relate to waiting times, where the services are available, and the actual buildings used.

Accident (Ch. 30). An unforeseen event or one with no apparent cause.

Acidosis (Ch. 8). Correctly known as acidaemia, an arterial blood pH of less than 7.35.

Active listening (Ch. 3). The careful use of communication skills where the focus of the helper's interaction with the client is to enable individuals examining an issue of significance to become aware of aspects, such as depth of feeling, which had until then been out of their awareness.

Acute liver failure (ALF) (Ch. 23). Breakdown of vital liver functions, usually caused by viral hepatitis.

Acute pain (Chs 7, 29). Temporary pain related to injury and which resolves during the appropriate healing period.

Addison's disease (Ch. 17). Deficient secretion of cortisol and aldosterone due to primary failure of the adrenal cortex.

Adduction (Ch. 27). Movement toward the midline of the body.

Adult nursing (Ch. 1 and all chapters). The branch of nursing that specializes in the care of adults and older adults in a variety of care settings.

Aerobic metabolism (Ch. 9). Production of energy in the form of adenosine triphosphate (ATP) from a fuel source such as glucose in the presence of oxygen.

Aetiology (Ch. 33 and all chapters). The study of factors involved in the development of a specific disease.

Afebrile (Ch. 5). Without fever. Having a normal body temperature.

Ageing (Ch. 32). Becoming old, to show the signs of increasing age.

Ageism (Ch. 32). Simple prejudice on the grounds of age. It may be at an individual or institutional level.

Aggression (Ch. 30). Hostile behaviour, either physical or verbal.

Albuminuria (Ch. 24). The presence of albumin in the urine.

Alkalosis (Ch. 8). Correctly known as alkalaemia, an arterial blood pH greater than 7.45.

Allergen (Ch. 28). An external substance which stimulates an immunological response.

Ambulation (Ch. 29). The process of walking, often used interchangeably with mobilization.

Amnesia (Ch. 14). Memory loss; may be partial or total.

Anabolic (Ch. 11). Describes the energy-requiring chemical reactions in the body where simple substances are used to make more complex molecules.

Anaemia (Ch. 18). The term used to describe the insufficient oxygen-carrying capacity of blood.

Anaerobic metabolism (Ch. 9). Production of energy from glucose without the presence of oxygen.

Anaesthesia (Ch. 29). Strictly defined as an absence of feeling. A drug-induced state of reduced sensation and awareness.

Analgesia (Ch. 7). The absence of pain in response to normally painful stimuli.

Anaphylactic shock (Ch. 9). Shock caused by an allergic reaction to an antigen, either ingested or injected.

Angina (Ch. 19). Chest discomfort caused by myocardial ischaemia. Typical angina is felt in the centre of the chest and frequently radiates to the left arm and lower jaw.

Anorexia (Ch. 22). Loss of appetite accompanied by a lack of interest in food.

Anosmia (Ch. 21). Absent sense of smell.

Anticipatory grief (Ch. 34). Starting the grieving process before a person has died.

Antimicrobial (Ch. 13). Against microbes.

Anuria (Ch. 24). The cessation of urine secretion by the kidneys; there is no urine output.

Anxiety (Chs 6, 30). State of tension or uneasiness as result of any perceived danger; apprehension.

Apheresis (Ch. 18). A technique whereby a single blood component is collected from a patient or donor.

Arrhythmia (Ch. 19). A disturbance in the rate, rhythm or conduction of the heart. Classified according to origin, mechanism or rate.

Arterial leg ulcers (Ch. 10). Ulcers on the lower leg or foot caused by inadequate arterial blood supply.

Arthroscopy (Ch. 27). Use of an intra-articular camera to assess, repair or reconstruct various tissues within and around joints.

Asepsis and infection control (Chs 13, 29). The absence of harmful bacteria. The methods of minimizing and preventing the spread of infection.

Assertiveness (Ch. 3). The ability to state one's views without violating the rights of others to state theirs and includes both verbal and non-verbal communication skills. It is based on the belief that everyone is worthy of respect and thus entitled to state his or her position and be heard.

Assessment (all chapters). Evaluation or judgement. The first stage of the nursing process at which patient problems and needs are identified.

Assessment of stress (Ch. 6). Methods used to assess stress include general observation (e.g. abnormal sweating), physiological measurements (e.g. heart rate), the use of various validated scales and self-reporting.

Astigmatism (Ch. 15). Uneven curvature of the cornea.

Ataxia (Ch. 14). Ill-timed and uncoordinated movements.

Atheroma (Ch. 19). A proliferation of smooth muscle cells and accumulation of lipid within the intima of the large arteries. When this occurs in the coronary arteries, it leads to coronary heart disease.

Audit (Ch. 2). Measuring quality and changing practice when improvement to care or treatment is required.

Aural toilet (Ch. 16). A procedure that is carried out to clean, dry and remove debris from the external auditory canal.

Avascular necrosis (Ch. 27). Death of tissue due to complete depletion of blood supply. Commonly seen with fractures of the femoral neck, leading to necrosis of the head of the femur.

Bacteria (Ch. 13). Single-celled microorganisms widely distributed in the environment. They can be pathogenic to humans, other animals and plants, or non-pathogenic. Pathogenic bacteria may be virulent and always cause infection, whereas others, known as opportunists, generally only cause infection when the host defences are reduced, such as during cancer chemotherapy. Non-pathogenic bacteria may become pathogenic if they move from their normal site, e.g. bowel bacteria causing cystitis.

Benchmarking (Ch. 2). A system of comparing an organization's standards against those of an external, but similar, organization, which is chosen especially for its excellence in quality.

Benign (Ch. 33). Describes a slow-growing tumour with the potential to become life-threatening depending on its anatomical position and its ability to generate metastases.

Bereavement (Ch. 34). The grief reactions following the death of a person. Also applied to the reactions occurring after other losses such as radical surgery.

Bile (Ch. 23). Alkaline fluid produced by hepatocytes, the main role of which is the emulsification of fats and absorption of fat-soluble vitamins and lipids.

Biliary colic (Ch. 23). Smooth muscle or visceral pain (severe) specifically associated with the passage of stones through the bile ducts.

Biliary system (Ch. 23). The pathway for bile flow from the canaliculi in the liver to the opening of the bile duct into the duodenum.

Bilirubin and biliverdin (Ch. 23). Bile pigments formed from the breakdown of red blood cells.

Biofeedback (Chs 12, 6). A technique by which information about a normally unconscious physiological process is presented to the patient and/or practitioner as a visual, auditory or tactile signal.

Biopsy (Ch. 33). A sample of tissue suspected of containing cancer cells.

Biopsychosocial (Ch. 7 and all chapters). Pertaining to the biological, psychological and social factors considered in a holistic approach.

Blanching erythema (Ch. 10). Reddening of the skin which goes white when light finger pressure is applied, a normal reaction to pressure.

Blister (Ch. 28). A fluid-filled lesion arising in the skin.

Body image (Chs 26, 33). How one perceives one's own body, and subjective sense of attractiveness. The view that each one of us presents about how we see ourselves in reality and as an ideal. It is strongly influenced by cultural norms and values, peer and media pressure.

Bone mineral density (Ch. 27). Bone mass; it is diminished in osteoporosis.

Bone marrow biopsy (Ch. 18). A diagnostic procedure that can take two forms: bone marrow aspirate or trephine. Biopsy samples are usually taken from the posterior iliac crest.

Bradykinesia (Ch. 14). Abnormally slow or retarded movement. There may be problems initiating and then stopping a movement; typically associated with Parkinson's disease.

Breast reconstruction (Ch. 26). The formation of a breast shape after a total mastectomy, using either an implant or a woman's own tissue (sometimes both).

Bronchoconstriction (Ch. 20). Narrowing of the airways.

Buffer (Ch. 8). A substance that minimizes changes in pH by accepting or donating a hydrogen ion.

Bulla (Ch. 28). A large watery blister (> 5 mm in diameter).

Burnout (Ch. 6). A state resulting from exposure to stressors, e.g. prolonged contact with very ill people. Stressors are often work-related and chronic, but burnout may occur as a response to an acute stressor. The adverse effects may be physical, intellectual, emotional, social or spiritual.

Cancer (Ch. 33). A term used to describe any malignant disease. It is characterized by genetic changes and inappropriate cell division and growth.

Carbohydrate (Ch. 11). A macronutrient. Carbohydrates are the major energy source used in the body. There are three major groups: sugars, starches and non-starch polysaccharides (NSP).

Carcinogen (Ch. 33). An agent or substance with the potential to cause cancer.

Cardiac output (Ch. 19). The amount of blood that is ejected from the heart in 1 minute. In the adult this is around 5 litres per minute.

Cardiac rehabilitation (Ch. 19). A process of helping the person with heart disease, e.g. coronary heart disease, to achieve optimal physical and social functioning and to reduce their risk of mortality and morbidity.

Cardiogenic shock (Ch. 9). Shock caused by cardiac failure.

Cast (Ch. 27). Made from plaster of Paris, resin-reinforced plaster bandages and water-activated polymerizable casts. They are used to immobilize the affected part until healing has occurred, so protecting against further damage.

Catabolic (Chs 11, 24). Describes the chemical reactions in the body where complex molecules are broken down into simpler substances to release energy.

Cataract (Ch. 15). An opacity of the crystalline lens.

Catheterization (Chs 12, 24). Insertion of a catheter, most usually into the urinary bladder, in order to drain urine or instil drugs.

Central venous catheters (Chs 11, 18). Long-term venous access devices that are used for patients undergoing intensive cytotoxic chemotherapy regimens, or parenteral nutrition.

Central venous pressure (CVP) (Chs 9, 19, 24, 31). A measurement of the pressure in the right atrium that can assist in fluid balance assessment.

Chemotherapy (Chs 18, 26, 33). The use of drugs to kill cells or slow growth. Usually describes drug treatment to kill cancer cells.

Chest pain (Ch. 19). Any form of pain in the chest not necessarily angina.

Cheyne–Stokes respiration (Ch. 20). Breathing characterized by rhythmic waxing and waning of the depth of respiration.

Cholangiography (Ch. 23). Rarely performed X-ray examination of the biliary system using opaque contrast medium.

Cholecystectomy (Ch. 23). Surgical removal of the gallbladder.

Cholecystitis (Ch. 23). Inflammation of the gallbladder.

Cholecystogram (Ch. 23). Rarely performed X-ray of the gallbladder after administration of opaque contrast medium. Superseded by CT and MRI.

Cholelithiasis (Ch. 23). Gallstones in the gallbladder.

Cholesteatoma (Ch. 16). Abnormally sited squamous epithelium in the middle ear.

Chronic illness (Ch. 35). An illness that exhibits one or more of the following qualities. It is permanent, is associated with irreversible change in the body's function or structure, requires extended rehabilitation, long periods of health care support or requires a major adaptation in the person's lifestyle. Most chronic illnesses exhibit more than one of these characteristics.

Chronic pain (Ch. 7). Pain that persists for more than 3 months or that outlasts the usual healing process.

Chronic wounds (Ch. 10). Wounds associated with prolonged healing times such as large burns, pressure ulcers and leg ulcers. Chronic wounds frequently produce large amounts of wound exudate.

Cilia (Chs 20, 21, 25). Tiny hairs found in the respiratory epithelium, which waft secretions continuously to the back of the nose. Also found in the epithelium lining the uterine tubes.

Circadian rhythm (Ch. 4). Describes a daily cycle.

Cirrhosis (Ch. 23). Chronic degenerative liver disease characterized by destruction of hepatocytes and the formation of dense fibrous scar tissue and fatty infiltration.

Clinical governance (Ch. 2). A system by which goals for quality health care and treatments are going to be set, delivered and monitored. Where quality falls short of the expected or agreed standards, clinical governance holds certain individuals to be ultimately responsible and answerable for it in any individual NHS Trust and provider of services.

Colloid (Ch. 8). A fluid containing solute particles that remain in the bloodstream because they are too large to pass through capillary membranes. Used intravenously to increase extracellular volume.

Colonization (Ch. 13). The presence of microorganisms in a specific environment, such as a body site with only minimal or no response. There is no disease or symptoms, but colonization provides a reservoir of microorganisms that may act as a source of infection.

Communication (all chapters). The delivery or exchange of information, ideas or feelings. Establishing social interaction.

Compliance (Ch. 24). Acting in accordance with a prescribed regimen of treatment such as drugs or diet.

Compression therapy (Ch. 10). A therapy used to reverse the effects of venous hypertension in people with venous leg ulcers. It is usually applied as bandages or hosiery, although other methods do exist.

Connective tissue (Ch. 10). A diverse group of tissues situated throughout the body. They are characterized by having a matrix containing fibres and cells. Examples include areolar, adipose, fibrous, elastic, bone, cartilage, and blood and haemopoietic tissue.

Consent (Ch. 29). To agree or grant permission for an action.

Constipation (Ch. 22). Infrequent, incomplete and often difficult evacuation of hard faeces.

Contamination (Ch. 13). Soiling or pollution of objects, food or water, or infection by pathogens.

Continence (Ch. 12). The ability to control the voiding of urine and faeces.

Continuous positive airways pressure (CPAP) (Ch. 31). A method of respiratory support in the spontaneously breathing patient, which can improve oxygenation and prevent alveolar collapse.

Contusion (Ch. 27). A bruise usually associated with trauma.

Cor pulmonale (Ch. 20). Right ventricular hypertrophy and failure due to vasoconstriction of the pulmonary circulation as a result of local hypoxia in the lungs.

Core temperature (Ch. 5). The temperature within the central cavities of the body (cranium, thorax and abdomen).

Coronary heart disease (Ch. 19). Atheroma of the coronary arteries that eventually may lead to angina, myocardial infarction or heart failure.

Corticosteroids (Ch. 17). Hormones secreted by the adrenal cortex: glucocorticoids, mineralocorticoids and sex hormones.

Counselling (Ch. 3). Verbal and non-verbal skills, which are used intentionally by helpers to enable the client or patient to increase their awareness of significant issues in their lives.

Crepitus (Ch. 27). Grinding noise or sensation within a joint. A symptom of a fracture.

Critical care continuum (Ch. 31). A model that reflects the dynamic nature of critical illness where not only the level of required care can change, but also the appropriateness of the clinical environment.

Cross-infection (Ch. 13). Infection caused when pathogens are transferred from one person to another.

Crust (Ch. 28). Outer layer consisting of dead cells and serum.

Crystalloid (Ch. 8). A clear solution that passes freely between the circulation and tissue fluid. Used to maintain fluid and electrolyte balance.

Culture (Ch. 3 and all chapters). The values and beliefs people or groups of people hold, which are manifest in their way of life and through which they make sense of existence, themselves and lived experiences. These are passed on explicitly and implicitly from generation to generation.

Cushing's disease (Ch. 17). A rare disease caused by excessive cortisol production by hyperplastic adrenal glands as a result of increased adrenocorticotrophic hormone (ACTH) secretion by a tumour or hyperplasia of the anterior pituitary gland. Cushing's syndrome is clinically similar to Cushing's disease but includes all causes of excessive cortisol secretion such as adrenal tumour, ectopic ACTH secretion by cancers elsewhere and due to treatment with glucocorticoids.

Cutaneous (Ch. 28). Pertaining to the skin.

Cyanosis (Ch. 20). Blueness of the skin and mucosa due to hypoxaemia.

Cycloplegic (Ch. 15). An agent/drug that paralyses the ciliary muscle of the eye.

Cytology (Ch. 33). The microscopic study of cells. Used to identify origin, structure and pathology of cells.

Day care surgery (Ch. 29). Surgery performed on an ambulatory basis not requiring an overnight hospital stay.

Debridement (Ch. 10). Removal of dead tissue or foreign bodies from a wound.

Deep vein thrombosis (Chs 19, 29). The formation of a clot or thrombus in a deep vein.

Dementia (Ch. 32). A term that means madness or insanity. A label that has been applied to a number of diseases which lead, not to madness, but to progressive loss of cognitive function, e.g. Alzheimer's disease, Lewy body disease and cerebrovascular dementia, amongst others.

Demography (Ch. 32). The study of populations and their characteristics, such as the age distribution.

Demyelination (Ch. 14). Loss of myelin surrounding nerve fibres.

Dermis (Ch. 28). The true skin; below the epidermis.

Detrusor muscle (Ch. 12). An expelling muscle such as that of the urinary bladder.

Diabetic ketoacidosis (Ch. 17). Acidosis due to accumulation of ketone bodies (e.g. 3-hydroxybutyrate) formed as fatty acids are incompletely oxidized when glucose is unavailable as an energy source. Dehydration, electrolyte imbalance and metabolic acidosis accompany severe hyperglycaemia.

Dialysis (Ch. 24). Process by which solutes are removed from solution by diffusion across a semi-permeable; requires the presence of a favourable solute gradient.

Diarrhoea (Ch. 22). Frequent loose stools.

Diathermy (Ch. 29). The application of heat via a high-frequency current to cut or coagulate tissue.

Differentiation (Chs 18, 33). The process by which cells and tissues develop the ability to perform specialized functions that distinguish them from other cell types. Malignant cells are graded by the degree of differentiation: well differentiated cancer cells resemble the original tissue, whereas poorly differentiated cancer cells are more primitive.

Diffusion (Ch. 8). The movement of a gas or solute from an area of high concentration to an area of lower concentration towards equilibrium.

Dignity (Ch. 29 and all chapters). Promoting the patient's sense of worth and self-respect.

Diplopia (Chs 14, 15). Double vision.

Disability (Ch. 35). The limitations which a person with impairment (e.g. a chronic disease or disfigurement) experiences in carrying out his or her normal functions.

Disc herniation (Ch. 27). Also termed disc prolapse or 'slipped disc'. Disruption to the normal integrity of the intervertebral disc, causing the nucleus pulposus to breach the annular fibres internally.

Discharge planning (Ch. 29). The process of preparation for return to a home environment.

Dislocation (Ch. 27). Displacement of articular surfaces within a joint, so that apposition is lost.

Disseminated intravascular coagulation (DIC) (Chs 9, 18). Results from the simultaneous overactivation of both the coagulation and fibrinolytic pathways, leading to widespread clotting and thrombus formation throughout the body. As clotting factors become exhausted, generalized bleeding can also occur.

Distress (Ch. 6). Negative stress. It is associated with adverse physical, psychological and social effects.

Diuretics (Ch. 24). Substances that increase urine secretion by the kidneys; they include diuretic drugs such as furosemide (frusemide), caffeine in drinks and alcohol.

Diurnal variation (Ch. 4). Describes the variations in physiological processes that occur within the daily pattern, e.g. hormone levels, body temperature, etc.

Diverticulosis (Ch. 22). A condition in which there are many diverticula (pouches), especially in the colon. Associated inflammation is known as diverticulitis.

Dysarthria (Ch. 14). Disorder of speech resulting from a problem in muscular control of speech mechanisms.

Dyspepsia (Ch. 22). Indigestion.

Dysphagia (Chs 11, 14, 22). Difficulty in swallowing.

Dysphasia (Ch. 14). A disorder of language; expressive and/or understanding.

Dyspnoea (Ch. 20). Difficulty breathing or breathlessness.

Dysuria (Ch. 24). Painful (or difficult) micturition.

Ecchymosis (Ch. 28). A large bruise.

Effectiveness (Ch. 2). Health care provision which results in beneficial patient outcomes.

Efficiency (Ch. 2). When services are cost-effective and delivered at as high a quality as possible within the resources available.

Effusion (Chs 20, 27). A collection of fluid in the tissues or body cavities, such as in a joint or a pleural effusion.

Electroencephalogram (EEG) (Chs 4, 14). The measurement of electrical activity in the brain by the use of electrodes placed on the skull.

Electrolyte (Ch. 8). A compound that dissociates into charged particles, called ions, in solution and can conduct an electric current.

Electromyogram (EMG) (Chs 4, 14, 27). The measurement of muscular movement and stimulation.

Electro-oculogram (EOG) (Ch. 4). The measurement of eye movements using electrodes placed near the eye on the temple.

Embryo (Ch. 25). Developing pregnancy from conception to the 8th week of gestation.

Emergency (Ch. 30). An unforeseen or sudden occurrence, requiring immediate action or intervention.

Emmetropia (Ch. 15). Normal vision.

Emollient (Ch. 28). Moisturizer which stays on the skin.

Empowerment (All chapters). The sharing of power and control; to have ownership over decision-making.

Encephalopathy (Chs 14, 23). Any abnormal condition of the structure or function of the brain tissues.

Endocrine gland/structure (Ch. 17). Ductless glands that produce hormones that pass directly into the blood or lymph. They include the pituitary, thyroid, parathyroids, adrenals, pancreas etc.

Endometriosis (Ch. 25). Presence of endometrial tissue outside the uterine cavity.

Endoscopic retrograde cholangiopancreatography (ERCP) (Ch. 23). Endoscopic examination of the pancreatic ducts and hepatobilary system.

Endoscopy (Chs 20, 21, 22, 23, 24, 25, 27). The examination of hollow tubular structures such as the gastrointestinal, urinary and respiratory tract, or body cavities using a flexible fibreoptic telescope (an endoscope). It also permits photography, biopsy and treatment.

Epidemiology (Ch. 33 and all chapters). The study of the distribution of diseases in populations. The incidence and prevalence of particular diseases such as cancer.

Epidermis (Ch. 28). The superficial layer of the skin.

Epistaxis (Ch. 21). Nosebleed. Usually minor but may be life-threatening.

Equity (Ch. 2). A dimension of quality in Maxwell's model which is about having services available to patients irrespective of their social, cultural or racial background. A patient's need for health care should be the paramount determinant of the appropriate provision.

Erectile dysfunction (ED) (Ch. 25). Can be defined as the inability of a man to gain an erection of sufficient quality for intercourse. This definition supersedes the older term of impotence.

Erythema (Ch. 28). Redness of the skin due to vascular congestion.

Erythrodermic (Ch. 28). A generalized redness of the skin at least 90% of total surface, associated with desquamation.

Eschar (Chs 10, 28). A collection of dehydrated exudate, fibrinogen and cellular debris that forms a hard, sometimes leathery, covering on the surface of a wound.

Ethics (Ch. 1 and all chapters). Relating to the study of moral knowledge and human behaviour, and what is considered by a society or a profession to be right, just and good.

Eustress (Ch. 6). Positive stress. It is associated with pleasurable excitement and euphoria. The long-term effects of eustress are less damaging than those from distress.

Evidence-based practice/nursing (Ch. 1 and all chapters). Professional practice that is based on the best available evidence regarding its effectiveness. Where there is insufficient research evidence, evidence-based care will be based on a consensus view of best practice.

Excoriation (Ch. 28). Loss of skin substance due to scratching.

Exfoliation (Ch. 28). Splitting off or separation of keratin and epidermal skin surface in scales or sheets.

Extension (Ch. 27). Straightening of a joint. The opposite of flexion or bending.

External auditory canal (Ch. 16). A bony and cartilaginous canal that allows the passage of sound from the pinna to the tympanic membrane.

External fixator (Ch. 27). External device used as an alternative treatment to internal fixation and the use of traction for certain fractures.

Exudate (Chs 10, 29). The serous fluid that is produced from the surface of a wound. It is a clear or straw-coloured secretion that varies in consistency from very runny to thick and viscous.

Faecal incontinence (Ch. 12). An inability to control the passage of faeces.

Fat (Ch. 11). A macronutrient. The main dietary fat is triacylglycerol (triglyceride). See Lipid.

Febrile (Ch. 5). Feverish; relating to a fever.

Fetus (Ch. 25). Developing pregnancy from the 9th week of gestation.

Fissure (Chs 22, 28). Cleft or split.

Fistula (Chs 22, 29). An abnormal opening or tract between two organs or structures.

Flaccid (Ch. 14). Soft and flabby, such as the loss of muscle tone due to disturbance of the lower motor neuron.

Flexion (Ch. 27). Bending at the joint. The opposite of extension or straightening.

Flexural (Ch. 28). Area of skin against skin, i.e. axilla, groin.

Fracture (Ch. 27). A break in the continuity of a bone.

Frailty (Ch. 32). Defies accurate definition but implies a lower than normal ability to withstand the physiological stresses which life imposes. Older people who are frail have disproportionately suffered from the process of ageing either due to lack of inherent ability to withstand the process of ageing or due to external factors such as environment.

Gallstones (Ch. 23). Stone-like masses (calculi) that form in the gallbladder.

Gastrointestinal tract/canal (Ch. 22). The whole digestive tract from mouth to anus. It comprises the mouth, oesophagus, stomach, small and large intestine (bowel).

Glasgow coma scale (Ch. 14). A 14-point scale for assessing conscious level by evaluating three behavioural responses: best verbal response, motor response and eye opening.

Glaucoma (Ch. 15). Condition occurring when the intraocular pressure (IOP) is high enough to damage the optic nerve as it leaves the eye and disrupt the visual field.

Glomerular filtration rate (GFR) (Ch. 24). The volume of plasma filtered by the kidneys in one minute.

Granulation tissue (Ch. 10). The term used to describe the growth of new capillary loops, and supporting collagen in the base of a wound during the proliferative phase of healing. Healthy granulation tissue is moist and red and is fragile.

Groups (Ch. 3). Any number of people together, whether purposefully or not.

Guttae (G) (Ch. 15). Prescription term for eye drops.

Gynaecomastia (Ch. 26). The growth of breast tissue in men.

Haematemesis (Ch. 22). Vomiting of blood from the gastrointestinal tract.

Haematuria (Ch. 24). Blood in the urine, either visible or microscopic.

Haemodynamic instability (Ch. 19). Unstable cardiac function, demonstrated through labile intracardiac pressures such as blood pressure or central venous pressure.

Haemoglobinopathy (Ch. 18). An inherited disorder of haemoglobin synthesis. Examples are sickle cell disease and thalassaemia.

Haemolysis (Ch. 18). The breakdown or destruction of red blood cells.

Haemopoiesis (Ch. 18). The process of blood cell formation within the bone marrow.

Haemopoietic growth factors (Ch. 18). Factors that regulate blood cell production by acting upon stem cells within the bone marrow, causing them to differentiate into specific cell types.

Haemopoietic stem cell transplantation (bone marrow transplantation) (Ch. 18). Enables normal blood cell production to be re-established in patients whose bone marrow function is inadequate or has failed as a result of disease or its treatment. The healthy stem cells are infused into the patient and serve to repopulate the bone marrow.

Haemoptysis (Ch. 20). Coughing up blood.

Haemostasis (Chs 18, 29). The process by which blood clots at the site of an injury to prevent excessive blood loss. It is often explained in terms of vasoconstriction, platelet plug formation, blood coagulation and fibrinolysis. Or the state of bleeding cessation following haemorrhage.

Haemostat (Ch. 29). A device, dressing or application which, when applied, stops bleeding.

Hand washing (Ch. 13 and all chapters). A vital activity in preventing and controlling infection in all settings. Local policies dictate situations where handwashing is undertaken both before and after a procedure or only after contact, and when gloves are worn and when antiseptic hand rubs are used.

Handicap (Ch. 35). A term used to indicate the limitations in social function caused by a disability. The term is rejected by many disability groups as it fails to acknowledge society's part in limiting the opportunities available to those with impairment.

Health (Ch. 1 and all chapters). A state of physical, emotional and social well-being. It is a personal construct.

Health education (Ch. 1 and all chapters). Provides education and enhances coping strategies, skills etc. to enable individuals to take charge of and improve their health and thus prevent them becoming patients. Measures used by health care professionals to enable people to adapt to changes in their health status, promote positive health behaviours, and support those wishing to change negative health behaviours.

Health promotion (Ch. 1 and all chapters). Describes the many diverse measures that aim to improve the health of individuals, specific communities or whole populations.

Helicobacter pylori (Ch. 22). Bacterium causing a common chronic infection found beneath the gastric mucosa, which affects gastric function and is now accepted as the cause of non-immune chronic gastritis and most peptic ulcers.

Hemiparesis (Ch. 14). Weakness on one side of the body.

Hemiplegia (Ch. 14). Paralysis on one side of the body.

Hepatitis (Ch. 23). Inflammation of the liver, usually associated with viral infections.

Hiatus hernia (Ch. 22). Occurs when a part of the stomach wall pushes up through a weakness in the diaphragm.

High-dependency unit (HDU) (Ch. 31). A designated clinical area that provides a level of care beyond what is possible or appropriate in a general ward/department.

Histology (Ch. 33). Microscopic study of tissues; used for the clarification of the characteristics of a cancer cell and the stage of the cancer.

Holistic care (Ch. 1 and all chapters). Health care that meets the physical, emotional and spiritual needs of patients and clients. Caring for the patient as a whole rather than individual problems.

Homeostasis (Ch. 24). The ability of cells to maintain a number of chemical and physical properties within a relatively narrow range.

Hormone (Ch. 17). A specific chemical messenger secreted by endocrine glands (and other structures) that is transported in the blood or lymph to regulate the functions of tissues and organs elsewhere in the body.

Hormone therapy (Ch. 26). The use of drugs which specifically inhibit the growth of hormone-responsive tumours.

Hospice (Ch. 34). A specialist unit caring for the palliative patient and family.

Hospital-acquired infection (HAI) (Ch. 13). Nosocomial infection. One that occurs in a patient who has been in hospital for at least 72 hours and did not have signs and symptoms of such infection on admission. The commonest HAI is urinary tract infection.

Hypercapnia (Ch. 20). Excess of carbon dioxide in arterial blood.

Hyperglycaemia (Ch. 17). Blood glucose level above normal.

Hypermetropia (Ch. 15). Long-sighted; near vision is blurred, whilst distance vision may be clear.

Hyperparathyroidism (Ch. 17). Overactivity of one or more parathyroid glands, usually due to parathyroid adenoma, and resulting in elevated serum calcium levels.

Hyperpyrexia (Ch. 5). Elevation in core body temperature above 40°C. In the majority of cases the cause is infection with microorganisms, but other causes include cancers and acute myocardial infarction. The thermoregulatory mechanisms are undamaged and the hypothalamus is functioning normally.

Hyperthermia (Ch. 5). Elevation in core body temperature due to loss of thermoregulatory control. There is dysfunction of the hypothalamus mainly due to brain injury.

Hyperthyroidism (Ch. 17). Thyrotoxicosis. A condition caused by excessive secretion of thyroid hormones. It results in increased metabolic rate.

Hyphaema (Ch. 15). The presence of blood in the anterior chamber of the eye.

Hypodermoclysis (Ch. 8). The subcutaneous infusion of fluids.

Hypoglycaemia (Ch. 17). Blood glucose level below normal.

Hypoparathyroidism (Ch. 17). Underactivity of the parathyroid glands resulting in decreased serum calcium levels, producing tetany.

Hypopyon (Ch. 15). The presence of pus in the anterior chamber of the eye.

Hyposmia (Ch. 21). A diminished sense of smell.

Hypothermia (Chs 5, 29). Decrease in core body temperature. Usually defined as less than 35°C but some authorities use less than 35.6°C.

Hypothyroidism (Ch. 17). Myxoedema. Condition caused by low circulating levels of one or both thyroid hormones; it results in decreased metabolic rate.

Hypovolaemia (Ch. 9). A reduction in the circulating blood volume.

Hypovolaemic shock (Ch. 9). Shock caused by a reduction in circulating blood volume.

Hypoxaemia (Chs 8, 9, 20). Lack of oxygen in the blood. Decreased arterial blood oxygen concentration.

Hypoxia (Ch. 9, 20). Lack of oxygen in the tissues.

Hypoxic respiratory drive (Ch. 20). The stimulus to breathe is driven by low levels of oxygen.

Hysterectomy (Ch. 25). Surgical removal of the uterus.

Hysteroscopy (Ch. 25). Surgical endoscopic investigation to view the uterine cavity.

Impairment (Ch. 35). A limitation in the function of a person's body or mind caused by disease or injury.

Infection (Ch. 13). The successful invasion, establishment and growth of microorganisms in the host tissues.

Infertility (Ch. 25). Also known as subfertility. Can be defined as the inability of a couple to conceive spontaneously.

Inflammatory bowel disease (IBD) (Ch. 22). Describes a range of inflammatory diseases that affect the gastrointestinal tract, e.g. Crohn's disease, ulcerative colitis, etc.

Inoculation injury (Ch. 13). An injury to the skin or mucosa that allows the entry of pathogens into the body such as a needlestick injury.

Inotrope therapy (Chs 31, 19). Inotropes are drugs that increase the force of contraction of the heart, thereby increasing blood pressure.

Insensible loss (Ch. 8). Normally occurring fluid losses through the skin and lungs of which the individual is not aware.

Insulin (Ch. 17). A polypeptide hormone produced by the pancreas. It influences the metabolism of carbohydrate, protein and fat. Commercially available insulin is used in the management of diabetes.

Intensive care unit (ICU) (Ch. 31). A designated clinical area that provides a level of care beyond what is possible or appropriate in the HDU.

Interdisciplinary care (Ch. 29). Collaborative care partnership involving two or more disciplines.

Intermittent (in/out) catheterization (Ch. 12). Drainage of the bladder with subsequent removal of the catheter.

Internal desynchronization (Ch. 4). Where the sensitive body rhythms do not match their 'normal' pattern for sleep and activity and become disordered.

Intestinal obstruction (Ch. 22). The intestine can be obstructed by something in the lumen, abnormality in the wall, or pressure from outside.

Intra-articular (Ch. 27). Within the joint.

Intracranial pressure (Ch. 14). Pressure inside the skull. Maintained within the normal range by the brain tissue, intracellular and extracellular fluid, cerebrospinal fluid and blood.

Ion (Ch. 8). An atom that has become electrically charged by gaining or losing an electron(s).

Irritable bowel syndrome (IBS) (Ch. 22). A common condition caused by abnormal contractions of the muscles of large intestine. Leads to recurring cramp-like or colicky abdominal pain and an altered bowel habit.

Ischaemia (Chs 9, 19). Lack of blood.

Isolation (Chs 13, 18, 33). Removal of a patient away from others. It may be to contain infection, protect immunocompromised individuals or isolate patients who are sources of microorganisms that may be transmitted from them to infect others.

Jaundice (Ch. 23). Yellow discoloration of the skin, sclera and mucous membranes, caused by increased serum bilirubin.

Jet lag (Ch. 4). Disturbance of physiological processes which normally follow a diurnal rhythm, occurs after travel through different time zones. May affect appetite, sleep, concentration, and cause tiredness.

Joint (Ch. 27). The articulation of two or more bones.

Keloid (Ch. 28). Elevated progressive scar formation without regression.

Kyphosis (Ch. 27). Exaggerated backward curvature of the spine, in the flexion/extension axis.

Laparoscopic cholecystecomy (Ch. 23). Surgical removal of the gallbladder using minimal access surgical techniques.

Laparoscopy (Ch. 25). Surgical endoscopic investigation using keyhole technique to view abdominal and pelvic organs.

Leukaemia (Ch. 18). A disorder that results from the uncontrolled proliferation of abnormal immature blood cells (blast cells) within the bone marrow.

Lipid (Ch. 11). A large diverse group of organic fat-like molecules that include triacylglycerols, phospholipids, fat-soluble vitamins, lipoproteins and prostaglandins.

Liver function tests (Ch. 23). A range of blood tests (e.g. bilirubin) to assist the diagnosis of various liver disorders.

Long-term care (Ch. 32). This type of care of older people takes place in four environments: the individual's own home, nursing homes, residential homes and hospitals. Apart from long-term care in hospital, the responsibility for long-term care in the community, which covers home, nursing and residential homes, rests with the local departments of social services.

Lymph nodes (Ch. 26). Accumulations of lymphoid tissue at strategic intervals, e.g. axilla. They filter lymph and remove extraneous particles such as microorganisms and cancer cells. Normally they are a site of B- and T-lymphocyte proliferation and antibody production.

Lymphoedema (Ch. 26). Swelling caused by a collection of lymph in the tissues, usually affecting the arm.

Lymphoma (Ch. 18). A diverse group of tumours that originate in lymphoid tissue. Divided into two groups: Hodgkin's lymphoma (Hodgkin's disease) and non-Hodgkin's lymphoma (NHL).

Macule (Ch. 28). Stain < 1 cm with a flat surface that does not blanch.

Malignant (Ch. 33). Cancer that has invaded the blood or lymphatic systems and/or surrounding tissue.

Mammogram (Ch. 26). An X-ray of the breast.

Mastalgia (Ch. 26). Breast pain.

Mastoid cavity (Ch. 16). An artificial cavity that is created by mastoid surgery and housed within the mastoid bone.

Mastoiditis (Ch. 16). An infective process that affects the air cells located in the mastoid bone.

Mechanical ventilation (Ch. 31). A mechanical ventilator can provide all or some of the breathing required in a patient with respiratory failure.

Melaena (Ch. 22). Describes black-coloured faeces that contain altered blood.

Men's health (Ch. 25). Can be defined using several components: biological –such as those diseases that affect men only; behavioural – the concept of risk and risk-taking; and social – context of sexuality. All three impact on men's perception of health and ill health.

Menorrhagia (Ch. 25). Heavy bleeding during the regular period, often accompanied by pain.

Menstrual cycle (Ch. 25). The hormonal cycle experienced by women from puberty to menopause, resulting in development and release of oocytes and menstruation.

Menstruation (Ch. 25). Shedding of endometrium causing bleeding during a period.

Metastases (Chs 26, 33, 34). The secondary deposits of cancer outside of the organ where the primary cancer exists. Spread occurs via the blood or lymphatic system, or across body cavities.

Microorganism (Ch. 13). Any microscopic cell. Often synonymous with bacterium but also includes protozoon, rickettsia, *Chlamydia*, fungus and virus.

Micturition (Chs 12, 24). Passing or voiding urine.

Mineral (Ch. 11). Inorganic mineral elements (e.g. sodium, calcium, iron and selenium). Micronutrients that function within the body and must be in the diet.

Miotic (myotic) (Ch. 15). A drug that decreases the size of the pupil (constricts).

Mixed urinary incontinence (Ch. 12). Involuntary leakage associated with urgency and also with exertion, effort, sneezing or coughing.

Monoclonal antibody (Ch. 18). Describes an antibody derived from a single cell. These highly specific antibodies are used to harness the body's natural immune system to destroy malignant cells by targeting specific antigens expressed on the surface of tumour cells.

Morbidity (all chapters). The state of being diseased.

Mortality (all chapters). Being mortal and subject to death, such as the number of people dying as a result of a certain disease or operative procedure. Mortality rate shows these statistically as the number occurring annually per unit of population.

Mucositis (Chs 18, 33). Inflammation of the oral or gastrointestinal mucosa.

Multidisciplinary team (all chapters). A team of health professionals working together to provide care for the patient and family.

Multiple organ dysfunction and failure (Ch. 9). Vital organs such as the kidney are unable to perform their usual functions, resulting in major derangements of metabolism and the need for organ support.

Mutagen (Ch. 33). A chemical with the potential to cause genetic changes in an embryo or within the first trimester of pregnancy.

Mydriatic (Ch. 15). A drug which increases the size of the pupil (dilates).

Myeloma (Ch. 18). A malignant disorder of the bone marrow that results from an uncontrolled proliferation of plasma cells.

Myopathy (Ch. 27). A disease of muscle.

Myopia (Ch. 15). Short-sighted. Distance vision is usually unclear, whilst near vision may be clear.

Necrosis (Ch. 10). Areas of tissue found in the wound bed that has become devitalized and has died due to ischaemia. Necrotic tissue often has a black or dark brown appearance; when moist it has a gelatinous appearance, and when dry, it has a hard leathery appearance (see 'eschar').

Neoplasm (Ch. 33). Any abnormal growth of tissue. Also referred to as a tumour. A neoplasm may be either benign or malignant.

Neuropathic pain (Ch. 7). Nerve injury or irritation is the source of pain, and pain persists long after the precipitating event.

Neutropenia (Ch. 18). The state of having too few neutrophils, usually defined as a neutrophil count of less than 1.0×10^9/L. This greatly increases the risk of systemic infection.

Nociception (Ch. 7). Perception of a potentially tissue damaging stimulus from the site of injury to the brain.

Nocturia (Chs 12, 24). Waking at night to pass urine.

Nodule (Ch. 28). Rounded, elevated solid lesion (> 1 cm).

Non-judgmental attitude (Ch. 25 and all chapters). Essential when nursing patients with any disorder but particularly so with those affecting the reproductive tract or sexual health in order to develop rapport when dealing with personal and sensitive issues.

Non-verbal communication (Ch. 3). The ways in which people consciously or unconsciously use physical expression, such as proximity, posture, gesture, facial expression, dress, time and space, to convey meaning.

Normal flora (Ch. 13). The microorganisms that normally colonize various areas of the body, e.g. *Escherichia coli* in the bowel.

Normothermia (Ch. 5). Normal body temperature.

Nosocomial infection (Ch. 13). Hospital-acquired infection.

Nursing and Midwifery Council (Ch. 1). The regulatory body for nursing and midwifery in the UK. It replaced the United Kingdom Central Council in April 2002.

Nursing models (Ch. 1 and all chapters). A conceptual framework designed to guide nurses in the assessment of patients' needs. Nursing models are based on a set of beliefs about four key issues: health, the patient/client, the environment and nursing.

Nursing process (Ch. 1 and all chapters). A systematic, problem-solving approach to nursing care that involves four stages: assessment, planning, implementation and evaluation.

Nutrition (Chs 11 and all chapters). The composition of food and the relationship between diet and health. In understanding nutritional needs, it is necessary to explore the physiological effects of nutrients and the sociological and psychological impact of eating.

Occulentum (Oc) (Ch. 15). Prescription term for ointment.

Ocular (Ch. 15). Pertaining to the eye.

Oedema (Ch. 8). The collection of excess tissue fluid.

Oesophageal varices (Ch. 23). Distended blood vessels caused by portal hypertension.

Olfaction (Ch. 21). The chemical sense of smell.

Oliguria (Ch. 24). Reduction in the amount of urine secreted by the kidneys; there is very little urine output.

Oncogenes (Ch. 33). Abnormal genes that cause unrestricted growth of cells and their descendants.

Oncology (Ch. 33). The study and treatment of cancer.

Oophorectomy (Ch. 25). Surgical removal of an ovary.

Ophthalmology (Ch. 15). The science that deals with the eye: structure, function, diseases and treatment.

Oral hypoglycaemic agents (Ch. 17). Drugs that reduce blood glucose (in a variety of ways).

Orthopnoea (Ch. 20). Ability to breathe freely only in the upright position.

Orthosis (Ch. 27). An external device utilized to correct, control or counteract the effect of an actual or developing deformity. They include braces, calipers and splints.

Osmosis (Ch. 8). The movement of a solvent, usually water, across a semi-permeable membrane from an area of high water concentration to one of low water concentration.

Osteoporosis (Ch. 27). A condition whereby the total amount of bone is reduced, with the bone becoming less dense. Common cause of fractures, particularly crush fractures of the spine, wrist and neck of femur fractures.

Otalgia (Ch. 16). Pain in or around the ear.

Otitis media (Ch. 16). An inflammatory process occurring in the middle ear.

Otorrhoea (Ch. 16). Discharge from the ear.

Otoscopy (Ch. 16). Examination of the tympanic membrane with an otoscope.

Outcome (Ch. 2). One of the criteria in Donabedian's Structure Process Outcome model and is the answer to the question: 'What do we need to achieve for patients?' For example, the result of a nursing procedure is an outcome.

Outreach team (Chs 9, 31). A team that offers a hospital-wide service to support the care of patients who have been discharged from critical care and to assist in the early identification of patients whose conditions are deteriorating.

Overactive bladder (Ch. 12). Frequency and urgency with/without nocturia and with/without urge incontinence.

Pain (Ch. 7). A unique subjective experience that the patient says hurts and has both a physiologic sensation and an emotional reaction to that sensation.

Pain and symptom management (Chs 7, 29, 34). Interventions used to control pain and associated symptoms, such as nausea, vomiting, constipation.

Pain assessment (Ch. 7). The subjective measurement of the patient's pain relying on the patient's report and not the perception of the health carer.

Pain threshold (Ch. 7). The lowest intensity at which a given stimulus is perceived as painful and is relatively constant across subjects for a given stimulus.

Pain tolerance (Ch. 7). The greatest level of pain that the individual is prepared to endure; this varies widely across subjects.

Palliation (Chs 26, 33, 34). Symptom relief, without a prospect of cure.

Palliative care (Ch. 34). Active total care of patients whose disease is not curable.

Palpitations (Ch. 19). A fluttering sensation that is felt in the chest. Usually caused by a fast or irregular heartbeat.

Pancreatitis (Ch. 23). Inflammation of the pancreas, may be acute or chronic.

Pancytopenia (Ch. 18). Describes a simultaneous reduction in red cell, white cell and platelet counts. It often occurs as a result of bone marrow disorder.

Papule (Ch. 28). Raised lesion or scaly, crusted, keratinized or macerated surface (< 1 cm).

Paracentesis (Ch. 23). Drainage of fluid, e.g. ascites from the peritoneal cavity.

Paraesthesia (Ch. 14). Any abnormal sensation such as tingling, burning or 'pins and needles'.

Paralinguistics (Ch. 3). The tone or modulation of the voice.

Paraplegia (Ch. 14). Paralysis affecting the trunk below the level of the spinal lesion, the lower limbs and usually the bladder and rectum.

Pathogenic (Ch. 13). Capable of producing disease, such as a microorganism.

Patient education (Ch. 29 and all chapters). The process of providing information to patients that seeks to enhance knowledge, attitudes and skills.

Pelvic floor (Ch. 12). The layers of muscles and connective tissue that support the pelvic organs.

Pelvic floor exercises (Ch. 12). Physiotherapy involving a series of pelvic floor contractions that may be used in conjunction with other aids, e.g. electrical stimulation or mechanical devices.

Penile cancer (Ch. 25). Cancer affecting the penis is usually squamous cell carcinoma. It is an uncommon cancer and is more common in men aged over 60 years. There are various types of pre-malignant lesions (chronic red or pale patches) that appear on the glans penis.

Peptic ulceration (Ch. 22). A non-malignant erosion in those parts of the digestive tract which are exposed to the gastric secretions; usually the stomach or duodenum but sometimes in the lower oesophagus, or jejunum following surgical anastomosis to the stomach.

Perforation of tympanic membrane (Ch. 16). A hole in the tympanic membrane.

Perfusion (Ch. 9). The flow of fluid (blood) through the tissues.

Perioperative care (Ch. 29). The entire surgical experience from pre-admission to discharge.

Peripheral temperature (Ch. 5). The temperature recorded at peripheral parts of the body, e.g. the limbs; temperature decreases with distance from the trunk (core temperature), i.e. the gradient between core and peripheral temperature increases.

Petechia (Ch. 28). Small, purple or red haemorrhagic spots.

Phonophobia (Ch. 14). Intolerance to noise.

Photophobia (Ch. 14). Intolerance to light.

Plaque (Ch. 28). Elevated, flat-topped lesions (> 1 cm).

Portal hypertension (hepatic portal hypertension) (Ch. 23). Increased vascular resistance within the hepatic portal vein, leading to the development of a collateral system, with back-flow into the veins of the stomach, spleen, intestines and oesophagus.

Post-anaesthetic recovery (Ch. 29). The emergence from the effects of anaesthesia in the immediate postoperative period.

Post-traumatic stress disorder (PTSD) (Ch. 6). A condition that occurs within 6 months of exposure to a triggering event. Defined by the WHO as: "A delayed and/or protracted response to a stressful event or situation (either short- or long-lasting) of an exceptionally threatening or catastrophic nature, which is likely to cause pervasive distress in almost anyone."

Power in nursing (Ch. 3). The ability to command and/or control situations where self and/or others are likely to have influence over or be influenced by, nursing practice. This may be intentional or unintentional, conscious or unconscious.

Preoperative assessment (Chs 25, 29). Holistic assessment of health status to ensure patients are fit to undergo general or local anaesthetic and surgery.

Pressure reducing equipment (Ch. 10). Equipment, usually beds, mattresses or chairs which, by distributing pressure over a greater surface area, reduces the pressure at any given point on the body. Examples include high-density foam mattresses, low air loss overlays.

Pressure-relieving equipment (Ch. 10). Equipment, usually mattresses or cushions, which completely removes the pressure from the body; this is usually in a cyclical method applying and removing the pressure in a given timed cycle.

Pressure ulcers (Ch. 10). Tissue damage (which may or may not involve a break in the skin) caused by direct application of pressure, shear or friction or a combination of these. Previously known as decubitus ulcers, pressure sores.

Primary intention (Ch. 10). Describes the process of healing when the two edges of a wound are held together by sutures, staples or other method of skin closure. Wounds healing by primary intention are characterized by minimal tissue loss such as surgical incisions, cuts or lacerations.

Process (Ch. 2). One of the criteria in Donabedian's Structure Process Outcome model and is the answer to the question: 'What do we need to do to achieve quality?' For example, how we provide care and services are process issues.

Pronation (Ch. 27). Turning of the palm of the hand downwards; the opposite of 'supination'.

Prosthesis (Ch. 27). An artificial device used to replace a particular body part, e.g. the use of a prosthetic limb following amputation.

Protein (Ch. 11). A macronutrient. Complex nitrogenous organic compounds formed from amino acids in different combinations and sequences. Essential for cellular function, growth and repair. They can be used as an energy source during catabolic states.

Proto-oncogenes (Ch. 33). Genes with the potential to undergo genetic change and transform into oncogenes.

Pruritus (Chs 23, 28). Intense itching; may be caused by accumulation of bile salts in the skin.

Pulmonary artery wedge pressure (PAWP) (Ch. 31). Pressure measured in the pulmonary circulation reflecting the pressures in the left side of the heart, which can contribute to the assessment of fluid balance and cardiopulmonary function.

Purpura (Chs 18, 28). Discoloration caused by the extravasation of blood into the skin or mucosae (see 'ecchymosis', 'petechia').

Pustule (Ch. 28). Pus-filled lesion (< 1 cm).

Pyloric stenosis (Ch. 22). Obstruction of the pylorus due to either spasm or scar tissue, leading to delayed gastric emptying, stomach distension and projectile vomiting.

Pyrexia (Ch. 5). Elevation of body temperature. Usually applied to temperatures between 37.5 and 40°C.

Quadriplegia (Ch. 14). See 'tetraplegia'.

Quality (Ch. 2 and all chapters). A generally agreed definition does not exist. One definition is excellence in what we do.

Quality assurance (Ch. 2). Generally accepted to be a planned, dynamic and cyclic system that is able to assure that problems can be identified through monitoring and measurement, options for solutions considered and the best one chosen to act on, thereby assuring quality.

Quality enhancement (Ch. 2). In effect, this means raising standards of care and treatment by health care providers.

RICE (Ch. 27). Acronym for *r*est, *i*ce, *c*ompression and *e*levation; used in acute injury management to limit inflammatory processes and to speed up the recovery process by eliminating swelling.

Radiotherapy (Chs 18, 26, 33, 34). The use of radiation to kill tumour cells. Used primarily in the treatment of cancer but sometimes used to treat non-malignant diseases.

Rapid/premature ejaculation (Ch. 25). Persistent or recurrent ejaculation with minimal sexual stimulation before, on or shortly after penetration and before the person wishes it.

Reflection/reflective practice (Ch. 1 and all chapters). The ability to review, during and in retrospect, one's professional thought, feelings and actions in order to learn from them, thus developing and adjusting practice so that improved or situationally appropriate services/care is delivered.

Refraction (Ch. 15). The bending of light rays as they pass through media of different densities. In normal vision (emmetropia), this allows the image to focus on the retina.

Rehabilitation (Chs 14, 19, 27, 33, 35). The restoration of a 'normal' or optimal state of health and the preparation of a disabled or disadvantaged person for employment by vocational counselling or training (Gender 1998, see Ch. 33).

Renal (Ch. 24). Pertaining to the kidney.

Renal failure (Ch. 24). May be acute or chronic. In either case, loss of normal renal function results in an inability to maintain fluid, electrolyte and acid–base homeostasis.

Renal replacement therapy (Chs 24, 31). A range of techniques that can provide key renal functions such as fluid, metabolic and electrolyte balance in acute or chronic renal failure.

Respiratory failure (Ch. 20). Inability to maintain adequate oxygenation and adequate carbon dioxide elimination.

Resuscitation (Ch. 30). The process of restoring to consciousness; intervention used to revive a patient.

Retinopathy (Ch. 15). A disease of the retina, e.g. diabetic retinopathy.

Rhinorrhoea (Ch. 21). Nasal discharge. May be clear, purulent (greenish-yellow) or bloodstained.

Rhinosinusitis (Ch. 21). Inflammation of the nose and air sinuses.

Safety (Ch. 29). Freedom from danger and risk.

Salpingectomy (Ch. 25). Surgical removal of one or both uterine (fallopian) tubes.

Scoliosis (Ch. 27). A lateral curvature of the spinal column. The cause may be structural, compensatory or protective.

Screening (Ch. 33). The process concerned with monitoring apparently healthy people with the aim of discovering previously undisclosed disease.

Secondary intention (Ch. 10). Chronic wounds that have large amounts of tissue loss, such as burns or pressure ulcers, cannot have their wound edges brought together. The term used to describe this type of healing is secondary intention. Healing by secondary intention is often slower than wounds healing by primary intention, as healing occurs from the wound base with the growth of new capillaries and connective tissue.

Seizure (Ch. 14). An electrical disturbance in the brain. The word 'fit' is not useful because seizures may not resemble the 'classic fit' of muscular convulsions and loss of consciousness.

Self-awareness (Ch. 3). The ability to be aware of one's own thoughts, feelings and actions and what motivates them, at any given time.

Senescence (Ch. 32). Visible signs of ageing; biological ageing.

Sepsis (Chs 9, 13). The state of being infected with pus-forming (pyogenic) microorganisms.

Septic shock (Ch. 9). Shock caused by overwhelming inflammatory response, resulting from infection.

Sexual health (Ch. 25). Health status of women and men related to internal and external reproductive structures.

Shift work (Ch. 4). Changing work hours can lead to internal desynchronization, whereby some biological rhythms are disordered. These include sleep-wake cycle, hormone secretion and metabolic processes.

Shock (Ch. 9). Inadequate or inappropriately distributed tissue perfusion resulting in generalized cellular hypoxia.

Skin closure (Ch. 29). Process of bringing wound edges together using sutures, clips, staples or surgical glue.

Skin preparation (Ch. 29). Preoperative removal of body hair and physical cleansing to minimize risk of sepsis and infection.

Skin turgor (Ch. 8). The elastic recoil of the skin when it is pinched.

Sleep (Ch. 4). A recurrent natural condition where consciousness is temporarily lost and bodily functions partly suspended. It is reversible, either by a natural return to consciousness or by external stimulation, e.g. by an alarm clock.

Sleep hygiene (Ch. 4). A ritual approach to settling known to promote sleep.

Sleep inversion (Ch. 4). Sleeping during the day and being awake at night.

Sleep latency (Ch. 4). Ability to fall asleep.

Slough (Ch. 10). Cellular debris and bacteria that collect on the surface of a wound. Slough is viscous and can be a variety of colours ranging from creamy white to yellow.

Somatic pain (Ch. 7). Pain that is well localized and consistent with the underlying lesion.

Somnambulance (Ch. 4). Sleep-walking.

Spastic (Ch. 14). Affected by spasm. Describes the increased muscle tone, rigidity and limb stiffness associated with disorders of upper motor neurons.

Standard (Ch. 2). A level of performance that is agreed in advance which should be measurable; quality is too all-encompassing a term and not directly measurable.

Stem cell (Ch. 18). Pluripotent stem cells are found within the bone marrow. They differentiate through several stages to become any type of blood cell.

Stenting (Chs 19, 23). The insertion of a stent to keep a duct or vessel patent.

Stoma (Chs 22, 24). The mouth, describes any opening, e.g. opening of the bowel or ureters on to the abdominal wall.

Stomatitis (Ch. 22). Embraces a number of conditions that are characterized by inflammation of the mouth.

Stress (Ch. 6). The response of an organism to any demand made upon it. It is generally associated with negative effects on health; however, a certain amount of stress is necessary for survival. Stress may be described as a negative (distress) or positive (eustress) phenomenon.

Stress management (Ch. 6). The measures taken to reduce the negative aspects of stress. They include pharmacological (orthodox and complementary) and non-pharmacological strategies such as dietary modification, exercise, time management, relaxation, counselling etc.

Stress urinary incontinence (Chs 12, 25). Involuntary leakage of urine on effort or exertion, or on sneezing or coughing.

Stressor (Ch. 6). Any stimulus that invokes the stress response; it follows that stressors encompass both physiological (e.g. blood loss, hunger, pain) and psychosocial (e.g. overwork, divorce, low income) phenomena.

Stress-related illness (Ch. 6). An illness that is related to maladaption to prolonged exposure to stress. The circulatory and immune systems are extremely susceptible to the destructive effects of prolonged stress. Other stress-related illnesses include tension headaches, peptic ulcer, worsening of asthma, anxiety and depression.

Stridor (Ch. 21). Harsh, noisy breathing. May occur on inspiration, expiration or both (biphasic).

Stroke volume (Ch. 19). The amount of blood ejected from the heart with each cardiac cycle. In the adult this is usually around 70 mL.

Structure (Ch. 2). One of the criteria in Donabedian's Structure Process Outcome model; it is the answer to the question: 'What do we need to have to be able to achieve quality?' For example, we need staff with appropriate skills and qualifications and in sufficient numbers to reach certain care standards.

Subluxation (Ch. 27). Partial dislocation of a joint.

Supination (Ch. 27). Turning of the hand so that the palm faces upward. Opposite of 'pronation'.

Suprapubic catheterization (Ch. 24). The insertion of a catheter into the bladder via an abdominal approach, above the level of the symphysis pubis.

Symptom control (Ch. 34). Relief of symptoms enabling patients to have an improved quality of life.

Syncope (Ch. 19). A sudden loss of consciousness, frequently caused by a sudden drop in blood pressure or a cardiac arrhythmia.

Tamoxifen (Ch. 26). An anti-oestrogen drug.

Teams (Ch. 3). Groups of people with different skills and/or roles, working together purposefully, in order to achieve a common aim.

Tendinitis (Ch. 27). Inflammatory condition of the tendon where active range of motion is often normal, but pain is experienced at the end of range.

Terminal care (Ch. 34). Care given to patients during the last few days of life.

Testicular cancer (Ch. 25). A relatively rare cancer but it is the most common malignancy in males under 35 years. However, it is one of the most curable solid tumours.

Tetraplegia/quadriplegia (Ch. 14). Paralysis affecting all four limbs.

Theory (Ch. 32). A supposition or set of logical ideas explaining something.

Therapeutic relationships (Ch. 3). Those where the processes of the relationships are used to focus on the individual or group of individuals needing emotional or physical help, to help improve their quality of life. Helpers develop and use this relationship through the skilful application of communication, technical and reflective skills.

Third space event (Ch. 8). Occurs in fluid volume deficit where there is loss of fluid from the extracellular fluid volume, e.g. into the peritoneal cavity or through the skin in burns.

Thrombocytopenia (Ch. 18). Describes an abnormally low platelet count below 150×10^9/L. Spontaneous bleeding tends to occur when the platelet count falls below 10×10^9/L.

Thyroidectomy (Ch. 17). Surgical removal of part or the whole of the thyroid gland.

Tracheostomy (Ch. 21). An opening into the trachea from the neck. May be temporary or permanent.

Traction (Ch. 27). A steady pull exerted on a body part. A form of treatment that is generally used to counteract the potential or actual problems caused by the pull of muscles on a damaged bone or joint.

Trauma (Ch. 30). An injury caused by an external force.

Tremor (Ch. 14). Involuntary rhythmic disorder of movement. May affect any part of the body but typically the hands, e.g. in Parkinson's disease.

Triage (Ch. 30). To sort and prioritize.

Triple assessment (Ch. 26). The use of three separate procedures in the diagnosis of primary breast cancer, namely clinical examination, mammography and needle biopsy.

Tumour lysis syndrome (TLS) (Chs 18, 33). Can result from the breakdown of tumour cells following cytotoxic treatments. There are metabolic problems, e.g. increased levels of potassium, uric acid (urate) and phosphate, and a reduction in calcium. TLS may cause renal failure and possible circulatory and respiratory failure.

Tympanic membrane (Ch. 16). A membrane that separates the middle ear from the external ear.

Type 1 diabetes mellitus (Ch. 17). Caused by an absolute deficiency of insulin. Previously known as juvenile-onset diabetes or insulin-dependent diabetes mellitus (IDDM).

Type 2 diabetes mellitus (Ch. 17). Due to varying degrees of insulin resistance, often due to obesity, and impaired insulin secretion.

Type 2 diabetes mellitus was previously known as maturity-onset diabetes or non-insulin-dependent diabetes mellitus (NIDDM).

Ultradian rhythm (Ch. 4). Sections of the cycle that forms a part of the circadian rhythm.

Universal precautions (Ch. 13 and all chapters). The routine infection control precautions taken during contact, or the possibility of contact, with blood and body fluids, such as wearing gloves and hand decontamination.

Uraemia (Ch. 24). Excessive amounts of urea and other nitrogenous waste material in the blood.

Uraemic syndrome (Ch. 24). Collection of symptoms that arise from loss of renal function.

Urge urinary incontinence (Ch. 12). Involuntary leakage accompanied by or immediately preceded by urgency.

Urinalysis (Chs 8, 24). Visual, physical, chemical, and possibly microbiological, examination of urine.

Urinary incontinence (Ch. 12). An inability to control the voiding of urine.

Urinary tract/system (Ch. 24). Comprises two kidneys, two ureters, the bladder and urethra. The kidneys produce urine; the ureters convey urine to the bladder, which stores it until there is a sufficient amount to elicit the desire to void urine, and then it passes through the urethra to the outside.

Venous leg ulcers (Ch. 10). Ulcers caused by chronic venous hypertension resulting from damage to the valves in the venous system of the lower leg.

Venous return (Ch. 19). Describes the blood returning to the right side of the heart.

Ventilation (Ch. 20). Maintenance of adequate oxygen and elimination of carbon dioxide.

Verbal communication (Ch. 3). The ways in which people consciously or unconsciously use words to convey meaning. This includes sign language.

Vesicle (Ch. 28). Small fluid-filled blister (< 5 mm in diameter).

Virus (Ch. 13). A microorganism that can only be visualized using electron microscopy. Viruses contain either DNA or RNA and can only replicate within the host cell. Viral diseases in humans include colds, influenza, measles, hepatitis, poliomyelitis and AIDS.

Visceral pain (Ch. 7). Pain that arises from distension of a hollow organ, often associated with autonomic sensations.

Vision (Ch. 15). Sight; the faculty of seeing.

Vision testing (Ch. 15). A series of tests/investigations used to assess the different aspects of vision.

Visual acuity (Ch. 15). Measure of the acuteness/fine detail of vision.

Visual impairment (Ch. 15). Any problem with vision affecting the ability to see near and distant objects clearly, the field of vision, ability to judge depth, discriminate colour and the ability to see one image at a time.

Vitamin (Ch. 11). Micronutrients. Organic compounds mainly consumed as part of the daily diet. However, some, such as vitamins K and D, are synthesized in the body. Vitamins are classified as either water-soluble or fat-soluble. They are found in both plant and animal foods and are named alphabetically and by their structure.

Whipple's procedure (Ch. 23). Radical resection of parts of the pancreas, duodenum and stomach for cancer of the head of pancreas.

Women's health (Ch. 25). The holistic health needs of women linked to their complex reproductive system. Problems may develop over a wide age range, from puberty to after the menopause. Many of these problems are not life-threatening but can adversely affect quality of life, having physical, psychological and social effects.

Wound care and drains (Ch. 29). The management of the surgical incision and any wound drainage system.

Index

Page numbers in *italics* indicate figures, boxes or tables; those in **bold** refer to main discussions.

A

A&E, *see* Accident and emergency (A&E) department
Abbreviated mental test, ten-item, 1060
ABC resuscitation system
  in cardiopulmonary resuscitation, **495–496**
  in shock, 162–166
ABCDE resuscitation system, in major trauma, 932–933
Abdomen
  acute, **603–604**
  'burst', 918
  distension, 598
  incision sites, *905*
  regions, *905*
Abdominal examination, 598
Abdominal pain, 597
  in acute abdomen, 603
  in cholecystitis, 640
  in early pregnancy, 726
  in ectopic pregnancy, 730
Abdominoperineal (AP) resection, 612
Abducens nerve, *279*
Aβ fibres, 113
ABO blood group system, **446–447**
  renal transplantation and, 694
Abortion, 725
  see also Miscarriage; Termination of pregnancy
Abortion Act (1967), 730–731
Abrasions, 934
Abscess
  breast, 779
  deep neck, **582**
  intracranial, 385, 517
  perianal, **617**
  perinephric, 674
  peritonsillar, **582**
  pulmonary, 517
  renal, **674**
Abuse, older adults, **981**
Acarbose, 418
Acceptability, social, *30*
Acceptance
  in helping relationships, 45
  stage, terminal illness, 1026
Access, to services, *30*
Accessory nerve, *279*
Accessory reproductive organs, male, 742–743
Accident and emergency (A&E) department, **923–945**
  caring in, 925
  challenging behaviour, 938
  emergency nurse practitioner, 929
  health promotion/accident prevention, 927–928

major disasters, 942–943
major trauma, 931–934
management, 928–929
mental health problems, 938–941
minor trauma, 934–936
nursing assessment, 925–927
prehospital care, 924–925
process of nursing, 925
resuscitation, 929–931
role, 924–925
social issues, 936–938
sudden death, 941–942
useful addresses, 944
users, 924
Accidents, **928**
  prevention, 288, 819, *820*, **927–928**
  spinal injuries, 324
  stress and, 104
  see also Falls; Trauma
Accommodation (of eye), **334–335**
Accountability
  registered nurses, 6, *7*
  student nurses, 7
ACE inhibitors, *see* Angiotensin-converting enzyme (ACE) inhibitors
Acetazolamide, *345*, 351, 356, 357
Acetylcholine (ACh), 275, 276
  receptor antibodies, in myasthenia gravis, 811
  and sleep, 61
Achalasia, 602
Achilles tendon
  problems, **827–828**
  tears, 827–828
  tendinitis, 827
Aciclovir, *345*, 855
Acid, 148, 149
  eye injuries, 360
Acid–base balance, **148–151**
  assessment of status, 149
  disorders, **149–151**
    blood gas values, *148*
    in chronic renal failure, 687
    mixed, 151
    see also Acidosis; Alkalosis
  in hypothermia, 90
  renal contribution, 149, **660–661**
  respiratory contribution, 149, **535**
Acid–base nomogram, Flenly, *150*
Acid phosphatase, serum, 671
Acidosis, *136*, 149–151
  blood gas values, *148*
  in hypothermia, 90
  in shock, 157, 161–162
  see also Lactic acidosis; Metabolic acidosis; Respiratory acidosis
Acne, 843, **851–852**
Acne Support Group, 875
Acoustic neuroma, 308, **389**
Acquired immune deficiency syndrome (AIDS), 764–765, 1047
  see also HIV infection

Acromegaly, **428–429**
Acromioclavicular (AC) separation, 825
ACTH, *see* Adrenocorticotrophic hormone
Action on ENT steering group, 368
Action potential, nerve, 275–276
Action on Smoking and Health (ASH), 530
Activated partial thromboplastin time (APTT), 450, 477, 526
Active listening, **48**, 49–50
Active transport, 136
Activities of daily living (ADL)
  assessment, 1059–1060
  in chronic illness and disability, 1056
  in fractures, 833, 836
  in respiratory disease, 539
  see also Disability; Functional status
Activities of living (ALs), 10–11
Activities of Living model of nursing (Roper), **10–11**, 1058–1059
Activity
  physical, *see* Physical activity
  in terminal illness, 1029
Activity theory of ageing, 972
Acupuncture, in overactive bladder, 242
Acute abdomen, **603–604**
Acute illness, 1048
Acute pain, 112
  adverse effects, 116–117
  assessment, **119–121**
    in older adults, *115*
    tools, 119–121
    validity and reliability, *119*
  management, *see* Pain management
  services, 121
  team, 121
  see also Postoperative pain
Acute renal failure, *see* Renal failure, acute
Acute respiratory distress syndrome (ARDS), 168
Acute tubular necrosis (ATN), 685
Adam's sign, *798*
Adaptation to chronic illness/disability, **1053–1054**
  facilitating, 1062–1063
  psychological, social and cultural factors, 1054
  stages, 1054
Addaction, 650
Addiction
  acute pain management, **128–129**
  see also Drug dependence; Substance misuse
Addison's disease, 437–438
Aδ fibres, 113
Adenohypophysis, 396–397
Adenoidal enlargement, 383, 384
Adenosine, and sleep, 61
Adenoviral infections, conjunctivitis, 361, 362
ADH, *see* Antidiuretic hormone
Adhesive capsulitis (frozen shoulder), **824**
Adhesive strips, wound closure, *936*
Adipose tissue, subcutaneous, 175

ADL, *see* Activities of daily living
Adolescents, 7
  chronic illness and disability, 1054
Adrenal cortex, 399
  adenomas/carcinomas, 438, 439, 440
  hypersecretion, **438–440**
  insufficiency, **437–438**
Adrenal crisis, 438
Adrenal glands, 394, **399–400**
  disorders, **437–441**
  stress responses, 400
Adrenal hyperplasia, congenital (CAH), **441**
Adrenal medulla, 399–400
Adrenalectomy, 439, **440**
Adrenaline (epinephrine), 400
  in anaphylaxis, 167
  during sleep, 62
  in heat generation, 77
  in local anaesthesia, 896
  in shock, 156, 157
  in stress, 96, 890
Adrenergic receptors, 276
Adrenocorticotrophic hormone (ACTH), 397,
    398
  in adrenal cortex insufficiency, 437, 438
  in congenital adrenal hyperplasia, 441
  in Cushing's syndrome, 438, 439
  deficiency, *430*, 437
  stimulation test, 402, 438
Adult nursing, 3–4, **7–8**
Adulthood, 7–8
  chronic illness and disability, 1054–1055
  see also Older adults
Advance directives, 18, **1027**
Advanced life support (ALS), 495, 496
Advanced Trauma Life Support (ATLS), 932
Advanced Trauma Nursing Course, 944
Adverse drug reactions (ADRs), 870
Advice, disguised, 49
Advocacy, patient, 51, 952, 1061
Aerobic metabolism, in shock, 154
Aetiology, 986
Afferent nerves, 274
After-drop, after rewarming in hypothermia, 89
Afterload, 165, 955
Age
  body water and, 134
  cancer risk and, 991
  defining 'old', 967–968
  fluid status and, 141
  gallstones and, 638
  minimum, to give consent, 892
  response to chronic illness and, 1054–1055
  sleep patterns and, 63–64
  testicular cancer and, 746
Age Concern, 1065
Age-related macular degeneration (AMD),
    353–354
Ageing, **967–969**
  back problems and, 814
  bone changes, 794
  consequences, **970–971**
  experience, **969–971**
  heterogeneity, **969**
  images, **969–970**
  implications of biological, **976**
  inequality and, **971**
  physiological changes, **975**
  population, 967, 969
  purpose, **969**
  skin changes, 175–176, *848*, 975, 976
  social, psychological and biological aspects,
    971–977
  successful, 969
  theories

biological, **974–975**
  cellular, 974–975
  hereditary, 974
  physiological, 974
  psychosocial, **972**
wound healing and, *179*
  see also Older adults
Ageism, **970**
Aggression, 51
  in A&E department, **938**, *939*
    causes, *939*
    handling, 938
  in mental illness, 940
  in stress, 97, 102
Agitation, terminal, 1039
Agnosia, *289*, *292*
AIDS, 764–765, 1047
  see also HIV infection
Air embolism, 147
Air-fluidized systems, 192, 193
Air travel
  deep vein thrombosis and, 526
  in diabetes, 415
Air ventilation systems
  filtered air, 264, 265, 267
  negative pressure, 264, 265
  operating theatre, 906
Airway(s)
  changes in asthma, 542
  lower, 533, *534*
  upper, 533, *534*
Airway maintenance devices (AMDs), 898–899
Airway management
  after tonsillectomy, 581
  after tracheostomy, 585
  in cardiopulmonary resuscitation, 495, 496
  in general anaesthesia, **898–899**
  immediate postoperative period, **908**
  in major trauma, 932
  in shock, 162, *163*
  unconscious patient, 290
Airway obstruction
  in COPD, 545
  measurement, 540–541
  partial, symptoms, 568
  postoperative, **908**
  reversibility testing, 541
  see also Bronchoconstriction
Airway pressure, mechanical ventilators, 961
Alanine, 400
Alanine aminotransferase (ALT), *625*
Alarm reaction, in stress response, 95–96
Albinism, **862–863**
Albumin
  plasma (serum), 215, 446, 600, *625*
    low, *see* Hypoalbuminaemia
  solutions, 165, 452
    in nephrotic syndrome, 684
  in urine, *see* Albuminuria; Microalbuminuria
Albuminuria, 656–657, 664–665
Alcohol
  drug interactions, 225
  hand rubs, 263
  -induced hepatitis, **633**
  wipes, in diabetes, 406
  withdrawal symptoms, 937
Alcohol consumption, 203
  A&E attenders, **936–937**
  assessment (CAGE questions), 624
  in atopic eczema, 849, 850
  cancer risk and, 990
  in cardiomyopathy, 518
  in diabetes, 414, *419*
  fluid status and, 141
  frostbite risk, 83

guidelines, *628*
  liver/pancreatic disease and, 627
  metronidazole and, 606, *607*
  osteoporosis and, 819
  road traffic accidents and, 288
  sleep and, 65
  stress and, 106
  urinary incontinence and, *236*
Alcohol misuse (including alcoholism), 104, 627
  in A&E attenders, 937
  acute pain management, 129
  advice and assistance, 636
  cirrhosis of liver, 633
  gastritis, 605
  homeless people, 938
  liver cancer, 637
  older adults, 627, *628*
  pancreatitis, 643, 644, 646, *647*
  thiamin deficiency, 208
Alcoholics Anonymous, 627, 636, 650
Aldosterone, **138**, 399, 658
  blood pressure regulation, 486
  in shock, 157
Aldosteronism, primary, **440**
Alkali, 148, 149
  eye injuries, 360
Alkaline phosphatase (ALP), serum
  in hepatic/pancreatic disorders, *625*, *647*
  in renal disease, 671
Alkalosis, *136*, 150, 151
  blood gas values, *148*
  see also Metabolic alkalosis; Respiratory
    alkalosis
Alkylating agents, 1006
All-trans-retinoic acid (ATRA), 477
Allergens
  avoidance, in atopic eczema, 850
  respiratory, 538
Allergic bronchopulmonary aspergillosis
    (APBA), 562
Allergic rhinitis, 571, *572*
Allergy
  blood transfusions, 454
  conjunctivitis, 361
  contact dermatitis, 851
  food, **219**
  investigations, 569
  i.v. infusions, 147
  patch testing, 848, 851
  preoperative assessment, 887
  urticaria, 854
  see also Anaphylaxis/anaphylactic shock
Allopurinol, 808
Alopecia (hair loss), **869**
  androgenic (male pattern), 869
  areata, 869
  chemotherapy-induced, 472
  scarring, 869
Alpha-1-antitrypsin deficiency, 545
Alpha-fetoprotein (AFP)
  in liver cancer, *625*, 637
  in testicular cancer, *745*, 747
Alpha glucosidase inhibitors, 418
Alprostadil, 754–755
Alveolar ventilation (V), 535, 955
Alveoli, 533, *534*
Alzheimer's disease, **322**
Amarant Trust, 767
Ambulance services, 925, 942
Ambulation
  postoperative, **919**
  see also Mobilization
Ambulatory surgery, 880
  see also Day surgery
Amenorrhoea, *717*

American Society of Anesthesiologists (ASA) grading, 882
Amino acid derivatives, 418
Amino acids, 203–204
    essential, 204, 217
    wound healing and, *218*
Aminosalicylates, 614
Amiodarone, 499, 500
Amlodipine, 512
Ammonia
    serum, *625*
    toxicity, *629*, 636
Amnesia, *289*
Ampulla of Vater, 623
Amputation
    in diabetes, 425
    limb prostheses, 802
    in peripheral arterial disease, 523, **524**
    stump bandaging, **802**, *803*
Amylase, serum, *625*, 645
Amylopectin, 205
Amylose, 205
Amyotrophic lateral sclerosis (ALS), *323*
Anaemia, **456–460**
    aetiology, 456
    after gynaecological surgery, *741*
    aplastic, **463–464**
    in cancer, 1013
    of chronic disease, 459, 687
    clinical presentation, 456–457
    in GI disorders, 600
    in glomerulonephritis, 683
    in gynaecological disorders, 715
    haemolytic, *see* Haemolytic anaemia
    haemorrhagic, 457
    investigations, 456
    iron deficiency, 210, 217, **457–458**
    in leukaemia, 468
    megaloblastic, 209, **458–459**
    in older adults, *456*
    pernicious, **458–459**
    sickle cell, 462
Anaerobic metabolism, in shock, 154, 157
Anaesthesia, **896–900**
    airway maintenance, 898–899
    in day surgery, 882–884
    fitness for, **885–887**
    general, **898–900**
    induction, 899–900
    maintenance, 900
    movement of patients during, 900–902
    premedication, 737, **894**
    recovery from, **907–910**
    reversal, 900
    as symptom, *289*
    triad, 897
    see also Local anaesthesia; Regional anaesthesia/analgesia
Anaesthetic agents, *884*
Anaesthetists
    ASA classification, 882
    assistant, 903–904
    in critical care, 951
Anal canal, 242, **596**
Anal cancer, **617**
Anal fissure, **617**
Anal fistulae, **617**
Anal sphincters, 242–243, 596
    damage, 243, *247*
    nerve damage, 243
Analgesia, **123–127**
    in burn injuries, 872, 873
    in cancer pain, 1017
    inhalation, 125
    in mucositis, 472

in pancreatitis, 645, 647
patient-controlled (PCA), **125–127**, 463, **910–911**
postoperative, *see* Postoperative analgesia
to promote sleep, 70
routes of administration, 125
in shock, 163
in terminal illness, 1032–1034
see also Pain management
Analgesic ladder, 1017, 1032–1034
Analgesic nephropathy, 684
Analgesics, **123–125**
    adjuvant, 1034
    non-opioid, 1033
    in older adults, *115*
    opioid, *see* Opioids
    oral administration, 125
    parenteral administration, 125, **1034–1035**
    rectal administration, 125
    transdermal administration, 125
Anaphylaxis/anaphylactic shock, 155
    management, **167**
    patients at risk, *159*
    transfusion-associated, 454
    see also Allergy
Anderson pressure ulcer risk score, *189*
Androgens
    ablation, in prostate cancer, 700–701
    adrenal, 399
    in polycystic ovary syndrome, 734
    testicular, 742
Aneurysm, aortic, **522–523**
Anger
    in chronic illness/disability, 1053
    in terminal illness, 1026
Angina pectoris, **503–505**
    in anaemia, 457
    nursing management, 504–505
    unstable, **505–506**
Angiogenic growth factors, 988
Angiography
    fluorescein, 338, **340–341**
    in neurological disease, 287
    in nose and throat disorders, 569
    in peripheral arterial disease, 523
    renal, **666**
Angiomas, cherry, *see* Telangiectasia
Angioplasty, percutaneous transluminal, 523
Angiotensin I, 138, 658
Angiotensin II, 138, 658
    blood pressure regulation, 486
    in shock, 156–157
Angiotensin II receptor antagonists, 682
Angiotensin-converting enzyme (ACE), 138
Angiotensin-converting enzyme (ACE) inhibitors, 138, 658
    in diabetes, 426, 682
    in heart failure, 511, 512
    in hypertension, 521
    side-effects, 512
Angular cheilitis, *859*
Angular stomatitis, 597, 600
Animal dander, 849, 850
Animals, avoidance, in respiratory allergy, *538*
Ankle
    fractures, **833**
    oedema, 144
    sprains, 822, 823, **828**
Ankle brachial pressure index (ABPI), 195, 198
Ankylosing spondylitis, **807**
Anorectal disorders, **616–617**
Anorexia, 213, **597**
    in heart failure, 511
    in terminal illness, **1037**
Anorgasmia, 757

Anosmia, *289*, 568
Anovulation, 734
Antacids, 225, *226*
Antegrade urography (pyelography), 667
Anterior chamber (eye), 333
Anterior cruciate ligament (ACL)
    reconstruction surgery, 827
    tears, 826
Anterior drawer test, *798*
Anthony Nolan Bone Marrow Trust, *474*
Anthropometry, **214**
Anti-androgens
    in acne, *852*
    in benign prostatic hyperplasia, 697
    in pancreatic cancer, 648
    in prostate cancer, 700–701
Anti-CD20 monoclonal antibodies, 470
Anti-D immunoglobulin, 447, 727, 730, 731
Anti-epileptic drugs (anticonvulsants), *314*, 315
    in brain tumours, *309*
    in diabetic neuropathy, 426
Anti-glomerular basement membrane (GBM) antibodies, 683
Anti-inflammatory agents
    in cystic fibrosis, 551
    ophthalmic, 345
    see also Corticosteroids; Non-steroidal anti-inflammatory drugs
Antibiotics
    in acne, *852*
    anti-tumour, 1007
    Clostridium difficile infections and, 255, 616
    in cystic fibrosis, 550–551
    in infective endocarditis, 517
    in meningitis, 311
    in neutropenia, 466
    ophthalmic, 345, 360
    in peritonitis, 692–693
    in pneumonia, 553
    preoperative, 894
    prophylactic
        immunosuppressed patients, 265
        infective endocarditis, 517
    resistance, 254, **255**
    in rheumatic fever, 514
    sensitivity testing, 254
    in sexually transmitted infections, 763, 764
    in sinusitis, 574
    topical
        in acne, *852*
        in wound management, 185, 186
    in tuberculosis, 555
    in urinary tract infections, 673
Antibodies, 447
Anticholinergics
    in Parkinson's disease, 320
    for premedication, 894
Anticholinesterases
    in myasthenia gravis, 811
    reversal of anaesthesia, *884*, 900
    urinary incontinence and, *236*
Anticoagulation
    in deep vein thrombosis, 526
    nursing management, 526
    prosthetic heart valves, 516
    surgical patients, 889
Anticonvulsants, *see* Anti-epileptic drugs
Antidepressants
    for stress, 105
    urinary incontinence and, *236*
Antidiuretic hormone (ADH, vasopressin), 138, 397
    deficiency, 431
    in oesophageal varices, 604
    renal function, 659–660

Antidiuretic hormone (continued)
in shock, 157
in stress, 890
Antiemetics, 1036
in chemotherapy-induced nausea and vomiting, 472, 1013
in opioid-treated patients, 124
surgical patients, 882–884, 911
Antifungal drugs
ophthalmic, 345
in tinea, 856
topical, 854
Antihistamines (H₁ antagonists)
in anaphylaxis, 167
eye drops/ointment, 345
nasal, 572
in nausea and vomiting, 1013, 1036
in urticaria, 854
Antihypertensive drugs, 521–522
in diabetes, 426, 427, 682
Antimetabolites, 1006
Antimicrobials, see Antibiotics
Antimuscarinics (muscarinic antagonists)
in asthma, 543
nasal, 572
in nausea and vomiting, 1036
nebulized, 547–548
ophthalmic, 344
in Parkinson's disease, 320
in urinary incontinence, 236, 242
Antipsychotics, urinary incontinence and, 236
Antipyretic agents, 80, 86, 164
Antiretroviral drugs, 765
post-exposure prophylaxis, 267, 268
Antiseptic soaps, 261, 262
Antiseptics, preoperative skin cleansing, 887
Antithyroid drugs, 432–433
Antituberculous drugs, 555, 675
Antiviral drugs
ophthalmic, 345
topical, 855
Antrochoanal polyps, 580
Antrostomy, 574
Anuria, 686
in acute pancreatitis, 644
Anus, 596
Anxiety
in blood disorders, 449
in fluid loss, 140
in gynaecological disorders, 712
management groups, 107
measurement, 104–105
nursing management, 890–891
pacemaker patients, 498
pain and, 118
perioperative, 737, 889–891
physiological effects, 890
in shock, 163
sleep problems, 65
state, acute, 940
stress and, 104
in terminal illness, 1039
see also Stress
Anxiolytics
for sleep promotion, 71
for stress, 105
Aorta
aneurysm, 522–523
coarctation, 528
dissection, 522–523
Aortic regurgitation, 515
Aortic stenosis, 515
Aortic valve, 483
Aphasia, 289, 292

Apheresis, 452, 475
Aphthous ulcers, 597, 601
Aplastic anaemia, 463–464
Apley test, 798
Apomorphine
in erectile dysfunction, 754, 756
in Parkinson's disease, 320, 321
Apoptosis, 987
Appendicectomy, 608
Appendicitis, 607–608
Appendix, 595, 607
Appetite, 597
in blood disorders, 449
drugs affecting, 225
see also Anorexia
Apprehension test, 798
Aprons, plastic, 263
Aqueous humour, 333–334
Arachidonic acid, 204
Arachis oil enemas, 1037
Arachnoid mater, 278
Arcuate arteries, 709
Arginine vasopressin (AVP), see Antidiuretic hormone
Aromatase inhibitors, 784
Aromatherapy, in palliative care, 1023
Arousal, 61, 890
curve (Hebb), 93, 94
Arrhythmias, 497–502
after myocardial infarction, 508
atrial, 497–501
in cardiogenic shock, 510
ECG monitoring, 490
electrophysiology studies, 492
in Guillain–Barré syndrome, 328
in hypothermia, 81, 90
in shock, 160
ventricular, 501–502
Arterial blood gases (ABG), 149
in acid–base disorders, 148
in critically ill patients, 958
normal values, 162
in respiratory failure, 557
in shock, 161–162
Arterial blood pressure, see Blood pressure
Arterial blood pressure monitoring, 488
in critically ill patients, 959
in shock, 160, 161–162
Arterial bypass surgery, 523
Arterial cannula, indwelling, 958, 959
Arterial embolization, in epistaxis, 576
Arterial injuries, in fractures, 829
Arterial (ischaemic) leg ulcers, 193, 194–195, 523
in diabetes, 427, 428
management, 197–198, 524
vascular assessment, 195–196
versus venous leg ulcers, 195
see also Peripheral arterial/vascular disease
Arterial ligation, in epistaxis, 576
Arterial pulses, see Pulses, arterial
Arteries, 485
Arterioles, 485
Arteriovenous fistula, haemodialysis patients, 691
Arthralgia, in rheumatic fever, 514
Arthritis
degenerative (osteoarthritis), 812–813, 830
in gout, 807–808
rheumatoid, 805–807, 815
septic (pyogenic), 812
Arthritis Care, 838
Arthrodesis, 805, 806
Arthroplasty, 805, 806
replacement, 812, 813

Arthroscopy, 798–799
in knee injuries, 827
Arthrotomy, 805, 806, 812
Artificial insemination, 760
Ascites (abdominal), 592, 625, 629
in cirrhosis, 634, 635
in ovarian cancer, 723
Ascorbic acid, see Vitamin C
Asepsis, 257
surgical, 905–906
in wound management, 915, 917
Aseptic (avascular) necrosis, 830
Aspartate aminotransferase (AST), 491, 625
Aspergillus fumigatus, 562
Aspiration, pulmonary, 893, 900
Aspiration cytology, 1001
Aspiration pneumonia, 553, 893
Aspirin, 226, 1033
in angina, 504
in myocardial infarction, 507
Assertive behaviour, 51
Assertiveness, 51–52
groups, 107
Assessment, see Nursing assessment; Pre-admission assessment; Preoperative assessment; other specific types of assessment
Assignments, reflective writing, 16
Assisted conception, 759, 760
Associate nurse, 12
Assumptions, 45–46
Asthma, 542–545
acute, levels of severity, 544
acute severe, 543–544
allergens and trigger factors, 538
in allergic bronchopulmonary aspergillosis, 562
chronic unresponsive, 545
deaths, risk factors, 544
epidemiology, 542
nasal polyps, 580
nursing management, 544–545
pathophysiology, 542
respiratory function tests, 540, 541
self-management plans, 544–545
sleep disturbances, 61, 71
stress and, 103
treatment, 542–543
Astigmatism, 335, 341
Astrocytes, 275
Astrocytomas, 308
Ataxia, 276, 289
Atelectasis, 953
Atheroma, 503, 523
Atheromatous plaque, 503
rupture, 505, 506
Athlete's foot (tinea pedis), 856, 858
Atopic eczema, 849–851, 855
Atopy, 538
Atracurium, 884
Atria, 482, 483
Atrial arrhythmias, 497–501
Atrial ectopic beats (extrasystoles), 500
Atrial fibrillation (AF), 499–500
Atrial flutter, 500
Atrial natriuretic peptide (ANP), 138
Atrial septal defect, 528
Atrial systole, 484, 485
Atrioventricular (AV) node, 483, 484
Atrioventricular (AV) valves, 482, 483
Atrophe blanche, 194
Atropine, 344, 884, 894
Attendance Allowance (AA), 1061
Audiometry, 373

Audit, **34–35**
　cancer services, 986
　clinical, 34
　definition, 34
　nursing, 34
　tools, 34–35, *35*
Auerbach's plexus, 592
Aura, epileptic, *314*
Aural toilet, 376
Auricle, *see* Pinna
Autoimmune diseases
　ageing and, 974
　blistering, **865–866**
　serum markers, *683*
Autoimmune haemolytic anaemia (AIHA), 460
Automated implantable defibrillators (AICDs), 502
Automatism, 315
Autonomic dysreflexia, **326**, *327*
Autonomic nervous system (ANS), 274
　control of micturition, 231, 661
　in shock, 156
　in stress, 95–96
Autonomic neuropathy, diabetic, 426–427
Autonomy
　older people in long-term care, 979
　respect for, 18
Avascular (aseptic) necrosis, 830
Axilla, temperature measurement, *84, 85*
Axillary dissection, in breast cancer, 783
Azathioprine, in inflammatory bowel disease, 614
Azelaic acid, *852*
Azelastine hydrochloride, *572*
Azidothymidine (AZT), 765

B

B cells, 446
Bacille Calmette-Guérin (BCG) vaccine, 555
　intravesical therapy, 679, *680*
Back pain, **814–816**
　causes, 814–815
　functional impact, 1050
　investigations, 815
　management, 815–816
　musculoskeletal, 814
　in myeloma, 465
　nursing management, 816
　in spinal cord compression, 1014–1015
Backache, stress and, 103
Baclofen, 810
Bacteria, **254**
　antibiotic resistance, 254, **255**
　antibiotic sensitivity testing, 254
　classification, 254
　commensal, *see* Microorganisms, normal flora
　culture, 254
　identification, 254
　pathogenic, 256, **257**
Bacterial infections
　eye, 359, 361, 362
　infective endocarditis, 516
　skin, 854–855
　tonsillitis, 581
Bacterial vaginosis, 732
Bacteriological tests, in skin conditions, 846
Bacteriuria, asymptomatic, 672
BACUP, *see* British Association of Cancer Patients
　　and their Families and Friends
Bad news, breaking, **52**, *53*
　in A&E department, 941
　emotional responses, 1010–1011,
　　1025–1026
　in learning disability, *1011*

Balance, 370
Balance disorders, *289*, **386–388**
　nursing management, 387–388
Balanitis xerotica obliterans, 751
Bandaging
　in atopic eczema, 850
　compression, 195, **196–197**, 528
　containment, in lymphoedema, 787
　in musculoskeletal disorders, **802**
　stump, **802**, *803*
Bankart lesion, 824
Barbiturates, 71
Bargaining response, terminal illness, 1026
Barium studies, **599–600**
　see also Contrast studies
Baroreceptor feedback mechanism, 156
Barthel index, **1059–1060**
Bartholin's glands, 711
Basal body temperature (BBT), 759
Basal cell carcinoma (BCC), 389, **868**
Basal metabolic rate (BMR), 203
　in spinal injuries, 325
　see also Hypermetabolic state
Basement membrane, skin, 174
Basophils, 446
Bath oils, medicated, 849, 850, 862
Bathing/showering
　maintaining healthy skin, 849
　patients in casts, 801
　preoperative, 737, 887
Battle's sign, *298*
BCG vaccine, *see* Bacille Calmette-Guérin (BCG)
　　vaccine
Becker muscular dystrophy (BMD), *809*
Bed rest
　in ankylosing spondylitis, 807
　in back pain, 815
　deep vein thrombosis and, 888
　in rheumatic fever, 514
　see also Immobility/immobilization; Rest
Bed sores, *see* Pressure ulcers
Bedding, sleep and, 69–70
Beds
　air-fluidized, 192, 193
　covers, in incontinence, 247
　low air loss systems, 192
　side rails, 290, *976*
Behavioural assessment
　critically ill patients, 957
　in terminal illness, 1031
Behavioural change, for smoking cessation,
　　536–537
Behavioural problems, 273, 277
　in Alzheimer's disease, 322
Belfast fixator, *804*
Beliefs, 44
Bell's palsy, **303–304**
Benchmarking, **27–28**
Beneficence, 18
Benefits, social security, 1031, *1061*
Benefits Agency, *1061*, 1065
Benefits Enquiry Line, *1061*
Benign paroxysmal positional vertigo (BPPV),
　　387
Benign prostatic hyperplasia (BPH), **696–699**
　clinical presentation, 235, 696
　management, 697–699
Benign tumours, **992–993**
Benzodiazepines
　to promote sleep, 70–71
　urinary incontinence and, *236*
Benzoyl peroxide, *852*
Bereavement, **1043–1044**
　in A&E departments, **941–942**
　counselling, 1044

in old age, **981**
　support organizations, 1044, 1045
Beri-beri, 208
Beta-2 agonists
　in asthma, *542*, 543
　nebulized, 547–548
Beta-adrenoceptor antagonists, *see* Beta-blockers
Beta-blockers, 276
　in angina, 504
　in heart failure, 512–513
　in hypertension, 521–522
　in hyperthyroidism, 433
　ophthalmic, *345*, 356, 357
　side-effects, 512–513
Betahistine, 387
Betamethasone sodium phosphate, *572*
Betaxolol, *345*, 356
Betel nut chewing, 597
Bicarbonate (HCO_3^-), *136*
　in acid–base disorders, *148*
　buffering system, 149
　excessive losses, 150
　in haemodialysis, 690
　homeostatic mechanisms, 149
　renal regulation, 661
Biceps tendon tear, **825–826**
Bier's block, 896
Biguanides, 418
Bilateral salpingo-oophorectomy (BSO), 718
Bile, 595, **622**
　concentration and storage, 623
Bile canaliculi, 622
Bile duct
　carcinoma, 643
　common, *see* Common bile duct
　T-tube drainage, 642, 643
Biliary colic, 638, 639
Biliary disorders, 621–622, **638–643**
　clinical characteristics, 627–629
　diagnostic tests and investigations, 625–626
　prevention and health education, 626–627
　useful addresses/websites, 650–651
Biliary system, *622*, *623*
　infections, 638
　tumours, **643**
　see also Gallbladder
Bilirubin, 622
　serum, *625*, 647
　urinary, *626*, *629*
Biliverdin, 622
Bimatoprost, *345*
Biofeedback
　in pain management, 128
　for stress, 108
　in stress incontinence, 240
Biological response modifiers (BRM),
　　1008–1009
Biological theories of ageing, **974–975**
Biomedical model of pain, 121
Biometry, 340
Biopsy
　bone marrow, **450–451**, 1002
　brain tumour, 309
　breast, 775, 1001
　brush, nose, 570
　cervix, 721
　endometrial, 718, 722, 759
　GI tract, 599
　heart, 518
　liver, **626**, 1002
　lymph node, 1001
　muscle, 799, 811
　in neurological disorders, 288
　renal, **667–668**
　skin, **848**, 1001

Biopsychosocial model of pain, 121
Biosurgery, wound debridement, 182
Biotechnology, in wound management, 186
Biotin, 209
Bipolar affective disorder, 940
Bisacodyl suppositories, 1037
Bisphosphonates, 736
Bites, *934, 935*
Bladder, **230, 661**
    chart/diary, 241
    emptying, *see* Micturition; Voiding
    exstrophy, 655
    function, 230, 231
    hypotonic/atonic, in diabetes, 426, 427, 428
    irrigation, continuous, 697, *698*, 699
    overactive, 235, **240–242**
    perforation, *740*
    retraining, 241
    spasms, painful, 1032
    ultrasound imaging, 666
Bladder cancer, 678, **679–681**, 994–995
    nursing management, 679–681
    screening, **1001**
Bladder neck, 230
Blanching erythema, 190
Bleaching, skin, 863
Bleeding, *see* Haemorrhage/bleeding
Blepharitis, **362–363**
Blepharospasm, 359
Blighted ovum, **727–728**
Blindness, 332
    registration, 342
    see also Visual impairment
Blistering skin disorders, **864–867**
    autoimmune, 865–866
    infective, 864–865
Blisters, 864
    aspiration, *865*
    see also Bullae
Blood, **445–449**
    clotting, *see* Coagulation
    compatibility for transfusion, 447, 452
    components for transfusion, 451–452
    donation, **451**
    leucocyte depletion, 451
    management of exposure to, 268
    pH, 149, 162, 535
    salvage/recycling, 454
    spillages, *631*
    supply, wound healing and, *179*
    whole, 451
Blood-borne infections, **267–268**, 627
    control measures, 268
    occupational transmission, 267–268
Blood–brain barrier, 277
Blood cells, **446**
Blood count, *see* Full blood count
Blood cultures, 491–492
Blood disorders, *see* Haematological disorders
Blood film, 450
Blood flow
    autoregulation, in shock, 156
    regulation, in shock, 156
Blood gases, arterial, *see* Arterial blood gases
Blood glucose, *see* Glucose, blood
Blood groups, **446–447**
Blood pressure (BP), **485–486**
    ambulatory recording, 522
    in critically ill patients, **955–956**, 959
    during sleep, 61
    in fluid balance assessment, 140, 663
    intra-arterial monitoring, *see* Arterial blood
        pressure monitoring
    measurement, **488**, 522
    in neurological assessment, 284

non-invasive monitoring (NIBP), 959
    preoperative assessment, 886
    regulation, 156–157, 485–486
    in shock, 156–157, 160
    supine and standing, 663
    see also Hypertension; Hypotension
Blood tests
    in cardiovascular disease, 491–492
    in endocrine disorders, 402
    in GI disorders, 600
    in gynaecological disorders, 715
    in haematological disorders, **450**
    in liver, biliary and pancreatic disorders, *625*
    in musculoskeletal disorders, 797
    in neurological disorders, 288
    normal values, *670*
    in skin conditions, 848
    in urinary system disorders, **669–671**
Blood transfusion, **451–455**
    alternatives to, 454–455
    in anaemia, 457
    autologous, 454
    blood group compatibility, 447, 452
    blood products for, 451–452
    complications, 452–454
        acute bacterial reactions, 454
        allergic reactions, 454
        circulatory overload, 454
        delayed, 454
        febrile reactions, 454
        incompatibility reactions, 453–454
    in hypovolaemia, 164
    in myelodysplasia, 464
    procedure, 452
    refusal, *455*
    safe administration, 452, *453*
    in thalassaemia, 461
Blood volume, 445
Body awareness, in cancer prevention, 991
Body clock, 61
Body fluids, management of exposure to, 268
Body image, altered, *681*
    in breast cancer, 784, 788
    in burn injuries, **874**
    cancer patients, **1015–1016**
    in inflammatory bowel disease, 616
    patients wearing orthoses, 802
    in penile cancer, 751
    stages of adaptation, 1054
    in terminal illness, 1031
    in testicular cancer, 748
    tracheostomy patients, 586
Body language (non-verbal communication),
        40–41, 175
Body map, skin lesions, 846, *847*
Body mass index (BMI), 214
    cancer and, 990
    in respiratory disease, 539
    wound healing and, *179*
    see also Obesity; Weight, body
Body surface area, burns assessment, 872, *873*
Boils, 854
Bone, **794**
    disorders, **818–820**
    effects of ageing, 794
    infections, 820
    medullary cavity, 794
    metastases, 821, 1032
    pain, 465, 1032
    tumours, **820–821**
        benign, 821
        malignant, 821
        metastatic, 821
Bone marrow, 447–448, 794
    aspiration/biopsy, **450–451**, 1002

disorders, **463–465**
donation, *474*
harvesting, for transplants, 475
suppression, 467, 471–472
transplantation, *see* Haemopoietic stem cell
    transplantation
Bone mineral density (BMD), 797
    see also Osteoporosis
Boundaries, **47**
Bovine spongiform encephalopathy (BSE), 313
Bowel disorders, **610–616**
Bowel function
    in inflammatory bowel disease, **615**
    in terminal illness, 1029
Bowel habit
    constipation and, 609
    in fluid balance disorders, 140
    in liver, biliary and pancreatic disorders, 624
Bowel obstruction, *see* Intestinal obstruction
Bowel perforation, *740*
Bowel preparation
    for barium enema, 599–600
    cleaning solutions, *610*
    preoperative, 611–612, 737, **894**
Bowel training, 246
Brachytherapy, 1005
Braden scale, 188, *189*
Bradycardia, sinus, **497–499**
Bradykinesia, *289*, 319
Braille, 343
Brain, **276–277**
    blood supply, 277, *278*
    'coning', 299
    herniation/shifts, **299**
    pain pathways, 113
Brain injury, **297–303**
    coup and contre-coup injury, 297
    primary, 297–298
    secondary, 298
    see also Head injury
Brain stem, 276
    blood pressure regulation, 156
    death, 289, *290*
    pain pathways, 113
Brain stem evoked responses (BSERs), 373
Brain tumours, **308–310**
    epidemiology and aetiology, 308
    investigations, 309
    medical/surgical management, 309
    nursing management, 309–310
BRCA-1 gene mutations, 776, 998
Breaking bad news, *see* Bad news, breaking
Breast, **771–772**
    abscess, 779
    augmentation, **790**
    awareness, 776, *777*
    benign tumours, **780**
    biopsy, 775, 1001
    cysts, 780
    developmental disorders, **779–780**
    fine-needle aspiration, 774
    hypoplasia, 779
    implants, 789, 790
    infections, **779**
    juvenile hypertrophy, 779, 780
    pain (mastalgia), **778**
    prostheses, 784
    reduction surgery, **790**
    self-examination, 999
    supernumerary, 779
Breast cancer, 771, **781–790**, 994
    aetiology and epidemiology, 781–782
    breast reconstruction after, 788–790
    clinical presentation, 782
    familial (high-risk patients), 776, *777*, 998

fungating lesions, 787–788
hormone replacement therapy and, 736
investigations, 782
lymphoedema, 785–787
male, 782, 784
medical/surgical management, 782–784
metastatic, 783, 785
nipple disorders, 781
nursing assessment, 772–773
nursing management, 784–785
in older women, 775
pathophysiology, 782
recurrent, 785
risk factors, 991
screening, 772, **775–776**, 777, 998–999
Breast care nurse (BCN), **773–774**
Breast disorders, **771–792**
benign, 778–781
congenital, **779–780**
diagnostic tests/investigations, 774–775
male, 772
nursing assessment, 772–773
one-stop clinics, 775
prevention/health education, 775–776
useful websites/addresses, 791–792
Breast-feeding
after breast reconstruction, 790
breast infections, 779
Breast reconstruction, **788–790**
flaps, 788–789
implants, 789
nursing management, 790
problems and complications, 790
Breast surgery
augmentation and reduction, 790
in breast cancer, **783**
conservative, 783
fungating lesions, 787
nursing management, 784
problems and complications, 790
see also Breast reconstruction; Mastectomy
Breath sounds, **958**
Breathing
assessment, see Respiratory assessment
in cardiopulmonary resuscitation, 495, 496
control, **534**, 954–955
depth, 538, 957
during sleep, 61
Kussmaul, 423, 957
in major trauma, 932
noisy, dying patients, 1042
problems, see Respiratory disorders
rescue, 496
rhythm, 538, 957
in shock, 162
techniques, in COPD, 548
Breathlessness/dyspnoea, 539
in anaemia, 457
in cardiovascular disease, 486
in COPD, 546
fluid balance and, 141
in heart failure, 511, 513
in lung cancer, 549–550
in motor neuron disease, 323
in nose and throat disorders, 568
in pneumonia, 554
in pneumothorax, 560
in shock, 157, 160
sleep disturbance, 65
smoking associated, 536
in terminal illness, 1028–1029, **1038–1039**
vicious cycle, 536
Breslow depth, 869
Brimonidine tartrate, 345, 356
Brinzolamide, 345, 356

Bristol Cancer Help Centre, 1010–1011
Bristol Stool Chart, 243, 244
British Allergy Foundation, 875
British Association of Cancer Patients and
their Families and Friends (BACUP),
310, 456, 650, 792, 1045
British Colostomy Association, 618
British Dermatology Nursing Group, 875
British Digestive Foundation, 618
British Heart Foundation, 530
British Liver Trust, 650
British Organ Donor Society, 530
British Society of Hearing Therapists, 391
British Standard (BS) 5750, **28**
British Thoracic Society (BTS)
asthma management guidelines, 542
COPD management guidelines, 548, 549
tuberculosis management guidelines, 555
Broad ligament, 709
Bromocriptine, in Parkinson's disease, 320
Bronchial hygiene, 961–962
Bronchiectasis, **552**
Bronchitis, chronic, 545
Bronchoalveolar lavage, 1001
Bronchoconstriction, 538
in asthma, 542, 544
Bronchodilation, 540
Bronchodilators
assessing response to, 540, 541
in asthma, 542, 543, 544
in cystic fibrosis, 551
Bronchoscopy, **542**, 1001
Bruch's membrane, 333, 353
Brudzinski's sign, 311
Brush biopsy, nose, 570
Bruxism, 67
BSE (bovine spongiform encephalopathy), 313
BT Age and Disability, 391
Buchanan bib, 584, 586
Budesonide, 572
Buffers, 149
Bulbourethral gland, 742
Bullae, 844, 864
see also Blisters
Bullous pemphigoid, **865**
Bullous Pemphigoid Support Group, 875
Bundle of His, 483, 484
Bunion (hallux valgus), 805, **813–814**
Bupivacaine, 884
Buprenorphine, 1034
Bupropion, 494, **536**
Burkitt's lymphoma, **470**
Burnout, **101–102**
causes, 101–102
in haematology units, 465
symptoms, 101
Burns, **871–874**
assessment, **871–872**, 873, 935
body image changes, 874
body surface area involved, 872, 873
depth, 871–872
first aid, 871
full-thickness, 872, 873, 874
initial management, 872–874
partial-thickness/deep dermal, 871, 873,
874
prevention, 871
superficial, 871, 873
surgical management, 874
types, 871
Burrows, 844, 859
Bursa, 795
Bursitis, **805**
Buschke–Löwenstein tumour, 751
Busulfan, 993

C

C fibres, 113
C-reactive protein (CRP), 600, 614
CA-125, serum, 715, 719, 723
Cachexia, 218, **1037**
Caecal volvulus, 604
Caecum, 595
Caffeine
restriction, 240, 241
sleep and, 65
in urinary incontinence, 240–241
CAGE questions, 624
Calcitonin, 398–399
Calcitriol (1,25-dihydroxycholecalciferol),
207, 399
Calcium (Ca^{2+}), 135
absorption, 661
deficiency, 209–210
dietary intake, 207, **209–210**
homeostasis, renal contribution, **661**
hormonal regulation, 399
imbalance disorders, 135
in chronic renal failure, 687
see also Hypercalcaemia; Hypocalcaemia
serum, 625, 671
in pancreatitis, 645
supplements, in hypoparathyroidism,
436, 437
Calcium channel blockers
in hypertension, 522
in Raynaud's phenomenon/disease, 525
urinary incontinence and, 236
'Calf pump', 485, 527
Calman-Hine report (1995), 986, 1004, 1018
Caloric tests, 372, 374
Calorie, 203
Camouflage, cosmetic, 863
Canal of Schlemm, 334
Cancer, **985–1019**
aetiology, 986–988
body image changes, 1015–1016
cells, 987–988
chemotherapy, see Chemotherapy
communication, 1009, **1011–1012**
deaths in women, 781
diagnostic procedures, 1001–1004
emotional responses to diagnosis, 1009–1011
epidemiology, 995
ethical dilemmas, 1017–1018
familial, 1004
grading, 1002, 1003
gynaecological, 712, **720–724**
invasive, 988
modes of spread, 989
natural history, 988–989
nursing management and interventions,
1010, 1011–1016
nutrition, 217–218
oncological emergencies, 1014–1015
pain, 1016–1017, **1032**
pain management, 1016–1017
patient teaching, 1012
predisposing factors, 989–991
prevention, 991–992
radiotherapy, see Radiotherapy
rehabilitation, 1016
screening and early detection, 996–1001
services, 986
staging, 1003–1004
stigmatization, 1053
support for family/friends, 1016
surgery, 1004
survival, 995, 1016

Cancer (continued)
  symptom control, 1012–1014
  symptoms, *1032*
  treatment modalities, 1004–1009
  warning signs, 992
  see also Palliative care; specific types of cancer
Cancer nurse
  gynaecological, 721–722, 723–724
  lead, 1017
  specialists, **1017**
Cancer in situ, see Carcinoma in situ
Cancerlink, 792
Candidiasis (thrush), *859*
  nails, 858, *859*, 870
  oesophageal, 601, 604–605
  oral, 601, *859*, 1035
  superficial, 858, *859*
  vaginal, 732, **762**
Cannabinoids, synthetic, 1013, 1036
Cannabis, 306
Capillaries, 485
  fluid shift, in shock, 156
  formation of new, in wound healing, 178
  tissue fluid formation, 136–137
Capillary permeability, increased, 137
Capillary refill, 486
Capsaicin cream, 426
Carbimazole, 432–433
Carbohydrate, 203, **205**
  in diabetes, *419*
Carbon dioxide (CO_2)
  in acid–base balance, 149
  in control of breathing, 534
  intracranial pressure and, *301*
  partial pressure in arterial blood ($Paco_2$), *148*,
    149, 161–162
  retention, see Hypercapnia
  transport, 446, **535**
Carbonic acid, 149, 660
Carbonic anhydrase inhibitors, *345*, 356
Carcinoembryonic antigen (CEA), 1000
Carcinogenesis, **988**
Carcinogens, 987, **989–990**, 991
Carcinoma, 989
Carcinoma in situ (CIS), 988, 989
  testicular, 746
Cardia, gastric, 593
Cardiac arrest, 495, 496, 502
  acid–base disorders, 151
  in hypothermia, 90
  see also Cardiopulmonary resuscitation
Cardiac arrhythmias, see Arrhythmias
Cardiac cycle, **484–485**
Cardiac enzymes, **491**, 507
Cardiac massage, external, 496
Cardiac output (CO), 485, **955**
  in critically ill patients, 955, 956
  measurement, 960
  in shock, *162*
Cardiac rehabilitation, 508–509
Cardiac surgery, **504**
  minimally invasive (MICS), 504
Cardiac tamponade, 510, **521**
  in pericarditis, 520, 521
Cardiogenic shock, 155, **510**
  aetiology, *159*, 510
  clinical presentation, 510
  medical management, **166–167**, 510
  nursing management, 510
Cardiomyopathy, **518–520**, 810
  dilated, *519*
  hypertrophic, *519*
  nursing management, 518
  restrictive, *519*
Cardiomyopathy Association, 518, 530

Cardiopulmonary arrest, 495
Cardiopulmonary bypass (CPB), 504
Cardiopulmonary resuscitation (CPR),
  495–496, 502
  ABC sequence, 495–496
  defibrillation, 496, 502
  steps, 496
Cardiovascular disease (CVD), **481–531**
  in chronic renal failure, 687
  in diabetes, 425, 426, 427
  diagnostic tests and investigations, 488–492
  fluid status, 141
  in Guillain–Barré syndrome, 328
  impaired wound healing, 178
  nursing assessment, 486–488
  in postmenopausal women, 735
  prevention and health education, 493–494,
    1059
  stress-related, 103
  useful addresses, 530
  see also Arrhythmias; Coronary heart disease;
    Heart failure; Stroke; *other specific*
    disorders
Cardiovascular monitoring and assessment,
  958–960, 962
Cardiovascular system, **481–486**
  critically ill patients, **955–956**
  during sleep, 61
  in multiple organ dysfunction, 168
  in shock, 156–157, 160
Cardioversion, direct current (DC), 499, **500**
Carditis, in rheumatic fever, 514
Care assistants, 12
Care homes
  standards of care, 27
  see also Nursing homes; Residential homes
Care Standards Act (2000), 27
Carers
  in Alzheimer's disease, 322
  assessment of well-being, 1060
  cancer patients, 1016
  feedback and satisfaction, **35**
  in incontinence, 232, 247
  involvement in care, 1060, 1061
  older adults, **980–981**
  palliative care, *1024*, 1027
  stress, **102–103**
  see also Family
Carers National Association, 1064
Caring about Carers (1999), 102
Carotene, 205, 842
Carotid arteries, 277, *278*
Carotid artery pulse, 487
Carotid endarterectomy, 292
Carotid sinus massage, 501
Carpal injuries, **835**
Carpal tunnel syndrome, **814**
Cartella shield, 350, 351
Cartilage, articular hyaline, 794, 795
Casts, **800–801**
Casualty, 924
Catabolic state, 159, 215, 217–218
  see also Hypermetabolic state
Cataract, **348–352**
  aetiology and epidemiology, 348
  clinical presentation, 348
  nurse practitioners, 332
  nursing management, 349–352
Cataract surgery, 332, **349**
  community management, 352
  complications, 349
  day case, 349
  discharge education/instructions, 351–352
  postoperative care, 350–351
  preoperative assessment, 349–350

  preoperative/intraoperative care, 350
Catecholamines, 400
  during sleep, 62
  in phaeochromocytoma, 440, 441
  in stress, 96
  see also Adrenaline; Noradrenaline
Catheterization, urinary, see Urinary
  catheterization
Caudal anaesthesia, 896
Caustic solutions, ingestion, 605
Celecoxib, 815
Cell cycle, *987*
Cell doubling theory, 974
Cells
  ageing, 974–975, 987
  division, 987
  growth, 987–988
  normal *versus* cancer, **987–988**
Cellulitis, 854–855
  breast, 779
  bullous, 864
Cellulose, 205
Centers for Disease Control (CDC), universal
  infection control precautions, 260,
  264–265
Central core disease, *809*
Central nervous system (CNS), 274, **276–279**
Central processing impairments, *289*
Central sensitization, 113
Central venous catheters, 960
  haemodialysis/haemofiltration, 691, *693*
  long-term, **470–471**
  parenteral nutrition, 224–225
  prevention of infection, *471*
  risks, 956
Central venous pressure (CVP), **488**
  critically ill patients, **959–960**
  in fluid balance assessment, 140, 663
  measurement, 161
  in shock, 161, 166
Centre for Reviews and Dissemination (York), *14*
Centronuclear myopathy, *809*
Cerebellopontine angle tumours, 389
Cerebellum, 276
Cerebral abscess, 385, 517
Cerebral contusions, 297
Cerebral cortex, 277
Cerebral oedema, 298, *301*
  in diabetic ketoacidosis, 423
  medical management, *309*
Cerebral perfusion pressure (CPP), 299
Cerebral thrombosis, 291
Cerebral venous sinus thrombosis, 291
Cerebrospinal fluid (CSF), **277–279**
  in meningitis, 311
  in multiple sclerosis, 305
  otorrhoea, *298*
  rhinorrhoea, *298*
  therapeutic removal, *301*
Cerebrovascular accident (CVA), see Stroke
Cerebrovascular disorders, **291–297**
Cerumen, see Ear wax
Ceruminous glands, 843
Cervical cancer, **721–722**, 994
  adjuvant chemotherapy, *999*
  aetiology, 721, 991
  investigations, 714–715, 721
  nursing management, 721–722
  screening, 714, 716, 721, **999–1000**
Cervical intraepithelial neoplasia (CIN), 715
Cervical mucus, 710
Cervical smear, **714**, 999–1000
Cervical spine control, in major trauma,
  932, *933*
Cervicitis, **732**

Cervix, uterine, 708, 709–710
  biopsy, 721
  colposcopic examination, 714–715
  speculum examination, 713, *714*
Chair covers, in incontinence, 247
Chalazion, **363**
Challenging behaviour
  in A&E department, **938**, *939*
  see also Aggression
Change management, **29**
Change model, 536–537
Changing Faces, 588
Chaperones, *713*
Charles Bonnet syndrome, 343
Charrier (Ch) size, urinary catheters, *675*
Chartered Society of Physiotherapy, 838
CHD, *see* Coronary heart disease
Cheilitis, angular, *859*
Chemical burns, 871
Chemical injury, eye, **360–361**
Chemicals, hepatotoxic, 627, 633
Chemoreceptor trigger zone (CTZ), 1035–1036
Chemoreceptors, 534, 954–955
Chemotherapy, 1004, **1006–1008**
  adjuvant, 1004
  in brain tumours, *309*
  in breast cancer, 783–785, 787
  in cervical cancer, *999*
  in haematological malignancy, **470–473**, 993
  -induced nausea and vomiting, 472, 1012–1013
  intravesical, bladder cancer, 679, *680*
  in leukaemia, 467, 468–469
  in lymphoma, 469–470
  in ovarian cancer, 723
  pathophysiology, 1006–1007
  safety issues, 1008
  side-effects, 471–473, 1007, *1008*
  stem cell transplant recipients, 475
  in testicular cancer, 748–749
  treatment schedules, 1007
  see also Cytotoxic drugs
Cherry angiomas, *see* Telangiectasia
Chest compressions, in cardiopulmonary resuscitation, 496
Chest drains, intercostal, **561**
Chest expansion test, *798*
Chest infections, **553–555**
  critically ill patients, 953
  postoperative, *740*, 889, **914**
  tracheostomy patients, 585
  see also Pneumonia; Respiratory tract infections
Chest movement, during breathing, 538–539
Chest pain, 486, **487–488**
  in angina, 503, 505, 506
  assessment, 487
  common causes, 488
  in myocardial infarction, 506, 508
  in sickle cell disease (chest crisis), 462, 463
Chest trauma, 560
Chest X-ray, 491
  in heart failure, 511
  in respiratory disorders, 541, 555, 560
Chewing gum, after tonsillectomy, 592
Chewing problems, 212–213, 222
CHI, *see* Commission for Health Improvement
Chickenpox, 855
Childbirth
  faecal incontinence and, 243
  urinary incontinence and, 232, 234
Children, in A&E department, 928
Chlamydia (trachomatis) infections, 732, **763**
  eye, 341, 361
  investigations, 714, 763

Chloasma, 863
Chloramphenicol eye drops/ointment, 360, 361, 363
Chlorhexidine, 261
  nasal, *572*
  preoperative skin cleansing, 887
Chloride (Cl⁻), *136*
  dietary, *207*, 210
  imbalance, *136*
Chlorpromazine, *226*, 1013
Chlorpropamide, 417–418
Cholangiocarcinoma, 643
Cholangiography, 626
Cholangitis, **641–643**
Cholecystectomy
  in cholecystitis, 640, 641
  laparoscopic, **639**, *640*
  open, **639–640**
Cholecystitis, 638
  acalculous, **641**
  acute, **640–641**
  chronic, **641**
Cholecystogram, 626
Cholecystokinin, 594, 595, 623
Choledochoduodenostomy, 648
Choledocholithiasis (bile duct stones), **641–643**
Choledochostomy with T-tube, 642, 643
Cholelithiasis, *see* Gallstones
Cholesteatoma, 372, 384
Cholesterol, 204, 493, 623
  gallstones, 638
  lowering drug therapy, 427, 494, 504
  lowering measures, 493–494
  serum, 216, *625*
    in diabetes, 427
    high, *see* Hypercholesterolaemia
  transport, 205
Cholestyramine, *226*
Cholinergic receptors, 276
Chondrosarcoma, 821
Chorda tympani, 369
Chordae tendinae, *482*, 483
Choriocarcinoma, *729*
Choroid, 333
Chromium, *207*, 211
Chronic illness, **1047–1065**
  adaptation to, 1053–1054
  anaemia of, **459**, 687
  assessment, 1058–1060
  care settings, 1056–1058
  common features, 1050–1051
  definitions, 1048
  developmental, psychological, social and cultural factors, 1051–1055
  impaired wound healing, 178–179
  long-term care, 1058
  multiple pathology, 1050
  new nursing roles, 1058
  nursing care, 1060–1063
  prevalence and impact, 1049–1051
  problems of daily living, 401
  rehabilitation, 1057
  social and role functions, 1060
  urinary incontinence, 233
  useful addresses, 1064–1065
  see also Disability
Chronic obstructive pulmonary disease (COPD), **545–548**
  acute exacerbations, management, 548, *549*
  causes/risk factors, 537, 545
  epidemiology, 545
  investigations, 541
  oxygen therapy, 546–547, 557
  pathophysiology, 545–546
  postoperative care, 908

  pulmonary rehabilitation, 548
  respiratory failure, 547, 548, 557
  treatment, 546–548
  trigger factors, 538
Chronic pain, 112
  back, 816
  non-malignant, **129–130**
Chronic renal failure, *see* Renal failure, chronic
Chronic venous insufficiency, 526, **527–528**
Chronotherapy, 1007
Chyme, 593, 594, 595
Ciclosporin, in psoriasis, 862
Cilia, respiratory tract, 533, 566
  see also Mucociliary clearance
Ciliary body, 333
Ciliary injection, 359
Cimetidine, *227*
Circadian rhythms, 60, 61–62
  body temperature, 61, 77, *78*, 84
  desynchronization, 63
  factors affecting, 63–64
  hormones, 62
Circle of Willis, 277, *278*
Circulating nurse, 904
Circulating volume
  in acute renal failure, 694
  assessment, 959–960
  in critically ill patients, 956
  increased, *see* Fluid volume excess
  loss of, *see* Hypovolaemia
  optimizing, in shock, 165–166
Circulation
  in cardiopulmonary resuscitation, 496
  in major trauma, 933
  postoperative assessment, **909**
  restricted, 78
  in shock, 162–163
Circulatory overload, *see* Fluid volume excess
Circulatory support, 949
Circulatory system, 481
  disorders, *see* Cardiovascular disease
  in stress, 96, **103**
  see also Cardiovascular system
Circumcision, 743, 752
  complications, *752*
  penile cancer and, 751, 752
Cirrhosis of liver, **633–636**
  aetiology and epidemiology, 633
  clinical presentation, 634
  investigations, 634
  medical management, 634
  nursing management, 634–636
  oesophageal varices, 604, 634–635
  pathophysiology, 634
  prognosis, 636
Cisplatin, in cervical cancer, 994
Cisternography, 287
Citizens Advice Bureau (CAB), *1061*
Clarifying, 48
Claudication, intermittent, 523
Clavicular fractures, **824–825**, 834
Cleansing
  preoperative skin, 887, 905
  wound, 181, 934
Cleft palate, ear syringing, *378*
Clients, *see* Patients
Climacteric, 735
  problems associated with, **735–736**
Clinical effectiveness, 24, 26, 33
Clinical governance, **25**
Clinical supervision, *101*, 106
Clippers, hair, 888
Clips, skin, 915
Clitoris, 711
Clomifene, *760*

Clonidine, 736
Clonus, *289*
Clonus test, *798*
Clostridium difficile diarrhoea
(pseudomembranous colitis),
255, *256*, **616**
Clothing
laundering soiled, 247
in major trauma, 933
protective, **263–264**, *631*
stroke patients, *294*
in sudden death, 942
surgical patients, 887
surgical personnel, **905–906**
Clotting, *see* Coagulation
Clubbing, finger, 539
Co-proxamol, 1033
Coagulation, 448–449
deep vein thrombosis and, 525
screen, 450, 492, 670
Coagulation factors, *448*, 623
recombinant products, *478*
replacement, in haemophilia, 452, 478
Coal tar, 862
Coarctation of aorta, *528*
Cobalamins, *see* Vitamin B$_{12}$
Cocaine hydrochloride, nasal, *572*
Cochlea, 370
Cochlear implant, *386*
Cochlear nerve, 370
Cochrane Library, *14*, 15
Code of professional conduct, 6, *7*
Codeine, 124
in faecal incontinence, 246
pupil constriction, 284
Coeliac disease, 219
Cognition, **285**
Cognitive behavioural therapy
in pain management, 128
in stress, 107
Cognitive function, assessment, 285
Cognitive impairment, *see* Dementia
Cognitive problems, 285, *289*
Cohort nursing, 264
Cold application
in back pain, 816
in hyperthermia, 86
in pain management, 128
Cold environments
angina and, 503
Raynaud's phenomenon/disease, 524–525
Cold injury, localized, *see* Frostbite
Cold sore, 855
Cold water
in hyperthermia, 86, 87
immersion, 81, 87
Colestipol, *226*
Colicky pain, 1032
Collagen
ageing changes, 175, 794, 974
skin, 175
Collecting duct, renal, 656, **659–660**
College of Occupational Therapists, 838
Colles' fracture, 835, *836*
Colloid solutions, 145
in hypovolaemia, 164, **165**
Colon, 595–596
ascending, 595–596
descending, 596
sigmoid, 596
transverse, 596
Colon Cancer Concern, 618
Colonization, 256
Colonoscopy, 599, 614, 1001
Colony-stimulating factors, 448, 1009

Colorectal cancer (CRC), **611–613**, 994
aetiology, 611, 990
screening, *1000*
Colostomy, 612
Colour vision, 335
testing, 340
Colpoperineorrhaphy, 725
Colporrhaphy, anterior, 725
Colposcopy, **714–715**, 721
Coma, 61
assessment, 280
hepatic, **636–637**
nursing interventions, 302
see also Consciousness, altered; Glasgow Coma
Scale
Comedones, *844*, 851
Comfort
in A&E department, *939*
in multiple sclerosis, 307
in pain management, 128
to promote sleep, 69–70
Commensal microorganisms, 257, 595, 843, 887
Commission for Health Improvement (CHI), 15, **25–26**
Common bile duct, 622, 623
stenting, 642, 648
stones (choledocholithiasis), **641–643**
Communicable Disease Surveillance Centre, 259
Communication, **39–56**
in A&E department, 925, *939*
after laryngectomy, 588
assessment, 1060
barriers to effective, 41
cancer patients, 1009, **1011–1012**
critically ill patients, 951
culture and, 41–42
erectile dysfunction as, 753
factors influencing, 41
in groups, 53–55
in hearing impairment, **375**, 385
Macmillan model, 40
in major disasters, 942
in motor neuron disease, 323
nature, 40–41
non-verbal, **40–41**, 175
oxygen therapy and, 559
in Parkinson's disease, 321
perioperative, 891, 895
personality theories and, 45–46
in resuscitation, 930–931
skills, 46, **47–53**
in spinal injuries, 325
in terminal illness, 1031
tracheostomy patients, 586
unconscious patient, 290–291
verbal, 40
in visual impairment, 342
Community
A&E department and, 924
nutritional interventions, 219
Community care
in chronic illness and disability, 1056
in incontinence, 233, 247–248
older adults, 979, 980–981
in terminal illness, **1024–1025**
see also Carers; Home
Community nurses, 12
in chronic illness and disability, **1057**
prescribing rights, 186, 248
see also District nurses; Practice nurses
Compartment syndrome, acute, 801, 829–830
Compensation
noise-induced hearing loss, 380
work-related stress, 102

Complaints, *7*
Complementary therapies
in pain management, *127*
in palliative care, *1023*
to promote sleep, 70
for stress, **105–106**
Compliance (concordance), *977*
in chronic renal failure, *689*
eye medication, 344–346
in heart failure, 512
mechanical ventilation, 961
in multiple sclerosis, 307
in older adults, **976–977**
in tuberculosis, 556
wound healing and, 180
Components of Life model, *926*
Compression bandaging, 195, **196–197**, 528
Compression hosiery/stockings
in chronic venous insufficiency, 526, 527
in deep vein thrombosis, 526
surgical patients, 889, 914
venous leg ulcers, *196*, **197**
Computed tomography (CT)
brain tumours, 309
in cancer diagnosis, 1002
in ear problems, 373
in endocrine disorders, 401
in head injury, 300
in liver, biliary and pancreatic disorders, 626
in musculoskeletal disorders, 797
in neurological disease, 287
in nose and throat disorders, 569
in urinary system disorders, 666
Concordance, *977*
see also Compliance
Concussion, 298
Condoms, 757, 761
Conduction, heat transfer by, 77
Conduction system, heart, **483–484**
Condylomata acuminata, 761, 855
Cones, 333, 335
Confidentiality, *7*
in cancer nursing, *1017*
Conflict, dealing with, 52
Confusion, **285**
assessment, *282*, 285
in fluid loss, 140
in terminal illness, 1039
Congenital adrenal hyperplasia (CAH), **441**
Congenital heart disease, **528**
'Coning', 299
Conjunctiva, 336
disorders, **361**
Conjunctivitis, **361**, *362*
Connective tissue
cutaneous, 175
formation, in wound healing, 178
Connective tissue disorders, **817–818**
Conn's syndrome, 440
Conscientious objection, 18, 731
Consciousness, 280
altered, **280**, *289*, 299
critically ill patients, 952
in diabetic ketoacidosis, 423
in head injury, 298
in hypoglycaemia, 421
in multiple organ dysfunction, 168
nursing management, **290–291**
nutritional status and, 213
in seizures, *314*
in shock, 157
versus sleep, 61
see also Coma
assessment, 280
in cardiopulmonary arrest, 495

postoperative period, **909**
see also Glasgow Coma Scale
Consent
  critically ill patients, **952**
  educated, 8
  good practice, *892*
  implied, 891
  informed, **8–9**, **19**, 891
  minimum age/capacity to give, 892
  preoperative, 737, **891–892**
  written, 891
Constipation, 242, 598, **609–610**
  assessment, 243, *244*
  brain tumours and, 310
  in cancer, *1013*
  causes, 609–610, 1037
  causing faecal incontinence, 243
  chemotherapy-induced, 472
  in critically ill patients, 953
  in diabetes, 426, 427, 428
  diagnostic criteria, 243
  enteral feeding and, *224*
  in fluid balance disorders, 140
  in Guillain–Barré syndrome, 328
  in heart failure, *513*
  in irritable bowel syndrome, 609
  management, 245, 246, 610, 1037
  in older adults, 978
  in Parkinson's disease, 322
  postoperative, 913–914
  prevention in hospital patients, *609*
  in terminal illness, **1037**
Contact dermatitis, **851**
Contact lenses, *361*
Contact tracing
  sexually transmitted infections, 761, 764
  tuberculosis, 556
Contamination, 257
Continence, **229–252**
Continence care, **246–249**
  advice and education, 247
  at home, 233
  in hospitals, 232–233
Continence Foundation, 250
  management of bowel problems, *247*
  pelvic floor exercises, 238, 239
Continence nurse specialists, 229, 246–247
Continence products, **247–249**
  appliances, 248–249
  pads, 247–248
  provision, *248*
Continuing professional development (CPD),
    6–7, 33
Continuity theory, ageing, 972
Continuous ambulatory peritoneal dialysis
    (CAPD), 428, 692
Continuous positive airway pressure (CPAP),
    961
  in respiratory failure, 559, *560*
  in sleep apnoea, 67
Contraception, **757–758**
  barrier methods, 757, 761
  breast cancer chemotherapy and, 784–785
  emergency hormonal, *758*
  methods available, 757
  in perimenopause, 736
Contractility, 955
  in shock, 156, 166
Contracts, making, 51
Contractures
  in burn injuries, 874
  in Guillain–Barré syndrome, 328
  in myopathies, 811
  in spinal injuries, 326
Contrast studies
  in liver, biliary and pancreatic disorders, 626

in neurological disease, 287
in throat disorders, 570
see also Barium studies
Contre-coup injury, brain, 297
Control, locus of, 94, 992
Control of infection *see* Infection control
Convection, heat transfer by, 77
Convective warming therapy, 89
Convulsions, *see* Seizures
Cooling blankets, 87, *164*
Cooling methods, **86–87**, *164*
Coombs' test, 450
COPD, *see* Chronic obstructive pulmonary disease
Coping
  assessment, 772–773, **1060**
  in chronic illness/disability, 1057
Copper, *207*, 210–211
  deposition, in Wilson's disease, 318
Cor pulmonale, 539
Cornea, 332, *333*
  abrasions, 360
  damage by foreign body, **359–360**
  disorders, **359–361**
  dystrophy, 359
  grafting, 359
  oedema, 349
  ulcers, **359**, *360*
Corneal topography, 340
Corneocytes, 842
Coronary angiography, **492**
Coronary angioplasty, *see* Percutaneous
    transluminal coronary angioplasty
Coronary arteries, 483
  atheromatous occlusion, 503
  spasm, 503
Coronary artery bypass graft (CABG), 504, 512
Coronary care unit (CCU), 947
Coronary circulation, **483**
Coronary heart disease (CHD), **503–509**
  aetiology and epidemiology, 503
  in diabetes, 427, 503
  diet and, **216**, 493, 494, 508
  investigations, 492
  pathophysiology, 503
  prevention and health education, *216*,
    493–494
  risk factors, 493
  stress and, 103
  see also Angina pectoris; Myocardial infarction
Coronary Prevention Group (CPG), 530
Coronary stents, PTCA, 504, 505
Coroner, 941, **1043**
Corpus cavernosum, 743
Corpus luteum, 707–708
Corticosteroids, 399
  in adrenal insufficiency, 438
  advice for patients on, 438
  in anaphylaxis, 167
  in aplastic anaemia, 464
  in asthma, 542, 543, 544
  in autoimmune blistering disorders, 865, 866
  in cancer symptom control, 1013, 1014
  in cystic fibrosis, 551
  in idiopathic thrombocytopenic purpura,
    476
  in inflammatory bowel disease, 614
  in inflammatory myopathies, 811
  local injections, 805, 824, 861
  nasal, *572*, 574
  for nasal polyps, 580
  in nausea and vomiting, 1036
  ophthalmic, *345*, 362
  in psoriasis, 862
  in rheumatoid arthritis, 806
  in spinal cord compression, 1015
  in tinea, 856

topical, 850, 854, 862
in vitiligo, 863
see also Glucocorticoids; Mineralocorticoids
Corticotrophin-releasing factor, hormone
    (CRF, CRH), *398*, *399*, 438
Cortisol, 399
  circadian rhythm, 62, 399
  excess, in Cushing's syndrome, 438, 439
  pharmacological, *see* Hydrocortisone
  in stress, 96–97, 890
Cosmetics, preoperative removal, 894
Cost
  continence appliances, 248
  and quality, **27**
Cough, 539
  in heart failure, 511
  in pneumonia, 553
  in terminal illness, **1038**
Cough reflex, 286
Counselling, 46, **47**
  bereavement, **1044**
  genetic, 289, 811
  skills, **46–47**
  in stress management, 106
  termination of pregnancy, 731
Count fingers (CF), in visual acuity testing, 339
Countercurrent exchange, in loop of Henle,
    658–659
Coup injury, brain, 297
Covering response, stigmatizing conditions, 1053
Cowper's gland, 742
Cox 2 inhibitors, in haemophilia, 478
CPAP, *see* Continuous positive airway pressure
CPR, *see* Cardiopulmonary resuscitation
Crackles, 958
Cranberry juice, 673
Cranial nerves, *279*
  disorders, **303–304**
  in Guillain–Barré syndrome, 327
Craniotomy, 310
Creatine kinase (CK), serum, 811
Creatine phosphokinase (CPK), 491
Creatinine, serum, **670**
Creatinine height index, 215
Creutzfeldt–Jakob disease (CJD), **313**
  sporadic, 313
  variant (vCJD), 313, 451, 906
Cricoid pressure, 900
Critical appraisal, 13–14
Critical care, 947
  averting admissions, 949
  continuum, 949
  development, 947–948
  early warning systems, 950–951
  enabling discharge, 949
  multidisciplinary team, **951–952**
  nurse training, 948
  outreach teams, *949*, *950*
  see also High-dependency unit; Intensive care
Critically ill patients, **947–965**
  assessment, 956–957
  classification, 948–951
  communication, 951
  decision-making and informed consent, 952
  effects of environment, 954
  inotrope therapy, 962–963
  mechanical ventilation, 960–962
  monitoring and assessment, 956–960
  nursing management, 951–953
  nutrition, 953
  personal care, 952–953
  physiological overview, 954–956
  relatives, 164, 951, 952
  renal replacement therapy, 963
  sleep disturbances, 64, 954
  stressors, 98, 954

Crohn's disease, 613
aetiology, 613–614
investigations, 614
medical/surgical management, 614–615
nursing management, 615–616
signs and symptoms, 614
Cromoglicate (cromoglycate)
eye drops/ointment, *345*, 361
nasal, *572*
Cross-infection, 257
mode of transmission, 256
prevention, **264–266**, 906
see also Infection control
Cross-linkage theory of ageing, 974
Crown–rump length (CRL), 728
CRUSE, 1045
Crush injury, *934*
Crusts, *844*
Crutches, **802–804**
Cryoprecipitate, 452
Crystalloid solutions, 145
in hypovolaemia, 164–165
CT, *see* Computed tomography
Cullen's sign, 644
Cultural differences, *42, 43*
adaptation to chronic illness, 1054
liver, biliary and pancreatic disorders, 624
pain perception, 116
sleep patterns, 64
stigmatization, 1053
Culture, **41–42**
A&E care and, 925
definition, **42**
disability and chronic illness and, 1051
dying patients, 1042
in nursing, **42**
nutrition and, 212
perioperative issues, *886*, 888
sudden death and, 941
wound healing and, 180
Culture media, 254
Cuscoe's speculum, 713, *714*
Cushing's disease, 438
Cushing's syndrome, **438–440**
aetiology and epidemiology, 438
clinical presentation, 438, 439
investigations, 439
medical/surgical management, 439
nursing management, 439–440
Cushions, *see* Mattresses/cushions
CVA (cerebrovascular accident), *see* Stroke
Cyanosis
in cardiovascular disease, 486
in critically ill patients, 957
in pigmented skin, *846*
postoperative, 908
in respiratory disease, 539
in shock, 157, 160
in terminal illness, 1029
Cyclizine, 388, *884*, 911
Cyclopentolate hydrochloride, *338, 344*, 350
Cyclophosphamide, 684
Cycloplegics, *344*, 350
Cyst, skin, *844*, **861**
Cystectomy
partial, 679
radical, with urinary diversion, **679–681**
Cystic fibrosis (CF), **550–552**
acute respiratory exacerbations, 550, **551**
end-stage management, 552
gene therapy, 552
nursing management, 551–552
Cystitis, **672–673**
clinical presentation, 672
'honeymoon', 672

and prostatitis, 750
Cystocele, *724, 725*
Cystography, **667**
Cystometry, 669
Cystoscopy, **668–669**
Cytology
aspiration, **1001**
cervical, **714**, 999–1000
Cytotoxic cross-matching, kidney donor and
recipient, 695
Cytotoxic drugs
administration, 471
long-term central venous catheters, 470–471
mechanisms of action, 1006–1007
in psoriasis, 862
see also Chemotherapy

D

Danazol, 734
Dantrolene sodium, 87
Dapsone, 866
Dark adaptation, 336
Darkness, promoting sleep, 69
Day centres, palliative care, **1023–1024**
Day surgery, **880–885**
benefits, 880–881
cataract, 349
discharge criteria, 885
eye problems, 332
gynaecological, 738
influences on suitability/acceptance, 882
medical selection, *883*
nasal septal surgery, *578*
older adults, 881
postoperative pain management, 884–885
pre-admission assessment and admission,
882–884
Daytime naps, 70
DDAVP, *see* Desmopressin
Deafness, *see* Hearing impairment
Death, **1042–1043**
brain stem, 289, *290*
follow-up support and counselling,
1043–1044
last offices, 1042
official aspects, 1042–1043
registration, 1043
reporting to coroner, 1043
sudden, *see* Sudden death
terminal care, **1041–1042**
viewing of body, 941
see also Bereavement; Dying; Terminal illness
Death certificate, 941, 942, 1043
Death rattle, 1042
DEBRA, 866, 875
Debridement, wound, 181–182
autolytic, 182
biosurgery, 182
in burn injuries, 874
enzymatic, 182
surgical, 181
Debrief, after major disasters, 942–943
Decision-making
in A&E triage, 927
critically ill patients, 952
Decubitus ulcers, *see* Pressure ulcers
Deep vein thrombosis (DVT), 485, **525–526**,
888–889
aetiology/risk factors, 525
in critically ill patients, 953
in Guillain–Barré syndrome, 328
nursing management, 526

postoperative, *740*, **914**
preoperative risk assessment, 888
prophylaxis, 526, 889, 902
Defecation, control of, **242–243**
Defence mechanisms, unconscious (mental),
45, **97**
Defibrillation, 496, 502
Defibrillators, 496
automated implantable (AICDs), 502
in public places, 496, 507
Deformity, physical, 1052
Degenerative neurological disorders,
318–323
Dehiscence, wound, 918–919
Dehydration, 139
in diabetic ketoacidosis, 423
enteral feeding and, 224
in heart failure, 512, 513
nursing assessment, 139, 140
in older adults, *138, 141*
predisposing factors, 140–142
prevention, 142
in pyrexia, 79, 86
terminal, *142*, **1028**
thirst and, 142
wound healing, *179*
see also Hypovolaemia
Deliberate self-harm, **940**
Delirium, 285
Dementia (cognitive impairment), **973**
in Alzheimer's disease, 322
in frail older people, 975–976
in multiple sclerosis, 307
paternalism *versus* risk, *979*
urinary incontinence, 234
Demographic change, 967, 969
Demyelinating disorders, **304–308**
Denial, 97
terminal illness, 1025–1026
Dental caps/crowns, 737, 894
Dentist, 221
Dentures, 602, 737, 894
Dependency
critically ill patients, 949, 952
older adults, 968–969, 975–976, 979
Depilatory creams, 737, 888
Depression
in A&E department, 940
measurement, 104–105
in old age, **974**
sleep problems, 65
stress and, 104
in terminal illness, 1026, 1039–1040
versus cognitive problems, 285
Dermal papillae, 175
Dermatitis
contact, **851**
seborrhoeic, **854**
see also Eczema
Dermatitis herpetiformis, **866**
Dermatomycoses, 855–859
prevention of infection/reinfection, *856*
Dermatomyositis (DM), 810, 811
Dermatophytes, 856
Dermatophytosis, *see* Tinea
Dermis, 174–175, 841–842
Dermoepidermal junction, 174
Dermoid cysts, 719, 861
Desferrioxamine, 454, 461
Desflurane, *884*
Desmopressin (DDAVP)
in diabetes insipidus, 431
in haemophilia, 478
in urinary incontinence, 242
Desmosomes, 174, 842

Despair
  Erikson's theory, 972
  in terminal illness, 1026
Desquamation, 842
Desynchronization, internal, 63
Detergent, for handwashing, 262
Detoxification, 623
Detrusor (muscle), 230, 661
  instability (overactive bladder), 235, **240–242**
  underactive/acontractile, 235
Developmental factors, chronic illness and
    disability, **1054–1055**
Dexamethasone
  brain tumours, *309*
  nasal, *572*
Dexamethasone suppression test, 402, 439
Dexterity, reduced, 141, 347
Dextran solutions, 165
Dextromoramide, 1034
Dextropropoxyphene, 124
Dextrose, *145*
  in diabetic ketoacidosis, 423
  in hypoglycaemia, 422
  in peritoneal dialysis fluid, 692
Diabetes complications, **421–428**, 1050
  acute, **421–424**
  long-term, 394, **424–428**
    aetiology and epidemiology, 424–425
    clinical presentation, 425–426
    investigations, 426
    medical management, 426–427
    nursing management, 427–428
    pathophysiology, 425
  macrovascular, 424, 425
  microvascular, 424, 425
  patient education, 414–415
  screening, 341, 352, 414
  see also specific complications
Diabetes Control and Complications Trial (DCCT),
    414, 421, 424
Diabetes insipidus (DI), 402, **431**
Diabetes mellitus, 394, **403–428**
  adaptation to, 1053
  alcohol intake, 414, *419*
  blood glucose monitoring (BGM), **409–410**,
    414, 420
  cataract surgery, 350
  in chronic pancreatitis, 646
  coronary heart disease, 427, 503
  in Cushing's syndrome, 440
  diagnosis, **402–403**
  driving, 410–411, 414
  foot care, 415
  gestational, 403, 416
  hearing loss, 374
  hypoglycaemia, 411, **421–422**
  impaired wound healing, 178
  insulin therapy, *see under* Insulin therapy
  nursing assessment, 401
  obesity and, 216
  perioperative care, 886
  preoperative fasting, 893
  prescription exemption, 413
  prevention and health education, 403
  psychological care, *402*, 405, 428
  secondary, 403
  smoking, 403, 414
  type 1, *see* Type 1 diabetes mellitus
  type 2, *see* Type 2 diabetes mellitus
  urinary incontinence, 234
  useful websites, 442
  work, 414
Diabetes National Service Framework (NSF),
    394, *395*
Diabetes specialist nurses, 394, 407, 409

Diabetes UK, 414, 415
Diabetic foot ulcers, 425, 427, 428
Diabetic ketoacidosis (DKA), 404, **422–424**
  clinical presentation, 414, 423
  management, 423–424
Diabetic nephropathy, **682–683**
  aetiology and epidemiology, 424–425, 682
  clinical presentation, 425, 682
  management, 426, 428, **682–683**
  pathophysiology, 425, 682
Diabetic neuropathy, 424, **425–426**
  medical management, 426–427
  nursing management, 428
Diabetic retinopathy, **352–353**
  aetiology and epidemiology, 352, 424
  background, 352
  clinical presentation, 425
  management, 352, 426, 427–428
  pre-proliferative, 352
  proliferative, 352, *353*
Diagnosis, nursing, 11–12
Dialysis, **689–694**
  before renal transplantation, 695
  decision to commence, 688–689
  in glomerulonephritis, 683
  in multiple organ dysfunction, 168
  nurse-led service, 653
  provision, 689
  see also Haemodialysis; Peritoneal dialysis
Diamorphine, 124, 1034
  epidural, 127
  in myocardial infarction, 507
  in unstable angina, 506
Diaphysis, 794
Diarrhoea, 598
  in cancer, 1013
  chemotherapy-induced, 472
  Clostridium difficile, *see* Pseudomembranous
    colitis
  diabetic, 426, 427
  enteral feeding and, *224*
  faecal incontinence in, 243
  in fluid balance disorders, 140
  in inflammatory bowel disease, 614, 615
  in irritable bowel syndrome, 609
  nutrition and, 214
  oral rehydration solutions, 142
  in stress, 96
Diary, reflective, 16, *17*
Diathermy, **904–905**
  bipolar, 904
  unipolar, 904
Diazepam, rectal, in status epilepticus, *316*
Diencephalon, 276–277
Diet
  advice on changing, 600
  after tonsillectomy, 581
  in atopic eczema, 850
  in autoimmune blistering disorders, 866
  cancer risk and, 990
  in cardiomyopathy, 518
  in cirrhosis, 636
  constipation and, 609
  coronary heart disease and, **216**, 493, 494,
    508
  dialysis patients, 688, 691, *693*
  elemental, 613–614
  elimination or exclusion, 219
  gallstones and, 638, *641*
  in haematological disorders, 455–456
  healthy, *see* Healthy eating
  in incontinence, 246, 247
  inflammatory bowel disease and, 613–614
  low-salt, 513
  in neutropenia, 466

  in osteoporosis, 819
  in pancreatic cancer, 648
  in pancreatitis, 646, 647
  sleep and, 65, 70
  stress and, 106
  in type 1 diabetes, 404, 409
  in type 2 diabetes, **419**
  weight-losing, 217
  see also Eating; Food; Nutrition
Dietary history, 214
Dietary reference values (DRVs), 202
Dietician, 219, 222, *223*, 225
  in amputation, 524
  in critical care, 952
  in diabetes, 409, 419
  renal, 691
  in Wilson's disease, 318
Differentiation, haemopoietic stem cells,
    447
Diffuse axonal injury, brain, 298
Diffusion, 134
Digestive Disorders Foundation, 650
Dignity, surgical patients, 902
Digoxin
  in atrial arrhythmias, 499, 500
  in heart failure, 512
  toxicity, 148, 500, 512
Dihydrocodeine, 124, 1033
1,25-Dihydroxycholecalciferol, 207, 399
Dilatation and curettage (D&C), 718, 731
'Dinner fork' deformity, 835, *836*
Diplopia, *289*
Direct antiglobulin test (DAT), 450
Direct current (DC) cardioversion, 499, **500**
Disability, **1047–1065**
  assessment, 1058–1060
  care settings, 1056–1058
  causes, 1049
  definitions, 1048, *1049*
  developmental, psychological, social and
    cultural factors, 1051–1055
  health policy, **1056**
  long-term care, 1058
  in major trauma, 933
  nursing care, 1060–1063
  prevalence and impact, 1049–1051
  social model, 1048, *1049*
  social and role functions, 1060
  useful addresses, 1064–1065
  see also Chronic illness; Mobility problems
Disability-adjusted life years (DALYs), 1049
Disability Living Allowance (DLA), *1061*
Disability Net, 1065
Disabled Living Foundation, 838
Disasters, major, **942–943**
Discharge
  after gynaecological surgery, *738, 739*
  day surgery unit, 884–885
  in minor trauma, 935–936
  planning, postoperative, **919**
  postoperative recovery unit, 909–910
Disease-modifying anti-rheumatic drugs
    (DMARDs), 806
Disengagement theory of ageing, **972**
Disinfection, surgical hand, 262
Disinhibited behaviour, 277
Dislocation, 823
  shoulder, **824**, 834
Displacement (psychological), *97*
Disregard, stigmatizing conditions, 1052
Disruptive patients, *607*
Disseminated intravascular coagulation (DIC),
    168, **477**
Distal convoluted tubule (DCT), 656, **659–660**
Distress, 94, 97

District nurses
    eye medication and, 346
    in palliative care, 1025
    postoperative cataract patient care, 352
    see also Community nurses
Disturbed behaviour
    in A&E department, 938–939
    assessment, 940
    causes, 939–940
    management in A&E, 940–941
Dithranol, 862
Diuretics
    adverse effects, 141–142
    in heart failure, 511, 512, 513
    in hypertension, 521
    in nephrotic syndrome, 684
    urinary incontinence and, 233, *236*
Diurnal variation
    body temperature, 61, 77, *78, 84*
    see also Circadian rhythms
Diverticular disease, **610–611**
Dizziness
    after ear surgery, 385, 386
    in anaemia, *457*
    in arrhythmias, 497, 500
    see also Vertigo
DNA
    alterations, in carcinogenesis, 987
    cytotoxic drug actions, 1006–1007
    radiation-induced damage, 1005
    in theories of ageing, 974
Documentation
    aggression in A&E, 938
    in major disasters, 942
    skin lesions, 846, *847*
    in sudden death, 942
    surgical patients, 895
Domestic violence, 937
Donabedian's structure–process–outcome model, 30, *31*
Donepezil hydrochloride, 322
Donor insemination (DI), *760*
Dopamine, 398
    after renal transplantation, 696
    in critically ill patients, 962–963
    in Parkinson's disease, 318–319
    and sleep, 61
Dopamine (D₂) receptor antagonists, 1013, 1036
Dopamine receptor agonists, in Parkinson's disease, 320
Dopaminergic drugs, in Parkinson's disease, 320
Doppler echocardiogram, 491
Doppler ultrasound
    in critically ill patients, 960
    leg ulcers, 193–194, *195*, 198
    oesophageal, in shock, 162
    in peripheral arterial disease, 523
Dorzolamide, *345*, 356
Doxapram, 559
Drains, wound, *see* Wound drains
Drapes, surgical, 906
Dreaming, 62
Dressing, stroke patients, *294*
Dressings, **182–187**
    alginate, *183*, 185
    in atopic eczema, 850–851
    burn injuries, 873, 874
    combination products, 186
    deodorizing, *183*, 185
    foam, *183*, 185
    hydrocolloid, *183*, 185
    hydrogel, *184*, 185
    ideal, 182
    interactive, 183

low adherent primary contact (medicated), *184*, 185
    older adults, *187*
    passive, 183
    polysaccharide bead (medicated), *184*, 186
    postoperative, **915**
    products available, 182–186
    selection of products, 186–187
    semipermeable film, *184*, 185
    silicone sheets/gels, *184*, 185
    wet wrap, 850–851
Dressler's syndrome, 520
Drinking
    helping patients with, 144, *145*
    in terminal illness, 1029
    see also Fluid intake
Drinkline, 650
Drinks
    at bedtime, 70
    in diabetes, *419*
    types, 144
Driving
    after gynaecological surgery, *739*
    in diabetes, 410–411, 414
    pacemaker patients, 498
    visual impairment and, 356
Drooling, in Bell's palsy, 303–304
Drop factor, 146
Drought, 140
Drug dependence
    A&E attenders, **937**
    acute pain management, 128–129
    viral hepatitis transmission, 627
Drug eruptions, **870–871**
    fixed, 870
Drug history, 596–597
Drugs/medications
    adverse reactions (ADRs), 870–871
    carcinogenic, 991
    causing constipation, 609
    causing erectile dysfunction, *753*
    causing hepatitis, *633*
    in chronic illness and disability, *1057*
    detoxification, 623
    disguising, *973*
    dying patients, 1042
    in hypothermia, 91
    nutrient interactions, **225**, *226–227*
    in older adults, **976–977**
    ophthalmic, **344–348**
    preoperative assessment, 886–887
    refusal to take, in dementia, 973
    in renal disease, 688–689
    self-poisoning, 940
    sleep disturbance, 65
    timing of regular, 70
    urinary incontinence and, *236*
    see also Pharmacokinetics
Dual energy X-ray absorptiometry (DXA), 797
Duchenne muscular dystrophy (DMD), 808, *809*
Ductal carcinoma in situ (DCIS), 782
Dumping syndrome, 606
Duodenal ulcers, 598, 606
Duodenoscopy, 599
Duodenum, 594
Dura mater, 277–278
DVT, *see* Deep vein thrombosis
Dying, **1041–1042**
    ethical issues, 289
    nursing care, 1041–1042
    in old age, **981**
    symptoms, *1041*
    see also Death; Terminal illness
Dynamic Standard Setting System (DySSSy), 31, 33

Dysarthria, 286
Dysfunctional uterine bleeding, *717*
Dysgeusia, *289*
Dyskaryosis, cervical, 715
Dyskinesia, dietary, 322
Dyslipidaemia, *see* Hyperlipidaemia
Dysmenorrhoea, 710, *717*
Dyspareunia, 735, 757
Dysphagia (swallowing difficulties), 212–213, 568, 602
    assessment flow chart, *213*
    fluid status and, 141
    in motor neuron disease, 323
    in neurological disease, 286
    nursing interventions, 222
    in oesophageal disorders, 602, 603, 604, 615
    in Parkinson's disease, 321
    in stroke, *292*, 293
Dysphasia, *289*
    in stroke, *292*
    swallowing problems and, 286
Dysplasia, 988
Dyspnoea, *see* Breathlessness/dyspnoea
Dyspraxia, *289*
Dystonia, *289*
Dysuria
    after intravesical therapy, 679
    in urinary tract infections, 672, 673

E

Ear, **368–370**
    anatomy, **368–370**
    'cauliflower', 381
    examination, **371–372**
    external, 367, **368**
        examination, 371–372
        tumours, **389**
    foreign bodies, 380, **381–382**
    glue, 372
    infections/inflammatory conditions, **382–386**
    inner, **369–370**
        tumours, **389**
    irritation (itching), *379*, 382
    microsuction, 376, *378*
    middle, 367, **368–369**
        tumours, **389**
        see also Otitis media
    trauma, **380–382**
    tumours, **389**
Ear canal, *see* External auditory canal
Ear and hearing problems, **367–391**, 565
    diagnostic tests and investigations, 372–374
    ear examination, 371–372
    history-taking, 370
    instruments used, *371*
    nursing assessment, 370–372
    prevention/health education, 374
    useful addresses, 391
    see also Nose and throat disorders
Ear surgery, 386
    discharge advice, 386
    nursing management, **385–386**
    pre- and postoperative care, 385
Ear syringing, 376–377, *379*
    contraindications, 377, *378*
    in otitis externa, 383
    procedure, *378*
    to remove foreign bodies, 382
Ear wax (cerumen), 368, 843
    excess, **376–377**
    in older adults, *376*

removal, 376–377
Eardrops, *377*
Eardrum, *see* Tympanic membrane
Early pregnancy assessment unit, 725, 726
Early warning systems, critical care, 950–951
Easi-breathe, *543*
Eating
  assistance with, *221*
  cultural influences, 212
  environment, 219–221
  healthy, *see* Healthy eating
  in mucositis, 472
  nursing interventions, 221
  in Parkinson's disease, 321
  sensory aspects, 211–212
  in terminal illness, 1029
  see also Diet; Feeding; Food; Nutrition
Eating disorders, 213
Ecchymosis, pigmented skin, *846*
ECG, *see* Electrocardiogram
Echocardiogram, **490–491**
  in heart failure, 511
  in infective endocarditis, 517
  in rheumatic fever, 514
Ectopic pregnancy, **729–730**
Ectropion, 364
Eczema
  atopic, **849–851**, *853*
  herpeticum, 864, 865
  stasis (gravitational or varicose), **851**
  see also Dermatitis
EEG, *see* Electroencephalogram
Effectiveness, *30*
  clinical, 24, 26, 33
Efferent fibres, 274
Efficiency, *27*, *30*
Ejaculation, rapid (premature), **756–757**
Ejaculatory duct, *742*
Elastin, 175
  ageing changes, 175
Elbow
  golfer's, *825*
  olecranon process fractures, 835
  tennis, 805, 825
Elderly, *see* Older adults
Electrical burns, 871
Electrical stimulation, in urinary incontinence, 240, 241–242
Electro-oculogram (EOG), 59, 60
Electrocardiogram (ECG), **488–490**
  12-lead, 490
  in atrial fibrillation, 499
  bedside monitoring, 490
  in cardiopulmonary arrest, 496
  in endocrine disorders, 402
  in heart failure, 511
  Holter monitoring, 490
  in hypothermia, 90
  leads, 489
  monitoring, critically ill patients, 958–959
  in myocardial infarction, 507, 508
  pacemaker patients, 498
  in shock, 160
  in unstable angina, 505
Electrocochleography (ECOG), 373, 374
Electroencephalogram (EEG), 59, **288**
  in epilepsy, 315
  in sleep, 60
Electrolaryngography, 570
Electrolyte balance, **133–148**
  disorders, *135–136*
    in chronic renal failure, 687
    diagnostic tests and investigations, 142–143
    in heart failure, 511

nursing assessment, 139–140
  nursing management and interventions, **147–148**
  predisposing factors, 140–142
  wound healing, *179*
  nursing assessment, **663**
  regulation, **137–138**, 658–660
Electrolytes, **134**, *135–136*
  movement, 134–136
  requirements, 146
  serum, *135–136*, 142, **670–671**
  see also specific electrolytes
Electromyography (EMG), 59, 288
  laryngeal muscles, 570
  in musculoskeletal disorders, 798, 811
Electrophysiology studies (EPS), 492
Elimination
  in motor neuron disease, 323
  in Parkinson's disease, 322
  in spinal injuries, 325
  in terminal illness, 1029
Emboli, 449
  in infective endocarditis, 516, 517
Embryo
  crown–rump length (CRL), 728
  transfer, IVF with, *760*
Emergencies, 924
  oncological **1014–1015**
  in palliative care, **1040**
  see also Accident and emergency (A&E) department
Emergency nurse practitioners (ENP), 924, **929**
Emergency services, in major disasters, 942
Emery-Dreifuss muscular dystrophy (EDMD), *809*
Emmetropia, 335
Emollients, 849
  in atopic eczema, 850
  in autoimmune blistering disorders, 865
  in psoriasis, 862
Emotional factors, in cancer development, **989**
Emotional responses
  cancer diagnosis, **1009–1011**
  terminal illness, **1025–1026**
Emotional support, *see* Psychological support
Empathy, 45, 47
Emphysema, 545
Employment, *see* Work
Empowerment
  bereaved relatives, 941
  patients, 35, 892
  staff, 34
Empyema
  gallbladder, 640
  pleural cavity, 553, 561
Encephalopathy, hepatic, *634*, 636–637
Enchondroma, 821
Endocarditis, infective (IE), 515, **516–517**
Endocardium, 482
Endocrine disorders, **393–443**
  diagnostic tests and investigations, 401–403
  myopathies, 810
  nursing assessment, 401
  prevention/health education, 403
  useful websites, 442
Endocrine glands/structures, 394–395
Endocrine system, **394–401**
  ageing changes, 975
  during sleep, 62
Endocrinology specialist nurses, 393
Endometrial ablation, **718**
Endometrial cancer, **722**
Endometrial polyps, 716, 718
Endometrial sampling (biopsy), 718, 722, 759
Endometriosis, **733–734**

Endometriosis Society, 767
Endometritis, 727, **732**
Endometrium, 709
  cyclical changes, 710–711
Endopelvic fascia, 230
Endophthalmitis, 349
  sympathetic, 358
Endoscopic retrograde cholangiopancreatography (ERCP), 626, 642–643, 1001
Endoscopic sinus surgery, 574
Endoscopic sphincterotomy, 639, 642
Endoscopy, 880
  cancer diagnosis, **1001–1002**
  day case, 880
  GI tract, **599**, 614, 1001
  see also Arthroscopy; Bronchoscopy; Cystoscopy; Laparoscopy
Endosteum, 772
Endotracheal intubation
  for anaesthesia, 899, 900
  communication problems, 951
  indications, 961
Endotracheal tube (ETT), 899, *962*
  nursing care, 961
Energy, **203**
  balance, **203**
  requirements, 203
  storage in liver, 623
Enflurane, *884*
ENT (ear, nose and throat) department, 370
Enteral feeding, **222–224**
  after laryngectomy, 587
  in cancer, 1004
  complications, 224
  critically ill patients, 953
  emergency regimens, 222, *223*
  in head injury, 302
  in multiple organ dysfunction, 169
  nursing management, 224
  post-surgical, 913
  regimens, 223
  routes, 222–223
Enterocele, *724*
Enterogastric reflex, 594
Entonox, 125
Entrapment neuropathy, 425–426, **814**
Entropion, 364
Enucleation, **358**
Environment
  A&E department, 925, *939*
  in atopic eczema, 850
  critical care, **954**
  dying patients, 1041
  liver, biliary and pancreatic disorders and, 624, 627
  in major trauma, 933
  mealtime, 219–221
  modification, in disability, 1063
  prehospital, 924–925
  resuscitation in A&E, 929
  surgical, **906**
  urinary incontinence and, 234–235
  in visual impairment, 343
Environmental pollution, cancer risks, 990
Eosinophils, 446
Ependymal cells, *275*
Ephedrine hydrochloride, *572*
Epicondylitis, **825**
  lateral, 825
  medial, 825
Epidermal inclusion cysts, 861
Epidermis, 174, **842**
  renewal and keratinization, 842
Epidermoid cysts, 861

Epidermolysis bullosa (EB), **866**
Epididymis, 742
Epididymitis, **750**, 763
Epidural anaesthesia/analgesia, **896–897**, *898*
    nursing management, 897
    in pain management, 124, **127**
    patient-controlled (PCEA), 127
    versus spinal anaesthesia, *897*
Epidural blood patch, 897
Epiglottis, 567
Epilepsy, **313–315**
    aetiology, 313–315
    clinical presentation, 315
    investigations, 315
    nursing management, 315
    stigma, 1053
    temporal lobe, *314*
Epinephrine, *see* Adrenaline
Epiphyseal plate, 794
Epiphysis, 794
Epistaxis, **574–577**
    medical/surgical management, 575–576
    nursing management, 576–577
    in older adults, *577*
Epithelial cells, 178, 989
Epley manoeuvre, 387
Epstein–Barr virus (EBV), 469, 470
Equity, *30*
ERCP (endoscopic retrograde
    cholangiopancreatography), 626,
    642–643, 1001
Erectile dysfunction (ED), **752–756**, 757
    aetiology, 752–753
    as communication, 753
    in diabetes, 426
    medical/surgical management, 754–756
    NHS treatment guidelines, 755–756
    nursing assessment, 753, *754*
    nursing management, 756
Erection, penile, 743–744
Erikson's theory of life span, **972**
Error catastrophe theory of ageing, 974
Erysipelas, 855
Erythema
    blanching, 190
    non-blanching, 190–191
    in pigmented skin, *846*
Erythema marginatum, 514
Erythrocyte sedimentation rate (ESR), 450,
    491–492
    in GI disorders, 600, 614
Erythrocytes, *see* Red cells
Erythroplasia of Queyrat, 751
Erythropoietin (EPO), 448, 455, 669–670
    in anaemia of chronic disease, 459
    in chronic renal failure, 687, *693*
    costs of therapy, *460*
Eschar, 181, 872
Escharotomy, 872
Escherichia coli, 672
Etanercept, 806
Ethambutol, 555, 675
Ethical issues, **16–19**
    in cancer nursing, **1017–1018**
    goodness or rightness, 18
    individual freedom, 19
    justice or fairness, 18–19
    in neurological problems, 289, *290*
    in palliative care, **1027–1028**
    truth-telling or honesty, 19
    value of life, 17–18
Ethmoidectomy, 580
Ethnic and racial differences
    cancer risk, 991
    inequality and ageing, 971

liver, biliary and pancreatic disorders, 624
    skin pigmentation, 842
    in testicular cancer, 746
Eulenberg's disease, *809*
European Pressure Ulcer Advisory Panel
    (EPUAP)
    classification tool, *191*
    risk assessment, 189
Eustachian tube, 369, 372
Eustress, 94, 97
Euthanasia, 18, **1028**
Evacuation of retained products of conception
    (ERPC), 727
Evaluation
    in nursing process, **13**
    quality of care, **34**
Evaporation, 77
'Evening types', 64
Evidence
    critical appraisal, 13–14
    sources, *14*
    systematic reviews, 26
    types, 13
Evidence-based Medicine, 14
Evidence-based nursing, **33**
Evidence-based Nursing, 14
Evidence-based practice, **13–15**, 24, **26**
Excoriation, 844
Exercise
    after gynaecological surgery, *739*
    after insulin injections, 409
    in back pain, 815, 816
    in blood disorders, 456
    in cardiovascular disease prevention, 494
    constipation and, 609
    in COPD, 548
    in heart failure, 513
    in hot environments, *81*
    in lymphoedema, 786
    older adults, 977–978
    in peripheral arterial disease, 523, 524
    postoperative, 914
    preventing dehydration, 142
    respiratory disorders and, *538*
    sleep and, 65, 70
    in stress management, 106
    in venous ulceration, *197*
    see also Physical activity
Exercise test treadmill, **490**, 505
Exfoliation, 842
Exhaustion, in stress, 97
Exostosis, ear canal, 372, 389
Explanation, **50–51**
Exposure, in major trauma, 933
Exposure-prone procedures (EPPs), 268
External auditory canal (EAC), 368
    exostosis, 372, 389
    see also Otitis externa
External fixators, **804**
External genitalia, female, 711
Extracapsular cataract extraction (ECCE), 349
Extracellular fluid (ECF), 134
    volume, *see* Circulating volume
Extradural haemorrhage, 297
Extraocular muscles, 336
Extravasation, intravenous fluids, 146
Exudate
    chronic wounds, 176
    venous leg ulcers, 194
    wound dressings, *183*, *184*, 185
Eye(s)
    anatomy and physiology, **332–336**
    dry, **363–364**
    enucleation, **358**
    examination, 337–338

foreign body (FB), 338, **359–360**
    infections, 359, 361, 362, 363
    injuries, **357–364**
        chemical, **360–361**
        prevention, 341
    light and dark adaptation, 336
    opening, assessing, 280, *282*
    prostheses, 358
    protection, 264, 341
    sunken, 140
Eye care
    in Bell's palsy, 303
    critically ill patients, **952**
    dying patients, 1042
    in multiple organ dysfunction, 169
    unconscious patients, *291*
Eye contact, 41, 927
Eye medications, topical (drops and ointment),
    344–348
    correct prescribing, *344*
    drugs available, *344–345*
    instillation problems, 346–348
    instillation technique, 346, *347*
Eye and vision problems, **331–366**
    diagnostic tests and investigations, 338–341
    in Graves' disease, 432
    in multiple sclerosis, 304
    in newly diagnosed diabetes, 406
    nursing assessment, 336–338
    painful and traumatic, 357–364
    painless, 348–357
    prevention/health education, 341
    useful addresses, 365
    see also Visual impairment
Eyeball, **332–334**
    accessory structures, 336
    layers, 332–333
Eyebrows, 336
Eyelashes, 336
Eyelids, 336
    age-related disorders, 364
    disorders, **362–364**
    steam treatment/hot compress, *363*

F

Face masks, 263, 906
Facial nerve, *279*
    palsy, 303–304, 385
Facial pain, in sinusitis, 573
Facioscapulohumeral muscular dystrophy, *809*
Factor VIII
    deficiency, 477
    treatment, 452, 478
Factor IX
    deficiency, 477
    treatment, 452, 478
Faecal collector pouches, 249
Faecal impaction
    management, 1037
    with overflow, 245, *247*
    urinary incontinence, 234, 240
Faecal incontinence, **243–246**
    assessment, 243, *244*
    causes, 243
    definition, 243
    management, 245–246, *247*
    nursing management, 246–249
    in spinal injuries, 325
Faecal occult blood (FOB) testing (FOBT), 600,
    1000
Faecal softeners, *610*
Faeces, 595

in jaundice, *629*
in liver, gallbladder and pancreatic disorders, 626
spillages, *631*
Fairness, **18–19**
Falciform ligament, 592
Fallopian tubes, *see* Uterine (fallopian) tubes
Fallot's tetralogy, *528*
Falls
  lower limb injuries, 830, 831, 832
  prevention, 819, *820*
  risk of older adults, **978**
  upper limb injuries, 824, 834, 835
Falx cerebri, 278
Familial (adenomatous) polyposis (FAP), **611**, 994, 1000
Familial hypercholesterolaemia, 216, 494
Family (and friends)
  abuse of older adults, 981
  anticipatory grief, 1026
  in chronic illness, 1051
  contacting absent, 941
  critically ill patients, 164, 951, 952
  dying patients, 1041
  in myocardial infarction, 508
  older adults, **971**
  palliative care, 1025
  in raised intracranial pressure, 302
  resuscitated patients, 196
  stress, 102–103
  support
    in bereavement, 941–942, 1042, **1043–1044**
    in cancer, **1016**
    in sudden death, **941–942**
    in terminal illness, **1026–1027**
  terminally ill patients, 1031
  viewing of deceased, 941
  witnessing resuscitation, 931, *932*
  see also Carers
Family planning, 758
Fanconi's anaemia, 463
Fanning, as cooling method, 86
Fasciculation, in motor neuron disease, 323
Fasciotomy, *805*, 830
Fasting
  effects of prolonged, 893
  fluid depletion, 140–141
  post-surgical, **913**
  preoperative, *141*, 218, 888, **892–894**
  restarting oral fluids after, 144
Fat embolism, 829
Fatigue
  in atopic eczema, 850
  in cancer patients, 1013
  chemotherapy-induced, 472–473
  in fluid loss, 140
  in haematological disorders, 449, 456, *457*
  in heart failure, 513
  in multiple sclerosis, 306, 307
  in myopathies, 810
Fats
  dietary, **204–205**, 216
    in diabetes, *419*
  as energy source, 203
  saturated, 204
  unsaturated, 204
Fatty acids, 204
  essential, 204
  monounsaturated, 204
  polyunsaturated (PUFA), *see* Polyunsaturated fatty acids
  short-chain (SCFAs), 205
  in stress, 96
  trans, 204

Fear
  paradoxical, 96
  terminal illness, 1026
  see also Anxiety
Feeding
  older adults, *980*
  patients, *221*
  sip, 222
  see also Eating; Enteral feeding; Nutrition
Female
  external genitalia, 711
  sex hormones, **707**
  see also Women
Female reproductive system, **706–711**
  benign tumours, **719–720**
  infections, **732–733**
  malignant tumours, 712, **720–724**
Femoral fractures
  distal, 831
  intertrochanteric, 831
  supracondylar, 831
Femoral neck fractures, **830–831**, *832*
  A&E care, *929*
  hip protectors to prevent, 831, 832
Femoral shaft fractures, **831**
Fentanyl, 124, *884*
  epidural, 127
  transdermal patches, 124, 125, 1034
Ferrous sulphate, 458
Fertilization, 758
Fetal demise, early, 728
Fetal heart, 726
Fetor hepaticus, 636
FEV$_1$, **540–541**
Fever, *see* Pyrexia
Fibre, dietary, 205, *419*
  constipation and, 609
  diverticular disease and, 610
  in irritable bowel syndrome, 609
Fibrin, 449
Fibroadenomas, breast, 780
Fibroblasts, 174, 178
Fibroids, uterine, 716, 718, 719
Fibular fractures, 832
Fight-or-flight response, *96*, 103
Filtration, 136
Financial problems
  assessment, 1060
  in terminal illness, 1031
  see also Poverty
Fine-needle aspiration (FNA), breast, 774
Finger clubbing, 539
Fire risk, oxygen therapy, 557
First aid, burns, **871**
Fissure, 844
Fissure in ano, **617**
Fistulae, postoperative, 915
Fits, *see* Seizures
Flaccid paralysis, *289*, 324, 327
Flaps, breast reconstruction, 788
Flatulence, 597
Fleet phospha-soda, *612*
Flenly acid–base nomogram, *150*
Flora, normal, 257, 595, 843, 887
Flotron boots, *902*
Flu vaccination, 553, 554
Fluid
  compartments, 134
  depletion, *see* Dehydration
  extracellular (ECF), 134
  intracellular (ICF), 134
  requirements, 146
  tissue, formation, **136–137**
  see also Circulating volume; Water

Fluid balance, **133–148**
  24-hour, 143
  charts, **143**, *144*, 663
  chemotherapy and, 473
  critically ill patients, 956, 959
  disturbances, **138–139**
    in chronic renal failure, 687
    diagnostic tests and investigations, 142–143
    isotonic, 138–139
    nursing assessment, 139–140
    nursing management and interventions, **143–147**
    osmolar, *138*, 139
    predisposing factors, 140–142
    see also Dehydration; Fluid volume excess; Hypovolaemia
  in head injury, 302
  nursing assessment, **663**
  in older adults, *957*
  postoperative, **912–913**
  regulation, **137–138**, 658–660
Fluid intake, 143, **144–145**, 671
  after period of fasting, 144
  constipation and, 609
  dialysis patients, 690–691, 692, *693*
  in evenings, 72
  in faecal incontinence, 246
  helping patients with, *144*, 145
  older people in long-term care, 980
  postoperative, 912
  in pyrexia, 86
  restriction, 145
  in sickle cell disease, 463
  types of oral fluids, 144
  in urinary incontinence, 235, 240–241
  in viral hepatitis, 632
  see also Drinking
Fluid losses (output), 143
  accurate measurement, 143
  insensible, 77, 143
  sensible, 143
  third space, 138
Fluid output, *see* Fluid losses
Fluid replacement
  intravenous infusions, *see* Intravenous (i.v.) infusions
  nasogastric tubes for, 145
  oral, **144**
  rectal infusion, 147
  subcutaneous infusion, 147
Fluid volume deficit, *see* Hypovolaemia
Fluid volume excess, *138*, 139
  blood transfusions, 454
  in chronic renal failure, 687
  in heart failure, 511, 513–514
  i.v. infusions, 147
  nursing assessment, 139–140
  postoperative, 913
Fluorescein
  angiography, 338, **340–341**
  eye staining, *345*, 360
5-Fluorouracil (5-FU), 1006, 1007
Flusinolide, *572*
Flutamide, in pancreatic cancer, 648
Foam mattresses, 191
Focal neurological deficits, 279, 284
  brain tumours, 308
  in raised intracranial pressure, 299
Focimetry, 340
Focusing, **334–335**
Folic acid (folate), *206*, **209**, 459
  deficiency, 209, 216, **459**
  serum levels, 600
  supplements, 209, 459

Follicle-stimulating hormone (FSH), 397, 398
  deficiency, 430
  in ovarian cycle, 707–708, 710
  ovulation induction, 760
Fomivirsen sodium, 345
Food
  allergy, **219**
  choice, **219**
  cultural aspects, 212
  drug interactions, **225**, 226–227
  fortification, **221**
  hygiene, 221, 466
  intake
    dying patients, 1041
    excess, 213
    factors affecting, 212–213
    history taking, 214
    insufficient, 213
    see also Eating
  intolerance, **219**, 850
  nutrients in, 202
  preferences, 211
  sleep and, 65, 70
  texture modification, 222
  see also Diet; Nutrition
Food-borne illness, outbreaks, 259
Foot
  athlete's (tinea pedis), 856, 858
  flat (pronated), 813
Foot care, in diabetes, 415, 427, 428
Foot drop, 328, 953
Foot ulcers
  diabetic, 425, 427, 428
  see also Leg ulcers
Footwear, surgical personnel, 906
Forced air heating systems, 903
Forearm fractures, 835
Foreign bodies (FB)
  ear, 380, **381–382**
  eye, 338, **359–360**
  nose, **580**
  oesophagus, 603
  swallowed, 594, 603
  wound healing and, 179
Foreskin (prepuce), 743, 752
Fortification, food, **221**
Fovea centralis, 333
Fractionation, 1005
Fracture dislocation, 823
Fractures, **828–836**
  classification, 828
  clinical presentation, 829
  complications, 829–830
  delayed union, 830
  descriptions, 828
  healing, 829
  lower limb, **830–833**
  malunion, 830
  management overview, 830
  non-union, 830
  nursing management, 833, 836, 837
  open (compound), 828
  osteoporotic, 799, 815, 819, 831
  palliative care, 1040
  pathological, 818, 819, 821, 828
  patterns, 829
  stress/fatigue, 828
  upper limb, **833–836**
Frailty, **975–976**
Freckles, **863–864**
Free radical theory of ageing, 974–975
Freedom, individual, **19**
Freezing, in Parkinson's disease, 319, 321
French gauge, urinary catheters, 675
Frequency of micturition, 235, 672, 696

Frequency-volume chart, 237
Fresh frozen plasma (FFP), 452
Freud, Sigmund, 45, 97
Friction, 188
Friends, see Family
Frontal lobe, 277
Frostbite, **83**
  nursing management, **91**
Frozen shoulder, **824**
Fruit and vegetables, 419
FSH, see Follicle-stimulating hormone
Full blood count (FBC), 450, 491–492, 715
Functional endoscopic sinus surgery (FESS), 574
Functional status
  assessment, **1059–1060**
  in chronic illness, 1049–1050
  see also Activities of daily living; Disability
Fundus examination, 333, 334
Funeral directors, **1043**
Fungal infections
  eye, 359
  infective endocarditis, 516
  investigations, 847, 848, 856
  meningitis, 311
  oral, 601
  skin, **855–859**
Fungating wounds, **787–788**, **1039**
Fungi, 254
Furosemide (frusemide), 226, 511, 684
Furuncles, 854
FVC, **540–541**

G

Gabapentin, in back pain, 816
Gag reflex, 286
Gain, secondary, 1053
Gait, festinating (shuffling), 319
Galactorrhoea, 430
Galantamine, 322
Gallbladder, 595, 622, 623
  disease, see Biliary disorders; Gallstones
  stasis, 638
  tumours, **643**
Gallstones (cholelithiasis), **638–640**
  aetiology and epidemiology, 216, 627, **638**
  common bile duct, see Choledocholithiasis
  complications, 640, 641, 643
  low-fat diet, 641
  medical/surgical management, 639
  nursing management, 639–640
  related pancreatitis, 644, 645
Gamete intrafallopian transfer (GIFT), 760
Gamma-aminobutyric acid (GABA), and sleep, 61
γ-glutamyl transferase (GGT), 625
Gas transport, **534–535**
Gastrectomy, 606
Gastric acid studies, **598**
Gastric cancer, 606
Gastric emptying, 593–594
Gastric-inhibiting peptide (GIP), 594
Gastric tonometry, in shock, 162
Gastric ulcers, 606
Gastrinomas, 598, **649**
Gastritis, **605**
Gastro-oesophageal reflux, 603, 605
Gastro-oesophageal sphincter, 593
Gastroenterostomy, 607
Gastrointestinal (GI) disorders, **591–619**
  chemotherapy-induced, 472
  in diabetes, 426, 427, 428
  diagnostic tests and investigations, **598–600**

  in multiple organ dysfunction, 168
  nursing assessment, **596–598**
  nutritional status, 214
  prevention and health education, 600
  signs and symptoms, **597–598**
  in spinal injuries, 325
  useful addresses, 618
Gastrointestinal (GI) tract, **591–596**
  ageing changes, 975
  endoscopy, **599**, 614, 1001
  lining, 591–592
  lower, disorders, **607–617**
  motility, critically ill patients, 953
  mucosa, 592
  in older adults, 597
  perforation, 603
  in stress, 96, **103**
  upper
    carcinoma, **605–606**
    disorders, **604–607**
    haemorrhage, **604**, **607**
Gastroparesis, diabetic, 426, 427, 428
Gastroscopy, 599
Gastrostomy, percutaneous endoscopic (PEG), 223, 953, 1004
Gate control theory, 112, 113
Gelatin solutions, 165
Gelofusine, 165
Gemeprost, 728, 731
Gender differences
  in body water, 134
  cancer risk, 991
  in gallstones, 638
  pain perception, 116
  sleep patterns, 64
  see also Men; Women
Gene therapy
  cystic fibrosis, 552
  myopathies, 808, 811
General adaptation syndrome (GAS), **94–97**, 103
General anaesthesia, **898–900**
General practitioners (GPs)
  in accidents and emergencies, 924, 938
  in palliative care, 1024–1025
Genetic counselling, 289, 811
Genetic screening, 537, **998**, 999
Genetics
  breast cancer, 776
  inflammatory bowel disease, 613
  myopathies, 808–810
  respiratory disorders, 537
  sleep patterns, 64
Genital herpes, **763**
Genital warts, **761–762**, 855
Genuineness, 45
Germ cell tumours, testicular, 746, 747
Gestational diabetes, 403, 416
Gestational trophoblastic disease, 729
GFR, see Glomerular filtration rate
GI, see Gastrointestinal
Giant cell arteritis, 317
Giant cell tumours, 821
Gigantism, **428–429**
Gingivitis, 601
Glasgow Coma Scale (GCS), **280**, 281, 933
  assessing eye opening, 280, 282
  assessing motor response, 280, 283
  assessing verbal response, 280, 282
  brain injury classification, 297
Glaucoma
  acute angle-closure, 548
  primary closed-angle (PCAG), 355, **357–358**
  primary open-angle, see Primary open-angle glaucoma

Glial cells, 274–275
Glibenclamide, *417*, 418
Glicazide, *417*
Glimepiride, *417*
Glioblastoma multiforme, 308
Gliomas, 275, **308–309**
Glipizide, *417*
Gliquidone, *417*
Glomerular capsule **656–658**
Glomerular filtration barrier, **656–658**
Glomerular filtration rate (GFR), 654–655, 656, 657–658
   age-related decline, 975
   estimation, 670
   in renal failure, 686
Glomerulonephritis, **683–684**
Glomerulus, **656–658**
   blood supply, 656
Glossitis, 601–602
Glossopharyngeal nerve, *279*
Glottis, 567
Gloves, **263**, 268
   sterile, 263
   surgical, **905**
   unsterile, 263
Glucagon, 400
   in glucose homeostasis, 400–401
   injection, in hypoglycaemia, 422
Glucocorticoids, **399**
   in adrenal insufficiency, 438
   in shock, 157
   see also Corticosteroids; Cortisol
Gluconeogenesis, 399, 400–401
Glucose, 205
   blood, *625*
      control, *see* Glycaemic control
      in diabetic ketoacidosis, 423, 424
      in hypothermia, 90
      meters, 409, 410
      monitoring (BGM), **409–410**, 414, 420
      see also Hyperglycaemia; Hypoglycaemia
   homeostasis, **400–401**
   intravenous, *see* Dextrose
   metabolism, in stress, 96
   oral, in hypoglycaemia, 422
   plasma, in diabetes diagnosis, 402, 403, 416
   renal reabsorption, 658
   renal threshold, 404
   urinary, 664
      monitoring, 420
      see also Glycosuria
Glucose regulators, non-sulphonylurea prandial, 418
Glue, surgical, *936*
Gluten intolerance, 219, 866
Glycaemic control
   assessment, 415
   hypoglycaemia risk and, 421
   long-term diabetes complications and, 424, 682
   targets, 409, 410, 414–415
Glycerine suppositories, 1037
Glycerol, 400
Glyceryl trinitrate (GTN, nitroglycerin)
   in angina, 504–505, 506
   in cardiogenic shock, 166
Glycogenesis, 400
Glycogenolysis, 400, 401
Glycolysis, 400
Glycopyrronium, *884*
Glycosuria, 143, 237, 404, 658, 664
Goal-setting, 12
   in chronic illness/disability, *1062*, 1063
Goitre
   in Hashimoto's disease, 435

simple (non-toxic), 435
   toxic multinodular, **434–435**
Goldmann applanation tonometry, 340
Golfer's elbow, 825
Gonadorelin analogues, in prostate cancer, 700
Gonadotrophin-releasing hormone (GnRH), 707, *708*
Gonadotrophins, 397, *398*
   deficiency, 430–431
Gonads, 394
Gonioscopy, 340
Gonorrhoea, 732, **763–764**
Goodness, **18**
Goodpasture's disease, 683
Goserelin, 784
Gosnell score, *189*
Gout, **807–808**
Governance
   clinical, **25**
   shared, 26, 34
Gowns, 263, 905
Graafian follicle, 707
Graft rejection, transplanted kidneys, 696, *697*
Graft-versus-host disease (GVHD), 475
      transfusion-associated (TA-GVHD), 267, 454, 475
Gram-negative organisms, 254, **255**
Gram-positive organisms, 254, **255**
Gram stain, **254**
Granulation, 178
Granulation tissue, 178
Granulocyte colony-stimulating factor (G-CSF), 448
Granulocyte-macrophage colony-stimulating factor (GM-CSF), 448
Granulocytes, 446
   transfusions, 451–452
Graves' disease, **432–434**
Gravitational eczema, **851**
Greenstick fractures, *829*
Greetings, **47–48**
Grey Turner's sign, 644
Grief, **1043–1044**
   abnormal, 1044
   anticipatory, 1026
   presentation of unresolved, 1044
Griseofulvin, *226*
Grommets, ear, 383, 384
Groups, **53–55**
   dynamics, 53–54
   roles, 54
   in stress, 107
   teaching, 54
   see also Team
Growth factors
   angiogenic, 988
   haemopoietic, *see* Haemopoietic growth factors
Growth hormone (GH), 397, *398*
   deficiency, 430–431
   oversecretion, 428–429
   sleep and, 62
Growth plate, 794
GTN, *see* Glyceryl trinitrate
Guedel oropharyngeal airway, 898, *899*
Guidance on Clinical Experience for Students (UKCC/NMC), 6, *7*
Guide dogs, 344
Guide Dogs for the Blind Association (GDB), 344, 365
Guidelines, care, **15**
Guillain–Barré syndrome (GBS), **327–328**
Gut, *see* Gastrointestinal (GI) tract
Guttae (G), 338
Gynaecological cancer, 712, **720–724**

Gynaecological disorders, **716–739**
   diagnostic tests and investigations, **712–715**
   nursing assessment, **711–712**
   prevention and health education, 715–716
Gynaecological examination, **713**
Gynaecological surgery, **736–739**
   for menstrual disorders, 718–719
   nursing management, 719
   postoperative care, 738–739
   postoperative complications, 739, *740–741*
   postoperative discharge advice, 739
   preoperative assessment, 736–737
   preoperative care, 737
Gynaecology oncology nurse, 721–722, 723–724
Gynaecomastia, 430, 779, 790

H

Haemaccel, 165
Haemangiomas, skin, **864**
Haematemesis, 598, 604
Haematocrit, 450
Haematological disorders, **445–480**
   bone marrow, 463–465
   diagnostic tests, 450–451
   haemoglobinopathies, 460–463
   haemostatic, 476–478
   lymphomas, 469–470
   nursing assessment, 449–450
   prevention and health education, 455–456
   red cells, 456–460
   in systemic lupus erythematosus, 817
   useful websites, 480
   white cells, 465–469
Haematological malignancy, **993**
   management, **470–476**
   see also Leukaemia; Lymphoma; Myeloma, multiple
Haematological system, **445–449**
Haematological tests, 450
Haematologists, in critical care, 952
Haematoma
   bilateral periorbital, *298*
   nasal septal, **579**
   pinna, **380–381**
   subdural, 279, 297–298
Haematuria, 142–143, 237, **664**
   after nephrostomy tube insertion, 677
   bladder cancer screening, 1001
   in urothelial tumours, 679
Haemodialysis, **690–691**
   in acute renal failure, **693–694**
   nutrition during, 688
   venous access for, 691, *693*
Haemodynamic instability, 521
Haemofiltration, 168
   in acute renal failure, **693–694**, 963
   vascular catheters for, *693*
Haemoglobin, 446, 535
   concentration
      in anaemia, 456
      in GI disorders, 600
      in urinary system disorders, 669–670
   glycosylated (HbA$_1$), 415
   sickle (HbS), 461–462
Haemoglobinopathies, **460–463**
Haemolysis, 454
   delayed, after blood transfusions, 454
Haemolytic anaemia, **460**
   autoimmune (AIHA), 460
   in sickle cell disease, 462
Haemophilia, 452, **477–478**
Haemophilus influenzae type b (Hib) vaccine, *312*

Haemopoiesis, **447–448**
Haemopoietic growth factors, 448, 471
  in aplastic anaemia, 464
  in chronic anaemia, 455
  in lymphoma, 470
  in myelodysplasia, 464
Haemopoietic stem cell transplantation,
    474–475
  allogeneic, 474, 475
  in aplastic anaemia, 464
  autologous, 474
  decision support, *474*
  in haemoglobinopathies, 461, 462
  in leukaemia, 467, 468, 469
  matched unrelated donor (MUD), 474
  in myelodysplasia, 464
  non-myeloablative, 475
Haemopoietic stem cells, 447
  differentiation, 447
  peripheral harvest, 475
Haemoptysis, 549, **561–562**
Haemorrhage/bleeding
  after gynaecological surgery, *740, 741*
  after pacemaker insertion, 498
  after renal angiography, 666
  after thyroidectomy, 433
  after tonsillectomy, 581
  anaemia from, *457*
  arrest, *see* Haemostasis
  fracture-associated, 829, 831
  in haemophilia, 477
  in liver and gallbladder disease, *629*
  in major trauma, 933
  nasal, *see* Epistaxis
  nursing management, 457
  oesophageal varices, 604, 607, 634–635
  palliative care, 1040
  postoperative, 909
  in thrombocytopenia, 476
  upper GI tract, **604**, **607**
Haemorrhoids, **617**
Haemostasis, **448–449**
  disorders, **476–478**
  intraoperative, **904–905**
Haemothorax, 560
Hair, **843**
  ageing changes, 975
  covering, surgical personnel, 906
  excessive, *see* Hirsutism; Hypertrichosis
  growth abnormalities, **869–870**
  loss, *see* Alopecia
  removal, preoperative, 737, **887–888**
  samples, 847
  terminal, 843
  vellus, 843
  washing, preoperative, 887
Hair follicles, 174, **843**
Halitosis, in terminal illness, 1035
Hallucinations, in visual impairment, 343
Hallux valgus (bunion), 805, **813–814**
Halothane, *884*
Hamstring strains, **826**
Hand(s)
  disinfection, surgical, 262
  fractures, 835
  as vehicles of infection, 256, 260, *261*
Hand movements (HM), in visual acuity testing,
    339
Hand rubs, alcohol, 263
Hand towels, 262
Handicap, definition, 1048, *1049*
Handwashing, **260–263**, *631*
  after removal of gloves, 263
  nurses' practices, *261*
  in postoperative care, 915, *917*

social, 262
  for surgery, 262, 905
  technique, 261, *262*
Hartmann's solution, *145*
Hartman's procedure, 611
Hashimoto's disease, 435
Hay fever, *571*
Head injury, **297–303**
  aetiology and epidemiology, 297
  clinical presentation, 298
  investigations, 300
  medical/surgical management, 300, *301*
  mild, discharge advice, *301*
  nursing assessment, 300
  nursing management, 300–303
  pathophysiology, 297–298
  raised intracranial pressure, 298–300
Headache, **316–318**
  brain tumours, 308, 309–310
  cluster, 316, *317*
  in head injury, 300, *301*
  nursing management, 316–318
  post-lumbar puncture, 897
  in raised intracranial pressure, *317*
  in sinusitis, 573
  stress and, 104
  tension, 104, 316, 318
  types, 316, *316–317*
Headway, 297, 303, 329
Headwear, surgical, 906
Heaf test, 555
Healing, *see* Wound healing
Health, **9–10**
  definition, 9
  older adults, **977–979**
  wound healing and, 178–179
Health care professionals
  education, *see* Staff education
  ending relationships, **53**
  handwashing, *see* Handwashing
  infected with blood-borne pathogens, 268
  occupational risk of infection, 267–268
  prevention of blood-borne infections, 268,
    631
  psychological support
    in A&E, 942–943
    in palliative care, 1026, **1027**
  stress and burnout, **100–102**, 1027
  see also Nurses
Health Development Agency, 530
Health policy, chronic illness and disability, **1056**
Health promotion, **9–10**
  in A&E, **927–928**
  in cancer prevention, **991–992**
  definition, 9
  nurse's role, 202–203
  older adults, **977–979**
  sharing information, 9–10
  see also Patient education (and information)
Health Quality Service, 34
Healthpromis, 1065
Healthy eating, 202
  in cardiovascular disease prevention, 493, 494
  in diabetes, *419*
  giving advice on, 202–203
Hearing, **370**
  ageing changes, 975
  assessment and tests, **373**
  problems, *see* Ear and hearing problems
Hearing aids, 375, *379*
  surgical patients, 737, 894, 909
  in tinnitus, 388
Hearing Concern, 391
Hearing impairment (loss), 289, **374–380**
  age-related (presbyaccusis), 377–379

communication, **375**, 385
  conductive, 374
  in Ménière's disease, 387
  noise-induced, 374, **380**
  sensorineural, 374
Heart, 481, **482–485**
  ageing changes, 975
  anatomy, 482–483
  biopsy, 518
  chambers, *482*, 483
  electrical conduction system, 483–484
  in stress, 96
  valves, *see* Valves, cardiac
Heart disease
  congenital, **528**
  coronary, *see* Coronary heart disease
  functional impact, 1050
  rheumatic, 514, *515*
  valvular, 514, **515–516**
Heart failure, **510–514**
  acute, 510
    see also Cardiogenic shock
  in anaemia, *457*
  in cardiomyopathy, 518
  chronic, **510–514**
    aetiology, 510
    clinical presentation, 511
    investigations, 511
    medical/surgical management, 511–512
    nursing management, 512–514
    pathophysiology, 510–511
    self-monitoring and self-management,
      513–514
  left-sided, 511
  in mitral regurgitation, 516
  in Paget's disease, 818
  right-sided, 511
  urinary incontinence, 233
Heart–lung transplantation, in cystic fibrosis,
    552
Heart rate
  in critically ill patients, 956, 958
  in shock, 156, 160
Heart rhythm, in critically ill patients, 956
Heart transplantation, **518–519**
Heartburn, 602, *603*, 605
Heat
  gain mechanisms, 77
  loss mechanisms, 77
  production, 77, 623
  regulation mechanisms, **76–77**
  transfer mechanisms, 76–77
Heat cramps, *80, 81*
Heat exhaustion, *80*
Heat stroke, *80*, 86–87
Heating, active cutaneous, 903
Hebb's arousal model, 93, *94*, 98
Helicobacter pylori, 605, 606
  urea breath test, 598–599
Help the Aged, 1045
Helping
  model, **43–44**
  relationships, 45
Hemi-inattention, *292, 293*
Hemianopia, *289, 292*, 335
Hemicolectomy, 612
Hemiplegia/hemiparesis, *289*, 796
  assessment, 284
  in head injury, 298
  in stroke, *292*
Henshaws Society for Blind People (HSBP),
    342, 343, 365
Heparin
  in deep vein thrombosis, 526
  low-molecular-weight (LMWH), 526

surgical patients, 889, 914
in unstable angina, 505–506
Hepatic artery, 622
Hepatic coma, **636–637**
Hepatic encephalopathy, *634*, 636–637
Hepatic portal vein, 622
Hepaticopancreatic ampulla, 623
Hepaticopancreatic sphincter (sphincter of
    Oddi), 594, 623
Hepatitis, **630–633**
    acute, 630
    alcohol-induced, **633**
    chronic, 630
    drug-induced, **633**
    toxic, 627, 633
    viral, *625*, **630–633**
      see also specific types
Hepatitis A (HAV), 627, 630, 633
Hepatitis B (HBV), **630–631**
    cancer risk, 991
    in drug users, 627
    infection control measures, 268, *631*
    nursing management, 632–633
    occupational transmission, 267–268
    sexual transmission, 627
    transfusion-associated transmission, 454
    vaccination/immunization, 268, *631*
Hepatitis C (HCV), 630, **631**
    control measures, 268
    in drug users, 627
    in haemophilia, *478*
    nursing management, 632–633
    occupational transmission, 267–268
    transfusion-associated transmission, 454
Hepatitis D (HDV), 627, 630, 631
Hepatitis E (HEV), 630, 631
Hepatitis G (HGV), 630, 631
Hepatolenticular degeneration, 318
Hepatorenal syndrome, 649
Herbal remedies, for stress, 105–106
Hereditary non-polyposis colorectal cancer
    (HNPCC), 994, 1000
Hering–Breuer reflex, 534
Hernia, **610**
Herpes labialis, 855
Herpes simplex virus (HSV), 855
    conjunctivitis, 361
    eczema herpeticum, 864
    genital, **763**, 855
    investigations, 846–847
    oesophageal, 604–605
    oral, 1035
Herpes zoster (shingles), **312–313**, 846, 855
Herpesviruses, 855
Hetastarch, 165
Hiatus hernia, 602, 610
Hiccups, 597–598
    in terminal illness, **1038**
Hickman lines, 470
High-density lipoproteins (HDLs), 205, 216, 493
High-dependency unit (HDU)
    development, 947, 948
    postoperative care, 907
High vaginal swabs (HVS), 714
Hill–Sachs lesion, 824
Hip flexor injury, **826**
Hip fractures, *see* Femoral neck fractures
Hip protectors, 831, *832*
Hip replacement, total (THR), 812, **813**
Hirsutism, 734, 735, **869–870**
Histamine, and sleep, 61
Histamine receptor (H₁) antagonists, *see*
    Antihistamines
History taking
    critically ill patients, 957

for triage in A&E, 927
HIV infection, 761, **764–765**
    as chronic disease, 1047
    clinical presentation, 765
    control measures, 268
    in haemophilia, *478*
    handicap, 1048
    lymphoma, 469, 470
    management, 765
    occupational transmission, 267–268
    sexual transmission, 716
    stigmatization, 1053
    transfusion-associated transmission, 454
    tuberculosis association, 674
HLA (human leucocyte antigens), 474, 694
HMG-CoA reductase inhibitors (statins), 427,
    494, 504
Hoarseness, 568, 587
Hodgkin's lymphoma, **469–470**
Holidays, in diabetes, 415
Holistic approach, 4, 9
    A&E department, 924
    critical care, 956
    palliative care, 1022, 1031
Holter monitoring, 490
Human's sign, 526
Homatropine, *344*, 360
Home
    adaptations, in visual impairment, 343
    continence care, 233
    long-term care of older people, 979, 980–981
    oxygen therapy, 546–547
    palliative care, **1024–1025**
    see also Community care
Home Responsibilities Protection, *1061*
Homeless people
    in A&E department, **938**
    tuberculosis, 555, 556
Homeostasis, ageing-related disturbances,
    974, 976
Homocysteine, plasma, 216
Honesty, **19**
Hordeolum, *338*, **363**
Hormonal therapy
    in breast cancer, 784, 785, 787
    in hypopituitarism, 431
    in prostate cancer, 700–701
Hormone replacement therapy (HRT),
    735–736, 819
Hormones, 394–395, **396**
    circadian rhythms, 62
    modes of action, 396
    regulation of secretion, 396
    see also individual hormones
Horseshoe kidney, *655*
Hosiery
    compression, *see* Compression
      hosiery/stockings
    containment, in lymphoedema, 787
Hospices, **1022–1023**, *1024*
    death in, 1043
    family support, 1026
Hospital-acquired infection (HAI, nosocomial
    infection), 253, 255, **257**
    pneumonia, 553
Hospital anxiety and depression scale, 104–105
Hospital at home schemes, 1057
Hospital Infection Control Practices Advisory
    Committee (HICPAC), 260, 264–265
Hospitals
    chronic illness and disability, **1056–1057**
    continence care, 232–233
    death in, 1041, 1043
    food choices, 219
    malnutrition in, 201–202, *211*

palliative care, **1023**, *1024*
    sleep problems, 63, 64, 65–66
Hot flushes, 735, 736
House dust mite, *538*, 850
Housemaid's knee, 805
Human chorionic gonadotrophin (β-hCG)
    in early pregnancy, 726, 728
    in ectopic pregnancy, 730
    in gestational trophoblastic disease, 729
    as tumour marker, 715, *745*, 747
Human immunodeficiency virus, *see* HIV
    infection
Human leucocyte antigens (HLA), 474, 694
Human papilloma virus (HPV), 761, 855
    cancer associations, 720, 721, 991
Humectant, 848
Humerus fractures
    proximal, **825**, 834
    shaft, 834
    supracondylar, 834
Humidification
    after tracheostomy, 558, 585, *586*
    oxygen, 558, 559
Humour, in pain management, 128
Hyaluronidase, 147
Hydatidiform mole, **729**
Hydralazine, *226*, 512
Hydration
    in head injury, 302
    older people in long-term care, 980
    skin, 848
Hydrocele, 750
Hydrochlorthiazide, *226*
Hydrocortisone
    in adrenal insufficiency, 438
    eye drops/ointment, *345*
    local injections, 805
    see also Cortisol
Hydrogen ions (H⁺), 148–149
    concentration ([H⁺]), in acid–base disorders,
    148
    excessive losses, 150
    homeostatic mechanisms, 149
    renal secretion, 661
Hydromorphone, 1034
Hydrostatic pressure, 136
    in capillaries, 136, 137
    in glomerular filtration, 657–658
Hydroxycobalamin, 459
Hydroxyethyl starch, 165
5-Hydroxytryptamine (serotonin), 61
5-Hydroxytryptamine receptor (5-HT₃)
    antagonists, 1036
    see also Ondansetron
Hydroxyurea (hydroxycarbamide), in sickle cell
    crises, 462
Hygiene, personal, *see* Personal hygiene
Hymen, 711
Hyoscine, *884*, 1036
Hypercalcaemia, *135*
    in hyperparathyroidism, 436–437
    of malignant disease, 1040
    in myeloma, 465
Hypercapnia (carbon dioxide retention), 557
    in critically ill patients, 958
    nursing assessment, 539
    oxygen therapy associated, 557
    respiratory stimulants, 559
Hyperchloraemia, *136*
Hypercholesterolaemia, **493–494**
    drug therapy, 494
    familial, 216, 494
    xanthomas, 870
    see also Hyperlipidaemia
Hyperemesis gravidarum, 729

Hyperglycaemia
in diabetes, 403, 404, 416
in diabetic ketoacidosis, 423
in hypothermia, 90
long-term complications, 424, 425
parenteral nutrition and, *225*
in septic shock, 167
Hypericum perforatum, 106
Hyperinsulinaemia, 416, 734
Hyperkalaemia, *135*, 148, 671
Hyperlipidaemia (dyslipidaemia), 427, 870
see also Hypercholesterolaemia
Hypermagnesaemia, *135*
Hypermetabolic state, 159, **217–218**, 302
see also Catabolic state
Hypermetropia, 335, 341
Hypernatraemia, *135*, 148
Hyperosmolar fluid imbalance, 139
Hyperosmolar non-ketotic hyperglycaemia
(HONKH), 416
Hyperparathyroidism, **436–437**
Hyperphosphataemia, *136*
Hyperpigmentation, 862
post-inflammatory, *846*, 853, 862
Hyperplasia, 988
Hyperprolactinaemia, 430
Hyperpyrexia, **78–79**, **86**
Hypertension, **521–522**
aetiology/risk factors, 210, 216, 521
in autonomic dysreflexia, 326
clinical presentation, 521
coronary heart disease risk, 494
in diabetes, 426, 427, 428, 682
diabetes complications and, 424
end-organ damage, 521, 522
essential, 521
impact, 1050–1051
medical management, 521–522
nursing management, 522
in phaeochromocytoma, 440, 441
prevention of complications, 1059
in renal disease, 683
secondary, 521
stress and, 103
Hyperthermia, **79–80**
malignant, *80*, 86–87
management, **86–87**
nutritional needs, 87
Hyperthyroid crisis (thyroid storm), 433
Hyperthyroidism, 431, 432
in Graves' disease, 432–434
myopathy, 810
signs and symptoms, *432*
in thyroiditis, 434
in toxic multinodular goitre/single adenoma,
434
Hypertonic solutions, 136, *145*, 146
Hypertrichosis, **870**
Hyperuricaemia, 807–808
Hyperventilation, 151
in critically ill patients, 958
in panic attacks, 940
in shock, 157
Hypervolaemia, *see* Fluid volume excess
Hyphaema, *338*, 349
Hypnotic drugs, **70–71**
urinary incontinence and, *236*
Hypo-osmolar fluid imbalance, 139
Hypoalbuminaemia, 215, 600, 684
Hypocalcaemia, *135*
in hypoparathyroidism, 436, 437
Hypocapnia, 958
Hypochloraemia, *136*
Hypodermis, 175
Hypodermoclysis, 147
Hypoglossal nerve, *279*

Hypoglycaemia
in diabetes, 411, **421–422**
explaining, *50*
in hypothermia, 90
in insulinoma, 649
signs and symptoms, 421
Hypogonadism, 430
Hypokalaemia, *135*
in heart failure, 512
in hypothermia, 90
management, 148
in primary aldosteronism, 440
Hypomagnesaemia, *135*
Hyponatraemia, *135*, 147
Hypoparathyroidism, 433–434, **436**
Hypopharynx, 566–567
Hypophosphataemia, *136*
Hypopigmentation, 862
Hypopituitarism, **430–431**
Hypopyon, *338*, 362
Hyposmia, 568
Hypostop, 422
Hypotension
in cardiogenic shock, 510
in critically ill patients, 955, 956
in epidural/spinal anaesthesia, 896–897
orthostatic (postural), 140, 663
in diabetes, 426, 428
in spinal injuries, 325
postoperative, 909
in septic shock, 155
in shock, 160, **166**
Hypothalamus, 394, **396**, *397*
damage, 78
in stress, 95
temperature regulation, 76, 77
Hypothermia, **81–83**
accidental, 81, 87–88
in burn injuries, 872
induced, 81
management, **87–91**
consequences of hypothermia, 90–91
fluid replacement, 89
monitoring and observations, 89–90
rewarming methods, 88–89
post-anaesthesia/postoperative, 82–83, 89
in surgical patients, 81–83, 89, **902–903**
temperature measurement, 84
therapeutic, 81–83
Hypothyroidism, 431, **435**
myopathy, 810
signs and symptoms, *435*
in thyroiditis, 434
Hypotonic solutions, 136, 146
Hypoventilation, 150–151
critically ill patients, 958
Hypovolaemia (fluid volume deficit), **138–139**
in burn injuries, 872
causes, 140–142, 147, *154*
management, **164–166**
nursing assessment, 139–140
pathophysiological effects, 156–157
see also Dehydration
Hypovolaemic shock, 154
management, **166**
patients at risk, *159*
postoperative, 909
Hypoxaemia, 149, 535, 557
in critically ill patients, 958
nursing assessment, 539
in shock, 157, 163
Hypoxia
cellular effects, 154
kidney damage, 656
nursing assessment, 539
postoperative, 908

in shock, **157**
in sickle cell disease, 462, 463
Hypoxic respiratory drive, 557
Hysterectomy, **718**
discharge advice after, *739*
nursing management, 719, 738
subtotal abdominal (STAH), 718
total abdominal (TAH), 718
vaginal, 718
Wertheim's (radical), 721–722
Hysterosalpingography, 714, 759
Hysteroscopy, 718, 722, 1002

I

ICP, *see* Intracranial pressure
Identification
self, 7
surgical patients, **895**
Idiopathic thrombocytopenic purpura (ITP),
476
Ileal conduit, for urinary diversion, 679–681
Ileocaecal valve, 594, 595
Ileostomy, 612
Ileostomy Association, 618
see also Stoma
Ileum, 594
Ileus, paralytic, **911–912**
Iliococcygeus muscle, 230, *231*
Iliopsoas injury, **826**
Imagery, in pain management, 128
Imaging
breast, 774–775
in cancer diagnosis, **1002**
ear, 373
in GI disorders, **599–600**
in gynaecological disorders, 713–714
in liver, biliary and pancreatic disorders,
626
in musculoskeletal disorders, 797
nervous system, 287–288
see also Computed tomography; Magnetic
resonance imaging; X-rays, plain
Imatinib, in chronic myeloid leukaemia, 468
Immobility/immobilization
anaesthetized patients, 900–902
in ankylosing spondylitis, 807
cast, 800–801
constipation and, 609
critically ill patients, **953**
deep vein thrombosis, 525
in frail older people, 975–976
in traction, 800
see also Bed rest; Mobility problems;
Mobilization; Rest
Immune cells, skin, 842, 843
Immune response, in SIRS, 158–159
Immune system
ageing, 974
and stress, 103
Immunity, impaired
in chronic renal failure, 687
in hypothermia, 90
impaired wound healing, 178–179
Immunization
health care professionals, 268
meningitis, *312*
Immunoglobulins, 447
Immunosuppressant drugs
in glomerulonephritis, 683, 684
in inflammatory bowel disease, 614
in psoriasis, 862
renal transplant recipients, 696
in rheumatoid arthritis, 806

Immunosuppressed patients, **267**
  protective isolation, 265, 267
  stem cell transplant recipients, 475
  wound healing, *179*
Immunotherapy, **1008–1009**
Impaired fasting glycaemia (IFG), 403
Impaired glucose tolerance (IGT), 403
Impairment
  assessment, **1059**
  definitions, 1048, *1049*
  see also Chronic illness; Disability
Impedance plethysmography (IPG), 525
Impetigo, 854, 855
  bullous, 864
Impingement syndrome (rotator cuff
      tendinitis/tears), 823–824
Impingement test, *798*
Implants
  breast, 789, 790
  cochlear, *386*
  intraocular lens (IOL), 349
  penile, 755, 756
  see also Prostheses
Implementation stage, nursing process,
  12–13
Impotence, *see* Erectile dysfunction
In vitro fertilization (IVF), *760*
Incapacity Benefit, *1061*
Incisional hernia, 610
Incisions, abdominal, *905*
Incontact, 247, 250
Incontinence, **229–252**
  fear of, 141
  in frail older people, 975–976
  functional, 292
  useful addresses, 250
  see also Faecal incontinence; Urinary
      incontinence
Incontinence pads, 247–248
Incus, 368, 369
Independence
  in visual impairment, 342–343
  see also Dependency; Self-care
Inequality, and ageing, **971**
Infection control, **253–270**
  categories of methods, 258
  chest drains, 561
  Creutzfeldt–Jakob disease, 313
  handwashing, 261–263
  in incontinence, 247
  intraoperative, **905–906**
  in neutropenia, 466
  preoperative measures, **887–888**
  principles, 257–258
  protective clothing, 263–264
  universal precautions, **260**, *261*, 264–265,
      268, 905
  useful websites, 269
  in viral hepatitis, 632
Infection control nurse (ICN), **258–259**
Infections
  after pacemaker insertion, 498
  in aplastic anaemia, 464
  biliary system, 638
  blood-borne, **267–268**
  bone, 820
  breast, **779**
  cancer causing, 991
  causes, **256–257**
  causing back pain, 815
  central venous catheters, *471*
  in cirrhosis, 636
  in diabetes, 404
  ear, **382–386**
  endogenous, 257

exogenous, 257
eye, 359, 361, 362, 363
female reproductive tract, **732–733**
hospital-acquired, *see* Hospital-acquired
    infection
host response, 256–257
inflammatory bowel disease and, 613
intravenous therapy and, 146, *225*
in leukaemia, 993
male reproductive tract, **750**
mode of transmission, 256
in multiple organ dysfunction, prevention,
  169
myocarditis, 518
nervous system, 289, **310–313**
in neutropenia, 465, 466
nose, 570–571
opportunistic, 257, 765
outbreaks, **258–259**
portal of entry, 256
postoperative, prevention, 887–888
prevention, **260–264**
pyrexia, 78, 79
renal transplant recipients, 696
reservoirs, 256
risks, critically ill patients, 956
in septic shock, 167
sexually transmitted/acquired (STIs/SAIs),
  732–733, **761–765**
skin, *see* Skin infections
skin defences, 842–843, 854
stress-related susceptibility, 103
subclinical, 256
surveillance, 258–259
Tenchkoff catheter exit site, 692
throat, **581–583**
wound, *see* Wound infections
see also Bacterial infections; Fungal infections;
    Viral infections; *specific infections*
Infectious diseases, 257
  isolation units, 265
  notifiable, *258*, 259
Infective endocarditis (IE), 515, **516–517**
Infertility (subfertility), **758–760**
  aetiology and epidemiology, 758
  chemotherapy-induced, 473
  in chronic renal failure, 688
  cyclophosphamide-induced, 684
  in hyperprolactinaemia, 430
  investigations, 758–759
  nursing management, 759–760
  in polycystic ovary syndrome, 735
  in testicular cancer, 748
  treatment, 759, *760*
  unexplained, *760*
Infestations, skin, **859–861**
Inflammation, 854
  pigmented skin, 846
  in SIRS, 158–159
  in wound healing, 177
Inflammatory bowel disease (IBD), **613–616**
  aetiology, 613–614
  investigations, 614
  medical management, 614–615
  nursing management, 615–616
  signs and symptoms, 614
  surgical management, 615
Inflammatory myopathies, 810, 811
Inflammatory skin disorders, **849–854**, 862
'Inflammatory soup', 113
Influenza (flu) vaccination, 553, *554*
Information
  in cancer care, 1012
  giving, **8–9**, 19
  for health promotion, 9–10

withholding, 19
  see also Patient education (and information)
Infusion control devices (pumps), 146, *963*
Inguinal hernia, 610
Inhalation analgesia, 125
Inhalation injury, 871
Inhaler delivery devices, *543*
Inhibin, 707, *708*
Inoculation injuries, 267, 268, *632*
Inotrope therapy, **962–963**
  nursing management, 963
  in shock, 166, 510
Insomnia, **65–66**
  causes, 65, *66*
  management, 65–66, 70–71
Instability, in frail older people, 975–976
Institutionalization, older people, 979
Instruments, surgical, *see* Surgical instruments
Insulation, passive, 903
Insulin, 400
  biphasic/mixed, 412
  bovine, 412
  deficiency, type 1 diabetes, 403–404
  delivery devices, 407–408
  functions, *401*
  in glucose homeostasis, 400–401
  human, 412
  intermediate-acting, 412
  isophane (NPH), *411*, 412
  lente, 412
  long-acting (ultralente), 412
  physiological profile, *413*
  porcine, 412
  resistance, 416
  secretion, in type 2 diabetes, 416
  short-acting (soluble), 411
  sources, 412
  storage, 409
  types, 411–412
Insulin analogues ('designer' insulins), 409,
    411–412
  regimens using, 412–413
Insulin dosers, 407, *408*
Insulin injections, **405–409**
  angle, 406
  equipment, 406, 407–408
  sites, 408–409
  timing, 409
  see also Insulin therapy
Insulin-like growth factor-I (IGF-I), 429
Insulin pens
  needle lengths, 408
  preloaded, 407, *408*
  reusable, 407, *408*
Insulin regimens, 412–413
  basal bolus, 412
  twice-daily, 413
Insulin sensitizers, 418
Insulin syringes, *407*
  drawing up insulin, 406, *407*
  needle lengths, 406
  sizes, 406
Insulin therapy
  in diabetic ketoacidosis, 423
  hypoglycaemia risk, 421
  in septic shock, 167
  sick day rules, 413–414
  in type 1 diabetes, 404, **405–409**, 411–413
  in type 2 diabetes, 417
  see also Insulin injections
Insulinomas, **649**
Integrated care pathways, 12
Integrity, Erikson's theory, 972
Intellectualization, *97*
Intelligence, effects of ageing, **972**

Intensive care, 947
  development, 947–948
Intensive care unit (ICU, ITU), 947
  bed shortages, 950
  postoperative care, 907
Interdigital candidosis, 858, 859
Interdisciplinary care
  surgical patients, 885, 895
  see also Team
Interferon, 79
  alpha, in chronic viral hepatitis, 631
  beta, in multiple sclerosis, 304, 305
  in cancer therapy, 1009
Interleukin-1 (IL-1), and sleep, 61
Interleukin-3, 448
Interleukin-6, 448
Interleukins, in cancer therapy, 1009
Intermediate care, 1056, 1057
Intermittent claudication, 523
Intermittent pneumatic compression system, 902
Internal desynchronization, 63
International Classification of Disease
    Impairment and Handicap (ICDIH),
    1048, 1049
International Classification of functioning
    disability and health (ICF), 1048
International Glaucoma Association (IGA),
    343, 365
International normalized ratio (INR), 450, 492,
    526, 625
Internet, 891
Interpreters, in visual impairment, 342
Interruptions, 50
Interstitial cell stimulating hormone (ICSH), 398
Interstitial lung diseases, 556–557
Interstitial nephritis, 684
Intertrigo, candidal, 859
Intertrochanteric fractures of femur, 831
Intervertebral disc
  degeneration, 814
  herniation (slipped disc), 814
  surgery (discectomy), 816
Intestinal ischaemia, 604
Intestinal obstruction, 604
  in terminal illness, 1038
Intra-aortic balloon pump (IABP), 167, 506
Intra-articular, 794
Intracellular fluid (ICF), 134
Intracerebral haemorrhage, 291, 298
Intracranial haemorrhage, traumatic, 297–298
Intracranial pressure (ICP), 277, 298–299
  raised, 279, 298–300
    altered consciousness, 280
    brain tumours, 308, 309
    clinical presentation, 299
    medical/surgical management, 300, 301,
      309
    nursing interventions, 302
    other observations, 284
    pathophysiology, 298–299
    pupillary response, 283
Intracytoplasmic sperm injection (ICSI), 760
Intraocular pressure (IOP)
  drugs to reduce, 356, 357
  in glaucoma, 355, 356, 357
  measurement, 340
  raised, 349, 351
Intraocular tumours, 358
Intraoperative care, 895–906
  anaesthesia, see Anaesthesia
  cataract surgery, 350
  hypothermia, 902–903
  patient dignity, 902
  patient movement and immobility, 900–902
  pressure ulcer prevention, 902

prevention of deep vein thrombosis, 902
  prevention of infection, 905–906
  procedural safety issues, 903–905
  sutures, 906–907
Intrauterine contraceptive devices (IUCDs or
    IUDs), 757
Intravenous catheters
  parenteral nutrition, 224–225
  site infection, 225
  see also Central venous catheters
Intravenous (i.v.) fluids, 145
Intravenous (i.v.) infusions, 145–147
  in burn injuries, 872
  complications, 146–147
  flow rate, 146
  in haemorrhage, 457
  in head injury, 302
  in hyperthermia, 87
  in hypothermia, 89
  in hypovolaemia, 164–166
  maintaining, 146
  in myocardial infarction, 508
  postoperative, 909, 912–913
  in pyelonephritis, 673
  in raised intracranial pressure, 301
  in shock, 163, 164–166
  in terminal illness, 1028
  unconscious patient, 290
Intravenous (i.v.) nurse specialist, 147
Intravenous urography (IVU), 667
Intrinsic factor, 209, 458, 606
  deficiency, 217, 458–459
Intubation, endotracheal, see Endotracheal
    intubation
Invalid Care Allowance, 1061
Iodine
  -based soaps, 261
  deficiency, 210, 435
  dietary intake, 207, 210
  radioactive (radio-iodine), 433, 434–435, 436
  in wound dressings, 185, 186
Ions, 134
Ipratropium bromide
  nasal, 572
  nebulized, 548
Iridotomy, laser, 357–358
Iris, 332–333
Iron, 207, 210, 446
  absorption, and vitamin C, 210, 225
  chelation therapy, 454, 461
  deficiency, 210, 217, 457–458
  overload, 454, 461
  serum levels, 600
  therapy, 458
Irritable bowel syndrome (IBS), 103, 608–609
Irritants
  in atopic eczema, 850
  contact dermatitis, 851
Ischaemia
  chronic, in peripheral arterial disease, 523
  in shock, 155, 157
Ischaemic leg ulcers, see Arterial (ischaemic)
    leg ulcers
Ishihara test, 340
Islet cell tumours, 649
Islets of Langerhans, 400
Isoflurane, 884
Isolation (of patients), 264–266
  confidentiality and, 265
  facilities, 265–266
  nursing categories, 266
  protective, 265, 267, 475, 1014
  psychological effects, 264
  single room, 265
  source, 264–265

Isolation (social)
  in chronic illness/disability, 1053
  older adults, 971
  in visual impairment, 342
Isoniazid, 226, 555, 675
Isosorbide dinitrate, 504
Isotonic solutions, 136, 145, 146
Isotope scanning, see Radionuclide scanning
Isotretinoin, 226, 852
Isovolumetric contraction, 484, 485
Isovolumetric relaxation, 484, 485
ISSUE, 767
Itching, see Pruritus

J

Jargon, 9, 42
Jarisch–Herxheimer reaction, 764
Jaundice, 598, 623, 628–629, 630
  in bile duct stones, 642
  obstructive, 626
  in pigmented skin, 846
  types and causes, 629
Jehovah's Witnesses, 455
Jejunostomy, feeding, 223
Jejunum, 594
Jet lag, 63, 72
Jewellery, 894
Johari window, 44, 44
Joint replacement surgery, 812, 813
Joints, 794–795
  disorders, 812–814
  injuries, 823
  movements, 795
  synovial, 794, 795
Joules, 203
Journal, reflective, 16, 17
Judgemental attitude, see Non-judgemental
    attitude
Jugular venous pressure (JVP), 140
Justice, 18–19
Juxtaglomerular apparatus (JGA), 657, 658

K

Kaposi's sarcoma, 765, 869
Keloids, 861
Keratin, 174, 842
  synthesis disorders, 861–862
Keratinization, 842
Keratinocytes, 842
Keratoconus, 340
Keratometry, 340
Kerion formation, 857
Kernig's sign, 311
Ketones
  in diabetic ketoacidosis, 423
  urinary (ketonuria), 143, 664, 665
    in diabetes, 404, 411
Ketostix, 411
Kidneys, 654, 655–661
  in acid–base balance, 149, 660–661
  agenesis, 655
  blood supply, 656
  in calcium and phosphate homeostasis,
    661
  congenital abnormalities, 655
  development and maturation, 654–655
  donation, 677–678, 694–695
  functions, 654
  horseshoe, 655

macroscopic structure, 655–656
malignant tumours, **677**, 679
nerve supply, 656
physiology, 656–661
ultrasound imaging, 665–666
in water and electrolyte balance, 137–138, 658–660
see also Renal
Knee
braces, 827
injuries, **826–827**, 831–832
replacement, total (TKR), 812, 813
Knowledge, types, **13–14**
Koebner phenomenon, 853, 861
Korsakoff's syndrome, 318
Kupffer cells, 622, 623
Kussmaul breathing, 423, 957
Kyphosis, 818

L

L-dopa, in Parkinson's disease, 320, 322
Labelling, 54–55
Labia majora, 711
Labia minora, 711
Laboratory
in outbreaks of infection, 259
specimens, safe collection and handling, 259, *260*
Labyrinth, 369–370
Labyrinthitis, 385
acute, **387**
Laceration, *934*
Lachman test, *798*, 826
Lacrimal system, 336
Lactate, 400
blood, 162
Lactate dehydrogenase (LDH), 491, *745*, 747, 811
Lactic acidosis, 150, 157
Lactose intolerance, 219
Landouzy–Dejerine muscular dystrophy, *809*
Langerhans' cells, 842, 843
Language
deficits, in stroke, *292*
difficulties, 9, 342
using appropriate, 9
Lanugo, 843
Laparoscopic cholecystectomy, **639**, *640*
Laparoscopy, **715**
in cancer diagnosis, 1002
in ectopic pregnancy, 730
in infertility, 759, *760*
Laparotomy, in ovarian cancer, 723
Large intestine (bowel), **595–596**
disorders, **610–616**
Large loop excision of transformation zone (LLETZ), 721
Larval therapy, 182
Laryngeal mask airway (LMA), 898–899
Laryngectomy, 587
nursing management, 587–588
protector (Buchanan bib), *584*, 586
Laryngitis, **583**
Laryngoscopy
endoscopic (direct), 569, **583**
indirect, 569
Laryngospasm, postoperative, 908
Larynx, 533, **567**
benign tumours, **587**
investigations of function, 570, 583
malignant tumours, **587–588**
obstruction, **583–584**

Lasegue's test, *798*
Laser treatment
diabetic retinopathy, 352
fungating breast lesions, 787
in glaucoma (iridotomy), 357–358
refractive errors (LASIK), 341
in rosacea, *852*, 853
Lashes, 336
Last offices, 1042
Latex allergy, 887, 905
Latissimus dorsi flap, breast reconstruction, 789
Laundry, 247, **266**
Laxatives, *610*, 1037
Lead cancer nurse, 1017
'League' tables, **29**
Learning disability
communication issues, *1011*
ear problems, 376, 381, 382
eye problems, 348, 349
Leave-taking, 53
Left ventricular assist devices (LVAD), **519–520**
Leg
arterial pulses, 487, 523
drainage bags, 249
see also Lower limb
Leg ulcers, **193–198**
arterial, *see* Arterial (ischaemic) leg ulcers
definition, 193
epidemiology and aetiology, 193
management principles, 196–198
management protocols, 198
mixed venous–arterial, 195, **198**
neuropathic, in diabetes, 425, 427, 428
patient assessment, 193–196
vascular assessment, 195–196
venous, *see* Venous leg ulcers
Legal issues, in neurological problems, 289
Leiomyomata (fibroids), uterine, 716, 718, 719
Lens
crystalline, *333*, 334
intraocular (IOL) implants, 349
Lentigines, **863–864**
Lethargy, *see* Fatigue
Let's Face It, 588
Leucocytes, *see* White cells
Leucopenia, 463
Leucopheresis, 452
Leucoplakia, 601
Leukaemia, 993
acute, **466–468**, **993**
lymphoblastic (ALL), 466, **467**
myeloid (AML), 466, **467**
nursing management, 467–468
promyelocytic, 477
chronic, **468–469**, **993**
lymphocytic (CLL), 468–469
myeloid (CML), 468, 993
nursing management, 469
Leukoplakia, penile, 751
Leukotriene antagonists, 543
Levator ani, 230, **231**
Levobunolol, *345*, 357
Levonorgestrel, 757, *758*
Leydig cell tumours, 746
Leydig cells, 742
LH, *see* Luteinizing hormone
Lice, **860–861**
body, 860–861
head, 860
pubic, 860–861
Lichen planus, **853**
Lichenification, *844*, 850
Lidocaine (lignocaine), *884*, 896
Life, value of, **17–18**
Life events, stressful, 98

Life-given experiences, 44
Life history approach, *973*
Life span, Erikson's theory, **972**
Lifestyle
advice, in coronary heart disease, 505
cancer risk and, 990
changes, coronary heart disease prevention, **494**
'disease', *647*
liver, biliary and pancreatic disorders and, 624, 627
wound healing and, 179–180
Ligaments, 794
injuries, 822
Light
sleep and, 64, 69
therapy, bright, 72
Light adaptation, 336
Lighting
skin examination, 844
in visual impairment, 343
Limb-girdle muscular dystrophy, *809*
Limb movement, **284**
Limb prostheses, 802
Limbic system, 95, 276–277
Limbus, 332
Linen disposal, **266**, *631*
Link Centre for Deafened People, 391
Linoleic acid, 204
Linolenic acid, 204
Lipid-lowering therapy, 427, 494
Lipids, 204
blood profile, 492
epidermal, 842
transportation, 204–205
see also Cholesterol; Fats
Lipodermatosclerosis, 194
Lipohypertrophy, 408, *409*
Lipoproteins, 204–205
Listening
in A&E triage, 927
active, **48**, 49–50
skills, 48
Lister, Joseph, 887, 893
Lithotripsy
bile duct stones, 642
renal calculi, 676
Litigation, after ear syringing, 377
Little's area, 566, 576
Liver, 595, **622–623**
anatomy, 622
biopsy, **626**, 1002
functions, 622–623
metabolic functions, 622–623
pain, in cancer, 1032
trauma, **638**
Liver disease, 621–622, **630–638**
clinical characteristics, 627–629
diagnostic tests and investigations, 625–626
end-stage, 631–632
nursing assessment, 623–625
prevention and health education, 626–627
useful addresses/websites, 650–651
Liver failure, 630, **636–637**
acute (ALF), fulminant, 636–637
nursing management, 637
Liver function tests, 600
Liver transplantation, 637
Liver tumours, **637–638**
benign, 637
malignant, 637
Living wills (advance directives), 18, **1027**
Local adaptation syndrome (LAS), 97
Local anaesthesia, 896
in acute pain management, 124–125, 127

Local anaesthesia (continued)
  adverse effects, 124–125
  cataract surgery, 349, 350, 351
  eye (topical), 338, 345
Local anaesthetic agents, 884, 896
Locus of control, 94, 992
'Log roll', 933
Loin pain, 673, 676
Loneliness, older adults, 971
Long-sightedness (hypermetropia), 335, 341
Long-term care
  in chronic illness and disability, **1058**
  in head injury, 303
  older adults, **979–980**
  in stroke, 296
Long-term illness, see Chronic illness
Loop of Henle, 656, **658–659**
  countercurrent exchange and multiplication,
    658–659
  exchange with vasa recta, 659, 660
Loperamide, 246, 1013
Lorazepam, 1013
Low air loss systems, 192
Low-density lipoproteins (LDLs), 205, 216, 493
Low vision aids, 343
Lower limb
  fractures, **830–833**
  sports injuries, 826–828
  see also Leg
Lower reference nutritional intake (LRNI), 202
Lower urinary tract
  anatomy and physiology, **229–231, 654–655**
  neurological control, 231
Ludwig's angina, **582–583**
Lugol's solution, 433
Lumbar puncture, 288
  in cancer diagnosis, 1002
  in meningitis, 311
  in multiple sclerosis, 305
Lund and Browder burn assessment chart,
    872, 873
Lung cancer, **549–550**, 993–994
  non-small cell (NSCLC), 549, 993–994
  risk factors, 549, 990
  screening, 998
  small cell (oat cell, SCLC), 549, 993–994
Lung cancer nurse specialists, 549–550
Lung transplantation, in cystic fibrosis, 552
Lungs
  in acid–base balance, 149, **535**
  ageing changes, 975
  collapse, see Pneumothorax
  heat loss, 77
  interstitial diseases, **556–557**
  stretch receptors, 534
  see also Pulmonary
Lupus erythematosus
  drug-induced, 817
  systemic (SLE), **817–818**
Lupus UK, 838
Luteinizing hormone (LH), 397, 398
  deficiency, 430
  in ovarian cycle, 707–708, 710
Lymph nodes
  biopsy, **1001**
  breast cancer involvement, 782, 783
  sentinel, in breast cancer, 783
Lymphadenopathy, in lymphoma, 469
Lymphatic drainage, impaired, 137
Lymphocytes, 446
Lymphoedema, 1014
  in breast cancer, **785–787**
  in vulval cancer, 720
Lymphoma, **469–470**
  Burkitt's, 470

clinical presentation, 469
Hodgkin's, 469–470
non-Hodgkin's (NHL), 469, **470**
relapsed, 470
testicular, 746–747

M

Macmillan Cancer Relief, 618
Macmillan model of communication, 40
Macmillan nurses, **1025**, 1040, 1041
Macronutrients, 202, **203–205**
Macrophages, 446
  skin, 174
  in wound healing, 177
Macula densa, 658
Macula lutea, 333
Macular degeneration, age-related (AMD),
    353–354
Macular Disease Society, 365
Macules, in pityriasis versicolor, 859
Maculopathy, diabetic, 352
Maggot (larval) therapy, 182
Magnesium (Mg^{2+}), 135
  dietary intake, 207, 210
  imbalance disorders, 135
  migraine and, 318
Magnetic resonance angiography (MRA), in
    urinary system disorders, 666–667
Magnetic resonance imaging (MRI)
  brain tumours, 309
  in cancer diagnosis, 1002
  in cardiovascular disease, 491
  contraindications, 797
  in ear problems, 373
  in endocrine disorders, 401, 429
  in liver, biliary and pancreatic disorders, 626
  in musculoskeletal disorders, 797
  in neurological disease, 287
  in nose and throat disorders, 569
Malabsorption, 214
  in chronic pancreatitis, 646, 647
  in cystic fibrosis, 551
Malassezia yeast infection, **858–859**
Male accessory reproductive organs, 742–743
Male reproductive tract, **741–744**
  infection and inflammation, 750
Malignant hyperthermia, 80, 86–87
Malignant tumours, **992–993**
Malleus, 368, 369
Mallory–Weiss syndrome, 607
Malnutrition
  in hospital, 201–202, 211
  nursing interventions, 221
  in older adults, 217, 978
  perioperative, 218, **888**
  protein energy (PEM), 206, 217, 218
  see also Nutrition
Mammary duct
  ectasia, 780, 781
  fistula, 779
  papillomas, 780
Mammography, **774–775**
  after breast reconstruction, 790
  screening, 772, 775–776, 998
Mannitol, 301, 357
Manual handling techniques, 900–901
Manual lymphatic drainage (MLD), 786
Marc's line, 869, 875
Marie Curie nurses, **1025**
Masks, 263, 906
Massage, 108
  in back pain, 816

in lymphoedema, 786
in palliative care, 1023
Mastalgia (breast pain), **778**
Mastectomy, 781, 783
  breast reconstruction after, **788–789**
  modified radical, 783
  nursing management, 784
  prophylactic, 776
  radical, 783
  simple, 783
  see also Breast surgery
Mastoid antrum, 369
Mastoidectomy, 386
Mastoiditis, 385
Mattresses/cushions
  foam, 191
  low air loss systems, 192
  operating table, 902
  pressure-relieving, 192, 193
  static overlays, 191–192
  warming, 903
Maturity-onset diabetes of the young (MODY),
    403
Maxillary antrum, proof puncture, 569
Maxwell's dimensions of quality, 30
McArdle's disease, 810
McMurray's test, 798
Mealtimes
  environment, 219–221
  staffing during, 221
Mean cell volume (MCV), 450
Mechanical stress, wound healing and, 179
Mechanical ventilation, see Ventilation,
    mechanical
Medial collateral ligament (MCL) tears, 826, 827
Medications, see Drugs/medications
Medicinal Products Prescription by Nurses,
    Midwives and Health Visitors Act (1992),
    186
Meditation, 107
Medley score, 189
Medulla oblongata, 276
Megaloblastic anaemia, 209, **458–459**
  folic acid deficiency, 459
  vitamin B$_{12}$ deficiency, 458–459
Meglitinides, 418
Meibomian cyst, 338
Meissner's plexus, 592
Melaena, 598, 607
Melanin, 842
Melanocytes, 842
Melanoma, malignant, 844, **868–869**
  risk factors, 990
Melatonin, 61, 72
Memory, age-related changes, **972–973**
Menarche, 716
Mendelson's syndrome (aspiration pneumonia),
    553, 893
Ménière's disease, **386–387**
Ménière's Society, 391
Meninges, **277–279**
Meningiomas, 308
Meningism, 311
Meningitis, **311–312**
  bacterial, 311–312
  immunization against, 312
  meningococcal, 263, 311
  pneumococcal, 312
  viral, 311
Meningococcal disease, 263, 311
Meningococcal group C vaccine, 312
Meniscectomy, 805, 827
Meniscus tears, 827
Menopausal symptoms, 735–736, 785
Menopause, 735–736

Menorrhagia, 458, 710, 716, *717*
  medical/surgical management, 716–719
  nursing management, 719
Men's health, 706, **741–757**
  breast cancer, 782, 784
  breast disorders, 772
  diagnostic tests and investigations, 744, *745*
  disease prevention and health promotion,
    744–745
  erectile dysfunction, 742, 744, 749,
    752–756
  nursing assessment, 744
  penile cancer, **751–752**
  pelvic floor exercises, 238–239
  sexual dysfunction, **752–756**
  testicular cancer, **745–749**
  urinary incontinence, 231, 235
  see also Gender differences
Menstrual cycle, **710–711**
  body temperature, 710–711, 759
  breast pain and, 778
  menstrual phase, 710
  proliferative phase, 710
  secretory phase, 710
  sleep and, 72
Menstrual disorders, **716–719**
  in hyperprolactinaemia, 430
Menstruation, 710, *733*
Mental capacity, to give consent, 892
Mental (unconscious) defence mechanisms,
  45, **97**
Mental Health Act (1983), 939
Mental health problems
  in A&E, **938–941**
  acute
    assessment, 940
    causes, 939–940
    management in A&E, 940–941
  sleep disturbance, 65
  stress and, **104**
  see also Psychological problems
Mental state
  critically ill patients, 957
  nutritional status and, 213
  in respiratory disease, **539**
Mesenteric plexus, 592
Mesentery, 592
Mesothelioma, 549
Metabolic acidosis, **150**
  blood gas values, *148*
  in chronic renal failure, 687
Metabolic alkalosis, *148*, **150**
Metabolic disorders
  musculoskeletal system, 807–808
  neurological, **318**
  see also Endocrine disorders
Metabolic myopathies, 810
Metabolism
  liver function, 622–623
  in skin, 175
  in spinal injuries, 325
  in systemic inflammatory response syndrome,
    159
  see also Hypermetabolic state
Metacarpal fractures, 835
Metaphysis, 794
Metastases, 988, 989
  bone, 821, 1032
  in breast cancer, 783, 785
  surgical treatment, 1004
Metformin, 418
Methicillin-resistant *Staphylococcus aureus*
  (MRSA), 255, 887
Methotrexate, 730, 862
Methyl-phenyl-tetrahydropyridine (MPTP), 319

Methylxanthines, 543
Metoclopramide, 1013, 1036
Metronidazole, in peptic ulceration, 606, *607*
Metrorrhagia, *717*
Microalbuminuria, in diabetes, 425, 682
Microbiologists, in critical care, 952
Microbiology, **254–255**
  in gynaecological disorders, 714
  in skin conditions, **846–848**
Microglia, *275*
Microlaryngoscopy, 569
Micronutrients, **205–211**
Microorganisms
  classification, 254
  normal flora (commensals), 257, 595, 843,
    887
  pathogenic, 256, **257**
  in respiratory disorders, 537
  transient, 887
  types, 254
  in urinary tract infections, 672
  see also Bacteria; Viruses
Micturition, 230, 662
  cycle, **231**
  neurological control, 231, 277, 662
  nursing assessment, 662
  see also Voiding
Mid-arm muscle circumference (MAMC), 214
Midazolam, *884*
Midbrain, 276
Middle-aged adults, chronic illness and disability,
  1054–1055
Mifepristone, 728, 731
Migraine, 104, *317*, 318
Milia, *844*
Mineral oil, 225, 227
Mineralocorticoids, 138, **399**
  see also Aldosterone
Minerals, 205, *207*, **209–211**
  patients on medication, *226–227*
Mini-Mental State Examination, 285
Minimally invasive cardiac surgery (MICS), 504
Minor injuries units (MIUs), 924, 934
  see also Trauma, minor
Minute volume, 957–958
Miosis, *see* Pupils, constriction
Miotics, *338*, *344*
Miscarriage, **725–727**
  complete, 726–727
  incomplete, 727
  inevitable, 726
  missed, 728
  recurrent, 728–729
  spontaneous, 725
  threatened, 725–726
Miscarriage Association, 727, 767
Misoprostol, 728
Mitomycin, intravesical therapy, 679, *680*
Mitral regurgitation, *515*, 516
Mitral stenosis, *515*
Mitral valve, 483
Mivacurium, *884*
Mobility aids
  in musculoskeletal disorders, **802–804**
  in visual impairment, 343
Mobility problems
  in cirrhosis, 636
  eye medication and, 347
  fluid intake and, 141
  nursing assessment, **796**
  nutrition and, 213
  in Parkinson's disease, 321
  in spinal injuries, 326
  in terminal illness, 1029
  urinary incontinence and, 233

  in visual impairment, 342
  see also Disability; Musculoskeletal disorders
Mobilization
  after joint replacement surgery, 813
  after myocardial infarction, 508
  critically ill patients, 953
  postoperative, 914, **919**
  stroke patients, 293–296
  see also Immobility/immobilization
Modernizing Social Services (1998), 1056
Moisturizers, *see* Emollients
Molar pregnancy (hydatidiform mole), **729**
Moles, malignant change, 868
Monitoring, 956
  in burn injuries, 872
  categories, 949
  critically ill patients, **956–960**
  quality of care, **34**
  see also specific types of monitoring
Monoamine-oxidase-B inhibitors, in Parkinson's
  disease, 320
Monoclonal antibodies, **475–476**
  anti-CD20, 470
Monocytes, 446
Mononeuropathies, in diabetes, 425
Monoparesis/monoplegia, *289*
Monosaccharides, 205
Montelukast, 543
Mood assessment, in terminal illness, 1031
Moon, 343
Moral issues, *see* Ethical issues
'Morning after pill', *758*
'Morning types', 64
Morphine, **123–124**, *884*, 1033
  epidural, 127
  patient information, *1034*
  side-effects, 123–124, 1033
Motor impairments, *289*
  in multiple sclerosis, 304
  in spinal injuries, 326
Motor nerves, 274
Motor neuron disease (MND), **323**
Motor response, assessing, 280, *283*
Motor vehicle accidents, *see* Road traffic accidents
Mouth, **592–593**
  assessment, *see* Oral assessment
  carcinoma, 600, *601*
  disorders, **600–602**
  dry (xerostomia), 139, 600–601
    critically ill patients, 953
    in terminal illness, 1035
  pain/discomfort, 139, 1035
  temperature measurement, *84*, 85
  white patches, 601
Mouth care, 601, 602
  after nasal packing/surgery, 577, 578
  in cancer, *1002*
  critically ill patients, **952–953**
  in diabetic ketoacidosis, 424
  dying patients, 1042
  in haematological malignancies, 472
  in multiple organ dysfunction, 169
  nutrition and, 221
  in oxygen therapy, 558–559
  in peritonsillar abscess, 582
  in terminal illness, **1035**
Mouth ulcers, 597, **601**, 1035
Movement
  anaesthetized patients, **900–902**
  critically ill patients, 957
  stroke patients, 293–296
MPTP (methyl-phenyl-tetrahydropyridine), 319
MRI, *see* Magnetic resonance imaging
MRSA (methicillin-resistant *Staphylococcus
  aureus*), 255, 887

Mucociliary clearance, 533, 566
  investigation, 570
  in sinusitis, *573*
Mucositis, 449, **472**, 1005, 1012
  oral, *see* Stomatitis
Mucous membranes (mucosa)
  in anaemia, *457*
  assessment of hydration, 663
  critically ill patients, 957
  gastrointestinal, 592
Muir and Barclay formula, 872
Müllerian-inhibiting hormone (MIH), 741
Multidisciplinary team, *see* Team
Multiple myeloma, **464–465**, 821
Multiple organ dysfunction, 154, **167–169**
  management, 168–169
  manifestations, 167–168
  mortality, 168, *169*
  pathophysiology, 157–159
Multiple sclerosis (MS), **304–308**
  clinical presentation, 304
  epidemiology and aetiology, 304
  investigations, 304–305
  medical management, 305–306
  nursing management, 306–308
  pathophysiology, 304
  specialist nurses, *306*
  urinary incontinence, 234, 304, 307
  waiting for a diagnosis, *305*
Mumps, 750
Mupirocin, *572*
Murphy's sign, 640
Muscarinic antagonists, *see* Antimuscarinics
Muscle(s)
  aches, in stress, 103
  agonists, *796*
  antagonists, *796*
  atrophy, 810, 953
  biopsy, 799, 811
  critically ill patients, 953
  disorders, **808–811**
  groups, *796*
  skeletal, **795–796**
  strains, 822–823
  synergists, *796*
  tone, in stress, 96, 103
  weakness, 810, 811
Muscle relaxants
  in anaesthesia, *884*
  in back pain, 816
Muscular dystrophies, 808, *809*
  congenital, *809*
  distal, *809*
Muscular Dystrophy Campaign, 838
Musculoskeletal disorders, **793–839**
  diagnostic tests and investigations,
    797–799
  inflammatory, 805–807
  metabolic, 807–808
  nursing assessment, **796**, 797
  nursing management principles, **799–804**
  origins, 796, *797*
  physical examination, 797, *798*
  prevention and health education, **799**
  in spinal injuries, 325
  surgical techniques, *805*
  useful addresses, 838
  wound healing, 178
  see also Mobility problems
Musculoskeletal system, **793–796**
  ageing changes, 975
MUSE (medicated urethral system for erections),
    754–755
Music, in pain management, 128
Mutagens, 987, 989–990

Myasthenia gravis, **811**
Mycobacterium tuberculosis, 555
  meningitis, 311
  multidrug resistant (MDR-TB), 255, 263,
    555–556
  see also Tuberculosis
Mycology, 254
  in skin conditions, 847
Mycoses, 855–859
  cutaneous, 856
  superficial, 855
  see also Fungal infections
Mydriasis, *see* Pupils, dilation
Mydriatics, *338*, *344*, 350
Myelin, 274, 275
Myelodysplasia/myelodysplastic syndrome
    (MDS), **464**
Myelography, 287
Myeloid cells, 446
Myeloma, multiple, **464–465**, 821
Myocardial contractility, *see* Contractility
Myocardial infarction (MI), **506–509**
  cardiac rehabilitation, 508–509
  clinical presentation, 506–507
  complications, 507, 508
  in diabetes, 425, 426
  discharge planning, 508
  epidemiology, 506
  functional impact, 1050
  immediate management, 507–508
  investigations, 491, 507
  later hospital care, 508
  medical management, 507
  nursing assessment, 508
  nursing management, 507–509
  pathophysiology, 506
  silent, 506
Myocardial revascularization, percutaneous, 504
Myocarditis, **518**
Myocardium, 482
  disorders, **517–520**
Myomectomy, 719
Myometrium, 709
Myopathies, **808–811**
  biochemical (metabolic), 810
  endocrine, 810
  inflammatory, 810, 811
  inherited genetic, 808–810, 811
  non-specific, 810
Myopia, 335, 341
Myotonia, 810, 811
Myotonia congenita, *809*
Myotonic dystrophy, *809*
Myotubular myopathy, *809*
Myringitis, bullous, 372
Myringoplasty, 384, *386*
Myxoedema, 431, 435
  pretibial, 432
  see also Hypothyroidism

N

Nail fold problems, **870**
Nails, 843
  candidosis, 858, *859*, 870
  clippings, 847
  fungal infection, 856, 858
  problems, **870**
Naloxone, 124, *884*, 900
Naps, daytime, 70
Narcolepsy, 66
Narcotics, *see* Opioids
Nasal cautery, in epistaxis, 575

Nasal discharge, 568
  see also Rhinorrhoea
Nasal drops, administration, *571*, 574
Nasal irritation, enterally fed patients, *224*
Nasal obstruction, 568, 577, **580**
Nasal packing
  complications, *576*
  in epistaxis, 575–576
  nursing management, 576–577
  postoperative, 578, 579
  removal, *576*, 578
Nasal polypectomy, 580
Nasal polyps, **580**
Nasal regurgitation, 286
Nasal septal surgery, **577–578**
  complications, 578
  in epistaxis, 576
  nursing management, 577–578
  in sinusitis, 574
Nasal septoplasty, 577
Nasal septum, 566
  deviation, **577–578**
  haematoma, **579**
  perforation, **579–580**
  submucosal resection, 577
Nasal surgery, postoperative care, 574
Nasal swabs, 569
Nasendoscope, 568
Nasoduodenal feeding tubes, 223
Nasogastric tubes, **145**
  enteral feeding, 222–223, 953
  postoperative aspiration, **911–912**
Nasojejunal feeding tubes, 223, 953
Nasopharyngeal airway, 898, *899*
Nasopharyngeal carcinoma, 383, 384
Nasopharynx, 533, 566–567
Nateglinide, 418
National Association of Bereavement Services,
    1045
National Association for Colitis and Crohn's
    Disease (NACC), 618
National Association of Laryngectomy Clubs,
    588
National Asthma Campaign, 545
National Cancer Research Institute (NCRI), 986
National Care Standards Commission (NCSC), 27
National Eczema Society, 875
National Health Service (NHS)
  changes, 25
  quality management, **24–29**
National Health Service and Community Care
    Act, 1056
National Institute for Clinical Excellence (NICE),
    14, 15, **25–26**
  Alzheimer's disease therapy, 322
  beta-interferon for multiple sclerosis, *305*
  cancer care, 986
  diabetes management, *405*, *415*
National Library for the Blind, 343, 365
National Osteoporosis Society, 767, 838
National Service Frameworks (NSFs), 15
  coronary heart disease, 493, 504
  diabetes, 394, *395*
  older people, 8, 967, *968*
Nausea and vomiting, 594, 597
  in acute pancreatitis, *644*
  in balance disorders, 387
  in cancer, *1010*, **1012–1013**, 1036
  chemotherapy-induced, 472, 1012–1013
  in diabetic ketoacidosis, 423
  enteral feeding and, *224*
  food intake and, 212
  in head injury, 298, 300
  non-pharmacological interventions, 1036
  opioid-induced, 123–124

pharmacological interventions, *see*
    Antiemetics
physiology, 1035–1036
postoperative, *see* Postoperative nausea and
    vomiting
in pyloric stenosis, 607
in terminal illness, **1035–1036**
Nebulizer therapy, **547–548**
Neck
    abscesses, deep, **582**
    lumps, palpable, 568
    palpation, 569
Necrosis, aseptic (avascular), 830
Necrotic tissue, wounds, *179*, 181–182
Need, relevance to, *30*
Needles
    suture, 906
    used in surgery, accounting for, 904
Needlestick injuries, 267, 268, *632*
Needs assessment, in chronic illness and
    disability, 1056
Neglect, *292*, 293
Negotiation, 52
Nemaline myopathy, *809*
Neomycin, nasal, *572*
Neoplasms, *see* Tumour(s)
Neostigmine, *884*, 900
Nephrectomy, 677
    discharge planning after, *678*
    nursing management, **677–678**
Nephrolithiasis (kidney stones), **676–677**, 953
Nephrolithotomy, 676
Nephron, **656–660**
    cortical, 656, *657*
    juxtamedullary, 656, *657*
Nephrostomy tube, 676
    nursing management, **676–677**
    urine specimen collection, *671*
Nephrotic syndrome, **684**
Nephroureterectomy, 679
Nerve entrapment, 425–426, **814**
Nerve impulse, **275–276**
Nerve injuries
    critically ill patients, 953
    in fractures, 829
Nervous system, **274–279**
    ageing changes, 975
    autonomic, *see* Autonomic nervous system
    central (CNS), 274, **276–279**
    functions, 274
    infections, 289, **310–313**
    peripheral (PNS), 274, 279
    somatic, 274
Neural tube defects, 209
Neuroglycopenia, 421
Neurohypophysis, 396, **397**
Neuroleptic malignant syndrome, *80*, 87
Neurological assessment, 279–286
    in head injury, 300
    in major trauma, 933
Neurological assessment/observation chart,
    280, *281*
    limb movement, 284
    other observations, 284
    pupillary response, 283–284
    see also Glasgow Coma Scale
Neurological problems, **273–330**
    categories of impairment, *289*
    cerebrovascular disorders, 291–297
    cranial nerve disorders, 303–304
    degenerative disorders, 318–323
    demyelinating (inflammatory) disorders,
        304–308
    diagnostic tests and investigations, 287–288
    in disc degeneration/herniation, 814
    ethical and legal issues, 289, *290*

faecal incontinence, 243, *247*
headache, *see* Headache
imaging, 287–288
infections, 310–313
in liver disease, *629*
in multiple organ dysfunction, 168
nursing assessment, *see* Neurological
    assessment
nutritional/metabolic, 318
in Paget's disease, 818
peripheral nerve disorders, 326–328
physical examination, 287
prevention/health education, 288–289
seizures and epilepsy, 313–315
in shock, 160
signs and symptoms, 279
spinal cord disorders, 323–326
in systemic lupus erythematosus, 817
trauma, *see* Head injury; Spinal injuries
tumours, *see* Brain tumours
urinary incontinence, 234, 235
useful websites, 329
Neurons, 274
Neuropathic pain, 112, 1032
Neurosurgery
    brain tumours, *309*
    nursing care after, 310
    in Parkinson's disease, 320–321
Neurotransmitters, *275, 276*
Neurovascular assessment
    in cast immobilization, 801
    in external fixation, 804
    fractured limbs, *830*, 834, 836
Neutropenia, 267, **465–466**, 1013
    aetiology, 465, 471
    in leukaemia, 467, 468, 993
    medical management, 465
    nursing management, 465–466, *1014*
    patient education and support, 456, 466
Neutrophils, 177, 446
The NHS Cancer Plan (2000), 986
NHS Centre for Reviews and Dissemination
    (York), *14*
The NHS Plan, 3–4
Niacin, *206*, **208–209**
NICE, *see* National Institute for Clinical
    Excellence
Nicotine, 536
    replacement therapy (NRT), 536
    sleep and, 65
    stress and, 104
    withdrawal symptoms, 536
    see also Smoking
Night shifts, 63
Nightmares, **66**
Nipples, 772
    discharge, 780–781
    disorders, **780–781**
    eczema, 781
    inversion, 780
    Paget's disease, 781
    reconstruction, 789
    supernumerary, 779
Nitrates
    in heart failure, 512, 513
    see also Glyceryl trinitrate
Nitrites, urinary, 665
Nitrogen balance, 24-hour, 215
Nitroglycerin, *see* Glyceryl trinitrate
Nitrous oxide, *884*
Nitrous oxide/oxygen (Entonox), 125
Nits, 860
Nociception, **113–114**
Nociceptive pain, 112
Nocturia, 65, **236**
    in benign prostatic hyperplasia, 696

in renal tuberculosis, 674
Nocturnal enuresis, **236**
Nodes of Ranvier, *274*, 275
Nodules, 851
Noise
    in critical care environments, 954
    induced hearing loss, 374, **380**
    sleep and, 64, 69
Non-assertive behaviour, 51
Non-blanching erythema, 190–191
Non-compliance, *see* Compliance
Non-Hodgkin's lymphoma (NHL), 469, **470**
Non-invasive positive pressure ventilation
    (NIPPV), 961
Non-invasive ventilation (NIV), 559–560, 961
Non-judgemental attitude
    in A&E department, 925
    sexually transmitted infections, 733, 761
    termination of pregnancy, 731
Non-maleficence, 18
Non-starch polysaccharides (NSP), 205
    see also Fibre, dietary
Non-steroidal anti-inflammatory drugs
    (NSAIDs), 124
    in back pain, 815
    in day surgery, 884
    in musculoskeletal disorders, 805
    routes of administration, 125
Non-verbal communication, **40–41**, 175
Noradrenaline (norepinephrine), 275, 276, 400
    during sleep, 62
    in heat generation, 77
    in shock, 156, 166, 167
    in sleep, 61, 62
    in stress, 890
North American Nursing Diagnosis Association
    (NANDA), 11–12
Norton Score, 14, 188, *189*
Nose, **566**
    drugs used, *572*
    examination, **568–569**
    foreign bodies, **580**
    fractures, **579**
    infection and inflammation, 570–571
    injuries, **579–580**
    investigations, **569–570**
    pain, 568
    signs and symptoms, 568
    tumours, 570, **587–588**
    see also Nasal
Nose and throat disorders, **565–589**
    diagnostic tests and investigations, 568–570
    general consideration, 570
    nursing assessment, 568
    nursing history, 568
    prevention and health education, 570
    tumours, **587–588**
    useful addresses, 588
Nosebleed, *see* Epistaxis
Nosocomial infection, *see* Hospital-acquired
    infection
NSAIDs, *see* Non-steroidal anti-inflammatory
    drugs
Nuclear imaging, *see* Radionuclide scanning
Nurse–client relationship, 43, **44–45**
    ending, 53
Nurse education programmes
    branches, 3
    requirements, 4–5, 5–6
Nurse Stress Index, *100*
Nurses
    attitudes
        older people, *see* Older adults, nurses'
            attitudes
        termination of pregnancy, 731, *732*
    back problems, 814

Nurses (continued)
  clinical supervision, 106
  in critical care team, 951
  critical care training, 948
  non-registered, 4
  prescribing rights, 186, 248
  reducing stress, 108
  role expansion, 3–4
  stress affecting, **100–102**
  see also Health care professionals
Nursing
  adult, 3–4, **7–8**
  definition, **4**
  meaning of, 4
  regulation, **4–6**
Nursing & Midwifery Council (NMC), 3, 6,
    33–34
Nursing assessment, **11–12**
  in A&E, **925–927**
  critically ill patients, 956–957
  see also under specific diseases and conditions
Nursing diagnosis, 11–12
Nursing homes
  in chronic illness and disability, 1056, 1058
  older adults, 979
  standards of care, 27
Nursing models, **10–11**
  A&E care, 925, 926
  in chronic illness and disability, 1058–1059
Nursing process, **11–13**
  in A&E, **925**
  assessment, 11–12
  evaluation, 13
  implementation, 12–13
  planning, 12
Nutrients, **202**
  altered metabolism, 214
  drug interactions, **225**, 226–227
  gastrointestinal losses, 214
  poor absorption, see Malabsorption
  see also specific nutrients
Nutrition, **201–228**
  in blood disorders, 449
  in burn injuries, 873
  in chronic renal failure, 687–688
  in cirrhosis, 636
  in COPD, 548
  critically ill patients, **953**
  in cystic fibrosis, 551
  definition, 202
  dialysis patients, 688, 691, 693
  enteral, see Enteral feeding
  in Guillain–Barré syndrome, 328
  in head injury, 302
  hypothermia and, 90–91
  in inflammatory bowel disease, **615–616**
  in liver, biliary and pancreatic disorders, 627
  in long-term care, **979–980**
  management flow chart, 220
  in multiple organ dysfunction, 169
  in multiple sclerosis, 308
  neurological disorders and, **318**
  nurse's role, 202–203
  nursing assessment, 211–214
  nursing interventions, 219–221
  older adults, **217**, 219, 220, **978–979**
  parenteral, **224–225**
  in Parkinson's disease, 321–322
  physiological aspects, 212–214
  post-surgical, 913, **913**
  psychological aspects, 211–212
  in pyrexia and hyperthermia, 87
  sociological aspects, 212
  in specific groups, 216–219

  in terminal illness, **1028**
  useful websites, 228
  in viral hepatitis, 632
  wound healing and, 179, **218**
  see also Diet; Eating; Food; Malnutrition
Nutrition nurse specialists, 219
Nutritional assessment, **214–216**
  anthropomorphic methods, 214
  biochemical indicators, 214–215
  chart, 215
  dietary history, 214
  in liver, biliary and pancreatic disorders, 624
  physical methods, 214
  preoperative, 888
  in respiratory disease, 539
Nutritional screening, 211
  tools, **215–216**
Nutritional supplements, **222**
Nutritional support, **222–225**
Nutritional teams, 216, 219
Nystagmus, 372

O

Obesity, **216–217**
  body water, 134
  gallstones and, 216, 627, 638
  in older adults, 978
  truncal (central), 415
  type 2 diabetes risk, 403, 415
  urinary incontinence, 234
  weight loss, 217
  in women, 715–716
  wound healing and, 179, 218
  see also Body mass index; Weight, body
Occipital lobe, 277
Occupational health hazards
  back pain, 814
  blood-borne infections, 267–268
  cancer, 990
  contact dermatitis, 851
  eye injuries, 341
  gastrointestinal disorders, 596
  hepatotoxic chemicals, 627
  noise-induced hearing loss, 374, 380
  nursing assessment, 539, 624
  stress, **100–102**
Occupational therapist (OT)
  in amputation, 524
  in back pain, 816
  in cognitive deficits, 285, 307
  in eating difficulties, 221
  older people, 980
  in palliative care, 1025
  in Parkinson's disease, 321
  stroke patients, 294
Octreotide, 429
Ocular problems, see Eye and vision problems
Oculentum (Oc), 360
Oculomotor nerve, 279
Oculopharyngeal muscular dystrophy, 809
Odour problems, in incontinence, 247
Odynophagia, 604
Oedema, **137**
  ankle, 144
  assessment tool, 486
  in cardiovascular disease, 486
  in heart failure, 511, 513
  in liver and gallbladder disease, 629
  in nephrotic syndrome, 684
  nursing assessment, 139–140, 662
  nursing management, 144

  in pigmented skin, 846
  pitting, 139, 625
  in respiratory disease, 539
  in stasis eczema, 851
  stump, 802
Oesophageal manometry, 570
Oesophageal spasm, diffuse, 602–603
Oesophageal varices, 594, **604**, 634
  bleeding, 604, 607, 634–635
Oesophagitis, **604–605**
  corrosive, 604, 605
  infective, 604–605
  reflux, 604, 605
Oesophagoscopy, 599
Oesophagus, **593**
  carcinoma, 605
  disorders, **602–603**
  diverticulum, 602
  foreign bodies, 603
  peptic ulceration, 606
  rings and webs, 603
Oestradiol, 707, 715
Oestriol, 707
Oestrogen, 227, 707
  adrenal, 399
  cancer risk and, 991
  cyclical changes, 707, 708, 710
  deficiency, 735
    urinary incontinence and, 234
  receptors (ER), in breast cancer, 782
  urinary incontinence and, 242
  see also Hormone replacement therapy
Oestrone, 707
Old age, definitions, 967–968
Older adults, 3, 8, **967–983**
  abuse, **981**
  alcohol misuse, 627, 628
  anaemia, 456
  bereavement and dying, **981**
  in breast cancer, 775
  cancer risk, 991
  cancer screening, 998
  cardiac rehabilitation, 509
  carers, **980–981**
  chronic illness/disability, 1055
  day surgery, 881
  dehydration, 138, 141
  demographic change, 967, 969
  depression, **974**
  drug therapy, **976–977**
  ear care, 374
  ear wax, 376
  epistaxis, 577
  eye tests, 341
  faecal incontinence, 243
  families, **971**
  fluid balance assessment, 957
  frail, **975–976**
  gastrointestinal changes, 597, 975
  health and health promotion, **977–979**
  hearing loss, 379
  hip (femoral neck) fractures, 830, 831, 832,
    929
  hypnotic drugs, 71
  hypothermia, 81, 87–88
  long-term care, **979–980**
  nurses' attitudes, 8, 970
    to pain, 115
    power and, 43, 44
  nursing management, **979–980**
  nutrition, **217**, 219, 220, **978–979**
  osteoarthritis, 812
  osteoporosis, 819
  pain perception/management, 115, 116

perioperative issues, *881–882*, 903
physical activity, *494*
preoperative assessment, 885
pressure ulcer risk, *187*, 976
renal function, 655
sexual health, 978
'single assessment process', 11
skin changes, 175–176, *848*, 975, 976
sleep, 63–64, *71*
spiritual aspects, **981**
stress response, *99*
tetanus immunization, 935
upper limb injuries, 833, 834
urinary incontinence, *see* Urinary
    incontinence
visual problems, 332, 975
wound dressings, *187*
wound healing, *179*
see also Ageing
Oldest old, 968, 969, **980**
Olecranon process fractures, 835
Olfaction, *see* Smell, sense of
Olfactometry, 570
Olfactory nerve, *279*
Oligodendrocytes, *275*
Oligodendrogliomas, 308
Oligomenorrhoea, *717*
Oliguria, 686
    in shock, 157, 510
Olive oil eardrops, *377*
Omentum
    greater, 592
    lesser, 592
'On–off effect', in Parkinson's disease, 320, 322
Oncogenes, 987
Oncological emergencies, **1014–1015**
Oncology nurse specialists, **1017**
    gynaecological, 721–722, 723–724
Ondansetron, *884*, 911, 1013, 1036
Onychomycosis (tinea unguium), 856, 858
Oocytes, 706, 707
Oogenesis, **707–708**
Oophorectomy, 718, 719
Openness, 45
Operating department assistant (ODA), 895
Operating department practitioner (ODP),
    895–896, 904
Ophthalmic medications, topical, *see* Eye
    medications, topical
Ophthalmic nurses, specialist, 332, 338
Ophthalmic problems, *see* Eye and vision
    problems
Ophthalmoscopy, 287, **338**
Opioid antagonist, 124
Opioids (narcotics), **123–124**
    addiction, 129
    in anaesthesia, *884*
    in back pain, 815
    in cancer pain, 1017
    in day surgery, 884
    endogenous, 113
    epidural, 127
    routes of administration, 125
    side-effects, 123–124
    strong, 1033–1034
    weak, 1033
Opportunistic infections, 257, 765
Optic chiasma, 335
Optic disc (blind spot), 333, *334*
Optic nerve, *279*, 333, *335*
Oral assessment, 139, **597**
    in haematological disorders, 449, 472
    in terminal illness, 1029
Oral cancer, 600, *601*

Oral care, *see* Mouth care
Oral contraceptive pill, *227*, 757
    in endometriosis, 734
Oral fluids, **144–145**
    see also Drinks; Fluid intake
Oral glucose tolerance test (OGTT), 402–403, 417
Oral hygiene, *see* Mouth care
Oral hypoglycaemic agents (OHAs), **417–418**,
    420
Oral rehydration solutions, 142
Orbit, 336
Orchid Cancer Appeal, 767
Orchidectomy
    nursing management, 747–749
    in prostate cancer, 700–701
    in testicular cancer, 747–748
Orchiopexy, 750
Orchitis, 750
Orem's self-care model, 1059
Organ of Corti, 370
Organ donation, 289, 1043
    kidney transplantation, 694–695
Organs
    ageing, **975**
    categories of monitoring and support, **949**
Orientation, assessment, *282*
Oropharyngeal airways, 898, *899*
Oropharynx, 566–567
Orthopaedic nurse specialist, *798, 799*
Orthopaedics, 793
    see also Musculoskeletal disorders
Orthoptic examination, 341
Orthotic devices (orthoses), **801–802**
Orthotist, 801
Osmolality, 136
    plasma, 397, 431
    urine, 431
Osmosis, 134–136
Osmotic diuretics, in raised intracranial pressure,
    301
Osmotic gradient, renal medulla, *658, 659*
Osmotic pressure, 136
    plasma, 136–137
Ossicles, auditory, 367, 369
Ossification, heterotopic, 325
Osteitis deformans (Paget's disease), **818**
Osteoarthritis (OA), **812–813**, 830
Osteocalcin, 208
Osteochondroma, 821
Osteogenesis imperfecta, **818–819**
Osteoidosteoma, 821
Osteomalacia, 208, **819**
Osteomyelitis, **820**
Osteophytes, 814
Osteoporosis, 210, 794, **819**
    aetiology and epidemiology, 819
    back pain, 815
    in critically ill patients, 953
    in Cushing's syndrome, 439
    fractures, 799, 815, 819, 831
    investigations, 797
    medical/surgical management, 819
    nursing management, 819, *820*
    postmenopausal, 735, 736
    prevention, 799
Osteosarcoma, 821
Osteotomy, *805*
Otalgia, 367, 368
    in ear infections, 382, 383
Otitis externa, 371, 372, **382–383**
    malignant, 382, 383
    nursing management, 383
Otitis media
    acute suppurative (ASOM), 372, **383–384**

chronic suppurative (CSOM), **384**
    complications, **385**
Otological diagnostic tests and investigations,
    372–374
Otorrhoea
    cerebrospinal fluid, *298*
    in ear infections, 383, 384
Otosclerosis, **379–380**
Otoscopy, **371–372**
Ottawa Charter (WHO 1986), 9
Outbreak control committee, 259
Outbreaks of infection, **258–259**
Outcome, 30
Outreach teams, critical care, **949**, *950*
Ovarian cancer, **722–724**, 991
Ovarian cycle, **707–708**, *710*
    follicular phase, 707
    luteal phase, 707–708
Ovarian cysts, 719–720
Ovarian drilling, 735
Ovarian follicles, 707
Ovaries, **706–708**
    surgical removal, 718, 719
    torsion, 719
Ovasites test, 848
Overactive bladder, 235, **240–242**
Overflow incontinence, 235, 696
Overlays
    low air loss, 192
    pressure-relieving, 192
    static, 191–192
Overweight
    type 2 diabetes risk, 403, 415
    see also Obesity
Ovulation, 707, 710
    body temperature change, 710–711
    induction, *760*
    investigations to confirm, 759
Ovum, blighted, **727–728**
Oxybuprocaine hydrochloride, 338
Oxygen (O_2)
    consumption
        during rewarming, 88
        measurement, 960
        myocardium, 483
    delivery, assessment, 960
    lack, *see* Hypoxia
    partial pressure in arterial blood (P_aO_2), 149,
        162, 535
    toxicity, 558
    transport, 446, **535**
Oxygen saturation
    assessment, 539
    critically ill patients, 958
    in hypothermia, 90
    postoperative monitoring, 908
    by pulse oximetry, 149, 541
    in shock, 161
Oxygen therapy, **557–559**
    in asthma, 544
    in COPD, 546–547, 557
    delivery devices, 558
    humidification of gases, 558, *559*
    long-term, 546–547
    monitoring, 557
    in myocardial infarction, 508
    nursing management, 558–559
    oxygen flow rates, 558
    in palliative care, 1039
    postoperative, **908**, 914
    problems, 557–558
    in shock, 163
    sleep and, 71
Oxytocin, 397, 772

P

P wave, 489
p53 gene, 988, 1004
Pacemakers, cardiac, 497–499
  permanent, 498–499
  temporary, 498
Pachymetry, 340
Packed cell volume (PCV), 450
Packed red cells, 451
$Paco_2$, 148, 149, 161–162
Paget's disease of bone, **818**
Paget's disease of nipple, 781
Pain, **111–131**
  acute, *see* Acute pain
  anatomy and physiology, 112–114
  assessment, **119–121**, 910
    in terminal illness, **1029–1030**
  biomedical model, 121
  biopsychosocial model, 121
  in blood disorders, 449
  bone, 465, 1032
  breast, **778**
  cancer, 1016–1017, **1032**
  central, 129
  chronic, *see* Chronic pain
  definitions, 111–112
  in liver disease, 635
  in liver, gallbladder and pancreatic disorders,
    629
  modulation, 113, *114*
  neuropathic, 112, 1032
  nociceptive, 112
  non-nociceptive, 112
  in pancreatitis, *644*, 645, 646
  perception, **112–113**, *114*
    factors affecting, 115–116
    mechanisms, 113
    modification, *114*
  phantom (limb), 112, 129, 524
  postoperative, *see* Postoperative pain
  psychogenic, 112
  referred, 112
  sleep disturbance, 65, 910
  somatic, 112
  spiritual, 112
  in terminal illness, **1032**
  threshold, 112
  tolerance, 112
  transduction, 113, *114*
  transmission, 113, *114*
  types, 112
  visceral, 112, 1032
Pain management, **123–128**
  in A&E department, *939*
  in back pain, 815
  barriers to effective, 117
  brain tumours, 309–310
  in burn injuries, 872, 873
  in cancer, **1016–1017**
  chronic non-malignant pain, 129–130
  in Guillain–Barré syndrome, 328
  in haemophilia, 478
  in myeloma, 465
  myths and misconceptions, 118
  non-pharmacological methods, 127–128,
    1017
  nursing standards, *122*
  in older adults, *115*, 116
  in pancreatic cancer, 648
  patient information and education, 118–119
  pharmacological methods, 123–127
  in pneumothorax, 561
  postoperative, *see* Postoperative analgesia

  in pre-existing substance misuse, 128–129
  recommendations and guidelines, 121–123
  requirements for effective, **117–123**
  in shock, 163
  in sickle cell crises, 462, 463
  staff education, 117–118
  structured approach, 121
  in terminal illness, **1032–1035**
  see also Analgesia; Analgesics
Painful stimuli
  to assess consciousness, 280, *282*
  assessing limb responses, 284
Palliative care, **1021–1046**
  20th century development, 1021–1022
  in breast cancer, 784, 787–788
  definition, 1022
  emergencies, 1040
  emotional support, 1026–1027
  ethical issues, 1027–1028
  in heart failure, 514
  historical background, 1021
  in leukaemia, 468
  in myeloma, 465
  nursing assessment, 1028–1031
  nursing management and interventions,
    1031–1040
  in ovarian cancer, 723–724
  radiotherapy, 1005
  settings, 1022–1025
  surgical treatment, 1004
  team, 1022
  in terminal stage, 1041–1042
  useful addresses, 1045
  see also Death; Dying; Terminal illness
Palliative care nurses, specialist, 1023,
    1040–1041
  referrals to, 1041
Pallor
  in pigmented skin, *846*
  see also Skin colour
Palpitations, 486
  in anaemia, *457*
  in arrhythmias, 499, 500, 501, 502
Pancreas, 400, 595, *622*, **623**
  endocrine, 394, **400–401**
    disorders, **403–428**
    in glucose homeostasis, 400–401
  exocrine, 623
  pseudocyst, 645
  tumours, **647–649**
Pancreatic cancer, **647–649**
Pancreatic disorders, 621–622, **643–649**
  clinical characteristics, 627–629
  diagnostic tests and investigations,
    625–626
  nursing assessment, 623–625
  prevention and health education, 626–627
  useful addresses/websites, 650–651
Pancreatic enzymes, 623
  supplements, 551, 646, 647, 648
Pancreatic islet cell tumours, **649**
Pancreatitis
  acute, **643–646**
    aetiology and epidemiology, 643
    clinical presentation, 644
    investigations, 644–645
    medical/surgical management, 645
    nursing management, 645–646
    pathophysiology, 643–644
  chronic, **646–647**
Pancreatoduodenectomy (Whipple's procedure),
    648–649
Pancytopenia, 463
  in cancer, 1013
  chemotherapy-induced, 467, 468, **471**

  see also Anaemia; Neutropenia;
    Thrombocytopenia
Panhypopituitarism, 430, 431
Panic attacks, 104, 151, 940
Panproctocolectomy, in inflammatory bowel
    disease, 615
Pantothenic acid, 209
Panuveitis, 362
P_aO_2, 149, 162, 535
Pap (cervical) smear, **714**, 999–1000
Papilloedema, 287, 333
Papules, 849, 851
  in lichen planus, 853
  in scabies, 859
Paracentesis, abdominal, 635
Paracetamol, 124, 884, 1033
  metabolism, 623
  overdose, 633
  rectal, 125
Paraesthesia, *289*, 328
Paralinguistics, **41**
Paralysis, *289*
Paralytic ileus, **911–912**
Paramedics, 925
Paramyotonia congenita, *809*, 810, 811
Paranasal sinuses, 566
  inflammation, *see* Sinusitis
  surgery, 574
  tumours, **587**
  washout, 573
Parapharyngeal abscess, 582
Paraphimosis, **752**
Paraphrasing, 48
Paraplegia, *289*, 1050
Paraquat, 319
Parasites Sellotape test, 848
Parathyroid glands, 394, **399**
  disorders, **436–437**
Parathyroid hormone (PTH), **399**, 436, 661
Parathyroidectomy, 437
Parenteral nutrition, **224–225**
  complications, 225
  nursing management, 225
  total (TPN), 224
Parenteral refeeding syndrome, *225*
Parenting, in chronic illness/disability, 1055
Paresis, *see* Weakness
Parietal lobe, 277
Parity, urinary incontinence and, 234
Parkinson's disease, **318–322**
  clinical presentation, 319, *320*
  epidemiology and aetiology, 319
  medical/surgical management, 319–321
  nursing management, 321–322
  pathophysiology, 319
Paronychia, **870**
Parotitis, 601
Paroxysmal atrial tachycardia (PAT), **501**
Partially sighted, registration, **342**
Partially Sighted Society, 365
Partnership in Action (1998), 102
Passing response, stigmatizing conditions,
    1053
Patch (skin) testing, 569, **848**, 851
Patellar apprehension test, *798*
Patellar fractures, 832
Paternalism, older people, 979
Paterson–Brown–Kelly syndrome, 603
Pathogens, 256, **257**
  conditional, 257
  conventional, 257
  opportunistic, 257
Pathologists, in critical care, 952
Patient allocation, 13
Patient-assisted transfer (PAT) slide, *900*, 901

Patient-controlled analgesia (PCA), **125–127**, 463, **910–911**
Patient-controlled epidural analgesia (PCEA), 127
Patient education (and information)
    acute pain management, 118–119
    in blood disorders, 455–456
    in cancer care, **1012**
    in chronic illness and disability, 1056, *1062*, 1063
    in COPD, 548
    in diabetes mellitus, **405–415**, 419–420
    for discharge, *920*
    eye medication, 346, *347*, 357
    preoperative, **890–891**
    stoma care, 612–613
    in urinary/faecal incontinence, 247
    viral hepatitis, 633
Patient-at-risk teams (PARTs), 949, *950*
Patients (clients)
    feedback and satisfaction, **35**
    labelling, 54–55
    stress affecting, **100**
    unpopular, *1052*
    wishes/choices, *7*, 18
Patient's Charter (1991), **28–29**
Peak expiratory flow rate (PEFR, peak flow), **540**
Peau d'orange, *782*
Pediculosis, **860–861**
Pellagra, 208–209
Pelvic adhesions, *760*
Pelvic floor, **230–231**
    assessment, 238
    biofeedback, 240
    dysfunction, 243
    education, **237–240**
    electrical stimulation, 240, 241–242
    neurological control, *231*
Pelvic floor exercises, 237, **238–239**, 672
    after transurethral resection of prostate, 697
    giving advice about, 716, 725
    for men, 238–239
    in overactive bladder, 241
    for women, 238
Pelvic inflammatory disease (PID), 716, **732–733**, 763
Pelvic nerve, 231
Pelvic surgery, deep vein thrombosis risk, *740*, 888
Pemphigoid, bullous, **865**
Pemphigus, **865**
Pemphigus Vulgaris Network, 875
Penectomy, 751–752
Penetrating wound, *934*
Penicillamine, 318
Penile cancer, **751–752**
Penile sheaths, 249
Penis, **743–744**
    erection, 743–744
    problems, **751–752**
    prostheses, 755, 756
    reconstructive surgery, 751–752
Pepsin, 593
Peptic ulceration, 103, **606**, *607*
Perception of light (PL), 339
Percutaneous endoscopic gastrostomy (PEG), 223, 953, 1004
Percutaneous myocardial revascularization, 504
Percutaneous transluminal angioplasty, 523
Percutaneous transluminal coronary angioplasty (PTCA), 504, 505
    in heart failure, 512
    in myocardial infarction, 507
Performance, relationship to stress, 93–94
Performance ('league') tables, **29**

Perfusion
    in multiple organ dysfunction, 167, 168
    peripheral, assessment, 160–161, 959
    pulmonary (Q), 535, 955
    in shock, 155, 157
Perianal abscess, **617**
Perianal care, in inflammatory bowel disease, 615
Pericardial effusion, 520
Pericardial rub, 520
Pericarditis, **520–521**
    constrictive, 520
Pericardium, 482
    disorders, **520–521**
Perichondritis, pinna, 381, **382**
Perimetrium, 709
Perimetry (visual field testing), 340
Perinephric abscess, 674
Perineum, 711
Periodic paralyses, familial, 808–810
Perioperative care, **879–922**
    older adults, *881–882*
    see also Intraoperative care; Postoperative care; Preoperative care; Surgery
Perioperative period, 879
Periorbital haematoma, bilateral, *298*
Periosteum, 794
Peripheral arterial/vascular disease (PAD/PVD), **523–524**
    clinical presentation, 194, 523
    in diabetes, 425
    see also Arterial (ischaemic) leg ulcers
Peripheral nerve disorders, **326–328**
Peripheral nervous system (PNS), 274, 279
Peripheral perfusion, assessment, 160–161, 959
Peripherally inserted central catheters (PICCs), parenteral nutrition, 224–225
Peristalsis, 592
Peritoneal cavity, 592
Peritoneal dialysis (PD), **691–693**
    automated (APD), 692
    continuous ambulatory (CAPD), 428, 692
    continuous cycling (CCPD), 692
    nutrition, 688
    sample regimen, *693*
Peritoneovenous shunt, 635
Peritoneum, **592**
Peritonitis, **608**
    acute, **603**
    in peritoneal dialysis patients, 692–693
Peritonsillar abscess, **582**
Pernicious anaemia, **458–459**
Persistent vegetative state, 61
Personal hygiene, 672
    after radioactive iodine therapy, 434
    critically ill patients, **952–953**
    during menstruation, *733*
    dying patients, 1041–1042
    in terminal illness, 1029
    unconscious patient, 290
Personal space, 40
Personality
    cancer-prone, 989
    effects of ageing, **972**
    self-awareness and, 45
    theories, and communication, **45–46**
    type A (stressful), 99, *100*, 107
    type B, 99
Petechia, *844*, *846*
Pethidine, 124, 127
Petrositis, 385
Peutz–Jeghers syndrome, 597
pH, 148–149
    arterial blood, 149, 162, 535
    regulation, 149

urine, 143, *664*, **665**
Phacoemulsification (phaco), 349
Phaeochromocytoma, **440–441**
Phagocytosis, 446
Phantom (limb) pain, 112, 129, 524
Pharmacokinetics
    in hypothermia, 91
    in older adults, **976**
    in renal dysfunction, *688*
Pharyngitis, **583**
Pharyngoscopy, 599
Pharynx, 566–567
Phenothiazines, *226*
Phenylephrine hydrochloride, ophthalmic, *344*, 350
Phenytoin, *226*
Philadelphia (Ph) chromosome, 468
Phimosis, 751, **752**
Phlebitis, 146, 527
Phonophobia, 311
Phosphate, *136*
    enemas, 1037
    homeostasis, renal contribution, **661**
    hormonal regulation, 399
    imbalance, *136*
        in chronic renal failure, 687
    serum, 671
Phosphofructosekinase deficiency, 810
Phospholipids, 204
Phosphorus, dietary, *207*, 210
Phosphorylase deficiency, 810
Photophobia, 311, 357, 362
    in albinism, 862
Photosensitivity, drug-induced, 871
Phototherapy, 862, 863
Phototypes (skin types), 846, *867*
Physical activity
    in blood disorders, 456
    cancer and, 990
    cardiovascular disease prevention, 494
    in chronic illness/disability, **1063**
    in diabetes, 428
    encouraging, in older people, *494*
    sleep and, 65, 70
    type 2 diabetes risk and, 416
    wound healing and, 180
    see also Exercise
Physical activity level (PAL), 203
Physical deformity, 1052
Physicians, in critical care, 952
Physiotherapists, in critical care, 952
Physiotherapy
    after nephrectomy, 678
    after renal transplantation, 696
    amputees, 524
    in back pain, 816
    in cystic fibrosis, 550
    in deep vein thrombosis, 526
    in inflammatory myopathies, 811
    in multiple sclerosis, 306
    patients in casts, 801
    postoperative, 914
    preoperative, 889
    in sports injuries, 823, 827
Pia, 278
Pigmentation
    changes, **846**
    disorders, **862–864**
    normal, **842**
    in pityriasis versicolor, 859
Piles (haemorrhoids), **617**
Pilocarpine eye drops, *338*, *344*
    in glaucoma, 356, 357
Piloerection, 77, 96
Pilonidal sinus, **617**

Pilosebaceous unit, **843**
Pin site care, *801*
Pineal body, 287, 394
Pinhole correction of vision, 339–340
Pinna, 368
  haematoma, **380–381**
  perichondritis, 381, **382**
  tumours, 389
Pioglitazone, 418
Pituitary gland, 394, **396–397**
  anterior, 396–397, *398*
    hyposecretion, **430–431**
  disorders, **428–431**
  posterior lobe, 396, 397
Pituitary tumours, 308, **428**
  ACTH-secreting, 438
  growth hormone-secreting, 428, 429
  hypopituitarism, 430, 431
  prolactinomas, 430
  surgical removal, 429
Pityriasis versicolor, **858–859**
Pityrosporum ovale, 854
Placebo response, **114**
Planning, care, **12**
Plaques, 844, 861
Plasma, **446**
  fresh frozen (FFP), 452
  osmolality, 397, 431
  osmotic pressure, 136–137
Plasma exchange, 452, *683*
Plasmapheresis, 452
Plaster of Paris casts, 800–801
Platelets, 446, 448
  counts, 476, *625*
  transfusions, 451, 457
Plethysmography, impedance (IPG), 525
Pleural cavity, 534
Pleural effusion, **561**, 723
Pleurectomy, 561
Pleuritic pain, 1032
Pleurodesis, 561
PLISSIT model, 1063
Plummer–Vinson syndrome, 603
Pneumatic compression system, intermittent, 902
Pneumococcal vaccine, *312*, 553
Pneumonia, **553–555**
  aspiration, 553, 893
  nosocomial, prevention, *961*
  see also Chest infections
Pneumothorax, **560–561**
  after central venous catheter insertion, 960
  after pacemaker insertion, 498
  postnephrectomy, 678
  spontaneous, 560
  tension, 560
  traumatic, 560
Podiatry
  in arterial leg ulcers, 524
  in diabetes, 427, 428
Podophyllin, 762
Police
  contacting absent relatives, 941
  in major disasters, 942
  in mental health problems, 939
  in rape and sexual assault, 937
Policies, 15
Pollution, cancer risks, 990
Polycystic kidney disease, **684–685**
  adult (APKD), 684–685
  autosomal recessive, *655*
Polycystic liver disease, 685
Polycystic ovary syndrome (PCOS), **734–735**
Polycythaemia, **459–460**
  primary proliferative (PPP), 459–460

secondary, 460
Polydipsia, 404, 431
Polymorphonuclear white cells, 446
Polymyositis (PM), 810, 811
Polyneuropathy, 327
Polysaccharides, 205
  non-starch (NSP), 205
Polyunsaturated fatty acids (PUFA), 204, 208
  coronary heart disease and, 216
  wound healing and, *218*
Polyuria, 404, 423, 431
Pons varolii, 276
PONV, *see* Postoperative nausea and vomiting
'Port wine' stain, 864
Portal circulation, 594
Portal hypertension, 594, 622, *629*, *634*
Portal vein, hepatic, 622
Portsmouth external fixation bar, *804*
Positioning
  in diabetic ketoacidosis, 424
  during eating, 221
  for epidural/spinal anaesthesia, 897, *898*
  immediate postoperative period, 908
  in pneumonia, 554
  in pressure ulcer prevention, 189–190
  in raised intracranial pressure, 302
  in retinal detachment, 354–355
  in shock, *163*
  sleep and, 70
  stroke patients, 293, *294*, *295*, 296
  surgical patients, **901–902**
  unconscious patient, 290
  in wound dehiscence, 918
Positron emission tomography (PET), 287–288, 1002
Post-anaesthetic recovery, **907–910**
Post-registration education and practice (PREP), **6–7**
Post-traumatic stress disorder (PTSD), **102**
Posterior chamber (eye), 333
Posterior cruciate ligament (PCL) tears, 826–827
Posterior drawer test, *798*
Post-herpetic neuralgia, 112, 312, 313
Postmenopausal women, **735–736**
  atrophic vaginitis, 732
  urinary incontinence, 234, 235, 242
  vaginal bleeding (PMB), 722
Postoperative analgesia, 125, *126*, **910–911**
  cataract surgery, 351
  cholecystectomy, 639, 640
  day surgery, **884–885**
  gynaecological surgery, 738
  nephrectomy, 678
  reasons for inadequate, 910
  in substance misusers, 129
  tonsillectomy, 581, 582
  see also Pain management
Postoperative care, **907–919**
  cataract surgery, 350–351
  discharge planning, 919
  ear surgery, 385
  fluid balance and monitoring, 912–913
  gynaecological surgery, 738–739
  immediate (recovery unit), 907–910
  joint replacement surgery, 813
  mobility and ambulation, 919
  nasal surgery, 574
  nutrition and fasting, 913
  orchidectomy, 748–749
  paralytic ileus/nasogastric intubation, 911–912
  radical cystectomy with urinary diversion, 681
  stoma surgery, 612–613, 681

tracheostomy, **585–586**
wound management, 914–919
see also Postoperative analgesia; Postoperative complications
Postoperative complications
  assessing potential for/prevention, **887–889**
  chest infection, *740*, 889, 914
  constipation, 913–914
  deep vein thrombosis, *740*, 914
  gynaecological surgery, 739, *740–741*
  renal/urinary, 913
Postoperative nausea and vomiting (PONV), *123*, 911, *912*
  after septal surgery, 578
  prophylaxis, 882–884, 892–893
Postoperative pain
  adverse effects, 117
  assessment, 119–121
  factors affecting, 115
  patient information and education, 118–119
  staff education, 118
Potassium (K$^+$), 134, *135*
  dietary intake, *207*, 210
  imbalance disorders, *135*
    in chronic renal failure, 687
    see also Hyperkalaemia; Hypokalaemia
  intravenous therapy, *148*, 423
  oral replacement therapy, 148
  renal regulation, 660
  serum, 669, 671
    in hypothermia, 90
Potassium iodide, 433
Potassium permanganate soaks/baths, 850, 865
Pouch of Douglas, *706*, 709
Poverty
  nutrition and, 212
  respiratory disorders and, 537
  in visual impairment, 342
  see also Financial problems
Power
  nurses and, **43**
  types, *43*
  see also Empowerment
Powerlessness, in chronic illness/disability, 1063
PR interval, 489
Practice nurses
  in chronic illness and disability, **1057**
  see also Community nurses
Pre-admission assessment, 885
  day surgery, 882–884
  musculoskeletal disorders, 796
  see also Preoperative assessment
Prednisolone eye drops, *345*, 362
Prednisone, *227*
Pregnancy
  asymptomatic bacteriuria, 672
  breast cancer, 782
  in cardiomyopathy, 518
  ectopic, **729–730**
  gestational diabetes, 403, 416
  iron deficiency anaemia, 458
  molar (hydatidiform mole), **729**
  nutrition, 217
  problems of early, **725–732**
  surgery and, 886
  termination, *see* Termination of pregnancy testing, 726
  in valvular heart disease, 516
Prehospital care, **924–925**
Prejudice, 1052
Preload, 165, 955
Premature atrial contraction (PAC), **500**
Premature ventricular contraction (PVC), 487, **501–502**
Premedication, 737, **894**

Premenstrual syndrome (PMS), *717*
Preoperative assessment, **885–889**
 cataract surgery, 349–350
 day surgery, 882–884
 fitness for surgery and anaesthesia, 885–887
 gynaecological surgery, 736–737
 musculoskeletal disorders, 796
 potential postoperative complications, 887–889
 see also Pre-admission assessment
Preoperative care, **885–895**
 cataract surgery, 350
 ear surgery, 385
 gynaecological surgery, **737**
 immediate measures, 894
 patient transfer, safety and identification, 895
 preventing postoperative complications, **887–889**
 psychological preparation, **889–891**
 radical cystectomy with urinary diversion, 679–681
 safety measures, **892–895**
 skin preparation, **887–888**
 stoma surgery, 612, 679–681
 see also Preoperative assessment
Prepuce (foreskin), 743, *752*
Presbyaccusis, **377–379**
Presbyopia, 341
Prescribing, nurse, 186, 248
Prescriptions exemption, in diabetes, 413
Pressure, 187, *188*
Pressure garments, burn injuries, 873–874
Pressure-reducing equipment, 191–192
Pressure-relieving equipment, 192
Pressure ulcers (sores), **187–193**
 in breathing difficulties, 72
 in cardiogenic shock, 510
 classification, 190–191
 in critically ill patients, 953
 epidemiology and aetiology, 187–188
 in Guillain–Barré syndrome, 328
 in multiple sclerosis, 307
 prevention, 189–190
  equipment, 191–193
  intraoperative, **902**
  see also Skin care
 risk assessment, 188–189
  in terminal illness, 1029
  tools, 188, *189*
 risk factors, 188
 risk in older patients, *187*, 976
 in spinal injuries, 325–326
 under casts, 801
 under orthotic devices, 802
Pretibial myxoedema, 432
Pretibial wound, *934*
Prevention, 991
 primary, 991
 secondary, 991, 1059
 tertiary, 991
Primary closed-angle glaucoma (PCAG), 355, **357–358**
Primary Ear Care Centre, 368, 375, 391
Primary intention, wound healing by, 176, 914
Primary lateral sclerosis (PLS), *323*
Primary nurse, 12
Primary nursing, 12
Primary open-angle glaucoma (POAG), 341, **355–357**
 medical/surgical management, *345*, 355–356
 nursing management, 356–357
Primary survey, **932–933**
Primidone, *226*
Prion proteins, 313
Private health care sector, quality in, **27**

Process, 30
Prochlorperazine, for vertigo, *385*, 386, 387, 388
Procidentia, complete, *724*
Proctoclysis, 147
Proctoscopy, 599
Professional conduct, code of, 6, *7*
Professional development, continuing (CPD), 6–7, 33
Professional misconduct, 6
Professional relationships, ending, **53**
Professional self-regulation, 33–34
Progesterone, *227*, 707
 cyclical changes, 707, *708*, 710
 serum, in infertility, 759
Progestogens
 contraceptive, 757
 in endometriosis, 734
Progressive bulbar palsy (PBP), *323*
Progressive muscular atrophy (PMA), *323*
Prohormone, 397
Proinsulin, 400
Projection (psychological), *97*
Prolactin (PRL), 397, *398*, 772
Prolactinomas, **430**
Prolapse, uterovaginal, **724–725**, 735
PromoCon, 250
Propofol, *884*, 899
Proprioception, loss of, *289*
Propionibacterium acnes, *852*
Propylthiouracil, 432–433
Prostaglandin analogues, *345*
Prostaglandin E₁, 754–755
Prostaglandins
 in menstruation, 710
 for termination of pregnancy, 728, 731
Prostate, 662, 742
 benign enlargement (hyperplasia) (BPH), 235, **696–699**
 disorders, **696–701**
 transurethral resection (TURP), **697–699**
Prostate cancer, **699–701**, 994
 management, 700–701
 screening, *700*, **1000–1001**
 stages, *700*
Prostate-specific antigen (PSA), *700*, 701, 1000–1001
Prostatectomy
 incontinence after, 238, 699, 701
 open, 697
 radical, 700, **701**
Prostatitis, 750
Prostheses
 breast, 784
 eye, 358
 joint replacement, 812
 nursing management, **802**
 penile, 755, 756
 surgical patients, 737, 894
 see also Implants
Prosthetic heart valves, 516
Protein energy malnutrition (PEM), 206, 217, 218
Proteins
 dietary, **203–204**
  dialysed patients, *688*, *693*
  in nephrotic syndrome, 684
  in Parkinson's disease, 322
 as energy source, 203
 serum (plasma), 215, 623
 in urine, *see* Proteinuria
Proteinuria, 142, **664–665**
 in diabetes, 424, 425
 in nephrotic syndrome, 684
 see also Albuminuria; Microalbuminuria

Prothrombin time (PT), 450, *625*
Proto-oncogenes, 987
Protocols, 15
Protozoa, 254
Proximal convoluted tubule (PCT), 656, **658**
Proximal humerus fractures, **825**, 834
Pruritus (itching), **853–854**
 aetiology, 853
 external auditory canal, *379*, 382
 in jaundice, 628, **629**
 management, 853–854
 nursing assessment, 844
 in scabies, 859
 in tinea, *857*, *868*
Pruritus ani, **616–617**, 853
Pseudo-addiction, 128–129
Pseudo-Cushing's syndrome, 439
Pseudogout, 807
Pseudohypoparathyroidism, 436
Pseudomembranous colitis (*Clostridium difficile* diarrhoea), 255, *256*, **616**
Pseudomonas aeruginosa infections, in cystic fibrosis, 551
Psoriasis, *379*, **861–862**
Psoriasis Association, 875
PSPS score, *189*
Psychiatric care, in A&E department, 940–941
Psychiatric liaison nurses, 941
Psycho-oncology, 1009
Psychological aspects
 ageing, 971
 cancer care, **1009–1011**
 disability and chronic illness, 1051, 1054
Psychological assessment
 in breast disorders, 772–773
 men, 744
 women, 737
Psychological problems
 in breast cancer, 785
 in incontinence, 232
 parenteral nutrition and, *225*
 in terminal illness, **1039–1040**
 in vitiligo, 863
 see also Anxiety; Depression; Mental health problems; Stress
Psychological support
 A&E staff, 942–943
 in brain tumours, 310
 in cancer, 1052
 in chronic illness/disability, **1062–1063**
 in diabetes, *402*, 405, 428
 family and friends, *see* Family, support
 in Guillain–Barré syndrome, 328
 in head injury, 302–303
 infertility treatment, 760
 in miscarriage, 726, 727, 728
 palliative care professionals, 1026, **1027**
 patients wearing orthoses, 802
 preoperative, **889–891**
 in resuscitation, 930–931
 surgical patients, 890–891
 in terminal illness, **1026–1027**
Psychosexual dysfunction, *see* Sexual dysfunction
Psychosexual therapy, 755
Psychosocial aspects
 ageing, 971, **972–974**
 brain tumours, 310
 pain perception/management, 115–116
 respiratory disease, 540, 548
 spinal injuries, 325
 see also Social factors
Psychosocial stressors, 98–99
Psychosocial theories of ageing, **972**
Psychotic episode, acute, 940

PTCA, *see* Percutaneous transluminal coronary angioplasty
Ptosis, **363**
Pubic hair, preoperative removal, 737
Public Health Laboratory Service, 259
Pubococcygeus muscle, 230, *231*
Puborectalis muscle, 230, *231*
Pudendal nerve, 231
Pudendum, 711
Pulmonary abscess, 517
Pulmonary artery, temperature, 85
Pulmonary artery catheters
    critically ill patients, **960**
    in shock, 162
Pulmonary artery occlusion/wedge pressures (PAOP/PAWP), 162, **488**, 960
Pulmonary circulation, 481
Pulmonary congestion, in heart failure, 511
Pulmonary embolism (PE), **526–527**
    i.v. infusions, 147
    in neurological problems, 290
    postoperative, *740*, 914
Pulmonary oedema
    in cardiogenic shock, 510
    in chronic renal failure, 687
    in heart failure, 511
Pulmonary perfusion (Q), 535, 955
    see also V/Q ratio
Pulmonary rehabilitation, **548**
Pulmonary stretch receptors, 534
Pulmonary valve, 483
Pulse
    critically ill patients, 958
    in fluid balance disorders, 140
    in heart failure, 511
    in neurological assessment, 284
    pacemaker patients, 498–499
    in shock, 160
    volume, 958
Pulse oximetry, 149, **541**
    critically ill patients, **958**
    postoperative, 908
    in respiratory disease, 539
    in shock, 161
Pulse pressure, 488
Pulses, arterial, **486–487**
    after renal angiography, 666
    legs (peripheral), 487, 523
Pulsus alternans, 511
Pupils, 333
    constriction (miosis), 333, 336
        in eye problems, 359, 362
        in neurological disorders, 284
    dilation (mydriasis), 333, 336
        in stress, 96
    fixed and dilated ('blown'), 283–284
    responses
        assessing, **283–284**, *338*
        in raised intracranial pressure, 299
Purkinje fibres, 483, 484
Purpura, *844*, *846*
Pus, 446
    swabs, 846, *847*
Pustules, *844*, 851
PUVA therapy, 862, 863
Pyelography, **667**
Pyelonephritis, **672–673**
    chronic, 673–674
    clinical presentation, 672
    management, 673
Pyloric stenosis, **607**
Pyloroplasty, 607
Pylorus, 593
Pyometria, 732
Pyrazinamide, 555, 675

Pyrexia, **78–79**
    in acute pancreatitis, *644*
    causes, 78
    in diabetic ketoacidosis, 423, 424
    in liver and gallbladder disease, *629*
    management, **86**
    in neutropenia, *1014*
    nutritional needs, 87
    risks and benefits, 79, *80*
    in shock, 164
    stages and patterns, 78–79
    transfusion-induced, 454
    water loss, 143
Pyridostigmine, 811
Pyridoxine, *see* Vitamin B$_6$
Pyruvate kinase (PK), serum, 811
Pyuria, sterile, 674

Q

QRS complex, 490
Quadriceps inhibition test, *798*
Quadriplegia, *289*, 796
Quality, 24
    audits, **34–35**
    cost and, **27**
    defining, **24**
    dimensions, **29–31**
    interventions, **32–33**
    models, **29–30**
    monitoring and evaluating, **34**
    in NHS, **24–26**
    in nursing care, **33–34**
    in private and voluntary sectors, **27**
    useful websites, 36
Quality assessment, 32
Quality assurance, 32
    cycle (spiral), 31
Quality circles, 32
Quality control, 32
Quality councils, 33
Quality enhancement, *31*, **32–33**
Quality improvement, 32
Quality improvement teams (QIT), 32–33
Quality of life
    in heart failure, 513–514
    as outcome of treatment, *997*
Quality management, **24–29**, 32
    total (TQM), 24, 30–31, 32
Quantitative ultrasound (QUS), 797
Questions, **48–50**
    closed, 49
    leading, 49
    multiple, 49
    open, 49
    open focused, 49
    rhetorical, 49
    value, 49–50
Quinsy (peritonsillar abscess), **582**

R

Racial differences, *see* Ethnic and racial differences
RADAR, 250, 838
Radial artery
    cannulation, 959
    pulse, 486–487
Radiant heating units, 903
Radiation
    exposure, cancer risk, **990**

heat transfer by, 76
Radioactive iodine therapy, 433, 434–435, 436
Radioallergosorbent test (RAST), 569, 848
Radiographers, in critical care, 952
Radiographs, plain film, *see* X-rays, plain
Radiology, *see* Imaging
Radionuclide scanning
    in cancer diagnosis, 1002
    in endocrine disorders, 402
    in GI disorders, 599
    in liver, biliary and pancreatic disorders, 626
    in renal disease, 667
Radiotherapy, 1004, **1005–1006**
    adjuvant, 1004
    brain tumours, *309*, 310
    in breast cancer, 784, 785, 787
    palliative, 1005
    pathophysiology, 1005
    in prostate cancer, 700
    safety issues, 1005–1006
    side-effects, 1005
    stem cell transplant recipients, 475
Radius fractures
    distal, 826, 835
    head of radius, 834–835
    shaft, 835
Range of motion (ROM), 794, 797
Range of motion (ROM) exercises
    in sports injuries, 823
    stroke patients, 293
Rape, **937**
Rash
    assessment in A&E, *935*
    distribution and configuration, **845**
    in meningitis, 311
    in rheumatic fever, 514
    in systemic lupus erythematosus, 817
Rationalization, *97*
Raynaud's phenomenon/disease, **524–525**
Re-registration, 6, 7
Reaction formation, *97*
Record-keeping, *see* Documentation
Recovery unit, postoperative, **907–910**, 947
Rectal bleeding, 598
Rectal examination, in urinary incontinence, 237
Rectal infusion, 147
Rectal prolapse, **617**
Rectocele, *724*, *725*
Rectovaginal pouch, *706*, 709
Rectum, 242, 596
    damage causing faecal incontinence, 243
    nerve damage, 243
    temperature measurement, *84*, 85
Recurrent laryngeal nerve paralysis, 586
Red cells (erythrocytes), **446**
    destruction in liver, 623
    disorders, **456–460**
    packed, 451
    sickling, 462
Reference nutritional intake (RNI), 202
Reflecting (in communication), 48
Reflection, **15–16**
    definition, 15
    models, 16
    written, 16
Reflective diary, 16, *17*
Reflective practice, **15–16**
Reflexes
    primitive, 286
    testing, 286, 287
    tonic neck, 294, 302
Reflux nephropathy, **673–674**
Refraction, **334–335**
Refractive errors, 335, 341

Regeneration, 176
Regional anaesthesia/analgesia, **896–897**
    in acute pain management, 124–125
    see also Epidural anaesthesia/analgesia
Register, professional, 6
Registration, requirements, 4–5, 5–6
Regression, 97
Regurgitation, 602, 605
    in anaesthesia, 900
    nasal, 286
Rehabilitation
    after joint replacement surgery, 813
    in cancer, **1016**
    cardiac, 508–509
    in chronic illness and disability, 1057
    in head injury, 303
    pulmonary, **548**
    settings, **1057**
    sports injuries, 823, 827, 828
    stroke, 293–296, 1057
    voice, 588
Rehydration, see Fluid replacement
Relaxation
    in pain management, 128
    progressive muscle, 107–108
    to promote sleep, 69–70
    in stress management, **107–108**
Relevance to need, 30
Reliability, definition, 119
Religious issues
    animal-derived insulins, 412
    in cancer care, 1012
    dying patients, 1042
    food acceptability, 212
    preoperative hair removal, 888
    in sudden death, 941
REM sleep, 60, 62
Renal abscess, **674**
Renal angiography, **666**
Renal arteries, 656
Renal biopsy, **667–668**
Renal blood vessels, congenital anomalies, 655
Renal calculi (nephrolithiasis), **676–677**, 953
Renal cell carcinoma, 677
Renal colic, 676
Renal disease, 653, **682–685**
    anaemia, 683, 687
    drugs and, 688–689
    fluid status, 141
    glomerulonephritis, 683–684
    nephrotic syndrome, 684
    reflux nephropathy, 673–674
    in systemic lupus erythematosus, 817
    tubulointerstitial, 684
    see also Diabetic nephropathy; Polycystic
        kidney disease
Renal failure, **685–696**
    acute (ARF), **685–686**
        aetiology, 685
        clinical presentation, 686
        investigations, 670, 671, 686
        management, 686
        in multiple organ dysfunction, 168
        pathophysiology, 685–686
        renal replacement therapy, 689, **693–694**,
            963
        in shock, 157
    chronic (CRF), **686–689**
        aetiology, 687
        blood tests, 670, 671
        clinical effects, 687–689
        patient compliance, 689
    end-stage (ESRF), 686–687
        breaking bad news, 668
        in diabetes, 425, 426, 428, 682–683

see also Renal replacement therapy
    in heart failure, 511
    in myeloma, 465
Renal function
    age-related decline, 655, 975
    in critically ill patients, 956
    decline, in chronic renal failure, 686,
        687–688
    investigations, 667, 669–671
    monitoring, in diabetes, 682
    physiology, **656–660**
    postoperative, **913**
Renal osteodystrophy, 687
Renal pelvis, 655–656
    transitional cell tumours, 679
Renal replacement therapy, **689–696**
    in acute renal failure, 689, **693–694**, 963
    in critically ill patients, **963**
    in diabetic nephropathy, 682–683
    in multiple organ dysfunction, 169
    see also Dialysis; Haemodialysis; Peritoneal
        dialysis; Renal transplantation
Renal support, 949
Renal transplantation, 690, **694–696**
    graft rejection, 696, 697
    nephrectomy of transplanted kidney, 677, 678
    nursing management, 695–696
    organ donation, 677–678, 694–695
Renal trauma, **677**
Renal tuberculosis, **674–676**
Renal tubule, 656
    distal convoluted (DCT), 656, **659–660**
    proximal convoluted (PCT), 656, **658**
    see also Collecting duct, renal; Loop of Henle
Renin, 658
Renin–angiotensin–aldosterone (RAA) system,
        658
    blood pressure regulation, 486
    in critically ill patients, 956
    in shock, 156–157
Repaglinide, 418
Repair, tissue, 176
Repression, 97
Reproducibility, definition, 119
Reproductive problems, **705–769**
    in chronic renal failure, 688
    useful addresses/websites, 767
Reproductive tract
    female, **706–711**
    male, **741–744**
Research, **13–15**
    action, 15
    cancer, **1018**
    critical appraisal, 14
    methods, 14–15
    purposes, 14
    qualitative, 14
    quantitative, 14
Reservoirs of infection, 256
Residential homes, 979, 1056
Resistance
    reaction, in stress response, 96–97
    to stigma, 1053
Respiration, see Breathing
Respiratory acidosis, **150–151**, 535
    blood gas values, 148
    in critically ill patients, 958
    in respiratory failure, 557
Respiratory alkalosis, **151**
    blood gas values, 148
    in critically ill patients, 958
Respiratory arrest, 495
Respiratory assessment, **538–540**
    critically ill patients, **957–958**
    in fluid balance disorders, 140

    in head injury, 300
    in major trauma, 932
    postoperative, **908**
    preoperative, 889
    in terminal illness, **1028–1029**
Respiratory centre, 534, 954
Respiratory depression, 124, 538
Respiratory disorders, **533–563**
    in acute pancreatitis, 644, 645–646
    causes/predisposing factors, 535–538, 539
    in chronic renal failure, 687
    critically ill patients, 955
    impaired wound healing, 178
    investigations, 540–542
    in myopathies, 810, 811
    nursing assessment, 538–540
    psychosocial factors, 540
    sleep effects, 62, **71–72**
    symptoms, 539
    in terminal illness, **1038–1039**
    trigger factors, 538
    useful websites, 562
    see also specific disorders
Respiratory failure, **557–560**, 958
    in COPD, 547, 548, 557
    in Guillain–Barré syndrome, 328
    mechanical ventilation, 961
    treatment, 557–560
    type I, 548, 557
    type II, 547, 548, 557
Respiratory function tests, **540–541**
Respiratory monitoring, basic, 949
Respiratory nurse specialists, 546, 547
Respiratory rate, **538**
    in critically ill patients, 957
    in neurological assessment, 284
    in shock, 157
Respiratory stimulants, 559
Respiratory support
    advanced, 949
    basic, 949
    in Guillain–Barré syndrome, 328
    see also Ventilation, mechanical
Respiratory system, **533–535**
    in acid–base balance, 149, 535
    anatomy, 533, 534
    critically ill patients, **954–955**
    during sleep, 61
    physiology, 534–535
    in shock, 157, 160
    in stress, 96, 103
Respiratory tract infections, **552–556**
    in cystic fibrosis, 550
    lower (LRTI), 553
        see also Chest infections; Pneumonia
    nursing assessment, 539
    in spinal injuries, 325
    sputum assessment, 541–542
    upper (URTI), 552–553
    see also Tuberculosis
Respite care, 981
Responsibility, student nurses, 7
Rest
    in unstable angina, 506
    in viral hepatitis, 632
    wound healing and, 179
    see also Bed rest; Immobility/immobilization
Rest pain, in peripheral arterial disease, 523,
        524
Restless legs, 65
Restlessness, dying patients, 1042
Restraint, acutely disturbed patients, 941
Results, waiting for, 100
Resuscitation
    in A&E department, **929–931**

Resuscitation *(continued)*
  in burn injuries, 872
  deciding not to, 496, *497*
  health and safety, 930
  in major trauma, 932–933
  psychological care, 930–931
  in shock, 162–163
  team, 930
  witnessed, 931, *932*
  see also Cardiopulmonary resuscitation
Resuscitation area, A&E department, 929
Retained products of conception, 727
Retching, 1035
Reteplase, 507
Reticular activating system (RAS), 59, 61
Reticulocyte count, 450
Retina, 333
  detachment, 349, **354–355**
  physiology, **335–336**
Retinal artery, central, 333
Retinoic acid, topical, *852*
all-trans-Retinoic acid (ATRA), 477
13-cis-Retinoic acid, *852*
Retinol, 205, 335
Retinopathy, diabetic, *see* Diabetic retinopathy
Retirement, 968, 971
Retrograde urography (pyelography), 667
Retroperitoneal (position), 592
Retropharyngeal abscess, 582
Revascularization
  percutaneous myocardial, 504
  peripheral arterial, 523, 524
Rewarming, **88–89**
  active external, 89
  active internal, 89
  in frostbite, 91
  guidelines, *88*
  passive external, 88–89
  shock, 90
  see also Warming
Rhesus blood group system, **447**
Rhesus sensitization, anti-D prophylaxis, 447,
  727, 730, 731
Rheumatic fever, acute, **514**
Rheumatic heart disease, 514, *515*
Rheumatoid arthritis (RA), **805–807**, 815
Rhinitis, **570–571**
  allergic, 571, *572*
  atrophic, 571
  vasomotor, 571, *572*
Rhinomanometry, 569
Rhinophyma, 852
Rhinorrhoea
  cerebrospinal fluid, *298*
  in sinusitis, 573
Rhinoscopy
  anterior, 568
  posterior, 568, *569*
Rhinosinusitis, chronic, *573*
Rhodopsin, 335
Rhythmic pattern disorders, **72**
Riboflavin, *see* Vitamin B₂
RICE regimen, 823, 826, 828
Rickets, 208, 819
Rifampicin, *226*, 555, 675
Rightness, **18**
Rigidity, *289*
  in Parkinson's disease, 319, 321
Rigor, 87
Ring pessary, in uterovaginal prolapse, 725
Ringer's lactate, *145*
Ringworm, *see* Tinea
Rinne's test, 373
Rivastigmine, 322
Road traffic accidents, 928

head injury, 297
  lower limb fractures, 830, 832
  prevention, 288, 799
Rod body disease, *809*
Rodent ulcer (basal cell carcinoma), 389, **868**
Rods, 333, 335
Rosacea, **852–853**
Rose bengal, *345*, 363
Rosiglitazone, 418
Rotator cuff tendinitis/tears, **823–824**
Rovsing's sign, 608
Roy adaptation model of nursing
  in chronic illness and disability, 1059
  nausea and vomiting in cancer, *1010*
  responses to altered body image, 1015
Royal College of Nursing (RCN), 944
  clinical effectiveness, 33
  standard-setting, 25, 31
Royal National Institute for the Blind (RNIB),
  342, 343, 365
Royal National Institute for the Deaf (RNID),
  375, 391
Royal Society for the Prevention of Accidents
  (RoSPA), 838, 944
Rule of nines, burns assessment, 872

S

Saccharin test, 570
Safe sex, promoting, 716, 757, *761*
Safety
  cytotoxic chemotherapy drugs, 1008
  intraoperative, **903–905**
  manual handling, 900–901
  older people with dementia, *979*
  preoperative measures, **892–895**
  radiation, 1005–1006
  resuscitation in A&E and, 930
  in visual impairment, 342–343
Salbutamol, 543
Salicylic acid, topical, 862
Saline solutions, *145*
Saliva, 593
  lack of, 600–601
Salmeterol, 543
Salpingectomy, 730
Salpingitis, **732–733**
Salpingo-oophorectomy, bilateral (BSO), 718
Salpingostomy, *760*
Salt (sodium) intake, *207*, 210, *419*
  in chronic renal failure, 687
  in heart failure, 513
Saltatory conduction, 275
Samaritans, 1045
Saphenous vein grafts, 504, 527
Saunders, Dame Cicely, 1022
Scabies, **859–860**
Scalds, 871, *935*
Scales, *844*
Scaphoid fractures, 835
Scars, *844*
  burn injuries, 873–874
  formation, 178
  hypertrophic, 861, 873–874
Schatzki ring, 603
Schizophrenia, 940
Schwann cells, *274*, 275
Sciatica, 814
Scintigraphy, *see* Radionuclide scanning
Sclera, 332, *333*
Scoliosis, *798*
Scoliosis Association, 838
Scottish Intercollegiate Guidelines Network, *14*

Scratching, 853
  in atopic eczema, 850
  nursing assessment, 844
  in scabies, 859
Screening
  cancer, **996–1001**
  genetic, *537*, **998**, *999*
  principles, 997–998
Scripting, 51–52
Scrotum, 741
Scrub nurse, 904
Seasonal affective disorder (SAD), 72
Sebaceous cysts, 861
Sebaceous glands, 174, **843**
Seborrhoeic dermatitis, **854**
Seborrhoeic keratosis, **867–868**
Sebum, 174, 843
Second messengers, 396
Secondary gains, 1053
Secondary intention, wound healing by, 176,
  914
Secondary survey, 933
Secretin, 594, 595
Security, sleep and, 70
Sedation
  acutely disturbed patients, 941
  critically ill patients, 952, 961
  preoperative, 894
Sedatives, urinary incontinence and, *236*
Seizures, **313–315**
  absence, *314*
  atonic, *314*
  brain tumours, 308
  myoclonic, *314*
  nursing management, 315
  partial, 313, *314*
  primary generalized, 313, *314*
  in terminal illness, 1040
  tonic-clonic, *314*
Selective oestrogen receptor modulator (SERM),
  736
Selegiline, in Parkinson's disease, 320
Selenium, *207*, **210**
  deficiency, 210
Self-awareness, **44–45**, 48
  cultural, *42*
  personality and, *45*
Self-care
  in chronic illness/disability, 1051, *1055*, *1059*
  postoperative, 919
  skin conditions, 841
Self-concept, 44
Self-disclosure, 48
Self-esteem
  assessment, 1060
  in inflammatory bowel disease, 616
Self-harm, deliberate, **940**
Self-help groups, 107
Self-image, *see* Body image
Self-inflicted conditions, stigma of, 1052
Sellick's manoeuvre, 900
Sellotape test, parasites, 848
Selye, Hans
  general adaptation syndrome (GAS), 94–97
  local adaptation syndrome (LAS), 97
  on stress, 93, 94
Semen, 742–743
  analysis, 759
Semi-circular canals, 370
Semilunar valves, *482*, 483
Seminal vesicles, 742
Seminoma, 746
Senescence, 969, 974, 987
Sengstaken–Blakemore oesophageal tube, 604
Sensation, cutaneous, 175

Sensory impairments, *289*
  in multiple sclerosis, 304
  in spinal injuries, 326
  in stroke, *292, 293*
Sensory nerves, 274
Sensory perception, critically ill patients, 954
Sentinel node, in breast cancer, 783
Sentinel piles (perianal skin tags), **617**
Sepsis, 158, 257
  hypotension in, 955
  nutrition, 217–218
Septic arthritis, **812**
Septic shock, 155, 158
  in cancer, **1014**
  defining criteria, *158*
  management, **167**
  mortality, 153
  patients at risk, *159*
  transfusion-associated, 454
Septicaemia
  i.v. infusions causing, 147
  meningococcal, 311
Sequestrectomy, *805, 820*
Serotonin, 61
Sertoli cell tumours, 746
Sertoli cells, 742
Serum, 446
Severe Disablement Allowance, *1061*
Sevoflurane, *884*
Sex differences, *see* Gender differences
Sex hormones
  adrenal cortical, 399
  female, **707**
  see also Androgens; Oestrogen; Progesterone
Sexual assault, **937**
Sexual dysfunction, 757
  in cancer, 473, 1016
  in chronic illness/disability, 1055, 1060,
    1063
  in chronic renal failure, 688
  in inflammatory bowel disease, 616
  male, **752–756**
  in spinal injuries, *325*
  in testicular cancer, 748
Sexual health, **757–760**
  older adults, 978
  promotion (safe sex), 716, 757, *761*
  useful addresses/websites, 767
  see also Contraception; Infertility
Sexual history-taking, 712, 758, *762*
Sexual intercourse
  after gynaecological surgery, *739*
  after transurethral resection of prostate, 699
  hepatitis B and D transmission, 627
Sexually transmitted (acquired) infections
    (STIs/SAIs), 732–733, **761–765**
Shared governance, 26, 34
Sharpey's fibres, 794
Sharps disposal, 267, *632*
  diabetic patients, 409
Shaving, preoperative, 737, 887
Shear, 188
Shearing injury, brain, 298
Sheath, urinary, 249
Shift work, 63
  in diabetes, 414
Shingles (herpes zoster), **312–313**, 846, 855
Shivering, 77, 81
  in hypothermia, 90
  postoperative, **908–909**
  in pyrexia, 164
Shock, **153–171**
  in acute pancreatitis, *644*
  anaphylactic, *see* Anaphylaxis/anaphylactic
    shock

cardiogenic, *see* Cardiogenic shock
compensated, 155
decompensated, 155, **157**
definition, 153–154
distributive, 155, *159*
guidelines for management, *163*
irreversible, 155–156
monitored signs, 160–162
neurogenic, 155, *159*
nursing assessment, 159–162
nursing management, 162–166
obstructive, 155, *159*
pathophysiological effects, 156–157
patients at risk, *159*
postoperative, **909**
progressive, 155
rewarming, 90
septic, *see* Septic shock
signs, 160–162
spinal, 155, *159*, 324
stages, 155–156
types, 154–155
  see also Multiple organ dysfunction; Systemic
    inflammatory response syndrome
Shock-wave lithotripsy, renal calculi, 676
Short-chain fatty acids (SCFAs), 205
Short-sightedness (myopia), 335, 341
Short stomach syndrome, 606
Shoulder
  acromioclavicular (AC) separation, 825
  dislocation, **824**, 834
  frozen, **824**
  rotator cuff tendinitis/tears, **823–824**
Showering, *see* Bathing/showering
Sialadenitis, 601
Sick day rules, type 1 diabetes mellitus, 413–414
Sickle cell crises, 462, 463
Sickle cell disease, **461–463**
Sigmoid colon, 596
Sigmoid sinus thrombosis, 385
Sigmoid volvulus, 604
Sigmoidoscopy, 599, 614, 1001
Sildenafil citrate (Viagra), 754
Silence
  in communication, 48
  promoting sleep, 69
Silicone breast implants, 789, 790
Sims speculum, 713, 714
'Single assessment process', older adults, 11
Sinoatrial (SA) node (sinus), 483, 484
Sinus bradycardia, **497–499**
  aetiology, 497
  medical management, 497
  nursing management, 497–499
Sinus rhythm, 488, 489
Sinus tachycardia, **499**
Sinuses, paranasal, *see* Paranasal sinuses
Sinusitis, **573–574**
  acute, 573, **574**
  chronic, 573
Sip feeding, 222
SIRS (systemic inflammatory response
    syndrome), **157–159**
Skeleton, **793–794**
Skene's glands, 711
Skills, teaching, 10
Skin, **173–176, 841–843**
  ageing, 175–176, *848, 975, 976*
  anatomy, 173–175
  appendages, **843**
  assessment, *176*, **844–846**
    in blood disorders, 449
    in cardiovascular disease, 486
    critically ill patients, 957
    in liver, biliary and pancreatic disorders, 625

  in terminal illness, 1029
  atrophy, *844*
  basement membrane, 174
  biopsy, **848**, 1001
  cleansing, preoperative, 887, 905
  commensal microorganisms, 843, 887
  cultured, 874
  cysts, *844*, **861**
  dry, 848
  drying technique, 849
  erythema, *see* Erythema
  functions, **175**, 842
  healthy, maintaining, **849**
  hydration, 848
  layers, 174–175
  maceration, *179*
  normal flora, 843
  patch testing, 569, **848**, 851
  pigmentation, *see* Pigmentation
  preparation, surgical patients, **887–888**, 905
  pressure damage, *see* Pressure ulcers
  protective role, 175, **842–843**, 854
  scrapings, 847
  swabs, 846, *847*
  thermoregulatory function, 77, 175
  turgor, *139, 486, 663, 957*
  types, 846, *867*
Skin cancer, **868–869**
  health promotion, *867*
  non-melanoma (NMSC), 868
  risk factors, 990
  see also Melanoma, malignant
Skin care
  amputees, 802
  in atopic eczema, 850–851
  dying patients, 1041–1042
  in incontinence, 247
  in liver disease, 632, 636
  in lymphoedema, 786
  patients in traction, 799, *801*
  principles, 176
  in spinal injuries, 325–326
  in venous ulceration, *197*
Skin colour
  in anaemia, *457*
  assessment, 846
  in cardiovascular disease, 486
  critically ill patients, 957
  in respiratory disease, 539
Skin grafts, 872, 874
Skin infections, **854–859**
  in atopic eczema, 850
  bacterial, 854–855
  blistering, 864–865
  fungal, 855–859
  viral, 855
  see also Infestations, skin
Skin infestations, **859–861**
Skin problems, **841–876**
  benign, **861**
  blistering disorders, **864–867**
  in Cushing's syndrome, 439, 440
  diagnostic tests and investigations, **846–848**
  disease prevention/health education,
    848–849
  distribution and configuration, **845**
  documentation, 846, *847*
  ear care, 374
  inflammatory, **849–854**, 862
  keratin synthesis disorders, **861–862**
  in liver disease, *629*
  nursing assessment, **843–846**
  stress-related, 103
  in systemic disorders, **870–871**
  useful addresses, 875

Skin problems (continued)
  vascular disorders, **864**
  in venous ulceration, 194
Skin rash, see Rash
Skin tags, perianal, **617**
Skin (peripheral) temperature, 76, 85–86
  in cardiovascular disease, 486
  core temperature difference, 76, 160–161,
    959
  critically ill patients, 957
  in fluid balance assessment, 663
  in shock, 160–161
Skin tumours, **867–869**
  benign, 867–868
  malignant, see Skin cancer
Skinfold thickness, 214
Skull fractures, 298
  basal, 298
Sleep, **59–74**
  assessment, 68
  common disorders affecting, 71–72
  critically ill patients, 64, 954
  deprivation, 62–63
  disorders, 65–67
  factors affecting normal, 63–64
  factors interrupting, 64–65, 910
  internal controls, 59–61
  latency, 65
  non-REM, 60
  physical changes during, 61–62
  physiology, 59–60
  promotion, 67–71
    non-pharmacological methods, 69–70
    nursing interventions, 67–70
    pharmacological methods, 69, 70–71
  purpose, 62–63
  REM, 60, 62
  in spinal injuries, 326
  stages, 60
  in terminal illness, 1030–1031
  useful websites, 73
  in viral hepatitis, 632
  wound healing and, 179
Sleep apnoea/hypopnoea, obstructive, **67**, 216
Sleep hygiene, 66
Sleep inversion, 157
Sleep paralysis, 60
Sleep terrors, **67**
Sleep–wake cycle, 59–60
  desynchronization, 63
  neurochemical controls, 60–61
Sleepwalking, **67**
Slides, patient-assisted transfer (PAT), 900, 901
Slit lamp examination, 339
Slough, debridement, 181–182
Small cell lung cancer (SCLC), 549, 993–994
Small intestine, **594–595**
SMART goals, 12
Smegma, 751
Smell, sense of (olfaction), 566
  assessment, 570
  loss of, 289, 568
Smith fracture, 835
Smoking, **535–537**
  in blood disorders, 456
  breast infections and, 779
  cancer risk, 990
  cessation, **536–537**, 716
  COPD and, 537, 545
  coronary heart disease risk, **494**
  in diabetes, 403, 414
  ectopic pregnancy and, 729–730
  history, 539
  inflammatory bowel disease and, 613

lung cancer and, 549
osteoporosis and, 819
pancreatic cancer and, 627
in peripheral arterial disease, 524
in Raynaud's phenomenon/disease, 524, 525
respiratory effects, 535–536, 537, 538
surgical patients, 889
urinary incontinence and, 234
see also Nicotine
Snellen chart, 339
Snoring, 67
Snuffbox, anatomical, 835
Soap
  for handwashing, 261, 262
  substitutes, 849, 850, 862
Social acceptability, 30
Social activity, in inflammatory bowel disease,
    616
Social assessment
  in breast disorders, 772
  in chronic illness and disability, 1060
  men, 744
  preoperative, 737
  in terminal illness, 1031
Social contact, 46, **47–53**
Social factors
  in adaptation to impairment, 1054
  in disability and chronic illness, 1051
  see also Psychosocial aspects
Social isolation, see Isolation (social)
Social problems, in A&E department, **936–938**
Social readjustment rating scale, 98–99, 105
Social security benefits, 1031, 1061
Social services
  in chronic illness and disability, 1056, 1061
  in visual impairment, 342, 343
Social skills groups, 107
Social workers
  in chronic illness and disability, 1060, 1061
  in palliative care, 1025
Socioeconomic factors
  cancer, 990
  constipation, 609
  liver, biliary and pancreatic disorders, 624
  see also Poverty
Sodium (Na+), 134, 135
  balance, regulation, 138
  dietary intake, see Salt (sodium) intake
  imbalance, 135
  replacement therapy, 147
  serum, 670–671
  urinary, in shock, 161
Sodium bicarbonate solutions, 145
Sodium–potassium (Na–K) pump, 136
Soft tissue injuries, 934, 935
Somatic pain, 112
Somatostatin, 398, 400
Somnambulance, **67**
Somnolence, excess, 66
Sorbitol, 425
Space
  intimate, 40
  personal, 40
Space blankets, 88
Spacers, large-volume, 543
Spasticity, 277, 289
  in multiple sclerosis, 306–307
  in myopathies, 810
  in spinal injuries, 326
  in stroke, 293
Specific gravity, urine, 143, **664**
Specimens, safe collection and handling, 259,
    260, 631
Spectacles, surgical patients, 737, 894, 909

Speculum examination, vagina and cervix, 713,
    714
Speech, 567
  rehabilitation, 588
  swallowing problems and, 212–213, 286
  in terminal illness, 1031
Speech and language therapist (SLT)
  in critical care, 952
  in Parkinson's disease, 321
  in swallowing problems, 213, 222, 286
  in throat problems, 586, 588
Spermatic cord, 741
Spermatogenesis, 742, 743
Spermatozoa, 742
  analysis in infertility, 759
  cryopreservation, 748
  production, 742, 743
Spermicides, 757
Spermiogenesis, 742, 743
Sphincter of Oddi (hepaticopancreatic
    sphincter), 594, 623
Sphincterotomy, endoscopic, 639, 642
Spinal anaesthesia, **896–897**, 898
  nursing management, 897
  total, 127
  versus epidural anaesthesia, 897
Spinal boards, 932, 933
Spinal cord, 276, 280
  degeneration, in B$_{12}$ deficiency, 209, 459
  disorders, **323–326**
  pain pathways, 113
  stimulation, 816
Spinal cord compression (SCC), 324,
    1014–1015, 1040
  effects of delayed diagnosis, 1015
  in myeloma, 465
Spinal fusion, 816
Spinal injuries, **324–326**
  aetiology, 324
  clinical presentation, 324
  common problems, 325–326
  management, 324
  nursing management, 324–326
Spinal Injuries Association, 325
Spinal manipulation, 816
Spinal micturition centre, 231
Spinal nerves, 279, 280
Spinal shock, 155, 159, 324
Spinal stenosis, **814–815**
Spinal surgery, 324
Spinal tumours, **324**, 815
Spiral arteries, 709, 710
Spiritual assessment
  preoperative, 737
  in terminal illness, 1031
Spiritual care
  cancer, **1011–1012**
  dying patients, 1042
  old age, **981**
Spiritual pain, 112
Spironolactone, in heart failure, 511
Splenectomy, 476
Sponging, tepid water, 86, 87
Sports injuries, **822–828**
  joints, 823
  lower limb, 826–828
  prevention, 799, 822
  sprains and strains, 822–823
  strapping, 802
  upper limb, 823–826
Sports participation, in stress management, 106
Sprains, **822**, 823
Sputum, **541–542**
  observation, 541–542

in tuberculosis, 555
Squamous cell carcinoma (SCC), 389, **868**
St John's wort, 106
ST segment, 490
    depression, 505
    elevation, 507, 520
Staff, *see* Health care professionals
Staff education
    to improve standards, 33–34
    in pain management, 117–118
    see also Nurse education programmes
Staffing, food intake and, 221
Staging, cancer, 1003–1004
Standards, **30–31**
    of care, **23–37**
    improving, **33**
    monitoring, evaluating and auditing,
        34–35
    setting, **30–31**
    structure–process–outcome approach, *31*
    triage in A&E, 926
    useful websites, 36
    using, *31*
Stapedectomy, 380
Stapes, *368*, *369*
Staphylococcus aureus
    breast infections, 779
    methicillin-resistant (MRSA), 255, 887
    osteomyelitis, 820
    toxic shock syndrome (TSS), 155, *733*
Staphylococcus epidermidis, 672
Staphylococcus saprophyticus, 672
Staples, skin, 915, *936*
Starch, 205
Starling's law of the heart, 165, 955
Stasis eczema, **851**
Static overlays, 191–192
Statins (HMG-CoA reductase inhibitors), 427,
        494, 504
Status epilepticus, *314*, *316*
Statutory Sick Pay (SSP), *1061*
Steam
    inhalations, after sinus surgery, 574
    treatment, chalazion, *363*
Steatorrhoea, 622, 623, 626, 646
Steinart's disease, *809*
Stem cell factor (SCF), *448*
Stem cell rescue, 474
Stem cell transplantation, *see* Haemopoietic stem
        cell transplantation
Stem cells, haemopoietic, *see* Haemopoietic stem
        cells
Stenting
    bile duct, 642, 648
    coronary artery, 504, 505
Stercobilinogen, 622
Sterilization, female, 757
Stevens–Johnson syndrome (SJS), **866–867**
Stigma, **1052–1053**
    cultural variations, 1053
    disability and chronic illness, 1048, 1051
    responses to, 1052–1053
    sexually acquired infections, 761
    types, 1052
Stings, *935*
Stitches, *see* Sutures
Stockings, compression, *see* Compression
        hosiery/stockings
Stoma
    adjusting to, *616*
    discharge advice, 613
    postoperative care, 612–613, 681
    preoperative care, 612, 679–681
Stoma nurse specialist, 612, 679–680, 681

Stomach, **593–594**
    carcinoma, 606
    functions, 593
    see also Gastric
Stomatitis (oral mucositis), 600, 602
    angular, 597, 600
    management, 472, *1002*
    in terminal illness, 1035
Stool form scale, Bristol, 243, *244*
Stools, abnormal, 598
Straight leg raising test, *798*
Strains, **822–823**
Strapping, **802**
Stratum basale, 174, 842
Stratum corneum, 174, 842
Stratum germinativum, 174
Stratum granulosum, 174, 842
Stratum lucidum, 174, 842
Stratum spinosum, 174, 842
Strawberry naevus, 864
Streptococcal throat infections, 514
Streptokinase, 507
Streptomycin, 555, 675
Stress, **93–109**
    in A&E department, 925
    in atopic eczema, 850
    cancer development and, **989**
    in carers, 102–103
    concepts, 93–94
    in haematology units, 465
    in health care professionals, 100–102, 1027
    inverted U hypothesis, 94
    management, 105–108
        complementary remedies, 105–106
        non-pharmacological methods, 106–108
        in nursing, 108
        pharmacological methods, 105
    measurement, 104–105
    models, 93–94
        engineering, 94, 99
        Hebb arousal curve, *93*, *94*, 98
    nursing assessment, 104–105
    nursing management, 890–891
    in patients, 100
    physiological effects, 890
    positive aspects, 94
    post-disaster, 943
    in Raynaud's phenomenon/disease, 524, 525
    in renal transplant recipients, 696
    responses, 94–97
        personality type and, 99, *100*
        physiological, 94–97, 400
        psychological, 97
        to surgery, 100, 890
    self-reporting, 105
    wound healing and, *179*, 180
    see also Anxiety
Stress incontinence, 235
    pelvic floor education, 237–240
    in uterovaginal prolapse, 724
Stress-related illness, **103–104**
Stressful life events, 98
Stressors, **98–99**
    critically ill patients, 98, 954
    in health care system, **100–103**
    physiological, 98
    psychosocial, 98–99
Stridor, 568, 583
    inspiratory, 586
    postoperative, 908
Stroke (cerebrovascular accident, CVA),
        291–296
    in atrial arrhythmias, 499, 500, 501
    chronic pain after, 129

clinical presentation, *292*
in diabetes, 425
disability, 1050
embolic, 291
epidemiology and aetiology, 291–292
haemorrhagic, 291
ischaemic, 291
medical/surgical management, 292
nursing management, 292–296
positioning after, *293*, *294*, *295*, 296
prevention/health education, 288, 493–494,
        1059
rehabilitation, 293–296, 1057
risk factors, 291–292
thrombotic, 291
Stroke volume (SV), 485
Structure, 30
Structure–process–outcome model
        (Donabedian), 30, *31*
Student nurses, 6
    UKCC/NMC guidance, 6, *7*
Stump bandaging, **802**, *803*
Stye, *338*, **363**
Subarachnoid haemorrhage (SAH), 291,
        296–297
    traumatic, 298
    versus subdural haematoma, 279
Subconjunctival haemorrhage, *298*
Subcutaneous infusions, **147**
Subdural haemorrhage/haematoma, *279*,
        297–298
Subfertility, *see* Infertility
Sublimation, *97*
Subluxation, 823
Submucosal plexus, 592
Substance misuse
    A&E attenders, 937
    acute pain management, **128–129**
    stress and, 104
    see also Alcohol misuse; Drug dependence
Sudden death, **941–942**
    in cardiovascular disease, 506
    caring for bereaved, 941–942
Sugars, 205
Suicide, 104
    attempted, 940
Sulphonylureas, **417–418**, *420*, 421
Summarizing, 48
Sun exposure
    cancer risk, 990
    health promotion, *867*
    pigmented lesions and, 863–864
    skin tumours and, 867, 868
Sunscreens, *867*
Superior mesenteric artery, 595
Superior vena cava obstruction (SVCO), 1040
Suprachiasmatic nucleus, 61
Supraorbital pressure, *282*
Suprapubic catheterization, 697, *698*
Supraspinatus isolation test, *798*
Supraventricular tachycardia (SVT), **501**
Surgeons
    assistants, 903–904
    in critical care team, 951
Surgery, **879–922**
    cancer, **1004**
    classification, 880
    context, 880
    day, *see* Day surgery
    fitness for, **885–887**
    hand disinfection, 262, 905
    hypothermia during/after, 81–83, *89*,
        902–903
    infection risks, 267–268

Surgery (continued)
nutritional intake and, 218
in palliative care, 1004
prophylactic, in familial cancer, 1004
stress response, 100, 890
technique, and wound healing, 179
terminology, 880
see also Intraoperative care; Postoperative care;
Preoperative care
Surgical assistant, 903–904
Surgical instruments
accounting for, 904
single-use/disposable, 906
sterile, 906
Surgical Materials Testing Laboratory, 200
Surgical scrub, 905
Surgical team, 903–904
Sutures, 906
absorbable and non-absorbable, 906, 907
minor wounds in A&E, 936
removal, 915
Suxamethonium, 884
Swabs
high vaginal (HVS), 714
nasal, 569
skin, 846, 847
surgical, accounting for, 904
wound, 918
Swallowing, 286, 567
assessment, 213, 286
difficulties, see Dysphagia
investigations, 570
Sweat, 843
Sweat glands, 843
apocrine, 843
eccrine, 843
Sweating, 843
abnormal, in diabetes, 426
fluid losses, 143
heat loss, 77
impaired, 78
in shock, 160
in stress, 96
Sympathetic nervous system, 400
blood pressure regulation, 955
in shock, 156
Sympathomimetics
nasal, 572
ophthalmic, 344, 345, 356
Symptom control
in cancer, 1012–1014
dying patients, 1041–1042
principles, 1032
in terminal illness, 1031–1040
see also Pain management; Palliative care
Synacthen (tetracosactrin) test, 402, 438
Synapses, 275–276
Syncope, 486, 500
Synovectomy, 805, 806
Synovial fluid, 795
Synovial joints, 794, 795
Syphilis, 764
Syringe drivers
management, 963, 1034
in palliative care, 1034
Systematic reviews, 26
Systemic circulation, 481
Systemic inflammatory response syndrome
(SIRS), 157–159
defining criteria, 158
pathophysiology, 158–159
patients at risk, 159
triggers, 158
Systemic lupus erythematosus (SLE), 817–818
Systemic vascular resistance (SVR), 485, 960

T

T cells, 446
HIV infection, 765
T-tube drainage, bile duct, 642, 643
T wave, 490
T₃, 398
T₄, see Thyroxine
Tachycardia
in anaemia, 457
in cardiogenic shock, 510
narrow complex, 501
paroxysmal atrial (PAT), 501
in shock, 160
sinus, 499
supraventricular (SVT), 501
ventricular (VT), 496, 502
Talking books, 343
Tamoxifen
in breast cancer, 784, 994
prophylactic, 776
Tampons, toxic shock syndrome and, 733
Tarui's disease, 810
Task allocation, 12, 13
Taste buds, 593
Taste disturbances, 212, 289
in terminal illness, 1035
Teaching
groups, 54
patient, see Patient education
skills, 10
Team, 54
A&E, 928–929, 942
acute pain, 121
care, in chronic illness/disability, 1061
critical care, 951–952
critical care outreach, 949, 949
nutritional, 216, 219
palliative care, 1022
patient-at-risk (PART), 949, 950
quality improvement (QIT), 32–33
resuscitation, 930
surgical, 903–904
wound management, 180, 186–187
Team leaders, 13, 930
Team nursing, 12–13
Tears, 336
artificial, 345, 364
deficiency, 363–364
Technical terms, using, 42
Technicians, in critical care, 952
Teeth
grinding during sleep, 67
loose or crowned, 737
Telangiectasia, 844, 852, 864
hereditary haemorrhagic, 864
Telephone advice lines, 924
Teletherapy, 1005
Telogen effluvium, 869
Telomeres, 987
Temazepam, 894
Temperature (body), 75–92
abnormal variations, 77–78
assessment, 83–86
equipment, see Thermometers
ritualized, 84
sites, 85–86
thermometer insertion times, 84–85
time of day, 84
axilla, 84, 85
basal (BBT), 758
core, 76
core–skin gradients, 82, 160–161, 959
in diabetic ketoacidosis, 423, 424

diurnal variation, 61, 77, 78, 84
during sleep, 61
factors affecting, 77–78
in menstrual cycle, 710–711, 759
in neurological problems, 284, 290
normal, 85
normal variations, 77, 78
oral, 84, 85
peripheral, see Skin (peripheral) temperature
postoperative monitoring, 908–909
pulmonary artery, 85
raised
cooling methods, 86–87
nursing management, 86–87
see also Hyperpyrexia; Hyperthermia;
Pyrexia
rectal, 84, 85
regulation, 76–78
disorders of, 75, 78–83
heat regulation mechanisms, 76–77
skin function, 77, 175
in shock, 160–161, 164
spermatogenesis and, 742
tympanic membrane, 84, 85
wound healing and, 179, 181
see also Frostbite; Hypothermia
Temperature (environmental)
in atopic eczema, 849, 850
bath water, 849
in burn injuries, 872
operating theatre, 903, 906
sleep and, 70
Temperature, pulse and respiration (TPR),
preoperative assessment, 886
Temporal arteritis, 317
Temporal bone, otitis media involving, 385
Temporal lobe, 277
epilepsy, 314
Tenchkoff catheter, 688, 689
Tendons, 796
strains, 822–823
Tenesmus, 598, 1032
Tennis elbow, 805, 825
Tenosynovectomy, 805, 806
Tenosynovitis, 805
Tenotomy, 805
Tentorium cerebelli, 278–279
Terbutaline, 543
Terminal care, 1041–1042
Terminal illness
in cystic fibrosis, 552
dehydration, 142, 1028
emotional responses, 1025–1026
ethical issues, 289
resuscitation, 496, 497
symptom control, 1031–1040
see also Death; Dying; Palliative care
Termination of pregnancy (TOP), 730–732
conscientious objection, 18, 731
ethical issues, 17–18
late, 731
nurse's attitude, 731, 732
nursing management, 731–732
Testes (testicles), 741–742
descent, 741
ectopic, 748
hormone production, 742
problems, 745–750
self-examination (TSE), 749, 1000
surgical removal, see Orchidectomy
torsion, 742, 750
trauma, 750
undescended, 750
Testicular cancer, 745–749, 994
aetiology and epidemiology, 745–746

clinical presentation, 747
investigations, 747
medical/surgical management, 747
non-seminoma germ cell, 746
nursing management, 747–749
pathophysiology, 746
screening, **1000**
secondary, 746–747
staging, *748*
stromal tumours, 746
Testosterone, 742
Tests, waiting for results, 100
Tetanus immunization, 935
Tetany, 433–434, 436
Tetracosactide (tetracosactrin) test, 402, 438
Tetracycline, *226*
Tetralogy of Fallot, *528*
Tetraplegia, *289*
Thalassaemia, **461**
major, 461
trait, 461
Theophylline, 543
Therapeutic relationship, **43–45**
Thermodilution cardiac output measurement, **960**
Thermogenesis, 77
Thermometers, **83–84**
electronic, 83
glass mercury, 83, 84
insertion times, 84–85
low-reading, 84
selection, 84
single-use chemical, 83, 84
tympanic membrane, 83–84, 85
Thermoregulation, **76–77**
skin function, 77, 175
Thiamin, *see* Vitamin B₁
Thiazolidinediones, 418
Thiopental sodium, *884*, 899
Thioridazine, *226*
'Third age', 968
Third space fluid losses, 138
Thirst, 137, 139
dehydration and, 142
inability to respond to, 140
Thomas' splint, 799, 831
Thomsen's disease, *809*
Thoracic cage, 533
Thoracocentesis, 560
Throat
disorders, *see* Nose and throat disorders
examination, **569**
infections and inflammation, **581–583**
investigations, 570
signs and symptoms, 568
sore (pain), 568
tumours, 570, **587–588**
Thrombin, 448–449
Thrombocytopenia, 463, **476–477**
in cancer, 1013
Thrombocytopenic purpura, idiopathic (ITP), 476
Thrombolytic therapy, 292
complications, 508
in myocardial infarction, 507
Thrombophlebitis, *225*, **527**
Thrombosis
deep vein, *see* Deep vein thrombosis
in polycythaemia, 460
Thrombus formation, 449
central venous catheters, 470–471
in myocardial infarction, 506
Thrush, *see* Candidiasis
Thymus gland, 394
Thyroglobulin, 398
Thyroid cancer, **435–436**

Thyroid disease, 402, **431–436**
Thyroid gland, 394, **397–399**
Thyroid hormones, 398–399
Thyroid nodule, toxic single, **434–435**
Thyroid-stimulating hormone (TSH), 397, 398
circadian rhythm, 62
deficiency, *430*
Thyroid storm, 433
Thyroidectomy, 433, 587
complications, 433, 436
nursing management, 433–434
Thyroiditis, **434**
Hashimoto's, 435
silent (painless), 434
subacute (de Quervain's), 434
Thyroplasty, 586
Thyrotoxic crisis *see* Thyroid storm
Thyrotoxicosis, 431, 432
see also Hyperthyroidism
Thyroxine (T₄), 398
in heat generation, 77
replacement therapy, 435
Tibial fractures, 832
Tibial plateau fractures, 832
Tidal volume, 957–958
Tilt table, 325
Time management, 106–107
Timolol maleate, *345*
Tinea, **856–858**
barbae, 856, *857*
capitis, 856, *857*, 858, 869
corporis, 856, *857*
cruris, 856, *857*
faciei, 856
manuum, 856, *857*, 858
pedis, 856, *858*
unguium, 856, 858
Tinnitus, 380, **388–389**
TIPSS (transluminal intrahepatic portosystemic stent shunt), 604
Tiredness, *see* Fatigue
Tissue fluid, formation, **136–137**
Tissue plasminogen activator (tPA), 507
Tissue repair, 176
see also Wound healing
Tissue typing, for renal transplantation, 695
Tissue viability, **173–199**
definition, 173
services, 173
Tissues, inadvertent i.v. fluid infusion, 146
Tizanadine, 816
TNM classification and grading system, 1003
Tobacco use
acute pain management, 129
cancer risk, **990**
see also Smoking
Tocopherols, 208
Toe temperature, 85–86
Tolbutamide, *417*
Tongue, **593**
coated, in terminal illness, 1035
disorders, **601–602**
Tonic neck reflexes, *294*, 302
Tonometry, Goldmann applanation, 340
Tonsillectomy, **581–582**
Tonsillitis, **581–582**
Tonsils, 567
Toothache, 139
Topical therapy
in acne, *852*
in atopic eczema, 850–851
in psoriasis, 862
Total Quality Management (TQM), 24, 30–31, 32

Touch
comatose patients, 302
critically ill patients, 954, 957
in visual impairment, 343
Towels, hand, 262
Toxic epidermal necrolysis (TEN), **866–867**
Toxic multinodular goitre, **434–435**
Toxic shock syndrome (TSS), 155, **733**
Toxic single (thyroid) adenoma, **434**
Trabeculectomy, 355, 356, 357
Trace elements, 205, *207*
Trachea, 567
Tracheal suction
after tracheostomy, 585
ventilated patients, 961–962
Tracheo-oesophageal feeding, 587
Tracheostomy, **584–586**
humidification of inspired air, 558, 585, 586
mechanical ventilation via, 961
nursing management, 584–586
postoperative care, **585–586**
tubes, 584, 585
wound and tube care, 585–586
Trachoma, 341, 361
Traction, **799–800**
pin site care, *801*
skeletal, 799, *800*
skin, *800*
Training, to improve standards, 33–34
TRAM flap, breast reconstruction, 788, *789*
Tramadol, 124, 815
Trans-rectus abdominus (TRAM) flap, breast reconstruction, 788, *789*
Transfers
resuscitated trauma patients, 933–934
stroke patients, 293–296
surgical patients, 894, 900–901
Transfusion, *see* Blood transfusion
Transfusion-associated graft-versus-host disease (TA-GVHD), 267, 454, 475
Transient ischaemic attack (TIA), 291
Transitional cell carcinoma, *see* Urothelial (transitional cell) tumours
Transluminal intrahepatic portosystemic stent shunt (TIPSS), 604
Transoesophageal echocardiogram (TOE), 491
Transoesophageal ultrasound, 960
Transport maximum (T$_m$), 658
Transurethral resection of prostate (TURP), **697–699**
Trauma, **821–836**
brain, *see* Head injury
chest, 560
in chronic venous insufficiency, 528
deep vein thrombosis and, 525
ear, **380–382**
eye, 357–364
fractures, 828
liver, **638**
major, **931–934**
assessment and management, 932–934
definitive care, 933–934
nursing roles, 932
primary survey, 932–933
secondary survey, 933
minor, **934–936**
assessment, 934, *935*
discharge advice, 935–936
management, 934–935, *936*
see also Sprains; Strains
nutritional needs, 217–218
preoperative assessment, 796
prevention, 799, 931
renal, **677**
sports-related, *see* Sports injuries

Trauma *(continued)*
   testicular, 750
   see also Accidents; Burns
Trauma Advisory Services, 944
Travel
   in diabetes, 415
   nursing history, 597
Treadmill exercise test, **490**, 505
Treatment
   refusal, 1027, *1028*
   withdrawing, *1027*, 1028
Tremor, *289*, 319
Trendelenburg test, *798*
Tretinoin, *852*
Triacylglycerol (triglycerides), 204
Triage, **925–927**
   scale, *927*
   skills required, 926–927
   standards, 926
Triceps skinfold (TSF) thickness, 214
Trichilemmal cysts, 861
Trichomoniasis, 732, **762–763**
Tricuspid valve, 483
Tricyclic antidepressants, 426, 816
Trigeminal nerve, *279*
Trigeminal neuralgia, 303, **304**
Trigger factors, respiratory disorders, 538
Trigone, 230, 661
Triiodothyronine (T_3), 398
Triple assessment, breast disorders, 775
Triple therapy, peptic ulcers, 606
Trochlear nerve, *279*
Trolleys, surgical patients, 895
Trophoblastic disease, gestational, 729
Tropicamide, *344*
Troponin I, 491
Truth-telling, **19**
Tryptophan, 209
TSH, *see* Thyroid-stimulating hormone
Tubal embryo transfer (TET), *760*
Tuberculin skin test, 555
Tuberculosis (TB), **555–556**
   adrenal cortex insufficiency, 437
   clinical presentation, 555, 675
   contact tracing, 556
   directly observed therapy (DOT), 556
   investigations, 541, 555, 675
   multidrug resistant (MDR-TB), 255, 263,
       555–556
   nursing management, 675–676
   pathophysiology, 555
   protective masks, 263
   renal, **674–676**
   treatment, 555–556, 675
   see also Mycobacterium tuberculosis
Tubulointerstitial disease, renal, **684**
Tumour(s), **992–995**
   benign, **992–993**
   cells, 987–988
   growth, 988
   invasion, 989
   malignant, **992–993**
   metastasis, *see* Metastases
   progression, 988
   solid, **993–995**
   see also Cancer
Tumour lysis syndrome (TLS), **473**, 476
Tumour Node Metastases (TNM) classification
       and grading system, 1003
Tumour suppressor genes, 987–988
Tuning fork tests, 373
TUR syndrome, 699
Turbinates, 566
   surgery, in sinusitis, 574
Turbohaler, *543*

Turgor, skin, 139, 486, 663, 957
TURP (transurethral resection of prostate),
       697–699
Tympanic membrane, 368–369
   otoscopic examination, 371, 372
   perforation, 372
       in otitis media, 383, 384
       traumatic, **381**
   surgical repair, 384, *386*
   thermometry, 83–84, 85
Tympanometry, 373
Tympanoplasty, *386*
Tympanosclerosis, 372, 384, 385
Type 1 diabetes mellitus, **403–415**, 1047
   aetiology and epidemiology, 403–404
   clinical presentation, 404
   diabetic ketoacidosis, 422
   'honeymoon period', 410
   hypoglycaemia, 411, 421
   investigations, 404
   long-term complications, 424
   medical management, 404
   nursing management, **404–415**
   pathophysiology, 404
   patient education, *405*
       at diagnosis, 405–411
       ongoing, 415
       over next 3 months, 411–415
   in-patient self-care, *406*
   prevention, 403
   sick day rules, 413–414
Type 2 diabetes mellitus, 403, **415–420**
   aetiology and epidemiology, 415–416
   clinical presentation, 416
   dietary management, 419
   hypoglycaemia, 421
   investigations, 416–417
   long-term complications, 424
   medical management, 417
   monitoring, 420
   nursing management, 418–420
   oral therapy, 417–418, 420
   pathophysiology, 416
   prevention/health education, 403
Tzanck smear, 847

U

UKCC, 6
Ulcerative colitis, 103, 613
   aetiology, 613–614
   investigations, 614
   medical/surgical management, 614–615
   nursing management, 615–616
   signs and symptoms, 614
Ulcers, 844
   see also specific types
Ulnar fractures
   distal, 826, 835
   olecranon process, 835
   shaft, 835
Ultradian rhythm, 60
Ultrasound imaging
   breast, 774–775
   Doppler, *see* Doppler ultrasound
   in gynaecological disorders, 713–714
   in infertility, 759
   in liver, biliary and pancreatic disorders, 626
   in neurological disorders, 288
   in nose and throat disorders, 569
   quantitative (QUS), 797
   renal, 665–666
   in urinary disorders, 665–666

Ultrasound therapy, in back pain, 816
Ultraviolet (UV) radiation
   cancer risk, 990
   psoriasis therapy, 862
   in sunlight, *867*
Umbilical hernia, 610
Unconditional positive regard, 45
Unconscious (mental) defence mechanisms,
       45, **97**
Unconscious patient
   nursing management, **290–291**
   see also Coma; Consciousness
Understanding
   accurate empathic, 45
   of terminal illness, assessing, 1031
Uniforms, 41, 42
United Kingdom Central Council for Nursing,
       Midwifery and Health Visiting (UKCC), 6
   see also Nursing & Midwifery Council
United Kingdom Prospective Diabetes Study
       (UKPDS), 424
Universal infection control precautions, **260**,
       261, 264–265, 268, 905
Unpopular patients, *1052*
Unsafe behaviour, and stress, 104
Unstable angina, **505–506**
Upper limb
   fractures and dislocations, **833–836**
   sports injuries, 823–826
Uraemia, 687–688
Uraemic syndrome, 685
Urea, serum, 142, **670**
Urea breath test, **598–599**
Ureteric colic, 676
Ureteric stents, 681
Ureters, **661**
   transitional cell tumours, 679
Urethra, **230, 661–662**
Urethral sphincter
   external, 230, 661
   internal, 661
Urethrocele, *724*
Urge incontinence, *see* Overactive bladder
Urgency of micturition, 235
Uric acid, 807–808
Urinalysis, 142–143, **663–664**
   preoperative, 886
   in urinary incontinence, 237
Urinary catheterization
   after gynaecological surgery, 738
   after prostatectomy, 699, 701
   choice of catheters, 249
   clean intermittent, 240
   continent urinary pouch, 681
   in head injury, 302
   in multiple organ dysfunction, 169
   postoperative, 913
   risks and benefits, 674
   in spinal injuries, 325
   suprapubic, 697, *698*
   unconscious patient, 290
   urine specimen collection, *671*
Urinary catheters
   for incontinence, 248–249
   indwelling, infections associated with, **674**
   selection, *675*
Urinary continence, mechanism, 230–231
Urinary diary, 241
Urinary disorders, **653–703**
   in diabetes, 426, 427, 428
   diagnostic tests and investigations, 665–671
   in multiple sclerosis, 307–308
   nursing assessment, 662–665
   physical examination, *665*
   in postmenopausal women, 735

prevention and health education, 671–672
sleep effects, **72**
in spinal injuries, 325
useful websites, 702
see also Specific disorders
Urinary diversion, **679–681**
postoperative care, 681
preoperative care, 679–681
Urinary incontinence, **231–242**
assessment, 234–235
causes, 233–234
childbirth and, 232, 234
definition, 229
drug therapy and, *236*
in hospitals, 232–233
impact, 232
investigations, 236–237
mixed, 235
in multiple sclerosis, 234, 304, 307
nursing management, 246–249
in older adults, 232–233
assessment, 234, *235*
treatment, 240, 242
overflow, 235, 696
in Parkinson's disease, 322
post-prostatectomy, 238, 699, 701
prevalence, 231–232
in spinal injuries, 325
treatment, *237–242*
types, 235–236
Urinary pouch, continent internal, 681
Urinary retention
acute, in benign prostatic hyperplasia, 697, 699
in multiple sclerosis, 307–308
postoperative, *740*, 913
Urinary system/tract, **654–662**
congenital abnormalities, *655*
development and maturation, 654–655
disorders, **672–685**
during sleep, 62
lower, 654, **661–662**
nursing assessment, 662–665
in shock, 157, 160
Urinary tract infections (UTIs), **672–673**
aetiology and epidemiology, 672
associated with urinary catheters, **674**
clinical presentation, 672
critically ill patients, 953
incontinence in, 234, 237
management, 676
postoperative, *740*
prevention, *673*
Urinary tract obstruction
acute renal failure, 685, 686
in benign prostatic hyperplasia, 696, 697
in nephrolithiasis, 676
overflow incontinence, 235
Urine
24-hour collection, 142
assessment, *see* Urinalysis
blood in, *see* Haematuria
catheter specimens (CSU), *671*
clean-catch specimen, *671*
concentration mechanism, 659–660
cytology, 671
early morning specimen (EMSU), 671
formation of hypo-osmotic or hyperosmotic, 658–659
leucocytes (white cells), *664*, 665
microscopy, 671
midstream specimen (MSSU), *671*
normal characteristics, *664*
osmolality, 431
pH, 143, *664* **665**
post-void residual volume, 237

specific gravity, 143, **664**
specimen collection, *671*
spillages, *631*
tests, 142–143, 671
Urine output
critically ill patients, 959
in fluid balance disorders, 140
in hypothermia, 90
postoperative, **913**
in shock, 157, 160, **161**
in stress, 96
Uro-sheaths, 249
Urobilinogen, 622
urinary, 626, *629*
Urodynamic investigations, 237, **669**
Uroflowmetry, 669
Urography, **667**
Urology, 653
Urostomy (ileal conduit for urinary diversion), 679–681
Urothelial (transitional cell) tumours, **678–681**
aetiology, 679
clinical presentation, 679
investigations, 679
medical/surgical management, 679
nursing management, 679–681
Urticaria, **854**
Uterine arteries, 709
Uterine cycle, *see* Menstrual cycle
Uterine (fallopian) tubes, **708**
ectopic pregnancy, 729–730
infection/inflammation, 732–733
patency testing, 714, 759
surgery, for infertility, 760
Uterovaginal prolapse, **724–725**, 735
Uterus, **708–711**
displacement, **724–725**
perforation, *740*
Uveal tract, 332–333
disorders, **362**
Uveitis, **362**
anterior, 362
posterior, 362

V

V/Q ratio, 535, 955
Vaccination, health care professionals, 268
Vacuum devices, for erectile dysfunction, 755
Vagina, **711**
Vaginal bleeding
in early pregnancy, 726, 727
in menopausal women, 735
postmenopausal, 722
see also Menstrual disorders
Vaginal cones, 239–240
Vaginal examination
bimanual, 713
speculum, 713, *714*
in urinary incontinence, 237
Vaginal swabs, high (HVS), 714
Vaginismus, 757
Vaginitis, **732**
atrophic, 732
Vagotomy, truncal, 607
Vagus nerve, *279*
Valerian, 106
Validity, definition, *119*
Valsalva manoeuvre, 501
Value for money (VFM), 25, 27
Values, 44, 45
Valves, cardiac, *482*, 483
prosthetic, 516

regurgitation (incompetence), 515
replacement surgery, **516**
stenosis, 515
Valvular heart disease, 514, **515–516**
Vancomycin-resistant *enterococcus* (VRE), 255
Varicella, 855
Varicella zoster virus (VSV), 312, 855
Varicocele, 750
Varicose eczema, **851**
Varicose veins, **525**
Varicosities, in liver and gallbladder disease, *629*
Vas deferens, 742
Vasa recta, 656, 659, *660*
Vascular disorders, **521–528**
skin, **864**
see also Peripheral arterial/vascular disease
Vascular system, **485–486**
Vasectomy, 757
Vasoconstriction, peripheral, 77
in hypothermia, 81, 90
in Raynaud's phenomenon/disease, 524
in shock, 156
in stress, 97
Vasoconstrictive drugs, in shock, 166
Vasodilatation, peripheral, 77
during rewarming in hypothermia, 89
Vasodilators
in cardiogenic shock, 166
in heart failure, 512
Vasomotor centre, 156
Vasopressin, *see* Antidiuretic hormone
Vecuronium, *884*
Vegans, 217, 456
Vegetables, *419*
Vegetarians, 217
Vegetations, endocardial, 516
Veins, **485**
varicose, **525**
Venesection, in polycythaemia, 460
Venography, 525
Venometer, 525
Venous access
devices, in thalassaemia, 461
for haemodialysis, 691, *693*
see also Central venous catheters; Intravenous catheters
Venous hydrostatic pressure, increased, 137
Venous hypertension, chronic, 194, 527
Venous insufficiency, chronic, 526, **527–528**, 851
Venous leg ulcers, 193, **194**, 527
compression bandaging, 195, **196–197**
management, **196–197**, *198*, *199*
prevention of recurrence, *197*
vascular assessment, 195
versus arterial leg ulcers, *195*
Venous return, 485, 527
Venous stasis, 525
Venous thrombosis, deep, *see* Deep vein thrombosis
Ventilation
alveolar (V), 535, 955
in major trauma, 932
mechanical, **960–962**
in Guillain–Barré syndrome, 328
indications, 961
nursing management, 961–962
patient compliance, 961
principles, 961
in raised intracranial pressure, *301*
in septic shock, 167
non-invasive (NIV), 559–560, 961
non-invasive positive pressure (NIPPV), 961
see also Breathing
Ventilation/perfusion (V/Q) ratio, 535, 955

Ventilation systems, air, *see* Air ventilation systems
Ventricles, brain, *278*
Ventricles, heart, *482*, *483*
Ventricular arrhythmias, **501–502**
Ventricular contraction, *484*, *485*
Ventricular ectopic beats (extrasystoles), **501–502**
Ventricular ejection, *484*, *485*
Ventricular fibrillation, 496, **502**
Ventricular filling, 484
Ventricular relaxation, *484*, *485*
Ventricular tachycardia (VT), 496, **502**
Ventriculography, 287
Venturi oxygen delivery systems, 558
Verbal communication, **40**
Verbal response, assessing, 280, *282*
Verrucae, 855
Vertebral artery, 277, *278*
Vertebral fractures, in osteoporosis, 815
Vertigo, 386
　after ear surgery, 385
　benign paroxysmal positional (BPPV), **387**
　ear testing and, 374
　in Ménière's disease, 387
　nursing management, 387–388
Vesicles, 844, 864
Vesicoureteric reflux (VUR), *655*, 673–674
Vestibular nerve, 370
Vestibular sedatives, 387
Vestibulocochlear nerve (VIII), *279*, 370
Viagra (sildenafil citrate), 754
Victim blaming, 101
Victim Support, 944
Video stroboscopy, larynx, 570
Videofluoroscopy, swallowing, 570
Vinca-alkaloids, 1007
Vincent's angina, 602
Violence
　in A&E department, **938**, *939*
　domestic, 937
　sexual, 937
　victims, **937**
Viral infections
　eye, 359, 361
　in haemophilia, 478
　hepatitis, *625*, **630–633**
　nervous system, 311, 312–313
　pyrexia, 79
　respiratory disorders, *538*
　skin, **854**
　transfusion-associated transmission, 454
　upper respiratory tract, 553
　see also specific infections
Virchow's triad, 525, 888
Virilization, in congenital adrenal hyperplasia, 441
Virology tests, in skin conditions, 846–847
Viruses, 254
　blood-borne, **267–268**, 627
　causing cancer, 991
　handwashing technique, 263
Visceral pain, 112, 1032
　secondary, 1032
Vision, 335
　ageing changes, 975
　problems, *see* Eye and vision problems
　testing, **339–340**
　tunnel, 355
Visitors, immunosuppressed patients, 267
Visual acuity (VA), **339–340**
Visual assessment
　in A&E triage, 927
　critically ill patients, 957
Visual cortex, 335

Visual fields, *335*
　loss, *289*, 341
　　in glaucoma, 355, 356
　　in stroke, *292*
　testing, 340
Visual impairment, 331–332, **341–344**
　communication, 342
　in diabetic retinopathy, 352–353
　instilling eye medication and, 347
　in neurological disorders, *289*
　nursing management, 342–344
　painless, **348–357**
　registration as blind/partially sighted, 342
　safety and independence, 342–343
　services and support, 343–344
Visual pathway, **335–336**
Vital signs
　in head injury, 300
　in hypothermia, 89–90
　postoperative, 738
Vitamin A, **205–207**, 335
　deficiency, 205, 206
　topical therapy, 862
　toxicity, 206–207
　wound healing and, *218*
Vitamin B$_1$ (thiamin), *206*, **208**
　deficiency, *206*, 208, 318
Vitamin B$_2$ (riboflavin), *206*, **208**
　deficiency, *206*, 208, 217
Vitamin B$_6$, *206*, **209**
　deficiency, *206*, 209
　toxicity, 209
Vitamin B$_{12}$, *206*, **209**, 456, 458
　deficiency, *206*, 209, **458–459**
　supplements, 606
Vitamin C, *206*, **209**
　deficiency, *206*
　iron absorption and, 210, 225
　wound healing and, *218*
Vitamin D, 205, *206*, **207–208**
　deficiency, *206*, 207–208, 980
　supplementation, 436, 437, 819
　synthesis, 175, 207
　topical therapy, 862
　toxicity, 208
Vitamin E, *206*, **208**, 216
Vitamin K, 205, *206*, **208**
　deficiency, *206*
　supplements, in liver disease, 632
Vitamins, **205–209**
　antioxidant, 216
　fat-soluble, 205
　patients on medication, *226–227*
　supplements, in cystic fibrosis, 551
　water-soluble, 205
Vitiligo, **863**
Vitiligo Society, 875
Vitreous, 333
Vocal cords (folds), 567
　paralysis, **586**
　polyps/nodules/papillomata, 587
Voice
　analysis, 570
　changes, 568, 586, 587
　production, 567
　rehabilitation, 588
　rest, after laryngoscopy, 583
Voiding
　inefficiency, 235, **240**
　preoperative, 894
　in terminal illness, 1029
Voluntary Euthanasia Society, 1027
Voluntary health care sector, quality in, **27**
Volvulus, intestinal, 604
Vomiting, **594**, 1035–1036

　projectile, 594
　see also Nausea and vomiting
Vomiting centre, 594, 1035–1036
Vulva, **711**
Vulval cancer, **720**
Vulvectomy, radical, 720

W

Waiting
　for results, 100
　times, A&E department, *927*, *939*
Waiting area, A&E department, 925
Waldeyer's ring, 567
Wales Council for the Blind, 365
Walking, to operating theatre, 895
Walsall pressure ulcer risk score, 188, *189*
Wandering, in dementia, 973
War Widows Association of Great Britain, 1045
Ward rounds, in critical care, 951
Wards
　managing infectious patients on, 266
　ultra-clean, 266
Warfarin, 208, *226*
　in cardiovascular disease, 492
　in deep vein thrombosis, 526
Warming
　cutaneous, 903
　see also Rewarming
Warts, 855
　genital, **761–762**, 855
Waste
　clinical, 266, 267
　disposal, 247, **266–267**, *631*
　domestic, 266
Water
　acute wound cleansing in A&E, *934*
　balance, *see* Fluid balance
　body, 134
　in burns first aid, 871
　cold, *see* Cold water
　depletion, *see* Dehydration
　distribution, **134**
　evaporation, 77
　intestinal absorption, 242
　movement, 134–136
　shortages, 140
　warm, in frostbite, 91
　see also Fluid
Water deprivation test, 431
Water excess (intoxication), 139
　see also Fluid volume excess
Waterlow score, 188, *189*
Weakness, *289*
　in anaemia, *457*
　assessing, 284
　in motor neuron disease, 323
　muscle, 810, 811
'Wear and tear' theory of ageing, 974
Weber's test, 373
Wegener's granulomatosis, 580
Weight, body
　cancer and, 990
　fluid balance assessment, 144, 663
　in haemodialysis, 690–691
　in heart failure, 513
　limits, pressure ulcer prevention devices, 192
　loss
　　in blood disorders, 449
　　in chronic pancreatitis, 646, 647
　　in diabetes, 404
　　in GI disorders, 597

in obesity, 217
nutritional assessment, 214, 888
sleep patterns and, 64
see also Body mass index; Obesity
Weil's disease, 596
Welfare benefits, 1031, *1061*
Well-being, assessment, **1060**
Wernicke–Korsakoff syndrome, 208, 318
Wernicke's encephalopathy, **318**
Wet wrap dressings, 850–851
Wheal, *844*
Wheelchairs, **804**
pressure ulcer prevention, *190*
Wheeze, 539, 958
Whipple's procedure, **648–649**
White blood cell count (WBC), 491, *625*
White cells (leucocytes), **446**
disorders, **465–469**
in urine, *664, 665*
White matter injury, brain, 298
Wigs, 472
Wilson's disease, **318**
'Wind up' phenomenon, 113
Women's health, 705, **706–739**
cancer deaths, *781*
cancer screening, 996
of child-bearing age
nutrition, 217
preoperative assessment, 886
disease prevention/health education,
715–716
faecal incontinence, 243
inequality of older, 971
nursing assessment, **711–712**
postmenopausal, *see* Postmenopausal women
psychological assessment, *712*
social assessment, *712*
urinary incontinence, 231, 232
causes, 234, 235
treatment, 238, 239–240, 242
see also Female; Gynaecological disorders;
Pregnancy
Wood's light examination, 848
Work
in cancer, 1016
in chronic illness/disability, 1055
in diabetes, 414
in inflammatory bowel disease, 616
nursing history, 596
-related hazards, *see* Occupational health
hazards
World Health Organization (WHO), 9
analgesic ladder, 1017, 1032–1034
definitions of disability, 1048
disability-adjusted life years (DALYs), 1049
Wound(s)
acute, *176*

management in A&E, **934–935**, *936*
management objectives, 180
types, *934*
assessment, 180, **181**, 915
chronic, **173–200**
characteristics, 176
management objectives, 180–181
see also Leg ulcers; Pressure ulcers
classification, 176, *918*
clean, *918*
clean contaminated, *918*
cleansing, 181, 934
closure methods in A&E, *936*
contaminated, *918*
contraction, 178
debridement, 181–182
dehiscence, 918–919
dirty/infected, *918*
drainage, 915
dressings, *see* Dressings
duration, *179*
fungating, **1039**
in breast cancer, **787–788**
location, *179*
malodorous, 185
measurement, 181
moisture, *179, 181, 182*
penetrating, *934*
size, *179*
swabs, 918
Wound Care Society, 200
Wound drains, **915–917**
after nephrectomy, 678
after open cholecystectomy, 640
closed systems, 915–917
nursing management, 917
open systems, 915
Wound healing, **176–180**
factors influencing/delaying, 178–180
inflammatory stage, 177
maturation stage, *177*, 178
nutrition and, *179*, **218**
physiology, 177–178
by primary intention, 176, *914*
proliferative stage, *177*, 178
by secondary intention, 176, *914*
tertiary, 915
Wound infections, **917–918**
breast surgery, 790
delayed wound healing, *179*
gynaecological surgery, *740*
nutrient demands, 218
preoperative preventative measures,
887–888
Wound management, **180–182**
acute wounds, 180
biotechnology, 186

burns, **873–874**
chronic wounds, 180–181
in Cushing's syndrome, 440
objectives, 180–181
postoperative, **914–919**
principles, 180
products, *see* Dressings
radical vulvectomy, 720
teams, 180, 186–187
useful websites, 200
Wright peak flow meter, 540
Wrist bands, 737, 895
Wrist fractures, 835, *836*

X

X-rays, plain
brain tumours, 309
in endocrine disorders, 401
in GI disorders, 599
in gynaecological disorders, 724
in head injury, 300
in inflammatory bowel disease, 614
in liver, biliary and pancreatic disorders,
626
in neurological disease, 287
in nose and throat disorders, 569
see also Barium studies; Chest X-ray; Contrast
studies
Xanthines, urinary incontinence and, *236*
Xanthomas, **870**
Xerostomia, *see* Mouth, dry

Y

Yeasts, 254
Young adults, chronic illness and disability,
1054–1055
Your Guide to the NHS (2001), 29

Z

Zafirlukast, 543
Zidovudine (AZT), 765
Zinc, *207*, **210**
deficiency, 210
wound healing and, *218*
Zollinger–Ellison syndrome, 649
Zyban (bupropion), 494, **536**
Zygote intrafallopian transfer (ZIFT), *760*